CONTENTS

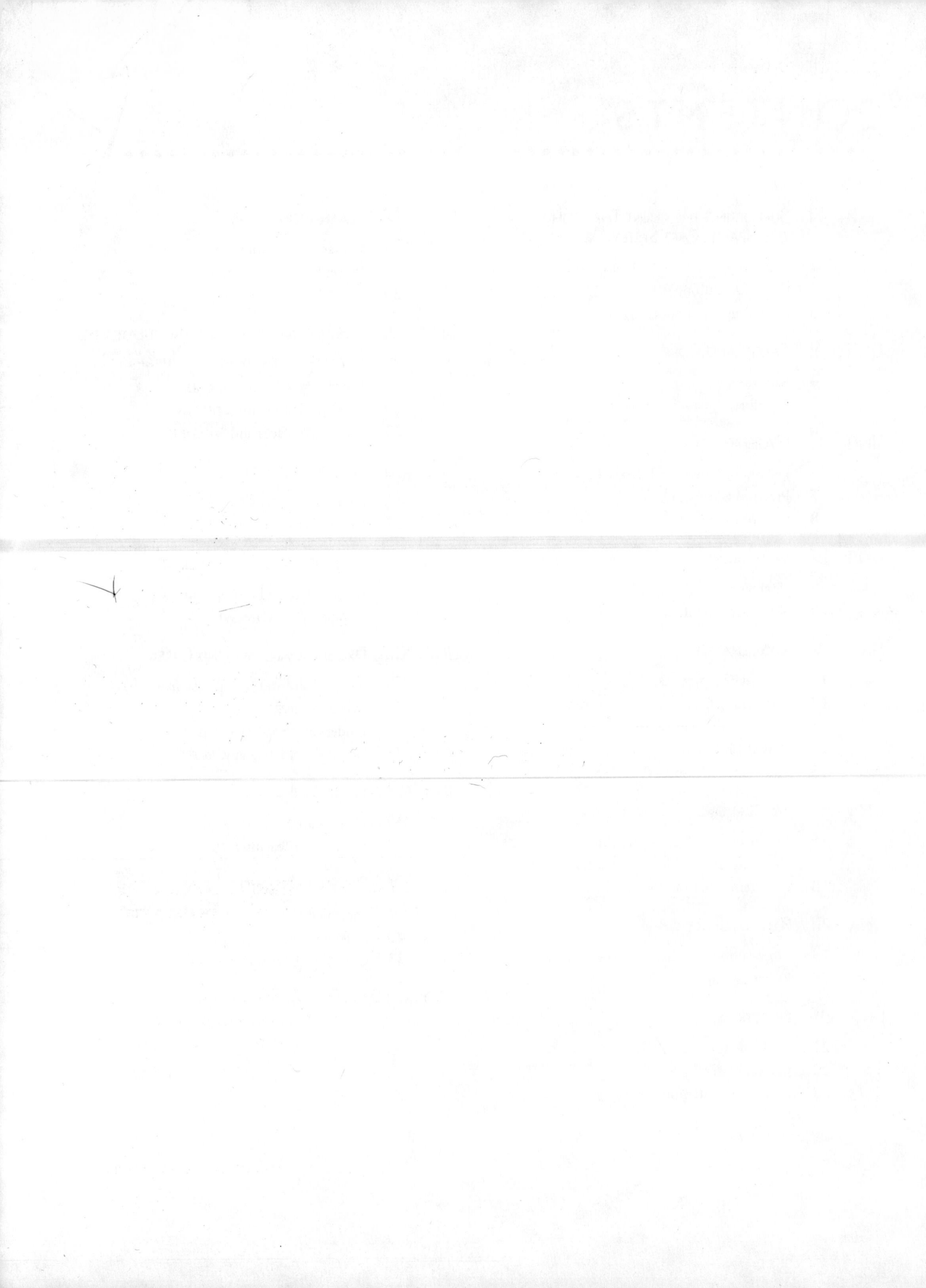

Clinical Nursing Skills & Techniques

Fifth Edition

Anne Griffin Perry, RN, MSN, EdD
Professor and Co-Coordinator, Adult Health Specialty
Saint Louis University Health Sciences Center
St. Louis, Missouri

Patricia A. Potter, RN, PhD(Cand.), CMAC
Nursing Research Scientist
Barnes-Jewish Hospital
St. Louis, Missouri

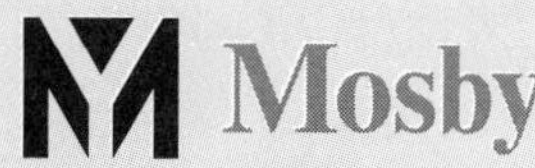

An Imprint of Elsevier Science

St. Louis London Philadelphia Sydney Toronto

With 1105 illustrations

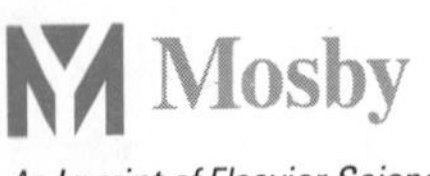

An Imprint of Elsevier Science

Vice President and Publishing Director, Nursing: *Sally Schrefer*
Executive Editor: *Susan Epstein*
Senior Developmental Editor: *Sharon Malchow*
Project Manager: *John Rogers*
Project Specialist: *Kathleen L. Teal*
Senior Production Editor: *Mary Turner*
Designer, Chapter and Cover Art: *Kathi Gosche*
Photography: *Rick Brady*

Fifth Edition

Pharmacology is an ever-changing field. Standard safety precautions must be followed, but as new research and clinical experience broaden our knowledge, changes in treatment and drug therapy may become necessary or appropriate. Readers are advised to check the most current product information provided by the manufacturer of each drug to be administered to verify the recommended dose, the method and duration of administration, and contraindications. It is the responsibility of the treating physician, relying on experience and knowledge of the patient, to determine dosages and the best treatment for each individual patient. Neither the Publisher nor the editor assumes any liability for any injury and/or damage to persons or property arising from this publication.

Mosby, Inc.
An Imprint of Elsevier Science
11830 Westline Industrial Drive
St. Louis, Missouri 63146

Printed in the United States of America

Library of Congress Cataloging in Publication Data

Perry, Anne Griffin.
Clinical nursing skills & techniques / Anne Griffin Perry, Patricia A. Potter.—5th ed.
p. ; cm.
Includes bibliographical references and index.
ISBN 0-323-01406-2
1. Nursing—Handbooks, manuals, etc. 2. Clinical medicine—Handbooks, manuals, etc.
I. Title: Clinical nursing skills and techniques. II. Potter, Patricia Ann. III. Title.
[DNLM: 1. Nursing Care—Handbooks. 2. Clinical Medicine—Handbooks. WY 49
P462c 2001]
RT51 .P365 2001
610.73—dc21

2001030649

02 03 04 05 GW / KPT 9 8 7 6 5 4 3 2

CONTRIBUTORS

Maureen Carty, MSN, OCN
Oncology Clinical Nurse Specialist
Genesis Medical Center
Davenport, Iowa

Mary F. Clarke, MA, RN
Informatics Nurse Specialist
Genesis Medical Center
Davenport, Iowa

Eileen Costantinou, RN, BSN, MSN
Professional Practice Consultant
Barnes-Jewish Hospital
St. Louis, Missouri

Wanda Cleveland Dubuisson, BSN, MN
Assistant Professor
University of Southern Mississippi, College of Nursing
Hattiesburg, Mississippi

Martha E. Elkin, RN, MSN
Lactation Counselor
Stephens Memorial Hospital
Norway, Maine

Amy Hall, PhD, MS, BSN, RN
Assistant Professor
Saint Francis Medical Center, College of Nursing
Peoria, Illinois

Marilee Kuhrik, RN, MSN, PhD
Associate Professor
Colorado Mountain College
Glenwood Springs, Colorado

Nancy S. Kuhrik, RN, MSN, PhD
Associate Professor
Colorado Mountain College
Glenwood Springs, Colorado

Ruth Ludwick, PhD, MSN, BSN, RNC, CNS
Associate Professor
Kent State University
Kent, Ohio

Rita Mertig, MS, BSN, RNC, CNS
Professor
John Tyler Community College
Richmond, Virginia

Jane Ruhland, RN, MSN, BSN
Education Coordinator
Barnes-Jewish St. Peters Hospital
St. Peters, Missouri

Jacqueline Raybuck Saleeby, PhD, RN, CS
Associate Professor
Jewish Hospital College of Nursing and Allied Health
St. Louis, Missouri

Julie Snyder, MSN, RNC
Faculty
Louise Obici, School of Nursing
Suffolk, Virginia

Anne Falsone Vaughan, MSN, BSN, CCRN
Clinical Instructor
Bellarmine College, Lansing School of Nursing
Louisville, Kentucky

Rita Wunderlich, PhD(Cand.), MSN(R), CCRN
Doctoral Candidate, Saint Louis University
Instructor
Clinical Nurse
Saint Louis University Hospital
St. Louis, Missouri

CLINICAL CONSULTANTS

Elizabeth A. Ayello, PhD, MS, BSN, RN, CS, CWOCN
Clinical Assistant Professor
New York University, Division of Nursing
New York, New York

Margaret Benz, RN, MSN, CSANP
Adjunct Assistant Professor
Saint Louis University
St. Louis, Missouri

Gale Carli, MSN, MHEd, BSN, RN
Assistant Professor
Ohlone College
Fremont, California

Ellen Carson, PhD, Clinical Specialist
Associate Professor
Pittsburg State University
Pittsburg, Kansas

Patricia A. Dettenmeier, MSN(R), BSN, CS, ANP
Adult Nurse Practitioner
Saint Louis University Health Sciences Center
St. Louis, Missouri

Martha E. Elkin, MSN
Lactation Counselor
Stephens Memorial Hospital
Norway, Maine

Susan Jane Fetzer, PhD, MBA, MSN, BSN, BA
Assistant Professor, Coordinator RN to BSN
University of New Hampshire
Durham, New Hampshire

Leah Frederick, MS, RN, CIC
Infection Control Consultant
Infection Control Consultants
Scottsdale, Arizona

Thelma Halberstadt, EdD, MS, BS, RN
Professor
Northern Essex Community College
Lawrence, Massachusetts

Amy Hall, PhD, MS, BSN, RN
Assistant Professor
Saint Francis Medical Center College of Nursing
Peoria, Illinois

Ruth Ludwick, PhD, MSN, BSN, RNC, CNS
Associate Professor
Kent State University
Kent, Ohio

Mary Kay Macheca, MSN(R), RN, CS, ANP, CDE
Certified Adult Nurse Practitioner and Certified Diabetes Educator
The Bortz Diabetes Control Center
Richmond Heights, Missouri

Mary K. Mantese, MSN, RN
Regulatory Compliance Manager
Barnes-Jewish West County Hospital
St. Louis, Missouri

Norma Metheny, PhD, MSN, BSN, FAAN
Professor and Dorothy A. Votsmier Chair in Nursing
Saint Louis University School of Nursing
St. Louis, Missouri

Sharon M.J. Muhs, MSN, RN
Registered Nurse
Saint Luke's Hospital
Chesterfield, Missouri

Elaine K. Neel, MSN, BSN
Nursing Instructor
Methodist Medical Center School of Nursing
Peoria, Illinois

Catherine A. Robinson, BA, RN
Clinical Nurse Manager
Barnes-Jewish Hospital

Sharon Souter, MSN, BSN
Director of Nursing Program
New Mexico State University at Carlsbad
Carlsbad, New Mexico

Patricia A. Stockert, RN, BSN, MS, PhD
Associate Professor
Saint Francis Medical Center College of Nursing
Peoria, Illinois

Pamela Becker Weilitz, MSN(R), RN, CS, ANP
Adult Nurse Practitioner
South City Health, LLC
St. Louis, Missouri

REVIEWERS

Marianne Adam, MSN, CRNP
Faculty
Meridan College and St. Luke's School of Nursing
Bethlehem, Pennsylvania

Marie H. Ahrens, MS
Clinical Instructor
University of Tulsa School of Nursing
Tulsa, Oklahoma

Tracy C. Babcock, BSN, MSN
Adjunct Assistant Professor
Montana State University College of Nursing
Bozeman, Montana

Sylvia Baird, RN, MM
Quality Improvement Coordinator
Spectrum Health
Grand Rapids, Michigan

Julie Baylor, MSN, RN
Doctoral Candidate
Saint Louis University
St. Louis, Missouri

Nichole Bethel, MSN, BSN
Nursing Faculty
Community College of Philadelphia
Philadelphia, Pennsylvania

Janice Boundy, PhD, RN
Professor
St. Francis College of Nursing
Peoria, Illinois

Margie E. Brown, RNC, MS, ANP
Staff Nurse, Retired Professor
St. Mary's Medical Center
Long Beach, California

Victoria M. Brown, RN, PhD, HNC
Professor
Georgia College & State University School of Health Sciences
Milledgeville, Georgia

Susan Burkett, MSN, CPN, CPNP
Administrator of TC Thompson Children's Hospital
Erlanger Health System
Chattanooga, Tennessee

Jeanie Burt, MSN, MA, BSN
Assistant Professor of Nursing
Harding University School of Nursing
Searcy, Arizona

Darlene Nebel Cantu, BSN, MSN, RNC
Director
Baptist Health System School of Professional Nursing
San Antonio, Texas

Gale Carli, MSN, MHEd, BSN, RN
Assistant Professor
Ohlone College
Fremont, California

Kathlyn Carlson, MA, BSN, CPAN
Registered Nurse Surgical Services
Abbott Northwestern Hospital
Minneapolis, Minnesota

Judy Chovanec-Toy, MSN, BSN
Assistant Professor
Kauai Community College
Lihue, Hawaii

Laura Clayton, MSN, RN, FNP
Assistant Professor
Shepherd College
Shepherdstown, West Virginia

Barbara P. Daniel, MS, MEd, CRNP
Professor
Cecil Community College
North East, Maryland

Carol A. deBlois, MA, BSN, RN, CNOR
Academic Affairs Manager
Bridgeport Hospital School of Nursing
Bridgeport, Connecticut

Amy Deutschendorf, MSN, AOCN
Senior Director Care Management, Education, and Practice; Faculty Associate
Johns Hopkins Bayview Medical Center
Baltimore, Maryland

Ingeborg Haug DiGiacomo, EdD
Professor
County College of Morris
Randolph, New Jersey

Patricia A. Eagan, MSN, BSN, RN
Retired
Pine Bluff, Arkansas

Sharon Eifried, PhD
Assistant Professor
Towson University
Towson, Maryland

Linda K. Evans, MSN, BSN
Instructor of Clinical Nursing
University of Missouri—Columbia
Columbia, Missouri

Linda Fasciani, MSN, BSN
Assistant Professor
County College of Morris
Randolph, New Jersey

Leah Frederick, MS, RN, CIC
Infection Control Consultant
Infection Control Consultants
Scottsdale, Arizona

Heidi Hahn, MHS, PT, CCS
Physical Therapist
Barnes-Jewish Hospital
St. Louis, Missouri

Lois Hamel, MS, ANP
Doctoral Candidate,
Assistant Adjunct Professor
MMC OB/GYN Associates
Scarborough, Maine

John Harper, MSN, RN, BC
Nurse Educator, Critical Care
Delaware County Memorial Hospital
Drexel Hill, Pennsylvania

Adrienne Henteman, MS, BSN
Registered Nurse, Administrative Associate
Spectrum Health
Grand Rapids, Michigan

Monica Hentemann, RN, BSN
Registered Nurse
Spectrum Health
Grand Rapids, Michigan

Dorothy G. Herron, PhD, RN, CS
Assistant Professor
University of Maryland School of Nursing
Baltimore, Maryland

Janice Hoffman, MSN, RN, CCRN
Doctoral Candidate
University of Maryland-Baltimore School of Nursing
Baltimore, Maryland

Beth Hogan-Quigley, MSN, BSN, CRNP
Clinical Lecturer
University of Pennsylvania School of Nursing
Philadelphia, Pennsylvania

Susan Junaid, MSN, ARNP
Assistant Professor
Allen College
Waterloo, Iowa

Linda L. Kerby, RNC, BSN, MA, BA
Consultant/Educator
Mastery Educational Consultations
Leawood, Kansas

Judith Ann Kilpatrick, MSN, BSN, RNC
DNSc Candidate,
Lecturer
Widener University School of Nursing
Chester, Pennsylvania

Christine R. Kuntz, ART, CRTT, RRT
Registered Respiratory Therapist
Memorial Medical Center
Springfield, Illinois

Maryanne Lachat, PhD, RNC
Associate Professor
Georgetown University
Washington, DC

Joan Anne Leach, ME, MS, CAGS
Professor of Nursing
Capital Community Technical College
Hartford, Connecticut

Virginia Lester, MSN, RN, CNS
Assistant Professor
Angelo State University
San Angelo, Texas

Rita G. Mertig, MS, BSN, RNC, CNS
Professor
John Tyler Community College
Richmond, Virginia

Ramona Reiber Midamba, MS, RN, CNM
Manager of Maternal-Child Department
Mission Hospital
Weslaco, Texas

Claudia L. Mitchell, MSN, BSN, RN
Professor of Nursing, ADN Program
Santa Barbara City College
Santa Barbara, California

Elizabeth Phillip, MSN
Instructor
St. Luke's Hospital School of Nursing
Bethlehem, Pennsylvania

Melissa Powell, MSN, RN
Assistant Professor
Eastern Kentucky University
Richmond, Kentucky

Elaine Princevalli, MS, BSN, RN
Instructor, Practical Nurse Education
State of Connecticut, Department of Education
Hamden, Connecticut

Marsha L. Ray, MSN, BSN, RN
Instructor
Shasta College
Redding, California

Robyn Rice, MSNR, RNC
Doctoral Candidate,
Clinical Associate Professor
Barnes College of Nursing
St. Louis, Missouri

Ruthie Robinson, MSN, RN, CNS, CCRN, CEN
Nursing Instructor
Lamar University
Beaumont, Texas

Alwilda Scholler-Jaquish, MN, MS, PhD, APRN, BC
Assistant Professor
Texas Tech University Health Sciences
Lubbock, Texas

Susan Scholtz, MN, BSN
DNSc Candidate,
Instructor and Faculty
St. Luke's Hospital School of Nursing and Moravian College
Bethlehem, Pennsylvania

Ruth Schumacher, MSN, BSN
Instructor, Maternal Child Nursing
University of Illinois—Chicago
Chicago, Illinois

Nancy Semenza, MS
Doctoral Candidate, Saint Louis University
Adjunct Faculty of Nursing
MacMurray College
Jacksonville, Illinois

Ellen Shannon, MSN
Doctoral Candidate,
Faculty
St. Luke's Hospital School of Nursing
Bethlehem, Pennsylvania

Ruth A. Shearer, BSN, RN, MS, MSN
Assistant Professor
Bethel College
Mishawaka, Indiana

Sharon Souter, MSN, RN
Director of Nursing Program
New Mexico State University at Carlsbad
Carlsbad, New Mexico

Kathleen G. Stilling, MS, BSN, RNC
Assistant Professor
Essex, Division of Allied Health and Human Performance
Baltimore, Maryland

Patricia A. Stockert, RN, BSN, MS, PhD
Associate Professor
Saint Francis Medical Center College of Nursing
Peoria, Illinois

Kathleen Upham, MSN, BSN, ONC
Assistant Professor
Coastal Georgia Community College
Brunswick, Georgia

Anne Vaughan, MSN, BSN
Clinical Instructor
Bellarmine College, Lansing School of Nursing
Louisville, Kentucky

Rosemary H. Wittstadt, EdD, MS, BS, RN
Professor
Retired, Towson University School of Nursing
Towson, Maryland

Thomas Worms, MSN
Associate Professor
Truman College, School of Nursing
Chicago, Illinois

CONTRIBUTORS TO PREVIOUS EDITIONS

WE WOULD LIKE TO ACKNOWLEDGE THE FOLLOWING PEOPLE, WHO PARTICIPATED IN EDITIONS THREE AND FOUR:

DELLA ARIDGE, RN, MSN
Clinical Nurse Specialist
Abdominal Organ Transplant Service
Saint Louis University Health Sciences Center
St. Louis, Missouri

ELIZABETH A. AYELLO, PHD, MS, BSN, RN, CS, CWOCN
Clinical Assistant Professor
New York University, Division of Nursing
New York, New York

LYNDAL GUENTHER BRAND, RN, BSN, MSN
Instructor, Missouri Baptist Medical Center
School of Nursing
St. Louis, Missouri

PEGGY BRECKINRIDGE, RN, BSN, MSN, FNP
Associate Professor of Nursing
College of Health Sciences
Roanoke, Virginia

VICTORIA M. BROWN, RN, BSN, MSN, PHD
Associate Professor, School of Nursing
Georgia College & State University
Milledgeville, Georgia

GINA BUFE, RN, BSN, MSN(R), PHD, CS
Psychiatric Clinical Nurse Specialist
Private Practice
Hyannis, Massachusetts

DOROTHY MCDONNELL COOKE, RN, PHD
Associate Professor of Nursing
Saint Louis University Health Sciences Center
St. Louis, Missouri

SHEILA A. CUNNINGHAM, RN, BSN, MSN
Assistant Professor of Nursing
Neumann College
Aston, Pennsylvania

RICK DANIELS, RN, BSN, MSN, PHD
Associate Professor of Nursing
Oregon Health Sciences University at Southern
Ashland, Oregon

MARDELL DAVIS, RN, MSN, CETN
School of Nursing
University of Alabama
Birmingham, Alabama

CAROLYN RUPPEL D'AVIS, RN, BSN, MSN
Director, Baccalaureate Program/Adjunct Assistant Professor
The Catholic University of America
Washington, DC

PATRICIA A. DETTENMEIER, RN, BSN, MSN(R), CCRN
Assistant Clinical Professor, School of Nursing
Instructor in Medicine, School of Medicine
Saint Louis University
St. Louis, Missouri

DEBORAH OLDENBURG ERICKSON, RN, BSN, MSN
Instructor, School of Nursing
Methodist Medical Center of Illinois
Peoria, Illinois

DEBRA FARRELL, BSN, CNOR
Operating Room Staff Nurse
Saint Anthony's Medical Center
St. Louis, Missouri

LINDA FASCIANI, RN, BSN, MSN
Assistant Professor of Nursing
County College of Morris
Randolph, New Jersey

SUSAN JANE FETZER, PHD, MBA, MSN, BSN, BA
Assistant Professor, Coordinator RN to BSN
University of New Hampshire
Durham, New Hampshire

MARLENE S. FOREMAN, BSN, MN, RNCS
Associate Professor of Nursing
Louisiana State University at Eunice
Eunice, Louisiana

Carol P. Fray, RN, MA
Associate Professor, Adult Health Nursing
College of Nursing
University of North Carolina at Charlotte
Charlotte, North Carolina

Paula Goldberg, RN, MS, MSN
Oncology Clinical Coordinator
Barnes Hospital
St. Louis, Missouri

Nancy C. Jackson, RN, BSN, MSN, CCRN
Pulmonary Clinical Nurse Specialist
St. Mary's Health Center
St. Louis, Missouri

Ruth L. Jilka, RD, CDE
Diabetes Educator
Barnes Hospital
St. Louis, Missouri

Teresa M. Johnson, RN, MSN, CCRN
Clinical Nurse Specialist
The Medical Center of Central Georgia
Macon, Georgia

Carl Kirton, RN, BSN, MA, CCRN, ACRN, ANP
Clinical Assistant, Professor of Nursing
New York University
New York, New York

Diane M. Kyle, RN, BSN, MS
Doctoral Candidate,
Supervisor of Clinical Services/Clinical Nurse Specialist
East Hartford Visiting Nurse Association, Inc.
East Hartford, Connecticut

Louise K. Leitao, RN(c), BSN, MA
Director of Clinical Services
East Hartford Visiting Nurses Association, Inc.
East Hartford, Connecticut

Gail B. Lewis, RN, MSN
Associate Professor
Barnes College
St. Louis, Missouri

Mary Kay Macheca, MSN(R), RN, CS, ANP, CDE
Certified Adult Nurse Practitioner and Certified Diabetes Educator
The Bortz Diabetes Control Center
Richmond Heights, Missouri

Jill Malen, RN, BSN, MS
Pulmonary Clinical Nurse Specialist
Barnes-Jewish Hospital at Washington University Medical Center
St. Louis, Missouri

Elizabeth Mantych, RN, MSN
Faculty, University of Missouri at St. Louis School of Nursing
St. Louis, Missouri

Mary Mercer, RN, MSN
Coordinator, Cardiac Rehabilitation
St. John's Mercy Medical Center
Creve Coeur, Missouri

Mary Dee Miller, RN, BSN, MS, CIC
Nurse Epidemiologist
Mercy Hamilton/Fairfield Hospitals
Hamilton, Ohio

Kathleen Mulryan, RN, BSN, MSN
Professor of Nursing
LaGuardia Community College
Long Island City, New York

Elaine K. Neel, RN, BSN, MSN
Instructor, School of Nursing
Methodist Medical Center of Illinois
Peoria, Illinois

Marsha Evans Orr, RN, BS, MS, CS
Zone Clinical Manager
Apria Healthcare
Phoenix, Arizona

Sharon Phelps, RN, BSN, MS
Nursing Practice Consultant
Barnes-Jewish Hospital
St. Louis, Missouri

Judith Roos, RN, MSN
Associate Professor
Jewish Hospital College of Nursing and Allied Health
St. Louis, Missouri

Jan Rumfelt, RNC, MSN, EdD
Associate Professor, School of Nursing
Southern Illinois University at Edwardsville
Edwardsville, Illinois

Linette M. Sarti, RN, BSN, CNOR
OR Charge Nurse
Bayfront Medical Center
St. Petersburg, Florida

April Sieh, RN, BSN, MSN
Assistant Professor
Delta College
University Center, Michigan

Marlene Smith, RN, BSN, M.Ed.
Staff Development Specialist
St. Louis Regional Medical Center
St. Louis, Missouri

Sharon Souter, RN, BSN, MSN
Director of Nursing Program
New Mexico State University at Carlsbad
Carlsbad, New Mexico

Martha A. Spies, RN, MSN
Assistant Professor
Deaconess College of Nursing
St. Louis, Missouri

Sandra Ann Szekely, RN, BSN
Director, Clinical & Infusion Services
Comfort Care of Michigan
Troy, Michigan

Pamela Becker Weilitz, MSN(R), RN, CS, ANP
Adult Nurse Practitioner
South City Health, LLC
St. Louis, Missouri

Laurel Wiersema, RN, MSN
Surgical Clinical Nurse Specialist
Barnes Hospital
St. Louis, Missouri

As always, this book is dedicated to my children,
Rebecca Lacey Perry and H. M. Perry IV.
It is my children who provide the
joys and richness in my life.
They are now young adults
beginning their careers,
and I'm very proud of who they are.
Anne Griffin Perry

To my many close friends,
who are my family.
You always encourage me,
brighten my day, and remind me
that there is so much to be thankful for.
Patricia A. Potter

PREFACE TO THE STUDENT

This book includes current, complete coverage of basic, intermediate, and advanced skills. The five-step nursing process provides the same overall framework that is used in most of your nursing textbooks. The clear two-column format is easy to read and includes rationales to explain why specific techniques are used. Each section and every feature was carefully developed to help you learn how to perform the skills and how to effectively care for your clients. This comprehensive resource will be invaluable as you take skills from the classroom to clinical practice. Check out some of these special features:

Over 1100 clear, high-quality **illustrations and photos** *show* you how steps are performed.

Critical Decision Points alert you to key information to consider *while* performing a skill.

Unexpected Outcomes and Related Interventions identify possible undesired results and provide appropriate actions.

Teaching Considerations tell you what to teach clients and families and how to evaluate learning.

Pediatric and Gerontological Considerations highlight specific needs of children and older adults.

Recording and Reporting provides guidelines for what to chart and report.

Home Care and Long-Term Care Considerations help you adapt skills for these settings.

Chapter 21 — Oral Nutrition

STEP	RATIONALE

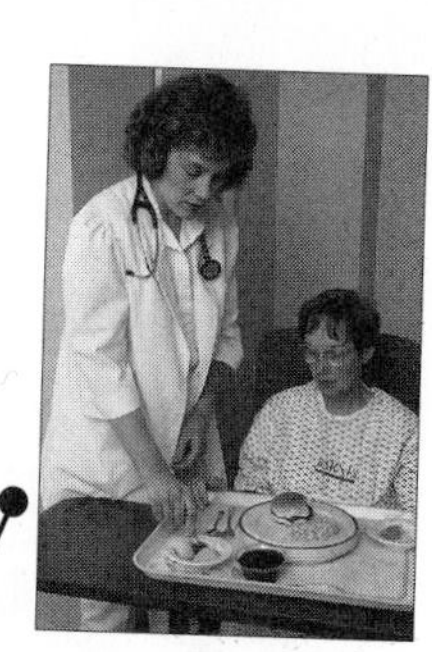

STEP **6** Nurse assisting client at mealtime.

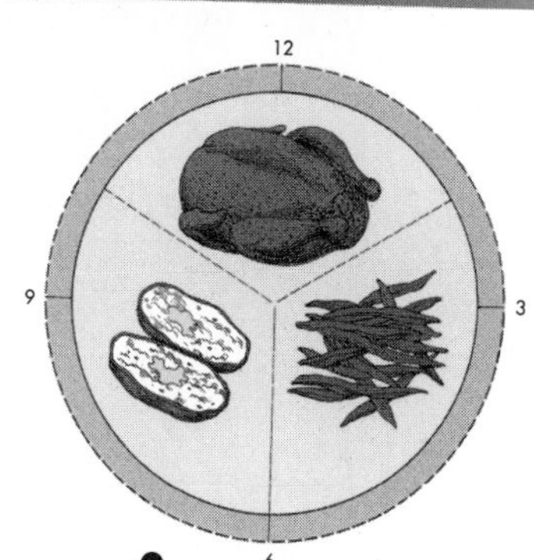

STEP **6a** For the visually impaired client: "The potatoes are at 9 o'clock." (From Elkin MK: *Nursing interventions and clinical skills*, ed 2, St. Louis, 1999, Mosby.)

STEP	RATIONALE
b. Neurologically impaired client: feed small amounts at a time and assess for ability to chew, manipulate tongue to form a bolus, and swallow. Give small amounts of thin liquids (soup, beverages) and assess for swallowing.	Clients with limited tongue strength and control may be unable to move bolus to back of mouth for swallowing. Checking for "pocketed" food in mouth prevents aspiration.

• *Critical Decision Point*
Clients with dysphagia who aspirate thin liquids may benefit from liquids thickened with commercial thickening products or from change in consistency of diet.

STEP	RATIONALE
c. Cancer client: check for food aversions before and during the meal.	May have strong, abnormal sense of taste and smell because of medications.
8. Provide fluids as requested. Do not allow client to drink all liquids at beginning of meal.	Assists with swallowing. Prevents client from filling up on liquids.
9. Talk with client during meal.	Meal should be a pleasant event. Conversation promotes so- ... Involve family if possible. ... occur whenever nurse and client are together.
	...fter meals helps prevent dental caries.
	...l tired after full meal. If client is prone to aspira- ...ead elevated 45 degrees for 30 minutes after meal. ...d of microorganisms.

Assisting the Adult Client With Oral Nutrition

STEP	RATIONALE
3. Determine client's tolerance to diet.	Overfeeding may cause nausea and vomiting. Underfeeding may leave client feeling hungry.
4. Monitor client's fluid and food intake.	Helps to determine whether client's nutritional and fluid needs are being met.
5. Observe client's ability to feed self.	Determines if client is gaining independence in feeding.

UNEXPECTED OUTCOMES AND RELATED INTERVENTIONS
- Client is unable to complete meal.
  - Determine why client is unable to finish meal (e.g., inadequate personnel for feeding assistance, ingestion of large volume of liquids immediately before meal, improper diet).
  - Determine if client's food preferences are met.
  - Determine if client is in pain or uncomfortable.
  - Assess for constipation.
- Client chokes on food.
  - Suction food and secretions from mouth and airway.
  - If choking occurs often, contact physician.
  - Make appropriate referrals (e.g., speech therapy).

RECORDING AND REPORTING
- Document in client's chart: client's tolerance of diet, amount eaten, and intake and output.
- If client is on calorie counts, record caloric intake on appropriate form; if intake and output are being evaluated, record fluid intake on appropriate form.
- If clients are receiving oral nutritional supplements (special foods or medical nutritionals such as Ensure, Isocal, and Resource), record the amount taken and communicate client tolerance (likes or dislikes, supplements to fill or replace meals) to the health care team to evaluate supplement effectiveness.
- Report any swallowing difficulties, food dislikes, refusal to eat to nurse in charge.

TEACHING CONSIDERATIONS
- Instruct client and family in required diet, including elimination of certain foods. Provide written instructions.
- Instruct client and family to maintain a nutritional balance of foods and to monitor intake of fluids, calories, fats, and salt.
- Teach family members to assist client in feeding self. Help client do as much as possible in feeding self.
- Instruct client and primary caregiver on importance of providing frequent mouth care.

HOME CARE CONSIDERATIONS
- Assess familiarity of client and primary caregiver with proper nutritional standards.
- Assess financial resources of client and family to determine if they are able to purchase proper foods for client.
- Assess priority given by client and family to provision of a balanced nutritional plan.
- Help client, family, and primary caregiver to make eating an enjoyable experience.

PEDIATRIC CONSIDERATIONS
- Infant feeding includes bottle or breast-feeding and the introduction of semisolid foods such as cereals at around 6 months; strained vegetables, meats, and fruits at around 8 months; and bite-size table foods at around 1 year. Cup feeding and finger foods are introduced as the child's fine motor skills develop (Wong, 1999).

LONG-TERM CARE CONSIDERATIONS
- Meals are part of the resident's social interaction with other residents and staff, and, as a result, residents rarely eat meals in their rooms.
- Meals in long-term care settings may be in a social dining program, where residents eat in a dining room and food is served as in a restaurant; family dining, in which residents serve themselves from a common serving bowl; or in an assistive dining program, in which residents can receive assistance with meals (Sorrentino and Gorek, 1999).

GERONTOLOGICAL CONSIDERATIONS
- Older adult clients may have diminished appetite because of loss of taste and smell and decreased number of taste buds.
- Interactions between nutrients and medicines may affect taste of foods or metabolism, absorption, digestion, or excretion of drugs (Lueckenotte, 2000).

person can lead to psychological problems and depression. It is important for the nurse to understand the psychological and social impact of altered ability to self-feed and to give the client as much choice, time, and independence as possible.

Dysphagia (difficulty swallowing) is the most common cause of aspiration in adults during oral feeding. Dysphagia can be caused by neurological and neuromuscular diseases and by trauma to or surgical procedures of the oral cavity or throat. The nurse should suspect the presence of dysphagia when the client coughs or gags during eating, exhibits multiple attempts at swallowing, complains of food "getting stuck" in the throat, or has poor lip and tongue control. **Aspiration** of food can lead to pneumonia and death. Nursing interventions for the dysphagic client can help to avoid aspiration, such as placing a "dysphagia" sticker on each client's chart or at the top of the client's bed.

Skill Performance Guidelines begin each chapter to help you identify principles that apply to all skills in the chapter.

Skill Performance Guidelines

1. Identify who are at risk for **malnutrition.** The nurse can provide preventive care and seek appropriate resources for intervention, for example, dietitian, nutritionist.
2. Be aware of the signs and symptoms of **malnutrition** (Table 21-1). Clients who are not thin and visibly malnourished may still have nutritional problems (e.g., the obese client with adequate fat reserves but depleted circulating protein reserves). Nutritional care should be provided for all clients.
3. Use a systematical and organized approach to nutritional assessment. This allows the nurse to obtain complete, essential information without being repetitive.
4. Be aware of the client's social history. Clients may be interested in healthy nutritional practices but may be unable to implement them (e.g., no refrigeration at home, lack of money to buy food or infant formula). The nurse needs to be aware of limitations and work with the client toward realistic goals.
5. Review the client's medical history. Certain diseases, medications, and medical problems can influence nutritional status. Clients with some medical problems or nonfunctioning GI tracts cannot be treated with oral nutrition. Parenteral therapies may be necessary (American Society for Parenteral and Enteral Nutrition [ASPEN], 1995).
6. Verify that the type of feeding ordered is what has been provided to the client at the proper temperature. Knowledge of the different types of oral diets (e.g., diabetic diet, lactose intolerant diet) helps the nurse properly plan and recommend changes to meet client needs.
7. Promote factors that improve client's appetite, such as encouraging client to select foods, small, frequent meals, and pleasant and comfortable surroundings.
8. An organized approach when feeding a client of any age helps the client feel more at ease, and appetite may increase in an unhurried atmosphere.
9. Be aware of the psychological impact on the adult client who cannot self-feed. Feeding in a timely, well paced, and understanding manner that allows maximal client independence can lessen the negative aspects of being fed by someone else. Instruct family members to provide a relaxed, social atmosphere when feeding the client and to al- low the clie[...] Assistive dev[...]
10. Recognize sy[...] swallow atte[...] that may inc[...]
11. Encourage c[...] from the hospital meal tray to use as a guide for preparing meals at home.

Tables organize key information for you.

Table 21-1 Clinical Signs of Nutritional Status

Body Area	Signs of Good Nutrition	Signs of Poor Nutrition
General appearance	Alert: responsive	Listless, apathetic, cachexia, cachectic appearance
Weight	Weight normal for height, age, body build	Obesity or underweight appearance (special concern for underweight)
Posture	Erect posture; straight arms and legs	Sagging shoulders; sunken chest; humped back
Muscles	Well-developed, firm muscles; good tone; [...] fat under	Flaccid appearance, poor tone, underdeveloped tone; tenderness; edema; wasted appearance; inability to walk properly
	[...]ness; nor-	Inattention; irritability; confusion; burning and tingling of hands and feet (paresthesia); loss of position and vibratory sense; weakness and tenderness of muscles (may result in inability to walk); decrease or loss of ankle and knee reflexes; absent vibratory sense
	[...]ation;	Anorexia; indigestion; constipation or diarrhea; liver or spleen enlargement

Continued

Skill 21-2 Assisting the Adult Client With Oral Nutrition

Assisting the adult with oral nutrition requires time, patience, knowledge, and understanding. Most people eat without assistance. However, with illness or trauma, the client may be physically unable to eat without assistance. Physical impairments that limit self-feeding include hemiplegia, fractured arm, quadriplegia, debilitating illness, or generalized weakness. The presence of intravenous (IV) catheters or tubings, dressings, and bandages can also limit self-feeding. In addition, some older adults tire quickly and may need to be assisted even though they can eat independently. Although adult feeding needs and techniques differ from those for infants, the adult who needs help to eat still needs compassion and understanding. Merely feeding the adult can be accomplished with common sense, but providing a socially meaningful mealtime requires education and experience on the part of the nurse.

Skill Performance Guidelines begin each chapter to help you identify principles that apply to all skills in the chapter.

Delegation Considerations for each skill guide you in delegating tasks to assistive personnel.

Delegation Considerations

The skill of assisting the client with oral nutrition can be delegated to unlicensed assistive personnel. Instruct care provider to help the client to a comfortable position in a chair or with the head of the bed elevated. Offer a washcloth and towel to client before the meal tray is provided. Instruct care provider to assist client with preparation of the tray or food, such as opening containers, cutting up meat, or pouring liquids. The tray should be at a comfortable height and distance from client. Instruct care provider to observe for any swallowing problems, such as coughing, gagging, or difficulty swallowing, and to notify nurse immediately. Clients with swallowing problems require the assistance of licensed personnel.

Equipment

- Two-handled cup with lid
- Plate with plate guard
- Utensils with splints
- Utensils with enlarged handles
- Towels

Equipment lists show specific items needed for each skill.

Step	Rationale
Assessment	
1. Assess that GI tract is functional, and determine what type of diet client can tolerate (Box 21-3).	Nurse's awareness of specific diet order provides appropriate nutrition.
2. Assess client's ability to swallow. In clients with neurological condition, assess **gag reflex.**	Some clients (those who have neurological diseases or are handicapped) may be at risk for dysphagia and aspiration and may not be able to tolerate a regular diet. Change in consistency of diet (thickened liquids, pureed, soft), swallow training, or alternative means of nutrition may be needed.
3. Place a tongue blade or an oral suction catheter tip on the back of client's tongue.	Clients who do not gag are at risk for aspiration (see Skill 21-3).
4. Determine to what extent client is able to self-feed. Assess physical motor skills, level of consciousness, visual acuity and peripheral vision, and mood.	Clients with any level of independence should not be totally fed by hospital staff. Thorough understanding of client's physical and cognitive limitations alerts the nurse to client's needs.
5. Assess client's appetite, tolerance of foods, cultural and religious preferences, and food likes and dislikes.	Awareness of client's needs before meals prevents misunderstanding and frustration for both nurse and client.
6. Assess whether client has food allergies.	Knowledge of client's food allergies prevents allergic reaction to food groups.

Rationales help you understand why steps are performed a certain way.

A convenient **two-column format** guides you step by step.

Nursing Diagnosis

Defining characteristics from the assessment data may reveal the following nursing diagnoses for clients requiring this skill:

- Risk for aspiration
- Risk for fluid volume deficit
- Feeding self-care deficit
- Sensory/perceptual alterations (gustatory)
- Impaired swallowing

Related factors are individualized based on client's condition or needs.

Chapter 21 Oral Nutrition

Box 21-3 Diet Progression of Hospitalized Clients

CLEAR LIQUID
Broth, bouillon, coffee, tea, carbonated beverages, clear fruit juices, gelatin, popsicles

FULL LIQUID
As above with addition of smooth textured dairy products, custards, refined cooked cereals, vegetable juice, pureed vegetables, all fruit juices

PUREED
All of above with addition of scrambled eggs, pureed meats, vegetables, fruits, mashed potatoes and gravy

MECHANICAL SOFT
All of above with addition of ground or finely diced meats, flaked fish, cottage cheese, cheese, rice, potatoes, pancakes, light breads, cooked vegetables, cooked or canned fruits, bananas, soups, peanut butter

SOFT
All of above with addition of moist tender meat, poultry, fish, soft casseroles, lettuce, tomatoes, soft fresh fruit, cake, cookies without nuts or coconut

From Grodner M, Anderson SL, DeYoung S: *Foundations and clinical applications of nutrition: a nursing approach,* ed 2, St. Louis, 2000, Mosby.

Boxes highlight important facts for your quick reference.

STEP	RATIONALE
PLANNING	
1. **Expected outcomes** following completion of procedure:	
▪ Client denies any gastric, swallowing, or chewing problems or food intolerances.	Indicates absence of gastric disturbance or food intolerance.
▪ Client's weight increases or remains the same over the time diet therapy is provided.	Nutritional intake exceeds or meets daily requirements.
▪ Client completes meal.	Prescribed dietary intake has been eaten; decreases risk of nutritional imbalances.
▪ Client is able to participate in independent feeding.	Enables client to be as independent as possible; provide assistive devices as needed to promote independence; involve family in mealtime if possible.
2. Prepare client's room for mealtime: a. Remove any unpleasant odors and sights (e.g., remove bedpans, bedside urinals, used dressings, trash).	Unsightly, odor-filled room can decrease client's appetite.
b. Clear overbed table.	
c. Set up chair for client and for nurse. Place bed in upright back position if client is unable to be up in the chair.	Certain conditions, such as pressure ulcer, traction, or spinal surgery, may prevent positioning with head elevated.
3. Prepare client for meal: a. Assist client with elimination needs.	Increases client's ... sult client's nu...
b. Help client wash hands.	Reduces spread o...
c. Assist client with mouth care. Clients with dysphagia or dry mouth may benefit from clear water rinsing or swabbing.	Oral hygiene imp...
d. Clients with stomatitis (irritation of oral mucosa) may benefit from rinsing with a solution containing ½ to 1 teaspoon of salt to 1 pint of water.	Clients may avoi... esophagitis.
e. Help client to put in dentures and put on eyeglasses or insert contact lenses if used. Check that dentures are	Enhances client's ... inhibit normal

Expected outcomes identify the anticipated client response to the skill.

Skill 21-2 Assisting

STEP	RATIONALE
f. Help client to comfortable sitting position. If client is unable to sit, turn client on side with the head of the bed elevated.	Minimizes risk o...
g. Obtain special devices and needed supplies to facilitate feeding (two-handled cup with lid, plate with plate guard, utensils with splints, utensils with enlarged handles, towels) before meal (see illustration).	Ensures organize...

Illustrations within skills are identified with the step number and legend to provide quick visual identification.

STEP **3g** Mealtime equipment. *Clockwise from upper left:* two-handled cup with lid, plate with plate guard, utensils with splints, and utensils with enlarged handles. (From Elkin MK: *Nursing interventions and clinical skills,* ed 2, St. Louis, 1999, Mosby.)

STEP	RATIONALE
IMPLEMENTATION	
1. Wash hands before preparing client's tray.	Reduces spread of microorganisms.
2. Assess tray for completeness and correct diet.	Prevents ingestion of incorrect or incomplete meal.
3. Prepare tray to meet client's needs: open cartons, remove lids, cut food, season food after asking client's preferences.	Clients with cognitive or physical impairments may not have the fine motor coordination needed to prepare tray for eating.
4. If client is able to eat independently, stop here. Return after 10 to 20 minutes.	Determines how well client is tolerating diet.
5. For client who cannot eat independently, begin feeding by assisting. ▪ Put yourself in a comfortable position. ▪ Ask client about any religious or cultural preferences before beginning feeding.	Sitting or standing close to client during feeding promotes psychologically comforting and caring environment, which may increase appetite. It is important that the caregiver be comfortable when feeding client, so as not to rush him or her through the meal.
6. Ask in what order client would like to eat, and cut food into bite-size pieces (see illustration).	Allows client more independence and control. Small pieces are easier to chew and minimize risk of aspiration.
a. It may be helpful for slightly confused, visually impaired, or easily fatigued clients to have food identified by location on plate as if the plate were a clock (see illustration).	
7. Feed client in a manner that facilitates chewing and swallowing. a. Older adult: feed small amounts at a time, assessing chewing, swallowing, and fatigue.	Decreased saliva production can impair swallowing in the older adult. Aspiration can result because of a decreased or absent gag reflex and relaxation of the lower esophageal sphincter (Williams, Hopper, 1999). Chewing and sitting up for feeding may accelerate onset of fatigue. Frequent rests may be helpful (White and others, 1991; Whitehouse, 1992).

An emphasis on **evidence-based practice** cites scientific research that supports techniques.

PREFACE TO THE INSTRUCTOR

Clinical Nursing Skills & Techniques is the book of choice in schools of nursing and health care agencies across the country.

Everything you have always loved about *Clinical Nursing Skills & Techniques* is here in the fifth edition, with new up-to-date content and improved features. It still offers complete coverage of more than 220 basic, intermediate, and advanced nursing skills, a nursing process framework that gives students a logical and consistent presentation, and a clear, two-column format with scientific rationales for steps. Plus, *new* skills and an increased focus on incorporating evidence-based practice, among many other new features, make this edition your number one choice.

CLASSIC FEATURES

- Current, comprehensive coverage of **more than 220 nursing skills** is included.
- **Five-step nursing process format** provides a consistent, clear presentation that helps students apply the process while learning each skill.
- Readable, easy-to-follow **two-column format** is used.
- Nearly **1100 large, clear photographs and drawings** provide visual understanding.
- **Rationales** are given for steps so students learn *why,* as well as how.
- **Critical Decision Points** focus the students' attention on key information to consider while performing skills to ensure safe and effective outcomes.
- **Expected Outcomes** identify the anticipated client response to the skill and reflect the outcome focus of current practice.
- **Current Centers for Disease Control and Prevention (CDC) infection control guidelines** are incorporated throughout.
- **Skill List, Objectives, and Key Terms** begin each chapter.
- **Skill Performance Guidelines** at the beginning of each chapter provide the student with guidelines applicable to all skills in the chapter.
- **Recording and Reporting** in each skill provides sample information on what to document and report.
- **Teaching Considerations** remind students to incorporate this essential nursing activity while performing skills.
- **Pediatric** and **Gerontologic Considerations** help students adapt a skill to the specific needs of children and older adults.
- **Home Care Considerations** teach students how to adapt skills in the home setting.
- **Critical Thinking Exercises,** based on realistic clinical situations, promote development of decision-making abilities regarding newly learned nursing skills.
- **Glossary** includes all key terms.

NEW FEATURES

- **Five new skills**
  - Using Small Volume Nebulizers
  - Placing a Client on a Rotokinetic Bed
  - Applying Pneumatic Compression Devices
  - Administering Continuous Subcutaneous Medications
  - Irrigating a Small-Bore Feeding Tube
- **New Shift Assessment chapter** includes those assessment areas most frequently used in the day-to-day, shift-to-shift care of the client.
- **Delegation Considerations** for each skill discuss the nurse's responsibility when assigning tasks to assistive personnel.
- An emphasis on **evidence-based practice** cites scientific research that supports the best practice approaches to skills.
- **Unexpected Outcomes and Related Interventions,** at the end of each skill, alert the student to possible undesired responses and outline appropriate nursing interventions.
- **Illustrations within skills are now identified with both step number and legend** to provide quick visual identification.
- **New Long-Term Care Considerations** highlight factors to consider when performing select skills in this setting.
- Contains **newest cardiopulmonary resuscitation (CPR) guidelines** from American Heart Association, September 2000.

TEACHING/LEARNING PACKAGE

- **Skills Performance Checklists** so both you and your students can evaluate skill performance. Students may purchase the checklists separately or at a special price when packaged with the text.
  Skills Performance Checklists: ISBN 0-323-01493-3
  Text and Checklist Package: ISBN 0-323-01497-6
- **Instructor's Resource Manual With NEW Test Bank.** Includes critical thinking exercises (from text) with answers, educational strategies, independent learning activities, cross curriculum guide, and multimedia resources. Test Bank contains over 500 completely new multiple choice questions in NCLEX format.
  ISBN 0-323-01413-5
- **MERLIN Website.** The unique passcode included in each copy of this text provides free access to MERLIN—Mosby's Electronic Resource Links and Information Network. This website was created especially for *Clinical Nursing Skills & Techniques* and features quarterly, updated links to annotated websites related to specific chapter content.

- **Mosby's Nursing Skills Video Series.** These innovative, action-packed videos give students a visual grasp of key skills. The series enhances classroom teaching as students observe actual nurses explaining procedures, performing skills, and interacting with clients. Contemporary concepts such as delegation, client rights, standard CDC precautions, and communication techniques are integrated throughout.

  Set I: Basic Nursing Skills: ISBN 0-323-01356-2

  Set II: Intermediate Nursing Skills: Coming Spring 2002. ISBN 0-323-01376-7

  Set III: Advanced Nursing Skills: Coming Fall 2002. ISBN 0-323-01387-2

ACKNOWLEDGMENTS

To the nursing editorial staff. We wish to acknowledge our editor, Suzi Epstein, for her attention to the trends that are influencing nursing today and recognizing the need to create innovative and well-designed textbooks. Suzi is a talented editor. She offers the guidance and support necessary to craft a text that we can be proud to publish.

To Shari Malchow, Senior Developmental Editor, who provides wise counsel in the review and critique of manuscript and who recognizes the elements of quality text. Her focus, direction, attention to detail, patience, and sense of humor ensure that we attend to the details necessary to develop an excellent product.

To our production team, Kathy Teal and Mary Turner. Their skill, expertise, and dedication to excellence ensure a publication that is logically, consistently and clearly presented. The countless hours spent and willingness to go above and beyond mark them as true professionals.

To Kathi Gosche, who designed this book inside and out. Her creativity brings a wonderful look and feel to the text, while ensuring that all elements are easy for the reader to identify.

To our contributors, excellent educators, and clinicians, who share their invaluable experiences and knowledge in the chapters they create. It is they who help us to achieve a "state-of-the-art" skills text.

To the professional nursing staffs and faculties at Barnes-Jewish Hospital, Jewish Hospital College of Nursing and Allied Health, and Saint Louis University. They continue to provide us with many ideas for the text as a result of their commitment to nursing. Their assistance has helped us achieve high quality for the textbook's photographic design.

To Rick Brady, for his excellent photography. Rick's photographic skills provide the richness of detail we try to show visually within the text.

To our clinical consultants, who willingly share their "state of the art" expertise and knowledge of evidence-based practice to assist us in the development of this text.

To our reviewers, for whose expertise and astute recommendations helped develop a text of high standards that reflects the current practice of nursing today.

To you, our readers, who continue to challenge us to make the very best textbook. We appreciate your insight, your ideas, and your continued desire to have the best information available for the care of your clients.

To our continued relationship as friends and co-authors. The experience of writing texts for over 20 years has taught us a great deal about one another. We look forward to continuing to collaborate so as to remain innovative and creative. The challenge is easier with the rewarding friendship that we have.

Anne Griffin Perry
Patricia A. Potter

CONTENTS

1

Admitting, Transfer, and Discharge

Skills

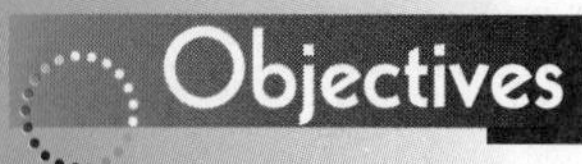

Objectives

Mastery of content in this chapter will enable the nurse to:

- Define the key terms listed.
- Describe the nurse's role in maintaining continuity of care through a client's admission, transfer, and discharge from an acute care facility.
- Explain the purpose and importance of advance directives.
- Identify clients in need of comprehensive discharge planning.
- Explain the importance of including the client's family in the admission, transfer, or discharge process.
- Describe the role of the nurse in discharge planning.
- Perform the following skills: admit a client to an agency, admit a client to a nursing division, transfer a client to a different agency, discharge a client.

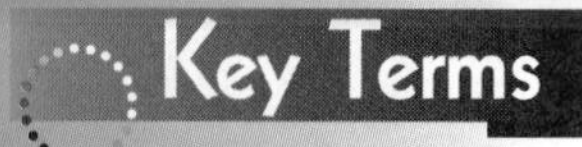

Key Terms

Advance directives
American Hospital Association (AHA)
Discharge planning
Joint Commission on Accreditation of Healthcare Organizations (JCAHO)
Nursing home (long-term care facility)
Patient Self-Determination Act
A Patient's Bill of Rights

A client often has numerous needs when entering the health care system. When these needs are complex, the client often requires multiple services from health care providers. In the acute care setting a variety of services are provided by multiple caregivers, and the nurse plays a key role in coordinating the client's care from admission to discharge. The nurse spends more time with clients than do other caregivers and thus is in the best position to understand the client's needs from a holistic perspective. The nurse coordinates the many resources required to ensure a smooth transition from the hospital to the next level of care. To separate the processes of admission and discharge is a critical error; the two are simultaneous and continuous. The nurse identifies clients' health care needs; anticipates physical, psychological, and social deficits that have implications for resuming normal activities; involves family and significant others in a plan of care; provides for health education; and assists in making health care resources available to the client. Ultimately the client and family should be prepared to understand the implications of any health problems and the responsibilities for continued care either in the home or next level of care setting.

Discharge planning is a process that facilitates a client's transition from a health care agency to the most independent level of care, whether that is home or another agency. The overall goal of discharge planning is to provide the best quality of care throughout all stages of the client's illness. Research has demonstrated, however, that nurses may be confused about discharge planning policies in their hospitals (Lowenstein and Hoff, 1994). The discharge planning process must be clearly stated so that all nurses are aware of its standards of practice and of their professional responsibility.

Federal requirements mandate all hospitals to have a discharge planning process (Box 1-1). Although the federal requirements were originally established for Medicare clients, they are generally applied to all clients within hospitals. The discharge planning process should be multidisciplinary and comprehensive.

Discharge from an agency can be stressful if a client and family members feel unprepared to resume normal activities or unable to adapt the hospital's therapeutic regimens to living at home. Before a client is discharged, the client and family members must know how to manage care in the home and what to expect in regard to any continuing physical problems. Without the necessary equipment and professional resources to care for continuing health problems, the client risks loss of any rehabilitation gains made before discharge. Failure to

Box 1-1 Federal Requirements for Discharge Planning Process

- Hospitals must identify at an early stage of hospitalization clients who are likely to suffer adverse health consequences upon discharge if there is no planning.
- The hospital must provide a discharge planning evaluation.
- A registered nurse, social worker, or other qualified person must develop or supervise development of the evaluation.
- Discharge planning must include an evaluation of the likelihood of needing post-hospital services and of the availability of the services.
- Discharge planning must include an evaluation of the likelihood of a client's capacity for self-care.
- Upon request of the client's physician, the hospital must arrange for development and implementation of the client's discharge plan.
- The evaluation must be completed on a timely basis so that appropriate arrangements for post-hospital care are made before discharge.
- The discharge planning evaluation must be in the client's medical record, and the results must be discussed with the client and/or significant others.

Modified from Discharge planning: conditions of participation, *Federal Register* 59:238, 1994. Healthcare Financing Administration, DHHS.

understand restrictions or implications of health problems may cause a client to develop complications after leaving the health care setting. For example, to control blood glucose levels, an adolescent newly diagnosed with diabetes mellitus must receive education on diabetes self-management, supplies (such as insulin, syringes, and a blood glucose monitor), and information regarding community resources. Without any one of these components, the adolescent is at risk for developing hyperglycemia, hypoglycemia, or long-term vascular complications associated with the disease. Poor discharge planning ignores the client's needs within the home and increases the chance of the client needing to reenter the health care system prematurely. An emphasis in current health care is to anticipate the client's discharge needs before the client enters the health care system.

Skill Performance Guidelines

1. Screen all clients upon admission to a health care setting for possible discharge needs.
2. Include the client, family, and relevant health care professionals in early planning for all moves through the health care system.
3. Consider the client's past experiences in health care settings.
4. Consider the client's cultural, socioeconomic, and educational background when discharge planning.
5. All appropriate health care providers who contribute to the client's care must collaborate in developing a plan of care for discharge.
6. Assist other health care personnel in assessing appropriate resources needed as clients move through the health care system.

Skill 1-1 Admitting Clients

A client can access the health care system in a variety of ways (e.g., hospital, emergent care center, clinic, or physician's office). Commonalities exist for the type of procedures used to admit clients to these settings (Box 1-2). However, each institution follows a different set of policies and procedures for admitting a client, and a client's condition determines the extent of the admitting procedure. For example, a client entering through the emergency department may not be in a condition to undergo the same interview process that takes place in a hospital admitting office. In this case family members provide pertinent information for the hospital's records while the client is transported directly to a nursing division. In contrast, an older adult client who can no longer attend to daily chores but who is still independent enough to perform some self-care undergoes extensive screening before being accepted as a **nursing home** resident.

Admitting officers, secretaries, and technicians are the personnel primarily involved with the preliminary admission procedures, such as interviewing clients and reviewing information about insurance, demographic data, and general agency procedures. Technicians can collect routine specimens and perform screening procedures such as electrocardiograms (ECGs). Some hospitals have a small satellite admitting office within the emergency department.

Box 1-2 Common Procedures for Admission to a Health Care Agency

- Placement of client in appropriate receiving area
- Assessment of client's health care problems and needs
- Determination of client's payment source for health care
- Explanation of client's rights and elements of advance directives
- Orientation to the health care agency's policies and procedures
- Preliminary testing and screening (specific for each agency and client's condition)
- Development of an individualized plan of care

Clients experience considerable anxiety about the admission process, so all personnel should treat them courteously and professionally. If a client is shown an uncaring attitude by just one individual, all personnel may be assumed to be uncaring and unprofessional. By making clients and families feel welcome, nurses and other staff members begin to establish a therapeutic relationship with the client.

Role of the Admitting Clerk or Secretary

The role of the admitting clerk or secretary includes specific activities such as initiating and maintaining a professional relationship with the client, providing for the client's safety, and providing for the client's legal rights. Each of these activities is an essential and important part of the admission process.

A courteous welcome by an admission clerk helps relieve the client's anxiety about a first encounter with agency personnel. Privacy can be maintained by escorting the client and family to an admitting interview area where important identifying information is collected (Figure 1-1). If the client does not speak English, an interpreter can be invaluable to ensure that correct information is gathered. If a client has a severe hearing impairment, an interpreter capable of using sign language may be called to assist during the admission procedure. Identifying information includes the client's full legal name, age, birth date, address, next of kin, physician, religious preference, occupation, and type of insurance. At this time, an identification (ID) band legibly stating the client's full legal

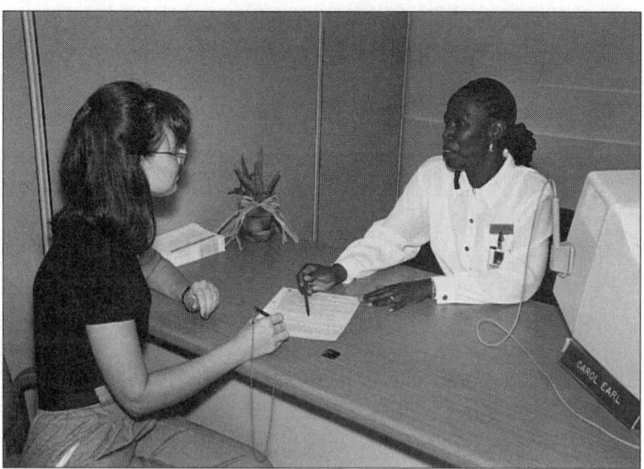

FIGURE **1-1** The admitting clerk gathers important information from client.

name, hospital or agency number, physician, and birth date should be applied securely to the client's wrist. The ID band serves to identify the client when therapies or procedures are performed. If a client is unconscious, identification may not be made until family members arrive. Also, a client who has been a victim of crime may be safer with an anonymous name under an agency's blackout procedure.

The admitting clerk or secretary should provide for the client's legal rights and instruct the client or legal guardian to read the general consent form for treatment, assess whether the form is understood, and request that the client or family member sign the form if there is agreement to be admitted for treatment. For the consent form to be valid, the client or guardian must be mentally and physically competent, be a legal adult, give voluntary consent, understand the risks and benefits of hospitalization, and have the opportunity to ask questions. Signature on the consent form will then give the agency the right to perform routine procedures and therapies, select room placement, and provide required nursing care.

Brochures pertinent to client rights and the activities that occur within the hospital should be provided to the client as part of the admission process. For instance, information pertaining to visiting hours and hospital services may be included in an admission packet. In addition, the **Patient Self-Determination Act,** effective December 1, 1991, requires all Medicare- and Medicaid-recipient hospitals to provide clients with information about their right to accept or reject medical treatment. In addition, clients must receive information about **advance directives** and be referred to appropriate resources if they want to discuss advance directives or receive help in completing an advance directive document (Burke, 1993) (Box 1-3). Many hospitals also provide clients the American Hospital Association's (AHA's) **"A Patient's Bill of Rights"** (Box 1-4), which cites the client's right to have access to information describing the purpose of the health care agency, organization, and policies and rules that affect the person's rights as a client.

Box 1-3 Advance Directives

- An advance directive is a document that gives a person's directions about future medical care or designates another person(s) to make medical decisions if the individual loses decision-making capacity.
- An advance directive conveys the client's choice in continuing medical care when the client is unable to speak or make decisions.
- Advance directives include a living will, power of attorney for health care, or a notarized handwritten document.
- The document should be available in the client's medical record.
- The attending physician is notified of the client's advance directive.
- Witnesses for an advance directive document should not be medical personnel, nor should they be related to the client or heirs to the client's estate.

Role of the Nurse

Nurses should be directly involved in assigning clients to rooms, completing a thorough nursing assessment, reviewing any advance directives, ensuring that necessary diagnostic testing is completed, and providing for continuity of care when the client is admitted through the emergency department. Admitting personnel should confer with nursing staff to ensure that a client's room is assigned based on the client's condition, health care needs, and personal preferences. For example, a client who is acutely ill and receiving multiple treatments may best be cared for in a room close to the nurse's station. Consideration of these factors during room selection minimizes the client's anxiety and prevents conflict with other clients.

When a client is admitted through the emergency department, the emergency department nurse should notify the nursing division in a report of the client's admission information, including the client's name, assigned room and bed, admitting physician, diagnosis, and pertinent information related to the client's condition (e.g., level of consciousness, intravenous fluid infusing, or need for oxygen). A full report ensures adequate preparation for the client's arrival and prompt treatment. The client and family members should be transported to the nursing division with an escort and introduced to the nurse assuming the client's care. Any pertinent observations about the client's behavior (e.g., anxiety or fear, or level of knowledge regarding need for health care) can be shared with the nursing staff at this time to foster continuity of care and assist the client and family in coping with a new environment and procedures.

Clients admitted the morning of a surgical procedure or treatment are called "same day" admissions. The nurse should provide them with basic instructions regarding the purpose of the surgery or treatment, preparatory procedures, and postsurgical or posttreatment care. Admission forms, consent forms, diagnostic tests, and instructions may be completed before the actual day of surgery. Informational booklets pertaining to the client's surgery or treatment are often available to clients well in advance of their surgery date.

Box 1-4 A Patient's Bill of Rights

Introduction

Effective health care requires collaboration between patients and physicians and other health care professionals. Open and honest communication, respect for personal and professional values, and sensitivity to differences are integral to optimal patient care. As the setting for the provision of health services, hospitals must provide a foundation for understanding and respecting the rights and responsibilities of patients, their families, physicians, and other caregivers. Hospitals must ensure a health care ethic that respects the role of patients in decision making about treatment choices and other aspects of their care. Hospitals must be sensitive to cultural, racial, linguistic, religious, age, gender, and other differences, as well as the needs of persons with disabilities.

The American Hospital Association presents *A Patient's Bill of Rights* with the expectation that it will contribute to more effective patient care and be supported by the hospital on behalf of the institution, its medical staff, employees, and patients. The American Hospital Association encourages health care institutions to tailor this bill of rights to their patient community by translating and/or simplifying the language of this bill of rights as may be necessary to ensure that patients and their families understand their rights and responsibilities.

Bill of Rights*

1. The patient has the right to considerate and respectful care.
2. The patient has the right to and is encouraged to obtain from physicians and other direct caregivers relevant, current, and understandable information concerning diagnosis, treatment, and prognosis.

   Except in emergencies when the patient lacks decision-making capacity and the need for treatment is urgent, the patient is entitled to the opportunity to discuss and request information related to the specific procedures and/or treatments, the risks involved, the possible length of recuperation, and the medically reasonable alternatives and their accompanying risks and benefits.

   Patients have the right to know the identity of physicians, nurses, and others involved in their care, as well as when those involved are students, residents, or other trainees. The patient also has the right to know the immediate and long-term financial implications of treatment choices, insofar as they are known.
3. The patient has the right to make decisions about the plan of care prior to and during the course of treatment and to refuse a recommended treatment or plan of care to the extent permitted by law and hospital policy and to be informed of the medical consequences of this action. In case of such refusal, the patient is entitled to other appropriate care and services that the hospital provides or transfer to another hospital. The hospital should notify patients of any policy that might affect patient choice within the institution.
4. The patient has the right to have an advance directive (such as a living will, health care proxy, or durable power of attorney for health care) concerning treatment or designating a surrogate decision maker with the expectation that the hospital will honor the intent of that directive to the extent permitted by law and hospital policy.

   Health care institutions must advise patients of their rights under state law and hospital policy to make informed medical choices, ask if the patient has an advance directive, and include that information in patient records. The patient has the right to timely information about hospital policy that may limit the hospital's ability to implement fully a legally valid advance directive.
5. The patient has the right to every consideration of privacy. Case discussion, consultation, examination, and treatment should be conducted so as to protect each patient's privacy.
6. The patient has the right to expect that all communications and records pertaining to care will be treated as confidential by the hospital, except in cases such as suspected abuse and public health hazards when reporting is permitted or required by law. The patient has the right to expect that the hospital will emphasize the confidentiality of this information when it releases it to any other parties entitled to review information in these records.
7. The patient has the right to review the records pertaining to medical care and to have the information explained or interpreted as necessary, except when restricted by law.
8. The patient has the right to expect that, within its capacity and policies, a hospital will make reasonable response to the request of a patient for appropriate and medically indicated care and services. The hospital must provide evaluation, service, and/or referral as indicated by the urgency of the case. When medically appropriate and legally permissible, or when a patient has so requested, a patient may be transferred to another facility. The institution to which the patient is to be transferred must first have accepted the patient for transfer. The patient must also have the benefit of complete information and explanation concerning the need for, risks, benefits, and alternatives to such a transfer.
9. The patient has the right to ask and be informed of the existence of business relationships among the hospital, educational institutions, other health care providers, or payors that may influence the patient's treatment and care.
10. The patient has the right to consent to or decline to participate in proposed research studies or human experimentation affecting care and treatment or requiring direct patient involvement, and to have those studies fully explained prior to consent. A patient who declines to participate in research or experimentation is entitled to the most effective care that the hospital can otherwise provide.
11. The patient has the right to expect reasonable continuity of care when appropriate and to be informed by physicians and other caregivers of available and realistic patient care options when hospital care is no longer appropriate.
12. The patient has the right to be informed of hospital policies and practices that relate to patient care, treatment, and responsibilities. The patient has the right to be informed of available resources for resolving disputes, grievances, and conflicts, such as ethnics committees, patient representatives, or other mechanisms available in the institution. The patient has the right to be informed of the hospital's charges for services and available payment methods.

These rights can be exercised on the patient's behalf by a designated surrogate or proxy decision maker if the patient lacks decision-making capacity, is legally incompetent, or is a minor.

A Patient's Bill of Rights was first adopted by the American Hospital Association in 1973. This revision was approved by the AHA Board of Trustees on October 21, 1992. American Hospital Association, 1999.

Continued

Box 1-4 A Patient's Bill of Rights—cont'd

Bill of Rights—cont'd

The collaborative nature of health care requires that patients, or their families/surrogates, participate in their care. The effectiveness of care and patient satisfaction with the course of treatment depend, in part, on the patient fulfilling certain responsibilities. Patients are responsible for providing information about past illnesses, hospitalizations, medications, and other matters related to health status. To participate effectively in decision making, patients must be encouraged to take responsibility for requesting additional information or clarification about their health status or treatment when they do not fully understand information and instructions. Patients are also responsible for ensuring that the health care institution has a copy of their written advance directive if they have one. Patients are responsible for informing their physicians and other caregivers if they anticipate problems in following prescribed treatment.

Patients should also be aware of the hospital's obligation to be reasonably efficient and equitable in providing care to other patients and the community. The hospital's rules and regulations are designed to help the hospital meet this obligation. Patients and their families are responsible for making reasonable accommodations to the needs of the hospital, other patients, medical staff, and hospital employees. Patients are responsible for providing necessary information for insurance claims and for working with the hospital to make payment arrangements, when necessary.

A person's health depends on much more than health care services. Patients are responsible for recognizing the impact of their lifestyle on their personal health.

Conclusion

Hospitals have many functions to perform, including the enhancement of health status, health promotion, and the prevention and treatment of injury and disease; the immediate and ongoing care and rehabilitation of patients; the education of health professionals, patients, and the community; and research. All these activities must be conducted with an overriding concern for the values and dignity of patients.

The nurse plays an active role in coordinating the client's movement through the admission process and on to a nursing division. As is the case with the initial admission process, a client's condition influences the extent and type of admission activities. When a critically ill client reaches a hospital's nursing division, the client must undergo extensive examination and treatment procedures almost immediately. Little time is available for the nurse to orient the client and family to the division or learn of their fears or concerns. When a client enters a hospital for elective treatment, the nurse may have more time to prepare the client psychologically for hospitalization. The client is less rushed through the admission process; however, surgery or diagnostic testing may be performed that same day. Early psychological preparation when the client is still at home can be very helpful in preparing clients for hospitalization.

The nurse must always be conscious of the client's level of fatigue and comfort. The admission process can be exhausting, especially when being delayed in the admitting office for a room assignment. When the client is experiencing physical or psychological symptoms, the nurse determines whether any portion of the admission process can be completed later.

Delegation Considerations

The skill of assessing clients during admission to a health care facility should not be delegated to assistive personnel. However, the following activities may be delegated: preparation of the client's room and equipment before admission, gathering and securing the client's personal care items, assisting with escorting and orienting the client and family to the nursing unit, and measuring vital signs and height and weight.

Equipment

- Bedpan and urinal
- Washbasin
- Bath towel and washcloth
- Toiletry times (e.g., soap, toothpaste, hand lotion; optional in some hospitals)
- Tissue paper
- Water pitcher and drinking cup
- Kidney or emesis basin
- Disposable thermometer (see agency policy)
- Sphygmomanometer
- Stethoscope
- Documentation forms

Step	Rationale
Room Preparation	
1. Wash hands and prepare room equipment and furniture. Prepare bed by adjusting it to lowest horizontal position. Turn down top sheet and spread. Arrange room furniture for easy access to bed.	Promotes client's comfort by preventing delays during care. Proper position of bed lessens likelihood of client falls and of back injuries to staff assisting the client into the bed.

STEP	RATIONALE
2. Be sure equipment is in working order. Then assemble any special equipment such as suction, oxygen supplies, or intravenous (IV) pole in client's room.	Prevents delays in delivering immediate treatment and provides for smooth transition between caregivers.

ASSESSMENT

STEP	RATIONALE
3. Greet client and family cordially. Introduce yourself by name and job title; explain your responsibilities in client's care. (Primary nurse may be assigned at this time.)	Reduces anxiety about admission and expedites client requests.
4. If client is not able to speak English or has a severe hearing impairment, arrange for a translation service so that a nursing assessment can be conducted.	Translation services are preferred over use of family members to ensure correct translation of medical terminology.
5. Assess client's general appearance, noting signs or symptoms of physical distress.	Provides baseline assessment.

• ***Critical Decision Point***
If client is having acute physical problems, postpone routine admission procedures until client's immediate needs are met.

STEP	RATIONALE
6. Escort client and family to assigned room. Introduce them to roommate if semiprivate room is assigned at this time.	Orientation begins with introduction to roommate.
7. Assess client's and family's psychological status by noting nonverbal behaviors and verbal responses to greetings and explanations.	Anxiety influences how well client adapts to a health care environment and retains instruction.
8. Assess vital signs (see Chapter 9) and height and weight (see Chapter 10).	Provides baseline measurement to compare future findings. Determines alterations from normal range.
9. Have family or friends leave room unless they choose to assist client with undressing. Close door and curtains. Help client undress and assist client into comfortable position.	Provides for privacy and prepares client for examination.
10. Obtain nursing history organized by standards or nursing care adopted by hospital (e.g., functional health patterns). Data will include: a. Client's perception of illness and health care needs b. Past medical history c. Presenting signs and symptoms	Joint Commission on Accreditation of Healthcare Organizations (JCAHO) (1999) requires each client to have an admission assessment prepared by an RN. Each institution must set time frame for completion of admission assessment (maximum time 24 hours).
d. Review of health status based on standards such as elimination, nutrition and metabolism, activity and exercise, self-concept, values and beliefs, cultural factors, social support, and cognitive function e. Risk factors for illness	A comprehensive health history provides a holistic view of client's health problems and response to those problems.
f. History of allergies, including type of substance and a description of the reaction client has previously experienced	Client may have a sensitivity to a drug or substance rather than a true allergy; this should be clarified. Specify all allergens to prevent accidental exposure.

• ***Critical Decision Point***
Provide client with allergy arm band listing allergies to foods, drugs, latex, or other substances; document allergies according to hospital policy.

STEP	RATIONALE
g. Risk factors for falling (e.g., neurological disorders, history of urinary urgency, use of sedatives and analgesics, history of unsteady gait, history of orthostatic hypotension)	Identification of risk factors may lead to placement of client on fall precautions (see agency policy).
h. Medication history, including prescribed, over-the-counter (OTC), and alternative therapies such as herbs and hormones	A complete medication history helps to assess potential for drug interactions and may explain client's presenting signs and symptoms.

Step	Rationale
i. Client's knowledge of health problems and expectations of care	
11. Conduct physical assessment of appropriate body systems (see Chapter 10). If not obtained in admitting, instruct client to provide a urine specimen. Inform client as to blood specimens to be collected or tests to be performed.	Provides objective data for identifying health problems. Preparation of client can relieve anxiety that is created when unannounced procedures are performed.
12. Check physician's orders for treatment measures that should be initiated immediately.	Delay can cause deterioration of client's condition.
13. Orient client to nursing division.	
a. Introduce staff members who enter room. Always introduce client by last name unless client indicates otherwise.	Helps client to recognize caregivers. Shows respect for client.
b. Tell client and family the name of head nurse or charge nurse of the division and explain that person's role in solving problems.	Provides means for client to communicate problems.
c. Explain visiting hours and their purpose.	Willingness to observe visiting hours policy ensures client will receive adequate rest.
d. Discuss smoking policy and identify smoking areas for client and family.	The JCAHO has a standard requiring dissemination and enforcement of a hospital-wide smoking policy that prohibits the use of smoking materials throughout the hospital. Exceptions are authorized for a client by a physician prescription (JCAHO, 1999).
e. Demonstrate use of equipment (e.g., bed, overbed table, lighting).	Client's safety depends on understanding correct use of equipment.
f. Show client how to use nurse call light and position it in a convenient place. Have client demonstrate use of light.	Ensures client knows how to call for assistance.
g. Escort client to bathroom (if able to ambulate).	Client's safety depends in part on understanding how to use toilet facilities.

- ***Critical Decision Point***

  Ensure that client knows how to call for assistance while in bathroom. (An emergency call light is installed in bathrooms.)

Step	Rationale
h. Explain hours for mealtime and nourishments to client and family.	Family may wish to visit during evening to assist with meals.
i. Describe services available (e.g., chaplain, beauty shop, activity therapy).	Offers client options for making decisions.

Nursing Diagnosis

Defining characteristics from the assessment data may reveal the following nursing diagnoses for clients requiring this skill:

- Anxiety
- Deficient knowledge regarding hospital procedures and planned therapies
- Fear
- Ineffective coping
- Powerlessness
- Risk for injury

Related factors are individualized based on client's condition or needs.

Planning

Step	Rationale
1. **Expected outcomes** following completion of procedure:	
▪ Client is able to explain purpose and schedule of planned treatments and procedures.	Understanding treatment plan gives client a better sense of control and reduces anxiety about the unknown.

Step	Rationale
▪ Client will demonstrate how to call for nurse when assistance is needed.	Falls commonly occur when clients attempt to reach toilet facilities or a chair without assistance.
▪ Client will be able to ambulate (if condition permits) in room free of obstacles and safely and efficiently use equipment in the room such as the bedside table, lights, and bed adjustment controls.	Equipment used in care of client can pose hazards.
▪ Client is able to verbalize understanding of smoking policy, visiting hours, mealtimes, and services available.	Knowledge of hospital policies assists client in adapting to the health care environment.

Implementation

Step	Rationale
1. Inform client about procedures or treatments scheduled for the next shift or day (e.g., visits by physician or dietitian). These vary based on nature of client's condition.	Client has right to be informed of any scheduled procedures or treatments. Being able to anticipate planned therapies minimizes anxiety.
2. Give client and family chance to ask questions about procedures or therapies. (If client is unresponsive or unable to understand, review with family.)	Provides opportunity to clarify expectations and misconceptions.
3. Collect valuables client chooses to keep at facility. Complete listing sheet (see agency policy) and have client or family member sign it. Place valuables in safe or send home with family.	Accounts for placement of valuables and prevents loss.
4. Ensure client and family have time together alone, if desired.	Admission can be stressful and fatiguing. Allows time for decision making.
5. Be sure call light is within easy reach and bed is in low position. (Check agency policy regarding use of side rails.)	Provides for client's safety. Side rails are typically used to reduce the chance of falls but can be considered a restraint if the side rail inhibits client's ability to get out of bed when desired (JCAHO, 1999).
6. Wash hands.	Reduces spread of microorganisms.

Evaluation

Step	Rationale
1. Confirm client's understanding of hospital policies, tests, and procedures through discussion and questions.	Learning and understanding are demonstrated through client feedback.
2. Observe client for nonverbal signs (e.g., restlessness, poor eye contact, facial tension).	Such signs may indicate anxiety.
3. Monitor client's ability to ambulate independently.	Provides data to judge client's ability to ambulate without injury.
4. Check client's room setup regularly.	Determines if care area is free of obstacles.

Unexpected Outcomes and Related Interventions

- Client denies understanding hospital policies or knowing purpose or schedule for tests and procedures.
  - Schedule a follow-up session with client.
  - Keep information focused and specific to client's situation. Include family if helpful.
- Client becomes restless, expresses concerns, or displays tension in body movements.
  - Give client time to discuss fears and concerns.
  - Show caring and compassion so that client becomes willing to communicate openly.
- Client falls or is injured.
  - Nurse must attend to client's immediate physical needs, inform physician of the injury or fall, reassess the client's environment, ensure that the environment is free of safety hazards, and complete incident report (see Chapter 3).
- Client develops respiratory distress, acute pain, vital signs alterations, or loss of consciousness during admission process.
  - Postpone admission procedure immediately, and intervene in response to client's presenting needs.

Recording and Reporting

- Record history and assessment findings on appropriate forms.

- If client has an advance directive, place copy in the medical record. In the absence of an actual advance directive, the substance of the directive is documented in the medical record (JCAHO, 1999).
- Notify physician of client's arrival; report any unusual findings. Secure admission orders if not previously provided.
- Begin to develop nursing plan of care. Confer with client and family as needed.

Teaching Considerations

- Explain to client that a different nurse provides care on each shift. Explain time frame for how assignments are made. When primary nursing is the method of care delivery, primary nurse introduces self to client and explains plan for coordination of care.
- Teaching can occur throughout the admission process. A nurse can provide information regarding physical assessment findings, planned diagnostic procedures, or hospital routines. A formal teaching plan should not begin until assessment is completed and a care plan is developed.
- Teaching begins early in a client's hospitalization. Nurse introduces instruction when client is able to be attentive and learn from the information. This can be difficult in an acute care setting. Information should be specific, focusing on topics such as the nature of client's illness, medications needed for treatment, and use of equipment in self-care (e.g., dressings, ambulatory devices).
- In an emergency situation instruct family members in the rationale for any procedures and routines to be used in client's care.

Pediatric Considerations

- Allow and encourage parental involvement in the child's care. Hospitalization is a major crisis for children with stress resulting from separation, loss of control, bodily injury, and pain. Separation anxiety is most evident from middle infancy throughout the toddler years, especially ages 16 to 30 months. The child experiences protest, despair, and detachment. Preschoolers are better able to tolerate brief periods of separation, but their protest behaviors are more subtle than those in younger children (e.g., refusal to eat, difficulty sleeping, withdrawing from others). School-age children are able to cope with separation but have an increased need for parental security and guidance (Wong and others, 1999). Allow parents to assist with routine care activities (e.g., bathing, eating) and when possible to remain with the child during procedures.
- The nurse can play an important role in making the hospital experience a chance for children to develop new socialization skills and to broaden their interpersonal relationships. The nurse fosters parent-child relationships, offers educational opportunities, and provides for socialization with other children (Wong and others, 1999).

Gerontological Considerations

- Hospitalized older adults with some functional disabilities often rapidly regress into a helpless state during hospitalization. Interventions that may help to retain functional status during an episodic illness include daily orientation cues for client, reassurance regarding probability of transient delirium, getting client up and out of room at least daily, using physical therapy (PT) and occupational therapy (OT) daily, keeping the environment pleasant and comfortable, and personalizing the environment (Wanich and others, 1992; Ebersole and Hess, 1998).
- Clients who characteristically fall in the hospital are those who have been recently admitted and are unfamiliar with surroundings, have several pathological conditions, take medications with sedative or tranquilizing effects, or have had multiple recent transfers. In addition, visual changes that occur with aging can lead to falls in hospitalized older adult clients (Ebersole and Hess, 1998).

Skill 1-2 Transferring Clients

Clients transfer to new patient care units and new agencies to receive different forms of therapy and services and to have care continued closer to home. When clients transfer, continuity of vital aspects of nursing care must be ensured. The argument is that better continuity of care ensures better client outcomes. However, the health care system creates barriers to continuity. Changes in care occur when the medical plan of treatment is revised by the physician assuming the client's care. In addition, the plan of care changes if the agency's policies and procedures differ from those of the previous institution. The client and family expect care to continue as smoothly as possible without interruptions in therapy that may hinder progress toward recovery.

The nurse who collaborates early with physicians and members of other health care disciplines plays an important role in ensuring efficient client transfer with good client outcomes. This is perhaps even more important when clients transfer from an intensive care unit (ICU) to a general nursing unit. Clients move from an ICU setting, where they are more closely supervised and receive continuous monitoring and treatment, to a general nursing unit with typically fewer staff and the significant challenge to maintain continuity of care. Usually physicians make transfer decisions with limited nurse input. Higgins (1999) argues that it is only through open recognition and valuing of the unique contributions of nurses and physicians to clinical judgment in critical care that the ultimate goal of enhancing client care can be realized.

When clients transfer from one agency to another, nurses from the two agencies have minimal opportunity to communicate. The client's plan of care must be documented thoroughly in the medical record and on the transfer form. It is particularly important for members of the receiving staff to have a clear understanding of the client's progress and current status. Primary nurses or charge nurses should take an active role in ensuring that the client's plan of care is clearly communicated either orally or in written form.

Delegation Considerations

Because of the related assessment and decision making, the skill of transferring clients should not be delegated to assistive personnel. However, the following activities may be delegated: dressing the client, preparation of the client's room before transfer, gathering and securing the client's personal care items and any equipment that may accompany the client, and assisting with escorting the client to the nursing unit.

Equipment

- Transfer forms
- Special equipment as needed: wheelchair or stretcher, emesis basin, bedpan and urinal, oxygen tank and tubing, intravenous (IV) pole, and cardiac monitor

Step	Rationale
Assessment	
1. In collaboration with physician, assess reason for client's transfer (e.g., change in condition, services available at agency, client or family preferences regarding client's location).	Client should have access to agency with best resources to meet health care needs. Physician determines client's physical stability for transfer.
2. Assess client's and family's willingness to consent to transfer. Explain purpose of transfer thoroughly and provide time to discuss client's and family's feelings about the change in care setting.	Transfers are sometimes planned quickly. Client requires adequate psychological preparation and must give consent to transfer.
3. Assess client's current physical condition and determine method for transport. When transferring to new agency, assess method of transport to transferring vehicle (e.g., wheelchair or stretcher) (consult agency policy).	Client's condition can change quickly and may influence stability for transfer and type of support needed during transport.

- ***Critical Decision Point***
  Determine if client's status and safety require life support equipment. Staff assisting with transfer should be trained in life support. When transporting to new agency, a vehicle equipped with life support equipment is necessary.

Step	Rationale
4. Assess if client requires pain relief or antiemetics before transfer.	Ensures client's comfort.
5. Assess whether client's family or significant others have been notified of transfer. (This applies when client is coherent and has consented to transfer.)	Provides adequate communication with family or significant others to assist with client's emotional and psychological adjustment to the transfer.

Nursing Diagnosis

Defining characteristics from the assessment data may reveal the following nursing diagnoses for clients requiring this skill:

- Anxiety
- Fear
- Deficient knowledge regarding transfer procedure
- Pain
- Powerlessness
- Risk for relocation stress syndrome

Related factors are individualized based on client's condition or needs.

STEP	RATIONALE
PLANNING	
1. **Expected outcomes** following completion of procedure:	
▪ Client's vital signs and physiological status are unchanged following transfer.	Treatments planned so as not to interrupt physical support of client during transfer.
▪ Client incurs no injury during transport procedures.	Safety measures are successful in transferring client from wheelchair or stretcher to transport vehicle.
▪ Client or family is able to explain purpose of transfer and procedure for transport.	Understanding provides client with sense of control.
▪ Receiving nursing staff acquires and confirms written plan of care.	
2. Arrange for client's transport to an agency by chosen vehicle (may require support from social worker).	Transfer should occur without delays so that client has access to all needed resources at all times.
3. Obtain transfer order from sending physician. Order should include name of receiving agency (when applicable), receiving physician's name, and statement of client's stability for transfer.	Physician is legally responsible for releasing client from medical care and arranging for receiving physician. Client has legal right to refuse transfer against medical advice.
4. When transfer is to a new agency, contact the agency and arrange for bed in appropriate setting. Confirm willingness of agency to accept client (may be completed by social worker or discharge coordinator).	Prevents delays when client arrives at destination. Receiving hospital must ensure that there is available space and qualified personnel to treat clients. Hospital must also agree in advance to transfer.
IMPLEMENTATION	
1. Review with client and family benefits and risks of transfer. Discuss reason for transfer, when it is to occur, and what procedures are planned. Encourage questions.	Benefits of transfer must outweigh risks. Explanation of transfer procedures minimizes client's and family's anxiety.
2. Make sure documentation in client's record is complete and accurate. Nursing care measures should be individualized based on client need.	Accurate information is necessary for receiving agency to assume client's care.
3. Obtain from client a signature on a release form giving permission to have a copy of medical record made for receiving agency (when applicable).	Medical personnel from receiving agency rely on client's medical record as primary resource in resuming client's care plan. Agency policies dictate the portion of a client's medical record to copy.

• ***Critical Decision Point***

Be sure client has signed release form. Information in client's record is confidential, and its use requires client's signed release.

STEP	RATIONALE
4. Complete nursing care transfer form according to agency policy. (When transfer is to a different nursing unit, entire medical record accompanies client.)	Form provides summary of client's pertinent nursing care needs to ensure continuity of care.
5. Gather client's personal care items, clothing, and valuables. Secure in suitcase or container.	Articles can be easily lost in transfer.
6. Anticipate problems client may develop just before or during transfer. Perform necessary nursing therapies such as suctioning or changing a dressing.	Ensures client's comfort and safety in transport.
7. Assist in transferring client to stretcher or wheelchair using proper body mechanics.	Client transported to outside agency is more easily moved by stretcher into transport vehicle.
8. Perform final assessment of client's physical stability.	Minimizes risk of client developing complications during transfer.

• ***Critical Decision Point***

Be sure to check vital signs, check for clear airway, inspect patency of intravenous lines, and note client's level of consciousness.

STEP	RATIONALE
9. When transfer is to an outside agency, accompany client to transport vehicle. Client's condition determines level of staff needed to transfer to new unit (see agency policy).	Ensures medically qualified personnel are in attendance until client leaves agency/unit.
10. Call receiving agency/unit and notify of impending transfer and client's status (check agency policy).	Notification of nurse in charge or nurse assuming care of client will ensure better continuity of care at time of client's arrival.

EVALUATION

1. During the final assessment compare data with previous findings.	Determines if client's condition is changing.
2. Inspect client's alignment and positioning on stretcher/wheelchair.	Proper alignment and positioning reduces risk of an injury occurring during transport.
3. Confirm client's understanding of transfer and procedures through discussion and questions.	Learning is demonstrated through client feedback.
4. Determine if receiving agency/nurse has questions about client's care.	Chart information can be misinterpreted.

UNEXPECTED OUTCOMES AND RELATED INTERVENTIONS

- Client's physical status deteriorates during preparation.
  - Call physician immediately.
  - Initiate necessary interventions to stabilize client's condition.
- Client sustains injury during transfer to wheelchair or stretcher.
  - Stabilize client and call physician.
  - Complete incident report.
- Client is confused or uncertain about transfer.
  - Provide clarification or additional explanation.
- Receiving staff misinterprets directions for client's care.
  - Sending agency should have representative nurse or physician call to confirm that there are no questions regarding client's care.

RECORDING AND REPORTING

- Sending nurse documents client's status, including vital signs and other assessment findings, nursing plan of care, time of transfer, and method of transport.
- Receiving nurse documents client's arrival at agency by recording date and time of arrival, reason for transfer, method of transport, client's condition, and care provided at time of arrival.

TEACHING CONSIDERATIONS

- A transfer can create anxiety for client and family members. It may become necessary for the nurse to carefully repeat instructions regarding transfer at a time when client and family can better attend to nurse's explanation.

PEDIATRIC CONSIDERATIONS

- Information sharing is critical whenever a child is transferred either within a hospital or between facilities. Children need their parents' comfort and security; thus parents need to be well informed. Older children need to be involved in any discussion regarding transfers.

GERONTOLOGICAL CONSIDERATIONS

- When older adult client is transferred to new facility, relocation is stressful. The nurse should ensure that significant support persons are still accessible and that client is thoroughly oriented to new surroundings, is allowed to take important memorabilia, and has opportunity to make decisions about care.

LONG-TERM CARE CONSIDERATIONS

- It is important that clients receive the level of services appropriate to their physical and mental health needs. Participation of social worker or discharge planner in transfer process will ensure that transfer to a long-term care facility is appropriate.
- Upon client's arrival at long-term care agency, nurse will complete resident assessment instrument (RAI). The RAI consists of the minimum data set (MDS), resident assessment protocols, and utilization guidelines specified in state operations guidelines (Lueckenotte, 2000).

Skill 1-3 Discharging Clients

Successful discharge planning is a centralized, coordinated, multidisciplinary process that ensures that the client has a plan for continuing care after leaving the hospital (American Hospital Association [AHA], 1983). This process should guarantee a prompt and well-coordinated discharge from acute care to ensure that adequate care is continued either in a client's home or in a restorative care setting. The discharge planning process has evolved from focusing on a single event—referral of a client to a community service or facility—to a process that has been expanded to numerous health care settings and whose goal is to ensure continuity of health care (Rorden and Taft, 1990). Discharge planning facilitates the transition of the client from one environment to another.

Probably the greatest challenge in effective discharge planning is communication. This is difficult when there are multiple service providers and when health care professionals are unwilling to be accountable for communicating with clients, family and friends, or the community-based service organizations. Anderson and Helms (1995) identified two major communication problems in discharge planning: pertinent data is not transmitted or it is of poor quality, and information concerning the client's care is late or often totally absent. The communication problem can be minimized when an organization has a discharge coordinator or case manager responsible for discharge planning. Staff in these roles are responsible for thoroughly assessing a client's health care needs at discharge, identifying available and needed resources, linking the client and family to the proper resources, coordinating services (as appropriate), and following up on the client's progress following discharge.

The AHA (1985) identified the following levels of outcomes for ensuring a client's successful discharge plan:

1. Client and family understand the diagnosis, anticipated level of functioning, discharge medications, anticipated medical follow-up, use of new equipment, diet and exercise regimens, and available support systems.
2. Specialized instruction or training is provided to the client and family to ensure proper care after discharge.
3. Community support systems are coordinated to enable the client to return home.
4. Relocation of the client and coordination of support systems or transfer to another health care facility are performed.

All caregivers who care for a client with a specific health problem must participate in discharge planning. Development of a plan with outcomes mutually accepted by the client and caregivers and ongoing communication about its progress are essential. Rorden and Taft (1990) described the discharge process as occurring in three phases: acute, transitional, and continuing care (Figure 1-2). In the acute phase medical attention dominates discharge planning efforts. During the transitional phase the need for acute care is still present, but its urgency declines and clients begin to address and plan for their future health care needs. In the continuing care phase the clients are able to participate in planning and implementing continuing care activities needed after discharge.

Reimbursement pressures have resulted in shorter hospital stays for clients. It is common for health care team members to direct more attention to the discharge needs of the severely debilitated client who requires continued health care in the home or another health care facility. However, even a client who is hospitalized only a few hours and who is without complications is often unprepared to resume a normal lifestyle immediately upon discharge. Can the client move about freely once home? Is the client able to prepare a meal? Every hospitalized client requires discharge planning. Certain conditions place clients at greater risk for being unable to meet continuing health care needs after discharge (Box 1-5). When a client has one of these conditions, it is especially important to coordinate referrals to appropriate outside agencies such as home health care or a rehabilitation agency.

Box 1-5 Client Risk Factors for Discharge Planning

- Lack of knowledge of treatment plan
- Altered cognition
- Newly diagnosed chronic disease
- Major or radical surgery
- More than three active medical problems
- Social isolation
- Emotional or mental instability
- Visual and hearing deficits
- Takes more than five drugs
- Lack of financial resources
- Lack of available or approximate referral sources
- Terminal illness
- Lack of in-home care provider

Data from Burgess W, Ragland EC: *Community health nursing: philosophy, process, practice,* Norwalk, Conn, 1983, Appleton-Century-Crofts and Blaylock A, Cason CL: Discharge planning predicting patients' needs, *J Gerontol Nurs* 18(7):8, 1992.

Delegation Considerations

The skill of discharging clients should not be delegated to assistive personnel. However, the following activities may be delegated: preparation of the client's room before discharge, gathering and securing the client's personal care items and any supplies that may accompany the client, and assisting with transporting the client to the discharge transport vehicle.

Equipment

- Wheelchair or stretcher

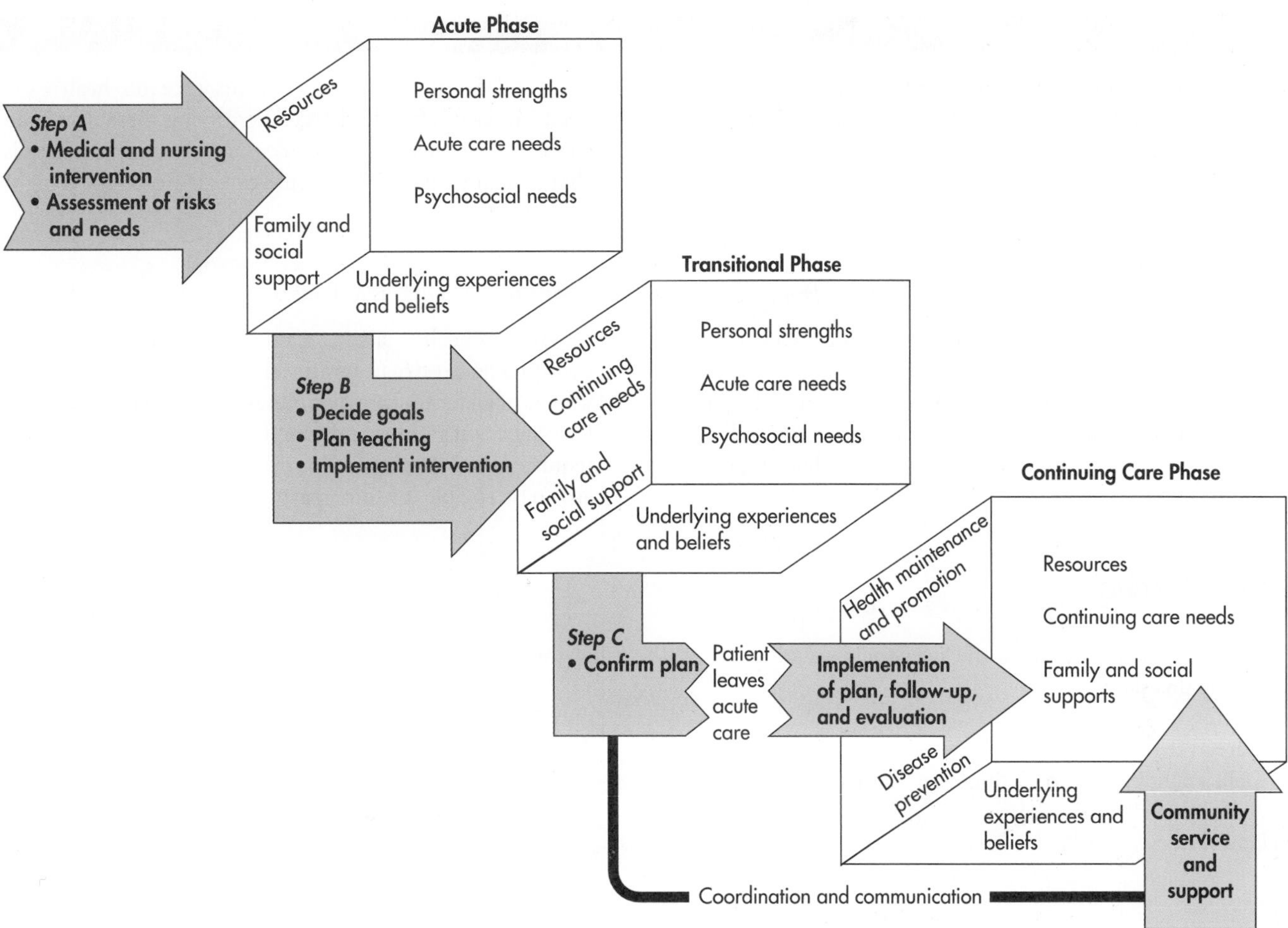

FIGURE 1-2 Phases of the discharge planning process. (Redrawn from Rorden JW, Taft E: *Discharge planning guide for nurses,* Philadelphia, 1990, Saunders.)

STEP	RATIONALE

ASSESSMENT

1. From time of admission, assess client's health care needs for discharge using nursing history and care plan; focus on ongoing assessments of client's physical health, functional status, psychosocial support system, financial resources, health values, cultural and ethnic background, level of education, and barriers to care (Clemen-Stone and others, 1997).

   Plan for discharge begins at admission and continues throughout client's stay in agency.

   Discharge planning interventions will focus on assisting clients to achieve maximal functioning.

2. Assess client's and family's need for health teaching related to how to perform home therapies, use of home medical equipment, restrictions resulting from health alterations, and possible complications.

   Improves understanding of health care needs and ability to achieve self-care at home. Inclusion of family member in teaching sessions provides client with available resource.

3. Assess with client and family any environmental factors within home that might interfere with self-care (e.g., size of rooms, doorway clearances, steps, bathroom facilities, availability of utilities). (A home health care nurse may be available on referral to assist with assessment.)

   May pose risks to safety as a result of limitation created by illness or need for certain therapies (see Chapter 39).

4. Collaborate with physician and staff in other disciplines (e.g., physical therapy) in assessing need for referral for skilled home health care services or extended care facility.

   Clients eligible for home health care are confined to home as result of illness, are under physician's care, and require skilled nursing care on intermittent basis. A multidisciplinary assessment ensures a comprehensive discharge plan.

Step	Rationale
5. Assess client's and family's perceptions of continued health care needs outside the hospital. Include an assessment of family caregiver's perceived ability to provide care to client.	Clients and family members may disagree on health care needs of client after discharge. Identifying these discrepancies early may help in more accurately developing the discharge plan (Bull, 1994). Family caregiving can be a highly stressful experience.

- ***Critical Decision Point***
  It may be necessary to talk with client and family separately to learn about true concerns or doubts.

Step	Rationale
6. Assess acceptance of health problems and related restrictions.	Acceptance of health status can affect willingness to adhere to therapies and restrictions after discharge.
7. Consult other health care team members about anticipated needs after discharge (e.g., dietitian, social worker, clinical nurse specialist, home health care nurse). Make appropriate referrals.	Members of all health care disciplines should collaborate to determine client's needs and functional abilities. Clients must require skilled nursing care or occupational or physical therapy to be eligible for third-party payment for home care.

Nursing Diagnosis

Defining characteristics from the assessment data may reveal the following nursing diagnoses for clients requiring this skill:

Anxiety	Interrupted family processes
Caregiver role strain	Fear
Deficient knowledge regarding home care restrictions	Self-care deficit: feeding, toileting, grooming, bathing/hygiene
Relocation stress syndrome	Impaired home-maintenance management

Related factors are individualized based on client's condition or needs.

Planning

Step	Rationale
1. **Expected outcomes** following completion of procedure:	
▪ Client or family caregiver is able to explain how health care is to continue in home (or other facility), what treatments or medications are needed, and when to seek medical attention for problems.	Increases likelihood of care not being interrupted in home (or other facility).
▪ Client is able to demonstrate self-care activities (or family member is able to administer care measures).	Feedback ensures learning.
▪ Obstacles to client's mobility and ambulation are removed in home setting. Items that are hazards because of client's health restrictions are removed.	Client may be physically weakened or have physical changes resulting from illness that predispose client to injury.

Implementation

Preparation Before Day of Discharge

Step	Rationale
1. Suggest ways to change physical arrangement of home to meet client's needs.	Client's level of independence and ability to retain function can be maintained within safe environment.
2. Provide client and family with information about community health care resources (e.g., medical equipment companies, Meals on Wheels, adult day care). Discharge coordinator can make referrals while client is in hospital.	Community resources may offer services client or family cannot provide.
3. After determining any barriers to learning and client's readiness to learn, conduct teaching sessions with client and family as soon as possible during hospitalization (e.g., signs and symptoms of complications, information regarding medications, use of medical equipment, follow-up care,	Gives client opportunities to practice new skills, ask questions, and obtain necessary feedback to ensure learning.

Step	Rationale
diet, exercise, restrictions imposed by illness or surgery). Pamphlets, books, or videotapes may be given to client. Client may also be referred to resources on the Internet.	

- ***Critical Decision Point***
  Different types of educational materials may be effective with different individual learning styles. Assess how client prefers to learn (e.g., read, watch video, listen to instructions). If printed material is to be used, be sure material at proper reading level is available.

Step	Rationale
4. Communicate client's and family's response to teaching and proposed discharge plan to other health care team members involved in client's care.	Facilitates development of individualized discharge plan.

Day of Discharge

- ***Critical Decision Point***
  If any of the following activities can be completed before day of discharge, planning will be more effective.

Step	Rationale
5. Let client and family ask questions or discuss issues related to home health care. A final opportunity to demonstrate learned skills may also be helpful.	Allows for final clarification of information previously discussed. Helps relieve anxiety.

- ***Critical Decision Point***
  Be sure to consider any variations in home setting (e.g., resources available, room setup in home) to be sure skills can be performed correctly.

Step	Rationale
6. Check physician's discharge orders for prescriptions, change in treatments, or need for special medical equipment. (Orders should be written as early as possible.)	Discharge is authorized only by physician. Early check of orders permits nurse to attend to any last-minute treatments or procedures well before discharge.
7. Determine whether client or family has arranged for transportation home.	Client's condition at discharge determines method of transport.
8. Offer assistance as client dresses and packs all personal belongings. Provide privacy as needed.	
9. Check all closets and drawers for belongings. Obtain copy of valuables list signed by client and have security or appropriate administrator deliver valuables to client.	Prevents loss of personal items. Client's signature verifies receipt of items. Relieves nursing department of liability for losses.
10. Provide client with prescriptions or pharmacy-dispensed medications ordered by physician. Offer a final review of any information needed to facilitate safe medication self-administration.	Review of drug information provides feedback to determine client's success in learning about medications.
11. Provide information on any follow-up appointments to the physician's office.	
12. Contact agency's business office to determine whether client needs to finalize arrangements for payment of bill. Arrange for client or family to visit office.	Source of concern for many clients is whether agency has accepted insurance or other payment forms.
13. Acquire utility cart to move client's belongings. Obtain wheelchair for clients unable to ambulate. Clients leaving by ambulance are transported on ambulance stretchers.	Provides for safe transport.
14. Assist client to wheelchair or stretcher using proper body mechanics and transfer techniques. Escort client to entrance of agency where source of transportation is waiting (see agency policy) (see illustrations). Lock wheelchair wheels. Assist client in transferring into automobile or transport vehicle. Help family place personal belongings in vehicle.	Prevents injury to nurse and client. Agency policy requires escort to ensure client's safe exit. Agency's liability ends once client is safely in vehicle.

A 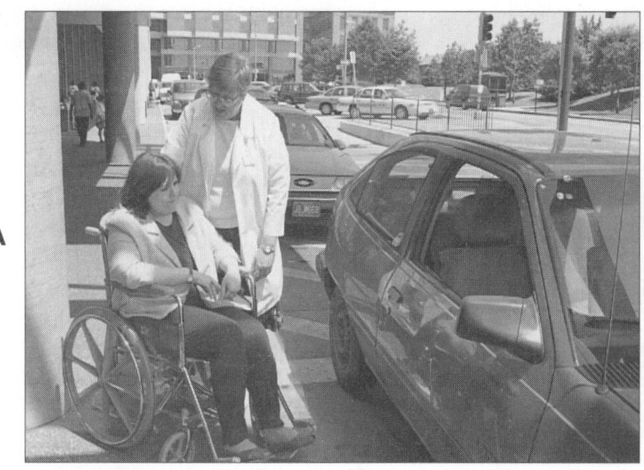

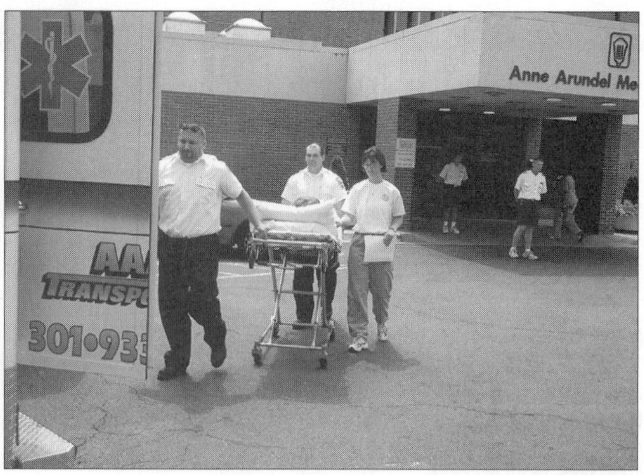

B

STEP **14** **A,** Nurse escorts client to transport vehicle at time of discharge via wheelchair. **B,** Many client are discharged via stretcher.

STEP	RATIONALE
15. Return to division and notify admitting or appropriate department of time of discharge. Notify housekeeping of need to clean client's room.	Allows agency to prepare for admission of next client.

EVALUATION

1. Ask client or family member to describe nature of illness, treatment regimens, and physical signs or symptoms to be reported to a physician.	Measures client's learning.
2. Have client or family member perform any treatments to be continued in the home.	Return demonstrations allow nurse to evaluate level of learning.
3. Home health nurse inspects home, identifies obstacles that pose risks for client, and recommends revisions.	Continuity of care is achieved.

UNEXPECTED OUTCOMES AND RELATED INTERVENTIONS

- Client or family is unable to explain self-care measures.
  - Provide immediate clarification or offer reinstruction.
- Client or family demonstrates treatment measures incorrectly.
  - Plan additional time to demonstrate treatment measures to client and family.
  - Ask client to explain what aspect of procedure is difficult to perform and why.
- Risks continue to be present in home.
  - Family or client may discount risk or may not have resources to make needed changes.
  - Home health nurse should attempt to problem solve and seek appropriate solution.
- Client or family resists discharge plans and refuses assimilation of new roles needed for home care.
  - Contact additional resources (e.g., social work, home health care, pastoral care) to assist client and family with home care needs.

RECORDING AND REPORTING

- Complete documentation of client's discharge on discharge summary form (Box 1-6). Client should receive signed copy of form.
- Document any unresolved problems and description of arrangements made for resolution in nurses' notes.
- Complete documentation in nurses' notes of status of client's health problems at time of discharge.

Box 1-6 Elements of a Written Discharge Summary Form

- Mode of discharge: ambulatory, wheelchair, stretcher
- Instructions for self-care activities: activity, diet, medications, special treatments such as wound care, self-catheterization, tracheostomy care
- Signs and symptoms of complications or drug reactions to be observant for
- Signs and symptoms that are normal for the individual
- Correct settings for any equipment required
- Planned follow-up appointment at physician's office, clinic
- Explanation of pertinent emergency procedures
- Client's signature, showing understanding of instructions

Teaching Considerations

- Assess client's fatigue and pain levels before undertaking any teaching activity. Keep focused on the important teaching topics to cover.
- Consider client's cultural, social, and educational background when developing a discharge teaching plan.
- Clients who have short stays in health care agency may not receive teaching until day of discharge. Include family or significant other as appropriate.
- Some prescriptions cannot be anticipated. Day of discharge may be only opportunity to teach client about medications. Some agencies have brochures or cards that provide specific information about individual drugs.

Pediatric Considerations

- Once family have learned how to perform any necessary caregiver skills, have them assume care before child returns home. Many hospitals incorporate a trial period requiring family to manage care before child's discharge home (Wong and others, 1999).
- The goal for home health care program for infants, children, or adolescents with chronic conditions is provision of comprehensive, cost-effective health care within a nurturing home environment. Environment should maximize capabilities of individual and minimize effects of disabilities (American Academy of Pediatrics, 1995).

Gerontological Considerations

- Research has demonstrated that older adults are vulnerable to poor outcomes during the first few weeks after discharge. This reinforces the importance of either telephone or home health care follow-up for older adults after discharge to address needs associated with functional decline and, in doing so, to prevent costly readmissions (Naylor and others, 1994).
- Older adults and their families may overestimate their ability to manage care after discharge. They may also disagree about what postdischarge care includes.

Home Care Considerations

- The AHA (1983) has recommended consideration of the following factors in planning for care at home:
  - Desire of client
  - Desire and capability of family to assume responsibility and to understand and follow treatment plan
  - Capabilities of resources in community for home health care services
  - Physical environment of home
  - Financial resources to provide adequate food and pay health care expenses
- Home health care nurses require detailed information about home environment, such as support systems and social and economic considerations that may modify and shape care, to develop complete and accurate care plans for client. Without such information home health care nurse may need to assess situation too quickly to develop a clear plan of care.
- Assess availability and skill of primary caregiver (e.g., spouse or neighbor): assess time availability, ability and willingness to give care, emotional and physical stamina, and knowledge of caregiving.
- Assess attitude of immediate family members: ability to adjust to demands of client care, impact of care demands on their lives (e.g., reducing noise levels in home and preparing special diets); and potential ongoing nature of client's needs. Family members who are not properly prepared for their role as caregivers may be overwhelmed by client's needs, which can lead to neglect or unnecessary hospital readmissions.
- Assess additional resources, including friends or neighbors who are available to help.
- Evaluate emergency preparations: call bell or phone within client's reach and appropriate written protocol.
- Assess referral for appropriateness of client admission to home health care agency based on the following admission criteria:
  - Client is confined to place of residence (homebound).
  - Client is under care of a physician.
  - Client needs part-time or intermittent skilled nursing services.
  - Reasonable expectation exists that client's medical, nursing, and social needs can be adequately met by home health care agency in client's place of residence.
  - Home health care services are necessary and reasonable for treatment of client's illness or injury.
- Obtain as much information as possible about client before nurse visits client in home setting, a visit to client and family during hospitalization is helpful.
- Document client intake information on home health care admission referral form. Ensure that information is complete. Discrepancies have been noted between information home health care nurses deem essential and information that they actually receive from agency discharging client (Anderson and Helms, 1995).
- Review information in conjunction with established home health care agency admission criteria.
- Inform client or family member and client's physician as to decision to accept or not accept client for admission to home health care agency.

Critical Thinking Exercises

1. An older adult is admitted to the hospital from a long-term care facility. The client has had an elevated temperature and is dehydrated. A new environment, coupled with the physiological stress of a fever, is causing the client to become restless and disoriented. How will this influence the assessment phase of the admission process?
2. Why is it important to have a client's advance directive available upon admission?

3. Describe ways the family can participate in the client's care during the discharge process.
4. Mr. Eisen has been in the hospital for only 2 days. He is 43 years old and owns his own business. Since having a workup for chest pain, he has not had the chance to talk with his physician. He is married, and his wife is available to help at home. Does Mr. Eisen have a risk factor that calls for discharge planning? If so, what is it?

References

American Academy of Pediatrics, Committee on Children with Disabilities: Guidelines for home care of infants, children, and adolescents with chronic disease, *Pediatrics* 96(1):161, 1995.

American Hospital Association: *A patient's bill of rights,* Chicago, 1999, The Association.

American Hospital Association: *Discharge planning standards: Society for Hospital Social Work Directors,* Chicago, 1985, American Hospital Publishing.

American Hospital Association: *Introduction to discharge planning for hospitals,* Chicago, 1983, American Hospital Publishing.

Anderson M, Helms L: Communication between continuing care organizations, *Res Nurs Health* 18(1):49, 1995.

Blaylock A, Cason CL: Discharge planning predicting patients' needs, *J Gerontol Nurs* 18(7):8, 1992.

Bull M: Elders' and family members' perspectives in planning for hospital discharge, *Appl Nurs Res* 7(4):190, 1994.

Burgess W, Ragland EC: *Community health nursing: philosophy, process, practice,* Norwalk, Conn, 1983, Appleton-Century-Crofts.

Burke M: Implementing the patient self-determination act, *Nurs Manage* 24(11):80, 1993.

Clemen-Stone S and others: *Comprehensive community health nursing,* ed 5, St. Louis, 1997, Mosby.

Discharge planning: conditions of participation, *Federal Register* 59:238, 1994. Health Care Financing Administration, DHHS.

Ebersole P, Hess P: *Toward healthy aging: human needs and nursing response,* ed 3, St. Louis, 1998, Mosby.

Health Care Financing Administration, Medicare and Medicaid programs; hospital conditions of participation: patients' rights, *Federal Register* 64(127):36081, 1999.

Higgins LW: Nurses' perceptions of collaborative nurse-physician transfer decision making as a predictor of patient outcomes in a medical intensive care unit, *J Adv Nurs* 29(6):1434, 1999.

Joint Commission on Accreditation of Healthcare Organizations: *Comprehensive accreditation manual for hospitals: the official handbook,* Chicago, 1999, The Commission.

Lowenstein A, Hoff P: Discharge planning: a study of nursing staff involvement, *J Nurs Adm* 24(4):45, 1994.

Lueckenotte AG: *Gerontologic nursing,* St. Louis, 2000, Mosby.

Naylor M and others: Comprehensive discharge planning for the hospitalized elderly: a randomized clinical trial, *Ann Intern Med* 120(12):999, 1994.

Rorden JW, Taft E: *Discharge planning guide for nurses,* Philadelphia, 1990, Saunders.

Wanich, CK, and others: Functional status outcomes of a nursing intervention in hospitalized elderly. *Image J Nurs Sch* 24(3):201, 1992.

Wong DL and others: *Whaley and Wong's nursing care of infants and children,* ed 6, St. Louis, 1999, Mosby.

2

COMMUNICATION

Skills

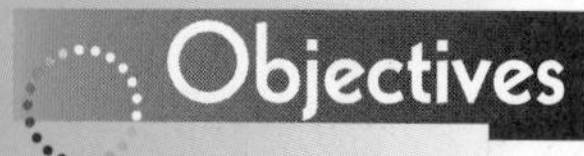

Mastery of content in this chapter will enable the nurse to:

- Define the key terms listed.
- Identify guidelines to use in therapeutic communication.
- Explain the communication process.
- Identify the purpose of therapeutic communication, communication in various phases of the nurse-client relationship, and special issues related to communication.
- Develop skills for therapeutic communication in various phases of the nurse-client relationship, and special situations related to communication.

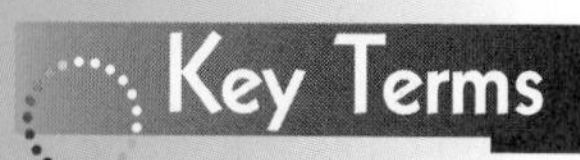

Active listening	Paraphrasing
Cadence	Reflecting
Clarifying	Restating
Comforting	Summarizing
De-escalation	Termination phase
Empathy	Therapeutic silence
Interviewing	Working phase
Orientation phase	

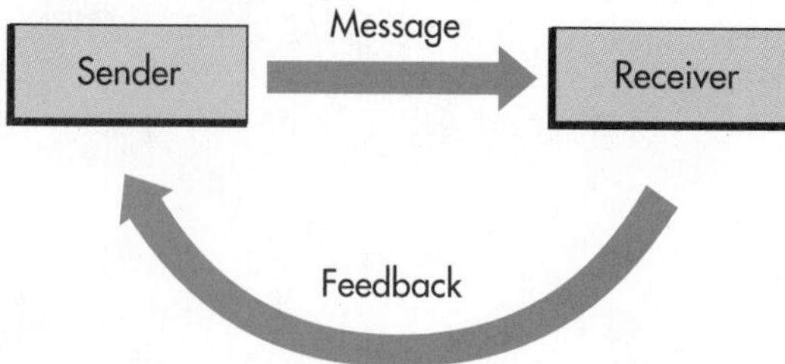

FIGURE **2-1** Communication is a two-way process.

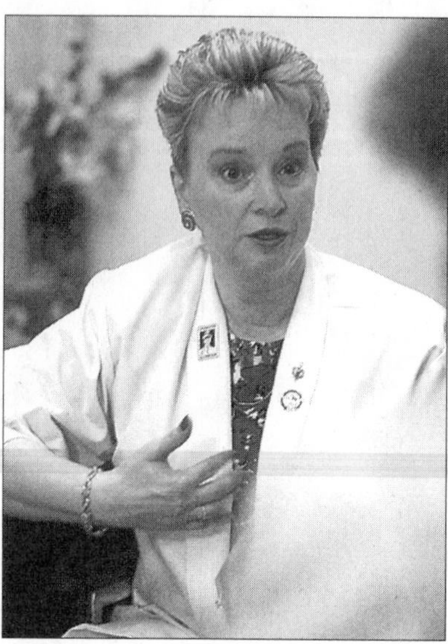

FIGURE **2-2** An open, relaxed posture conveys interest.

Effective communication extends beyond the client to include family members/significant others and members of the health care team. Therefore nurses must possess effective communication skills as a part of their fundamental nursing knowledge base. This chapter does not intend to give a complete introduction to the complicated process of communication. Rather, the purpose of this chapter is to provide a framework by which nurses can develop a repertoire of therapeutic skills that are essential to the communication process.

Communication is an interaction between two or more persons that involves the exchange of information between a sender and a receiver (Figure 2-1). It is an essential component of the human experience, involving the expression of emotions, ideas, and thoughts through verbal (words or written language) and nonverbal (behaviors) exchanges. Therapeutic communication is an application of the process of communication to promote the well-being of the client.

Verbal communication includes both spoken word and written word. The sender of verbal communication through the spoken word must be aware of the tone, volume, and **cadence** (pace or rate) of voice to send an accurate message. The sender of verbal communication through both the spoken and written word also must be aware of cultural differences between sender and receiver, such as the use of jargon or slang. Other issues the sender must consider with written communication include barriers such as cognitive and visual impairments of the receiver. In addition, the developmental perspectives of the client should be taken into consideration, because these may influence the method of communication used.

Nonverbal communication describes all behaviors that convey messages without the use of verbal language. This type of communication includes body movement, physical appearance, personal space, and touch. The sender of nonverbal communication must be aware of body language, which includes the sender's posture, body position, gestures, eye contact, facial expression, and movement (Figure 2-2). For clarity, nonverbal communication should be consistent with the spoken word. When assessing the needs of the client, one should assess the nonverbal messages received from the client and validate them; for example, if the client is observed to be wringing his or her hands and sighing often, the nurse may ask, "You seem anxious today. Is there anything on your mind?" Problems in language behavior can be avoided through the consistent use of clear, mutually understood verbal terminology and nonverbal gestures. A nurse must be aware of any cultural norms or values (e.g., eye contact) to which the client may adhere to avoid misinterpretation of nonverbal cues.

Communication is essential to nursing. Nurses use communication skills in caring for clients by providing information, providing comfort, promoting understanding, clarifying misinformation, assisting in developing plans of care, and facilitating wellness through client teaching. Through the relationship the nurse has with the client, a connection is made that is an essential component of the healing process. There are several key components of effective communication. One such component is self-awareness. Both the nurse and the client must be aware of the feelings they have about themselves and others, as well as the feelings about the content of the messages sent and received. Genuineness, empathy, and respect are key elements for the nurse to possess. Other components that may affect therapeutic nurse-client communication include nonverbal cues, culture, and previous experience. When initially interviewing the client, the nurse assesses personal, family, and community strengths and resources. Special situations with clients that may hinder the communication process include the noncommunicative client, the hostile/aggressive client, and the noncompliant client.

Skill Performance Guidelines

1. Listen to what and how the client communicates, that is, content and verbal and nonverbal messages. Some clients express themselves clearly without difficulty. Often, however, indirect and nonverbal cues communicate a client's needs.
2. Nonverbal communication involves transmission of messages without the use of words. Personal appearance, tone of voice, facial expression, posture, gait, gestures, and touch are ways to convey nonverbal messages.
3. Know your own attitudes toward the client or situation. Being unaware of personal feelings can lead to negative consequences of communication. To control what and how one communicates, one must be aware of personal feelings.
4. Control external factors in both the environmental setting and the psychological setting that influence or hinder communication. If the nurse is talking with the client about the client's personal concerns, privacy is important. If teaching, the nurse may want to have a family member/significant other present with whom to reinforce the content of the instruction. If the client is experiencing subjective distress in the form of pain or anxiety, measures should be taken to minimize these subjective experiences. Controlling noise level and interruptions may also be important.
5. Establish and understand the purpose of interaction. This is an essential quality of effective communication. Without this quality, communication is casual and superficial.
6. Guide the interaction depending on the client's condition and response. Client needs remain the focus of the interaction. For example, a nurse establishes that the purpose of the interaction is client teaching; however, the client just heard of the death of a loved one and expresses the need to talk about the death. The nurse assists the client with grieving and thus remains flexible and creative in the interaction.

Skill 2-1 Establishing the Nurse-Client Relationship

A therapeutic nurse-client relationship is planned and client centered and involves goal-directed interactions using therapeutic communication skills. The primary goal of effective therapeutic communication for the nurse is to promote wellness and growth in clients. Therapeutic communication empowers clients to make decisions but differs from social communication in that it is client centered and goal directed with limited disclosure from the professional. Social communication involves equal opportunity for personal disclosure, and both participants seek to have personal needs met (Keltner, Schwecke, and Bostrom, 1999). Nurses do not share intimate details of their personal lives with clients. Personal self-disclosure by the nurse should occur only if it may be of help to the client, such as helping the client focus on key issues. Skills that are essential to therapeutic communication include **active listening, clarifying, comforting,** focusing, genuineness, informing, **interviewing,** paraphrasing, **reflecting, restating, summarizing,** suggesting, use of **therapeutic silence,** and use of open-ended statements/questions. Some of these skills are defined with case illustrations identifying therapeutic and nontherapeutic examples of their use (Box 2-1). In addition to the skills presented in Box 2-1, **paraphrasing** involves restating the client's original message by transforming the message into the nurse's own words without losing the meaning. Empathy in communication is achieved through the use of the aforementioned skills. **Empathy** is objective and nonjudgmental and consists of insightful awareness of the feelings, emotions, and behavior of another person. It differs from sympathy in that sympathy is nonobjective and noncritical. Barriers to therapeutic communication include giving an opinion, offering false reassurance, being defensive, showing approval or disapproval, stereotyping, and asking "why?" The therapeutic nurse-client relationship is goal directed, with the client moving toward productive modes of interpersonal functioning. The nurse-client relationship, believed to be the crux of nursing, is characterized by three overlapping phases: orientation, working, and termination. The **orientation phase** involves

Box 2-1 Therapeutic Communication Techniques

Technique: Listening
Definition: An active process of receiving information and examining one's reaction to messages received
Example: Maintaining eye contact and receptive nonverbal communication
Therapeutic value: Nonverbally communicates nurse's interest and acceptance to client
Nontherapeutic threat: Failure to listen, interrupting client

Technique: Broad Openings
Definition: Encouraging client to select topics for discussion
Example: "What are you thinking about?"
Therapeutic value: Indicates acceptance by nurse and value of client's initiative
Nontherapeutic threat: Domination of interaction by nurse; rejecting responses

Technique: Restating
Definition: Repeating main thought client has expressed
Example: "You say that your mother left you when you were 5 years old."
Therapeutic value: Indicates nurse is listening and validates, reinforces, or calls attention to something important that has been said
Nontherapeutic threat: Lack of validation of nurse's interpretation of message; being judgmental; reassuring; defending

Technique: Clarification
Definition: Attempting to put into words vague ideas or unclear thoughts of client to enhance the nurse's understanding or asking client to explain what he or she means
Example: "I'm not sure what you mean. Could you tell me again?"
Therapeutic value: Helps to clarify client's feelings, ideas, and perceptions and to provide an explicit correlation between them and the client's actions
Nontherapeutic threat: Failure to probe; assumed understanding

Technique: Reflection
Definition: Directing back to client ideas, feelings, questions, or content
Example: "You're feeling tense and anxious, and it's related to a conversation you had with your sister last night?"
Therapeutic value: Validates nurse's understanding of what client is saying and signifies empathy, interest, and respect for client
Nontherapeutic threat: Stereotyping client's responses, inappropriate timing of reflections; inappropriate depth of feeling of reflections; inappropriate to the cultural experience and educational level of the client

Technique: Humor
Definition: Discharge of energy through comic enjoyment of the imperfect
Example: "This gives a whole new meaning to 'Just relax.'"
Therapeutic value: Can promote insight by making conscious repressed material, resolving paradoxes, tempering aggression, revealing new options, and is a socially acceptable form of sublimation
Nontherapeutic threat: Indiscriminate use; belittling client; screen to avoid therapeutic intimacy

Technique: Informing
Definition: Skill or information giving
Example: "I think you need to know more about how your medication works."
Therapeutic value: Helpful in health teaching or client education about relevant aspects of client's well-being and self-care
Nontherapeutic threat: Giving advice

Technique: Focusing
Definition: Questions or statements that help client expand on a topic of importance
Example: "I think that we should talk more about your relationship with your father."
Therapeutic value: Allows client to discuss central issues related to problem and keeps communication process goal directed
Nontherapeutic threat: Allowing abstractions and generalizations; changing topics

Technique: Sharing Perceptions
Definition: Asking client to verify nurse's understanding of what client is thinking or feeling
Example: "You're smiling, but I sense that you are really very angry with me."
Therapeutic value: Conveys nurse's understanding to client and has potential for clearing up confusing communication
Nontherapeutic threat: Challenging client; accepting literal responses; reassuring; testing; defending

Technique: Theme Identification
Definition: Underlying issues or problems experienced by client that emerge repeatedly during nurse-client relationship
Example: "I've noticed that in all the relationships that you have described, you've been hurt or rejected by the man. Do you think this is an underlying issue?"
Therapeutic value: Allows nurse to best promote client's exploration and understanding of important problems
Nontherapeutic threat: Giving advice; reassuring; disapproving

Technique: Silence
Definition: Lack of verbal communication for a therapeutic reason
Example: Sitting with client and nonverbally communicating interest and involvement
Therapeutic value: Allows client time to think and gain insights, slows the pace of the interaction, and encourages client to initiate conversation, while conveying nurse's support, understanding, and acceptance
Nontherapeutic threat: Questioning client: asking for "why" responses; failure to break a nontherapeutic silence

Technique: Suggesting
Definition: Presentation of alternative ideas for client's consideration relative to problem solving
Example: "Have you thought about responding to your boss in a different way when he raises that issue with you? For example, you could ask him whether a specific problem has occurred."
Therapeutic value: Increases client's perceived options or choices
Nontherapeutic threat: Giving advice, inappropriate timing; being judgmental

Modified from Stuart GW, Laraia M: *Principles and practice of psychiatric nursing,* ed 6, St. Louis, 1998, Mosby.

learning about the client and any initial concerns and needs. In the orientation phase, roles of the nurse or other health care provider are clarified, information is collected, goals are established, misunderstandings are clarified, and rapport is established between the nurse and the client. When the strategies of the orientation phase are successful and the client is ready, the work toward effective goal attainment can begin with the **working phase** of the nurse-client relationship. The **termination phase** consists of evaluation and summary of progress toward prescribed goals. Preparation for termination generally begins at the beginning of the relationship. The nurse must communicate effectively with clients throughout all three phases of the nurse-client relationship.

Delegation Considerations

Therapeutic communication is a goal of all client interactions, delegated or not. Establishing therapeutic communication is a skill that can be delegated to assistive personnel following appropriate instruction. However, before delegation of this skill assistive personnel must be informed of the proper way to interact verbally and nonverbally with the client and of environmental considerations, such as privacy and confidentiality. The following skills should be reviewed: communicating with the cognitively or sensorially impaired client, the older client, the pediatric client, the anxious client, and the potentially violent client if warranted according to the nursing assessment.

Step	Rationale
Assessment	
1. First contact nurse has with client occurs during the orientation phase. Nurse determines that nurse-client relationship is in orientation phase by assessing the following behaviors: client's needs, coping strategies, defenses, and adaptation styles.	Recurrent themes in client's responses help to identify problem areas related to health status (e.g., avoidance of questions, request for information, expression of a loss).
2. Determine client's need to communicate (e.g, client who constantly uses call light; client who is crying; client who does not understand an illness; client who has just been admitted to the hospital or nursing home).	Clients in need of support, comfort, knowledge, or encouragement can benefit from meaningful communication.
3. Assess reason client needs health care.	Nature of illness can affect client's coping ability and effectiveness in communicating needs and concerns.
4. Assess factors about self and client that normally influence communication: perceptions, values and beliefs; emotions; sociocultural background; severity of illness; knowledge; age; verbal ability; roles and relationships; environmental setting; physical comfort or discomfort (Figure 2-3).	Communication is a dynamic process influenced by interpersonal and intrapersonal processes. By assessing factors that influence communication nurse can more accurately assess experiences of client.

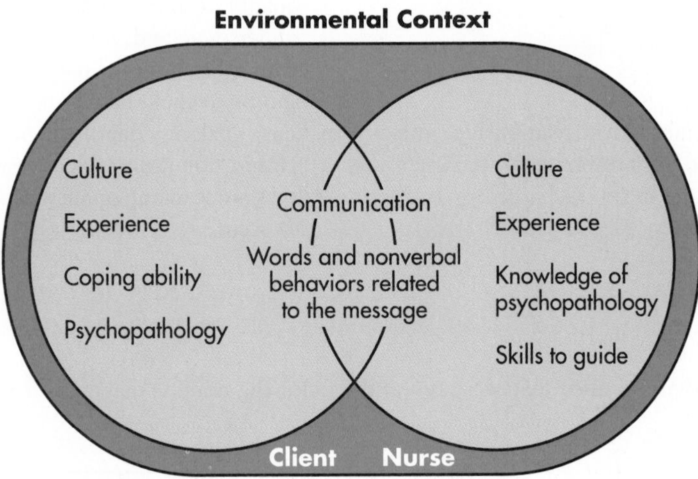

FIGURE 2-3 Essential and influencing variables of the therapeutic communication environment. (Modified from Keltner N, Schwecke L, Bostrom C: *Psychiatric nursing*, ed 3, St. Louis, 1999, Mosby.)

STEP	RATIONALE

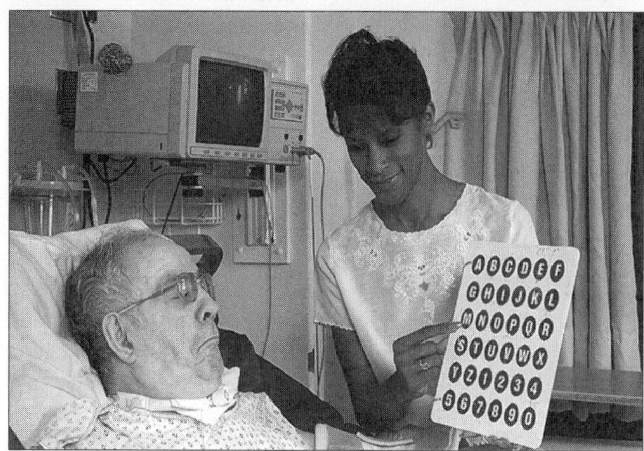

FIGURE 2-4 Tracheostomy interferes with speech.

STEP	RATIONALE
5. Nurse assesses own barriers to communication with client (e.g., bias toward client's condition, anxiety from inexperience).	Barriers prevent nurse from conveying empathy and caring.
6. Assess client's language and ability to speak. Does client have difficulty finding words or associating ideas with accurate word symbols? Does client have difficulty with expression of language and/or reception of messages? What is client's primary language?	Assessment determines need for special communication techniques (e.g., picture boards; aids, such as an interpreter) (Figure 2-4).
7. Observe client's pattern of communication and verbal or nonverbal behavior (e.g., gestures, tone of voice, eye contact).	Client's patterns of communication may determine type of and manner of communication used by nurse.
8. Assess resources available in selecting communication methods:	
a. Review information available through chart, care plan, past experience, nursing assessment, client interview.	
b. Consult with family, physician, and other health care team members concerning client's condition, problems, impression.	Relying totally on information from client can restrict quality of interaction. Additional resources provide insight into best methods to communicate. The greater amount or quality of information nurse has, the greater the ability to understand and communicate with client. Collaboration with other health care team members facilitates nurse's response to client based on integration of knowledge.
9. Before working phase of nurse-client relationship, nurse assesses client's readiness to work toward goal attainment.	Client's goals are identified and agreed upon by effective communication skills such as restating and clarifying.
10. Consider when client is due to be discharged or transferred from health care agency.	Allows nurse to anticipate when termination of relationship is to occur.

NURSING DIAGNOSIS

Defining characteristics from the assessment data may reveal the following nursing diagnoses for clients requiring this skill:

- Anxiety
- Impaired verbal communication
- Ineffective coping (specify)
- Decisional conflict (specify)
- Fear
- Deficient knowledge (specify)
- Noncompliance (specify)
- Impaired social interaction

Related factors are individualized based on client's condition or needs.

Step	Rationale
Planning	
1. **Expected outcomes** following completion of procedure:	
▪ A therapeutic relationship is established between nurse and client.	Trust is established.
▪ Client is able to express ideas, fears, and concerns clearly and openly with relief of anxiety.	Once clients are able to talk directly about emotions, the focus can be on coping more effectively with them (Keltner, Schwecke, and Bostrom, 1999).
▪ Client goals are identified and achieved.	Interaction remains client focused.
▪ Client understands information communicated by nurse.	This provides a means to build trust and develop a knowledge base for client to make decisions.
2. Prepare for communication during orientation phase by providing a warm and accepting environment, establishing trust, formulating individualized client goals, considering time allocation, formulating initial questions, and mentally preparing to keep one's mind clear of other concerns or distractions.	Preparation is part of planned process that facilitates communication and interaction. Planning for orientation phase assists in identifying actual or potential problems, current health status, and experience. Without understanding purpose of interaction, allowing adequate time, or preparing for communication, a greater risk exists of casual non–goal-oriented communication that may fail to assist client in reaching a greater potential toward physical, psychological, social, and spiritual health.
3. Prepare client and environment physically by providing a quiet environment conducive to interaction, maintaining privacy, reducing distractions or interruptions, and taking care of client's physical needs before beginning discussion.	Certain environments are more conducive to therapeutic interactions than others. Privacy is less threatening to client and promotes freer expression of feelings. Distractions and interruptions hinder adequate reception of the message. Taking care of basic needs decreases client distractions.
4. Prepare for communication during working phase by identifying strategies to achieve established goals, which includes development of a realistic plan to meet identified health goals of clients.	Preparation promotes goal attainment and avoids risk of misinterpretation.
5. Prepare for communication during termination phase by identifying methods of summarizing and synthesizing information pertinent for aftercare.	Effective communication by summarizing and synthesizing information reinforces behavior change.
Implementation	
Orientation Phase	
1. Create a climate of warmth and acceptance. Maintain a supportive environment, considering both environmental factors (temperature of room, noise level) and emotional and physical state of client (presence of pain or anxiety). Be aware of nonverbal cues that are both sent and received.	This facilitates open exchange without fear or anxiety.
2. Provide an introduction by addressing client by name and introducing self and role on health care team ("Hello, my name is Sally and I am the registered nurse assigned to take care of you today . . ."). Use clear, specific communication (verbal and nonverbal) to provide information and clarify concerns.	Congruent verbal and nonverbal communication conveys warmth and respect and helps to establish rapport. Clear, specific communication decreases confusion and anxiety.
3. Use appropriate nonverbal behaviors (e.g., good eye contact, open relaxed position, sitting eye level with client [see Figure 2-2]).	This facilitates communication by providing a nonverbal message that conveys nurse is interested in what client has to say.
4. Observe client's nonverbal behaviors. Actively listen to client. If client's verbal behaviors do not match nonverbal behaviors, nurse should seek clarification.	Congruence between client's verbal and nonverbal behaviors ensures correct message is received by nurse.

Step	Rationale
5. Explain purpose of interaction when information is to be shared.	Information and explanation can decrease anxiety about the unknown.

- ***Critical Decision Point***
  Establish a therapeutic environment in which client feels at ease, as well as conveying empathy to client while gathering data and helping client to identify the problem.

Step	Rationale
6. Identify client's expectations in seeking health care.	This conveys a level of interest in client's needs.
7. Encourage client to ask for clarification at any time during the communication.	This gives client a sense of control and keeps channels of communication open.
8. Use therapeutic communication techniques when interacting with client (refer to Box 2-1).	Techniques serve to establish a greater understanding of messages sent and received.

Working Phase

Step	Rationale
9. Use effective communication skills such as restating, reflecting, and paraphrasing to identify and clarify strategies for attainment of mutually agreed-upon goals.	Effective communication ensures clear understanding on part of client and improves ability of client to participate in care.
10. Problem areas are discussed and prioritized.	Client's anxiety is minimized through the nurse's nonjudgmental, supportive approach.
11. Provide information to client and help client express needs and feelings.	Client is able to respond to help and fully participates in realistic plan to attain health-related goals. This helps client develop workable solutions based on goals that have meaning to client and that are supportive of client well-being.

- ***Critical Decision Point***
  Use questions carefully and appropriately. Ask one question at a time, and allow sufficient time to answer. Use direct questions. Avoid asking questions about information that may not have yet been disclosed to the client (e.g., human immunodeficiency virus [HIV] status). Avoid asking "why" questions; this may cause increased defensiveness in the client and may hinder communication.

Step	Rationale
12. Avoid communication barriers as discussed earlier in this chapter.	Communication breakdown occurs when a message is not received, is distorted, or is not understood. Communication may be hindered by nontherapeutic responses.

Termination Phase

Step	Rationale
13. Use effective communication skills to discuss discharge/termination issues and to guide discussion related to specific client changes in thoughts and behaviors.	Effective communication skills reinforce behaviors/skills learned during working phase of relationship.
14. Summarize with client what was discussed during interaction, including goal achievement.	Summary signals close of interaction, allows nurse and client to depart with same idea, and provides a sense of closure at completion of discussion. It mutually confirms understanding.

Evaluation

Step	Rationale
1. Observe client's verbal and nonverbal responses to your communication, noting client's willingness to share information and concerns during orientation phase.	Both verbal and nonverbal feedback reveal client's interest and willingness to communicate and reflect client's ability to form a therapeutic relationship with nurse.
2. Note your response to client and client's response to you. Evaluate effectiveness of therapeutic techniques used in establishing rapport with client. Consider use of alternative techniques if previous skills were ineffective.	Sensitivity to one's own ability at using therapeutic communication skills can improve ability to adjust techniques when necessary.
3. During working phase, evaluate client's ability to work toward identified goals. Elicit feedback (verbal and nonverbal) to determine success of goal attainment. Evaluate client's health status in relation to identified goals. Reevaluate and identify barriers if client goals are not met.	Feedback is an essential step in evaluating new behaviors. Modifications must be made if goals cannot be met.

STEP	RATIONALE
4. During termination phase, use communication skills such as summarizing and restating. Client's strengths are reinforced, issues still requiring work are outlined, and an action plan is developed.	Client progress is evaluated, and recommendations are communicated. Health status of client is evaluated in terms of attainment of mutually agreed-upon goals.

UNEXPECTED OUTCOMES AND RELATED INTERVENTIONS

- Client continues to verbally and nonverbally express feelings of anxiety, fear, anger, confusion, distrust, and helplessness. Client may be responding to internal and external factors and cues. Client may speak a different language.
  - Assess client's level of anxiety, fear, and distrust.
  - Repeat message to client at a later time.
  - Use a caring tone of voice and facial expression to help alleviate fears of client who may speak a different language.
- Feedback between nurse and client reveals a lack of understanding. Barriers to communication exist. Nurse may have let own personal issues interfere with establishment of a therapeutic nurse-client relationship. Nonverbal cues (e.g., poor eye contact, facial expressions, and gestures) indicate ineffective communication, which may be due to misunderstanding, cultural issues, pain, or other health-related issues. Client may speak a different language.
  - Assess for barriers to communication.
  - Make appropriate adjustments to communication style. Use special approaches for clients who speak a different language, for example, use of gestures, pictures, and play-acting to help client understand.
  - Consider cultural normal associated with eye contact, use of touch, personal space, and nonverbal behaviors.
  - Repeat message in different ways if necessary.
  - Avoid using medical terms that client may not understand.
  - Be alert to words client seems to understand and use them frequently.
- Nurse is unable to acquire information about client's ideas, fears, and concerns. Techniques used by nurse fail to promote client's willingness to communicate openly. Trust is not established. Goals are not identified and therefore cannot be achieved.
  - Use alternative communication techniques to promote client's willingness to communicate openly.
  - Offer another professional for client to talk with to obtain necessary information.

RECORDING AND REPORTING

- Record in nurses' notes communication pertinent to client's health, response to illness or therapies, and responses that demonstrate understanding or lack of understanding (include verbal and nonverbal cues).
- Report any pertinent information obtained through client's verbal and nonverbal behaviors to members of health care team.

TEACHING CONSIDERATIONS

- Client's readiness to communicate and understand teaching conducted by nurse should be assessed.
- Be aware of cultural and gender differences when interacting with clients. Plan for identified communication difficulties associated with culture, language, age, and gender. Use gestures, pictures, and playacting to help client understand. Be alert to literacy status. Be alert to words client seems to understand and use them frequently.
- Client teaching should be individually tailored to meet needs of client. Teaching should always be conducted toward meeting client's learning needs with consideration for client's preferred methods for learning. This may include, but is not limited to, communicating through return demonstrations, computer-assisted learning tools, written information, audiovisual media, and checklists.

PEDIATRIC CONSIDERATIONS

- Communicating with children requires an understanding of feelings and thought processes from the child's perspective, (Wong and others, 1999).
- Nurse must use vocabulary that is familiar to child, based on child's level of understanding. Nurse must evaluate child's usual patterns of communication.
- Nurse needs to understand child's cognitive, developmental, and functional level to select most appropriate communication techniques. Some age-appropriate communication techniques include storytelling and drawing (Wong and others, 1999).

GERONTOLOGICAL CONSIDERATIONS

- Be aware of any cognitive or sensory impairment. Each client must be assessed individually, and nurse must avoid stereotyping older adults as having cognitive or sensory impairments.
- Nurse should speak face-to-face with hard-of-hearing client and assess whether or not client hears and understands words. Have client use hearing aid if appropriate.
- It is important to understand the value of good communication skills and importance of history and personality within older adult population in terms of providing both human and therapeutic responses. Regression to earlier defenses is normal and adaptive with this population, particularly when facing illness (Sherrell and Buckwalter, 1998).
- Nurse should make sure older client with visual impairments uses assistive devices such as eyeglasses and large-print reading material to aid in communication (Elkin, Perry, and Potter, 2000).

HOME CARE CONSIDERATIONS

- Identify primary caregiver for client. This individual may be family member, friend, or neighbor.
- Assess level of understanding of client and primary caregiver regarding client's condition.
- Avoid making unnecessary changes in client's lifestyle, and incorporate client's daily habits into communication event (e.g., bathing and dressing client).

Skill 2-2 Communicating With the Anxious Client

Clients in the health care setting may experience anxiety for a variety of reasons; a newly diagnosed illness, separation from loved ones, threat associated with diagnostic tests or surgical procedures, and expectations of life changes are just a few factors that can cause anxiety. How successfully a client copes with anxiety depends in part on previous experiences, the presence of other stressors, the significance of the event causing anxiety, and the availability of supportive resources. The nurse can be a support to the client. The nurse can help to decrease anxiety through effective communication. Communication methods reviewed in this skill assist the nurse in helping the anxious client clarify factors causing anxiety and to cope more effectively.

DELEGATION CONSIDERATIONS

Communication with an anxious client is best managed by a professional nurse. However, therapeutic communication is important in all client interactions. Communicating effectively with the anxious client is a skill that assistive personnel must be able to perform. However, before delegation of this skill the assistive personnel must be informed of the proper way to interact verbally and nonverbally with the client and the staff member must understand why the client is anxious. The skills necessary for communicating with the anxious client should be reviewed with assistive personnel.

STEP	RATIONALE
ASSESSMENT	
1. Assess for physical, behavioral, and verbal cues that indicate client is anxious, such as dry mouth, sweaty palms, tone of voice, frequent use of call light, difficulty concentrating, wringing of hands, and statements such as "I am scared."	Anxiety can interfere with usual manner of communication and thus interfere with client's care and treatment. Extreme anxiety can interfere with comprehension, attention, and problem-solving abilities.
2. Assess for possible factors causing client anxiety (e.g., hospitalization, unknown diagnosis, or fatigue).	Client's feeling of anxiety may be unknown to nurse. Understanding the source of anxiety can assist nurse in client support and communication.
3. Assess factors influencing communication with client (e.g., environment, timing, presence of others, values, experiences, need for personal space because of heightened anxiety).	Understanding factors that influence communication helps nurse identify effective communication strategies (Morse and Intrieri, 1997).
4. Assess own level of anxiety and make a conscious effort to remain calm.	Anxiety is highly contagious, and one's own anxiety can exacerbate client's anxiety.
5. Nurse may need to confer with family members about possible causes of client's anxiety.	Gathering information about client from a family perspective is useful because family may shed new light on situation (Keltner, Schwecke, and Bostrom, 1999).

NURSING DIAGNOSIS

Defining characteristics from the assessment data may reveal the following nursing diagnoses for clients requiring this skill:

- Anxiety
- Impaired verbal communication
- Ineffective coping (specify)
- Decisional conflict (specify)
- Fear
- Deficient knowledge (specify)
- Impaired social interaction

Related factors are individualized based on client's condition or needs.

Planning

Step	Rationale
1. **Expected outcomes** following completion of procedure:	
▪ Client's anxiety is reduced through use of effective communication techniques.	Client is given resource to cope with stressor(s).
2. Prepare for communication by considering the following: client goals, time allocation, and resources.	Effective communication allows client to establish rapport, to achieve a sense of calm, and to begin to analyze source of anxiety.
3. Recognize and control own anxiety (breathe slowly and deeply). Be aware of nonverbal cues that indicate own anxiety (e.g., body language, posture, and cadence of speech).	Nurse's own anxiety can increase client's anxiety.
4. Prepare environment physically by providing a quiet, calm area, allowing ample personal space.	Decreasing stimuli can have a calming effect. Invasion of personal space is known to increase anxiety.

• ***Critical Decision Point***

First acknowledge and take care of anxious client's physical and emotional discomfort, but avoid dwelling on physical complaints. Focus on understanding client, providing feedback and assisting in problem solving, and providing atmosphere of warmth and acceptance.

Implementation

Step	Rationale
1. Provide brief, simple introduction; introduce yourself and explain purpose of interaction.	Anxiety may limit amount of information client can understand.
2. Use appropriate nonverbal behaviors and active listening skills, such as staying with client at bedside.	Nonverbal messages to client convey nurse's interest and help to alleviate anxiety.
3. Use appropriate verbal techniques that are clear and concise to respond to anxious client. Use brief statements that both acknowledge current feeling state and provide direction to client.	Appropriate techniques and statements provide reassurance and prevent further escalation of anxiety.
4. Help client acquire alternate coping strategies, such as progressive relaxation, slow deep-breathing exercises, and visual imagery (see Chapter 5).	Coping mechanisms provide foundation for effective communication so that client can explore causes of anxiety and steps to alleviate anxious feelings.
5. Minimize noise in physical setting.	A less stimulating environment can create a calming, stress-free atmosphere that reduces anxiety.
6. Provide necessary comfort measures.	Pain can heighten client's anxiety.

Evaluation

Step	Rationale
1. Observe for continuing presence of physical signs and symptoms or behaviors reflecting anxiety.	Observation determines extent to which planned interaction relieved client's anxiety.
2. Have client discuss ways to cope with anxiety in the future and make decisions about own care.	This measures client's ability to assume more health-promoting behavior.
3. Evaluate client's ability to discuss factors causing anxiety.	Evaluation measures client's ability to attend or focus on area of concern.

Unexpected Outcomes and Related Interventions

- Physical signs and symptoms of anxiety continue. Nurse's interaction may have increased client's anxiety, or source of anxiety is not resolved.
  - Utilize refocusing or distraction skills, such as relaxation or imagery, to reduce anxiety (Fortinash and Holoday-Worret, 2000).
- Client displays difficulty in decision making, and preparation of facts may be altered. Client avoids nurse's efforts at focusing discussion or is unable to discuss real concerns. Anxiety continues to prevent client from problem solving.
  - Be clear and direct when communicating with client to avoid misunderstanding.

- Touch, when used appropriately, may help control feelings of panic. Touch is an integral part of human behavior, and clients respond positively to touch as a warm, caring nursing approach (Routasalo, 1999).
- Anxiety continues to escalate.
  - Continue to use previous steps.
  - Be very direct and clear when making requests. If client needs to deal with stimulus causing anxiety, reintroduce when client is less anxious.
  - Touch, while therapeutic, requires individualized assessment of client's anxiety level and need for personal space. When used appropriately, reassurance through human touch may help control feelings of panic.
  - As a last resort, administer an antianxiety medication (per orders).

Recording and Reporting

- Record in nurses' notes cause of client's anxiety and any exhibited signs and symptoms of behaviors.
- Report methods used to relieve anxiety and client's response to ensure continuity of care between nurses.

Teaching Considerations

- Teaching client to identify possible sources of anxiety, such as illness, hospitalization, knowledge deficits, or other known stressors, gives client knowledge of anxiety and increases client's sense of control over anxiety.

Pediatric Considerations

- Children often demonstrate anxiety through physical and behavioral signs but are unable to express anxiety verbally. Children may express anxiety through restless behavior, physical complaints, or behavioral regression. It is important to note any changes in child's behavior that occur during illness or hospitalization (Wong and others, 1999).

Gerontological Considerations

- Anxiety is one of the most common symptoms seen in older adults. Clients often become ritualistic and intent on performing activities a certain way. Anxiety can develop as a result of a specific event or a general pattern of change (e.g., decline in health) (Lueckenotte, 2000).

Home Health Considerations

- Anxiety may been seen in home care settings and should be managed based on client's presenting behaviors with a consideration of any cognitive/physical impairments.

Long-Term Care Considerations

- Anxiety may be seen in long-term care settings, such as residential care facilities and assisted living facilities, and should be managed based on client's presenting behaviors with consideration of any cognitive/physical impairments.
- Psychosocial factors such as anxiety and confusion, lack of mobility, and spacial organization of long-term care institution are factors that decrease social contacts, thus hindering communication with both peers and health care providers. This leads to further feelings of isolation, boredom, and increased anxiety (Morse and Intrieri, 1997).

Skill 2-3 Verbally De-escalating the Potentially Violent Client

Anger is the common underlying factor associated with potential for violence. A client can become angry for a variety of reasons. The anger may be directly related to a client's experience with illness, or it can be associated with problems that existed before the client entered the health care setting. In the health care setting, the nurse has frequent contact with a client and thus often becomes the target of the client's anger. It is important for the nurse to understand that in many cases the client's ability to express anger is important to recovery. For example, when a client has experienced a significant loss, anger becomes a means to help cope with grief. A client may express anger toward the nurse, but the anger often hides a specific problem or concern. For example, a client diagnosed as having cancer may voice displeasure with the nurse's care instead of expressing a fear of dying.

It can be very stressful for a nurse to deal with an angry client. Anger can represent rejection or disapproval of the nurse's care. A nurse's efforts at satisfying the needs of one angry client can result in a failure to meet the priorities of other clients.

The nurse must allow the client to express anger openly, and the nurse must not feel threatened by the client's words. However, the client's anger should not be allowed to compromise care. Skills for communicating with an angry client or a potentially violent client allow a nurse to assist the client in dealing with anger constructively and in refocusing emotional energy toward effective problem solving. **De-escalation** skills are useful techniques that can be used to manage the potentially violent client; these skills range from using nonthreatening verbal and nonverbal messages to safely disengaging and controlling the aggressor physically (Fortinash and Holoday-Worret, 2000).

Delegation Considerations

De-escalation is a skill best performed by a professional nurse. However, assistive personnel must be able to communicate effectively with the potentially violent client, provided that communication with this type of client is not beyond the skill level of the assistive personnel. Before delegation of this skill, assistive personnel must be informed of the proper way to interact verbally and nonverbally with the client. The skills for communicating with the potentially violent client and methods of de-escalation should be reviewed with assistive personnel, as well as approaches that have previously been successful and unsuccessful.

Step	Rationale

Assessment

Step	Rationale
1. Observe for behaviors that indicate client is angry (e.g., pacing, clenched fist, loud voice, throwing objects) and/or expressions that indicate anger (e.g., repeat questioning of nurse, nonadherence to requests, belligerent outbursts, and threats).	Anger is a normal expression of frustration or response to feeling threatened. However, its expression can interfere with or block communication and interactions.
2. Assess factors that influence communication of angry client, such as refusal to comply with treatment goals, use of sarcasm or hostile behavior, having a low frustration level, or being emotionally immature.	Allows nurse to accurately assess situation or experiences of client that can hinder or facilitate communication.
3. Consider resources available to assist in communicating with potentially violent client, such as members of health care team or family members.	May assist in clarifying cause and intervention required to deal with client's anger.

- ***Critical Decision Point***

  With some violent behaviors (e.g., physical aggression) nurse may be unable to de-escalate the situation. When this potential exists, nurse must know whom to call for assistance (e.g., trained techs, security staff).

Nursing Diagnosis

Defining characteristics from the assessment data may reveal the following nursing diagnoses for clients requiring this skill:

- Anxiety
- Impaired verbal communication
- Ineffective individual coping (specify)
- Decisional conflict (specify)
- Fear
- Risk for violence: self-directed or directed at others
- Impaired social interaction

Related factors are individualized based on client's condition or needs.

Planning

Step	Rationale
1. **Expected outcomes** following completion of procedure:	
▪ Client no longer exhibits verbal and nonverbal expressions of anger.	De-escalation techniques successfully allow client to express anger in a constructive way.
2. Prepare for interaction with angry client:	
a. Pause to collect own thoughts, feelings, and reactions.	Awareness and control of your own reaction and responses can facilitate more constructive interaction.
b. Determine what client is saying.	
c. Attempt a calm, firm, assertive approach. Attempt to talk in comfortable, reassuring voice.	
3. Prepare environment to de-escalate potentially violent client.	Potentially violent client needs to be in an environment with decreased stimuli and to have protection from injury to self or against others.
a. Encourage other people, particularly those who provoke anger, to leave room or area.	Encourages client's expression of anger rather than provokes it.

Step	Rationale
b. Maintain adequate distance.	Avoids pressuring client; the nurse maintains safe distance if anger becomes out of control.
c. Maintain open exit. Position self closest to the door to facilitate escape from a potentially violent situation. Do not block exit so client feels escape is unattainable; this may potentiate a violent outburst.	Prevents feeling of being trapped for both nurse and client.
d. Make sure gestures are slow and deliberate rather than sudden and abrupt.	Less chance of misinterpretation of message and less threatening.
e. When anger begins to disturb others, close door. This is particularly important if client is becoming agitated.	Agitation and anxiety can spread to others. Some hospital rooms may be equipped with security windows or cameras to allow for observation of client.
f. Reduce disturbing factors in room (e.g., noise, drafts, inadequate lighting).	Reduces irritating factors.
g. Take care of client's physical and emotional needs and discomforts (e.g., offer analgesic for pain).	Physical and emotional needs may be factors in client's anger; sometimes client is not aware of these needs.

Implementation

Step	Rationale
1. Create climate of acceptance for client. Maintain nonthreatening verbal and nonverbal communication skills when interacting with angry or potentially violent client.	A relaxed atmosphere may prevent further escalation.
2. Respond to the potentially violent client.	
a. Use therapeutic silence and allow client to ventilate feelings.	Often de-escalates anger because anger expends emotional and physical energy; client runs out of momentum and energy to maintain anger at high level.
b. Answer questions as appropriate; if client asks power-struggle type of question, redirect and set limits by giving clear, concise expectations. Inform client of potential consequences and follow through with consequences if behaviors are not altered.	By setting limits on power-struggle questions, structure is provided, and anger is diffused.
c. If client is making verbal threats to harm others, remain calm yet professional and continue to set limits with inappropriate behavior.	Angry client loses ability to process information rationally and therefore may impulsively express anger through intimidation.

- ***Critical Decision Point***

  If strong likelihood of imminent harm to others is present upon discharge, nurse should notify proper authorities (e.g., nurse manager).

Step	Rationale
d. Maintain personal space and safety with client who is making verbal threats of violence directed at others. Maintain nonthreatening nonverbal behaviors, including body language.	Avoiding sudden movements and loud tones prevents nurse from giving the appearance of an attack (Maier, 1996).

- ***Critical Decision Point***

  The potentially violent client can be impulsive and explosive, and therefore nurse must keep personal safety skills in mind. In this case touch should be avoided (Maier, 1996).

Step	Rationale
e. If client appears to be calm and anger is diffused, explore alternatives to situation or feelings of anger.	Processing with client may prevent future explosive outbursts and teach client effective ways of dealing with anger.

Evaluation

Step	Rationale
1. Observe for continuing behaviors of verbal expressions of anger.	Indicates success of communication efforts.
2. Note client's ability to answer questions and problem solve.	Determines whether anger has lessened so that client can focus on alternative coping skills.

Unexpected Outcomes and Related Interventions

- Client continues to demonstrate behaviors or verbal expression of anger or violence. Nurse is unable to assist client in relieving source of anger or in expressing anger openly without violent acts. Fellow staff should be available to assist if necessary.
  - Reassess factors contributing to anger. Also remove or alter factors contributing to anger.
  - Take charge with calm, firm directions. Give as-needed (prn) medications as ordered for agitation/escalating behaviors. Direct client to a quiet area for a "time out."

Recording and Reporting

- Record in nurses' notes cause of client's anger (if determined) and behaviors client exhibits.
- Record and report technique used to de-escalate and client's response.

Teaching Considerations

- Clients experiencing emotionally charged situations may not comprehend message. Focus on understanding client, providing feedback and assisting in problem solving, and providing an atmosphere of safety, warmth, and acceptance.
- Teaching client to identify possible factors that contribute to angry outbursts, such as inadequate coping skills, low frustration levels, illness, hospitalization, knowledge deficits, or other known stressors, may give client a sense of control over situation. As well, one should teach client new adaptive methods of coping with anger.

Pediatric Considerations

- Limit setting for inappropriate behaviors exhibited by child that are applied immediately are effective, especially because children tend to have less internal control over their own behaviors (Wong and others, 1999).

Gerontological Considerations

- Clients who have cognitive impairments may exhibit tantrumlike behaviors in response to real or perceived frustration. Nurse can use distraction techniques to remove cognitively impaired older adult client from disturbing stimuli, or nurse can use redirection to activity that is pleasurable to client (Lueckenotte, 2000).

Home Care Considerations

- Personal safety for nurse against potentially violent client or family member extends to all health care settings, including client's home. Nurse may be in potentially dangerous situation while giving care to client at home; nurse may give care to client without support from other staff members.
- Be aware of physical surroundings, including possible exits.
- Maintain nonthreatening position, including body language, position, and cadence, when interacting with angry or potentially violent client. Nurse should attempt to de-escalate client. If de-escalation does not occur and nurse feels safety may be threatened, nurse should call for assistance or remove self from situation.

Long-Term Care Considerations

- The nurse may be in a potentially dangerous situation while giving care to client in long-term care facility, due to staffing conditions and physical organization of institution. (Morse and Intrieri, 1997).
- Nurse must be cognizant of verbal and nonverbal cues of client that are indicative of escalating anger.
- Maintain nonthreatening position, including body language, position, and cadence, when interacting with angry or potentially violent client. Nurse should attempt to de-escalate client. If de-escalation does not occur and nurse feels safety may be threatened, nurse should call for assistance. (Maier, 1996).

Critical Thinking Exercises

1. Discuss which therapeutic communication techniques can be best used during the orientation phase of the nurse-client relationship (formulating an assessment and plan of care for client).
2. Mr. X is an angry young adult client recently admitted to your nursing division for surgery to a broken leg from a skiing accident. His angry behavior is escalating, and he is making violent threats against you and all hospital staff. His roommate has become fearful of him. How would you defuse this situation?
3. Mrs. J is a new resident of the long-term care facility in which you are working. She displays behaviors consistent with a client suffering from progressive dementia. She appears frightened at times, because she does not recognize any familiar faces among the staff and other residents. She is hard of hearing and has recently misplaced her eyeglasses. How would you manage this client?

References

Elkin M, Perry A, Potter P: *Nursing interventions and clinical skills,* ed 2, St. Louis, 2000, Mosby.

Fortinash K, Holoday-Worret P: *Psychiatric mental health nursing,* ed 2, St. Louis, 2000, Mosby.

Keltner N, Schwecke L, Bostrom C: *Psychiatric nursing,* ed 3, St. Louis, 1999, Mosby.

Lueckenotte A: *Gerontologic nursing,* ed 2, St. Louis, 2000, Mosby.

Maier G: Managing threatening behavior: the role of talk up and talk down, *J Psychosoc Nurs Ment Health Serv* 33:25, 1996.
Morse J, Intrieri R: "Talk to me": patient communication in a long-term care facility, *J Psychosoc Nurs Ment Health Serv* 35:34, 1997.
Routasalo P: Physical touch in nursing studies: a literature review, *J Adv Nurs* 30(4):843, 1999.
Sherrell K, Buckwalter K: Therapeutic approaches with the physically ill elderly: the value of listening, history, and personality, *J Gerontol Nurs,* 24:54, 1998.
Stuart G, Laraia, M: Stuart and Sundeen's *Principles and practice of psychiatric nursing,* ed 6, St. Louis, 1998, Mosby.
Wong DL and others: *Whaley and Wong's nursing care of infants and children,* ed 6, St. Louis, 1999, Mosby.

3

Recording and Reporting

Skills

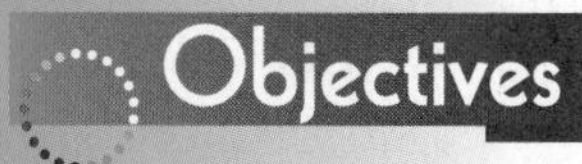

Mastery of content in this chapter will enable the nurse to:

- Define the key terms listed.
- Describe guidelines for effective documentation and reporting.
- Describe a change-of-shift report given to a nursing team.
- Complete an incident report accurately.
- Write a nurse's progress note using SOAP, SOAPE, PIE, and focus charting formats.
- Describe information found in a patient care profile and nursing Kardex.
- Complete a nursing flow sheet.
- Explain guidelines used in documentation of home health care and long-term care.
- Describe the role of critical pathways in multidisciplinary documentation.
- Discuss the role of computerization in documentation.

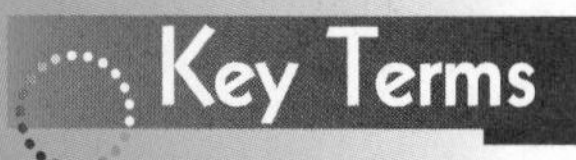

Acuity charting
Case management
Charting by exception
Consultation
Critical pathways
Evidence-based practice
Flow sheet
Focus charting
Incident report
Kardex
Negligence
Objective data
Patient care profile (PCP)
PIE
Problem-oriented medical record (POMR)
Residents
SOAP
Standardized care plan
Subjective data
Variance

Nursing documentation continues to be an essential component of health care delivery. Documentation has become a vital link between the provision and evaluation of health care (Iyer and Camp, 1995). One of the most challenging nursing issues is how to document quality client care within the constraints imposed by regulations, limited resources, and finances.

Quality documentation depends on members of the health care team being able to communicate effectively with one another in both written and spoken word. Furthermore, technology has increased the variety and methods of documentation, which potentially heightens the productivity and scope of nursing practice (Mathews and Zadak, 1993). Nurses are accountable for their actions, and, as a result, written information must be clear and logical, exactly describing all client care delivered.

Nursing documentation is becoming increasingly more important because of its fiscal connection in determining the cost of client care. If information regarding client care is not recorded, organizations may not be able to recover their costs. The medical record has basically become a client's health care bill. Documentation is also a major indicator of quality for health care organizations. Accreditation agencies such as the Joint Commission on Accreditation of Healthcare Organizations (JCAHO) establish standards for nurses (and other health care providers) in the monitoring and evaluation of the quality and appropriateness of client care (JCAHO, 2000). An organization's success in meeting JCAHO standards largely depends on the quality of documentation.

Multidisciplinary Communication Within the Health Care Team

An optimum level of client care requires proficient communication among the members of the health care team (Figure 3-1). Records and reports communicate specific information about a client's health status and the interventions that all health care team members contribute toward improving the client's health. When information is communicated clearly and accurately in a timely way, health care is more efficient and the client benefits.

Reports are oral or written exchanges of information shared between caregivers in a number of ways. Reports can include information about a client's clinical status, observations made about the client's behavior, data pertaining to diagnostic tests, and directions for changes in therapy. For example, after completing a work shift, nurses give a verbal or

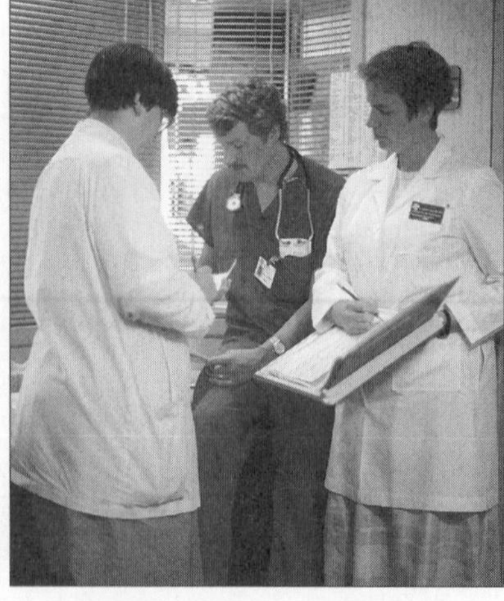

FIGURE **3-1** Communication among members of the health care team.

taped report to nurses on the next shift (Skill 3-1). The report is detailed so that the oncoming nurse can assume the client's care efficiently. A physician may call a nursing unit to receive a verbal report on a client's progress for the day. The laboratory submits written reports summarizing diagnostic test results for inclusion in the medical record.

A medical record is a permanent, legal, written document that communicates information relevant to a client's health care management. Members of all health care disciplines who deliver client care (e.g., nurses, social workers, dietitians, physical therapists, and physicians) make entries in the medical record. An example is a clinic record or chart. After each clinic visit, information about the client's health care is recorded. With each successive visit the record is available to the physician and other members of the health care team. It is a continuing account of the client's health status and needs, the treatments delivered, results of diagnostic tests, and the client's response to therapy.

Another way that information is communicated is through discussions among health care team members. They allow for a review of information so that problems are identified and solutions are recommended. An example is a discharge planning conference, in which members of several disciplines meet to discuss the client's progress toward discharge goals. **Consultations** are another form of discussion whereby one professional caregiver provides formal advice about the care of a client. For example, a dietitian may consult with the nurse on the best foods to meet a client's dietary restrictions. Consultations and conferences should be documented in a client's record so that all caregivers benefit from the information and plan the client's care accordingly.

Guidelines for Quality Documentation and Reporting

Quality documentation and reporting enhance efficient, individualized client care and can be achieved through the use of standard guidelines (Table 3-1).

Factual. A factual record or report contains descriptive, objective information about what a nurse sees, hears, feels, and smells. The nurse discriminates between **objective** and **subjective data.** An objective data description (e.g., "Pulse 78 beats per minute, regular; wound is 2 cm deep") is the result of direct observation and measurement. Factual information is less likely to be misleading or cause misinterpretation. Vague words such as *fair, good, stable, appears,* or *seems* and phrases such as *within normal limits* are not acceptable because they lead to inferences or conclusions that cannot be supported by objective information. If a nurse makes inferences or conclusions without factual information, errors in care can occur.

Records and reports can also include subjective information (data verbalized by the client). If a client gives information to the nurse, it should be recorded as a subjective entry in the client's own words. For example, "Client states, 'I feel helpless since I can't do anything for myself.'" The nurse can then add objective findings that more clearly describe the client's emotional problem, such as crying or loss of appetite. The description "the client seems depressed" does not communicate helpful information. The description does not tell another caregiver whether the client is withdrawing from conversation or threatening self-injury. A record or report clearly explains the nurse's observations of the client's behaviors and not an interpretation of those observations.

Accurate. A client's record must be accurate so that precise documentation is achieved. The use of exact measurements such as "intake, 220 ml of water" rather than "client drank an adequate amount of fluid" is essential. Measurements are used to determine whether a client's condition improves or deteriorates. Use of an institution's accepted abbreviations, symbols, and system of measures (e.g., metric) ensures that all staff members use the same language in reports and records.

Correct spelling is also important for accurate documentation and reporting. Terms can easily be confused or misinterpreted (e.g., *dysphagia* versus *dysphasia*). Simple spelling mistakes can cause serious treatment errors. It is particularly important to spell medication names correctly on administration records because of the potential of a medication administration error.

Accurate documentation of nursing interventions involves making entries in the record after an intervention is completed. For example, a nurse charts medication administration only after drugs ordered for a time or occasion have been given. An accurate entry in a record must reflect what nurses do during the time frame of the entry. **Nurses never document before administering therapies, and they never chart**

Table 3-1 Guidelines for Correct Recording

Guideline	Correct Action
Do not erase, apply correction fluid, or scratch out errors made while recording.	Draw a single line through the error, write the word "error" above it, and sign your name or initials. Then record the note correctly.
Do not leave blank spaces in nurses' notes.	Draw a line horizontally through the space and sign your name at its end.
Record all entries legibly and permanently.	Use black or blue ink for all entries (check agency policy for type of ink preferred); never use pencil, which can be erased.
Begin each entry with the time and end with your signature and title (students may be required to sign an abbreviation of their school).	Sign using first initial, complete last name, and title (C. Robinson, RN *or* T. Wallace, SN, U of I).

Box 3-1 Criteria to Report for Select Situations and Activities

Symptom (e.g., pain, nausea, headache, dizziness)
- Description of episode
- Location of symptom
- Severity
- Onset
- Precipitating factors
- Frequency and duration
- Aggravating and relieving factors
- Associated symptoms

Sign (e.g., rash, tenderness on palpation of body part, decreased breath sounds)
- Location of sign
- Description or quality of findings
- Aggravating or relieving factors
- Onset

Nursing care measures (e.g., enema, bath, dressing change)
- Time administered
- Equipment used if appropriate
- Client's response (positive [+] or negative [−])
- Nurse's observations

Client behavior (e.g., anxiety, confusion, hostility)
- Onset
- Behaviors exhibited
- Precipitating factors
- Nursing response or action
- Client's response

Medication administration
- Time administered
- Any required preliminary observations (e.g., pulse rate, blood pressure)
- Client's response or effect of medication (positive [‡] or negative [−−])
- Nursing measures taken for negative response

Client teaching
- Information or topic presented
- Method of instruction (e.g., discussion, role playing, demonstration)
- Resources used (e.g., videotape, booklet)
- Evidence that client understands instruction (e.g., return demonstration, change in behavior)

Discharge planning
- Client goals or expected outcomes
- Progress toward goals
- Need for referrals or resources
- Client's involvement in care plan

+, For example, client denied pain during dressing change.
−, For example, client experienced severe abdominal cramping during enema.
‡, For example, client reports that pain is reduced after analgesic.
−−, For example, rash is noted over lower abdomen.

for anyone else or let anyone chart for them. The exception is when nurses who have left the work site call their units to report on medication or therapy they had not charted while on duty. All nurses should be familiar with agency policy and procedure so as to know how to document such exceptions.

Late entries can be made in special situations. A common example is when the medical record is not available when the nurse needs it. A client may be relocated for a diagnostic test. A medication must be entered for the time it was actually given. Late progress notes are recorded by the actual time and date of entry, but information within the note refers to actual time of occurrence or when the entry should have been made. Often the nurse may determine that important information should be added after a progress note has been completed. The nurse simply enters a follow-up progress note. Finally, a late entry may also involve a situation in which the nurse omits a progress note and later realizes the need to add information. It is important to follow agency policy when writing a late entry.

Another way to ensure accuracy is to correctly sign and countersign entries. Any descriptive entry in a record ends with the caregiver's full name and title (e.g., Romero Hernandez, RN). In many institutions the first initial is accepted. Nicknames are not used. Nursing students sign their name and identify themselves as students, for example, "S. Caldwell, OHSU nursing student." RNs or nurse educators may countersign a note entered into the record by a nursing student. When a nurse countersigns, it means that the entry was reviewed and the care given was approved. When a nurse countersigns an entry, it is important that the person administering care is clearly identified. If the record is inaccurate, both nurses can share liability for any client injury. Different agencies may have specific countersigning policies.

Complete. The information within a recorded entry or verbal report should be complete, containing concise information about a client. Lengthy notes are difficult to read. Sketchy or abbreviated notes may leave an impression that nursing care was hurried or incomplete. A long verbal report wastes time and is often boring. A brief, well-written note or report avoids unnecessary words and irrelevant detail. Criteria are standardized for complete communication of certain health problems or nursing activities (Box 3-1).

Whenever it becomes necessary for a nurse to notify the nurse in charge, a supervisor, or a physician of information about a client, it is important that the information be completely documented in the record. The nurse documents the time of the call, the person notified, and the information reported (e.g., "1900 Dr. Abernathy notified of BP 90/60, pulse 116, urticaria present over trunk and extremities in reaction to IV morphine sulfate, S. Jackson, RN"). To further illustrate, a negative example using this same scenario is "1900 Dr. notified of an allergic reaction to morphine sulfate." The obvious lack of completeness demonstrates its importance in documentation.

Current. Timely entries are essential in the client's ongoing care. Delays in recording or reporting can result in serious omissions and untimely delays for needed care. Legally a late entry in a chart may be interpreted as **negligence** (an omission of care). Ongoing decisions about client care must be based on currently reported information. Activities that must be communicated *at the time they occur* include administration of medications or treatments; vital signs; clinical or physical assessment; preparation for diagnostic tests or surgery; change in a client's status and resulting treatment, if any; and admission, transfer, discharge, or death of a client. Routine activities such as bathing or giving oral hygiene do not need to be charted immediately. This information is often entered on flow sheets. The institution's accepted time system, military or civilian (Figure 3-2), should be used for reporting or documenting information. Note that military time begins at one minute after midnight and is recorded as 0001. Each minute is incrementally added until 1:00 AM is recorded as 0100, and so on. For example, 2:22 AM is recorded 0222.

Organized. The nurse communicates information in a chronological and logical format. A health care team member will better understand information reported or recorded in the order in which it occurred, for example, changes that occur in a client's status, followed by tests ordered, treatments started, and the client's response. If an institution uses a format for written notes (e.g., SOAP or PIE), follow the format according to institution standards. Another guideline for organized charting is use of the cephalocaudal (head-to-toe) approach in recording assessment findings. Describe findings beginning with the client's head and neck, progressing down the thorax, abdomen, and lower extremities.

Confidential. A confidential communication is information given by one person to another with trust and confidence that such information will not be inappropriately disclosed. The law protects information about clients that is gathered by examination, observation, conversation, or treatment. Nurses are legally and ethically obligated to keep information about clients' illnesses and treatments confidential. Only staff members who are directly involved in a client's care have legitimate access to the client's records. A record cannot be photocopied for anyone's personal use. Clients do have the legal right to read their own medical record (check agency policy).

Development of computerized systems creates the need for preventing unauthorized access to client information (Styffe, 1997). This can be accomplished by user-access codes and transaction logs. For example, a nurse who works on one nursing unit may be restricted from accessing client records on other units, depending on how the organization has set up its security program. Set levels of authorization according to the role of the user for client care is now technologically available (JCAHO, 2000).

Legible. Recorded notes that are illegible can cause treatment errors. If a nurse's script is not legible, entries should be printed. Most institutions require the use of black or blue ink. The use of checklists and computerized documentation limits handwritten recorded entries. When mistakes are made, erasures or scratching out errors are not allowed (see Table 3-1). There may be a time when there is a need to clarify the error with the nurse, so the initial entry must be legible. In testifying for legal cases nurses must be able to read their notes, often years after the questionable event.

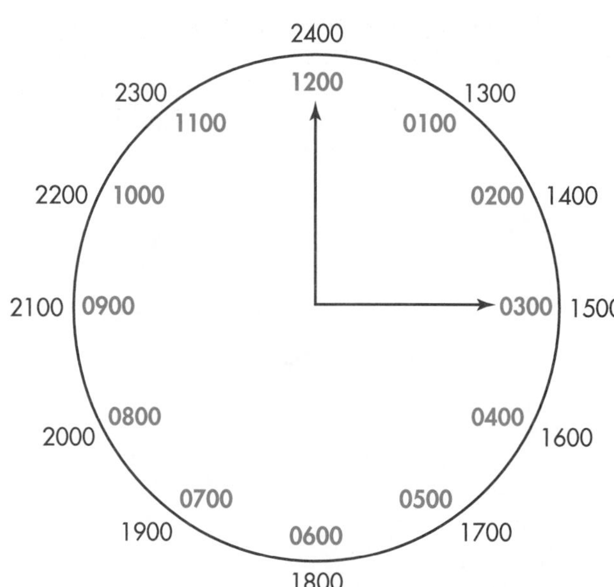

FIGURE 3-2 Military time clock. Instead of two 12-hour cycles, the military clock is one 24-hour time cycle, e.g., 3 PM is 1500 military time.

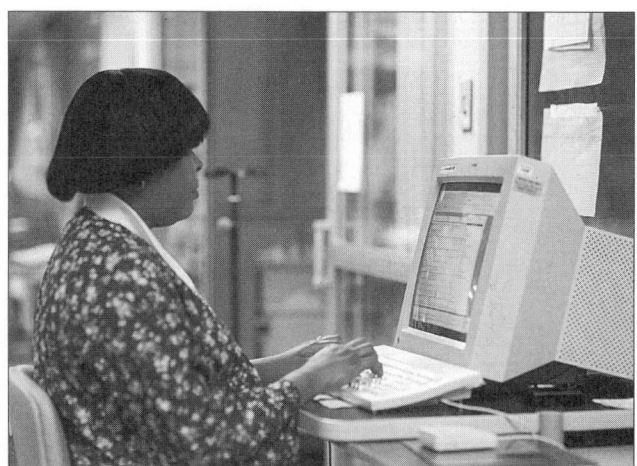

FIGURE 3-3 Computerized documentation provides many benefits.

Computerized Records

Computers are used in health care facilities in a variety of ways, including computerized documentation systems (Figure 3-3). There are many benefits to computerized documentation, such as reduction of transcription errors, standardization of nursing care, increased nursing productivity and efficiency, and easier monitoring for quality improvement. Computerization of data provides complete legibility of information and offers a structure for software design that reinforces standards of nursing care. Despite the convenience of computerization and the rapid availability of data, computerized documentation should never prevent nurses from recording thorough and detailed client care information.

Computerized documentation continues to change drastically with the introduction of new technologies. Notebook-sized computers with pen-based reading functions, handwriting recognition capabilities, and automated speech-recognition systems are examples. Nurses and physicians within more progressive institutions work closely together in the design and refinement of software programs that offer innovative approaches to enter and track clinical information.

Common Record-Keeping Forms and Formats

Nurses practice in a variety of settings, and different facilities use a variety of documentation forms and formats for entering data. Many forms eliminate the need to duplicate repeated data in the nursing notes. The forms present special types of information in a format more accessible than the compilation of all progress notes. Most of the forms are self-explanatory as to the type of information required from the nurse.

Nursing History and Assessment Forms. A nursing history and assessment form is completed at the time a client is ad-

Ashland Community Hospital

ADMIT FORM

Part I: Admission Routine

Date Time | Temp. Pulse Resp.
Mode ☐ amb. ☐ gurney ☐ wc ☐ other | B/P
Via ☐ admitting ☐ ER ☐ other | Height Actual Weight
Admitting Physician: | **Family Physician:**
Admitting Diagnosis:
Most Recent Adm. (hosp./date/reason)
Patient's Statement (of present complaint)

IMMUNIZATION STATUS
☐ CURRENT ☐ NOT CURRENT PHYSICIAN NOTIFIED

Allergies:
Type of Reaction

Medications Patient's significant other understands purpose ☐ yes ☐ no

Medication and strength	freq.	time last dose	Medication and strength	freq.	time last dose	**Disposition of meds:**
1.			6.			☐ did not bring
2.			7.			☐ patient has
3.			8.			☐ family has
4.			9.			☐ pharmacy
5.			10.			

Valuables List: (jewelry, clothing, etc.)

☐ glasses ☐ contact lenses ☐ dentures– ☐ bridge/partial ☐ other
Oriented to ☐ room ☐ bed ☐ phone ☐ call light/TV ☐ visiting hours ☐ safety/smoking policy
☐ doctor's orders ☐ armband

Part II: Patient/Family History

Patient History (major illnesses/operations/major injuries) include endocrine history/problems—past pregnancies

1	4	7
2	5	8
3	6	9

Use of tobacco ☐ no ☐ yes Type Daily amount
Use of alcohol ☐ no ☐ yes Type Daily amount
Organ donor ☐ no ☐ yes Living will ☐ no ☐ yes If yes, copy at ACH ☐ no ☐ yes
Other pertinent information:
Family History ☐ heart disease ☐ stroke ☐ hypertension ☐ asthma ☐ TB ☐ diabetes ☐ cancer
☐ kidney disease ☐ allergy ☐ epilepsy ☐ blood disorder ☐ mental disorder ☐ other
Socio/Economic Religion: Marital status: ☐ single ☐ married ☐ divorced ☐ widowed
Family ☐ lives with ☐ lives alone ☐ no family **Lives in** ☐ house ☐ apt. ☐ other
Occupation ☐ full time ☐ part time ☐ retired ☐ other
ADL ☐ independent ☐ needs assist with (specify what kind of help is needed and who provides it)

Anticipated Discharge Needs: ☐ self care ☐ community agency ☐ discharge planner ☐ other
Comments/plan:
Notify in emergency: relation phone
Nearest relative: relation phone
Info obtained from ☐ patient ☐ family ☐ other **Admitting Nurse:**

ACH 144

FIGURE 3-4 Nurse admission form. (Courtesy Ashland Community Hospital, Ashland, Ore.)

mitted for nursing care. Nurse practice acts designate the RN to be responsible for documenting client assessment. The form usually contains basic biographical data (e.g., age, method of admission, and physician), the admitting medical diagnosis or chief complaint, a brief medical-surgical history (e.g., previous surgeries or illnesses, allergies, and medication history), the client's perceptions about illness or hospitalization, and a physical assessment of all body systems (Figure 3-4). The form provides a guide that the admitting nurse uses to make a thorough assessment to identify relevant nursing diagnoses or client problems. Information on history forms provides baseline data that can be compared with changes in the client's condition. The JCAHO (2000) requires that a nursing assessment be completed by an RN for each client at the time of admission to a health care agency.

Part III: System Assessment

Place an "X" in area of abnormality. If unable to assess, indicate reason.

Assess eyes, ears, nose, throat for abnormality. ☐ No problem

EENT							(other)
impaired vision	blind	pain	reddened	drainage	gums		
hard of hearing	deaf	burning	edema	lesion	teeth		

Explain:

Assess chest configuration, resp. rate, rhythm, depth, pattern, breath sounds, comfort. ☐ No problem

RESP							(other)
asymmetric	tachypnea	apnea	rales	cough	absent		
barrel-chest	bradypnea	shallow	rhonchi	sputum	diminished		
dyspnea	orthopnea	labored	wheezing	pain	cyanotic		

Explain:

Assess heart sounds, rate, rhythm, pulse, blood pressure, circulation, fluid retention, comfort. ☐ No problem

CV							(other)
arrhythmia	tachycardia	rub	numbness	dimin. pulses	edema		
irregular	bradycardia	murmur	tingling	absent pulses			
pain	S_3 or S_4	fatigue					

Explain:

Assess weight, abdomen, bowel habits, swallowing, bowel sounds, comfort. ☐ No problem

Home diet/food habits/caffeine amount— stool color

GI							(other)
weight loss	N or V	anorexia	diarrhea	distention	hypoactive BS	mass	
obese	thirst	dysphagic	constipation	rigidity	hyperactive BS	pain	

Explain:

Assess urine freq., control, color, consistency, odor, comfort/Gyn—bleeding, discharge, pregnancy. ☐ No problem

Birth control method last menses last Pap smear

GU and GYN							(other)
pain	hesitancy	oliguria	dysuria	urine color	vaginal bleeding		
frequency	incontinent	nocturia	hematuria	discharge	pregnancy		

Explain:

Assess motor function, sensation, LOC, strength, grip, gait, coordination, orientation, speech, vision. ☐ No problem

NEURO							(other)
weakness	numbness	headache	paralysis	stuporous	pupils		
unsteady	tingling	seizures	lethargic	comatose	speech		
vertigo	pain	tremors	confused	vision	grip		

Explain:

Assess mobility, motion, gait, alignment, joint function/Skin color, texture, turgor, integrity. ☐ No problem

MS and SKIN					
appliance	stiffness	itching	petechiae	hot	drainage
prosthesis	swelling	lesion	poor turgor	cool	
deformity	wound	rash	skin color	flushed	
atrophy	pain	eochymosis	diaphoretic	moist	

Explain:

Date:__________Time:__________ R.N. Signature__________

FIGURE 3-4, cont'd Nurse admission form.

Graphic Sheets and Flow Sheets. **Flow sheets** and graphic sheets are forms that allow nurses to document assessment findings and routine care activities that are performed repeatedly. Common entries on flow sheets are vital signs, physical assessment findings, intake and output, laboratory data, fall risk criteria, and skin and pain assessments. The assessment flow sheet facilitates a thorough assessment by providing a framework for entries, instead of using open-ended narrative charting (O'Brien and Landstrom, 1994). It is unnecessary to chart a narrative progress note each time that vital signs are checked, a bath is given, or a drug is administered. The flow sheet is a quicker and more efficient way to record information. Figure 3-5 shows an example of a nursing flow sheet.

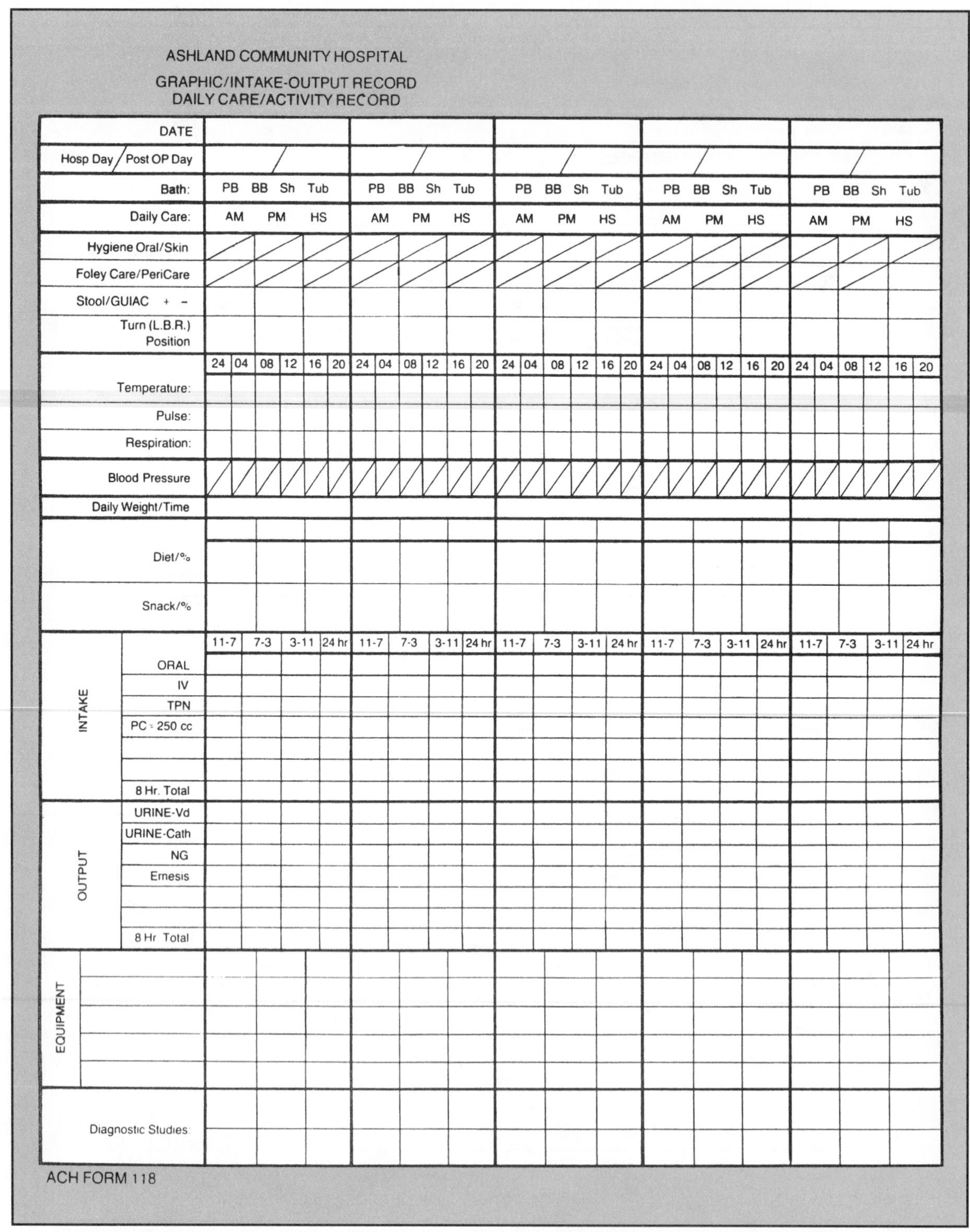

ASHLAND COMMUNITY HOSPITAL
GRAPHIC/INTAKE-OUTPUT RECORD
DAILY CARE/ACTIVITY RECORD

DATE					
Hosp Day / Post OP Day	/	/	/	/	/
Bath:	PB BB Sh Tub	PB BB Sh Tub	PB BB Sh Tub	PB BB Sh Tub	PB BB Sh Tub
Daily Care:	AM PM HS	AM PM HS	AM PM HS	AM PM HS	AM PM HS
Hygiene Oral/Skin					
Foley Care/PeriCare					
Stool/GUIAC + -					
Turn (L.B.R.) Position					
	24 04 08 12 16 20	24 04 08 12 16 20	24 04 08 12 16 20	24 04 08 12 16 20	24 04 08 12 16 20
Temperature:					
Pulse:					
Respiration:					
Blood Pressure					
Daily Weight/Time					
Diet/%					
Snack/%					
INTAKE	11-7 7-3 3-11 24 hr	11-7 7-3 3-11 24 hr	11-7 7-3 3-11 24 hr	11-7 7-3 3-11 24 hr	11-7 7-3 3-11 24 hr
ORAL					
IV					
TPN					
PC = 250 cc					
8 Hr. Total					
OUTPUT: URINE-Vd					
URINE-Cath					
NG					
Emesis					
8 Hr Total					
EQUIPMENT					
Diagnostic Studies:					

ACH FORM 118

FIGURE **3-5** Graphic intake-output record. (Courtesy Ashland Community Hospital, Ashland, Ore.)

In some agencies, flow sheets are included within computer software programs. Nurses are able to enter data, which later can be printed out as a flow sheet. The computer provides continuous storage of flow sheet data, eliminating the need to review multiple pages of forms.

When completing a flow sheet, the nurse carefully reviews previous entries to identify changes in the client's progress or condition. A trend on a graphic vital sign flow sheet, for example, can reveal a client's slow deterioration. When caregivers review flow sheets, the expectation follows that ongoing data are meaningful and relevant to the client's care.

Patient Care Profile or Nursing Kardex. A **patient-care profile (PCP)** is a report that is automatically updated each shift within a computerized medical record. A PCP can be generated for an individual client or group of clients and may include current orders, demographic data, diagnostic tests ordered, nursing and medical therapies, and information related to activities of daily living (ADLs). Agencies that have not converted to computerized nursing records use a nursing Kardex. The **Kardex** is a flip card or notebook page, usually kept at the nurses' station, that includes the same kind of information as the PCP on a separate form for each client. Both the PCP and Kardex can be used by the nurses during a change-of-shift report. The forms facilitate access to current information without having to access the client's entire record. A PCP or Kardex may also include standardized or individualized nursing care plans. These records may not become a permanent part of the client's record, because they often function as work sheets. Refer to agency policy.

Discharge Summary Forms. The nurse, the social worker, and other members of the health care team prepare a clinical summary of a client's condition and health care needs at the time of discharge (see Chapter 1). The reason for hospitalization, significant findings, client's status, and any specific teaching plan are included on discharge summary forms (JCAHO, 2000). Often a copy of the discharge form is given to the client's family member or home health care nurse. This ensures better continuity of care as the client transfers to another inpatient facility, home, respite care, or long-term care.

Charting by Exception. **Charting by exception** is an approach to streamline documentation by reducing repetition and time spent in charting (Iyer and Camp, 1995). It is a method for documenting normal findings and routine care based on clearly defined standards of practice and predetermined criteria for nursing assessments and interventions. With standards integrated into documentation forms, such as predefined normal assessment findings or predetermined interventions for a specific situation, a nurse needs only to document significant findings or exceptions to the predefined norms. In other words, the nurse writes a descriptive note on the form or a progress note only when the standardized statement on the form is not met (Figure 3-6). Assessments are standardized on forms so that all caregivers evaluate and document findings consistently.

The assumption with charting by exception is that all standards are met with a normal or expected response unless otherwise documented. When nurses see entries in the chart, they know that something out of the ordinary has been observed or has occurred. For that reason, it is easy to track when changes in a client's condition have developed. Any exception should be described thoroughly so that staff can monitor and intervene appropriately. The exception is recorded consistently until it is resolved.

Acuity Charting. **Acuity charting** or documentation requires nursing staff to document each client's level of acuity. Acuity is typically determined by the types of nursing care activities a client requires (e.g., simple versus complex medications, simple versus complex wound care, frequency of vital sign monitoring). Acuity reports are either developed by health care agencies themselves or by various proprietary companies. Many agencies use computerized systems that rapidly compute acuity levels for nursing units. Nurse staffing patterns are determined for each nursing unit, each shift, on the basis of overall client acuity. Acuity systems work from the principle that the higher the client acuity, the more nursing staff required. For this reason, it is important for acuity reports to be accurate.

Documenting Standards of Care

Standardized Care Plans. The JCAHO requires clients in health care organizations to have a nursing plan of care. The plan of care may be communicated in a variety of ways, through a problem-oriented medical record (POMR) (see Skill 3-2), nurses' progress notes, and the use of standardized care plans. **Standardized care plans** are developed by staff and help to provide a format to integrate evidence-based practice into nursing care. **Evidence-based practice** includes recommended nursing interventions that have been shown to be effective when tested in clinical research. The standardized plans are based on an institution's standards of nursing practice, are preprinted, and specify the recommended care measures for clients who have similar health problems. Most standardized care plans also allow the nurse to individualize the written plan. Any modifications in implementation and desired outcomes of care may be documented. The nurse remains responsible for individualizing the approach to client care.

Standardized Outcomes. Standardized language is becoming recognized as the means by which nurses can communicate consistent information to describe a clinical situation (Micek and others, 1996). When nurses use the same language to identify client problems and plan client outcomes, nursing care becomes more effective and appropriate to client needs. There are classification systems that provide standardized language. The North American Nursing Diagnosis Association (NANDA) (2000) has developed standardized nursing diagnoses to describe clients' responses to health problems. The *Nursing Interventions Classification (NIC)* provides a label name, a definition, and a list of activities that a nurse might do to carry out the intervention (McCloskey and Bulechek, 2000). Use of these standardized labels in documentation may prove useful to communicate client care needs more clearly.

Working Copy

BARNES-JEWISH HOSPITAL

Nursing Shift Assessment C-6

Requested by: CAROL

789651458 X
Collins, Phil

S.S.

Dr.

Unit: Bed:

Search Interval From: 05-Dec-1999 at 07:00
To: 06-Dec-1999 at 14:51

Patient Assessment

		Monday 12/06 07:00
N/S	**NEUROSENSORY STANDARD** Alert and awake. If asleep awakens to name. Verbal appropriate, clear, and understandable. Swallows without coughing. Oriented to time, place, person and situation. Behavior is appropriate to situation. Moves all extremities well, ambulates with steady gait.	Within Normal Limits
RESP	**RESPIRATORY STANDARD** Respirations are even and unlabored. Nailbeds and mucous membranes are pink. Patent airway. Lung sounds clear to auscultation. No cough noted	Within Normal Limits
CARD	**CARDIOVASCULAR STANDARD** Regular palpable pulses. Skin pallor within patient's norm. Skin warm and dry. No edema.	Within Normal Limits
SKIN	**SKIN INTEGRITY STANDARD** Skin and mucous membranes intact without notable lesions or impaired integrity. Mucous membranes moist and pink. Braden Score greater than 17.	* Exception as noted below
	Braden Risk Assessment	Mobility: Slightly Limited (3) Sensory: Slightly Limited (3) Moisture: Occasionally Moist (3) Activity: Walks Occasionally (3) Nutrition: Adequate (3) Friction/Shear: Potential Problem (2) Total Score 17
	Casts, Splints, Braces Type: Fiberglass Cast Site: Right Lower Leg	Maintains correct anatomical position No pressure areas noted Distal extremity pink warm to touch Palpable distal pulse Capillary Refill <3 seconds Sensation normal Able to move distal phalanges.
	VASCULAR ACCESS STANDARD IV SITE: Site free of redness, swelling, pain, bleeding, drainage, IV patent, dressing occlusive and intact.	
NUTR	**NUTRITION STANDARD** Tolerating prescribed diet without nausea and vomiting. Eating at least 75% of each meal without difficulty. Feeds self.	Within normal limits
	Diet Type	Regular
GI	**GASTROINTESTINAL STANDARD** Abdomen soft. Bowel sounds active all 4 quadrants. No pain with palpation. Having bowel movements within patient's normal pattern, consistency, and color.	Within Normal Limits
GU	**GENITOURINARY STANDARD** Continent of urine. Urine clear and yellow to amber color.	Within Normal Limits
PSYCH	**PSYCHOSOCIAL STANDARD** Accepts situation and facial expressions are appropriate. family support available and patient receives visitors. Able to communicate without assistance.	Within Normal Limits
EDU	Health Status Teaching	
	Tests/Procedures/Therapies	
	Medication Teaching	
	Nutrition Teaching	
	Medical Equipment Teaching	
HMGT	Equipment	
Charted By		cl

Signatures:
cl C. Logan, RN

Printed: 06-Dec-1999 at 14:51

FIGURE **3-6** Charting by exception—assessment form. (Courtesy Barnes-Jewish Hospital, BJC Health System, St. Louis.)

Another standard form of language being used throughout health care is client outcomes. The *Nursing Outcomes Classification (NOC)* provides an outcome label, a definition, and a list of interventions that might result in the outcome (Johnson, Maas, and Moorhead, 2000). The use of outcomes is essential when evaluating the achievement of the quality and appropriateness of client care. "An outcome is defined as a desired health state, condition, or behavior" (Micek and others, 1996). Three levels of care can be used in defining client outcomes. Prevention and promotion outcomes involve maintaining the client's health and self-care ability. Maintenance outcomes involve preventing decline of the client. Restorative outcomes focus on returning the client to a minimum level of health. Many clients have outcomes of each type, even during acute hospitalization. For example, a client may be admitted for treatment of a fractured hip resulting from a fall. The maintenance outcome could relate to maintaining skin integrity and range of motion. The prevention and promotion outcome could relate to helping the client and family plan for providing a safe home environment that minimizes risk for falls. The restorative outcome would focus on the client's rehabilitation activities.

Outcome statements require a target date for completion, which can vary greatly depending on the outcome desired. Once the date is established, nurses evaluate the client's progress toward achievement at the prescribed intervals. Each evaluation of progress determines if the client's problem or diagnosis is resolved or if the plan must be revised or extended. In some cases a different plan needs to be implemented. Each outcome is individualized for the particular client using specific measurement criteria. Such a process promotes continuity of care across the continuum of a client's care and centers on the client's and family's ability to restore, maintain, or improve the client's health.

Case Management and Critical Pathways. The **case management** model of delivering care involves a caregiver (e.g., primary nurse or case manager) to coordinate the client's care from admission to discharge. Case management programs use a multidisciplinary plan of care that is often summarized into **critical pathways.** These are usually one- to two-page formats that include key interventions and expected outcomes that allow the health care team to follow integrated care plans for client problems specific to a medical condition or surgical procedure (Figure 3-7). The documentation is minimal because the nurse charts on a standardized form, specific to the pathway of an individual client.

The critical paths are used on each shift of care to direct and monitor the flow of client care (Anders, Tomai, and Clute, 1997). Due to the nature of human responses, there are variances in outcomes as the client deviates from the critical path plan. For example, a client may not progress with ambulation as projected or a client may have a drainage tube removed earlier than expected. These variances refer to either the negative or positive changes in a client's progression toward expected outcomes (Acord-Szczesny, 1994). A **variance** analysis is necessary to review the data for trends and developing and implementing an action plan to respond to the identified client problems. Critical pathways place all care providers on the same page so that they can coordinate client care together.

Home Health Care Documentation

In the home setting, documentation is the crucial element for continuity of nursing care; it represents the evidence of achieving nursing standards and provides the basis for reimbursement for home health care services. Because Medicare has specific guidelines for eligibility for home care reimbursement, documentation that fulfills these guidelines is essential. Both quality of care and justification for financial reimbursement depend on effective documentation (Braunstein, 1993). Because some parts of the medical record are needed in the home, whereas other parts are needed in the caregiver's office, methods are being developed for "electronic home visits," including the use of modems and laptop computers (Miller, 1995).

In home care the nurses' notes should clearly identify the necessity of the nursing visit. The nurses' notes must be able to justify to the reader, usually a reimbursement reviewer, that the care provided is commensurate with the care plan of the overall health care team, the client requires the care in the home, and a necessary service is provided.

Long-Term Care Documentation

Resident assessment is a critical part of long-term care documentation. Clients in long-term care facilities are called **residents** because the long-term facility is their home. The Omnibus Budget Reconciliation Act of 1987 (OBRA '87) has prescribed the method of resident assessment and care plan development in an instrument known as the resident assessment instrument (RAI) (Lueckenotte, 2000). The RAI consists of the minimum data set (MDS), resident assessment protocols, and utilization guidelines specified by the Health Care Financing Administration (HCFA) (1995). The MDS includes a comprehensive resident assessment with criteria such as cognitive and communication patterns, physical functioning, mood, behavior, psychosocial well-being, and skin, nutritional, and dental status. State regulations define when each portion of the MDS and the plan of care must be completed. An interdisciplinary functional assessment is required.

The challenges of caring for residents in long-term care are very different from the acute care setting, which creates significant differences in documentation (Iyer and Camp, 1999). For example, acute care charting includes frequent physical assessment findings (e.g., vital signs and head-to-toe assessment), in some case using an hourly format, or at least every shift. For stable long-term care residents these entries may be made weekly or monthly. Outside agencies, for example, the state department of health, determine the standards and policies for long-term care documentation. The RN is responsible for identifying episodic changes that may require more intensive nursing intervention and documentation for residents who become ill.

BARNES

CARE PATH®
501
LUNG TRANSPLANT EVALUATION

1

SERVICE	PHYSICIAN	
PRIMARY NURSE	PRIMARY NURSE	
DC DATE	ADM DATE	DATE OF SURGERY

A-8

Problem Number	PATIENT PROBLEMS / NURSING DIAGNOSES
#1	LACK OF KNOWLEDGE R/T LUNG TRANSPLANT EVALUATION EXPERIENCE
#2	DECREASE IN EXERCISE CAPACITY R/T IMPAIRED OXYGENATION/VENTILATION/DECONDITIONING
#3	POTENTIAL FOR ALTERATION IN COPING R/T SITUATIONAL CRISIS/TRANSITION
#4	POTENTIAL FOR ALTERATION IN FAMILY PROCESSES R/T SITUATIONAL CRISIS/TRANSITION
#5	POTENTIAL FOR ALTERATION IN NUTRITION R/T INAPPROPRIATE INTAKE/DYSPNEA
#6	IMPAIRED GAS EXCHANGE R/T ALVEOLAR-CAPILLARY MEMBRANE CHANGE/ALTERED BLOOD FLOW *IF APPROPRIATE

#	1 - 12	1 - 12	1 - 2, 6 - 8, 12	2, 10, 12	1
	ASSESSMENT / MONITORING	CONSULTS	PROCEDURES / TEST	TREATMENT	ACTIVITY
PRE ADMIT		Transplant office to preschedule following as needed for pt.: 2-D Echo, Quant. V-Q, Resting RVG, PFTs, MRI, Cardiac Cath, Chest CT, Transesophageal echocardiogram			
DAY 1	Braden scale Respiratory status Fall prevention Assess/individualize pt. problem list	Notify consults as per orders. Check with transplant P.A. for additional tests which may be needed. SMA 6 and 12, CBC, CMV, HSV, EBV, Vz titers, HbsAq, HbsAb, HIV, Hep. A, Hep. C titers, T & S, PT, PTT HLA (A,B,C,DR) Typing, incl. cytotoxic screen, u/a - routine & micro, CXR-AP & lat EKG	Apply skin tests 07 Nursing, Pulm. Rehab., 08 & H.O. 09 10 11 12 Psychologist 13 14 CDL 15 16 PFTs 17 Chaplain 18 19 Cardiology Consult 20	Appropriate bed surface for Braden scale O_2 • At rest ______ • Activity ______ CPT x1 x2 x3 x4 by Nursing, Physical Therapy, family Aerosols x1 x2 x3 x4 (Self)	Continue activity as done at home

SIGNATURE	INIT.	SIGNATURE	INIT.	SIGNATURE	INIT.

3100-45 (REV. 10/93)

501

FIGURE 3-7 Critical pathway. (Courtesy Barnes-Jewish Hospital, BJC Health System, St. Louis.)

2

BARNES

CARE PATH®
501
LUNG TRANSPLANT EVALUATION

CNS	DIETARY	RT
HOME HEALTH	OT	OTHER
PT	SW	OTHER

A-8

Problem Number	PATIENT PROBLEMS / NURSING DIAGNOSES
#7	POTENTIAL FOR INEFFECTIVE AIRWAY CLEARANCE R/T EXCESSIVE SECRETIONS/FATIGUE
#8	INEFFECTIVE BREATHING PATTERN R/T INCREASED WORK OF BREATHING
#9	POTENTIAL FOR INFECTION R/T ALTERED NUTRITION/CHRONIC DISEASE
#10	POTENTIAL FOR INJURY R/T PHYSICAL DECONDITIONING
#11	SPIRITUAL DISTRESS R/T CHALLENGED BELIEF AND VALUE SYSTEM
#12	POTENTIAL FOR ALTERED SKIN INTEGRITY R/T POOR NUTRITION/DECREASED MOBILITY

1	1, 5, 9, 12	1 - 12	1 - 12	1, 2, 4, 11	
MEDS / IVS	NUTRITION	PATIENT / FAMILY EDUCATION	DISCHARGE PLANNING	PSYCHOSOCIAL/ EMOTIONAL/ SPIRITUAL NEEDS	INITIALS (SEE KEY AT BOTTOM)
		Give LTE manual, 6200 pt. letter.			
Pt. to do self meds.; Initiate IV access within 2 hrs. of admission	Continue home diet	Lung transplant evaluation Review tests for day 1 & 2 Personalize instruction to pts. individual learning needs. **Pt./family able to verbalize purpose and any special preparation for follow-up care for tests.**	Plan of care has been mutually set with pt./ family. Educational and DC planning needs will be assessed. **Pt./family verbalizes understanding of care path.**	Allow pt./ family to verbalize concerns and questions and relate problems back to appropriate discipline.	

SIGNATURE	INIT.	SIGNATURE	INIT.	SIGNATURE	INIT.

FIGURE **3-7, cont'd** Critical pathway.

Skill 3-1 Giving a Change-of-Shift Report

In addition to written documentation, nurses report information about their assigned clients to the nurses working the next shift. The purpose of the report is to provide continuity of care for the client. A change-of-shift report may be given orally in person, by audiotape recording, or with walking rounds from client to client. Oral reports are given in a conference room with nurses from both shifts participating. When an audiotape is used, the report is recorded before the end of the shift. This allows the nurses who are preparing to leave to finish last-minute tasks while the oncoming staff listens to the report. It is very beneficial to allow time for clarification or updates before the previous nurses leave the unit. Reports given in person or on rounds allow immediate feedback when questions are raised. Confidentiality must be maintained in all forms of reports.

Delegation Considerations

The skill of change-of-shift report should not be delegated to assistive personnel. However, assistive personnel should know what to report to the nurse to whom they are assigned so that any pertinent information can be included (after validation) in the report.

Equipment

- Worksheets, nursing Kardex (or patient care profile), nursing care plan or multidisciplinary treatment plan or critical pathway
- Tape recorder (according to agency policy)

Step	Rationale
Assessment	
1. Gather information from worksheets, assistive personnel report, or other relevant documents.	Nurse will not read forms during report that the next nurse can easily read independently. However, data used in reports must be current and reflect an overview of client's progress during shift.
Planning	
1. Prioritize information based on client's needs and problems; for example, report on immediate treatment planned for newly admitted client, report on educational progress of client about to be discharged home	Data reported need to reflect changes during shift and be pertinent, specific, and accurate.
• ***Critical Decision Point*** *Report only relevant information to next shift to ensure staff's timely responsiveness.*	
Implementation	
1. Develop an organized format for delivering report that includes a description of client's needs and concerns. For each client the following information may be included:	
a. *Background information*—Include client's name, sex, age, current primary reason for hospitalization, and brief history. Also include any known allergies, code status (i.e., do not resuscitate), and special needs as related to any physical challenges (e.g., blind, hearing deficit, amputee).	Data are organized based on priorities and individualized by reporting nurse.

STEP	RATIONALE
b. *Assessment data*—Provide objective observations and measurements made by nurse during shift. Describe client's condition and emphasize any recent changes. Include any *relevant* information reported by client, family, or health care team members, such as laboratory data and diagnostic test results.	Oncoming nurse will use data as baseline for comparison during next shift.
c. *Nursing diagnoses*—Include nursing diagnoses appropriate for client.	This clarifies client's current responses to health problems.
d. *Interventions, outcomes, and evaluation*—(steps can be combined in a report).	
(1) Describe therapies or treatments administered during shift and expected outcomes (e.g., relief of pain, improved airway patency). Specify how interventions are uniquely implemented for this client. Explain client's response and whether outcomes are met. Format of evaluation could be a critical pathway and use of variance documentation.	Staff learn the effect interventions are having on client's recovery and progress.
(2) Describe instructions given in teaching plan and client's ability to demonstrate learning.	Continuity of teaching is ensured, minimizing repetition, but communicating any needs for reinforcement.
e. *Family information*—Report on family visitation or involvement, specifically as it influenced client. Explain if family members were included in care procedures or instruction.	Report informs staff as to level of involvement family members have assumed in client's care.
f. *Discharge plan*—Client's progress toward discharge is reviewed during each change-of-shift report. Discharge plan identifies interventions and outcomes needed to allow client to have a smooth transition from hospital or health care facility to home. This plan also identifies health care referrals, roles and responsibilities of multidisciplinary team, and their follow-up visits.	All team members collaborate to follow plan of care that promotes discharge.
g. *Current priorities*—Explain clearly the priorities to which oncoming nurse must attend.	Provides for continuity of care.
2. *Clarify*—Ask staff from oncoming shift if they have any questions regarding information reported.	This allows for clarification of misinterpretation and discussion of additional areas of interest.

• ***Critical Decision Point***

Find specific nurses from next shift who will be directly providing care to clients for whom report was given.

Skill 3-2 Documenting Nurses' Progress Notes

A medical record is a comprehensive descriptive document of a client's health status and needs and the services provided for a client's care. Accurate documentation reflects the quality of care and provides evidence of each health care team member's accountability in giving care. The purpose of the client's record is to provide information for communication, education, assessment, research, financial billing, auditing, and legal documentation (Table 3-2).

Nurses involved in the direct care of clients are responsible for recording assessments of a client's condition, changes in a client's condition, a detailed accounting of nursing interventions, and an evaluation of the client's progress toward established outcomes. The nursing department of each health care agency selects the method used for documentation of client care. The method should reflect the philosophy of the nursing service and incorporate the standards of care and practice for the de-

Table 3-2 Purposes of Records

PURPOSE	DESCRIPTION
Communication	The record is a means for health care team members to communicate processes in the client's *care* (e.g., individual therapies, client education, use of referrals) and the client's *progress* (e.g., response to therapies). Anyone reading the record should have a clear understanding of the plan of care.
Education	The record contains a variety of information, including medical and nursing diagnoses, successful and unsuccessful therapies, and diagnostic findings. Students of nursing, medicine, and other health-related disciplines use records as educational resources.
Assessment	Records provide data that nurses use to identify and support nursing diagnoses and plan proper interventions for care. Information from records adds to the nurse's own observations and assessment. Information in medical progress notes allows the nurse to anticipate the status of the client and to conduct an assessment that augments, validates, or confirms physician findings.
Research	Statistical data relating to the frequency of clinical disorders, complications, use of specific medical and nursing therapies, deaths, and recovery from illness can be gathered from client records. Records describe characteristics of the client populations in a health care agency.
Financial billing	The medical record is a document that shows the extent to which hospitals should be reimbursed for services. For the facility to obtain full reimbursement, the record must show that all physicians' orders were completed adequately and correctly, and it must reflect results of those orders.
Auditing	A regular review of information in client records gives a basis for evaluation of the quality and appropriateness of care provided in an institution. The JCAHO requires health care institutions to establish quality assessment and improvement programs to conduct objective, ongoing reviews of client care. Review of records can reveal information about the processes and outcomes of care.
Legal documentation	A medical record must be accurate because it is a legal document. In the case of a lawsuit, the medical record, not the nursing care, is on trial. Nursing care may have been excellent; however, care not documented is care not done as far as a court of law is concerned.

partment. For example, if a nursing department's standards of practice use nursing diagnosis or a framework such as Gordon's functional health patterns (1994), the documentation system uses diagnoses or health patterns in care plans and other forms.

The **problem-oriented medical record (POMR)** is a format for documentation that places emphasis on the client's problems. Data are organized by problem or diagnosis, and narrative notes include assessment, planning, intervention, and evaluative information specific to the client's health status. In a true POMR system, all caregivers contribute to a single list of identified client problems. Most institutions use a modified POMR system whereby nursing staff contribute to a single list of nursing diagnoses or problems. Clients benefit from a POMR charting method because all health care team members can contribute to a common plan of care. A POMR has a database, problem list, care plan, and progress notes.

The database contains all available assessment information about the client (e.g., the physician's report of the physical examination and medical history, the nurse's admission history, the clinical or physical assessment, and the dietitian's assessment). The database remains active and current, with revisions made as new data become available.

The problem list should include each of the client's problems or diagnoses, listed in the order in which each problem was identified. The list is comprehensive, including physiological, psychosocial, cultural, spiritual, environmental, and developmental needs. Usually the problem list is in a selected location (e.g., in front of the record), so that it is easy to find and can serve as an organizer or table of contents.

Care plans are developed for each problem. These plans may be diagnostic, therapeutic, or educational and often have a multidisciplinary approach. In a diagnostic plan the physician indicates diagnostic studies to be performed. A therapeutic plan may include specific medical therapies ordered by the physician, or if the therapeutic plan is based on a nursing diagnosis, the nurse outlines proposed interventions. An educational plan includes the types of information or skills required by a client to assume self-care or adapt to any health-related problems. In a POMR all team members have access to the various plans of care so that care can be better coordinated.

Progress notes are a form of recording that document a client's progress. Often these notes follow a special format so that information about each client problem is documented and communicated clearly (Box 3-2). The various formats used for progress notes include **SOAP** (acronym for Subjective data, Objective data, Assessment, and Problem); SOAPE (acronym for Subjective data, Objective data, Assessment, Plan, and Evaluation); **PIE** (acronym for Problem, Intervention, and Evaluation); APIE (acronym for Assessment, Plan, Intervention, and Evaluation); and the format used in **focus charting,** DAR (Data, Action, and Response). The nurse uses the same format whenever a progress note is entered. It then becomes easy for staff to find notes referring to each problem. Any caregiver should be able to read a progress note and understand what type of problem a client has, the level of care provided, and the results of interventions.

Box 3-2 Formats for Recording Progress Notes

PIE (Acronym for Problem, Intervention, and Evaluation)

Problem-oriented system in which progress notes are written based on a list of identified problems, and detailed data may be entered by any member of the health care team.

Example:

P (Problem): Client states, "I am dreading this surgery because last time I had a terrible reaction to the anesthesia and had such terrible pain when they made me get out of bed." Noted muscle tension and loud, agitated voice.

I (Intervention): Notified anesthesiologist, Dr. M, of client's prior experience. Discussed alternatives for anesthesia and pain-control options. Stressed importance of activity for circulation/healing. Encouraged to keep nurses informed of pain level/need for medication and that pain may be present, but manageable.

E (Evaluation): Client stated she was "very relieved." Stated she would tell the nurses about pain.

SOAP (Acronym for Subjective data, Objective data, Assessment, and Plan)

Usually based on a numbered list of problems or nursing diagnoses.

Example:

S (Subjective data—the client's statements regarding the problem): Client states, "I am dreading this surgery because last time I had a terrible reaction to the anesthesia and had such terrible pain when they made me get out of bed."

O (Objective data—observations that support or are related to subjective data): Noted muscle tension and loud, agitated voice.

A (Assessment/analysis—conclusions reached based on data): Fear related to pain/anesthesia.

P (Plan—the plan for dealing with the situation): Notified anesthesiologist, Dr. M, of client's prior experience. Discussed alternatives for anesthesia/pain control options. Stressed importance of activity for circulation/healing. Encouraged to keep nurses informed of pain level/need for medication and that pain may be present, but manageable.

Focus or DAR Charting

A way to organize progress notes to make them more clear and organized.

Example:

D (Data): Client states, "I am dreading this surgery because last time I had a terrible reaction to the anesthesia and had such terrible pain when they made me get out of bed." Noted muscle tension and loud, agitated voice.

A (Nursing Action): Notified anesthesiologist, Dr. M, of client's prior experience. Discussed alternatives for anesthesia and pain-control options. Stressed importance of activity for circulation/healing. Encouraged to keep nurses informed of pain level/need for medication and that pain may be present, but manageable.

R (Client Response): Client stated she was "very relieved." Stated understanding of the importance of informing the nurses about pain.

NOTE: Some agencies add P (Plan) and refer to this as DARP charting.

Example:

P (Plan): Assess pain level at least every 4 hours postoperatively. Provide nonpharmacological pain management techniques and administer medication as needed.

Narrative Note

Describes client data in a narrative paragraph.

Example:

Client states, "I am dreading this surgery because last time I had a terrible reaction to the anesthesia and had such terrible pain when they made me get out of bed." Noted muscle tension and loud, agitated voice. Notified anesthesiologist, Dr. M, of client's prior experience. Discussed alternatives for anesthesia and pain-control options. Stressed importance of activity for circulation/healing. Encouraged to keep nurses informed of pain level/need for medication and that pain may be present, but manageable.

Delegation Considerations

Charting progress notes should not be delegated to assistive personnel. Assistive personnel may be allowed to document repetitive care activities on flow sheets (e.g., I&O, height and weight). The RN is responsible for any follow-up to validate client outcomes.

Equipment

- Progress note forms (manual or computer)
- Pen

Step	Rationale
Assessment	
1. Review all necessary assessments and nursing interventions required by client. Evaluate client's response and status of each diagnosis.	Nursing process organizes nursing care and directs care toward appropriate client problems.

STEP	RATIONALE
IMPLEMENTATION	
1. Identify forms to be maintained and their location.	Comprehensive documentation requires proper information be entered on all necessary forms.
a. Forms at bedside or on chart holder just outside door may include graphic chart for vital signs, intake and output record, checklist or flow sheet for routine care or a critical pathway, medication administration record, and nurses' progress notes.	Accurate clinical decisions are often based on information completed in correct format.
b. Other nursing forms that may be included: intravenous (IV) flow sheets; diabetic record; pain management flow sheet; admission, transfer, and discharge forms; and teaching forms. Follow guidelines for charting (see Table 3-1) to ensure quality documentation.	
2. After each client contact, identify information that needs to be documented. Consider: a. Abnormal findings b. Changes in status c. New problems identified	Prompt documentation increases accuracy and promotes effective communication to other members of health care team.
3. Document in a timely fashion without leaving open spaces between notes and include date and time.	Prompt documentation provides accurate record of client status and avoids omissions resulting from unexpected events.
4 Using agency format, determine the most effective way to include significant changes, including the following: a. Pertinent factual objective data b. Selected subjective data that validates or clarifies c. Nursing actions taken d. Client responses to actions taken e. Additional plans needing to be implemented f. To whom information has been reported, including name and status	When additional follow-up is needed, documenting to whom this has been reported shares responsibility with that individual.
5. Sign progress note with full name or first initial and last name and status according to agency policy. Do not leave an open space between this note and the previously written note. Students are usually required to indicate their level of education and school affiliation.	Signatures identify persons accountable for client care.

Skill 3-3 Incident Reporting

An incident is any event not consistent with the routine operation of a health care unit or routine care of a client. The client, visitor, or employee may be at risk when anything unusual occurs in a health care area. Examples of incidents include a client fall, accidental needle-stick injury, medication administration error, a visitor experiencing symptoms of illness, or carelessness in performance of a procedure that leads to actual or potential client injury. When an incident occurs, the nurse involved or the nurse who witnessed the incident completes an **incident report.** Reporting of incidents helps in the identification of high-risk trends in nursing care or daily unit operations that warrant correction. The report is completed even if an injury does not occur or is not apparent. The information from incident reports helps nursing staff find solutions to prevent repeated incidents. The reports are an important part of a unit's quality improvement program (Table 3-3). Incident reports are not a part of the permanent medical record, but they are kept by the facility to track reoccurring or high-risk problems so as to develop appropriate policies.

Table 3-3 Examples of Incident Report Entries

Proper Entry	Incorrect Entry
6 PM Client found on floor at foot of bed; able to respond to name when called. 2-cm abrasion noted across left forehead. Vital signs stable. Dr. Smith notified and arrived on floor at 6:15 PM. Placed client on fall-prevention protocol.	Client found on floor at foot of bed, probably fell on way to bathroom. Small abrasion over left forehead. Dr. Smith notified. Client instructed to use call light when needing to go to bathroom.
Administered morphine sulfate 10 mg at 4 PM; 6 mg morphine sulfate ordered. Monitored vital signs q 15 minutes; called Dr. Jones; vital signs remain stable.	Administered 10 mg morphine sulfate at 4 PM without checking order before administering. 6 mg morphine sulfate ordered.
Needle stick to right index finger, caused minimal bleeding. Notified employee health department.	Needle stick to right index finger, likely due to needle left in bed linen after blood drawing. Notified employee health.

Delegation Considerations

Incident reporting often involves assistive personnel who actually find the client in the situation that must be reported. Caregivers need to know their responsibility in actions to take, in reporting what they have found, and in explaining their actions to resolve the situation. Overall, writing incident reports should not be delegated to assistive personnel.

Equipment

- Incident report form, pen

Step	Rationale
Assessment	
1. Be observant when witnessing an incident: note exactly the sequence of events involved in incident, including time and type of incident; injury to client, nurse, or other staff; and observation of factors that may have contributed to incident (e.g, wet floor discovered in area of client fall, loose needle in client's bed linen).	Report must include objective, chronological information in the event incident leads to a lawsuit or investigation into institutional policy and procedure. Nurse who witnessed incident or who found client at time of incident files report.
• ***Critical Decision Point*** *Prepare an incident report on any questionable event. Do not avoid incident reporting based on the notion that punitive actions are taken whenever incident reports are filed.*	
2. Assess extent of any injury to client or others, including client's subjective report and objective physical examination findings.	Indicates type of treatment or action needed.
Implementation	
1. If incident involves an injury, take steps to restore individual's safety, such as stabilizing client's position after a fall and assessing for further injuries.	A priority is to stabilize any injury to prevent worsening of individual's condition.
2. When client sustains an injury, call a physician immediately.	Ensures prompt medical attention.
3. When visitor or staff member sustains an injury, refer to emergency department or appropriate treatment setting.	
4. Complete incident report form.	Prompt recording ensures accurate data.
• ***Critical Decision Point*** *Document on incident report form as quickly as possible. The closer to the event, the more accurate the recording. (NOTE: This also necessitates that staff readily know where incident forms are kept and which forms to use for clients, visitors, staff.)*	

Step	Rationale
a. Record time of incident and describe exactly what occurred or was observed, using objective findings and observations (see Table 3-3).	Prevents inferences and misinterpretation.

• ***Critical Decision Point***
It is extremely important to use words that are objective in nature and to use language that does not allow for subjective interpretation. Do not include personal opinions or feelings. Direct quotes by victim can be documented as victim's interpretation of incident.

Step	Rationale
b. Describe objectively client's or staff member's condition when incident was discovered or observed.	Establishes baseline for comparison with any later changes.
c. Describe measures taken by any caregivers at time of incident.	Provides standard in determining appropriateness of therapies.
d. Send completed report to designated department.	Data are used for facility's risk management and quality improvement programs.
5. When client is involved, document events of incident in client's chart.	
a. Do not duplicate all information from incident report.	Incident report can include factors nurse observed that may be contrary to policy and procedure. Client's chart should include only objective description of incident.
b. Do not record that incident report was completed.	Client's chart is legally recoverable and can be used in court. Incident reports are property of institution but are recoverable through subpoena.
c. Simply enter objective description of what happened.	Medical record is for purpose of documenting client's health status and medical care, not to blame or justify events of incident.
d. Record any assessment and intervention activities initiated as a result of incident.	
6. If client was injured, implement any ordered therapies and begin routine assessment of body systems influenced by injury.	Ensures continuity of client care and ongoing assessment of client needs.

Critical Thinking Exercises

1. During your assessment of Mr. Summers, you note a skin rash on the lower abdomen. The charting by exception assessment form has the standard entry "Skin intact, clear, without rashes, excoriations, or lesions." How would you document your findings on Mr. Summers?
2. You are the RN working with a patient care technician who approaches you to report on Mrs. Dye. The technician tells you, "When I turned Mrs. Dye to her right side she began to complain of pain in her back. She became restless and said, 'The pain is killing me.' I wanted to let you know as soon as I could." How would you evaluate the technician's report? In what way could it be improved?
3. Ms. Nyway is scheduled to be discharged from the hospital tomorrow. You spend time with her to instruct her on how to administer a metered-dose inhaler. The client has not had previous experience in using an inhaler. You explain the purpose of the inhaler and the importance of not using it more than the recommended doses per day. You demonstrate how the inhaler works and then observe Ms. Nyway administer her first dose. Ms. Nyway struggles a bit with grasping the inhaler. Then when she inhales the drug, she begins to swallow. Ms. Nyway says, "It's difficult to take a breath to inhale. I feel like swallowing the medication." You clarify the importance of inhaling the aerosolized medication. Write your nursing documentation of this interaction using both the SOAP and DAR formats for progress notes.

References

Acord-Szczesny J: Computer tracking of critical path variations, *Inside Case Manage* 1(2):1, 1994.

Anders RL, Tomai JS, Clute RM: Development of a scientifically valid coordinated care path, *J Nurs Adm* 27(5):45, 1997.

Braunstein ML: The electronic patient records solution, *Caring* 12(7):30, 1993.

Gordon M: *Nursing diagnosis: process and application,* ed 3, St. Louis, 1994, Mosby.

Health Care Financing Administration: *Resident assessment instrument training manual and resource guide,* Baltimore, 1995, The Administration.

Iyer PW, Camp NH: *Nursing documentation: a nursing process approach,* ed 2, St. Louis, 1995, Mosby.

Iyer PW, Camp NH: *Nursing documentation: a nursing process approach,* ed 3, St. Louis, 1999, Mosby.

Johnson M, Maas M, Moorhead S: *Iowa Outcomes Project. Nursing Outcomes Classification (NOC),* ed 2, St. Louis, 2000, Mosby.

Joint Commission on Accreditation of Healthcare Organizations: *Accreditation manual for hospitals,* Chicago, 2000, The Commission.

Lueckenotte AG: *Gerontologic nursing,* ed 2, St. Louis, 2000, Mosby.

Mathews J, Zadak K: Managerial decisions for computerized patient care planning, *Nurs Manage* 24:7, 1993.

McCloskey J, Bulechek GM: *Nursing Interventions Classification (NIC),* ed 3, St. Louis, 2000, Mosby.

Micek WT and others: Patient outcomes: the link between nursing diagnoses and interventions, *J Nurs Adm* 26(11):29, 1996.

Miller K: Home health care update 95, *Nursing* 25:7, 1995.

North American Nursing Diagnosis Association: *Nursing diagnoses: definitions and classification 1999-2000,* Philadelphia, 2000, The Association.

O'Brien K, Landstrom G: Using system integration to revise documentation, *Nurs Manage* 25:2, 1994.

Styffe EJ: Privacy, confidentiality, and security in clinical information systems: dilemmas and opportunities for the nurse executive, *Nurs Adm Q* 21(3):21, 1997.

4

SAFETY

Skills

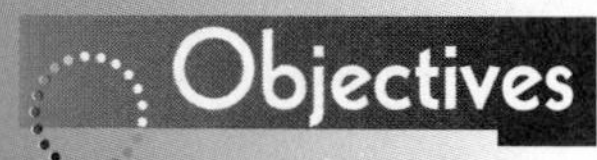

Mastery of content in this chapter will enable the nurse to:

- Define the key terms listed.
- Discuss methods to reduce physical and environmental hazards in all health care settings.
- Identify nursing diagnoses associated with a client's safety.
- Develop expected outcomes for clients whose safety is threatened.
- Discuss specific risks to safety as they pertain to the older adult client.
- Describe nursing interventions specific for reducing the risk of falls.
- Describe steps in the design of a restraint-free environment.
- Describe nursing interventions for a client who experiences generalized seizures.
- Describe methods to evaluate interventions designed to maintain or promote a client's safety.

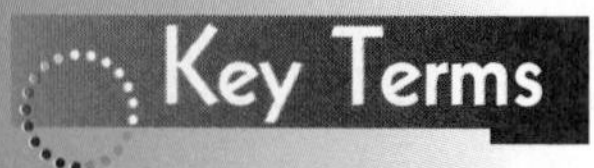

Aspiration
Belt restraints
Extremity restraints
Jacket restraints
Mitten restraints
Mummy restraints
Physical restraint
Seizure
Seizure precautions

Health promotion and illness prevention involve maintaining the client's safety. Maintenance of a client's safety in the home, community, and health care environment is essential. Promoting client safety reduces the length and cost of treatment, the frequency of treatment-related accidents, the potential for lawsuits, and the number of work-related injuries to personnel. In addition, a safe environment encourages clients to assume a more active role in their health care practices.

Threats to an adult client's safety are frequently related to lifestyle habits. The client who abuses alcohol has a greater risk than other persons for motor vehicle accidents. Likewise, the long-term smoker has a greater risk of cardiovascular or pulmonary disease than does the nonsmoker. The adult experiencing a high level of stress is more likely to have an accident because of the impact of stress on decision making. High levels of stress can also cause headaches, gastrointestinal disorders, and infection.

Accidents are the primary threats to the safety of older adults. Beginning at about age 70, the death rate from falls increases dramatically, and the rate continues to increase with age. The National Center for Health Statistics estimates that falls were the fourth most frequent type of death among older adults in 1997. Falls are a leading cause of injury in hospitalized older adult clients as well. Injuries to older adults can be related to psychogenic factors, physiologic changes occurring because of the aging process, pathological conditions, medications, and/or environmental hazards. Ebersole and Hess (1998) identify the following areas for nurses to consider when attempting to provide a safe environment for the older adult: housing, relocation stress, institutionalization, migration patterns, transportation and mobility, community and neighborhood supports, adaptational capacity of the aged, and environmental safety and convenience.

A client's safety can be maintained by preventing client self-injury. These accidents are classified as client-inherent accidents. Examples are self-inflicted cuts, injuries, and burns; ingestion or injection of foreign substances; self-mutilation or setting fires; and pinching fingers in drawers or doors. Client-inherent accidents can occur in both oriented and disoriented clients of all ages.

Measures designed to promote client safety are the result of individualized assessment findings. Often it is the conclusion of the nurse that a client's safety is at risk, and subsequent nursing interventions are implemented. Assessment of a client's safety should occur in the home, health care facility, and community environment.

A safe environment is one in which clients' basic needs are met, physical hazards are reduced or eliminated, transmission of microorganisms is reduced, and sanitary measures are carried out. Physical hazards, especially those implicated in falls, can be minimized by adequate lighting, removing clutter, and installing safety features, such as grip bars and nonslip floor surfaces. In addition, in the hospital or long-term care setting, safety is enhanced by the presence of call lights or other signaling devices, side rails, and electronic devices that trigger an audio alarm to alert staff to clients who may need assistance.

Clients at risk for injury from falling or other injuries may need restraints temporarily. Restraints are not a solution for a client problem; they are a temporary means to control behavior. Restraints do not necessarily prevent falls. In fact, it has been shown that clients may suffer fewer injuries if left unrestrained (Capezuti and others, 1996; Patterson, Strumpf, and Evans, 1995). Many complications are associated with the use of restraints, the most severe resulting in client death. There are many alternatives to the use of restraints, and all should be employed before using restraints. Ideally nurses should collaborate to design fall prevention programs and a restraint-free environment for clients. When restraints are necessary for client safety, the nurse must follow agency-specific policies. A physician's time-limited order is needed, and the appropriate restraint must be used and applied correctly. The client or family member's informed consent is necessary in the long term care setting. In addition, measures to prevent the hazards of immobility and other complications must be instituted.

A client with a unique risk for injury is one who suffers a seizure disorder. Certain forms of seizures involve sudden, violent, involuntary muscle contractions along with loss of consciousness. During a seizure clients can injure themselves from falls or when their bodies convulsively strike hard surfaces. Nurses caring for clients who have a seizure disorder must be familiar with seizure precautions to provide adequate protection to the client. Nursing interventions are designed to protect a client from traumatic injury, maintain a patent airway, and maintain a positive sense of self-esteem.

Another source of environmental hazard in health care settings is the use of radioactive materials in the diagnosis and treatment of clients, such as during x-ray procedures or radioactive implants. The Nuclear Regulatory Commission strictly regulates safe handling, use, and disposal of radioactive materials. Care providers need to be familiar with agency policies governing use of these materials. Safety measures relating to time, distance, and shielding must be instituted with the goal of reducing exposure of clients, visitors, and staff to radiation (Box 4-1).

Box 4-1 General Guidelines for Reducing Radiation Exposure

- Explain treatment plan to client and family, including activity limitation, side effects, safety regulations, and time and distance limits.
- Provide private room, and place sign on the door indicating radioactive materials are in room.
- A badge or dosimeter indicating extent of exposure may be indicated for staff who work in areas where radiation is used frequently.
- Rotate care providers and avoid exposure of women in early pregnancy.
- Wear a protective shield (lead apron or gloves) when providing care. Wash gloves before removing, and dispose of in designated waste container. Wash hands thoroughly after removing gloves.
- Wrap all nondisposable items that have come in contact with the radioactive material, and send to department responsible for decontamination.
- Identify needed requirements relating to laboratory specimens, dietary tray, dressings, linens, trash, secretions, and excretions.
- Request a discharge survey by radiation safety officer to ensure that all sources of radiation have been removed at the completion of treatment.

Skill Performance Guidelines

1. Know the client's age, level of awareness, orientation, ability to assimilate information and make judgments, ability to communicate, sensory and motor status, usual activity patterns, and activities of daily living.
2. Know the client's medical history and present therapies. Certain illnesses, such as stroke, and medications, such as tranquilizers, can cause physical or cognitive impairment that increases the risk of injury.
3. Be aware of environmental conditions that can affect the client's safety and increase risk of injury due to falls, restraint use, or a seizure.
4. Know the proper indications for and use of physical restraints for a client receiving nursing care in a hospital or extended care facility.

Skill 4-1 Fall Prevention

It is estimated that about 30% of the population 65 years and older living in the community falls at least once each year (Clinical News, 1995) and that falls account for up to 90% of all reported hospital incidents, with the risk for the older adult being significantly greater (Brady and others, 1993). It is therefore essential for nurses to accurately assess clients and their environment for risk factors. In this way measures may be instituted to reduce and/or eliminate hazards before client injury occurs. In the home older clients are more likely to fall in the bedroom, bathroom, and kitchen. These falls most often occur while transferring from beds, chairs, and toilets; getting into or out of bathtubs; tripping over carpet edges or doorway thresholds; slipping on wet surfaces; and descending stairs (Tideiksaar, 1989). Therefore it is important to carefully assess the environment and to inform the client of potential hazards (Box 4-2). In the hospital setting a tool, such as the RISK for falls assessment tool, may be used to identify a client at risk for falling (Box 4-3). The client's physical status, mental status, medications, and devices used to ambulate are assessed to determine the degree of risk. Based on an individual client's condition and environment, nursing measures are instituted to ensure safety. The call light/intercom system (Figure 4-1) should be explained to the client and family. Be sure side rails are used appropriately. A full set of raised side rails is considered a physical restraint. Raising only the two top side rails gives client's room to exit a bed safely and to maneuver within the bed. Beds and wheelchairs are locked, and beds are left in the low position (Figure 4-2). Clients may be placed in a Geri chair, or a wedge cushion (Figure 4-3) may be used on the chair or wheelchair to hinder unassisted ambulation. Seating in lounges or dayrooms should be arranged to encourage client interaction. Various types of seating should be available, such as lounge chairs and recliners. Wheelchairs should be used only to transport clients. Visual cues, such as color-coded arm bands or signs on the door or at the bedside, have been found to be effective in easily identifying risk-prone clients within an institution, so that staff know which clients may need special assistance.

For clients who continue to attempt to ambulate without necessary assistance, electronic bed and chair alarm devices

Box 4-2 Home Hazard Assessment

Home Exterior

Are sidewalks uneven?
Are steps in good repair?
Do steps have securely fastened handrails?
Is there adequate lighting?
Is outdoor furniture sturdy?

Home Interior

Do all rooms, stairways, and halls have adequate lighting?
Are night-lights available?
Are area rugs secured?
Are wooden floors nonslippery?
Is furniture placed appropriately to permit mobility?
Is furniture sturdy enough to provide support for getting up and down?
Are temperature and humidity within normal range?
Are there any steps or thresholds that may pose a hazard?
Are step edges clearly marked with colored tape?
Are handrails available and secure?
Are extension cords used appropriately?
Are smoke, fire, and carbon monoxide detectors installed?

Kitchen

Are hand-washing facilities available?
Is the pilot light on for the gas stove?
Are the dials on the stove readable?
Are storage areas within easy reach?
Are cleaning fluids, bleach, etc., in original containers and stored properly?
Is the water temperature within normal range?
Are there clean areas for food storage and preparation?
Is refrigeration adequate?
Are appliances in good working order?
Are electrical appliances located away from water sources?
Are electrical cords in good condition?

Bathroom

Are hand-washing facilities available?
Are there skidproof strips or surfaces in the tub or shower?
Are bath mats secured?
Does the client need grip bars near the bathtub and toilet?
Does the client need an elevated toilet seat?
Is the medicine cabinet well lighted?
Are medications in their original containers?
Have outdated medications been discarded?

Bedroom

Are beds of adequate height to allow getting on and off easily?
Is day and night lighting adequate?
Are floor coverings nonskid?
Does the client have a telephone nearby?
Are emergency numbers visible near the phone?

Modified from Tideiksaar R: Home safe home: practical tips for fall-proofing, *Geriatr Nurs* 11(6):280, 1989 and Ebersole P, Hess P: *Toward healthy aging: human needs and nursing process,* ed 5, St. Louis, 1998, Mosby.

Box 4-3 Risk for Falls Assessment Tools

Tool 1: RISK Assessment Tool for Falls

Directions: Place a check mark in front of elements that apply to your client. The decisions of whether a client is at risk for falls is based on your nursing judgment. Guideline: A client who has a check mark in front of an element with an asterisk (*) or four or more of the other elements would be identified as at risk for falls.

General Data

___ Age over 60
___ History of falls before admission*
___ Postoperative/admitted for surgery
___ Smoker

Physical Condition

___ Dizziness/imbalance
___ Unsteady gait
___ Diseases/other problems affecting weight-bearing joints
___ Weakness
___ Paresis
___ Seizure disorder
___ Impairment of vision
___ Impairment of hearing
___ Diarrhea
___ Urinary frequency

Mental Status

___ Confusion/disorientation*
___ Impaired memory or judgment
___ Inability to understand or follow directions

Medications

___ Diuretics or diuretic effects
___ Hypotensive or central nervous system suppressants (e.g., narcotic, sedative, psychotropic, hypnotic, tranquilizer, antihypertensive, antidepressant)
___ Medication that increases gastrointestinal motility (e.g., laxative, enema)

Ambulatory Devices Used

___ Cane
___ Crutches
___ Walker
___ Wheelchair
___ Geriatric (Geri) chair
___ Braces

Tool 2: Reassessment Is Safe "KARE" (RISK) Tool

Directions: Place a check in front of any element that applies to your client. A client who has a check mark in front of any of the first four elements would be identified as at risk for falls. In addition, when a high-risk client has a check mark in front of the element "Use of a wheelchair," the client is considered to be at greater risk for falls.

___ Unsteady gait/dizziness/imbalance
___ Impaired memory or judgment
___ Weakness
___ History of falls
___ Use of a wheelchair

Modified from Brians LK and others: The development of the RISK tool for fall prevention, *Rehabil Nurs* 16(2):67, 1991.

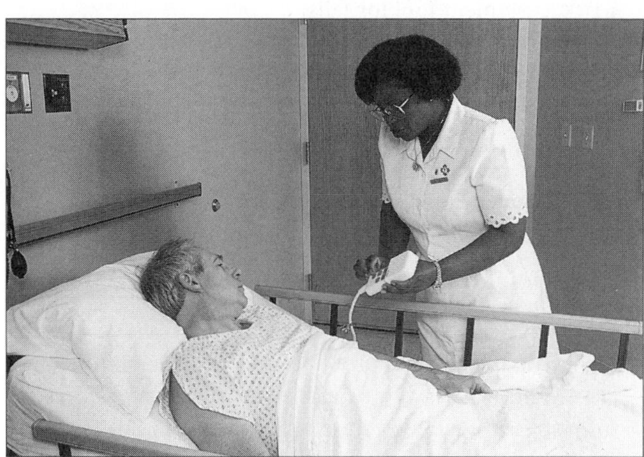

FIGURE 4-1 The nurse demonstrates the use of the call light to the client and secures it in an accessible position.

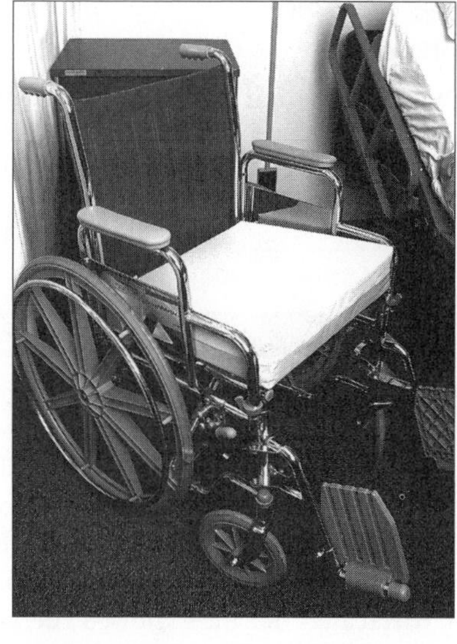

FIGURE 4-3 A wedge pillow on the seat is thicker at the front, deterring the client from getting up without assistance.

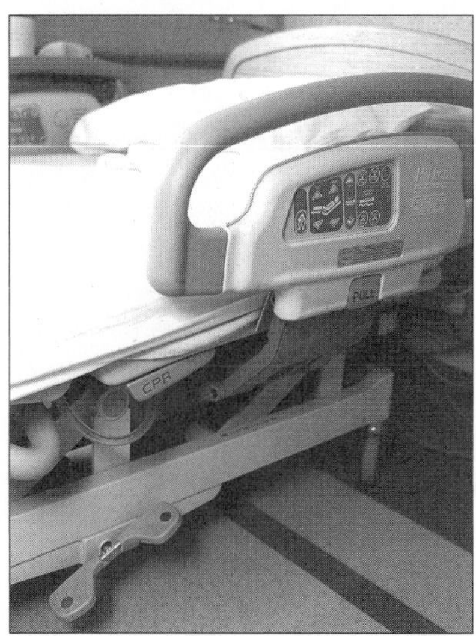

FIGURE 4-2 The hospital bed should have the wheels locked, be kept in the low position, and have the side rails up (when appropriate).

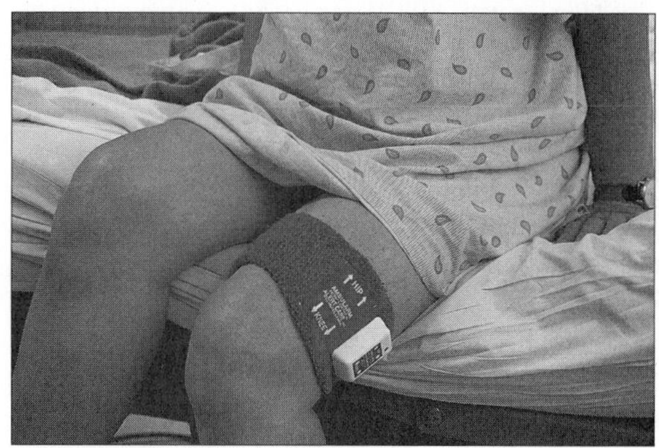

FIGURE 4-4 Position-sensitive switch triggers an audio alarm when client approaches a near vertical position when getting out of bed. (Courtesy Alert Care, Mill Valley, Calif.)

may be utilized. These devices are designed to warn nursing staff that a client is attempting to leave the bed or a chair unassisted. A variety of devices are available and include the use of a knee band that sounds an alarm when the client reaches a near vertical position (Figure 4-4), pressure-sensitive strips placed beneath the client and under the buttocks (Figure 4-5), and a tether alarm that is clipped to the client's garment. These devices alert staff that a fall situation is occurring. In this way staff can respond to the client in a timely fashion and provide needed assistance.

At home or in the health care setting it is very important that clients have adequate footwear when ambulating. Clients should have well-fitting, sturdy shoes with nonskid rubber soles. A walking shoe or sneaker is recommended. In addition, clients should wear cotton socks, which absorb moisture and prevent friction.

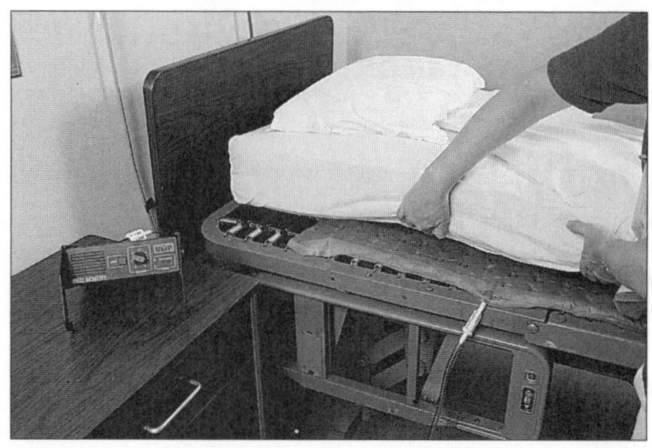

FIGURE 4-5 Pressure-sensitive pad triggers an audio alarm when client's weight is removed from the bed. (From Sorrentino SA: *Assisting with patient care,* St. Louis, 1999, Mosby.)

Delegation Considerations

Assessment of a client's risk for falling should not be delegated to assistive personnel. However, the skills necessary to prevent falls can be delegated. Inform the care provider of the risks identified and any client-specific measures to minimize risks.

Equipment

- Home hazard assessment
- A risk assessment tool for falls
- Hospital bed with side rails
- Call light

Step	Rationale
Assessment	
1. Assess older adult directly, and review medical history for physiological changes common to aging process that increase risk of falling: osteoporosis, decreased hearing, decreased night vision, cataracts or glaucoma, orthostatic hypotension, decreased balance, slowed nervous system response, osteoarthritis.	Physiological alterations predispose client to falls (e.g., postmenopausal woman is prone to osteoporosis and therefore at risk of breaking hip or ankle when walking: fall results from stress fracture; fracture is not caused by fall).
2. Review client's medication history for medications that may cause physical or cognitive impairment and lead to falls.	Antihypertensive medications and diuretics may cause hypotension. Narcotics and tranquilizers may cause drowsiness.
3. Assess risk factors in home, health care facility, and/or community that pose a threat to older adult's safety (e.g., improperly lighted stairways, obstructed walkway, throw rugs).	Provides opportunity to decrease risk of accidents.
4. Determine client's actual or risk of injury as a result of motor, sensory, or cognitive changes (e.g., visual acuity, unsteady gait, confusion).	Provides opportunity to identify factors that increase older adult's risk of injury.

Nursing Diagnosis

Defining characteristics from the assessment data may reveal the following nursing diagnoses for clients requiring this skill:

- Risk for injury
- Deficient knowledge related to safety precautions
- Impaired physical mobility
- Disturbed perception (visual)

Related factors are individualized based on client's condition or needs.

Planning

Step	Rationale
1. **Expected outcomes** following completion of procedure:	
▪ Client's environment is free of hazards.	Environmental hazards predispose client to potential injury.
▪ Client or family member is able to identify safety risks.	Client awareness of risks promotes cooperation and an understanding of treatment plan.
▪ Client does not suffer a fall or injury.	An injury due to a fall can be life threatening, causing dependency or immobilization.

Implementation

Home or Health Care Facility

Step	Rationale
1. Provide adequate, nonglare lighting throughout.	Reduces likelihood of falling over objects or bumping into them. Glare is a major problem for older adults.
2. Remove unnecessary objects from rooms, hallways, and stairs.	Eliminates potential hazards.
3. Arrange necessary objects in a logical way, placing them consistently in easy-to-reach locations.	Placing items such as eyeglasses, dentures, hearing aid, and telephone allows client to carry out self-care activities safely.

Step	Rationale

- ***Critical Decision Point***
  Clients who follow a consistent routine feel more secure, are less confused, and can better recognize safety hazards.

4. Install secure, easily visible grip bars or handrails in hallways and bathrooms (see illustration) and raised toilet seats. — Provides support when stepping out of tub, rising from toilet, or walking down hall.
   a. Place smooth but slip-resistant handrails at least 2 inches from wall. — Allows client to grasp handrail firmly for support.
   b. Secure handrail firmly so that user's weight can be supported, especially at bottom and top of a stairway. — Greatest risk of falling is at top and bottom stairs because center of gravity is being shifted and balance is unstable.

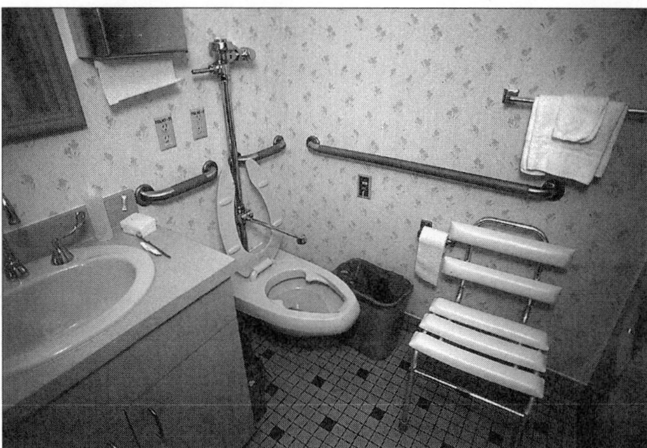

STEP **4** Grip bars should be installed in bathrooms.

5. Stairs:
   a. Within home or facility install treads with uniform depth of 9 inches and 9-inch risers (vertical face of steps). — Eliminates need to continually adjust vision.
   b. Install uniform textured or plain-colored surfaces on each tread, and mark edge of tread with easy-to-see contrasting color. — Provides obvious visual clue to end of step. Uniform texture or color helps to decrease vertigo. Older adults can see certain colors more clearly than others.
   c. Ensure proper lighting of each tread. Block sun or lightbulb glare with translucent shades or screens or use lower wattage bulbs. — Older client's vision is unable to quickly adjust to changes in lighting.
   d. Ensure adequate headroom so users do not have to duck to use stairs. — Sudden changes in head position may result in dizziness.
   e. Remove protruding objects from staircase walls. — Decreased peripheral vision may prevent client from seeing objects.
   f. Keep outdoor walkways and stairs in good condition (free of holes, cracks, and splinters) and well lighted. Paint edge of stairs with contrasting color (e.g., bright yellow). — Decreased visual acuity can prevent older client from seeing structural defect.
6. Floors:
   a. Secure all carpeting, mats, and tile; place nonskid backing under area rugs. — Ability to regain balance after tripping and preventing a fall is reduced in older adults.

   - ***Critical Decision Point***
     Area rugs can cause a hazard because they create an uneven walking surface, making tripping a risk. Reduce use of area rugs as much as possible.

   b. Dry spills on floors immediately. — Slipping occurs more readily on wet surfaces.
   c. Do not wax floors to a high sheen. — Waxing can cause glare. Older adults are very sensitive to glare and experience reduced visual acuity.

Step	Rationale
Health Care Facility	
7. Identify client by checking arm band and having client state name.	Prevents client care errors.
8. Introduce self to client, including both name and title or role, and explain what you plan to do.	Reduces client anxiety and promotes cooperation.
9. Gather equipment and wash hands.	Promotes organization and reduces transmission of microorganisms.
10. Provide privacy. Position and drape client as needed.	Prevents lowering of client's self-esteem.
11. Adjust bed to proper height, and lower side rail on side of client contact.	Allows for proper body mechanics and prevents injury.
12. Call light/intercom system (see Figure 4-1):	
a. Explain and demonstrate how to turn call light/intercom system on and off at bedside and in bathroom.	Knowledge of location and use of call light is essential to client safety.
• ***Critical Decision Point*** *Observe client return demonstration to ensure learning has taken place.*	
b. Consistently secure call light/intercom system to an accessible location.	Prevents client from searching for device, overreaching, and possibly falling out of bed.
13. Side rails (see Figure 4-2):	
a. Explain to client and family the two main reasons for using side rails: preventing falls and turning self in bed.	Promotes client and family cooperation.
b. Check agency policies regarding side rail use.	Side rails may be considered a restraint device when used to prevent ambulatory client from getting out of bed (Health Care Financing Administration [HCFA], 1999).
c. Keep top two side rails up and bed in low position with bed wheels locked when client care is not being administered and client is an older adult, weak, confused, sedated, or sleeping.	Prevents client from falling out of bed. With bed in low position, if client climbs over side rails and falls, trauma may be reduced.
d. Leave one side rail up and one down on side where oriented and ambulatory client gets out of bed.	Getting into bed is easier; client can use side rail to position self once in bed.
14. Provide clear instructions to client and family regarding any mobility restrictions, ambulation and transfer techniques.	Promotes client independence and understanding of treatment plan.
15. Explain to client specific safety measures to prevent falls (e.g., wear well-fitting, flat footwear with nonskid soles, dangle feet for a few minutes before standing, walk slowly, and ask for help if dizzy or weak) (see Chapter 27).	Promotes client understanding and cooperation. Dangling provides adjustment to orthostatic hypotension, allowing blood pressure to stabilize before ambulating.
16. Make sure ambulatory client's pathway to bathroom facilities is clear.	Eliminates potential hazards and promotes client independence.

Evaluation

Step	Rationale
1. Observe that client's living environment is modified for safety in relation to cognitive and motor needs.	Determines which modifications are needed within home or health care agency environment so client's safety is increased.
2. Evaluate the need for assistive devices such as walker, cane, or bedside commode.	Assistive device may provide more stability and help client assume a more active role.
3. Ask client or family member to identify safety risks.	Ensures client is able to identify risks to safety.
4. Reassess motor, sensory, and cognitive status to determine client's response to modification of potential risks. Determine that no falls or injuries occur.	Determines degree to which nursing interventions have been effective in reducing actual or potential threats to client's safety.

Unexpected Outcomes and Related Interventions

- Client is unable to identify safety risks.
  - Reinforce identified risks with client, or involve family member/friend and review safety measures needed to prevent a fall.
- Client suffers a fall. Safety measures were unsuccessful.
  - Nurse must attend to client's immediate physical needs, inform physician of fall and any apparent injury, reassess client's environment to ensure that environment is free of safety hazards, complete incident report, and communicate to other care providers that client is at risk for falls.

Recording and Reporting

- Record specific risks to client safety and interventions to reduce them on risk assessment tool or nurses' notes.
- Report to all health care personnel specific risks to client's safety and measures taken to minimize risks.
- Document relevant information related to instructions given to client and family and other safety measures employed (e.g., side rails, call light, electronic monitoring device).
- If client suffers a fall, inform physician. Document what occurred, including description of fall as given by patient or witness. Be sure to include any injuries noted, tests or treatments given, follow-up care, and additional safety precautions taken after fall.

Teaching Considerations

- Client should be instructed to have yearly vision and hearing examinations. Adaptive devices, such as a hearing aid or glasses, may be needed or modified.
- In a health care facility, client and family should be thoroughly oriented to surroundings, with special emphasis given to call lights and/or intercom devices.
- Emphasize the need to always look ahead when ambulating and to use good posture.

Gerontological Considerations

- Older adults, especially postmenopausal women, are at risk for fractured hips. Fractures can cause independent clients to become more dependent or immobilized (Lueckenotte, 2000).
- Older adult clients with short-term memory loss or cognitive dysfunction may be unable to follow directions and may attempt to climb out of bed or get up from chair unassisted.

Home Care Considerations

- Home environment should be assessed carefully.
- Night-lights, grip bars, handrails, raised toilet seats, and skid-proof strips or surfaces for tub or shower should be used.
- Items in home should be kept in their familiar positions and within easy reach.
- Client may need hospital bed, with side rails, and bell to signal caregiver or family, especially at night.

Long-Term Care Considerations

- Clients who wander from a facility are at risk for injury. Specific interventions such as electronic wandering devices can be used to reduce this risk.

Skill 4-2 Designing a Restraint-Free Environment

For clients who are at risk of falling or wandering, physical restraints should be the last resort and used only when reasonable alternatives have failed. When necessary, clients may need to be restrained to prevent serious injury due to falling and wandering, to protect from self-injury (e.g., pulling out tubes, removing dressings), and to prevent violence toward others.

Recently the public, the media, and the United States Congress have grown increasingly concerned about the need to ensure basic protections for client health and safety in health care facilities, especially with regard to the use of restraints and seclusion. In August 1999 the Health Care Financing Administration (HCFA) revised its standards regarding the use of restraints, which all hospitals must meet to participate in Medicare and Medicaid programs. The Health Care Financing Administration defines clients' rights and choices regarding restraints, and the reasons for the use of physical restraint are clearly stated. The use of mechanical or physical restraints must be part of the prescribed medical treatment, all less restrictive interventions must be tried first, other disciplines must be used, and supporting documentation must be provided (HCFA, 1999). For example, a nurse caring for a client who is attempting to dislodge a tube must try less restrictive measures first, such as a mitten or diversional activity. If the alternatives fail, the nurse may consider use of a restraint to prevent injury. A face-to-face assessment by the physician is required, and a physician's order is necessary before a restraint device is placed on the client.

A restraint-free environment should be the goal for all clients, whether in a health care facility or home. Measures can be taken to ensure safety for those clients who are at risk for self-injury by interrupting therapy and those who may inflict injury on others.

Delegation Considerations

The skills necessary to assess client behaviors and make decisions about less restrictive interventions should not be delegated to assistive personnel. Promoting a safe environment and monitoring client behavior for risk of injury may be delegated to assistive personnel.

Equipment

- Visual or auditory stimuli (e.g., calendar, clock, radio, television, pictures)
- Diversional activities (e.g., puzzle, game, music, stuffed animal, dummy tube)

Step	Rationale

Assessment

1. Assess client's physical and mental status, such as orientation; level of consciousness; ability to understand, remember, and follow directions; balance; gait; vision; hearing; bowel/bladder routine; level of pain; laboratory values; and presence of orthostatic hypotension.
   Rationale: Accurate assessment helps to identify safety risks and physiological causes for behavior and ensures proper interventions.

   - ***Critical Decision Point***
     Inability to understand or follow directions indicates client needs constant supervision.

2. Review prescribed medications (e.g., sedatives, hypnotics).
   Rationale: Medication interactions or side effects often contribute to falling or altered mental status.
3. Assess client's knowledge of condition and treatment.
   Rationale: Knowledge of treatment protocols and rationales may increase client's cooperation.

Nursing Diagnosis

Defining characteristics from the assessment data may reveal the following nursing diagnoses for clients requiring this skill:

Risk for injury
Deficient knowledge (specify area; e.g., alternatives to restraints)
Risk for trauma

Related factors are individualized based on client's condition or needs.

Planning

1. **Expected outcomes** following completion of procedure.
   - Client will be injury free and/or will not inflict injury on others while in a restraint-free environment.

Implementation

1. Orient client and family to surroundings, introduce to staff, and explain all treatments and procedures.
   Rationale: Promotes client understanding and cooperation.
2. Encourage family and friends to stay with client. Sitters or companions may be utilized. In some institutions, volunteers can be effective companions.
   Rationale: Reduces client anxiety and increases safety when one person provides care and supervision is constant.
3. Place client in a room that is easily accessible to caregivers.
   Rationale: Allows for frequent observation.
4. Provide appropriate visual and auditory stimuli. Clock, calendar, radio, television, and family pictures may be indicated.
   Rationale: Orients client to day, time, and physical surroundings.

   - ***Critical Decision Point***
     Stimuli must be individually selected for client to ensure appropriateness.

Step	Rationale
5. Meet client's needs as quickly as possible.	Toileting needs, relief of pain, and other activities of daily living, provided in a timely fashion, decrease client discomfort and anxiety.

- ***Critical Decision Point***
  Getting out of bed for toileting purposes is one of the most common events leading to a client's fall, especially during evening or night hours when rooms may be darkened.

Step	Rationale
6. Approach client in a calm, nonthreatening, professional manner.	Reduces tension in the environment.
7. Provide the same caregivers to the extent possible.	Provides stability of routine care and consistency in approach.

- ***Critical Decision Point***
  A sufficient number of staff should be readily available quickly for emergency situations.

Step	Rationale
8. Provide scheduled ambulation, chair activity, and toileting. Organize treatments so client has long uninterrupted periods throughout the day.	Provides for sleep and rest periods. Constant activity may irritate client.
9. Position intravenous (IV) catheters, urinary catheters, tubes/drains out of client view, or use camouflage by wrapping IV site with bandage or stockinet, placing undergarments on client with urinary catheter, or covering abdominal feeding tubes/drains with loose abdominal binder.	Facilitates medical treatment and reduces client access to tubes/lines.
10. Stress reduction techniques, such as back rub, massage, and imagery, may be employed (see Chapter 5).	Reduced stress allows client energy to be channeled more appropriately.
11. Utilize diversional activities such as puzzles, games, books, folding towels, drawing/coloring, or an object to hold. Be sure it is an activity client consents to.	Meaningful diversional activities provide distraction, help to reduce boredom, and provide tactile stimulation.
12. Various disciplines should be utilized in client's care.	Physical therapy, speech therapy, and occupational therapy may assist client to focus on appropriate actions.
13. Review medications frequently, and confer with physician if changes are needed.	Idiosyncratic reactions and drug interactions may cause changes in client behavior.

Evaluation

Step	Rationale
1. Observe client for any injuries.	Client should be injury free.
2. Observe client's behavior toward staff, visitors, and other clients.	Client's behavior should not cause injury to others.
3. Determine need for continuation of invasive treatments such as IV catheters, urinary catheters, and feeding tubes and whether less invasive treatment can be substituted.	Eliminates cause and reason for restraint.

Unexpected Outcomes and Related Interventions

- Client may continue to be at risk for injury, disrupt therapy, or commit violent acts toward others.
  - Intensify supervision of client, and notify physician. Restraints or medication may be indicated.

Recording and Reporting

- Record restraint alternatives attempted, client behaviors, and interventions to mediate these behaviors.

Teaching Considerations

- Clients and family members should be familiar with all medications and their possible side effects.

Gerontological Considerations

- Older clients who become confused and attempt to disrupt therapy or become violent may be suffering from effects of multiple drug administration, may be hypoxic, or may have fluid and electrolyte imbalance. Laboratory reports, signs and symptoms of fluid and electrolyte disturbances, and possible side effects of medications and interactions of all medications must be assessed (Brenner and Durnin-Duffy, 1998).

HOME CARE CONSIDERATIONS

- Clients at risk for self-injury or violence to others need intensive supervision. Family and/or caregiver must recognize this and be able to provide it.

LONG-TERM CARE CONSIDERATIONS

- For clients who are wanderers, exercise the person as ordered. Adequate exercise often reduces wandering. Do not argue with person who wants to leave. Go with person who insists on going outside. Make sure he or she is properly dressed. Guide person inside after a few minutes (Sorrentino, 2000).
- Reminisce with person to help maintain orientation.

Skill 4-3 Applying Physical Restraints

Clients at risk for injury may need to be temporarily restrained. A **physical restraint** is any device, garment, material, or object that restricts a person's freedom of movement or access to one's body. The restraint must be clinically justified and a part of the prescribed medical treatment and plan of care, and all other less restrictive measures must be employed first (see Skill 4-2).

The use of restraints has been associated with several serious complications. The Food and Drug Administration (FDA), which regulates restraints as medical devices and requires manufacturers to label them "prescription only," estimates that hundreds of restraint-related injuries occur each year, approximately 100 of them resulting in client death. Most client deaths have resulted from suffocation from a vest or jacket restraint (Lambert, 1992).

In addition, pressure ulcer formation, hypostatic pneumonia, constipation, incontinence, contractures, and neurovascular impairment can result from enforced immobility. Altered sensory perception and altered thought processes may also result. Humiliation, fear, anger, and a decreased sense of self-esteem may occur (Weick, 1992).

When the use of restraints is the only appropriate intervention to maintain the client's safety, both the client and the family should be informed that the restraint is temporary and protective. As with other procedures, the nurse must follow specific agency guidelines when using restraints. Most institutions require a physician's order (Figure 4-6), which should specify the type of behavior requiring restraint, the type of restraint, and time limitations. Orders should be renewed according to agency policy and based upon reassessment and reevaluation of the restrained client.

DELEGATION CONSIDERATIONS

Assessment of client's behavior, level of orientation, need for restraints, appropriate type to use, and specific assessments related to oxygenation, skin integrity, and neurovascular status should not be delegated to assistive personnel. However, the following aspects of the skill may be delegated to assistive personnel: correct placement of the restraint; observing for constriction of circulation, skin integrity, adequate breathing; when and how to change position; providing range of motion (ROM) and skin care, toileting, and opportunities for socialization.

EQUIPMENT

- Proper restraint
- Padding

Holy Family Hospital and Medical Center
Methuen, Massachusetts

PHYSICIAN RESTRAINT ORDER SHEET

ALLERGIES (FOOD AND/OR DRUG): ☐ NKA

HEIGHT: WEIGHT:

DIAGNOSIS(ES):

DATE	MEDICATION ORDERS	ALL OTHER ORDERS
	A physician's order is required for the use of restraint and/or seclusion. The order must be written or the telephone order countersigned by the ordering or "covering" physician within 24 hours of the order being given. "Restrain p.r.n." orders are not permitted. Orders must include a time limit not to exceed 24 hours. Physicians must review the use of restraints and reissue medical orders every 24 hours.	
		1) Restrain patient according to hospital policy.
		2) Behavior requiring restraint:
		☐ Confusion/disorientation/combative
		☐ Self harm
		☐ Harm to others/surroundings
		☐ Removing medical devices
		☐ Other
		3) Length of time (may not exceed 24 hrs):
		☐ 24 hours; ☐Other
		4) Type of restraint to be used:
		5) Additional instructions if any:
	Signature:	

✓ ORDERS CARRIED OUT (ALLERGIES, HT, WT, & DIAGNOSIS(ES) MUST BE COMPLETED ON ALL ADMISSION ORDERS AND UPDATED AS NECESSARY)

6/95 MF#682

Caritas Christi • A Catholic Health Care System • Member

A

FIGURE **4-6** **A,** Restraint order form. (Courtesy Holy Family Hospital and Medical Center, Methuen, Mass.)

Continued

B

Holy Family Hospital and Medical Center
70 East Street, Methuen, MA 01844

BEHAVIORAL RESTRAINT FLOW SHEET

Behavior Requiring Restraint: (Check all that apply)
- ☐ Confusion/disorientation/combative
- ☐ Self Harm
- ☐ Harm to others/surroundings
- ☐ Removing medical devices
- ☐ Other: ____________

Less Restrictive Measures Attempted: (Check all that apply)
- ☐ Pain/comfort measures
- ☐ Schedule position changes
- ☐ Schedule toileting
- ☐ Place closer to Nursing Station
- ☐ Reorient
- ☐ Encourage family/friends to visit
- ☐ Other: ____________

Physician order obtained: ☐ Yes; ☐ No

Type of Restraint: (Check all that apply)
- ☐ Soft wrist/ankle
- ☐ Halter type vest
- ☐ Seat Belt
- ☐ Mitts
- ☐ Leather
- ☐ Other: ____________

Patient/Family Informed: ☐ Yes; ☐ No

If no, Comment: ____________

Date Restraint Applied: ____________ **Time:** ________

Date Restraint Ended: ____________ **Time:** ________

Date: Time:am/pm	12	2	4	6	8	10	12	2	4	6	8	10
1. Hydration/Nutrition/Elimination												
2. Skin condition												
3. Range of motion/turn & position												
4. Communication (call light in reach)												
5. Circulation/Neurovascular Changes												
6. Assess chg. in clinical condition/behavior												
7. Assess for early release												
8. Restraint reduced/removed*												
9. Behavioral/Safety Check done q15"												
10. Vital Signs (if applicable)**												
Initials of assessor:												

Initials/Signature: Initials/Signature: Initials/Signature:

Comments:

* New order required when restraint removed or reduced. ** Temperature not required unless indicated.

KEY: ✓ = Observation / Intervention; NN = Nurses' Notes; O = Patient Off Unit; R = Restraint Removed

Note: It is not necessary to document the Behavioral/Safety Check every 15 minute but nurse must note every 2 hours in the assessment documentation #7 that the observation was performed. ***Any changes in behavior require an assessment.***

Caritas Christi · A Catholic Health Care System · Member

Written: 7/95; Revised: 16. August 1996

FIGURE **4-6, cont'd** B, Behavioral restraint flow sheet. (Courtesy Holy Family Hospital and Medical Center, Methuen, Mass.)

Step	Rationale
Assessment	
1. Determine client's need for restraint if other less restrictive measures fail to prevent interruption of therapy or injury to self or others.	Restraints may be needed when other less restrictive measures fail to prevent interruption of therapy such as traction, IV infusions, or nasogastric tube feedings; to prevent the confused or combative client from removing Foley catheters, surgical drains, or life support equipment; to reduce risk of injury to others by client; and at times to reduce risk of client falling out of bed or wheelchair.
2. Assess client's behavior, such as confusion, disorientation, agitation, restlessness, combativeness, or inability to follow directions.	If client's behavior continues despite attempts to eliminate cause of behavior, use of physical restraint may be needed.
3. Review agency policies regarding restraints. Check physician's order for purpose of restraint and type, location, and duration of restraint. Determine if signed consent for use of restraint is needed.	Physician's order is necessary to apply restraints. The least restrictive type of restraint should be ordered. Because restraints limit client's ability to move freely, nurse must make clinical judgments appropriate to client's condition and agency policy. If nurse restrains client in emergency situation because of violent or aggressive behavior that presents an immediate danger, a face-to-face physician assessment within 1 hour is needed (HCFA, 1999).
4. Review manufacturer's instructions for restraint application before entering client's room.	Nurse should be familiar with all devices used for client care and protection. Incorrect application of restraint device may result in client injury or death.
5. Inspect area where restraint is to be placed. Assess condition of skin underlying area on which restraint is to be applied.	Restraints may compress and interfere with functioning of devices or tubes. Assessment provides baseline to monitor client's skin integrity

- ***Critical Decision Point***
  Restraints should not interfere with equipment such as IV tubes. They should not be placed over access devices, such as an arteriovenous (AV) dialysis shunt.

Step	Rationale
6. Introduce self to client and family and assess their feelings about restraint use. Explain that it is temporary and designed to protect client from injury.	Client and family must be informed about use of restraint.

Nursing Diagnosis

Defining characteristics from the assessment data may reveal the following nursing diagnoses for clients requiring this skill:

- Impaired physical mobility
- Risk for impaired skin integrity
- Risk for peripheral neurovascular dysfunction
- Anxiety
- Self-care deficit
- Risk for situational low self-esteem
- Risk for violence: self-directed or other-directed
- Risk for injury

Related factors are individualized based on a client's condition or needs.

Planning

Step	Rationale
1. **Expected outcomes** following completion of procedure:	
▪ Client remains free from injury.	Injury can be life threatening, cause dependency or immobilization, and increase length of stay.
▪ Client's therapy (e.g., IV tube, catheters) is uninterrupted.	Disruption of therapy can cause client injury, pain, or discomfort and increase risk of infection.
▪ Client's self-esteem and dignity are maintained.	Physical restraints can have a detrimental effect on psychosocial well-being of client.

STEP	RATIONALE
IMPLEMENTATION	
1. Identify client by checking arm band and having client state name, if possible.	Prevents client care errors.
2. Approach client in a calm, confident manner. Explain what you plan to do.	Reduces client anxiety and promotes cooperation.
3. Gather equipment and wash hands.	Promotes organization and reduces transmission of microorganisms.
4. Provide privacy. Position and drape client as needed.	Prevents lowering of client's self-esteem.
5. Adjust bed to proper height and lower side rail on side of client contact.	Allows nurse to utilize proper body mechanics and prevent injury.
6. Be sure client is comfortable and in correct anatomical position.	Prevents contractures and neurovascular impairment.
7. Pad skin and bony prominences (if necessary) that will be under the restraint.	Reduces friction and pressure from restraint to skin and underlying tissue.
8. Apply selected restraint: **Always refer to manufacturer's directions.**	
a. **Jacket (Vest or Posey) restraint:** Apply jacket or vest over gown, pajamas, or clothes. Jacket restraints have sleeves. They close in back with zippers or hook and loop. Vest restraints should have front and back of garment labeled as such (see illustration). Criss-cross vest in front; one side of jacket restraint crosses over other side across chest, and straps are placed at client's hips.	Restrains client while lying or reclining in bed and while sitting in chair or wheelchair. Criss-crossing in back can cause risk of death from strangulation. Clothing or gown prevents friction against skin.
b. **Belt restraint:** Have client in a sitting position. Apply over clothes, gown, or pajamas. Remove wrinkles or creases from front and back of restraint while placing it around client's waist. Bring ties through slots in belt. Help client lie down if in bed. Avoid placing belt too tightly across client's chest or abdomen (see illustrations).	Restrains center of gravity and prevents client from rolling off stretcher or sitting up while on stretcher or from falling out of bed. Tight application may interfere with ventilation.

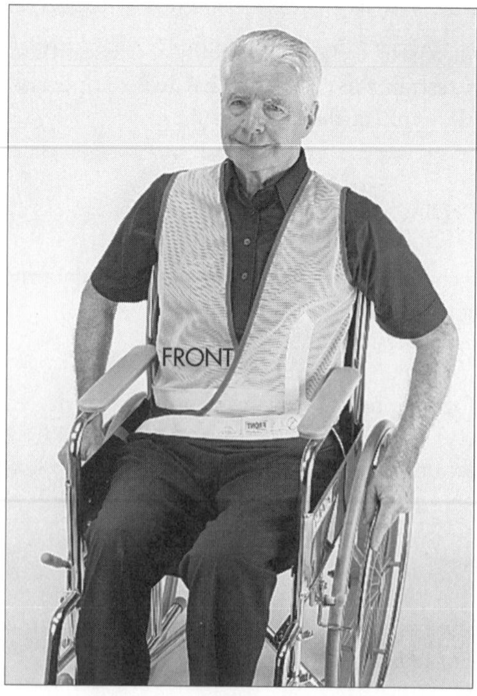

STEP **8a** Jacket (vest or Posey) restraint. (From Sorrentino SA: *Mosby's Textbook for Nursing Assistants*, ed. 5, St. Louis, 2000, Mosby; Courtesy J.T. Posey Co., Arcadia, Calif.)

STEP	RATIONALE
c. **Extremity (ankle or wrist) restraint:** restraint designed to immobilize one or all extremities. Commercially available limb restraints are composed of sheepskin with foam padding (see illustration). Limb restraint is wrapped around wrist or ankle with soft part toward skin and secured snugly in place by Velcro straps.	Maintains immobilization of extremity to protect client from injury from fall or accidental removal of therapeutic device (e.g., IV tube or Foley catheter). Tight application may interfere with circulation.

- ***Critical Decision Point***

  Client with wrist and ankle restraints is at risk for aspiration if placed in supine position. Place client in lateral position rather than supine.

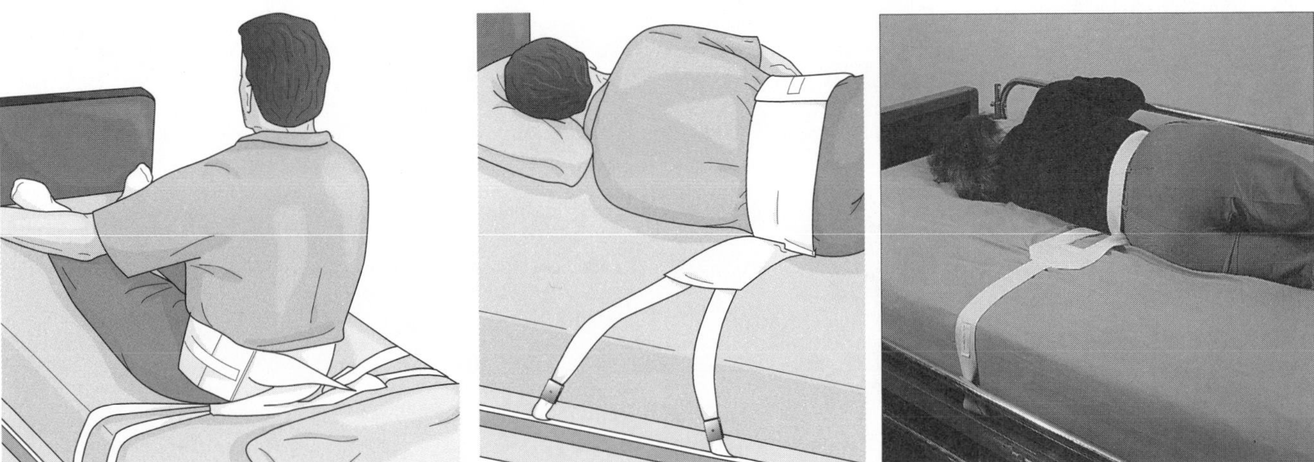

STEP **8b** Roll belt restraint tied to the bed frame and to an area that does not cause the restraint to tighten when the bed frame is raised or lowered. (From Sorrentino SA: *Mosby's Textbook for Nursing Assistants*, ed 5, St. Louis, 2000, Mosby.)

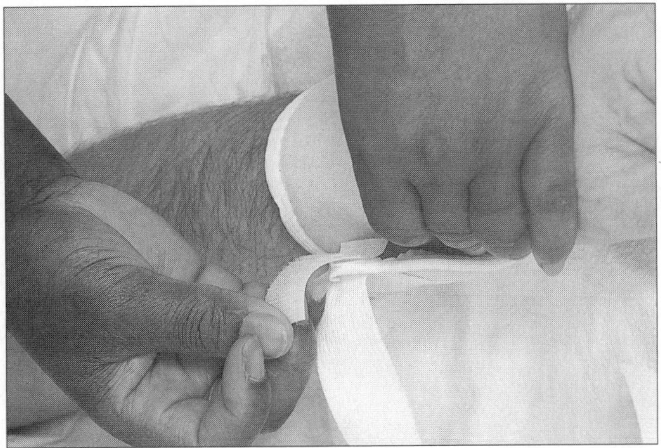

STEP **8c** Securing an extremity restraint. (Courtesy J.T. Posey Co., Arcadia, Calif.)

STEP	RATIONALE
d. **Mitten restraint:** thumbless mitten device to restrain client's hands (see illustration).	Prevents clients from dislodging invasive equipment, removing dressings, or scratching, yet allows greater movement than a wrist restraint.
9. Attach restraint straps to bed frame when head of bed is raised or lowered (see illustration). **Do not attach to side rails.** Restraint may also be attached with client in chair or wheelchair to chair frame.	Client may be injured if restraint is secured to side rail and it is lowered.
10. When client is in a wheelchair, jacket restraint should be secured by placing ties under armrests and securing at back of chair (see illustration).	Prevents client from sliding and being choked by restraint.

- ***Critical Decision Point***
  If ties are not under armrests, clients may be able to slide ties up the back of the chair and free themselves.

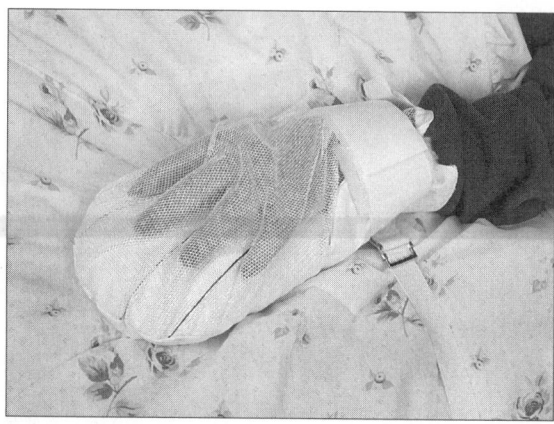

STEP **8d** Mitten restraint. (From Sorrentino SA: *Assisting with patient care,* St. Louis, 1999, Mosby.)

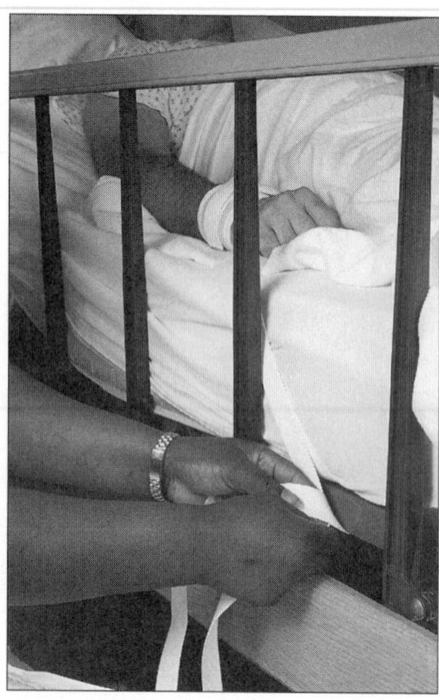

STEP **9** Restraints should be tied to the bed frame and to an area that does not cause the restraint to tighten when the bed frame is raised or lowered.

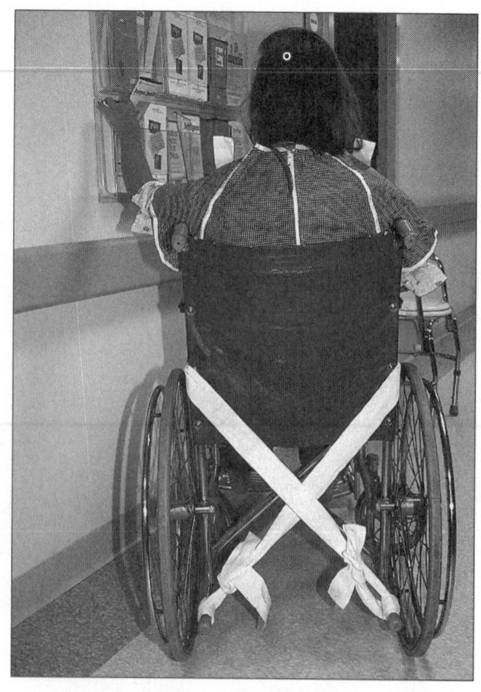

STEP **10** Jacket restraint secured to back of wheelchair.

STEP	RATIONALE
11. Secure restraints with a quick-release tie (see illustrations).	Allows for quick release in an emergency.
12. Insert two fingers under secured restraint (see illustration).	Checking for constriction prevents neurovascular injury.

- ***Critical Decision Point***
  A tight restraint may cause constriction and impede circulation.

13. Proper placement of restraint, skin integrity, pulses, temperature, color, and sensation of the restrained body part should be assessed **at least every hour** or according to agency policy.	Frequent assessments prevent complications, such as suffocation, skin breakdown, and impaired circulation.
14. Restraints should be removed at least every 2 hours (Joint Commission on Accreditation of Healthcare Organizations [JCAHO], 1999). If client is violent or noncompliant, remove one restraint at a time and/or have staff assistance while removing restraints.	Provides opportunity to change client's position, perform full ROM, toileting, and exercise and to provide food or fluids.

- ***Critical Decision Point***
  Violent or aggressive client should not be left unattended while restraints are off.

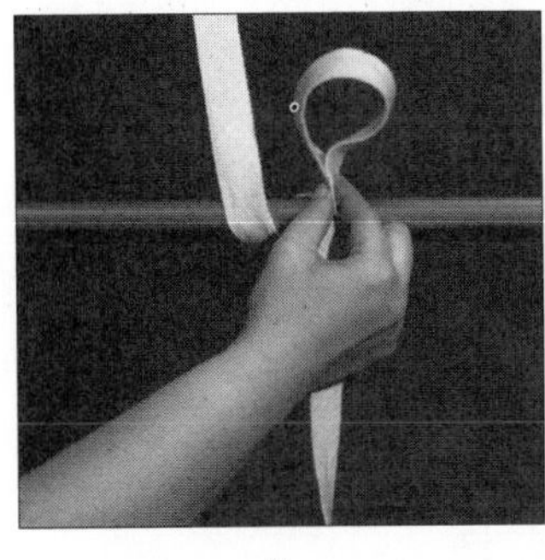
A

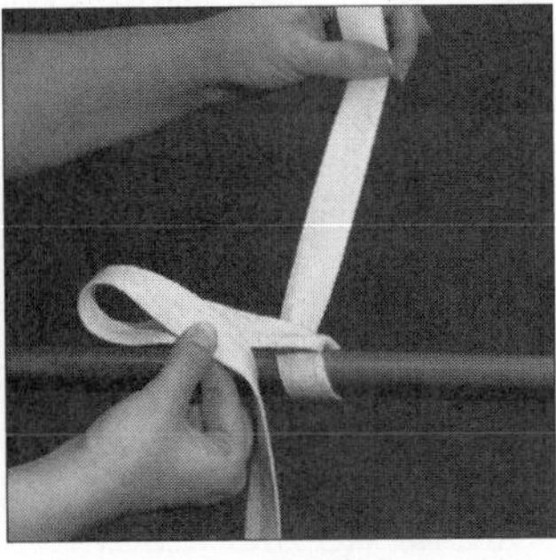
B

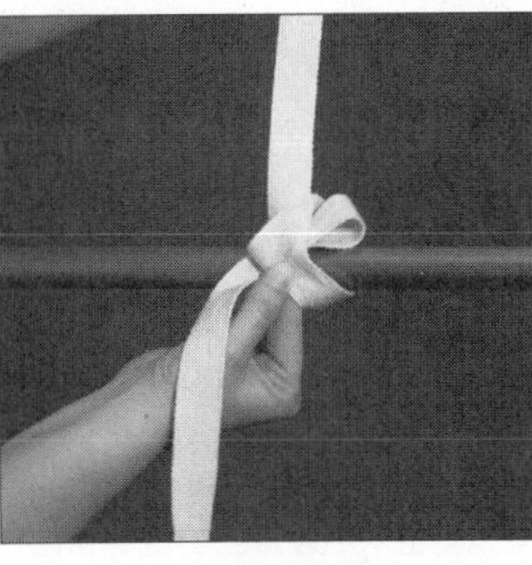
C

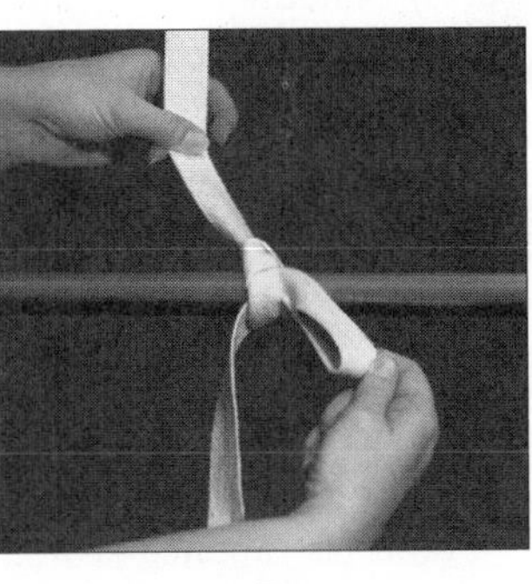
D

STEP **11** The Posey quick-release tie. (Courtesy J.T. Posey Co., Arcadia, Calif.)

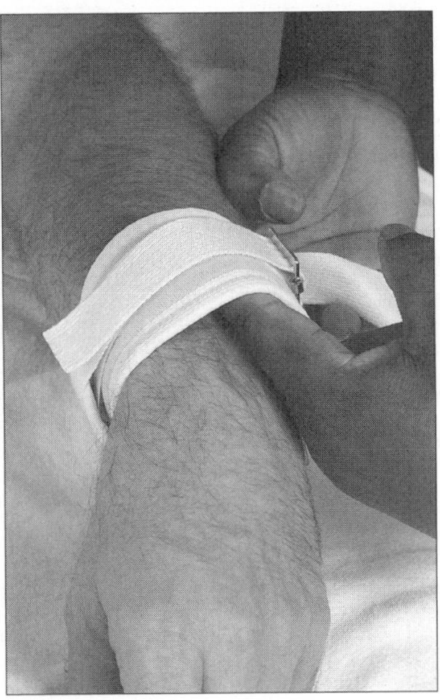

STEP **12** The nurse checks restraints for constriction by inserting two fingers under the restraint.

Step	Rationale
15. Secure call light or intercom system within reach.	Allows client, family, or caregiver to obtain assistance quickly.

- ***Critical Decision Point***
  Restraints restrict movement, making clients unable to perform their activities of daily living without assistance. Providing food/fluids and assisting with toileting and other activities is essential.

Step	Rationale
16. Leave bed or chair with wheels locked. Bed should be in the lowest position.	Locked wheels prevent bed or chair from moving if client attempts to get out. If client falls when bed is in lowest position, chances of injury are reduced.
17. Wash hands.	Reduces transmission of microorganisms.

Evaluation

Step	Rationale
1. Inspect client for any injury, including all hazards of immobility, while restraints are in use.	Client should be free of injury and not exhibit any signs of immobility complications.
2. Observe IV catheters, urinary catheters, and drainage tubes to determine that they are positioned correctly.	Reinsertion can be uncomfortable and can increase risk of infection or interrupt therapy.
3. Reassess client's need for continued use of restraint at least every 24 hours with the intent of discontinuing restraint at the earliest possible time (JCAHO, 1999).	Face-to-face reassessment by physician is required and new order obtained if restraint is to be continued.

Unexpected Outcomes and Related Interventions

- Client experiences impaired skin integrity related to improper or prolonged use of restraint.
  - Reassess need for continued use of restraint and if other alternative measures can be employed. If restraint is needed to protect client or others from injury, ensure restraint is applied correctly and provide adequate padding.
  - Check skin under restraint for abrasions, and remove restraints more frequently.
  - Change wet or soiled restraints to prevent skin maceration.
- Client has altered neurovascular status of an extremity, such as cyanosis, pallor and coldness of skin, or complaints of tingling, pain, or numbness.
  - Remove restraint immediately, and notify physician.
- Client exhibits increased confusion and disorientation.
  - Evaluate cause for altered behavior, and attempt to eliminate cause.
  - Provide appropriate sensory stimulation, reorient as needed, and attempt restraint alternatives.
- Client releases restraint and suffers a fall or other traumatic injury.
  - Attend to client's immediate physical needs, inform physician of fall or injury, and reassess type of restraint and its correct application.

Recording and Reporting

- Record nursing interventions employed to ensure client's safety prior to use of restraints.
- Record client's behavior before restraints were applied, level of orientation, and client's or family member's understanding of purpose of restraint and consent for application.
- Record in nurses' notes or restraint flow sheet type and location of restraint applied, time restraint was applied, and specific assessments related to oxygenation, skin integrity, musculoskeletal system, and peripheral vascular integrity.
- Record client's behavior after restraints were applied, times client was assessed while restraints were on and findings, attempts to utilize alternatives to restraint and client's response, times restraint is released (temporarily and permanently), and client's response when restraints were removed.

Teaching Considerations

- Explain thoroughly the use of restraint. Caution family against removing, repositioning, or retying restraint.

Pediatric Considerations

- When a child needs to be restrained for a procedure, it is best that person applying restraint not be child's parent or guardian.

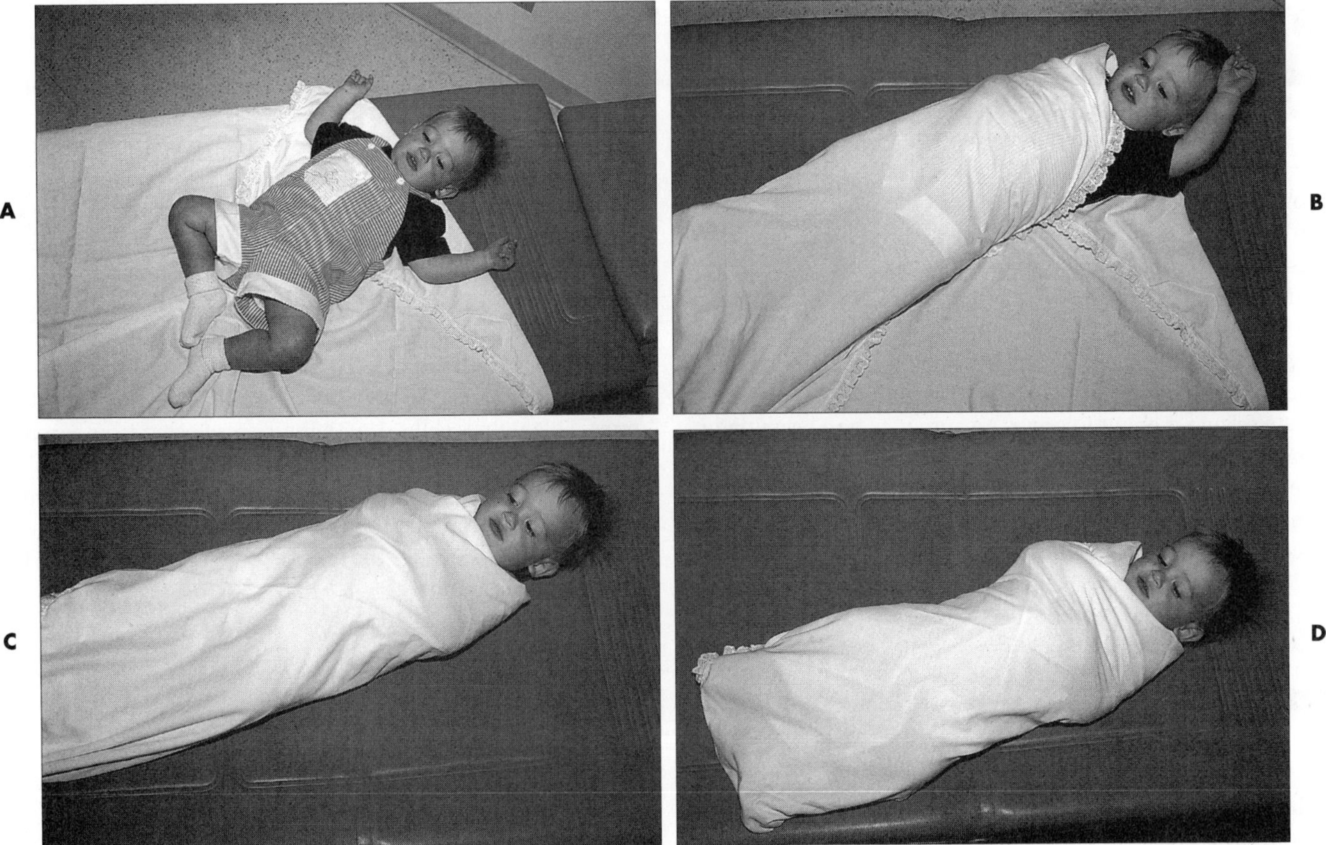

FIGURE 4-7 Mummy restraint.

- A **mummy restraint** is a safe, efficient, short-term method to restrain small child or infant for examination or treatment. Open a blanket and fold one corner toward the center. Place child on blanket with shoulders at fold and feet toward opposite corner (Figure 4-7, *A*).
- With child's right arm straight down against body, right side of blanket is pulled firmly across right shoulder and chest and secured beneath left side of body (Figure 4-7, *B*). Left arm is placed straight against side, and left side of blanket is brought across shoulder and chest and locked beneath child's body on right side (Figure 4-7, *C*). Lower fold is folded and brought over body and tucked or fastened securely with safety pins (Figure 4-7, *D*) (Wong and others, 1999).

Gerontological Considerations

- Advanced age is not in itself an indication for use of restraints. Promoting functional restoration by performing individual assessment of risk factors, orienting client as needed, modifying the environment, teaching muscle strengthening exercises, and meeting older client's needs in activities of daily living will help prevent falls and other traumatic injuries (Ebersole and Hess, 1998).

Home Care Considerations

- A physical restraint is a device that requires a physician order. It should not be sent home with family unless device is needed to protect client from injury. If client's family wishes to use restraint at home, a physician's order is required and clear instructions should be given regarding proper application, care needed while in restraints, and complications to look for.

Long-Term Care Considerations

- Unnecessary restraint is false imprisonment. The person must understand reason for restraint. The person is told how restraint will help planned medical treatment and risk of restraint use.
- Restraints are not used to discipline a person or for staff convenience (Sorrentino, 2000).

Skill 4-4 Seizure Precautions

A **seizure** is a hyperexcitation of neurons in the brain leading to a sudden, violent, involuntary series of muscle contractions that may be paroxysmal and episodic, as in a seizure disorder, or transient and acute, as after a head injury. A generalized tonic-clonic or grand mal seizure lasts from 1 to 2 minutes (no longer than 5 minutes) and is characterized by a cry, loss of consciousness, tonicity (rigidity), clonicity (jerking), and incontinence. Prior to a convulsive episode, a few clients may report an aura, which serves as a warning or sense that a seizure is about to occur. An aura may be a bright light, smell, or taste (Shantz and Spitz, 1993). Following the seizure, there is a postictal phase, during which the client may have amnesia, confusion, and may fall into a deep sleep (Seizure recognition and observation, 1992).

Status epilepticus consists of generalized tonic-clonic seizures that last longer than 5 minutes or are followed quickly by subsequent seizures. This constitutes a medical emergency and requires intensive monitoring and treatment.

Seizure precautions include all nursing interventions to protect the client from traumatic injury, side-lying position for adequate ventilation and drainage of secretions, providing privacy, and providing support following the seizure. It is recommended that objects not be placed in a client's mouth to avoid injury to the oral cavity. It has been found that significant injury to the mouth is rare during a seizure, even the most violent ones (Ellis, 1993). Injury may occur from forcing an object into the mouth and from teeth biting down on a hard object. Even soft objects may come apart and be aspirated. It is important that the nurse observe the client carefully before, during, and after the seizure so that the episode can be documented accurately.

Delegation Considerations

Assessment of a client's need to be placed on seizure precautions cannot be delegated to assistive personnel. Setting up seizure precautions and protecting clients at risk for seizures may be delegated to assistive personnel. Measures to emphasize if a client is at risk for a seizure include the following: the importance of protecting the client from a fall, avoiding attempts to restrain, and not placing anything in the client's mouth.

Equipment

- Oral airway
- Padding for side rails and headboard
- Suction machine
- Oral suction equipment
- Clean disposable gloves

Step	Rationale
Assessment	
1. Assess seizure history, noting frequency of seizures, presence of aura, and sequence of events, if known. Use family as resource if necessary	Knowledge about seizure history enables nurse to anticipate onset of seizure activity.
2. Assess for medical and surgical conditions that may lead to seizures or exacerbate existing seizure condition.	Neurological conditions and surgery may precipitate seizures.
3. Assess medication history and client's adherence.	Seizure medications must be taken as prescribed and not stopped suddenly. This may precipitate seizure activity.
4. Inspect client's environment for potential safety hazards if seizure occurs.	An airway, suction apparatus, clean gloves, and pillows should be visible for immediate use in hospital setting for clients with history of seizures.

Nursing Diagnosis

Defining characteristics from the assessment data may reveal the following nursing diagnoses for clients requiring this skill:

- Risk for aspiration
- Ineffective airway clearance
- Situational low self-esteem
- Noncompliance
- Deficient knowledge regarding safety precautions during seizure activity

Related factors are individualized based on a client's condition or needs.

STEP	RATIONALE

PLANNING

1. **Expected outcomes** following completion of procedure:
   - Client remains free of traumatic injury while experiencing seizure. — Injury from a fall or from jerking may occur as a result of onset of seizure activity.
   - Client's airway remains patent during seizure activity. — Airway occlusion and aspiration are potential complications of seizure activity.
   - Client does not experience a lowered sense of self-esteem following seizure episode. — Loss of bowel or bladder control is common in tonic-clonic seizures, causing client to feel embarrassment or shame.

IMPLEMENTATION

1. Position client safely. If standing or sitting at time of seizure, guide client to floor and protect head by cradling in nurse's lap or placing pillow under head. Clear surrounding area of furniture. If client is in bed, raise side rails, pad, and put bed in low position.
   Position protects client from traumatic injury, especially head injury.
2. If possible, provide privacy. Have staff control flow of visitors in area.
   Embarrassment is common after a seizure, especially if others witnessed the seizure.
3. If possible, turn the client on side, with head flexed slightly forward.
   Position prevents tongue from blocking airway and promotes drainage of secretions, thus reducing risk of aspiration.
4. Do not restrain client. Loosen clothing.
   Prevents musculoskeletal injury.
5. Do not force any objects into client's mouth.
   Prevents injury to mouth and prevents possible aspiration.

- ***Critical Decision Point***
  Injury may result from forcible insertion of hard object. Soft objects may break or come apart and be aspirated.

6. Stay with client, observing sequence and timing of seizure activity.
   Accurate, specific observations will assist in documentation, diagnosis, and treatment of seizure disorder.
7. After seizure is over, explain what happened, and answer client's questions.
   Informing clients of type of seizure activity experienced will assist them in participating knowledgeably in their care.
8. For clients experiencing status epilepticus, put on clean gloves and insert an oral airway (see illustration) when jaw is relaxed between seizure activity. Hold airway with curved side up, insert downward until airway reaches back of throat, then rotate and follow natural curve of tongue.
   Intensive monitoring and treatment are required for this medical emergency. Frequently an oral airway must be inserted and suctioning performed (see Chapters 14 and 16). Clean gloves prevent nurse from coming in contact with client's saliva.

- ***Critical Decision Point***
  Do not place fingers near or in client's mouth. Client may inadvertently bite nurse's fingers during a seizure. Do not forcibly insert airway if client's teeth are still clenched.

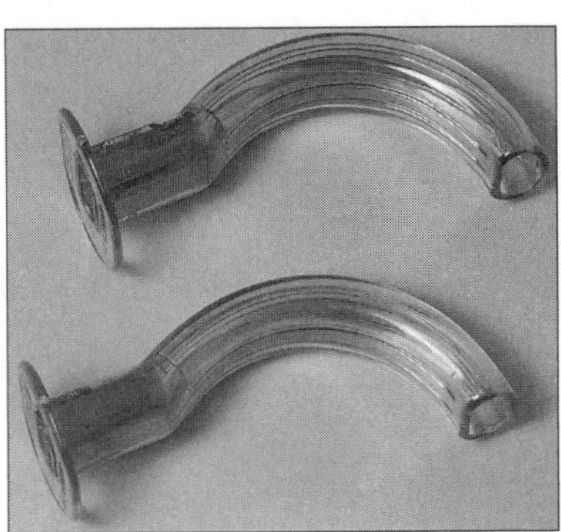

STEP **8** Oral airways.

STEP	RATIONALE
9. Pad side rails and headboard (see illustration).	Traumatic injury may be reduced. Avoid use of pillows to pad side rails because suffocation could occur.

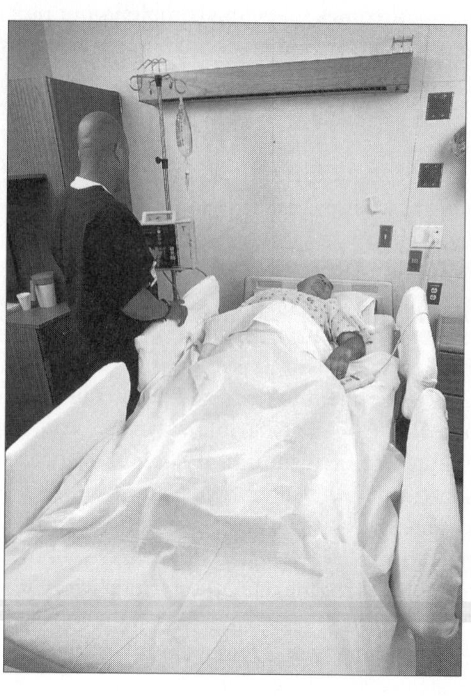

STEP 9 Padded side rails and headboard.

10. Following seizure, assist client to position of comfort in bed with padded side rails up and bed in lowest position. Place call light or intercom system within reach and provide a quiet nonstimulating environment.	Provides for continued safety. Clients are often confused and sleepy following a seizure.
11. Offer psychosocial support, stay with client to explain what has occurred. Foster an atmosphere of acceptance and respect, and provide time for client to express feelings and concerns.	Clients who accept the reality of a disease and integrate this reality into their own self-concept experience higher levels of self-esteem.
12. Wash hands.	Reduces transmission of microorganisms.

EVALUATION

1. Assess client for traumatic injury during and after seizure episode.	Injury may occur during seizure activity.
2. Assess client's mental status after seizure (level of consciousness, confusion, hallucinations).	Temporary mental status changes are common following a seizure.
3. Assess for bowel or bladder incontinence.	Loss of bowel or bladder control can increase client anxiety and risk of skin breakdown.

- ***Critical Decision Point***
  Inspect oral cavity for breaks in mucous membrane due to bites and broken teeth.

4. Observe client's color and respiratory rate and pattern during and after seizure.	Client may experience shallow irregular breathing during seizure, but normal color and respirations should be apparent following the episode.
5. If possible, ask client to verbalize feelings after seizure.	Therapeutic interaction may enable client to recognize feelings associated with having a seizure disorder. Client self-esteem is maintained.

Unexpected Outcomes and Related Interventions

- Client suffers traumatic injury.
  - Nurse must attend to client's immediate physical needs, inform physician of injury, reassess client's environment to ensure that environment is free of safety hazards, complete incident report, and communicate to other care providers measures taken to reduce risk for further injury.
- Client's airway becomes occluded, and materials are aspirated.
  - Insert oral airway, and apply suction to maintain patent airway.
- Client verbalizes negative feelings following a seizure.
  - Offer support to client, and allow for verbalization of feelings.

Recording and Reporting

- Record timing of seizure activity and sequence of events.
- Record presence of aura (if any), level of consciousness, posture, color, movements of extremities, incontinence, and client's status immediately following seizure.
- Report to physician immediately as seizure begins. Status epilepticus is an emergency situation requiring immediate medical therapy.

Teaching Considerations

- Clients should be thoroughly familiar with prescribed medications. Medication should never be stopped suddenly because this may precipitate seizures.
- Alcohol should be avoided because it may be incompatible with anticonvulsive medications. It may intensify central nervous system depression.
- Proper oral hygiene and frequent dental care are necessary when client takes phenytoin (Dilantin) long term, because gingival hyperplasia is a side effect (Skidmore-Roth, 2000).
- Client should wear a medical alert bracelet or carry identification card noting presence of seizure disorder and listing medications taken.
- Hypoglycemia, fatigue, stress, and illness have potential to initiate seizure activity (Beare and Myers, 1994). Therefore clients should eat a balanced diet at regular intervals, get enough sleep, and consult their doctor promptly when ill.
- A seizure condition usually imposes driving limitations. It is recommended that a waiting period of 1 seizure-free year elapse before client attempts to drive or operate dangerous equipment (Phipps and others, 1999).
- Some antiepileptic medications (AEDs) may interfere with effectiveness of oral contraceptives, making pregnancy a possibility. In addition, taking a single AED causes a threefold increase in risk of birth defects. Although pregnancy is rarely contraindicated, client should be counseled about potential effects (Rolak, 1998).

Pediatric Considerations

- Benign febrile seizures occur in 3% to 5% of children under the age of 5 with no cause for the seizure other than a high fever. It is important, however, that benign febrile convulsions be differentiated from epilepsy (Rolak, 1998).

Gerontological Considerations

- Older adults may have many various symptoms that can impede the recognition of a seizure disorder. Confusion lasting several days, receptive and expressive language problems, and unusual behaviors may be the result of a seizure (Lannon, 1995).
- Older adults tend to metabolize anticonvulsants more slowly; therefore drugs may accumulate, resulting in toxicity. Many anticonvulsants have known blood levels for therapeutic ranges, so blood levels should be monitored carefully (McKenry and Salerno, 1999).
- If client has dentures, do not try to remove them during a seizure. If they loosen, tilt head slightly forward and remove after seizure (Lannon, 1995).

Home Care Considerations

- Family members need to be familiar with care of client experiencing a seizure.
- Client's home should be assessed for environmental hazards in light of seizure condition.
- Until seizure condition is well controlled (usually for at least 1 year), client should not take a tub bath or engage in activities such as swimming unless knowledgeable family member is present.
- Referral to the Epilepsy Foundation or a similar group may help to improve client's self-esteem and coping ability

Critical Thinking Exercises

1. A pleasantly confused 83-year-old nursing home resident is admitted to your medical unit. Based on her admission, she was identified to be at fall risk due to a history of falls, confusion, and an unsteady gait. What fall prevention measures can you take to ensure your client's safety?
2. You have been assigned to care for Jason, a 17-year-old client who was just admitted for evaluation of his new-onset tonic-clonic seizures. What safety measures will you implement to prevent client injury if a seizure were to occur? Why are these measures indicated? What teaching consideration will be important for Jason and his family before discharge?
3. You are caring for a 40-year-old mother of two who has recently been diagnosed with breast cancer that has spread to her lungs. Although morphine has been effective in relieving her pain, she is agitated and restless and at risk for removing her IV catheter. Attempts to soothe and calm her have been ineffective. What measures can be taken to prevent the use of restraints in this client?
4. Assistive care personnel report increased agitation and restlessness of a client after placing a chest vest restraint on the client. What actions should the nurse take after receiving this report?

References

Beare P, Myers J: *Principles and practice of adult health nursing,* ed 2, St. Louis, 1994, Mosby.

Brady R and others: Geriatric falls: prevention strategies for the staff, *J Gerontol Nurs* 19(9):26, 1993.

Brenner Z, Durnin-Duffy K: Toward restraint free care, *Am J Nurs* 98(12):16f, 1998.

Brians LK and others: The development of the RISK tool for fall prevention, *Rehabil Nurs* 16(2):67, 1991.

Capezuti E and others: Physical restraint use and falls in nursing home residents, *J Am Geriatr Soc* 44(6):627, 1996.

Clinical News: falls in the home—the price of prevention, *Am J Nurs* 95(2):10, 1995.

Ebersole P, Hess P: *Toward healthy aging: human needs and nursing process,* ed 5, St. Louis, 1998, Mosby.

Ellis C: Nursing assessment and intervention for the patient experiencing seizures: a structured approach, *Clin Nurs Pract Epilepsy* 1(2):4, 1993.

Health Care Financing Administration: *Federal Register* 64(127), 1999.

Joint Commission on Accreditation of Healthcare Organizations: *Comprehensive accreditation manual for hospitals,* Chicago, January 1999, The Association.

Lambert V: Patient Restraints, *FDA Consumer* 26(8):9, 1992.

Lannon S: Epilepsy in the elderly, *Clin Nurs Pract Epilepsy* 2(2):5, 1995.

Lueckenotte AG: *Gerontologic nursing,* St. Louis, 2000, Mosby.

McKenry L, Salerno E: *Mosby's pharmacology in nursing,* ed 20, St. Louis, 1999, Mosby.

Patterson JE, Strumpf NE, Evans LK: Nursing consultation to reduce restraints in a nursing home, *Clin Nurse Specialist* 9(4):231, 1995.

Phipps W and others: *Medical-surgical nursing: concepts and clinical practice,* ed 6, St. Louis, 1999, Mosby.

Rolak LA: *Neurology secrets,* ed 2, Philadelphia, 1998, Hanley & Belfus.

Seizure recognition and observation: a guide for allied health professionals, ed 2, Landover, Md, 1992, Epilepsy Foundation of America.

Shantz D, Spitz M: What you need to know about seizures, *Nursing* 23(11):34, 1993.

Skidmore-Roth L: *Mosby's drug guide for nurses,* St. Louis, 1996, Mosby.

Sorrentino SA: *Mosby's textbook for nursing assistants,* St. Louis, 2000, Mosby.

Sorrentino SA: *Assisting with patient care,* St. Louis, 1999, Mosby.

Tideiksaar R: Home safe home: practical tips for fall-proofing, *Geriatric Nurs* 11(6):280, 1989.

Weick M: Physical restraints: an FDA update, *Am J Nurs* 92(11):74, 1992.

Wong DL and others: *Whaley & Wong's nursing care of infants and children,* ed 6, St. Louis, 1999, Mosby.

5

COMFORT

Skills

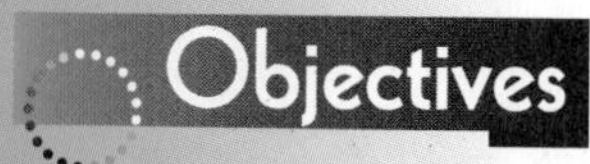

Mastery of content in this chapter will enable the nurse to:

- Define the key terms listed.
- Identify various nonpharmacological pain relief measures.
- Identify skills appropriate for relieving a client's specific pain complaint.
- Assess a client's level of comfort.
- Plan care based on a client's history and physical assessment.
- Assist a client in positioning and splinting to achieve pain relief.
- Discuss mechanisms by which nonpharmacological measures relieve pain.
- Assist a client in the use of nonpharmacological measures to relieve pain.
- Deliver medication through a patient-controlled analgesia (PCA) device.
- Teach a client to use a PCA device.
- Monitor and manage the client receiving intraspinal analgesia.
- Evaluate the effectiveness of pain-management techniques.

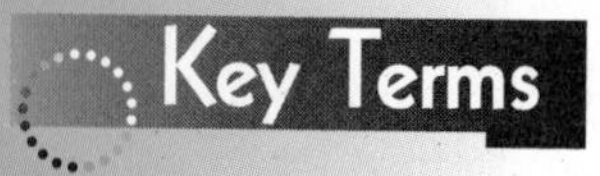

Acute pain
Addiction
Anticipatory guidance
Cancer pain
Chronic nonmalignant pain
Cutaneous stimulation
Distraction
Effleurage
Epidural
Friction
Guided imagery
Intraspinal
Intrathecal
Massage
Nonopioids
Nonpharmacological
Opioids
Pain intensity
Pain tolerance
Patient-controlled analgesia (PCA)
Pétrissage
Pharmacological agents
Physical dependence
Relaxation
Splinting
Tolerance

Pain is a complex phenomenon that is much more than a single sensation caused by a specific stimulus. The stimulus for pain can be physical and/or mental in nature. Pain is subjective and highly individualized. It involves the individual's behavioral and emotional responses to the pain experience. Pain is tiring and demands a person's energy. It can interfere with personal relationships and influence the meaning of life. Certain types of pain create predictable signs and symptoms, but the nurse can only assess pain by relying on the client's report and behavior. The client is the only one who knows whether pain is present and what the experience is like. According to McCaffery (1968) "Pain is whatever the experiencing person says it is, existing when she/he says it does" (AHCPR, 1992). It is not the responsibility of clients to convince the nurse that they have pain; it is the nurse's responsibility to believe them. The International Association for the Study of Pain defined pain as "an unpleasant sensory and emotional experience associated with actual or potential tissue damage, or an experience described in terms of such damage" (National Institute of Nursing Research, 1994).

Pain is often difficult to precisely categorize. The literature commonly identifies three types of pain:

Acute pain is pain occurring from a time-limited illness or a recent event such as acute injury, medical procedures, or surgery that:

- Has a rapid onset
- Varies in intensity
- Usually lasts less than 6 months (National Institute of Nursing Research, 1994)

Chronic nonmalignant pain is pain that:

- Is prolonged
- Varies in intensity
- Lasts longer than 6 months (McCaffery and Pasero, 1999)

Cancer pain is pain that:

- May be due to tumor progression and its related pathologic state and/or treatment modalities (McCaffery and Pasero, 1999)
- May have a rapid or prolonged onset
- Varies in intensity
- Can last less than or longer than 6 months

The nurse may use several approaches to manage pain. Because an individual's experiences are quite personal, pain management requires an individualized approach. The most common approach involves administration of **pharmacological agents: nonopioids** and **opioids** (Table 5-1). Timely administration before a client's pain becomes severe is crucial to ensure that the client gains optimal relief. In some circumstances, administration of pharmacological agents at regular intervals "around the clock" rather than on an "as-needed" (prn) basis is preferable. This pain approach is useful in managing pain before it becomes severe (e.g., during the early postoperative period) and can facilitate an earlier recovery (Acute Pain Management Guideline Panel, 1992; Jacox and others, 1994). Often a combination of nonopioids and opioids is effective in managing pain. Although caregivers may fear that frequent administration of pain medications will result in the client's psychological and physiological dependence on the medication, such dependence is actually rare (Ferrante, 1996). According to a study by Paice, Toy, and Shott (1998), clients also report being concerned about **addiction** and tolerance. Therefore it is important for the nurse to understand the differences between addiction, **physical dependence,** and **tolerance** (Box 5-1) in order to reassure the client (McCaffery and Ferrell, 1999).

Other approaches for pain relief use complementary **nonpharmacological** interventions for the client in pain. These interventions provide an opportunity for the client to assume an active role in achieving a higher level of comfort, and, in some instances, freedom from pain. When a single therapy cannot provide relief for the client, it is recommended that an integrated approach that considers both pharmacological and nonpharmacological therapies in managing pain be utilized.

Promoting comfort with nonpharmacological interventions, as with pharmacological agents, requires careful attention to assessment and planning. The experience of pain is influenced by a client's age; level of cognition; personality; culture and ethnicity; coping style; emotional, physical, and spiritual needs; state of health; and past pain experiences. The effectiveness of any therapy will be minimal if clients do not receive what they perceive as helpful. It is important for clients to actively participate in any attempts to alleviate discomfort, because they are the best authority on their pain (Jacox and others, 1994; McCaffery and Pasero, 1999).

The concept of clients as authoritative participants makes pain control an ethical and legal issue. Pain can dehumanize, destroy autonomy, and create a sense of hopelessness and powerlessness in the client, yet the treatment of pain is regularly and systematically inadequate (McCaffery and Ferrell, 1999). Although pain experience is primarily subjective and qualitative, it is often treated objectively and quantitatively by health care providers who inadequately assess, underprescribe, and often undermedicate clients (McCaffery and Ferrell, 1999). Pain that is caused or allowed as a result of nurses' or physicians' attitudes and outdated practices therefore becomes a matter of ethics—for example, a nurse who does not believe that clients have pain because they are watching TV or

Table 5-1 Two Analgesic Groups: Examples Within Each Group

NONOPIOIDS TWO GROUPS ARE:	OPIOIDS TWO GROUPS ARE:
a. *Acetaminophen* (Tylenol)	a. *Mu agonists* (full agonists, pure agonists, morphine-like)
b. *NSAIDs*	Examples:
Examples:	Codeine (as in Tylenol No. 3)
Aspirin	Fentanyl (Duragesic patch)
Carprofen (Rimadyl)	Hydrocodone (as in Lortab, Vicodin)
Choline magnesium trisalicylate (Trilisate)	Hydromorphone (Dilaudid)
Choline salicylate (Arthropan)	Levorphanol (Levo-Dromoran)
Diflunisal (Dolobid)	Meperidine (Demerol)
Etodolac (Lodine)	Methadone
Fenoprofen calcium (Nalfon)	Morphine
Ibuprofen (Motrin, Advil)	Oxycodone (OxyContin; as in Percocet)
Ketorolac (Toradol)	Propoxyphene (Darvon)
Ketoprofen (Orudis)	b. *Agonist-antagonists*
Meclofenamate sodium (Meclomen)	Examples:
Mefenamic acid (Ponstel)	Buprenorphine (Buprenex)
Nabumetone (Relafen)	Butorphanol (Stadol)
Naproxen (Naprosyn)	Dezocine (Dalgan)
Naproxen sodium (Anaprox, Aleve)	Nalbuphine (Nubain)
Piroxicam (Feldene)	Pentazocine (Talwin)
Salsalate (Disalcid)	

Modified from McCaffery M, Pasero C: *Pain: clinical manual,* St. Louis, 1999, Mosby.

Box 5-1 Definitions Related to the Use of Opioids in Pain Treatment

The Committee on Pain of the American Society of Addiction Medicine recognizes the following definitions as appropriate and clinically useful definitions and recommends their use when assessing the use of opioids in the context of pain treatment.

PHYSICAL DEPENDENCE

Physical dependence on an opioid is a physiologic state in which abrupt cessation of the opioid, or administration of an opioid antagonist, results in a withdrawal syndrome. Physical dependency on opioids is an expected occurrence in all individuals in the presence of continuous use of opioids for therapeutic or for nontherapeutic purposes. It does not, in and of itself, imply addiction.

TOLERANCE

Tolerance is a form of neuroadaptation to the effects of chronically administered opoids (or other medications), which is indicated by the need for increasing or more frequent doses of the medication to achieve the initial effects of the drug. Tolerance may occur both to the analgesic effects of opioids and to the unwanted side effects such as respiratory depression, sedation, or nausea. The occurrence of tolerance is variable, but it does not, in and of itself, imply addiction.

ADDICTION

Addiction in the context of pain treatment with opioids is characterized by a persistent pattern of dysfunctional opioid use that may involve any or all of the following:

- Adverse consequences associated with the use of opioids
- Loss of control over the use of opioids
- Preoccupation with obtaining opioids despite the presence of adequate analgesia

From McCaffery M, Pasero C: *Pain: clinical manual,* St. Louis, 1999, Mosby; modified from Hoffman NG, Halikas J, Mee-lee Y: *Patient placement criteria for the treatment of psychoactive substance use disorders,* Chevy Chase, Md, 1991, American Society of Addiction Medicine.

Table 5-2 Misconceptions: Barriers to the Assessment and Treatment of Pain

MISCONCEPTION	CORRECTION
1. The best judge of the existence and severity of a client's pain is the physician or nurse caring for the client.	The client's self-report is the most reliable indicator of the existence and intensity of pain.
2. Clinicians should use their personal opinions and beliefs about the truthfulness of the client to determine the client's true pain status.	Allowing each clinician to act on personal beliefs presents the potential for different pain assessments by different clinicians, leading to different interventions from each clinician. This results in inconsistent and often inadequate pain management. It is essential to establish the client's self-report of pain as the standard for pain assessment.
3. Visible signs, either physiologic or behavioral, accompany pain and can be used to verify its existence and severity.	Even with severe pain, periods of physiologic and behavioral adaptation occur, leading to periods of minimal or no signs of pain. Lack of pain expression does not necessarily mean lack of pain.
4. The pain rating scale preferred for use in daily clinical practice is the visual analog scale (VAS).	For clients who are verbal and can count from 0 to 10, the NRS pain rating scale is preferred. It is easy to explain, measure, and record, and it provides numbers for setting pain-management goals.
5. Cognitively impaired elderly clients are unable to use pain rating scales.	When an appropriate pain rating scale (e.g., 0-10) is used and the client is given sufficient time to process information and respond, many cognitively impaired elderly can use a pain rating scale.

Modified from McCaffery M, Pasero C: *Pain: clinical manual,* St. Louis, 1999, Mosby.

Box 5-2 JCAHO Pain Standards

The new JCAHO standards call upon health care organizations to:

- Recognize the right of patients to appropriate assessment and management of pain
- Assess pain in all patients
- Record the assessment in a way that facilitates regular reassessment and follow-up
- Educate providers/patients and families
- Establish policies that support appropriate prescription or ordering of pain medicines
- Include patient needs for symptom control in discharge planning
- Collect data to monitor effectiveness and appropriateness of pain management

From Joint Commission on Accreditation of Healthcare Organizations: *Comprehensive accreditation manual for hospitals: the official handbook,* Oak Brook Terrace, Ill, 2000, The Commission.

visiting with friends or a physician who orders only Demerol for a dying client with intractable pain. McCaffery and Pasero (1999) have identified common misconceptions about pain that health care professionals need to consider when planning client care (Table 5-2). Managing a client's pain can be challenging and rewarding if the health care team is knowledgeable about the nature of pain and how it might best be treated. Freedom from pain is not always a realistic goal. In these clients pain management may have to be directed toward pain control rather than complete pain relief.

In the early 1990s the Agency for Health Care Policy and Research (AHCPR) issued guidelines for effective pain management for clients with acute and cancer pain (Acute Pain Management Guideline Panel, 1992; Jacox and others, 1994). These guidelines are designed to help caregivers, clients, and clients' families understand the nature and treatment of pain. In 1999 the Joint Commission on Accreditation of Healthcare Organizations (JCAHO), which accredits 80% of the nation's hospitals encompassing 98% of hospital beds, set standards for the assessment and treatment of clients in pain. Organizations are being called on to confront and overcome institutional barriers that may prevent adequate pain management for clients (Box 5-2). The first and last skill in this chapter focus on nonpharmacological comfort measures. Administration of medications through patient-controlled analgesia and an intraspinal catheter are the focus of the last two skills. These skills may be used alone or in combination, depending on a client's needs. Many of the measures discussed can be taught to the client and family for use in the home.

Skill Performance Guidelines

1. Know the client's past and current medical history, type of therapy, and current medications.
2. Determine the client's perception of the pain experience. A thorough assessment of factors contributing to the client's pain will enable the nurse to select appropriate therapies. In addition, assess the effects of pain on self-care abilities, quality of life, and sleep.
3. Demonstrate respect for the client's evaluation of the quality and quantity of pain experienced and the response to methods of pain management. It is important to assess the client's acceptable level of comfort so that both client and nurse are striving for the same outcome.
4. Control environment factors that may influence the client's response to discomfort, such as too much stimuli or fatigue, as well as the effectiveness of comfort measures used.

5. Decide the frequency for assessing a client's comfort. It is the nurse's responsibility to assess the client's response to comfort measures and expression of discomfort. The collection of data leading to establishment of pain trends and a comparison of changes in pain patterns is useful in making therapeutic decisions.
6. Communicate to the physician significant changes in the client's comfort level and possible need for changes in pain-management regimen. There is no firm guide for the best time to report changes in comfort. However, the nurse who knows the client well and listens to a client's response to the pain-management interventions can identify along with the client when comfort measures are no longer effective or no longer necessary and when the type and quality of pain have changed.

Skill 5-1 Removing Painful Stimuli

After assessment of an individual's pain or discomfort, removal of the painful stimulus may be a quick and effective approach to help a client gain relief. Although this is a seemingly simple, even obvious, solution, removal of a painful stimulus is often overlooked in the search for a more complicated reason for the pain. Common sources of discomfort are damp, wet, or constrictive dressings, wrinkled bed linens, environmental irritants such as the noise of a television, and activity in excess of the individual's tolerance. Maintaining an uncomfortable position for a prolonged period is another common source of discomfort, particularly for dependent clients.

If a client is fatigued or anxious, even mild irritations can become significant sources of pain. The nurse should always remain observant during any contact with the client for potential sources of painful stimuli. Removal of painful stimuli, careful repositioning, and teaching splinting and breathing techniques during coughing or movement can afford clients considerable relief for extended periods of time. The client can often suggest the most comfortable position to assume. The nurse must judge whether any position is contraindicated on the basis of the client's health status.

Delegation Considerations

The nurse, in collaboration with the client, is responsible for the assessment, planning, initial implementation, and evaluation of needed comfort measures. When delegating skills to assistive personnel, consider the following: report changes in client's condition; identify and eliminate environmental conditions that might enhance pain; provide the client maximum rest periods; turning, positioning, and reducing environmental stimuli are important for comfort and pain control.

Equipment

- Pillows
- Dressings

Step	Rationale
Assessment	
1. Assess client's risk for pain or discomfort (e.g., postoperative clients, those with open wounds or burns, cancer clients, those undergoing invasive procedures or dental procedures, anxious clients, those suffering headache or flu, clients with chronic low back pain, clients in labor).	Allows nurse to anticipate client's needs and to intervene in a timely manner.
2. Assess for physical, behavioral, and emotional signs and symptoms of acute pain or discomfort.	Combination of signs and symptoms may help reveal source and nature of pain.
a. Verbalization that pain is present	
b. Moaning, crying, whimpering	
c. Facial expressions (e.g. grimace, clenched teeth)	
d. Changes in heart rate, increased or irregular respirations, changes in blood pressure, dilated pupils	Signs of sympathetic nervous system stimulation (which elicits fight-or-flight response) are often, but not universally, observed in clients experiencing acute pain (Acute Pain Management Guideline Panel, 1992).
e. Pallor	

Step	Rationale
f. Increased blood glucose level	The stress of unrelieved pain causes the endocrine system to release excessive amounts of hormones and decrease insulin levels. The metabolic responses can include hyperglycemia (McCaffery and Pasero, 1999).
g. Diaphoresis	
h. Change in mental status (e.g., confusion)	
i. Decreased gastrointestinal (GI) motility, nausea, and vomiting	Signs and symptoms typically occur with pain originating from involvement of visceral organs and result from stimulation of the parasympathetic nervous system.
j. Muscle tension, restlessness, exhaustion	Continued stimulation of sympathetic nervous system depletes energy stores.
k. Powerlessness, stoicism, anxiety, fear	Responses typical when acute pain continues unrelieved.
3. Assess for physical, behavioral, and emotional signs and symptoms of chronic pain: a. Verbalization that pain is present b. Fatigue, insomnia, anorexia, impaired mobility, distorted posturing, weight changes, depression, hopelessness, anger, fear, social withdrawal	Clients with chronic pain often do not show overt signs and symptoms of pain. Signs and symptoms reflect physiological adaptation and decreased sympathetic nervous system response. Psychological and emotional distress can be seen in clients with chronic pain.

- ***Critical Decision Point***
  Sustained physiological responses could cause serious harm if pain is unrelieved. Most people reach a level of adaptation in which physical signs return to normal. Be aware that if pain has been prolonged a client will not always exhibit physical signs and symptoms.

Step	Rationale
4. Assess characteristics of pain:	Guides clinician in collecting information about client's pain experience.
a. Onset and duration	Helps to determine length of time client has been in pain.
b. Location	Allows nurse to identify possible causative factors from client's description of pain.
c. **Pain intensity:** Using a visual analog scale (VAS) ask client to rate pain on a scale of 0 to 10 (0, no pain; 10, worst pain)	Pain is a subjective experience; therefore client's evaluation should be accepted. The pain rating scale is regarded as the most reliable indicator of pain intensity (see illustration) (McCaffery and Pasero, 1999).
d. Quality (e.g., use open-ended questions such as, "Tell me what your pain feels like" or "Describe how you fell.")	Assists in identifying the underlying pain mechanism (e.g., somatic or neuropathic pain) (McCaffery and Pasero, 1999).

- ***Critical Decision Point***
  Pain should be described in the client's words. Only if client cannot describe the pain, offer examples, such as sharp, dull, pricking, burning, stabbing, gnawing, aching, and pounding.

Step	Rationale
e. Pain pattern (environmental): Assess environment for factors that worsen pain experience (e.g., movement, eating, position).	Environmental stimuli, such as loud noises, bright lights, strong odors, or temperature extremes, can alter client's response to pain.

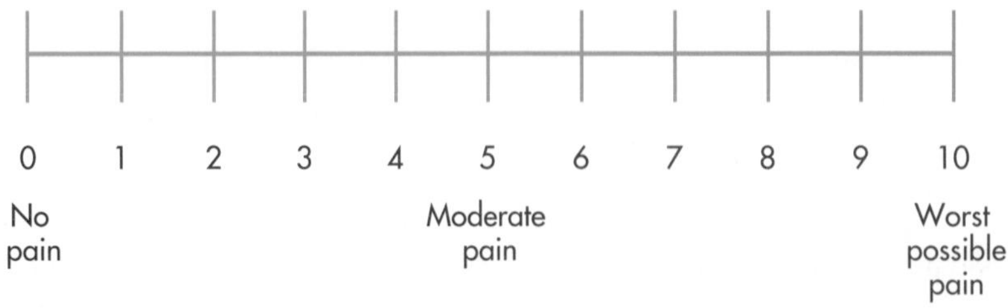

STEP **4c** Pain rating scale. (From McCaffery M, Pasero C: *Pain: clinical manual,* St. Louis, 1999, Mosby.)

STEP	RATIONALE
f. Pain pattern (physical): Assess factors that precipitate or aggravate pain or discomfort (e.g., movement, eating, position).	Certain types of pain may be precipitated or aggravated by select factors. Allows nurse to identify the nature and source of discomfort.
g. Relief measures: Ask client to identify previous methods that are effective in relieving pain (e.g., positioning, heat or cold, ritualistic behaviors, medications).	No single approach is right for every client. A combination of interventions is often the most effective approach to pain relief (Acute Pain Management Guideline Panel, 1992).
h. Concomitant symptoms: symptoms that often occur with pain (e.g., headache, constipation, restlessness).	Signs and symptoms of sympathetic nervous system stimulation caused by stress and unrelieved pain (McCaffery and Pasero, 1999).
i. Effects of pain on client's lifestyle (e.g., inability to work, engage in sex, socialize).	Unrelieved pain may affect client's quality of life and interfere with activities of daily living.
5. Examine site of client's pain or discomfort. Include inspection (discoloration, swelling, drainage), palpation (change in temperature, area of altered sensation, painful area, areas that trigger pain, areas that reduce pain), and range of motion of involved joints (if applicable).	Clinical observations clarify information from client. Site of discomfort may direct nurse to specific types of pain-relief measures.

• ***Critical Decision Point***

Examination may require temporary removal of dressing followed by reapplication (see Chapter 36).

6. Check physician's orders for position restrictions.	Client's physical condition may prohibit certain positions used to relieve pain.

NURSING DIAGNOSIS

Defining characteristics from the assessment data may reveal the following nursing diagnoses for clients requiring this skill:

- Activity intolerance
- Anxiety
- Fear
- Ineffective coping
- Deficient knowledge
- Pain (acute, chronic)
- Powerlessness

Related factors are individualized based on client's condition or needs.

PLANNING

1. **Expected outcomes** following completion of procedure:	
▪ Client verbalizes full or partial relief from pain.	Removing painful stimulus may result in near immediate relief.
▪ Nonverbal behaviors may reflect that comfort is attained.	Pain may be controlled but not absent, depending on its cause.
2. Prepare client's environment:	
a. Temperature suited to client	Temperature extremes can alter client's response to pain.
b. Lighting	Bright or very dim lighting can aggravate pain sensation.
c. Sound	Loud or irritating sounds can aggravate pain.
d. Activity	Prevent unnecessary interruptions, coordinate activities, and allow for rest periods. Fatigue reduces tolerance for pain.
e. Close room door or curtain.	Provides privacy and reduces stimuli that may increase pain.
3. Explain to client that **splinting** with pillows and positioning can reduce pain.	Promotes clients understanding and cooperation with procedure.
4. Explain steps to be taken to minimize pain stimuli.	Reduces fear and anxiety.

IMPLEMENTATION

1. Wash hands. Apply gloves if exposure to body fluids or blood is likely.	Reduces transmission of infection.

STEP	RATIONALE
2. Assess client's need for pharmacological interventions.	Assess need for more immediate pain relief before initiating interventions.
3. Remove painful stimulus:	
a. Assist client to a position that fully exposes area of discomfort.	Improves access to area and minimizes client's need to move.
b. Move bed linen aside to expose only area of discomfort and maintain client's privacy.	
c. Remove wet dressing, if applicable.	Minimizes irritation to wound and surrounding skin.
d. Smooth wrinkles in bed linens.	Reduces pressure and irritation to skin.
e. Loosen any constrictive bandage or device (e.g., blood pressure cuff, elastic wrap bandages, upper band of elastic hose, intravenous (IV) dressings, identification bands).	Bandage or device encircling extremity may restrict circulation.

- ***Critical Decision Point***
  In case of casts or pressure bandages, physician's order will be needed to loosen or adjust.

STEP	RATIONALE
f. Remove underlying tubes, wires, or equipment.	Objects apply pressure directly on dependent skin surfaces.
4. Apply splinting (e.g., pillow or folded blanket):	
a. Explain purpose of splinting to client.	Promotes client's cooperation.
b. Assist client to place hands firmly over area of discomfort (see illustration).	Splinting immobilizes painful area.
c. Assist client to splint during coughing, deep breathing, and turning.	Splinting decreases movement and subsequent pain during activity.
d. Assist client to attain comfortable position within normal body alignment.	Turning and repositioning reduce stimulation of pain and pressure receptors.
e. Use pillow to support body position.	
5. Remove and dispose of gloves. Wash hands.	Reduces transmission of infection.

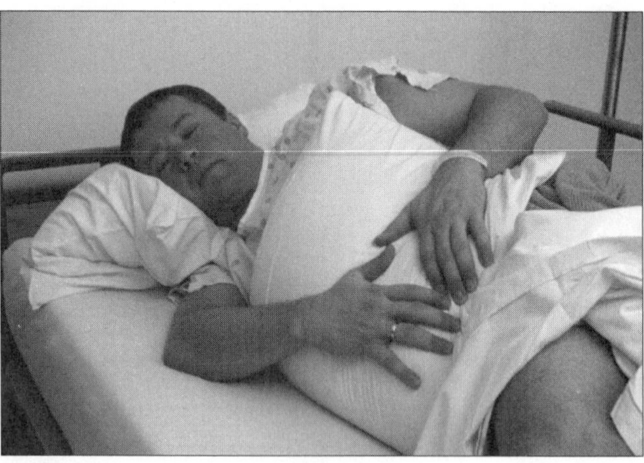

STEP 4b Client splinting area of discomfort.

EVALUATION

1. Evaluate client's comfort level, using original assessment criteria (e.g., severity, quality).	Determines client's response to interventions in a timely manner after each intervention.

UNEXPECTED OUTCOMES AND RELATED INTERVENTIONS

- Client verbalizes continued discomfort or describes worsening of pain.
  - Reassess and implement additional pain-relief measures.
- Client continues to display nonverbal behaviors reflecting pain.
  - Reassess and implement additional pain-relief measures.

Recording and Reporting

- Report change in pain assessment findings, presence of bright red blood saturating dressing, constriction of casted extremity, or change in vital signs to physician. If findings indicate worsening of client's condition, physician should be notified so that appropriate medical treatment can be initiated.
- Record findings of ongoing assessment, interventions completed (including notification of physician, if done), and client's response to interventions. Documents client's response and provides improved continuity of care for future pain experiences.

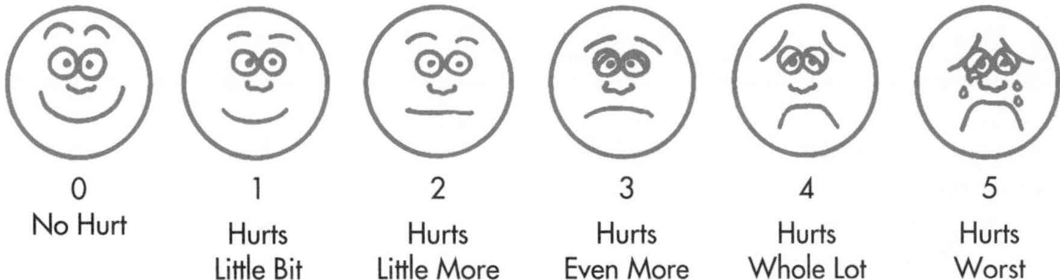

FIGURE **5-1** Wong-Baker FACES Pain Rating Scale. (From Wong DL and others: *Whaley and Wong's nursing care of infants and children,* ed 6, St. Louis, 1999, Mosby.)

Teaching Considerations

- Review client's technique when using coughing and deep-breathing exercises. Use demonstration if necessary.
- Explain to client and family about behavioral changes that can be caused by medication.

Pediatric Considerations

- Although validity and reliability scores of pain rating scales generally increase with age, some rating tools can be used with a child as young as 3 years of age (Wong and others, 1999).
- Children may be reluctant to report pain because they may have misconceptions about the cause of their pain or they may fear the consequences (e.g., another painful procedure or an injection).
- Infants and children experience pain but may respond to pain differently than adults do because of their different developmental levels. For example, they may cry and thrash about, have sleep disturbances, have a shortened attention span, suck or rock, refuse to eat or play, or be quiet and withdrawn. Still others become active when they are in pain; variations in activity levels are related to the child's personality, developmental level, and previous pain experiences (Wong and others, 1999).
- Parents can be a helpful source of information when assessing a child's pain and when planning pain-relief therapies. Most parents know how their child exhibits pain and which pain-relief interventions have been successful or unsuccessful.
- Children can rate their level of pain on the Wong-Baker FACES Pain Rating Scale (Figure 5-1) or the Oucher Pain Scale (Figure 5-2).

Gerontological Considerations

- Many older clients tend to have inadequately managed pain because of concerns regarding adverse effect of pharmacological treatments (Gagliese and Melzack, 1997).

OUCHER®

100 — 90 — 80 — 70 — 60 — 50 — 40 — 30 — 20 — 10 — 0 —

FIGURE **5-2** African-American version of the Oucher Pain Scale. (© Denyes, Villarruel, 1990. Used with permission.)

- Older adults may require more time for repositioning.
- Pain is not a natural occurrence of aging or chronic disease. Such a belief can lead to underreporting of pain (Hicks, 1999).

HOME CARE CONSIDERATIONS

- Home living conditions, such as type of bed, stairs, and environmental stimuli, should be considered. Supportive bed and quiet environment will enhance sleep and promote pain management.

Skill 5-2 Patient-Controlled Analgesia (PCA)

Causes of pain are numerous, particularly in the acute care setting. Parenteral administration of opioids is the method of choice when acute or severe pain exists, when high doses of oral drugs are ineffective, or when clients have obstructive or absorptive gastrointestinal (GI) alterations. One of the advances in pain-control modalities is **patient-controlled analgesia (PCA),** which allows clients to self-administer small continuous doses of intravenous (IV) or subcutaneous opioids (usually morphine) as they feel the need.

Patient-controlled analgesia is used extensively in postoperative, obstetrical, oncological, and trauma clients and in those experiencing sickle cell crises. The two variations of PCAs are the electronic computerized pump, which is attached to an IV pole (Figure 5-3) or to the client's pajamas by a waist belt, and the nonelectronic, non–battery operated pump, which may be attached to an IV pole or placed in a "sleeve" and attached to the client's gown or around the client's wrist. The latter is lightweight, less costly, and more portable. However, measurement of the total, cumulative dosage is more difficult with the nonelectronic pump.

A PCA consists of three parts: an infusion pump with a chamber that houses a prefilled syringe (infuser), a timing unit linked to a switch or button that is activated by the client to deliver a preset dose of medicine (patient-control module), and tubing that delivers the medication from the infuser through the patient-control module to an indwelling IV line. Computerized PCAs can be programmed to deliver specific physician-prescribed doses of medication in a number of ways: as predetermined interval doses, as a bolus dose, as a continuous infusion (basal rate), or as a combination of the three. Overdosing is prevented by interposing a preprogrammed delay time or "lockout" (usually 5 to 10 minutes) between client-initiated doses as ordered by the physician.

The PCA has several advantages. It allows more constant serum levels of the opioid and therefore avoids the peaks and troughs of large bolus. Because the blood level is maintained within a narrow range of the minimum effective analgesia concentration for the individual, pain relief is enhanced and the incidence of side effects, such as sedation and respiratory depression, is decreased (Nossel, 1996). A second advantage is that fewer postoperative complications may occur as a result of sedation, probably because of diminished sedation, which can lead to cardiovascular and respiratory complications associated with immobility. Earlier and easier ambulation may also help minimize postoperative complications. Increased client control and independence are other advantages of PCA. Because the device provides medication on demand as soon as the client feels the need, the total amount of opioid use can be reduced. PCA allows the client to manage pain with minimal nursing intervention and therefore also saves nursing time. Clients are not as dependent on the nursing staff for pain medications as they are with the more conventional oral or intramuscular (IM) and subcutaneous (SQ) injectable medications. A final advantage is that PCA offers a more ethical approach to pain control: clients have some control over the frequency and timing of the administration of their pain medication and are less dependent on the attitudes and values of health care providers.

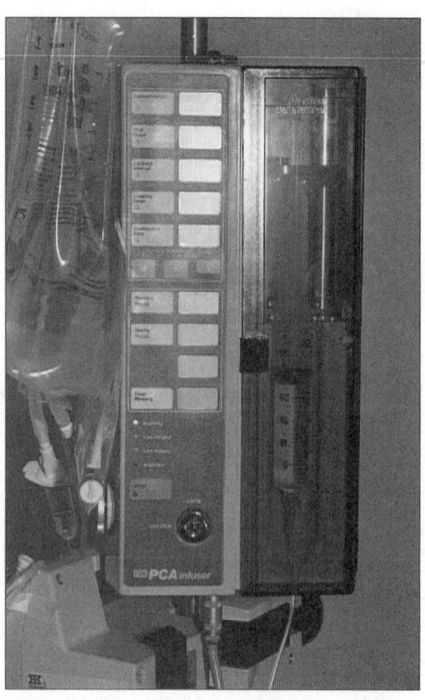

FIGURE 5-3 Patient-controlled analgesia (PCA) device.

Delegation Considerations

The administration of PCA should not be delegated to assistive personnel. However, assistive personnel should know the signs of unrelieved pain and report them when they occur. Assistive personnel should *never* administer a PCA dose for the client.

Equipment

- PCA system
- Identification label and time tape (may already be attached and completed by pharmacy)
- 18- or 20-gauge needle
- Alcohol swab
- Adhesive tape
- Disposable gloves

Step	Rationale
Assessment	
1. Assess client's current medical-surgical history.	Allows nurse to anticipate type of pain client may experience.
2. Assess for physical, behavioral, and emotional signs and symptoms of pain or discomfort (see Skill 5-1, Assessment steps 2 and 3).	Combination of signs and symptoms may reveal source and nature of pain.
3. Assess characteristics of pain (see Skill 5-1, Assessment step 4).	Guides clinician in collecting information about client's pain experience.
4. Assess environment for factors that contribute to pain.	
5. If client has had surgery, inspect incision.	Can reveal evidence of tissue trauma or damage, which stimulates peripheral pain receptors to transmit impulses to cortex to create conscious awareness of pain (McCaffery and Pasero, 1999).
6. Assess patency of existing IV infusion line (see Chapter 19).	IV line must be patent for medication to reach venous circulation.
7. Assess venipuncture site for infiltration or inflammation (see Chapter 19).	Confirmation of placement of IV needle or catheter and integrity of surrounding tissues ensures medication is administered safely.
8. Assess knowledge and effectiveness of previous pain-management strategies.	Response to pain-control strategies assists in identifying learning needs and affects client's willingness to try therapy.
9. Check physician's order for name of medication dose and frequency of medication.	Opioid medication administration is a dependent nursing function and requires physician's prescription. Commonly prescribed medications such as morphine sulfate, fentanyl citrate (Sublimaze), hydromorphone, and buprenorphine hydrochloride (Buprenex) can be used for PCA.
10. Check client's history of drug allergies.	Avoids placing client at risk for allergic reaction.

Nursing Diagnosis

Defining characteristics from the assessment data may reveal the following nursing diagnoses for clients requiring this skill:

- Activity intolerance
- Anxiety
- Fear
- Ineffective coping
- Deficient knowledge regarding patient-controlled analgesia.
- Pain (acute, chronic)
- Powerlessness
- Risk for infection

Related factors are individualized based on client's condition or needs.

Planning

Step	Rationale
1. **Expected outcomes** following completion of procedure:	
▪ Client verbalizes pain relief.	Drug is given safely and is effective in providing pain control.

STEP	RATIONALE
▪ Client exhibits relaxed facial expression and body position.	
▪ Client remains alert and oriented.	
▪ Client increasingly participates in self-care activities.	
▪ Client correctly operates PCA device.	Demonstrates learning.
2. Explain purpose and demonstrate function of PCA:	Effective explanations allow client participation in care and independence in pain control. Preoperative education about PCA therapy has been shown to improve postoperative pain relief (Knoerl, 1999).
a. Device is designed to deliver specific type and dose of pain medication that promotes comfort yet minimizes drowsiness.	

• ***Critical Decision Point***
Be sure client is alert, attentive, and able to manipulate PCA button.

STEP	RATIONALE
b. Device allows client to push medication demand button on timing unit instead of calling nurse.	Gives client control of pain. Client does not have to call and wait for nurse to prepare and deliver medication.
c. Provides lockout time between dose to prevent overdosage. Client can tell when timing unit is ready to deliver another dose.	System has built-in safeguards to help prevent accidental administration of doses or overdosing. No medication can flow between pushes unless a basal rate is programmed.
d. Infuser will be on IV pole or attached to bed clothing or wrist.	
e. Device administers balanced amount of medication to provide comfort and minimize drowsiness.	Balanced dosing with client-controlled administration produces constant serum drug levels rather than peaks and troughs associated with prn nurse-administered therapy (Nossel, 1996).

• ***Critical Decision Point***
Instruct client to check with nurse or physician with questions and concerns, or if medication is not controlling pain. A "rescue" dose may need to be given for breakthrough pain, or dosage may need to be adjusted.

STEP	RATIONALE
3. Check infuser and patient-control module for accurate labeling or evidence of leaking.	Avoids medication error. Damage to system can occur in shipping and handling; inspect to avoid injury or harm to client, self, or others.
4. Program computerized PCA pump to deliver prescribed medication dose and lockout interval.	Ensures safe, therapeutic drug administration.
5. Draw curtains around client's bed or close door to room.	Maintains client's privacy.
6. Position client comfortably for procedure. Maintain any postoperative position restrictions. Venipuncture or central line site needs to be accessible.	Comfortable position enhances effectiveness of analgesia.

IMPLEMENTATION

STEP	RATIONALE
1. Wash hands.	Reduces transmission of microorganisms.
2. Follow the "five rights" to be sure of correct medication (see Chapter 16). Check client's identification band and call client by name.	Minimizes risk of medication error and harm to client.
3. Apply gloves.	Reduces potential contact with blood when working with IV line.
4. Attach 18- or 19-gauge needle to exit tubing adapter of patient-control module or attach needleless system adapter.	Adapter used to connect with IV line.
5. Wipe injection port of IV line with alcohol if closed port is being used.	Alcohol is a topical antiseptic that minimizes entry of surface microorganisms during needle insertion.
6. If using needle, insert needle into injection port nearest IV site. Connect exit tubing adapter to port nearest IV site.	Establishes route for medication to enter main IV line.
7. Secure connection and immobilize PCA tubing.	Prevents dislodging of needle from port. Facilitates ambulation.
8. Administer loading dose of analgesia as prescribed.	A one-time dose may be given manually by nurse or programmed into PCA pump.

STEP	RATIONALE
9. Discard gloves and supplies in appropriate containers. Wash hands.	Reduces transmission of infection.
10. If client is experiencing pain, demonstrate use of PCA system; if not, have client repeat instructions given earlier (see illustrations).	Repeating instructions reinforces learning. Checking client's understanding through return demonstration helps nurse determine client's level of understanding and ability to manipulate device.
11. Dispose of empty cassette or syringe in compliance with institutional policy.	If PCA is discontinued before device is completely empty, record drug wastage on PCA medication record per institutional policy. Note date, time, amount of drug wasted, and reason for wastage. Wastage must be witnessed and record signed by two registered nurses. Control and dispensation of opioids are regulated by the Controlled Substances Act.

EVALUATION

1. Use pain rating scale to evaluate client's pain intensity.	Determines response to PCA. Documenting "PCA in use" or "PCA effective" is not an adequate record of the client's pain level.
2. Observe for signs of adverse reactions.	Intravenous medications produce rapid effects.
3. Periodically check infusion rate and condition of site (follow protocol of institution). Infusion rate may be checked by observing movement of volume indicator on infuser.	Intravenous site must remain patent for proper drug administration. Infiltration requires discontinuation of infusion.
4. Have client demonstrate dose delivery.	Evaluates skill in use of PCA.

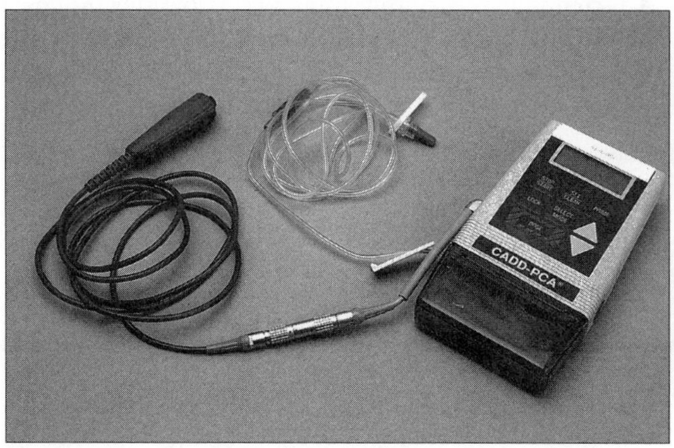

A

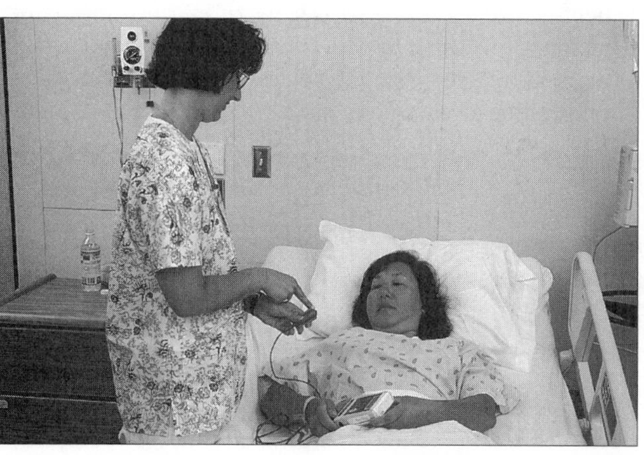

B

STEP **10** **A,** PCA system. **B,** Nurse demonstrates use of PCA system.

UNEXPECTED OUTCOMES AND RELATED INTERVENTIONS

- Client verbalizes discomfort is still present or pain intensity is worse. Underlying medical or postsurgical condition may have changed, or client may be undermedicated.
    - Consult with physician regarding ordered dose.
- Client displays nonverbal behaviors reflective of pain.
    - Evaluate effectiveness of current PCA settings.
- Client is sedated and not readily arousable.
    - Client may be oversedated and may need to have dose stopped or reduced (Box 5-3) or needs a reversal agent.

Box 5-3 Sedation Scale

S = Sleep, easy to arouse
1 = Awake and alert
2 = Slightly drowsy, easily aroused
3 = Frequently drowsy, arousable, drifts off to sleep during conversation
4 = Somnolent, minimal or no response to physical stimulation

From McCaffery M, Pasero C: *Pain: clinical manual,* St. Louis, 1999, Mosby.
Box 5-3 illustrates a scale that can be used to assess sedation levels in patients receiving opioid analgesia.

- Client is unable to manipulate PCA device to maintain pain control.
  - Alternative medication routes may be needed.

RECORDING AND REPORTING

- Record drug, dose, and time begun on appropriate medication record. Specify concentration and dilutent. Note lockout time.
- Record regular periodic assessments of client status on PCA medication record, in the narrative notes, pain assessment flow sheet or the documentation tool used in the institution. Forms may vary from institution to institution, but information recorded is similar. Indicate vital signs, if appropriate; sedation status; pain rating; status of vascular access site; amount of solution infused; amount of solution remaining; amount of drug received.

TEACHING CONSIDERATIONS

- Instructions are best given during pain-free or pain-reduced states and before initiating therapy. If preoperative client, instruct before surgery.
- Encourage client to push button on timing unit whenever pain is felt. Tell client not to delay interval if there is pain.
- Explain regimen to family so that they can support and assist client.
- Inform client of pain-management strategies that may supplement or enhance pharmacological intervention.
- The subcutaneous route can be used with a PCA (basal and/or demand) when the client is unable to take oral medications or intravenous access is very limited.
- Intermittent subcutaneous dosing through an indwelling subcutaneous catheter can be taught to family (Letizia, Shenk, and Jones, 1999) (see Chapter 18).

PEDIATRIC CONSIDERATIONS

- Patient-controlled analgesia can be an effective means of pain control in children who can understand the concept. When selecting pediatric candidates for PCA use, consideration must be given to developmental level, cognitive level, and motor skills. PCA use was found to be safe and effective for clients as young as 7 years (Acute Pain Management Guideline Panel, 1992). From a developmental perspective, use of PCA is particularly effective with adolescents, because it leads to feeling of control.
- Pharmacological pain support is safe and effective in pediatric clients when dose is calibrated according to child's weight. As with adults, doses may need adjusting after initiation of medication to obtain analgesia with minimal side effects (Acute Pain Management Guideline Panel, 1992).
- It is important that family members be reminded not to push the button for the pediatric client unless they have been designated as the primary pain manager.

GERONTOLOGICAL CONSIDERATIONS

- Older clients appear more sensitive to analgesic properties, especially opioids (American Geriatric Society, 1998).
- If confusion occurs while using a PCA, lowering the dose or switching to one family member responsible for pushing the button or nurse-activated around-the-clock dosing is recommended (McCaffery and Pasero, 1999).

Skill 5-3 Intraspinal Analgesia

The use of **epidural** and **intrathecal** opioids is becoming an accepted technique for management of acute postoperative, traumatic, labor, cancer, nonsurgical, and intractable chronic nonmalignant pain (Rawal, 1999). Small doses of medication can produce deep, prolonged analgesia with less systemic adverse effects. The term **intraspinal** is often used when referring to both the epidural and intrathecal routes of administration (McCaffery and Pasero, 1999). The epidural space and the intrathecal space are not the same. The epidural space surrounds the spinal cord and the intrathecal space. This potential space contains a network of veins and nerves that travel outward from the spinal cord. The intrathecal space surrounds the spinal cord. It contains cerebral spinal fluid that bathes the spinal cord.

The brain and spinal cord are covered by three meninges, or membranes. The dura mater is the outermost protective membrane. The epidural space lies between the dura mater and the vertebral column. When an opioid is injected into the epidural space, it binds to opiate receptors located on the dorsal horn of the spinal cord and blocks the transmission of pain impulses to the cerebral cortex of the brain. Because the opioid does not cross the blood-brain barrier, pain relief results from drug levels in the spinal cord rather than in the plasma, with little central or systemic distribution of the drug.

For placement of an epidural or intrathecal catheter, the client should be placed in the lateral decubitus or sitting position with shoulders and hips squared and hips and head flexed (Naber, Jones, and Halm, 1994). The anesthesiologist or client's attending physician places a catheter into the epidural space (Figure 5-4), generally in the lower lumbar region, to administer analgesics. However, thoracic epidurals are becom-

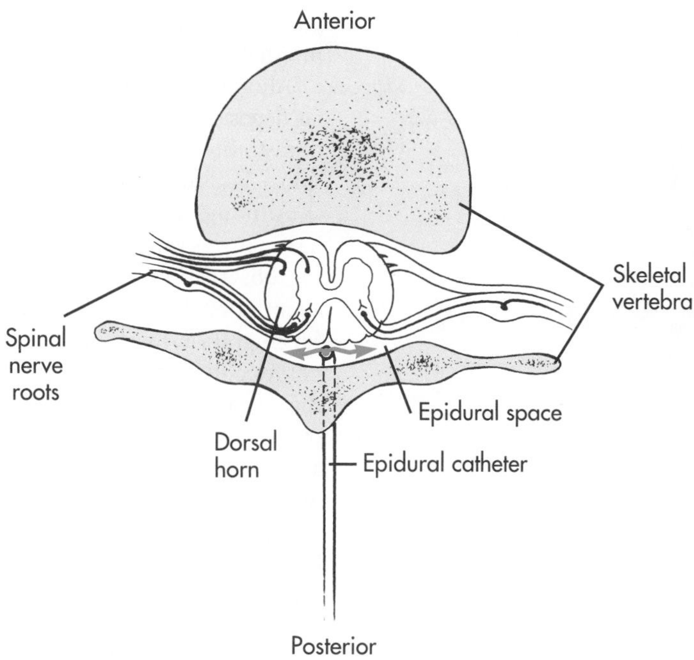

FIGURE 5-4 Anatomical drawing of epidural space.

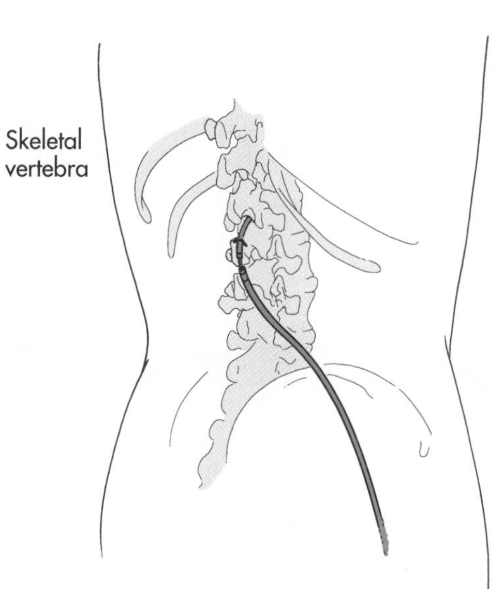

FIGURE 5-5 External epidural catheter.

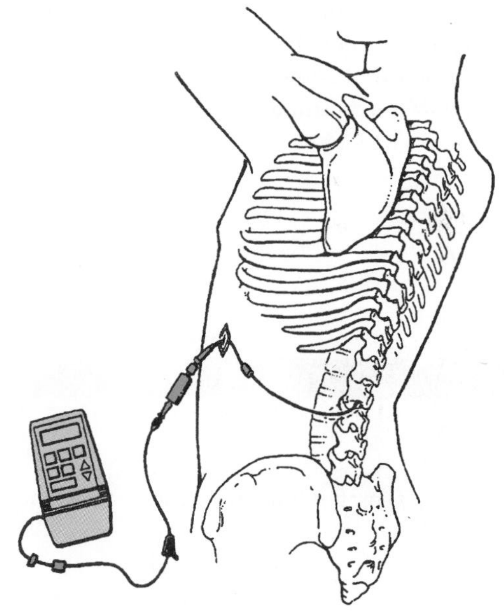

FIGURE 5-6 External catheter and ambulatory infusion pump. (Courtesy SIMS Deltec, Inc., St. Paul, Minn.)

ing increasingly common. When the catheter is intended for temporary or short-term use, it may not be sutured in place and exits from the insertion site on the back (Figure 5-5). By contrast, a catheter intended for permanent or long-term use is "tunneled" subcutaneously and exits on the side of the body or on the abdomen (Figure 5-6). Tunneling decreases the chance of infection or dislodging of the catheter. In both cases the catheter is covered with a sterile occlusive dressing (Figure 5-7) and secured to the client. Epidural/intrathecal medication can be administered either intermittently by bolus injection or

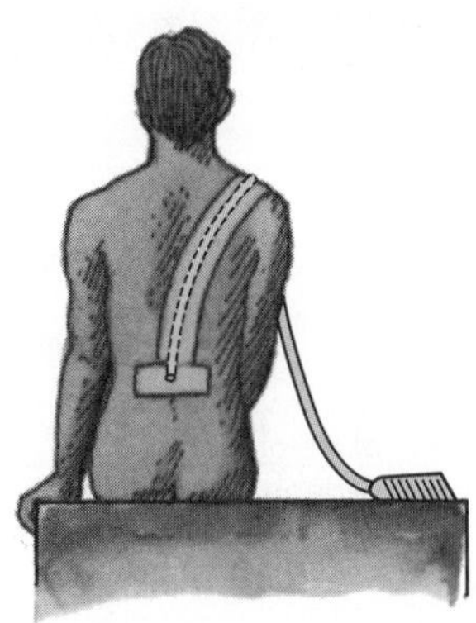

FIGURE **5-7** Epidural catheter taped in place. (Courtesy Astra Zeneca Pharmaceuticals, Wilmington, Del.)

continuously by a controlled delivery system such as an infusion pump (see Chapter 20). Registered nurses, as regulated by their State Boards of Nursing are allowed to administer bolus injections and infusion of analgesics into the epidural space. Bolus dosing of any medication into the intrathecal space is generally not allowed. It is important for the nurse to follow internal and external policy.

Although epidural administration is influenced by epidural fat deposition and systemic opioid absorption, intrathecal administration can produce almost immediately high cerebral spinal fluid concentrations of the drug that are dose dependent.

Although the use of intraspinal opioids for pain control has many advantages for the client, it requires astute nursing observation and care. The catheter poses a threat to client safety because of its anatomical location, its potential for migration through the dura, and its proximity to spinal nerves and vessels. An epidural catheter migration through the dura can produce medication levels too high for intrathecal use. Epidural and intrathecal doses are *not* equivalent. Intrathecal doses are more potent, and therefore doses are much smaller than epidural doses. As an example, the epidural dose of morphine is 10 to 20 times greater than that required for an intrathecal dose (Rawal, 1999). Assisting the client in obtaining pain control or relief, evaluating the analgesic effect, and intervening appropriately in the event of a complication or occurrence of side effects are the responsibilities of the nurse caring for these clients.

Delegation Considerations

Administration of intraspinal anesthesia should not be delegated to assistive personnel. **Administration of medication via the intraspinal route must be in compliance with individual State Board of Nursing standards.** Staff must be instructed in how to reposition clients to prevent disruption of the catheter.

Equipment

- Disposable gloves
- Prediluted preservative-free opioid as prescribed by physician and prepared for use in IV infusion pump (usually prepared by pharmacy)
- Infusion pump
- Infusion pump and compatible tubing without Y-ports. Some infusion pumps have tubing color coded for intraspinal use.
- Tape
- Label (for tubing)

Step	Rationale
Assessment	
1. Assess client's comfort level and presenting medical/surgical condition.	Certain conditions may make intraspinal analgesia the method of choice for pain control: postoperative states, clients with trauma or advanced cancer that is not responsive to other pain management modalities, and those predisposed to cardiopulmonary complications because of preexisting medical condition or surgery.

- ***Critical Decision Point***

  Contraindications to epidural analgesia include coagulopathies, abnormal clotting studies, history of multiple abscesses, sepsis (McCaffery and Pasero, 1999). Additional contraindications may include skeletal or spinal abnormalities.

Step	Rationale
2. Assess for physical, behavior, and emotional signs and symptoms of pain (see Skill 5-1, Assessment step 2).	Combination of signs and symptoms provides baseline to later determine efficacy of analgesia.
3. Assess characteristics and intensity of pain (see Skill 5-1, Assessment step 4).	Serves as a baseline to later determine efficacy of analgesia.
4. Assess environment for factors that may be contributing to pain.	Nurses can eliminate environmental stimuli that aggravate client's response to pain.

Step	Rationale
5. Assess sedation level of client by assessing for level of orientation, motor functioning, and drowsiness.	Establishes a baseline before first dose.
6. Check client's history of drug allergies.	Avoids placing client at risk for allergic reaction.
7. Assess rate, pattern, and depth of respirations.	Establishes baseline.
8. Assess blood pressure.	Vasodilatation can occur, and hypotension, including orthostatic hypotension, is common. Assist the client when changing positions.
9. Assess mobility and motor and sensory function (see Chapter 10) before assisting client into or out of bed. Check for:	Opioids can be given as a solo agent or in combination with other medications such as low-dose anesthetic agents (Rawal, 1999). Subanesthetic doses work synergistically with intraspinal opioids to provide better analgesia at lower doses. Bupivacaine (Marcaine) and ropivicaine (Naropin) are common anesthetics used for epidural analgesia.
a. Motor weakness or numbness and tingling of lower extremities (paresthesias)	The goal of adding low-dose anesthetic agents is for analgesia not anesthesia. Factors such as catheter placement, medication dose, and individual client response can result in unwanted motor and sensory deficits.
10. Check to see if catheter is secured to client's skin.	Aids in preventing dislodging or migration of catheter.
11. Assess catheter insertion site for:	
a. Redness, warmth, tenderness, swelling	Local inflammation and superficial skin infection at insertion site can occur.
b. Drainage	Purulent drainage is sign of infection. Clear drainage may indicate puncture of dura, causing medication to be delivered into subarachnoid space or causing cerebrospinal fluid leakage. Bloody drainage may indicate catheter entered blood vessel.
12. Check physician's order for medication, dosage, and infusion method.	Medication administration is dependent nursing function and requires physician's prescription.
13. If continuous infusion, check infusion pump for proper calibration and operation.	Ensures client will obtain prescribed analgesic dose. Be mindful of catheter placement, either epidural or intrathecal, because there is a substantial difference in dosage according to the route.
14. If continuous infusion, check patency of tubing.	Kinked tubing will interrupt analgesic infusion.
15. Keep a patent IV in place until 24 hours after epidural analgesia has ended.	Allows for IV access in case IV medications have to be given to counteract adverse reactions.

Nursing Diagnosis

Defining characteristics from the assessment data may reveal the following nursing diagnoses for clients requiring this skill:

- Pain (acute, chronic)
- Activity intolerance
- Anxiety
- Fear
- Deficient knowledge regarding intraspinal analgesia
- Powerlessness
- Risk for injury
- Risk for infection

Related factors are individualized based on client's condition or needs.

Planning

Step	Rationale
1. **Expected outcomes** following completion of procedure:	
▪ Client verbalizes pain relief.	Indicates drug and dose are effective in relieving pain, catheter is intact, and equipment is functioning properly in compliance with physician order.

Step	Rationale
▪ Catheter and injection cap or infusion pump tubing are securely taped and labeled.	Closed, intact system prevents entry of pathogens and disruption of flow of medication.
▪ Client remains normotensive, and heart rate stays in normal range.	Indicates absence of potential side effects of epidural opioids.
▪ Client is alert and oriented.	Indicates absence of excessive sedation.
▪ Respirations are regular, unlabored, and equal to or greater than 8 breaths per minute.	Indicates absence of respiratory depression.
▪ Client does not experience headache.	Indicates catheter in epidural space.
▪ Epidural dressing is dry and intact.	No cerebrospinal fluid leakage.
▪ Catheter and infusion tubing are free of knots and kinks.	Helps to ensure that system is patent.
▪ No redness, warmth, exudate, tenderness, or swelling is evident at catheter insertion site. Client is afebrile.	Indicates absence of inflammation or infection.
▪ Client voids without difficulty and in adequate amounts.	Indicates absence of urinary retention (a potential side effect).
▪ Client has no or minimal pruritus and no paresthesias of lower extremities.	Indicates absence of potential side effect of epidural medications.
2. Identify client by checking arm band and asking client's name.	Ensures correct client receives ordered drug.
3. Explain purpose and function of epidural analgesia and expectations of client during procedure. For example, ask client to call for assistance before getting out of bed.	Proper explanation enhances client cooperation and effective results.
4. Attach "epidural line" label to tubing.	Labeling helps to ensure medication analgesic is administered into correct line and into epidural space.
5. Use tubing *without* Y-ports for continuous infusions.	Use of tubing without Y-ports prevents accidental injection or infusion of other medication meant for vascular space into epidural space.
6. Draw curtains around client's bed or close door to room.	Maintains client's privacy.

Implementation

Step	Rationale
1. Wash hands and apply gloves.	Reduces transmission of microorganisms.
2. Administer continuous infusion:	
a. Attach container of diluted preservative-free medication to infusion pump tubing and prime (see Chapter 20).	Tubing should be filled with solution and free of air bubbles to avoid air embolus.
b. Attach proximal end of tubing to pump and distal end to epidural catheter. Tape all connections. Start infusion. (See Chapter 19 for use of infusion pump.)	Infusion pumps propel fluid through tubing. Taping maintains a secure, closed system to help prevent infection. A filter may be needed on tubing depending on institutional policy.
c. Check infusion pump for proper calibration and operation. Many institutions have two nurses check settings.	Maintains patency and ensures client is receiving proper dose and pain relief.
3. Remove and dispose of gloves. Wash hands.	Reduces transmission of microorganisms.

Evaluation

Step	Rationale
1. Evaluate comfort level and compare with original assessment data.	Determines if response to analgesia has been effective and if catheter is securely in place.
2. Observe for signs of adverse reactions to epidurally administered opioid.	Although pain is relieved with smaller doses and side effects are less severe with epidural opioid analgesia, side effects can still occur.
3. Observe respiratory rate, rhythm, and pattern; sedation level; and skin color.	Respiratory depression may result from epidural opioid use as long as 24 hours after initiation. Respiratory rate should be monitored at least every 1 to 2 hours depending on institutional policy.

Step	Rationale

- ***Critical Decision Point***
  Keep an ampule of naloxone (Narcan), 0.4 mg, a strong opioid antagonist, at the bedside to use in case of emergency to counteract adverse reactions. Give naloxone in incremental doses to improve respiratory function. Reversal of analgesic effect may result in acute withdrawal and pain (Jacox and others, 1994).

Step	Rationale
4. Monitor blood pressure and pulse.	Postural hypotension and heart rate changes may occur.
5. Monitor intake and output. Assess for bladder distention. Observe for frequency or urgency.	Urinary retention may occur as a result of effects of medication on spinal nerves innervating the bladder.
6. Observe for pruritus, especially of face, head, neck, and torso.	Itching is the most common side effect when opioids are delivered via the intraspinal route (McCaffery and Pasero, 1999).
7. Observe for nausea and vomiting.	Nausea and vomiting can begin 4 to 6 hours after a bolus because of time needed for drug to reach chemoreceptor trigger zone. Nausea from epidural analgesia is exacerbated by movement.
8. Check insertion site for clear or bloody drainage. Assess for complaints of headache.	Headache and cerebrospinal fluid leakage can occur from a dural puncture. Bloody drainage may occur if catheter has migrated into a vessel.
9. Monitor temperature. Observe insertion site for signs of inflammation.	Infection can occur from poor sterile technique or systemic bacteremia.
10. Evaluate for paresthesias.	Excessive analgesia, infusion of drugs toxic to central nervous system, or contact of catheter with neural tissue may cause sensory deficits (Acute Pain Management Guideline Panel, 1992).

Unexpected Outcomes and Related Interventions

- Client states pain is still present. Primary causes are insufficient drug dose or catheter blockage, breakage, or improper position. With continuous infusion, pump may be malfunctioning or tubing may not be patent.
  - Check all tubing, connections, medication doses and pump settings.
- Client is lethargic or not easily aroused.
  - Stop epidural infusion. Administer a reversal agent such as Narcan per physician order.
- Client experiences periods of apnea or respirations are less than 8 breaths per minute, shallow, or irregular.
  - Stop or reduce rate of epidural infusion. Notify physician.
- Client suddenly complains of headache. Clear drainage is present on epidural dressing or more than 1 ml of fluid can be aspirated from catheter.
  - Possible indication that catheter has migrated and punctured the dura.
  - Stop the medication, and notify physician.
- Blood is present on epidural dressing or can be aspirated from catheter. Probable indication that catheter has punctured a vessel.
  - Stop the infusion and notify physician.
- Redness, warmth, tenderness, swelling, or exudate is noted at catheter insertion site. Client is febrile.
  - Notify the physician.
- Client experiences minimal urinary output, urinary frequency or urgency, bladder distention, pruritus, and nausea and vomiting.
  - These are side effects of medication. Dosage needs to be altered or side effects managed by other treatments or medications.

Reporting and Recording

- Record drug, dose, and time begun and ended on appropriate medication record. Specify concentration and dilutent.
- Record any supplemental analgesic requirements.
- Review pump settings and usage with the next shift.
- Record regular periodic assessments of client's status in nurses' notes or on appropriate flow sheets or in narrative notes. Indicate vital signs, intake and output, sedation level, pain status, neurological status, status of epidural site, presence or absence of adverse reactions to medication, and presence or absence of complications results from placement and maintenance of epidural catheter.
- Report any adverse reactions or complications to physician.

Teaching Considerations

- Describe catheter placement and use to client as appropriate. Drawing or showing pictures helps.
- Teach client the purpose, action, and signs and symptoms of adverse reactions to opioid to be administered. Teach client to report pain level using pain scale and to report any side effects.

- Inform client of other pain-management strategies that may supplement or enhance pharmacological intervention (e.g., imagery, distraction, relaxation).
- Explain that pain relief begins within 30 to 60 minutes of initiation of epidural infusion.
- Explain therapy to family or significant others so that they can support and assist client.
- Some clients may feel so much better after obtaining pain relief that they attempt to ambulate without assistance or to overdo their activities. Caution them to begin slowly to avoid injury and call for nurse to assist.

PEDIATRIC CONSIDERATIONS

- The use of epidural analgesia has increased in children.
- EMLA cream can be applied to the site 2 hours before catheter insertion. Because the same analgesics are administered to children as are given to adults, children are at risk for the same side effects and adverse reactions (McCaffery and Pasero, 1999).

GERONTOLOGICAL CONSIDERATIONS

- Supplemental IV or IM dosages of opioids used for breakthrough pain or inadequate analgesia must be given and titrated carefully because of possibility of additive or synergistic interactions, especially in older adults (Jacox and others, 1994).

HOME CARE CONSIDERATIONS

- Clients needing long-term or permanent therapy are discharged with a tunneled catheter. Before consideration of catheter placement in preparation for discharge and care in the home, several variables need to be assessed, including fine motor skills, cognitive ability, stage of disease and prognosis, and degree of involvement of family or significant others.
- Teach client and caregiver proper dosage and administration of medication. Evaluating client's technique for catheter care and administering medication, as well as reinforcing instructions, are priorities.
- Explain pain assessment based on pain scale and available drug and dosage for breakthrough pain. Inform client how to contact clinician for increase in dosage if highest level prescribed is ineffective.
- Teach client and caregiver aseptic technique for opioid administration as needed and for all catheter care procedures, including dressing changes. Instruct client to change dressing every week (policy will vary with home care agency). Teach signs and symptoms of infection, and instruct client to report to nurse or physician immediately should signs and symptoms appear.
- Teach client and caregiver about signs and symptoms of adverse reactions to medication being used and interventions to alleviate side effects.
  - Urinary retention: Teach how to perform straight catheterization.
  - Pruritus: Advise client to wear clean, lightweight cotton clothing; keep room cool; use cool moist compresses; lubricate skin; apply cornstarch.
- Teach client and caregivers about medications to control side effects.
- Give phone numbers of clinicians to contact in emergency.
- Teach client about resources in the community.
- Arrange for home care services in the community.

Skill 5-4 Nonpharmacological Aids to Promote Comfort

There are a variety of nonpharmacological interventions that assist in lessening pain and can be used in acute care and in the home and restorative care settings. These pain relief measures can also be used in combination with pharmacological interventions, thus improving the level of pain relief. Nondrug techniques may diminish the physical effects of pain, alter the client's perception of pain, and provide the client with a greater sense of control. Distraction, relaxation, guided imagery, and cutaneous stimulation such as massage and accupressure are examples of effective nonpharmacological pain relief measures. The AHCPR guidelines for acute pain management (1992) cite nonpharmacological interventions to be appropriate for clients who find such interventions appealing, express anxiety or fear, may benefit from avoiding or reducing drug therapy, and have incomplete pain relief after use of pharmacological interventions.

Clients often must undergo a number of painful diagnostic and therapeutic procedures. The degree of discomfort depends on large part on a client's knowledge and perceptions of the experience. Because perception is greatly influenced by higher centers in the brain, the pain experience is a product of a person's past pain experiences, values, cultural expectations, and emotions. The nurse has an excellent opportunity to assist clients in learning to control their anxieties and fears. **Anticipatory guidance** is a cognitive strategy that involves use of descriptive sensory words and phrases the client is familiar with (Wilkie and Boss, 1996). The client gains an understanding of what to expect during a procedure. Clients should have the opportunity to ask questions about the procedure and their role during the procedure. The nurse makes the client as comfortable as possible to eliminate potential irritants. The client thus is able to direct full attention to the procedure, with the result of improved **pain tolerance.**

Cutaneous Stimulation

Massage

Modifying the perception of pain, as well as minimizing the reaction to pain, provides a client considerable pain relief. A gentle **massage,** a form of **cutaneous stimulation,** is the application of touch and movement to muscles, tendons, and ligaments without manipulation of the joints (Haldeman and Hooper, 1999). A proper massage not only blocks perception of pain impulses but also helps relax muscle tension and spasm that otherwise might increase. Massage of a body part is often an instinctual response to pain or discomfort and thus is a basic but highly effective means of control. A massage of the back, shoulders, and lower part of the neck is sometimes referred to as a back rub. A nurse should offer a back rub after a bath or before a client prepares for sleep to promote relaxation and comfort, to relieve muscle tension, and to stimulate circulation. An effective back rub takes 3 to 5 minutes and is an important intervention for decreasing pain and improving sense of well-being.

Heat/Cold

Heat and cold applications (see Chapter 38) relieve pain and promote healing. The selection of heat versus cold varies with client preference and the client's condition. Heat produces vasodilation, reduced blood viscosity, reduced muscle tension, and increased tissue metabolism. Cold produces vasoconstriction, reduced cell metabolism, and increased blood viscosity. Although the physiological responses to heat and cold may differ, superficial heat and superficial cold applications may provide comfort in similar conditions such as muscle spasms, strains, and localized joint pain. Caution should be exercised in using heat or cold applications with clients who are unconscious or have impaired sensation. Frequent skin assessment should be performed.

Relaxation

Relaxation is a cognitive strategy that provides mental and physical pain relief or reduces pain to an acceptable level. By teaching clients the use of progressive relaxation techniques, the nurse offers the client a sense of self-control when pain occurs. Progressive relaxation may be used independently or with other pain-relief measures. The nurse should be available to assist the client in performing relaxation techniques and in timing procedures (such as dressing changes) so that the technique can be most beneficial. The client's full participation and cooperation are necessary for progressive relaxation to be effective. The techniques are particularly effective for chronic pain, labor pain, and relief of procedure-related pain.

Guided Imagery

Guided imagery is a creative sensory experience that can effectively reduce pain perception and minimize reaction to pain. It draws on internal experience of memories, dreams, fantasies, and visions; explores the inner world of experience; protects the privacy of the client; and fosters the imagination. The goal of imagery is to have the client use one or several of the senses to create an image of the desired result. This image creates a positive psychophysiological response (Dossey, 1995). Thus focus of the imagination helps clients change their perceptions about their disease, treatment, and healing ability, which may help relieve pain, tension, or stress. Choosing images that clients find pleasant requires a careful assessment by the nurse. Otherwise, the nurse may mistakenly describe images of objects or things that the client fears or dislikes. For example, a scene of rolling waves at the seashore may be restful to one client but desolate or frightening to another. Imagery may be used with progressive relaxation or massage or as a distraction.

Distraction

Distraction is a technique that diverts an individual's attention away from the pain sensation. By introducing meaningful stimuli, the nurse helps the client refocus attention. The client's pain tolerance increases as distraction lowers awareness of pain (Wilkie and Boss, 1996). Typically distraction is most effective for mild to moderate pain, but with intense concentration even acute pain can be moderated. In most cases the pain relief lasts only as long as the distraction; when the distraction is removed, the client may have a heightened awareness of pain. Examples of distraction include music, visitors, television, breathing exercises, or active listening.

Delegation Considerations

The nurse is responsible for the assessment, planning, initial implementation, and evaluation of nonpharmacological comfort measures. When delegating to assistive personnel: explain the expected client response, have staff reinforce the use of individualized nonpharmacological interventions for prevention and relief of pain, and have staff report a worsening of client's pain.

Equipment

- Massage: lotion or oil, folded sheet, bath towel
- Relaxation: relaxation tape and tape player
- Distraction: based on type of distraction (e.g., tape player, assorted music tapes, puzzles, video games, other games).

Step	Rationale

Assessment

Step	Rationale
1. Have client identify intensity of pain or discomfort.	Pain is a subjective experience. Numerical pain rating scale allows client freedom to identify pain perception and is therefore considered the most reliable indicator of pain intensity (McCaffery and Pasero, 1999).
2. Assess physiological, behavioral, and emotional responses to pain or discomfort (see Skill 5-1, Step 2).	Physiological responses of individuals vary with severity and duration of pain. Responses serve as means to evaluate effectiveness of pain-relief measures. Overt signs and symptoms may not be present with chronic pain. Physical signs and symptoms may indicate change in comfort level.
3. Assess characteristics of pain and underlying probable cause (see Skill 5-1, Step 4).	Determines if nonpharmacological approaches are appropriate. Massage is contraindicated in cases of muscle, bone, or joint injury.

- ***Critical Decision Point***
  It may be helpful the first time to administer an analgesic so that client can gain a level of comfort needed to practice noninvasive approaches.

Step	Rationale
4. Examine site of client's pain or discomfort. Include inspection (discoloration, swelling, drainage), palpation (change in temperature, area of altered sensation, painful area, areas that trigger pain, areas that reduce pain), and range of motion of involved joints (if applicable).	Clinical observations clarify information from client. Site of discomfort may direct nurse to specific types of pain-relief measures.
5. Assess client's willingness to receive nonpharmacological pain-relief measures.	Clients have the right to decide about their own care. Participation increases effectiveness. If client is reluctant to try activity, accept this uncertainty and provide information about suggested therapy so that client can make decision.
6. Assess activities client participates in at home that may serve as distraction (e.g., jigsaw puzzles, crocheting or knitting, board games, music, imagery, and relaxation tapes).	Doing these activities in health care setting increases likelihood that client will participate.
7. Assess client's language level and identify descriptive terms that will be used when employing relaxation, guided imagery, anticipatory guidance.	Provides clarification of information.

Nursing Diagnosis

Defining characteristics from the assessment data may reveal the following nursing diagnoses for clients requiring these skills:

- Activity intolerance
- Anxiety
- Fear
- Ineffective coping
- Deficient knowledge regarding nonpharmacological methods of pain control
- Pain (acute, chronic)
- Powerlessness

Related factors are individualized based on client's condition or needs.

Planning

Step	Rationale
1. **Expected outcomes** following completion of procedure:	
▪ Client is relaxed and comfortable after technique or diagnostic procedure as evidenced by slow, deep respirations; calm facial expressions; calm tone of voice; relaxed muscles; relaxed posture.	Effective guidance before and during procedure assists client to relax and experience less discomfort. Physiological response to relaxation procedures and massage is deep relaxation. Distraction promotes comfort by diverting attention from one situation to another.

STEP	RATIONALE
▪ Client verbalizes pain relief.	Although objective physiological indicators to determine pain intensity or relief exist, they are not as reliable as client's subjective expression (Acute Pain Management Guideline Panel, 1992).
▪ Client demonstrates and describes pain-relief measures.	Demonstrates client learning.
2. Explain purpose of technique and what will be expected of client during activity. If diagnostic or therapeutic procedure is to be performed, plan to explain procedure in advance.	Proper explanation of activity results in enhanced client participation. Client will have time to understand nurse's explanations, avoiding anxiety associated with confusion or misunderstanding.
3. Plan to perform technique before or after client's rest period.	Use 2-hour intervals for rest between pain-relief activities whenever possible to maximize effects.
4. Assist client to use bathroom before performing technique, if needed.	Techniques may take 20 to 30 minutes. Client comfort enhances relaxation and decreases distraction.
5. Prepare environment by:	
a. Controlling lighting in room	Darkened room can be relaxing.
b. Controlling distractions by visitors or staff	Distractions prevent client from attending to pain-reduction or pain-control techniques.
c. Maintaining comfortable room temperature (sheet or light blanket prevents chilling)	Temperature extremes can alter client's response to pain.
d. Closing curtains around client's bed or closing door	Maintains client's privacy, helps control lighting, and reduces anxiety.
6. Assist client to comfortable position for technique chosen, such as semi-Fowler's or Sims' position.	Client comfort enhances relaxation and participation in skills.

IMPLEMENTATION

Anticipatory Guidance

STEP	RATIONALE
1. Use descriptive terms to explain steps of procedure in detail to client. Respect client's listening limitations.	Knowing what to expect helps client cope with painful or uncomfortable procedures.
2. Explain to client approximate length of time procedure will take (e.g., 10 to 20 minutes). Warn client that delays may occur (e.g., in preparing treatment room, transporting client, waiting for physician).	Knowing how long procedure will take helps eliminate anxiety.
3. Prepare by describing sensations client can anticipate during steps of procedure (e.g., pressure, cold, needle prick).	Nurse cannot assure client there will be no pain. Ability to anticipate sensation minimizes actual discomfort.
4. Verbally guide client through procedure using terms identified previously (e.g., "Physician is going to clean your skin with a cool liquid." "Now you will feel a needle stick." "It will feel like someone is pinching your skin.").	Repetition of explanation of steps during procedure helps orient client to progress.
5. Assist client in returning to comfortable position.	Some procedures require uncomfortable or immobile position; when possible, reposition client for comfort.

Massage

STEP	RATIONALE
1. Wash hands.	Reduces transmission of microorganisms.
2. Adjust bed to high, comfortable position and lower upper side rail if raised.	Ensures proper body mechanics and prevents strain on nurse's back muscles.
3. Place client in comfortable position such as prone or side-lying position.	Enhances relaxation and exposes area to be massaged.

- ***Critical Decision Point***
  Clients with respiratory difficulties may lie on side with head of bed elevated.

STEP	RATIONALE
4. Drape client to expose only area to be massaged.	Maintains client's privacy and warmth.
5. Warm lotion in hands or in basin of warm water.	Warm lotion is soothing, and warmth helps to produce local muscle relaxation.

STEP	RATIONALE
6. Choose stroke technique based on desired effect:	
a. **Effleurage** (see illustrations)	Gliding stroke, used without manipulating deep muscles, smoothes and extends muscles, increases nutrient absorption, improves lymphatic and venous circulation (Meintz, 1995).
b. **Pétrissage** (see illustration)	Use on tense muscle groups to "knead" muscles, promote relaxation, and stimulate local circulation.
c. **Friction**	Strong circular strokes bring blood to surface of skin, thereby increasing local circulation and loosening tight muscle groups.

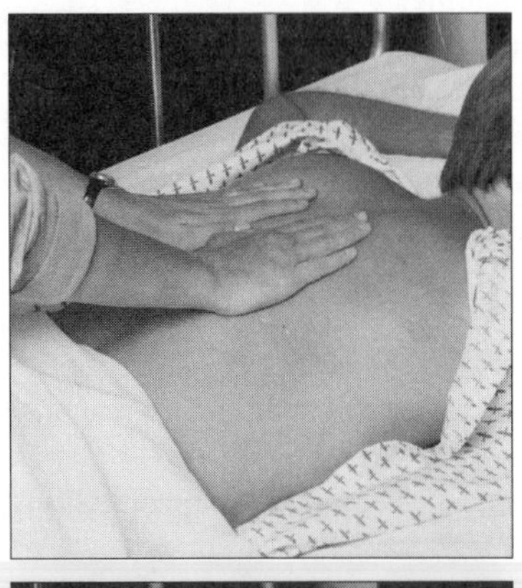

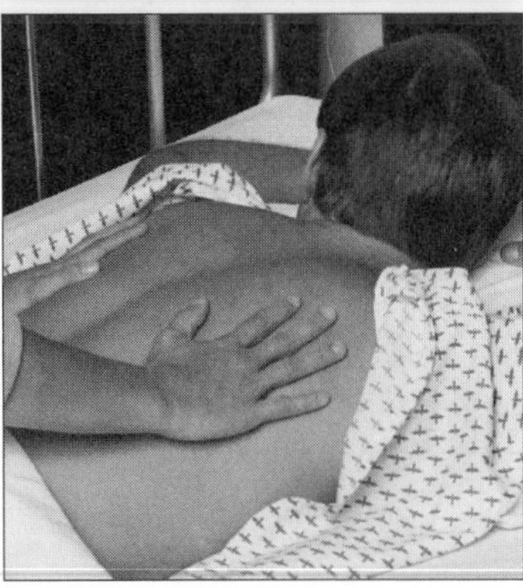

STEP **6a** Effleurage.

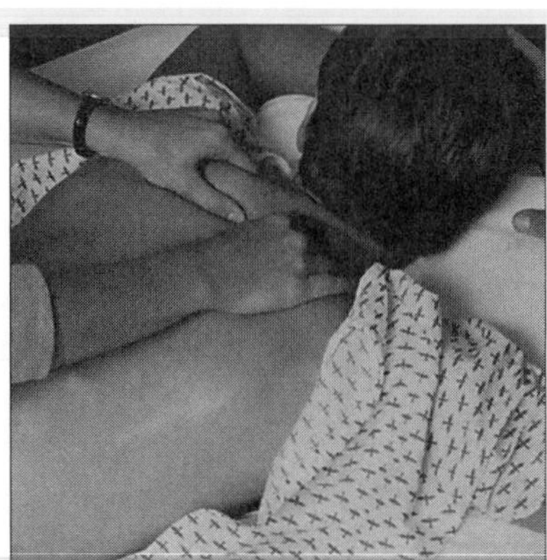

STEP **6b** Pétrissage.

STEP	RATIONALE
7. Encourage client to breathe deeply and relax during massage.	Potentiates effects of massage.
8. Standing behind client, stimulate scalp and temples.	
9. Supporting client's head, rub muscles at base of head.	Strong circular strokes (friction) stimulate local circulation and relaxation.
10. Massage hands and arms, as appropriate:	Releases tension in hands and arms. Studies indicate that anxious behaviors may be significantly reduced with hand massage.
a. Support hand and apply friction to palm using both thumbs.	
b. Support base of finger and work each finger in corkscrewlike motion.	
c. Complete hand massage using effleurage strokes from fingertips to wrist.	
d. Knead muscles of forearm and upper arm between thumb and forefinger, as appropriate.	Encourages relaxation; enhances circulation and venous return.

STEP	RATIONALE
11. Massage neck, as appropriate:	
a. Place client in prone position unless contraindicated.	Provides access to neck muscles.
b. Knead each neck muscle between thumb and forefinger.	Reduces tension that often localizes in neck muscles.
c. Gently stretch neck by placing one hand on top of shoulders and other at base of head and gently move hands away from each other.	Helps relax muscle body.
12. Massage back, as appropriate:	
a. Keep client in prone postition unless contraindicated; side lying postion is an option.	
b. Do not allow hands to leave client's skin.	Continuous contact with skin's surface is soothing and stimulates circulation to tissues. Breaking contact with skin can startle client.
c. Apply hands first to sacral area; massage in circular motion (see illustration). Stroke upward from buttocks to shoulders. Massage over scapulas with smooth, firm stroke. Continue in one smooth stroke to upper arms and laterally along sides of back down to iliac crests. Continue massage pattern for 3 minutes.	Gentle firm pressure applied to all muscle groups promotes relaxation.

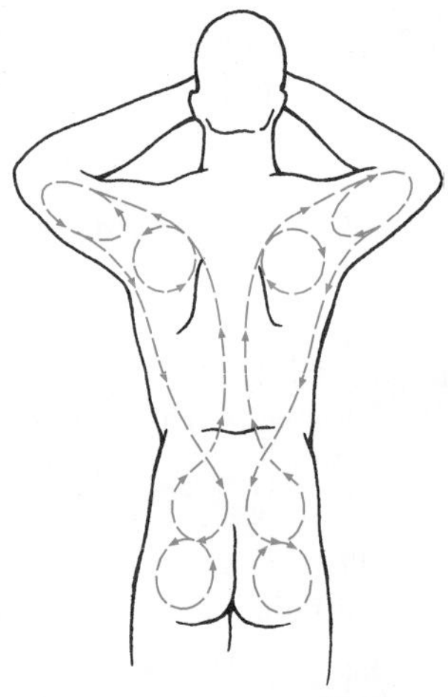

STEP **12c** Circular massage.

- ***Critical Decision Point***

  Be certain to massage muscular region, not bruised, swollen, or inflamed areas or bones of the spine (Meintz, 1995).

STEP	RATIONALE
d. Use long, gliding strokes along muscles of spine in upward and outward motion.	Massage follows distribution of major muscle groups.
e. Knead muscles of each shoulder toward front of client.	Area often tightens because of tension.
f. Use palms in upward and outward circular motion from lower buttocks to neck.	
g. Knead muscles of upper back and shoulder between thumb and forefinger.	These muscles are thick and can be vigorously massaged.
h. Use both hands to knead muscles up one side of back, then other.	
i. End massage with long stroking movements.	Most soothing of massage movements.
13. Massage feet, as appropriate:	
a. Place client in supine position.	Returns client to comfortable anatomic position.
b. Hold foot firmly. Support ankle with one hand or support sides of foot with each hand while performing massage.	Maintains joint stability during massage.
c. Make circular motions with thumb and fingers around bones of ankle and top of foot.	Relaxes muscles.

Step	Rationale
d. Trace space between tendons with firm finger pressure, moving from toe to ankle.	
e. Massage sides and top of each toe.	
f. Use top of fist to make circular motions on bottom of foot.	
g. Knead sides of foot between index finger and thumb.	
h. Conclude with firm, sweeping motions over top and bottom of foot.	Light strokes may tickle.
14. Tell client you are ending massage.	Informs and prepares client for inhalation and exhalation (next step).
15. When procedure is complete, instruct client to inhale deeply, exhale, and then initially move about slowly after resting a few minutes.	Returns client to more awake and alert state. When deeply relaxed, client may experience dizziness on arising too rapidly.
16. Wipe excess lotion or oil from client's back with bath towel.	Excess lotion or oil can irritate skin and lead to breakdown.
17. Return bed to low position and raise side rails as appropriate when massage is finished. Wash hands.	Reduces spread of microorganisms.

Relaxation

Step	Rationale
1. Instruct client to take several slow, deep breaths.	Increased oxygen can lessen anxiety and prevent shortness of breath with relaxation. Breaths should be diaphragmatic and deep to avoid hyperventilation.
2. Have client close eyes, if desired.	Client may be less easily distracted.
3. Instruct client to follow verbal cues for relaxation; use calm, soft voice.	Relaxation is guided verbally or by tape until individual is comfortable with sequence and no longer needs verbal guidance.
a. Begin series of alternating tightening and relaxing muscle groups if not contraindicated: (1) clench right fist, relax; (2) clench left fist, relax; (3) clench both fists, relax; (4) tighten right biceps, relax; (5) tighten left biceps, relax.	Alternating tension and relaxation in muscle groups allows client to feel difference.

- ***Critical Decision Point***

  Tension of each muscle group is maintained for 5 to 7 seconds except for the feet. Allows time to focus on the muscle group; cramps can easily occur in the feet.

Step	Rationale
b. As each muscle group is completed, ask client to enjoy relaxed feeling and allow mind to drift and think how nice it is to be relaxed; ask client to breathe deeply.	Distracts client from perceiving pain. Enhances the relaxation response. Breathing deeply prevents Valsalva response, which can increase intrathoracic pressure and compromise cardiac function.
c. Instruct client to repeat each step two times: (1) reach with right arm, relax; (2) reach with left arm, relax; (3) reach with both arms, relax; (4) wrinkle forehead, relax; (5) squint eyes, relax; (6) tighten jaw muscles, relax; (7) press head into pillow, relax; (8) bring right shoulder to earlobe, relax; (9) bring left shoulder to earlobe, relax; (10) bring both shoulders to earlobe, relax; (11) tighten abdominal muscles, relax; (12) tighten hips and buttocks, relax; (13) press right leg into mattress, relax; (14) press left leg into mattress, relax; (15) point right toes and stretch, relax; (16) point left toes and stretch, relax; (17) stretch right leg, relax; (18) stretch left leg, relax; (19) stretch both legs, relax; (20) flex right foot, relax; (21) flex left foot, relax; (22) flex both feet, relax; (23) tense right leg, relax; (24) tense left leg, relax; (25) tense both legs, relax; (26) tense entire body, relax.	Relaxation is integrated response associated with diminished sympathetic nervous system arousal; decreased muscle tension is desired outcome. Relaxation decreases pulse and respiration rates and blood pressure and reduces anxiety.

Step	Rationale
• ***Critical Decision Point*** *If muscle group tightens after relaxation has proceeded to other muscles, return to that group and repeat tension-relaxation until relaxation is achieved.*	
d. Calmly explain during exercise that client may feel sensations of tingling, heaviness, floating, or warmth as relaxation occurs.	Prevents anxiety should sensation occur without warning.
e. Ask client to continue slow, deep breaths.	Allows opportunity to enjoy feelings of relaxation.
4. When exercise is complete, instruct client to inhale deeply, exhale, and then initially move about slowly after resting a few minutes.	Returns client to more awake and alert state. When deeply relaxed, client may experience dizziness on arising too rapidly.
Guided Imagery	
1. Direct client through guided imagery exercise:	
a. Instruct client to imagine that inhaled air is ball of healing energy.	Development of specific images assists in removal of pain perception.
b. Imagine inhaled air travels to area of pain.	Client's ability to concentrate decreases pain perception.
2. Alternatively nurse may direct imagery:	
a. Suggest client think about going to pleasant place such as beach or mountains.	Directs imagery after selection of restful place by nurse and client.
b. Direct client to experience all sensory aspects of restful place (e.g., for beach: warm breeze, warm sand between toes, warmth of sunshine, rhythmic sound of waves, smell of salt air, gulls gliding and swooping in air).	Helps client concentrate and relax.
c. Continue deep, slow, rhythmic breathing.	Promotes relaxation.
d. Count to three, inhale, and open eyes. Move about slowly initially.	
3. Provide client time to practice exercise without interruption.	Guided imagery requires an intense level of concentration that may take time to achieve.
Distraction	
1. Direct client's attention away from pain with distraction techniques.	Redirection of attention alters emotional or cognitive aspects of pain.
2. Ask client to close eyes or to focus on single object in room.	Directs attention inward and protects client from external distraction.
3. Instruct client to concentrate on slow, rhythmic breathing. Guide breathing or instruct client to control and concentrate on breathing by thinking: "in, one, two; out, one, two."	Promotes full relaxation.
4. Continue distraction using chosen activity.	Focusing on an activity diverts attention from painful sensation.
a. Use music of client's choosing. Emphasize listening to rhythm and adjust volume as pain increases or decreases.	
b. Direct client to give detailed account of an event or story.	Stress details of event to enhance distraction from pain stimulus.
c. Engage client in conversation; encourage participation of family members and visitors.	Visitors can help direct attention away from mild to moderate pain.

Evaluation

Step	Rationale
1. Evaluate client's physiological and behavioral response to technique. Observe character of respirations, body position, facial expression, tone of voice, mood, mannerisms, verbalization of discomfort.	Determines effectiveness of procedure, level of relaxation, degree of pain relief achieved, and which procedures were most effective.
2. Use pain rating scale to evaluate comfort level.	Objectively measures change in pain intensity.
3. Observe client perform pain-control measures.	Confirms learning.

Unexpected Outcomes and Related Interventions

- Client is uncomfortable during diagnostic or therapeutic procedure, requiring procedure to be delayed or stopped.
  - Focus on helping client to relax and to answer any questions or concerns.
- Client may be unable to concentrate on technique because of intense pain.
  - Attempt relaxation or distraction techniques.
- Client indicates continued discomfort: tense posture or muscles, increased pulse, increased or shallow respirations, splinting or holding painful body part, facial grimacing, restlessness or irritability, verbalized discomfort.
  - Evaluate effectiveness of nonpharmacological interventions.
  - May need a combination of nonpharmacological and pharmacological interventions.
- Client is unable to describe or use pain-relief measures.
  - Assess for behavioral signs of pain (e.g., moaning, grimacing, or crying) and provide pain-relief measures for the client.
- Discomfort increases.
  - Need to determine causal factors.

Recording and Reporting

- Record in nurses' notes client's assessment findings, procedure and technique, preparation given to client, client's response to procedure or technique, and further comfort needs related to event. Incorporate pain-relief technique into nursing care plan.
- Record alterations in client's condition (e.g., changes in blood pressure, pulse, respiration, condition of client's skin, complaints of dizziness).
- Report client's response to nonpharmacological interventions to the staff at change to shift.
- Report any unusual responses to techniques (e.g., uncontrolled or aggravated pain) to nurse in charge or physician. Unexpected findings or occurrences during procedure should be reported because additional assistance or time with client may be needed.

Teaching Considerations

- Clients need information about different pain therapies because participation is essential to successful outcome.
- Techniques may require more practice before results are achieved. Pharmacological intervention may be required to lessen pain so that client can achieve relaxation and to augment other methods of pain control.
- Teach client to rest between periods of activity because fatigue increases pain perception.
- Discuss and practice with client possible techniques to use at home.
- If appropriate, teach family member how to perform massage (if not contraindicated) as part of home care (Meintz, 1995).

Pediatric Considerations

- A number of nonpharmacological pain-management therapies can be used successfully with children. Distraction and relaxation strategies work for all ages. The technique or device used will need to be suitable to the developmental level of the child (e.g., a pacifier can be used for the infant, reading or playing a recording of a favorite story is appropriate for the preschooler, listening to music on a portable cassette or CD player with headphones may work for a teenager).
- Because children have an active imagination, relaxation can be a powerful adjuvant in pain control.
- Play therapy and art can also be effective.
- Parents can be very helpful in providing pain relief. They often provide comfort, for example, by their presence, by their conversation, and by holding and cuddling their child (Acute Pain Management Guideline Panel, 1992; Jacox and others, 1994; Wong and others, 1999).

Gerontological Considerations

- Pain may be difficult to assess in older adults. Cognitive impairment or dementia may affect their ability to report pain severity on a visual analog scale or numerical scale. Behavioral observations (e.g., agitation, restlessness, groaning) for pain may be confused with signs of dementia (Acute Pain Management Guideline Panel, 1992).
- Visual, hearing, cognitive, and motor impairments may make it difficult for older adults to be able to effectively use procedures such as distraction, relaxation, or guided imagery (Acute Pain Management Guideline Panel, 1992).

Home Care Considerations

- Family members may need to collaborate planning time to reduce noise and other stimuli in the home to promote client's relaxation.

Critical Thinking Exercises

1. There are multiple physical, behavioral, and emotional signs and symptoms of pain. What is the single most reliable factor that indicates a client has pain?
2. Nonpharmacological interventions are useful in reducing the physical effects of pain. What other benefits are there from these interventions?
3. Identify potential complications you might see in the individual receiving epidural analgesia.
4. What teaching considerations would be appropriate for an individual receiving analgesia via PCA?

References

Acute Pain Management Guideline Panel: *Acute pain management: operative or medical procedures and trauma.* Clinical practice guideline, AHCPR Pub No 92-0032, Rockville, Md, 1992, Agency for Health Care Policy and Research, Public Health Service, U.S. Department of Health and Human Services.

American Geriatrics Society Guidelines, *Journal of the American Geriatrics Society* 46:635-651, 1998.

Dossey B: Using imagery to help your patient heal *AJN* 95(6)40-46, 1995.

Ferrante MF: Principles of opioid pharmacotherapy: practical implications of basic mechanisms, *J Pain Symptom Manage* 11(5):265, 1996.

Gagliese L, Melzack R: Chronic pain in elderly people, *Pain* 70:3, 1997.

Haldeman S, Hooper PD: *Mobilization, manipulation, massage and exercise for the relief of musculoskeletal pain.* In Wall PD, Melzack: *Textbook of pain,* ed 4, London, 1999, Churchill Livingstone.

Hicks TJ: Pain among the elderly: an action plan, *Nurs Case Manage* 4(3):145, 1999.

Jacox A and others: *Management of cancer pain.* Clinical practice guideline No 9, Rockville, Md, 1994, Agency for Health Care Policy and Research, Public Health Service, U.S. Department of Health and Human Services.

Joint Commission on Accreditation of Healthcare Organizations: *Comprehensive accreditation manual for hospitals: the official handbook.* Oak Brook Terrace, Ill, 2000, The Commission.

Knoerl D and others: Preoperative PCA teaching program to manage postoperative pain, *Medsurg Nurs* 8(1):25, 1999.

Letizia M, Shenk J, Jones TD: Intermittent subcutaneous injections of pain medication: effectiveness, manageability, and satisfaction, *Am J Hosp Palliat Care* 16(4):585, 1999.

McCaffery M, Ferrell BR: Opioids and pain management, what do nurses know? *Nursing* 29(3):48, 1999.

McCaffery M, Pasero C: *Pain: clinical manual,* ed 2, St. Louis, 1999, Mosby.

Meintz S: Whatever became of the back rub? *RN* 58(4):49, 1995.

Naber L, Jones G, Halm M: Epidural analgesia for effective pain control, *Critical Care Nurse* 14(5):69, 77, 1994.

National Institute of Nursing Research: *Symptom management: acute pain,* Bethesda, Md, 1994, Public Health Service, National Institutes of Health, U.S. Department of Health and Human Services.

Nossel M: Chronic nonmalignant pain management. In Salerno E, Willens J: *Pain management handbook: an interdisciplinary approach,* St. Louis, 1996, Mosby.

Paice JA, Toy C, Shott S: Barriers to cancer pain relief: fear of tolerance and addiction, *J Pain Symptom Manage* 16(1):1, 1998.

Rawal N: Epidural and spinal agents for postoperative analgesia, *Surg Clin North Am* 79(2):313, 1999.

Wilkie D, Boss B: Pain: nursing assessment and role in management. In Lewis S, Collier I, Heitkemper M: *Medical-surgical nursing: assessment and management of clinical problems,* ed 4, St. Louis, 1996, Mosby.

Wong DL and others: *Whaley and Wong's nursing care of infants and children,* ed 6, St. Louis, 1999, Mosby.

6

Personal Hygiene and Bed Making

Skills

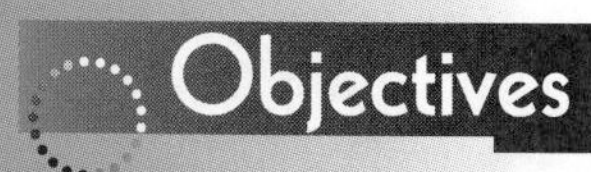

Objectives

Mastery of content in this chapter will enable the nurse to:

- Define the key terms listed.
- Discuss guidelines used to provide hygiene care to clients.
- Identify principles of aseptic technique applied while administering a bed bath.
- Administer a complete bed bath.
- Explain precautions to take while assisting clients with a tub bath or shower.
- Record pertinent observations made while bathing clients.
- Administer perineal care to male and female clients.
- Identify guidelines to follow when administering mouth care.
- Explain differences in providing oral care to dependent versus unconscious clients.
- Administer oral hygiene correctly to a client.
- Discuss precautions used to prevent breakage of dentures.
- Identify guidelines for administering hair, nail, and foot care.
- Comb and brush a client's hair.
- Shampoo the hair of a bedridden client.
- Shave a male or female client.
- Identify risk factors for foot and nail problems.
- Safely administer nail care.

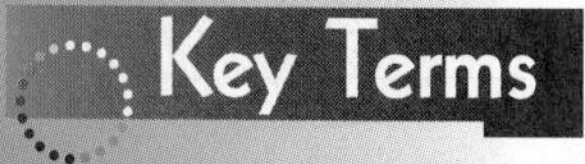

Key Terms

Alopecia
Aspiration
Buccal
Cerumen
Cheilosis
Cuticle
Dental caries
Dentifrice
Dermatitis
Flossing
Gag reflex
Gingivae
Gingivitis
Halitosis
Hygiene
Maceration
Mastication
Necrotic
Neuropathy
NPO
Periodontal
Periodontitis
Plaque
Podiatrist
Pruritus
Sebaceous gland
Sebum
Stomatitis
Tartar
Tepid
Vellus

Many clients require assistance with personal hygiene or must learn hygiene techniques. **Hygiene** is the science of health. Maintenance of personal hygiene is necessary for an individual's health, comfort, safety, and sense of well-being.

Hygiene practices are congruent with health promotion. The nurse's role is to maintain or assist the client to maintain the integrity of skin surfaces so that skin cells receive the nutrition and hydration needed to resist injury and disease. To provide skin care, the nurse should understand the structure and function of the skin.

Bathing and Skin Care

An active organ, the skin's functions include protection, secretion, excretion, temperature regulation, and sensation. Three primary layers make up the skin: the epidermis, dermis, and subcutaneous tissue. The skin covers the entire surface of the body and is continuous with mucous membranes of the mouth, eyes, ears, nose, vagina, and rectum. Thorough hygiene is essential for the integrity and function of each skin layer.

The epidermis, or outer skin layer, contains several thin layers of cells undergoing different stages of maturation. The innermost layer continually produces new cells that migrate to the outer layer, the stratum corneum, where dead cells are shed from the epidermal surface.

Bacteria reside on the skin's outer surface. These resident bacteria are normal flora that do not cause disease but inhibit multiplication of disease-causing microorganisms. Transient bacteria that arise from objects coming in contact with the skin are also present. Bathing removes dead cells and bacteria and helps maintain skin integrity.

The dermis contains bundles of collagen and elastic fibers to support the epidermis. Nerve fibers, blood vessels, sweat glands, **sebaceous gland,** and hair follicles are found in the dermis. Sebaceous glands secrete **sebum,** an oily, odorous fluid, into the hair follicles. Sebum lubricates skin and hair. Two types of sweat glands, the eccrine and the apocrine glands, are distributed over the skin's surface. Eccrine glands secrete a watery fluid (sweat) that assists in temperature control through evaporation. The apocrine glands secrete sweat in the axillary and genital areas. Bacterial decomposition of sweat from the apocrine glands causes body odor.

The subcutaneous tissue layer contains blood vessels, nerves, lymph tissue, and loose connective tissue filled with fat cells. Fatty tissue insulates the body. Subcutaneous tissue also provides support for upper skin layers.

Because a portion of the skin is usually exposed to environmental irritants and because the skin is an active organ sensitive to physiological changes within the body, some skin problems commonly occur (Table 6-1). The nurse should look for the presence of such conditions while providing hygiene and should suggest measures to alleviate these conditions. The client is always the best resource to explain the nature and course of skin problems as they develop. Skin problems can cause changes that affect a client's appearance and body image. The nurse should be sensitive to the client's feelings while attempting to care for a skin problem.

Table 6-1 Common Skin Problems

PROBLEM	CHARACTERISTICS	IMPLICATIONS	INTERVENTIONS
Dry skin	Flaky, rough texture on exposed areas such as hands, arms, legs, or face.	Skin may become infected if epidermal layer is allowed to crack.	Bathe less frequently. Use superfatted soap (e.g., Dove) for cleansing (Hardy, 1990). Rinse body of all soap well, because residue left can cause irritation and breakdown. Add moisture to air through use of humidifier. Increase fluid intake when skin is dry. Use moisturizing lotion to aid healing process; lotion forms protective barrier and helps maintain fluid within skin. Use creams to clean skin that is dry or irritated by soaps and detergents.
Acne	Inflammatory, papulopustular skin eruption, usually involving bacterial breakdown of sebum; appears on face, neck, shoulders, and back.	Infected material within pustule can spread if area is squeezed or picked. Permanent scarring can result.	Wash hair and skin each day with hot water and soap to remove oil. Use cosmetics sparingly because oily cosmetics or creams accumulate in pores and tend to make condition worse. Dietary restrictions may need to be implemented. Foods found to aggravate condition should be eliminated from diet. Exposure to ultraviolet rays, either from sunshine or heat lamp, may help control acne; use caution to prevent burning of skin. Use prescribed topical antibiotics for severe acne.
Hirsutism	Excessive growth of body and facial hair, especially in women.	Hirsutism may cause negative body image by giving female a male appearance.	The following may be used to remove unwanted hair: depilatories (can cause infection, rashes, or dermatitis), shaving (safest method), electrolysis (permanently removes hair by destroying hair follicles), tweezing (lasts temporarily), and bleaching (lasts temporarily).
Skin rashes	Skin eruption that may result from overexposure to sun or moisture or from allergic reaction; may be flat or raised, localized or systemic, pruritic or nonpruritic.	If skin is continually scratched, inflammation and infection may occur. Rashes can also cause discomfort.	Wash area thoroughly and apply antiseptic spray or lotion to prevent further itching and aid healing process. Warm soaks may relieve inflammation.
Contact dermatitis	Inflammation of skin characterized by abrupt onset with erythema, pruritus, pain, and appearance of scaly oozing lesions; seen on face, neck, hands, forearms, and genitalia.	Dermatitis is often difficult to eliminate because person is usually in continual contact with substance causing skin reaction. Substance may be hard to identify.	Condition usually disappears when exposure to causative agents (e.g., cleansers, soaps) is avoided.
Abrasion	Scraping or rubbing away of epidermis; may result in localized bleeding and later weeping of serous fluid.	Infection occurs easily as result of loss of protective skin layer.	Nurses should always be careful not to scratch clients with their jewelry or fingernails. Wash abrasions with mild soap and water. Dressing or bandage could increase risk of infection because of retained moisture.

Mouth Care

The oral cavity, which is lined with a normally moist, intact mucous membrane, contains the teeth and gums. The membranous lining, composed of both epithelial and connective tissue, protects underlying organs, secretes mucus to keep the oral cavity lubricated, and absorbs water, salts, and other solutes. Saliva, a clear viscous fluid secreted by the mucous and salivary glands of the mouth, moistens the oral cavity, initiates digestion of starches, provides a means for removing cellular and bacterial debris, and aids in the chewing and swallowing of food. The buffer capacity of saliva protects the gums and teeth. Normally the mucosa is light pink and moist.

The teeth are organs of chewing, or **mastication.** Dentin, a hard, ivory-like substance that surrounds the pulp cavity, forms the major part of a tooth (Figure 6-1). A layer of enamel, visible in the oral cavity, covers the upper portion of the tooth, or crown. The **periodontal** membrane, just below the gum margins, surrounds the tooth root and holds it firmly in place. A tooth receives its blood, lymph, and nerve supply from the base of the tooth socket within the jaw. Healthy teeth are smooth, shiny, and properly aligned.

The gums, or **gingivae,** are mucous membranes with underlying supportive fibrous tissue. They encircle the necks of

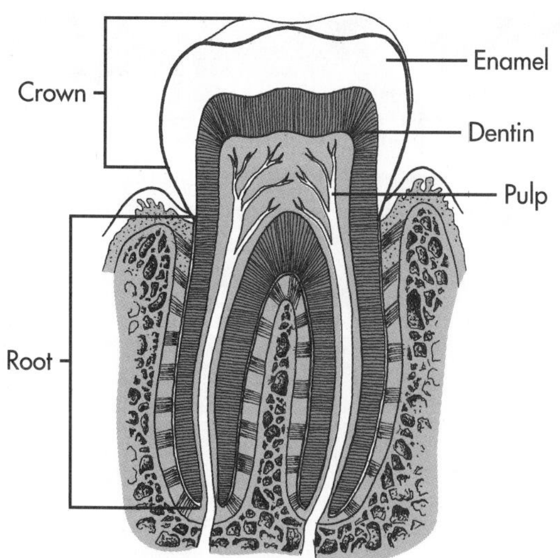

FIGURE 6-1 Normal tooth.

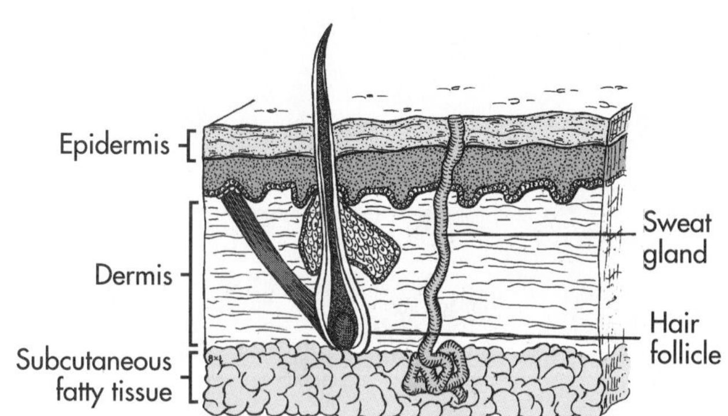

FIGURE 6-2 Cross section of hair follicle and supporting structures.

erupted teeth to hold them firmly in place. The gums are normally pink, moist, firm, and relatively inelastic.

Structures of the oral cavity must receive regular hygiene to remain healthy for a person's comfort, sense of well-being, maintenance of nutrition, and protection from infection (Beighton and others, 1999). Even a minor alteration of the oral cavity, such as inflammation of the gums, can create a significant health problem. Appetite is diminished, and the discomfort from inflammation can become an annoying irritant. Thorough oral hygiene maintains the integrity of oral cavity structures.

The nurse needs to assist clients in maintaining good oral hygiene by teaching correct techniques or by actually performing hygiene for weakened or disabled clients. Educating clients about common gum and tooth disorders and methods of prevention may motivate them to follow good oral hygiene practices (Fellona and DeVore, 1999). It may be necessary for the nurse to refer clients to a dentist for problems requiring special care.

Hair Care

Hair grows from follicles located within the dermis of the skin (Figure 6-2). Tiny blood vessels supply each follicle with nourishment necessary for normal hair growth. Each hair has a shaft extending from the follicle. Sebaceous glands secrete sebum, an oily substance, into each follicle, which lubricates the hair and scalp. The hair shaft is normally shiny and pliant and is not excessively oily, dry, or brittle.

The primary function of hair is protection. For example, hair protects the scalp from injury and the sun's rays. Eyebrows and eyelashes protect the eyes from foreign particles.

Two types of hair cover the body. Terminal hair is the long, coarse, thick hair that is easily visible on the scalp, axillae, and pubic area. Special hair care practices focus primarily on care of terminal hair. **Vellus** is the soft, fine hair that covers the entire body except for the palms of the hands, fingertips, soles of the feet, tips of the toes, and part of the genitalia. Hair growth, distribution, and pattern can be indicators of a person's health status. Hormonal changes, emotional and physical stress, aging, gender, race, nutrition, infection, and certain diseases can affect hair characteristics. The hair shaft is an inert structure; any change in its color or condition occurs as a result of hormonal activity and nutrient supply to the hair follicle. For example, a reduction in the serum protein level will result in hair becoming dry and brittle.

A person's appearance and sense of well-being often depend on the way the hair looks and feels. Illness or disability may prevent clients from maintaining daily hair care. An immobilized client's hair soon becomes tangled if not brushed or combed regularly. Dressings may leave sticky adhesive, blood, or antiseptic solutions on the hair. Diaphoresis leaves hair oily and unmanageable. Proper hair care is important to a person's body image. Brushing, combing, shampooing, and shaving are basic hygiene measures.

When caring for clients from different cultures, it is important to learn as much as possible about the client's cultural customs and beliefs. Ask the client about preferred hair care methods or any cultural restrictions. For example, African-Americans' hair is quite dry. Special conditioners may be needed to maintain conditioning.

Skill Performance Guidelines

1. Consider clients' cultural preferences in regard to grooming techniques. For example, women of some cultures shave the hair on their legs, whereas others prefer to keep their legs unshaven.

2. Consider clients' normal grooming routines. Individualize plan of care to reflect client's normal schedule of activities of daily living (ADLs).
3. Bathe body parts as soon as they become soiled. Problems such as incontinence, wound drainage, or excessive diaphoresis may require bathing several times a day.
4. Attempt to provide baths during the time of day that the client prefers.
5. Protect clients from injury by assessing and controlling the bath water temperature.
6. Wear gloves whenever there is risk of contacting body fluids.
7. Control environmental factors that may alter skin integrity, such as moisture, heat, and external sources of pressure (wrinkled bed linen, improperly placed drainage tubing).
8. Encourage clients and involve family or significant other to participate in bathing and skin care.
9. Establish a regular oral hygiene routine that the client can easily follow at home. Ideal dental hygiene requires brushing after every meal and before bed and flossing at least once a day, the ideal being after each meal.
10. Respect clients' preferences for grooming products. However, the nurse may have opportunities to caution against use of products that can damage skin or teeth or injure hair and nails.
11. Remember that dental hygiene can be a means for improving the client's comfort level. Persons who are mouth breathers, are using oxygen, are unable to eat or drink, have nasogastric tubes inserted, or have had trauma or surgery of the mouth will benefit from frequent oral care.
12. Use the time spent providing mouth care to teach clients about factors that increase the incidence of dental or gum disease and the techniques that ensure good oral hygiene.

Skill 6-1 Bathing a Client

Nurses provide two categories of baths: cleansing and therapeutic. Cleansing baths are usually given in the morning before scheduled tests or procedures. However, some clients may prefer bathing in the evening or during the night shift. In addition to cleansing the skin, the bath stimulates circulation and reduces body odor by removing secretions, perspiration, and bacteria from the skin. Self-image is therefore restored. While bathing the client, the nurse can get to know the client better and interact therapeutically. Further assessments can be made, and joint range-of-motion (ROM) exercises can be performed.

The type of cleansing bath a nurse provides depends on the client's physical capabilities and the degree of hygiene required. The nurse is responsible for assessing what type of bath is most appropriate for the client's needs.

Bathing of skin surfaces affords a client considerable comfort. However, depending on the condition of the hair and nails, the client may not feel completely clean. When a person is unable to perform personal care during illness or disability, it becomes the nurse's responsibility to assist with cleaning and grooming hair, shaving, and soaking and trimming nails. Many of the procedures can be done during or immediately after a bath. Clients may appreciate having their hair combed or feet soaked any time during the day to maintain an attractive appearance or to promote comfort. The client should be encouraged to make decisions regarding need and frequency of hygienic care.

Types of cleansing baths include:

1. Complete bed bath—Administered to clients who are totally dependent. The nurse gives the bath with the client in bed.
2. Partial bed bath—Consists of bathing only body parts that would cause discomfort if left unbathed, such as hands, face, axillae, and perineal area. Dependent clients in need of partial hygiene or self-sufficient bedridden clients who are unable to reach all body parts receive a partial bed bath.
3. Tub bath—Client is immersed in a tub of water. The tub bath allows more thorough washing and rinsing than a bed bath. Client may still require the nurse's assistance. Some institutions have tubs equipped with lifting devices that facilitate positioning dependent clients in the tub.
4. Shower—Client sits or stands under a continuous stream of water. The shower provides more thorough cleansing than a bed bath.

Therapeutic baths are generally ordered by physicians for a specific effect, such as soothing the skin or promoting healing. Types of therapeutic baths include:

1. Sitz bath—Cleanses and reduces pain and inflammation of perineal and anal areas. Used for client who has undergone rectal or perineal surgery or childbirth or has local irritation from hemorrhoids or fissures. The client sits in a special tub or basin.
2. Medicated bath (oatmeal, cornstarch, sodium bicarbonate, Aveeno, Burow's solution)—Aids in relief of skin irritation and creates an antibacterial and drying effect. Oatmeal has added effect of softening and lubricating the skin.

Delegation Considerations

Skills of bathing can be delegated to assistive personnel. It is important to provide caregivers information about the importance of not massaging reddened skin areas, early signs of impaired skin integrity, and when to report changes in the skin to the nurse.

Equipment

- Two washcloths
- Two bath towels
- Bath blanket
- Soap and soap dish
- Toiletry items (deodorant, powder, lotion, cologne)
- Warm water
- Clean hospital gown or client's own pajamas or gown
- Laundry bag
- Disposable gloves (when risk for contacting body fluids)
- Washbasin

Step	Rationale
Assessment	
1. Assess client's tolerance for activity, discomfort level, cognitive ability, musculoskeletal function, and the presence of equipment (e.g., intravenous [IV] or oxygen tubing) that may interfere with bathing-hygiene.	Determines client's ability to perform bathing and level of assistance required from nurse. Also determines type of bath to administer (e.g., tub bath, partial bed bath).
• ***Critical Decision Point*** *Clients whose levels of independence and mobility change frequently may require more or less assistance during bathing.*	
2. Assess client's bathing preferences: frequency of and time of day bathing preferred, type of hygiene products used, and other factors related to cultural diversity.	Client participates in plan of care. Promotes client's comfort and willingness to cooperate.
3. Ask if client has noticed any problems related to condition of skin.	Provides nurse with information to direct physical assessment of skin during bathing.
4. Identify risks for skin impairment: a. Immobilization (e.g., clients who have paralysis, immobilized extremities, traction; weakened or disabled clients) b. Reduced sensation (e.g., paresthesias, circulatory insufficiency, neuropathies) c. Nutritional and hydration alterations d. Excessive moisture secretion or excretion on skin, particularly on skin surfaces that rub against each other (e.g., under breasts, in perineal area) e. Vascular insufficiency f. External devices applied to or around skin (e.g., casts, braces, restraints, dressings, catheters, tubes) g. Older adult clients h. Friction (sliding down in bed) i. Incontinence (bowel or bladder) j. Allergies	Risk factors increase the likelihood of injury to the skin because of pressure, impaired tissue synthesis, softening of or friction on tissues, and impaired circulation (see Chapter 7).
5. Assess client's knowledge of skin hygiene in terms of its importance, preventive measures to take, and common problems encountered (see Table 6-1).	Determines client's learning needs.
6. Check physician's therapeutic bath order for type of solution, length of time for bath, body part to be attended.	Therapeutic baths are ordered for specific physical effect, which may include promotion of healing or soothing effect.
7. Review orders for specific precautions concerning client's movement or positioning.	Prevents accidental injury to client during bathing activities. Determines level of assistance required by client.

Step	Rationale

Nursing Diagnosis

Defining characteristics from the assessment data may reveal the following nursing diagnoses for clients requiring this skill:

- Activity intolerance
- Bathing/hygiene self-care deficit
- Impaired skin integrity
- Deficient knowledge regarding skin care
- Risk for impaired skin integrity

Related factors are individualized based on client's condition or needs.

Planning

Step	Rationale
1. **Expected outcomes** following completion of procedure:	
▪ Skin is clean, dry, elastic, well hydrated, and without areas of local inflammation.	Indicates intact integument.
▪ Previous skin lesions are cleaner, with less drainage.	Sizes of lesions do not change after one bathing.
▪ Joint range of motion (ROM) remains same or improves from previous measurement.	Important measure for bed rest clients prone to contractures.
▪ Client expresses sense of comfort and relaxation.	Bath relaxes client and removes sources of discomfort.
▪ Client tolerates bath without fatigue or chilling.	Fatigue during bathing can indicate worsening of chronic cardiopulmonary conditions.
▪ Client describes benefits and techniques of proper hygiene and skin care.	Demonstrates learning.
2. Explain procedure and ask client for suggestions on how to prepare supplies. If partial bath, ask how much of bath client wishes to complete.	Promotes client's cooperation and participation.
3. Adjust room temperature and ventilation, close room doors and windows, and draw room divider curtain.	Warm room that is free of drafts prevents rapid loss of body heat during bathing. Privacy ensures client's mental and physical comfort.
4. Prepare equipment and supplies.	Avoids interrupting procedure or leaving client unattended to retrieve missing equipment.

Implementation

Complete or Partial Bed Bath

Step	Rationale
1. Offer client bedpan or urinal. Provide towel and washcloth.	Client will feel more comfortable after voiding. Prevents interruption of bath.
2. Wash hands.	Reduces transmission of microorganisms.

- ***Critical Decision Point***
  Apply gloves if there is an actual or a risk for drainage or secretions on client's skin.

Step	Rationale
3. Lower side rail closest to you and assist client in assuming comfortable supine position, maintaining body alignment. Bring client toward side closest to you. Place hospital bed in high position.	Aids nurse's access to client. Maintains client's comfort throughout procedure. Nurse does not have to reach across bed, thus minimizing strain on back muscles.
4. Loosen top covers at foot of bed. Place bath blanket over top sheet. Fold and remove top sheet from under blanket. If possible, have client hold bath blanket while withdrawing sheet.	Removal of top linens prevents them from becoming soiled or moist during bath. Blanket provides warmth and privacy.
5. If top sheet is to be reused, fold it for replacement later. If not, dispose in laundry bag, taking care not to allow linen to contact uniform.	Proper disposal prevents transmission of microorganisms.

STEP	RATIONALE
6. Remove client's gown or pajamas. If an extremity is injured or has reduced mobility, begin removal from *unaffected* side. If client has intravenous (IV) access, remove gown from arm *without* IV first. Then remove gown from arm with IV. Remove IV from pole, and slide IV tubing and bag through the arm of client's gown. Rehang IV container and check flow rate (see illustrations).	Provides full exposure of body parts during bathing. Undressing unaffected side first allows easier manipulation of gown over body part with reduced ROM.
7. Pull side rail up. Fill washbasin two-thirds full, with warm water. Check water temperature and also have client place fingers in water to test temperature tolerance. Place plastic container of bath lotion in bathwater to warm, if desired.	Raising side rail maintains client's safety as nurses leaves bedside. Warm water promotes comfort, relaxes muscles, and prevents unnecessary chilling. Testing temperature prevents accidental burns. Bathwater warms lotion for application to client's skin.
8. Lower side rail and remove pillow if allowed, and raise head of bed 30 to 45 degrees. Place bath towel under client's head. Place second bath towel over client's chest.	Removal of pillow makes it easier to wash client's ears and neck. Placement of towels prevents soiling of bed linen and bath blanket.
9. Fold washcloth around fingers of nurse's hand to form mitt (see illustration). Immerse mitt in water and wring thoroughly.	Mitt retains water and heat better than loosely held washcloth; keeps cold edges from brushing against client, and prevents splashing.
10. Inquire if client is wearing contact lenses. If so, perform eye care as described in Chapter 8. Wash client's eyes with plain warm water. Use different section of mitt for each eye. Move mitt from inner to outer canthus (see illustra-	Soap irritates eyes. Use of separate sections of mitt reduces infection transmission. Bathing eye from inner to outer canthus prevents secretions from entering nasolacrimal duct. Pressure can cause internal injury.

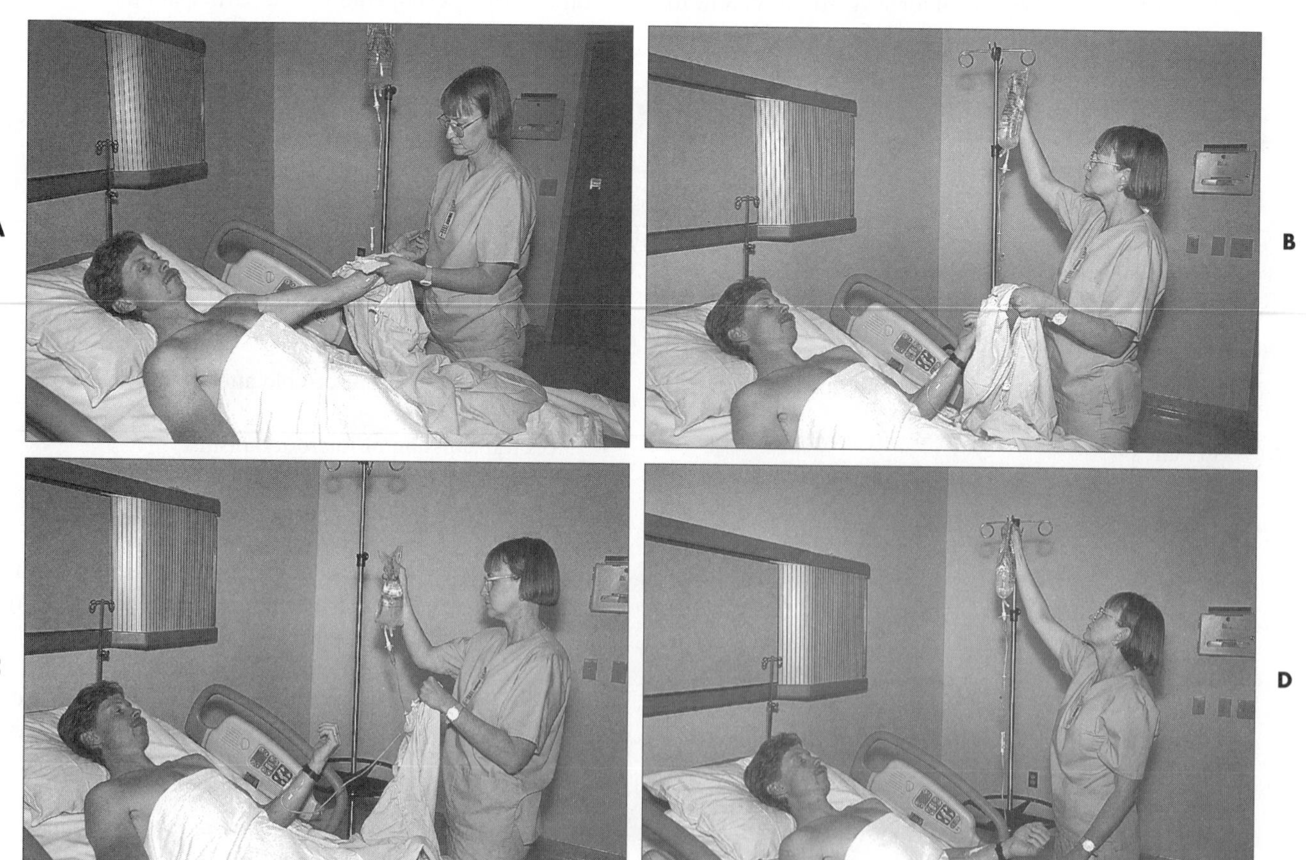

STEP 6 **A,** Remove client's gown. **B,** Remove IV from pole. **C,** Slide IV tubing and bag through arm of client's gown. **D,** Rehang IV bag.

STEP	RATIONALE
tion). Soak any crusts on eyelid for 2 to 3 minutes with damp cloth before attempting removal. Dry eye thoroughly but gently.	
11. Ask if client prefers to use soap on face. Wash, rinse, and dry well forehead, cheeks, nose, neck, and ears. (Men may wish to shave at this point or after bath.)	Soap tends to dry face, which is exposed to air more than other body parts.
12. Remove bath blanket from client's arm that is farthest from you. Place bath towel lengthwise under arm. Raise side rail and move to other side to wash arm if desired.	Bathing far side first prevents reaching over clean area.
13. Bathe arm with soap and water using long, firm strokes from distal to proximal areas (fingers to axilla). Raise and support arm above head (if possible) while thoroughly washing axilla.	Soap lowers surface tension and facilitates removal of debris and bacteria when friction is applied during washing. Long, firm strokes stimulate circulation. Movement of arm exposes axilla and exercises joint's normal ROM.
14. Rinse and dry arm and axilla thoroughly. If client uses deodorant, apply it.	Alkaline residue from soap discourages growth of normal skin bacteria (Barnes, 1987). Excess moisture causes skin maceration, or softening. Deodorant controls body odor.
15. Fold bath towel in half and lay it on bed beside client. Place basin on towel. Immerse client's hand in water. Allow hand to soak for 3 to 5 minutes before washing hand and fingernails (see Skill 6-6). Remove basin and dry hand well.	Soaking softens cuticles and calluses of hand, loosens debris beneath nails, and enhances feeling of cleanliness. Thorough drying removes moisture from between fingers.
16. Raise side rail and move to other side of bed. Lower side rail and repeat Steps 12 through 15 for other arm.	

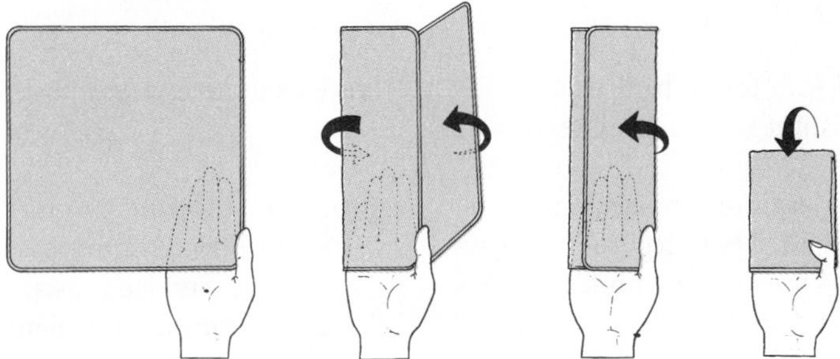

STEP **9** Steps for folding washcloth to form a mitt.

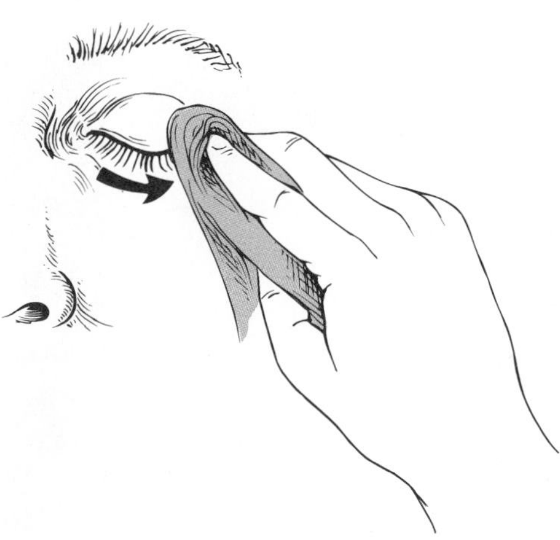

STEP **10** Wash eye from inner to outer canthus.

Step	Rationale
17. Check temperature of bathwater and change water if necessary.	Warm water maintains client's comfort.

- ***Critical Decision Point***
  If client is at risk for falling, be sure top two side rails are up before obtaining fresh water. Note: All four side rails raised may be considered a restraint.

Step	Rationale
18. Cover client's chest with bath towel and fold bath blanket down to umbilicus. With one hand, lift edge of towel away from chest. With mitted hand, bathe chest using long, firm strokes. Take special care to wash skinfolds under female client's breasts. It may be necessary to lift breast upward while bathing underneath it. Keep client's chest covered between wash and rinse periods. Dry well.	Draping prevents unnecessary exposure of body parts. Towel maintains warmth and privacy. Secretions and dirt collect easily in areas of tight skinfolds. Skinfolds are susceptible to excoriation if breasts are pendulous.
19. Place bath towel lengthwise over chest and abdomen. (Two towels may be needed.) Fold blanket down to just above pubic region.	Prevents chilling and exposure of body parts.
20. With one hand, lift bath towel. With mitted hand, bathe abdomen, giving special attention to bathing umbilicus and abdominal folds. Stroke from side to side. Keep abdomen covered between washing and rinsing. Dry well.	Moisture and sediment that collect in skinfolds predispose skin to **maceration** and irritation.
21. Apply clean gown or pajama top.	Maintains client's warmth and comfort. Dressing affected side first allows easier manipulation of gown over body part with reduced ROM.

- ***Critical Decision Point***
  *If one extremity is injured or immobilized, always dress affected side first.**

Step	Rationale
22. Cover chest and abdomen with top of bath blanket. Expose near leg by folding blanket toward midline. Be sure perineum is draped.	Prevents unnecessary exposure.
23. Bend client's leg at knee by positioning nurse's arm under leg. While grasping client's heel, elevate leg from mattress slightly and slide bath towel lengthwise under leg. Ask client to hold foot still. Place bath basin on towel on bed and secure its position next to foot to be washed.	Towel prevents soiling of bed linen. Support of joint and extremity during lifting prevents strain on musculoskeletal structures. Sudden movement by client could spill bath water. (Omit this step if client is unable to hold leg in basin.)
24. With one hand supporting lower leg, raise it and slide basin under lifted foot. Make sure foot is firmly placed on bottom of basin. Allow foot to soak while washing leg. If client is unable to hold leg, do not immerse; simply wash with washcloth (see illustration).	Proper positioning of foot prevents pressure being applied from edge of basin against calf. Soaking softens calluses and rough skin.

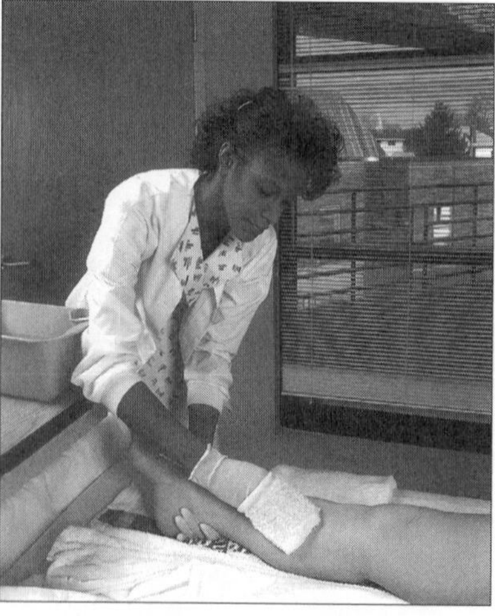

STEP **24** Wash client's leg.

*This step may be omitted until completion of bath; gown should not become soiled during remainder of bath.

Step	Rationale
25. Unless contraindicated, use long, firm strokes in washing from ankle to knee and from knee to thigh. Dry well.	Promotes venous return.
• ***Critical Decision Point*** *Clients with history of deep vein thromboses or blood-clotting disorders should not have their lower extremities washed with long, firm strokes. Use short, light strokes.*	
26. Cleanse foot, making sure to bathe between toes. Clean and clip nails as needed (see Skill 6-6). Dry well. If skin is dry, apply lotion.	Secretions and moisture may be present between toes. Lotion helps retain moisture and soften skin.
• ***Critical Decision Point*** *Do not massage any reddened area on client's skin.*	
27. Raise top side rail and move to other side of the bed. Lower side rail and repeat Steps 22 through 26 for other leg and foot.	
28. Cover client with bath blanket, raise side rail for client's safety, and change bathwater.	Decreased bathwater temperature can cause chilling. Clean water reduces microorganism transmission.
29. Lower side rail. Assist client in assuming prone or side-lying position (as applicable). Place towel lengthwise along client's side.	Exposes back and buttocks for bathing.
30. Keep client draped by sliding bath blanket over shoulders and thighs. Wash, rinse, and dry back from neck to buttocks using long, firm strokes. Pay special attention to folds of buttocks and anus. Give a back rub, and change the bathwater.	Maintains warmth and prevents unnecessary exposure. Skinfolds near buttocks and anus may contain fecal secretions that harbor microorganisms. Clean water reduces microorganism transmission.
31. Apply disposable gloves if not done previously.	Prevents contact with microorganisms in body secretions.
32. Assist client in assuming side-lying or supine position. Cover chest and upper extremities with towel and lower extremities with bath blanket. Expose only genitalia. (If client can wash, covering entire body with bath blanket may be preferable.) Wash, rinse, and dry perineum (see Skill 6-2). Pay special attention to skinfolds. Apply water-repellant ointment to area exposed to moisture.	Maintains client's privacy. Clients capable of performing partial bath usually prefer to wash their own genitalia. Water-repellant ointments (e.g., A and D, Pericare) protect skin from moisture (Agency for Health Care Policy and Research, 1992).
33. Dispose of gloves in receptacle.	Prevents transmission of infection.
34. Apply additional body lotion or oil as desired.	Moisturizing lotion prevents dry, chapped skin.
35. Assist client in dressing. Comb client's hair. Women may want to apply makeup.	Promotes client's body image.
36. Make client's bed (see Skill 6-7 and Procedural Guidelines Box 6-3).	Provides clean environment.
37. Remove soiled linen and place in dirty-linen bag. Clean and replace bathing equipment. Replace call light and personal possessions. Leave room as clean and comfortable as possible.	Prevents transmission of infection. Clean environment promotes client's comfort. Keeping call light and articles of care within reach promotes client's safety.
38. Wash hands.	Reduces transmission of microorganisms.
Tub Bath or Shower	
1. Consider client's condition and review orders for precautions concerning client's movement or positioning.	Prevents accidental injury to client during bathing.
2. Schedule use of shower or tub.	Prevents unnecessary waiting that can cause fatigue.
3. Check tub or shower for cleanliness. Use cleaning techniques outlined in agency policy. Place rubber mat on tub or shower bottom. Place disposable bath mat or towel on floor in front of tub or shower.	Cleaning prevents transmission of microorganisms. Mats prevent slipping and falling.
4. Collect all hygienic aids, toiletry items, and linens requested by client. Place within easy reach of tub or shower.	Placing items close at hand prevents possible falls when client reaches for equipment.

STEP	RATIONALE
5. Assist client to bathroom if necessary. Have client wear robe and slippers to bathroom.	Assistance prevents accidental falls. Wearing robe and slippers prevents chilling.
6. Demonstrate how to use call signal for assistance.	Bathrooms are equipped with signaling devices in case client feels faint or weak or needs immediate assistance. Clients prefer privacy during bath if safety is not jeopardized.
7. Place "occupied" sign on bathroom door.	Maintains client's privacy.
8. Fill bathrub halfway with warm water. Check temperature of bath water, then have client test water, and adjust temperature if water is too warm. Explain which faucet controls hot water. If client is taking shower, turn shower on and adjust water temperature before client enters shower stall. Use shower seat or tub chair and provide if needed (see illustration).	Adjusting water temperature prevents accidental burns. Older adults and clients with neurological alterations (e.g., spinal cord injury) are at high risk for burns as a result of reduced sensation. Use of assistive devices facilitates bathing and minimizes physical exertion.

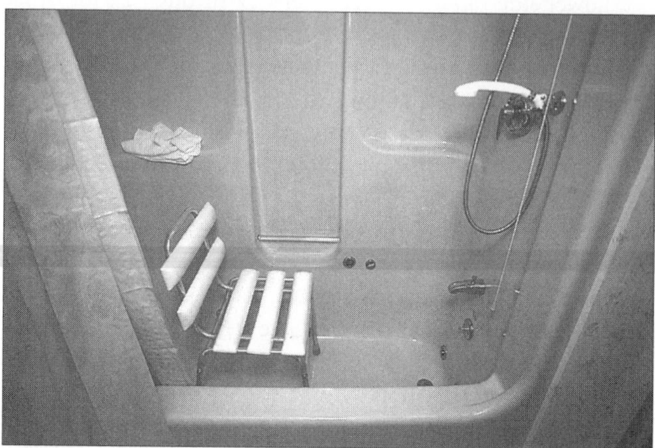

STEP **8** Shower seat for client safety.

STEP	RATIONALE
9. Instruct client to use safety bars when getting in and out of tub or shower. Caution client against use of bath oil in tub water.	Prevents slipping and falling. Oil causes tub surfaces to become slippery.
10. Instruct client not to remain in tub longer than 20 minutes. Check on client every 5 minutes.	Prolonged exposure to warm water may cause vasodilation and pooling of blood, leading to light-headedness or dizziness.
11. Return to bathroom when client signals, and knock before entering.	Provides privacy.
12. For client who is unsteady, drain tub of water before client attempts to get out of it. Place bath towel over client's shoulders. Assist client in getting out of tub as needed and assist with drying.	Prevents accidental falls. Client may become chilled as water drains.

- ***Critical Decision Point***

  Weak or unstable clients need extra assistance in getting out of a tub. Planning for additional personnel is essential before attempting to assist the client from the tub.

STEP	RATIONALE
13. Assist client as needed in donning clean gown or pajamas, slippers, and robe. (In home setting client may put on regular clothing.)	Maintains warmth to prevent chilling.
14. Assist client to room and comfortable position in bed or chair.	Maintains relaxation gained from bathing.
15. Clean tub or shower according to agency policy. Remove soiled linen and place in dirty-linen bag. Discard disposable equipment in proper receptacle. Place "unoccupied" sign on bathroom door. Return supplies to storage area.	Prevents transmission of infection through soiled linen and moisture.
16. Wash hands.	Reduces transfer of microorganisms.

STEP	RATIONALE
EVALUATION	
1. Observe skin, paying particular attention to areas that were previously soiled, reddened, or showed early signs of breakdown.	Techniques used during bathing should leave skin clean and clear.
2. Observe ROM during bath.	Measures joint mobility.
3. Ask client to rate level of comfort.	Determines if bath achieves relaxation.
4. Ask if client feels fatigued.	Determines client's tolerance of bathing activities.
5. Ask client to explain proper hygiene techniques.	Evaluates client's knowledge level.

UNEXPECTED OUTCOMES AND RELATED INTERVENTIONS

- Areas of excessive dryness, rashes, or pressure ulcers appear on skin.
  - Review agency skin care policy regarding moisturizing lotions.
  - Limit frequency of complete baths.
  - Complete pressure ulcer assessment (see Chapter 7).
  - Obtain special bed surface if client is at risk for skin breakdown.
- Joint ROM decreases.
  - Increase ROM exercises (unless contraindicated).
  - Encourage more self-care by client.
- Client becomes excessively fatigued and unable to cooperate or participate in bathing.
  - Reschedule bathing to a time when client is more rested.
  - Clients with breathing difficulties require pillow or elevated head of bed during bath.
  - Notify physician if this is a change in client's fatigue level.
- Client seems unusually restless or complains of discomfort.
  - Schedule client rest periods.
  - Consider analgesia if client complains of pain or discomfort before the bath.

RECORDING AND REPORTING

- Record bath on flow sheet. Note level of assistance required.
- Record condition of skin and any significant findings (e.g., reddened areas, bruises, nevi, or joint or muscle pain).
- Report evidence of alterations in skin integrity to nurse in charge or physician.

TEACHING CONSIDERATIONS

- Clients with decreased sensation need to be cautious when entering hot bathwater. Whenever possible they need to use unaffected extremity to test water temperature to avoid accidental scalding.
- Family members caring for clients in the home should be included in discussions about hygiene.
- Instruct clients on how to inspect surfaces between skinfolds for signs of irritation or breakdown.

PEDIATRIC CONSIDERATIONS

- Adolescents may require and/or prefer more frequent bathing as a result of more active sebaceous glands.
- Child may prefer to have parent or family help with bath.

GERONTOLOGICAL CONSIDERATIONS

- Consider conditions of older adult's skin when planning hygiene routine. Because of the aging process, more moisture is needed; client's skin can be rehydrated with lotions and fluids (Lueckenotte, 2000).
- Older adults with urinary incontinence need meticulous skin care to reduce skin irritation from urine and feces (see Chapters 7 and 24).
- Older adults may require less frequent baths, more frequent application of skin lotion.

HOME CARE CONSIDERATIONS

- In home setting, set up equipment according to established routines. Client is best resource for what works in terms of convenience and saving time.
- Clients at risk for falls may wish to have grab bars installed around tub and have bathroom floor carpeted. Client also may use portable shower seat.
- The types of bath for the homebound client are the complete bed bath; the abbreviated bed bath, during which only parts of the body are washed that, if neglected, might cause illness, odor, or discomfort; and the partial bath, which may take place at the sink, in the tub, or in the shower.
- Type of bath chosen depends on assessment of the home, availability of running water, and condition of bathing facilities.
- If beds do not have side rails, positioning may be accomplished with pillows or by placing bed against wall.
- Never leave bathing client unattended. Adhesive strips on bottom of tub or shower, handrails, chairs, or stools in tub or shower will further protect client.
- Determine if there is need to have home health aide or other assistance after discharge. Contact social service or appropriate department within hospital to obtain referral to home health agency.

LONG-TERM CARE CONSIDERATIONS

- Tubs in long term care settings frequently come equipped with electronic thermometers to measure water temperature.
- Skin related problems in long-term care settings may include methicillin-resistant staphylococcus aureus (MSRA) infections, pressure ulcers, circulatory ulcers, **dermatitis,** skin cancers, herpes zoster (shingles) (Lueckenotte, 2000).
- Residents in long-term care facilities should be encouraged to do as much personal care as possible and to wear their own street clothes (Sorrentino, 1999).

Skill 6-2 Providing Perineal Care

Perineal care involves thorough cleansing of the client's external genitalia and surrounding skin. A client routinely receives perineal care during a bath. Clients most in need of perineal care are at greatest risk for acquiring an infection, such as clients with indwelling Foley catheters, clients who are incontinent, and clients recovering from rectal or genital surgery or childbirth.

"Pericare" is important in promoting the client's comfort and cleanliness. Special attention is given to cleansing the skin around the genitals, because secretions can accumulate and cause skin breakdown and infection of the skin and urinary or reproductive systems. The nurse retains responsibility for doing this procedure if the client is unable to do so and determines the client's understanding of the importance of basic perineal hygiene.

Gloves must be worn during the procedure because of the risk of contacting infectious microorganisms, such as human immunodeficiency virus (HIV) or herpesvirus, from perineal drainage. Certain clients require perineal care at times other than during a bath (e.g., because of fecal incontinence or as part of Foley catheter care). In addition, pericare promotes healing after perineal surgery or vaginal deliveries.

To minimize embarrassment for both the nurse and the client, it helps for the nurse to be of the same sex as the client. Embarrassment should not cause the nurse to overlook the client's hygiene needs.

DELEGATION CONSIDERATIONS

Skills of perineal care can be delegated to assistive personnel. It is important to inform and assist care providers in proper way to position male and female clients and to provide instructions as to proper positioning of an indwelling catheter during perineal care. In addition, assistive personnel must have sufficient information about signs and symptoms of infection, excoriation, perineal drainage, and the need to report to the nurse any changes in the client's perineal area.

EQUIPMENT

- Washbasin
- Soap dish with soap
- Two or three washcloths
- Bath towel
- Bath blanket
- Waterproof pad or bedpan
- Toilet tissue or diaper wipes
- Disposable gloves
- Additional supplies are needed when pericare is given other than during a bath: cotton balls or swabs, a solution bottle or container filled with warm water or prescribed rinsing solution, waterproof bag

STEP	RATIONALE
ASSESSMENT	
1. Identify clients at risk for developing infection of genitalia, urinary tract, or reproductive tract (e.g., uncircumcised male, perineal surgery, presence of indwelling catheter, fecal incontinence).	Secretions that accumulate on surface of skin surrounding female and male genitalia act as reservoir for infection. Tissues traumatized by surgery or by presence of foreign object provide route for introduction of infectious organisms.
2. Assess client's cognitive and musculoskeletal function.	Determines client's ability to perform self-care and determines level of assistance required from nurse.
3. Assess genitalia for signs of inflammation, skin breakdown, or infection (see Chapter 7).	Determines extent of perineal care required by client.
4. Assess client's knowledge of importance of perineal hygiene.	Clients at risk for infection in perineal area may be unaware of importance of cleanliness. Reflects client's need for education.

STEP	RATIONALE

NURSING DIAGNOSIS

Defining characteristics from the assessment data may reveal the following nursing diagnoses for clients requiring this skill:

- Bathing/hygiene self-care deficit
- Impaired skin integrity
- Deficient knowledge regarding hygienic care
- Risk for impaired skin integrity
- Risk for infection
- Impaired physical mobility

Related factors are individualized based on client's condition or needs.

PLANNING

1. **Expected outcomes** following completion of procedure:
   - Skin and surrounding genitalia are clean, intact, and without redness or drainage. — Skin is free of irritation or infection.
   - Client expresses sense of cleanliness and denies irritation. — Perineum is clean.
   - Client is able to describe or perform steps of perineal hygiene. — Client acquires self-care skills.
2. Explain procedure and its purpose to client. — Helps minimize anxiety during procedure that is often embarrassing to nurse and client.
3. Prepare necessary equipment and supplies. — Used when administering a bed bath.

IMPLEMENTATION

1. Pull curtain around client's bed or close room door. Assemble supplies at bedside. — Maintains client's privacy and ensures orderly procedure.
2. Raise bed to comfortable working position. Lower side rail and assist client in assuming side-lying position, placing towel lengthwise along client's side and keeping client covered with bath blanket. — Facilitates good body mechanics. Provides easy access to genitalia.
3. Apply disposable gloves. — Reduces transmission of microorganisms.
4. If fecal material is present, enclose in a fold of underpad or toilet tissue and remove with disposable wipes. Cleanse buttocks and anus, washing front to back (see illustration). Cleanse, rinse, and dry area thoroughly. If needed, place an absorbent pad under client's buttocks. Remove and discard underpad and replace with clean one. — Cleansing reduces transmission of microorganisms from anus to urethra or genitalia.

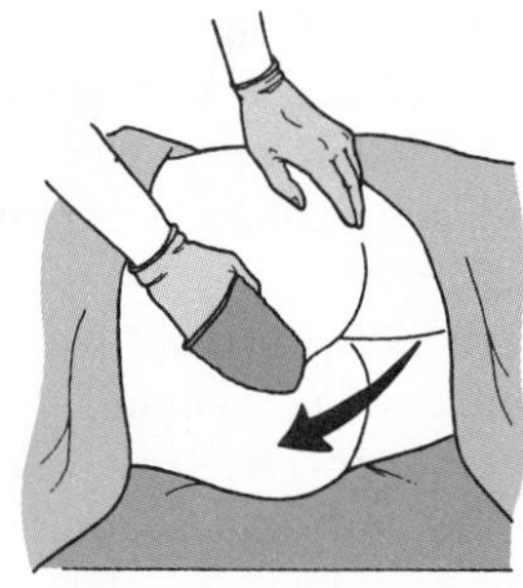

STEP 4 Cleanse buttocks from front to back.

5. Change gloves when they are soiled.
6. Fold top bed linen down toward foot of bed and raise client's gown above genital area. — Exposes perineal area for easy accessibility.
   a. "Diamond" drape client by placing bath blanket with one corner between client's legs, one corner pointing toward each side of bed, and one corner over client's chest. Tuck side corners around client's legs and under hips. — Prevents unnecessary exposure of body parts and maintains client's warmth and comfort during procedure.
   b. Raise side rail. Fill washbasin with warm water. — Prevents client from falling. Proper water temperature prevents burns to perineum.

STEP	RATIONALE
c. Place washbasin and toilet tissue on overbed table. Place washcloths in basin.	Equipment placed within nurse's reach prevents accidental spills.
7. Provide perineal care.	
a. Female perineal care:	
(1) Assist client to dorsal recumbent position.	Provides easy access to genitalia.
(2) Lower side rail and help client flex knees and spread legs. Note restrictions or limitations in client's positioning.	Provides full exposure of female genitalia. Minimize degree of abduction in female if position causes pain because of arthritis or contracture or in older adults with decreased mobility.
(3) Fold lower corner of bath blanket up between client's legs onto abdomen. Wash and dry client's upper thighs.	Minimizes transmission of microorganisms. Keeping client draped until procedure begins minimizes anxiety. Buildup of perineal secretions can soil surrounding skin surfaces.
(4) Wash labia majora. Use nondominant hand to gently retract labia from thigh; with dominant hand, wash carefully in skinfolds. Wipe in direction from perineum to rectum (front to back). Repeat on opposite side using separate section of washcloth. Rinse and dry area thoroughly.	Skinfolds may contain body secretions that harbor microorganisms. Wiping from perineum to rectum (front to back) reduces chance of transmitting fecal organisms to urinary meatus.
(5) Separate labia with nondominant hand to expose urethral meatus and vaginal orifice. With dominant hand, wash downward from pubic area toward rectum in one smooth stroke (see illustration). Use separate section of cloth for each stroke. Cleanse thoroughly around labia minora, clitoris, and vaginal orifice.	Cleansing method reduces transfer of microorganisms to urinary meatus. (For menstruating women or clients with indwelling urinary catheters, cleanse with cotton balls.) 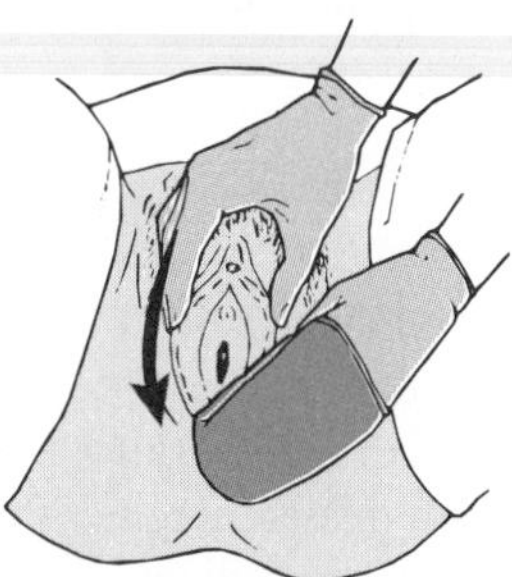 STEPS **7a(5)** Cleanse from perineum to rectum (front to back).
(6) If client uses bedpan, pour warm water over perineal area. Dry perineal area thoroughly, using front-to-back method.	Rinsing removes soap and microorganisms more effectively than wiping. Retained moisture harbors microorganisms.
(7) Fold lower corner of bath blanket back between client's legs and over perineum. Ask client to lower legs and assume comfortable position.	
b. Male perineal care:	
(1) Lower side rails and assist client to supine position. Note restriction in mobility.	Provides full exposure of male genitalia.
(2) Fold lower corner of bath blanket up between client's legs and onto abdomen. Wash and dry client's upper thighs.	Minimizes transmission of microorganisms. Keeping client draped until procedure begins minimizes anxiety. Buildup of perineal secretions can soil surrounding skin surfaces.
(3) Gently raise penis and place bath towel underneath. Gently grasp shaft of penis. If client is uncircumcised, retract foreskin. If client has an erection, defer procedure until later.	Towel prevents moisture from collecting in inguinal area. Gentle but firm handling reduces chance of client having an erection. Secretions capable of harboring microorganisms collect underneath foreskin.
(4) Wash tip of penis at urethral meatus first. Using circular motion, cleanse from meatus outward (see illustration). Discard washcloth and repeat with clean cloth until penis is clean. Rinse and dry gently.	Direction of cleansing moves from area of least contamination to area of most contamination, preventing microorganisms from entering urethra.

STEP	RATIONALE
(5) Return foreskin to its natural position.	Tightening of foreskin around shaft of penis can cause local edema and discomfort.

- ***Critical Decision Point***

  After administering perineal care, the nurse needs to make sure the foreskin is in its natural position. This is extremely important in those clients with decreased sensation in their lower extremities.

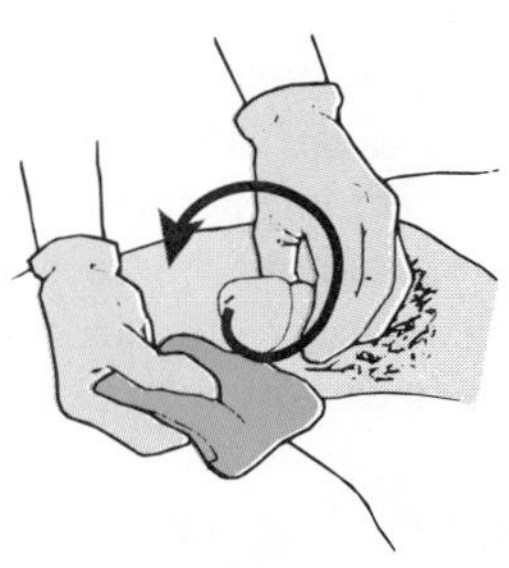

STEP **7b(4)** Use circular motion to cleanse tip of penis.

STEP	RATIONALE
(6) Wash shaft of penis with gentle but firm downward strokes. Pay special attention to underlying surface of penis. Rinse and dry penis thoroughly. Instruct client to spread legs apart slightly.	Vigorous massage of penis can lead to erection, which can embarrass client and nurse. Underlying surface of penis may have greater accumulation of secretions. Abduction of legs provides easier access to scrotal tissues.
(7) Gently cleanse scrotum. Lift it carefully and wash underlying skinfolds. Rinse and dry.	Pressure on scrotal tissues can be painful to client. Secretions collect between skinfolds.
(8) Fold bath blanket back over client's perineum and assist client in turning to side-lying position.	Draping promotes comfort and minimizes client's anxiety. Side-lying position provides access to anal area.
8. If client has had urinary or bowel incontinence, apply thin layer of skin barrier containing petrolatum or zinc oxide over anal and perineal skin.	Protects skin from excess moisture and toxins from urine or stool (Maklebust and others, 1995). Clients who are incontinent or who are exposed to body secretions need more frequent skin assessment to determine risk for pressure ulcer development. Fully assess exposed skin before repositioning.
9. Remove disposable gloves and dispose in proper receptacle.	Moisture and body secretions on gloves can harbor microorganisms.
10. Assist client in assuming a comfortable position and cover with sheet.	Client's comfort helps to minimize stress of procedure.
11. Remove bath blanket and dispose of all soiled bed linen. Return unused equipment to storage area.	Reduces transmission of microorganisms.

EVALUATION

1. Inspect surface of external genitalia and surrounding skin after cleansing.	Thick secretions may cover underlying skin lesions or areas of breakdown. Evaluation determines need for additional hygiene.
2. Ask if client feels sense of cleanliness.	Determines client's comfort level.
3. Observe client's ability to perform hygiene and ask questions about its importance.	Determines client's self-care ability and knowledge level.

UNEXPECTED OUTCOMES AND RELATED INTERVENTIONS

- Skin and genitalia may be inflamed, with localized tenderness, swelling, and presence of foul-smelling discharge.
  - Bathe area frequently to keep clean and dry.
  - Obtain an order for a Sitz bath.
  - Apply protective barrier.
  - Indicates infection or maceration of skin layers. Physician may need to order specific antibacterial, antifungal ointment.

- Client expresses discomfort.
  - Perineal area is not fully cleansed; perform perineal hygiene again.
- Client is unable to describe or perform perineal hygiene.
  - Further instruction is required at a later time.

Recording and Reporting

- Record procedure and presence of any abnormal findings (e.g., character and amount of discharge, condition of genitalia).
- Record appearance of suture line, if present.
- Report any break in suture line or presence of abnormalities to nurse in charge or physician.

Teaching Considerations

- Clients most at risk for infection of perineum are taught signs and symptoms of early infection, as well as principles and techniques for cleansing perineum correctly.
- Clients who are physically unable to perform hygiene and who rely on family members for care must have family instructed on hygiene techniques.

Pediatric Considerations

- Young adolescent girls should learn basic perineal hygiene measures and know why they are predisposed to urinary tract infections.

Gerontological Considerations

- Older adults with limited mobility need assistance in perineal care. Using a side-lying position increases client's comfort and provides nurse with opportunity to provide perineal care and inspect surrounding skin as well.

Home Care Considerations

- For clients who require bathing, assess perineum at every visit because of risk for infection and skin breakdown.

Skill 6-3 Brushing Teeth

Brushing, flossing, and irrigation are necessary for proper cleansing of teeth. Brushing removes food particles, loosens plaque, and stimulates gums. **Plaque** is the cause of dental caries. **Flossing** removes **tartar** that collects at the gum line. Irrigation removes dislodged food particles and excess toothpaste. When a client becomes ill, a regular dental hygiene routine is often difficult, if not impossible, to follow. The nurse offers oral hygiene assistance as required, from preparing needed supplies to actually brushing the client's teeth.

The nurse's responsibility also includes determining the frequency with which clients require brushing. Certain conditions resulting from illness or therapy cause the oral cavity to become excessively dry or irritated. For example, clients with food or fluid restrictions often develop thick, foul-tasting secretions in the mouth because of reduced hydration. Frequent oral hygiene provides considerable relief. Frequency of care should be based on the condition of the oral cavity and the client's level of comfort. Oral hygiene may be required as often as every 1 to 2 hours.

Clients who wear dentures should be encouraged to continue to care for them, and to provide this care as frequently as with natural teeth. Routine denture care reduces the risk of gingival infection. However, when clients are unable to care for their own dentures, the nurse must provide this care (Procedural Guidelines Box 6-1). Dentures are the client's personal property and should be handled with care because they can be easily broken. Dentures should be stored in an enclosed, labeled cup for soaking or when dentures are not worn, such as during surgery or diagnostic procedures. Once clients are returned from their procedure, most prefer to have their dentures inserted as soon as possible.

Delegation Considerations

Skills of brushing teeth can be delegated to assistive personnel. The care provider must be able to recognize impaired integrity of oral mucosa and report it to nurse properly.

Equipment

- Soft-bristled toothbrush (hard toothbrush damages enamel and gums)
- Nonabrasive fluoride toothpaste or dentifrice (abrasive toothpastes wear down enamel)
- Dental floss
- Water glass with cool water
- Normal saline or fluoride mouthwash (optional; follow client's preference)
- Emesis basin
- Face towel
- Paper towels
- Disposable gloves

Box 6-1 Procedural Guidelines

Cleaning Dentures

Equipment: Soft-bristled toothbrush, denture toothbrush, emesis basin or sink, denture dentifrice or toothpaste, water glass, 4 × 4 inch gauze, washcloth, denture cup, disposable gloves

1. Clean dentures for client during routine mouth care. Dentures need to be cleansed as often as natural teeth.
2. Fill emesis basin with tepid water. (If using sink, place washcloth in bottom of sink, and fill sink with approximately 1 in of water.)
3. Remove dentures: If client is unable to do this independently, apply gloves, grasp upper plate at front with thumb and index finger wrapped in gauze, and pull downward. Gently lift lower denture from jaw, and rotate one side downward to remove from client's mouth. Place dentures in emesis basin or sink.
4. Apply dentifrice or toothpaste to denture, and brush surfaces of dentures (see illustration). Hold dentures close to water. Hold brush horizontally, and use back-and-forth motion to cleanse biting surfaces. Use short strokes from top of denture to biting surfaces of teeth to clean outer tooth surface. Hold brush vertically, and use short strokes to clean inner tooth surfaces. Hold brush horizontally, and use back-and-forth motion to clean undersurface of dentures.
5. Rinse dentures thoroughly in tepid water.
6. Return dentures to client, or store in tepid water in denture cup. Keep denture cup inside bedside cabinet.

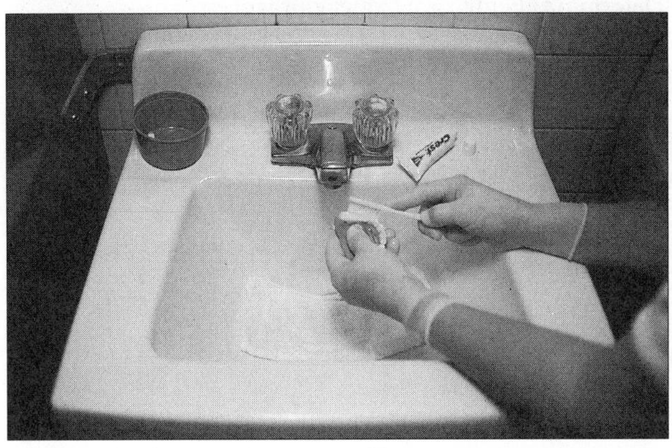

STEP **4** Brushing surface of denture.

STEP	RATIONALE
ASSESSMENT	
1. Wash hands and apply disposable gloves.	Reduces transmission of microorganisms. Gloves prevent contact with microorganisms in blood or saliva.
2. Inspect integrity of lips, teeth, **buccal** mucosa, gums, palate, and tongue (see Chapter 10).	Determines status of client's oral cavity and extent of need for oral hygiene.
3. Identify presence of common oral problems:	Helps determine type of hygiene client requires and information client requires for self-care.
a. **Dental caries**—chalky white discoloration of tooth or presence of brown or black discoloration	
b. **Gingivitis**—inflammation of gums	
c. **Periodontitis**—receding gum lines, inflammation, gaps between teeth	
d. **Halitosis**—bad breath	
e. **Cheilosis**—cracking of lips	
f. **Stomatitis**—inflammation of the mouth	
4. Remove gloves and wash hands.	Prevents spread of microorganisms.
5. Assess risk for oral hygiene problems:	Certain conditions increase likelihood of impaired oral cavity integrity and need for preventive care.
a. Dehydration, inability to take fluids or food by mouth **(NPO)**	Causes excess drying and fragility of mucous membranes; increases accumulation of secretions on tongue and gums.
b. Presence of nasogastric or oxygen tubes; mouth breathers	Causes drying of mucosa (Harrell and Damon, 1989).
c. Chemotherapeutic drugs	These drugs kill rapidly multiplying cells, including cancerous tumors and cells lining oral cavity and gastrointestinal tract. Drug effects can lead to stomatitis (Dudjak, 1987).
d. Radiation therapy to head and neck	Reduces salivary flow and lowers pH of saliva; can lead to stomatitis and tooth decay (Danielson, 1988).

Step	Rationale
e. Presence of artificial airway	Increases irritation to gums and mucosa. Excess secretions accumulate on teeth and tongue.
f. Blood-clotting disorders (e.g., leukemia, aplastic anemia)	Predisposes to inflammation and bleeding of gums.
g. Oral surgery, trauma to mouth	Break in mucosa increases risk of infection. Vigorous brushing can disrupt suture lines.
h. Aging	With advancing age, mucosa becomes thin and less elastic.
i. Diabetes mellitus	Prone to dryness of mouth, gingivitis, periodontal disease, and loss of teeth.
6. Determine client's oral hygiene practices:	Allows nurse to identify errors in technique, deficiencies in preventive oral hygiene, and client's level of knowledge regarding dental care.
a. Frequency of toothbrushing and flossing	
b. Type of toothpaste or **dentifrice** used	
c. Last dental visit	
d. Frequency of dental visits	
e. Type of mouthwash or moistening preparation	Lemon-glycerine preparations can be detrimental. Glycerine is an astringent that dries and shrinks mucous membranes and gums. Lemon exhausts salivary reflex and can erode tooth enamel (Adams, 1996; Fitch, 1999). Mouthwash provides pleasant aftertaste but can dry mucosa after extended use if it has an alcohol base.
7. Assess client's ability to grasp and manipulate toothbrush. Assessment determines level of assistance required from nurse.	Older adult clients or persons with musculoskeletal or nervous system alterations may be unable to hold toothbrush with firm grip or manipulate brush.

Nursing Diagnosis

Defining characteristics from the assessment data may reveal the following nursing diagnoses for clients requiring this skill:

Impaired oral mucous membrane
Bathing/hygiene self-care deficit
Deficient knowledge regarding oral hygiene care

Related factors are individualized based on client's condition or needs.

Planning

Step	Rationale
1. **Expected outcomes** following completion of procedure:	
▪ Client expresses feeling of cleanliness.	Hygiene measures remove secretions and thickened musosa.
▪ Oral cavity structures have normal characteristics.	If client had degree of alteration before brushing, condition should not be worse after brushing.
• Oral mucosa is moist, intact, and of normal color.	Mucosa and gums are moist and intact.
• Gums are pink, firm, and adherent to neck of teeth.	
• Teeth are clean, smooth, and shiny.	
• Tongue is pink and without secretions or coating.	
▪ Client describes correct oral hygiene techniques and necessary frequency.	Demonstrates understanding of nurse's instructions.
▪ Client makes choices regarding hygiene procedure and assists by flossing and brushing.	Client is able to manage self-care.
2. Prepare equipment at bedside.	

Step	Rationale
3. Explain procedure to client and discuss preferences regarding use of hygienic aids.	Some clients feel uncomfortable about having the nurse care for their basic needs. Client involvement with procedure minimizes anxiety.

Implementation

Step	Rationale
1. Place paper towels on overbed table and arrange other equipment within easy reach.	Creates organized workspace.
2. Raise bed to comfortable working position. Raise head of bed (if allowed) and lower side rail. Move client or help client move closer. Side-lying position can be used.	Raising bed and positioning client prevent nurse from straining muscles. Semi-Fowler's position helps prevent client from choking or aspirating.
3. Place towel over client's chest.	
4. Apply gloves.	Prevents contact with microorganisms or blood in saliva.
5. Apply toothpaste to brush, holding brush over emesis basin. Pour small amount of water over toothpaste.	Moisture aids in distribution of toothpaste over tooth surfaces.
6. Client may assist by brushing. Hold toothbrush bristles at 45-degree angle to gum line (see illustration). Be sure tips of bristles rest against and penetrate under gum line. Brush inner and outer surfaces of upper and lower teeth by brushing from gum to crown of each tooth. Clean biting surfaces of teeth by holding top of bristles parallel with teeth and brushing gently back and forth (see illustration). Brush sides of teeth by moving bristles back and forth (see illustration).	Angle allows brush to reach all tooth surfaces and to clean under gum line where plaque and tartar accumulate. Back-and-forth motion dislodges food particles caught between teeth and along chewing surfaces.

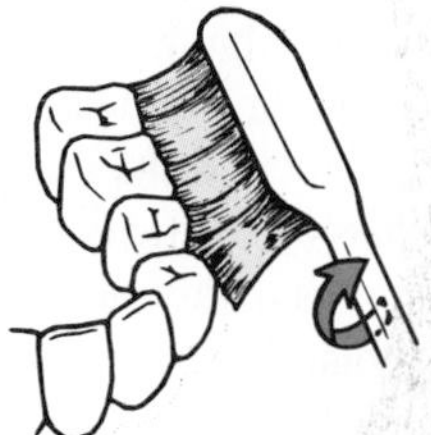
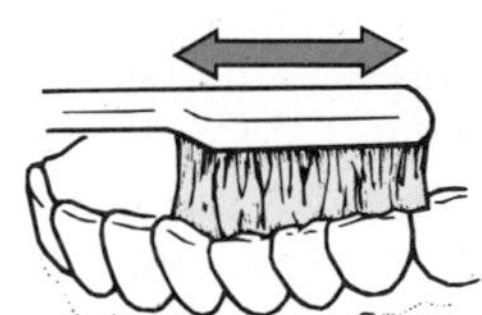
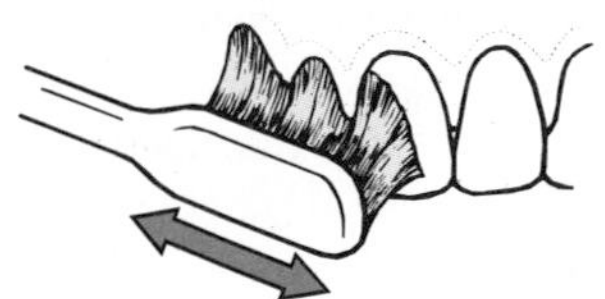

STEP **6** Direction for toothbrush placement.

Step	Rationale
7. Have client hold brush at 45-degree angle and lightly brush over surface and sides of tongue. Avoid initiating gag reflex.	Microorganisms collect and grow on tongue's surface and contribute to bad breath. Gagging may cause aspiration of toothpaste.
8. Allow client to rinse mouth thoroughly by taking several sips of water, swishing water across all tooth surfaces, and spitting into emesis basin.	Irrigation removes food particles.
9. Allow client to gargle or rinse mouth with mouthwash as desired.	Mouthwash leaves pleasant taste in mouth.
10. Assist in wiping client's mouth.	Promotes sense of comfort.
11. Allow client to floss.	Reduces tartar on tooth surfaces.
12. Allow client to rinse mouth thoroughly with cool water and spit into emesis basin. Assist in wiping client's mouth.	Irrigation removes plaque and tartar from oral cavity.
13. Assist client to comfortable position, remove emesis basin and bedside table, raise side rail, if appropriate, and lower bed to original position.	Provides for client comfort and safety.
14. Wipe off overbed table, discard soiled linen and paper towels in appropriate containers, remove soiled gloves, and return equipment to proper place.	Proper disposal of soiled equipment prevents spread of infection.
15. Wash hands.	Reduces transmission of microorganisms.

STEP	RATIONALE
EVALUATION	
1. Ask client if any area of oral cavity feels uncomfortable or irritated.	Pain indicates more chronic problem.
2. Apply gloves and inspect condition of oral cavity.	Determines effectiveness of hygiene and rinsing.
3. Ask client to describe proper hygiene techniques.	Evaluates client's learning.
4. Observe client brushing.	Evaluates client' ability to use correct technique.

UNEXPECTED OUTCOMES AND RELATED INTERVENTIONS

- Mucosa is dry and inflamed.
  - Increase client's hydration.
  - Apply protectant to client's lips.
- Gum margins are retracted from teeth, with localized areas of inflammation. Bleeding occurs around gum margins.
  - Report findings because client may have an underlying bleeding tendency.
  - Switch to a soft-bristled toothbrush.
  - Avoid too vigorous brushing and flossing.
  - A swab stick containing an aqueous solution of sorbitol, sodium, carboxymethylcellulose, and electrolytes may be used.
- Teeth show signs of dental caries.
  - Refer client to dentist.
- Tongue continues to have thick coating.
  - Special care and tongue brushing are needed.

RECORDING AND REPORTING

- Record procedure on flow sheet. Note condition of oral cavity in nurses' notes.
- Report bleeding or presence of lesions to nurse in charge or physician.
- Client is unable to describe correct oral hygiene techniques or brush properly.
  - Further instruction is required.

TEACHING CONSIDERATIONS

- Educate clients about methods to prevent tooth decay (e.g., reduce intake of carbohydrates, especially sweet snacks between meals; brush within 30 minutes of eating sweets; rinse mouth thoroughly with water or eat acid-containing fruit such as an apple; use fluoridated water) (Fellona and DeVore, 1999).
- Cheilosis can be prevented by applying lip ointment or lubricant and avoiding licking of lips.

PEDIATRIC CONSIDERATIONS

- As soon as teething begins, clean an infant's gum pads and teeth with a small piece of gauze twice a day (after breakfast and after the last meal of the day). This practice eliminates decay-producing plaque.
- Teach parents that a bottle given to a child at bedtime should contain only water. Falling asleep with a bottle of milk or juice or while breast-feeding bathes the teeth in a carbohydrate-rich fluid that can cause cavities and tooth discoloration.
- Parents and caregivers need to be responsible for the child's oral hygiene for about the first 8 years, because the child does not develop the neural patterns and muscular coordination needed for performing mouth care until that age.
- Unless problems occur earlier, dental visits should begin about age 2. After the first visit, dental checkups every 6 months are encouraged (Wong and others, 1999).

GERONTOLOGICAL CONSIDERATIONS

- A number of normal age-related changes occur in the oral cavity. Thinning of the oral mucosa and decreased vascularity of the gingivae predispose older adults to injury and periodontal disease. Loss of tissue elasticity and decreased mass and strength of the muscles make chewing more difficult. Resorption of the alveolar bone can loosen natural teeth. The number of taste buds declines. In an attempt to enhance the taste of food, the older adult may choose salty and sugary foods, which erode tooth enamel and expose dentin (Pettigrew, 1989).
- Even with these changes, most mouth problems are preventable with good oral hygiene practices and regular dental checkups.

HOME CARE CONSIDERATIONS

- During the initial admission visit, document the condition of the client's mouth, teeth, and gums, thus providing a baseline for assessment of the client's ability to comply with special diets and fluid intake and to carry out oral hygiene practices.

Skill 6-4 Performing Mouth Care for the Unconscious or Debilitated Client

Unconscious or debilitated clients pose challenges because of their risk for having alterations of the oral cavity and because of their total dependence on the nurse for oral care. Critically ill and unstable clients may have so many physiological problems that oral hygiene is not a priority (Fitch and others, 1999). The nurse should recognize that these clients may not eat or drink orally; frequently they are mouth breathers or they have artificial airways, and they often have nasogastric or oxygen therapy. All of these factors contribute to drying of the mucosa and the formation of secretions and crusts on the tongue and mucous membranes. Some clients require mouth care as often as every 1 to 2 hours until the mucosa returns to normal. Many unconscious clients have no **gag reflex** as a result of neurological injury. The accumulation of salivary secretions in the mouth can easily lead to **aspiration.** Because oral secretions usually contain gram-negative bacteria, aspiration may lead to pneumonia. Proper oral hygiene requires keeping the oral mucosa moist and removing secretions that can lead to infection. Preventing deterioration of oral health is an important part of nursing care of the unconscious or debilitated client.

Delegation Considerations

Skills of brushing teeth of an unconscious or debilitated client can be delegated to assistive personnel. However, the nurse must first assess the client's gag reflex and then inform the assistive personnel of the proper way to position clients for mouth care. For this skill, assistive personnel must be able to safely use the oral suction catheter for clearing oral secretions (see Skill 13-1). As with all mouth care, care providers must know how to recognize impaired integrity of oral mucosa.

Equipment

- Antiinfective solution (e.g., diluted hydrogen peroxide) that loosens crusts
- Small soft-bristled toothbrush
- Sponge toothette or tongue blade wrapped in single layer of gauze
- Padded tongue blade
- Face towel
- Paper towels
- Emesis basin
- Water glass with cool water
- Water-soluble lip lubricant
- Small-bulb syringe (optional)
- Suction machine equipment (optional)
- Disposable gloves

Step	Rationale

Assessment

Step	Rationale
1. Wash hands. Apply disposable gloves.	Reduces transmission of microorganisms in blood or saliva.
2. Test for presence of gag reflex by placing tongue blade on back half of tongue.	Reveals whether client is at risk for aspiration.

- ***Critical Decision Point***
  Clients with impaired gag reflex require oral care as well. The nurse must determine the type of suction apparatus needed at the bedside to protect the client's airway against aspiration.

Step	Rationale
3. Inspect condition of oral cavity (see Chapter 10).	Determines condition of oral cavity and need for hygiene.
4. Remove gloves. Wash hands.	Prevents spread of infection.
5. Assess client's risk for oral hygiene problems (see Skill 6-3).	Certain conditions increase likelihood of alterations in integrity of oral cavity structures. May require more frequent care.

Nursing Diagnosis

Defining characteristics from the assessment data may reveal the following nursing diagnoses for clients requiring this skill:

Impaired oral mucous membrane
Risk for aspiration
Risk for injury

Related factors are individualized based on client's condition or needs.

Step	Rationale

Planning

1. **Expected outcomes** following completion of procedure:
   - Buccal mucosa and tongue are pink, moist, and intact. Gums are moist and intact. Teeth are cleaner, smooth, and shiny. Tongue is pink and without coating. Lips are moist, smooth, and without cracks. — Degree of improvement in condition of oral cavity structures will depend on extent of secretions or changes that existed before care.
   - Debilitated client expresses feeling of cleanliness. — Comfort achieved.
   - Oral pharynx remains patent. — Secretions removed, thus avoiding aspiration.
2. Unless contraindicated (e.g., head injury, neck trauma), position client on side (Sims' position) with head turned well toward dependent side and head of bed lowered. Raise side rail. — Allows secretions to drain from mouth instead of collecting in back of pharynx. Prevents aspiration.
3. Explain procedure to client. — Allows debilitated client to anticipate procedure without anxiety. Unconscious client may retain ability to hear.

Implementation

1. Wash hands and apply disposable gloves. — Reduces transfer of microorganisms.
2. Place paper towels on overbed table and arrange equipment. If needed, turn on suction machine and connect tubing to suction catheter. — Prevents soiling of table top. Equipment prepared in advance ensures smooth, safe procedure.
3. Pull curtain around bed or close room door. — Provides privacy.
4. Raise bed to its highest horizontal level; lower side rail. — Use of good body mechanics with bed in high position prevents injury.
5. Position client close to side of bed; turn client's head toward mattress. — Proper positioning of head prevents aspiration.
6. Place towel under client's head and emesis basin under chin. — Prevents soiling of bed linen.
7. Carefully separate upper and lower teeth with padded tongue blade by inserting blade, quickly but gently, between back molars. Insert when client is relaxed, if possible. Do not use force (see illustration). — Prevents client from biting down on nurse's fingers and provides access to oral cavity.

   • ***Critical Decision Point***
   Never use fingers to separate client's teeth.

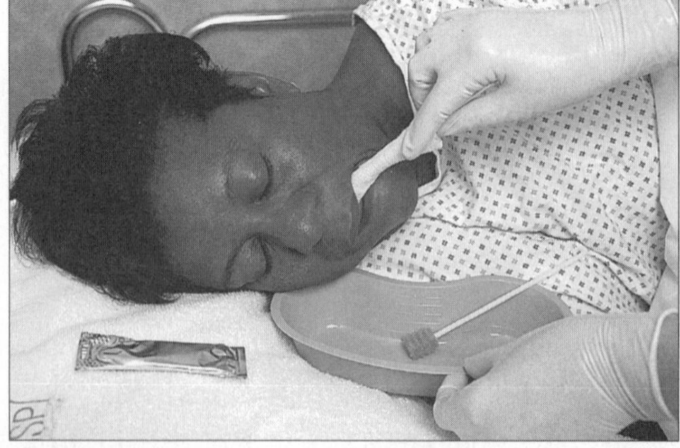

STEP **7** Separate upper and lower teeth with padded tongue blade.

8. Clean mouth using brush or sponge toothettes moistened with peroxide and water. Clean chewing and inner tooth surfaces first. Clean outer tooth surfaces. Swab roof of mouth, gums, and inside cheeks. Gently swab or brush tongue but avoid stimulating gag reflex (if present). Moisten — Brushing action removes food particles between teeth and along chewing surfaces. Swabbing helps remove secretions and crusts from mucosa and moistens mucosa. Repeated rinsing removes peroxide that can be irritating to mucosa.

STEP	RATIONALE
clean swab or toothette with water to rinse. (Bulb syringe may also be used to rinse.) Repeat rinse several times.	
9. Suction secretions as they accumulate, if necessary.	Suction removes secretions and fluid that can collect in posterior pharynx.
10. Apply thin layer of water-soluble jelly to lips (see illustration).	Lubricates lips to prevent drying and cracking.

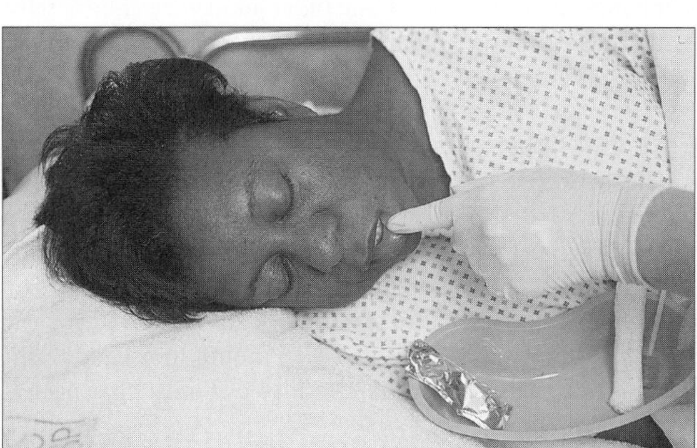

STEP **10** Application of water-soluble moisturizer to lips.

STEP	RATIONALE
11. Inform client that procedure is completed.	Provides meaningful stimulation to unconscious or less responsive client.
12. Raise side rails as appropriate. Remove gloves and dispose in proper receptacle.	Prevents transmission of microorganisms.
13. Reposition client comfortably and return bed to original position.	Maintains client's comfort and safety.
14. Clean equipment and return to its proper place. Place soiled linen in proper receptacle.	Proper disposal of soiled equipment prevents spread of infection.
15. Wash hands.	Reduces transmission of microorganisms.

EVALUATION

STEP	RATIONALE
1. Apply gloves and inspect oral cavity.	Determines efficacy of cleansing. Once thick secretions are removed, underlying inflammation or lesions may be revealed.
2. Ask debilitated client if mouth feels clean.	Evaluates level of comfort.
3. Assess client's respirations on an ongoing basis.	Ensures early recognition of aspiration.

UNEXPECTED OUTCOMES AND RELATED INTERVENTIONS

- Secretions or crusts remain on mucosa, tongue, or gums.
  - More frequent oral hygiene is needed.
  - A pediatric-size toothbrush may provide better hygiene (Fitch and others, 1999).
- Localized inflammation of gums or mucosa is present.
  - More frequent oral hygiene with soft-bristled toothbrush is needed.
  - Apply OralBalance moisturizing gel to mucosa and massage (Fitch and others, 1999).
  - Chemotherapy and radiation can cause stomatitis. Clients should rinse mouth before and after meals and at bedtime using normal saline or solution of ½ to 1 teaspoon of salt or baking soda to 1 pint of **tepid** water. To loosen and remove thick mucus, use one part of hydrogen peroxide to four parts of normal saline followed by warm water or saline rinse (Greifzu, Radjeski, and Winnick, 1990).
- Lips are cracked or inflamed.
  - Apply OralBalance moisturizing gel to lips or water soluble lubricant.
- Client aspirates secretions.
  - If present, suction oral airways as secretions accumulate to maintain patent airway (see Chapter 13).

RECORDING AND REPORTING

- Record procedure, including pertinent observations (e.g., presence of bleeding gums, dry mucosa, ulcerations, crusts on tongue).
- Report any unusual findings to nurse in charge or physician.

Teaching Considerations

- Family members may care for debilitated client in the home. Instruction in mouth care is needed so that family understands how to protect client from aspirating, while thoroughly cleansing oral cavity.

Pediatric Considerations

- As soon as teething begins, clean an infant's gum pads and teeth with a small piece of gauze twice a day (after breakfast and after the last meal of the day). This practice eliminates decay-producing plaque.
- Teach parents that a bottle given to a child at bedtime should contain only water. Falling asleep with a bottle of milk or juice or while breast-feeding bathes the teeth in a carbohydrate rich fluid that can cause cavities and tooth discoloration.
- Parents and caregivers need to be responsible for the child's oral hygiene for about the first 8 years, because the child does not develop the neural patterns and muscular coordination needed for performing mouth care until that age.
- Unless problems occur earlier, dental visits should begin about age 2. After the first visit, dental checkups every 6 months are encouraged (Wong and others, 1999).

Gerontological Considerations

- A number of normal age-related changes occur in the oral cavity. Thinning of the oral mucosa and decreased vascularity of the gingivae predispose older adults to injury and periodontal disease. Loss of tissue elasticity and decreased mass and strength of the muscles make chewing more difficult. Resorption of the alveolar bone can loosen natural teeth. The number of taste buds declines. In an attempt to enhance the taste of food, the older adult may choose salty and sugary foods, which erode tooth enamel and expose dentin (Pettigrew, 1989).

Home Care Considerations

- Irrigate oral cavity with bulb syringe; if unavailable, substitute gravy baster or large syringe.
- Encourage primary caregiver to cleanse client's mouth at least twice a day. If client breathes through mouth, gauze or soft linen may be wrapped around tongue blade, moistened, and used every 1 to 2 hours to keep mouth moist and fresh.
- A solution to use for oral care, available at most pharmacies, is carbamide peroxide.

Skill 6-5 Hair Care

Personal hygiene needs of the client also include hair care. Hair care consists of shampooing and shaving.

Shampooing a Client's Hair

The frequency of shampooing depends on condition of the hair and the person's daily routines. Hair condition may have gender and racial variations. Dry hair, which commonly results from aging and protein deficiency, requires less frequent shampooing than oily hair or the hair of people who exercise actively.

The nurse should remind hospitalized clients that staying in bed, excess perspiration, or treatments that leave blood or solutions in the hair may require more frequent shampoos. In a hospital setting it may be necessary to transport a client by stretcher to a special facility where a spray nozzle and sink are available for shampooing.

Clients who are allowed to sit in a chair usually can be shampooed in front of a sink. The individual should be positioned facing away from the sink, with the head and neck hyperextended over the sink's edge. A folded towel placed under the neck on the edge of the sink provides added comfort. If the client must sit at the bedside, it is possible to shampoo the hair as the client leans forward over a wash basin. Caution is needed with clients who have suffered neck injuries, since flexion and hyperextension of the neck could cause further injury.

Delegation Considerations

The skill of shampooing can be delegated to assistive personnel. Before delegation inform and assist care provider in proper way to position clients with head or neck mobility restrictions and review any procedures for use of medicated shampoo for lice; stress the steps to take to prevent transmission to other clients.

If the client cannot sit in a chair or be transferred to a stretcher, shampooing must be done with the client in bed (Procedural Guidelines Box 6-2). This may be done after the bath (common in the care of infants) or later as a separate procedure.

Box 6-2 Procedural Guidelines

Shampooing Hair of Bed-Bound Client

Equipment: Bath towels, washcloths, shampoo and hair conditioner (optional), water pitcher, plastic shampoo trough, washbasin, bath blanket, waterproof pad, clean comb and brush, hair dryer (optional)

1. Before washing client's hair, determine that there are no contraindications to this procedure. Certain medical conditions, such as head and neck injuries, spinal cord injuries, and arthritis, could place the client at risk for injury during shampooing because of positioning and manipulation of client's head and neck.
2. Inspect the hair and scalp before initiating the procedure. This determines the presence of any conditions that may require the use of special shampoos or treatments (e.g., for dandruff or the removal of dried blood) (Table 6-2).
3. Place waterproof pad under client's shoulders, neck, and head (see illustration). Position client supine, with head and shoulders at top edge of bed. Place plastic trough under client's head and washbasin at end of trough. Be sure trough spout extends beyond edge of mattress.
4. Place rolled towel under client's neck and bath towel over client's shoulders.
5. Brush and comb client's hair.
6. Obtain warm water.
7. Ask client to hold face towel or washcloth over eyes.
8. Slowly pour water from water pitcher over hair until it is completely wet (see illustration). If hair contains matted blood, apply gloves, apply peroxide to dissolve clots, and then rinse hair with saline. Apply small amount of shampoo.
9. Work up lather with both hands. Start at hairline, and work toward back of neck. Lift head slightly with one hand to wash back of head. Shampoo sides of head. Massage scalp by applying pressure with fingertips.
10. Rinse hair with water. Make sure water drains into basin. Repeat rinsing until hair is free of soap.
11. Apply conditioner or cream rinse if requested, and rinse hair thoroughly.
12. Wrap client's head in bath towel. Dry client's face with cloth used to protect eyes. Dry off any moisture along neck or shoulders.
13. Dry client's hair and scalp. Use second towel if first becomes saturated.
14. Comb hair to remove tangles, and dry with dryer if desired.
15. Apply oil preparation or conditioning product to hair, if desired by client.
16. Assist client to comfortable position, and complete styling of hair.

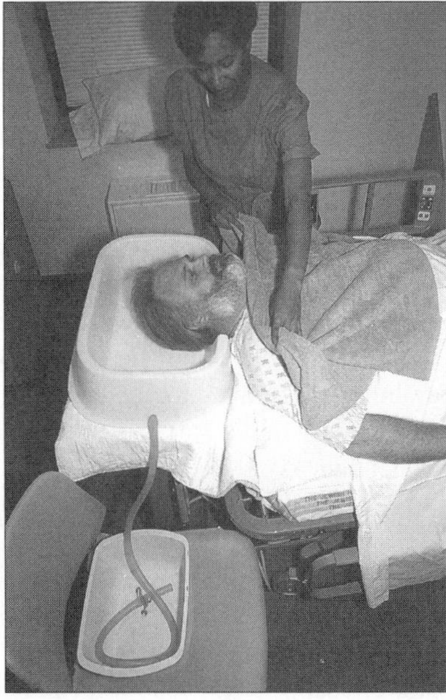

STEP **3** Client with waterproof pad under shoulders, neck, and head.

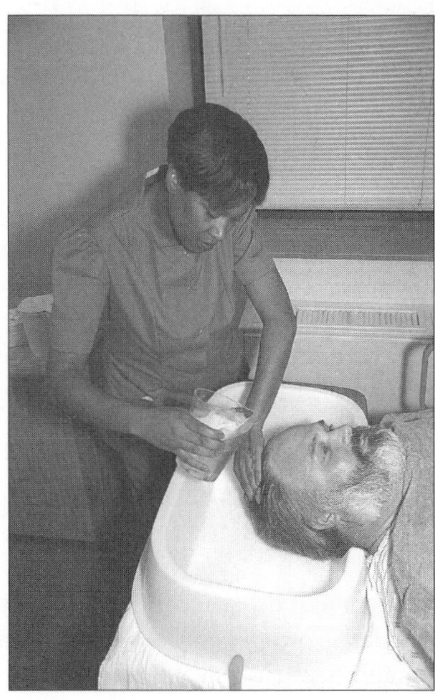

STEP **8** Pour water over hair.

Table 6-2 Hair and Scalp Problems

PROBLEM	CHARACTERISTICS	IMPLICATIONS	INTERVENTIONS
Dandruff	Scaling of the scalp accompanied by itching; in severe cases, dandruff on eyebrows.	Dandruff causes embarrassment; if dandruff enters eyes, conjunctivitis may develop.	Shampoo regularly with medicated shampoo; in severe cases seek physician's advice.
Ticks	Small gray-brown parasites that burrow into skin and suck blood.	Ticks transmit several diseases to people; most common are Rocky Mountain spotted fever, Lyme disease, and tularemia.	Do not pull ticks from skin because sucking apparatus remains and may become infected; placing drop of oil or ether on tick or covering it with petrolatum eases removal; oil suffocates tick.
Pediculosis capitis (head lice)	Tiny grayish white parasitic insects that attach to hair strands; eggs look like oval particles, resemble dandruff; bites or pustules may be observed behind ears and at hairline.	Head lice are difficult to remove and if not treated may spread to furniture and other people.	Use medicated shampoo for eliminating lice; repeat 12 to 24 hours later; change bed linens, using isolation precautions required by agency.
Pediculosis corporis (body lice)	Tend to cling to clothing so may not be easily seen; body lice suck blood and lay eggs on clothing and furniture.	Client itches constantly; scratches on skin may become infected; hemorrhagic spots may appear on skin where lice are sucking blood.	Client should bathe or shower thoroughly; after skin is dried, apply lotion for eliminating lice; after 12 to 24 hours another bath or shower should be taken; bag infested clothing or linen until laundered.
Pediculosis pubis (crab lice)	Found in pubic hair; crab lice are grayish white with red legs.	Lice may spread through bed linen, clothing, or furniture or sexual contact.	Shave hair off affected area; cleanse as for body lice; if lice were sexually transmitted, partner must be notified.
Alopecia	Occurs in all races. Balding patches in periphery of hairline, hair becomes brittle and broken; caused by improper use of hair curlers and picks, tight braiding, hot styling tools, certain diseases.	Patches of uneven hair growth and loss alter client's appearance.	Stop hair care practices that damage hair.

Shaving a Client

Shaving of facial hair can be done after a bath or shampoo. Most men prefer to do this task for themselves. However, when a client is physically unable to shave, the nurse should be able to perform the procedure as quickly and comfortably as possible. Men without beards usually shave daily. Clients with mustaches and beards require daily grooming. Keeping these areas clean is important because food particles collect easily in the hair. The beard or mustache should be trimmed, combed, or washed as needed or at the client's request. The nurse should never shave off a mustache or beard without client consent. Some religions and cultures forbid cutting or shaving any body hair (e.g., the Sikh religion) (Galanti, 1991).

Some women may wish to shave the hair under their arms or on their legs. Generally, it is not necessary for women to shave each day, but some may prefer it. The technique used to shave a woman's axillary or leg hair is the same as that for the male client's facial hair.

Delegation Considerations

The skill of shaving can be delegated to assistive personnel. Instruct care provider in proper way to position clients with head or neck mobility restrictions. Review any individualized skin care guidelines.

Equipment

- Disposable razor: razor with new blade, disposable gloves (optional), bath towel(s), mirror, washcloth, washbasin, shaving cream or soap, aftershave lotion (if client desires)
- Electric razor: razor (with clean cutting heads), bath towel, skin or beard conditioner, mirror, aftershave lotion (if client desires)
- Mustache care: scissors, brush or comb, bath towel, gooseneck lamp or overhead light, mirror

STEP	RATIONALE

ASSESSMENT

Step	Rationale
1. Assess if client has bleeding tendency. Review medical history or laboratory values (e.g., platelet counts, prothrombin time).	Determines need to use electric razor for client's safety.

• ***Critical Decision Point***
Clients receiving anticoagulant therapy should use an electric razor.

Step	Rationale
2. Assess client's ability to manipulate razor.	Determines level of assistance required.
3. Assess client's preferences for shaving products (e.g., after-shave lotion, skin conditioner, shaving cream).	Promotes client's independence through decision making.

NURSING DIAGNOSIS

Defining characteristics from the assessment data may reveal the following nursing diagnoses for clients requiring this skill:

Dressing/grooming self-care deficit
Impaired physical mobility
Risk for injury

Related factors are individualized based on client's condition or needs.

PLANNING

Step	Rationale
1. **Expected outcomes** following completion of procedure:	
▪ Client expresses sense of comfort, with sensation of face feeling clean and refreshed.	Hair and soap lather are removed.
▪ Skin surface is smooth, well hydrated, and free of cuts.	Client is free from injury.
▪ Client assists with procedure.	Participation provides sense of control.
2. While performing actual procedure, ask client to explain steps he or she uses to shave. Ask client to indicate if shave becomes uncomfortable.	Client can become apprehensive about being accidentally cut.

IMPLEMENTATION

Disposable Razor

Step	Rationale
1. Arrange supplies at bedside table and adjust lighting.	Easy access to supplies prevents interruption of procedure. Lighting provides clear view of client's face.
2. Assist client to sitting or supine position with head of bed elevated.	Provides easy access to all sides of client's face.
3. Place bath towel over client's chest and shoulders.	Prevents shaving cream or water from soiling gown.
4. Run warm water in washbasin. Check water temperature.	Warm water will soften beard. Proper temperature prevents accidental burns.
5. Place washcloth in basin and wring out thoroughly. Apply cloth over client's entire face for several seconds.	Warm cloth helps soften skin and beard. Sensation of warmth can be relaxing.

• ***Critical Decision Point***
If client has sores, open lesions, or a tendency to bleed, the nurse should apply disposable gloves.

Step	Rationale
6. Apply shaving cream or soap to client's face. Smooth cream evenly over sides of face, chin, and under nose.	Cream creates additional softening effect and lubricates skin for application of razor.

STEP	RATIONALE
7. Hold razor in dominant hand at 45-degree angle to the client's skin. Begin by shaving across one side of client's face. Use nondominant hand to gently pull skin taut while shaving.	Use short, firm strokes in direction hair grows (see illustration). Short downward strokes work best over upper lip. Holding skin taut prevents razor cuts and discomfort during shaving.

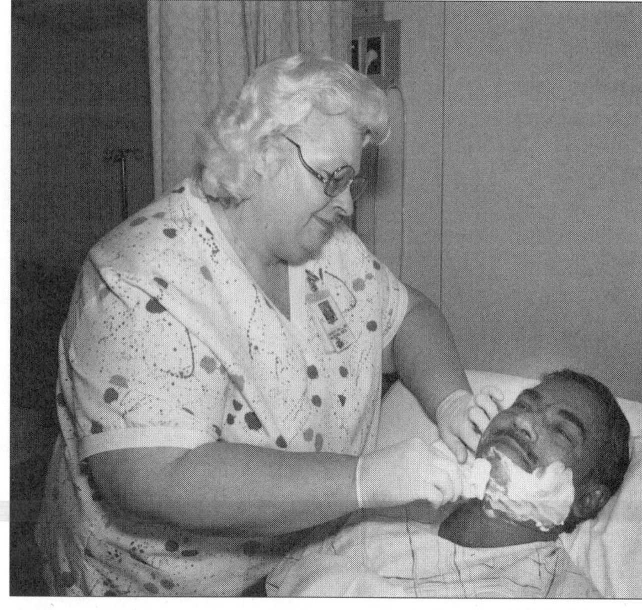

STEP 7 Shaving a client using short, firm strokes.

STEP	RATIONALE
8. Dip razor blade in water as shaving cream accumulates on blade's edge.	Keeps cutting surface of razor blade clean.
9. After all facial hair is shaved, rinse face thoroughly with moistened washcloth.	Prevents accumulation of shaving cream, which can cause drying of skin.
10. Dry face thoroughly and apply aftershave lotion if desired.	Retained moisture may cause chapping of skin.
11. Assist client to comfortable position.	
12. Return equipment to proper place. Discard soiled linen in hamper. Wash hands.	Maintains cleanliness of client's environment and reduces transmission of infection.

Electric Razor

STEP	RATIONALE
1. Perform Steps 1 through 3 for disposable razor.	
2. Apply skin conditioner or preshave preparation.	Softens skin and beard to reduce friction from razor head.
3. Turn razor on and begin by shaving across side of face. Gently hold skin taut while shaving over skin's surface. Use gentle downward stroke of razor in direction of hair growth.	Prevents pulling of beard and skin.
4. After completing shave, apply aftershave lotion as desired.	Stimulates and lubricates skin.
5. Perform Steps 11 and 12 for disposable razor.	

Mustache and Beard Care

STEP	RATIONALE
1. Perform Steps 1 through 3 for disposable razor.	
2. If necessary, gently comb mustache or beard.	Straightens hair that requires trimming.
3. Allow client to use mirror and direct areas to trim with scissors.	Allows client to make decisions about care; maintains sense of independence.

EVALUATION

STEP	RATIONALE
1. Inspect condition of shaved area and skin underneath beard or mustache.	Nurse looks for areas of localized bleeding from cuts and for areas of dryness.
2. Ask client if face feels clean and comfortable.	Evaluates level of client's comfort.
3. Ask if client is satisfied with degree of participation.	Client maintains sense of control.

Unexpected Outcomes and Related Interventions

- Small isolated nicks or cuts may appear on skin.
  - Obtain a new disposable razor or change the blade.
  - Change technique so as to glide razor over the client's skin.
- Skin surface may appear dry.
  - This is a result of soap drying skin; use a moisturizing shaving foam.
  - Apply moisturizing lotion to client's skin after shave.

Recording and Reporting

- It is not necessary to record shaving procedure unless it is included on the agency's checklist.

Teaching Considerations

- Shaving is a simple procedure that can be taught to a family member. Instruct primary caregiver in safety precautions for shaving, especially if client is receiving anticoagulant therapy.
- Instruct family member in technique to follow in the event the client is accidentally nicked.

Pediatric Considerations

- Usually the facial hair of adolescents does not grow quickly, and thus a shave might not be necessary each day.

Gerontological Considerations

- Usually the facial hair of older clients does not grow quickly, and a shave might not be necessary each day.

Home Care Considerations

- Provide adequate towels around client's neck to avoid spilling shaving cream or water on chest or bed.
- Provide adequate lighting for procedure.
- Perform procedure in comfortable setting, such as bathroom or bedroom.

Skill 6-6 Performing Nail and Foot Care

Feet and nails often require special care to prevent infection, odors, and injury to soft tissues. Often people are unaware of foot or nail problems until discomfort or pain occurs. Common foot and nail problems are listed in Table 6-3. Foot disorders, including **neuropathy,** infection, and ulceration, are a constant threat to the independence of a client with diabetes or vascular conditions (Slovenkai, 1998). Problems often result from abuse or poor care of the feet and hands, such as biting nails or trimming them improperly, exposure to harsh chemicals, or wearing ill-fitting shoes. Changes in the shape, color, and texture of nails may result from various nutritional, infectious, and circulatory disorders.

The feet are important to a person's physical and emotional health. Foot pain may cause a person to change gait, resulting in strain on different muscle groups. If job performance requires a person to walk or stand comfortably, a foot disorder can become a serious problem.

Nails are epithelial tissues that grow from the root of the nail bed located in the skin at the nail groove. A normal healthy nail is transparent, smooth, and convex. Color includes variations of pink with translucent white tips. Pigment deposits or bands are common in nail beds of clients with dark skin. The nail bed angle should measure 160 degrees. The nail is surrounded by a **cuticle,** which slowly grows over the nail and must be regularly pushed back. The skin around the nail beds and cuticles should be smooth and without inflammation.

Nail and foot care should be included in a client's daily hygiene; the best time is during the client's bath.

Delegation Considerations

The skill of nail and foot care of the nondiabetic client can be delegated to assistive personnel. Inform and assist care provider in proper way to use nail clippers, and caution the care provider to use warm water.

Equipment

- Washbasin
- Emesis basin
- Washcloth
- Bath or face towel
- Nail clippers
- Orange stick (optional)
- Emery board or nail file
- Body lotion
- Disposable bath mat
- Paper towels
- Disposable gloves

Table 6-3 Common Foot and Nail Problems

CONDITION	CHARACTERISTICS	IMPLICATIONS	INTERVENTIONS
Callus	Thickened portion of epidermis, consisting of mass of horny, keratotic cells; usually flat, painless, and found on undersurface of foot or on palm of hand; caused by local friction or pressure.	Foot calluses may cause discomfort when wearing tight-fitting shoes.	Advise client to wear gloves when using tools or objects that may create friction on palms. Encourage client to wear comfortable shoes. Soak callus in warm water and Epsom salts to soften cell layers. Use pumice stone to remove callus after it softens. Applications of creams or lotions can reduce re-formation. Use of orthotic devices (e.g., foam insoles, metatarsal pads, various cushioning devices) redistributes weight and pressure away from callus area.
Corns	Keratosis caused by friction and pressure from shoes; mainly on toes, over bony prominence; usually come shaped, round, and raised. Calluses with painful core.	Conical shape compresses underlying dermis, making it thin and tender. Pain is aggravated by tight-fitting shoes. Tissue can become attached to bone if allowed to grow. Clients may suffer alteration in gait because of pain.	Surgical removal may be necessary, depending on severity of pain and size of corn. Use oval corn pads carefully, since they increase pressure on toes and reduce circulation.
Plantar warts	Fungating lesion that appears on sole of foot; caused by Papillomavirus.	Warts may be contagious, are painful, and make walking difficult.	Refer client to podiatrist.
Athlete's foot (tinea pedis)	Fungal infection of foot; scaliness and cracking of skin between toes and on soles of feet; small blisters containing fluid may appear, apparently induced by constricting footwear (e.g., sneakers).	Athlete's foot can spread to other body parts, especially hands. It is contagious and frequently recurs.	Feet should be well ventilated. Drying feet well after bathing and applying powder help prevent infection. Wearing clean socks or stockings reduces incidence. Physician may order application of griseofulvin, miconazole nitrate, or tolnaftate.
Ingrown nails	Toenail or fingernail growing inward into soft tissue around nail; results from improper nail trimming, poor shoe fit, or heredity.	Ingrown nails can cause localized pain when pressure is applied.	Treatment is frequent warm soaks in antiseptic solution and removal of portion of nail that has grown into skin. Instruct client on proper nail trimming techniques. Professional debridement of offending nail border or removal of affected nail margin may be necessary.
Ram's horn nails	Unusually long curved nails.	Attempt by nurse to cut nails may damage nail bed and/or cause infection.	Refer client to podiatrist.
Paronychia	Inflammation of tissue surrounding nail after hangnail or other injury; occurs in people who frequently have their hands in water; common in diabetic clients.	Area can become infected.	Treatment is hot compresses or soaks and local application of antibiotic ointments. Paronychia can be prevented by careful manicuring.
Foot odors	Result of excess perspiration promoting microorganism growth. Faulty foot hygiene or improper footwear may also contribute.		Frequent washing, use of foot deodorants and powders, and clean footwear will prevent or reduce this problem.

STEP	RATIONALE
ASSESSMENT	
1. Inspect all surfaces of fingers, toes, feet, and nails. Pay particular attention to areas of dryness, inflammation, or cracking. Also inspect areas between toes, heels, and soles of feet.	Integrity of feet and nails determines frequency and level of hygiene required. Heels, soles, and sides of feet are prone to irritation from ill-fitting shoes. Proper footwear is essential in reducing the risk of injury and subsequent ulcer formation (Armstrong and Lavery, 1998).

• ***Critical Decision Point***

Clients with peripheral vascular diseases, diabetes mellitus, older adults, and clients whose immune system is suppressed may require nail care from a specialist to reduce the risk for infection.

STEP	RATIONALE
2. Assess color and temperature of toes, feet, and fingers. Assess capillary refill of nails. Palpate radial and ulnar pulse of each hand and dorsalis pedis pulse of foot; note character of pulses.	Assesses adequacy of blood flow to extremities. Circulatory alterations may change integrity of nails and increase client's chance of localized infection when break in skin integrity occurs (Strauss, Hart, and Winant, 1998).
3. Observe client's walking gait. Have client walk down hall or walk straight line (if able).	Painful disorders of feet can cause limping or unnatural gait (Armstrong and Lavery, 1998).
4. Ask female clients about whether they use nail polish and polish remover frequently.	Chemicals in these products can cause excessive dryness.
5. Assess type of footwear worn by clients: Are socks worn? Are shoes tight or ill fitting? Are garters or knee-high nylons worn? Is footwear clean?	Types of shoes and footwear may predispose client to foot and nail problems (e.g., infection, areas of friction, ulcerations).
6. Identify client's risk for foot or nail problems:	Certain conditions increase likelihood of foot or nail problems.
a. Elderly	Poor vision, lack of coordination, or inability to bend over contribute to difficulty among elderly in performing foot and nail care. Normal physiological changes of aging also result in nail and foot problems.
b. Diabetes	Vascular changes associated with diabetes reduce blood flow to peripheral tissues. Break in skin integrity places diabetic at high risk for skin infection. Lower extremity complications of diabetes can involve nerves, muscles, bone, and vasculature, therefore making assessment of and management of foot problems complex (Cooppan and Habershaw, 1995).
c. Heart failure, renal disease	Both conditions can increase tissue edema, particularly in dependent areas (e.g., feet). Edema reduces blood flow to neighboring tissues.
d. Cerebrovascular accident, stroke	Presence of residual foot or leg weakness or paralysis results in altered walking patterns. Altered gait pattern causes increased friction and pressure on feet.
7. Assess type of home remedies clients use for existing foot problems:	Certain preparations or applications may cause more injury to soft tissue then initial foot problem.
a. Over-the-counter liquid preparations to remove corns	Liquid preparations can cause burns and ulcerations.
b. Cutting of corns or calluses with razor blade or scissors	Cutting of corns or calluses may result in infection caused by break in skin integrity.
c. Use of oval corn pads	Oval pads may exert pressure on toes, thereby decreasing circulation to surrounding tissues.
d. Application of adhesive tape	Skin of older adult is thin and delicate and prone to tearing when adhesive tape is removed.
8. Assess client's ability to care for nails or feet: visual alterations, fatigue, musculoskeletal weakness.	Extent of client's ability to perform self-care determines degree of assistance required from nurse.
9. Assess client's knowledge of foot and nail care practices.	Level of client's knowledge determines client's need for health teaching.

STEP	RATIONALE

NURSING DIAGNOSIS

Defining characteristics from the assessment data may reveal the following nursing diagnoses for clients requiring this skill:

- Ineffective tissue perfusion
- Dressing/grooming self-care deficit
- Impaired physical mobility
- Impaired skin integrity
- Deficient knowledge regarding foot and nail care
- Risk for infection
- Risk for injury

Related factors are individualized based on client's condition or needs.

PLANNING

1. **Expected outcomes** following completion of procedure:
   - Nails are smooth. Cuticles and tissues surrounding nail are clear and of normal color. Surfaces of feet are smooth. — Excess skin layers are removed. Nail integrity and cleanliness are maintained.
   - Client walks freely, without pain or unusual gait. — Sources of pressure or irritation are removed (Slovenkai, 1998).
   - Client explains or demonstrates nail care correctly. — Client learns skill.
2. Explain procedure to client, including fact that proper soaking requires several minutes. — Client must be willing to place fingers and feet in basins for 10 to 20 minutes. Client may become anxious or fatigued.
3. Obtain physician's order for cutting nails if agency policy requires it. — Client's skin may be accidentally cut. Certain clients are more at risk for infection, depending on their medical condition.

IMPLEMENTATION

1. Wash hands. Arrange equipment on overbed table. — Easy access to equipment prevents delays.
2. Pull curtain around bed or close room door (if desired). — Maintaining client's privacy reduces anxiety.
3. Assist ambulatory client to sit in bedside chair. Help bedfast client to supine position with head of bed elevated. Place disposable bath mat on floor under client's feet or place towel on mattress. — Sitting in chair facilitates immersing feet in basin. Bath mat protects feet from exposure to soil or debris.
4. Fill washbasin with warm water. Test water temperature. — Warm water softens nails and thickened epidermal cells, reduces inflammation of skin, and promotes local circulation. Proper water temperature prevents burns and injury (Armstrong and Lavery, 1998).
5. Place basin on bath mat or towel and help client place feet in basin. Place call light within client's reach. — Clients with muscular weakness or tremors may have difficulty positioning feet. Client's safety is maintained.
6. Adjust overbed table to low position and place it over client's lap. (Client may sit in chair or lie in bed.) — Easy access prevents accidental spills.
7. Fill emesis basin with warm water and place basin on paper towels on overbed table. — Warm water softens nails and thickened epidermal cells.
8. Instruct client to place fingers in emesis basin and place arms in comfortable position. — Prolonged positioning can cause discomfort unless normal anatomical alignment is maintained.
9. Allow client's feet and fingernails to soak for 10 to 20 minutes. Rewarm water after 10 minutes. — Softening of corns, calluses, and cuticles ensures easy removal of dead cells and easy manipulation of cuticle.

   • ***Critical Decision Point***
   Diabetic clients should never soak hands and feet.

10. Clean gently under fingernails with orange stick while fingers are immersed (see illustration). Remove emesis basin and dry fingers thoroughly. — Orange stick removes debris under nails that harbors microorganisms. Thorough drying impedes fungal growth and prevents maceration of tissues.
11. With nail clippers, clip fingernails straight across and even with tops of fingers (see illustration). Shape nails with emery board or file. If client has circulatory problems, do not cut nail; file the nail only. — Cutting straight across prevents splitting of nail margins and formation of sharp nail spikes that can irritate lateral nail margins. Filing prevents cutting nail too close to nail bed (Strauss, Hart, and Winant, 1998).

STEP	RATIONALE

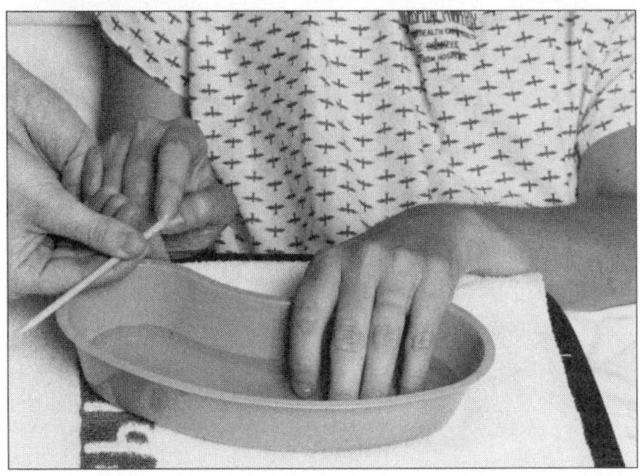

STEP 10 Cleanse under fingernails with orange stick.

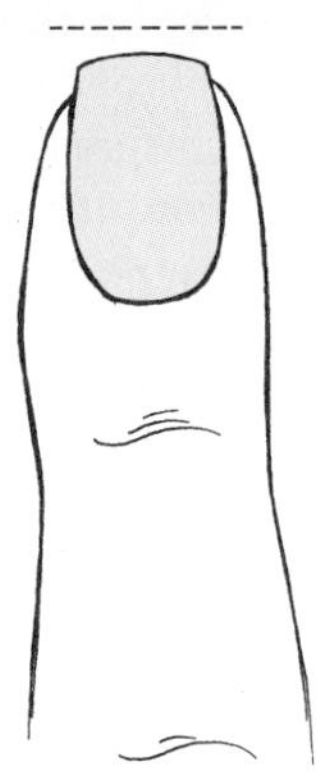

STEP 11 Nails are trimmed straight across.

A

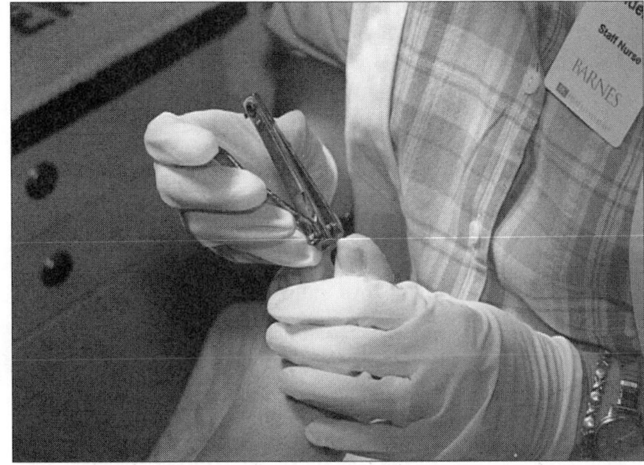

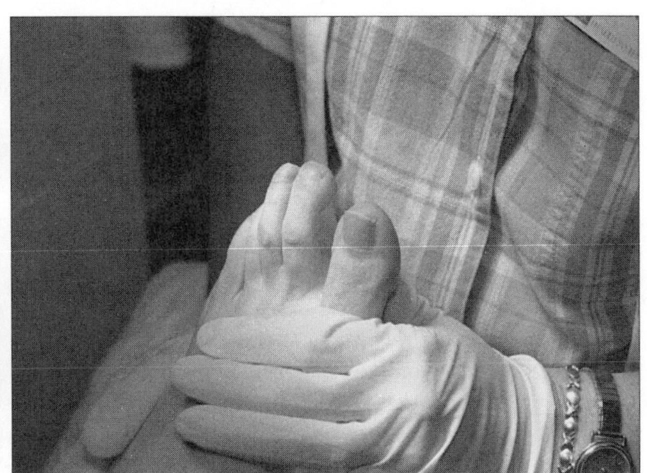

B

STEP 16 **A,** Trim toenails straight across. **B,** Toenail after trimming.

STEP	RATIONALE
12. Push cuticle back gently with orange stick.	Pushing back cuticles reduces incidence of inflamed cuticles.
13. Move overbed table away from client.	Provides easier access to feet.
14. Apply disposable gloves and scrub callused areas of feet with washcloth.	Gloves prevent transmission of fungal infection. Friction removes dead skin layers.
15. Clean gently under nails with orange stick. Remove feet from basin and dry thoroughly.	Removal of debris and excess moisture reduces chances of infection.
16. Clean and trim toenails using procedures in Steps 11 and 12 (see illustrations). Do not file corners of toenails.	Shaping corners of toenails may damage tissues (Strauss, Hart, and Winant, 1998).
17. Apply lotion to feet and hands and assist client back to bed and into comfortable position.	Lotion lubricates dry skin by helping to retain moisture.
18. Remove disposable gloves and place in receptacle. Clean and return equipment and supplies to proper place. Dispose of soiled linen in hamper. Wash hands.	Reduces transmission of infection.

Evaluation

1. Inspect nails and surrounding skin surfaces.	Inspection enables nurse to evaluate condition of skin and nails and allows nurse to note any remaining rough nail edges.
2. Ask client to explain or demonstrate nail care.	Demonstration allows nurse to evaluate client's level of learning techniques.
3. Observe client's walk after toenail care.	Observation allows nurse to evaluate level of comfort and mobility achieved.

Unexpected Outcomes and Related Interventions

- Nails discolored, rough, and concave or irregular in shape.
  - Continue hygiene practice because a single hygiene measure will not improve nail condition.
- Cuticles and surrounding tissues may be inflamed and tender to touch. Localized areas of tenderness may occur on feet with calluses or corns at point of friction.
  - Repeated nail care is needed.
  - Referral to **podiatrist** may be needed.
- Ulcerations involving toes or feet may remain.
  - Institute wound care policies.
  - Consult with wound care specialist and/or podiatrist.
- Client unable to explain or perform foot care.
  - Provide client teaching and demonstration of foot care.
  - Use return demonstration to document client learning.
- Client complains of pain while walking and has unsteady gait.
  - Pressure or irritation on foot is still present; client may need referral to podiatrist.

Recording and Reporting

- Record procedure and observations (e.g., breaks in skin, inflammation, ulcerations).
- Report any breaks in skin or ulcerations to nurse in charge or physician.

Teaching Considerations

- Instruct nondiabetic client to wash and soak feet daily using lukewarm water. Thoroughly pat feet dry and dry well between toes.
- Caution client against cutting corns or calluses or using commercial removers. Consult physician or podiatrist.
- If feet tend to perspire, apply mild foot powder.
- Encouraging client to wear absorbent liners with nylon stockings will also help reduce perspiration and foot odors. Seamless white socks are preferred, since they are more absorbent (Strauss, Hart, and Winant, 1998).
- If dryness is noted along feet or between toes, apply lanolin, baby oil, or even corn oil and rub gently into skin.
- Teach client to avoid wearing elastic stockings or constricting garters and to avoid crossing legs. Both impair circulation to lower extremities.
- Inspect feet daily: tops and soles, heels, and area between toes. Use mirror to check soles and heels.
- Encourage client to wear clean socks or stockings daily (change twice a day if feet perspire a lot).
- Check for holes or darns that might cause pressure.
- Caution client against walking barefoot. Clients with impaired foot circulation should wear protective footwear at all times and check inside of shoes daily for pebbles, foreign objects, and tears in inner liner (Osterman and Stuck, 1990).
- Encourage client to wear proper-fitting shoes. Soles of shoes should be flexible and nonslipping. Shoes should have porous uppers and be sturdy, closed in, and not restrictive to the feet (Slovenkai, 1998).
- Minor cuts should be washed immediately and dried thoroughly. Only mild antiseptics (e.g., Neosporin ointment) should be applied to the skin. Avoid iodine or merbromin.

Gerontological Considerations

- Changes in aging skin include thinning of epidermis and subcutaneous fat and dryness because of decreased activity of oil and sweat glands. These changes can be seen in the feet. In addition, nails become opaque, tough, scaly, brittle, and hypertrophied.
- A lifetime of limited exercise can result in laxity of foot ligaments and musculature and lead to instability and impaired mobility.
- Common foot problems of older adults include heel pain caused by tearing of plantar fascia and foot musculature, metatarsalgia (pain beneath metatarsal head), hammer toes and claw toes, corns and calluses, pathological nail conditions (e.g., ingrown toenails, fungal infections), arthritis, and neuropathies that cause diminished sensation in foot (Lueckenotte, 2000).
- Older persons are also more vulnerable to bunions because feet tend to spread with aging. Young people are rarely affected, although bunions sometimes occur in individuals as young as 10 to 13 years of age (Luekenotte, 2000).

Home Care Considerations

- Alternative therapies: moleskin applied to areas of feet that are under friction is less likely to cause local pressure than corn pads; spot adhesive bandages can guard corns against friction but do not have padding to protect against pressure; wrapping small pieces of lamb's wool around toes reduces irritation of soft corns between toes (Beuscher, 1998).

Skill 6-7 Care of the Client's Environment

When caring for clients who need to remain in or near their bed for an extended period, it is important to try to make that environment as comfortable as possible. A calm, comfortable restorative environment can be maintained in a hospital, in an extended care facility, or in the client's home.

Rooms should be comfortable, safe, and large enough to allow clients, visitors, and care providers to move about freely. The care provider should be able to control temperature, ventilation, noise, and odors easily.

A room in a typical hospital, extended care, or long-term care facility contains the following basic pieces of furniture: overbed table, bedside stand, storage space, chairs, lights, and bed with call light. These furnishings provide a setting for the client to rest, as well as safe and convenient access to all client care supplies. Behind each bed is a wall unit that may contain various power outlets and receptacles for connecting oxygen and suction equipment. In most hospitals a mercury sphygmomanometer with cuff is attached to the wall. Special intensive care units often have poles extending from the ceiling on which to hang intravenous (IV) fluid bags. The room is generally designed so that all necessary supplies and equipment are easily accessible for the nurse and physician's use.

When care is provided in the client's home, special equipment and adaptations to the client's home may be necessary. If a client is to receive home oxygen, then oxygen tanks are needed, and with some oxygen equipment, the client may need additional electrical wiring in the home. Clients and their families may need to order a hospital bed and overbed table so that physical care can be given easily. In addition, the client's bathroom is adapted with safety equipment for ease in toileting and getting into and out of the tub and shower.

Room Equipment

Chairs

Most hospital rooms contain an armless, straight-back chair and an upholstered lounge chair with arms. When clients are recovering from surgery or illnesses resulting in abdominal pain, they often prefer the straight-back chair because less effort is needed to get into or out of it. Straight-back chairs are convenient when temporarily transferring the client from the bed, for example, during bed making. The straight-back chair is also easier to maneuver than the heavy lounge chair. However, the straight-back chair may be more uncomfortable and less safe for certain clients than the deeper lounge chair. The lounge chair often has a deeper seat and may require more effort on the part of the client to sit comfortably.

Lights

Each room has an overbed light that focuses on the client's bed. The light controls are usually on the call light apparatus. Each room also has a floor or table lamp. Special examination lights may extend over the bed from the wall or ceiling. These lights are useful during procedures such as a dressing change. They are often moveable and should be positioned for easy reach but moved aside when not in use. Portable lamps provide extra illumination for bedside procedures. These are especially useful to focus light on hard-to-reach areas, for example, during urinary catheter insertion.

A call light is at each client's bedside. When a client presses a button located on the side rail of the bed or at the end of an extension cord, a light goes on at the nurses' station or outside the client's room. The call light signal indicates that a client needs assistance and is "calling" the nurse. In addition to call lights, most hospitals have intercom systems that allow clients to talk to a staff person at the nurses' station (Figure 6-3). Many hospital units also have emergency signal lights, particularly in the client's bathroom, which nurses use to call for assistance when clients are in trouble. Clients may also be instructed to use the emergency signal lights if an emergency situation arises when they are in the bathroom alone.

Overbed Tables

The overbed table is a long, narrow table with wheels. It can be adjusted to various heights over the client's bed or chair. It usually contains two storage drawers. The table provides ideal working space for the nurse and serves as a surface on which to place meal trays, toiletry items, and objects frequently used by the client.

Bedside Stand

The bedside stand or table is a small table or cabinet located next to the bed. It is used to store the client's personal articles and hygiene equipment such as the bath basin, towels, or an emesis basin. Each table usually contains a drawer above and a cupboard below. The telephone, water pitcher, facial

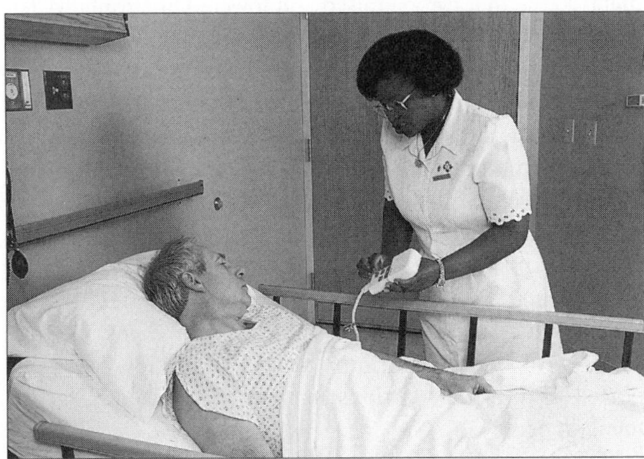

FIGURE 6-3 Nurse teaching client how to use intercom to nurses' station.

Table 6-4 Common Bed Positions

Position	Description	Uses
Fowler's	Head of bed raised to angle of 45 to 90 degrees or more; semisitting position (knees raise on most beds approximately 15 degrees).	Preferred while client eats; used during nasogastric tube insertion and nasotracheal suction; promotes lung expansion.
Semi-Fowler's	Head of bed raised approximately 30 to 45 degrees; incline is less than Fowler's position (knees raise on most beds approximately 15 degrees).	Promotes lung expansion; relieves strain on abdominal muscles.
Trendelenburg's	Entire bed frame tilted, with head of bed down.	For postural drainage; facilitates venous return in clients with poor peripheral perfusion.
Reverse Trendelenburg's	Entire bed frame tilted, with foot of bed down.	Used infrequently; promotes gastric emptying and prevents esophageal reflux.
Flat	Entire bed frame parallel with floor.	For clients with vertebral injuries and in cervical traction. Position used for clients who are hypotensive, and generally preferred by clients for sleeping.

tissues, and drinking cup are commonly placed on the bedside table.

Beds

Because the bed is the piece of equipment used most by the client, it should be designed for comfort and safety, and it should be adaptable to various positions.

The typical hospital bed consists of a firm mattress on a metal frame that can be raised and lowered horizontally. The frame is divided into three sections so that the operator can raise and lower the head and foot of the bed separately, in addition to inclining the entire bed with the head up or down. Table 6-4 lists common bed positions. Most beds are powered by electric motors, but some beds operate manually or by hydraulic power.

Hospital beds come in two different lengths. Standard length is approximately 6 feet (a longer bed is available for taller clients). Each bed sits on four rollers, or casters, that allow the nurse to move the bed easily. Often clients who are critically ill or who are immobilized in traction are transported to different locations, such as the radiology department, in bed.

The position of a bed is usually changed by electric controls built into the side of the bed, at the foot of the bed, or on a bedside cable. Clients can thus raise or lower sections of the bed without expending much energy. It is important for nurses to instruct clients on the proper use of the controls and to caution them against positions that might cause harm. A hospital bed is usually 65 to 70 cm (26 to 28 inches) above the floor at its lowest level. In the home most beds are 50 to 55 cm (20 to 22 inches) high. The greater height of a hospital bed prevents undue musculoskeletal strain on the nurse and the client. It is unnecessary for the nurse to reach across or bend down while caring for clients, and clients can move from the bed to a chair with minimal stress on hips and knees.

Beds contain a number of safety features. Locks located on the wheels, casters, or at the center of the bed frame (Figure 6-4) should be used whenever the bed is stationary to prevent accidental movement during performance of a procedure (e.g., transferring the client from bed to a stretcher). Side rails, located on both sides of a bed, help clients position themselves and provide upper extremity support as a client gets out of bed. Caution must be used in raising siderails. Research suggests that the risk of client falls is greater when all four siderails are raised because clients try to climb over the rails to exit the bed. Raising the two upper rails gives clients an exit route if they are able to move inde-

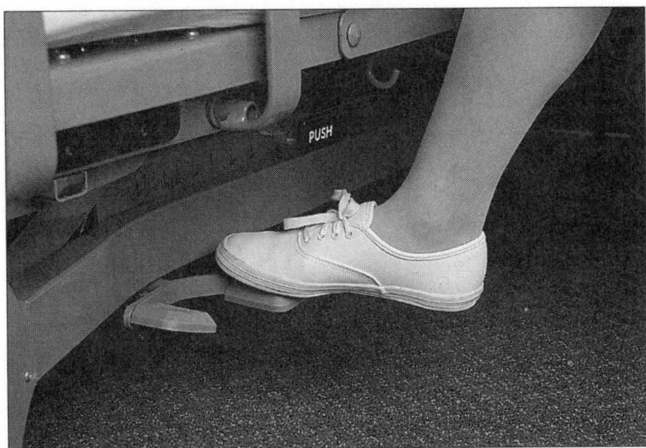

FIGURE 6-4 Lock on bed wheels.

pendently. Use of all four siderails is considered a physical restraint (see Chapter 4). Side rails are adjustable metal frames that can be raised and lowered by pushing or pulling a knob. When a side rail has been lowered the nurse never leaves the bedside with the client still in bed. Each bed also has a special headboard that is removable. This feature is important in emergency situations when the medical team must have easy access to the client's head during cardiopulmonary resuscitation (see Chapter 15).

Mattresses

Most beds have firm, water-repellent mattresses. A mattress should have an even surface for the client's comfort. Most mattresses have handles on the sides to be used when the mattresses are removed or turned over. A rubber or plastic surface permits easy cleaning. Special mattresses provide extra comfort and support for clients and relieve pressure on bony prominences. Chapter 30 reviews a variety of special mattresses and indications for their use.

Special Equipment

There is special equipment that may be added to a bed or room. Examples of equipment available are listed in Box 6-3. The nurse is responsible for knowing how to use all equipment safely.

Box 6-3 Special

Foot Boots

Boots made of a smooth substance such as foam or sheepskin to support the foot in dorsiflexion (Figure 6-5) may be preferred over foot boards because dorsiflexion is maintained while positioning the client in nonsupine positions. The boot stays secured with Velcro strips. Daily removal and inspection of the foot are required.

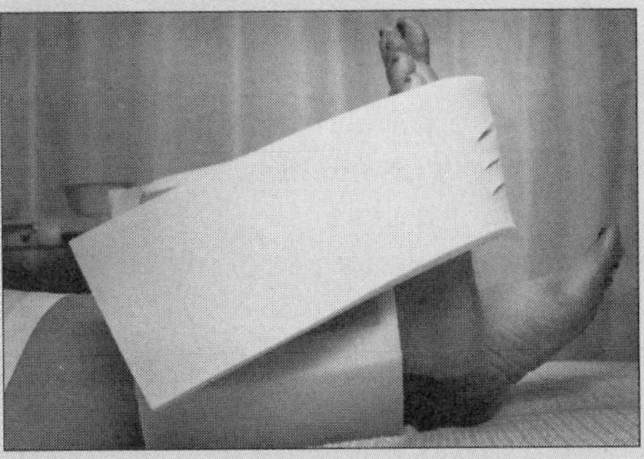

FIGURE 6-5 Foam foot boot supporting foot in dorsiflexion.

Bed Board

A long wooden or plexiglass board, the length of a regular bed mattress, that is placed under a mattress to provide added support. Clients with back pain frequently use bed boards. The boards are hinged so that the foot or end of the bed can be elevated.

Intravenous (IV) Pole

A metal pole or stand that supports an IV fluid container while fluid is administered to a client. The rod may fit into the metal frame of a client's bed, stand on the floor, or attach to an overhead track (Figure 6-6).

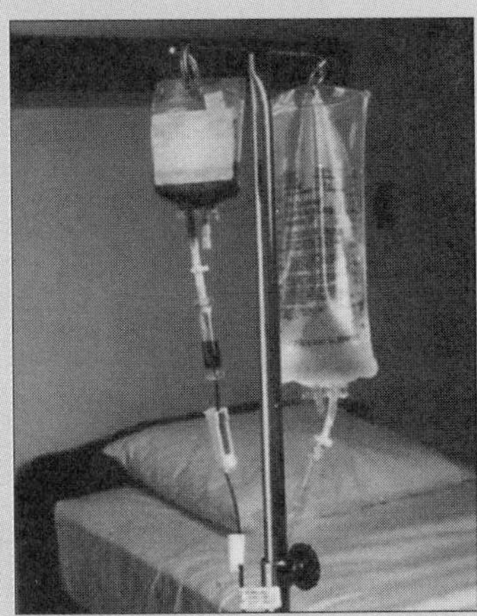

FIGURE 6-6 Intravenous pole supporting IV fluid container.

Skill Performance Guidelines

1. Keep the environment as comfortable as possible by controlling ventilation and temperature. Depending on a client's age and physical condition, room temperature should be maintained between 20° C and 23° C (68° F and 74° F). Infants, older adults, and the acutely ill may need a warmer temperature. However, certain critically ill clients require cooler room temperatures to lower the body's metabolic demands. Controlling drafts and eliminating lingering odors from draining wounds, vomitus, bedpans, or urinals will also improve a client's comfort. Most hospitals now prohibit smoking in clients' rooms.
2. Control extraneous noises in a client's room. Ill clients are sensitive to noises in a hospital environment. A nurse should try to control noise level by handling equipment

Box 6-4 Procedural Guidelines

Making an Unoccupied Bed

Equipment: Linen bag, mattress pad (change only when soiled), bottom sheet (flat or fitted), drawsheet (optional), top sheet, blanket, bedspread, waterproof pads (optional), pillowcases, bedside chair or table, disposable gloves (if linen is soiled), washcloth, and antiseptic cleanser.

1. Determine if client has been incontinent or if excess drainage is on linen. Gloves will be necessary.
2. Assess activity orders or restrictions in mobility in planning if client can get out of bed for procedure. Assist to bedside chair or recliner.
3. Lower side rails on both sides of bed and raise bed to comfortable working position.
4. Remove soiled linen and place in laundry bag. Avoid shaking or fanning linen.
5. Reposition mattress and wipe off any moisture using a washcloth moistened in antiseptic solution. Dry thoroughly.
6. Apply all bottom linen on one side of bed before moving to opposite side.
7. Be sure fitted sheet is placed smoothly over mattress. To apply a flat unfitted sheet, allow about 25 cm (10 in) to hang over mattress edge. Lower hem of sheet should lie seam down, even with bottom edge of mattress. Pull remaining top portion of sheet over top edge of mattress.
8. While standing at head of bed, miter top corner of bottom sheet (see Skill 6-7, Step 15)
9. Tuck remaining portion of unfitted sheet under mattress.
10. Optional: Apply drawsheet, laying center fold along middle of bed lengthwise. Smooth drawsheet over mattress and tuck excess edge under mattress, keeping palms down.
11. Move to opposite side of bed and spread bottom sheet smoothly over edge of mattress from head to foot of bed.
12. Apply fitted sheet smoothly over each mattress corner. For an unfitted sheet, miter top corner of bottom sheet (see Step 8) making sure corner is taut.
13. Grasp remaining edge of unfitted bottom sheet and tuck tightly under mattress while moving from head to foot of bed. Smooth folded drawsheet over bottom sheet and tuck under mattress, first at middle, then at top, and then at bottom.
14. If needed, apply waterproof pad over bottom sheet or drawsheet.
15. Place top sheet over bed with vertical center fold lengthwise down middle of bed. Open sheet out from head to foot, being sure top edge of sheet is even with top edge of mattress.
16. Make horizontal toe pleat; stand at foot of bed and fan fold in sheet 5 to 10 cm (2 to 4 in) across bed. Pull sheet up from bottom to make fold approximately 15 cm (6 in) from bottom edge of mattress.
17. Tuck in remaining portion of sheet under foot of mattress. Then place blanket over bed with top edge parallel to top edge of sheet and 15 to 20 cm (6 to 8 in) down from edge of sheet. (Optional: Apply additional spread over bed.)
18. Make cuff by turning edge of top sheet down over top edge of blanket and spread.
19. Standing on one side at foot of bed, lift mattress corner slightly with one hand, and with other hand tuck top sheet, blanket, and spread under mattress. Be sure toe pleats are not pulled out.
20. Make modified mitered corner with top sheet, blanket, and spread. After triangular fold is made, do not tuck tip of triangle (see illustration).

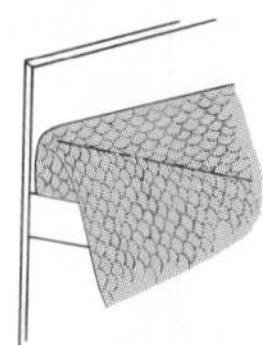

STEP **20** Modified mitered corner.

21. Go to other side of bed. Spread sheet, blanket, and spread out evenly. Make cuff with top sheet and blanket. Make modified corner at foot of bed.
22. Apply clean pillowcase.
23. Place call light within client's reach on bed rail or pillow and return bed to height allowing for client transfer. Assist client to bed.
24. Arrange client's room. Remove and discard supplies. Wash hands.

properly; making sure equipment is in proper working order; controlling voice volume; and, unless contraindicated, closing the client's room door.

3. Make the environment as safe as possible. Keep all personal care items within the client's reach. When the head of the bed is raised, the bedside stand is usually not within easy reach and must be moved forward. If the client must leave the bed to go to the bathroom, be sure there are no objects obstructing the way.
4. Make the environment personal for the client. A picture of family members, some get well cards, or a small radio may help the client to relax. However, do not clutter the client's

room with unnecessary equipment and supplies. Whenever possible remove equipment and supplies after treatments are complete.

5. Be sure the client is easily accessible to the health care team. Often a client will have numerous IV lines and drainage tubes connected to portable poles and suction machines. At times of emergency, the health care team must reach the client easily and quickly. Keep IV poles and portable equipment in positions that do not obstruct access to the client.

Making an Unoccupied Bed

Clients spend much of their time in bed, eating, bathing, using bedpans or urinals, and undergoing numerous therapeutic procedures. It is essential that the nurse keep the bed as clean and comfortable as possible. Frequent inspections are necessary to be sure that the linen is clean, dry, and wrinkle free. Bed linen that becomes wet or soiled should be changed immediately.

Whenever possible the nurse should make the bed while it is unoccupied. Having the client get out of bed is an ideal way to promote ambulation. The nurse usually makes a bed in the morning after the client's bed bath or while the client is up bathing and showering. Another convenient time for bed making is when the client is out of the room for tests or procedures.

By making an unoccupied bed the nurse can ensure that the linen is smooth and free of wrinkles. It is also easier to insert any extra waterproof pads or special foam rubber mattresses (see Chapter 32) when bed is unoccupied (Procedural Guidelines Box 6-4).

Making an Occupied Bed

At times it is necessary to make a bed that is occupied by a client. The client may be too weak to get out of bed; the illness may prohibit sitting up; or the client may be restricted to bed because of postprocedure precautions, traction, or heavy body or leg casts. If a client is confined to bed, bed making should be done in a way that conserves time and the client's energy. The nurse also tries to keep the client as comfortable as possible. In cases where a client experiences severe pain, an analgesic administered 30 to 60 minutes before the procedure is helpful in controlling pain and maintaining comfort.

Even though the client is unable to get out of bed, the nurse encourages self-help as much as possible. For example, the client can turn, assist in moving up in bed, or hold top sheets while linen is applied. These activities help maintain the client's strength and mobility and allow participation in hygiene care.

Making an occupied bed poses some difficulties. It is harder to prevent transfer of organisms from soiled linens to clean linens and to keep newly applied linen smooth and wrinkle-free. The procedure can be done quickly, however, if the nurse is organized.

Delegation Considerations

The skill of making an occupied bed can be delegated to assistive personnel. Before delegating this skill, review any precautions or activity restrictions for the client. Inform the care provider how to properly position clients during occupied bed-making procedure. Be sure assistive personnel know what to do if wound drainage, dressing material, drainage tubes, or IV tubing becomes dislodged or is found in the linens. Instruct the care provider in what to do if client becomes fatigued.

Equipment (Figure 6-7)

- Linen bag(s)
- Mattress pad (needs to be changed only when soiled)
- Bottom sheet (flat or fitted)
- Drawsheet
- Top sheet
- Blanket
- Bedspread
- Waterproof pads and/or bath blankets (optional)
- Pillowcases
- Bedside chair or table
- Disposable gloves (optional)
- Towel
- Disinfectant

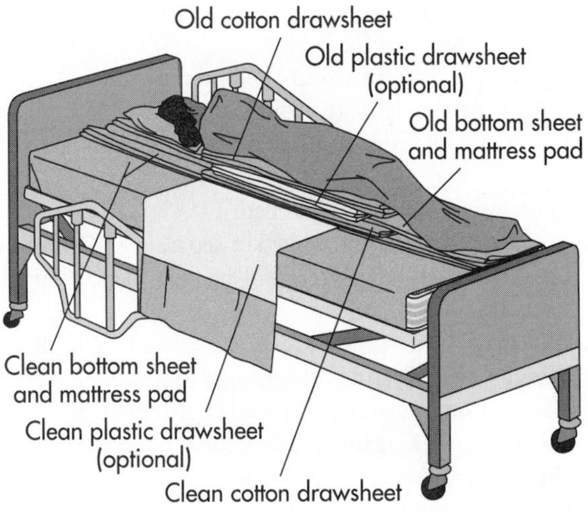

FIGURE 6-7 Equipment for making occupied bed.

STEP	RATIONALE

ASSESSMENT

Step	Rationale
1. Assess potential for client incontinence or for excess drainage on bed linen.	Determines need for protective waterproof pads or extra bath blankets on bed.
2. Check chart for orders or specific precautions concerning movement and positioning.	Ensures client safety and use of proper body mechanics.

NURSING DIAGNOSIS

Defining characteristics from the assessment data may reveal the following diagnoses for clients requiring this skill:

- Activity intolerance
- Impaired physical mobility
- Impaired skin integrity and risk for
- Pain (acute, chronic)
- Bathing/hygiene self-care deficit

Related factors are individualized based on client's condition or needs.

PLANNING

Step	Rationale
1. **Expected outcomes** following completion of procedure:	
▪ Client's skin remains free from breakdown.	Bed linen is smooth and without wrinkles.
▪ Client expresses feeling of relaxation and comfort.	
▪ There are no areas of redness from bed linen irritation.	
2. Explain procedure to the client, noting that the client will be asked to turn on side and roll over linen.	Minimizes anxiety and promotes cooperation.

IMPLEMENTATION

Step	Rationale
1. Wash hands and apply gloves (gloves are worn only if linen is soiled or there is risk for contact with body secretions).	Reduces transmission of microorganisms.
2. Assemble equipment and arrange on bedside chair or table. Remove unnecessary equipment such as a dietary tray or items used for hygiene.	Assembling all equipment provides for smooth procedure and assists in increasing client's comfort. Placing linen on clean surface minimizes spread of infection.
3. Draw room curtain around bed or close door.	Maintains client's privacy.
4. Adjust bed height to comfortable working position. Lower any raised side rail on one side of bed. Remove call light.	Minimizes strain on back. It is easier to remove and apply linen evenly to bed in flat position. Provides easy access to bed and linen.
5. Loosen top linen at foot of bed.	Makes linen easier to remove.
6. Remove bedspread and blanket separately. If spread and blanket are soiled, place them in linen bag. Keep soiled linen away from uniform.	Reduces transmission of microorganisms.
7. If blanket and spread are to be reused, fold them by bringing the top and bottom edges together. Fold farthest side over onto nearer bottom edge. Bring top and bottom edges together again. Place folded linen over back of chair.	Folding method facilitates replacement and prevents wrinkles.
8. Cover client with bath blanket in the following manner: unfold bath blanket over top sheet. Ask client to hold top edge of bath blanket. If client is unable to help, tuck top of bath blanket under shoulder. Grasp top sheet under bath blanket at client's shoulders and bring sheet down to foot of bed. Remove sheet and discard in linen bag.	Bath blanket provides warmth and keeps body parts covered during linen removal.

STEP	RATIONALE
9. With assistance from another nurse, slide mattress toward head of bed.	If mattress slides toward foot of bed when head of bed is raised, it is difficult to tuck in linen. In addition, it is uncomfortable for the client because the client's feet may be pressed against or hang over the foot of the bed.
10. Position client on the far side of the bed, turned onto side and facing away from you. Be sure side rail in front of client is up. Adjust pillow under client's head.	Turning client onto side provides space for placement of clean linen. Side rail ensures client's safety from forward falls from the bed surface and helps client in moving.
11. Loosen bottom linens, moving from head to foot.	Prepares for removal of all bottom linen simultaneously.
12. With seam side down (facing the mattress), fanfold bottom sheet and drawsheet toward client—first drawsheet, then bottom sheet. Tuck edges of linen just under buttocks, back, and shoulders. Do not fanfold mattress pad if it is to be reused (see illustration).	Provides maximum workspace for placing clean linen. Later, when client turns to other side, soiled linen can be removed easily.
13. Wipe off any moisture on exposed mattress with towel and appropriate disinfectant.	Reduces transmission of microorganisms.
14. Apply clean linen to exposed half of bed:	
a. Place clean mattress pad on bed by folding it lengthwise with center crease in middle of bed. Fanfold top layer over mattress. (If pad is reused, simply smooth out any wrinkles.)	Applying linen over bed in successive layers minimizes energy and time used in bed making.
b. Unfold bottom sheet lengthwise so that center crease is situated lengthwise along center of bed. Fanfold sheet's top layer toward center of bed alongside the client. Smooth bottom layer of sheet over mattress, and bring edge over closest side of mattress. Allow edge of sheet to hang about 25 cm (10 in) over mattress edge. Lower hem of bottom sheet should lie seam down and even with bottom edge of mattress (see illustration).	Proper positioning of linen on one side ensures that adequate linen will be available to cover opposite side of bed. Keeping seam edges down eliminates irritation to client's skin.

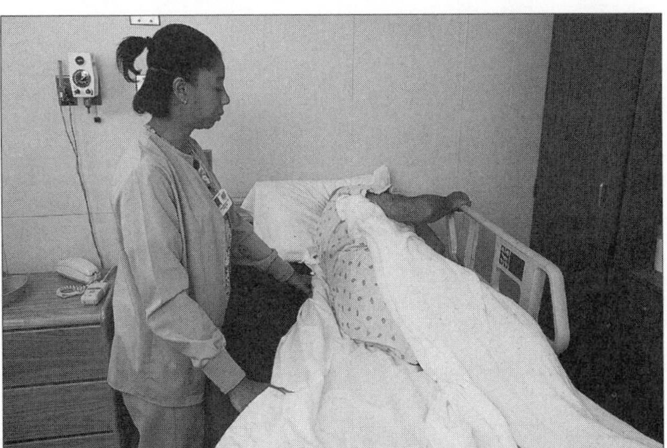

STEP **12** Old linen-tucked client.

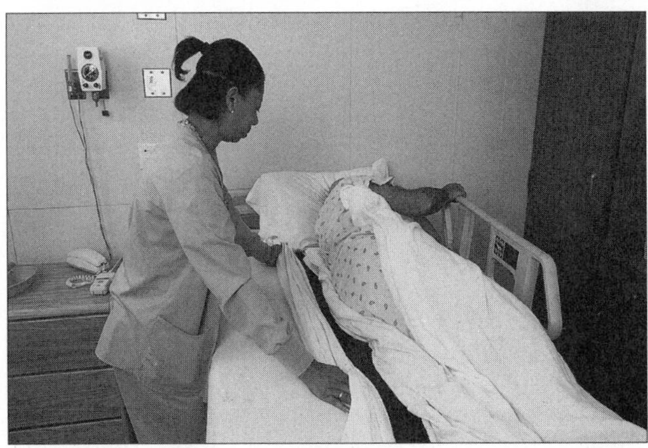

STEP **14b** Clean linen applied to bed.

15. Miter bottom sheet at head of bed:
    a. Face head of bed diagonally. Place hand away from head of bed under top corner of mattress, near mattress edge, and lift.
    b. With other hand, tuck top edge of bottom sheet smoothly under mattress so that side edges of sheet above and below mattress would meet if brought together.
    c. Face side of bed and pick up top edge of sheet at approximately 45 cm (18 in) from top of mattress (see illustration)

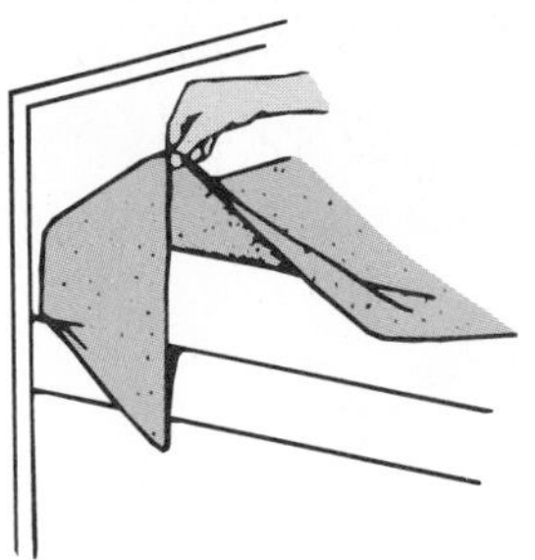

STEP **15c** Top edge of sheet picked up.

STEP	RATIONALE
d. Lift sheet, and lay it on top of mattress to form a neat triangular fold, with lower base of triangle even with mattress side edge (see illustration).	
e. Tuck lower edge of sheet, which is hanging free below the mattress, under mattress. Tuck with palms down, without pulling triangular fold (see illustration).	
f. Hold portion of sheet covering side of mattress in place with one hand. With the other hand, pick up top of triangular linen fold and bring it down over side of mattress (see illustration). Tuck this portion under mattress (see illustrations).	Mitered corner cannot be loosened easily even if client moves frequently in bed.

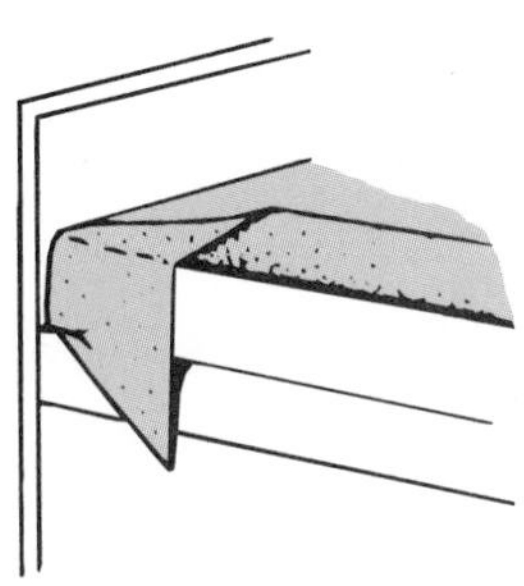
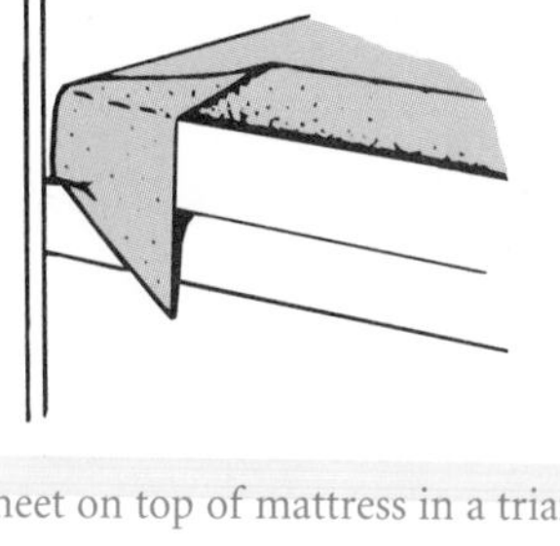

STEP **15d** Sheet on top of mattress in a triangular fold.

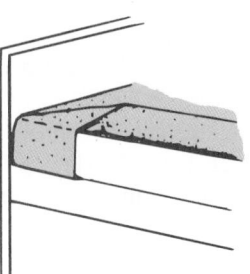

STEP **15e** Lower edge of sheet tucked under mattress.

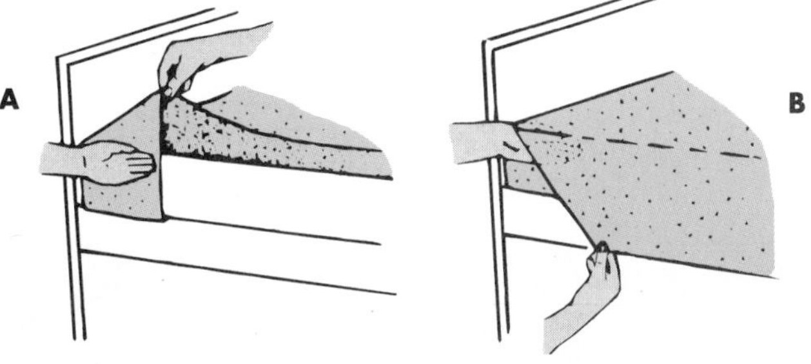

STEP **15f(A)** and **(B)** Triangular fold placed over side of mattress.

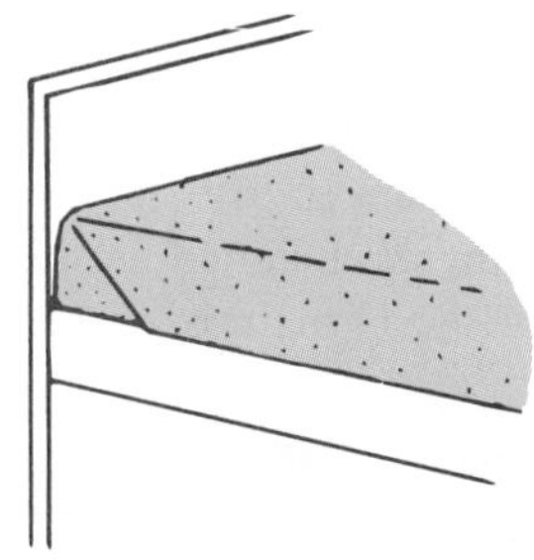

STEP **15f(3)** Linen tucked under mattress.

STEP	RATIONALE
16. Tuck remaining portion of sheet under mattress, moving toward foot of bed. Keep linen smooth.	Folds of linen are source of irritation.
17. (Optional) Open drawsheet so that it unfolds in half. Lay centerfold along middle of bed lengthwise, and position sheet so that it will be under the client's buttocks and torso (see illustration). Fanfold top layer toward client, with edge along client's back. Smooth bottom layer out over mattress, and tuck excess edge under mattress (keep palms down).	Drawsheet is used to lift and reposition client. Placement under client's torso distributes most of client's body weight over sheet.

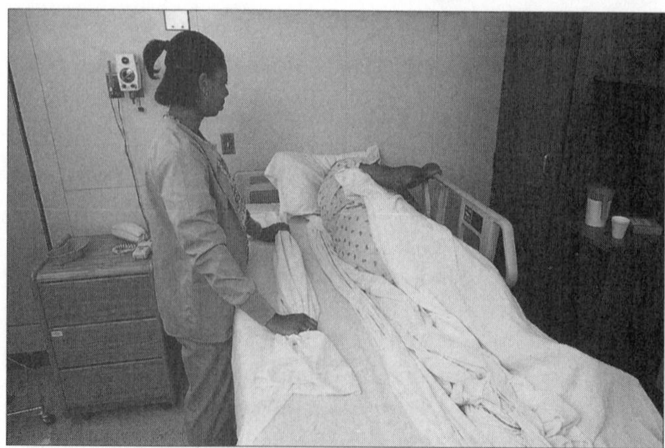

STEP **17** Optional drawsheet.

STEP	RATIONALE
18. Place waterproof pad over drawsheet, with centerfold against client's side. Fanfold top layer toward client.	Protects bed linen from being soiled.
19. Have client roll slowly toward you, over the layers of linen (see illustration). Raise side rail on working side and go to other side.	Positions client for removal and placement of linens. Maintains client's safety and body alignment during turning.

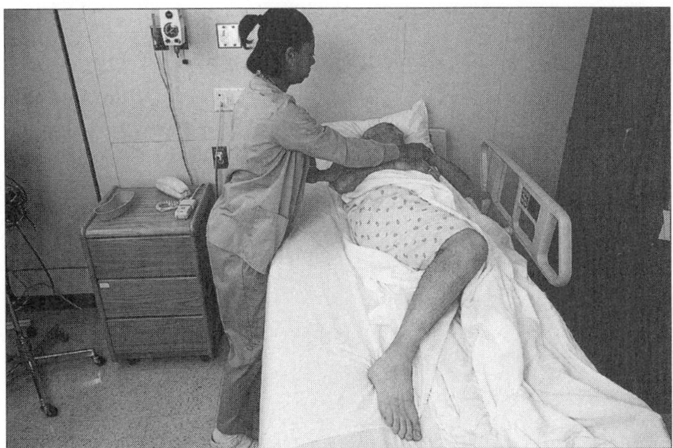

STEP **19** Client rolling over layers of linen.

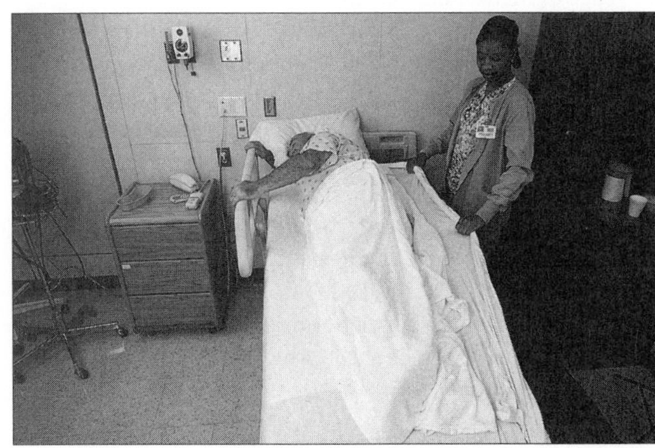

STEP **20** Loosen edges of soiled linen.

STEP	RATIONALE
20. Lower side rail. Assist client in positioning on other side, over folds of linen. Loosen edges of soiled linen from under mattress (see illustration).	Exposes opposite side of bed for removal of soiled linen and placement of clean linen. Makes linen easier to remove.
21. Remove soiled linen by folding it into a bundle or square, with soiled side turned in. Discard in linen bag. If necessary, wipe mattress with antiseptic solution, and dry mattress surface before applying new linen.	Reduces transmission of microorganisms.
22. Pull clean, fanfold linen smoothly over edge of mattress from head to foot of bed.	Smooth linen will not irritate client's skin.
23. Assist client in rolling back into supine position. Reposition pillow.	Maintains client's comfort.
24. Miter top corner of bottom sheet (see Step 15). When tucking corner, be sure that sheet is smooth and free of wrinkles.	Wrinkles and folds can cause irritation to skin.
25. Facing side of bed, grasp remaining edge of bottom sheet. Lean back; keep back straight; and pull while tucking excess linen under mattress. Proceed from head to foot of bed. (Avoid lifting mattress during tucking to ensure fit.)	Proper use of body mechanics while tucking linen prevents injury.
26. Smooth fanfolded drawsheet out over bottom sheet. Grasp edge of sheet with palms down; lean back; and tuck sheet under mattress. Tuck from middle to top and then to bottom.	Tucking first at top or bottom may pull sheet sideways, causing poor fit.
27. Place top sheet over client with centerfold lengthwise down middle of bed. Open sheet from head to foot, and unfold over client.	Sheet should be equally distributed over bed by correctly positioning centerfold.
28. Ask client to hold clean top sheet, or tuck sheet around client's shoulders. Remove bath blanket and discard in linen bag.	Sheet prevents exposure of body parts. Having client hold sheet encourages client participation in care.
29. Place blanket on bed, unfolding it so that crease runs lengthwise along middle of bed. Unfold blanket to cover client. Top edge should be parallel with edge of top sheet and 15 to 20 cm (6 to 8 in) from top sheet's edge.	Blanket should be placed to cover client completely and provide adequate warmth.

Step	Rationale
30. Place spread over bed according to Step 29. Be sure that top edge of spread extends about 2.5 cm (1 in) above blanket's edge. Tuck top edge of spread over and under top edge of blanket.	Gives bed neat appearance and provides extra warmth.
31. Make cuff by turning edge of top sheet down over top edge of blanket and spread.	Protects client's face from rubbing against blanket or spread.
32. Standing on one side at foot of bed, lift mattress corner slightly with one hand and tuck top linens under mattress. Top sheet and blanket are tucked under together. Be sure that linens are loose enough to allow movement of client's feet. Making a horizontal toe pleat is an option.	Makes neat-appearing bed. Pressure ulcers can develop on client's toes and heels from feet rubbing against tight-fitting bed sheets.
33. Make modified mitered corner with top sheet, blanket, and spread (see illustration):	
a. Pick up side edge of top sheet, blanket, and spread approximately 45 cm (18 in) from foot of mattress. Lift linen to form triangular fold, and lay it on bed.	
b. Tuck lower edge of sheet, which is hanging free below mattress, under mattress. Do not pull triangular fold.	

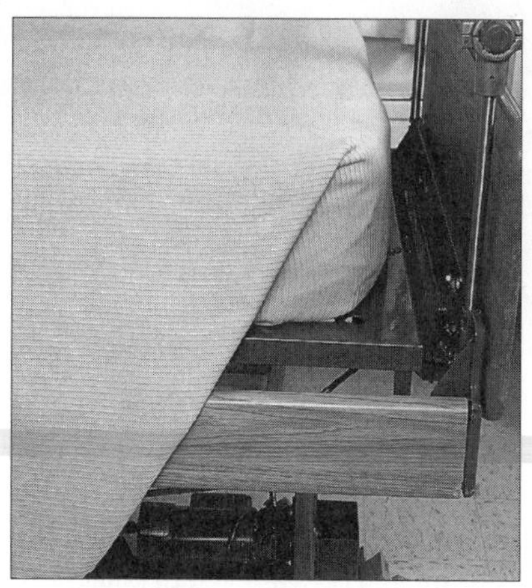

STEP **33** Mitered corner.

Step	Rationale
c. Pick up triangular fold, and bring it down over mattress while holding linen in place along side of mattress. Do not tuck tip of triangle.	Secures top linen but keeps even edge of blanket and top sheet draped over mattress.
34. Raise side rail. Make other side of bed; spread sheet, blanket, and bedspread out evenly. Fold top edge of spread over blanket and make cuff with top sheet (see Step 31); make modified mitered corner at foot of bed (see Step 33).	Side rail protects client from accidental falls.
35. Change pillowcase:	
a. Have client raise head. While supporting neck with one hand, remove pillow. Allow client to lower head.	Support of neck muscles prevents injury during flexion and extension of neck.
b. Remove soiled case by grasping pillow at open end with one hand and pulling case back over pillow with the other hand. Discard case in linen bag.	Pillows slide out easily, thus minimizing contact with soiled linen.
c. Grasp clean pillowcase at center of closed end. Gather case, turning it inside out over the hand holding it. With the same hand, pick up middle of one end of the pillow. Pull pillowcase down over pillow with the other hand.	Eases sliding of pillowcase over pillow.
d. Be sure pillow corners fit evenly into corners of pillowcase. Place pillow under client's head.	Poorly fitting case constricts fluffing and expansion of pillow and interferes with client comfort.
36. Place call light within client's reach and return bed to comfortable position.	Ensures client safety and comfort.
37. Open room curtains, and rearrange furniture. Place personal items within easy reach on overbed table or bedside stand. Return bed to a comfortable height.	Promotes sense of well-being.
38. Discard dirty linen in hamper or chute and wash hands.	Prevents transmission of microorganisms.

STEP	RATIONALE
EVALUATION	
1. Ask if client feels comfortable.	Bed lines clean and smooth.
2. Inspect skin for areas of irritation.	
3. Observe client for signs of fatigue, dyspnea, pain, or discomfort.	Provides nurse with data about client's level of activity tolerance and ability to participate in other procedures.

Unexpected Outcomes and Related Interventions

- Client feels discomfort from linen fold.
  - Tighten sheets.
  - Change client's position frequently.
- Client's skin shows signs of breakdown.
  - Institute skin care measures to reduce risk of pressure ulcer (see Chapter 7).
  - Change client's position frequently.

Recording and Reporting

- Making an occupied bed need not be recorded.

Teaching Considerations

- Explain steps of procedure involving client's participation.

Critical Thinking Exercises

1. You are helping a family care for an older adult relative in the home. What instruction would you provide for foot care?
2. Describe how you might instruct a daughter to perform perineal care for her mother, who has arthritis of the hips.
3. What assessment data would you collect when caring for the foot of a 67-year-old diabetic client whose foot was cut while walking barefoot in the backyard?

References

Adams, R: Qualified nurses lack adequate knowledge of oral health, resulting in inadequate oral care of patients on mechanical ventilation, *Journal of Advanced Nursing,* vol. 24:552-560, 1996.

Agency for Health Care Policy and Research: *Pressure ulcers in adults: prediction and prevention,* Pub Nos 92-0047, 92-0050, Rockville, Md, 1992, Public Health Service, U.S. Department of Health and Human Services.

Armstrong DG, Lavery LA: Diabetic foot ulcers: prevention, diagnosis and classification, *Am Fam Physician* 57(6):1325, 1998.

Barnes SH: Patient and family education for the patient with a pressure necrosis, *Nurs Clin North Am* 22:463, 1987.

Beighton D and others: The influence of specific foods and oral hygiene on the microflora of fissures and smooth surfaces of molar teeth: a 5-day study, *Caries Res* 33(5):349, 1999.

Beuscher TL: Community outreach foot care for the elderly: a winning proposition, *Home Healthc Nurse* 16(1):37, 1998.

Cooppan R, Habershaw G: Preventing leg and foot complications, *Patient Care* 29(3):35, 1995.

Danielson KH: Oral care and older adults, *J Gerontol Nurs* 14:6, 1988.

Dudjak LA: Mouth care for mucositis due to radiation therapy, *Cancer Nurs* 10:131, 1987.

Fellona MO, DeVore LR: Oral health services in primary care nursing centers: opportunities for dental hygiene and nursing collaboration, *J Dent Hyg* 73(2):69, 1999.

Fitch JA, Munro CL, Glass CA and Pellegrini JM: Oral care in the adult intensive care unit, *American Journal of Critical Care,* 8(2): 314, 1999.

Galanti G: *Caring for patients from different cultures,* Philadelphia, 1991, University of Pennsylvania Press.

Greifzu S, Radjeski D, Winnick B: Oral care is part of cancer care, *RN* 53:43, 1990.

Hardy M: A pilot study of the diagnosis and treatment of impaired skin integrity: dry skin in older persons, *Nurs Diagn* 90:60, 1990.

Harrell JS, Damon JF: Prediction of patients' need for mouth care, *West J Nurs Res* 11:748, 1989.

Joyner M: Hair care in the black patient, *J Pediatr Health Care* 2:281, 1988.

Kahn R: Renewing the commitment to oral hygiene, *Geriatr Nurs* 7:244, 1986.

Lueckenotte AG: *Gerontologic Nursing,* ed 2, St. Louis, 2000, Mosby.

Maklebust J: Pressure ulcer update, *RN* 41(12):56, 1991.

Maklebust J, Margolis D: Pressure ulcers: definition and assessment parameters—NPUAP proceedings 1995, *Adv Wound Care* 7(4):28, 1995.

Meckstroth RL: Improving quality and efficiency in oral hygiene, *J Gerontol Nurs* 15:38, 1989.

Moss SJ: Preventive techniques in infant dental care, *Nurse Pract* 13:37, 1988.

Osterman HM, Stuck FM: The aging foot, *Orthopaedic Nursing* 9:43, 1990.

Pettigrew D: Investing in mouth care, *Geriatr Nurs* 10:22, 1989.

Slovenkai NP: Getting and keeping a leg up on diabetes-related food problems, *J Musculoskeletal Med* 15(12):46, 1998.

Sorrentino SA: *Assisting with patient care,* St. Louis, 1999, Mosby.

Strauss MB, Hart JD, Winant DM: Preventive foot care: a user friendly system for patients and physicians, *Postgrad Med* 103(5):233, 1998.

Wong DL, Hockenberry-Eaton M, Wilson D, Winkelstein ML, Ahmann E, DeVito-Thomas P: *Whaley & Wong's nursing care of infants and children,* ed 6, St. Louis, 1999, Mosby.

7

Pressure Ulcer Care

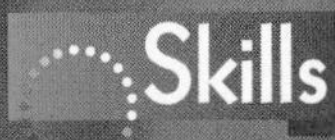

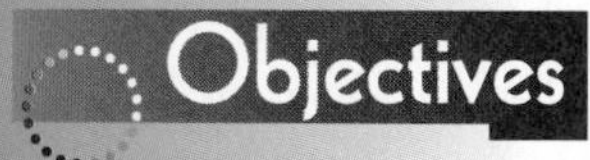

Objectives

Mastery of content in this chapter will enable the nurse to:

- Define the key terms listed.
- Describe guidelines to follow in preventing pressure ulcer formation.
- Identify risks for development of pressure ulcers.
- Identify outcome criteria for clients at risk for pressure ulcers or impaired skin integrity.
- Discuss the meaning of risk assessment scores for four commonly used pressure ulcer risk assessment scales.
- Describe characteristics of the entire client, as well as the pressure ulcer itself, to include in an assessment.
- Discuss indications for the use of topical agents in the treatment of pressure ulcers.
- Apply topical agents correctly to a pressure ulcer.
- Discuss teaching needs of the client and family regarding pressure ulcers.

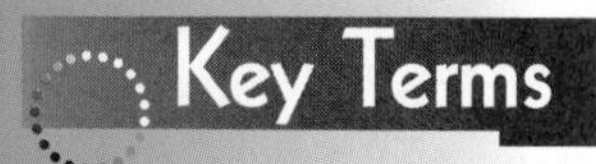

Key Terms

Astringent
Capillary closing pressure
Colonized
Debridement
Erythema
Eschar
Excoriation
Exudate
Ischemia
Maceration
Necrosis
Pressure ulcer
Shearing force
Slough
Topical agents
Undermining

Pressure ulcers (formerly called decubitus ulcers, pressure sores, or bed sores) are "localized areas of tissue **necrosis** that develop when soft tissue is compressed between a bony prominence and an external surface for a prolonged period of time" (National Pressure Ulcer Advisory Panel [NPUAP], 1989). Ischemia develops when pressure on the skin (32 mm Hg, or **capillary closing pressure**) is greater than the pressure inside the small, peripheral blood vessels supplying blood to the tissue. Fat and muscle tissue do not tolerate decreased blood flow and are therefore less resistant to pressure than skin (Maklebust and Sieggreen, 1996). Maklebust and Sieggreen (1996) describe the two models of **pressure ulcer** formation that have been proposed. The traditional model is that the tissue destruction first occurs in the epidermis of the skin and then later in the deeper layers of tissue. The other model suggests that the tissue nearest to the bone or muscle is injured first, before signs of tissue damage can be seen on the skin surface. Ischemia may be evident by skin discoloration such as redness or **erythema** in clients with light skin or purple in clients with darkly pigmented skin. If pressure is unrelieved or repeated, tissues will continue to break down relative to the client's general health and tolerance for pressure. This pressure, if not relieved, can cause irreversible tissue damage in as little as 90 minutes (Kosiak, 1959).

Pressure points over bony prominences where pressure ulcers occur are shown in Figure 7-1. The most common sites are the sacrum, heels, elbows, lateral malleoli, greater trochanters, and ischial tuberosities (Barczak and others, 1997). Pressure ulcers can occur on any area of skin subjected to pressure. Nonbony locations include the nares, with pressure ulcers resulting from nasogastric (NG) tubes or oxygen cannulas; the ears, with ulcers resulting from oxygen cannulas; or the genitalia, with ulcers resulting from Foley catheter tension.

Shearing force also contributes to pressure ulcer formation. **Shearing force** is any tension that stretches the skin during turning or moving in bed. This force causes reduced blood flow to the tissues in the region. In addition, this circulatory impairment often is compounded by the altered body metabolism and negative nitrogen balance that commonly occur in immobilized clients.

Pressure ulcers pose serious risks to a client's health. A break in the skin, seen in stages II to IV pressure ulcers (Table 7-1), eliminates the body's first line of defense against infection. When an ulcer extends into the subcutaneous tissues, protein- and electrolyte-rich body fluids are lost through the wound. With large ulcers, serious electrolyte imbalances can occur. A pressure ulcer can prolong morbidity and interfere with the rehabilitative and supportive care the client receives.

Significant numbers of clients are at risk for or suffering from pressure ulcers; it is critical that nurses respond with an aggressive preventive approach. Care is complex because of the many variables involved in each client's risk for developing pressure ulcers. Even high-risk clients who receive thorough nursing care may develop ulcers in spite of the nurse's efforts. When a pressure ulcer develops, the nurse must explore the possible precipitating factors, vigorously attempt to minimize the effects of these variables, and propose wound care treatment using current wound healing principles in the management of the ulcer (see Chapter 35 and 36).

Skill Performance Guidelines

1. Adequate nutrition is important in the prevention and treatment of pressure ulcers (AHCPR, 1994). A diet high in protein with enough calories, vitamins, and minerals can maintain normal tissue status and promote healing

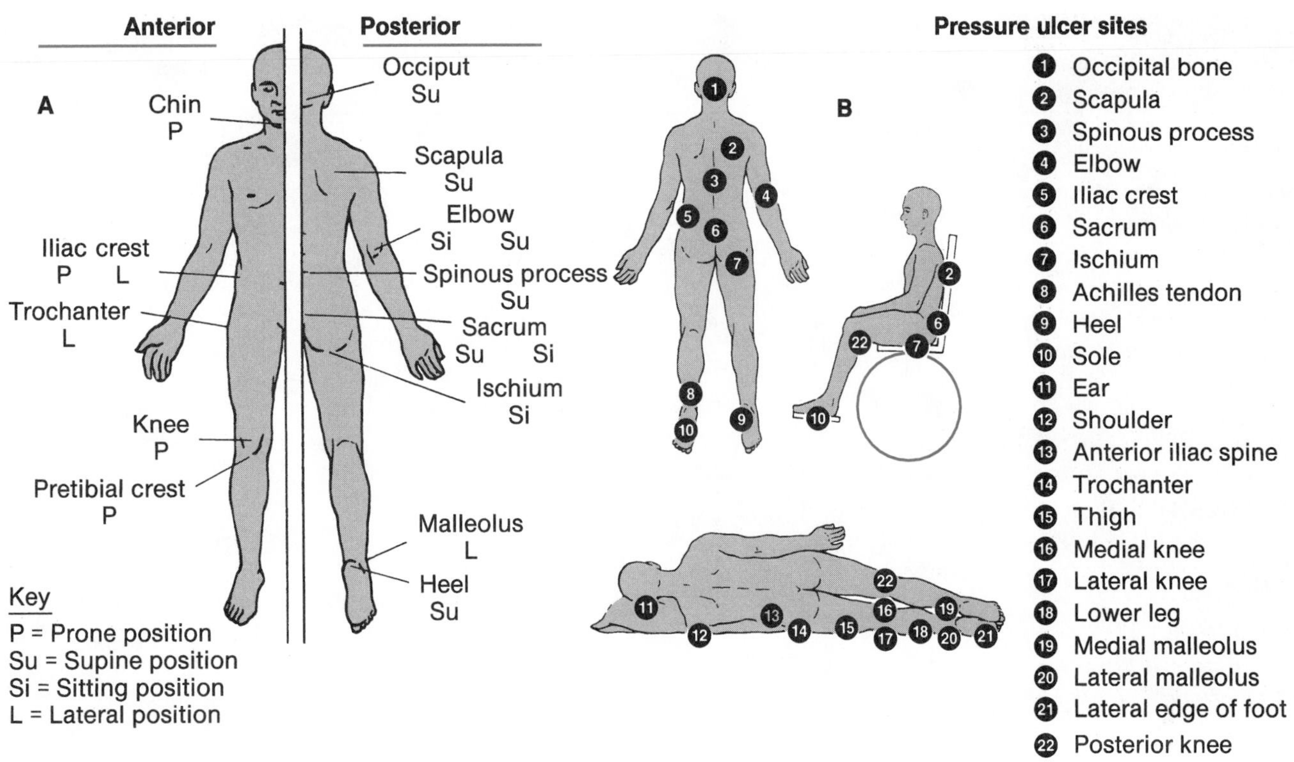

FIGURE **7-1** **A,** Bony prominences most frequently underlying pressure sores. **B,** Pressure ulcer sites. (From Trelease CC: Developing standards for wound care, *Ostomy Wound Manage* 26:50, 1988.)

(AHCPR, 1994). For most clients the goal of positive nitrogen balance can be achieved by a dietary intake of 30 to 35 kcal/kg/day and 1.25 to 1.50 g of protein/kg/day (AHCPR, 1994). Clients who are suspected of having or who have actual vitamin and/or mineral deficiencies will need supplementation (AHCPR, 1994).

2. Frequently turn and position client to relieve pressure around superficial capillaries and allow tissues to compensate for temporary **ischemia.** Classic research (Kosiak, 1959) found that tissue ischemia begins within 1 to 2 hours after onset of pressure in paraplegic animals. Turning clients every 1 to 2 hours and properly positioning them will help minimize formation of pressure ulcers (see Chapter 27).
3. Specialized beds and mattresses (see Chapter 30) distribute pressure on dependent body parts more evenly. Clients at high risk for pressure ulcer formation should be placed on these devices as soon as possible.
4. Use chair cushions to reduce pressure when client is seated. Encourage small movement shifts every 15 to 30 minutes while client is seated.
5. Do not expose client's skin to moisture or increased temperature. Incontinence, diaphoresis, and wound drainage are factors that promote **maceration** of superficial skin layers. Thorough washing and drying will help maintain skin integrity.
6. Frequently inspect linen and bedclothes to be sure they are clean, dry, and wrinkle free. Uneven underlying bed linen or bedclothes can create pressure against skin layers.
7. Eliminate anything that may contribute to ischemic damage, such as massage and "donuts" (air-filled or foam rings) (AHCPR, 1992, 1994).

Carefully monitor the pressure ulcer with regard to the process of healing. Changes in therapy are frequently indicated. Prescribed treatment for a client's pressure ulcer will vary, depending on the extent of the ulcer and the client's underlying condition.

Skill 7-1 Risk Assessment and Prevention Strategies

The optimal treatments for pressure ulcers are the early identification of the at-risk client and the implementation of prevention strategies. The following three populations are known to be at risk for pressure ulcers: (1) clients with a neurological impairment that decreases sensation, (2) chronically ill long-term care clients, and (3) orthopedic clients. Although these groups can be readily identified, *any* client exposed to the right conditions for pressure ulcer development may be at risk.

Table 7-1 Staging of Pressure Ulcers

Staging Definition*

Stage I

A stage I pressure ulcer is an observable pressure related alteration of intact skin whose indicators as compared to an adjacent or opposite area on the body may include changes in one or more of the following:

- Skin temperature (warmth or coolness)
- Tissue consistency (firm or boggy feel)
- Sensation (pain, itching)

The ulcer appears as defined area of persistent redness in a lightly pigmented skin whereas in darker skin tones, the ulcer may appear with persistent red, blue or purple hues.

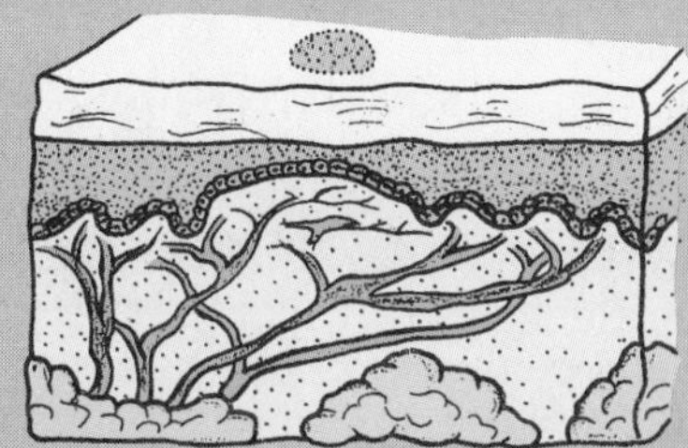

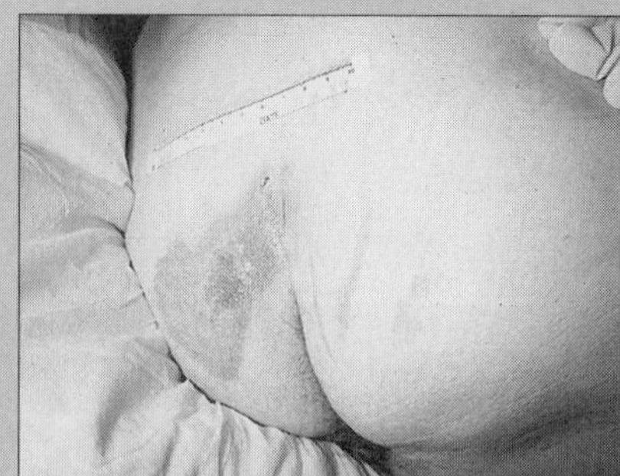

Stage II

Partial-thickness skin loss involving epidermis and/or dermis. The ulcer is superficial and presents clinically as an abrasion, blister, or shallow crater.

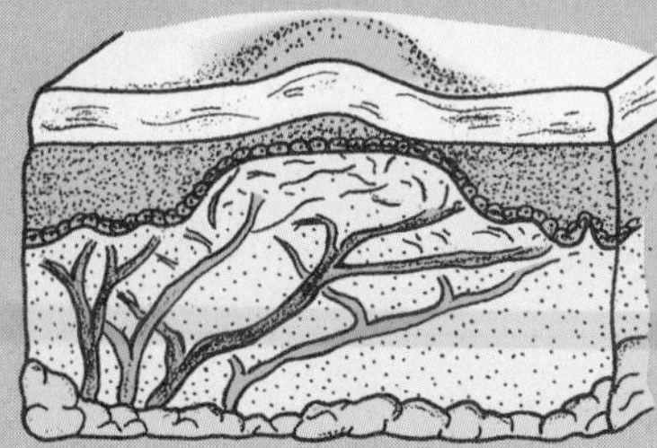

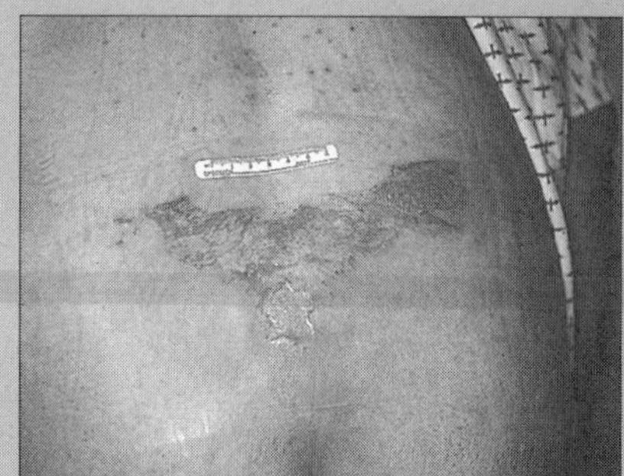

Stage III

Full-thickness skin loss involving damage or necrosis of subcutaneous tissue that may extend down to, but not through, underlying fascia. The ulcer presents clinically as a deep crater with or without undermining of adjacent tissue.

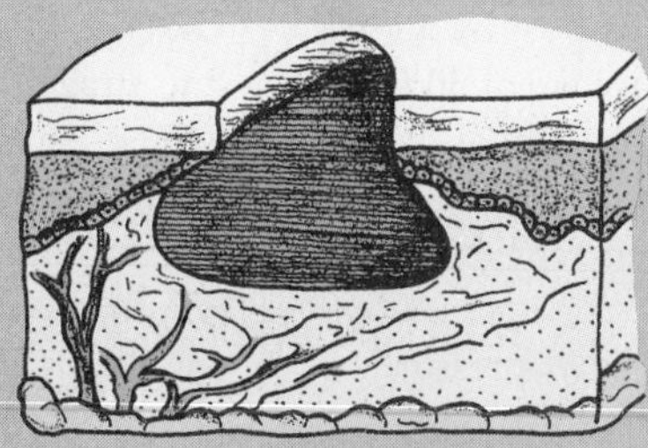

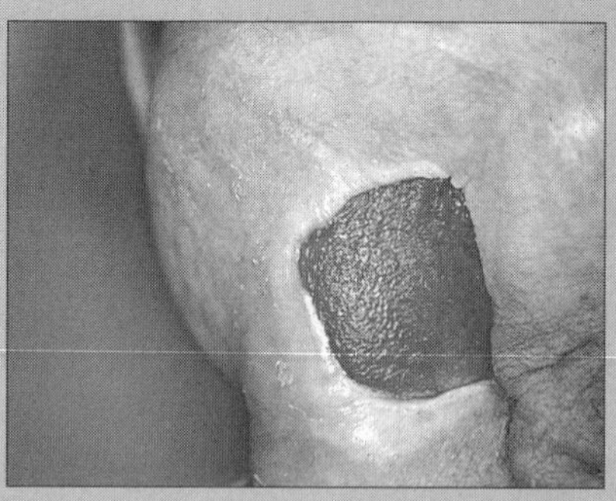

Stage IV

Full-thickness skin loss with extensive destruction, tissue necrosis, or damage to muscle, bone, or supporting structures, for example, tendon or joint capsule. (NOTE: Undermining and sinus tracts may also be associated with stage IV pressure ulcers.)

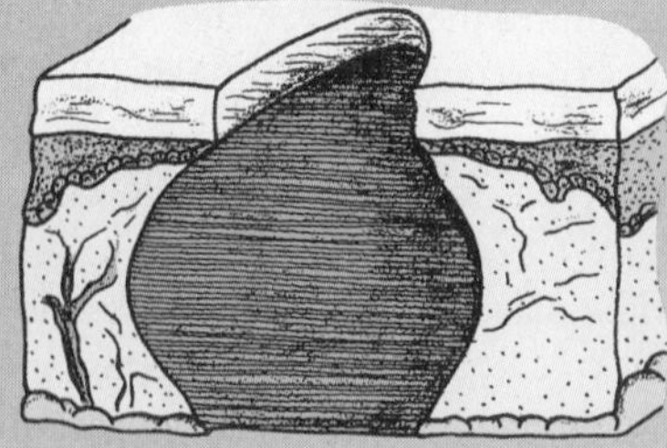

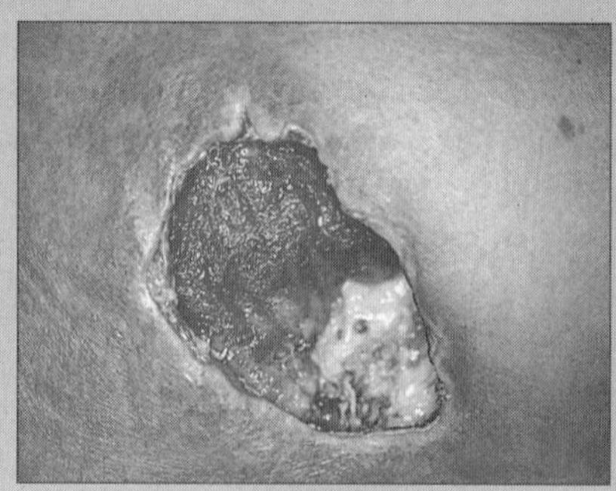

From AHCPR Panel for the Treatment of Pressure Ulcers in Adults: *Treatment of pressure ulcers.* Clinical practice guideline No. 15, Pub No. 95-0653, Rockville, Md, 1994, Public Health Service, U.S. Department of Health and Human Services.

*Staging definitions recognize these assessment limitations:

1. Identification of stage I pressure ulcers may be difficult in patients with darkly pigmented skin.
2. When eschar is present, accurate staging of the pressure ulcer is not possible until the eschar has sloughed or the wound has been debrided.
3. It may be difficult to assess pressure ulcers in persons with casts, other orthopedic devices, or support stockings.

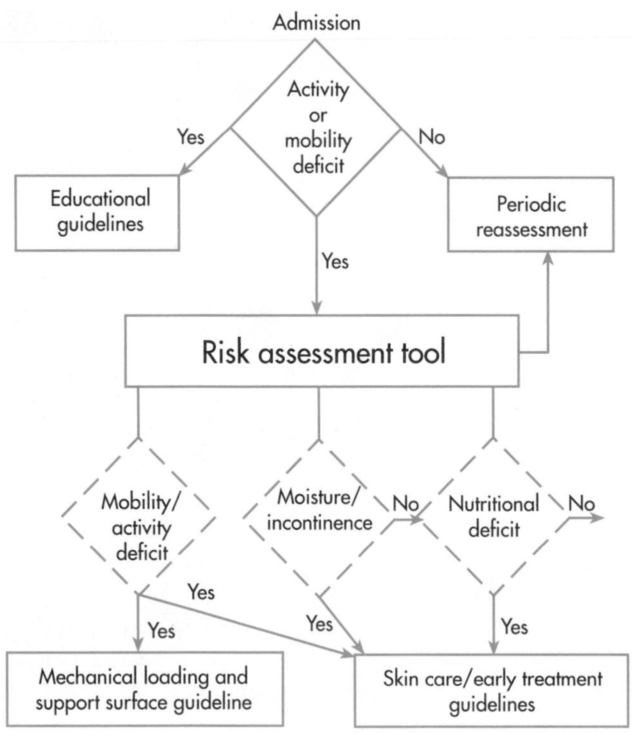

FIGURE 7-2 Risk assessment tool. (Modified from Panel for the Prediction and Prevention of Pressure Ulcers in Adults, *Pressure ulcers in adults: prediction and prevention.* Clinical practice guideline No 3, Pub No 92-0047, Rockville, Md, 1992, Agency for Health Care Policy and Research, Public Health Service, U.S. Department of Health and Human Services.)

The Agency for Health Care Policy and Research [AHCPR] panel developed clinical guidelines for pressure ulcer prevention and treatment of stage I pressure ulcers in 1992. The guidelines recommended that clients who are bed or chair bound or who have an impaired ability to reposition should be assessed for pressure ulcer risk. The AHCPR 1994 guidelines state that additional factors that may put a client at risk for developing pressure ulcers include immobility, incontinence, nutritional factors such as inadequate dietary intake and impaired nutritional status, and altered level of consciousness. Clients with advanced age, excess body heat, and diminished sensation may also be at risk for developing pressure ulcers. Friction and shear can also contribute to pressure ulcer development.

The AHCPR 1992 panel recommended that a valid and reliable risk assessment tool be used on admission and at periodic intervals after admission for all clients found to have a mobility deficit (Figure 7-2). The panel suggested the use of risk assessment tools such as the Braden scale or the Norton scale. The earliest reported scale was in 1962 the Norton scale, which has the following five risk factors: physical condition, mental state, activity, mobility, and incontinence (Norton and others, 1962). The Braden scale (Table 7-2) has the following six parameters: sensory perception (recognition of pressure), friction and shear, ability to change and control body position, skin moisture, nutritional intake, and physical activity (Bergstrom, Demuth, and Braden, 1987). Risk cutoff scores may also vary for specific client populations (Table 7-3). Although not mentioned in the AHCPR guidelines, other risk

Table 7-2 Braden Scale for Predicting Pressure Ulcer Risk*

	1 Point	2 Points	3 Points	4 Points
Sensory Perception Ability to respond meaningfully to pressure-related discomfort	*Completely limited:* Unresponsive (does not moan, flinch, or grasp) to painful stimuli due to diminished level of consciousness or sedation. OR Limited ability to feel pain over most of body surface.	*Very limited:* Responds only to painful stimuli. Cannot communicate discomfort except by moaning or restlessness. OR Has a sensory impairment which limits the ability to feel pain or discomfort over half of body.	*Slightly limited:* Responds to verbal commands but cannot always communicate discomfort or need to be turned. OR Has some sensory impairment which limits ability to feel pain or discomfort in 1 or 2 extremities.	*No impairment:* Responds to verbal commands. Has no sensory deficit that would limit ability to feel or voice pain or discomfort.
Moisture Degree to which skin is exposed to moisture	*Constantly moist:* Skin is kept moist almost constantly by perspiration, urine, etc. Dampness is detected every time patient is moved or turned.	*Very moist:* Skin is often, but not always, moist. Linen must be changed at least once a shift.	*Occasionally moist:* Skin is occasionally moist, requiring an extra linen change approximately once a day.	*Rarely moist:* Skin is usually dry, linen requires changing only at routine intervals.

From Barbara Braden, PhD, RN, Creighton University School of Nursing, Omaha, Neb.

*Score client in each of the six subscales. Maximum score is 23, indicating little or no risk. A score of ≤16 indicates "at risk"; ≤9 indicates high risk.

Continued

Table 7-2 Braden Scale for Predicting Pressure Ulcer Risk—cont'd

	1 POINT	2 POINTS	3 POINTS	4 POINTS
ACTIVITY Degree of physical activity	*Bedfast:* Confined to bed.	*Chairfast:* Ability to walk severely limited or nonexistent. Cannot bear down weight and/or must be assisted into chair or wheelchair.	*Walks occasionally:* Walks occasionally during day, but for very short distances, with or without assistance. Spends majority of each shift in bed or chair.	*Walks frequently:* Walks outside the room at least twice a day and inside room at least once every 2 hours during waking hours.
MOBILITY Ability to change and control body position	*Completely immobile:* Does not make even slight changes in body or extremity position without assistance.	*Very limited:* Makes occasional slight changes in body or extremity position but unable to make frequent or significant changes independently.	*Slightly limited:* Makes frequent though slight changes in body or extremity position independently.	*No limitations:* Makes major and frequent changes in position without assistance.
NUTRITION Usual food intake pattern	*Very poor:* Never eats a complete meal. Rarely eats more than one third of any food offered. Eats 2 servings or less of protein (meat or dairy products) per day. Takes fluids poorly. Does not take a liquid dietary supplement. OR Is NPO and/or maintained on clear liquids or IVs for more than 5 days.	*Probably inadequate:* Rarely eats a complete meal and generally eats only about half of any food offered. Protein intake includes only 3 servings of meat or dairy products per day. Occasionally will take a dietary supplement. OR Receives less than optimal amount of liquid diet or tube feeding.	*Adequate:* Eats over half of most meals. Eats a total of 4 servings of protein (meat, dairy products) each day. Occasionally will refuse a meal, but will usually take a supplement if offered. OR Is on a tube-feeding or TPN regimen that probably meets most of nutritional needs.	*Excellent:* Eats most of every meal. Never refuses a meal. Usually eats a total of 4 or more servings of meat and dairy products. Occasionally eats between meals. Does not require supplements.
FRICTION AND SHEAR	*Problem:* Requires moderate to maximum assistance in moving. Complete lifting without sliding against sheets is impossible. Frequently slides down in bed or chair; repositioning with maximal assistance. Spasticity, contractions, or agitation leads to almost constant friction.	*Potential problem:* Moves feebly or requires minimal assistance. During a move skin probably slides to some extent against sheets, chair, restraints, or other devices. Maintains relatively good position in chair or bed most of the time but occasionally slides down.	*No apparent problem:* Moves in bed and in chair independently and has sufficient muscle strength to sit up completely during move. Maintains good position in bed or chair at all times.	

Table 7-3 Pressure Ulcer Braden Risk Cutoff Scores by Client Population

CLIENT POPULATION	RISK CUT SCORES
General population	≤16
Intensive care unit (ICU) patients	≤15
Elderly patients	≤18
Black and Latino patients	≤18

Data from Braden BJ, Bergstrom N: Clinical utility of the Braden scale for predicting pressure sore risk, *Decubitus* 2(3):44, 1989; Jiricka MK and others: Pressure ulcer risk factors in an ICU population, *Am J Crit Care* 4(5):361, 1995; Lyder CH and others: Validating the Braden scale for the prediction of pressure ulcer risk in Black and Latino/Hispanic elders: a pilot study, *Ostomy/Wound Manage* 44(suppl 3A):42s, 1998.

assessment tools used clinically are the Gosnell (1973) scale and the Knoll scale (which was developed by Abruzzese [1982] in 1975). It is important to understand how to interpret the meaning of the client's total score on whatever scale you use.

Delegation Considerations

This skill should not be delegated to assistive personnel.

Equipment

- Risk assessment tool
- Documentation record
- Body chart or tracing film and/or camera
- Lanolin-based lotion
- Pressure-relief mattress, bed, and/or chair cushion
- Positioning aids

Step	Rationale
Assessment	
1. Identify any client characteristic that might be risk factors for pressure ulcer formation.	Determines need to administer preventive care in addition to use of topical agents for existing ulcers.
a. Paralysis, paresis, or immobilization caused by restrictive devices	Client is unable to turn or reposition independently to relieve pressure.
b. Sensory loss	When sensory loss is present the client feels no discomfort from pressure and does not independently change position.
c. Circulatory disorders	Disorders reduce perfusion of skin's tissue layers.
d. Fever	Increases metabolic demands of tissues. Accompanying diaphoresis leaves skin moist.
e. Anemia	Decreased hemoglobin reduces oxygen-carrying capacity of blood and amount of oxygen available to tissues.
f. Malnutrition	Inadequate nutrition can lead to weight loss, muscle atrophy, and reduced tissue mass. Less tissue is available to serve as a pad between skin and underlying bone. Poor protein, vitamin, mineral, and caloric intake limit wound-healing capabilities.
g. Incontinence	Skin becomes exposed to moist environment containing bacteria. Moisture causes skin maceration.
h. Heavy sedation and anesthesia	Client is not mentally alert and does not turn or change position independently. Sedation can also alter sensory perception.
i. Age	Older skin is less elastic and drier; tissue mass is reduced.
j. Dehydration	Results in decreased skin elasticity and turgor.
k. Edema	Edematous tissues are less tolerant of pressure, friction, and shear.
l. Existing pressure ulcers	Limits surfaces available for position changes, placing available tissues at increased risk.
m. History of pressure ulcer	Tensile strength of the skin from a previously healed pressure ulcer is about 80%; therefore this area cannot tolerate pressure as much as undamaged skin.
2. Select one of the risk assessment tools.	A valid and reliable risk assessment tool should be used to evaluate client's risk for developing a pressure ulcer (AHCPR, 1992).
3. Identify additional risks for pressure ulcer formation by assessing the factors that are found on the selected risk assessment tool.	To prevent pressure ulcers, individuals at risk must be identified so that risk factors can be reduced through intervention (AHCPR, 1992).
4. Obtain "risk score" (see Tables 7-2, 7-3, and 7-4) and evaluate its meaning based on client's unique characteristics.	The risk cutoff score will depend on the instrument used and the client's age or skin pigmentation; it predicts client's need for preventive care.
5. Assess condition of client's skin over regions of pressure (see Figure 7-1). Body weight against bony prominences places underlying skin at risk for breakdown. Look for areas of:	"Skin inspection is fundamental to any plan for preventing pressure ulcers" (AHCPR, 1992).
a. Skin discoloration (redness in light-tone skin; purplish or bluish in darkly pigmented skin) and temperature changes (warmth or coolness) (Bennett, 1995; Henderson and others, 1997). See Box 7-1 for cultural considerations in assessing clients with darkly pigmented skin.	May indicate that tissue was under pressure; hyperemia is a normal physiological response to hypoxemia in tissues.

Table 7-4 Guidelines for Pressure Ulcer Risk Assessment

Level of Care	Initial	Reassessment
Acute care	On admission	• 48 hrs after admission • ICU patients 24-48 hrs • Whenever a major change in patient's condition occurs • Intervals will vary depending upon how rapid patient's condition is changing
Long-term care	On admission	• Weekly for first 4 weeks after admission • Routinely on quarterly basis
Home care	On admission	• Every RN visit

From Braden B: Risk assessment in pressure ulcer prevention. In Krasner D, Kane D: *Chronic wound care: a clinical source book for health care professionals,* ed 2, Wayne, Pa, 1997, Health Management Publications.

Box 7-1 Cultural Considerations for Skin Assessment for Pressure Ulcers: The Client With Darkly Pigmented Skin

Color—Assess Localized Skin Color Changes

Any of the following may appear:

- Skin color changes are different from usual skin tone.
- Color is darker than surrounding skin—purplish, bluish, eggplant.

Importance of lighting for skin assessment:

- Use natural or halogen light.
- Avoid fluorescent lamps, which can give the skin a bluish tone.
- Avoid wearing tinted lenses when assessing skin color.

Tissue Consistency

- Assess for edema, presence of nonpitting, swelling.
- Assess for firm or boggy feel.

Sensation

- Assess for pain or changes in skin sensation such as itching.

Skin Temperature

- Initially skin in the area of pressure ulcer may feel warmer than surrounding skin.
- Subsequently skin may feel cooler than surrounding skin.
- Use back of your hand and finger and, if client condition permits, no gloves when doing this assessment.

Data from Bennett MA: Report of the Task Force on the Implications for Darkly Pigmented Intact Skin in the Prediction and Prevention of Pressure Ulcers, *Adv Wound Care* 8(6):34, 1995; Henderson CT and others: Draft definition of stage I pressure ulcers: inclusion of persons with darkly pigmented skin, *Adv Wound Care* 10(5):16, 1997.

Step	Rationale
b. Blanching	Blanching is normal, expected response in clients with lightly pigmented skin. Blanching is not present in skin damaged from pressure.
c. Induration or hardiness, boggyness	Localized edema beneath the skin surface, induration commonly occurs with abnormal hyperemia (Pires and Mueller, 1991).
d. Pallor and mottling	Persistent hypoxia in tissues that were under pressure; an abnormal physiological response.
e. Absence of superficial skin layers	Represents early pressure ulcer formation.
f. Skin temperature	Palpation of differences in temperature between the area of a stage I pressure ulcer and adjacent skin area may be an initial indicator of ischemia.
g. Spasticity	Spasticity may result in pressure ulcer development in atypical locations such as between the buttocks.
6. Assess client for additional areas of potential pressure.	Clients at high risk have multiple sites for pressure necrosis, in addition to bony prominences.
a. Nares: nasogastric (NG) tube, oxygen cannula	
b. Tongue and lips: oral airway, endotracheal (ET) tube	
c. Ears: oxygen cannula, pillow	
d. Intravenous (IV) sites (especially long-term access sites)	Stress on catheter at exit site.

STEP	RATIONALE
e. Drainage tubes	Stress against tissue at exit site.
f. Wound drainage	Wound drainage is caustic to skin and underlying tissues, thereby increasing risk for skin breakdown.
g. Indwelling urethral (Foley) catheter	For female clients, the catheter can put pressure on the labia, especially when edematous. For male clients, pressure from a catheter not properly anchored can put pressure on the tip of the penis and urethra.
h. Orthopedic and positioning devices	Improperly fitted or applied devices have the potential to cause pressure on adjacent skin and underlying tissue.

- ***Critical Decision Point***
  Inspect skin around and beneath orthopedic devices, such as cervical collar, braces, or cast.

7. Observe client for preferred positions when in bed or chair.	Preferred positions result in weight of body being placed on certain bony prominences. Presence of contractures may result in pressure exerted in unexpected places.
8. Observe ability of client to initiate and assist with position changes.	Potential for friction and shear increases when client is completely dependent on others for position changes.

- ***Critical Decision Point***
  Assess client's and support persons understanding of risks for pressure ulcers. This provides an opportunity to begin prevention education using the AHCPR consumer booklets on pressure ulcers.

NURSING DIAGNOSIS

Defining characteristics from the assessment data may reveal the following nursing diagnoses for clients requiring this skill:

- Risk for impaired skin integrity.
- Impaired skin integrity
- Imbalanced nutrition: less than body requirements
- Impaired tissue perfusion
- Impaired physical mobility
- Deficient knowledge related to pressure ulcer prevention

Related factors are individualized based on client's condition or needs.

PLANNING

1. **Expected outcomes** following completion of procedure:	
▪ Skin is intact without discoloration (such as erythema [redness] or purplish [eggplant] color) or breakdown.	Prevention strategies are successful.
▪ Client is able to change positions independently.	Turning schedule has not disrupted sleep pattern.
▪ Peripheral circulation is maintained as evidenced by absence of pallor, mottling, or redness.	Adequate blood flow is maintained.
2. Explain procedure(s) and purpose to client and family.	Relieves anxiety and provides opportunity for education.
3. Wash hands and prepare equipment and supplies.	Reduces transmission of microorganisms.

IMPLEMENTATION

1. Implement the National Pressure Ulcer Advisory Panel [NPUAP] pressure ulcer prevention points (see Box 7-2), which are based on the AHCPR clinical guidelines.	Using these may prevent the client from developing a pressure ulcer.
2. Close room door or bedside curtain.	Maintains client privacy.
3. If client has open, draining wounds, use disposable gloves.	Use of standard precautions prevents accidental exposure to body fluids.

Box 7-2 Pressure Ulcer Prevention Points

A. Risk assessment
1. Consider all bed-bound or chair-bound persons, or those whose ability to reposition is impaired, to be at risk for pressure ulcers.
2. Select and use a method of risk assessment, such as the Norton Scale or the Braden Scale, that ensures systematic evaluation of individual risk factors.
3. Assess all at-risk clients at the time of admission to health care facilities and at regular intervals thereafter.
4. Identify all individual risk factors (decreased mental status, moisture, incontinence, nutritional deficits) to direct specific preventive treatments. Modify care according to the individual factors.

B. Skin care and early treatment
1. Inspect the skin at least daily, and document assessment results.
2. Individualize bathing frequency. Use a mild cleansing agent. Avoid hot water and excessive friction.
3. Assess and treat incontinence. When incontinence cannot be controlled, cleanse skin at time of soiling, use a topical moisture barrier, and select underpads or briefs that are absorbent and provide a quick drying surface to the skin.
4. Use moisturizers for dry skin. Minimize environmental factors leading to dry skin such as low humidity and cold air.
5. Do not massage over bony prominences.
6. Use proper positioning, transferring, and turning techniques to minimize skin injury caused by friction and shear forces.
7. Use dry lubricants (cornstarch) or protective coverings to reduce friction injury.
8. Identify and correct factors compromising protein/caloric intake, and consider nutritional supplementation/support for nutritionally compromised persons.
9. Institute a rehabilitation program to maintain or improve mobility/activity status.
10. Monitor and document interventions and outcomes.

C. Mechanical loading and support surfaces
1. Reposition bed-bound persons at least every 2 hours, chair-bound persons every hour.
2. Use a written repositioning schedule.
3. Place at-risk persons on a pressure-reducing mattress/chair cushion. Do not use donut-type devices.
4. Consider postural alignment, distribution of weight, balance and stability, and pressure relief when positioning persons in chairs or wheelchairs.
5. Teach chair-bound persons, who are able, to shift weight every 15 minutes.
6. Use lifting device (e.g., trapeze or bed linen) to move rather than drag persons during transfer and position changes.
7. Use pillows or foam wedges to keep bony prominences such as knees and ankles from direct contact with each other.
8. Use devices that totally relieve pressure on the heels (e.g., place pillows under the calf to raise the heels off the bed).
9. Avoid positioning directly on the trochanter when using the side-lying position (use the 30-degree lateral inclined position).
10. Elevate the head of the bed as little (maximum 30-degree angle) and for as short a time as possible.

D. Education
1. Implement educational programs for the prevention of pressure ulcers that are structured, organized, comprehensive, and directed at all levels of health care providers, clients, family, and caregivers.
2. Include information on:
   a. Etiology of and risk factors for pressure ulcers
   b. Risk assessment tools and their application
   c. Skin assessment
   d. Selection/use of support surfaces
   e. Development/implementation of individualized programs of skin care
   f. Demonstration of positioning to decrease risk of tissue breakdown
   g. Accurate documentation of pertinent data
3. Include built-in mechanisms to evaluate program effectiveness in preventing pressure ulcers.

Modified from National Pressure Ulcer Advisory Panel, 1989.

Step	Rationale
4. Assist client to change position. Use the following positions:	See Chapters 27 and 28 for specifics. Avoid positions that place client directly on an area of existing ulceration. It may be helpful to use a schedule for position changes.
a. Supine	Protects shoulders, trochanter, and malleolus.
b. Prone	Used only in clients who can tolerate, breathing difficulty is normal.

STEP	RATIONALE
c. 30-degree lateral (see illustration)	Achieved with one pillow under shoulder and one pillow under leg on the same side. Protects sacrum and trochanters. The 30-degree lateral and prone positions may be useful at night to prolong the time between position changes, resulting in less sleep disruption for the client and caregiver.

• ***Critical Decision Point***

Observe for skin discoloration in area that was under pressure. In light-skin clients, redness from initial flushing is expected. In darkly pigmented clients, skin may appear purplish or bluish (Bennett, 1995; Henderson and others, 1997). Bennett also suggests using natural or halogen light sources when assessing for discoloration on clients with darkly pigmented skin. Avoid using fluorescent lighting because it can give a bluish tint to skin that can interfere with accurate assessment of skin coloring (see Box 7-1).

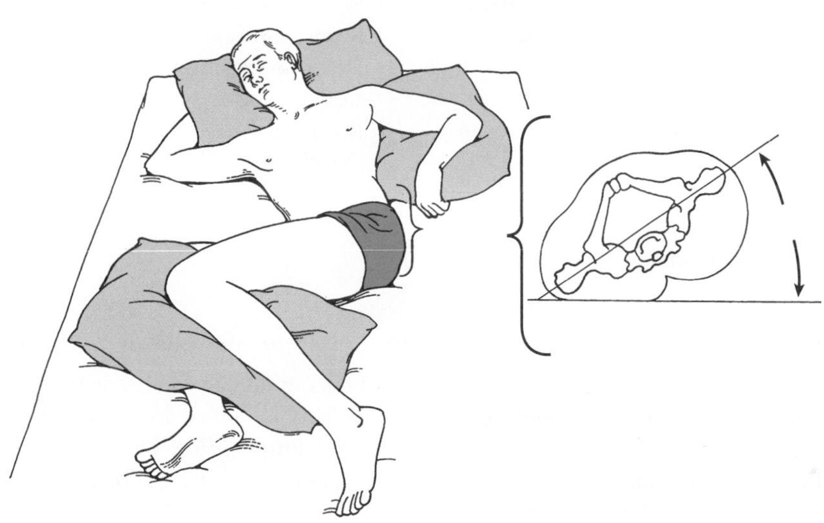

STEP **4c** 30-degree lateral position.

STEP	RATIONALE
5. Palpate any area of discoloration or mottling. Skin temperature changes may be an important early indicator of a stage I (see Table 7-1) pressure ulcer in clients with darkly pigmented skin (Bennett, 1995; Henderson and others, 1997) (see Box 7-1).	Early detection of pressure indicates need for more frequent position changes. A hard or boggy area may characterize early tissue injury.
6. Monitor length of time any area of discoloration persists.	Redness usually persists for 50% of the time hypoxia occurred.
a. Determine appropriate turning interval.	If turning interval is 2 hours, a redness lasts 15 minutes, then hypoxia was approximately 30 minutes.
b. When a turning interval of less than $1^1/_2$ to 2 hours is necessary, a pressure-relief device may be needed (Knox, 1999) (see Chapter 30).	Recommended turning interval should be the turning interval minus hypoxia time: 2 hr − 30 min = $1^1/_2$ hr. Inadequate blood flow is an important mechanism affecting skin breakdown. Use of dynamic support surfaces has shown an increase in tissue perfusion (Mayrovitz and Smith, 1999).

• ***Critical Decision Point***

If client requires a pressure-relief surface for the bed, an appropriate pressure-relief surface should also be considered for the chair.

STEP	RATIONALE
7. Remove gloves, discard appropriately, and wash hands.	Reduces spread of microorganisms.

Step	Rationale

Evaluation

Step	Rationale
1. Observe a client's skin for areas at risk for change in color or texture.	Enables nurse to evaluate success of prevention techniques.
2. Observe tolerance of client for position change.	Position changes may interfere with client's sleep and rest pattern.
3. Compare subsequent risk assessment scores.	Provides ongoing comparison of client's risk level to facilitate appropriateness of plan of care.

Unexpected Outcomes and Related Interventions

- Skin becomes mottled, reddened, purplish, or bluish.
  - Document and communicate interval for reevaluation of risk assessment score.
  - Obtain physician's order (when needed) for identified consults such as physical therapist, dietitian, clinical nurse specialist (CNS), and enterostromal therapy nurse.
  - Reevaluate position changes.
- Client reports sense of fatigue and inability to sleep.
  - Modify client's positioning and turning schedule to promote sleep.
- Areas under pressure develop persistent discoloration, induration, or temperature changes.
  - Document and communicate interval for reevaluation of risk assessment score.
  - Obtain physician's order (when needed) for identified consults such as physical therapist, dietitian, CNS, and enterostomal therapy nurse.

Recording and Reporting

- Record client's risk score.
- Record appearance of skin under pressure.
- Describe positions, turning intervals, pressure-relieving support devices, and other prevention measures.
- Report any need for additional consultations for the high-risk client.

Teaching Considerations

- Review the AHCPR 1992 and 1994 consumer booklets on pressure ulcers with client and family (Ayello, 1993, 1995).
- Explain risks of pressure ulcer formation.
- Assist client (and family) to understand multiple factors involved in preventing and treating pressure ulcers.
- Explain and demonstrate positioning options to achieve pressure relief.
- Explain the purpose and maintenance of pressure-relief devices.
- When teaching clients to change position for pressure relief, suggest using television programming and commercial intervals or a watch with an alarm as reminders.

Gerontological Considerations

- In older adults, a risk score of 17 or 18 (rather than the usual score of 16) may be a more efficient prediction of pressure ulcer risk on the Braden scale (Bryant and others, 1992; Bergstrom, 1994; Braden, 1997).
- Sitting posture and position need to be reevaluated because body weight and muscle tone change with age.
- In the older client, the epidermal-dermal junction becomes flatter, putting client at increased risk for epidermal peel as a result of shearing forces (Loescher, 1995).
- Older adult clients have specialized teaching needs that can be best identified by a thorough learning assessment that takes into consideration normal aging process and its impact on learning (Ayello, Mezey, and Amella, 1997).

Home Care Considerations

- The 30-degree lateral and prone positions may be useful at night to prolong the time between position changes, resulting in less sleep disruption for client and caregiver.
- Identify community resources, such as neighbors and relatives, for assistance should client need help with position changes, including after a fall.
- Pressure-relief maneuvers must be customized to the independent client. The individual may find a watch with a timer, even or odd hours, and television commercials helpful in remembering to complete pressure-relief techniques.
- Home care clients older than 60 years old should be closely monitored for pressure ulcer development if they have any of the following risk factors: wheelchair dependence, incontinence, anemia, fracture, oxygen use, skin drainage, or adult child as primary caregiver (Berquist and Frantz, 1999).

Skill 7-2 Treatment of Pressure Ulcers

Treatment of clients with pressure ulcers requires a holistic approach that uses the expertise of the multidisciplinary health care team (Agency for Health Care Policy and Research [AHCPR], 1994). It involves not only assessment and local care of the pressure ulcer but also assessment and care of the entire client (AHCPR, 1994). Pressure ulcer treatment includes local care of the wound and supportive measures such as pressure relief and adequate nutrition. The basis for the development of an effective pressure ulcer treatment plan is a thorough assessment of the client and the ulcer (Figure 7-3) (AHCPR, 1994). Local wound care principles are wound **debridement** (if the ulcer is necrotic), cleaning, and dressing application (see also Chapters 35 and 36).

The best solution to use to clean most pressure ulcers is normal saline (AHCPR, 1994). **Astringents** such as alcohol and witch hazel can harm skin layers through excessive drying and vasoconstriction, which can reduce local blood flow to tissues. It is also important to avoid using topical agents such as povidone-iodine, iodophor, sodium hypochlorite solution (Dakin's solution), hydrogen peroxide, or acetic acid, which kill the cell fibroblasts that are necessary for wound healing (AHCPR, 1994).

Local treatment of pressure ulcers includes the use of a variety of dressings, which are selected on the basis of the ulcer's characteristics. Occlusive dressings are used with increasing frequency to treat pressure ulcers. Occlusive dressings (transparent dressings, hydrocolloid dressings, and hydrogels) may be used alone or in combination with topical agents (see Chapter 36). All pressure ulcers are considered **colonized;** therefore the AHCPR (1994) suggests that clean dressings and gloves, rather than sterile, be used. Swab cultures only detect surface organisms, and therefore using them routinely to detect wound infection is not recommended (AHCPR, 1994). The AHCPR panel (1994) does recommend quantitative methods of wound culture such as tissue biopsy and wound fluid aspiration.

Current research may determine additional methods useful in treating pressure ulcers. Some ongoing areas of research include topically applied growth factors, electrical stimulation (Itoh and others, 1991), and hyperbaric oxygen therapy (Surman, 1996). Growth factors occur naturally in wound fluid and may stimulate both granulation and epithelialization when applied topically. Pulsed electrical stimulation is a procedure that can be performed by physical therapists with the goal of increased wound healing. Although controversial, hyperbaric oxygen therapy uses increased amounts of pressurized oxygen delivered to clients in a variety of specialized methods (Surman, 1996).

Delegation Considerations

This skill should not be delegated to assistive personnel.

Equipment

- Disposable gloves (clean)
- Goggles and cover gown
- Plastic bag for dressing disposal
- Measuring device (tape measure)
- Cotton-tipped applicators
- Camera and tracing film (optional)
- Topical agent (as ordered)
- Cleansing agent (normal saline)
- Sterile solution container
- Washbasin, washcloths, towels
- Dressing of choice
- Skin protectant
- Hypoallergenic tape (if needed)
- 35-ml syringe with 19-gauge needle
- Documentation records (e.g., graph paper)

Step	Rationale
Assessment	
1. Assess the client's level of comfort and need for pain medication (AHCPR, 1994; Dallam and others, 1995).	Dressing change procedure is better tolerated if pain is controlled.
2. Determine if client has allergies to **topical agents.**	Topical agents contain elements that may cause localized skin reactions.
3. Review prescriber's order for topical agent or dressing (in many cases physician follows nurse's recommendations for pressure ulcer care).	Ensures that proper medication and treatment are administered.

- ***Critical Decision Point***
  Determine if the order is consistent with established wound care guidelines (such as AHCPR). If the order is not consistent with guidelines or varies from guidelines, review the order with the prescriber.

Step	Rationale
4. Wash hands, and apply clean gloves. Close room door or bedside curtains.	Reduces transmission of microorganisms and prevents accidental exposure to body fluids.

Step	Rationale
5. Position client to allow dressing removal and position plastic bag for dressing disposal.	Area should be accessible for dressing change. Proper disposal of old dressing promotes proper handling of contaminated waste.
6. Assess each of the client's pressure ulcer(s) and surrounding skin to determine ulcer characteristics, including its stage (see Table 7-1).	Staging is a way of classifying a pressure ulcer. It is based on the depth of destruction of the tissue. All pressure ulcer staging systems are based on the depth of the tissue destroyed. The nurse must be able to see the type of tissue on the bottom of the pressure ulcer bed. Therefore a pressure ulcer that is covered with necrotic tissue (**eschar,** which is black, hard necrotic tissue) or slough (yellow, stringy necrotic tissue) cannot be staged (AHCPR, 1994).

- ***Critical Decision Point***

To correctly stage a pressure ulcer, the nurse must be able to see its base. Therefore pressure ulcers that are covered with necrotic tissue cannot be staged until the eschar is debrided (AHCPR, 1994). Debridement of the pressure ulcer can be accomplished by several methods (Mosher and others, 1999). Do not use reverse staging to describe a pressure ulcer as it heals. *It is incorrect to say that a stage IV pressure ulcer that begins to heal is now a stage III.*

Step	Rationale
7. Another way to classify pressure ulcers is by the color of the wound bed. Known as the *red-yellow-black color system,* it is quick and easy to use (Krasner, 1995). Wounds that are necrotic are classified as *black wounds;* wounds that have exudate and yellow **slough** are classified as *yellow wounds;* and wounds that are in the active healing phase and are clean with pink to red granulation and epithelial tissue are classified as *red wounds* (Krasner, 1995).	The color of the wound identifies the healing phase of the wound. Fluctuance is the "wavelike" motion, indicative of the presence of fluid, used to describe the appearance of wound tissue" (AHCPR, 1994). Necrotic heel pressure ulcers should be assessed daily to monitor for changes in wound healing. If the wound progresses or the wound bed changes color, debridement may be necessary (AHCPR, 1994).
8. Minimum pressure ulcer characteristics to include in assessing the wound are as follows: location, stage, size, sinus tracts, exudate, necrotic tissue (black, hard tissue is called **eschar,** granulation tissue, and epithelization. Consider using either the Bates-Jensen (1990) Pressure Sore Status Tool (Figure 7-3) or Ayello's Assessment Mnemonic (1996) (Box 7-3). All pressure ulcers should be reassessed at least weekly (AHCPR, 1994).	Wound volume also can be calculated by covering the pressure ulcer with a transparent membrane dressing and then filling the wound with a measured amount of normal saline. After determining the amount of fluid needed to "fill" the wound, it is important to remove the saline and dressing and then proceed with the client's dressing protocol.

Box 7-3 Ayello's Assessment Mnemonic

Anatomical location, age	A	Chronic wounds heal slower.
Size, shape, stage	S	Staging of the wound will help in selecting the appropriate healing treatments and dressing. Measuring guides can assist in determining the length and width of the ulcer. A sterile cotton-tipped application can be used to measure the depth of the ulcer.
Sinus tract	S	Gently use a sterile cotton-tipped applicator tip to locate any sinus tracts.
Exudate	E	Wound drainage must be contained to protect the surrounding skin.
Sepsis	S	Systemic infections must be treated. Routine swab culturing of pressure ulcers for local infection is not recommended (AHCPR, 1994).
Surrounding skin	S	Protect the surrounding skin from breakdown from moisture.
Margins, maceration	M	Identify condition of wound margins and if they are contracting. Evaluate for maceration; if present, institute measures to protect skin.
Erythema, epithelization, eschar	E	Evaluate for wound healing, as evidenced by these changes in the ulcer. Erythema in clients with dark skin tone is best assessed with good lighting. Skin may have a purplish hue (Graves, 1990).
Necrotic, nose, neovascularization	N	Necrotic tissue must be removed to stage and heal the ulcer.
Tissue bed, tenderness to touch, tension, temperature, treatments	T	Identify tissue bed and prior ulcer treatment and medicate for pain (Bergstrom and others, 1994).

Courtesy Elizabeth Ayello. See Ayello EA: Keeping pressure ulcers in check, *Nursing* 26(10):62, 1996.

STEP	RATIONALE
a. Note color, temperature, edema, moisture, and appearance of skin around the ulcer and of the ulcer itself. Remember to modify the assessment technique based on the client's individual skin color (see Box 7-1).	Skin condition may indicate progressive tissue damage. Retained moisture causes maceration, which should prompt the clinician to consider the adequacy of the dressing in controlling wound exudate.

PRESSURE SORE STATUS TOOL NAME________________

Complete the rating sheet to assess pressure sore status. Evaluate each item by picking the response that best describes the wound and entering the score in the item score column for the appropriate date.

Location: Anatomic site. Circle, identify right (R) or left (L) and use "X" to mark site on body diagrams:

____ Sacrum & coccyx ____ Lateral ankle
____ Trochanter ____ Medial ankle
____ Ischial tuberosity ____ Heel Other Site ____

Shape: Overall wound pattern; assess by observing perimeter and depth.
Circle and date appropriate description:

____ Irregular ____ Linear or elongated
____ Round/oval ____ Bowl/boat
____ Square/rectangle ____ Butterfly Other Shape ____

Item	Assessment	Date	Date	Date
		Score	**Score**	**Score**
1. **Size**	1 = Length x width < 4 sq cm 2 = Length x width 4-16 sq cm 3 = Length x width 16.1-36 sq cm 4 = Length x width 36.1-80 sq cm 5 = Length x width > 80 sq cm			
2. **Depth**	1 = Non-blanchable erythema on intact skin 2 = Partial thickness skin loss involving epidermis &/or dermis 3 = Full thickness skin loss involving damage or necrosis of subcutaneous tissue; may extend down to but not through underlying fascia; &/or mixed partial & full thickness &/or tissue layers obscured by granulation tissue 4 = Obscured by necrosis 5 = Full thickness skin loss with extensive destruction, tissue necrosis or damage to muscle, bone or supporting structures			
3. **Edges**	1 = Indistinct, diffuse, none clearly visible 2 = Distinct, outline clearly visible, attached, even with wound base 3 = Well-defined, not attached to wound base 4 = Well-defined, not attached to base, rolled under, thickened 5 = Well-defined, fibrotic, scarred or hyperkeratotic			
4. **Under-mining**	1 = Undermining < 2 cm in any area 2 = Undermining 2-4 cm involving < 50% wound margins 3 = Undermining 2-4 cm involving > 50% wound margins 4 = Undermining > 4 cm in any area 5 = Tunneling &/or sinus tract formation			
5. **Necrotic Tissue Type**	1 = None visible 2 = White/grey non-viable tissue &/or non-adherent yellow slough 3 = Loosely adherent yellow slough 4 = Adherent, soft, black eschar 5 = Firmly adherent, hard, black eschar			
6. **Necrotic Tissue Amount**	1 = None visible 2 = < 25% of wound bed covered 3 = 25% to 50% of wound covered 4 = > 50% and < 75% of wound covered 5 = 75% to 100% of wound covered			

FIGURE 7-3 Bates-Jensen Pressure Sore Status Tool. (Courtesy Barbara Bates-Jensen.)

Continued

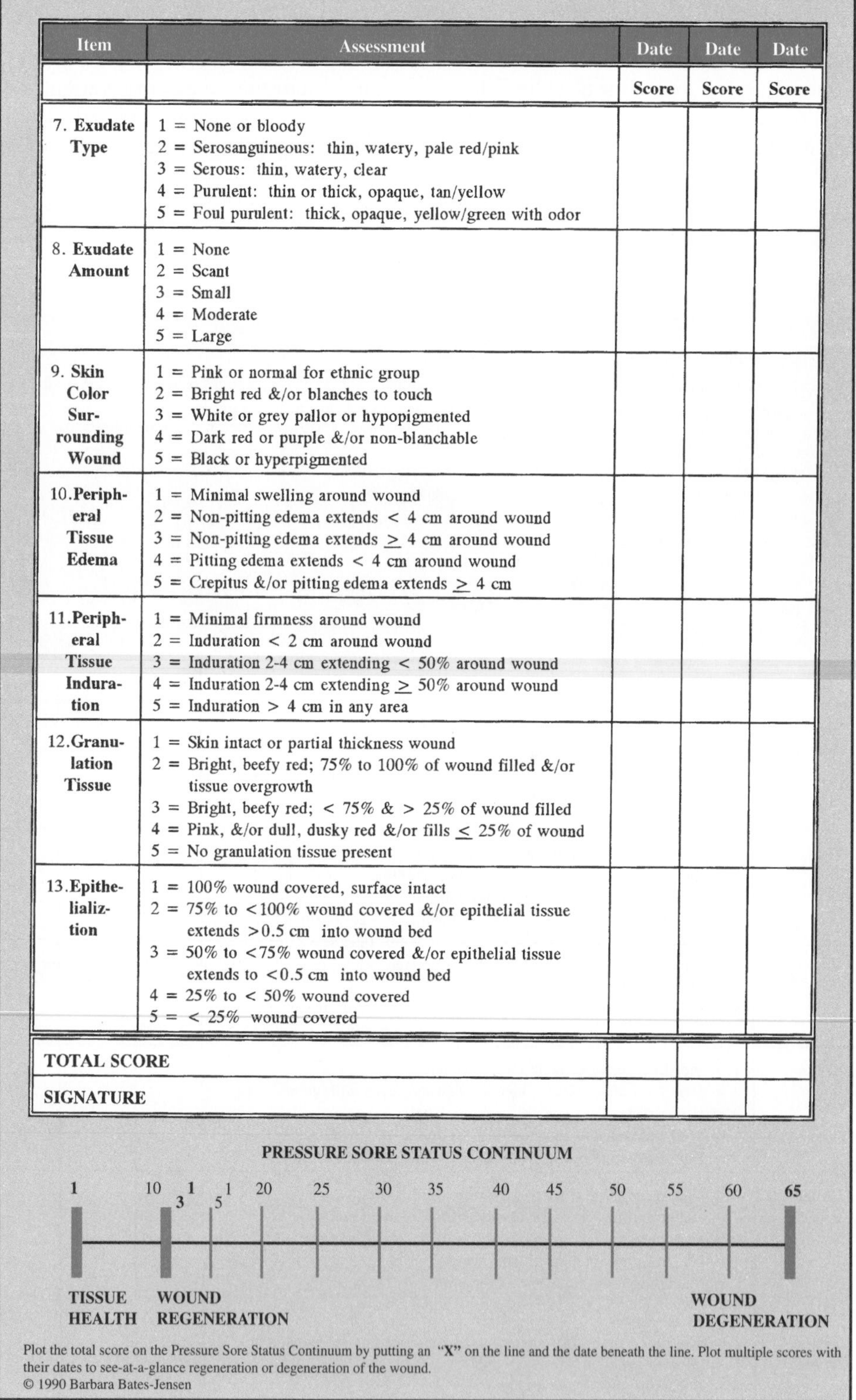

Item	Assessment	Date	Date	Date
		Score	Score	Score
7. **Exudate Type**	1 = None or bloody 2 = Serosanguineous: thin, watery, pale red/pink 3 = Serous: thin, watery, clear 4 = Purulent: thin or thick, opaque, tan/yellow 5 = Foul purulent: thick, opaque, yellow/green with odor			
8. **Exudate Amount**	1 = None 2 = Scant 3 = Small 4 = Moderate 5 = Large			
9. **Skin Color Sur-rounding Wound**	1 = Pink or normal for ethnic group 2 = Bright red &/or blanches to touch 3 = White or grey pallor or hypopigmented 4 = Dark red or purple &/or non-blanchable 5 = Black or hyperpigmented			
10. **Periph-eral Tissue Edema**	1 = Minimal swelling around wound 2 = Non-pitting edema extends < 4 cm around wound 3 = Non-pitting edema extends ≥ 4 cm around wound 4 = Pitting edema extends < 4 cm around wound 5 = Crepitus &/or pitting edema extends ≥ 4 cm			
11. **Periph-eral Tissue Indura-tion**	1 = Minimal firmness around wound 2 = Induration < 2 cm around wound 3 = Induration 2-4 cm extending < 50% around wound 4 = Induration 2-4 cm extending ≥ 50% around wound 5 = Induration > 4 cm in any area			
12. **Granu-lation Tissue**	1 = Skin intact or partial thickness wound 2 = Bright, beefy red; 75% to 100% of wound filled &/or tissue overgrowth 3 = Bright, beefy red; < 75% & > 25% of wound filled 4 = Pink, &/or dull, dusky red &/or fills ≤ 25% of wound 5 = No granulation tissue present			
13. **Epithe-lializ-tion**	1 = 100% wound covered, surface intact 2 = 75% to <100% wound covered &/or epithelial tissue extends >0.5 cm into wound bed 3 = 50% to <75% wound covered &/or epithelial tissue extends to <0.5 cm into wound bed 4 = 25% to < 50% wound covered 5 = < 25% wound covered			
TOTAL SCORE				
SIGNATURE				

PRESSURE SORE STATUS CONTINUUM

Plot the total score on the Pressure Sore Status Continuum by putting an "X" on the line and the date beneath the line. Plot multiple scores with their dates to see-at-a-glance regeneration or degeneration of the wound.

FIGURE **7-3, cont'd** Bates-Jensen Pressure Sore Status Tool. (Courtesy Barbara Bates-Jensen.)

PRESSURE SORE STATUS TOOL

Instructions for use

General Guidelines:

Fill out the attached rating sheet to assess a pressure sore's status after reading the definitions and methods of assessment described below. Evaluate once a week and whenever a change occurs in the wound. Rate according to each item by picking the response that best describes the wound and entering that score in the item score column for the appropriate date. When you have rated the pressure sore on all items, determine the total score by adding together the 13-item scores. The HIGHER the total score, the more severe the pressure sore status. Plot total score on the Pressure Sore Status Continuum to determine progress.

Specific Instructions:

1. **Size**: Use ruler to measure the longest and widest aspect of the wound surface in centimeters; multiply length x width.

2. **Depth**: Pick the depth, thickness, most appropriate to the wound using these additional descriptions:
   - 1 = tissues damaged but no break in skin surface.
   - 2 = superficial, abrasion, blister or shallow crater. Even with, &/or elevated above skin surface (e.g., hyperplasia).
   - 3 = deep crater with or without undermining of adjacent tissue.
   - 4 = visualization of tissue layers not possible due to necrosis.
   - 5 = supporting structures include tendon, joint capsule.

3. **Edges**: Use this guide:

Indistinct, diffuse	=	unable to clearly distinguish wound outline.
Attached	=	even or flush with wound base, <u>no</u> sides or walls present; flat.
Not attached	=	sides or walls <u>are</u> present; floor or base of wound is deeper than edge.
Rolled under, thickened	=	soft to firm and flexible to touch.
Hyperkeratosis	=	callous-like tissue formation around wound & at edges.
Fibrotic, scarred	=	hard, rigid to touch.

4. **Undermining**: Assess by inserting a cotton tipped applicator under the wound edge; advance it as far as it will go without using undue force; raise the tip of the applicator so it may be seen or felt on the surface of the skin; mark the surface with a pen; measure the distance from the mark on the skin to the edge of the wound. Continue process around the wound. Then use a transparent metric measuring guide with concentric circles divided into 4 (25%) pie-shaped quadrants to help determine percent of wound involved.

5. **Necrotic Tissue Type**: Pick the type of necrotic tissue that is <u>predominant</u> in the wound according to color, consistency and adherence using this guide:

White/gray non-viable tissue	=	may appear prior to wound opening; skin surface is white or gray.
Non-adherent, yellow slough	=	thin, mucinous substance; scattered throughout wound bed; easily separated from wound tissue.
Loosely adherent, yellow slough	=	thick, stringy, clumps of debris; attached to wound tissue.
Adherent, soft, black eschar	=	soggy tissue; strongly attached to tissue in center or base of wound.
Firmly adherent, hard/black eschar	=	firm, crusty tissue; strongly attached to wound base <u>and</u> edges (like a hard scab).

FIGURE 7-3, cont'd For legend, see facing page.

6. **Necrotic Tissue Amount**: Use a transparent metric measuring guide with concentric circles divided into 4 (25%) pie-shaped quadrants to help determine percent of wound involved.

7. **Exudate Type**: Some dressings interact with wound drainage to produce a gel or trap liquid. Before assessing exudate type, gently cleanse wound with normal saline or water. Pick the exudate type that is predominant in the wound according to color and consistency, using this guide:

Bloody	=	thin, bright red
Serosanguineous	=	thin, watery pale red to pink
Serous	=	thin, watery, clear
Purulent	=	thin or thick, opaque tan to yellow
Foul purulent	=	thick, opaque yellow to green with offensive odor

8. **Exudate Amount**: Use a transparent metric measuring guide with concentric circles divided into 4 (25%) pie-shaped quadrants to determine percent of dressing involved with exudate. Use this guide:

None	=	wound tissues dry.
Scant	=	wound tissues moist; no measurable exudate.
Small	=	wound tissues wet; moisture evenly distributed in wound; drainage involves ≤ 25% dressing.
Moderate	=	wound tissues saturated; drainage may or may not be evenly distributed in wound; drainage involves > 25% to ≤ 75% dressing.
Large	=	wound tissues bathed in fluid; drainage freely expressed; may or may not be evenly distributed in wound; drainage involves > 75% of dressing.

9. **Skin Color Surrounding Wound**: Assess tissues within 4 cm of wound edge. Dark-skinned persons show the colors "bright red" and "dark red" as a deepening of normal ethnic skin color or a purple hue. As healing occurs in dark-skinned persons, the new skin is pink and may never darken.

10. **Peripheral Tissue Edema**: Assess tissues within 4 cm of wound edge. Non-pitting edema appears as skin that is shiny and taut. Identify pitting edema by firmly pressing a finger down into the tissues and waiting for 5 seconds, on release of pressure, tissues fail to resume previous position and an indentation appears. Crepitus is accumulation of air or gas in tissues. Use a transparent metric measuring guide to determine how far edema extends beyond wound.

11. **Peripheral Tissue Induration**: Assess tissues within 4 cm of wound edge. Induration is abnormal firmness of tissues with margins. Assess by gently pinching the tissues. Induration results in an inability to pinch the tissues. Use a transparent metric measuring guide with concentric circles divided into 4 (25%) pie-shaped quadrants to determine percent of wound and area involved.

12. **Granulation Tissue**: Granulation tissue is the growth of small blood vessels and connective tissue to fill in full thickness wounds. Tissue is healthy when bright, beefy red, shiny and granular with a velvety appearance. Poor vascular supply appears as pale pink or blanched to dull, dusky red color.

13. **Epithelialization**: Epithelialization is the process of epidermal resurfacing and appears as pink or red skin. In partial thickness wounds it can occur throughout the wound bed as well as from the wound edges. In full thickness wounds it occurs from the edges only. Use a transparent metric measuring guide with concentric circles divided into 4 (25%) pie-shaped quadrants to help determine percent of wound involved and to measure the distance the epithelial tissue extends into the wound.

FIGURE **7-3, cont'd** Bates-Jensen Pressure Sore Status Tool. (Courtesy Barbara Bates-Jensen.)

STEP	RATIONALE
b. Measure two maximum perpendicular diameters. It is important to have the client in the same position each time pressure ulcer measurements are taken. This will provide consistency so that subsequent measurements can be compared for changes in size. Obtain the wound's length first and then its width (Surface area = Length × Width). Use either a tape or circular pressure ulcer measuring device (see illustration).	Provides an objective measure of wound size. May influence size and type of dressing selected. Wound measurement techniques may have different results when used by different clinicians, thus decreasing the accuracy of repeated wound measurements for comparison purposes (Langemo and others, 1998).

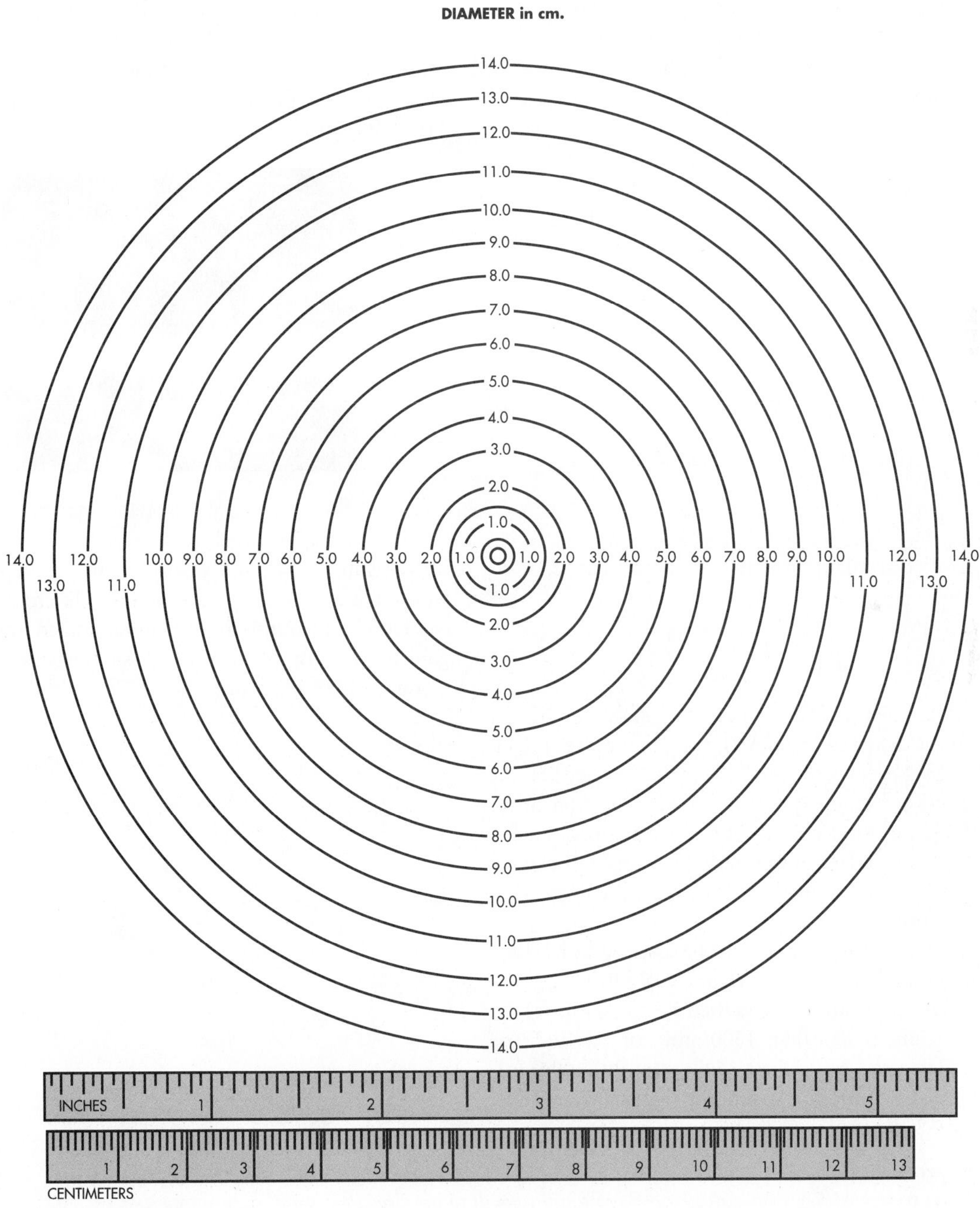

STEP **8b** Measuring guide. Center over wound to be measured. (Modified from Maklebust J, Sieggreen M: *Pressure ulcers: guidelines for prevention and nursing management,* ed 2, Springhouse, Pa, 1996, Springhouse.)

STEP	RATIONALE
c. Measure the depth of the pressure ulcer using a sterile saline–moistened, cotton-tipped applicator or other device that will allow measurement of wound depth. Place the applicator *gently* into the pressure ulcer until it touches the bottom. Mark the place on the applicator where it reaches the top of the wound, and then remove the applicator from the ulcer. Measure the distance from the tip of the applicator to the mark using a measuring tape or ruler to determine the depth of the pressure ulcer (Volume = $2[L \times D] + [W \times D] + [L + D]$).	Depth measure is important for determining wound volume. Although surface area adequately represents tissue loss in stage I and II ulcers, volume more adequately represents tissue loss in deeper stage III and IV wounds.
d. Measure depth (D) of undermining skin by lateral tissue necrosis. Use a cotton-tipped applicator, and gently probe under skin edges.	Undermining represents the loss of the underlying tissues (subcutaneous and muscle) to a greater extent than the skin (see illustration). Undermining may indicate progressive tissue necrosis.

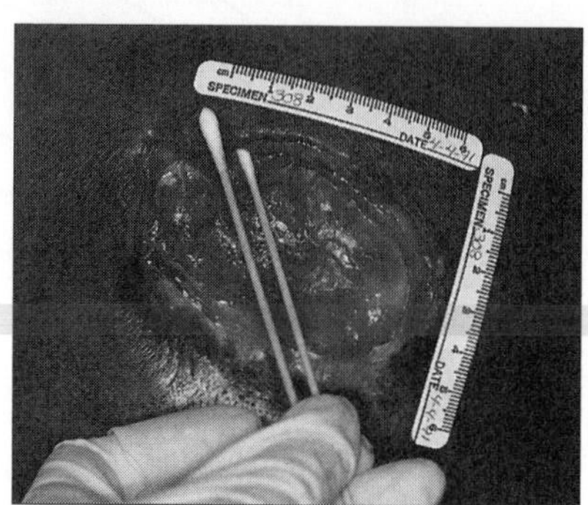

STEP **8d** Measuring depth of undermining of skin.

STEP	RATIONALE
9. Remove gloves, discard appropriately, and wash hands.	Reduces transmission of microorganisms. Repeated hand washing is necessary as nurse assesses different pressure areas. Different wounds may be contaminated by different organisms. Failure to repeatedly wash hands can cause cross-wound contamination.
10. Assessment of the entire client is necessary in developing a pressure ulcer treatment plan. According to the AHCPR (1994), this assessment should include (a) a complete history and physical examination, (b) the identification of complications and comorbid conditions, (c) a nutritional assessment, (d) an assessment of pain, (e) a psychosocial assessment, and (f) an evaluation of the individual's risks for additional pressure ulcers.	
11. The client's nutritional status should be assessed at least every 3 months. Clinically significant malnutrition is present if (a) serum albumin is less than 3.5 g/100 ml, (b) lymphocyte count is less than 1800/mm^3, or (c) body weight has decreased more than 15% (AHCPR, 1994). Observe the client's mouth and skin for signs of vitamin and mineral deficiencies.	

• ***Critical Decision Point***

When malnutrition is suspected, consider a nutritional consult to modify client's diet to promote wound healing.

STEP	RATIONALE
12. Assess client's and support persons' understanding of pressure ulcer characteristics and purpose of treatment (AHCPR, 1994).	Explanations relieve anxiety and promote cooperation during procedure.

STEP	RATIONALE

NURSING DIAGNOSIS

Defining characteristics from the assessment data may reveal the following nursing diagnoses for clients requiring this skill:

Impaired skin integrity
Pain (acute, chronic)
Impaired nutrition: less than body requirements
Impaired tissue perfusion
Impaired physical mobility
Deficient knowledge regarding pressure ulcer treatment plan

Related factors are individualized based on client's condition or needs.

PLANNING

Step	Rationale
1. **Expected outcomes** following completion of procedure:	
▪ Ulcer drainage decreases.	Wound bed of ulcer begins to heal.
▪ Ulcer measurements and tracings are progressively smaller.	
▪ Skin surrounding ulcer remains healthy and intact.	Ulcer does not progress in size.
2. Nutrition is adequate to compensate for wound fluid losses and wound repair (see illustration).	
3. Skin surrounding the ulcer is protected from trauma.	Wound fluids and agents used in treatment may be irritating to intact skin.
4. Client's overall skin is protected from further breakdown.	Client may remain at risk for further breakdown while existing ulcer heals.
5. Explain procedure and its purpose to client and family. Use the AHCPR (1994) consumer booklet *Treating Pressure Sores* (Ayello, 1995). Individualize the teaching plan for older adult clients, taking into account the normal aging changes that affect learning (Ayello, Mezey, and Amella, 1997).	Preparatory explanations relieve anxiety, correct any misconceptions about the ulcer and its treatment, and offer an opportunity for client and family education.
6. Prepare the following necessary equipment and supplies:	
a. Washbasin, warm water, soap, washcloth, and bath towel.	Used to bathe surrounding skin.
b. Normal saline or other wound-cleansing agent in sterile solution container. Use a 19-gauge needle or angiocath with a 35-ml syringe for wound irrigation.	Ulcer surface must be cleansed before the application of topical agents and a new dressing.

• ***Critical Decision Point***
Use only noncytotoxic agents to clean ulcers.

Step	Rationale
c. Prescribed topical agent:	
(1) Enzymatic agents: Santyl (collagenase), Accuzyme (papain-urea). Make sure the manufacturer's specific directions for the frequency of application are followed.	Enzymes debride dead tissue to clean ulcer surface.

• ***Critical Decision Point***
If using an enzymatic debriding agent, do not use wound-cleansing agents with metals.

Step	Rationale
d. Dressing (Table 7-5) (see Chapter 36).	
(1) Select an appropriate dressing based on the pressure ulcer characteristics, purpose for which the dressing is intended, and client care setting.	The dressing should maintain a moist environment for the wound while keeping the surrounding skin dry (AHCPR, 1994).
(2) Gauze type: 4 × 4 pads, fluffs	Applied over ulcers treated with enzymes, mechanical debridement with a wet to dry normal saline dressing, or dextranomer beads.

• ***Critical Decision Point***
Make sure the dressing's absorbency is adequate for the amount of wound drainage. Check that wound does not dry out or that surrounding skin does not become macerated.

STEP	RATIONALE
(3) Transparent membrane dressings.	Applied over superficial ulcers and skin subjected to shear.

- ***Critical Decision Point***
  Transparent membrane dressings can also be used for autolytic debridement of noninfected pressure ulcers.

(4) Hydrocolloid	Maintains moist environment to facilitate wound healing.

- ***Critical Decision Point***
  Hydrocolloid can also be used to protect skin from friction and shear injury. Some of the brands have custom shapes available for specific anatomical parts, such as heels, elbows, and sacrum. Monitor this dressing when it is near the anus to make sure it is intact (AHCPR, 1994).

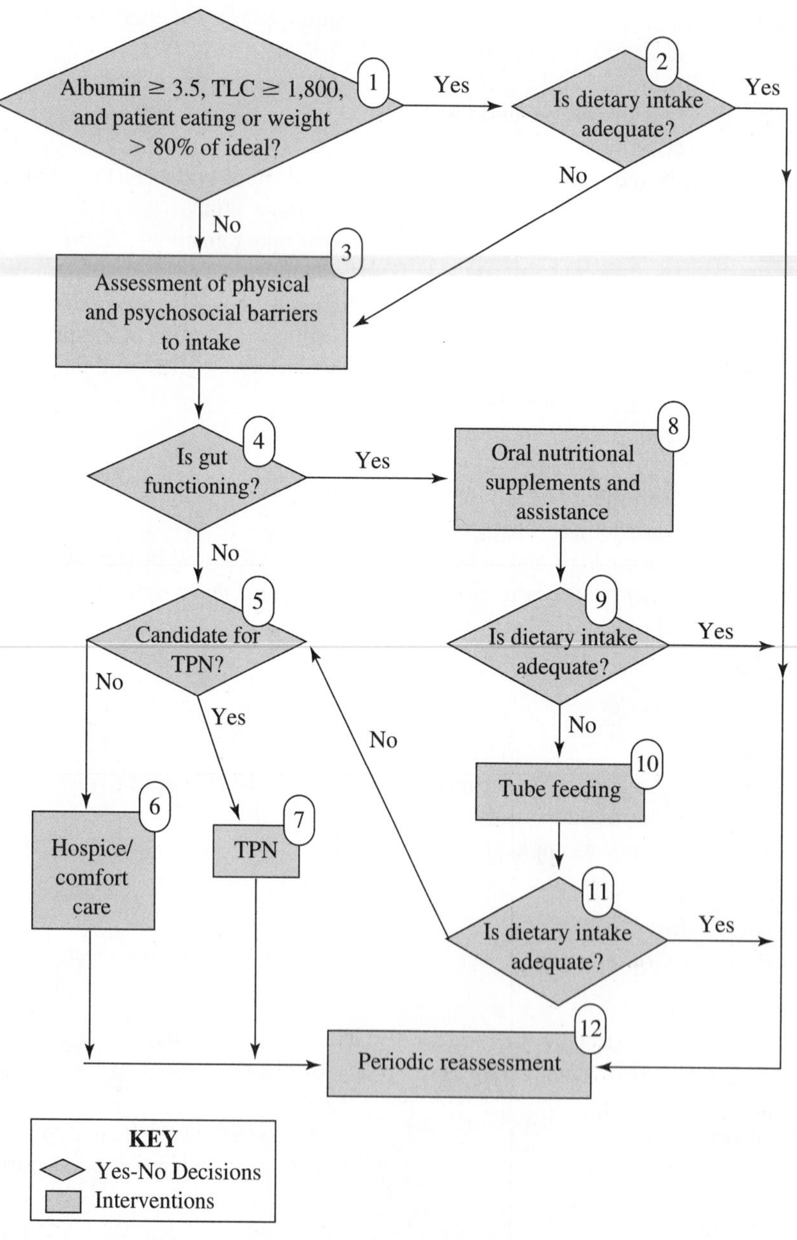

STEP **2** Nutritional assessment and support. (From Bergstrom N and others: *Treatment of pressure ulcers,* AHCPR Pub No. 95-0652, Rockville, Md, 1994, Agency for Health Care Policy and Research, Public Health Service, U.S. Department of Health and Human Services.)

STEP	RATIONALE
(5) Hydrogel	Maintains moist environment to facilitate wound healing. Very soothing to clients with painful wounds.
(6) Calcium alginate	Highly absorbent of wound **exudate** in heavily draining wounds.

- ***Critical Decision Point***

  Some alginate dressings give off a "low tide" odor when they interact with the wound exudates. This is not to be equated with the foul odor associated with wound infections.

Table 7-5 Treatment Options by Ulcer Stage

ULCER STAGE	ULCER STATUS	DRESSING	COMMENTS*	EXPECTED CHANGE	ADJUVANTS
I	Intact	None	Allows visual assessment.	Resolves slowly without epidermal loss over 7 to 14 days.	Turning schedule. Support hydration. Nutritional support. Silicone-based lotion to decrease shear. Pressure-relief mattress or chair cushion.
		Film, adherent	Protects from shear.		
		Hydrocolloid	May not allow visual assessment.		
II	Clean	Composite film	Viasorb film, plus telfa, Exudry. Limits shear.	Heals through reepithelialization and epithelial budding.	See previous stage. Manage incontinence.
		Hydrocolloid	Change every 7 days if occlusive seal.		
		Hydrogel sheet	Absorbent, requires secondary dressing of gauze or adherent film.		
III	Clean	Hydrocolloid	See stage II.	Heals through granulation and reepithelialization. (NOTE: does not become a stage II ulcer as it heals.)	See previous stages. Electrical stimulation. Evaluate pressure-relief needs.
		Hydrogel foam	Apply ¼-inch thick, cover with gauze or hydrocolloid.		
		Exudate absorbers calcium alginate wound pastes	Change when strike through is noted on secondary dressing. Cover with gauze or hydrocolloid.		
		Gauze, fluffy	Use with normal saline.		
		Growth factors	Use with gauze.		
IV	Clean	Hydrogel	See stage III Clean.	Heals through granulation and reepithelialization.	Surgical consult for closure. See stages I, II, and III Clean.
		Hydrocolloid plus hydrocolloid paste/beads	See stage III Clean; critical to treat areas of undermining.	Because of contraction, surface may close more rapidly than base, leaving wound cavity.	
		Calcium alginate	See stage III Clean.		
		Gauze	Pack deeply undermined ulcers.		
		Growth factors	Use with gauze.		
	Eschar	Adherent film	Will facilitate softening of eschar.	Eschar will lift at the edges as healing progresses. Cross-hatching central area of eschar with a small blade will facilitate release from center.	See previous stages. Surgical consult for debridement. Enzymes covered with gauze dressing may be used to debride ulcer.
		Hydrocolloid	Will facilitate softening of eschar.		
		Gauze plus ordered solution	Absorb drainage and control odor if Dakin's is used.		
		None	Rarely, if eschar is dry and intact, no dressing is used, allowing eschar to act as physiological cover.		

*As with *all* occlusive dressings, wounds should *not* be clinically infected.

Step	Rationale
(7) Exudate absorbers	Highly absorbent of wound exudate.
(8) Foam	Protective and will prevent wound dehydration; also absorbs small to moderate amounts of drainage.
e. Hypoallergenic tape or adhesive dressing sheet (Hypofix).	Used to secure nonadherent dressing. Prevents skin irritation and tearing.

Implementation

Step	Rationale
1. Assemble needed supplies at beside. Close room door or bedside curtains. Wash hands, and apply gloves. Open sterile packages and topical solution containers. (Goggles and moistureproof cover gown should be worn if potential for contamination from spray exists when cleansing the wound.)	Maintains client privacy. Supplies should be ready for easy application so that nurse can use supplies without contaminating them; reduces transmission of microorganisms.
2. Remove bed linen and client's gown to expose ulcer and surrounding skin. Keep remaining body parts draped.	Prevents unnecessary exposure of body parts.
3. Gently wash skin surrounding ulcer with warm water and soap.	Cleansing of skin surface reduces bacteria.
4. Rinse area thoroughly with water.	Soap can be irritating to skin.
5. Gently dry skin thoroughly by patting lightly with towel.	Retained moisture causes maceration of skin layers.
6. Wash hands and change gloves.	Aseptic technique must be maintained during cleansing, measuring, and application of dressings. Refer to institutional policy regarding use of clean or sterile gloves.
7. Cleanse ulcer thoroughly with normal saline or prescribed wound-cleansing agent. Use an adequate amount of pressure (measured in pounds per square inch [psi]) to effectively clean the wound, but do not use so much pressure that you injure the wound tissue. In a nonnecrotic wound, between 4 and 15 psi is considered safe and effective for cleaning a pressure ulcer (AHCPR, 1994).	Irrigation under proper pressure removes exudate and dead tissue.
a. Use a 19-gauge needle (or angiocath) with a 35-ml syringe to clean most pressure ulcers, especially deep ulcers.	The pressure of this type of wound-cleaning system is 8 psi, which will not harm the fragile healing tissue in the pressure ulcer (AHCPR, 1994).
b. Cleansing in the shower may be done with a handheld shower head.	Refreshing to client and provides thorough cleansing.
8. Whirlpool treatments may be used to assist with wound debridement. Keep the wound directly away from the water jets.	Removes wound debris. Previously applied enzymes may require soaking for removal. Whirpool should not be used on clean granulating wounds.
9. Apply topical agents, if prescribed.	
a. Enzymes:	Follow manufacturer's directions for frequency of application. Be aware of what solutions inactivate the enzymes, and avoid their use in wound cleaning.
(1) Using a wooden tongue blade, apply a small amount of enzyme debridement ointment directly to the necrotic areas on the base of pressure ulcer. Avoid getting the enzyme on the surrounding skin. The amount of enzyme should be the same as the amount of butter you would spread on bread. A thick layer of ointment is not necessary; a thin layer absorbs and acts more effectively. Cross-hatching of the eschar areas may be needed in some necrotic pressure ulcers. Do not apply enzyme to surrounding skin.	Proper distribution of ointment ensures effective action. Some enzymes can cause burning, paresthesia, and dermatitis to surrounding skin.

Step	Rationale
(2) Place gauze dressing directly over ulcer, and tape it in place. Follow specific manufacturer's recommendation for type of dressing material to use to cover a pressure ulcer when using enzymatic agent.	Protects wound and prevents removal of ointment during turning or repositioning.
b. Hydrogel agents:	
(1) Cover surface of ulcer with hydrogel using applicator or gloved hand.	Provides maintenance of wound humidity while absorbing excess drainage. May be used as carrier for topical agents.
(2) Apply a secondary dressing, such as dry gauze, hydrocolloid, or transparent dressing over gel to completely cover ulcer.	Holds hydrogel against wound surface because hydrogel amphorous form or sheet form does not adhere to the wound and requires a secondary dressing to hold it in place.
c. Calcium alginates:	Provide maintenance of wound humidity while absorbing excess drainage. Use in heavily draining wounds.
(1) Pack wound with alginate using applicator or gloved hand.	
(2) Apply a secondary dressing, such as dry gauze, foam, or hydrocolloid over alginate.	Holds alginate against wound surface.
10. Reposition client comfortably off pressure ulcer.	Avoids accidental removal of dressings.
11. Remove gloves, and dispose of soiled supplies. Wash hands.	Reduces transmission of microorganisms.

Evaluation

Step	Rationale
1. Observe skin surrounding ulcer for inflammation, edema, and tenderness.	A clean pressure ulcer should show evidence of some healing within 2 to 4 weeks. Contact dermatitis may result from exposure to certain topical agents. Without proper preventive care, ulcer can spread to involve neighboring tissue.
2. Inspect dressings and exposed ulcers, observing for drainage, foul odor, and tissue necrosis. Monitor client for signs and symptoms of infection, including fever and elevated white blood cell (WBC) count.	Ulcers can become infected.
3. Compare subsequent ulcer measurements.	Allows comparison of serial measurements to assess wound healing. It is helpful to plot surface area and volume measurements on graph paper (see illustration).

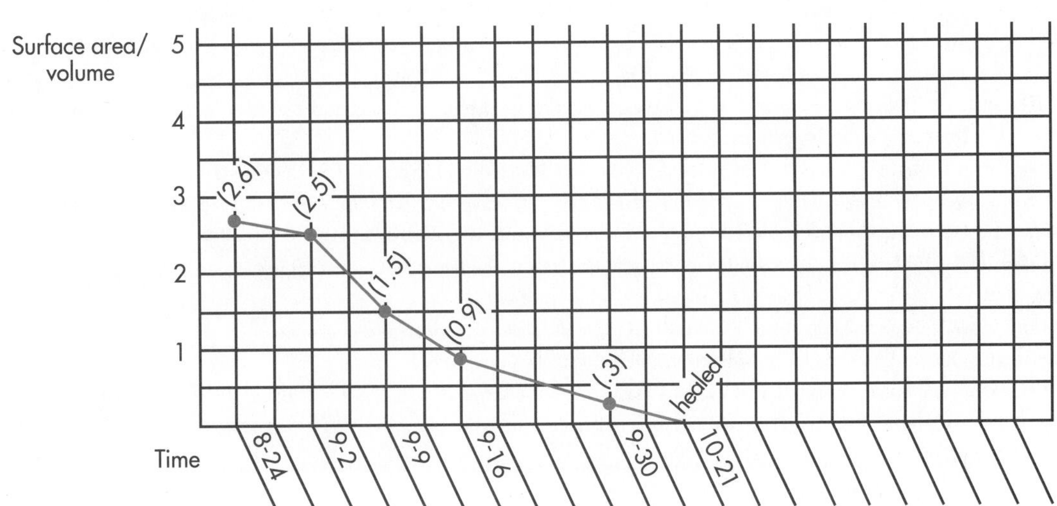

STEP 3 Graph of wound surface area or volume measurements over time.

STEP	RATIONALE
4. Use one of the scales designed to measure wound healing, such as the PUSH Scale (Table 7-6) (NPUAP, 1999) (Thomas and others, 1997) or the PSST (Bates-Jensen, 1990).	Allows for objective measure of sound healing progress.
Do not use the pressure ulcer staging system to measure pressure ulcer healing (NPUAP, 1995).	Use of the staging system to measure healing rather than its intended use for depth of tissue destruction is inappropriate (NPUAP, 1995).

- ***Critical Decision Point***
  Deterioration of the client's or the ulcer's condition indicates the need for reevaluation of the treatment plan (AHCPR, 1994).

Table 7-6 PUSH Tool 3.0

Patient Initials: ______________ Study ID#: ______________

Study Day #: ______________ Date: ______________

DIRECTIONS:

Observe and measure the pressure ulcer. Categorize the ulcer with respect to surface area, exudate, and type of wound tissue. Record a sub-score for each of these ulcer characteristics. Add the sub-scores to obtain the total score. A comparison of total scores measured over time provides an indication of the improvement or deterioration in pressure ulcer healing.

Length	0 0 cm^2	1 <0.3 cm^2	2 0.3-0.6 cm^2	3 0.7-1.0 cm^2	4 1.1-2.0 cm^2	5 2.1-3.0 cm^2	
× Width		6 3.1-4.0 cm^2	7 4.1-8.0 cm^2	8 8.1-12.0 cm^2	9 12.1-24.0 cm^2	10 >24.0 cm^2	Sub-score
Exudate amount	0 None	1 Light	2 Moderate	3 Heavy			Sub-score
Tissue type	0 Closed	1 Epithelial tissue	2 Granulation tissue	3 Slough	4 Necrotic tissue		Sub-score
							Total score

Length × Width: Measure the greatest length (head to toe) and the greatest width (side to side) using a centimeter ruler. Multiply these two measurements (length × width) to obtain an estimate of surface area in square centimeters (cm^2). Caveat: Do not guess! Always use a centimeter ruler and always use the same method each time the ulcer is measured.

Exudate amount: Estimate the amount of exudate (drainage) present after removal of the dressing and before applying any topical agent to the ulcer. Estimate the exudate (drainage) as none, light, moderate, or heavy.

Tissue type: This refers to the types of tissue that are present in the wound (ulcer) bed. Score as a "4" if there is any necrotic tissue present. Score as a "3" if there is any amount of slough present and necrotic tissue is absent. Score as a "2" if the wound is clean and contains granulation tissue. A superficial wound that is reepithelizing is scored as a "1". When the wound is closed, score as a "0".

4-Necrotic Tissue (Eschar): black, brown, or tan tissue that adheres firmly to the wound bed or ulcer edges and may be either firmer or softer than surrounding skin.

3-Slough: yellow or white tissue that adheres to the ulcer bed in strings or thick clumps, or is mucinous.

2-Granulation Tissue: pink or beefy red tissue with a shiny, moist, granular appearance.

1-Epithelial Tissue: for superficial ulcers, new pink or shiny tissue (skin) that grows in from the edges or as islands on the ulcer surface.

0-Closed/Resurfaced: the wound is completely covered with epithelium (new skin).

Version 3.0: 9/15/98 National Pressure Ulcer Advisory Panel.

Unexpected Outcomes and Related Interventions

- Skin surrounding ulcer becomes macerated.
  - Reduce exposure of surrounding skin to topical agents and moisture.
  - Select a dressing that has increased moisture-absorbing capacity.
- Ulcer becomes deeper with increased drainage and/or development of necrotic tissue.
  - Review current wound care management.
  - Consult with multidisciplinary team regarding changes in wound care regimen.
  - Obtain wound cultures (see Chapter 42).
- Pressure ulcer extends beyond original margins.
  - Monitor for systemic signs and symptoms of poor wound healing, such as abnormal laboratory results (WBC, hemoglobin/hematocrit, serum albumin, serum prealbumin, total proteins), weight loss, and fluid imbalances.
  - Assess and revise current turning schedule.
  - Consider further pressure-reducing devices (see Chapter 30).

Recording and Reporting

- Record appearance of ulcer in client's record.
- Describe type of topical agent used, dressing applied, and client's response.
- Report any deterioration in ulcer appearance to nurse in charge or physician.

Teaching Considerations

- Discuss treatment and identify individual(s) who will assist in care at home.
- Discuss process of wound healing and expected wound appearance, for example, client's and support persons' perception about appearance of the pressure ulcer. An eschar may look like a scab that indicates wound healing to the client or support persons.
- Discuss with client and support persons perceptions about size of pressure ulcer. Lay people may think that a "bedsore" is small, about the size of a wedding ring. Some of the larger wounds, especially after debridement, may be very troublesome to the client and support persons.
- Discuss with client and support persons perceptions about treatment. Client and support persons may believe it is cruel for staff to keep turning and positioning the client every 2 hours. They may misunderstand some dressing change techniques such as pulling out the dried gauze dressing used for mechanical debridement.
- Identify the signs, symptoms, and four stages of ulcers to report to the health care team.
- Review prevention guidelines to halt further breakdown.
- Discuss options for maintaining good nutrition.

Gerontological Considerations

- Wound healing may be slower in the older adult (Lueckenotte, 2000).
- The normal reduction in the Langerhans' cells in the older adult's epidermis causes a decrease in T-cell function and immunity (Loescher, 1995).
- Because older skin has a slower and less intense inflammatory reaction, older clients must be monitored more closely for altered responses to skin irritants (Loescher, 1995).

Home Care Considerations

- Consider caregiver time when selecting a dressing. In the home care setting, caregivers may choose more expensive dressing materials to reduce the frequency of dressing changes (AHCPR, 1994).
- Cost can also be a factor. Some clients have more time than financial resources. They may choose a less expensive treatment option such as dressing material, especially if there is no third-party reimbursement. Another example might be teaching the family to make a normal saline rather than buying it premade.
- Disposal of contaminated dressings in the home should be done in a manner consistent with local regulations (AHCPR, 1994).
- Identify clean storage area for dressing supplies.
- Determine availability of required supplies.
- Discuss need for home health nurse.
- Discuss need for home pressure-relief surface or bed.
- Identify adaptive equipment needed to care for client at home.
- Medicare regulations limit reimbursement of some types of pressure-relief equipment for stage III and IV pressure ulcers.

Long-Term Care Considerations

- Rehabilitation units may use a variety of position-relief devices and beds.
- Clients may be discharged to long-term care facilities that specialize in pressure ulcer and wound care.

Critical Thinking Exercises

1. A 72-year-old African-American man is admitted to the hospital with a diagnosis of left cerebral vascular accident (CVA). He has right-sided weakness and cannot turn or walk without using his walker and one person's assistance. He also has difficulty swallowing and is incontinent of urine. What risk factors, if any, for pressure ulcers does this client have?
2. On admission to the nursing home, an 86-year-old Irish woman needs a pressure ulcer risk assessment score done using the Braden scale. Using the following client assessment data, determine her pressure ulcer risk assessment score: Client responds to verbal commands but cannot communicate her need to be turned. She walks occasionally during the day, but only for short distances. Her mobility is slightly limited, and she can make frequent but slight changes in her extremities independently. She has sufficient strength to sit up completely and maintains a good position in the bed or chair at all times. Her skin is thin, dry, and intact, and only routine linen changes are needed. Her appetite is excellent, and she eats most of the meals offered to her. What is her risk score? One week later, her score on the Braden scale is 16. Explain the clinical significance of each of these findings. What plan of care is indicated at this time?
3. In assessing your 66-year-old Latino client, you find he has a 3 × 2 cm wound on his sacrum that is 1-inch deep. The wound extends into his subcutaneous tissue but not through it. The tissue bed is pink to red, and there is scant serous exudate. What stage is this pressure ulcer? What other assessments should the nurse do of this pressure ulcer? What type of wound care would you expect?

References

Abruzzese R: The effectiveness of an assessment tool in specifying nursing care to prevent decubitus ulcers. In *PRN: the Adelphi report—project for research in nursing,* 1982, Adelphi University Library, New York.

AHCPR Panel for the Prediction and Prevention of Pressure Ulcers in Adults: *Pressure ulcers in adults: prediction and prevention.* Clinical practice guideline No. 3, Pub No. 92-0047, Rockville, Md, 1992, Public Health Service, U.S. Department of Health and Human Services.

AHCPR Panel for the Treatment of Pressure Ulcers in Adults: *Treatment of pressure ulcers.* Clinical practice guideline No. 15, Pub No. 95-0653, Rockville, Md, 1994, Public Health Service, U.S. Department of Health and Human Services.

Ayello EA: Teaching the assessment of patients with pressure ulcers, *Decubitus* 5(4):53, 1992.

Ayello EA: A critique of the AHCPR's Preventing pressure ulcers: a patient's guide as a written instructional tool, *Decubitus* 6(3):44, 1993.

Ayello EA: Critique of AHCPR's Consumer guide: treating pressure sores, *Adv Wound Care* 8(5):18, 1995.

Ayello EA: Keeping pressure ulcers in check, *Nursing* 26(10):62, 1996.

Ayello EA, Mezey M, Amella EJ: Educational assessment and teaching of older clients with pressure ulcers, *Clin Geriatr Med* 13(3):483, 1997.

Barczak CA and others: Fourth national pressure ulcer prevalence survey, *Adv Wound Care* 10(4):18, 1997.

Barczak C and others: Fourth national pressure ulcer prevalence survey, *Adv Wound Care* 12(7):339, 1999.

Bates-Jensen B: New pressure ulcer status tool, *Decubitus* 3(3):14, 1990.

Bennett MA: Report of the Task Force on the Implications for Darkly Pigmented Intact Skin in the Prediction and Prevention of Pressure Ulcers, *Adv Wound Care* 8(6):34, 1995.

Bergstrom N, Demuth PJ, Braden BJ: A clinical trial of the Braden scale for predicting pressure sore risk, *Nurs Clin North Am* 22(2):417, 1987.

Bergstrom N and others: *Treatment of pressure ulcers.* AHCPR Pub No. 95-0652, Rockville, Md, Public Health Service, U.S. Department of Health and Human Services, Agency for Health Care Policy and Research, 1994.

Berquist S and Frantz R: Pressure ulcers in community-based older adults receiving home health care, *Adv Wound Care,* 12(7):339, 1999.

Braden B: Risk assessment in pressure ulcer prevention. In Krasner D, Kane D: *Chronic wound care: a clinical source book for health care professionals,* ed 2, Wayne, Pa, 1997, Health Management Publications.

Braden BJ, Bergstrom N: Clinical utility of the Braden scale for predicting pressure sore risk, *Decubitus* 2(3):44, 1989.

Braden BJ, Bergstrom N: Predictive utility of the Braden scale for predicting pressure sore risk, *Res Nurs Health* 17:459, 1994.

Bryant RA and others: Pressure ulcers. In Bryant RA, editor: *Acute and chronic wounds: nursing management,* St. Louis, 1992, Mosby.

Dallam L and others: Pressure ulcer pain: assessment and quantification, *J Wound Ostomy Continence Nurs* 22(5):211, 1995.

Fowler EM: Equipment and products used in management and treatment of pressure ulcers, *Nurs Clin North Am* 22(7):449, 1987.

Gosnell DJ: An assessment tool to identify pressure sores, *Nurs Res* 22:55, 1973.

Graves DJ: Stage I in ebony complexion, *Decubitus* 3(4):4, 1990 (letter).

Henderson CT and others: Draft definition of stage I pressure ulcers: inclusion of persons with darkly pigmented skin, *Adv Wound Care* 10(5):16, 1997.

Itoh M and others: Accelerated wound healing of pressure ulcers by pulsed high peak power electromagnetic energy (Diapulse), *Decubitus* 4(1):24, 1991.

Jiricka MK and others: Pressure ulcer risk factors in an ICU population, *Am J Crit Care* 4(5):361, 1995.

Knox DM: Core body temperature, skin temperature, and interface pressure: relationship to skin integrity in nursing home residents, *Adv Wound Care* 12(5):246, 1999.

Kosiak M: Etiology and pathology of decubitus ulcers, *Arch Phys Med Rehabil* 40:62, 1959.

Krasner D: Wound care how to use the red-yellow-black system, *Am J Nurs* 5:44, 1995.

Langemo DK and others: Two-dimensional wound measurement: comparison of 4 techniques, *Adv Wound Care* 11(7):337, 1998.

Loescher LJ: The dynamics of aging skin. *Progressions* 7(20):3, 1995.

Lueckenotte AG: *Gerontologic nursing,* ed 2, St. Louis, 2000, Mosby.

Lyder CH and others: Validating the Braden scale for the prediction of pressure ulcer risk in Black and Latino/Hispanic elders: a pilot study, *Ostomy Wound Manage* 44(suppl 3A):42s, 1998.

Maklebust J, Sieggreen M: *Pressure ulcers: guidelines for prevention and nursing management,* ed 2, Springhouse, Pa, 1996, Springhouse.

Mayrovitz HN, Smith SR: Adaptive skin blood flow increases during hip-down lying in elderly women, *Adv Wound Care* 12(6):295, 1999.

Mosher BA and others: Outcomes of 4 methods of debridement using a decision analysis methodology, *Adv Wound Care* 12(2):81, 1999.

National Pressure Ulcer Advisory Panel (NPUAP): Pressure ulcer prevalence, cost and risk assessment: consensus development conference statement, *Decubitus* 2(2):24, 1989.

National Pressure Ulcer Advisory Panel (NPUAP): NPUAP position on reverse staging of pressure ulcers, *Adv Wound Care* 8(6):32, 1995.

Norton D, McLaren R, Exon-Smith AN: *An investigation of geriatric nursing problems in hospital, 1962.* Reissue, Edinburgh, 1975, Churchill Livingstone.

Pires M, Mueller A: Detection and management of early tissue pressure indicators: a pictorial essay, *Progressions* 3(3):3, 1991.

Surman MW: An introduction to hyperbaric oxygen therapy for the ET nurse, *J Wound Ostomy Continence Nurs* 23(2):80, 1996.

Thomas DR and others: Pressure ulcer scale for healing: derivation and validation of the PUSH Tool, *Adv Wound Care* 10(5):96, 1997.

Trelease CC: Developing standards for wound care, *Ostomy Wound Manage* 26:50, 1988.

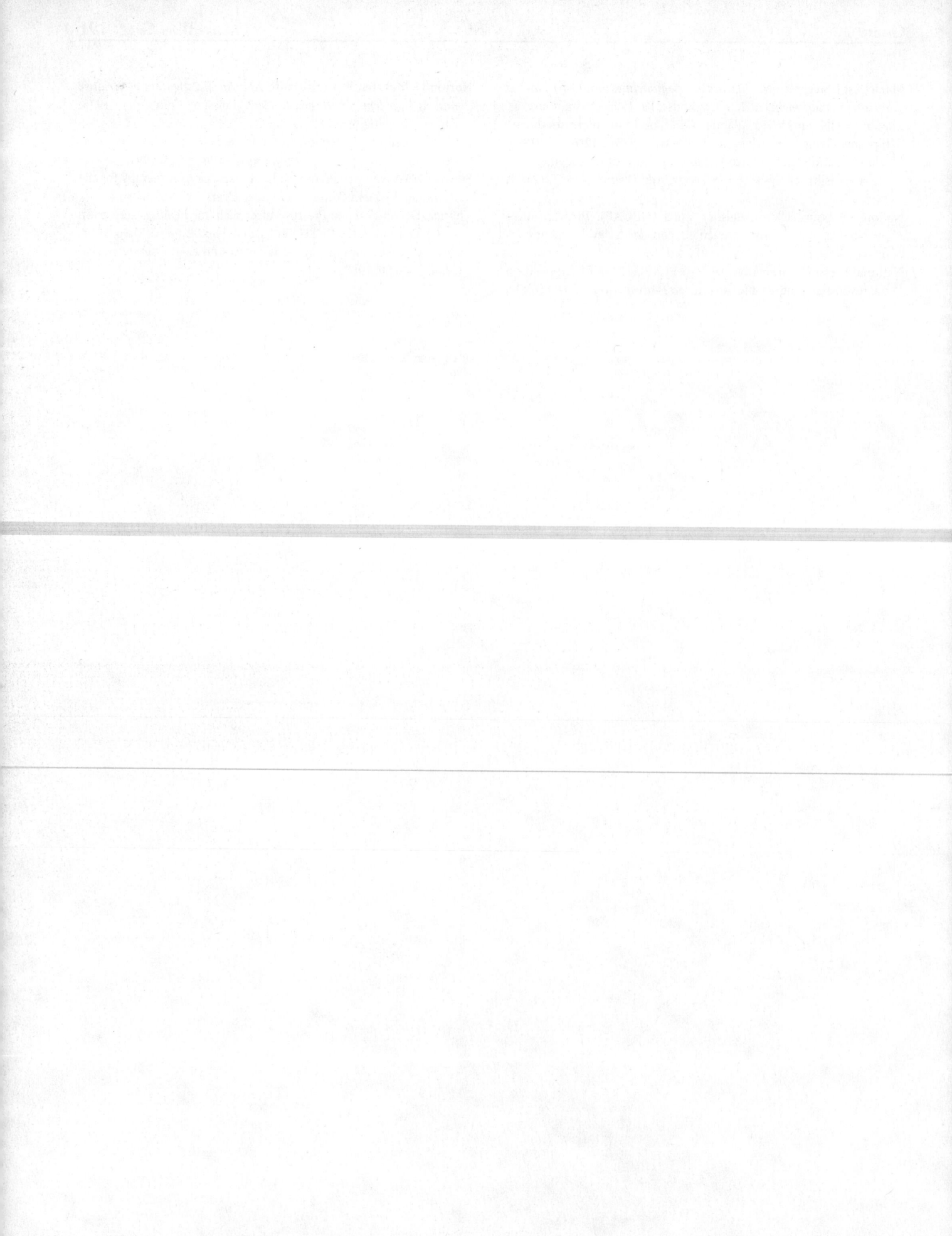

8

CARE OF EYE AND EAR PROSTHESES

Skills

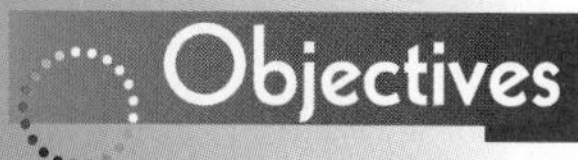

Objectives

Mastery of content in this chapter will enable the nurse to:

- Define the key terms listed.
- Explain why proper care of prostheses is important to a client's self-esteem.
- Identify guidelines used in caring for lenses and prostheses.
- Explain differences in the care of soft and rigid contact lenses.
- Correctly remove, store, cleanse, and insert a contact lens.
- Explain the rationale for maintaining aseptic technique during care of an artificial eye.
- Describe techniques that determine whether a hearing aid functions properly.
- Correctly remove, cleanse, and reinsert a hearing aid.

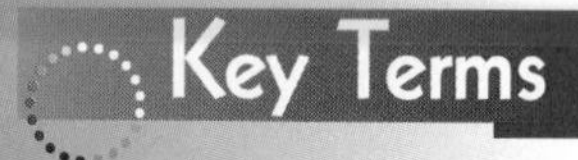

Key Terms

Audiologist	Optometrist
Contact lens	Presbycusis
Enucleation	Presbyopia
Myopia	Prosthesis
Ophthalmologist	Refractive errors

Many clients rely on artificially constructed devices to replace or restore lost or impaired body functions. Eyeglasses and contact lenses help to restore visual loss, and hearing aids can improve sound reception. Clients often depend on these devices to maintain an attractive appearance, as well as to improve sensory function. Artificial eyes in particular help clients maintain a normal appearance when an eye has been lost as the result of injury or disease. Prostheses and contact lenses must fit and function properly so that clients can function normally within their environment. Clients can be extremely sensitive about lenses or prosthetic care. Accidental breakage or malfunction can seriously impair sensory function and threaten self-esteem when a client becomes dependent on others for assistance.

Lenses and prostheses must be cleaned regularly to ensure proper function. Most clients have an established routine for cleaning their contact lenses or prostheses. When clients are unable to care for themselves, the nurse must understand the correct way to clean, handle, and store contact lenses and prostheses. Clients usually show great interest in the manner in which the nurse performs cleaning and maintenance procedures. Careful handling of lenses, artificial eyes, and hearing aids is vital to avoid damage to these devices or to clients' eyes or ears.

Skill Performance Guidelines

1. Let the client be a resource in the care of each device. Unless receiving lenses or a prosthesis for the first time, a client is likely to have an established routine for care and maintenance and has adapted special care techniques as well. It is the nurse's responsibility to be sure clients are not damaging the devices or injuring themselves.
2. Always protect the device from breakage. Replacement can be costly.
3. When a sensory loss exists, use techniques that facilitate interaction with the client. For example, if a client wears a hearing aid, the nurse should use communication techniques, such as message boards and paper and pencil, that improve the client's ability to interact successfully. If visual function is reduced, the nurse should provide visual aids to improve the client's interaction with the environment.
4. Encourage clients to express feelings about changes in body image, such as feeling unusual or different, because of reliance on an artificial device for function or appearance. For example, clients with hearing impairments are often treated as though they are mentally impaired because they do not understand what is said to them. Family members become frustrated when they cannot communicate with the client whose hearing aid malfunctions. The nurse can be supportive and demonstrate understanding when communicating with these clients and can teach families methods for interacting more effectively.

Skill 8-1 Taking Care of Contact Lenses

A **contact lens** is a thin, transparent, circular disk that fits directly over the cornea of the eye. Contact lenses are designed specifically to correct **refractive errors** of the eye or abnormalities in the cornea's shape. They are relatively easy to apply and remove.

There are three basic types of contact lenses: rigid (hard), soft, and rigid gas permeable (RGP), also known as oxygen permeable. They differ in size, material, and amount of oxygen flow they permit to the eye's surface. Rigid contact lenses are made of firm, durable plastic and are smaller than the cornea. These lenses ride on the tear film layer of the cornea and are held in place by surface tension. Blinking causes the tear film to move under and over the contact lens, providing oxygen to the cornea. Soft contact lenses are made of soft, flexible plastic, and because they cover the entire cornea and a small rim of the sclera, they do not ride on the corneal tear film. The cornea receives oxygen through the soft lens, which is oxygen permeable. Rigid gas-permeable lenses are similar to the rigid lens, but the plastic lens allows oxygen to pass through to the cornea. All three lenses are available as clear (untinted) or tinted.

Contact lenses are also available as daily wear, extended wear, and disposable. All lenses must be removed periodically to prevent ocular infection and corneal ulcers or abrasions. Daily-wear lenses should be removed overnight for cleaning and disinfection and should not be worn for more than 10 to 14 hours daily. It is recommended that all extended-wear lenses be worn no longer than 7 consecutive nights without cleaning and disinfecting (Farley, 1998). Disposable lenses are available for daily wear and extended wear and are usually replaced every 1 to 2 weeks. Pain, tearing, discomfort, and redness of the conjunctivae may be symptoms of lens overwear. Persistence of symptoms even after lens removal is abnormal, however, and may indicate serious ocular damage.

As contact lenses are worn, they accumulate secretions and foreign matter. This material deteriorates and then irritates the eye, causing distorted vision and risk for infection. Once removed, reusable contact lenses should be cleaned and thoroughly disinfected.

Care of contact lenses includes proper cleaning, insertion and removal, and storage. Many clients wear contact lenses today. It is extremely important that nurses determine whether clients wear contact lenses, particularly when clients are admitted to hospitals or agencies in unresponsive or confused states. If a seriously ill client is wearing contact lenses and this fact goes undetected, severe corneal injury can result.

Clients usually have a preferred method for caring for their lenses. When it is necessary for the nurse to assist with lens care, the client's preferences should be considered. In addition, the nurse needs to be aware that some disinfecting solutions do not mix with one another and can cause damage to the contact lens surface.

Delegation Considerations

The skill of caring for contact lenses can be delegated to assistive personnel. It will be necessary to inform and assist the care provider in the proper way to care for the client's specific type of contact lens. Be sure to stress to the care provider that careful handling of the contact lens is of utmost importance to prevent physical injury to the client and damage to the lenses. Instruct the care provider to explain the steps of the procedure to the client as the procedure progresses and to use appropriate communication techniques to ensure smooth completion of the task at hand. Also be sure to inform the care provider of the types of findings to report (e.g., eye pain, redness, or eye drainage).

Equipment

- Clean lens storage container
- Bath towel
- Suction cup (optional)
- Sterile saline solution
- Sterile lens cleaning solution
- Sterile lens rinsing solution
- Sterile lens disinfectant
- Sterile enzyme solution (depends on care regimen)
- Sterile wetting solution (depends on care regimen)
- Cotton ball or cotton-tipped applicator
- Emesis basin
- Disposable gloves

Step	Rationale
Assessment	
1. Place towel just below client's face.	Catches lens if one should accidentally fall from eye.
2. Stand at client's side. Inspect eye or ask client if contact lens is in place.	Lenses are generally comfortable to wear, and client may forget they are in place. Prolonged wear may cause injury to eye.

- ***Critical Decision Point***
  Unconscious or confused clients entering the health care setting should be carefully assessed; lenses are often difficult to assess if clear (untinted).

STEP	RATIONALE
3. Ask if client feels any eye discomfort and assess length of time client normally wears lenses.	Scratched lens can cause corneal irritation and abrasion. Accumulation of dust or debris between lens and cornea causes irritation. Continuous wearing of certain types of lenses can irritate cornea.
4. Ask if client is able to manipulate and hold contact lens.	Determines level of assistance required in care.

- ***Critical Decision Point***
  May need to assess level of assistance required later after lenses have been removed and if client has eyeglasses available.

STEP	RATIONALE
5. Assess client for any unusual visual signs/symptoms (reduced visual acuity, blurred vision, halos, photophobia).	May indicate underlying visual alteration or need to change lens prescription. A reduction of visual acuity calls for referral.
6. Assess types of medications prescribed for client: sedatives, hypnotics, muscle relaxants, antihistamines, anticholinergics, and antidepressants.	Sedatives, hypnotics, and muscle relaxants reduce blink reflex and thus reduce lubrication of cornea. Antihistamines, anticholinergics, and antidepressants can reduce tear production.
7. After lenses are removed (see Implementation), inspect eye for signs of corneal irritation (e.g., redness, pain, swelling of eyelids and conjunctivae, discharge, excess tearing).	Signs/symptoms indicate corneal irritation or abrasion.

- ***Critical Decision Point***
  If pain persists or worsens after removal of lenses, an immediate referral to the ophthalmologist should be made. Severe pain may indicate corneal epithelium disruption or infection (Cheng and others, 1999).

NURSING DIAGNOSIS

Defining characteristics from the assessment data may reveal the following nursing diagnoses for clients requiring this skill:

- Bathing/hygiene self-care deficit
- Deficient knowledge regarding contact lens care
- Pain (acute, chronic)
- Risk for infection
- Risk for injury
- Disturbed sensory perception (visual)

Related factors are individualized based on client's condition or needs.

PLANNING

STEP	RATIONALE
1. **Expected outcomes** following completion of procedure:	
▪ Client verbalizes comfort after removal and/or reinsertion of lenses.	Lenses are removed or inserted properly.
▪ Client's eye shows no signs of ocular infection (e.g., redness, pain, swelling, discharge, blurred vision, photophobia) or injury (e.g., irritation, foreign body sensation, tearing).	Indicates that there is no infection or injury from removal or insertion of lenses.
▪ Client verbalizes improved visual perception after lens cleaning.	Lenses cleaned and positioned correctly.
▪ Client demonstrates the proper technique for removing, cleaning, and reinserting lenses.	Learning achieved.
2. Discuss procedure with client.	Client can assist in planning by explaining technique that may aid removal and insertion. Client may be anxious as nurse retracts eyelids and manipulates lenses.
3. Have client assume supine or sitting position in bed or chair.	Provides easy access for nurse while retracting eyelids and manipulating lenses.

- ***Critical Decision Point***
  Client may assume side-lying position if movement and position are restricted for this procedure.

STEP	RATIONALE
4. Assemble supplies at bedside.	Provides easy access to supplies.

Step	Rationale

Implementation

Removing Soft Lenses

1. Wash hands. Apply disposable gloves if there are cuts, scratches, or dermatological lesions on nurse's hands. — Reduces transmission of microorganisms. Standard precautions apply to lesions when they contain visible blood.
2. Place towel just below client's face. — Catches lens if one should accidentally fall from eye.
3. Add 2 to 3 drops of sterile saline solution to client's eye. — Lubricates eye to facilitate lens removal.
4. Tell client to look straight ahead. — Eases tipping of lens during removal.
5. Using middle finger, retract lower eyelid. — Exposes lower edge of lens.
6. With pad of index finger of same hand, slide lens off cornea onto white of eye. — Positions lens for easy grasping. Use of finger pad (rather than fingernail) prevents injury to cornea and damage to lens.
7. Pull upper eyelid down gently with thumb of other hand and compress lens slightly between thumb and index finger. — Causes soft lens to double up. Air enters underneath lens to release suction.
8. Gently pinch lens and lift out. — Protects lens from damage. Avoid allowing lens edges to stick together. Soft lenses consist primarily of water and can be easily torn.

- ***Critical Decision Point***
  If lens edges stick together, place lens in palm and soak thoroughly with sterile saline solution. Gently roll lens with index finger in back-and-forth motion. If gentle rubbing does not separate edges, soak lens in sterile saline solution, which assists in returning lens to normal shape.

9. Clean and rinse lens (see Cleansing and Disinfecting Contact Lenses). Place lens in proper storage case compartment: "R" for right lens and "L" for left lens (see illustration). — Ensures proper lens will be reinserted into correct eye. Proper storage prevents crackling or tearing.

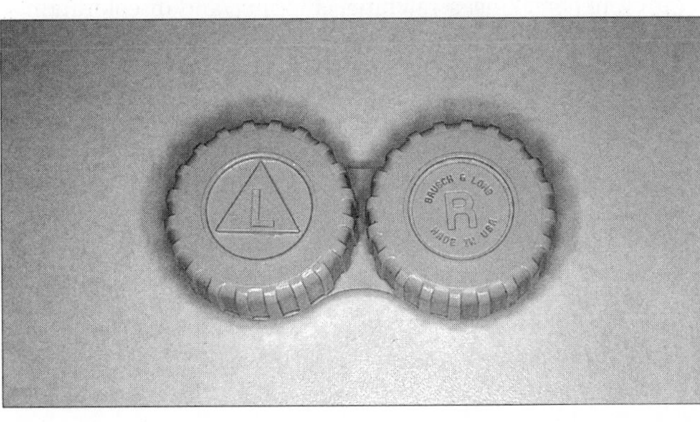

STEP **9** Contact lens storage case.

10. Repeat Steps 3 through 9 for other lens. Secure cover over storage case. Label with client's name and room number. — Proper storage prevents damage to or loss of lenses.
11. Assess appearance and condition of eyes after lenses are removed. — Provides baseline data (e.g., redness, tearing, complaints of pain) regarding condition of eye following removal of lenses.
12. Dispose of towel, remove gloves, and wash hands. — Reduces transmission of infection.

Removing Rigid Lenses

1. Wash hands and apply gloves if needed. — Reduces transmission of microorganisms.
2. Place towel just below client's face. — Catches lens if one should accidentally fall from eye.
3. Be sure lens is positioned directly over cornea. — Correct position of lens allows easy removal from eye.

- ***Critical Decision Point***
  If lens is not positioned directly over cornea, have client close eyelids, place index and middle fingers of one hand on eyelid just beside the lens and beneath, and gently but firmly massage lens back into place.

4. Place index finger on outer corner of client's eye and draw skin gently back toward ear (see illustration). — Tightens eyelid against eyeball.

STEP	RATIONALE

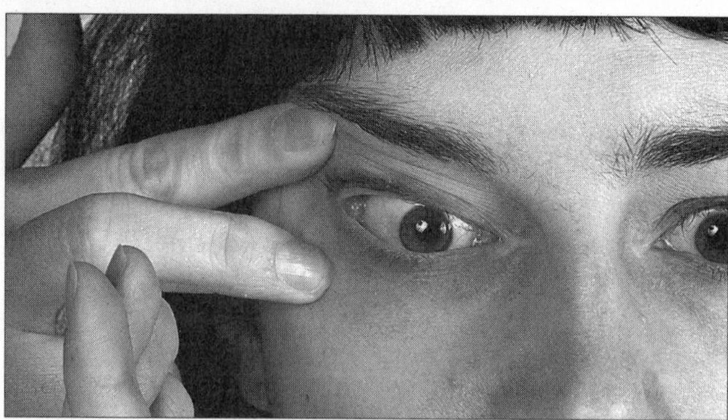

STEP 4 Finger placement for removal of rigid contact lens.

STEP	RATIONALE
5. Tell client to blink. Do not release pressure on eyelid until blink is completed.	Maneuver should cause lens to dislodge and pop out. Lid margins must clear top and bottom of lens until the blink.
6. If lens fails to pop out, gently retract eyelid beyond edges of lens. Press lower eyelid gently against lower edge of lens.	Pressure causes upper edge of lens to tip forward.

• ***Critical Decision Point***

A lens suction cup can be used to remove lenses from the eyes of confused or unconscious clients. Gently apply suction cup to lens surface and lift out.

STEP	RATIONALE
7. Allow both eyelids to close slightly and grasp lens as it rises from eye. Cup lens in hand.	Maneuver causes lens to slide off easily. Protects lens from breakage.
8. Clean and rinse lens (see Cleansing and Disinfecting Contact Lenses). Place lens in proper storage case compartment: "R" for right lens and "L" for left lens. Center lens in storage case, convex side down.	Both lenses may not have the same prescription. Proper storage prevents breaking, scratching, chipping, and discoloration.
9. Repeat Steps 3 through 8 for other lens. Secure cover over storage case. Label with client's name and room number.	Proper storage prevents damage to or loss of lenses.
10. Dispose of towel, remove gloves, and wash hands.	Reduces spread of infection and keeps client's environment neat.

Cleansing and Disinfecting Contact Lenses

STEP	RATIONALE
1. Wash hands.	Reduces transmission of microorganisms.
2. Assemble supplies at bedside. Place towel over work area.	Provides easy access to supplies. Towel catches lens if accidentally dropped and avoids breakage, scratching, and tearing.

• ***Critical Decision Point***

Check expiration dates of all solutions and discard outdated solutions to avoid adverse effects or infections.

STEP	RATIONALE
3. Open lens container carefully, taking care not to flip lens caps open suddenly.	Prevents lenses from being accidentally spilled or flipped out of case.
4. After removing one lens from case, apply one or two drops of cleaning solution to lens in palm of hand (use cleanser recommended by lens manufacturer or eye care practitioner).	Removes tear components, including mucus, lipids, and proteins that collect on lens.
5. Rub lens gently but thoroughly on both sides for 20 to 30 seconds. Use index finger (soft lenses) or little finger or cotton-tipped applicator soaked with cleaning solution (rigid lenses) to clean inside lens. Be careful not to touch or scratch lens with fingernail.	It is easier to manipulate and clean lens using fingertips. Cleans microorganisms from all surfaces. Nails of care provider should be cut short to prevent scratching or tearing of lens.
6. Holding lens over emesis basin, rinse thoroughly with manufacturer-recommended rinsing solution (soft lenses) or cold tap water (rigid lenses).	Removes debris and cleaning solution from lens surface. Rinsing methods and solutions differ for each type of lens.

Step	Rationale
7. Place lens in proper storage case compartment and fill with storage solution recommended by manufacturer or eye care practitioner.	Disinfects lens, removes residue, enhances wetability of lens, and prevents scratches to lens that can be caused by a dry case.
8. Repeat Steps 3 through 7 for other lens.	

Inserting Soft Lenses

Step	Rationale
1. Wash hands thoroughly with mild noncosmetic soap, rinse well, and dry with clean lint-free towel or paper towel. Apply gloves if needed.	Lint or film left on hands from towels or cosmetic or deodorant soaps can be transferred to lens and irritate eye.
2. Place towel over client's chest.	Catches lens if accidentally dropped and avoids breakage, scratching, and tearing.
3. Remove right lens from storage case and rinse with recommended rinsing solution; inspect lens for foreign materials, tears, and other damage.	Removes disinfectant solution. Prevents irritation or damage to eye. Always begin with right lens to avoid placing wrong lens in eye.
4. Check that lens is not inverted (inside out).	Soft lens is inverted if bowl has a lip; it is in proper position if curve is even from base to rim.
5. Using middle or index finger of opposite hand, retract upper lid until iris is exposed.	Soft lenses do not adhere as easily as hard lenses. Separating lids as much as possible allows room for lens to completely contact cornea without touching lids or lashes.
6. Using middle finger of the hand holding the lens, pull down lower lid.	Provides full response of cornea.
7. Instruct client to look straight ahead "through" the lens and finger; then gently place lens directly on cornea and release lids slowly, starting with lower lid.	Ensures secure fit and comfort.
8. If lens is on sclera rather than cornea, tell client to slowly close eye and roll it toward the lens. Sometimes it helps to put very gentle pressure on the closed eyelid to aid in centering the lens on the cornea.	Centers soft lens over cornea.
9. Tell client to blink a few times.	Ensures lens is centered, free of trapped air, and comfortable.
10. Be sure lens is centered properly by asking client to open eyes and note if vision is blurred.	If lens slips to side of cornea or into conjunctival sac, vision will blur.
11. Repeat Steps 3 through 10 for left eye.	
12. Assist client to comfortable position after lens is inserted.	
13. If client's vision is blurred:	
a. Retract eyelids.	
b. Locate position of lens.	
c. Ask client to look in direction opposite lens, and with index finger, apply pressure to lower eyelid margin and position lens over cornea.	
d. Have client look slowly toward lens.	Repositions lens over center of cornea as client looks toward lens.
14. Discard soiled supplies and solution from storage case, rinse case thoroughly and allow to air dry, and wash hands.	Reduces transmission of microorganisms.

Inserting Rigid Lenses

Step	Rationale
1. Wash hands thoroughly with mild noncosmetic soap, rinse well, and dry with clean lint-free towel or paper towel. Apply gloves if needed.	Lint or film left on hands from towels or cosmetic or deodorant soaps can be transferred to lens and irritate eye.
2. Place towel over client's chest.	Catches lens if accidentally dropped and avoids breakage and scratching.
3. Remove right lens from storage case; attempt to lift lens straight up (see illustration).	Sliding lens out of case can cause scratches on the surface. Always begin with right lens to avoid placing wrong lens in eye.

Step	Rationale

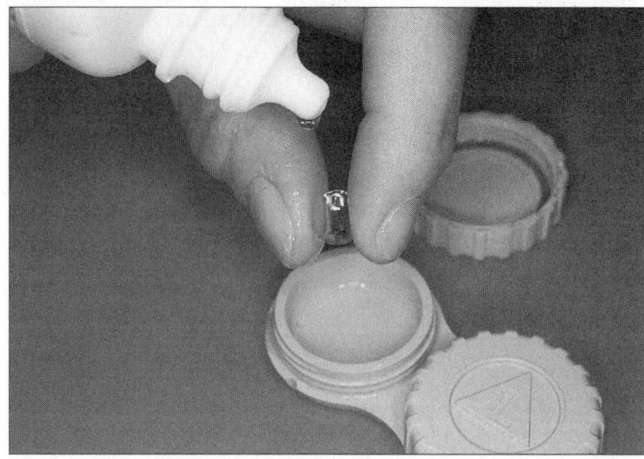

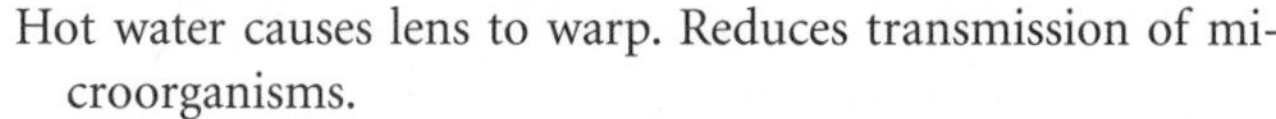

STEP **3** Removal of rigid lens from storage case.

Step	Rationale
4. Rinse with cold tap water.	Hot water causes lens to warp. Reduces transmission of microorganisms.
5. Wet lens on both sides using prescribed wetting solution.	Lubricates lens so that it slides easily and adheres to cornea.
6. Place lens concave side up on tip of index finger of dominant hand (see illustration).	Proper manipulation of lens ensures easy insertion. Inner surface of lens should face up so that it is applied against cornea.
7. Instruct client to look straight ahead while retracting lower eyelid; place lens gently over center of cornea (see illustration).	Rigid lens can be placed as client looks straight ahead. Retraction of lids promotes easy insertion between lid margins.

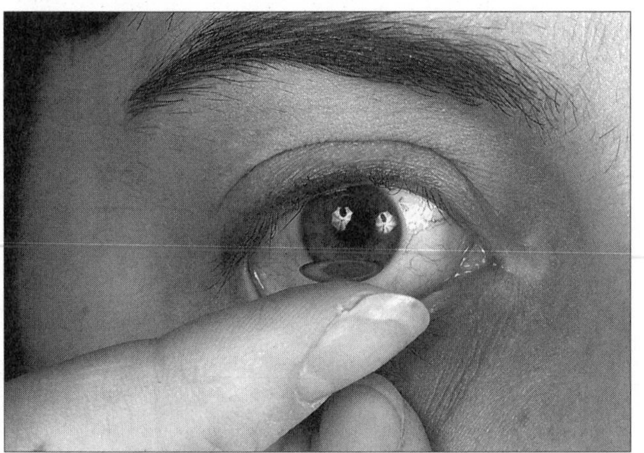

STEP **6** Placement of lens on fingertip.

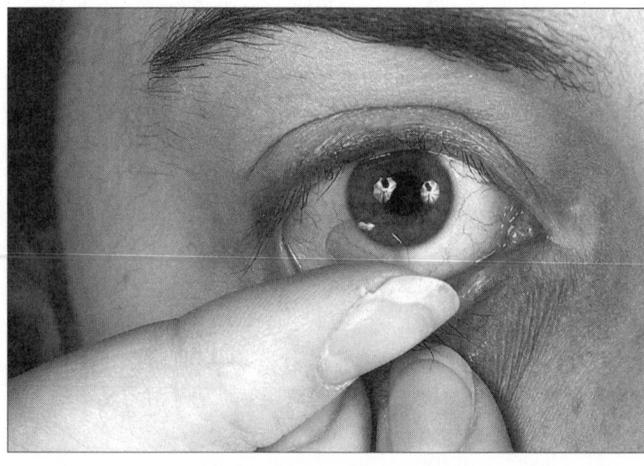

STEP **7** Retraction of lower eyelid, immediately before placement of lens on cornea.

Step	Rationale
8. Ask client to close eyes briefly and to avoid blinking.	Helps to secure position of lens.
9. Be sure lens is centered properly by asking client to open eyes and note if vision is blurred.	If lens slips to side of cornea or into conjunctival sac, vision will blur.
10. Repeat Steps 3 through 9 for left eye.	
11. Assist client to comfortable position.	
12. Discard soiled supplies and solution from storage case, rinse case thoroughly and allow to air dry, and wash hands.	Reduces transmission of microorganisms.

Evaluation

Step	Rationale
1. Ask client if lens feels comfortable after removal and reinsertion of lenses.	Determines if any debris is caught between lens and cornea. Lens should be removed if client experiences discomfort.

STEP	RATIONALE
2. Inspect eye (over time) for signs of ocular infection.	Demonstrates efficacy of lens care over time.
3. Assess client's visual acuity (see Chapter 10).	Determines improvement in visual perception.
4. Observe client for signs of eye injury.	Determines if procedure performed safely.
5. Observe client demonstrating technique for lens care.	Evaluates client's understanding of techniques.

UNEXPECTED OUTCOMES AND RELATED INTERVENTIONS

- Client complains of burning, pain, or foreign body sensation.
  - Remove lenses.
  - Clean lenses using appropriate technique.
  - Rest eyes.
  - If symptoms continue, consult vision care specialist.
- Client develops blurred vision.
  - Check for correct placement of contact lenses.
  - If off center, gently guide contact towards center with client's eye partially closed.
  - Lens may need to be removed and reinserted.
- Client develops inflammation of conjunctiva, pain, discharge, excess tearing, or reduced vision.
  - Remove lens.
  - If symptoms continue, notify vision care specialist.
- Client is unable to perform lens care correctly.
  - Teach client appropriate skills of cleaning, disinfecting, inserting, and removing lenses.
  - Provide written instructions and brochures with needed information.

RECORDING AND REPORTING

- Record or report any signs/symptoms of visual alterations noted during procedure.
- Record on nursing care plan or Kardex times of lens insertion and removal if client is going to surgery or special procedure.
- When client is going to a special procedure or to the operating room, record if contact lenses are in or stored at the client's bedside.

TEACHING CONSIDERATIONS

- Special heat-resistant cases can be placed in electric heating units for soft lens sterilization; however, units usually are not available in health care institutions.
- Wearers of soft and extended-wear lenses are at risk for ocular infections and corneal ulcers. Common infectious agents are *Pseudomonas aeruginosa* and staphylococci. Infection by *Acanthamoeba* organisms is rare but can cause a more serious infection and may ultimately result in blindness (Cheng and others, 1999). Adherence to recommended methods of lens care should be emphasized. Advise client against using saliva, homemade saline solution, or tap water as wetting solutions because they can cause infection.
- Some women experience discomfort with contact lens wear during menstrual periods, pregnancy, menopause, or while taking oral contraceptives. Hormonal-related fluid retention may cause corneal swelling and result in ill-fitting lenses.
- Nurse should encourage client to see a vision care specialist (**ophthalmologist** or **optometrist**) regularly: every 3 to 5 years before age 40, every 2 years after age 40, and yearly after age 65.
- Encourage client to remember the mnemonic RSVP: *R*edness, *S*ensitivity, *V*ision problems, and *P*ain. If one of these problems occurs, remove contact lenses immediately. If problems continue, contact vision care specialist (Lewis, Heitkemper, and Dirksen, 2000).
- Disposable or planned replacement lenses should be thrown away after prescribed wearing period.
- Use aerosol products (e.g., hair spray, cologne, deodorants) before lenses are inserted.
- Apply makeup after lenses are inserted and use water-based or water-soluble eyeliners only; cosmetics trapped under a lens can cause irritation.
- Do not use eye drops or medications without consulting an eye care practitioner.

PEDIATRIC CONSIDERATIONS

- Parents and/or older children can learn how to care for lenses.

GERONTOLOGICAL CONSIDERATIONS

- When checking for visual impairment during a nursing history, consider age of client. Some symptoms occur in people in one age-group and not in another. The incidence of **myopia,** or nearsightedness, tends to increase up to the third decade of life. On the other hand, **presbyopia,** or farsightedness, resulting from loss of elasticity of the lens, occurs with advancing age; it begins to affect people in their mid-40s (Ebersole and Hess, 1998).
- Other visual changes that normally occur with aging include reduced visual fields, decreased visual acuity, delayed dark-light adaptation, impaired night vision, impaired accommodation to near objects, impaired color vision, impaired depth perception, presence of floaters, presence of opacities, and increased glare sensitivity. As a result of these changes, the older client's environment should be assessed for potential hazards (see Chapter 39) and adapted to the client's visual needs (Ebersole and Hess, 1998).
- Caregivers need to be alert for common visual changes (e.g., loss of night vision, changes in functional ability, decreased socialization, increased frequency in bumping into objects,

slowness when descending stairs) (Kavanaugh and Tate, 1996).

HOME CARE CONSIDERATIONS

- Rigid lenses and daily-wear soft lenses should be removed for sleeping, sunbathing, swimming, and showering.
- Clients in the home setting should be cautioned against working over sink unless towel is placed in sink or sink stopper is in place.
- Lenses must be both cleaned and disinfected. One procedure does not replace the other.
- If client develops an eye infection (e.g., conjunctivitis) the affected lens may have to be replaced. The client should notify the eye practitioner.
- Do not wear lenses in presence of noxious or irritating vapors or fumes because they can cause damage to contact lens surface.

Skill 8-2 Taking Care of an Artificial Eye

As a result of tumor, infection, congenital blindness, or severe trauma to the eye, clients may have to undergo **enucleation,** a procedure involving the complete removal of the eyeball. Surgery is indicated when there is danger of an infectious or malignant process spreading to the neighboring eye or brain tissue or when trauma has caused disruption of the entire globe of the eye. All that remains after enucleation is the socket and eyelids. For obvious cosmetic purposes, clients who have undergone enucleation are often fitted with an artificial eye, or **prosthesis.** Artificial eyes are made of plastic and sometimes glass. The common plastic prosthesis is smooth and assumes the shape of the normal eyeball's anterior curvature. The prosthesis fits just behind the client's eyelids. Each prosthesis is designed to have the appearance of the client's natural iris, pupil, and sclera. Prostheses are relatively easy to remove and insert and can be worn day and night. Cleansing with soap and water can be done daily or any time up to several months based on client's preference.

DELEGATION CONSIDERATIONS

The skill of caring for a prosthetic eye can be delegated to assistive personnel.

Inform and assist the care provider in the proper way to care for eye prostheses. Also stress to the care provider that careful handling of the prosthetic eye is of utmost importance to prevent physical injury to the client and damage to the prosthesis. Have the care provider protect the client's privacy when inserting or removing artificial assistive devices (e.g., artificial eye). Also be sure to teach the care provider to explain steps of the procedure to the client as the procedure progresses and to inform the care provider of types of findings to report (e.g., pain or eye socket drainage).

EQUIPMENT

- Soft washcloth or cotton gauze square
- Washbasin with warm water or saline
- 4 × 4 inch gauze pads
- Mild soap
- Facial tissues
- Bath towel
- Suction device (e.g., rubber bulb syringe, medicine dropper bulb) (optional)
- Disposable gloves
- Covered plastic storage case

STEP	RATIONALE
ASSESSMENT	
1. Determine which eye is artificial.	
• ***Critical Decision Point*** *Care provider must avoid showing any revulsion during procedure.*	
2. Inspect surrounding tissues of eyelid and eye socket for inflammation, tenderness, swelling, and drainage. (Inspect socket after removal of prosthesis.)	Infection can spread easily to neighboring eye, underlying sinuses, or brain tissue.
3. Assess client's routine for prosthetic care: frequency and methods of cleaning.	Determines compliance with and knowledge of self-care.
4. Assess client's ability to remove, clean, and reinsert prosthesis.	Determines level of assistance required during care.

STEP	RATIONALE

NURSING DIAGNOSIS

Defining characteristics from the assessment data may reveal the following nursing diagnoses for clients requiring this skill:

- Bathing/hygiene self-care deficit
- Risk for infection
- Risk for injury
- Deficient knowledge regarding eye prosthesis care
- Pain (acute, chronic)
- Disturbed sensory perception (visual)

Related factors are individualized based on client's condition or needs.

PLANNING

STEP	RATIONALE
1. **Expected outcomes** following completion of procedure:	
▪ Client verbalizes feelings regarding prosthesis removal and care.	Reflects level of acceptance conveyed by nurse.
▪ Client's eyelid margins are clean and of normal pink color, with lashes turned away from prosthesis.	Eyelids are cleaned and positioned correctly.
▪ Client demonstrates no signs of infection, such as redness, tenderness, swelling, or discharge from socket or eyelid margins.	Eyelid margins and socket are free of infection.
▪ Client verbalizes that prosthetic eye fits comfortably.	Prosthesis is inserted correctly.
▪ Client demonstrates the proper technique for removing, cleaning, and reinserting prosthesis.	Learning is achieved.
2. Discuss procedure with client.	Allows client opportunity to suggest further ideas about procedure.
3. Assist client to sitting or supine position with head elevated.	Position facilitates removal of prosthesis with less chance of breakage.

IMPLEMENTATION

STEP	RATIONALE
1. Wash hands. Apply disposable gloves.	Reduces transmission of microorganisms.
2. With thumb, gently retract lower eyelid against lower orbital ridge (see illustration).	Exposes lower edge of eye prosthesis.
3. Exert slight pressure below eyelid and slide prosthesis out (see illustration). If prosthesis does not slide out, use moistened rubber bulb syringe or medicine dropper bulb to apply direct suction to prosthesis.	Breaks suction, causing prosthesis to rise and slide out of socket (Bocking and others, 1990).

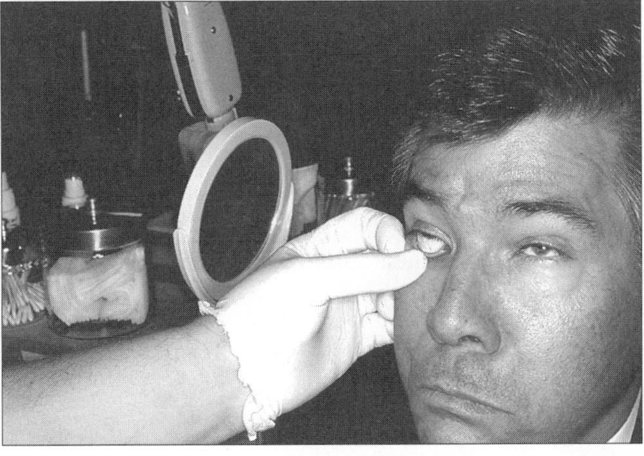

STEP 2 Retraction of lower lid to aid removal of eye prosthesis.

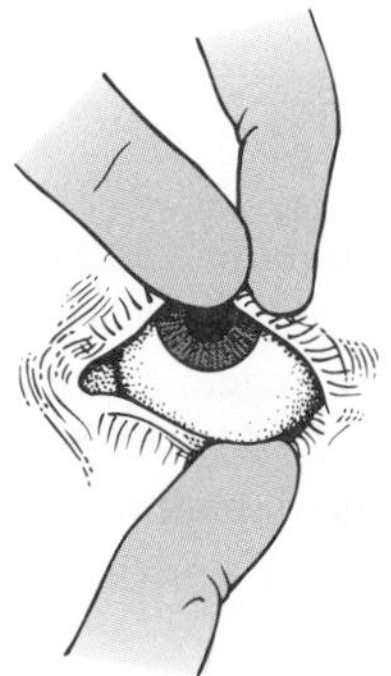

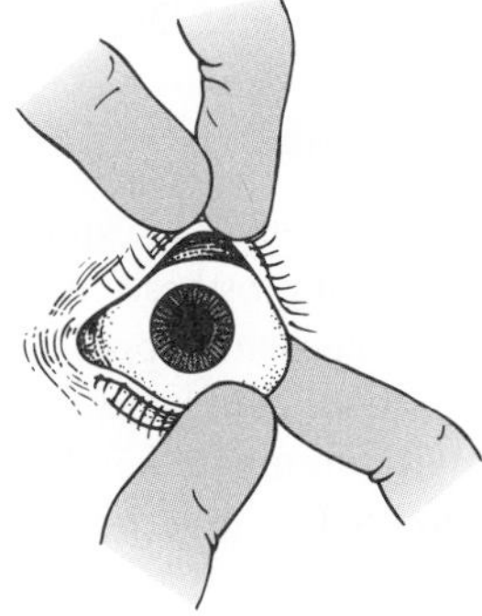

STEP 3 Exertion of pressure below eyelid and removal of prosthesis.

Step	Rationale
4. Place prosthesis in palm of hand.	Protects prosthesis from breakage.
5. Clean prosthesis:	
a. Wash with mild soap and warm water or plain saline solution by rubbing well between thumb and index finger.	Tears and secretions containing microorganisms may have collected on surface of prosthesis. Soap is less irritating than detergents.
b. Rinse well under running tap water (see illustration).	Removes soap and residue.

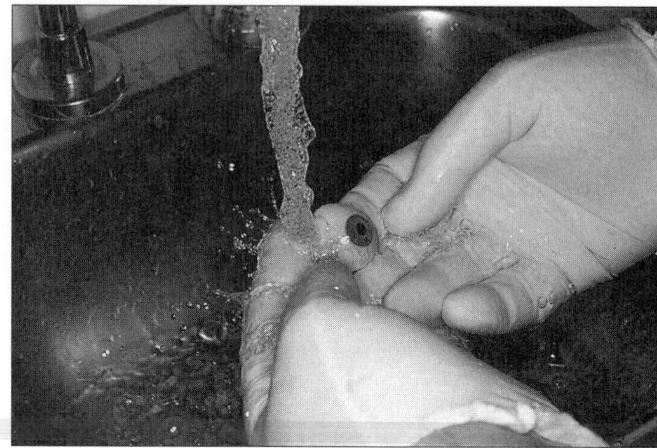
STEP 5b Rinsing of eye prosthesis.

Step	Rationale
6. Dry and polish prosthesis with soft washcloth or facial tissue.	Maintains shiny appearance of prosthesis to resemble normal eye.

• ***Critical Decision Point***
Inspect prosthesis for rough edges, which may abrade tissue surfaces.

Step	Rationale
7. If client is not to have prosthesis reinserted, store in sterile saline solution or water in plastic storage case. Label container and place in bedside stand.	Maintains integrity of prosthesis during storage.
8. Clean eyelid margins and socket:	
a. Retract upper and lower eyelid margins with thumb and index finger.	Exposes eye socket.
b. Wash socket with clean washcloth or gauze square moistened with warm water or saline solution.	Removes secretions that contain microorganisms. Soap is not used when cleaning socket because it is difficult to rinse thoroughly and may cause irritation to tissues.
c. Remove excess moisture with gauze pads.	Removes moisture that can harbor microorganisms.
d. Wash eyelid margins with mild soap and water. Wipe from inner to outer canthus using a clean section of cloth with each wipe.	Prevents secretions from entering tear duct in inner canthus.

• ***Critical Decision Point***
If crusts are difficult to remove, place moistened cloth over eyelids for several minutes during cleaning. This helps to loosen all crusts.

Step	Rationale
e. Dry eyelids by wiping from inner to outer canthus.	
9. Moisten prosthesis in water.	Water lubricates prothesis, making insertion easier.
10. Retract client's upper eyelid with index finger or thumb of nondominant hand.	Eases prosthesis insertion.
11. With dominant hand, hold prosthesis so that notched or pointed edge is positioned toward nose and iris faces outward.	Ensures proper fit (Bocking and others, 1990).

STEP	RATIONALE
12. Slide prosthesis up under upper eyelid as far as possible and then push down lower lid to allow prosthesis to slip into place (see illustration). • ***Critical Decision Point*** *Do not force prosthesis into socket.*	Prosthesis will fit evenly into socket.

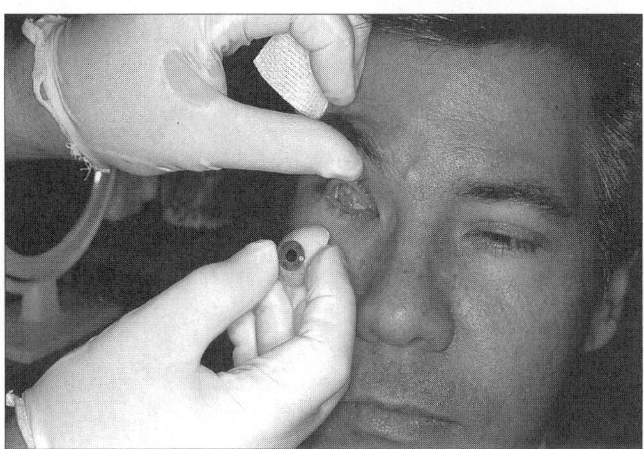

STEP **12** Replacement of eye prosthesis into eye socket.

STEP	RATIONALE
13. Gently wipe away excess fluid if necessary. Wipe toward nose to prevent dislodgement.	
14. Help client assume comfortable position.	Maintains client's comfort.
15. Dispose of soiled supplies, remove gloves, and wash hands.	Reduces transmission of microorganisms.

EVALUATION

STEP	RATIONALE
1. Ask client about feelings regarding prosthesis removal and care.	Evaluates client's self-concept.
2. Inspect condition of eyelids and socket.	Evaluates cleanliness and position of eyelids and presence of infection. Artificial eye will not move in socket nor will pupil respond to light reflex or accommodation.
3. Ask client if prosthesis fits comfortably.	Determines comfort level and assists in determining the client's ability to perform techniques.
4. Have client demonstrate prosthetic care.	Evaluates client's ability to perform procedure.

UNEXPECTED OUTCOMES AND RELATED INTERVENTIONS

- Client states prosthesis feels uncomfortable.
  - Reposition prosthesis.
  - If uncomfortable sensation remains, remove prosthesis and inspect for any sharp or rough edges.
- Signs of inflammation develop in tissues of socket or lid margins.
  - Remove prosthesis for a few days.
  - Provide client with comfortable eye patch until inflammation subsides.
- Excessive, purulent, or foul drainage develops.
  - Instruct client on proper hand washing and use of clean hand towels to help prevent infection.
  - Contact physician for possible use of broad-spectrum antibiotic.
  - Reinsert prosthesis after infection has subsided.
- Client reports increased mucus discharge.
  - Artifical tears may need to be used.
  - Consult with physician/prosthetist.
  - Encourage client to visit prosthetist annually to have artificial eye cleaned and polished.
- Client is unable to explain or perform prosthetic care.
  - Teach prosthetic eye care to client and significant other.
  - Provide literature/brochures regarding prosthetic eye care.
  - Provide demonstration and have client and significant other perform a return demonstration.

Recording and Reporting

- Record removal of prosthesis and storage location for client going to surgery.
- Record or report any alterations in integrity of tissues surrounding eye (e.g., purulent or foul drainage).

Teaching Considerations

- Never use alcohol, chemicals, or any solvents for cleaning; these agents can damage plastic prostheses (Bocking and others, 1990).
- Look for rough edges on prosthesis after removal, which may abrade tissue surfaces.
- Instruct primary caregiver not to force artificial eye into socket.
- If rubbing the prosthetic eye, rub toward the nose. Wiping away from the nose may cause the eye to fall out.
- Wear a protective patch or goggles when swimming, diving, or water skiing, or remove the prosthesis and store it.

Pediatric Considerations

- Young children, even infants and toddlers, are able to be fitted with an artificial eye. Parents must be taught how to care for the prosthesis until the child is able to independently perform care.

Gerontological Considerations

- Assess the manual dexterity of the older adult client. The nurse will need to assist with removal and insertion if dexterity is diminished.

Home Care Considerations

- Assess level of understanding of client and primary caregiver regarding client's condition and need for a prosthesis.
- Assess ability and willingness of client and primary caregiver to administer eye care.
- Assess physical condition for which client is receiving home care and determine special precautions necessary.
- Assess ability of client to cooperate with procedures.
- Client in home setting should use available equipment (e.g., clean washcloth). Procedure need not be sterile.
- Some clients may wear a prosthesis for several months before removing or cleaning. Excess tearing or crusting indicates need to clean eye and socket.

Skill 8-3 Taking Care of an In-the-Ear Hearing Aid

Hearing is vital for normal communication and orientation to sounds in the environment. For people with hearing loss, hearing aids improve the ability to hear and understand spoken words. Hearing aids amplify so that sound is heard at a more effective level. All aids have four basic components:

1. A microphone, which receives and converts sound into electrical signals
2. An amplifier, which increases the strength of the electrical signal
3. A receiver, which converts the strengthened signal back into sound
4. A power source (batteries), which energizes the components

In addition, programmable (analog and digital) hearing aids are on the market. These aids input signals rather than just amplifying the sounds. They are programmed by an audiologist with the use of a computer specific to a client's hearing impairment. These aids are adjusted to accommodate the range of the client's residual hearing. Programmable aids independently amplify high-frequency (soft-spoken consonants) from low-frequency (loudly spoken vowels) sounds; this process occurs rapidly and continuously. Programmable hearing aids also contain a remote control that has two user-selected programs (e.g., everyday listening and "special situations"); this remote also contains the volume control (ReSound Corporation, 1994, 1995). There are several styles of hearing aids available to clients today:

1. An in-the-canal (ITC) aid fits entirely in the ear canal (Figure 8-1). It has cosmetic appeal, is easy to manipulate and place in the ear, does not interfere with the wearing of eyeglasses or use of the telephone, and can be worn during most physical exercise. However, obtaining a proper fit is more difficult, and cerumen tends to plug this model more than others.
2. An in-the-ear (ITE or intra-aural) aid fits into the external auditory ear and allows more fine-tuning (Figure 8-2). It is more powerful and therefore is useful for a wider range

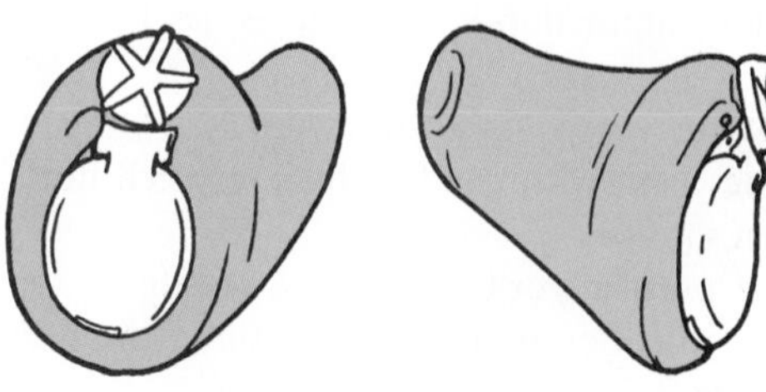

FIGURE 8-1 In-the-canal hearing aid.

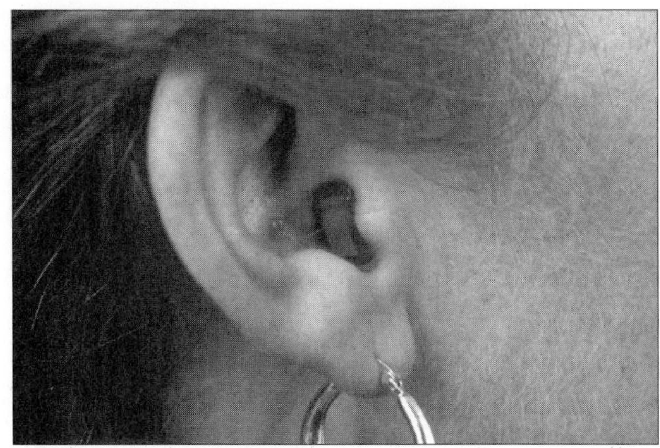
A

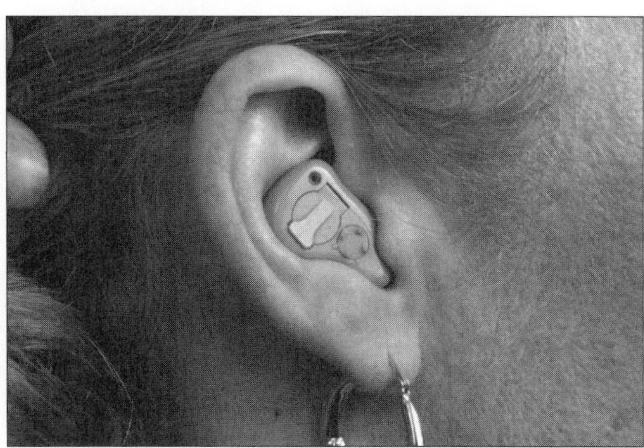
B

FIGURE 8-2 An in-the-ear hearing aid.

of hearing loss than the ITC aid. It is easy to position and adjust and does not interfere with eyeglass wearing. However, it is slightly more noticeable than the ITC aid and is not recommended for persons with moisture or skin problems in the ear canal. It is the most common type worn today.

3. A behind-the-ear (BTE or postaural) aid hooks around and behind the ear and is connected by a short, clear, hollow plastic tube to an ear mold inserted into the external auditory canal (Figure 8-3). It is useful for clients with rapidly progressive hearing loss or manual dexterity difficulties and those who find partial ear occlusion intolerable. Disadvantages are that it is more visible, may interfere with eyeglasses and telephone use, and is more difficult to keep in place during physical exercise.
4. The eyeglass aid is a hearing aid that fits in the ear canal and attaches to a battery located on the arm of the eyeglass frame. The frame must be bulky to accommodate the equipment; therefore style selection is limited.

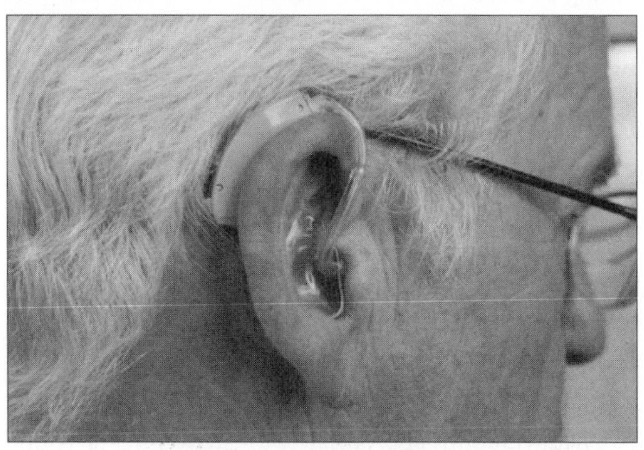

FIGURE 8-3 A behind-the-ear hearing aid.

Hearing aid devices can be tailored to a client's specific amplification need. Anyone caring for a client with a hearing aid should know that the device is delicate and must be protected from moisture, heat, and breakage.

Delegation Considerations

The skills of caring for a hearing aid can be delegated to assistive personnel.

Inform and assist the care provider in the proper way to care for the hearing aid. Stress to the care provider that careful handling of this device is of utmost importance to prevent physical injury to the client and damage to the device. Instruct the care provider to explain the steps of the procedure to the client as the procedure progresses and to use appropriate communication techniques to ensure smooth completion of the task. Also inform the care provider of the types of findings to report (e.g., ear pain, increased cerumen, or changes in the client's level of hearing).

Equipment

- Soft towel and washcloth
- Brush or wax loop
- Storage case
- Disposable gloves (if drainage present)

Step	Rationale
Assessment	
1. Assess client's knowledge of and routines for cleaning and caring for hearing aid.	Determines client's understanding and need for health education. Nurse will adapt method of care to client's procedure.
2. Determine whether client can hear clearly with use of aid by talking slowly and clearly in normal tone of voice.	Inability to hear may indicate faulty function of hearing aid.

Step	Rationale
3. Assess whether hearing aid is working by removing it from client's ear (see manufacturer's directions). Close battery case and turn volume slowly to high. Cup hand over hearing aid. If squealing or a whistling sound (feedback) is heard, it is working. If no sound is heard, replace batteries and test again.	Determines need for new battery. Feedback squeal will cause harsh whistling sound.
4. Inspect ear mold for cracked or rough edges.	Can cause irritation to external ear canal.
5. Inspect for accumulation of cerumen around aid and plugging of opening in aid.	Prevents clear sound reception and transmission.

Nursing Diagnosis

Defining characteristics from the assessment data may reveal the following nursing diagnoses for clients requiring this skill:

- Impaired verbal communication
- Deficient knowledge regarding hearing aid care
- Risk for injury
- Disturbed sensory perception (auditory)

Related factors are individualized based on client's condition or needs.

Planning

Step	Rationale
1. **Expected outcomes** following completion of procedure:	
▪ Client hears conversation spoken in normal tone of voice and responds appropriately.	Batteries are operational. Aid is secure and unobstructed.
▪ Client demonstrates proper care of hearing aid.	Demonstrates learning.
▪ Client responds appropriately to environmental sounds.	Client is able to hear warning sounds of danger.
▪ Client states that aid fits comfortably.	Aid is positioned correctly.
2. Have client suggest any additional tips for care; explain that next step is to clean and reinsert hearing aid.	Client becomes uncomfortable when unable to hear clearly. Explain all steps before removing aid to minimize confusion and anxiety.

Implementation

Cleaning Hearing Aid

Step	Rationale
1. Wash hands. Apply disposable gloves only if drainage present.	Reduces transmission of microorganisms.
2. Assemble supplies at bedside table or sink area.	Procedure can be performed without delays.
3. Wipe aid with dry, soft washcloth. Use wax loop or brush (supplied with aid) or tip of syringe needle to clean the holes in the aid. Hold hearing aid so that canal faces the floor.	Wax prevents clear sound reception and transmission. Holding hearing aid canal toward the floor allows wax particles to fall out the openings of the device (McConnell, 1996).

- ***Critical Decision Point***
  Do not jam wax deeper into holes because this could cause damage to the aid.

Step	Rationale
4. Wash ear canal with washcloth moistened in soap and water. Rinse and dry.	Removes cerumen from ear canal.
5. If hearing aid is to be stored, place it in dry, safe storage case and/or a container that has a desiccant material.	Protects hearing aid against damage, moisture, and breakage.
6. Open battery door and allow it to air dry. When hearing aid is not in use, be sure hearing aid is turned off or remove or disconnect battery.	Increases battery life and allows moisture to evaporate (Olson, 1995).
7. Label case with client's name and room number.	Helps to prevent loss of client's personal belongings.

- ***Critical Decision Point***
  If client uses two aids, note right or left ear when labeling case.

STEP	RATIONALE
Inserting Hearing Aid	
1. Check batteries (see Assessment) and replace batteries (if necessary) over soft surface (e.g., towel).	Necessary for proper sound amplification. Protects hearing aid against damage and breakage (Olson, 1995).
2. Turn aid off and turn volume control down.	Will protect client from sudden exposure to feedback sounds.
3. Hold the aid so that the canal—the long portion with the hole(s)—is at the bottom. Guiding the aid along client's cheek, bring it to the ear.	Proper orientation is important for hearing aid insertion.
4. Insert canal portion of aid into the ear first. Use other hand to pull down and back on outer ear. Gently push the aid into ear until it is in place and fits snugly in the midline.	Opens up ear canal for easier insertion (Olson, 1995).
5. If hearing aid has volume control, gradually adjust volume to comfortable level for talking to client in regular voice at 3 to 4 feet away. Rotate volume control toward the nose to increase volume and away from the nose to decrease volume.	Gradual adjustment prevents exposing client to harsh squeal or feedback. Client should hear nurse comfortably.

- ***Critical Decision Point***
  Programmable aids have the volume control located on the remote. For most clients, hearing aids work best at lower volume settings.

6. Remove soiled equipment from bedside. Dispose of used supplies. Wash hands.	Maintains clean environment and reduces risk of infection.

EVALUATION

1. Converse with client in normal tone of voice and observe response.	Determines improvement in auditory function.
2. Observe client performing hearing aid care.	Demonstrates client's understanding of techniques.
3. Observe client's response to environmental sounds.	Inability to hear environmental sounds may indicate faulty function of hearing aid.
4. Question client about comfort after insertion of hearing aid.	Determines client's comfort level.

UNEXPECTED OUTCOMES AND RELATED INTERVENTIONS

- Client is unable to hear conversations or environmental sounds clearly.
  - Remove hearing aid and evaluate whether ear canal is obstructed.
  - Make sure battery type is correct and it was inserted correctly.
  - If no obstruction is noted and battery is correct, hearing aid may be malfunctioning. Follow up with an **audiologist** or manufacturer of hearing aid.
  - Manipulate volume slowly to determine whether or not aid is functioning properly.
- Client's verbal responses are inappropriate.
  - Assess functioning of hearing aid.
- Client is unable to clean or insert hearing aid.
  - Teach and demonstrate how to clean and insert hearing aid to client and significant other (see Implementation).
  - Provide appropriate literature demonstrating these skills.
- Client complains of ear discomfort and may complain of whistling sound.
  - Reposition hearing aid—make sure that aid is secured and free from wax.
  - Adjust volume control on aid or remote.

RECORDING AND REPORTING

- Document that aid is removed and stored if client is going for surgery or special procedure.
- Report to nursing staff and document on plan of care the difficulties client has in communicating.

TEACHING CONSIDERATIONS

- Nurse should discuss with client the guidelines for hearing aid use and tips for self-care.
- Never use alcohol or other chemicals as cleaning agents because they can cause cracking and drying of the mold.
- A hearing aid specialist or audiologist must clean actual hearing aid device.
- Suggest assistive listening devices for specific situations (e.g., telephone or television amplifiers).
- Teach client some methods for managing the environment through improved listening techniques (e.g., speech reading, listening in a quiet environment, close proximity to the speaker).
- Teach family additional communication techniques.

Pediatric Considerations

- As children grow older, they can become self-conscious of a hearing aid (Wong, 1999). The aid can be made less conscious with hair styling, selection of attractive frames for glasses (over the ear aid), and placement of the on-the-body type where it is not seen.
- Child is given responsibility to care for device as soon as child is able.

Gerontological Considerations

- Hearing aids are small, and that fact together with age-related neuromuscular changes (i.e., stiff fingers, enlarged joints, decreased sensory perception) often make the care and handling of the hearing aid a difficult and frustrating experience for the older adult. Clients with these hearing conditions should contact their hearing aid specialist or audiologist for assistance.
- **Presbycusis,** hearing loss associated with aging, results in high-pitched sounds becoming inaudible, thus hearing becomes increasingly restricted to low-frequency sounds. High-frequency sounds include the consonants *f, p, t, k, ch, sh,* and *st;* these sounds are increasingly difficult for the older adult to hear. Because consonants are the letters by which spoken words are recognized, the ability of the older adult with presbycusis to understand the spoken word is greatly affected.
- Nurses need to be alert for cues of hearing loss such as inappropriate responses in conversing or responding, postural behavior, social withdrawal, volume level of radio and television, and family perception of the client's hearing ability (Cavendish, 1998; Jupiter and Spivey, 1997).

Home Care Considerations

- Assess level of understanding of client and primary caregiver regarding care required for the hearing aid.
- Assess willingness and ability of client or primary caregiver to perform necessary care of hearing aid.
- Assess physical conditions for which client is receiving home care and determine necessary special precautions.
- Assess ability of client to cooperate with procedures to care for hearing aid.
- Avoid exposure of aid to extreme heat or cold. Do not leave aid in its case near stove, heater, or sunny window. Do not use with hair dryer on hot settings or with sunlamp. In humid climate, a storage case containing silica gel is ideal for absorbing moisture.
- Remove aid for bathing or when visiting a hair stylist.
- Hair spray tends to clog the aid; therefore apply hair spray *before* fitting the aid.
- Store batteries in cool, dry place.
- Keep spare batteries on hand (especially around holidays). Batteries can last a few days to a few weeks depending on the type of battery, frequency of use, volume setting, and power of the aid. Dispose of used batteries properly because they are harmful if swallowed.
- Various brands of aids use different sizes of batteries, and thus batteries are not interchangeable. Insert batteries only when aid is turned off.

Critical Thinking Exercises

1. You are working in an acute care setting. A client enters with report of a chemical splash into his left eye. He is a contact lens wearer. What is your priority of care? How will you remove the lens?
2. Kathy Jones is a 19-year-old college student who comes to the student health clinic with an eye infection. She is a contact lens wearer, and this is her third infection in 3 months. What would you tell a client with contact lenses to do to prevent ocular infections or corneal abrasions?
3. The Lopez family is in a pediatric clinic for the first visit for the 18-month-old daughter, who is being fitted for an eye prosthesis. What will you teach the parents about the care of the prosthesis?
4. You are caring for Mr. Kyle, who is 76 years old and has been wearing a hearing aid for 1 year. On this home visit he complains about gradually losing ability to hear with this aid. What assessments will you make on the client and the hearing aid?

References

Bocking H and others: Making sense of artificial eyes, *Nurs Times* 86(18):40, 1990.

Cavendish R: Adult hearing loss, *Am J Nurs* 98(8):50, 1998.

Cheng KH and others: Incidence of contact-lens-associated microbial keratitis and its related morbidity, *Lancet* 354(9174):181, 1999.

Cohen E, Krachmer J: Red eyes and contact lenses, *Patient Care* 26(9):143, 1992.

Ebersole P, Hess P: *Toward healthy aging: human needs and nursing response,* ed 5, St. Louis, 1998, Mosby.

Farley D: Keeping an eye on contact lenses, *FDA Consumer,* March-April 1998.

Jupiter T, Spively V: Perception of hearing loss and hearing handicap on hearing aid use by nursing home residents, *Geriatr Nurs* 18(5):201, 1997.

Kavanaugh K, Tate B: Recognizing and helping older persons with vision impairments, *Geriatr Nurs* 17(2):68, 1996.

Lewis S, Heitkemper M, Dirksen S: *Medical-surgical nursing: assessment and management of clinical problems,* ed 5, St. Louis, 2000, Mosby.

McConnell E: Handling your patient's hearing aid, *Nursing* 26(7):22, 1996.

Olson R: Now hear this! *RN* 58(8):43, 1995.

ReSound Corporation: *Hear what you've been missing,* Redwood City, Calif, 1994, ReSound Corporation.

ReSound Corporation: ReSound hearing health care, *Hearing J* 48(7):53, 1995.

Wong DL: *Whaley and Wong's nursing care of infants and children,* ed 6, St. Louis, 1999, Mosby.

9

VITAL SIGNS

Skills

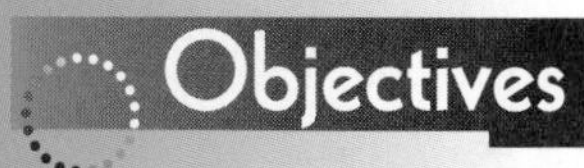

Objectives

Mastery of content in this chapter will enable the nurse to:

- Define the key terms listed.
- Correctly record vital signs.
- Identify when it is appropriate to assess each vital sign.
- Correctly assess a client's oral, rectal, axillary, and tympanic membrane temperatures.
- Identify factors to assess in determining potential alterations in body temperature.
- Discuss factors in selecting temperature measurement sites.
- Correctly assess a client's radial and apical pulse.
- Identify factors to assess in determining potential alterations in pulse character.
- Explain implications of a pulse deficit.
- Correctly assess a client's respirations.
- Identify factors to assess in determining potential alterations in respirations.
- Correctly measure a client's blood pressure (BP) using techniques of auscultation and palpation.
- Discuss factors in selecting an extremity to measure blood pressure.
- Identify factors to assess in determining potential alterations in BP.
- Correctly assess a client's oxygenation status using pulse oximetry.
- Identify factors to assess in determining potential alterations in oxygen saturation.

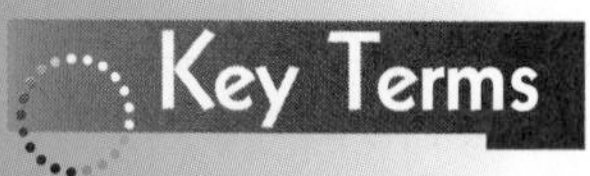

Key Terms

Antipyretic
Apical pulse
Axillary
Bradycardia
Bradypnea
Cardiac output
Centigrade
Core temperature
Diastolic pressure
Dyspnea
Dysrhythmia
Fahrenheit
Febrile
Fever
Heatstroke
Hypertension
Hyperthermia
Hypotension
Hypothermia
Orthopnea
Orthostatic hypotension
Oximetry
Oxygen saturation
Postural hypotension
Premature ventricular contraction (PVC)
Pulse deficit
S_1
S_2
Sphygmomanometer
Stroke volume (SV)
Systolic pressure
Tachycardia
Tachypnea
Thermoregulation
Tympanic
Vasoconstriction
Vasodilation
Vital signs

Temperature, pulse, blood pressure (BP), oxygen saturation, and respiration are the most frequent measurements obtained by health care practitioners. These measurements indicate if the circulatory, pulmonary, neurological, and endocrine body systems are functioning normally. Because of their importance as indicators of the body's physiological status and response to physical, environmental, and psychological stressors they are referred to as **vital signs.** Vital signs may reveal sudden changes in a client's condition, as well as changes that occur progressively over a lengthy period of time. Any difference between a client's normal baseline measurement and present vital signs can be an indication for the nurse to initiate appropriate nursing therapies and to pursue necessary medical interventions.

A fifth vital sign, pain assessment, is rapidly becoming a standard of care in health care settings. There are few clients who do not experience some level of discomfort or pain. Frequently pain is the symptom that leads clients to seek health care. For this reason, assessment of a client's pain status is critical to understanding a client's clinical status and progress. Chapter 5 summarizes pain assessment.

Vital signs are included in a routine physical assessment (Chapter 10). The nurse's findings aid in determining whether it is necessary to assess specific body systems more thoroughly. For example, during a routine vital sign measurement the nurse notes an abnormal respiratory rate; the nurse then auscultates lung sounds. Vital sign assessment may be limited to measurement of a single vital sign for the purpose of reviewing a specific aspect of a client's condition. For example, after administering an antipyretic medication, the nurse measures the client's temperature to evaluate the drug's effects. Part of the nurse's clinical judgment involves deciding which vital signs to measure, when measurements should be made, and the frequency of assessment (Box 9-1). The nurse should always obtain a baseline measurement of vital signs upon first contact with a client to provide a means for comparison with subsequent vital sign measurements.

Skill Performance Guidelines

1. The nurse caring for a client is responsible for vital signs measurement. Although measurement of select vital signs

Box 9-1 When to Take Vital Signs

1. On a client's admission to a health care facility
2. In a hospital or care facility on a routine schedule according to a physician's order or institution's standards of practice
3. When assessing the client during home health visits
4. Before and after a surgical or invasive diagnostic procedure
5. Before and after the administration of medications or application of therapies that affect cardiovascular, respiratory, and temperature control functions
6. When the client's general physical condition changes (e.g., loss of consciousness or increased severity of pain)
7. Before, during, and after nursing interventions influencing a vital sign (e.g., before and after a client previously on bed rest ambulates, before and after the client performs range-of-motion exercises)
8. When the client reports specific symptoms of physical distress (e.g., feeling "funny" or "different")

can be delegated to assistive personnel, the nurse must analyze and interpret their significance and make decisions about appropriate interventions.

2. Equipment used to measure vital signs must be functional and chosen based on a client's condition and characteristics to ensure accurate findings.
3. Knowing the normal range for all vital signs enables the nurse to detect deviations from normal.
4. A client's usual range for vital signs may differ from the standard range for age or physical state. Acceptable values for a client serve as a baseline for comparing later findings; thus a nurse detects changes in condition over time.
5. The nurse knows the client's medical history, therapies, and prescribed medications. Some illnesses or treatments cause predictable vital sign changes. Most medications affect at least one of the vital signs.
6. The nurse controls or minimizes environmental factors that may affect vital signs. Measuring a client's BP after exercise or an emotional upset may yield values that are not clear indicators of the client's current status.
7. An organized, systematic (step-by-step) approach when taking vital signs ensures accuracy of findings.
8. Based on the client's condition the nurse collaborates with the physician to decide the minimum frequency of vital sign assessment. The nurse may judge independently if more frequent assessments are needed. If a client's physical condition begins to worsen, the nurse takes vital signs more often, sometimes as often as every 5 to 10 minutes. After a client returns from surgery or a major diagnostic examination, such as cardiac catheterization, frequent measurements are taken until the vital signs stabilize back to the acceptable range before the procedure. Changes or trends in vital signs are useful in making therapeutic decisions for client care.
9. The nurse analyzes results of vital sign measurements and incorporates all the clinical findings about a client in determining nursing diagnoses. Vital signs are not assessed in isolation. The nurse assesses physical signs or symptoms, as well as vital signs, to be aware of the client's ongoing health status.
10. The nurse verifies and communicates significant changes in vital signs. Baseline measurements allow a nurse to identify changes in vital signs. When vital signs appear abnormal, it may help to have another nurse repeat the measurement. The nurse informs the physician when vital signs become abnormal and reports any changes to the nurse in charge.
11. In an outpatient setting, vital signs are taken before the health care provider examines the client.

Skill 9-1 Measuring Body Temperature

Body temperature is the difference between the amount of heat produced by the body processes and the amount of heat lost to the external environment. The **core temperature,** or temperature of the deep body tissues, is under control of the hypothalamus and is maintained within a narrow range. Skin or body surface temperature rises and falls as the temperature of the surrounding environment changes and can fluctuate dramatically.

The body tissues and cells function best within a relatively narrow temperature range, from 36° C to 38° C (96.8° F to 100.4° F), but no single temperature is normal for all people. An acceptable temperature range for adults depends on age, gender, range of physical activity, and state of health (Figure 9-1).

Many factors affect the body temperature. Physiological and behavioral control mechanisms act to maintain a constant core temperature. For example, peripheral **vasodilation** increases blood flow to the skin, which increases the amount of heat radiated to the environment. Control mechanisms have failed when heat produced by the body is not equal to heat lost to the environment. For example, clients who lack sweat gland function are unable to tolerate warm temperatures because they cannot cool themselves adequately. **Fever** occurs when heat loss mechanisms are unable to keep pace with excess heat production, resulting in an abnormal rise in body temperature. When an individual has a **febrile** condition, pyrexia, the nurse initiates temperature-control measures such as controlling environmental temperatures, remov-

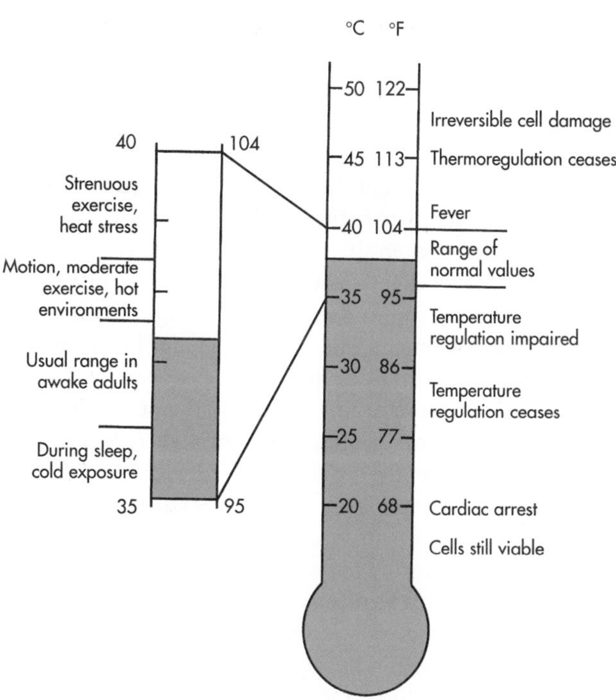

FIGURE 9-1 Ranges of normal temperature values and physiological consequences of abnormal body temperature. (Modified from Thibodeau GA, Patton KT: *Anatomy and physiology,* ed 3, St. Louis, 1996, Mosby.)

Box 9-2 Core and Surface Temperature Measurement Sites

Core	Surface
Rectum	Skin
Tympanic membrane	Oral
Esophagus	Axilla
Pulmonary artery	
Urinary bladder	

ing external coverings, and administering ordered **antipyretics** to achieve better temperature control.

The measurement of body temperature is aimed at obtaining a representative average temperature of core body tissues. Average usual temperature varies depending on the measurement site used. Research findings from numerous studies are contradictory; however, it is generally accepted that rectal temperatures are usually 0.5° C (0.9° F) higher than oral temperatures, and **axillary** and **tympanic** temperatures are usually 0.5° C (0.9° F) lower than oral temperatures (Holtzclaw, 1998). Sites reflecting core temperature are more reliable indicators of body temperature than sites reflecting surface temperatures (Box 9-2).

To ensure accurate temperature readings each site must be measured correctly (Irvin, 1999). The same site should be used when repeated measurements are necessary or temperature measurements are compared over time. Each site has advantages and disadvantages (Box 9-3). The nurse chooses the safest and most accurate site for the client.

Three types of thermometers measure body temperature: mercury-in-glass, electronic, and chemical single use or reusable. The mercury-in-glass thermometer has been a standard device for temperature measurement for many years. It continues to be widely used in the home. However, because of the risk of mercury exposure from accidental breakage, many health care settings are eliminating mercury thermometers. Mercury is highly permeable through the skin and mucous membranes; inhaled vapors diffuse rapidly into the blood and are transported to body tissues. When a mercury-in-glass thermometer breaks, staff must take immediate action to protect themselves from exposure.

The mercury-in-glass thermometer consists of a glass tube sealed at one end with a mercury-filled bulb at the other. Exposure of the bulb to heat causes the mercury to expand and rise in the enclosed tube. The length of the thermometer is marked with either **Fahrenheit** or **centigrade** calibrations (Figure 9-2). Three types of mercury-in-glass thermometers are available: oral or slim-tipped; stubby, and pear-shaped

Box 9-3 Advantages and Disadvantages of Select Temperature Measurement Sites and Methods

MERCURY-IN-GLASS

Advantages

Easy to store.

Low cost.

Three-minute measurement remains gold standard for temperature measurement.

Disadvantages

Risk of breakage, which can result in mercury exposure. Many states and pharmacy companies are banning sales.

ELECTRONIC THERMOMETER

Advantages

Plastic sheath unbreakable; ideal for children.

Very rapid measurement (4 seconds).

Expensive

Disadvantages

May be less accurate by axillary route.

Risk of transferring nosocomial clostridium infection by rectal route.

Box 9-3 Advantages and Disadvantages of Select Temperature Measurement Sites and Methods—cont'd

Chemical Thermometer

Advantages

Disposable, easy to store.
Used for clients in isolation.

Disadvantages

Some types difficult to read.
Have been shown to underestimate temperature (Erickson, 1996).

Tympanic Membrane Sensor

Advantages

Easily accessible site.
Can be used for tachypneic clients.
Provides accurate core reading.
Very rapid measurement (2 to 5 seconds).
Can be obtained without disturbing, waking, or repositioning client.
Eardrum close to hypothalamus; sensitive to core temperature changes.
Unaffected by oral intake of food or fluids or smoking.

Disadvantages

Hearing aids must be removed before measurement.
Cerumen impaction can lower readings (Hasel and Erickson, 1995).
Otitis media can distort readings.
Should not be used with clients who have had surgery of the ear or tympanic membrane.
Measurement accuracy in newborns has been questioned (Bliss-Holtz, 1995).
Requires disposable probe cover.
Expensive.

Rectal

Advantages

Argued to be more reliable when oral temperature cannot be obtained.

Disadvantages

May lag behind core temperature during rapid temperature changes.
Should not be used for clients with diarrhea, clients who have had rectal surgery, a rectal disorder, or decreased platelets.
May be source of client embarrassment and anxiety.
Risk of body fluid exposure.
Should not be used for routine vital signs in newborns (Cusson, Madonia, and Taekman, 1997).

Oral

Advantages

Accessible—requires no position change.
Comfortable for client.
Provides accurate surface temperature reading.
Reflects rapid change in core temperature.

Disadvantages

Causes delay in measurement if client recently ingested hot/cold fluids or foods, smoked, or receives oxygen by mask/cannula (Holtzclaw, 1998).
Should not be used with clients who have had oral surgery, trauma, history of epilepsy, or shaking chills.
Should not be used with infants, small children, or confused, unconscious, or uncooperative clients.
Risk of body fluid exposure.

Axilla

Advantages

Safe and noninvasive.
Can be used with newborns and unconscious clients.

Disadvantages

Long measurement time.
Requires continuous positioning by nurse.
Measurement lag behind core temperature during rapid temperature changes.
Not recommended in infants and young children (Haddock and others, 1996).

Skin

Advantages

Inexpensive.
Provides continuous reading.
Safe and noninvasive.
Can be used for neonates.

Disadvantages

Lags behind other sites during temperature changes, especially during hyperthermia.
Diaphoresis or sweat can impair adhesion.
Unreliable during chill phase of fever (Holtzclaw, 1998).
Can be affected by environmental temperature.

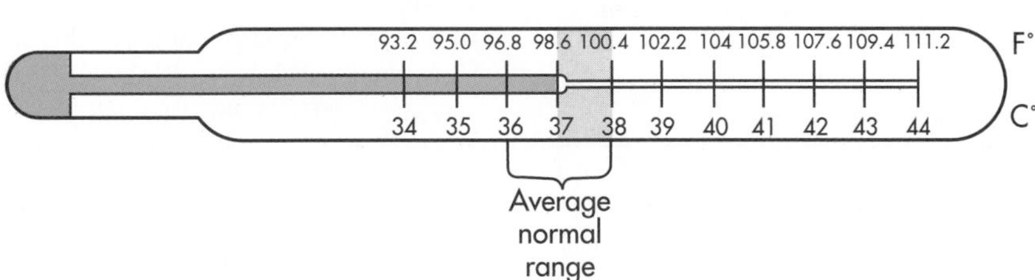

FIGURE 9-2 Comparison of Fahrenheit and centrigrade calibrations.

Box 9-4 Procedural Guidelines

Measuring Body Temperature With a Mercury-in-Glass Thermometer

A. Oral Temperature Measurement

1. Apply disposable gloves.
2. Hold end (if color coded, tip will be blue) of glass thermometer with fingertips.
3. Read mercury level while gently rotating thermometer at eye level (see illustration). If mercury is above desired level, grasp tip of thermometer securely, stand away from solid objects, and sharply flick wrist downward. Continue shaking until reading is below 35.5° C (96° F).

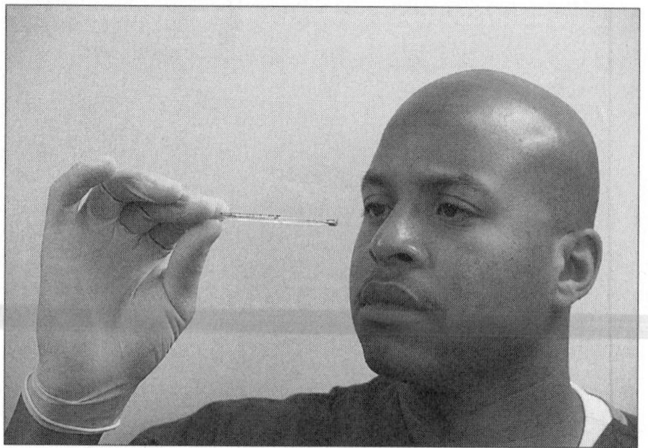

STEP **A3** Nurse reading mercury thermometer at eye level.

4. Insert thermometer into plastic sleeve cover (if available at institution).
5. Ask client to open mouth and gently place thermometer under tongue in posterior sublingual pocket lateral to center of lower jaw (see illustration).

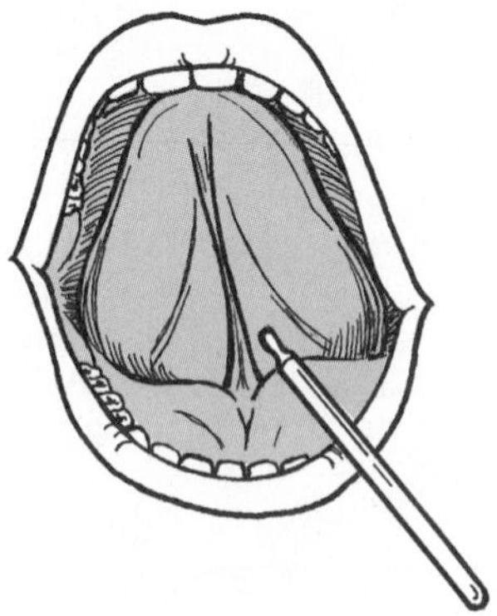

STEP **A5** Sublingual area of oral cavity.

6. Ask client to hold thermometer with lips closed. Caution against biting down on thermometer, moving mouth, or repositioning thermometer (see illustration).

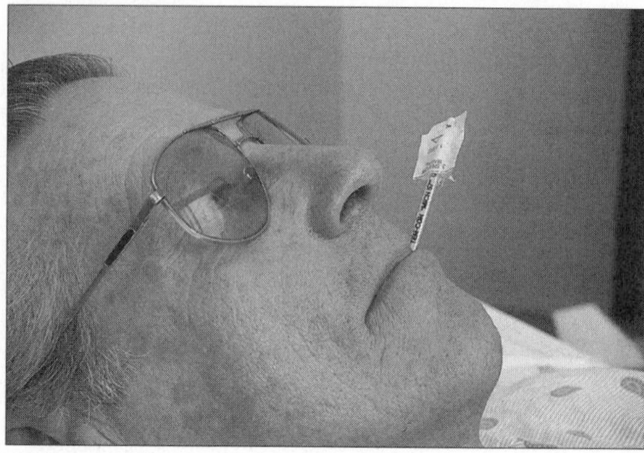

STEP **A6** Client holding glass thermometer with lips closed.

7. Leave the thermometer in place for 3 minutes.
8. Carefully remove thermometer, remove and discard plastic sleeve cover in appropriate receptacle, and wipe off any remaining secretions with clean tissue. Wipe in rotating fashion from fingers toward bulb. Dispose of tissue in appropriate receptacle.
9. Read at eye level. Gently rotate until scale appears.

B. Rectal Temperature Measurement

1. Draw curtain around bed and/or close room door. Assist client to side-lying Sims' position with upper leg flexed. Move aside bed linen to expose only anal area. Keep client's upper body and lower extremities covered with sheet or blanket.
2. Apply disposable gloves.
3. Hold end (if color-coded, tip will be red) of glass thermometer with fingertips.
4. Read mercury level while gently rotating thermometer at eye level. If mercury is above desired level, grasp tip of thermometer securely, stand away from solid objects, and sharply flick wrist downward. Continue shaking until reading is below 35.5° C (96° F).
5. Insert thermometer into plastic sleeve cover (if available).
6. Squeeze liberal portion of lubricant on tissue. Dip thermometer's blunt end into lubricant, covering 2.5 to 3.5 cm (1 to $1^1/_2$ inches) for adult.

rectal (Figure 9-3). Procedural Guidelines Box 9-4 summarizes the procedure for measuring body temperature with a mercury-in-glass thermometer.

The electronic thermometer consists of a rechargeable, battery-powered display unit, a thin wire cord, and a temperature-processing probe covered by a disposable plastic sheath (Figure 9-4). The electronic thermometer has become the most common type found within health care settings. Separate probes are available for oral and rectal use. The oral probe has a blue tip, and the rectal probe has a red tip. Electronic thermometers are designed to provide 4-second predictive temperatures and 3-minute standard

Box 9-4 Procedural Guidelines—cont'd

Measuring Body Temperature With a Mercury-in-Glass Thermometer—cont'd

7. With nondominant hand, separate client's buttocks to expose anus. Ask client to breathe slowly and relax.
8. Gently insert thermometer into anus in direction of umbilicus 3.5 cm ($1^1/_2$ inches) for adult. Do not force thermometer.
9. If resistance is felt during insertion, withdraw thermometer immediately. Never force thermometer. Consider alternative site.
10. Hold thermometer in place for 2 minutes or according to agency policy. Never leave client unattended when thermometer is in place.
11. Carefully remove thermometer, remove and discard plastic sleeve cover in appropriate receptacle, and wipe off any remaining secretions with clean tissue. Wipe in rotating fashion from fingers toward bulb. Dispose of tissue in appropriate receptacle.
12. Read at eye level. Gently rotate until scale appears.
13. Wipe client's anal area with soft tissue to remove lubricant or feces and discard tissue. Assist client in assuming a comfortable position.

C. Axillary Temperature Measurement

1. Prepare thermometer as you did for the oral temperature measurement. Be sure client's axillary area is dry, and insert thermometer into center of axilla, with lower arm over thermometer, and place arm across client's chest (see illustrations).
2. Hold thermometer in place for 3 minutes.
3. Remove thermometer, remove and discard plastic sleeve cover in appropriate receptacle, and wipe off any remaining secretions with clean tissue. Wipe in rotating fashion from fingers toward bulb. Dispose of tissue in appropriate receptacle.
4. Read thermometer at eye level. Gently rotate until scale appears.

After Measuring Body Temperature

- Store thermometer at bedside in appropriate protective storage container.
- Remove and dispose of gloves in appropriate receptacle. Wash hands.
- Discuss findings with client as needed.

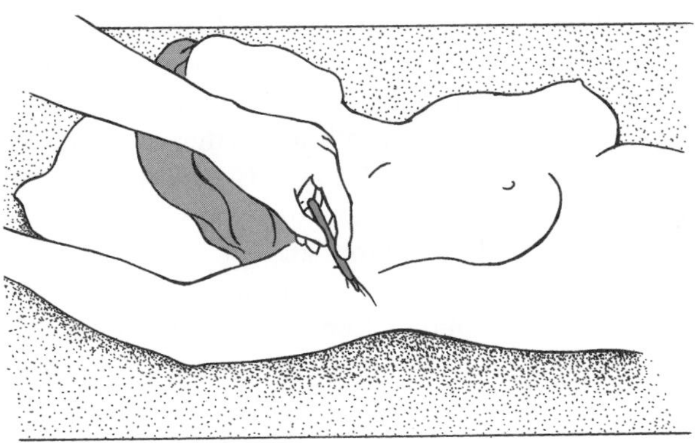

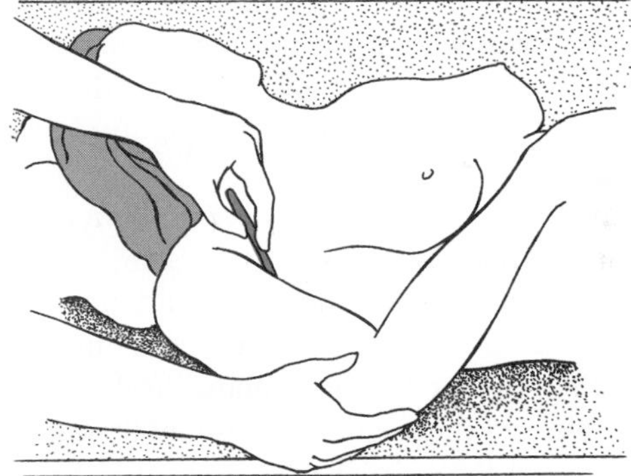

STEP **C1** Inserting axillary thermometer.

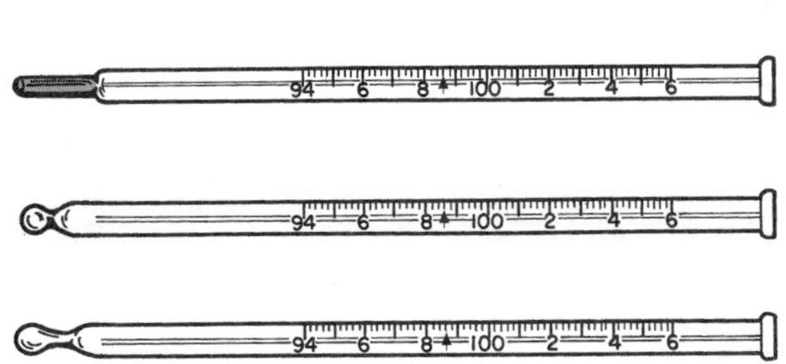

FIGURE **9-3** *Top to bottom:* comparison of oral (axillary is appropriate as well); stubby (any site); and rectal thermometers.

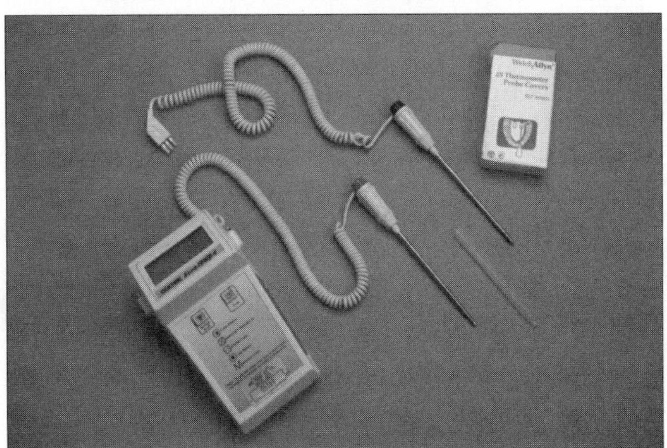

FIGURE **9-4** Electronic thermometer with disposable plastic sheath.

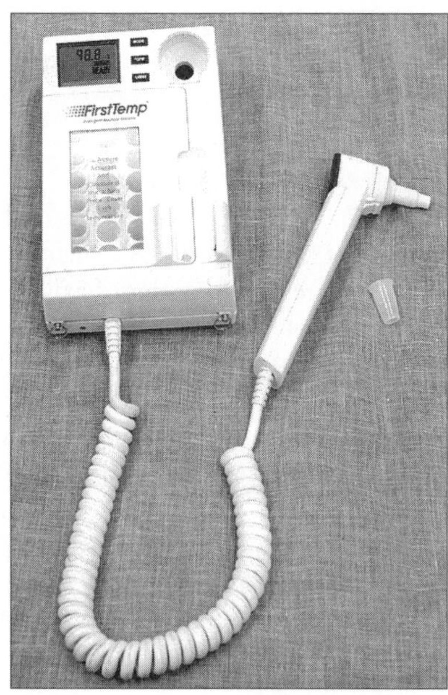

FIGURE 9-5 Tympanic membrane thermometer.

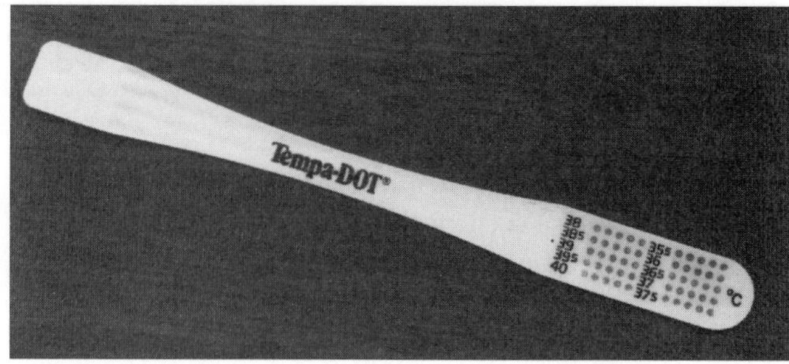

FIGURE 9-6 Disposable, single-use thermometer.

temperatures. In day-to-day clinical situations, the 4-second predictive is most commonly used.

Another form of electronic thermometer is used exclusively for tympanic temperature. An otoscope-like speculum with an infrared sensor tip detects heat radiated from the tympanic membrane of the ear (Figure 9-5). Within 2 to 5 seconds after placement in the auditory canal and depressing the scan button, a value appears on the display unit. A sound signals when the peak temperature reading has been measured.

An electronic thermometer is not necessarily more accurate than a mercury-in-glass thermometer, factors that influence oral temperature measurements affect all types of thermometers. The advantages of electronic thermometers are that their readings appear within seconds, they are easy to read, they are safe, and client discomfort is minimized.

Chemical dot single-use or reusable thermometers are disposable thin strips of plastic with a temperature sensor at one end. The sensor consists of a matrix of chemically impregnated dots that are formulated to change color at different temperatures. In the Celsius version there are 50 dots, each representing temperature increments of 0.1° C over a range of 35.5° C to 40.4° C. The Fahrenheit version has 45 dots with increments of 0.2° F and a range of 96.0° F to 104.8° F (Erickson and others, 1996). Chemical dots on the thermometer change color to reflect temperature reading, usually within 60 seconds. Most are designed for single use (Figure 9-6); however, there is a brand now available that can be reused for a single client. The chemical dots in the reusable thermometer return to the original color within a few seconds. The chemical dots thermometers are most commonly used for oral temperatures, particularly with children. They can also be used at axillary or rectal sites, covered by a plastic sheath at the latter, with a placement time of 3 minutes (PyMaH, 1994). Chemical dot thermometers are useful for screening temperatures, especially in infants, but may be less appropriate for measuring temperature in acutely ill clients. Erickson and colleagues (1996) found that chemical dot thermometers may underestimate oral temperature by 0.4° C or more in 50% of adults measured and thus lack sensitivity to screen for fever.

Delegation Considerations

The skill of temperature measurement can be delegated to assistive personnel. Inform the caregiver if any precautions are needed in positioning the client during measurement and advise the caregiver of the appropriate route and device. Also be sure to inform the caregiver of the frequency of temperature measurement, the client's usual values, and the need to report abnormalities.

Equipment

- Appropriate thermometer
- Soft tissue
- Lubricant (for rectal measurements only)
- Pen, pencil, vital sign flow sheet or record form
- Disposable gloves, plastic thermometer sleeve, or disposable probe cover
- Towel

Step	Rationale
Assessment	
1. Determine need to measure client's body temperature.	
a. Note client's risks for temperature alterations: expected or diagnosed infection, open wounds or burns, white blood cell count below 5,000 or above 12,000, immuno-	Certain conditions place clients at risk for temperature alterations and may require more frequent temperature measurement and nursing assessment.

STEP	RATIONALE
suppressive drug therapy, injury to hypothalamus, exposure to temperature extremes, blood product infusion, hypothermia or hyperthermia therapy, or postoperative status.	
b. Assess for signs and symptoms that may accompany temperature alteration: **Fever:** (depending on stage) pale or flushed skin; skin warm or hot to touch; skin dry or diaphoretic; dry mucous membranes; shivering with chills; piloerection or "gooseflesh" of skin; tachycardia; malaise with muscle or joint pain; nausea, vomiting, or diarrhea; feeling hot or cold; restlessness. **Hyperthermia:** decreased skin turgor, tachycardia; hypotension; decreased venous filling; concentrated urine. **Heatstroke:** hot, dry skin; tachycardia; hypotension; excessive thirst; muscle cramps; visual disturbances; confusion or delirium. **Hypothermia:** pale skin; skin cool or cold to touch; bradycardia and dysrhythmias; uncontrollable shivering; reduced level of consciousness; shallow respirations.	Physical signs and symptoms may alert nurse to alteration in body temperature.
2. Assess for factors that normally influence temperature:	Allows nurse to accurately assess for presence and significance of temperature alteration.
a. Age	Older adults have a narrower range of temperature than do younger adults.

- ***Critical Decision Point***
  No single temperature is normal for all people. A temperature within an acceptable range in an adult may reflect a fever in an older adult. Undeveloped temperature control mechanisms in infants and children can cause temperature to rise and fall rapidly.

STEP	RATIONALE
b. Exercise	Muscle activity raises heat production.
c. Hormones	Women have wider temperature fluctuations than men because of menstrual cycle hormonal changes; body temperature change can vary during menopause.
d. Stress	Stress elevates temperature.
e. Environmental temperature	Infants and older adults are more sensitive to environmental temperature changes.
f. Medications	Drugs may impair or promote sweating, vasoconstriction, vasodilation, or interfere with the ability of the hypothalamus to regulate temperature.
g. Daily fluctuations	Body temperature normally changes 0.5 to 1° C during a 24-hour period. Temperature is lowest during early morning. Most clients have maximum temperature elevation around 6 PM; temperature falls gradually during night (Beaudry, VandenBosch, and Anderson, 1996).
3. Assess site most appropriate for clients' temperature measurement (see Box 9-3).	Determines if client's status contraindicates selection of a specific method or site.

- ***Critical Decision Point***
  Know contraindications for each site.

STEP	RATIONALE
a. Oral b. Rectum c. Axilla d. Tympanic membrane	
4. Determine previous baseline temperature and measurement site (if available) from client's record.	Allows nurse to assess for change in condition. Provides comparison with future temperature measurements.

STEP	RATIONALE

NURSING DIAGNOSIS

Defining characteristics from the assessment data may reveal the following nursing diagnoses for clients requiring this skill:

- Risk for imbalanced body temperature
- Hyperthermia
- Hypothermia
- Ineffective thermoregulation

Related factors are individualized based on client's condition or needs.

PLANNING

1. **Expected outcomes** following completion of procedure:
   - Body temperature is within acceptable range for client's age-group. — **Thermoregulation** is maintained.
   - Body temperature returns to baseline range following therapies for abnormal temperature. — Nurse controls for environmental factors that could alter temperature.
2. Explain to client the way temperature will be measured and importance of maintaining proper position until reading is complete. — Promotes client cooperation and increases compliance. Clients are often curious about their temperatures and should be cautioned against prematurely removing the thermometer to read results.

IMPLEMENTATION

1. Wash hands. — Reduces transmission of microorganisms.
2. Assist client to comfortable position that provides easy access to temperature measurement site. — Ensures both client's comfort and accuracy of temperature reading.
3. Obtain temperature reading
   a. Oral temperature measurement with electronic thermometer
      (1) Apply disposable gloves (optional). — Use of an oral probe cover, which can be removed without physical contact, minimizes need to wear gloves.
      (2) Remove thermometer pack from charging unit. Attach oral probe (blue tip) to thermometer unit. Grasp top of probe stem, being careful not to apply pressure on the ejection button. — Charging provides battery power. Ejection button releases plastic cover from probe.
      (3) Slide disposable plastic probe cover over thermometer probe until cover locks in place (see illustration). — Soft plastic cover will not break in client's mouth and prevents transmission of microorganisms between clients.

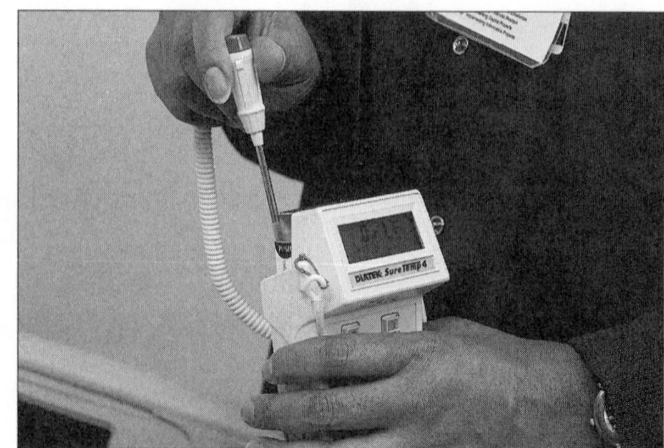

STEP **3a(3)** Nurse inserts electronic thermometer probe into probe cover. Cover snaps in place.

Step	Rationale
(4) Ask client to open mouth; then gently place thermometer probe under tongue in posterior sublingual pocket lateral to center of lower jaw.	Heat from superficial blood vessels in sublingual pocket produces temperature reading. With electronic thermometer, temperatures in right and left posterior sublingual pocket are significantly higher than in area under front of tongue.
(5) Ask client to hold thermometer probe with lips closed.	Maintains proper position of thermometer during recording.
(6) Leave thermometer probe in place until audible signal occurs and client's temperature appears on digital display; remove thermometer probe from under client's tongue.	Probe must stay in place until signal occurs to ensure accurate reading.
(7) Push ejection button on probe stem to discard plastic probe cover into appropriate receptacle.	Reduces transmission of microorganisms.
(8) Return thermometer stem to storage position of thermometer unit.	Protects probe from damage. Returning probe automatically causes digital reading to disappear.
(9) If gloves worn, remove and dispose in appropriate receptacle. Wash hands.	Reduces transmission of microorganisms.
(10) Return thermometer to charger.	Maintains battery charge.
b. Rectal temperature measurement with electronic thermometer	
(1) Draw curtain around bed and/or close room door. Assist client to side-lying Sim's position with upper leg flexed. Move aside bed linen to expose only anal area. Keep client's upper body and lower extremities covered with sheet or blanket.	Maintains client's privacy, minimizes embarrassment, and promotes comfort.
(2) Apply disposable gloves.	Maintains standard precautions when exposed to items soiled with body fluid.
(3) Remove thermometer pack from charging unit. Attach rectal probe (red tip) to thermometer unit. Grasp top of probe stem, being careful not to apply pressure on the ejection button.	Charging provides battery power. Ejection button releases plastic cover from probe.
(4) Slide disposable plastic probe cover over thermometer probe until cover locks in place.	Probe cover prevents transmission of microorganisms between clients.
(5) Squeeze liberal portion of lubricant on tissue. Dip thermometer's blunt end into lubricant, covering 2.5 to 3.5 cm (1 to $1^1/_2$ inches) for adult.	Lubrication minimizes trauma to rectal mucosa during insertion. Tissue avoids contamination of remaining lubricant in container.
(6) With nondominant hand, separate client's buttocks to expose anus. Ask client to breathe slowly and relax.	Fully exposes anus for thermometer insertion. Relaxes anal sphincter for easier thermometer insertion.
(7) Gently insert thermometer into anus in direction of umbilicus 3.5 cm ($1^1/_2$ inches) for adult. Do not force thermometer.	Ensures adequate exposure against blood vessels in rectal wall.
(8) If resistance is felt during insertion, withdraw immediately. Never force thermometer.	Prevents trauma to mucosa.
(9) Leave thermometer probe in place until audible signal occurs and client's temperature appears on digital display; remove thermometer probe from anus (see illustration).	Probe must stay in place until signal occurs to ensure accurate reading.
(10) Push ejection button on probe stem to discard plastic probe cover into appropriate receptacle.	Reduces transmission of microorganisms.
(11) Return thermometer probe to storage position of recording unit.	Protects probe from damage. Returning probe automatically causes digital reading to disappear.

Step	Rationale
STEP **3b(9)** Probe removed smoothly from anus.	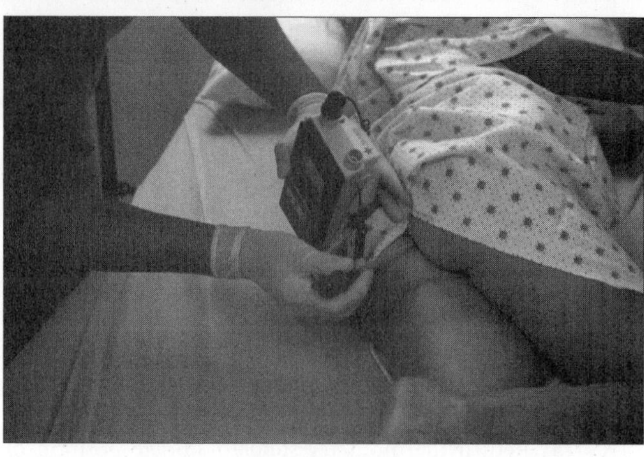
(12) Wipe client's anal area with soft tissue to remove lubricant or feces and discard tissue. Assist client in assuming a comfortable position.	Provides for comfort and hygiene.
(13) Remove and dispose of gloves in appropriate receptacle. Wash hands.	Reduces transmission of microorganisms.
(14) Return thermometer to charger.	Maintains battery charge.
c. Axillary temperature measurement with electronic thermometer	
(1) Draw curtain around bed and/or close room door. Assist client to supine or sitting position. Move clothing or gown away from shoulder and arm.	Maintains client's privacy, minimizes embarrassment, and promotes comfort. Exposes axilla for correct thermometer placement.
(2) Remove thermometer pack from charging unit. Attach oral probe (blue tip) to thermometer unit. Grasp top of probe stem, being careful not to apply pressure on the ejection button.	Charging provides battery power. Ejection button releases plastic cover from probe.
(3) Slide disposable plastic probe cover over thermometer probe until it locks in place.	Probe cover prevents transmission of microorganisms between clients.
(4) Raise client's arm away from torso, dry axilla if excess perspiration is present.	May interfere with accurate reading.
(5) Insert thermometer probe into center of axilla, lower arm over probe, and place arm across client's chest.	Maintains poor position of thermometer against blood vessels in axilla.
(6) Hold thermometer in place until audible signal occurs and client's temperature appears on digital display, remove probe from axilla.	Probe must stay in place until signal occurs to ensure accurate reading.
(7) Push ejection button on thermometer probe stem to discard plastic probe cover into appropriate receptacle.	Reduces transmission of microorganisms.
(8) Return thermometer probe to storage position of recording unit.	Protects probe from damage. Returning probe automatically causes digital reading to disappear.
(9) Assist client in assuming a comfortable position, replacing linen or gown.	Restores comfort and sense of well-being.
(10) Wash hands.	Reduces transmission of microorganisms.
(11) Return thermometer to charger.	Maintains battery charge.
d. Tympanic membrane temperature with electronic thermometer	
(1) Assist client in assuming comfortable position with head turned toward side, away from nurse. If client lies on one side, use upper ear.	Ensures comfort and exposes auditory canal for accurate temperature measurement. Heat trapped in down ear will cause false high temperature reading.

STEP	RATIONALE

• ***Critical Decision Point***
Right-handed persons should obtain temperature from client's right ear, left-handed persons should obtain temperature from client's left ear. The less acute angle of approach, the better the probe position.

STEP	RATIONALE
(2) Note if there is an obvious presence of ear wax in the client's ear canal.	Lens cover of speculum must not be impeded by earwax to ensure clear optical pathway. Switch to other ear or select alternate measurement site.
(3) Remove thermometer handheld unit from charging base, being careful not to apply pressure on the ejection button.	Base provides battery power. Removal of handheld unit from base prepares it to measure temperature. Ejection button releases plastic probe cover from thermometer tip.
(4) Slide disposable speculum cover over otoscope-like tip until it locks into place. Be careful not to touch lens cover.	Soft plastic probe cover prevents transmission of microorganisms between clients. Lens cover must be unimpeded by dust, fingerprints, or earwax to ensure clear optical pathway.
(5) Insert speculum into ear canal following manufacturer's instructions for tympanic probe positioning (see illustration): (a) Pull ear pinna backward, up and out for an adult. (b) Move thermometer in a figure-eight pattern. (c) Fit probe snug in canal and do not move. (d) Point toward nose.	Correct positioning of probe with respect to ear canal ensures accurate readings. The ear tug straightens the external auditory canal, allowing maximum exposure of tympanic membrane. Some manufacturers recommend movement of speculum tip in a figure-eight pattern that allows sensor to detect maximum tympanic membrane heat radiation. Gentle pressure seals ear canal from ambient air temperature, which can alter readings as much as 2.8° C or 5° F (Braun and others, 1998).

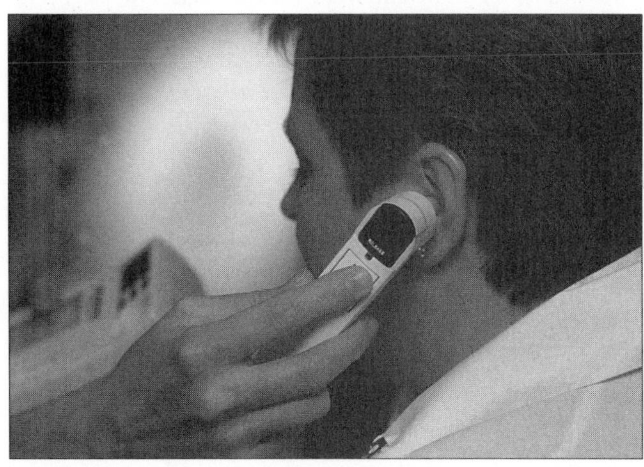

STEP **3d(5)** Tympanic membrane thermometer with probe cover placed in client's ear.

STEP	RATIONALE
(6) As soon as probe is in place, depress scan button on handheld unit. Leave thermometer probe in place until audible signal occurs and client's temperature appears on digital display.	Depression of scan button causes infrared energy to be detected. Otoscope tip must stay in place until signal occurs to ensure accurate reading.
(7) Carefully remove speculum from auditory meatus.	
(8) Push ejection button on handheld unit to discard plastic probe cover into appropriate receptacle.	Reduces transmission of microorganisms. Automatically causes digital reading to disappear.
(9) Return handheld unit to charging base.	Protects sensor tip from damage.
(10) Assist client in assuming a comfortable position.	Restores comfort and sense of well-being.
(11) Wash hands.	Reduces transmission of microorganisms.
4. Discuss findings with client as needed.	Promotes participation in care and understanding of health status.

STEP	RATIONALE

EVALUATION

Step	Rationale
1. If temperature is assessed for the first time, establish temperature as baseline if it is within acceptable range.	Used to compare future temperature measurements.
2. Compare temperature reading with client's previous baseline and acceptable temperature range for client's age-group.	Body temperature fluctuates within narrow range; comparison reveals presence of abnormality. Improper placement or movement of thermometer can cause inaccuracies. Second measurement confirms initial findings of abnormal body temperature.
3. If client has fever, temperature should be taken approximately 30 minutes after administering antipyretics, and every 4 hours until temperature stabilizes.	Will determine if temperature begins to fall in response to therapy.

- ***Critical Decision Point***
  If temperature is abnormal, repeat measurement. (With tympanic membrane temperature, measure other ear or wait 2 to 3 minutes to repeat.) If indicated, select an alternative site or instrument.

UNEXPECTED OUTCOMES AND RELATED INTERVENTIONS

- Body temperature is above acceptable range.
  - Initiate measures to lower body temperature; cool room environment, reduce bed covers, keep clothing and bed linen dry, limit physical activity, administer antipyretics as ordered. Increase fluid intake to at least 3 L daily (unless contraindicated).
  - Prevent or control spread of infection through wound care, pulmonary hygiene, adequate urinary elimination.
- Body temperature is below acceptable range.
  - Initiate measures to increase body temperature, heat room environment, cover with warm blankets, close room doors or control drafts.
  - Encourage warm liquids.
- Thermometer does not register (not uncommon with chemical dot thermometers).
  - Reassess correct placement, or choose alternate site.

RECORDING AND REPORTING

- Record temperature and route on vital sign flow sheet (Figure 9-7) or computer printout. Also record in nurses' notes any signs or symptoms of temperature alterations.
- Report abnormal findings to nurse in charge or physician.

TEACHING CONSIDERATIONS

- Identify client's ability to initiate preventive health measures and recognize alteration in body temperature. Educate clients and family members about measures to prevent body temperature alterations.
- Educate clients about risk factors for hypothermia and frostbite: fatigue, malnutrition; hypoxemia; cold, wet clothing; alcohol intoxication.
- Educate clients about risk factors for heatstroke: strenuous exercise in hot humid weather; tight-fitting clothing in hot environments; exercising in poorly ventilated areas; sudden exposures to hot climates; poor fluid intake before, during, and after exercise.
- Educate clients regarding the importance of taking and continuing antibiotics as directed until course of treatment for infection is completed.

PEDIATRIC CONSIDERATIONS

- Axillary temperature cannot be relied on to detect fevers in infants and young children (Haddock and others, 1996).
- Children may assume prone position for rectal temperature measurement.
- Axillary or skin temperature is safest for newborns. In an infant or young child it may be necessary to hold arm against child's side when assessing axillary temperature.
- Smith (1998) recommends a 5-minute axillary temperature for children.
- Temperature may be taken as the last vital sign with children who cry or become restless.
- Infants are very sensitive to slight changes in environmental temperatures.

GERONTOLOGICAL CONSIDERATIONS

- The temperature of older adults is at the lower end of the normal temperature range: 36° C (96.8° F).
- Temperatures considered within normal range may reflect a fever in an older adult.
- Older adults are very sensitive to slight changes in temperature.
- Edentulous adults or older adults with poor muscle control may be unable to close their mouth tightly enough to obtain accurate oral temperature readings.

VITAL SIGN / I & O / PAIN RECORD

DATE ______________________

HOUR	00	01	02	03	04	05	06	07	08	09	10	11	12	13	14	15	16	17	18	19	20	21	22	23
TEMP: *R = Rectal* *A = Axillary* *T = Tympanic*			36^8						37^2				37^2				37^4							
METHOD																								
PULSE			82						84				86				80							
RESPIRATION			16						16		18		20				16							
BP SYSTOLIC / DIASTOLIC			140/80						146/80		140/78		146/82				140/80							

FREQUENT VITAL SIGNS	TIME	BP	PULSE	RESP	TEMP	TIME	BP	PULSE	RESP	TEMP	TIME	BP	PULSE	RESP	TEMP	TIME	BP	PULSE	RESP	TEMP

WEIGHT *SCALE KEY:* ❑ BED ❑ STANDING ❑ W/CHAIR ❑ SLING **WT** ______________________ ❑ LB ❑ KG

PAIN

PAIN RATING SCALES

❑ Verbal *

0 1 2 3 4 5 6 7 8 9 10

No pain — Moderate pain — Worst possible pain

❑ Faces * *

0 2 4 6 8 10

❑ Non-verbal

0 1 2 3 4 5 6 7 8 9 10

Sleeping/Calm — Grimacing w/movement — Moaning w/movement — Restless — Constant moaning w/o stimuli

TARGET / LOCATION	00	01	02	03	04	05	06	07	08	09	10	11	12	13	14	15	16	17	18	19	20	21	22	23
PAIN INTENSITY 10 X = SITE 1 5 0 = SITE 2 0																								
TYPE *SEE KEY																								
INTERVENTION *SEE KEY																								
RELIEF ACCEPTABLE (Y / N)																								
LEVEL OF CONSCIOUSNESS																								

KEY

TYPE OF PAIN:

Aching, **AC**ute, **AG**itation, **AN**xiety, **B**urning, **CO**nstant, **C**ramping, **CR**-Chronic, **CS**-Crushing, **D**ull, **H**eavy, **I**ntermittent, **R**adiating, **S**harp, **ST**-Stabbing, **T**ender, **TH**robbing, Other: ______________

INTERVENTION:

1 - Medication, 2 - Relaxation, 3 - Touch, 4 - Guided imagery, 5 - Heat, 6 - Cold, 7 - Pastoral care, 8 - Music, 9 - Prayer, 10 - Massage, 11 - Other ______________

LEVEL OF CONSCIOUSNESS: 1 = Wide awake 2 = Drowsy 3 = Dozing intermittently 4 = Only awakens when aroused 5 = Difficult to arouse

SIGNATURE/TITLE	HRS WORKED	SIGNATURE/TITLE	HRS WORKED	SIGNATURE/TITLE	HRS WORKED

31000130

ADDRESSOGRAPH / LABEL

SSM HEALTH · CARE℠

VITAL SIGN / I & O / PAIN RECORD

SLM-1000-035 (6/2000) 10 FRONT

FIGURE **9-7** **A,** Temperature, pulse, and respiration recording on vital signs flow sheet. (Courtesy St. Mary's Health Center, St. Louis.) Form courtesy SSM Health Care, St. Mary's Health Center, St. Louis, MO. (*Pain Rating Scale from McCaffery M, Pasero C: Pain clinical manual, ed. 2, St. Louis, 1999, Mosby; **Wong-Baker FACES Pain Rating Scale from Wong DL and others: Wong's Essentials of Pediatric Nursing, ed. 6, St. Louis, 2001, Mosby.)

- Older adults are sensitive to environmental temperature change because their thermoregulatory systems are not as efficient.
- With aging, cerumen tends to be drier and cilia become stiff, contributing to buildup of cerumen impaction, which can interfere with accurate tympanic temperature measurement.

Home Care Considerations

- Assess temperature and ventilation of client's environment to determine existence of any environmental conditions that may affect client's temperature.
- Assess safe storage of mercury-in-glass thermometers to protect from breakage and mercury spills.
- Because pharmacies are reducing their sales of mercury thermometers, clients may need to obtain other thermometers for home use.

Skill 9-2 Assessing Radial Pulse

The ejection of blood from the heart distends the walls of the aorta. Because of the force of the blood exiting the heart, aortic distention creates a pulse wave that travels rapidly toward the extremities. When the pulse wave reaches a peripheral artery, it can be felt by palpating the artery lightly against underlying bone or muscle. The pulse is the palpable bounding of the blood flow. The number of pulsing sensations occurring in 1 minute is the pulse rate.

Assessing the client's peripheral pulse sites offers valuable data for determining the integrity of the cardiovascular system. Pulse rate, rhythm, and strength indirectly evaluate the heart's **cardiac output** (CO). An abnormally slow, rapid, or irregular pulse may indicate the heart's inability to deliver an adequate cardiac output. The strength or amplitude of a pulse reflects the volume of blood ejected against the arterial wall with each heart contraction, also called **stroke volume** (SV). If the heart's stroke volume decreases, the pulse often becomes weak and difficult to palpate. In contrast, a full bounding pulse is an indication of increased stroke volume.

The integrity of peripheral pulses indicates the status of blood perfusion to the area distributed by the pulse (Table 9-1). For example, assessment of the right femoral pulse determines whether blood flow to the right leg is adequate. If a peripheral pulse feels weak on palpation, the volume of blood reaching tissues distal to the pulse site may be inadequate.

Table 9-1 Pulse Sites

Site	Location	Rationale for Selection
Temporal	Over temporal bone of the head, above and lateral to the eye	Easily accessible site to assess pulse in children
Carotid	Along medial edge of sternocleidomastoid muscle in the neck	Easily accessible site to assess character of peripheral pulse; used during physiological shock or cardiac arrest when other sites are not palpable.
Apical	Fourth to fifth intercostal space at left midclavicular line	Site for auscultation of heart sounds
Brachial	Groove between biceps and triceps muscles at the antecubital fossa	Site used to assess status of circulation to lower arm Site used to auscultate blood pressure
Radial	Radial (thumb) side of forearm at the wrist	Common site to assess character of peripheral pulse; assesses status of circulation to hand
Ulnar	Ulnar side of forearm at the wrist	Site used to assess status of circulation to ulnar side of hand; used to assess Allen's test
Femoral	Below the inguinal ligament, midway between symphysis pubis and anterior superior iliac spine	Site used to assess character of pulse during physiological shock or cardiac arrest when other pulses are not palpable; assesses status of circulation to the leg
Popliteal	Behind the knee in popliteal fossa	Site used to assess status of circulation to the lower leg
Posterior tibial	Inner side of each ankle, below medial malleolus	Site used to assess status of circulation to the foot
Dorsalis pedis	Along top of foot between extension tendons of great and first toe	Site used to assess status of circulation to the foot

An inefficient contraction of the heart that fails to transmit a pulse wave to the peripheral pulse site creates a pulse deficit. Pulse deficits are frequently associated with dysrhythmias and warn of potential alteration of cardiac output. To assess for a **pulse deficit,** the nurse and a colleague assess a peripheral pulse rate and the apical pulse rate (Skill 9-3) simultaneously and compare the measurements. The difference between the rates is the pulse deficit.

The radial artery pulse is the most common peripheral site for pulse rate assessment (Figure 9-8). The carotid artery site is also commonly used when the radial pulse is weak or difficult to palpate. Assessment of other peripheral pulse sites, such as the brachial or femoral artery, is unnecessary when routinely obtaining vital signs. Other peripheral pulses are assessed when a complete physical is conducted or when the radial artery is not available for assessment because of surgery, trauma, or impaired blood flow.

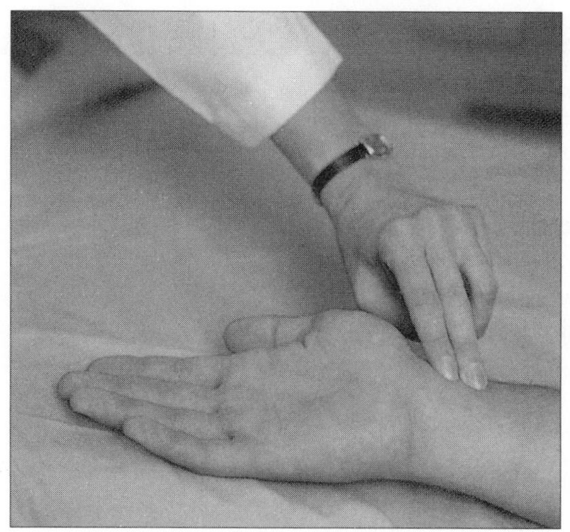

FIGURE **9-8** Location of right radial pulse site.

Delegation Considerations

The skill of radial pulse measurement can be delegated to assistive personnel unless the client is considered unstable. Inform caregiver if the client has a history of or risk for irregular pulse or abnormally slow or rapid pulse, and advise the caregiver if it is necessary to assess the pulse more frequently than standard practice. Be sure the caregiver is aware of the client's usual baseline pulse rate, and instruct the caregiver to report any abnormalities that should be reconfirmed.

Equipment

- Wristwatch with second hand or digital display
- Pen, pencil, vital sign flow sheet or computer record form

Step	Rationale
Assessment	
1. Determine need to assess radial pulse:	
a. Note risk factors for alterations in pulse.	Certain conditions place clients at risk for pulse alterations: a history of heart disease, cardiac dysrhythmia, onset of sudden chest pain or acute pain from any site, invasive cardiovascular diagnostic tests, surgery, sudden infusion of large volume of intravenous (IV) fluid, internal or external hemorrhage, or administration of medications that alter cardiac function. A history of peripheral vascular disease can alter pulse rate and quality.
b. Note signs and symptoms of altered SV and CO, such as dyspnea, fatigue, chest pain, orthopnea, syncope, palpitations (person's unpleasant awareness of heartbeat), jugular venous distention, edema of dependent body parts, cyanosis or pallor of skin.	Physical signs and symptoms may indicate alteration in cardiac function, which affects radial pulse rate and rhythm.
c. Client has signs and symptoms of peripheral vascular disease such as pale, cool extremities; thin, shiny skin with decreased hair growth; thickened nails.	Physical signs and symptoms may indicate alteration in local arterial blood flow.
2. Assess for factors that influence radial pulse rate and rhythm: age, exercise, position changes, fluid balance, medications, temperature, sympathetic stimulation.	Allows nurse to accurately assess presence and significance of pulse alterations.

STEP	RATIONALE
3. Determine client's previous baseline pulse rate (if available) from client's record.	Allows nurse to assess for change in condition. Provides comparison with future pulse measurements.

NURSING DIAGNOSIS

Defining characteristics from the assessment data may reveal the following nursing diagnoses for clients requiring this skill:

- Activity intolerance
- Ineffective cardiopulmonary tissue perfusion
- Decreased cardiac output
- Risk for imbalanced fluid volume
- Ineffective peripheral tissue perfusion

Related factors are individualized based on client's condition and needs.

PLANNING

STEP	RATIONALE
1. **Expected outcomes** following completion of procedure:	
▪ Radial pulse is palpable, within acceptable range for client's age.	Adults average 60 to 100 beats per minute.
▪ Rhythm is regular.	Cardiac status is stable.
▪ Radial pulse is strong, firm, and elastic.	Radial artery is patent.
2. Explain to client that radial pulse rate (HR) is to be assessed. Encourage client to relax as much as possible. If client has been active, wait 5 to 10 minutes before assessing pulse.	Anxiety or activity can cause elevation in heart rate. Radial pulse rate should be assessed at rest to allow for objective comparison of values.

IMPLEMENTATION

STEP	RATIONALE
1. Wash hands.	Reduces transmission of microorganisms.
2. If necessary, draw curtain around bed and/or close door.	Maintains privacy and minimizes embarrassment.
3. Assist client to assume a supine or sitting position.	Provides easy access to pulse sites.
4. If supine, place client's forearm straight alongside or across lower chest or upper abdomen with wrist extended straight (see illustration). If sitting, bend client's elbow 90 degrees and support lower arm on chair or on nurse's arm. Slightly extend or flex wrist with palm down until strongest pulse is noted.	Relaxed position of lower arm and extension of wrist permits full exposure of artery to palpation.

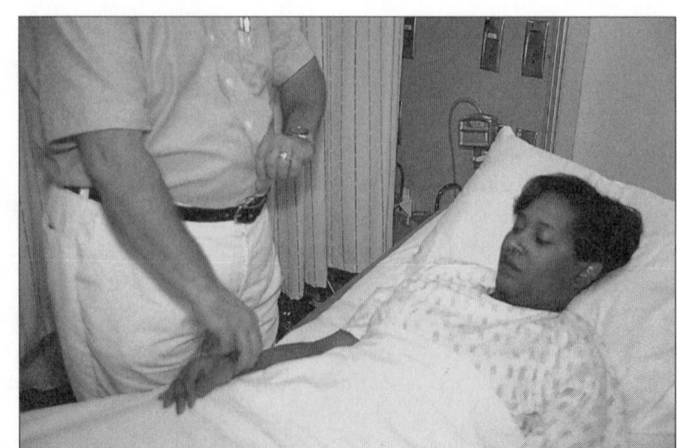

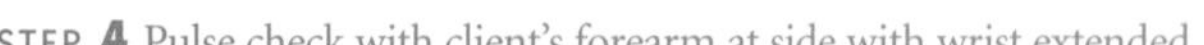
STEP 4 Pulse check with client's forearm at side with wrist extended.

STEP	RATIONALE
5. Place tips of first two or middle three fingers of hand over groove along radial or thumb side of client's inner wrist (see illustration).	Fingertips are most sensitive parts of hand to palpate arterial pulsation. Nurse's thumb has pulsation that may interfere with accuracy.

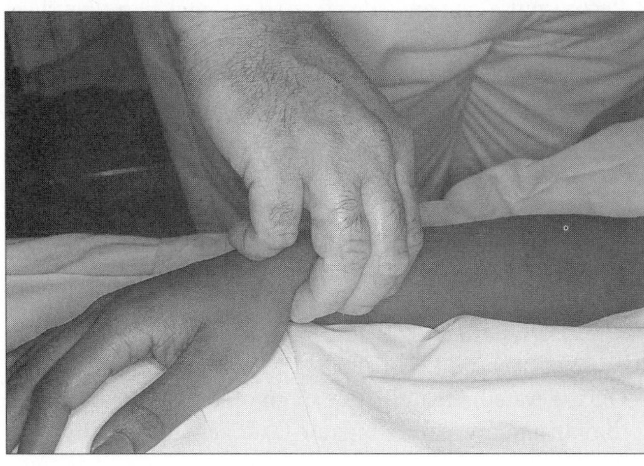

STEP **5** Hand placement for pulse checks.

STEP	RATIONALE
6. Lightly compress against radius, obliterate pulse initially, and then relax pressure so pulse becomes easily palpable.	Pulse is more accurately assessed with moderate pressure. Too much pressure occludes pulse and impairs blood flow.
7. Determine strength of pulse. Note whether thrust of vessel against fingertips is bounding, strong, weak, or thready.	Strength reflects volume of blood ejected against arterial wall with each heart contraction.
8. After pulse can be felt regularly, look at watch's second hand and begin to count rate: when sweep hand hits number on dial, start counting with zero, then one, two, and so on.	Rate is determined accurately only after nurse is assured pulse can be palpated. Timing begins with zero. Count of one is first beat palpated after timing begins.
9. If pulse is regular, count rate for 30 seconds and multiply total by 2.	A 30-second count is accurate for rapid, slow, or regular pulse rates.
10. If pulse is irregular, count rate for 60 seconds. Assess frequency and pattern of irregularity.	Inefficient contraction of heart fails to transmit pulse wave, interfering with CO, resulting in irregular pulse. Longer time period ensures accurate count.
11. When pulse is irregular, compare radial pulses bilaterally.	A marked inequality may indicate arterial flow is compromised to one extremity and action should be taken.

- ***Critical Decision Point***

  If pulse is irregular, assess for pulse deficit. Count apical pulse (Skill 9-3) while a colleague counts radial pulse. Begin pulse count by calling out loud simultaneously when to begin measuring pulses. If pulse count differs by more than 2, a pulse deficit exists, which may indicate alterations in CO.

STEP	RATIONALE
12. Assist client in returning to comfortable position.	Promotes comfort and sense of well-being.
13. Discuss findings with client as needed.	Promotes participation in care and understanding of health status.
14. Wash hands.	Reduces transmission of microorganisms.

EVALUATION

STEP	RATIONALE
1. If pulse is assessed for the first time, establish radial pulse as baseline if it is within acceptable range.	Used to compare future pulse assessments.
2. Compare pulse rate and character with client's previous baseline and acceptable range for client's age.	Allows nurse to assess for change in client's condition and for presence of cardiac alteration.

UNEXPECTED OUTCOMES AND RELATED INTERVENTIONS

- Pulse rate for an adult is under 60 beats per minute (**bradycardia**), over 100 beats per minute (**tachycardia**), or pulse rhythm is irregular.
  - Confer with physician and be prepared to order/obtain an electrocardiogram.
  - For irregular rhythm assess apical pulse for pulse deficit.
- Radial pulse may be weak and difficult to palpate.
  - Assess for swelling in surrounding tissues or any encumberance (e.g., dressing or cast) that may impede blood flow.
  - Obtain Doppler or ultrasound stethoscope to detect low-velocity blood flow.
- Pulse deficit is present.
  - Report findings to physician.

RECORDING AND REPORTING

- Record pulse rate and site assessed on vital sign flow sheet (see Figure 9-7) or nurses' notes. Also record any accompanying signs and symptoms of pulse alterations.
- Report abnormal findings to nurse in charge or physician.

TEACHING CONSIDERATIONS

- Clients taking certain prescribed cardiotonic or antidysrhythmic medications should learn to assess their own pulse rates to detect side effects of medications. Clients undergoing cardiac rehabilitation should learn to assess their own pulse rates to determine their response to exercise (see Chapter 28).
  - Monitoring carotid pulse rate is taught to clients taking heart medications or starting a prescribed exercise regimen.

PEDIATRIC CONSIDERATIONS

- Apical or brachial pulse is best site for assessing infant's or young child's HR and rhythm.

GERONTOLOGICAL CONSIDERATIONS

- It is often difficult to palpate the pulse of an older adult or obese client. A Doppler ultrasound stethoscope provides a more accurate reading.
- The arteries of an older adult may feel stiff and knotty because of decreased elasticity.
- Once elevated, the pulse rate of an older adult takes longer to return to normal resting rate (Lueckenotte, 2000).

Skill 9-3 Assessing Apical Pulse

Each ventricular contraction ejects approximately 60 to 70 ml (stroke volume) of blood into the aorta. The heart rate is the number of ejections occurring in 1 minute. The volume of blood pumped by the heart during 1 minute is the **cardiac output (CO).** The cardiac output equals the product of the amount of blood pumped by the ventricle per stroke, or the **stroke volume (SV),** and the heart rate (HR) for 1 minute. The apical pulse is the most reliable noninvasive way to assess cardiac function. The **apical pulse** rate is the assessment of the number and quality of apical sounds in 1 minute. Each apical pulse is the combination of two sounds. S_1 and S_2. $\mathbf{S_1}$ is the sound of the tricuspid and mitral valves closing at the end of ventricular filling, just before systolic contraction begins. $\mathbf{S_2}$ is the sound of the pulmonic and aortic valves closing at the end of ventricular ejection.

A stethoscope is used to auscultate sound waves of the apical pulse (Figure 9-9). It is a closed cylinder that amplifies sound waves as they reach the body's surface. The four major parts of the stethoscope are the earpieces, binaurals, tubing, and chestpiece.

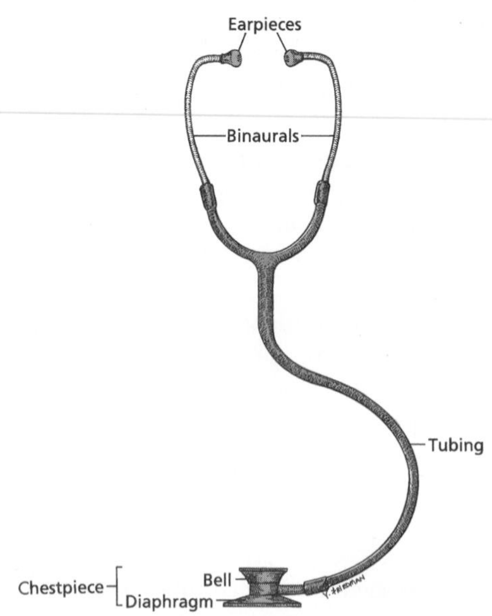

FIGURE 9-9 Acoustic stethoscope.

The plastic or rubber earpieces should fit snugly and comfortably in the nurse's ears. Binaurals should be angled and strong enough so the earpieces stay firmly in place without causing discomfort. The earpieces follow the contour of the ear canal, pointing toward the face when the stethoscope is in place.

The polyvinyl tubing should be flexible and 30 to 40 cm (12 to 18 inches) in length; longer tubing decreases sound transmission. The tubing should be thick walled and moderately rigid to eliminate transmission of environmental noise and to prevent kinking.

The chestpiece consists of a bell and diaphragm. The diaphragm is a circular flat-surfaced portion of the chestpiece covered with a plastic disk. It transmits high-pitched sounds created by high-velocity movement of air and blood. The diaphragm is positioned to make a tight seal against the client's skin. Enough pressure is exerted to complete the seal and should leave a temporary red ring on the client's skin when the diaphragm is removed.

The bell is the cone-shaped portion of the chestpiece usually surrounded by a rubber ring to avoid chilling the client. It transmits low-pitched sounds created by the low-velocity movement of blood. The bell is held lightly against the skin for sound amplification. The bell and diaphragm are rotated into position on the chestpiece depending on which part the nurse chooses to use. To test, lightly tap to determine which side is functioning.

Delegation Considerations

Often the apical pulse is measured when the nurse suspects an irregularity in the radial pulse or the client's condition warrants a more accurate assessment. In this situation, delegation of pulse assessment is inappropriate. When measurement of apical pulse is a routine practice, it can be delegated to assistive personnel. Be sure the caregiver is aware of the usual values for the client, and inform the caregiver to report any abnormalities that should be reconfirmed.

Equipment

- Stethoscope
- Wristwatch with second hand or digital display
- Pen, pencil, vital sign flow sheet or record form
- Alcohol swab

Step	Rationale
Assessment	
1. Determine need to assess apical pulse:	
a. Note risk factors for alterations in apical pulse.	Certain conditions place clients at risk for pulse alterations: heart disease, cardiac dysrhythmias, onset of sudden chest pain or acute pain from any site, invasive cardiovascular diagnostic tests, surgery, sudden infusion of large volume of intravenous (IV) fluid, internal or external hemorrhage, and administration of medications that alter heart function.
b. Assess for signs and symptoms such as dyspnea, fatigue, chest pain, orthopnea, syncope, palpitations (person's unpleasant awareness of heartbeat), jugular venous distention, edema of dependent body parts, cyanosis or pallor of skin.	Physical signs and symptoms may indicate alteration in cardiac output or stroke volume.
2. Assess for factors that normally influence apical pulse rate and rhythm:	Allows nurse to accurately assess presence and significance of pulse alterations.
a. Age	Infant's heart rate at birth ranges from 100 to 180 beats per minute at rest; by age 2, pulse rate slows to 70 to 110 beats per minute, by adolescence, rate varies between 60 and 100 beats per minute and remains so throughout adulthood; no changes occur in older adults at rest and in absence of disease.
b. Exercise	Physical activity requires an increase in CO that is met by an increased HR and SV; a well-conditioned client may have a slower-than-usual resting HR and returns more quickly to resting rate after exercise.
c. Position changes	Heart rate increases temporarily when changing from lying to sitting or standing position.

STEP	RATIONALE
d. Medications	Antidysrhythmics, sympathomimetics, and cardiotonics affect rate and rhythm of pulse; large doses of narcotic analgesics can slow HR; general anesthetics slow HR; central nervous system stimulants such as caffeine can increase HR.
e. Temperature	Fever or exposure to warm environments increases HR; HR declines with hypothermia.
f. Sympathetic stimulation	Emotional stress, anxiety, or fear results in stimulation of the sympathetic nervous system, which increases HR.
3. Determine previous baseline apical rate (if available) from client's record.	Allows nurse to assess for change in condition. Provides comparison with future apical pulse measurements.

NURSING DIAGNOSIS

Defining characteristics from the assessment data may reveal the following nursing diagnoses for clients requiring this skill:

Ineffective cardiopulmonary tissue perfusion

Decreased cardiac output

Related factors are individualized based on client's condition or needs.

PLANNING

1. **Expected outcomes** following completion of procedure:	
▪ Apical heart rate is within acceptable range.	Adults average 60 to 100 beats per minute.
▪ Rhythm is regular.	Cardiovascular status is stable.
2. Explain to client that apical pulse rate is to be assessed. Encourage client to relax as much as possible. Ask client not to speak while assessing pulse. If client has been active, wait 5 to 10 minutes before assessing pulse.	Anxiety or activity can cause elevation in HR. Client's speech interferes with nurse's ability to hear sounds when apical pulse is measured. Apical pulse rate should be assessed at rest to allow for objective comparison of values.

IMPLEMENTATION

1. Wash hands.	Reduces transmission of microorganisms.
2. Draw curtain around bed and/or close door.	Maintains privacy and minimizes embarrassment.
3. Assist client to supine or sitting position. Move aside bed linen and gown to expose sternum and left side of chest.	Exposes portion of chest wall for selection of auscultatory site.
4. Locate anatomical landmarks to identify the point of maximal impulse (PMI), also called the apical impulse. Heart is located behind and to left of sternum with base at top and apex at bottom. Find Angle of Louis just below suprasternal notch between sternal body and manubrium, can be felt as a bony prominence (see illustrations). Slip fingers down each side of angle to find second intercostal space (ICS). Carefully move fingers down left side of sternum to fifth ICS and laterally to the left midclavicular line (MCL). A light tap felt within an area 1 to 2 cm ($^1/_2$ to 1 inch) of the PMI is reflected from the apex of the heart.	Use of anatomical landmarks allows correct placement of stethoscope over apex of heart. This position enhances ability to hear heart sounds clearly. If unable to palpate the PMI, reposition client on left side. In the presence of serious heart disease, the PMI may be located to the left of the MCL or at the sixth ICS.
5. Place diaphragm of stethoscope in palm of hand for 5 to 10 seconds.	Warming of metal or plastic diaphragm prevents client from being startled and promotes comfort.
6. Place diaphragm of stethoscope over PMI at the fifth ICS, at the left MCL, and auscultate for normal S_1 and S_2 heart sounds (heard as "lub-dub") (see illustrations).	Allow stethoscope tubing to extend straight without kinks that would distort sound transmission. Normal sounds S_1 and S_2 are high pitched and best heard with the diaphragm.

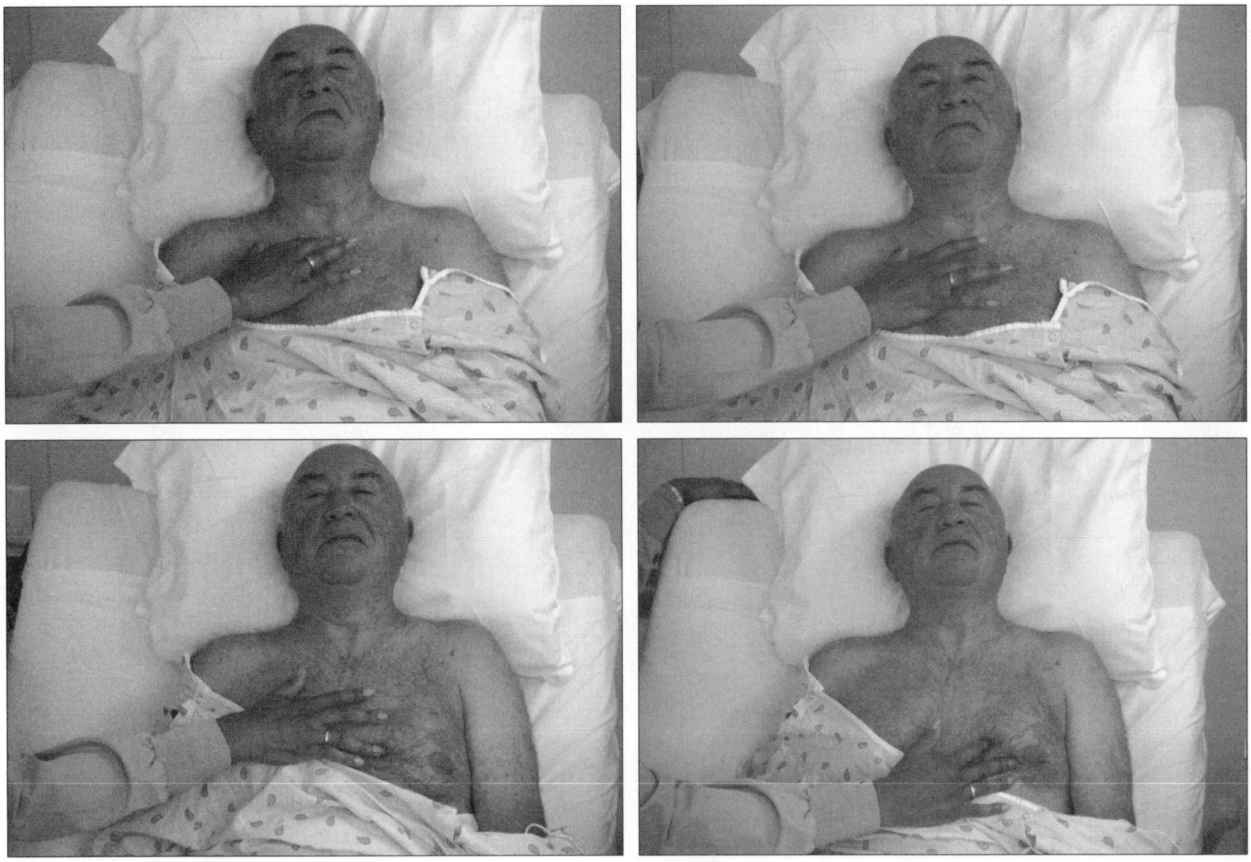

A B

C D

STEP 4 **A,** Nurse locates sternal notch. **B,** Nurse locates second intercostal space. **C,** Nurse locates fifth intercostal space. **D,** Nurse locates PMI at intercostal space at the midclavicular line.

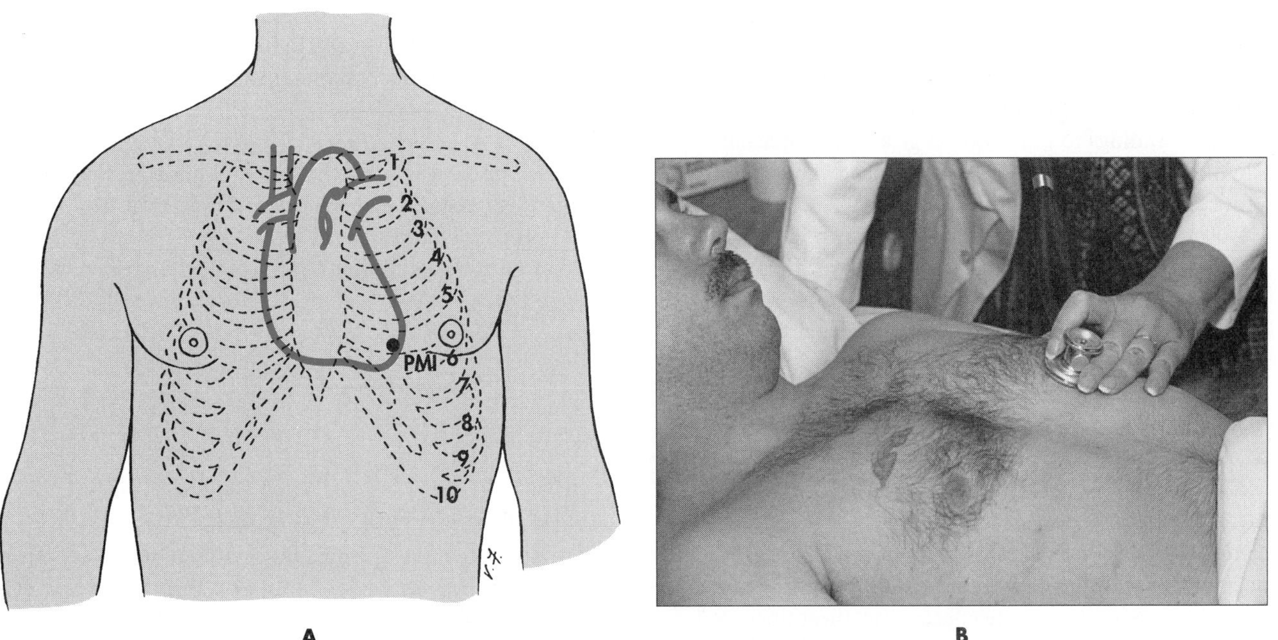

STEP 6 **A,** Location of PMI in adult. **B,** Stethoscope over PMI.

STEP	RATIONALE
7. When S_1 and S_2 are heard with regularity, use watch's second hand and begin to count rate: when sweep hand hits number on dial, start counting with zero, then one, two, and so on.	Apical rate is determined accurately only after nurse is able to auscultate sounds clearly. Timing begins with zero. Count of one is first sound auscultated after timing begins.
8. If apical rate is regular, count for 30 seconds and multiply by 2.	Regular apical rate can be assessed within 30 seconds.
9. If heart rate is irregular, or client is receiving cardiovascular medication, count for 1 minute (60 seconds).	Irregular rate is more accurately assessed when measured over longer interval.
10. Note regularity of any **dysrhythmia** (S_1 and S_2 occurring early or later after previous sequence of sounds; for example, every third or every fourth beat is skipped).	Regular occurrence of dysrhythmia within 1 minute may indicate inefficient contraction of heart and alteration in cardiac output.
11. Replace client's gown and bed linen; assist client in returning to comfortable position.	Restores comfort and promotes sense of well-being.
12. Discuss findings with client as needed.	Promotes participation in care and understanding of health status.
13. Wash hands.	Reduces transmission of microorganisms.
14. Clean earpieces and diaphragm of stethoscope with alcohol swab routinely after each use.	Stethoscopes are frequently contaminated with microorganisms. Regular disinfection can control nosocomial infections (Embrey and others, 1998).

EVALUATION

1. If pulse is assessed for the first time, establish apical rate as baseline if it is within an acceptable range.	Used to compare future pulse assessments.
2. Compare apical rate and character with client's previous baseline and acceptable range of heart rate for client's age.	Allows nurse to assess for change in client's condition and for presence of cardiac alteration.

- ***Critical Decision Point***
  If apical rate is abnormal or irregular, repeat measurement or have another nurse conduct measurement. Original measurement may result from error by assessor. Second measurement confirms initial findings of abnormal HR.

UNEXPECTED OUTCOMES AND RELATED INTERVENTIONS

- Apical rate under 60 (bradycardia) or over 100 (tachycardia), indicating potential poor cardiac output.
  - Report findings to nurse in charge and/or physician.
- Rhythm is irregular, indicating a potential for inefficient ventricular ejection and poor CO.
  - Notify nurse in charge and physician. An electrocardiogram may be ordered to detect conduction alterations.
- Occasional **premature ventricular contractions (PVCs)** are common in most persons. However, frequency of PVCs increases with heart disease. Nurse will hear premature sequence of S_1 and S_2 and then short pause before normal S_1 and S_2 return.
  - Numerous PVCs or PVCs that alternate with a normal heartbeat repeatedly should be reported to physician.

RECORDING AND REPORTING

- Record apical rate and rhythm on vital sign flow sheet or computer record (see Figure 9-7). Record any signs or symptoms of alterations in CO in nurses' notes.
- Report abnormal findings to nurse in charge or physician.

TEACHING CONSIDERATIONS

- Caregivers of clients taking certain prescribed cardiotonic or antidysrhythmic medications should learn to assess apical pulse rates to detect side effects of medications.

PEDIATRIC CONSIDERATIONS

- Children often have a sinus dysrhythmia, which is an irregular heart beat that speeds up with inspiration and slows down with expiration.

- Point of maximal impulse of an infant is usually located at the third to fourth ICS near the left sternal border.
- Apical pulse is best site for assessing infant's or young child's HR and rhythm.
- Breath holding in an infant or child affects apical pulse rate.

GERONTOLOGICAL CONSIDERATIONS

- The PMI may be difficult to palpate in an older adult because the anterior-posterior diameter of the chest increases with age, and the heart becomes repositioned as a result of left ventricular enlargement.
- When assessing older adult women with sagging breasts, the breast tissue is gently lifted and the stethoscope placed at the fifth ICS or the lower edge of the breast.
- Heart sound may be muffled or difficult to hear in older adults because of an increase in air space in the lungs.

HOME CARE CONSIDERATIONS

- Assess home environment to determine which room affords a quiet environment for auscultation of apical rate.

Skill 9-4 Assessing Respirations

The mechanism of respiration exchanges oxygen (O_2) and carbon dioxide (CO_2) between cells of the body and the atmosphere. Three processes are involved in respiration: *ventilation,* mechanical movement of gases into and out of the lungs; *diffusion,* movement of O_2 and CO_2 between the alveoli and the red blood cells; and *perfusion,* distribution of red blood cells to and from the pulmonary capillaries. The nurse directly assesses ventilation by observing the rate, depth, and rhythm of respiratory movements. Accurate assessment of respiration depends on recognizing normal thoracic and abdominal movements. Normal breathing is active and passive. On inspiration the diaphragm contracts, causing abdominal organs to move downward and forward, thereby increasing the vertical size of the chest cavity. At the same time, the ribs lift upward and outward and the sternum lifts outward to aid the transverse expansion of the lungs. On expiration the diaphragm relaxes upward, the ribs and sternum return to their relaxed position, and the abdominal organs return to their original position (Figure 9-10). During quiet breathing the chest wall gently rises and falls. More energy is required during inspiration than during expiration. Little energy is needed to expire air out of the lungs. Expiration is an active process only during exercise, voluntary hyperventilation, and certain disease states.

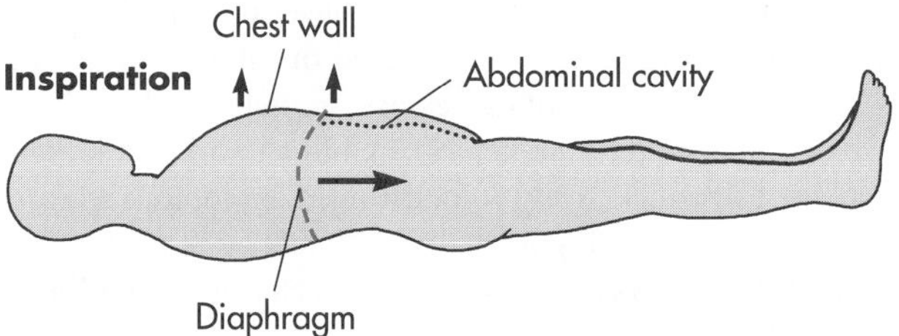

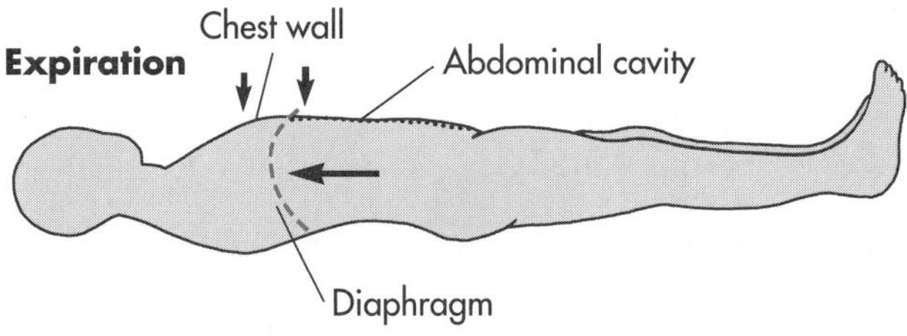

FIGURE 9-10 Illustration of diaphragmatic and chest wall movement during inspiration and expiration.

DELEGATION CONSIDERATIONS

The skill of respiration measurement can be delegated to assistive personnel unless the client is considered unstable. Inform the care provider if the client is at risk for increased or decreased respiratory rate or irregular respirations. Also be sure that the care provider is aware of the usual values for the client, and advise the care provider to report any abnormalities.

EQUIPMENT

- Wristwatch with second hand or digital display
- Pen, pencil, vital sign flow sheet or record form

STEP	RATIONALE
ASSESSMENT	
1. Determine need to assess client's respirations:	
a. Note risk factors for respiratory alterations.	Conditions that place client at risk for ventilatory alterations detected by changes in respiratory rate, depth, and rhythm: fever, pain and anxiety, diseases of chest wall or muscles, constrictive chest or abdominal dressings, presence of abdominal incisions, gastric distention, chronic pulmonary disease (emphysema, bronchitis, asthma), traumatic injury to chest wall with or without collapse of underlying lung tissue, presence of a chest tube, respiratory infection (pneumonia, acute bronchitis), pulmonary edema and emboli, head injury with damage to brain stem, and anemia.
b. Assess for signs and symptoms of respiratory alterations, such as bluish or cyanotic appearance of nail beds, lips, mucous membranes, and skin; restlessness, irritability, confusion, reduced level of consciousness; pain during inspiration; labored or difficult breathing; orthopnea; use of accessory muscles; adventitious breath sounds (Chapter 10), inability to breathe spontaneously; thick, frothy, blood-tinged, or copious sputum produced on coughing.	Physical signs and symptoms may indicate alterations in respiratory status related to ventilation.
2. Assess for factors that influence character of respirations:	Allows nurse to accurately assess for presence and significance of respiratory alterations.
a. Exercise	Respirations increase in rate and depth to meet the need for additional oxygen and rid the body of CO_2.
b. Anxiety	Respirations increase in rate and depth as a result of stimulation by the sympathetic nervous system.
c. Acute pain	Pain alters rate and rhythm of respirations; breaths become shallow.
d. Smoking	Chronic smoking changes pulmonary airways, resulting in an increased respiratory rate at rest.
e. Medications	Narcotic analgesics, general anesthetics, and sedative hypnotics depress rate and depth; amphetamines and cocaine may increase rate and depth, bronchodilators cause dilation of airways that ultimately can slow respiratory rate.
f. Postural changes	Standing or sitting erect promotes full ventilatory movement and lung expansion; stooped or slumped posture impairs ventilatory movement; lying flat prevents full chest expansion.
g. Neurological injury	Damage to the brain stem impairs the respiratory center and inhibits rate and rhythm.
h. Anemia	Decreased hemoglobin levels lower the amount of oxygen carried in the blood, which results in increased respiratory rate to increase oxygen delivery.
3. Assess pertinent laboratory values:	
a. Arterial blood gases (ABGs) (values may vary slightly within institutions): pH 7.35 to 7.45 $PaCO_2$ 35 to 45 mm Hg PaO_2 80 to 100 mm Hg SaO_2 94% to 98%	Arterial blood gases measure arterial blood pH, partial pressure of O_2 and CO_2, and arterial O_2 saturation, which reflects client's oxygenation status.

STEP	RATIONALE
b. Pulse oximetry (SpO_2): normal SpO_2 90% to 100%; 85% to 89% may be acceptable for certain chronic disease conditions; less than 85% is abnormal (Skill 9-6).	SpO_2 less than 85% is often accompanied by changes in respiratory rate, depth, and rhythm.
c. Complete blood count (CBC): normal CBC for adults (values may vary within institutions): hemoglobin: 14 to 18 g/100 ml, males; 12 to 16 g/100 ml, females (Hematocrit: 40% to 54% , males; 38% to 47%, females. Red blood cell count: 4.6 to 6.2 million/mm^3, males; 4.2 to 5.4 million/mm^3, females (see Chapter 43).	Complete blood count measures red blood cell count, volume of red blood cells, and concentration of hemoglobin, which reflects client's capacity to carry O_2.
4. Determine previous baseline respiratory rate (if available) from client's record.	Allows nurse to assess for change in condition. Provides comparison with future respiratory measurements.

NURSING DIAGNOSIS

Defining characteristics from the assessment data may reveal the following nursing diagnoses for clients requiring this skill:

- Activity intolerance
- Impaired gas exchange
- Impaired spontaneous ventilation
- Ineffective airway clearance
- Ineffective breathing pattern

Related factors are individualized based on client's condition or needs.

PLANNING

STEP	RATIONALE
1. Expected outcomes following completion of procedure:	
▪ Respiratory rate is within acceptable range.	Adults average 12 to 20 respirations per minute.
▪ Respirations are regular and of normal depth.	Respiratory status is stable.
2. If client has been active, wait 5 to 10 minutes before assessing respirations.	Exercise increases respiratory rate and depth. Respirations should be assessed at rest to allow for objective comparison of values.
3. Assess respirations after pulse measurement in adult.	Inconspicuous assessment of respirations immediately after pulse assessment prevents client from consciously or unintentionally altering rate and depth of breathing.
4. Be sure client is in comfortable position, preferably sitting or lying with the head of the bed elevated 45 to 60 degrees.	Sitting erect promotes full ventilatory movement. Position of discomfort may cause client to breathe more rapidly.

• ***Critical Decision Point***

Clients with difficulty breathing ***(dyspnea)*** *such as those with congestive heart failure or abdominal ascites or in late stages or pregnancy should be assessed in the position of greatest comfort. Repositioning may increase the work of breathing, which will increase respiratory rate.*

IMPLEMENTATION

STEP	RATIONALE
1. Draw curtain around bed and/or close door. Wash hands.	Maintains privacy. Prevents transmission of microorganisms.
2. Be sure client's chest is visible. If necessary, move bed linen or gown.	Ensures clear view of chest wall and abdominal movements.
3. Place client's arm in relaxed position across the abdomen or lower chest, or place nurse's hand directly over client's upper abdomen (see illustration).	A similar position used during pulse assessment allows respiratory rate assessment to be inconspicuous. Client's or nurse's hand rises and falls during respiratory cycle.

Step	Rationale

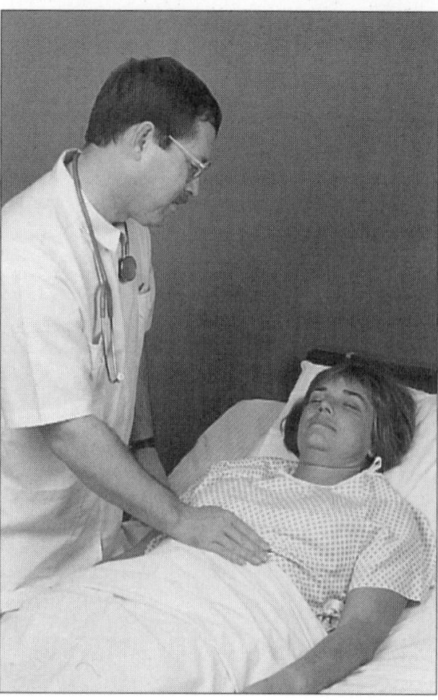

STEP 3 Nurse's hand over client's abdomen to check respiration.

Step	Rationale
4. Observe complete respiratory cycle (one inspiration and one expiration).	Rate is accurately determined only after nurse has viewed respiratory cycle.
5. After cycle is observed, look at watch's second hand and begin to count rate: when sweep hand hits number on dial, begin time frame, counting one with first full respiratory cycle.	Timing begins with count of one. Respirations occur more slowly than pulse; thus timing does not begin with zero.
6. If rhythm is regular, count number of respirations in 30 seconds and multiply by 2. If rhythm is irregular, less than 12, or greater than 20, count for 1 full minute.	Respiratory rate is equivalent to number of respirations per minute. Suspected irregularities require assessment for at least 1 minute.
7. Note depth of respirations, subjectively assessed by observing degree of chest wall movement while counting rate. Nurse can also objectively assess depth by palpating chest wall excursion or auscultating the posterior thorax after rate has been counted (Chapter 10). Depth is shallow, normal, or deep.	Character of ventilatory movement may reveal specific disease state restricting volume of air from moving into and out of the lungs.
8. Note rhythm of ventilatory cycle. Normal breathing is regular and uninterrupted. Sighing should not be confused with abnormal rhythm. Periodically people unconsciously take single deep breaths or sighs to expand small airways prone to collapse.	Character of ventilations can reveal specific types of alterations.
9. Replace bed linen and client's gown.	Restores comfort and promotes sense of well-being.
10. Wash hands.	Reduces transmission of microorganisms.
11. Discuss findings with client as needed.	Promotes participation in care and understanding of health status.

Evaluation

Step	Rationale
1. If respirations are assessed for the first time, establish rate, rhythm, and depth as baseline if within acceptable range.	Used to compare future respiratory assessment.

STEP	RATIONALE
2. Compare respirations with client's previous baseline and usual rate, rhythm, and depth.	Allows nurse to assess for changes in client's condition and for presence of respiratory alterations.
3. Correlate respiratory rate, depth, and rhythm with data obtained from pulse oximetry and arterial blood gas measurements if available.	Evaluation of ventilation, perfusion, and diffusion are interrelated.

UNEXPECTED OUTCOMES AND RELATED INTERVENTIONS

- Respiratory rate is below 12 **(bradypnea)** or above 20 **(tachypnea).** Rhythm may be irregular (Table 9-2). Depth of respirations increased or decreased.
  - Be sure client is in a comfortable Fowler's or high-Fowler's position that allows for full expansion of chest wall.
  - Check for tight dressings or other encumberances to ventilation.
  - Notify physician if alteration continues, and be prepared to initiate oxygen therapy as needed. An ABG test or chest x-ray examination may be ordered to evaluate nature of respiratory problem.
  - Maintain patency of any existing artificial airway.
- Client demonstrates Kussmaul's, Cheyne-Stokes, or Biot's respirations (see Table 9-2).
  - Notify physician, and anticipate immediate therapy will be ordered.

RECORDING AND REPORTING

- Record respiratory rate on vital sign flow sheet or computer record (see Figure 9-7). Record abnormal depth and rhythm in narrative form in nurses' notes.
- Indicate type and amount of oxygen therapy, if used, in nurses' notes.
- Report abnormal findings to nurse in charge or physician.

TEACHING CONSIDERATIONS

- Clients who demonstrate decreased ventilation may benefit from being taught deep-breathing and coughing exercises (Chapter 33).
- Instruct family caregiver to contact home care nurse or physician if unusual fluctuations in respiratory rate occur.

PEDIATRIC CONSIDERATIONS

- Acceptable average respiratory rate (breaths per minute) for newborns is 35 to 40; infant (6 months) is 30 to 50; toddler (2 years) is 25 to 32; and child is 20 to 30.
- Infant's respirations are primarily diaphragmatic and thus observed by abdominal movement.
- Infants tend to breathe less regularly.
- Nurse can simply observe infant or young child while chest and abdomen are exposed.
- The young child may breathe slowly for a few seconds and then suddenly breathe more rapidly.
- Apnea monitors may be used for infants or newborns who are at risk for respiratory compromise or arrest.

GERONTOLOGICAL CONSIDERATIONS

- Aging causes ossification of costal cartilage and downward slant of ribs, resulting in more rigid rib cage, which reduces chest wall expansion. Kyphosis and scoliosis that can occur in older adults may also restrict chest expansion.
- Depth of respirations tend to decrease with aging.
- Older adults may depend more on accessory abdominal muscles during respiration than weakened thoracic muscles.

HOME CARE CONSIDERATIONS

- Assess for environmental factors in the home that may influence client's respiratory rate such as secondhand smoke, poor ventilation, or gas fumes.

Table 9-2 Alterations in Breathing Pattern

ALTERATION	DESCRIPTION
Bradypnea	Rate of breathing is regular but abnormally slow (less than 12 breaths per minute).
Tachypnea	Rate of breathing is regular but abnormally rapid (greater than 20 breaths per minute).
Hyperpnea	Respirations are increased in depth. Occurs normally during exercise.
Apnea	Respirations cease for several seconds. Persistent cessation results in respiratory arrest.
Cheyne-Stokes respiration	Respiratory rate and depth are irregular, characterized by alternating periods of apnea and hyperventilation. Respiratory cycle begins with slow, shallow breaths that gradually increase to abnormal rate and depth. The pattern reverses, breathing slows and becomes shallow, climaxing in apnea before respiration resumes.
Kussmaul's respiration	Respirations are abnormally deep but regular. Common in diabetic ketoacidosis.
Biot's respiration	Respirations are abnormally shallow for two to three breaths followed by irregular period of apnea.

Skill 9-5 Assessing Arterial Blood Pressure

Blood pressure (BP) is the force exerted by the blood against the vessel walls. During a normal cardiac cycle, BP reaches a peak that is followed by a trough, or low point, in the cycle. The peak pressure occurs when the heart's ventricular contraction, or systole, forces blood under high pressure into the aorta. When the ventricles relax, the blood remaining in the arteries exerts a minimum or diastolic pressure. **Diastolic pressure** is the minimal pressure exerted against the arterial wall at all times.

The standard unit for measuring BP is millimeters of mercury (mm Hg). The measurement indicates the height to which the BP can sustain the column of mercury. The most common technique of measuring BP is auscultation using a sphygmomanometer and stethoscope. As the sphygmomanometer cuff is deflated, the five different sounds heard over an artery are called Korotkoff phases. The sound in each phase has unique characteristics (Figure 9-11). Blood pressure is recorded with the systolic reading (first Korotkoff sound) before the diastolic (beginning of the fifth Korotkoff sound). The difference between **systolic pressure** and diastolic pressure is the pulse pressure. For a BP of 120/80, the pulse pressure is 40.

Blood pressure, reflects various interrelated hemodynamic factors within the circulatory system: cardiac output, peripheral resistance, blood volume, blood viscosity, and vessel wall elasticity. Blood pressure has a direct relationship to cardiac output (CO) and peripheral vascular resistance (R):

$$BP = CO \times R$$

As CO increases, more blood is pumped into the arterial system, causing systolic BP to rise. When the size of the arteries and arterioles decreases, the resistance (R) to blood flow increases, causing the BP to rise. In contrast, as vessels dilate and vascular resistance falls, BP drops. The volume of blood circulating within the vascular system affects BP. Normally blood volume remains constant: 5000 ml in an adult. However, if volume increases, such as after a rapid intravenous (IV) infusion, pressure exerted against arterial walls rises. When circulating blood volume falls, as in the case of hemorrhage or dehydration, BP falls. When the thickness or viscosity of the blood increases, the heart must contract more forcefully to move the blood through the circulatory system and BP rises. When vessel walls are elastic, they are easily distensible and can accommodate changes in pressure. Arteriosclerotic

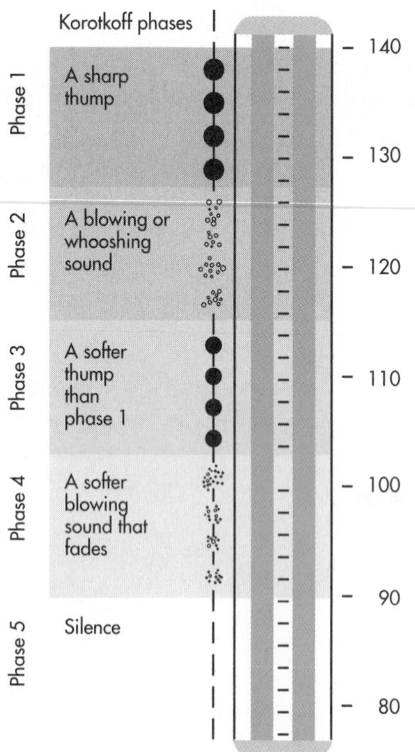

FIGURE 9-11 The sounds auscultated during blood pressure measurement can be differentiated into five Korotkoff phases. In this example, the blood pressure is 140/90.

Table 9-3 Classification of Blood Pressure for Adults Age 18 Years and Older*

Category	Systolic (mm Hg)		Diastolic (mm Hg)
Optimal†	<120	and	<80
Normal	<130	and	<85
High normal	130-139	or	85-80
Hypertension‡			
Stage 1	140-159	or	90-99
Stage 2	160-179	or	100-109
Stage 3	≥180		≥110

From National Institutes of Health, National High Blood Pressure Education Program; National Heart, Lung and Blood Institute: *The sixth report of the Joint National Committee on Prevention, Detection, Evaluation and Treatment of High Blood Pressure,* NIH Pub No 98-4080, Bethesda, Md., 1997, NIH.

*Not taking antihypertensive drugs and not acutely ill. When systolic and diastolic blood pressures fall into different categories, the higher category should be selected to classify the individual's blood pressure status. For example, 160/92 mm Hg should be classified as stage 2 hypertension, and 174/120 mm hg should be classified as stage 3 hypertension. Isolated systolic hypertension is defined as SBP of 140 mm Hg or greater and DBP below 90 mm Hg and staged appropriately (e.g., 170/82 mm Hg is defined as stage 2 isolated systolic hypertension). In addition to classifying stages of hypertension on the basis of average blood pressure levels, clinicians should specify presence or absence of target organ disease and additional risk factors. This specificity is important for risk classification and treatment.

†Optimal blood pressure with respect to cardiovascular risk is below 120/80 mm Hg. However, unusually low readings should be evaluated for clinical significance.

‡Based on the average of two or more readings taken at each of two or more visits after an initial screening.

vessels lose their elasticity, no longer yield to pressure, and the BP rises.

Hypertension

Hypertension is a major factor underlying death from heart attack and stroke in the United States and Canada. **Hypertension** is defined as systolic blood pressure (SBP) of 140 mm Hg or greater, diastolic blood pressure (DBP) of 90 mm Hg or greater, or taking antihypertensive medication National Institutes of Health [NIH], 1997). The Joint National Committee on Prevention, Detection, Evaluation, and Treatment of High Blood Pressure has set criteria for determining categories of hypertension (Table 9-3). The diagnosis of hypertension in adults is made on the average of two or more readings taken at each of two or more visits after an initial screening. One BP recording revealing a high SBP or DBP does not qualify as a diagnosis of hypertension. However, if the nurse assesses a high reading (for example, 150/90 mm Hg), the client should be encouraged to return for another checkup within 2 months (Table 9-4).

Hypotension

Hypotension is generally considered present when the systolic blood pressure falls to 90 mm Hg or below. Although some adults have a low blood pressure normally, for the majority of people, low blood pressure is an abnormal finding associated with illness (e.g., hemorrhage or myocardial infarction). **Orthostatic hypotension,** also referred to as **postural hypotension,** occurs when a normotensive person develops symptoms (e.g., light-headedness or dizziness) and low blood pressure when rising to an upright position. In severe cases, loss of consciousness may occur. Normally, when a healthy individual changes from a lying to sitting or standing position, the peripheral blood vessels in the legs constrict, the heart rate and contractility increase, and blood pressure remains adequate to perfuse the heart and brain (Roper, 1996). Orthostatic changes in vital signs are good indicators of blood volume depletion.

Blood Pressure Equipment

Arterial blood pressure may be measured either directly (invasively) or indirectly (noninvasively). The direct method requires electronic monitoring equipment and the insertion of a thin catheter into an artery. The risks of invasive blood pressure monitoring require use in an intensive care setting.

The more common noninvasive method requires use of the sphygmomanometer and stethoscope. A **sphygmomanometer** includes a pressure manometer, an occlusive cloth or disposable vinyl cuff that encloses an inflatable rubber bladder, and a pressure bulb with a release valve that inflates the bladder (Figure 9-12). There are two types of manometers: aneroid and mercury. The aneroid manometer has a glass-enclosed circular gauge containing a needle that registers millimeter calibrations. Metal parts in the aneroid manometer are subject to temperature expansion and contraction; thus the instrument is not as reliable as a mercury manometer.

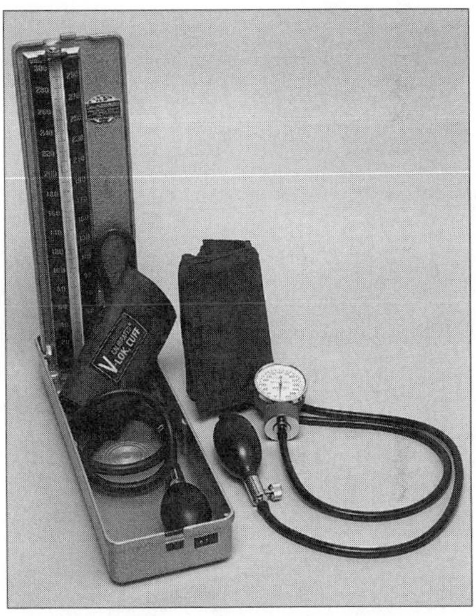

FIGURE **9-12** Mercury and aneroid sphygmomanometers.

Table 9-4 Recommendations for Follow-up Based on Initial Blood Pressure Measurements for Adults

Initial Blood Pressure (mm Hg)*		
Systolic	Diastolic	Follow-up Recommended†
<130	<85	Recheck in 2 years
130-139	85 to 89	Recheck in 1 year‡
140-159	90 to 99	Confirm within 2 months‡
160-179	100 to 109	Evaluate or refer to source of care within 1 month
≥180	≥110	Evaluate or refer to source of care immediately or within 1 week depending on clinical situation

National Institutes of Health, National High Blood Pressure Education Program; National Heart, Lung and Blood Institute: *The sixth report of the Joint National Committee on Prevention, Detection, Evaluation, and Treatment of High Blood Pressure,* NIH Pub No 98-4080, Bethesda, Md, 1997, NIH.

*If systolic and diastolic categories are different, follow recommendations for shorter time follow-up (e.g., 160/86 mm Hg should be evaluated or referred to source of care within 1 month).

†Modify the scheduling of follow-up according to reliable information about past blood pressure measurements, other cardiovascular risk factors, or target organ disease.

‡Provide advice about lifestyle modifications.

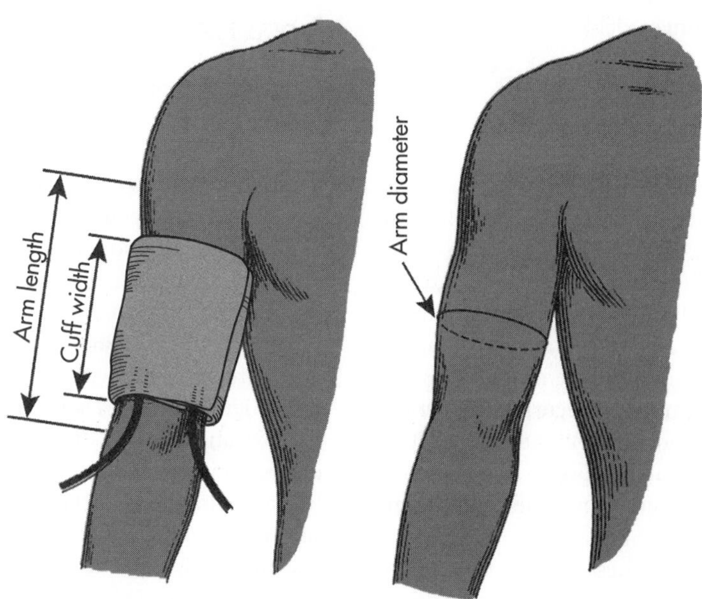

FIGURE **9-13** Guidelines for proper blood pressure cuff size. Cuff width = 20% more than upper arm diameter, or 40% of circumference and two thirds of arm length.

Table 9-5 Common Mistakes in Blood Pressure Assessment

ERROR	EFFECT
Bladder or cuff too wide	False low reading
Bladder or cuff too narrow	False high reading
Cuff wrapped too loosely or unevenly	False high reading
Deflating cuff too slowly	False high diastolic reading
Deflating cuff too quickly	False low systolic and false high diastolic reading
Arm below heart level	False high reading
Arm above heart level	False low reading
Arm not supported	False high reading
Stethoscope that fits poorly or impairment of the examiner's hearing, causing sounds to be muffled	False low systolic and false high diastolic reading
Stethoscope applied too firmly against antecubital fossa	False low diastolic reading
Inflating too slowly	False high diastolic reading
Repeating assessments too quickly	False low systolic reading
Inaccurate inflation level	Inaccurate interpretation of systolic and diastolic readings
Multiple examiners using different Korotkoff sounds for diastolic readings	False high systolic and low diastolic reading

Aneroid manometers must be recalibrated regularly. Before using the aneroid manometer, the nurse must be sure the needle points to zero.

The mercury manometer is an upright tube containing mercury. Pressure created by inflation of the bladder moves the column of mercury upward against the force of gravity. Millimeter calibrations mark the height of the mercury column. The mercury manometer is the gold standard for measuring blood pressure and is considered the most accurate of the sphygmomanometers. To ensure accurate readings, the mercury column should fall freely when pressure is released and always be at zero when the cuff is deflated. Mercury manometers may be wall mounted or portable.

The release valves of both mercury and aneroid sphygmomanometers should be clean and freely moveable in either direction. The valve, when closed, should hold the mercury or pressure constant. A sticky valve makes pressure cuff deflation hard to regulate. The pressure bulb and tubing should be airtight.

Cloth or disposable vinyl compression cuffs contain an inflatable bladder and come in several different sizes. The size selected is proportional to the circumference of the limb being assessed (Figure 9-13). Ideally the width of the cuff should be 40% of the circumference (or 20% wider than the diameter) of the midpoint of the limb on which the cuff is to be used (National Institutes of Health, 1997). The bladder enclosed within the cuff should encircle at least 80% of the arm (NIH, 1997). Many adults require a large adult cuff. A regular-size cuff holds a bladder in the width of 12 to 13 cm (4.8 to 5.2 inches) and the length of 22 to 23 cm (8.5 to 9 inches). An improperly fitting cuff produces inaccurate BP readings (Table 9-5).

Delegation Considerations

The skill of blood pressure measurement can be delegated to assistive personnel unless the client is considered unstable. Inform the caregiver if the client's blood pressure has been abnormal and if it is necessary to assess blood pressure more frequently than standard practice. Be sure the caregiver is aware of the usual values for the client, and inform the care provider if the client has alterations affecting the appropriate limb for blood pressure measurement. Also inform the care provider if the client is at risk for orthostatic hypotension and verify how to measure.

Equipment

- Mercury or aneroid sphygmomanometer (NOTE: Be sure aneroid is calibrated to a mercury sphygmomanometer annually.)
- Cloth or disposable vinyl pressure cuff of appropriate size for client's extremity
- Stethoscope
- Alcohol swab
- Pen, pencil, vital sign flow sheet or record form

Step	Rationale
Assessment	
1. Determine need to assess client's BP:	
a. Note risk factors for alteration in BP.	Certain conditions place clients at risk for BP alteration: history of cardiovascular disease, renal disease, diabetes, circulatory shock (hypovolemic, septic, cardiogenic, or neurogenic), acute or chronic pain, rapid IV infusion of fluids or blood products, increased intracranial pressure, postoperative, toxemia of pregnancy.
b. Presence of signs and symptoms of BP alterations: Hypertension is often asymptomatic until pressure is very high. In clients at risk for High Blood Pressure (HBP), assess for headache (usually occipital), flushing of face, nosebleed, and fatigue in older adults. Hypotension is associated with dizziness; mental confusion; restlessness; pale, dusky, or cyanotic skin and mucous membranes; cool, mottled skin over extremities.	Physical signs and symptoms may indicate alterations in BP.
2. Assess for factors that influence BP:	
a. Age	Normal average BP varies throughout life (see Pediatric and Gerontologic Considerations).
b. Gender	During and after menopause women can have higher blood pressures than men of same age.
c. Daily (diurnal) variation	Blood pressure varies throughout day, pressure is lowest in early morning, rises during morning and afternoon, and peaks in late afternoon or evening.
d. Position	Blood pressure can fall as person moves from lying to sitting or standing position; normally, postural variations are minimal.
e. Exercise	Increases in oxygen demand by the body for activity increases BP.
f. Sympathetic stimulation	Pain, anxiety, or fear stimulates the sympathetic nervous system to increase heart rate (HR), CO, and vascular resistance, causing BP to rise.
g. Medications	Antihypertensives, diuretics, beta-adrenergic blockers, vasodilators, calcium channel blockers, angiotensin-coverting enzyme (ACE) inhibitors, and antidysrhythmics lower BP; narcotic analgesics and general anesthetics can also cause hypotension.
h. Smoking	Smoking results in **vasoconstriction,** a narrowing of blood vessels, causing BP to rise.
i. Race	Rate of hypertension is higher in urban African-Americans than in European-Americans. African-Americans tend to develop more severe hypertension at an earlier age and have twice the risk for the complications of hypertension (Brashers, 1998).

STEP	RATIONALE
3. Determine best site for BP assessment. Avoid applying cuff to extremity when intravenous fluids are infusing, an arteriovenous shunt or fistula is present, breast or axillary surgery has been performed on that side, or if extremity has been traumatized, diseased, or requires a cast or bulky bandage. The lower extremities may be used when the brachial arteries are inaccessible.	Inappropriate site selection may result in poor amplification of sounds, causing inaccurate readings. Application of pressure from inflated bladder temporarily impairs blood flow and can further compromise circulation in extremity that already has impaired blood flow.
4. Determine previous baseline BP and site (if available) from client's record.	Allows nurse to assess for change in condition. Provides comparison with future BP measurements.

NURSING DIAGNOSIS

Defining characteristics from the assessment data may reveal the following nursing diagnoses for clients requiring this skill:

- Ineffective cardiopulmonary tissue perfusion
- Decreased cardiac output
- Ineffective peripheral tissue perfusion
- Deficient knowledge regarding medication adherence for BP control
- Deficient fluid volume
- Excess fluid volume

Related factors are individualized based on client's condition or needs.

PLANNING

1. **Expected outcomes** following completion of procedure:	
▪ Blood pressure is within acceptable range for client's age.	Cardiovascular status is stable.
2. Exlain to client that BP is to be assessed. Have client rest at least 5 minutes before measurement (NIH, 1997). Ask client not to speak when BP is being measured.	Reduces anxiety that can falsely elevate readings. Exercise can cause false elevations in BP as well. Talking to a client when the BP is being assessed increases readings 10% to 40% (Thomas and others, 1993).
3. Be sure client has not ingested caffeine or smoked for 30 minutes before assessment of BP (NIH, 1997).	Caffeine or nicotine can raise BP reading.
4. Have client assume sitting or lying position. Be sure room is warm, quiet, and relaxing.	Maintains client's comfort during measurement. The client's perceptions that the physical or interpersonal environment is stressful affect the BP measurement (Thomas & DeKeyser, 1996).
5. Select appropriate cuff size.	Use of improper size cuff can cause false low or false high reading.
6. Wash hands.	Reduces transmission of microorganisms.

IMPLEMENTATION

Assessing Blood Pressure by Auscultation—Upper Extremities

1. With client sitting or lying, position client's forearm, supported if needed at heart level, with palm turned up (see illustration)	If arm is unsupported, client may perform isometric exercise that can increase diastolic pressure 10%. Placement of arm above the level of the heart causes false low reading.
2. Expose upper arm fully by removing constricting clothing.	Ensures proper cuff application.

STEP	RATIONALE

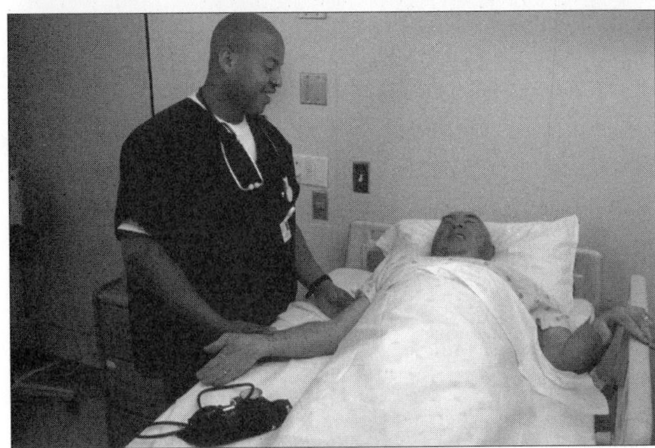

STEP 1 Client's forearm supported on bed.

A

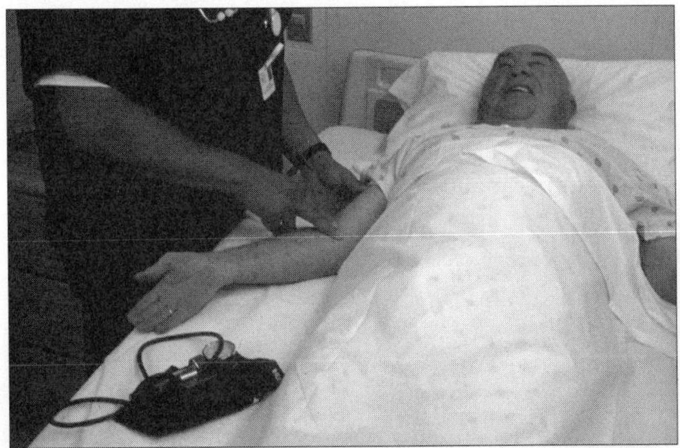

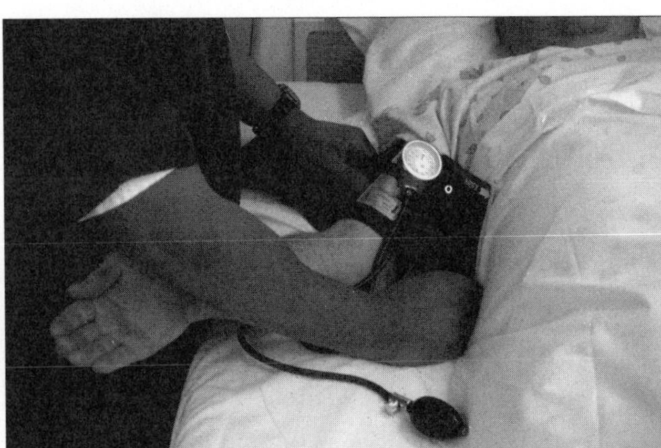

B

C

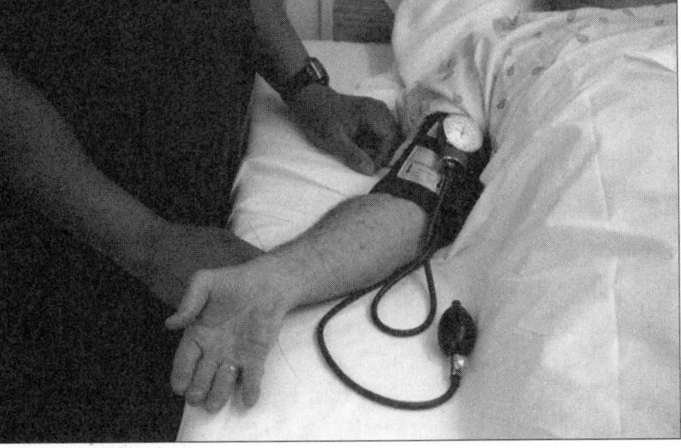

STEP 3 **A,** Nurse palpating client's brachial artery. **B,** Center bladder of cuff above artery. **C,** Blood pressure cuff wrapped around upper arm.

STEP	RATIONALE
3. Palpate brachial artery (see illustration *A*). Position cuff 2.5 cm (1 inch) above site of brachial pulsation (antecubital space). Apply bladder of cuff above artery by centering arrows marked on cuff over artery (see illustration *B*). If there are not any center arrows on cuff, estimate the center of the bladder and place this center over artery. With cuff fully deflated, wrap cuff evenly and snugly around upper arm (see illustration *C*).	Inflating bladder directly over brachial artery ensures proper pressure is applied during inflation. Loose-fitting cuff causes false high readings.

STEP	RATIONALE
4. Position manometer vertically at eye level. Observer should be no farther than 1 m (approximately 1 yard) away.	Accurate readings are obtained by looking at the meniscus of the mercury at eye level. The meniscus is the point where the crescent-shaped top of the mercury column aligns with the manometer scale. Looking up or down at the mercury results in distorted readings.
5. Measure blood pressure.	
a. Two-Step Method:	
(1) Relocate brachial pulse. Palpate artery distal to the cuff with fingertips of nondominant hand while inflating cuff. Note point at which pulse disappears and continue to inflate cuff to a pressure 30 mm Hg above that point. Note the pressure reading. Slowly deflate cuff and note point when pulse reappears. Deflate cuff fully and wait 30 seconds.	Estimating systolic pressure prevents false-low readings, which may result in the presence of an auscultatory gap. Maximal inflation point for accurate reading can be determined by palpation. If unable to palpate artery because of weakened pulse, an ultrasonic stethoscope can be used. Deflating cuff prevents venous congestion and false high readings.
(2) Place stethoscope earpieces in ears and be sure sounds are clear, not muffled.	Each earpiece should follow angle of ear canal to facilitate hearing.
(3) Relocate brachial artery and place diaphragm of stethoscope over it. Do not allow chestpiece to touch cuff or clothing (see illustration).	Proper stethoscope placement ensures optimal sound reception. Stethoscope improperly positioned causes muffled sounds that often result in false low systolic and false high diastolic readings.
(4) Close valve of pressure bulb clockwise until tight.	Tightening of valve prevents air leak during inflation.
(5) Quickly inflate cuff to 30 mm Hg above client's estimated systolic pressure (see illustration).	Inflation ensures accurate measurement of systolic pressure.

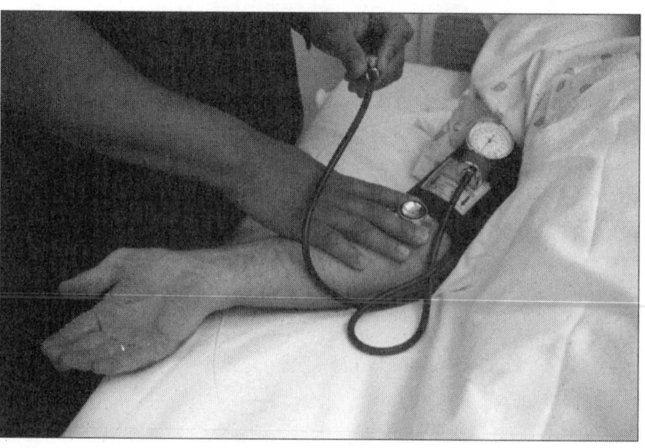

STEP **5a(3)** Stethoscope over brachial artery to measure BP.

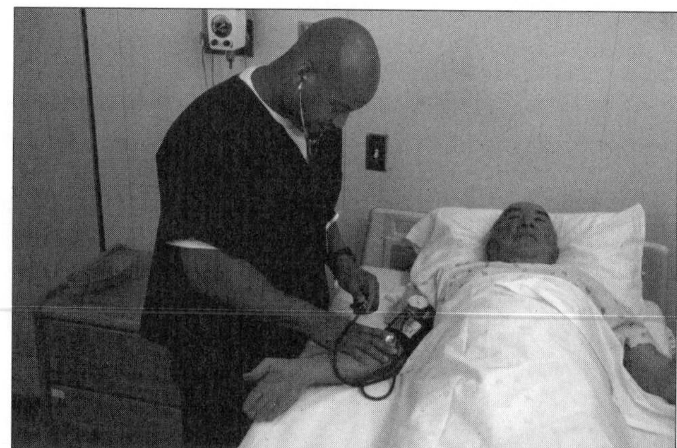

STEP **5a(5)** Inflating BP cuff.

STEP	RATIONALE
(6) Slowly release pressure bulb valve and allow mercury or needle of aneroid to fall at rate of 2 to 3 mm Hg/sec.	Too rapid or slow a decline in mercury level can cause inaccurate readings.
(7) Note point on manometer when first clear sound is heard. The sound will slowly increase in intensity.	First Korotkoff sound indicates systolic pressure.
(8) Continue to deflate cuff gradually, noting point at which sound disappears in adults. Note pressure to nearest 2 mm Hg. Listen for 20 to 30 mm Hg after the last sound and then allow remaining air to escape quickly.	Beginning of the fifth Korotkoff sound is recommended by American Heart Association (1993) as indication of diastolic pressure in adults. Fourth Korotkoff sound involves distinct muffling of sounds and is recommended by the American Heart Association as indication of diastolic pressure in children.
b. One-Step Method:	
(1) Place stethoscope earpieces in ears and be sure sounds are clear, not muffled.	Earpieces should follow angle of ear canal to facilitate hearing.

Step	Rationale
(2) Relocate brachial artery and place diaphragm of stethoscope over it. Do not allow chestpiece to touch cuff or clothing.	Proper stethoscope placement ensures optimal sound reception.
(3) Close valve of pressure bulb clockwise until tight.	Tightening of valve prevents air leak during inflation.
(4) Quickly inflate cuff to 30 mm Hg above client's usual systolic pressure.	Inflation above systolic level ensures accurate measurement of systolic pressure.
(5) Slowly release pressure bulb valve and allow mercury or needle of aneroid manometer to fall at rate of 2 to 3 mm Hg/sec.	Too rapid or slow a decline in mercury level can cause inaccurate readings.
(6) Note point on manometer when first clear sound is heard. The sound will slowly increase in intensity.	Record as systolic pressure.
(7) Continue to deflate cuff gradually, noting point at which sound disappears in adults. Note pressure to nearest 2 mm Hg. Listen for 20 to 30 mm Hg after the last sound and then allow remaining air to escape quickly.	Beginning of the fifth Korotkoff sound is recommended by American Heart Association (1993) as indication of diastolic pressure in adults. Fourth Korotkoff sound involves distinct muffling of sounds and is recommended by the American Heart Association as indication of diastolic pressure in children.
6. It is a good idea to obtain two sets of BP measurements, 2 minutes apart. Use the second set as your baseline.	Helps to prevent false positives based on the client's sympathetic response (alerting reaction). Minimizes effect of anxiety, which often causes a first reading to be higher than subsequent measures (Roper, 1996).
7. Remove cuff from client's arm unless measurement must be repeated.	Continuous cuff inflation causes arterial occlusion, resulting in numbness and tingling of client's arm.
8. If this is first assessment of client, repeat procedure on other arm.	Comparison of BP in both arms detect circulatory problems. (Normal difference of 5 to 10 mm Hg exists between arms.)
9. Assist client in returning to comfortable position and cover upper arm if previously clothed.	Restores comfort and provides sense of well-being.
10. Discuss findings with client as needed.	Promotes participation in care and understanding of health status. Makes client accountable for follow-up assessment.
11. Wash hands.	Reduces transmission of microorganisms.
12. Clean earpieces and diaphragm of stethoscope with alcohol swab as needed (optional).	Controls transmission of microorganisms when nurses share stethoscope.

Assessing Blood Pressure by Auscultation—Lower Extremities

Step	Rationale
1. Assist client to prone position. If unable to assume position, assist client to supine position with knee slightly flexed.	Prone position provides best access to popliteal artery.
2. Move aside bed linen and any constrictive clothing from leg.	Ensures proper cuff application.
3. Locate popliteal artery behind knee.	Artery palpation site lies just below client's thigh, in back of knee in popliteal space.
4. Apply large leg cuff 2.5 cm (1 inch) above artery around posterior aspect of middle thigh. Center arrows marked on cuff over artery (see illustration).	Proper cuff size is necessary for accurate reading. Cuff must be wide and long enough to allow for larger girth of the thigh. Narrow cuff causes false high readings.
5. Position manometer vertically at eye level. Observer should be no farther than 1 m (approximately 1 yard) away.	Accurate readings are obtained by looking at the meniscus of the mercury at eye level. The meniscus is the point where the crescent-shaped top of the mercury column aligns with the manometer scale. Looking up or down at the mercury results in distorted readings.
6. Using popliteal artery, follow Step 5b for auscultation of upper extremity.	
7. If this is first assessment of client, repeat procedure on other leg.	Comparison of BP in both legs detects circulatory problems.
8. Assist client in returning to comfortable position, and cover leg if previously clothed.	Restores comfort and promotes sense of well-being.

STEP	RATIONALE

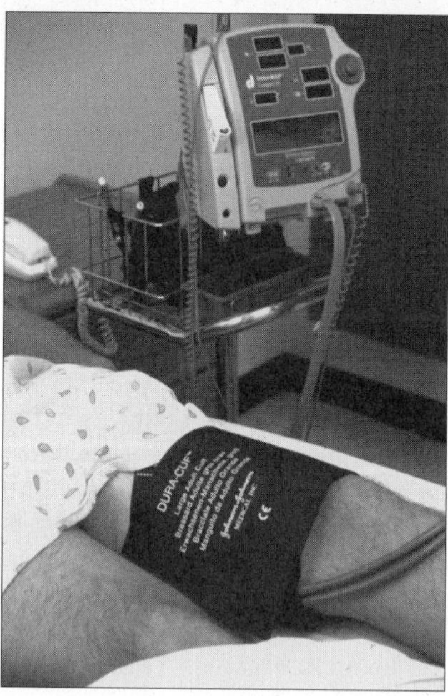

STEP 4 Leg cuff applied around thigh.

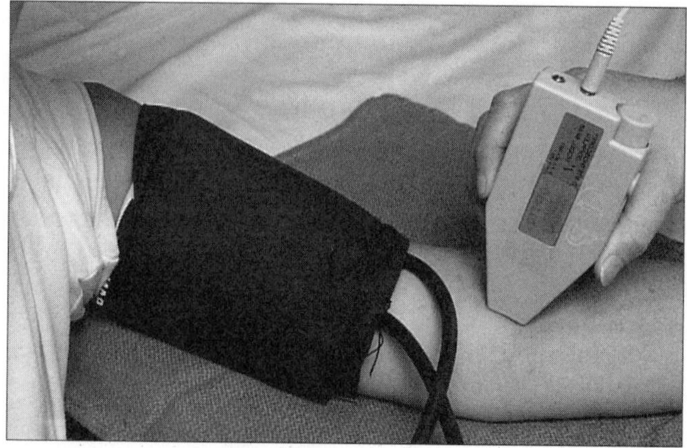

STEP 2 Doppler stethoscope over brachial artery to measure BP.

STEP	RATIONALE
9. Discuss findings with client as needed.	Promotes participation in care and understanding of health status. Makes client accountable for follow-up assessment.
10. Wash hands.	Reduces transmission of microorganisms.
11. Clean earpieces and diaphragm of stethoscope with alcohol swab as needed (optional)	Controls transmission of microorganisms when nurses share stethoscope.

Assessing Blood Pressure by Palpation

STEP	RATIONALE
1. Follow Steps 1 through 4 of auscultation method for upper extremity.	
2. Continually palpate brachial, radial, or popliteal artery with fingertips of one hand. Inflate cuff to a pressure 30 mm Hg above point at which pulse can no longer be palpated.	Ensures accurate detection of true systolic pressure once pressure valve is released.

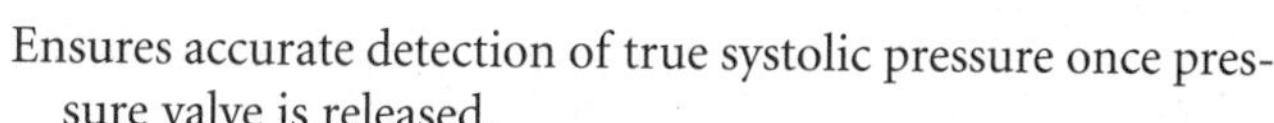

- ***Critical Decision Point***

  If unable to palpate artery because of weakened pulse, a Doppler ultrasonic stethoscope can also be used (see illustration).

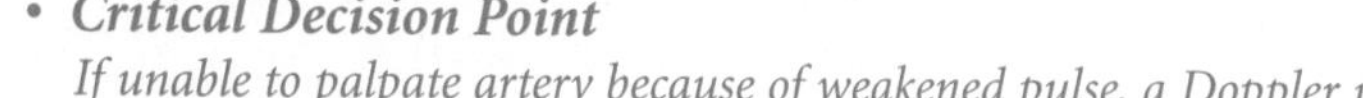

STEP	RATIONALE
3. Slowly release valve and deflate cuff, allowing mercury to fall at rate of 2 mm Hg/sec.	Too rapid or slow a decline in mercury level can result in inaccurate readings.
4. Note point on manometer when pulse is again palpable.	Palpation can identify the systolic pressure only.
5. Deflate cuff rapidly and completely. Remove cuff from client's extremity unless measurement must be repeated.	Continuous cuff inflation causes arterial occlusion, resulting in numbness and tingling of client's arm.
6. Assist client in returning to comfortable position and cover upper arm if previously clothed.	Restores comfort and promotes sense of well-being.
7. Discuss findings with client as needed.	Promotes participation in care and understanding of health status.
8. Wash hands.	Reduces transmission of microorganisms.

EVALUATION

STEP	RATIONALE
1. If BP is assessed for the first time, establish BP as baseline if it is within acceptable range.	Used to compare future BP measurements.
2. Compare BP reading with client's previous baseline and usual BP for client's age.	Allows nurse to assess for change in condition. Provides comparison with future BP measurements.

Unexpected Outcomes and Related Interventions

- Blood pressure is above or below acceptable range for client's age.
  - Repeat measurement or have RN colleague repeat measurement in 1 to 2 minutes.
  - Report abnormal findings to physician.
- Blood pressure is inaudible or difficult to obtain.
  - Repeat measurement in 1 to 2 minutes, using alternative site or using an ultrasound stethoscope.
- A difference of more than 10 mm Hg between BP measurements on upper extremities.
  - Report abnormal finding to physician.
- Client experiences orthostatic hypotension.
  - Return to safe position in bed or chair.
  - Restrict activity that may drop BP further.

Recording and Reporting

- Record BP and site assessed on vital sign flow sheet (see Figure 9-7) or nurses' notes. Also record any signs or symptoms of BP alterations.
- Report abnormal findings to nurse in charge or physician.

Teaching Considerations

- Educate client about risks for hypertension. Persons with family history of hypertension, premature heart disease, lipidemia, or renal disease are at significant risk. Obesity, cigarette smoking, heavy alcohol consumption, high blood cholesterol and triglyceride levels, and continued exposure to stress from psychosocial and environmental conditions are factors linked to hypertension (NIH, 1997).
- Primary prevention of hypertension includes lifestyle modifications (e.g., lose weight, exercise daily, reduce sodium and saturated fat intake, and maintain adequate intake of dietary potassium and calcium). Cigarette smoking is a powerful risk factor, and tobacco should be avoided in any form (NIH, 1997).
- Instruct primary caregiver to take BP at same time each day and after client has had a brief rest. Take BP sitting or lying down; use same position and arm each time pressure is taken.
- Instruct primary caregiver that if the pressure is difficult to hear, it may be that the cuff is too loose, not big enough, or too narrow; the stethoscope is not over arterial pulse, cuff was deflated too quickly or too slowly; or cuff was not pumped high enough for systolic readings.

Pediatric Considerations

- Blood pressure is not a routine part of assessment in children under 3 years.
- Blood pressure measurement can frighten children. Prepare child for squeezing feeling of inflated BP cuff by comparing sensation to elastic band on finger or a tight hug on the arm.
- Obtain BP in child before anxiety-producing tests or procedures are performed. At times it may be unrealistic to wait 5 minutes to assess BP. In emergency situations, do not wait.
- Average width of cuff bladder for infant is 2.4 to 3.2 inches; average length of cuff bladder for child is 4.8 to 5.4 inches.
- When a child reaches adolescence, BP varies by body size. Normal range for 10- to 19-year-olds at the 90th percentile is 124 to 136/77 to 84 for boys and 124 to 127/63 to 74 for girls.

Gerontological Considerations

- Older adults, especially frail older adults, have lost upper arm mass, requiring special attention to selection of BP cuff size.
- Hypertension is extremely common in older adults. An older adult's BP range is usually 140 to 160/80 to 90. Systolic blood pressure is a better predictor of events (coronary heart disease, cardiovascular disease, heart failure, stroke, end-stage renal disease) than is diastolic blood pressure (National High Blood Pressure Education Working Group, 1994).
- Older adults often experience a fall in BP after eating.
- Older adults are instructed to change position slowly and wait after each change to avoid postural hypotension and to prevent injuries.

Home Care Considerations

- Assess home noise level to determine the room that will provide the quietest environment for assessing BP.
- Assess family's financial ability to afford a sphygmomanometer for performing BP evaluations on a regular basis. Validated electronic devices or aneroid sphygmomanometers that have proven to be accurate according to standard testing are recommended, along with appropriate-size cuffs. Finger monitors are inaccurate (NIH, 1997).

Skill 9-6 Measuring Oxygen Saturation (Pulse Oximetry)

Pulse **oximetry** is the noninvasive measurement of arterial blood oxygen saturation—the percent to which hemoglobin is filled with oxygen. A pulse oximeter is a probe with a light-emitting diode (LED) connected by cable to an oximeter. Light waves emitted by the LED are absorbed and then reflected back by oxygenated and deoxygenated hemoglobin molecules. The reflected light is processed by the oximeter, which calculates pulse oxygen saturation (SpO_2). SpO_2 is a reliable estimate of arterial oxygen saturation (SaO_2) (Tittle and Flynn, 1997). For this reason, the use of oximetry can judiciously reduce the need to collect arterial blood gas (ABG) specimens for oxygen saturation analysis. In adults the oximeter probe can be applied to the earlobe, finger, toe, or bridge of the nose, because a highly vascular area is needed to detect the degree of change in the transmitted light (Box 9-5).

The measurement of SpO_2 is simple, painless, and has few of the risks associated with more invasive measurements of SaO_2 such as arterial blood gas sampling. However, the measurement of SpO_2 is affected by factors that affect light transmission, such as outside light sources or client motion. Avoid direct sunlight or fluorescent lighting when using an oximeter. Light reflection from hemoglobin molecules can be influenced by carbon monoxide in the blood, jaundice, and intravascular dyes. Conditions that decrease arterial blood flow such as peripheral vascular disease, hypothermia, pharmacological vasoconstrictors, hypotension, or peripheral edema affect accurate determination of SpO_2.

Because light reflected from hemoglobin molecules is processed to determine SpO_2, any abnormality in the type or amount of hemoglobin affects oxygen saturation and SpO_2 values. The more hemoglobin that is saturated by oxygen, the higher the **oxygen saturation.** Normally SpO_2 is greater than 90%. Pulse oximetry is clinically indicated in clients who have an unstable oxygen status or are at risk for alterations in oxygenation.

Box 9-5 Characteristics of Pulse Oximeter Sensor Probes and Sites

REUSABLE PROBE

Digit Probe

Readings more accurate (Carroll, 1997b, Grap, 1998)
Easy to apply, conforms to various sizes
Yields strong correlation with SaO_2

Earlobe

Clip-on smaller and lighter though more positional than digit probe
Greater accuracy at lower saturations (Tittle and Flynn, 1997)
Good when uncontrollable or rhythmic movements (e.g., hand tremors), exercise are present (Carroll, 1997a)
Least affected by decreased blood flow (Grap, 1998)

DISPOSABLE SENSOR PAD

Can be applied to a variety of sites: earlobe of adult, nose bridge, palm or sole of infant
Less restrictive for continuous SpO_2 monitoring
Expensive
Contains latex
Skin under adhesive may become moist and harbor pathogens
Available in variety of sizes, pad can be matched to infant weight (Hanna, 1995)

DELEGATION CONSIDERATIONS

The skill of oxygen saturation measurement can be delegated to assistive personnel. Inform the care provider of appropriate sensor site for measurement of oxygen saturation, based on client's condition. Also be sure to inform the care provider of the frequency of oxygen saturation measurements, and instruct the care provider to notify the nurse immediately of any reading lower than SpO_2 of 90% or any emergent readings physician prescribes for client. Also caution the care provider to *not* use pulse oximetry as assessment of heart rate since because irregular rhythm may not be detected.

EQUIPMENT

- Oximeter
- Oximeter probe appropriate for client and recommended by manufacturer
- Acetone or nail polish remover
- Pen, pencil, vital sign flow sheet or record form

STEP	RATIONALE

ASSESSMENT

Step	Rationale
1. Determine need to measure client's oxygen saturation:	
a. Note risk factors for alteration of oxygen saturation.	Certain conditions place clients at risk for decreased oxygen saturation: acute or chronic compromised respiratory function, recovery from general anesthesia or conscious sedation, traumatic injury to chest wall with or without collapse of underlying lung tissue, ventilator dependence, changes in O_2 therapy.
b. Assess for signs and symptoms of alterations in oxygen saturation: altered respiratory rate, depth, or rhythm; adventitious breath sounds (Chapter 10); cyanotic appearance of nail beds, lips, mucous membranes, and skin; restlessness, irritability, confusion; reduced level of consciousness; labored or difficulty breathing.	Physical signs and symptoms may indicate abnormal oxygen saturation.
2. Assess for factors that influence measurement of SpO_2 such as oxygen therapy, hemoglobin level, hypotension, and temperature.	Allows nurse to accurately assess oxygen saturation variations. Peripheral vasoconstriction related to hypothermia can interfere with SpO_2 determination.
3. Consult agency's policy or review client's medical record for physician's order for pulse oximetry.	Medical order may be required to assess oxygen saturation with pulse oximetry.
4. Determine previous baseline SpO_2 (if available) from client's record.	Allows nurse to assess for change in condition. Provides comparison with future temperature measurements.
5. Assess site most appropriate for sensor probe placement (e.g., finger, earlobe, bridge of nose). a. Site must have adequate local circulation and be free of moisture. b. Artificial nails and certain nail polish colors will alter readings; place probe on finger free of polish or artificial nail. c. If client has tremors or is likely to move, use ear lobe. d. If client is obese, clip-on probe may not fit properly, obtain a single use (tape-on) probe.	Sensor requires pulsating vascular bed to identify hemoglobin molecules that absorb emitted light. Changes in SpO_2 are reflected in the circulation of finger capillary bed within 30 seconds and the capillary bed of ear lobe within 5 to 10 seconds. Moisture impedes ability of sensor to detect SpO_2 levels. Motion artifact is most common cause of inaccurate readings (Carroll, 1997b).

NURSING DIAGNOSIS

Defining characteristics from the assessment data may reveal the following nursing diagnoses for clients requiring this skill:

- Dysfunctional ventilatory weaning response
- Activity intolerance
- Impaired gas exchange
- Impaired spontaneous ventilation
- Ineffective airway clearance
- Ineffective breathing pattern

Related factors are individualized based on client's condition or needs.

PLANNING

Step	Rationale
1. **Expected outcomes** following completion of procedure:	
▪ Client's SpO_2 remains between 90% and 100%.	Indicates adequate oxygenation.
▪ Client's oxygenation therapies are adjusted without invasive measures.	Oximetry provides accurate SpO_2 measurement.
2. Obtain appropriate equipment and place at bedside.	Mixing probes from different manufacturers can result in burn injury to client. Clip-on ear probes are convenient, quicker to apply, but more susceptible to movement interference.
3. Explain purpose of procedure to client and how oxygen saturation will be measured.	Promotes client cooperation and increases compliance.

Step	Rationale
Implementation	
1. Wash hands.	Reduces transmission of microorganisms.
2. Position client comfortably. If finger is chosen as monitoring site, support lower arm.	Ensures probe positioning and decreases motion interferences with signal.
3. Instruct client to breathe normally.	Prevents large fluctuations in minute ventilation and possible error in SpO_2 readings.
4. If finger is to be used, remove fingernail polish with acetone from digit to be assessed.	Ensures accurate readings. Opaque coatings decrease light transmission; nail polish containing blue pigment can absorb light emissions and falsely alter saturation.
5. Attach sensor probe to monitoring site (see illustration). Instruct client that clip-on probe feels like a clothespin on the finger but will not hurt.	Select sensor site based on peripheral circulation and extremity temperature. Peripheral vasoconstriction can alter SpO_2. Pressure of sensor probe's spring tension on a finger or ear lobe may be uncomfortable.

- ***Critical Decision Point***

  Do not attach probe to finger, ear, or bridge of nose if area is edematous or skin integrity is compromised. Do not attach probe to fingers that are hypothermic. Select ear or bridge of nose if client has a history of peripheral vascular disease. Do not use disposable adhesive probes if client is allergic to latex.

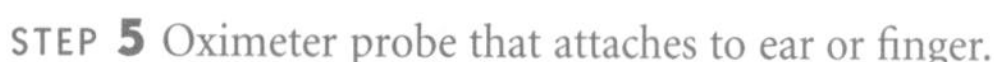

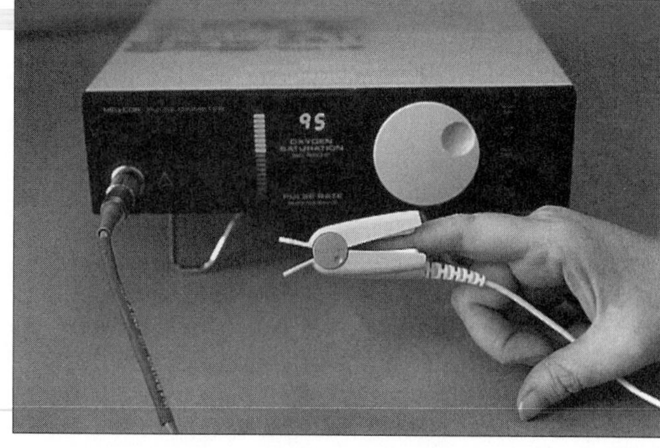

STEP **5** Oximeter probe that attaches to ear or finger.

Step	Rationale
6. Turn on oximeter by activating power. Observe pulse waveform/intensity display and audible beep. Correlate oximeter pulse rate with client's radial pulse.	Pulse waveform/intensity display enables detection of valid pulse or presence of interfering signal. Pitch of audible beep is proportional to SpO_2 value. Double checking pulse rate ensures oximeter accuracy.

- ***Critical Decision Point***

  Oximeter pulse rate, client's radial pulse, and apical pulse should be equivalent. Differences requires reevaluation of oximeter probe placement and may require reassessment of pulse rates.

Step	Rationale
7. Inform client that oximeter will alarm if probe falls off or if client moves probe. Read SpO_2 on digital display.	
8. Leave probe in place until oximeter readout reaches constant value and pulse display reaches full strength during each cardiac cycle. Read SpO_2 on digital display.	Reading may take 10 to 30 seconds depending on site selected.
9. Discuss findings with client as needed.	Promotes participation in care and understanding of health status.
10. If continuous SpO_2 monitoring is planned, verify SpO_2 alarm limits and alarm volume, which are preset by the manufacturer at a low of 85% and a high of 100%. Limits for SpO_2 and pulse rate should be determined as indicated by client's condition. Verify that alarms are on. Assess skin integrity under sensory probe and relocate sensor probe regularly.	Alarms must be set at appropriate limits and volumes to avoid frightening clients and visitors. Spring tension of sensor probe or sensitivity to disposable sensor probe adhesive can cause skin irritation and lead to disruption of skin integrity.

STEP	RATIONALE
11. Remove probe and turn oximeter power off.	Batteries can be depleted if oximeter left on.
12. Assist client in returning to comfortable position.	Restores comfort and promotes sense of well-being.
13. Wash hands.	Reduces transmission of microorganisms.

EVALUATION

1. If oxygen saturation is assessed for the first time, establish SpO_2 as baseline if it is within acceptable range.	Used to compare future assessments of oxygen saturation.
2. Compare SpO_2 with client's previous baseline and acceptable SpO_2. Note use of oxygen therapy.	Allows nurse to assess for change in client's condition and presence of respiratory alteration.
3. For continuous monitoring, assess skin integrity underneath probe routinely, based on client's peripheral circulation.	Prevents tissue ischemia.

UNEXPECTED OUTCOMES AND RELATED INTERVENTIONS

- Client's SaO_2 is less than 95%.
  - Reposition probe and reevaluate. If SaO_2 is unacceptable, notify physician.
  - Position client in high-Fowler's or semi-Fowler's position. Be prepared to initiate or adjust oxygen therapy.
  - Implement measures to reduce energy consumption. An arterial blood gas level may be obtained to validate oximetry reading.
- Pulse waveform/intensity display is weak.
  - Locate different peripheral vascular bed, and reposition pulse oximeter probe.
  - Use another sensor if available.
  - Assess apical and radial pulse to evaluate cardiovascular status.

RECORDING AND REPORTING

- Record SpO_2 on vital sign flow sheet or nurses' notes, indicating type and amount of oxygen therapy used by client during assessment. Assessment of O_2 saturation after administration of specific therapies should be documented in narrative form in nurses' notes. Also record any signs and symptoms of oxygen desaturation in nurses' notes.
- Report abnormal findings to nurse in charge or physician.
- Correlate SpO_2 with SaO_2 obtained from arterial blood gas measurements if available. Documents reliability of noninvasive assessment.
- Record in nurses' notes client's use of continuous or intermittent pulse oximetry. Documents use of equipment for third-party payers.

TEACHING CONSIDERATIONS

- Teach client significance of monitoring oxygen saturation.
- Teach client signs and symptoms of hypoxemia: headache, somnolence, confusion, dusky color, shortness of breath, dyspnea.
- Teach client effect of high-risk behaviors, such as cigarette smoking, on oxygen saturation.

PEDIATRIC CONSIDERATIONS

- Infant and toddler sensors attached to adhesive sensor pads are available and conform to fingers, palm of hand, and sole of foot.
- Ear lobe and bridge-of-nose sensors are not used for infants and toddlers.

GERONTOLOGICAL CONSIDERATIONS

- Identifying an acceptable pulse oximeter probe site may be difficult on older adults because of likelihood of peripheral vascular disease, decreased carbon dioxide level, cold-induced vasoconstriction, and anemia.

HOME CARE CONSIDERATIONS

- Pulse oximetry is used in home care to noninvasively monitor oxygen therapy or changes in oxygen therapy.

Critical Thinking Exercises

1. A nurse assistant has obtained a blood pressure reading for one of your assigned clients. He tells you that the client's blood pressure is 140/90. The last BP reading for the client was 120/70. What should you do?
2. Mrs. Lee is an 80-year-old client who has a history of a cerebrovascular accident (stroke). She has drooping on the right side of her mouth. When you attempt to place an oral thermometer in her mouth she is unable to keep it positioned in the sublingual pocket. What should you do?
3. Mr. Becker is experiencing acute pain after returning from a surgical procedure to correct a fracture in his right leg. When you enter his room, he is restless, complaining of pain in his leg, and he is diaphoretic. What effects do you anticipate pain will have on his vital signs?

References

American Heart Association: *Recommendations for human blood pressure determination by sphygmomanometers.* Dallas, 1993, The Association.

Beaudry M, VandenBosch T, Anderson J: Research utilization: Once-a-day temperatures for afebrile patients, *Clin Nurse Spec* 10(1):21, 1996.

Bliss-Holtz J: Methods of newborn infant temperature monitoring: a research review, *Issues Comp Pediatr Nurs* 18:287, 1995.

Braun SK and others: Getting a better read on thermometry, *RN* 61(3):57, 1998.

Brashers *Clinical application of pathophysiology,* St. Louis, 1998, Mosby.

Carroll P: Using pulse oximetry in the home, *Home Healthcare Nurse* 15(2):89, 1997a.

Carroll P: Pulse oximetry at your fingertips, *RN* vol. 60(2):22, 1997b.

Cusson P, Madonia JA, Taekman JB: The effect of environment on body site temperatures in full term neonates, *Nurs Res* 46(4):202, 1997.

Embrey JP and others: Stethoscope hygiene: a potential vector of nosocomial infections, *J Am Assoc Nurse Anesth* 66(5):491, 1998.

Erickson RS and others: Accuracy of chemical dot thermometers in critically ill adults and young children, *Image J Nurs Sch* 28:23, 1996.

Grap MJ: Pulse oximetry, *Critic Care Nurse* 18(1):94, 1998.

Haddock BJ and others: The falling grace of axillary temperatures, *Pediatr Nurs* 22(2):121, 1996.

Hanna D: Equipment guidelines for pulse oximetry use in pediatrics. *J Pediatric Nurse* 10(2):124, 1995.

Hasel KL, Erickson RS: Effect of cerumen on infrared ear temperature measurement, *J Gerontol Nurs* 21(2):6, 1995.

Holtzclaw BJ: New trends in thermometry for the patient in ICU, *Crit Care Nurs Q* 21(4):12, 1998.

Irvin SM: Comparison of the oral thermometer versus the tympanic thermometer, *Clin Nurs Spec* 13(2):85, 1999.

Leicke-Rude M, Bloom LF: A comparison of temperature taking methods in neonates, *Neonatal Net* 17(5):21, 1998.

Lueckenotte AG: *Gerontologic nursing,* ed 2, St. Louis, 2000, Mosby.

National High Blood Pressure Education Program Working Group: National High Blood Pressure Education Program Working Group report on hypertension in the elderly, *Hypertension* 23:275, 1994.

National Institutes of Health, National High Blood Pressure Education Program; National Heart, Lung and Blood Institute: *The sixth report of the Joint National Committee on Prevention, Detection, Evaluation and Treatment of High Blood Pressure,* NIH Pub No 98-4080, Bethesda, Md., 1997, NIH.

PyMaH Corporation. Tempa-DOT single-use clinical thermometer: technical Information, Flemington, NJ, 1994.

Roper M: Back to basics: assessing orthostatic vital signs, *Am J Nurs* 98(8):43, 1996.

Smith J: Are electronic thermometry techniques suitable alternatives to traditional mercury in glass thermometry techniques in the paediatric setting? *J Adv Nurs* 29(5):1030, 1998.

Thibodeau GA, Patton KT: *Anatomy and physiology,* ed 3, St. Louis, 1996, Mosby.

Thomas SA and others: Nursing blood pressure research, 1980-1990: a bio-psycho-social perspective, *Image J Nurs Sch* 25(2):157, 1993.

Thomas SA, DeKeyser R: Blood pressure. *Annual Review of Nursing Research,* 14:3, 1996.

Tittle M, Flynn MB: Correlation of pulse oximetry and co-oximetry. *Dimensions in Critical Care Nursing* 16(2):88, 1997.

10

SHIFT ASSESSMENT

Skills

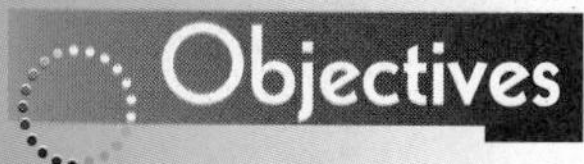

Objectives

Mastery of content in this chapter will enable the nurse to:

- Define the key terms listed.
- Discuss purposes of shift assessment.
- Describe the techniques used with each assessment skill.
- Describe proper positioning for the client during each phase of the examination.
- Discuss the importance of understanding cultural diversity when assessing clients.
- List techniques to promote the client's physical and psychological comfort during an examination.
- Make environmental preparations before an assessment.
- Identify information to collect from the nursing history before a physical assessment.
- Discuss normal physical findings for clients across the life span.
- Discuss ways to incorporate health promotion and health teaching into an assessment.
- Identify self-screening assessments commonly performed by clients.
- Successfully complete a shift assessment.
- Document assessment findings on appropriate forms.

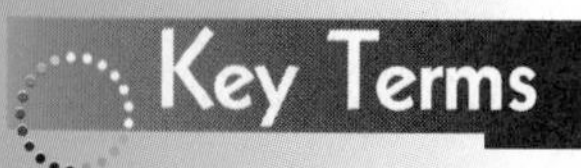

Key Terms

Atrophy
Auscultation
Bruit
Cardiomegaly
Cerumen
Conjunctiva
Costovertebral angle (CVA) tenderness
Crackles
Cyanosis
Dorsum
Edema
Erythema
Friction rub
Inspection
Integument
Intercostal spaces
Mucopurulent
Nares
Olfaction
Orthostatic hypotension
Pallor
Palpation
Percussion

Periodic systematic assessments are done on a regular basis in nearly every health care setting, that is, hospitals, home health, and nursing homes. In acute care settings a brief assessment is done at the beginning of each shift to identify changes in the client's status compared with the previous assessment. This routine assessment takes 10 to 15 minutes and reveals information that supplements the database for the client. In nursing homes and home health similar assessments are done weekly or monthly and more frequently when a change in health status occurs.

A more comprehensive assessment is done on admission to a health care agency. This assessment involves a detailed review of a client's condition, with the nurse collecting a nursing history and performing a behavioral and physical examination. The health history involves an interview with a client to gather subjective data about any presenting conditions. A physical assessment is a head-to-toe review of each body system that offers objective information about the client. The client's condition and response affect the extent of the examination. Once data are gathered, the nurse groups significant findings into patterns of data that reveal actual or potential nursing diagnoses (Table 10-1). Each abnormal finding directs the nurse to gather additional data. Information gathered during an initial assessment and examination provides the baseline for a client's functional abilities and serves as a comparison for future assessment findings. In addition, the information helps the nurse select the best nursing measures to manage the client's health problems.

Nurses are often the first to detect changes in clients' conditions, regardless of the setting. For this reason the ability to think critically and interpret client behaviors and physiological changes is essential. The skills of physical assessment are powerful tools with which to detect subtle as well as obvious changes in a client's health.

Assessment Techniques

Inspection, palpation, percussion, auscultation, and olfaction are assessment techniques that enable the nurse to collect a broad range of physical data about clients. **Inspection** is the process of visual examination of body parts. An experienced nurse learns to make many observations, almost simultaneously, while becoming very perceptive of abnormalities. The secret is to always pay attention to the client. Watch all movements and look carefully at any body part being inspected. It is important to recognize normal physical characteristics of clients of all ages before trying to distinguish abnormal findings.

Experience is needed to recognize normal variations among clients, as well as ranges of normal for individual clients. Cultural diversity is also recognized as one of the factors that influences both normal variations and potential alterations. It is extremely important for the nurse to methodically take the time necessary to carefully assess each body part. If the nurse becomes hurried, significant signs may be overlooked and incorrect conclusions may be made about a client's condition.

Table 10-1 Development of Individualized Nursing Diagnoses

Assessment Method	Findings	Patterns	Nursing Diagnosis
Inspection of skin	Skin along sacral area is intact. There is 3-cm area of redness around coccyx; skin blanches on palpation. No skin lesions are observed.	There is pressure area around coccyx.	Risk for impaired skin integrity
Palpation of skin	Skin is moist from diaphoresis. There is tenderness to palpation around sacral area. There is good skin turgor.	Skin moisture promotes maceration.	
Historical data	Client suffered fractured left leg. Client is immobilized due to left leg traction.	Continued pressure is exerted over sacrum.	

Inspection requires good lighting and full exposure of body parts. Each area is inspected for size, shape, color, symmetry, position, and the presence of abnormalities. If possible, each area inspected is compared with the same area on the opposite side of the body. When necessary, use additional light, such as a penlight, to inspect body cavities such as the mouth and throat. *Do not hurry. Pay attention to detail.* Verify and clarify all abnormalities with subjective client data. In other words, ask the client for further information about each abnormality or change.

Palpation involves use of the sense of touch. Through palpation the hands can make delicate and sensitive measurements of specific physical signs, including resistance, resilience, roughness, texture, temperature, and mobility. Palpation is often used with or after visual inspection. The nurse uses different parts of the hand to detect specific characteristics. For example, the **dorsum** (back) of the hand is sensitive to temperature variations. The pads of the fingertips detect subtle changes in texture, shape, size, consistency, and pulsation of body parts. The palm of the hand is especially sensitive to vibration. The nurse measures position, consistency, and turgor by lightly grasping the body part with the fingertips.

Assist the client to be relaxed and positioned comfortably because muscle tension during palpation impairs the nurse's ability to palpate correctly. Asking the client to take slow, deep breaths enhances muscle relaxation. Tender areas are palpated last. The nurse asks the client to point out areas that are more sensitive and notes any nonverbal signs of discomfort. Clients appreciate warm hands, short fingernails, and a gentle approach. Palpation may be either light or deep and is controlled by the amount of pressure applied with the fingers or hand. Light palpation precedes deep palpation. The nurse must consider the client's condition, the area being palpated, and the reason for using palpation. For example, when a client is admitted to the emergency department following an automobile accident the nurse should consider the factors surrounding the client's injury and inspect the chest wall carefully before performing any palpation around the area of the ribs.

To palpate, the nurse applies pressure slowly, gently, and deliberately, depressing about 1 cm (½ inch). Tender areas are examined further using light intermittent pressure. After light palpation, deeper palpation may be used to examine the condition of organs. The nurse depresses the area being examined approximately 2 cm (1 inch). Caution is the rule. Bimanual palpation involves one hand placed over the other while pressure is applied. The upper hand exerts downward pressure as the other hand feels the subtle characteristics of underlying organs and masses. A student nurse seeks the assistance of a qualified instructor before attempting deep palpation.

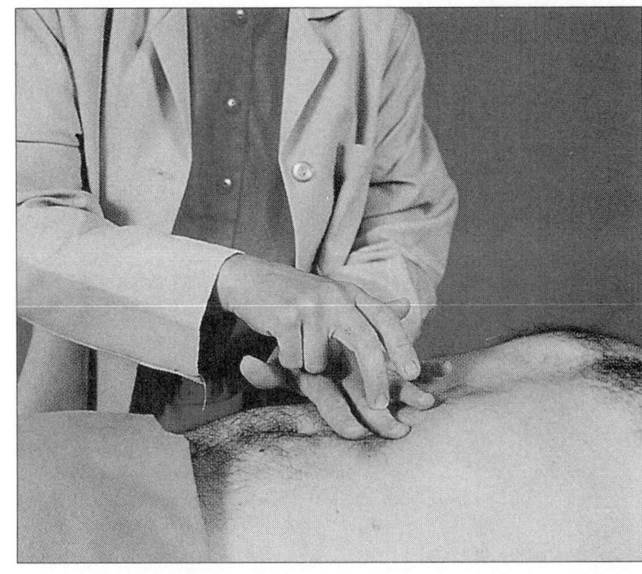

FIGURE **10-1** Indirect percussion of the abdomen. (From Barkauskas VH and others: *Health and physical assessment,* ed 2, St. Louis, 1998, Mosby.)

Percussion involves tapping the body with the fingertips to evaluate the size, borders, and consistency of body organs and to discover fluid in body cavities (Figure 10-1). It requires practice and skill. Percussion helps identify the location, size, and density of underlying structures. The nurse strikes the body's surface with a finger to create a vibration, and sound waves are heard as percussion tones arising from vibrations in body tissues (Seidel and others, 1999). The character of sound depends on the density of underlying tissues. For example, the

Table 10-2 Sounds Produced by Percussion

Sound	Intensity	Pitch	Duration	Quality	Common Location
Tympany	Loud	High	Moderate	Drumlike	Enclosed, air-containing space; gastric air bubble, puffed-out cheek
Resonance	Moderate to loud	Low	Long	Hollow	Normal lung
Hyperresonance	Very loud	Very low	Longer than resonance	Booming	Emphysematous lung
Dullness	Soft to moderate	High	Moderate	Thudlike	Liver, spleen, gallbladder
Flatness	Soft	High	Short	Flat	Muscle

Box 10-1 Learning to Use a Stethoscope

1. Place earpieces in both ears with tips of earpieces turned toward the face. *Lightly* blow into the stethoscope's diaphragm. Again place earpieces in both ears, this time with ends turned toward the back of the head. *Lightly* blow into the stethoscope's diaphragm. The earpiece should follow the contour of the ear canal. After learning the right fit for the loudest sound, wear the stethoscope the same way each time.
2. Put the stethoscope on and *lightly* blow into the diaphragm. If sound is barely audible, *lightly* blow into the bell. Sound is carried through only one part of the chestpiece at a time. If sound is greatly amplified through the diaphragm, the diaphragm is in position for use. If sound is barely audible through the diaphragm, the bell is in position for use.
3. Listen while moving the diaphragm lightly over the hair on your arm. The bristling sound created by rubbing of hair against the diaphragm mimics a sound heard in the lungs. Also, always be sure to keep the diaphragm stationary and firm to reduce extraneous sounds.
4. Place the stethoscope on and gently tap tubing. The sound can distract from being able to hear sounds created by body organs. Always avoid stretching or moving the tubing; it should hang freely.

normal lung transmits sounds with high intensity and low pitch, whereas the solid liver transmits a high-pitched sound of soft intensity.

There are two methods of percussion: direct and indirect. The direct method involves striking the body surface directly with one or two fingers. The indirect technique is performed by placing the middle finger of the examiner's nondominant hand firmly against the body surface. With palm and fingers remaining off the skin, the tip of the middle finger of the dominant hand strikes the base of the distal joint of the finger. The examiner uses a quick, sharp stroke, keeping the forearm stationary. The wrist remains relaxed to deliver the proper blow. Once the finger has struck, the wrist snaps back. If the blow is not sharp, if the hand is held loosely, or if the palm rests on the body surface, the sound is softened and the nurse cannot detect the presence of underlying structures. A light, quick blow produces the clearest sounds. Table 10-2 describes the five different percussion sounds.

Auscultation is listening to sounds produced by the body with a stethoscope. To auscultate correctly, listen in a quiet environment both for the presence of sound and its characteristics. The nurse is more successful in auscultation after knowing normal sounds from each body structure, including the passage of blood through an artery, heart sounds, and movement of air through the lungs. These sounds vary according to the location in which they can most easily be heard. Likewise, the nurse becomes familiar with areas that normally do not emit sounds. It is important for a student to listen to many normal sounds in order to recognize abnormal sounds when they arise.

To auscultate, the nurse needs good hearing acuity, a good stethoscope, and knowledge of how to use the stethoscope properly (Box 10-1). Nurses with hearing disorders may purchase stethoscopes with greater sound amplification and may need to ask colleagues to verify some findings through auscultation. It is more effective to place the stethoscope directly on client's naked skin because clothing obscures and changes sound.

Through auscultation the nurse notes the following characteristics of sound:

Frequency—Number of sound wave cycles generated per second by a vibrating object. The higher the frequency, the higher the pitch of a sound and vice versa.

Loudness—Amplitude of a sound wave. Auscultated sounds are described as loud or soft.

Quality—Sounds of similar frequency and loudness from different sources. Terms such as blowing or gurgling describe quality of sound.

Duration—Length of time that sound vibrations last. Duration of sound is short, medium, or long. Layers of soft tissue dampen the duration of sounds from deep internal organs.

A nurse cannot be successful at auscultation without knowing how to use a stethoscope properly. Chapter 9 describes the parts of the acoustic stethoscope and use of the bell and diaphragm.

Olfaction is using the sense of smell to detect abnormalities that go unrecognized by any other means. Some alterations in body function and certain bacteria create characteristic odors (Table 10-3).

Table 10-3 Assessment of Characteristic Odors

ODOR	SITE OR SOURCE	POTENTIAL CAUSES
Alcohol	Oral cavity	Ingestion of alcohol; diabetes
Ammonia	Urine	Urinary tract infection
Body odor	Skin, particularly in areas where body parts rub together (e.g., under arms, breasts, perineal area)	Poor hygiene, excess perspiration (hyperhidrosis), foul-smelling perspiration (bromhidrosis)
Feces	Wound site	Wound abscess
	Vomitus	Bowel obstruction
	Rectal area	Fecal incontinence
Foul-smelling stools in infant	Stool	Malabsorption syndrome
Halitosis	Oral cavity	Poor dental and oral hygiene, gum disease
Sweet, fruity ketones	Oral cavity	Diabetic acidosis
Stale urine	Skin	Uremic acidosis
Sweet, heavy, thick odor	Draining wound	*Pseudomonas* (bacterial) infection
Musty odor	Casted body part	Infection inside cast
Fetid, sweet odor	Tracheostomy or mucous secretions	Infection of bronchial tree (*Pseudomonas* bacteria)

Preparation for Assessment

The shift assessment begins the moment you see the client and continues each time you encounter the client. It is important to have as much awareness as possible of the client's health history and the reason for care. Also be alert for any changes or problems that may have developed since the last assessment.

Preparation of the environment, equipment, and client promotes a smooth assessment. To promote client comfort and efficiency it is essential to provide privacy for the client (e.g., a separate room; curtains or dividers to enclose the client's bed; or in the home, a bedroom can be used); a warm, comfortable temperature; a loose-fitting gown or pajamas for the client; adequate direct lighting; control of outside noises; and precautions to prevent interruptions by visitors or other health care personnel. The bed should be at the nurse's waist level if possible.

Preparing the Client

To facilitate an accurate assessment, prepare the client both physically and psychologically. A tense, anxious client may have difficulty understanding or following directions or cooperating with the nurse's instructions. To prepare the client the nurse needs to:

1. Provide for the client's physical comfort by allowing the opportunity to empty the bowel or bladder (a good time to collect needed specimens).
2. Provide privacy.
3. Minimize client's anxiety and fear by conveying an open, receptive, and professional approach. The nurse thoroughly explains what will be done, what the client should expect to feel, and how the client can cooperate, using simple terms.
4. Provide access to body parts while draping areas that need not be exposed.
5. Eliminate drafts, control room temperature, and provide warm blankets.
6. Help the client assume positions during the assessment (Table 10-4) so that body parts are accessible and the client stays comfortable. A client's ability to assume positions will depend on physical strength and limitations. Some positions are uncomfortable or embarrassing; keep a client in position no longer than is necessary.
7. Pace assessment according to the client's physical and emotional tolerance.
8. Use relaxed voice tone and facial expressions to put client at ease.
9. Encourage the client to ask questions and report discomfort felt during the examination.
10. Have a family member or a third person of the client's gender in the room during assessment of genitalia. This prevents the client from accusing the nurse of behaving in an unethical manner.

Physical Assessment of Various Age-Groups

Children and Adolescents

1. Routine examinations of children have a focus on health promotion and illness prevention, particularly for care of well children with competent parenting and no serious health problems (Wong and others, 1999). The focus is on growth and development, sensory screening, dental examination, and behavioral assessment.
2. Children who are chronically ill, disabled, in foster care, or foreign-born adopted may require additional assessment.
3. When obtaining histories of infants and children, gather all or part of the information from parents or guardians.
4. Parents may think they are being tested or judged by the examiner. Offer support during examination, and do not pass judgment.
5. Call children by their preferred name, and address parents as "Mr. and Mrs. Brown" rather than by first names.

Table 10-4 Positions for Physical Assessment

POSITION	AREAS ASSESSED	RATIONALE	LIMITATIONS
Sitting 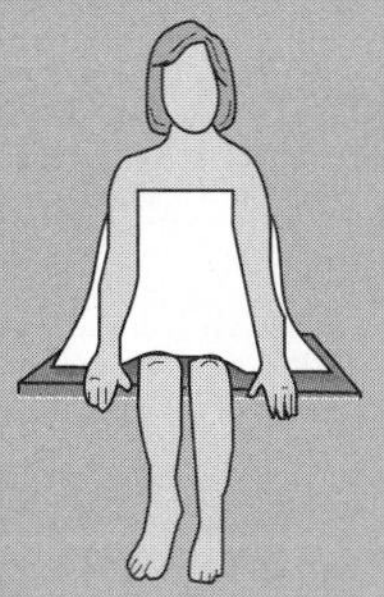	Head and neck, back, posterior thorax and lungs, anterior thorax and lungs, breasts, axillae, heart, vital signs, and upper extremities	Sitting upright provides full expansion of lungs and provides better visualization of symmetry of upper body parts.	Physically weakened client may be unable to sit. Examiner should use supine position with head of bed elevated instead.
Supine 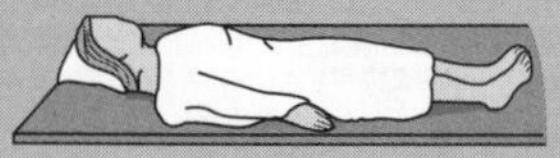	Head and neck, anterior thorax and lungs, breasts, axillae, heart, abdomen, extremities, pulses	This is most normally relaxed position. It provides easy access to pulse sites.	If client becomes short of breath easily, examiner may need to raise head of bed.
Dorsal recumbent 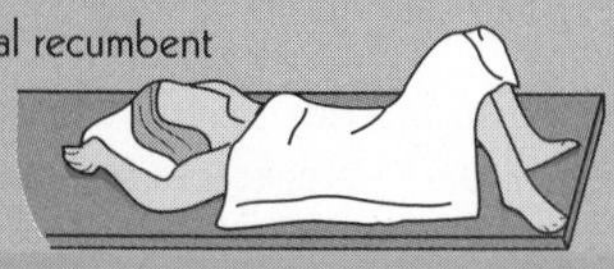	Head and neck, anterior thorax and lungs, breasts, axillae, heart, abdomen	Position is used for abdominal assessment because it promotes relaxation of abdominal muscles.	Clients with painful disorders are more comfortable with knees flexed.
Lithotomy* 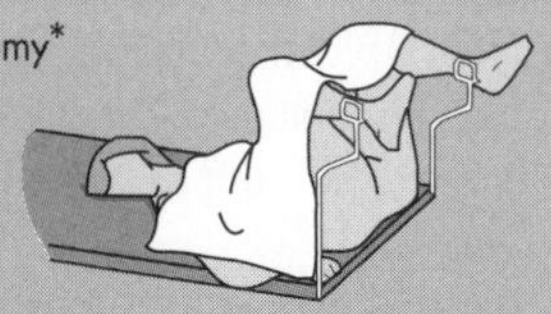	Female genitalia and genital tract	This position provides maximal exposure of genitalia and facilitates insertion of vaginal speculum.	Lithotomy position is embarrassing and uncomfortable, so examiner minimizes time that client spends in it. Client is kept well draped.
Sims' 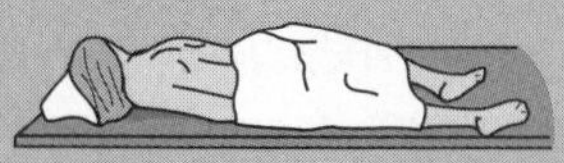	Rectum and vagina	Flexion of hip and knee improves exposure of rectal area.	Joint deformities may hinder client's ability to bend hip and knee.
Prone 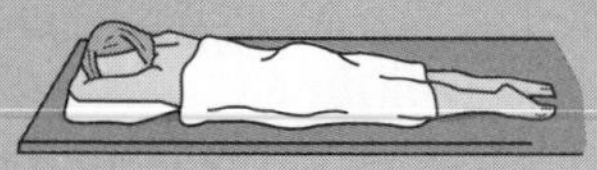	Musculoskeletal system	This position is used only to assess extension of hip joint.	This position is poorly tolerated in clients with respiratory difficulties.
Lateral recumbent 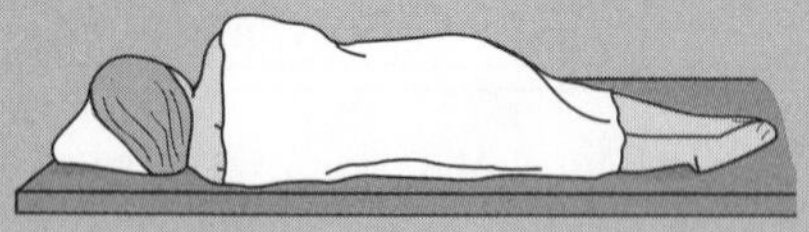	Heart	This position aids in detecting murmurs.	This position is poorly tolerated in clients with respiratory difficulties.
Knee-chest* 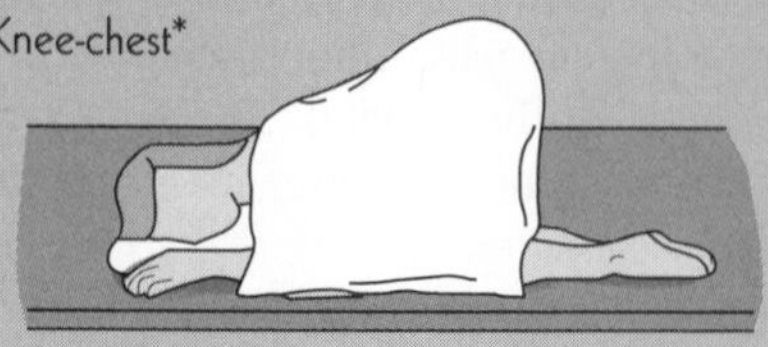	Rectum	This position provides maximal exposure of rectal area.	This position is embarrassing and uncomfortable.

*Clients with arthritis or other joint deformities may be unable to assume this position.

6. Open-ended questions often allow parents to share more information and to describe more of the child's problems.
7. Older children and adolescents tend to respond best when treated as adults and individuals and often can provide details about their health history and severity of symptoms.
8. The adolescent has a right to confidentiality. After talking with parents about historical information, the nurse arranges to be alone with the adolescent to speak further privately and to perform the examination.

Older Adults

1. Do not assume that aging is always accompanied by illness or disability. Most older adults are able to adapt to change and maintain functional independence (Lueckenotte, 2000).
2. Allow extra time and be patient, relaxed, and unhurried with older adults.
3. Provide adequate space for an examination, particularly if the client uses a mobility aid.
4. Plan the history and examination; taking into account the older adult's energy level, physical limitations, pace, and adaptability. More than one session may be needed to complete the assessment (Lueckenotte, 2000).
5. Measure performance under the most favorable conditions. Take advantage of natural opportunities for assessment (e.g., during bathing, grooming, mealtime) (Lueckenotte, 2000).
6. Sequence an examination to keep position changes to a minimum. Be efficient throughout the examination to limit client movement.
7. Be sure an examination of an older adult includes review of mental status.

Box 10-2 Cultural Awareness of Touch During Physical Examination

Physical contact with a client can convey a variety of meanings, depending on the client's cultural background. Consider these guidelines, but remember that each client is an individual and may respond differently.

Hispanics
- Highly tactile
- Very modest (men and women)
- May ask for health care provider of same gender
- Women may refuse to be examined by male health care provider

Asians/Pacific Islanders
- Avoid touching (patting head is strictly taboo)
- Touching during an argument equals loss of control (shame)
- Public display of affection toward members of same gender is permissible (but not toward members of opposite gender)

African-Americans
- May not like to be touched without permission
- May exercise level of distrust or caution initially in care provider

Native Americans
- Shake hands lightly
- May not like to be touched without permission
- Nonverbal communication is important

Data from Lueckenotte A: *Gerontologic nursing*, ed 2, St. Louis, 2000, Mosby, Seidel HM and others: *Mosby's guide to physical examination*, ed 4, St. Louis, 1999, Mosby.

Skill Performance Guidelines

1. Set priorities for assessment based on a client's presenting signs and symptoms or health care needs. For example, a client who develops sudden shortness of breath should first undergo an assessment of the lungs and thorax. If a client is acutely ill, the nurse may choose to assess only the involved body systems. The nurse's judgment is needed to ensure that an examination is relevant and inclusive.
2. Organize the examination. Compare both sides of the body for symmetry. If a client becomes fatigued, offer rest periods. Perform painful procedures near the end of the examination.
3. Use a head-to-toe approach. Follow the sequence of inspection, palpation, percussion, and auscultation (except for abdominal assessment). This sequence facilitates an effective assessment.
4. Encourage the client to be an active participant. Clients are usually knowledgeable about their physical condition. Often the client can let the nurse know when certain findings are normal or when actual changes have occurred.
5. Respect the client's race, gender, age, and cultural beliefs. These important variables often influence assessment findings and approaches to use. A client's health beliefs, use of alternative therapies, nutritional habits, relationships with family, and comfort with close physical contact during an assessment must be considered (Box 10-2).
6. Follow standard precautions for infection control. Assessments may require the nurse to have contact with body fluids and discharge. When there are breaks in the skin, lesions, or wounds, gloves must be worn. In some circumstances the nurse must wear a gown.
7. Consider the possibility of latex allergy. The incidence of serious allergic reaction to latex has increased dramatically (Seidel and others, 1999).
8. Record quick notes to facilitate accurate documentation.
9. Continue to use assessment skills during each contact, including activities such as bathing, administration of medications, or other therapies or while conversing with a client.
10. Integrate health promotion and education into physical assessment activities. There are "teachable moments" when the nurse can share findings and educate clients about health promotion.
11. Record summary of the assessment using appropriate medical terminology and in the sequence that findings are gathered. Use commonly accepted medical abbreviations to keep notes concise.

Skill 10-1 General Survey

The general survey begins a review of the client's primary health problems, and it includes assessment of the client's vital signs, height and weight, general behavior, and appearance. The survey provides information about characteristics of an illness, a client's hygiene, skin and body image, emotional state, recent changes in weight, and developmental status. The survey can reveal important information about the client's behavior that can influence how the nurse communicates instructions to the client and continues the assessment.

Delegation Considerations

The general survey should not be delegated to assistive personnel. However, the following activities may be delegated: measuring height and weight, oral intake, urinary output, and vital signs and reporting a client's subjective signs and symptoms. All monitoring data must be reported.

Stethoscope
Sphygmomanometer and cuff
Thermometer
Digital watch or wristwatch with second hand
Tape measure
Clean nonlatex gloves

Step	Rationale
Assessment	
1. Note if client has had any acute distress: difficulty breathing, pain, anxiety. If such signs are present, defer general survey until later.	Signs establish priorities regarding what part of the examination to conduct first.

• ***Critical Decision Point***
Findings may change the direction of the examination. Any client in acute distress will require an immediate assessment of the body system(s) affected.

Step	Rationale
2. Review graphic sheet for temperature, pulse, respirations, and blood pressure and consider factors or conditions that may alter reading of vital signs (see Chapter 9).	Provides baseline and historical data regarding client's vital signs.
3. Determine client's primary language. If need for an interpreter is identified, determine availability of family members.	Facilitates the presence of interpreters if needed. If possible, have interpreters of the same gender and one who is older. Have the interpreter translate verbatim if possible.
4. Reconfirm (after reviewing history) primary reason client has sought health care.	Keeps assessment focused on client to ensure that client's expectations are addressed.
5. Identify client's normal height and weight. If a sudden gain or loss in weight has occurred, determine amount of weight change and period of time in which it occurred. Assess if client has recently been dieting or following exercise program.	Generally, weight of 15% to 20% above standard indicates excess body fat; however, fluid retention is one factor that must be ruled out. A person's weight can fluctuate daily because of fluid loss or retention (1 L of water weighs 1 kg, or 2.2 pounds).
6. Review client's past fluid intake and output (I&O) records.	Fluid and electrolyte balance maintains health and function in all body systems. Intake includes all liquids taken orally, by feeding tube, and parenterally. Liquid output includes urine, diarrhea stool, fistulas, vomitus, drainage from gastric suction, and drainage from postsurgical tubes, such as chest tubes or Jackson-Pratt drains.
7. Identify client's general perceptions about personal health.	Assessment of client's general appearance coupled with client's own perceptions may reveal specific problem areas.
8. Assess for evidence of latex allergy, which may include contact dermatitis or systemic reactions.	Gloves will be worn during certain aspects of the assessment. Repeated exposure may result in more serious reactions, including asthma, itching, and anaphylaxis (Seidel and others, 1999).

STEP / **RATIONALE**

PLANNING

1. **Expected outcomes** following completion of procedure:
   - Client demonstrates alert, cooperative behaviors without evidence of physical or emotional distress during assessment.

     Nurse uses calm and confident approach during assessment. Client has no abnormal findings.
   - Client provides appropriate subjective data related to physical condition.

     Client able to cooperate with assessment.
2. Prepare client: Tell the client you will be doing a routine process to check for areas of concern. Ask client to tell you if any area you examine hurts when touched.

   Understanding promotes client's cooperation. Pain is an important finding during assessment.

IMPLEMENTATION

1. Throughout assessment note client's verbal and nonverbal behaviors. Determine the level of consciousness and orientation by observing and talking to client (Box 10-3).

   Behaviors may reflect specific physical abnormalities. Dementia and level of consciousness influences ability to cooperate. Timing of recent medications, especially pain medication and sedatives, may alter assessment data.
2. Obtain temperature, pulse, respirations, and blood pressure unless taken within last 3 hours or a serious potential change is noted (e.g., change in level of consciousness or difficulty breathing) (see Chapter 9). Inform client of vital signs.

   Vital signs provide important information regarding physiological changes in relation to oxygenation and circulation (Elkin, Perry, and Potter, 2000).
3. Observe the following aspects of appearance: gender, race, and age. Note the client's physical features.

   Gender influences type of examination performed and manner in which assessments are made. Different physical characteristics and predisposition to illnesses are related to gender and race.
4. If uncertain whether client understands a question, rephrase or ask a similar question.

   Inappropriate response from a client may be caused by language or deterioration of mental status, preoccupation with illness, or decreased hearing acuity.

Box 10-3 Symptoms That May Indicate Dementia

LEARNING AND RETAINING NEW INFORMATION

Trouble remembering recent conversations, events, and appointments

Frequently misplaces objects

HANDLING COMPLEX TASKS

Difficulty following a complex train of thought

Difficulty performing tasks that require many steps

REASONING ABILITY

Unable to develop plan to address problems at work or home

Displays uncharacteristic disregard for rules of social conduct

SPATIAL ABILITY AND ORIENTATION

Difficulty driving

Difficulty in organizing objects around the house

Difficulty finding way around familiar places

LANGUAGE

Increasing difficulty with expressing self

Difficulty following conversations

BEHAVIOR

Appears more passive and less responsive

More irritable and suspicious than usual

Misinterprets visual and auditory stimuli

Data from Agency for Health Care Policy and Research: *Recognition and initial assessment of Alzheimer's disease and related dementias,* 1996, Rockville, Md, Agency for Health Care Policy and Research.

STEP	RATIONALE
5. If a client's responses are inappropriate, ask short, to-the-point questions regarding information the client should know, for example: "Tell me your name." "What is the name of this place?" "Tell me where you live." "What day is this?" "What month is this?" or "What season of the year is this?"	Measures client's orientation to person, place and time. This may be noted in documentation as "Oriented × 3." If disoriented in any way, include subjective and/or objective data rather than just documenting disoriented.
6. If client is unable to respond to questions of orientation, offer simple commands, for example, "Squeeze my fingers" or "Move your toes."	Levels of consciousness exist along a continuum including full responsiveness, inability to consciously initiate meaningful behaviors, and unresponsiveness to stimuli.
7. Assess posture and position, noting alignment of shoulders and hips while client stands and sits. Observe whether the client has a slumped, erect, or bent posture (see illustration).	May reveal musculoskeletal problem, mood, or presence of pain.

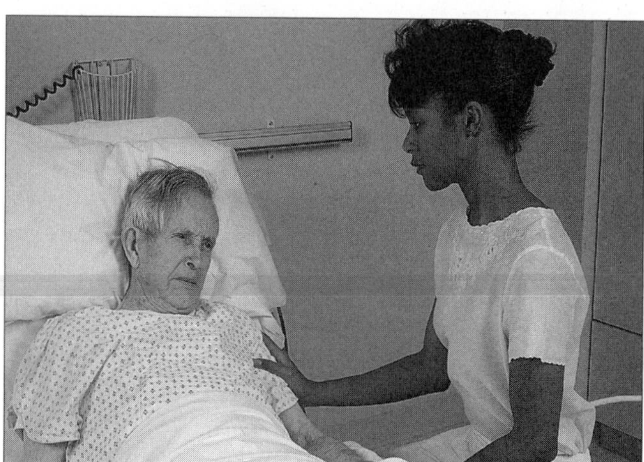

STEP **7** Observe client's position and posture. (From Elkin M, Perry A, Potter P: *Nursing interventions and clinical skills,* ed 2, St. Louis, 2000, Mosby.)

STEP	RATIONALE
a. Body movements. Are they purposeful? Are there tremors of the extremities? Are any body parts immobile?	May indicate neurological or muscular problem or emotional stress.
b. Note if movements are coordinated or uncoordinated.	
8. Assess speech. Is it understandable and moderately paced? Is there an association with the person's thoughts?	May reflect neurological impairment, injury or impairment of mouth, improperly fitting dentures, or differences in dialect and language.
9. Observe hygiene and grooming for presence or absence of makeup, type of clothes (hospital or personal), and cleanliness.	Grooming may reflect activity level prior to examination, resources available to purchase grooming supplies, client's mood, and self-care practices. May also reflect culture, lifestyle, economic status, and personal preferences.
a. Observe the color, distribution, quantity, thickness, texture, and lubrication of hair.	Changes in hair distribution may reflect hormonal changes, changes from aging, poor nutrition, or use of certain hair care products.
b. Inspect the condition of nails.	Changes may indicate inadequate nutrition or grooming practices, nervous habits, or systemic diseases.
c. Assess the presence or absence of body odor.	Body odor may result from physical exercise, deficient hygiene, or physical or mental abnormalities. Inadequate oral hygiene or unhealthy teeth may cause bad breath.
10. Assess the eyes.	
a. Inspect position of eyes, color, condition of **conjunctiva,** and movement.	Asymmetrical positioning or eye movement may reflect trauma or tumor growths. Differences in color may be congenital; changes in color of conjunctiva may be due to local infection or symptomatic of another abnormality, (e.g., pale conjunctiva is associated with anemia).

STEP	RATIONALE
b. Note client's near vision (ability to read newspaper or magazines) and far vision (follow movement, ability to read the clock, television, or signs at a distance).	If client has visual acuity or visual field loss, make adjustments to support self-care measures (e.g., feeding, bathing and hygiene, dressing) and teaching.
c. Inspect pupils for size, shape, and equality (see illustration).	Normal pupils are round, clear, and equal in size and shape.
d. Test pupillary reflexes. To test reaction to light, dim room lights. If lights can not be dimmed, cup hand over eye to temporarily shield the light. As client looks straight ahead, move penlight from side of client's face and direct light on pupil. Observe pupillary response of both eyes, noting briskness and equality of reflex (see illustrations).	Darkened room normally ensures brisk response of pupils to light. Pupil that is illuminated constricts. Pupil in other eye should constrict equally (consensual light reflex).

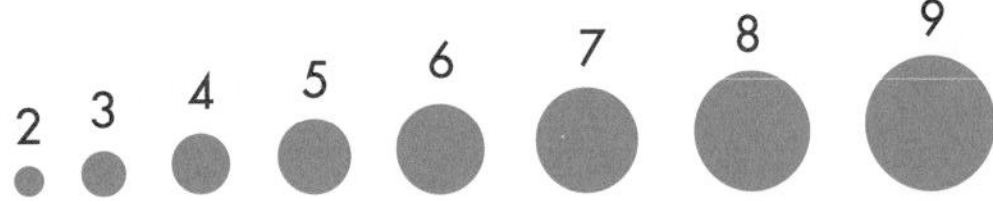

STEP **10c** Pupil sizes in millimeters.

A 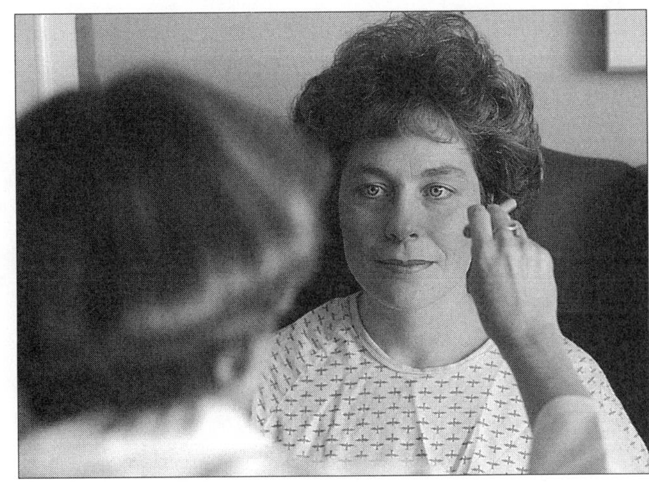

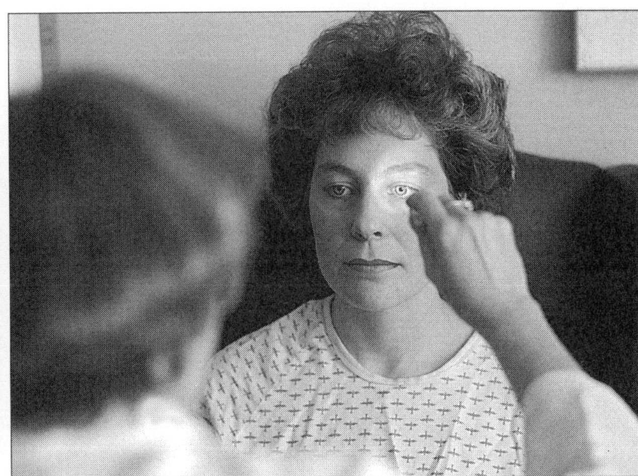 B

STEP **10d** **A,** Holding penlight to side of client's face. **B,** Illumination of pupil causes pupillary constriction.

11. Assess hearing. Note the client's response to questions and the presence/use of a hearing aid. If hearing loss is suspected, ask client to repeat random numbers with two equally accented syllables (e.g., nine, four). Repeat gradually increasing voice intensity until client correctly repeats the numbers.

Seidel and others (1999) report that clients normally hear numbers clearly when whispered, responding correctly at least 50% of the time. For client with obvious hearing impairment, speak clearly and concisely, stand so that client can see face, and toward client's good ear, speak in low pitch, and avoid yelling.

- ***Critical Decision Point***
  If hearing deficit is present, inspect client's ears because impaired hearing may be due to impacted ***cerumen,*** *external otitis, or swelling in ear canal due to allergic reactions to materials in hearing aids (Meador, 1995).*

12. Inspect nose externally for shape, skin color, alignment, and presence of deformity or inflammation. Note color of mucosa and any lesions, discharge, swelling, or presence of bleeding.

Character of discharge and inflammation indicate allergy or infection. Perforation and erosion of the septum and puffiness and/or increased vascularity of the mucosa can indicate habitual use of intranasal cocaine and opioids.

Step	Rationale
13. In clients with a nasogastric, nasointestinal, or nasotracheal tube, inspect **nares** for excoriation or inflammation. Stabilize tube as needed.	Swallowing or coughing reflex causes movement of tubes against nares and pressure against tissues and mucosa can result in tissue erosion.
14. Assess the mouth. Inspect oral mucosa, tongue, teeth, and gums for hydration, discoloration, and obvious lesions (see illustration). Determine if client wears dentures or retainers and if they are comfortable. Dentures may be removed to visualize and palpate gums.	Ill-fitting dentures and retainers chronically irritate mucosa and gums and may pose risk for mouth cancer.
15. Ask if client has noted any changes in the skin, including: **a.** Pruritus, oozing, bleeding **b.** Change in the appearance of a bump or nodule; a change in sensation; itchiness, tenderness, or pain **c.** Petechiae (tiny, pinpoint-size, red or purple spots on the skin caused by small hemorrhages in the skin layers).	Incidence of melanoma, an aggressive form of skin cancer, has increased significantly. It is more than 10 times higher in whites than in African Americans (American Cancer Society, 1999). The cancer can spread to other parts of the body quickly. Early detection and prompt treatment are critical. (Box 10-4) Petechiae may indicate serious blood clotting disorder, drug reaction, or liver disease.

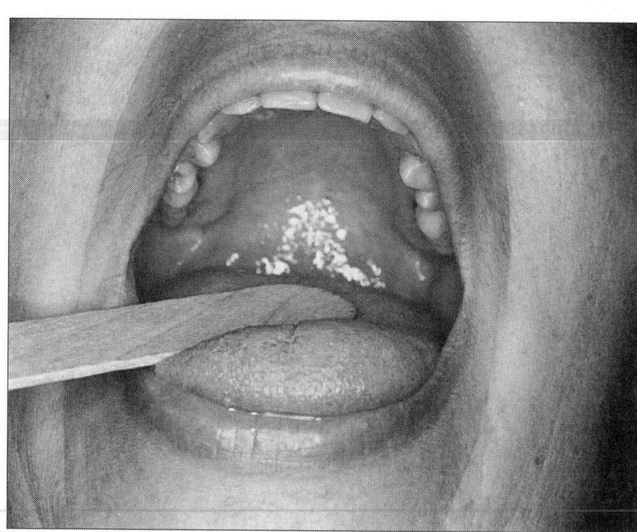

STEP **14** Inspect mouth.

Box 10-4 Malignant Melanoma

MNEMONICS

The ABCD Rule of Melanoma

Here is a simple way to remember the characteristics that should alert you to the possibility of malignant melanoma.

A *A*symmetry of lesion
B *B*orders; irregular
C *C*olor blue/black or variegated
D *D*iameter > 6 mm

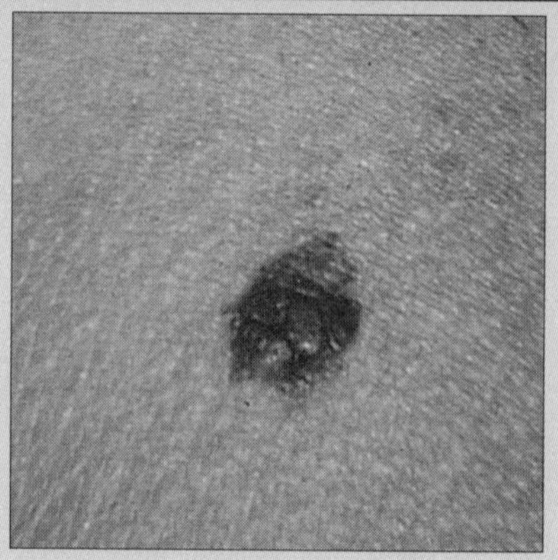

Malignant melanoma. (Courtesy Walter Tunnessen, MD, University of Pennsylvania, Philadelphia.)

STEP	RATIONALE
16. Inspect skin surfaces, comparing color of symmetrical body parts. Scan the entire body, noting areas unexposed to sun. Look for any patches or areas of skin color variation.	Changes in color can be indicative of pathological alterations (Table 10-5). Bluish discoloration of mucosa at base of tongue (central **cyanosis**) indicates low oxygen saturation, seen in lung disease and congenital heart defects of children. Peripheral cyanosis (bluish discoloration of lips and nail beds) results from low cardiac output or local vasoconstriction.

• ***Critical Decision Point***
Be alert for basal cell carcinomas, often seen in sun-exposed areas. Frequently these occur in a background of sun-damaged skin.

17. Carefully inspect color of face, oral mucosa, lips, conjunctiva, sclera, and nail beds.	Nurse can more readily identify abnormalities in areas of body where melanin production is lowest.

• ***Critical Decision Point***
When assessing the skin of a client with bandages, cast, restraints, or other restrictive devices, note areas of ***pallor*** *and decreased temperature, which may indicate impaired circulation. Immediate release of pressure from the restrictive device may be necessary.*

18. Use ungloved fingertips to palpate skin surfaces to feel moisture of intact skin.	Moisture is directly related to degree of hydration and condition of outer lipid layer of the skin surface. Older adults are prone to xerosis, which is evident as dry, scaly skin (Lueckenotte, 2000).
a. Stroke skin surfaces lightly with fingertips to detect texture of skin's surface. Note whether skin is smooth or rough, thick or thin, tight or supple and if localized areas of hardness or lesions are present.	Localized texture changes result from trauma, surgical wounds, or lesions.
b. Palpate any areas that appear irregular in texture.	Allows nurse to detect localized areas of hardness and/or tenderness within subcutaneous skin layers.

• ***Critical Decision Point***
If client receives routine injections (e.g., insulin or heparin), develop a plan to rotate injection sites systematically. Localized areas of hardness from repeated injections may be found over injection sites. Local skin changes from repeated injections can be prevented by site rotation (Hauner, 1996).

Table 10-5 Skin Color Variations

COLOR	CONDITION	CAUSES	ASSESSMENT LOCATIONS
Bluish (cyanosis)	Increased amount of deoxygenated hemoglobin (associated with hypoxia)	Heart or lung disease, cold environment	Nail beds, lips, mouth, skin (severe cases)
Pallor (decrease in color)	Reduced amount of oxyhemoglobin	Anemia	Face, conjunctivae, nail beds, palms of hands
	Reduced visibility of oxyhemoglobin resulting from decreased blood flow	Shock	Skin, nail beds, conjunctivae, lips
Loss of pigmentation	Vitiligo	Congenital or autoimmune condition causing lack of pigment	Patchy areas on skin over face, hands, arms
Yellow-orange (jaundice)	Increased deposit of bilirubin in tissues	Liver disease, destruction of red blood cells	Sclera, mucous membranes, skin
Red (erythema)	Increased visibility of oxyhemoglobin caused by dilation or increased blood flow	Fever, direct trauma, blushing, alcohol intake	Face, area of trauma, sacrum, shoulders, other common sites for pressure ulcers
Tan-brown	Increased amount of melanin	Suntan, pregnancy	Areas exposed to sun: face, arms; areolae, nipples

STEP	RATIONALE
19. Using clean gloves, inspect character of any secretions; note color, odor, amount, and consistency (e.g., thin and watery or thick and oily).	Character of secretions from skin lesions helps to indicate type of lesion.
20. Using dorsum (back) of hand, palpate for temperature of skin surfaces (nurse may remove a glove temporarily if worn). Compare symmetrical body parts. Compare upper and lower body parts. Note distinct temperature differences. Note localized areas of warmth.	Increased or decreased skin temperature reflects increase or decrease in blood flow. Skin on dorsum of hand is thin, which allows detection of subtle temperature changes. A stage I pressure ulcer may cause warmth and **erythema** (redness) of an area. The temperature of the environment and anxiety may also affect skin temperature.
21. Assess skin turgor by grasping fold of skin on the sternal area with the fingertips. Release skinfold and note ease and speed with which skin returns to place (see illustration).	With reduced turgor, skin remains suspended or "tented" for a few seconds before slowly returning to place. This indicates decreased elasticity and possible dehydration (Elkin, Perry, and Potter, 2000). With altered turgor it is essential to provide measures for prevention of pressure ulcers.

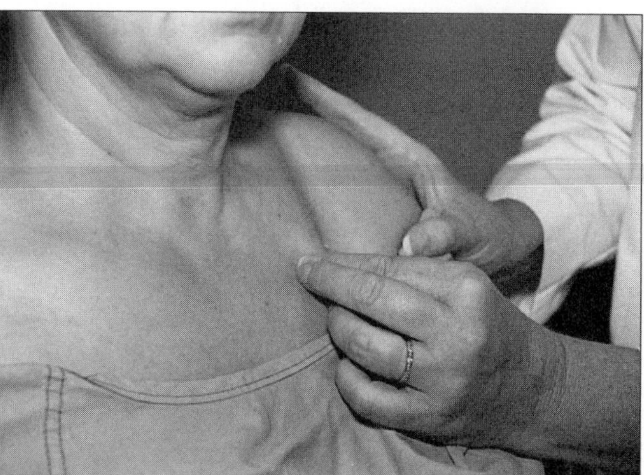

STEP **21** Checking skin turgor.

STEP	RATIONALE
22. Assess condition of skin for pressure areas, paying particular attention to regions of pressure (e.g., sacrum, greater trochanter, heels, occipital area, clavicles). If areas of redness are noted, place fingertip over area and apply gentle pressure, then release.	Normal reactive hyperemia (redness) is visible effect of localized vasodilation, body's normal response to lack of blood flow to underlying tissue. Affected area of skin will blanch with fingertip pressure.

• ***Critical Decision Point***

Evidence of normal reactive hyperemia on pressure points should result in repositioning of client and development of turning schedule if client is dependent (see Chapter 7).

STEP	RATIONALE
23. When lesion is detected, with adequate lighting inspect color, location, texture, size, shape, type (Box 10-5). Note also grouping (e.g., clustered or linear) and distribution (localized or generalized).	Certain skin lesions can be identified by a characteristic pattern of features.
a. Gently palpate any lesion to determine mobility, contour (flat, raised, or depressed), and consistency (soft or hard). If lesion is moist or draining, apply disposable gloves before palpation.	Gentle palpation prevents accidental rupture of underlying cysts. Gloves reduce transmission of microorganisms.
b. Note if client reports tenderness during palpation.	Tenderness may be indicative of inflammation or pressure on body part.
c. Measure size of lesion (height, width, depth) with centimeter ruler.	Provides for baseline to assess changes in lesion over time.

Box 10-5 Types of Primary Skin Lesions

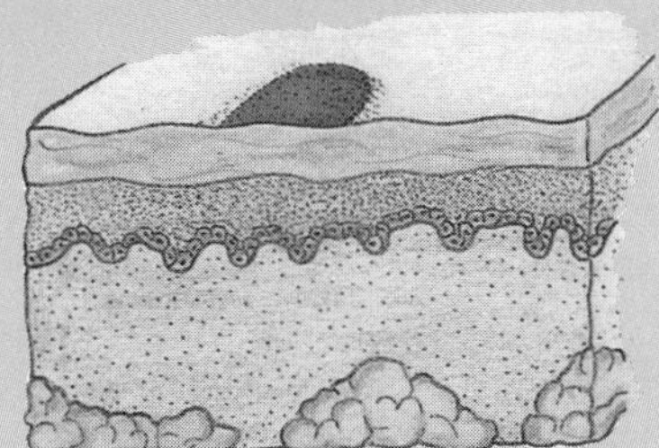

Macule: flat, nonpalpable change in skin color, smaller than 1 cm (e.g., freckle, petechia)

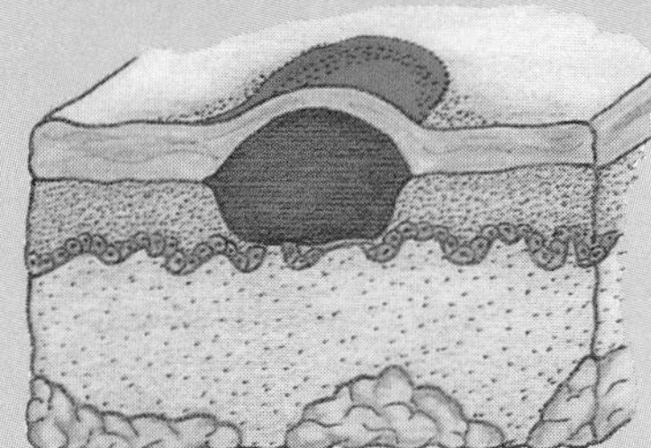

Papule: palpable, circumscribed, solid elevation in skin, smaller than 0.5 cm (e.g., elevated nevus)

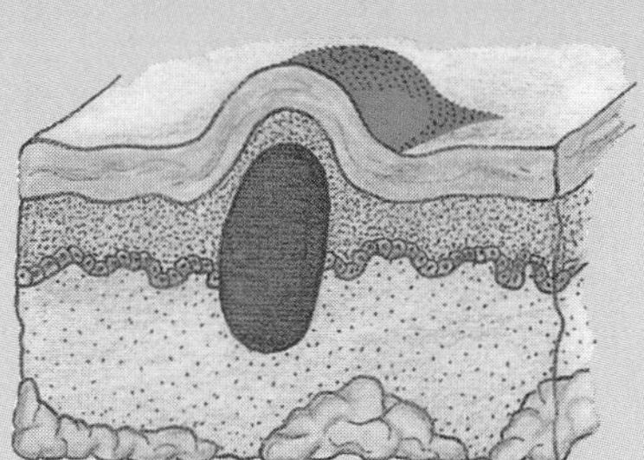

Nodule: elevated solid mass, deeper and firmer than papule, 0.5-2.0 cm (e.g., wart)

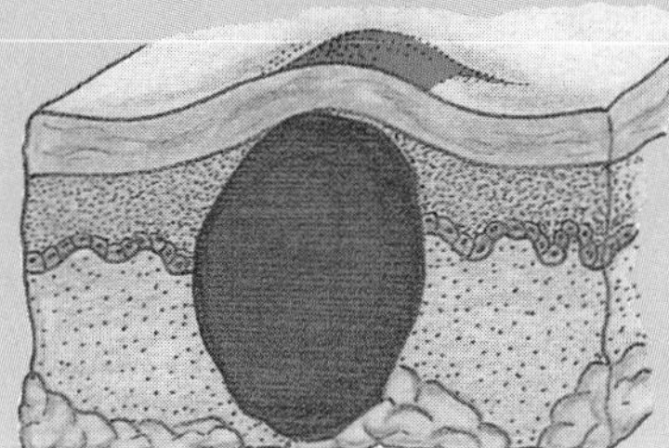

Tumor: solid mass that may extend deep through subcutaneous tissue, larger than 1-2 cm (e.g., epithelioma)

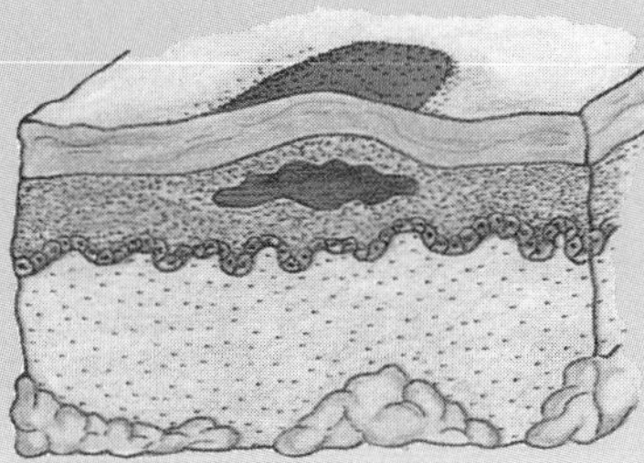

Wheal: irregularly shaped, elevated area or superficial localized edema, varies in size (e.g., hive, mosquito bite)

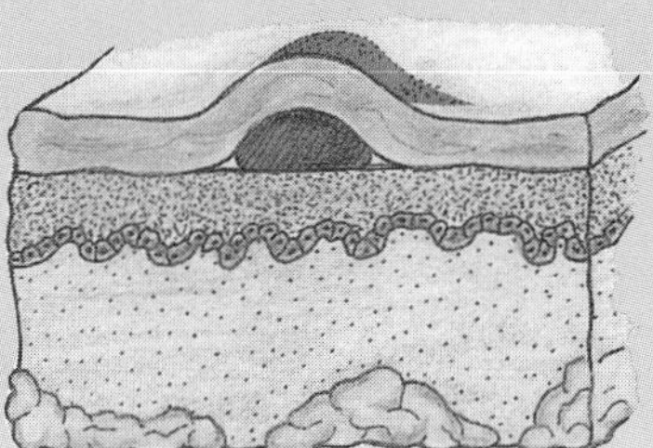

Vesicle: circumscribed elevation of skin filled with serous fluid, smaller than 0.5 cm (e.g., herpes simplex, chickenpox)

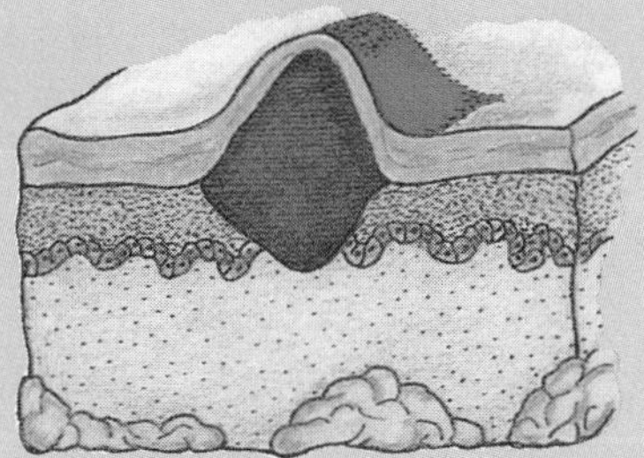

Pustule: circumscribed elevation of skin similar to vesicle but filled with pus, varies in size (e.g., acne, staphylococcal infection)

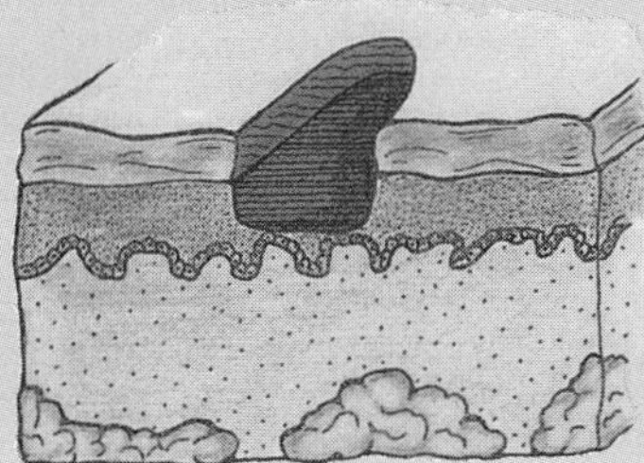

Ulcer: deep loss of skin surface that may extend to dermis and frequently bleeds and scars, varies in size (e.g., venous stasis ulcer)

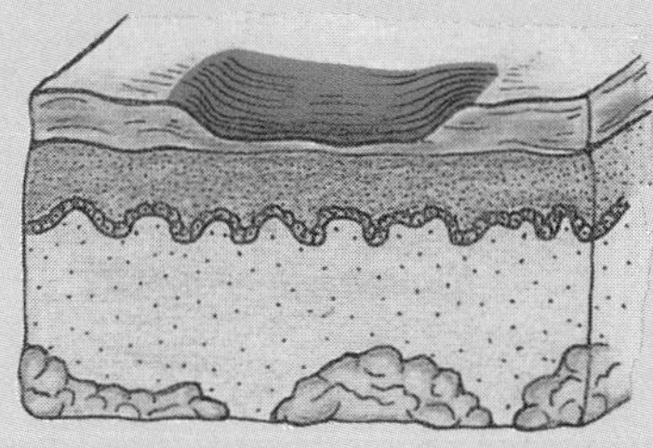

Atrophy: thinning of skin with loss of normal skin furrow with skin appearing shiny and translucent, varies in size (e.g., arterial insufficiency)

Step	Rationale
24. Using clean gloves, inspect and palpate intravenous (IV) site (see illustration) for evidence of inflammation (redness, heat, swelling, drainage, or tenderness) or infiltration (puffiness, pallor and coolness). Note when site is due to be changed.	Presence of infiltration or phlebitis requires IV to be discontinued. Agency policy dictates frequency of site change.
25. Use the "five rights" to check IV fluids and medications, including type of fluids and rate of infusion. Note expiration date of fluids and tubing.	Infusion rate that is too rapid may result in fluid volume excess; a rate too slow can result in inadequate fluid replacement. Changing the fluids and tubing according to agency policy helps prevent IV-related infections (Pugliese, 1997).

STEP	RATIONALE

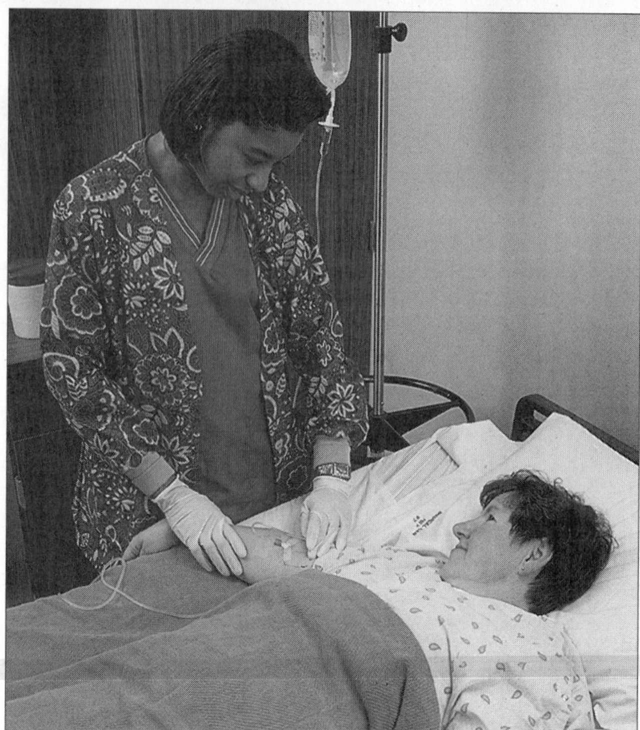

STEP **24** Palpating IV site for tenderness.

STEP	RATIONALE
26. Assess affect and mood: note if verbal expressions match nonverbal behavior and if appropriate to situation.	Reflects client's mental status, consciousness, feelings, and emotional status.
27. Observe client interaction with spouse or partner, older adult child, or caregiver. Be alert for indications of fear, hesitancy to report health status, or willingness to let caregiver control assessment interview. Does partner or caregiver have a history of violence, alcoholism, or drug abuse? Is the person unemployed, ill, or frustrated with caring for client? Note if client has any obvious physical injuries.	Abuse may first be suspected in clients who have suffered obvious physical injury or neglect, show signs of malnutrition, or have bruises on the extremities or trunk. Partners or caregivers may have history of abusive or addictive behaviors.

- ***Critical Decision Point***

  Be discrete in how interview is handled. It may be necessary to delay assessment to a later time, when the partner or caregiver is not present. Asking a partner or caregiver to leave during an assessment may create an awkward situation.

STEP	RATIONALE
28. Observe for signs of abuse:	
a. For a child: Blood on underclothing, pain in genital area, difficulty sitting or walking.	Indicative of child sexual abuse.
b. For a female client: Injury or trauma inconsistent with reported cause, obvious injuries to face or neck (black eyes, broken nose, lip lacerations, broken teeth, strangulation marks, burns).	Indicates domestic abuse.
c. For an older adult: Injury or trauma inconsistent with reported cause, injuries in unusual locations (such as neck or genitalia), pattern injuries (left when an object with which a person is struck leaves an imprint), parallel injuries (such as bilateral bruises on the upper arms suggesting the client was held and shaken), and burns (shaped like a cigarette, iron, rope, or immersion with a clear line of demarcation).	Prolonged interval between injury and time medical care was sought are signs indicative of older adult abuse or neglect (Lynch, 1997).

STEP	RATIONALE

- ***Critical Decision Point***
  A pattern of findings indicating abuse usually mandates a report to a social service center (refer to state guidelines). Nurse should obtain immediate consultation with physician, social worker, and other support staff to facilitate placement in a safer environment.

EVALUATION

1. Observe throughout the assessment for evidence of physical or emotional distress.	Interaction during assessment can reveal emotional problems. Maneuvers used during physical exam can reveal presence of physical problems.
2. Compare assessment findings with previous observations.	Determines if change has occurred.
3. Ask the client if there is information about physical condition that has not been discussed.	Clients may feel they are bothering the nurse by asking questions unless the opportunity for questions is provided.

UNEXPECTED OUTCOMES AND RELATED INTERVENTIONS

- Client demonstrates acute distress (e.g., respiratory distress, acute pain, or severe anxiety).
  - Respond immediately to identified need (repositioning, oxygen, or medication as appropriate).
  - Obtain vital signs.
  - Notify physician.
- Client has abnormal skin condition (dry texture, reduced turgor, lesions).
  - Identify contributing factors and prevent continued irritation or damage as appropriate (see Chapter 7).
- Client is unwilling or unable to provide adequate information relating to identified concerns.
  - Seek information from family members if present.
  - Review client's record for baseline data.

NURSING DIAGNOSIS

Defining characteristics from the assessment data may reveal the following nursing diagnoses for clients requiring this skill. (Confirmation of any one diagnosis will usually require more data gathering during assessment.)

Imbalanced nutrition: less than body requirements or more than body requirements
Deficient fluid volume or excess fluid volume
Anxiety or fear
Bathing/hygiene self-care deficit
Impaired physical mobility
Impaired wheelchair mobility
Impaired bed mobility
Impaired skin integrity
Ineffective breathing pattern
Ineffective peripheral tissue perfusion
Pain (acute, chronic)
Dysfunctional family processes: alcoholism
Caregiver role strain

Related factors are individualized based on client's condition or needs.

RECORDING AND REPORTING

- Record client's vital signs on vital sign flow sheet.
- Record description of alterations in client's general appearance.
- Describe client's behaviors using objective terminology. Include client's self-report of signs and symptoms.
- Report abnormalities and acute symptoms to nurse in charge or physician.

TEACHING CONSIDERATIONS

- During general survey, inform client about normal range of vital signs for age and physical condition and normal weight for height and body frame.
- Explain that it is best to weigh self in the morning after voiding and before food or drink is taken.
- If client is on established diet, discuss any problems client has in diet preparation or food selection. The best form of weight reduction is to achieve gradual weight loss by increasing exercise and decreasing caloric intake. Refer to clinical dietitian for specific information.
- Instruct client to prevent skin cancer by avoiding overexposure to the sun. Protective clothing (e.g., wide-brimmed hats and long sleeves) and sunscreen should be worn. Apply sunscreen with sun protection factor (SPF) greater than or equal to 15 approximately 15 minutes before going into the sun and after swimming or perspiring. Avoid exposure to the sun's ultraviolet rays at midday (10 AM to 3 PM), when

the rays are the strongest. Do not use indoor sun lamps or tanning salons. Medications such as oral contraceptives and antibiotics can make skin more sensitive to sun.

- Common visual changes with aging include reduced acuity (presbyopia), loss of or reduction in peripheral vision, reduced tearing, sensitivity to glare or bright lights.
- Measurement of visual acuity and visual fields helps nurse determine level of assistance client requires with daily living activities and ability of client to safely ambulate and function independently within home. Client and family may need to make adjustments in how rooms are arranged at home and in obtaining self-help aids.

Pediatric Considerations

- Measurement of physical growth is a key element in evaluation of a child's health status. An effort sponsored by the World Health Organization has resulted in the revision of growth charts for young children from birth to 5 years. This will be constructed from an international longitudinal study including breastfed infants (Garza and De Onis, 1999).
- Infants are weighed nude. Children may be weighed in light underclothes or gown.
- A child's interactions with parents provide valuable information regarding the child's behavior.

Gerontological Considerations

- An older adult's presenting signs and symptoms can be deceiving. An older adult has a diminished physiological reserve that may mask the usual, or "classic," signs and symptoms of a disease. In older adults signs and symptoms are often blunted or atypical (Lueckenotte, 2000).
- Nutritional problems are frequently noted in older adults. Skipping meals is a common practice. The amount of nutrition becomes questionable. The following factors pose risks for malnutrition in older adults: limited income, loneliness, abuse of alcohol and other central nervous system depressants, forgetfulness, inability to feed self, reduced strength and mobility, and decreased vision (Ebersole and Hess, 1998).
- Common skin changes with aging include dryness, wrinkling, reduced elasticity, and "liver spots" in areas exposed to sun. Common lesions include seborrheic keratosis (pigmented macular-papular lesion that can be warty, scaly, or greasy); cherry angioma (bright, ruby-red or purplish papular lesion); skin tags (soft pinkish-tan to light-brown pedunculated lesions); and senile lentigines (gray-brown irregular macular lesions on sun-exposed areas) (Lueckenotte, 2000). Inspection of the feet is critically important in the presence of impaired circulation, impaired vision, and diabetes. Common podiatric conditions include ulceration, fungal infection, calluses, bunions, and plantar warts (Sitzman 1999).

Home Care Considerations

- In the home the focus may be on the client's ability to perform basic self-care tasks. The nurse should ensure that the home assessment builds on all health concerns identified in other settings.

Long-Term Care Considerations

- The minimum data set (MDS) is a tool that includes a comprehensive assessment of residents in the long-term care setting. It is meant to provide a total picture of a resident and to provide an ongoing comprehensive assessment of each resident, emphasizing functional ability and both a physical and a psychosocial profile. Only an RN can function as the assessment coordinator. Contributions are made by licensed vocational or practical nurses, the dietary supervisor, social worker, recreational therapist, physical and occupational therapist (Lueckenotte, 2000).

Skill 10-2 Assessing the Thorax and Lungs

Assessment of respiratory function is one of the most critical assessments because alterations can quickly become life threatening. Routine shift assessment is essential because changes in respiration can occur quickly as a result of a variety of factors, including immobility, infection, and fluid overload. Alteration in pulmonary function usually affects other body systems. For example, reduced blood oxygenation can cause changes in mental alertness because of the brain's sensitivity to lowered oxygen levels. Thus the nurse must carefully assess findings from all body systems when determining the nature of pulmonary problems.

Shift assessment of the lungs includes auscultation, which assesses the movement of air through the tracheobronchial tree. Recognizing the sounds created by normal airflow allows the nurse to detect sounds caused by obstruction of the airways. Assessment also includes inspection, palpation, and percussion.

To perform a lung assessment accurately, the nurse needs to be familiar with the anatomical landmarks of the chest wall (Figure 10-2). This assists in identifying findings in relation to the location of the lobes of the lung (Figure 10-3) and the position of each rib. To locate the position of each rib anteriorly, the nurse begins by finding the Angle of Louis at the manubriosternal junction. The angle is a visible and palpable protrusion of the sternum at the point at which the second rib articulates with the sternum. The nurse counts the ribs and **intercostal spaces** from this point. The number of each intercostal space corre-

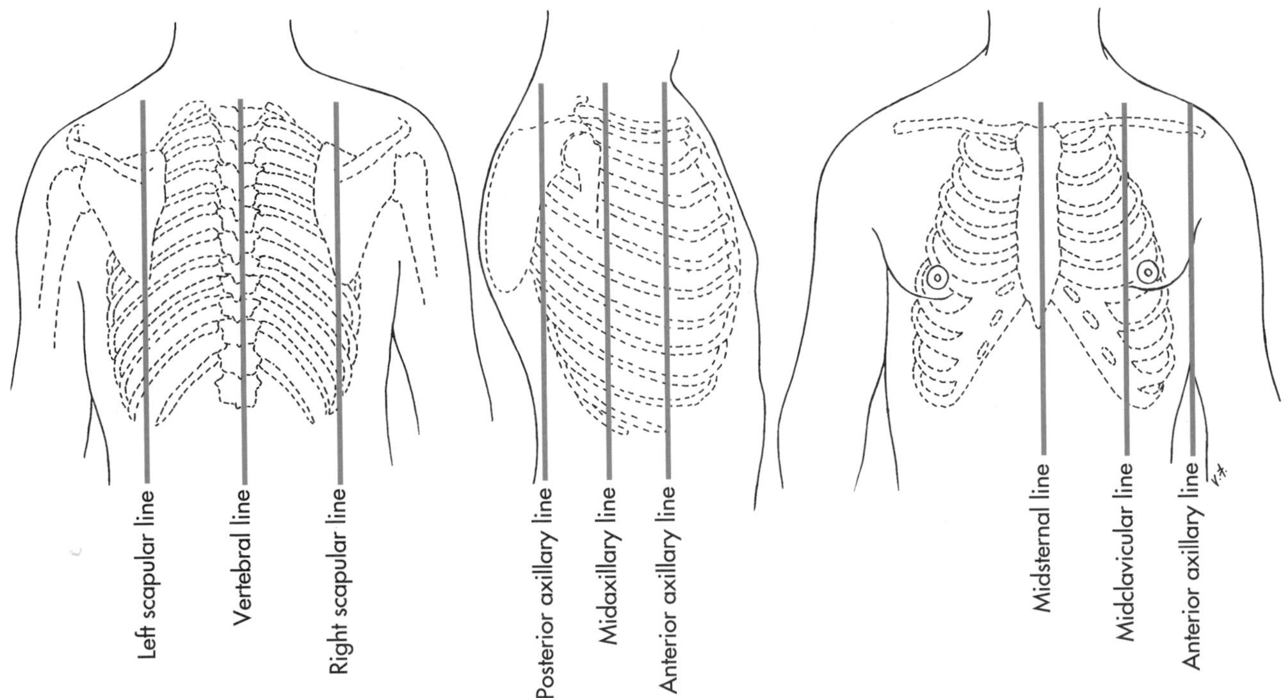

FIGURE **10-2** Anatomical landmarks of chest wall. **A,** Posterior view. **B,** Lateral view. **C,** Anterior view.

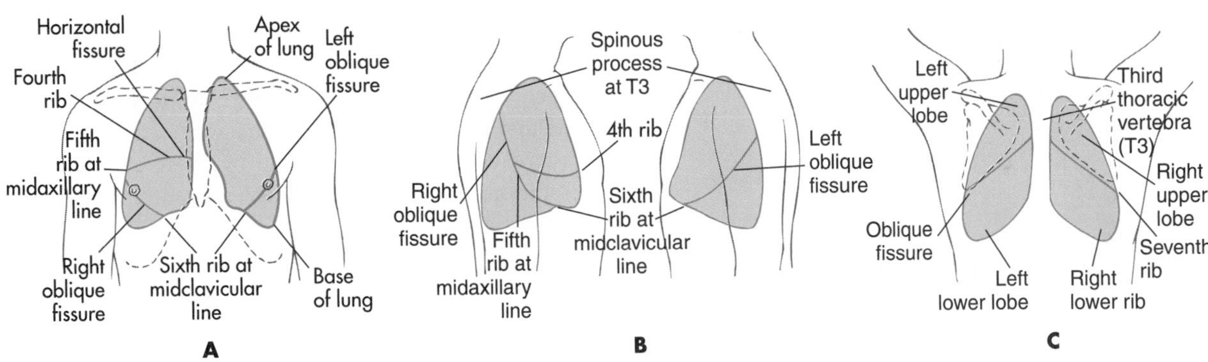

FIGURE **10-3** Position of lung lobes in relation to anatomical landmarks. **A,** Anterior. **B,** Lateral. **C,** Posterior.

sponds to that of the rib just above it. Intercostal spaces are not always visible and are difficult to palpate in some individuals.

Examination of the lungs and thorax is most effective when the client is undressed to the waist. Begin with the client sitting for assessment of the posterior and lateral chest. The client may sit or lie down for examination of the anterior chest. A female client may keep a gown draped loosely over her chest while the posterior chest is examined. Good lighting is essential. The nurse needs to assess the client's ability to tolerate position changes and level of distress. Often a client confined to bed rest or the client with chest pain has limited lung expansion.

Delegation Considerations

Assessment of the lung and thorax should not be delegated to assistive personnel. However, the following activities may be delegated: monitoring status of client's respirations and reporting distress and changes in rate and depth.

Equipment

- Stethoscope
- Disposable gloves

STEP	RATIONALE
ASSESSMENT	
1. Assess history of tobacco or marijuana use, including type of tobacco, duration, and amount in pack years. (Pack years = Number of years smoking times the number of packs per day.) If client has quit, determine the length of time since smoking stopped.	Smoking is a risk factor linked with the incidence of lung cancer, heart disease, and chronic lung disease (emphysema and chronic bronchitis). Smoking is responsible for 87% of all lung cancers in the United States (American Cancer Society, 1999).
2. Ask if client experiences any of the following: persistent cough (productive or nonproductive), sputum production, chest pain, shortness of breath, orthopnea, dyspnea during exertion, activity intolerance, and recurrent attacks of pneumonia or bronchitis.	Symptoms indicative of respiratory alterations may help nurse localize any objective findings.
3. Determine if client works in environment containing pollutants such as asbestos, coal dust, or chemical irritants. Does client have exposure to secondhand cigarette smoke?	Clients with chronic respiratory disease, particularly asthma, have symptoms aggravated by change in temperature and humidity, irritating fumes or smoke, emotional stress, and physical exertion.
4. Review history for known or suspected human immunodeficiency virus (HIV) infection, substance abuse, low income, and residence in nursing home.	Known risk factors for exposure to and/or development of tuberculosis.
5. Ask if client has history of cough, hemoptysis, weight loss, fatigue, night sweats, and/or fever.	Signs and symptoms for both tuberculosis and HIV infection.
6. Assess for history of allergies to pollen, dust, or other airborne irritants, as well as to any foods, drugs, or chemical substances.	Symptoms client demonstrates may be caused by allergic response to allergen: choking feeling, bronchospasm with respiratory stridor, wheezing on auscultation, dyspnea, cyanosis, and diaphoresis.
7. Review family history for cancer, tuberculosis, allergies, or chronic obstructive pulmonary disease (COPD).	The most common symptom of pulmonary tuberculosis is a cough. Initially cough is nonproductive. If untreated, it becomes productive with mucoid or **mucopurulent** sputum. Other symptoms include night sweats and weight loss. The condition may be diagnosed by chest x-ray examination, sputum for acid-fast bacillus, and sputum for culture and sensitivity.
PLANNING	
1. **Expected outcomes** following completion of procedure:	
▪ Respirations are passive, diaphragmatic or costal, and regular (12 to 20 per minute in adult) with symmetrical expansion.	Characteristics of normal respirations.
▪ Breath sounds are clear to auscultation and equal bilaterally.	Air flows without interference or obstruction. Corresponding sites side to side should sound the same.
▪ Client is able to describe factors that predispose to lung disease.	Awareness of risks can improve compliance with healthful behavior.
▪ Client assumes appropriate posture for best ventilation.	Client can learn about benefits of good posture as examination maneuvers are performed.
IMPLEMENTATION	
1. Position client sitting upright. For bedridden client, elevate head of bed 45 to 90 degrees.	Promotes full lung expansion during examination.
a. If unable to tolerate sitting, supine position and side-lying positions are used.	Clients with chronic respiratory disease will likely need to sit up throughout the examination because of shortness of breath. Assistance of another caregiver may be required to position unresponsive clients.

STEP	RATIONALE
b. Remove gown or drape first from posterior chest, keeping legs covered. As examination progresses, remove gown from area being examined.	Avoids unnecessary exposure and provides full visibility of thorax. Allows direct placement of diaphragm or bell on the client's skin, which enhances clarity of sounds.
c. Explain all steps of procedure, encouraging client to relax and breathe normally through the mouth.	Anxiety may alter respiratory function. Breathing through the mouth decreases extraneous sounds from air passing through the nose.
2. POSTERIOR THORAX: If possible, stand behind client to inspect thorax for shape, deformities, position of the spine, slope of the ribs, retraction of intercostal spaces during inspiration, and bulging of intercostal spaces during expiration.	Allows for identification of any factors that may impair chest expansion and any symptoms of respiratory distress. In a child, shape of chest is almost circular, with anterioposterior (AP) diameter in 1:1 ratio. In adult, chest is twice as wide as deep with 1:2 AP diameter. Chronic lung disease results in 1:1 ratio. This is referred to as a "barrel chest." Clients with breathing problems assume postures that improve ventilation.

- ***Critical Decision Point***
  Localized chest pain may be evidenced by the client holding the chest wall during breathing. Assess the nature of pain, including onset, precipitating factors, quality, region, and radiation.

STEP	RATIONALE
3. Determine the rate and rhythm of breathing (see Chapter 9).	This is a good time to count respirations, with client relaxed and unaware of inspection. Awareness could alter respirations.
4. Systematically palpate posterior chest wall, costal spaces, and intercostal spaces, noting any masses, pulsations, unusual movement, or areas of localized tenderness (see illustration). If suspicious mass or swollen area is detected, palpate for size, shape, and typical qualities of lesion (see Skill 10-1). Do not palpate painful areas deeply.	Palpation assesses further characteristics and confirms or supplements findings from assessment. Localized swelling or tenderness may indicate trauma to ribs or underlying cartilage. A fractured rib fragment could be displaced.

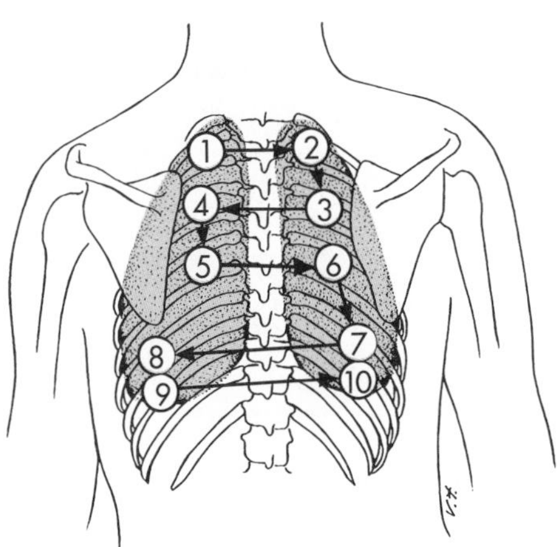

STEP **4** Pattern for assessment of posterior thorax.

STEP	RATIONALE
5. Standing behind client, place thumbs along the spinal processes at the tenth rib, with the palms lightly contacting the posterolateral surfaces (see illustration *A*). The nurse's thumbs should be about 2 inches (5 cm) apart, with the thumbs pointing toward the spine and the fingers pointing laterally. Press hands toward client's spine to form small skinfold between thumbs. After exhalation, client takes deep breath. Note movement of thumbs (see illustration *B*) and note symmetry of chest wall movement. Normally thumbs separate 3 to 5 cm (1 ½ to 2 inches) during chest excursion.	Palpation of chest excursion assesses depth of client's breathing. This technique is good measure to evaluate client's ability to perform deep-breathing exercises (see Chapter 33). Limited movement on one side may indicate that client is voluntarily splinting during ventilation because of pain. Avoid allowing the hands to slide over the skin, which gives a false measure of excursion.

A B

STEP 5 **A,** Position of hands for palpation of posterior thorax excursion. **B,** As client inhales, movement of chest excursion separates nurse's thumbs.

Table 10-6 Normal Breath Sounds

DESCRIPTION	LOCATION	ORIGIN
VESICULAR		
Vesicular sounds are soft, breezy, and low pitched. Inspiratory phase is 3 times longer than expiratory phase.	Best heard over lung's periphery (except over scapula)	Created by air moving through smaller airways
BRONCHOVESICULAR		
Bronchovesicular sounds are medium-pitched and blowing sounds of medium intensity. Inspiratory phase is equal to expiratory phase.	Best heard posteriorly between scapulae and anteriorly over bronchioles lateral to sternum at first and second intercostal spaces	Created by air moving through large airways
BRONCHIAL		
Bronchial sounds are loud and high pitched with hollow quality. Expiration lasts longer than inspiration (3:2 ratio).	Best heard over trachea	Created by air moving through trachea close to chest wall

STEP	RATIONALE
6. Percuss the chest wall moving from side to side and top to bottom following the same pattern as with palpation (see Step 4). Using indirect percussion, percuss intercostal spaces over symmetrical areas of the lungs. Compare percussion notes for all lung lobes.	Determines density of underlying lung tissue. Ask client to fold arms forward across chest. This position separates scapulas to expose more lung tissue to assessment.
7. Ausculate breath sounds. Have client take slow deep breaths with the mouth slightly open. For adult, place diaphragm of stethoscope firmly on chest wall over intercostal spaces (see illustration). Listen to entire inspiration and expiration at each stethoscope position. Systematically compare breath sounds over right and left sides (see Step 6). If sounds are faint, ask client to breathe a little deeper temporarily.	Assesses movement of air through tracheobronchial tree (Table 10-6). Recognition of normal airflow sounds allows detection of sounds caused by mucus or airway obstruction. Sounds are characterized by length of inspiratory and expiratory phases.

STEP	RATIONALE

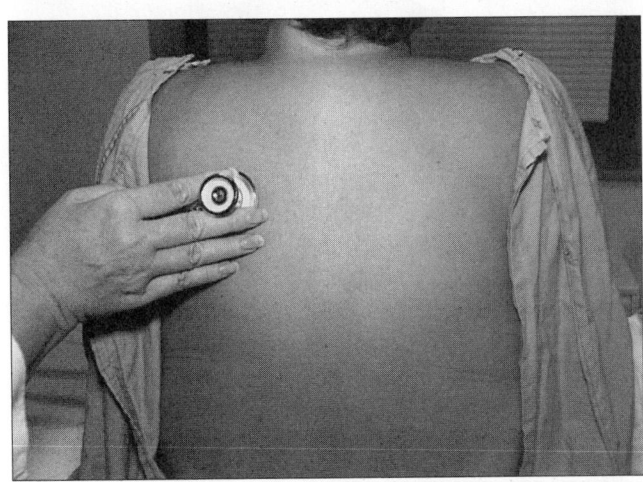

STEP 7 Use of diaphragm of stethoscope to auscultate breath sounds.

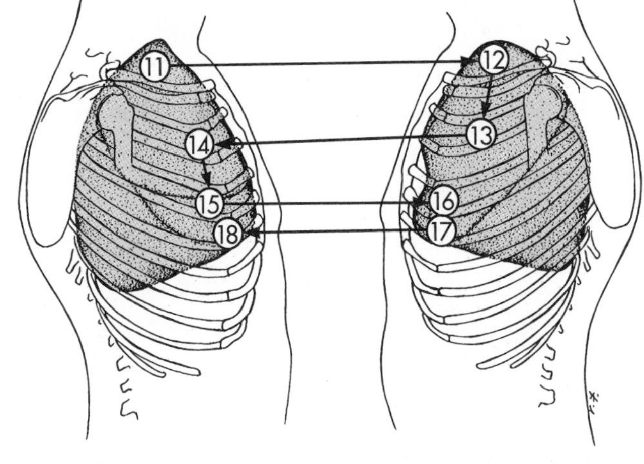

STEP 9 Pattern for assessment of lateral thorax.

8. LATERAL THORAX: Instruct client to raise arms and inspect chest wall for same characteristics as reviewed for posterior chest.

   Improves access to lateral thoracic structures.

9. Extend palpation, percussion, and auscultation of posterior thorax to lateral sides of chest, except for excursion measurement (see illustration).

   Allows for location of abnormalities in lateral lung fields.

10. ANTERIOR THORAX: Inspect accessory muscles of breathing: sternocleidomastoid, trapezius, and abdominal muscles, noting effort to breathe.

    Extent to which accessory muscles are used reveals degree of effort to breathe. Generally these muscles are not used for breathing.

11. Inspect width or spread of angle made by costal margins and tip of sternum. Angle is usually larger than 90 degrees between margins.

    Indicates congenital, acquired, or traumatic alterations that may influence client's chest expansion.

12. Observe the client's breathing pattern, observing symmetry and degree of chest wall and abdominal movement. Respiratory rate and rhythm are more often assessed on the anterior chest wall.

    Assesses client's effort to breathe; symmetrical, passive movement indicates no respiratory distress.

13. Palpate anterior thoracic muscles and ribs for lumps, masses, tenderness, or unusual movement.

    Localized swelling or tenderness may indicate trauma to underlying ribs or cartilage.

14. Palpate anterior chest excursion. Place hands over each lateral rib cage, with thumbs approximately 5 cm (2 inches) apart and angled along each costal margin. Thumbs are pushed toward client's midline to create skinfold between thumbs. As client inhales deeply, thumbs should normally separate approximately 3 to 5 cm (1 ½ to 2 inches), with each side expanding equally.

    Assesses depth of client's breathing and ability to perform deep-breathing exercises. Certain abnormalities are evident if expansion is not symmetrical.

15. Percuss anterior thorax between intercostal spaces with client lying or sitting (procedure is easier if client lies down). Begin above clavicles; move across and then down as during palpation (see illustration).

    Lying position facilitates ability to deliver sharp blow to chest wall to elicit clear sound. Percussion over anterior thorax enables nurse to locate position of liver, heart, and lung. Normal lung is resonant. Underlying liver, heart, and stomach create percussion notes different from that of lung (see illustration).

16. With client sitting, auscultate anterior thorax following same pattern as for percussion. If adventitious sounds are auscultated (Table 10-7), have client cough. Listen with stethoscope to determine if sound has disappeared.

    Using a systematic pattern of assessment comparing sides helps to identify abnormal sounds. Rhonchi often are eliminated or altered by coughing. **Crackles** and wheezes are not.

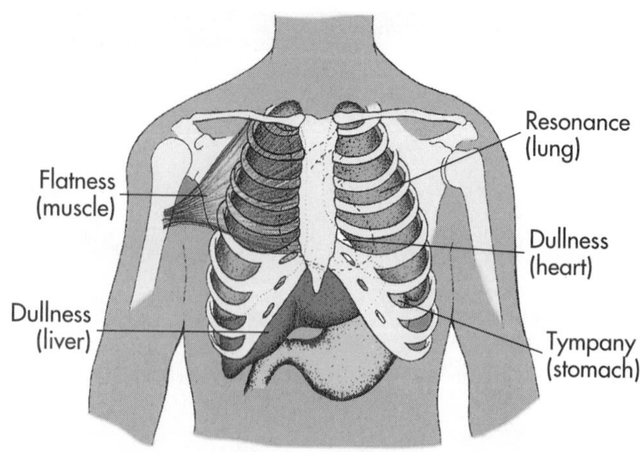

STEP **15** Variations in percussion notes in normal thorax and upper abdomen.

Table 10-7 Adventitious Breath Sounds

Sound	Site Auscultated	Cause	Character
Crackles (previously called rales)	Most commonly heard in dependent lobes: right and left lung bases	Random, sudden reinflation of groups of alveoli; also related to increase in fluid in small airways	Fine crackles are high-pitched fine, short, interrupted crackling sounds heard during end of inspiration, usually not cleared with coughing Moist crackles are lower, more moist sounds heard during middle of inspiration; not cleared with coughing
Rhonchi	Primarily heard over trachea and bronchi; if loud enough, can be heard over most lung fields	Muscular spasm, fluid, or mucus in larger airways, causing turbulence	Loud, low-pitched, rumbling coarse sounds heard most often during inspiration or expiration; may be cleared by coughing
Wheezes	Can be heard over all lung fields	High-velocity air flow through severely narrowed bronchus	High-pitched, continuous musical sounds like a squeak heard continuously during inspiration or expiration; usually louder on expiration; do not clear with coughing
Pleural friction rub	Heard over anterior lateral lung field (if client is sitting upright)	Inflamed pleura, parietal pleura rubbing against visceral pleura	Dry, grating quality heard best during inspiration; does not clear with coughing; heard loudest over lower lateral anterior surface

STEP	RATIONALE
EVALUATION	
1. Compare findings with normal assessment characteristics for thorax and lungs.	Determines presence of abnormalities.
2. Have client identify factors leading to lung disease.	Demonstrates learning.

UNEXPECTED OUTCOMES AND RELATED INTERVENTIONS

- Chest contour is abnormal, with anteroposterior diameter in 1:1 ratio.
  - Barrel-shaped chest is caused by aging and chronic lung disease.
- Posturing is observed, with client leaning over table or splinting side of chest with hand.
  - Indicates breathing difficulties (chronic lung disease and pain, respectively).
  - Assist client into a position to improve lung expansion (e.g., high Fowler's position).
- Respirations are rapid or slow and irregular (see Chapter 9) and bulging of intercostal spaces may be present.
  - Position client.
  - Auscultate lungs for abnormal sounds.
  - Notify physician.
- Chest excursion is reduced.
  - Depth of breathing is reduced by pain, postural deformity, or fatigue.
  - Reposition client.
  - Administer analgesic if appropriate.
- Percussion note is dull or flat over lung tissue. Dullness occurs over the scapula, ribs, sternum, or spine. Dullness over lung tissue may be created by presence of fluid.
  - Have client cough and deep breathe.
  - Notify physician.
  - Obtain chest x-ray examination if needed.
- Abnormal breath sounds (adventitious sounds) are auscultated over one or both lungs.
  - Have client cough to determine if clear.
  - Notify physician.
- Client is unfamiliar with risks for lung disease.
  - Education is necessary.
- Client does not assume preferred posture for optimal ventilation.
  - This is difficult to change quickly; may require exercise and further discussion.

NURSING DIAGNOSIS

Defining characteristics from the assessment data may reveal the following nursing diagnoses for clients requiring this skill:

Ineffective airway clearance
Ineffective breathing pattern
Impaired gas exchange
Pain (acute, chronic)
Fatigue
Risk for infection

Related factors are individualized based on client's condition or needs.

RECORDING AND REPORTING

- Record observations and findings in nurses' notes or assessment flow sheet.
- Record respiratory rate and character on vital signs flow sheet.
- Report abnormalities to nurse in charge or physician.
- If client has a productive cough and mucus is purulent, obtaining a specimen is appropriate. Record amount, color, consistency and odor of mucus.

TEACHING CONSIDERATIONS

- The risk of lung cancer declines about 30% to 50% after remaining cigarette free for 10 years. With further abstinence the risk continues to decline (American Cancer Society, 1999).
- Exposure to radiation, arsenic, and asbestos from occupational, medical, and environmental sources, air pollution, tuberculosis, and passive smoke contribute significantly to lung cancer.
- Discuss warning signs of lung cancer such as a persistent cough, sputum streaked with blood, chest pains, and recurrent attacks of pneumonia or bronchitis.

PEDIATRIC CONSIDERATIONS

- Children younger than age 6 exhibit noticeable abdominal or diaphragmatic movement.

- Older children and adults exhibit more costal or thoracic movement (Wong and others, 1999).
- Use bell to auscultate breath sounds in children. Breath sounds are louder in children because of their thin chest walls.

GERONTOLOGICAL CONSIDERATIONS

- Older adults have a costal angle (anteriorly) of slightly less than 90 degrees. The anteroposterior diameter may be increased from kyphosis.
- In older adults chest expansion is reduced because of calcification of rib cartilage and partial contraction of inspiratory muscles.
- Older adults should be vaccinated against the flu in the early fall (Lueckenotte, 2000).

Skill 10-3 Assessing the Heart and Neck Vessels

A client who has signs or symptoms of heart (cardiac) problems, such as chest pain, may be suffering a life-threatening condition requiring immediate attention. In this situation the nurse acts quickly and decides on the portions of the examination that are absolutely necessary. When a client's condition is stable, a more thorough assessment can reveal baseline heart function and any risks for heart disease. Clients tend to seek information about heart disease because it remains a leading cause of death in the United States. The heart and neck vessels can be assessed together because the two systems work in unison and are in close proximity.

The nurse may begin assessment of the heart after examining the lungs because the client is already in a suitable position with the chest exposed. Assessment then proceeds to the neck vessels. The nurse uses inspection, palpation, auscultation, and percussion during the examination.

DELEGATION CONSIDERATIONS

Comprehensive heart and neck vessel assessment should not be delegated to assistive personnel. Assistive personnel can be trained to assess apical pulse and peripheral pulses correctly. Assessment of peripheral pulses is important for all staff to know, particularly in specialty areas such as vascular surgery and orthopedics, where the skill is performed frequently. The staff member must be familiarized with the importance of measuring peripheral pulses in specific clients. Assistive personnel need to be instructed to recognize temperature and color changes along with changes in peripheral pulses.

EQUIPMENT

- Stethoscope
- Doppler stethoscope (optional)
- Conducting gel (if a doppler is used)

STEP	RATIONALE
ASSESSMENT	
1. Assess client for history of smoking, alcohol intake, caffeine intake (coffee, tea, soft drinks, chocolate), use of "recreational" drugs, exercise habits, and dietary patterns and intake.	These can contribute to risk factors for cardiovascular disease.
2. Determine if client is taking medications for cardiovascular function (e.g., antidysrhythmics, antihypertensives, antianginals) and if client knows their purpose, dosage, and side effects.	Allows nurse to assess client's compliance with and understanding of drug therapies. Medications for cardiovascular function cannot be taken intermittently.
3. Ask if client has experienced dyspnea, chest pain or discomfort, palpitations, excess fatigue, cough, leg pain or cramps, **edema** of the feet, cyanosis, fainting, and orthopnea. Ask if symptoms occur at rest or during exercise.	These are the cardinal symptoms of heart disease. Cardiovascular function may be adequate during rest but not during exercise.

STEP	RATIONALE
4. If client reports chest pain, determine onset (sudden or gradual), precipitating factors, quality, region, severity, and if it radiates. Anginal pain is usually a deep pressure or ache that is substernal and diffuse, radiating to one or both arms, neck, or jaw.	Symptoms may reveal myocardial infarction or coronary artery disease.
5. Assess family history for heart disease, diabetes, high cholesterol levels, hypertension, stroke, or rheumatic heart disease.	Family history of heart problems increases risk for heart and vascular disease, as do these other factors.
6. Ask client about a history of heart trouble (e.g., heart failure, congenital heart disease, coronary artery disease, dysrhythmias, murmurs), heart surgery, or vascular disease (hypertension, phlebitis, varicose veins).	Knowledge reveals client's level of understanding of condition. A preexisting condition influences examination techniques used by nurse and expected findings.

PLANNING

Expected outcomes following completion of procedure:

▪ Heart rate is between 60 to 100 beats per minute (adolescent through adult) and without extra sounds or murmurs.	Indicates normal rhythm and rate, normal sinus rhythm (NSR).
▪ Point of maximal impulse (PMI) is palpable at fifth intercostal space at left midclavicular line in adult.	
▪ Client describes changes in own behavior that reduce risks for heart disease and/or may improve cardiovascular function.	Information may improve client's health care habits.
▪ Client describes schedule, dosage, purpose, and benefits of medications being taken for cardiovascular function.	Information related to health benefits may improve compliance with therapy.
▪ Blood pressure is within normal limits for client (see Chapter 9).	Normal cardiovascular function.
▪ Carotid pulse is localized, strong, elastic, and equal bilaterally. No change occurs during inspiration or expiration without carotid **bruit** present.	Vessel is patent.
▪ Jugular veins distend when client lies supine and flatten when client is in sitting position.	Venous pressure is normal.

IMPLEMENTATION

1. Assist client to be as relaxed and comfortable as possible.	An anxious or uncomfortable client can have mild tachycardia that may lead the nurse to confounding findings.
2. Have client assume semi-Fowler's or supine position.	Provides adequate visibility and access to left thorax and mediastinum. Client with heart disease often experiences shortness of breath while lying flat.
3. Explain procedure. Avoid facial gestures reflecting concern.	Client with previously normal cardiac history may become anxious if nurse shows concern.
4. Be sure that room is quiet.	Subtle, low-pitched heart sounds are difficult to hear.
5. Form a mental image of the exact location of the heart (see illustration). The base of the heart is the upper portion, and the apex is the bottom tip. The surface of the right ventricle comprises most of the heart's anterior surface.	Visualization improves ability to assess findings accurately and determine possible source of abnormalities.
6. Find the angle of Louis felt as a ridge just below the suprasternal notch (see Skill 9-3) (between the sternal body and manubrium). Slip fingers down each side of angle to feel adjacent ribs. The intercostal spaces are just below each rib.	Anatomic point used to locate intercostal spaces to assess corresponding heart sounds.

STEP	RATIONALE

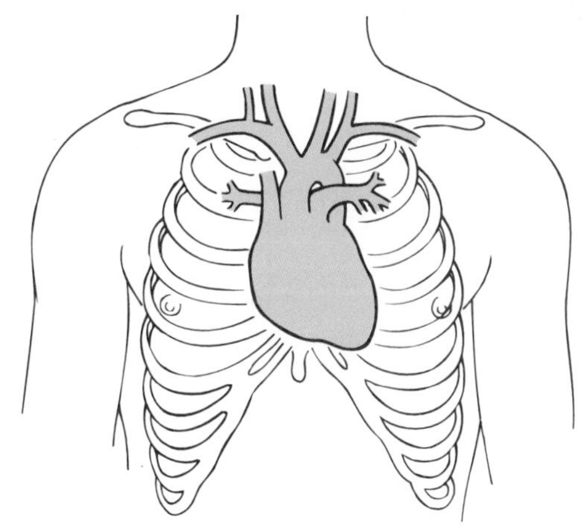

STEP **5** Anatomical position of the heart.

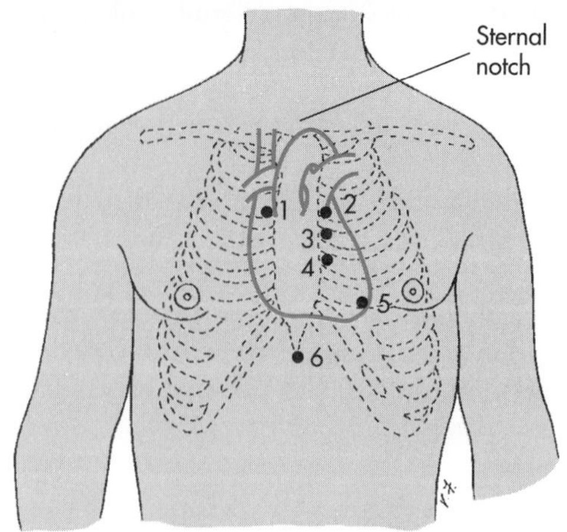

STEP **7** Areas for examination of the heart (note location of bony landmarks).

7. Find the following anatomical landmarks (see illustration):
   a. The aortic area is at the second intercostal space on the client's right (1).
   b. The pulmonic area is at the second intercostal space on left (2).
   c. The second pulmonic area is found by moving down left side of sternum to the third intercostal space (3), also referred to as Erb's point.
   d. The tricuspid area (4) is located at the fourth left intercostal space along the sternum.
   e. The mitral area is found by moving fingers laterally to client's left to locate fifth intercostal space at left midclavicular line (5).
   f. The epigastric area (6) is at the inferior tip of the sternum.

Familiarity with landmarks allows nurse to describe findings more clearly and ultimately may improve assessment.

8. Stand to the client's right and look first at the precordium with the client supine. Note any visible pulsations and more exaggerated lifts at the anatomical landmarks. Inspect closely at the area of the apex.

May reveal size and symmetry of the heart. The apical impulse is normally visible at the midclavicular line in the fifth intercostal space. The apical impulse (PMI) may become visible only when the client sits up, bringing the heart closer to the anterior wall. It is easily obscured by obesity.

• ***Critical Decision Point***

Presence of a thrill is not normal and may indicate a disruption of blood flow caused by a defect in closure of a heart valve or atrial septal defect.

9. Locate the PMI by palpating with fingertips along fifth intercostal space in midclavicular line (see illustration). Note a light, brief pulsation in an area 1 to 2 cm (½ to 1 inch) in diameter at the apex.

In the presence of serious heart disease, the PMI will be located to the left of the midclavicular line related to enlarged left ventricle. In chronic lung disease the PMI may be to the right of the midclavicular line as a result of right ventricular enlargement.

• ***Critical Decision Point***

A stronger than expected impulse may be a heave or lift, which may indicate increased cardiac output or left ventricular hypertrophy.

10. If palpating PMI is difficult, turn client onto left side.

Maneuver moves the heart closer to the chest wall.

11. Inspect the epigastric area and palpate the abdominal aorta. Note a localized strong beat.

Rules out reduced blood flow or diffuse pulse, which may indicate a number of abnormalities.

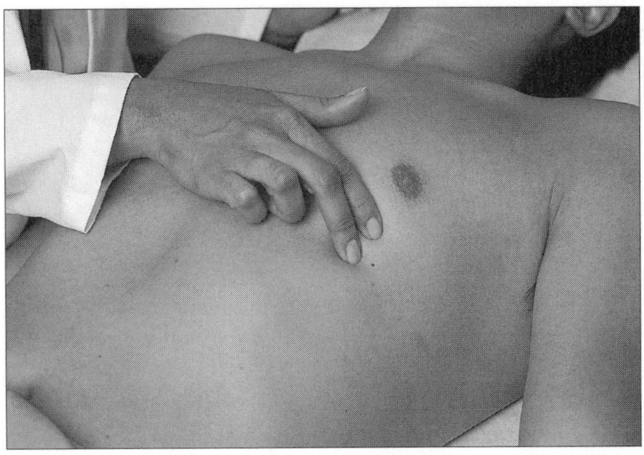

STEP **9** Palpation of PMI.

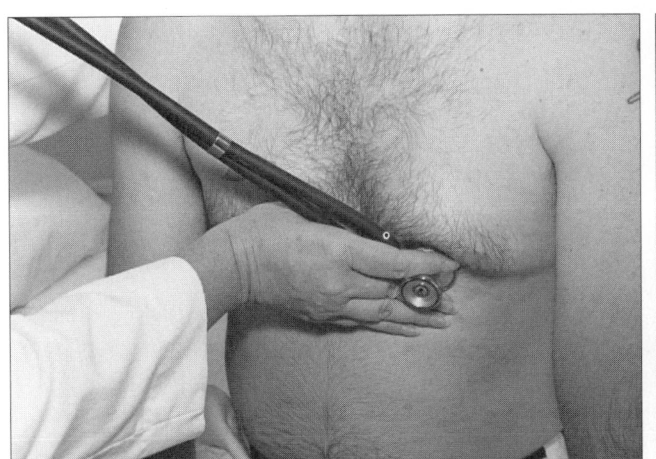

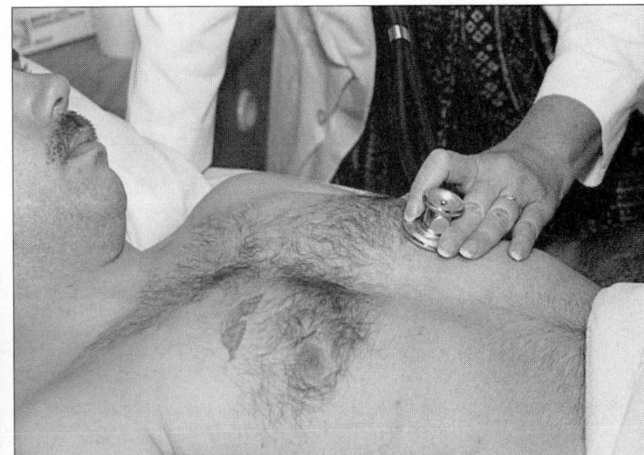

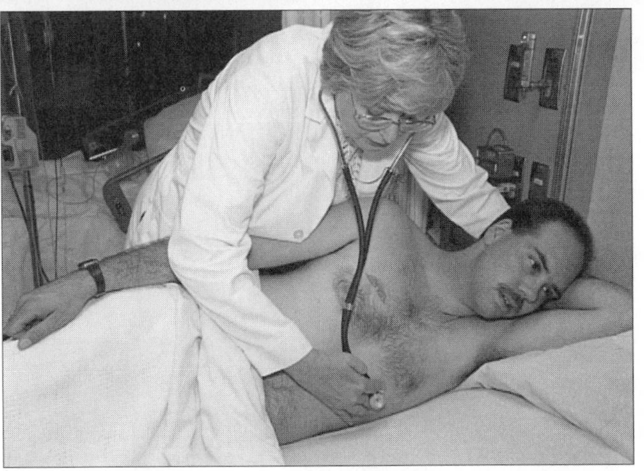

STEP **12** Client positions for auscultation of heart sounds. **A,** Sitting. **B,** Supine. **C,** Left lateral.

STEP	RATIONALE
12. Auscultate heart sounds. Begin by having client sit up and lean slightly forward; then have client lie supine; and end the examination with client in a left lateral recumbent position (see illustrations). In a female client it may be necessary to lift the left breast to hear heart sounds more effectively.	Different positions help to clarify type of sounds heard. Sitting position is best to hear high-pitched murmurs (if present). Supine is common position to hear all sounds. Left lateral recumbent is best position to hear low-pitched sounds.

STEP	RATIONALE
13. While auscultating sounds at each anatomical landmark: ask client not to speak but to breathe comfortably. Begin with the diaphragm of the stethoscope; then alternate with the bell. Use very light pressure for the bell. Inch the stethoscope along; avoid jumping from one area to another. Do not try to hear all heart sounds at once.	Auscultation requires the examiner to isolate each heart sound at all auscultation sites.
a. Begin at the apex or PMI; then move systematically to the tricuspid area, second pulmonic area, and pulmonic and aortic areas. (NOTE: Some examiners use reverse sequence.) S_1 is best heard at the apex and is simultaneous with the carotid pulse.	At normal slow rates S_1 is high pitched and dull in quality and sounds like a "lub." This sound precedes the systolic phase of heart contraction.
b. Listen for S_2 at each site. It precedes the diastolic phase and sounds like "dub." This sound is best heard at the aortic area. Heart sounds will vary by pitch, loudness, and duration, depending on the auscultatory site (Table 10-8).	Normal sounds S_1 and S_2 are high pitched and best heard with diaphragm.
c. After both sounds are heard clearly as "lub-dub," count each combination of S_1 and S_2 as one heartbeat. Count the number of beats for 1 minute.	Determines apical pulse rate.
d. Assess heart rhythm by noting the time between S_1 and S_2 (systole) and then the time between S_2 and the next S_1 (diastole). Listen to the full cycle at each auscultation area. Note regular intervals between each sequence of beats. There should be a distinct pause between S_1 and S_2.	Failure of heart to beat at regular intervals is a dysrhythmia, which interferes with heart's ability to pump effectively.
e. When heart rate is irregular, compare apical and radial pulses (Table 10-9). Auscultate the apical pulse and then immediately palpate the radial pulse. A colleague can assess the radial pulse while you assesses the apical.	Determines if a pulse deficit (radial pulse is slower than apical) exists. Deficit indicates that ineffective contractions of the heart fail to send pulse waves to the periphery.

Table 10-8 Heart Sounds According to Auscultatory Area

	AORTIC	PULMONIC	SECOND PULMONIC	MITRAL	TRICUSPID
Pitch	$S_1 < S_2$	$S_1 < S_2$	$S_1 < S_2$	$S_1 < S_2$	$S_1 < S_2$
Loudness	$S_1 < S_2$	$S_1 < S_2$	$S_1 < S_2$*	$S_1 > S_2$†	$S_1 > S_2$
Duration and others	$S_1 > S_2$	$S_1 > S_2$	$S_1 > S_2$	$S_1 > S_2$	$S_1 > S_2$

Modified from Seidel HM and others: *Mosby's guide to physical examination,* ed 4, St. Louis, 1999, Mosby.
*S_1 is relatively louder in second pulmonic area than in aortic area.
†S_1 may be louder in mitral area than in tricuspid area.

Table 10-9 Common Types of Dysrhythmias

DEFINITION	CAUSE
Sinus dysrhythmia: Pulse rate changes during respiration, increasing at peak of inspiration and declining during expiration.	Blood is momentarily trapped in lungs during inspiration, causing fall in heart's stroke volume.
Sinus tachycardia: Pulse rhythm is regular, but rate is accelerated to more than 100 beats/min.	Exercise, emotional stress, and caffeine or alcohol ingestion are common factors that cause increased firing of sinoatrial node.
Sinus bradycardia: Pulse rhythm is regular, but rate is slower than normal at 40 to 60 beats/min.	Sinoatrial node fires less frequently. This is common in well-conditioned athletes and with use of antidysrhythmic medications.
Premature ventricular contraction: Premature beat occurs before regularly expected heart contraction.	Ventricle contracts prematurely because of electrical impulse bypassing normal conduction pathway. It may occur so early that it is difficult to detect as second beat. It may be followed by a pause.
Atrial fibrillation: Rapid, random contractions of atria cause irregular ventricular beats at 130 to 150 beats/min.	Atria discharge very rapidly, with some impulses not reaching ventricles. This condition occurs in rheumatic heart disease and mitral stenosis. It causes reduced cardiac output.

STEP	RATIONALE
14. Continue to auscultate for extra heart sounds at each site. If any abnormal sounds are heard, note pitch, loudness, duration, and timing (when in relation to the cardiac cycle). Note location on the chest wall.	Abnormal sounds include murmurs. Characteristics of murmurs help to identify contributing factors.
a. Use the bell of the stethoscope and listen for low-pitched extra heart sounds such as S_3 and S_4 gallops, clicks, and rubs. S_3, or a ventricular gallop, occurs just after S_2 at the end of ventricular diastole. It may sound like "lub-dub-ee" or "Ken-tuc-ky." S_4, or an atrial gallop, occurs just before S_1 or ventricular systole. It sounds like "dee-lub-dub" or "Ten-nes-see."	Gallops may be caused by premature rushes of blood into a ventricle that is stiff or dilated or an atrial contraction pushing against a ventricle that is not accepting blood.
b. Listen for clicks as short, high-pitched extra sounds.	Clicks are caused by abnormalities such as mitral valve prolapse or prosthetic valves.
c. With client leaning forward or lying on the left side, listen for **friction rubs** as squeaky or rubbing sounds. Instruct client to hold breath as you continue to listen.	Rubs may result from lungs or inflamed visceral and parietal layers of the pericardium of the heart rubbing against one another. If the sound is present only while the client is breathing, the origin of the rub is pulmonary rather than cardiac.
15. Auscultate for heart murmurs over each of the auscultation sites.	Murmurs are sustained swishing or blowing sounds heard at the beginning, middle, or end of systole or diastole. They are caused by increased blood flow through a normal valve, forward flow through a stenotic valve or into a dilated vessel or chamber, or backward flow through a valve that fails to close.
16. When a murmur is detected, listen carefully to note where the murmur can be heard best. Note the intensity of the murmur:	Intensity is related to rate of blood flow through the heart or the amount of blood regurgitated. A thrill is a continuous palpable sensation like the purring of a cat. A thrust is the upward lift felt when palpating the chest wall.
17. Note if the murmur is low, medium, or high in pitch, using the bell for low-pitched sounds.	Pitch depends on velocity of blood flow through the valves.
18. Assess carotid arteries: Have client remain in sitting position.	Allows easier mobility of neck to expose artery for inspection and palpation.
19. Inspect neck on both sides for obvious pulsations of artery. Ask client to turn head slightly away from artery being examined. Sometimes pulse wave can be seen.	Carotids are the only sites to assess quality of pulse wave (see illustration). Experience is required to evaluate wave in relation to events of cardiac cycle.

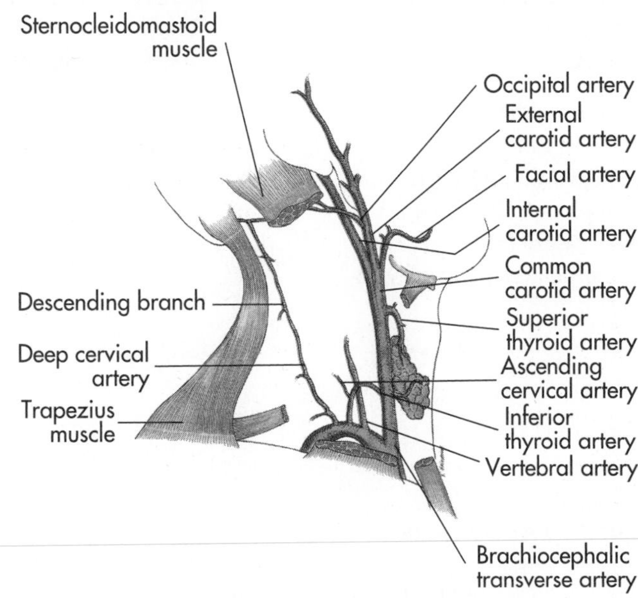

STEP **19** Anatomical position of carotid artery.

STEP	RATIONALE
20. Palpate each carotid artery separately with index and middle fingers around medial edge of sternocleidomastoid muscle. Ask client to raise chin slightly, keeping the head straight (see illustration). Note rate and rhythm, strength, and elasticity of artery. Also note if pulse changes as client inspires and expires.	If both arteries were occluded simultaneously, client could lose consciousness from reduced circulation to brain. Turning head improves access to artery. Change may indicate a sinus dysrhythmia.

• ***Critical Decision Point***

Do not vigorously palpate or massage the artery. Stimulation of carotid sinus may cause a reflex drop in heart rate and blood pressure.

STEP	RATIONALE
21. Place bell of stethoscope over each carotid artery, auscultating for blowing sound (bruit) (see illustration).	Narrowing of carotid artery's lumen by arteriosclerotic plaques causes disturbance in blood flow. Blood passing through narrowed section creates turbulence and emits blowing or swishing sound.

• ***Critical Decision Point***

Observing a client in the Fowler's position with an obvious visible jugular pulsation suggests need for immediate treatment. Observe for cyanosis (bluish discoloration) of lips, mouth, conjunctiva, or nail beds.

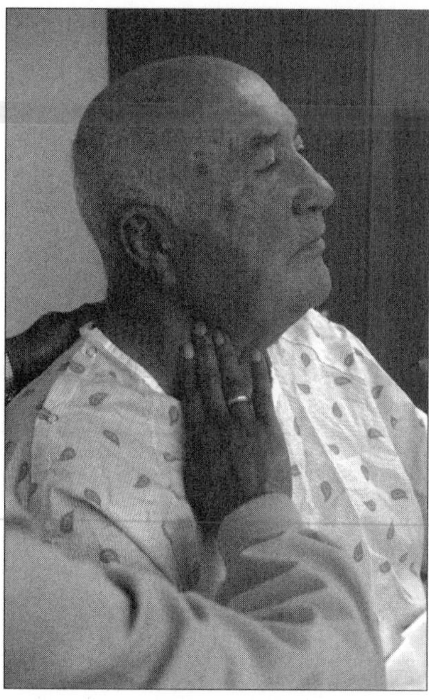

STEP **20** Palpate each carotid artery separately.

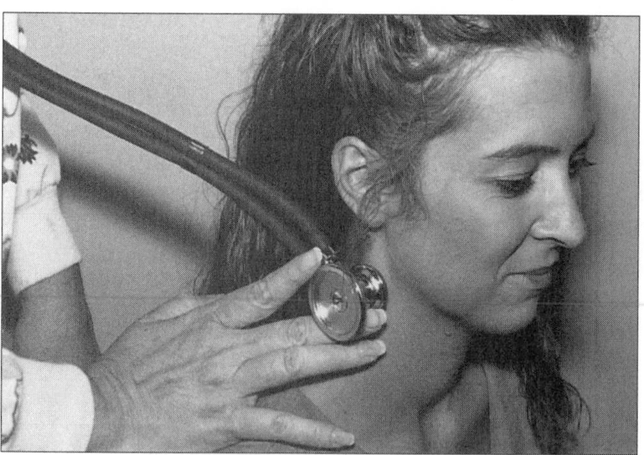

STEP **21** Auscultation for carotid artery bruit.

STEP	RATIONALE
22. To assess venous pressure have client sit at a 45-degree angle and slowly recline into the supine position, avoiding neck hyperextension or flexion. Measure the distance between the angle of Louis and the highest point of vein pulsation (see illustration).	Normal veins are flat when client is sitting, and pulsations become evident as client's head is lowered. A height of pulsation greater than 2.5 cm indicates fluid overload.

EVALUATION

STEP	RATIONALE
1. Compare findings with normal assessment characteristics of heart and vascular system.	Determines presence of abnormalities.
2. If heart sounds are not audible or if pulses are not palpable, ask another nurse to confirm assessment.	Abnormal assessment findings should be validated by another professional nurse.
3. Ask client to describe behaviors that increase risk for heart and vascular disease.	Demonstrates learning.

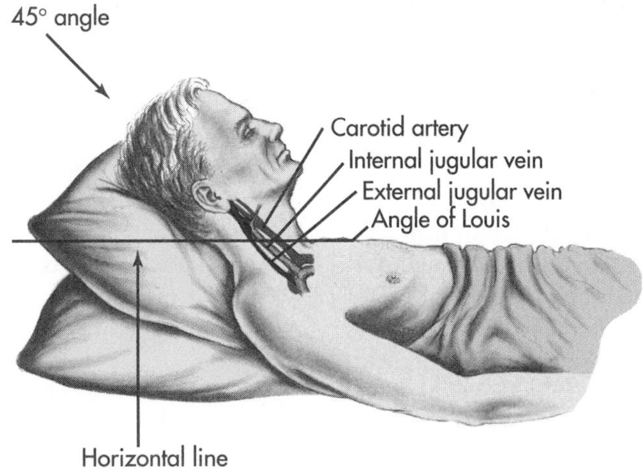

STEP **22** Position for assessment of jugular vein distention. (From Thompson JM and others: *Mosby's manual of clinical nursing,* ed 3, St. Louis, 1993, Mosby.)

Unexpected Outcomes and Related Interventions

- Abnormal findings that are new to the assessment data require physician notification. These include:
  - Pulsations, vibrations, or both are palpable. These are result of valvular problem, murmur, or both.
  - Point of maximal impulse is found to left of midclavicular line, which is the result of **cardiomegaly.**
  - Extra heart sounds S_3 or S_4 are auscultated. Extra sounds indicate atrial or ventricular gallop.
  - Murmur is auscultated. Impaired blood flow through heart may indicate need for immediate medical attention. Some murmurs are benign.
  - Jugular venous pressure is elevated. This is a sign of right-sided heart failure.
- Heart rate is irregular, with rate less than 60 beats per minute or more than 100 beats per minute.
  - Check blood pressure. If low, dysrhythmia may be contributing to inadequate cardiac output.
  - Observe for sensations or reports of dizziness or feeling "faint."
  - Notify physician.
- Pulse deficit is noted. There is risk for inadequate cardiac output.
  - Obtain vital signs.
  - Notify physician.
- Client is unable to explain risks for heart or vascular disease.
  - Additional education is needed.

Nursing Diagnosis

Defining characteristics from the assessment data may reveal the following nursing diagnoses for clients requiring this skill:

Activity intolerance
Ineffective peripheral tissue perfusion
Decreased cardiac output
Pain (acute, chronic)
Deficient knowledge regarding risks for heart disease

Related factors are individualized based on client's condition or needs.

Recording and Reporting

- Record all findings for heart and vascular assessment in nurses' notes or flow sheet.
- Record any instruction provided to client and client's response.
- Report immediately to physician any irregularities in heart function and indications of impaired arterial blood flow.
- Clients with dysrhythmias or pulse deficits may require an electrocardiogram or Holter monitor per physician's order.

Teaching Considerations

- Explain risk factors for heart disease: high dietary intake of saturated fat or cholesterol, lack of regular aerobic exercise, smoking, excess weight, stressful lifestyle, hypertension, and family history of heart disease.
- Refer client (if appropriate) to resources available for controlling or reducing risks (e.g., nutritional counseling, exercise class, and stress reduction programs).
- Explain that research shows clinical benefit from reducing dietary intake of cholesterol and saturated fats. Tell client

that about 70% to 75% of saturated fatty acids come from meats, poultry, fish, and dairy products and that the one-step diet recommended by the National Institutes of Health includes an intake of total fat less than 30% of calories, saturated fatty acids less than 10% of calories, and cholesterol less than 300 mg/100 ml (Krauss, 1996).

- Encourage client to have regular measurement of total blood cholesterol levels and triglycerides. More than one cholesterol measurement is needed to assess the blood cholesterol level accurately. Low-density lipoprotein (LDL) cholesterol is the major component of atherosclerotic plaques. Separate measurement of LDL cholesterol is wise in a client with high total blood cholesterol levels. An LDL cholesterol level of 160 mg/100 ml or higher indicates high risk.
- Advise client to avoid cigarette smoking because nicotine causes vasoconstriction.

Pediatric Considerations

- Perform cardiac assessment on infant or toddler while quiet, before more uncomfortable procedures.
- Point of maximal impulse is at third or fourth intercostal space at left midclavicular line in infant or child.
- It is not uncommon for children to have third heart sounds (S_3). Sinus dysrhythmia occurs normally in many children. (Wong and others, 1999).
- Children have louder, higher-pitched heart sounds because of their thin chest walls.

Gerontological Considerations

- Point of maximal impulse may be difficult to find in an older adult because anteroposterior diameter of the chest deepens.
- Accidental massage of the carotid sinus during palpation of the carotid artery can be a particular problem for older adults, causing a sudden drop in heart rate from vagal nerve stimulation (Lueckenotte, 2000).
- Older adults with hypertension may benefit from regular monitoring of blood pressure (daily, weekly, or monthly). Home monitoring kits are available. Teach client how to use them.

Skill 10-4 Assessing the Abdomen

Abdominal assessment is complex because of the multiple organs located within and near the abdominal cavity. This area of the body is associated with many health complaints, and many people are embarrassed by bowel or bladder dysfunction, reproductive or urinary elimination problems. Abdominal pain is one of the most common symptoms clients report when seeking medical care. Abdominal pain could be caused by alterations in organs such as the stomach, gallbladder, or intestines; or the pain may be the result of spinal or muscular injury. An accurate assessment requires matching the client's history with a careful assessment of the location of physical symptoms (Table 10-10).

To perform an effective abdominal assessment the nurse needs a detailed knowledge of the underlying structures involved, including the lower pelvis, kidneys, rectum, genitalia, liver, gallbladder, stomach spleen, intestines, and reproductive organs (Figure 10-4). An abdominal assessment is routine after abdominal surgery and for any client who has undergone invasive diagnostic tests of the gastrointestinal tract (see Chapter 42).

Table 10-10 Common Causes for Abdominal Pain

Conduction	Physical Alteration	Physical Signs and Symptoms
Appendicitis	Obstruction of the appendix associated with inflammation, perforation, and peritonitis.	Sharp pain directly over the irritated peritoneum 2-12 hours after onset. Often pain localizes at McBurney's point in the right lower quadrant between the anterior iliac crest and the umbilicus. Associated with rebound tenderness.
Cholecystitis	Obstruction of the cystic duct causing inflammation or distention of the gallbladder.	Murphy's sign: Apply gentle pressure below the right subcostal arch and below the liver margin. Sharp pain and inspiratory arrest occur when the client takes a deep breath (Wright, 1997).
Constipation	Disruption in normal bowel pattern, which may occur with narcotic use or inadequate fiber and fluid intake.	Generalized discomfort accompanied by distention and palpation of a hard mass in the left lower quadrant. Nausea and vomiting may begin after several days.
Crohn's disease	A chronic inflammatory lesion of the ileum. Cause is unknown.	Steady colicky pain in the right lower quadrant, with cramping, tenderness, flatulence, nausea, fever, and diarrhea. Often associated with bloody stools, weight loss, weakness, and fatigue.

Table 10-10 Common Causes for Abdominal Pain—cont'd

CONDUCTION	PHYSICAL ALTERATION	PHYSICAL SIGNS AND SYMPTOMS
Gastroenteritis	Inflammation of the stomach and intestinal tract.	Generalized abdominal discomfort accompanied by nausea, vomiting, diarrhea.
Intestinal obstruction	Blockage of the lumen of the intestine.	Colicky pain, nausea, vomiting, constipation, and abdominal distention. Bowel sounds are hyperactive with a rushing sound or absence of bowel sounds.
Pancreatitis	Inflammation of the pancreas associated with alcoholism and gallbladder disease.	Steady epigastric pain close to the umbilicus radiates to the back. Associated with abdominal rigidity and vomiting. Pain is unrelieved by vomiting.
Paralytic ileus	Obstruction of the small bowel that occurs after abdominal surgery or use of anticholinergic medications.	Generalized severe abdominal distention, nausea, and vomiting.
Peptic ulcers	Damage of gastrointestinal (GI) mucosa at any area of the GI tract. May be caused by bacterial infection or nonsteroidal antiinflammatory drugs. Believed to be unrelated to stress. Aggravated by smoking and excessive alcohol use.	Localized midepigastric pain with heartburn that develops 2 hours or more after meals, when the stomach is empty. Eating may relieve the pain. Acidic liquid, such as orange juice or coffee, may aggravate the pain (Daly, 1997).

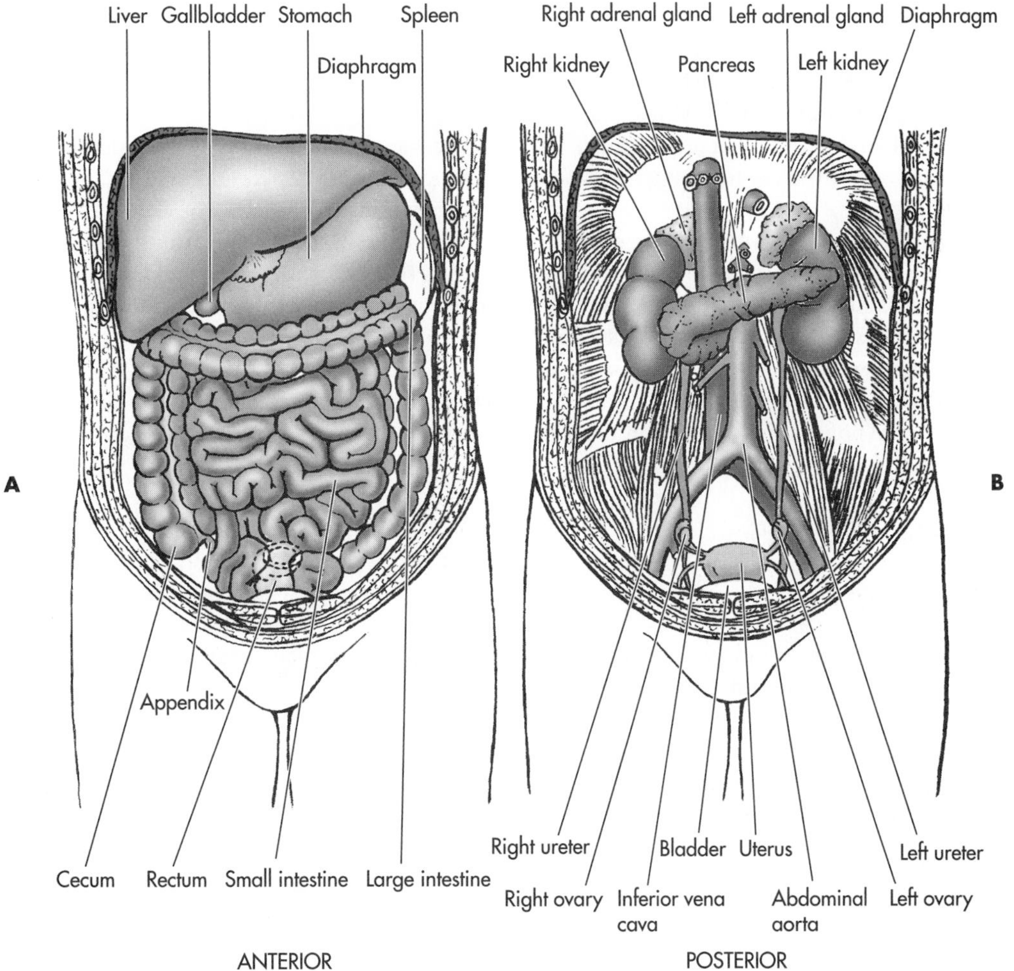

FIGURE **10-4** Location of organs in the abdomen. **A,** Anterior. **B,** Posterior. (From *Mosby's expert ten minute physical examinations,* St. Louis, 1997, Mosby.)

Delegation Considerations

This skill should not be delegated to assistive personnel. However, assistive personnel should know to report the development of abdominal pain or changes in the client's bowel habits or dietary intake.

The order of an abdominal assessment differs from that of other assessments. The nurse begins with inspection and follows with auscultation. It is important to auscultate before palpation and percussion since these maneuvers may alter the frequency and character of bowel sounds.

Equipment

- Stethoscope
- Tape measure
- Examination light
- Marking pen

Step	Rationale
Assessment	
1. If client has abdominal or low back pain, assess the character of pain in detail (location, onset, frequency, precipitating factors, aggravating factors, type of pain, severity, course).	Knowing pattern of characteristics of pain helps determine its source.
2. Carefully observe client's movement and position, such as: a. Lying still with knees drawn up. b. Moving restlessly to find a comfortable position. c. Lying on one side or sitting with knees drawn up to chest.	Positions assumed by the client may reveal nature and source of pain (e.g., peritonitis, renal stone, and pancreatitis).
3. Assess client's normal bowel habits: frequency of stools; character of stools; recent changes in character of stools; measures used to promote elimination, such as laxatives, enemas, dietary intake; and eating and drinking habits.	These data, compared with information from physical assessment, may help to identify cause and nature of elimination problems.
4. Determine if client has had abdominal surgery, trauma, or diagnostic tests of the gastrointestinal tract.	Surgical or traumatic alterations of abdominal organs may cause adhesions in expected findings (e.g., position of underlying organs). Diagnostic tests may change character of stool.
5. Assess if client has had any nausea, vomiting, or cramping, especially in last 24 hours.	Changes may indicate alterations in upper gastrointestinal tract (e.g., stomach or gallbladder) or lower colon.
6. Assess for difficulty in swallowing, belching, flatulence, bloody emesis (hematemesis), black or tarry stools (melena), heartburn, diarrhea, or constipation.	Indicative of gastrointestinal alterations.
7. Determine if client takes antiinflammatory medications (e.g., aspirin, steroids, and nonsteroidal antiinflammatory drugs), or antibiotics.	These pharmacological agents may cause gastrointestinal upset or bleeding.
8. Inquire about family history of cancer, kidney disease, alcoholism, hypertension, or heart disease.	Data may reveal risk for significant abdominal alterations. Chronic alcohol ingestion can cause gastrointestinal and liver problems.
9. Determine if female client is pregnant.	Pregnancy may cause nausea and vomiting, as well as changes in abdominal shape and contour.
10. Review client's history for health care occupation, hemodialysis, intravenous drug use, household or sexual contact with hepatitis B virus (HBV) carrier, sexually active (heterosexual person more than one sex partner in previous 6 months), sexually active homosexual or bisexual man, international traveler in area of high HBV prevalence.	These are risk factors for HBV exposure.
Planning	
1. **Expected outcomes** following completion of procedure:	
▪ Abdomen is soft and symmetrical with smooth and even contour. No mass, distention, or tenderness is palpable. No forceful visible pulsations are noted.	Normal findings.

STEP	RATIONALE
▪ Bowel sounds are active and audible in all four quadrants.	
▪ No **costovertebral angle (CVA) tenderness** is present.	No inflammation of kidney.
▪ Client denies discomfort or worsening of existing discomfort following examination.	Nurse uses proper examination procedures.
▪ Client is able to list warning signs of colon cancer.	Demonstrates learning.

IMPLEMENTATION

STEP	RATIONALE
1. Prepare client:	
a. Ask if client needs to empty bladder or defecate.	Palpation of full bladder can cause discomfort and feeling of urgency and make it difficult for client to relax.
b. Keep upper chest and legs draped.	Maintains client's comfort during examination, promoting relaxation.
c. Be sure that room is warm.	Promotes clients' comfort.
d. Expose area from just above the xiphoid process down to the symphysis pubis.	Provides full visualization of abdomen.
e. Have client lie supine or in a dorsal recumbent position with arms down at sides and knees slightly bent. A small pillow may be placed under client's knees.	Placing the arms under the head or keeping knees fully extended can cause the abdominal muscles to tighten. Tightening of muscles prevents adequate palpation.

• ***Critical Decision Point***

Observe respirations as position is changed. If abdomen is distended lying flat may result in increased respiratory difficulty due to pressure on the diaphragm (Daly, 1997).

STEP	RATIONALE
f. Maintain conversation during assessment except during auscultation. Explain steps calmly and slowly.	Client's ability to relax during assessment improves accuracy of findings.
g. Ask client to point to tender areas.	Painful areas are assessed last. Manipulation of body part can increase client's pain and anxiety and make remainder of assessment difficult to complete.
2. Identify landmarks that divide abdominal region into quadrants; from the tip of xiphoid process to symphysis pubis crosses line intersecting umbilicus, dividing abdomen into four equal sections (see illustration).	Location of findings by common reference point helps successive examiners to confirm findings and locate abnormalities. Normal ventilation involves rhythmic movement of abdomen as diaphragm descends and rises and a slight pulsation of aorta with each beat of systole.

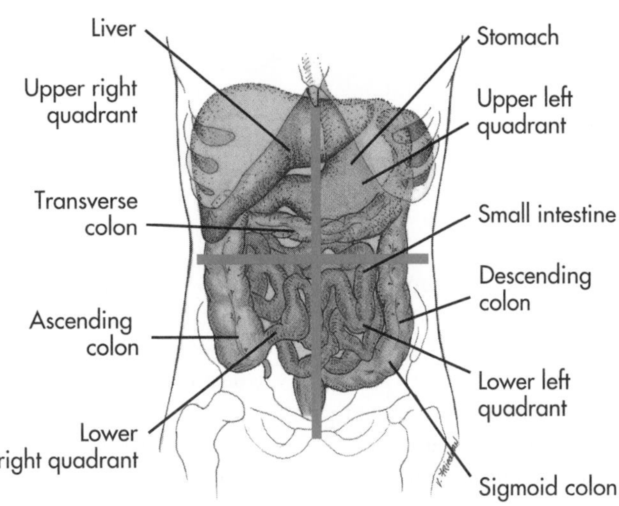

STEP **2** Division of abdomen into quadrants.

Step	Rationale
3. Inspect skin of abdomen's surface for color, scars, venous patterns, rashes, lesions, silvery white striae (stretch marks), and artificial openings. Observe lesions for characteristics described in Skill 10-1.	Scars reveal evidence that client has had past trauma or surgery. Striae indicate stretching of tissue from growth, obesity, pregnancy, ascites, or edema. Venous patterns may reflect liver disease (portal hypertension). Artificial openings indicate bowel or urinary diversion (see Chapter 26).
4. If bruising is noted, ask if client self-administers injections (e.g., heparin or insulin).	Frequent injections can cause bruising and hardening of underlying tissues.

- ***Critical Decision Point***

Bruising may also indicate physical abuse, accidental injury, or bleeding disorders.

Step	Rationale
5. Inspect the contour, symmetry, and surface motion of the abdomen. Note any masses, bulging, or distention. (Flat abdomen forms a horizontal plane from xiphoid process to symphysis pubis. Round abdomen protrudes in convex sphere from horizontal plane. Concave abdomen sinks into muscular wall. All are normal.)	Changes in symmetry or contour may reveal underlying masses, fluid collection, or gaseous distention. An everted (pouch extends outward) umbilicus may indicate distention. A hernia can also cause the umbilicus to protrude upward.
6. If abdomen appears distended, note if distention is generalized. Look at the flanks on each side.	Distention may be caused by the six Fs (fat, flatus, feces, fluids, fibroid, and fetus). If gas causes distention, flanks do not bulge. If fluid causes distention, flanks bulge. Tumor may cause a more unilateral bulging or distention. Pregnancy causes symmetrical bulge in lower abdomen.
7. If distention is suspected, measure size of abdominal girth by placing tape measure around abdomen at level of umbilicus (see illustration). Use the marking pen to indicate where tape measure was applied.	Consecutive measurements will show any increase or decrease in abdominal distention. All subsequent measurements are taken at same level of umbilicus to provide objective means to evaluate changes. A water-based pen can be used to make a mark on abdomen for subsequent measurements.

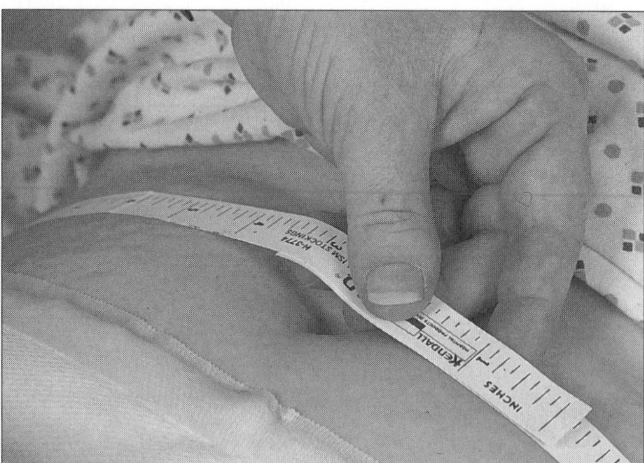

STEP **7** Measuring abdominal girth at the level of the umbilicus.

Step	Rationale
8. If nasogastric or intestinal tube is connected to suction, turn off momentarily.	Sound of suction machine obscures bowel sounds.
9. To auscultate bowel sounds place the diaphragm of the stethoscope lightly over each of the four abdominal quadrants. Ask client not to talk. Listen until repeated gurgling or bubbling sounds are heard in each quadrant (minimum of once in 5 to 20 seconds). Describe sounds as normal, hyperactive, hypoactive or absent. Listen 5 minutes over each quadrant before deciding that bowel sounds are absent.	Normal bowel sounds occur irregularly every 5 to 15 seconds. Absence of sounds indicate cessation of gastric motility. Hyperactive bowel sounds not related to hunger or a recent meal may indicate diarrhea or early intestinal obstruction. Hypoactive or absent bowel sounds may indicate paralytic ileus or peritonitis (Daly, 1997). It is common for bowel sounds to be hypoactive postoperatively for 24 hours or more, especially following abdominal surgery.

STEP	RATIONALE

- ***Critical Decision Point***

Severe paralytic ileus may be accompanied by nausea and vomiting, increasing distention, and inability to pass flatus.

10. Place the bell of the stethoscope over the epigastric region of the abdomen and each quadrant. Auscultate for vascular (whooshing) sounds.

Determines presence of turbulent blood flow (bruit) through thoracic or abdominal aorta.

- ***Critical Decision Point***

If aortic bruit is auscultated, suggesting presence of an aneurysm, stop assessment and notify physician immediately. Do not percuss or palpate a suspected area where a bruit is heard.

11. With client supine gently percuss each of four abdominal quadrants systematically. Note areas of tympany and dullness.

Reveals presence of air or fluid in stomach and intestines. Normal percussion is tympanic because of swallowed air in gastrointestinal tract. Presence of fluid or underlying masses is revealed by dull percussion.

12. To determine if distention is caused by fluid or air, percuss for a fluid wave:
    a. Ask another person to assist by pressing gently and firmly at the midline of the abdomen (see illustration).
    b. Place your fingertips along the sides of the lower abdomen in the lumbar region and thrust quickly into the client's side with your dominant hand, keeping the nondominant hand in place.
    c. Feel for a fluid wave with the nondominant hand.

If no fluid wave is felt the distention is caused by air. Presence of a fluid wave indicates ascites, found in cirrhosis, peritonitis, metastatic carcinoma, ovarian carcinoma, and pancreatitis. Ascites from liver congestion is often accompanied by jaundice, pruritus, dependent edema, and enlarged superficial abdominal veins (Daly, 1997).

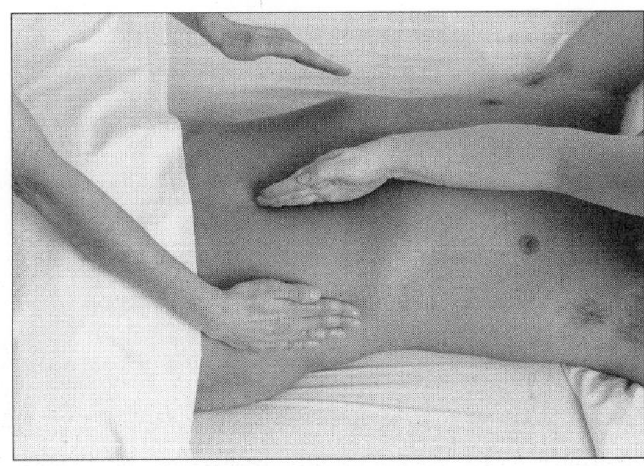

STEP **12a** Testing for fluid wave.

13. Ask client if abdomen feels unusually tight and determine if this is a recent development.

Continued sensation of fullness helps to detect distention. A feeling of fullness after a heavy meal causes only temporary destention. Tightness is not felt with obesity.

14. With client sitting, gently but firmly percuss over each costovertebral angle along scapular lines (see illustration *A*). Use ulnar surface of fist to percuss directly against client's skin or indirectly by placing nondominant hand flat against costovertebral angle and percuss with dominant hand (see illustration *B*). Note if client experiences pain.

Determines presence of kidney inflammation.

15. Lightly palpate over each abdominal quadrant, laying the palm of the hand with fingers extended and approximated lightly on the abdomen. Keep the palm and forearm horizontal. The pads of the fingertips depress the skin approximately 1 cm ($\frac{1}{2}$ inch) in a gentle dipping motion (see illustration).

Detects areas of localized tenderness, degree of tenderness, and presence and character of underlying masses. Palpation of sensitive area causes guarding (voluntary tightening of underlying abdominal muscles).

    a. Note muscular resistance, distention, tenderness, and superficial masses or organs while observing client's face for signs of discomfort.

Client's verbal and nonverbal cues may indicate discomfort from tenderness. Firm abdomen may indicate active obstruction with fluid or gas building up.

    b. Note if abdomen is firm or soft to touch.

Soft abdomen is normal or reveals that obstruction is resolving.

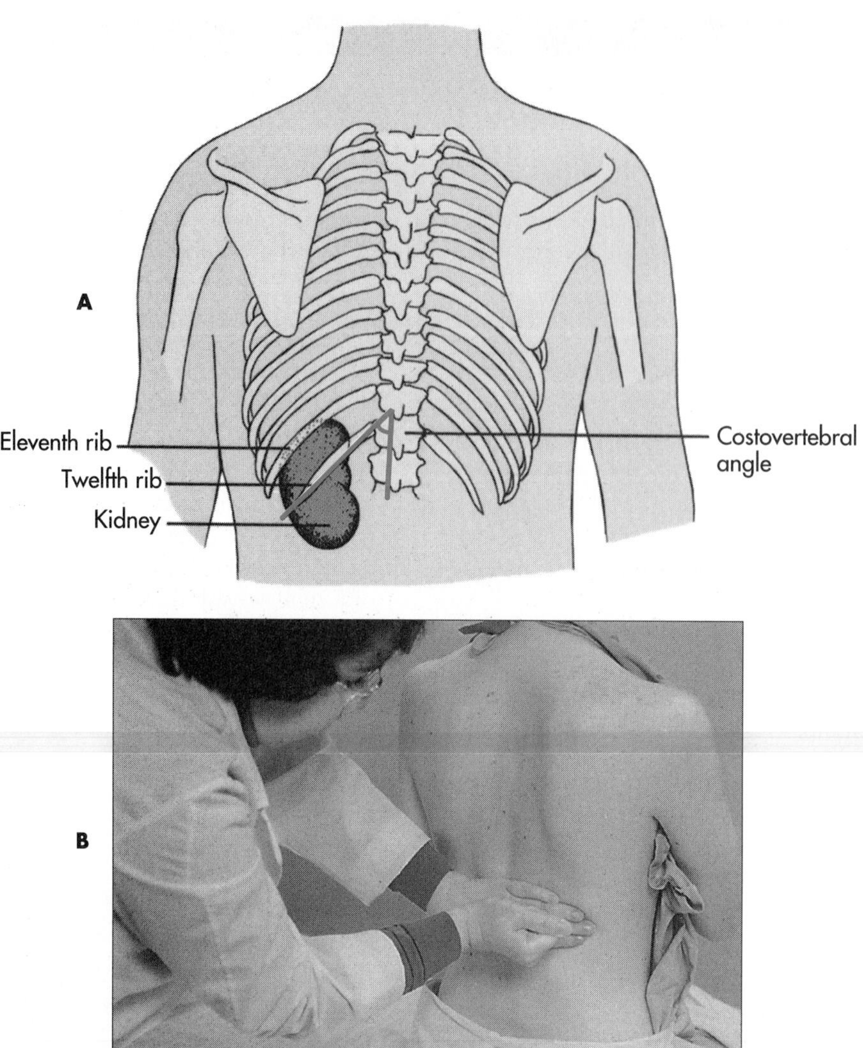

STEP **14** **A,** Assessing for CVA tenderness. **B,** Percussion of the kidney. (From Seidel HM and others: *Mosby's guide to physical examination,* ed 4, St. Louis, 1999, Mosby.)

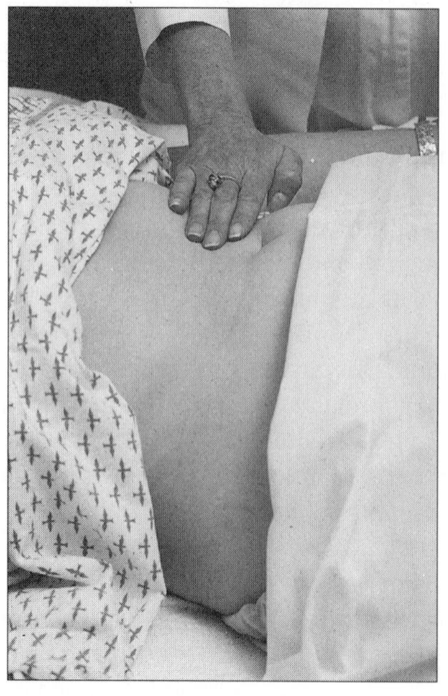

STEP **15** Light palpation of the abdomen.

STEP	RATIONALE
16. Just below umbilicus and above symphysis pubis, palpate for a smooth, rounded mass. While applying light pressure, ask if client has sensation of need to void.	Detects presence of dome of distended bladder.

- ***Critical Decision Point***

  Routinely check for distended bladder if client has been unable to void, client has been incontinent, or an indwelling Foley catheter is not draining well.

STEP	RATIONALE
17. If masses are palpated, note size, location, shape, consistency, tenderness, mobility, and texture.	Descriptive characteristics help to reveal type of mass.
18. When tenderness is present, press one hand slowly and deeply into the involved area and then let go quickly. Note if pain is aggravated.	Tests for rebound tenderness. Results are positive if pain increases.
19. Perform deep palpation, being sure the client is relaxed. Depress the palm and fingers approximately 2.5 to 7.5 cm (1 to 3 in) into the abdomen (see illustration).	Detects less obvious masses and delineates abdominal organs.

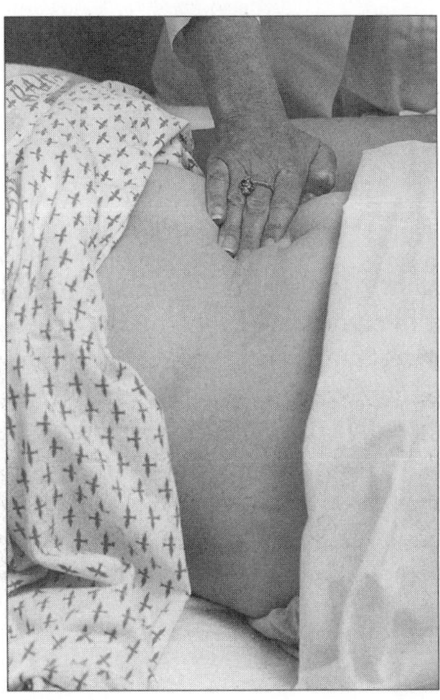

STEP **19** Deep palpation of the abdomen.

EVALUATION

▪ Compare assessment findings with normal assessment characteristics of abdomen.	Determines presence of abnormalities.
▪ Ask client to describe signs and symptoms of colon cancer.	Demonstrates learning.

UNEXPECTED OUTCOMES AND RELATED INTERVENTIONS

- Abdomen is asymmetrical, with palpable mass, and dull to percussion.
  - Report to the physician because findings may indicate enlarged liver, spleen, or tumor.
- Abdomen protrudes symmetrically, with skin taut, client complains of tightness, and/or bowel sounds are absent. Gastrointestinal motility has ceased. Client is vomiting.
  - Keep client on nothing by mouth (NPO) status, and encourage ambulation.
  - Notify physician.
    - Gastric decompression may become necessary.
- Hyperactive bowel sounds are evident with gastrointestinal motility. Commonly they result from anxiety, diarrhea, overuse of laxatives, inflammation of the bowel, or reaction of the intestines to certain foods.
  - Client may need to be NPO.
    - Client may need antidiarrheal medication.
- Rebound abdominal tenderness is found. Results from peritoneal irritation (e.g., appendicitis, or pancreatitis) (Wright, 1997).
  - Avoid palpating area.
  - Notify physician if this is a new finding.
    - Place client on NPO status.

- Bladder is palpable over symphysis pubis. Bladder is distended.
  - Facilitate voiding.
    - If unable to void, urinary catheterization may be necessary.
- Internal organs (liver, spleen) are enlarged.
  - Notify physician.
  - Do not continue to palpate area.
    - Place client on NPO status.
- Abdominal girth is increased, accompanied by a fluid wave. Fluid has built up within peritoneal cavity.
  - Notify physician.
  - Place client on NPO status.
- Client is unable to describe signs and symptoms of colon cancer.
  - Additional education is necessary.

Nursing Diagnosis

Defining characteristics from the assessment data may reveal the following nursing diagnoses for clients requiring this skill:

Imbalanced nutrition: less than body requirements
Constipation
Diarrhea
Pain (acute, chronic)
Anxiety

Related factors are individualized based on client's condition or needs.

Recording and Reporting

- Record results of assessment in nurses' notes or flow sheet.
- Record content of any client instruction.
- Report serious abnormalities, such as absent bowel sounds, presence of mass, or acute pain, to nurse in charge and physician.

Teaching Considerations

- Long-term progressive weight loss (late symptom), change in bowel habits, and blood in stools are signs of colon cancer.
- Explain that factors such as diet, regular exercise, limited use of over-the-counter drugs causing constipation, establishment of regular elimination schedule, and good fluid intake promote normal bowel elimination (see Chapter 25).
- Caution client about dangers of excessive use of laxatives or enemas.
- If client has acute pain, explain activities or positions to avoid.
- Explain to client the need to have a controlled weight reduction program when attempting to lose weight.
- If client is a health care worker or has contact with blood or body fluids of affected persons, encourage client to receive series of three hepatitis B vaccine doses.

Pediatric Considerations

- Most common palpable mass in child is feces, usually felt in right lower quadrant (Wong and others, 1999).
- Have a child stand erect and then lie supine during inspection of abdominal surface. Normal abdomen of infants and young children is cylindrical in erect position and flat in supine position.
- In infants and children skin is usually taut and without wrinkles or creases.

Gerontological Considerations

- Older adult often lacks abdominal tone; underlying organs are more easily palpable.
- A weakened intestinal musculature and decreased peristalsis affect the large intestine.
- Constipation along with nausea, flatulence, and heartburn are common.
- Stress to older adults importance of adequate fluid intake, regular exercise, and a diet with at least 4 servings daily of fresh fruit and vegetables and high-fiber foods to promote normal defecation.

Skill 10-5 Assessing the Extremities and Peripheral Circulation

The nurse's assessment of the extremities and peripheral circulation uses inspection and palpation. Initial assessment involves a general inspection of gait, posture, and body position. A more thorough assessment of major bone, joint, and muscle groups is indicated in the presence of abnormalities. Much of the assessment can be performed while the nurse examines other body systems; for example, while assessing neck structures, the nurse can also assess neck range of motion

(ROM). It is effective for the nurse to integrate assessment into routine activities of care, for example, while bathing or positioning the client. Assessment is especially important when the client reports pain or loss of joint or muscle function. Neurological assessment is often conducted simultaneously because muscles may be weakened as a result of nerve involvement.

Prolonged illness or immobility may result in muscle weakness and **atrophy.** Hospitalized clients may experience altered peripheral circulation as a result of high or low blood pressure or constriction of the extremities with dressings or a cast (Elkin, Perry, and Potter, 2000).

Inadequate tissue perfusion results in an inadequate delivery of oxygen and nutrients to cells, a condition called ischemia. This can be caused by constriction of vessels or by occlusion (blockage) from clot formation. The effects of ischemia depend on the duration of the problem and the metabolic needs of the tissues. Ischemia results in pain. If lack of oxygen to tissues is unrelieved, tissue necrosis (death) occurs. An embolus is a blood clot that breaks loose and travels through the circulation. If the clot obstructs circulation to the lungs or the brain, it can be life threatening.

Delegation Considerations

Physical examination of musculoskeletal function should not be delegated to assistive personnel. However, assistive personnel may assist clients with ambulation, transfer, and positioning and should recognize problems with gait and ROM. Assistive personnel should be instructed to report any problems noted in ROM or muscle strength and precautions relating to the importance of gentleness during ROM to avoid forcing a joint beyond the client's current ROM. Assistive personnel should be informed of clients at risk for falls and should be provided with instructions for clients with muscular weakness who require special assistance with transfer and ambulation.

Equipment

- Tape measure
- Doppler
- Reflex hammer

Step	Rationale
Assessment	
1. Review client history (particularly with female clients) for heavy alcohol use, cigarette smoking, constant dieting, calcium intake less than 500 mg daily, thin and light body frame, females who have never been pregnant, occurrence of menopause before age 45, postmenopause, bilateral oophorectomy (ovary removal), family history of osteoporosis, or European American, Asian, or Native American race.	These are risk factors for osteoporosis.
2. Ask client to describe history of bone, muscle, or joint function (e.g., recent fall, trauma, lifting heavy objects, bone or joint disease with sudden or gradual onset) and location of alteration.	Assists in assessing nature of musculoskeletal problem.
3. Assess nature and extent of client's pain: location, duration, severity, predisposing and aggravating factors, relieving factors, and type of pain. If pain or cramping is reported in the lower extremities, ask if it is relieved or aggravated by walking. Assess the distance walked and characteristics of pain before, during, and after activity.	Alterations in bone, joints, or muscle are frequently accompanied by pain, which has implications not only for comfort but also ability to perform activities of daily living. Pain caused by certain vascular conditions tends to increase with activity.
4. Determine how client's alteration influences ability to perform activities of daily living (e.g., bathing, feeding, dressing, toileting, and ambulating) and social functions (e.g., household chores, work, recreation, sexual activities).	Level of nursing care is determined by extent to which client can perform self-care. Type and degree of restriction in continuing social activities influence topics for client education.
5. Assess height decrease of woman older than 50 by subtracting current height from recall of height at age 30.	A loss of height more than 2 inches from the height at age 30 strongly suggests the presence of osteoporosis (American Medical Directors Association, 1998).

STEP	RATIONALE

PLANNING

1. **Expected outcomes** following completion of procedure:
   - Client demonstrates erect posture, strong grasp, steady gait, with arms swinging freely at side. — Indicates normal alignment, gait, and muscle strength.
   - There is bilateral symmetry of extremities in length, circumference, alignment, position, and skinfolds (Seidel and others, 1999).
   - Full active ROM is present in all joints with good muscle tone and absence of contractures, spasticity, or muscular weakness. — Indicates normal ROM of joints.
   - Peripheral pulses are equal and strong (3+), extremities are warm and pink, with capillary refill less than 3 seconds. There is no dependent edema. — Peripheral circulation intact.

IMPLEMENTATION

1. Prepare client:
   a. Integrate musculoskeletal assessment during other portions of physical assessment or during nursing care. As in assessment of **integument,** nurse can conduct assessment of musculoskeletal system as client moves in bed, rises from chair, walks, or goes through movements required during complete physical examination. — The nurse can conduct assessment of the musculoskeletal system as client moves in bed, rises from chair, or goes through movements required during complete physical examination. Integration saves time for both nurse and client.
   b. Plan time for short rest periods during assessment. — Movement of body parts and various maneuvers may fatigue client. It is especially important to consider rest periods with older adult and very ill clients.
2. Observe ability to use arms and hands for grasping objects (see illustration). — Assess coordination and muscle strength.
3. Assess muscle strength of upper extremities by applying gradual increase in pressure to muscle group. — Upper and lower extremity on client's dominant side is normally stronger than that on nondominant side. Pain, rather than weakness, may cause reduced muscle strength; however, long-term pain can lead to muscle weakening.

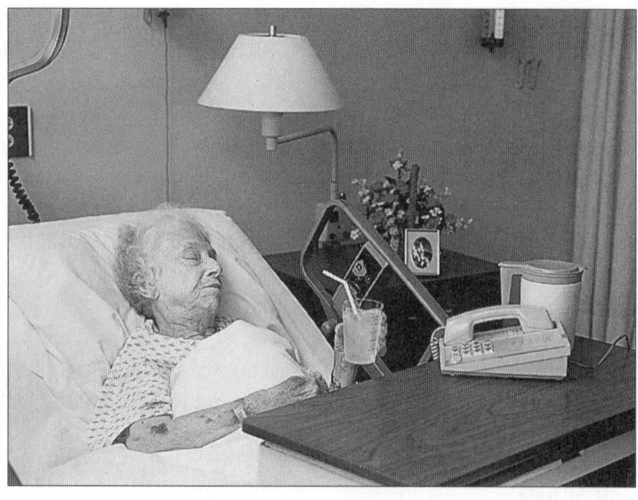

STEP **2** Observe use of arms and hands.

STEP	RATIONALE
4. To assess hand grasp strength, cross your hands, and have the client grasp the fingers of both of your hands and squeeze them as hard as possible. To avoid discomfort, the nurse may cross index and middle fingers (see illustration).	It is common for the client's dominant hand to be slightly stronger than the nondominant hand. By crossing hands clients' right hand grasps your right hand.

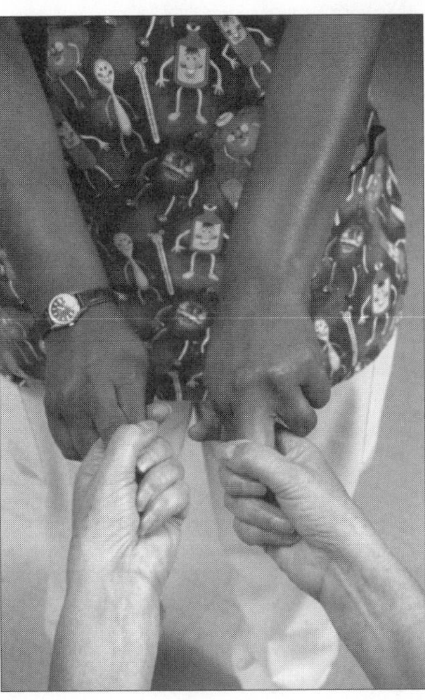

STEP 4 Assessing strength of hand grasps comparing sides.

STEP	RATIONALE
5. Have client resist pressure applied by attempting to move against resistance (e.g., flex elbow). Have client maintain resistance until told to stop. Compare symmetrical muscle groups. Note weakness, and compare right with left.	Compares symmetrical muscle groups for strength on the following scale. Rate muscle strength on scale of 0 to 5: Grade as follows: 0 No voluntary contraction 1 Slight contractility, no movement 2 Full range of motion, passive 3 Full range of motion, active 4 Full range of motion against gravity, some resistance 5 Full range of motion against gravity, full resistance
6. If muscle weakness is identified, measure muscle size with tape measure placed around body of muscle. Compare with same muscle on opposite side of body.	Indicates degree of atrophy.
7. Observe position for sitting, supine, prone, or standing. Muscles and joints should be exposed and free to move to allow for accurate measurement.	Each joint or muscle group may require different position for measurement.
8. Inspect gait as client walks and stands. Observe for foot dragging, shuffling or limping, balance, presence of obvious deformity in lower extremities, and position of the trunk in relation to the legs.	Gait is more natural if client is unaware of nurse's observation.
9. Stand behind client and observe postural alignment (position of hips relative to shoulders). Look sideways at cervical, thoracic, and lumbar curves (see illustration).	Abnormal curves of posture include lordosis (swayback, increased lumbar curvature), kyphosis (hunchback, exaggerated posterior curvature of thoracic spine), and scoliosis (lateral spinal curvature). Postural changes may indicate muscular, bone, or joint deformity; pain; or muscular fatigue. Head should be held erect.

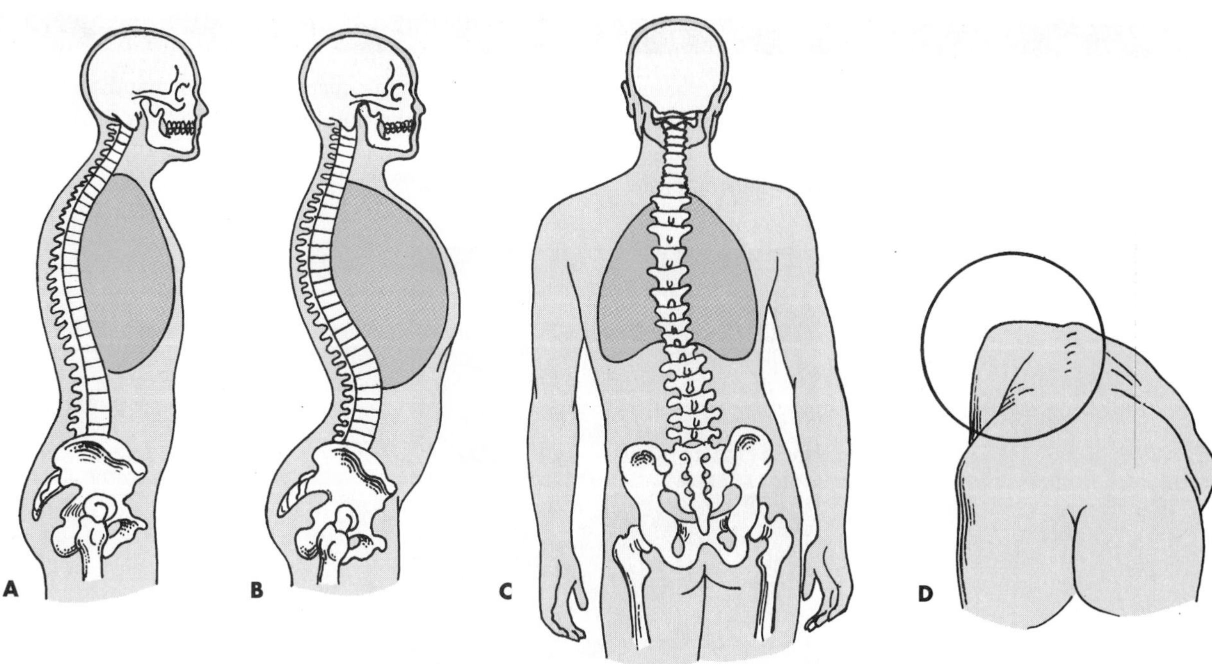

STEP 9 Spinal deformities. **A,** Kyphosis. **B,** Lordosis. **C,** Scoliosis. **D,** Scoliosis with client bending forwards.

STEP	RATIONALE
10. Make a general observation of the extremities. Look at overall size, gross deformity, bony enlargement, alignment, and symmetry.	General review helps to pinpoint areas requiring in-depth assessment.
11. Gently palpate bones, joints, and surrounding tissues in involved areas. Note any heat, tenderness, edema, or resistance to pressure.	May reveal changes resulting from trauma or chronic disease. Do not attempt to move joint when fracture is suspected or when joint is apparently "frozen" by lack of movement over a long period of time.
12. Ask client to put major joint through its full ROM (Table 10-11). Observe equality of motion in same body parts:	Assessment of client's normal ROM provides baseline for assessing later changes after surgery or inactivity. Clients with deformities, reduced mobility, joint fixation, or weakness may require passive motion assessment.
a. Active motion: (Client needs no support or assistance and is able to move joint independently.) Instruct client in moving each joint through its normal range. It may be necessary to demonstrate movements and ask client to mimic your movements.	Identifies muscle strength, as well as detecting altered strength or limited range of motion.
b. Passive motion (joint has full ROM but client does not have the strength to move it independently): Have client relax and move the same joints passively until the end of the range is felt. Support extremity at joint. Do not force the joint if there is pain or muscle spasm.	Determines ability to perform joint motion in the presence of muscle weakness. Forcing joint may cause injury and pain.
13. Palpate joint for swelling, stiffness, tenderness, and heat; note any redness.	Indicates acute or chronic inflammation. Range of motion may cause pain or injury.
14. Assess muscle tone in major muscle groups. Normal tone causes mild, even resistance to movement through entire ROM.	If muscle has increased tone (hypertonicity), any sudden movement of joint is met with considerable resistance. Hypotonic muscle moves without resistance. Muscle feels flabby.
15. Inspect lower extremities for changes in color and condition of the skin (Table 10-12). Note skin and nail texture, hair distribution, venous patterns, edema, and scars or ulcers. Compare skin color lying and standing.	Changes may reflect impaired peripheral circulation.
16. Palpate edematous areas, noting mobility, consistency, and tenderness.	Assists in determining extent of edema.

Table 10-11 Assessing Range of Motion (ROM)*

Body Part	Assessment Procedure	ROM
Upper Extremities		
Shoulders	Raise both arms to a vertical position at the sides of the head.	Flexion.
	Place both hands behind the neck, with elbows out to the sides.	External rotation and abduction.
	Place both hands behind the small of the back (internal rotation).	Internal rotation.
	Have client make small circles with hands with arms extended at shoulder level.	Circumduction.
Elbows	Bend and straighten the elbows.	Flexion and extension.
	Place hands at waist with elbows flexed.	
Wrist	Flex and extend wrist.	Flexion and extension.
	Bend wrist to radial then ulnar side—radial and ulnar deviation.	
	Turn palm upward, then downward.	Supination and pronation.
Hand	Make a fist with both hands.	Flexion and extension.
	Extend and spread fingers and thumb.	Adduction and abduction.
Lower Extremities		
Hips (with client supine)	With knees extended, raise one leg upward.	Flexion: Expect 90 degrees.
	Repeat with knee flexed.	
	Swing legs laterally.	Abduction: Expect 45 degrees. Adduction: Expect 30 degrees.
	With knee flexed hold the ankle and rotate the leg inward and outward.	Internal and external rotation: Expect 40-45 degrees.
Knees (with client sitting)	Raise the foot, keeping the knee in place.	Extension: Expect full extension and up to 15 degrees hyperextension.
Ankle	With foot held off the floor, point toes, then bring toes back toward the knee.	Plantar flexion: Expect 45 degrees Dorsiflexion: Expect 20 degrees.
	Turn foot inward and then outward.	Inversion and eversion: Expect to reach 5 degrees.
Toes	Bend toes down and back.	Expect to reach 40 degrees.

*This may be done actively by the client (AROM) or passively by the nurse (PROM).

Table 10-12 Comparison of Venous and Arterial Insufficiency

Assessment	Arterial	Venous
Pain	Burning, throbbing, cramping, increases with exercise	Aching, increases in evening and with dependent position
Paresthesia	Numbness, tingling, decreased sensation	None
Temperature/color	Cool to touch, pale when elevated	Warm, flushed, cyanotic, brown discolorations on ankles
Capillary refill	>3 seconds	Not applicable
Pulses	Diminished or absent	Present
Ulcerations	Deep, well defined at site of trauma or tips of toes	Shallow ulcers around ankles (chronic venous stasis); edema apparent

Step	Rationale
17. Assess for pitting edema by pressing area firmly with thumb for 5 seconds, then releasing. Depth of indentation determines severity (see illustration). 2 mm: 1+ edema 4 mm: 2+ edema 6 mm: 3+ edema 8 mm: 4+ edema	Edema results from fluid in tissues. Inadequate venous return causes edema in the sacrum if client is confined to bed or in the feet and ankles if sitting. In some settings a tape measure may be used to measure the circumference of the extremity (Galindo-Ciocon, 1995).

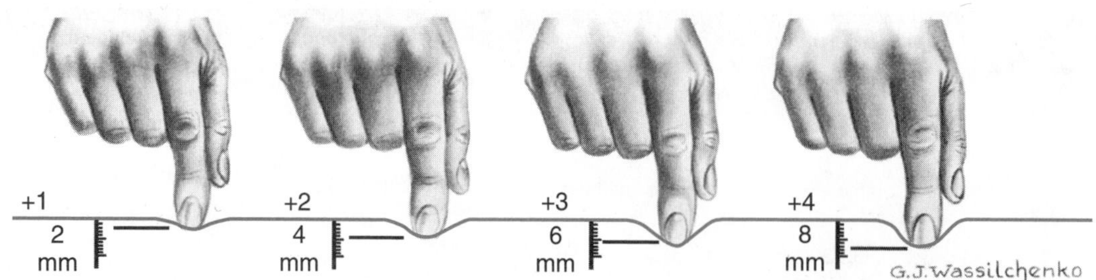

STEP 17 Pitting edema. (From Seidel HM and others: *Mosby's guide to physical examination,* ed 4, St. Louis, 1999, Mosby.)

STEP	RATIONALE
18. Grasp client's fingernail or toenail and note color of nail bed. Next, apply gentle, firm pressure to the nail bed. Release quickly, watching for color change. Circulation is restored and normally returns to pink color in less than 3 seconds.	Assess capillary refill. Cold environmental temperature, with vasoconstriction and vascular disease can delay refill. Local pressure from a cast or bandage may also deter refill.
19. Ask if the client experiences tenderness, and palpate for heat, firmness, or localized swelling of the calf muscle.	Signs of phlebitis or deep venous thrombosis (DVT). If there is a strong suspicion of DVT, testing for Homans' sign is contraindicated. Clients who have been immobilized for several days and those who have bone or joint disease, surgical correction of joint or bone, or pain are at risk for altered tissue perfusion (Breen, 2000).
20. If calf appears normal, test for Homans' sign by supporting the leg while flexing the foot in dorsiflexion (see illustration). Ask if the client experiences pain in the calf.	If pain is apparent, a positive Homans' sign is noted and the possibility of deep venous thrombosis needs to be considered. However, Homans' sign is absent in nearly half of known cases and may be present in other conditions as well (Breen, 2000).
21. Starting at the most distal part of each extremity, palpate each peripheral artery for equality, comparing side to side; elasticity of vessel wall: depress and release artery, noting ease with which it springs back to shape and strength of pulse (force of blood against arterial wall) using the following rating scale (Seidel and others, 1999). 0 No pulse palpable 1+ Pulse is difficult to palpate, weak and thready, and easy to obliterate 2+ Stronger than 1+, located with light pressure 3+ Easy to palpate and not easily obliterated 4+ Strong, bounds against fingertips, and cannot be obliterated	Comparison of both arteries allows nurse to determine any localized obstruction or disturbance in blood flow. Pulses should be symmetrical side to side. If asymmetry is noted, look for other factors related to impaired circulation.

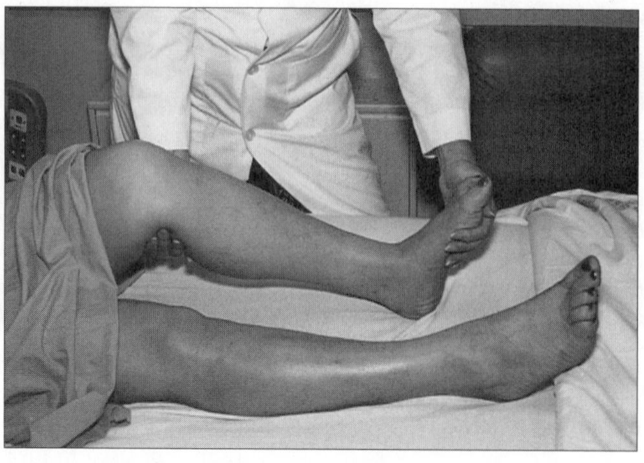

STEP 20 Dorsiflexion to test Homans' sign.

STEP	RATIONALE
22. Palpate radial pulse by lightly placing tips of first and second fingers in groove formed along radial side of forearm, lateral to flexor tendon of wrist (see illustration).	Pulse is relatively superficial and should not require deep palpation.
23. Palpate ulnar pulse by placing fingertips along ulnar side of forearm (see illustration).	Palpated when arterial insufficiency to hand is expected or when nurse assesses effects that radial occlusion (e.g., during arterial blood gas sampling) might have on circulation to hand (Chapter 41).
24. Palpate brachial pulse by locating groove between biceps and triceps muscles above elbow at antecubital fossa (see illustration). Place tips of first two fingers in muscle groove.	Artery runs along medial side of extended arm, requiring moderate palpation.
25. Have client lie supine with feet relaxed, and palpate dorsalis pedis pulse. Gently place fingertips between great and first toe; slowly move fingers along groove between extensor tendons of great and first toe until pulse is palpable (see illustration).	Artery lies superficially and does not require deep palpation. Pulse may be congenitally absent.

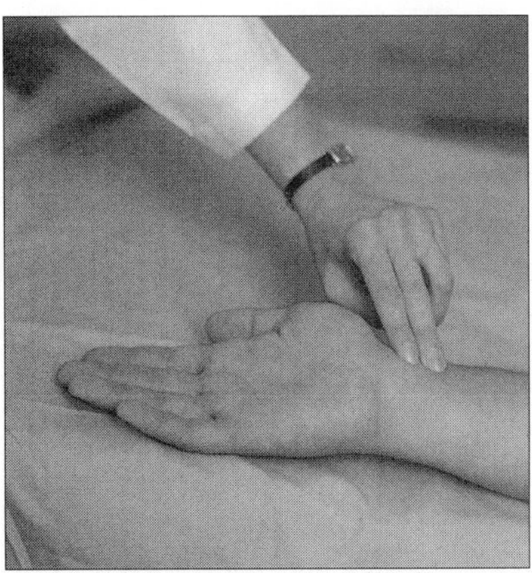

STEP 22 Palpation of radial pulse.

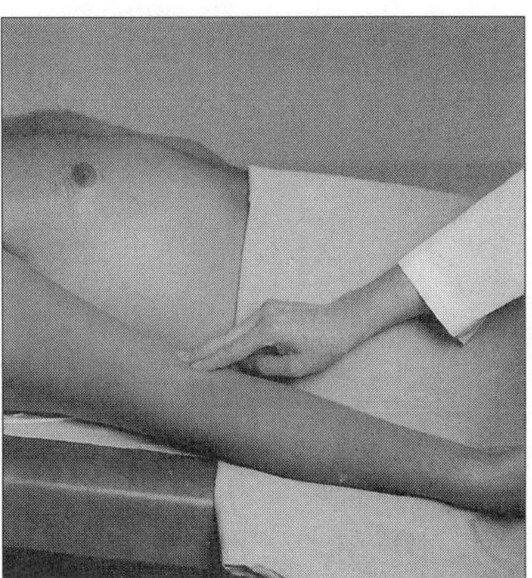

STEP 24 Palpation of brachial pulse.

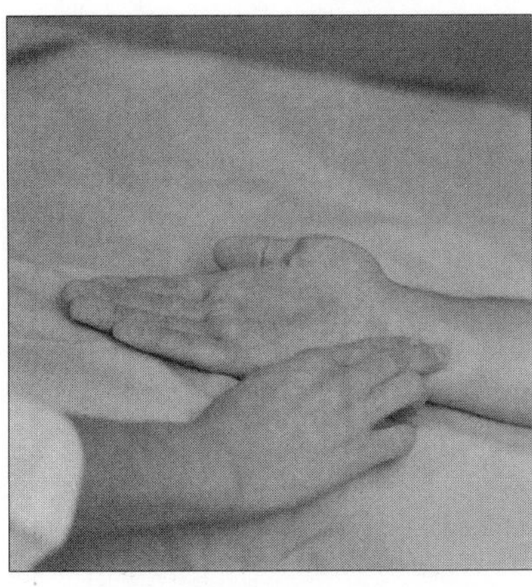

STEP 23 Palpation of ulnar pulse.

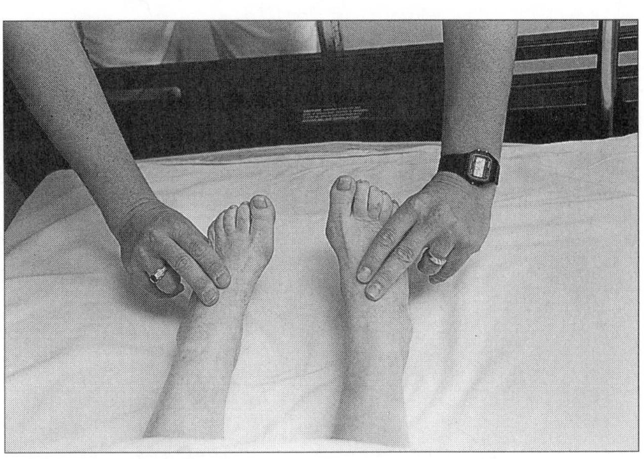

STEP 25 Palpation of pedal pulses.

Step	Rationale
26. If the pedal pulse is difficult to palpate pulse or it is not palpable, use a Doppler instrument over the pulse site: a. Apply conducting gel to the client's skin over the pulse site or onto transducer tip of probe. b. Turn doppler on. Gently apply ultrasound probe to the skin, altering angle until pulsation is audible. Adjust volume as needed (see illustration).	Doppler amplifies sounds, allowing nurse to hear low-velocity blood flow through peripheral arteries.
27. Palpate posterior tibial pulse by having client relax and slightly extend feet. Place fingertips behind and below medial malleolus (ankle bone) (see illustration).	Artery is easily palpable with foot relaxed.
28. Palpate popliteal pulse by having client slightly flex knee with foot resting on table or bed. Instruct client to keep leg muscles relaxed. Palpate deeply into popliteal fossa with fingers of both hands placed just lateral to midline. Client may also lie prone to achieve exposure of artery (see illustration).	Flexion of knee and muscle relaxation improve accessibility of artery. Popliteal pulse is one of the more difficult pulses to palpate.
29. With client supine, palpate femoral pulse by placing first two fingers over inguinal area below inguinal ligament, midway between pubic symphysis and anterosuperior iliac spine (see illustration). *If drainage or secretions are present, apply gloves.*	Supine position prevents flexion in groin area, which interferes with artery access.

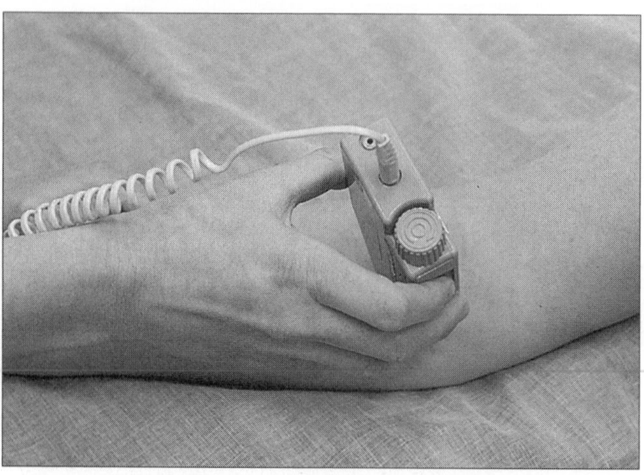

STEP **26b** Use of doppler for brachial pulse.

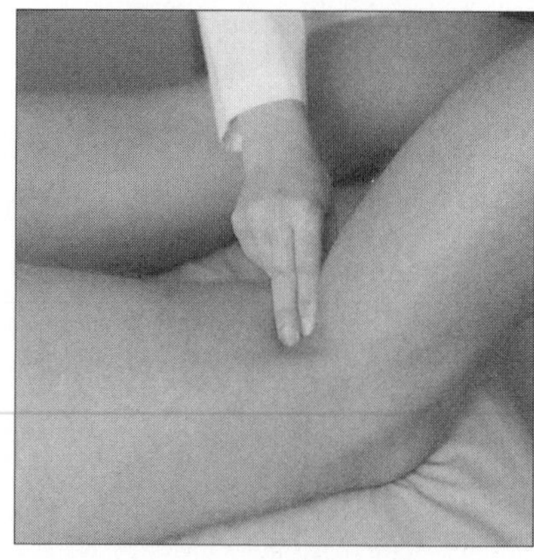

STEP **28** Palpation of popliteal pulse with client prone.

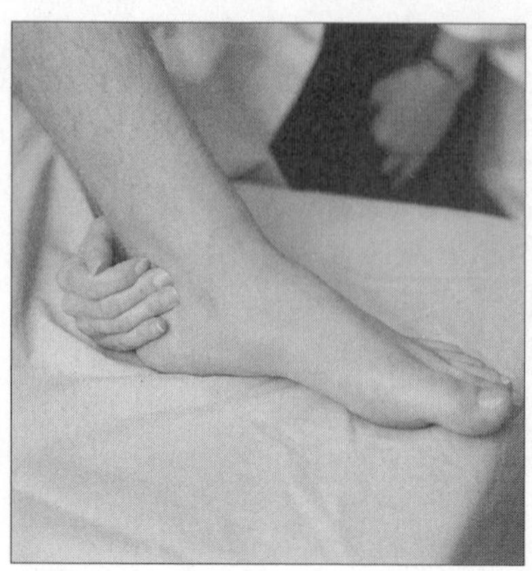

STEP **27** Palpation of posterior tibial pulse.

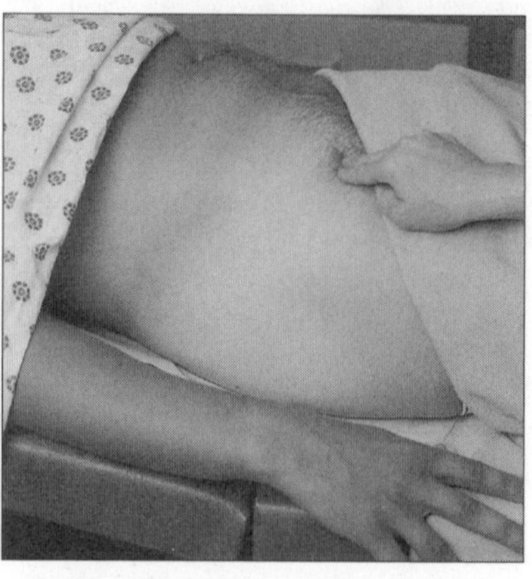

STEP **29** Palpation of femoral pulse.

STEP	RATIONALE
30. In clients with back pain or surgery, a cerebrovascular accident, or spinal cord compression it is appropriate to monitor deep tendon reflexes (DTR) (McHugh and McHugh, 1990). In many settings this is not part of the routine shift assessment.	Muscle spasticity and hyperactive reflexes may result from disorders such as stroke and paralysis. Diminished DTRs and muscle weakness may suggest lower motor neuron disorders such as amyotrophic lateral sclerosis (ALS) or Guillian-Barré syndrome.
31. If indicated, test DTR: For each reflex tested, compare sides and assign a grade on the following scale: 0 No response 1+ Sluggish or diminished response 2+ Normal, active, or expected response 3+ More brisk than expected; slightly hyperactive 4+ Very brisk; hyperactive, with clonus	Reflexes normally are equal bilaterally. Clonus is described as repeated spasms of repeated muscular contraction and relaxation. The severity of clonus is often noted based on counting the number of spasms.
a. Knee reflex: Palpate the patellar tendon just below the patella. Tap the pointed end of the reflex hammer briskly on the tendon. The normal response is knee extension (see illustration).	
b. Plantar response (Babinski's reflex): Using the handle end of the reflex hammer, stroke the lateral aspect of the sole, from the heel to the ball of the foot. The toes should flex inward and downward (see illustration).	This is usually considered abnormal in adults.
c. If Babinski's reflex is present, which is normal in a newborn, the great toe will dorsiflex, accompanied by fanning of the other toes.	
d. Ankle clonus: If reflexes seem hyperactive, testing ankle clonus is indicated. Support the knee in a slightly flexed position, and move the forefoot in a circular motion several times, ending with a sharp dorsiflexion of the foot. Maintain that position while watching and feeling for rhythmic oscillations (see illustration).	Sustained clonus with continued repeated movement indicates a pathologic condition.

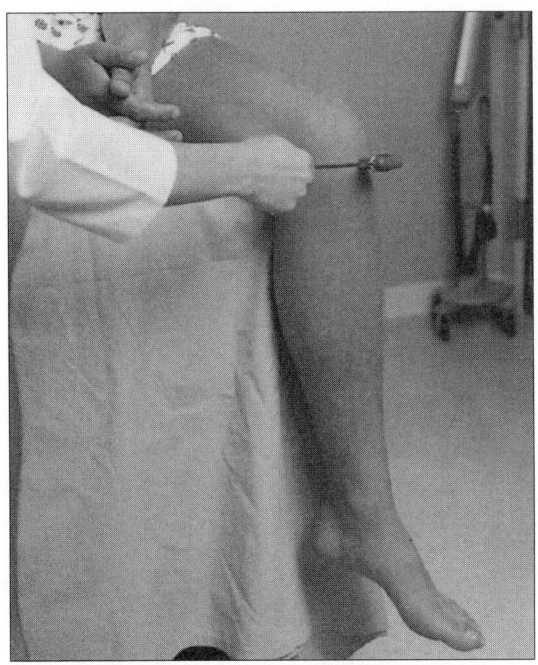

STEP **31a** Testing DTR with reflex hammer. (From *Mosby's expert ten minute physical examinations,* St. Louis, 1997, Mosby.)

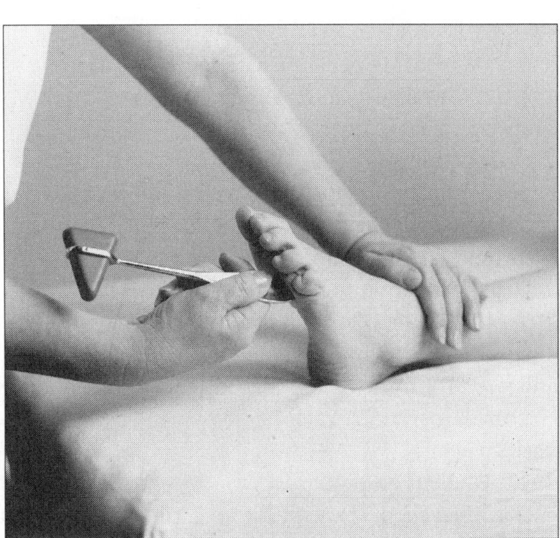

STEP **31b** Testing Babinski's reflex. (From *Mosby's expert ten minute physical examinations,* St. Louis, 1997, Mosby.)

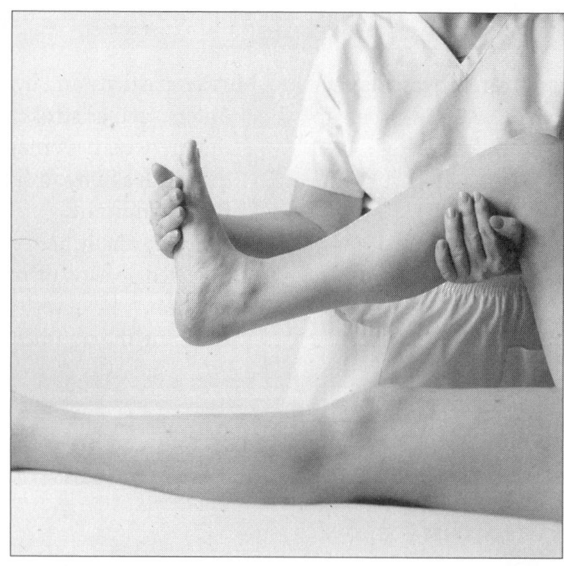

STEP **31d** Testing clonus. (From *Mosby's expert ten minute physical examinations,* St. Louis, 1997, Mosby.)

STEP	RATIONALE
EVALUATION	
1. Compare muscle strength and range of motion with previous shift assessment.	Determines presence of abnormalities.
2. Compare pulses and capillary refill bilaterally with previous shift assessment.	
3. Compare presence and extent of edema with previous shift assessment.	
4. Evaluate level of client's discomfort following procedure.	Determines if manipulation of musculoskeletal structures intensifies client's discomfort.

UNEXPECTED OUTCOMES AND RELATED INTERVENTIONS

- Previously palpable pedal pulses are diminished or absent, indicating circulatory compromise.
  - Notify physician.
  - Elevate extremity.
- Client's lower extremities have pale, cool, thin, and shiny skin, with reduced hair growth and thickened nails, indicating chronic arterial insufficiency.
  - Instruct client on proper foot care.
  - Refer to podiatrist for nail trimming.
  - Inspect feet for signs of impaired skin integrity.
- Joints are prominent, swollen, and tender with nodules or overgrowth of bone in distal joints, indicating signs of arthritis.
  - Instruct client on proper ROM.
  - Determine client's knowledge regarding antiinflammatory medications.
- Reduced ROM in one or more major joints—shoulder, elbow, wrist, fingers, knee, hip.
  - Assess for pain during movement, with joint unstable, stiff, painful, or swollen or with obvious deformity.
  - Notify physician.
  - Reduce mobility in extremity until cause of abnormal joint motion is determined.
- Client demonstrates weakness in one or more major muscle groups, or gait demonstrates unsteady balance with shuffling or stumbling of feet.
  - Assess client's musculoskeletal and neurological functioning.
  - Provide for client safety when ambulating.

Nursing Diagnosis

Defining characteristics from the assessment data may reveal the following nursing diagnoses for clients requiring this skill:

- Disturbed body image
- Risk for injury
- Impaired physical mobility
- Pain (acute, chronic)
- Ineffective peripheral tissue perfusion

Related factors are individualized based on client's condition or needs.

Recording and Reporting

- Record all findings in nurses' notes or appropriate assessment flow sheet.
- Report to nurse in charge or physician acute pain or sudden muscle weakness, which may be indicative of condition requiring immediate treatment.
- Report changes in peripheral circulation evidenced by edema or diminished or absent pulses or capillary refill, which may indicate circulatory compromise that can result in permanent nerve damage or tissue death if untreated.

Teaching Considerations

- Instruct client about correct postural alignment. Consult with physical therapist to provide client with exercises for improving posture.
- To reduce bone demineralization, instruct older adult client on a proper weight-bearing exercise program (e.g., walking, low-impact aerobics) to be followed three or more times a week.
- Also encourage intake of calcium to meet recommended daily allowance. Increased vitamin D aids calcium absorption.
- In women, recommended calcium supplements are 1000 mg before menopause and 1500 mg after menopause. Encourage female client to consult with physician regarding use of estrogen replacement.
- Explain to clients with low back pain that they can benefit from modification of work factors (e.g., lifting heavy weights, use of protective equipment), regular aerobic exercise, and exercises that strengthen the back and increase trunk flexibility.

Pediatric Considerations

- Infants must be carefully examined for musculoskeletal anomalies resulting from genetic or fetal insults. An examination includes review of posture, generalized movement, symmetry and skin creases of the extremities, muscle strength, and hip alignment.
- Normally the back of a newborn is rounded or C-shaped from the thoracic and pelvic curves.
- Scoliosis, lateral curvature of the spine, is an important childhood problem, especially in females, apparent at puberty. (For closer examination, have child stand erect, wearing only underclothes. Observe from behind, looking for asymmetry of shoulders and hips. Then observe from the back as the child bends forward.) Uneven dress hems or pant leg hems or uneven fit of clothing at the waist may be noted.
- The shape of bones may vary in children. Most conditions are benign, for example, valgus of the lower legs (lateral bowing of tibia), which is common in toddlers until they have well-developed lower back and leg muscles; varus of the knee (opposite of valgus) is normal in children from age 2 to 7 years (Wong and others, 1999). If either of these conditions is excessive, further evaluation is needed.
- Watching a child during play can reveal information about musculoskeletal function.

Gerontological Considerations

- Instruct older adults about fall prevention. Modifications can be made in the home environment to reduce the risk of falls (see Chapter 39).
- Older adult's gait normally has smaller steps and a wider base of support.
- Functional assessment is a measurement of older person's ability to perform basic self-care tasks (Lueckenotte, 2000). When client is unable to perform self-care easily, determine the need for assistive devices (e.g., zippers on clothing instead of buttons, elevation of chairs to minimize bending of knees and hips). Creativity by the nurse is often needed (Kee, 2000).
- Instruct older adult client to pace activities to compensate for loss in muscle strength.
- Older adults tend to assume a stooped, forward-bent posture, with hips and knees somewhat flexed and arms bent at the elbows and the level of the arms raised (Ebersole and Hess, 1998).
- In older adults joints often become swollen and stiff, with reduced ROM resulting from cartilage erosion and fibrosis of synovial membranes.
- Older adults may develop kyphosis because of osteoporosis.

Skill 10-6 Assessing Intake and Output

Measuring and recording intake and output (I&O) during a 24-hour period helps to complete the assessment data base for fluid and electrolyte balance. The nurse is responsible for recording all intake (liquids taken orally, by feeding tube, and parenterally) and all output (urine, diarrhea, vomitus, gastric suction, and drainage from surgical tubes). When possible, assistance from the alert client or family facilitates accuracy, independence, and a sense of participation in the plan of care.

Monitoring I&O may be an independent or a dependent nursing intervention. Keeping records of I&O is appropriate if a client has a fever, has edema, is receiving intravenous or diuretic therapy, or is placed on restricted fluids. It is also important when a client has electrolyte losses associated with vomiting, diarrhea, gastrointestinal drainage, or extensive open wounds such as burns. General monitoring of I&O should be evaluated for all clients, although measuring and documentation on the chart is not required in some situations.

When indicated, I&O is totalled and evaluated at the end of each shift or at specified times, usually 8 hours. Significant alterations are apparent by comparing 24-hour totals over several days. Because fluid imbalance may occur at any time, awareness of intake and output should be maintained for all clients, even when documentation is not required.

Delegation Considerations

Evaluation of I&O totals at the end of each shift and comparing 24-hour totals over several days, monitoring and recording of intravenous therapy, wound or chest tube drainage, and tube feedings should not be delegated to assistive personnel. The skill of measuring and recording oral intake and urinary output can be delegated to assistive personnel. Emphasize the importance of standard precautions relating to body fluids, accuracy in measuring and recording I&O, and the use of the metric system with standard containers. Clarify information that should be reported, including significant alteration in intake or changes in color, amount, or odor of output. Caution assistive personnel to be sensitive to the privacy needs of the client.

Equipment

- Sign alerting all personnel of I&O measurement
- Daily I&O record
- Graduated measuring container
- Bedpan, urinal, bedside commode, or urine "hat" (a receptacle that fits under the toilet seat)
- Disposable clean gloves

Step	Rationale
Assessment	
1. Identify clients with conditions that can increase fluid loss:	
a. Fever	Prolonged fever diminishes body fluids by increasing insensible water losses from lungs through increased respiratory rate and from diaphoresis.
b. Diarrhea and/or vomiting	Diarrhea and vomiting may lead to fluid and electrolyte imbalances, especially in the very young and frail older adults. Loss of potassium and chloride ions and excretion of hydrogen ions alter acid-base balance.
c. Surgical wound drainage or chest tube drainage	Wound drainage represents plasma or whole blood loss. If significant amounts are lost, fluid loss must be replaced.
d. Gastric suction	Hydrochloric acid, potassium, and fluids from the stomach are removed.
e. Major burns	Fluid volume loss is directly proportional to amount and depth of injury. Major fluid shifts can occur at specific intervals following severe burns.
f. Severe trauma (especially crushing injuries)	Hyperkalemia results from release of intracellular potassium from injured cells.
g. Endocrine imbalance	
(1) Cushing's disease	Corticosteroids can cause sodium and water retention with potassium excretion.

STEP	RATIONALE
(2) Addison's disease	Deficiency of corticosteroids causes sodium and water excretion.
(3) Diabetic ketoacidosis	Osmotic diuresis from increased blood glucose levels causes fluid volume deficit.
2. Identify clients with the following conditions: (clients with impaired swallowing, unconscious clients, clients with impaired mobility).	Have risk of insufficient fluid intake.
3. Identify clients who are taking medications that can influence fluid balance, including diuretics and steroids.	Symptoms of fluid imbalance may be present in clients receiving synthetic steroid preparations such as prednisone.
4. Assess signs and symptoms of dehydration and fluid overload.	Signs of dehydration result from reduction of fluid within tissues and circulatory system. Compensation for overhydration results in a fluid shift into tissues, causing edema.
5. Weigh clients daily, and observe for dehydration or fluid volume excess: Mild dehydration: 2% to 5% loss Moderate dehydration: 6% to 9% loss Severe dehydration: 10% to 14% loss Life threatening: 20% loss Mild fluid overload: 2% to 4% gain Moderate overload: 5% to 7% gain	Kidneys attempt to excrete excess fluid during periods of overhydration and conserve body water during periods of dehydration.

- ***Critical Decision Point***
  Daily weights must be obtained with the same scale, same time of day, and with comparable articles of clothing.

STEP	RATIONALE
6. Monitor laboratory reports: a. Urine specific gravity (normal is 1.010 to 1.030). b. Hematocrit (Hct) (normal range is 38% to 47% for females and 40% to 54% for males). (1) Increased hematocrit suggests dehydration. (2) Low hematocrit suggests blood loss/hemorrhage.	Clients' condition and therapies such as parenteral fluid replacement, can alter laboratory values.
7. Assess client and family's knowledge of the purpose and process of I&O measurement.	Improves cooperation in reporting intake and output to nurse.

PLANNING

STEP	RATIONALE
1. **Expected outcomes** following completion of procedure:	
▪ Oral intake is 600 to 900 ml greater than output and at least 1500 ml per 24 hours.	Normal oral intake maintained.
▪ Weight remains within 2% of baseline.	
▪ Hematocrit and urine specific gravity are within normal limits (WNL).	Normal hydration achieved without fluid alterations.
2. Post sign alerting personnel that I&O measurement is required.	Ensures that all sources of intake and output will be measured by staff.
3. Place I&O record in established location at the bedside or at the door.	

IMPLEMENTATION

STEP	RATIONALE
1. Explain to client and family the reasons I&O are important.	Encouraging fluids is a nursing responsibility. Any client not restricted in total fluid intake should be encouraged to consume at least 1500 ml/day. Postoperative clients are frequently prescribed clear liquid diets and advanced to solid foods as the nurse determines that they are able to tolerate it.

STEP	RATIONALE
2. Measure and record all intake of fluid:	
a. Liquids with meals, gelatin, custards, ice cream, popsicles, sherbets, ice chips (recorded as 50% of measured volume [e.g., 100 ml of ice chips equals 50 ml of water]).	Provides comprehensive and accurate assessment.
b. Liquid medicines such as antacids are counted as fluid intake, as are fluids with medications.	
c. Tube feedings (See Chapter 22)	
d. Parenteral fluids, blood components, and total parenteral nutrition (See Chapter 23)	

- ***Critical Decision Point***
  Intake should be recorded as soon as it is measured to maintain accuracy. If more than one client is in the same room, each must have urine receptacles labeled with name and bed location.

STEP	RATIONALE
3. Instruct client and family to call nurse to empty contents of urinal, urine hat, or commode each time it is used (see illustration). Incontinence, vomiting, and excessive perspiration also need to be monitored and reported to the nurse.	Urine leakage on a pad can be weighed (1 ml of urine weighs 1 g, and the number of pads used in 24 hours can be counted (Moore, 1998).
4. Inform client and family that Foley catheter drainage bag and wound, gastric, or chest tube drainage are closely monitored, measured, and recorded and that the nurse or assistive personnel are responsible for this. Each client must have a graduated container clearly marked with name and bed location and used only for the client indicated.	Prevents client or family from disrupting drainage systems.
5. Observe color and characteristics of urine in Foley tubing. Sometimes hourly urine output is measured using a special device (see illustration).	Drainage in the tubing is representative of current output. Characteristics of drainage in the bag are often very noticeably different based on changes over time.

- ***Critical Decision Point***
  In adults urine output less than 30 ml/hr can indicate decreased renal perfusion and should be reported. When output is low, a special device that facilitates measuring hourly output should be used (see illustration).

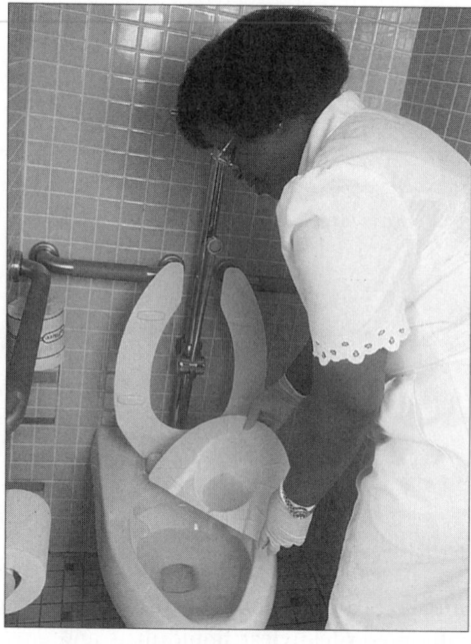

STEP **3** Measuring and emptying the urine "hat."

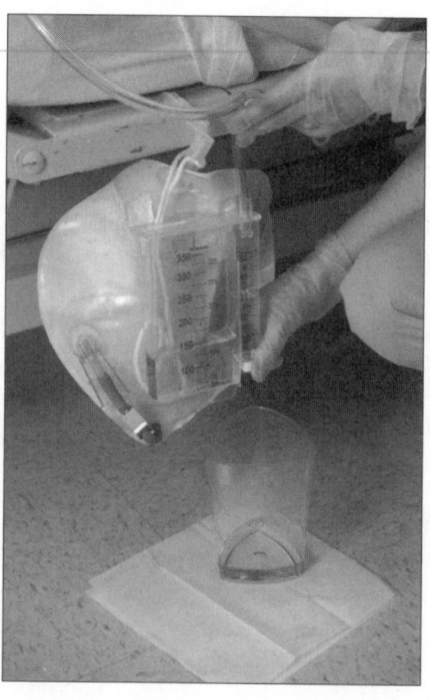

STEP **5** Device for monitoring hourly urine output.

STEP	RATIONALE
6. Measure drainage at the end of the shift, using appropriate containers and noting color and characteristics:	Provides comprehensive and accurate assessment.
a. Chest tube drainage is measured by marking and recording the time on the collection chamber at specified intervals (see illustration).	

- ***Critical Decision Point***
  Chest tube drainage is emptied ONLY when container is nearly full. A closed system is necessary to maintain lung reexpansion.

STEP	RATIONALE
b. Measure Jackson-Pratt drainage using a medicine cup (see illustration).	Drainage is usually less than 30 ml in volume.
c. Measure larger drainage pouches with graduated cup with a 240-ml capacity (see illustration).	

- ***Critical Decision Point***
  Disposable clean gloves must be worn to measure urine and wound drainage and to handle related equipment. If splashing is anticipated, wear mask, eye protection, and gown.

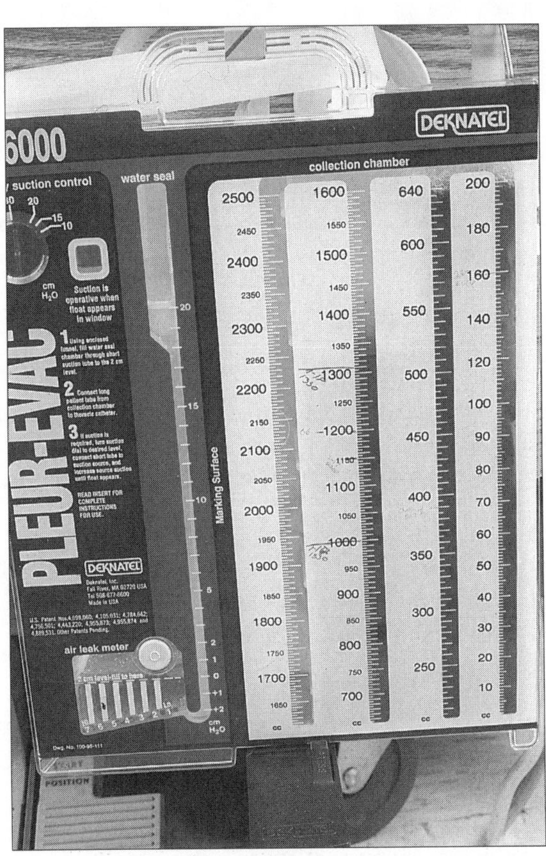

STEP **6a** Measuring chest tube drainage.

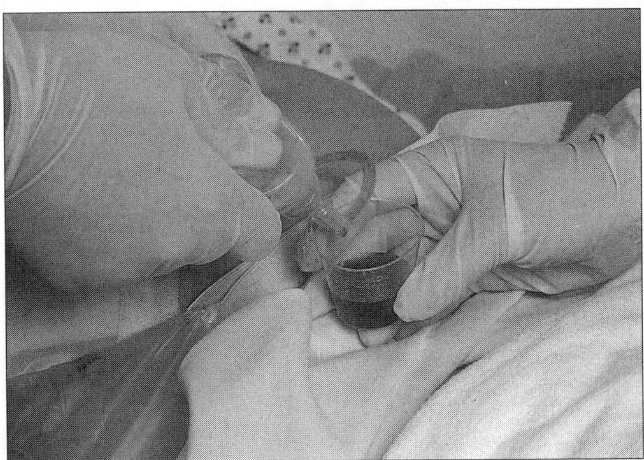

STEP **6b** Measuring wound drainage thought a Jackson-Pratt drain.

EVALUATION

1. Observe condition of skin and mucous membranes.	Condition reflects hydration status.
2. Observe color, characteristics, and amount of urine and wound drainage.	Presence of sudden increase in bright red blood may contribute to hypovolemic shock.
3. Note I&O balance or imbalance (see Table 10-13).	Indicates client's overall fluid status.

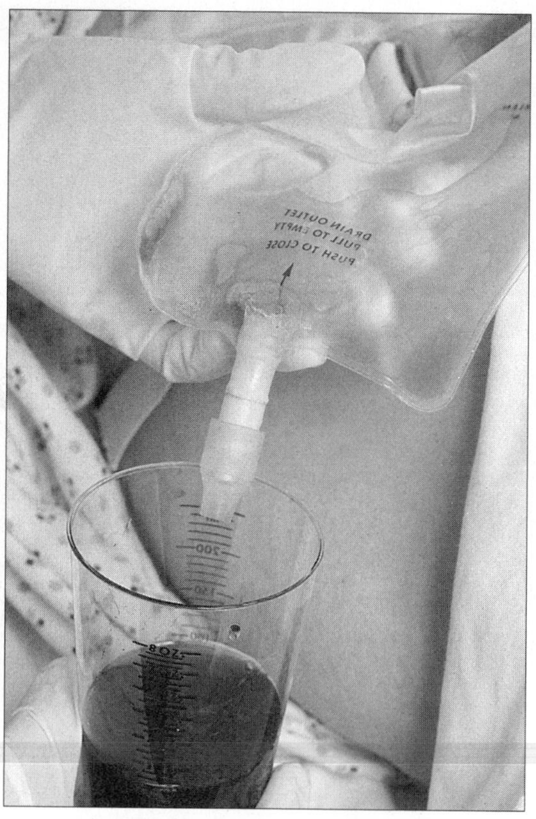

STEP **6c** Measuring drainage from large drainage pouch.

Table 10-13 Assessing for Fluid Imbalances

Fluid Volume Deficit	Fluid Volume Excess
• Output greater than intake	• Intake greater than output
• Decreased blood pressure	• Crackles (pulmonary edema)
• Increased pulse	
• Fever	• Bounding pulse
• Flat neck veins when supine	• Jugular venous distention (JVD)
• Slow venous filling of dependent hands	
• Rapid weight loss >5%	• Rapid weight gain
• Dry mouth	• Pitting edema
• Dry skin	
• Tenting	

Unexpected Outcomes and Related Interventions

- Prolonged fluid loss without adequate replacement of fluid as evidenced by output greater than intake, weight loss greater than 2% over 24 to 48 hours, and an increased hematocrit value.
  - Obtain frequent vital signs.
  - Observe for **orthostatic hypotension** when sitting client up in bed or assisting with ambulation (see Chapter 9).
  - Administer fluid replacement as ordered.
  - Notify physician of changes in client's physical assessment status.
- Chemical or physiological imbalance results in fluid retention evidenced by intake greater than output.
  - Notify physician.
  - Weigh client.
  - Place client on fluid restrictions.
  - Administer diuretics as ordered.

Nursing Diagnosis

Defining characteristics from the assessment data may reveal the following nursing diagnoses:

Deficient fluid volume
Excess fluid volume
Urinary retention
Incontinence (functional, stress, reflex, or urge)
Diarrhea

Related factors are individualized based on client's condition or needs.

Recording and Reporting

- At specified time according to agency policy calculate total intake and output on the specified intake and output record at the bedside or at the door.
- Document the total on the client's record (Figure 10-5).
- Report immediately to physician any urine output less than 30 ml/hr or significant changes in daily weight, which suggest fluid volume deficit or excess.

VITAL SIGN / I & O / PAIN RECORD

Date ______________ **INTAKE** *KEY:* **C**ontinent / **I**ncontinent **OUTPUT**

	Parenteral				Oral / Tube Feedings			Urine		Other				
Type:					Oral	TF	Flush							BM
To Count:					Amt	Amt	Amt	Amt	Amt	Amt	Amt	Amt	Amt	Amt/Freq
2300					120									
2400								325		Chest Tube 75				
0100		50												
0200														
0300														
0400														
0500														
0600														
8 hr Sub Totals		50			120			325		75				
8 hr Total Parenteral / 8 hr total Oral/tube / 8 hr Shift Intake					170			8 hr Shift's Output					400	
To Count:														
0700					650									
0800								500						
0900														
1000		50								75				
1100														
1200														
1300														
1400														
8 hr Sub Totals		50			650			500		75				
8 hr Total Parenteral / 8 hr total Oral/tube / 8 hr Shift Intake					700			8 hr Shift's Output					575	
To Count:														
1500					650			600						
1600														
1700										75				
1800														
1900		50												
2000														
2100														
2200														
8 hr Sub Totals		50			650			600		75				
8 hr Total Parenteral / 8 hr total Oral/tube / 8 hr Shift Intake					700			8 hr Shift's Output					675	
Twenty-four hour Total					1570			Twenty-four hour Total					1650	

FLUID EQUIVALENTS

1 oz	30cc	8 oz (1 cup)	240cc
4 oz (1/2 cup)	120cc	12 oz (soda-1 can)	360cc
6 oz (3/4 cup)	180cc		

ADDRESSOGRAPH / LABEL

SSM HEALTH · CARE℠

VITAL SIGN / I & O / PAIN RECORD

SLM-1000-035 (6/2000) 10 BACK

FIGURE **10-5** Intake and output summary. (Courtesy SSM Health Care, St. Mary's Health Center, St. Louis, MO.)

TEACHING CONSIDERATIONS

- Some clients who are able to ambulate need to be reminded of need to measure and record all liquid intake and output.
- Severely ill or disoriented clients may be unable to understand reasons for I&O measurement or participate in measuring and recording. Family members often are able to help maintain accurate records.
- Clients who have fluid restriction (e.g., renal failure, congestive heart failure) may need *strict* I&O because fluid imbalance can quickly result in serious physiological changes.

PEDIATRIC CONSIDERATIONS

- Infants and young children have a greater need for water and are more vulnerable to alterations in fluid and electrolyte balance (Wong and others, 1999).
- Fluid and electrolyte imbalances occur more rapidly with vomiting and diarrhea than they do in the adult population (Wong and others, 1999).
- Infants need to ingest a greater amount of fluid per kilogram of body weight than do older children (Wong and others, 1999).

GERONTOLOGICAL CONSIDERATIONS

- With age, bladder capacity decreases, the prevalence of involuntary bladder contractions increases, and more urine is produced at night (Lueckenotte, 2000).
- Urinary incontinence is not a function of age and should be thoroughly evaluated (Lueckenotte, 2000).
- Clients with chronic illness and/or older than age 60 are at greater risk of fluid and electrolyte imbalances secondary to gastroenteritis.
- Older adults are more susceptible to fluid and electrolyte imbalances with prolonged fever.

HOME CARE CONSIDERATIONS

- Have client and caregiver practice measuring I&O correctly using I&O chart and available containers. Provide more appropriate measuring devices if needed.
- Instruct client and caregiver regarding daily weights as an important adjunct to monitoring I&O. Stress the importance of using the same scale, same time of day, and similar clothing.

Critical Thinking Exercises

1. Sara Williams, age 36, was admitted yesterday with right lower quadrant abdominal pain. Describe the most important points to include relating to her pain in her morning shift assessment. List the assessment techniques to be used in the order of priority.
2. A postoperative client is becoming more distended and refuses breakfast. It is the second postoperative day following a cholecystectomy (removal of gallbladder). What additional assessment data should be gathered during your initial shift assessment?
3. As you begin your shift assessment of Jane Jacobs, a 45-year-woman recovering from a hysterectomy, she reports discomfort at her intravenous site. How would you proceed with your assessment?
4. Jim Lewis, a 76-year-old man with arthritis who lives alone at home, reports difficulty walking. What physical assessments could you perform while he is in bed in relation to this concern?

References

Agency for Health Care Policy and Research: *Recognition and initial assessment of Alzheimer's disease and related dementias,* Rockville, Md, 1996, Agency for Health Care Policy and Research.

American Cancer Society: *Cancer facts and figures 1999,* Atlanta, 1999, The Society.

American Medical Directors Association: *Osteoporosis: clinical practice guidelines,* 1998 (http://www.amda.com).

Barkauskas VH and others: *Health and physical assessment,* ed 2, St. Louis, 1998, Mosby.

Breen P: DVT: What every nurse should know, *RN* 63(4):58, 2000.

Daly S: *Expert 10 Minute Physical Examinations,* St. Louis, 1997, Mosby.

Ebersole P, Hess P: *Toward healthy aging: human needs and nursing response,* ed 5, St. Louis, 1998, Mosby.

Elkin M, Perry A, Potter P: *Nursing interventions and clinical skills,* ed 2, St. Louis, 2000, Mosby.

Galindo-Ciocon D: Nursing care of elders with leg edema, *J Gerontol Nurs* 21(7):7, 1995.

Garza C, De Onis M: A new international growth reference for young children, *Am J Clin Nutr* 70(1):1695, 1999.

Hauner H, Stockamp B, Haastert B: Prevalence of lipohypertrophy in insulin-treated diabetic patients and predisposing factors, *Exp Clin Endocrinol Diabetes* 104(2):106, 1996.

Kee C: Osteoarthritis: manageable scourge of aging, *Nurs Clin North Am* 35(1):199, 2000.

Krauss RM: Dietary guidelines for healthy Americans approved by the American Heart Association Science Advisory and Coordinating Committee, *Circulation* 94:1795, 1996.

Lueckenotte A: *Gerontologic nursing,* ed 2, St. Louis, 2000, Mosby.

Lynch SH: Elder abuse: what to look for, how to intervene, *Am J Nurs* 97(1):27, 1997.

McHugh J, McHugh W: How to assess deep tendon reflexes, *Nursing* 20(8):62, 1990.

Meador JA: Cerumen impaction in the elderly, *J Gerontol Nurs* 21(12):43, 1995.

Moore K: Weigh the evidence, *Nurs Times* 94(42):65, 1998.

Mosby's expert ten minute physical examinations, St. Louis, 1997, Mosby.

Pugliese G: Reducing risks of infection during vascular access, *J Intraven Nurs* 20(6 suppl):511, 1997.

Seidel HM and others: *Mosby's guide to physical examination,* ed 4, St. Louis, 1999, Mosby.

Sitzman K: Feet first, *Home HealthC Nurse* 17(5):328, 1999.

Thompson JM and others: *Mosby's manual of clinical nursing,* ed 3, St. Louis, 1993, Mosby.

Wong DL and others: *Whaley and Wong's nursing care of infants and children,* ed 5, St. Louis, 1999, Mosby.

Wright JA: Seven abdominal assessment signs every emergency nurse should know, *J Emerg Nurs,* 23(5):446, 1997.

11

Oxygen Therapy

Skills

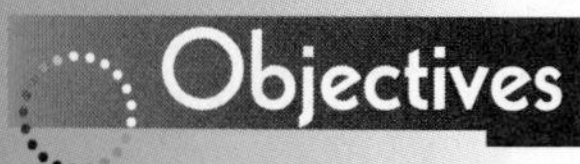

Objectives

Mastery of content in this chapter will enable the nurse to:

- Define the key terms listed.
- Discuss indications for oxygen therapy.
- Discuss methods for administering oxygen therapy.
- Demonstrate applying a nasal cannula and an oxygen mask.
- Demonstrate administering oxygen therapy to a client with an artificial airway.
- Demonstrate proper use of incentive spirometry.
- Demonstrate using continuous positive airway pressure (CPAP).
- Demonstrate administering mechanical ventilation.
- Demonstrate how to measure a peak expiratory flow rate (PEFR).

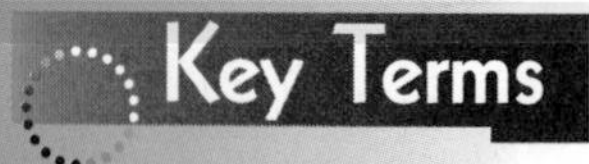

Key Terms

Cyanosis
Hypercapnia
Hypoxemia
Hypoxia
Incentive spirometry
Nasal cannula
Negative-pressure ventilation
Oxygen mask
Oxygen therapy
Peak expiratory flow rate
Positive-pressure ventilation
Pressure-cycled ventilation
T tube
Tidal volume
Tracheostomy collar
Volume-cycled ventilation

Box 11-1 Assessment of Signs and Symptoms Associated With Hypoxia

ACUTE CHANGES
- Apprehension
- Anxiety
- Decreased level of consciousness (LOC)
- Increased pulse rate
- Increased rate and depth of respiration
- Decreased lung sounds
- Elevated blood pressure
- Dyspnea
- Use of accessory muscles of respiration
- Cardiac dysrhythmias

INSIDIOUS CHANGES
- Pallor
- Increased fatigue
- Decreased ability to concentrate
- Dizziness
- Behavioral changes
- Cyanosis
- Clubbing
- Adventitious lung sounds

Oxygen therapy is the administration of supplemental oxygen (O_2) to a client to prevent or reduce **hypoxia,** a condition in which there is insufficient oxygen to meet the metabolic demands of the tissues and cells. Hypoxia results from **hypoxemia,** a deficiency of arterial blood oxygen. Hemoglobin carries oxygen and carbon dioxide (CO_2) to and from the cells. The presence of decreased hemoglobin levels reduces the amount of oxygen transported to the cells and CO_2 transported away from the cells. Hemoglobin levels and acid-base status have direct effects on oxygenation. A state of acidemia increases the ability of hemoglobin to release oxygen to the tissues. Alkalemia prevents the hemoglobin from easily releasing oxygen to the tissues.

Various disease states require the use of oxygen therapy to correct impaired gas exchange and the resultant hypoxemia. An example of such a disease state is pneumonia. Pneumonia results in impaired gas exchange because of fluid and secretions in the lung, causing a decrease in oxygen diffusion from the lungs to the arterial blood supply. A client with chronic bronchitis, a form of chronic obstructive pulmonary disease (COPD), may have normal arterial oxygen levels during the day but may experience oxygen desaturation, a reduction in the arterial oxygen level during sleep, requiring oxygen at night to prevent hypoxemia. A client with emphysema, another type of COPD, may experience low oxygen levels all the time or in association with increased activity, a condition called exercise-induced hypoxia. Clients with COPD and carbon dioxide retention are at risk for developing CO_2 narcosis induced by administration of high levels of oxygen. The chemoreceptors monitor CO_2 levels. In the individual with healthy lungs the chemoreceptors are sensitive to small changes in CO_2 levels and effectively regulate ventilation. When the CO_2 level rises to a certain level, the person inhales air. In the client with COPD, the chemoreceptors are not sensitive to small changes in CO_2 and regulate ventilation poorly, resulting in CO_2 retention. Therefore in these clients, changes in the oxygen level stimulate changes in ventilation. If high levels of oxygen are administered, their stimulus to breathe is extinguished. Administration of oxygen therapy is not without possible complications (Box 11-1).

Clients with cardiovascular disease, such as left ventricular failure, may not be able to supply oxygen to the tissues due to decreased cardiac output. Supplemental oxygen helps decrease the work of the left ventricle and increase oxygen delivery to the tissues.

Before administering oxygen assess the client for a temporary or permanent abnormal chest wall configuration. Temporary abnormalities that can affect ventilation and the delivery of oxygen include obesity, pregnancy, and chest trauma. Congenital musculoskeletal abnormalities such as kyphosis affect oxygenation because of decreased lung expansion. The nursing assessment of a client requiring supplemental oxygen therapy may reveal many findings associated with hypoxia. Presenting symptoms depend on the client's age, level of health, present disease process, and the presence of chronic illnesses. Anxiety, confusion, and restlessness are early signs of hypoxia. Additional assessment findings include changes in blood pressure, cardiac dysrhythmias such as premature ventricular contractions (PVCs), tachycardia, tachypnea, dyspnea, drowsiness, headaches, disorientation, forgetfulness, and nausea. The pulse may become rapid and irregular because of cardiac dysrhythmias.

Initially blood pressure is elevated. If hypoxia remains uncorrected, hypotension may develop. Respiratory rate and depth are increased. As hypoxia worsens, the client's activity tolerance decreases, and the client may become confused, with loss of short-term memory. Worsening of a hypoxic state may lead to a decreased level of consciousness and coma.

Cyanosis, a bluish discoloration of the skin and mucous membranes, is a late sign of hypoxia. Cyanosis is caused by vasoconstriction of the peripheral blood vessels or decreased oxyhemoglobin. It can be seen in clients who are very cold or have decreased peripheral circulation because of vascular disease and in those with a decreased level of circulating oxyhemoglobin. The nurse never assumes a lack of cyanosis means adequate oxygenation. Cyanosis caused by hypoxia is assessed in the oral mucosa, the conjunctiva of the eye, and around the lips, known as circumoral cyanosis.

Oxygen Systems

The oxygen delivery system selected depends on the level of oxygen support the client needs, based on the severity of the hypoxia and the disease process. Other factors considered include the client's age, level of health and orientation level, the presence of an artificial airway, whether the setting is in the hospital or the home, the type of home environment, and the type of support and care given after discharge.

Oxygen is available in a number of systems. Oxygen provided in a hospital or institutional setting is a bulk liquid oxygen system designed to store the oxygen at −34° C (−29° F) and deliver it as a gas at wall outlets in the client's room. An oxygen flowmeter is required to regulate the flow rate in liters of oxygen delivered (Figure 11-1).

Compressed oxygen is available in gas cylinders and exists as a nonliquefied gas at 1800 to 2400 pounds per square inch (psi) at 21° C (70° F). Oxygen cylinders used in hospitals include the large "H" size, holding about 6600 L of oxygen, and the small "E" size, holding 625 L of oxygen. An oxygen regulator/flowmeter controls the flow rate of oxygen delivered from the cylinder. The H size is used as a main source, because the tank is not easily portable. The E size is smaller and allows portability (Figure 11-2).

Skills presented in this chapter focus on administration of oxygen therapy and respiratory maneuvers to improve oxygenation and promotion of lung expansion. The nursing care measures used are based on specific assessment findings.

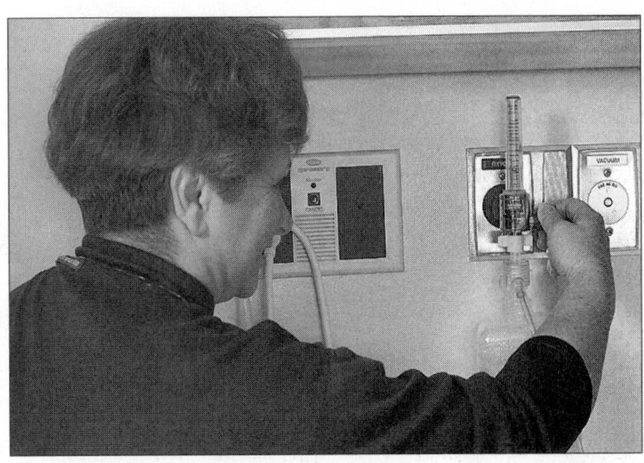

FIGURE **11-1** Flowmeter attached to oxygen source.

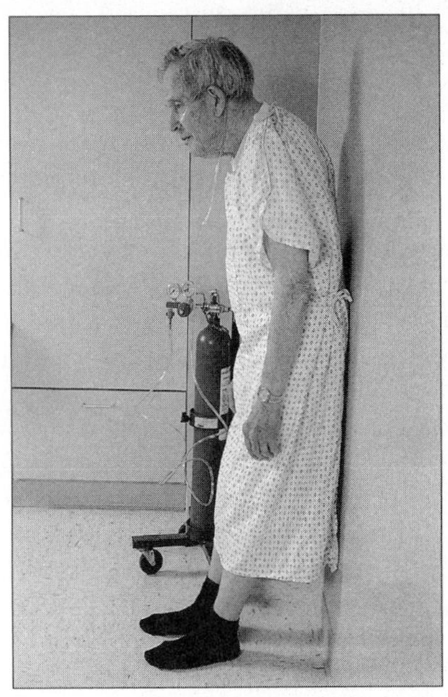

FIGURE **11-2** Smaller E tank for portability.

Skill Performance Guidelines

1. Know the client's normal range of vital signs. Hypoxia can affect the client's vital signs.
2. Know the client's usual behavioral pattern. The nurse, friends, and family may notice behavioral changes such as restlessness, agitation, anxiety, apprehension, and inability to concentrate.
3. Know the client's medical history. It is important to be aware of the client with COPD who is a carbon dioxide retainer. High inspired oxygen concentrations may result in severe side effects such as respiratory depression.
4. Be aware of environmental conditions. Clients with chronic respiratory diseases have difficulty maintaining optimal oxygen levels in polluted environments. If a client

Box 11-2 Oxygen Safety Guidelines

- Oxygen is a medication and should not be adjusted without a physician's order.
- An "Oxygen in Use" sign must be placed on the client's door and in the client's room. If oxygen is used at home, a sign is placed on the door of the house.
- Oxygen delivery systems must be kept 10 feet from any open flames.
- Oxygen supports combustion; however, it will not explode.
- No smoking should be allowed on the premises.
- A "No Smoking" sign is placed on the client's door and in the client's home. If oxygen is used at home, a sign is placed on the door of the house.
- When oxygen cylinders are used, they must be secured so that they will not fall over. Oxygen cylinders are stored upright, chained, or in appropriate holders.

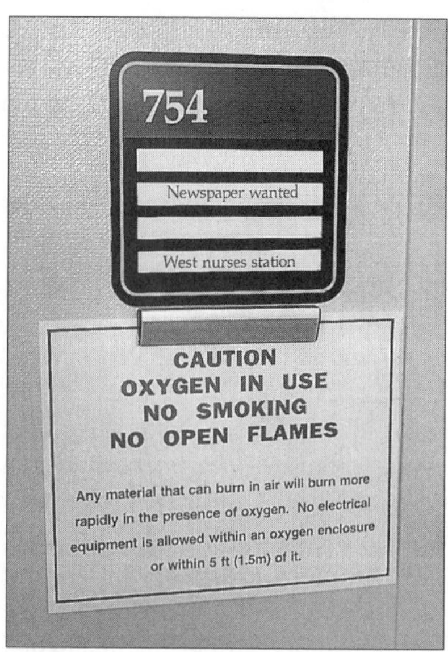
754
Newspaper wanted
West nurses station
CAUTION
OXYGEN IN USE
NO SMOKING
NO OPEN FLAMES
Any material that can burn in air will burn more rapidly in the presence of oxygen. No electrical equipment is allowed within an oxygen enclosure or within 5 ft (1.5m) of it.

FIGURE 11-3 Proper display for oxygen in use sign.

is to receive home oxygen therapy, an environmental assessment is completed to determine respiratory hazards in the home such as the use of gas stoves or kerosene space heaters or the presence of smokers in the home.

5. Document the client's smoking history. Smoking damages the lungs' mucociliary clearance mechanism and paralyzes the ciliary action, resulting in a decreased ability to clear mucus from the airways. Mucus pools in the airways create an environment for the development of infections. Accumulation of mucus may lead to the development of chronic bronchitis. Long-term chronic bronchitis ultimately results in hypoxia.
6. Know the client's most recent hemoglobin values.
7. Know the client's past and current arterial blood gas (ABG) values.
8. Know the client's cardiac output. Estimate the cardiac output by the blood pressure. If the client is hypotensive, the cardiac output is low or inadequate and oxygen delivery to the tissues will be reduced.
9. Oxygen is regarded as a medication. Increasing the oxygen liter flow rate for shortness of breath is similar to doubling heart medication.
10. It is important to provide education to the client and family about home oxygen therapy so that the client and family understand proper use of the equipment. Safety measures for oxygen use are very important (Box 11-2). These measures are taught to the client and caregivers to ensure proper use. In the hospital setting, signage is used to alert caregivers and visitors that oxygen is in use (Figure 11-3).

Skill 11-1 Applying a Nasal Cannula or Oxygen Mask

Nasal Cannula

A **nasal cannula** is a simple, comfortable device for delivering oxygen to a client (Figure 11-4). The two tips of the cannula, about 1.5 cm (½ inch) long, protrude from the center of a disposable tube and are inserted into the nostrils. Oxygen is delivered via the cannula at a flow rate from 0.5 to 6 L/min. Higher flow rates dry airway mucosa and do not increase the inspired oxygen concentration (FIO_2). Humidification is not used for rates less than 4 L/min. At flow rates greater than 4 L/min, humidification helps prevent drying of nasal and oral mucous membranes. Approximate FIO_2 can be estimated by the flow rate (Table 11-1). The delivered oxygen percentage will vary, depending on the rate and depth of the client's breathing.

A nasal cannula is an effective mechanism for oxygen delivery. It allows the client to breathe through the mouth or nose, is available for all age-groups, and is adequate for short-term or long-term use. Cannulas are inexpensive, disposable, generally comfortable, and easily accepted by most clients.

Oxygen Mask

An **oxygen mask** is shaped to fit snugly over the client's mouth and nose and is secured in place with a strap. The two primary

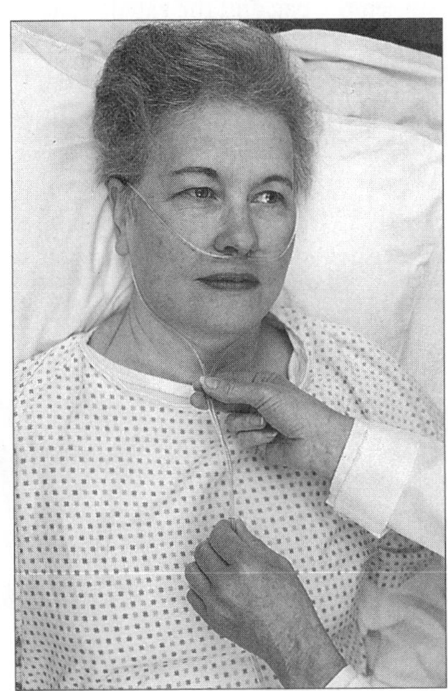

FIGURE 11-4 Nasal cannula is useful for low oxygen concentration (2 L/min) for clients with chronic lung disease.

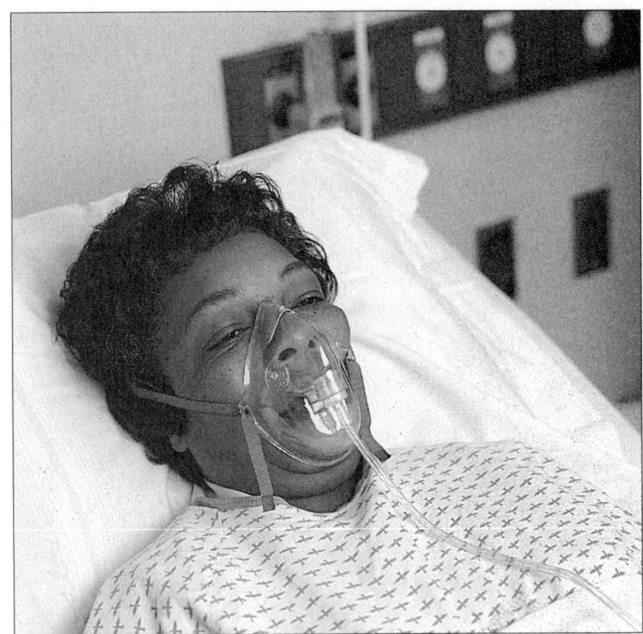

FIGURE 11-5 Simple face mask can deliver concentrations of 35% to 50% using flow rates of 6 to 10 L/min.

Table 11-1 Flow Rate and Approximate FIO_2

Flow (L/min)	FIO_2
Nasal Cannula	
1	21%-24%
2	24%-28%
3	28%-32%
4	32%-36%
5	36%-40%
6	40%-44%
Face Mask	
5-6	40%
6-7	50%
7-10	60%

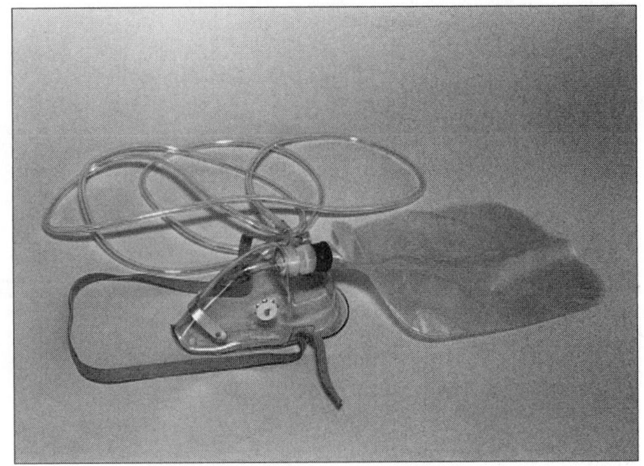

FIGURE 11-6 Nonrebreathing mask.

types of masks are those delivering a low FIO_2 and those delivering a high FIO_2.

A simple face mask is a flexible, cone-shaped device with a metal strip to mold the mask to the nose, an adjustable head strap, and multiple exhalation ports (Figure 11-5). The mask is contraindicated for clients who retain carbon dioxide (CO_2). The percentage of oxygen that can be delivered with a simple face mask ranges from 40% to 60%, depending on the liter flow and depth of respirations (see Table 11-1).

A nonrebreathing mask is a flexible, cone-shaped device with a reservoir bag attached. A one-way flap valve is between the bag and mask to allow for inhalation of oxygen and prevent accumulation of expired CO_2. A one-way flap valve covers the exhalation ports to prevent dilution of oxygen with inhaled room air (Figure 11-6). A nonrebreathing mask is used for severe hypoxia. Flow rates of 10 L/min can produce an FIO_2 of 80% to 95%, depending on the client's respiratory rate and depth. To ensure the client's inspiratory demands are being met, observe the reservoir bag; it should not collapse during inspiration.

A partial rebreathing mask is a flexible, cone-shaped device with a reservoir bag attached (Figure 11-7). This mask differs from the nonrebreathing mask because there are no one-way

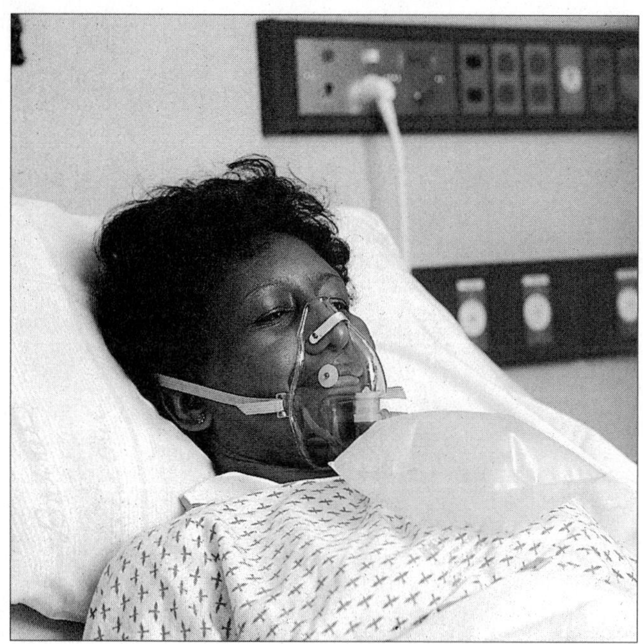

FIGURE **11-7** Partial rebreathing mask can deliver concentrations of 60% to 90% using flow rates of 6 to 10 L/min.

flap valves between the bag and the exhalation ports. The partial rebreathing bag is indicated for clients with severe hypoxia and delivers an FiO_2 of 60% to 90%.

A Venturi mask is a cone-shaped device with entrainment ports of various sizes at the base of the mask (Figure 11-8). The entrainment ports are adjustable to permit regulation of FiO_2 from 24% to 50%. This mask is useful because it delivers a more precise concentration of oxygen to the client (Table 11-2).

Table 11-2 Venturi Mask Systems

FiO_2 Setting	Minimal O_2 Flow Rate (L/min)
24%	4
28%	4
31%	6
35%	8
40%	8
50%	10

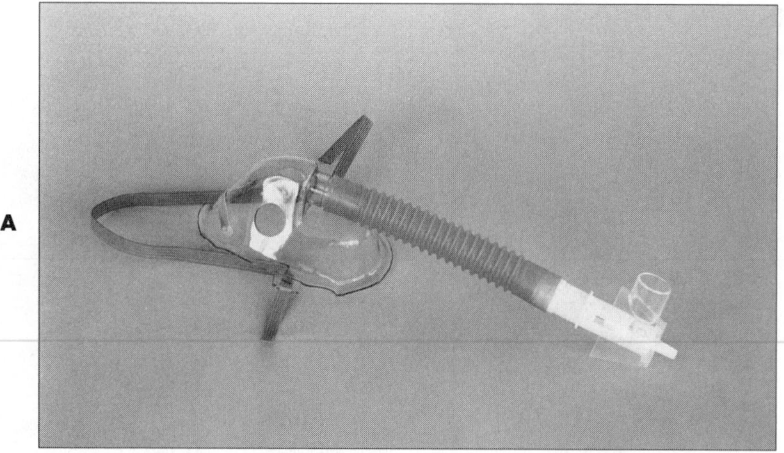

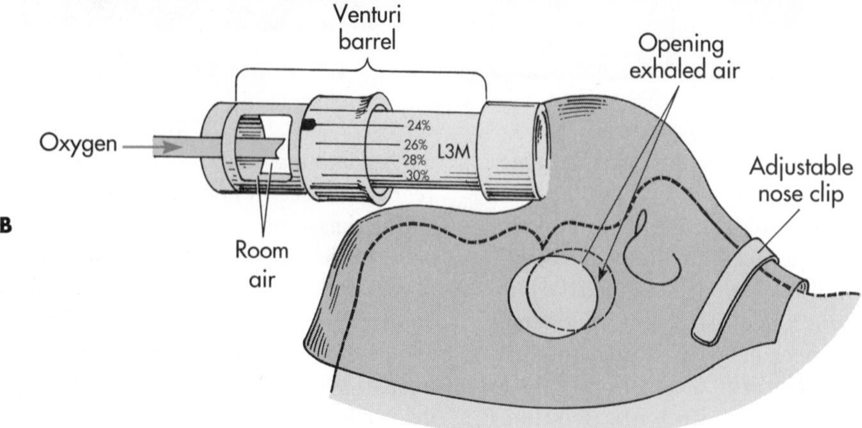

FIGURE **11-8** **A,** Venturi mask. **B,** Turning Venturi barrel sets percentage of oxygen delivered from 24% to 50% at preset intervals.

The face tent is a shieldlike device that fits under the client's chin and sweeps around the face (Figure 11-9). Oxygen concentrations of 21% to 50% may be delivered. A concentration of 21% is delivered if the device is used with compressed air for aerosol purposes only, because atmospheric air contains 21% oxygen. When higher oxygen concentrations are desired, the flow rate is set at 10 L/min. The actual concentration of oxygen delivered will be affected by the rate and depth of the client's respirations.

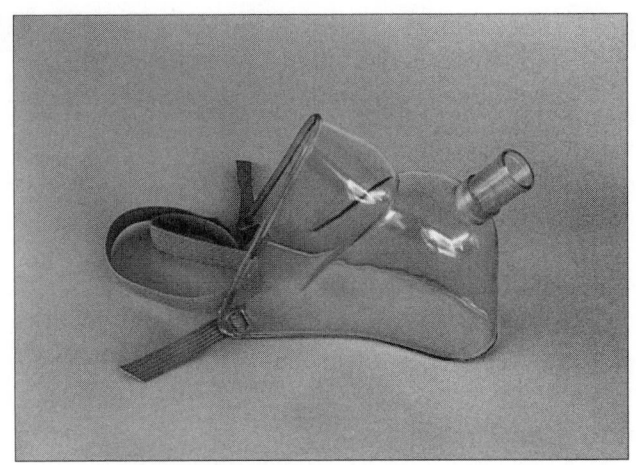

FIGURE 11-9 Face tent for oxygen delivery.

Delegation Considerations

The skills of setting up and applying a nasal cannula or an oxygen mask can be delegated to appropriately trained assistive personnel. The device setup and client should be assessed and checked by a nurse. The care provider should be instructed in proper way to set up and apply the oxygen delivery device, about any unexpected outcomes associated with the oxygen delivery device, and about the need to report them if any occur.

Equipment

- Nasal cannula or oxygen mask
- Oxygen tubing
- Humidifier, if indicated
- Sterile water for humidifier
- Oxygen source
- Oxygen flowmeter
- Appropriate room signs

Step	Rationale
Assessment	
1. Observe for signs and symptoms associated with hypoxia (see Box 11-1)	Assessment provides the nurse with baseline data.
• ***Critical Decision Point*** *Clients with sudden changes in their vital signs, LOC, or behavior may be experiencing profound hypoxia.*	
2. Observe for patent airway, and remove airway secretions by having client cough and expectorate mucous or by suctioning (see Chapter 13).	Secretions can plug the airway, decreasing the amount of oxygen that is available for gas exchange in the lungs.
3. If available, note client's most recent arterial blood gas (ABG) results or pulse oximetry value.	Objectively documents the client's pH, arterial oxygen, arterial CO_2, or arterial oxygen saturation.
• ***Critical Decision Point*** *Note if the current oxygen therapy has been meeting the client's oxygenation needs. Determine what factors have changed, resulting in the new assessment findings.*	
4. Review client's medical record for the medical order for oxygen, noting delivery method, flow rate, and duration of oxygen therapy.	Ensures safe and accurate O_2 administration.
5. Complete respiratory system assessment.	Determines presence of respiratory abnormalities impeding oxygenation.

STEP	RATIONALE

NURSING DIAGNOSIS

Defining characteristics from the assessment data may reveal the following nursing diagnoses for clients requiring this skill:

Impaired gas exchange
Ineffective breathing pattern

Related factors are individualized based on client's condition or needs.

PLANNING

Step	Rationale
1. **Expected outcomes** following completion of procedure:	
▪ Client's signs of hypoxia are reduced or eliminated. ▪ Client's vital signs will return to baseline. ▪ Client's work of breathing will decrease. ▪ Client will experience increased lung expansion. ▪ Client's LOC will return to baseline. ▪ Arterial blood gas values or oxygen saturation will return to normal or baseline.	Client demonstrates improved oxygenation.
▪ Client's nares and nasal mucosa remain intact.	Oxygen cannula applied correctly.
2. Explain the procedure to client and family.	Increases compliance and cooperation of the client and family.

IMPLEMENTATION

Step	Rationale
1. Wash hands.	Reduces transmission of microorganisms.
2. Attach nasal cannula or oxygen mask to oxygen tubing and attach oxygen tubing to flowmeter.	
3. Adjust oxygen flow rate to prescribed dosage, usually between 1 and 6 L/min.	Ensures correct O_2 delivery.
4. Apply oxygen delivery device and adjust elastic headband or plastic slide until it fits snugly and comfortably. Allow sufficient slack on oxygen tubing and secure to client's clothes.	Directs flow of oxygen into client's upper respiratory tract. Client is more likely to keep apparatus in place if it fits comfortably.
5. Observe for proper function of oxygen delivery device: a. Nasal cannula: Cannula is positioned properly in the nares. b. Nonrebreathing mask: Reservoir bag should fill on exhalation and not collapse on inhalation. c. Partial rebreathing mask: Reservoir should fill on exhalation and not collapse on inhalation. d. Venturi mask: Percentage of FiO_2 should correlate with flow rate (see Table 11-2). e. Face tent: Mist should always be present. f. Assess flowmeter and oxygen source for proper setup and prescribed flow rate.	Ensures patency of delivery device and accuracy of oxygen flow rate.
6. Monitor clients response to changes in the oxygen flow rate with pulse oximetry (see Chapter 9).	Monitoring with pulse oximetry allows for noninvasive, cost-effective trending of the client's arterial oxygen saturation and pulse rate.

• ***Critical Decision Point***

Collaborate with physician for a plan of ongoing monitoring of oxygenation with ABG levels or trending pulse oximetry.

Step	Rationale
7. Wash hands.	Reduces transmission of microorganisms.

STEP	RATIONALE
EVALUATION	
1. Observe for decreased anxiety, improved level of consciousness and cognitive abilities, decreased fatigue, absence of dizziness, decreased pulse with regular rhythm, decreased respiratory rate, return to normal blood pressure, improved color, and return to client's baseline vital signs.	Evaluates effectiveness of interventions.
2. Monitor arterial blood gas levels or observe pulse oximetry for oxygen saturation.	Documents client's level of oxygenation.
3. Assess adequacy of oxygen flow each shift.	Ensures patency of the oxygen delivery device.
4. Observe client's external ears, nares, and nasal mucous membranes for evidence of skin breakdown.	Oxygen therapy can cause drying of nasal mucosa. The delivery device can cause skin breakdown where the device comes in contact with the face, neck, and ears.

UNEXPECTED OUTCOMES AND RELATED INTERVENTIONS

- Client experiences skin breakdown, irritation, drying of nasal mucosa, sinus pain, or epistaxis.
  - Increase humidification to oxygen delivery system.
  - Provide appropriate skin care.
- Client experiences continued hypoxia.
  - Obtain physician's orders for follow-up pulse oximetry monitoring or ABG determinations.
  - Notify the physician about the continued hypoxia.
  - Consider measures to improve airway patency, coughing techniques, oropharyngeal or oratracheal suctioning.

RECORDING AND REPORTING

- Record the respiratory assessment findings; method of oxygen delivery, flow rate, client's response; any adverse reactions or side effects; change in physician's orders.
- Report any unexpected outcome to physician or nurse in charge.

TEACHING CONSIDERATIONS

- Begin discharge teaching if client is to continue oxygen therapy after discharge.
- Teach the client and family the importance of and rationale for oxygen therapy.
- Discuss safety precautions for oxygen use (see Box 11-2) with the client and family.
- Discuss signs of oxygen toxicity and CO_2 retention (e.g., confusion, headache, decreased LOC, somnolence, CO_2 narcosis, respiratory arrest) (see Box 11-1).

GERONTOLOGICAL CONSIDERATIONS

- The arterial oxygen pressure (PO_2) falls 4 mm Hg per decade of life. A 70-year-old will have a normal arterial PO_2 between 75 and 80 mm Hg (Weilitz, 2000).
- The older adult has a reduced oxygen-carrying capacity (Hgb × 1.34, the amount in cubic centimeters of oxygen each hemoglobin molecule can carry) because of a decreased hemoglobin level.

HOME CARE CONSIDERATIONS

- The client and family must know how to use the oxygen delivery system (e.g., cylinders, concentration, liquid oxygen) and delivery device.
- Teach family members what changes the client may demonstrate that indicate worsening hypoxia.
- Oxygen tubing in the home setting is available in lengths of 15 m (50 feet).
- Oxygen-conserving devices that administer oxygen during inhalation are often used in the home care setting. These help reduce the use and cost of long-term oxygen therapy (Rice, 2000).

Skill 11-2 Administering Oxygen Therapy to a Client With an Artificial Airway

Clients with an artificial airway require constant humidification to the airway. An artificial airway bypasses the normal filtering and humidification process of the nose and mouth. The two devices that supply humidified gas to an artificial airway are a T tube and a tracheostomy collar.

The **T tube,** also called a Briggs adaptor, is a T-shaped device with a 15-mm (3/5-inch) connection that connects an oxygen source to an artificial airway such as an endotracheal (ET) tube or tracheostomy (Figure 11-10). The recommended flow rate is 10 L/min with a nebulizer set to the appropriate inspired oxygen concentration (FIO_2).

A **tracheostomy collar** is a curved device with an adjustable strap that fits around the client's neck (Figure 11-11). There are two ports: an exhalation port that remains patent at all times and the port that connects to the oxygen source with large-bore tubing. The flow rate is set at 10 L/min with a nebulizer set to the appropriate FIO_2 that provides humidification to the lower airways via the tracheostomy tube opening.

Delegation Considerations

The skills of setting up and applying a T tube or a tracheostomy collar to a client with an artificial airway can be delegated to appropriately trained assistive personnel. The device setup and the client should be assessed by a nurse.

The care provider should be informed and assisted in proper way to set up and apply T tube or tracheostomy collar and instructed about any unexpected outcomes associated with the oxygen delivery device and the need to report them if any occur.

Equipment

- T tube or tracheostomy collar
- Large-bore oxygen tubing
- Nebulizer
- Sterile water for nebulizer
- Oxygen or gas source
- Gloves
- Goggles (if splash risk exists)
- Flowmeter
- "Oxygen in use" sign

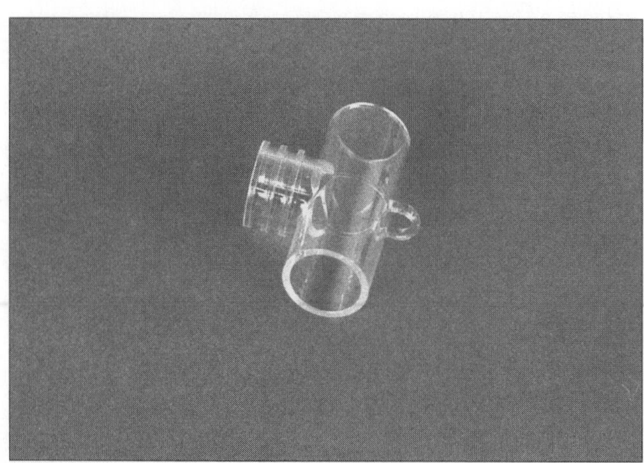

FIGURE **11-10** T tube.

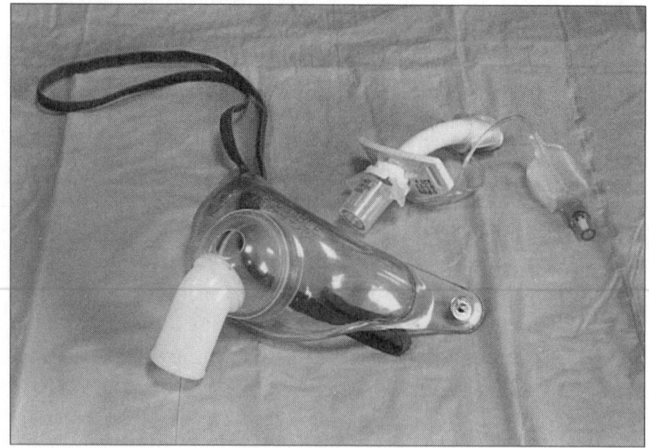

FIGURE **11-11** Tracheostomy collar.

Step	Rationale
Assessment	
1. Observe for signs and symptoms associated with hypoxia (see Box 11-1).	Assessment provides the nurse with baseline data.

- ***Critical Decision Point***
  Clients who demonstrate changes over time may have a worsening of a chronic or an existing condition or a new medical problem. For example, clients with a decreased hemoglobin level may have decreased oxygenation because the hemoglobin cannot carry enough oxygen to meet physiological needs.

Step	Rationale
2. Observe for patent airway, and remove airway secretions by suctioning (see Chapter 13).	Secretions can plug the airway, decreasing the amount of oxygen that is available for gas exchange in the lung. Secretions can also occlude the T tube or tracheostomy collar, impeding oxygen delivery to the client.

STEP	RATIONALE
3. If available, note client's most recent arterial blood gas (ABG) results or arterial oxygen saturation.	Objectively documents the client's pH, arterial oxygen, arterial carbon dioxide (CO_2), or arterial oxygen saturation.

- ***Critical Decision Point***
  Note if the current oxygen therapy has been meeting the client's oxygenation needs. Determine what factors have changed, resulting in the new assessment findings.

STEP	RATIONALE
4. Review client's medical record for the medical order for oxygen, noting delivery method, flow rate, and duration of oxygen therapy.	Ensures safe and accurate O_2 administration.
5. Complete total respiratory system assessment (see Chapter 10).	Determines presence of respiratory abnormalities impeding oxygenation.

NURSING DIAGNOSIS

Defining characteristics from the assessment data may reveal the following nursing diagnoses for clients requiring this skill:

Impaired gas exchange
Ineffective breathing pattern
Ineffective airway clearance

Related factors are individualized based on client's condition or needs.

PLANNING

STEP	RATIONALE
1. **Expected outcomes** following completion of procedure:	
▪ Signs of hypoxia are reduced or eliminated.	Client experiences improved oxygenation.
▪ Client's vital signs will return to baseline.	
▪ Client's work of breathing will decrease.	
▪ Client will experience increased lung expansion.	
▪ Client's level of consciousness (LOC) will return to baseline.	
▪ Arterial blood gas values or arterial oxygen saturation will return to normal or baseline.	
2. Explain the purpose of the T tube or tracheostomy collar to the client and family.	Explanation decreases the client's anxiety and reduces oxygen consumption.

IMPLEMENTATION

STEP	RATIONALE
1. Wash hands, apply gloves, apply goggles, and consider use of barrier gown.	Reduces transmission of microorganisms and prevents contact with pulmonary secretions.

- ***Critical Decision Point***
  Clients with excessive secretions or forceful productive coughs place the caregiver at risk for contact with pulmonary secretions.

STEP	RATIONALE
2. Attach T tube or tracheostomy collar to large-bore oxygen tubing and to humidified room air or oxygen source, if indicated.	Provides supplemental humidification to avoid drying of the airway.
3. If oxygen is ordered, adjust flow rate to 10 L/min or as ordered, adjust nebulizer to proper FIO_2 setting, and attach T tube or tracheostomy collar to endotracheal or tracheostomy tube.	Flow rate ensures humidification; nebulizer regulates FIO_2.
4. Monitor client's response to changes in the oxygen flow rate with pulse oximetry (see Chapter 9).	Monitoring with pulse oximetry allows for noninvasive, cost-effective trending of the client's arterial oxygen saturation and pulse rate.

STEP	RATIONALE

- ***Critical Decision Point***
  Collaborate with physician for plan of ongoing monitoring of oxygenation with ABG levels or trending pulse oximetry.

STEP	RATIONALE
5. Observe that T tube does not pull on endotracheal or tracheostomy tube. Observe for secretions within T tube or tracheostomy collar and suction as necessary (see Chapter 13).	Pulling effect can increase client's discomfort and cause pressure to side of client's mouth or tracheal stoma. Maintains patent airway.
6. Observe oxygen tubing frequently for accumulation of fluid. If fluid is present, drain tube away from client and discard fluid in proper receptacle.	Excess water is medium for bacterial growth. Draining contaminated water into proper receptacle prevents contamination of entire humidifying unit.
7. Set up suction equipment at client's bedside.	Client may experience increased airway secretions resulting from humidification.
8. Remove gloves and goggles; wash hands.	Reduces transmission of microorganisms and contamination with pulmonary secretions.

EVALUATION

STEP	RATIONALE
1. Observe for decreased anxiety, improved LOC and cognitive abilities, decreased fatigue, absence of dizziness, decreased pulse with regular rhythm, decreased respiratory rate, return to normal blood pressure, improved color, and return to client's baseline vital signs.	Evaluates effectiveness of interventions.
2. Observe the position of the oxygen delivery device to ensure that it is not pulling on the artificial airway.	Pulling on the artificial airway may result in damage to the oral cavity or stoma.
3. Monitor arterial blood gas levels or observe pulse oximetry.	Documents client's level of oxygenation.

UNEXPECTED OUTCOMES AND RELATED INTERVENTIONS

- Client experiences stoma irritation; thick, tenacious secretions; pressure areas on neck or near stoma site.
  - Implement measures to maintain skin integrity (see Chapter 7).
  - Increase frequency of airway care.
  - Suction secretions from artificial airway and lungs as indicated.
- Client experiences continued hypoxia.
  - Determine if the cause of the continued hypoxia is the oxygen delivery device, plugging of the airway, the oxygen flow rate, or a new clinical problem.
  - Notify physician of continued or worsening hypoxia.

RECORDING AND REPORTING

- Record the respiratory assessment findings; method of oxygen delivery, flow rate, client's response; any adverse reactions or side effects; change in physician's orders.
- Report any unexpected outcome to physician or nurse in charge.

TEACHING CONSIDERATIONS

- Teach the client and family alternative communication techniques (Chapter 2) to enhance communication with caregivers and to reduce frustration.
- Teach the client and family the importance of and rationale for the oxygen therapy.
- Teach the client and family safety precautions for oxygen use (see Box 11-2).
- Teach the client and family signs and symptoms of oxygen toxicity and CO_2 retention (e.g., confusion, headache, decreased LOC, somnolence) (see Box 11-1).

HOME CARE CONSIDERATIONS

- The client with an artificial airway who is at home may have a permanent tracheostomy, as well as a T tube or a tracheostomy collar.
- The client or caregiver should be able to perform tracheostomy care and suctioning techniques (see Chapter 13).

Skill 11-3 Using Incentive Spirometry

Incentive spirometry assists the client in deep breathing. An incentive spirometer (IS) is most often used following abdominal or thoracic surgery to help reduce the incidence of postoperative pulmonary atelectasis. Postoperative deep breathing and coughing have been shown to be as effective as using an incentive spirometer when performed frequently. The advantage of the IS is the visual feedback to clients about the depth of their breaths. The two types of spirometers are flow oriented and volume oriented.

Flow-oriented ISs have one or more plastic chambers with freely movable, colored balls. As the client inhales slowly, the balls are elevated to a premarked area (Figure 11-12). The goal is to keep the balls elevated for as long as possible to ensure maximal sustained inhalation, not to snap the balls to the top of the chamber with a rapid, very brief, low-volume breath. Even if a very slow inspiration does not elevate the balls, this pattern may achieve greater lung expansion. The advantage of a flow-oriented IS is the slow, steady expansion of the lung.

Volume-oriented ISs have a bellows that the client must raise to a predetermined volume by inhaling slowly (Figure 11-13). An achievement light or counter is used to provide feedback to the client. Some devices have a marker that moves up as the client inhales. The advantage of the volume-oriented IS is that a known inspiratory volume can be achieved and measured with each breath.

The use of the IS encourages clients to breathe deeply and achieve their normal inspiratory capacity. Incentive spirometry is used most often with postoperative clients. It is helpful to determine the client's baseline preoperative inspiratory capacity. An inspiratory volume one half to three quarters of baseline is an acceptable postoperative volume. Clients benefiting from incentive spirometry include those using it preoperatively, especially before abdominal, cardiac, or orthopedic surgery; clients with a history of smoking, pneumonia, or chronic respiratory disease; and clients with atelectasis.

Delegation Considerations

The skill of assisting a client with incentive spirometry can be delegated to appropriately trained assistive personnel. The device setup and the client should be assessed and checked by a nurse following implementation. The care provider should be informed in the proper way to set up and use the IS and aware of the client's target goal for spirometry.

Equipment

- Flow-oriented IS or volume-oriented IS

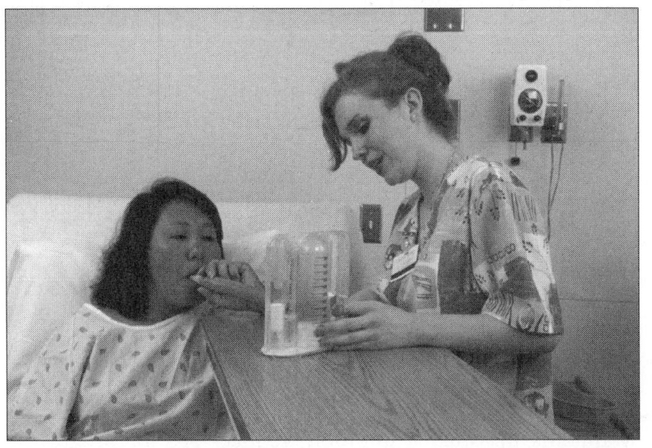

FIGURE **11-12** Flow-oriented incentive spirometer.

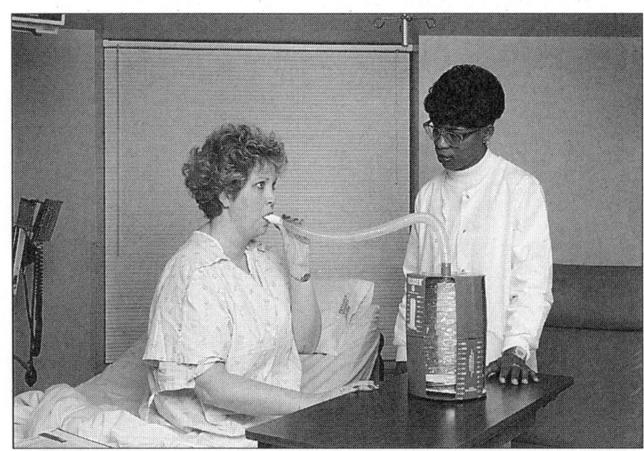

FIGURE **11-13** Volume-oriented incentive spirometer.

Step	Rationale

Assessment

1. Identify clients who would benefit from incentive spirometry. — Alerts health care personnel to those clients at risk for respiratory complications during illness or postoperatively.

• ***Critical Decision Point***
Clients with flail chest require other respiratory maneuvers to correct asymmetrical chest wall motion. Clients who may experience difficulty with incentive spirometry include those who are confused, malnourished, or cognitively impaired and those who lack necessary motor skills.

2. Assess client's respiratory status, including symmetry of chest wall expansion, respiratory rate and depth, sputum production, and lung sounds (see Chapter 10). — Decreased chest wall movement, crackles or decreased lung sounds, increased respiratory rate, or increased sputum production can indicate a need for incentive spirometry or other respiratory maneuvers to improve lung expansion.
3. Review the physician's order for incentive spirometry. — Health care institutions frequently require a medical order for incentive spirometry in order to receive third-party reimbursement for the spirometer.

Nursing Diagnosis

Defining characteristics from the assessment data may reveal the following nursing diagnoses for clients requiring this skill:

Impaired gas exchange
Ineffective breathing pattern
Ineffective airway clearance

Related factors are individualized based on client's condition or needs.

Planning

1. **Expected outcomes** following completion of procedure:
   - Client will demonstrate correct use of the IS. — Demonstrates learning.
   - Client achieves target volume and number of repetitions per hour. — Demonstrates increased lung expansion.
   - Client has normal breath sounds.
2. Explain the procedure to the client and family. — Understanding the purpose of incentive spirometry and its proper use will improve compliance with use.

Implementation

1. Wash hands. — Reduces transmission of microorganisms.
2. Position client in a semi-Fowler's or high-Fowler's position. — Promotes optimal lung expansion during respiratory maneuver.
3. Instruct client to place lips completely over mouthpiece. — Showing client to correctly place mouthpiece is a reliable technique for teaching psychomotor skill and enables client to ask questions.
4. Instruct client to inhale slowly and maintain a constant flow, like pulling through a straw. When maximal inspiration is reached, client should hold breath for 2 to 3 seconds and then exhale slowly. — Maintains maximal inspiration; reduces risk of progressive collapse of individual alveoli.

• ***Critical Decision Point***
Allow clients to rest between IS breaths to prevent hyperventilation and fatigue.

5. Have client repeat the maneuver until goals are achieved. — Ensures correct use of the spirometer and client's understanding of use.
6. Wash hands. — Reduces transmission of microorganisms.

STEP	RATIONALE
EVALUATION	
1. Observe client's ability to use incentive spirometry by return demonstration.	Determines client's ability to perform breathing exercise correctly.
2. Assess if the client is able to achieve the target volume or frequency.	Measures compliance with therapy and lung expansion.
3. Auscultate chest during respiratory cycle.	Documents lung wall expansion, identifies any abnormal lung sounds, and determines if airways are clear.

UNEXPECTED OUTCOMES AND RELATED INTERVENTIONS

- Client is unable to achieve incentive spirometry target volumes and frequency independently.
  - Encourage client to attempt IS more frequently followed by rest periods.
  - Teach cough-control exercises.
  - Teach client how to splint and protect incision sites.
- Client has decreased lung expansion and/or abnormal breath sounds.
  - Teach client cough-control exercises.
  - Provide assistance with suctioning if clients cannot effectively cough up their secretions.

RECORDING AND REPORTING

- Record the lung sounds before and after incentive spirometry, the frequency of use, the volumes achieved, and any adverse effects.
- Report any changes in respiratory assessment or client's inability to use IS

TEACHING CONSIDERATIONS

- Teach client to examine sputum for consistency, amount, and color changes.
- Identify learning objectives for preparing client to use the IS: correctly places the mouthpiece; achieves satisfactory maximal inspiration; repeats the maneuver the required number of times; and understands the rationale for performing incentive spirometry.

GERONTOLOGICAL CONSIDERATIONS

- Older adults may have difficulty coordinating the use of the IS. They may require additional time to learn the procedure; however, once they understand and learn the procedure, they will be very capable of continuing with the plan.
- The older adult has an increased respiratory rate, between 16 and 25 breaths per minute. Observe closely for hyperventilation and fatigue.

HOME CARE CONSIDERATIONS

- Have client return demonstrate correct procedure for use before discharge.

Skill 11-4 Administering Mechanical Ventilation

Clients requiring mechanical ventilation need support for ventilation and/or oxygenation. Clinical problems such as respiratory failure, exacerbation of chronic obstructive lung disease, status asthmaticus, Guillain-Barré syndrome, spinal cord trauma, respiratory muscle paralysis, and pneumonia may require mechanical ventilation support. Clients requiring acute mechanical ventilation are most often cared for in an intensive care unit. An endotracheal tube (ETT) or a tracheostomy tube will need to be placed to attach the ventilator.

There are two types of mechanical ventilation: positive pressure and negative pressure. Positive pressure ventilation is the usual method of ventilation. **Positive-pressure ventilation** delivers a positive pressure to inflate the lungs. The increased positive intrathoracic pressure may impede venous return to the right side of the heart, resulting in a decreased cardiac output, tachycardia, and hypotension. The nurse must be alert for these side effects.

Negative-pressure ventilation is used for clients with primary neuromuscular illnesses that interfere with normal respiratory muscle function, such as multiple sclerosis, muscular dystrophy, and early stages of chronic obstructive pulmonary disease (COPD). The client is fitted with a poncho or shell that is connected to the ventilator. Air is removed from between the client's chest wall and the interior wall of the poncho or shell, causing the client to inhale. The client using negative pressure ventilation does not need an artificial airway.

Many types of mechanical ventilators are available for acute care use. Mechanical ventilators are available in pressure-cycled and volume-cycled machines. **Pressure-cycled ventilation** delivers a specified pressure to the client, achieving a **tidal volume,** or amount of air, in milliliters, per breath (Figure 11-14). **Volume-cycled ventilation** delivers a specified tidal volume. Volume-cycled ventilators are most often used in the clinical setting. Clients using pressure-cycled ventilators are at higher risk for development of pneumothorax, hypotension, and decreased cardiac output as a result of the ventilator's achieving the prescribed pressure without regard for lung compliance. Volume-cycled ventilators achieve tidal volume with preset pressure limits and are more sensitive to lung compliance. Time-cycled ventilators provide an inspiratory phase until a preset time is reached. This often results in varying tidal volumes.

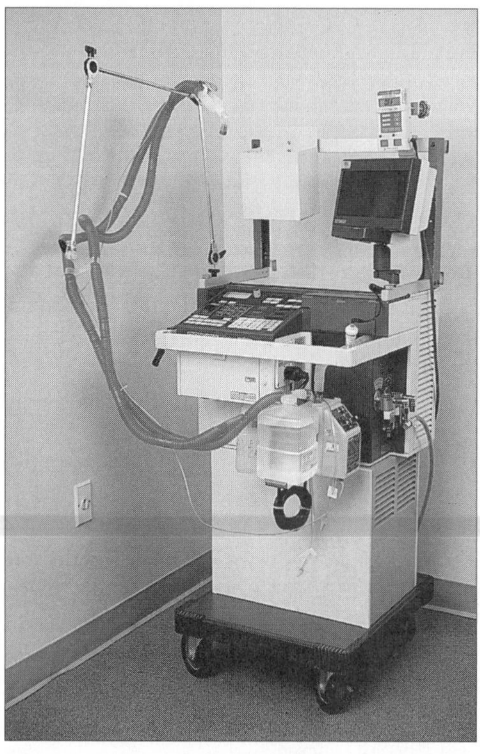

FIGURE **11-14** A mechanical ventilator.

MODES OF VENTILATION

There are many different modes of mechanical ventilation to support different conditions and physiological processes. Modes of ventilation include control mode (CM), continuous mandatory ventilation (CMV), synchronized intermittent mandatory ventilation (SIMV), and pressure support ventilation (PSV). The more frequently used modes of ventilation are CMV, SIMV, and PSV. They support oxygenation and provide varying levels of ventilatory support that can be adjusted to meet the client's needs (Table 11-3). Continuous mandatory ventilation provides continuous ventilation to the client, maintaining the respiratory rate and tidal volume. Synchronized intermittent mandatory ventilation attempts to synchronize the ventilator breaths with the client's spontaneous breathing. This reduces competition between the ventilator and the client.

Pressure support ventilation is actually a spontaneous breathing mode, because the ventilator does not deliver a preset

Table 11-3 Modes of Mechanical Ventilation

MODE	DEFINITION	INDICATIONS	COMMENTS
Control mode (CM)	Preset tidal volume and preset rate delivered to the client regardless of the client's respiratory effort. Client cannot initiate breaths or change the ventilatory pattern.	Neuromuscular disease Drug overdose Reduction of work of breathing	Client may require sedation to reduce competition with the ventilator. Rarely used.
Continuous mandatory ventilation (CMV)	Preset tidal volume at preset rate is delivered to the client. The client can initiate breaths that are delivered at the preset tidal volume.	Reduction of work of breathing Respiratory muscle fatigue COPD Postanesthesia	Client may need sedation to reduce spontaneous breaths.
Synchronized intermittent mandatory ventilation (SIMV)	Preset tidal volume at preset rate is synchronized with the client's spontaneous breathing to reduce competition between machine-delivered and client-spontaneous breaths.	Primary ventilatory mode Used to wean clients from mechanical ventilation	Client synchrony with the ventilator is improved. Rates ≤6 breaths per minute can result in increased work of breathing.
Pressure support ventilation (PSV)	Provides positive pressure during the inspiratory cycle of a spontaneous inspiratory effort (Weilitz, 2000).	Weaning clients with COPD Primary ventilatory mode in higher pressures	There is no preset respiratory rate. The nurse must assess for respiratory muscle fatigue and periods of apnea. Decreases work of breathing by overcoming resistance of airway and ventilatory circuit.

tidal volume or rate. It provides a preset pressure to augment the inspiratory process and help overcome the initial work of breathing. It is used both for ventilation and to assist in weaning the client. Clients on PSV need to be assessed frequently for respiratory muscle fatigue and potential periods of apnea.

Positive end-expiratory pressure (PEEP) and continuous positive airway pressure (CPAP) are adjuncts to ventilation used to increase oxygenation. Positive end-expiratory pressure is positive airway pressure maintained at the end of exhalation. This allows more time for gas exchange and opens small airways and closed alveolar units, thus improving oxygenation. Continuous positive airway pressure is the maintenance of a positive airway pressure above atmospheric pressure during inspiration and expiration in the spontaneously breathing client. It improves oxygenation in the same manner as PEEP.

Alarms and Settings

The mechanical ventilator has a number of settings to adjust the amount of oxygen delivered, the amount of tidal volume, the time for inspiration and expiration, and the pressure at which each breath is delivered. The tidal volume, the amount of air per breath, is usually set at 10 to 15 ml/kg body weight. The respiratory rate is usually set at 10 to 16 breaths per minute. Initially the oxygen may be set at 100% if the reason for intubation and ventilation was cardiopulmonary arrest. The goal of providing oxygenation is to maintain an arterial oxygen pressure (PO_2) of greater than or equal to 60 mm Hg using an inspired oxygen concentration (FIO_2) of 50% or less. Table 11-4 lists the ventilator parameters the nurse must become familiar with to care for a client on mechanical ventilation.

There are a number of alarms on the ventilator to ensure client safety. Each ventilator is a little different; however, the basic alarms are similar. Alarms common to all ventilators include high-pressure, low-pressure, low–exhaled volume, and oxygen alarms (Table 11-5). The nurse must know how to respond to the ventilator alarms and what nursing actions may be required to preserve the client's respiratory status. The two most frequent alarms are the high-pressure and low-pressure alarms. The high-pressure alarm is usually set at 10 to 15 cm greater than the peak airway pressure. When this alarm sounds, it indicates the ventilator has met resistance to delivering the tidal volume and requires more pressure to inflate the lungs. The client may have coughed during the inspiratory cycle, may need suctioning, or may have changed position. More acute problems that require immediate nursing intervention include the development of a pneumothorax or displacement of the ETT or tracheostomy tube. The low-pressure alarm sounds when the ventilator has no resistance to inflating the lung. The client may be disconnected from the ventilator, or a leak has developed in the ventilator circuit.

Once the condition for which the client required mechanical ventilation is corrected, the weaning process is initiated. Weaning from mechanical ventilation is the gradual reduction of ventilation and oxygenation support until the client is breathing spontaneously and can be oxygenated with a low-flow oxygen device. Many clients who are unable to wean from the mechanical ventilator may be transferred to subacute nursing care for continued care or in preparation for home mechanical ventilation. Generally these clients are hemodynamically stable; however, they require continual ventilatory support.

Table 11-4 Ventilator Parameters

Parameter	Definition	Ventilator Setting
Tidal volume (V_T)	Amount of air inspired and expired with each breath	10 to 15 ml/kg of body weight
Respiratory rate (R or RR)	Number of breaths delivered per minute	10 to 16 breaths per minute
Fraction of inspired oxygen (FIO_2)	Amount of oxygen the client receives	21% to 100% to maintain PaO_2 60 to 80 torr
PEEP	Positive pressure applied at end expiration to improve oxygenation	+3 to 5 cm H_2O may be used to approximate physiological PEEP* May require higher levels (>5 cm H_2O) in respiratory failure (e.g., adult respiratory disease syndrome)
Sigh	Larger than normal breath to provide hyperinflation; helps prevent atelectasis	Usually twice the tidal volume breath; about 10 to 15 ml/kg Rate is usually set at 10 to 15 times per hour
Sensitivity	Determines the inspiratory effort required to trigger the ventilator	Set to respond to an inspired volume of less than 1% of the client's tidal volume
Peak airway pressure	The maximal pressure level required to deliver the desired tidal volume	<40 cm H_2O
I:E ratio	Comparison of inspiratory (I) to expiratory (E) time	Normally set 1:1, 1:2, or 1:3 Example: inspiration 2 seconds, expiration 4 seconds; then I:E = 1:2
Exhaled minute ventilation (V_E)	Measures the exhaled minute ventilations in liters	Alarm set at 15% greater than client's average V_E

*Some clinicians believe that the ETT with inflated cuff creates a closed system with the ventilator and does not require 3 to 5 cm of PEEP.

Table 11-5 Troubleshooting Mechanical Ventilation

Ventilator Alarm	Possible Cause	Nursing Interventions
Sudden increase in peak airway pressure (high-pressure alarm)	Coughing Airway plugging	Clear secretions by suctioning.
	Changes in client position	Reposition client.
	Pneumothorax	Assess breath sounds and chest wall movement.
	Incorrect ETT position	Verify placement of ETT. Assess breath sounds. Verify cm level of ETT.
	Kinked ventilator circuit	Check circuit; unkink tubing.
	Excessive water in ventilator circuit	Drain ventilator tubing.
Gradual increase in peak airway pressure	Decreasing lung compliance	Evaluate breath sounds; suction.
	Exacerbation of acute process	Check for reversible causes: airway plugging, bronchospasm.
Sudden decrease in peak airway pressure (low-pressure alarm)	Client disconnected from ventilator	Check for disconnection.
	Leak in ventilator circuit	Evaluate circuit connections; tighten loose connections.
Change in minute ventilation or tidal volume	Leak in ETT cuff	Check cuff seal.
Decrease	Airway secretions	Suction excessive secretions.
	System leak	Check circuit connections.
	Increased respiratory rate	Evaluate respiratory rate.
Increase	Hypoxia	Evaluate for signs of hypoxia. Evaluate need to obtain ABG sample or monitor pulse oximetry.
Change in respiratory rate	Client anxiety	Reassure client.
	Increased metabolic demand	Evaluate body therapy, heart rate, and rhythm.
	Hypoxia	Obtain ABG levels or monitor pulse oximetry.

The mechanical ventilator also has settings to regulate the temperature of the water in the humidifier, known as the cascade. The temperature of the heater in the cascade is set at or just below normal body temperature. This provides warm, moistened air for delivery to the airway. The cascade is a potential source of contamination of the ventilator circuit if the water that collects in the ventilator tubing is drained back into the cascade unit.

Home Mechanical Ventilation

The client on mechanical ventilation can be successfully managed in the home. Neuromuscular disease such as amyotrophic lateral sclerosis (ALS), muscular dystrophy, brain and spinal cord diseases, chest wall disease, central hypoventilation syndrome, and advanced COPD are just a few of the diseases for which clients are managed at home on mechanical ventilators. Many factors determine if a client and family are candidates for home ventilation. Assessment criteria include the desire of the client and family, the client's acceptance of ventilator dependence, the client's and family's ability to understand and perform daily care procedures, the home environment, personnel resources, monetary resources, and resources and technologies for support in the community.

The goals of long-term ventilator care should include extension of life, enhancement of the quality of life, provision of an environment that enhances individual potential, reduction of morbidity, improvement of physical and physiological function, and cost-effectiveness. Clients and families who are candidates for home mechanical ventilation should be prepared for discharge by a multidisciplinary team including representatives of nursing, medicine, dietary service, social service, the home health nurse, and the home care durable medical equipment company. The nurse in the hospital must be familiar with the home ventilator to assist the client with discharge planning and education.

Delegation Considerations

The skill of administering mechanical ventilation should not be delegated to assistive personnel.

Equipment

- Appropriate mechanical ventilator
- 50 psi oxygen source
- Ventilator circuit
- Humidification source
- Heated passover system
- Artificial nose
- Heated wire system
- Ambu-bag with oxygen connecting tubing and flowmeter
- Gloves
- Goggles (if splash risk exists)

STEP	RATIONALE

ASSESSMENT

1. Observe for signs and symptoms associated with hypoxia (see Box 11-1). — Assessment provides the nurse with baseline data.
2. Observe for patent airway and remove airway secretions by suctioning (see Chapter 13). — Secretions can plug the airway, decreasing the amount of oxygen that is available for gas exchange in the lung. Secretions can also occlude the T tube or tracheostomy collar, impeding oxygen delivery to the client.
3. If available, note client's most recent arterial blood gas (ABG) results or arterial oxygen saturation. — Objectively documents the client's pH, arterial oxygen, arterial CO_2, or arterial oxygen saturation.

- ***Critical Decision Point***
  Evaluate if the current ventilation therapy is meeting the client's oxygenation and ventilation needs. Determine what factors have changed, resulting in the new assessment findings.

4. Review client's medical record for the medical order for mechanical ventilation, noting mode of ventilation, respiratory rate, oxygen setting, and tidal volume. — Mechanical ventilation usually requires a physician's order.
5. Complete total respiratory system assessment (see Chapter 10). — Determines presence of respiratory abnormalities impeding oxygenation and ventilation.

NURSING DIAGNOSIS

Defining characteristics from the assessment data may reveal the following nursing diagnoses for clients requiring this skill:

- Impaired gas exchange
- Ineffective breathing pattern
- Ineffective airway clearance
- Impaired spontaneous ventilation
- Dysfunctional ventilatory weaning response
- Risk for infection
- Impaired verbal communication

Related factors are individualized based on client's condition or needs.

PLANNING

1. **Expected outcomes** following completion of procedure:
   - Client will have increased lung expansion. — Client experiences improved oxygenation and ventilation.
   - Client will maintain ABG levels and oxygen saturation within normal range or at baseline.
   - Client experiences reduction in feelings of dyspnea and work of breathing.
   - Client uses communication board, paper and pencil, or computer to state needs. — Appropriate communication system matches clients abilities.
2. Explain to client and family the purpose and reasons for initiation of mechanical ventilation. — Helps client to express fears and wishes. Plays a role in the weaning process (Moody and others, 1997).

IMPLEMENTATION

1. Wash hands; apply gloves and goggles. Apply barrier gown if secretions are projectile. — Reduces transmission of microorganisms and exposure to pulmonary secretions.
2. Attach mechanical ventilator to ETT or tracheostomy tube. Observe for proper functioning of mechanical ventilator. — Ensures client is receiving proper mechanical ventilation.

- ***Critical Decision Point***
  The mechanical ventilator requires programming of accurate settings before attaching to the client. This is most often the responsibility of the respiratory therapist; however, it may also be a collaborative responsibility of the nurse.

STEP	RATIONALE
3. Verify that the ETT or tracheostomy tube is properly positioned by listening to both lungs and assessing chest wall symmetry.	Properly placed artificial airway will ensure that both lungs are equally ventilated. Improper airway placement may lead to unilateral lung ventilation.
4. Observe client for synchronization with mechanical ventilation and response to therapy.	Ensures client is comfortable using ventilator and has not experienced any adverse hemodynamic effects.
5. Monitor heart rate, blood pressure, respiratory rate, and cardiac rhythm.	Implementation of mechanical ventilation can result in decreased venous return and associated hemodynamic changes.
6. Secure ventilator tubing to reduce pull on tracheostomy or ET tube.	Prevents accidental dislodging of artificial airway.
7. Note the level of the ETT at the lips or nares.	Provides a baseline for depth of tube placement.
8. Set up suction equipment.	Need to provide airway care and suctioning as needed of ET or tracheostomy tube to prevent plugging of the airway and to reduce the risk of infection.

- ***Critical Decision Point***
  Determine if the client will need an oral suction setup, as well as endotracheal suctioning.

9. Position client to promote best oxygenation and ventilation.	Positioning can affect oxygenation and ventilation (Gawlinski and Dracup, 1998; Manning and others, 1999).
10. Collaborate with the physician frequently about the status of the client and the response to therapy and ongoing monitoring to assess oxygenation status and continued need for mechanical ventilation.	
11. Remove gloves and goggles; wash hands.	Reduces transmission of microorganisms and exposure to pulmonary secretions.

EVALUATION

1. Evaluate client's response to mechanical ventilation. Observe for decreased anxiety; improved LOC and cognitive abilities; decreased fatigue; absence of dizziness; decreased pulse, regular rhythm; decreased respiratory rate and work of breathing; return to normal blood pressure; improved color.	Hypoxia and **hypercapnia** are reduced or corrected.
2. Monitor ABG levels—observe pulse oximetry.	Documents client's level of oxygenation.
3. Observe integrity of client ventilator system.	Ensures adequate delivery of mechanical ventilation.

UNEXPECTED OUTCOMES AND RELATED INTERVENTIONS

- Client experiences stiff, noncompliant lung; alveolar edema; pulmonary congestion; chest pain; intraalveolar hemorrhage; substernal chest pain; pneumothorax; continued decrease in blood pressure related to use of positive pressure.
  - Notify physician.
  - Remain with client.
  - Conduct a complete cardiac and pulmonary assessment.
- Client experiences hypoxia
  - Notify physician.
  - Assess client.
  - Assess integrity of ventilator system.
- Client experiences hypercapnia
  - Notify physician.
  - Assess client.
  - Assess integrity of ventilator system.

RECORDING AND REPORTING

- Record in progress notes:
  - Respiratory assessment findings
  - Mode of mechanical ventilation
  - Oxygen level, actual client tidal volume, ordered tidal volume, actual client respiratory rate, ordered respiratory rate, peak airway pressure
  - Client's response to mechanical ventilation
  - Level of the ETT, any adverse reactions or side effects
  - Change in the physician's orders
- Report to nurse in charge or physician:
  - Sudden change in client's respiratory status
  - Ventilator-associated problems

Teaching Considerations

- Teach the client and family about the rationale for mechanical ventilation.
- Teach client and family about the alarms and what they mean.
- Teach client and family alternative communication techniques to reduce frustration and fear.

Home Care Considerations

- Clients requiring home mechanical ventilation need to be taught complete care of the mechanical ventilator system, suctioning, and artificial airway care. Skills include assembling the ventilator circuit, cleaning the circuit, and daily equipment maintenance (Rice, 2000).
- Client and family should have a thorough knowledge of the operation of the home ventilator, the knobs and settings, and the power sources.
- Use a checklist for ensuring consistency of care for the client on a ventilator.
- Evaluate the following areas during each visit: oxygen flow, alarm system, inspiratory pressure, high-pressure alarm, tidal volume setting, humidifier, respiratory rate, tubing, temperature, resuscitation bag, tracheostomy care, breath sounds, suctioning, and tubing changes.
- The durable medical equipment provider, the home health nurse, and the primary care nurse should develop a teaching plan to ensure that client and family have a complete working knowledge of the ventilator before discharge.
- Instruct client and primary caregiver in what to do in case of respiratory distress or power failure. Check to determine availability of emergency batteries.
- Instruct family in use of the Ambu-bag (see Chapter 15).

Long-Term Care Considerations

- Clients who require long-term mechanical ventilation may be transferred to a chronic ventilator facility or a long-term ventilator dependency floor within the hospital. The purpose of such a transfer is to aggressively rehabilitate the client through physical therapy, occupational therapy, and speech therapy. The overall goal is to effectively wean client from the mechanical ventilator.
- Prepare client and family for long-term care and the role of client and family for successful rehabilitation.
- If possible have family visit facility before client discharge.

Skill 11-5 Measuring Peak Expiratory Flow Rates

Pulmonary function studies are essential for diagnosis of pulmonary disease. For clients with chronic airflow obstruction such as asthma, measurement of the **peak expiratory flow rate** (PEFR) gives objective data about the severity of the airway obstruction. The PEFR is the maximum flow rate, in liters, that can be generated during a forced expiratory maneuver using a peak flowmeter. Benefits to measuring the PEFR are that it is simple, quantitative, reproducible, and inexpensive, and it correlates well with forced expiratory volume at 1 second (FEV_1). The PEFR is a more objective measure of severity than symptoms such as wheezing and shortness of breath. Peak expiratory flow rate measures are used to assess asthma severity, monitor response to therapy, both acutely and chronically, diagnose exercise-induced asthma, detect asymptomatic deterioration in lung function, and assess the degree of airflow obstruction during health care visits.

A plan of action is developed with the client and the physician to address changes in the PEFR. When the PEFR drops, the client has a specific plan of action that includes changes in medication, when to notify the physician, and changes in the medical therapy. It is important that the client and caregiver know and understand the specific plan, the expected change in the PEFR, and when to notify the physician or go to the emergency department.

The disadvantage of PEFR is that it is effort dependent. The client must be willing and cooperative with the procedure to obtain accurate and reliable measurements. Because PEFR measures only large airway function, clients with mild asthma may be underdiagnosed.

Delegation Considerations

The skill of measuring peak expiratory flow rates should not be delegated to assistive personnel.

Equipment

- Peak flowmeter

STEP	RATIONALE

ASSESSMENT

Step	Rationale
1. Observe for signs of airway obstruction: shortness of breath, wheezing, use of accessory muscles of respiration, cyanosis, and nasal flaring.	Indicates client is in distress. Airway obstruction can be life threatening and demands immediate intervention.
2. Observe for patent airway and the need for removal of any secretions.	Secretions increase airway resistance and may plug the airway.
3. Complete respiratory assessment.	Provides objective baseline data.
4. Review client's medical record for the order to measure PEFR and expected rate to be achieved by the client.	Provides client outcome measure when treatment is at effective levels.

NURSING DIAGNOSIS

Defining characteristics from the assessment data may reveal the following nursing diagnoses for clients requiring this skill:

Impaired gas exchange
Ineffective breathing pattern
Deficient knowledge regarding measuring PEFR

Related factors are individualized based on client's condition or needs.

PLANNING

Step	Rationale
1. **Expected outcomes** following completion of procedure:	
▪ Client's PEFR will remain within 20% of personal best.	PEFR less than 80% of personal best indicates the need for more aggressive therapy and continual daily monitoring.
▪ Client correctly uses PEFR.	Demonstrates learning. Correct use of PEFR is essential to determine adequacy of expiratory airflow in clients with airway reactivity.
2. Explain the procedure to the client and family.	Promotes client and family cooperation.

IMPLEMENTATION

Step	Rationale
1. Place indicator at base of the numbered scale (see illustration).	Starts reading from zero.
2. Have client stand up.	Increases lung expansion and promotes deep breathing.

• ***Critical Decision Point***

If clients are unable to stand, have them sit on a chair or on the edge of the bed or in high-Fowler's position.

Step	Rationale
3. Have client take a deep breath.	Maximal effort is required for an accurate reading.
4. Have client place the meter in the mouth and close the lips around the mouthpiece (see illustration).	Increases the accuracy of measurement, and the exhalation will be directed through the peak flowmeter.
Be sure that client has not obstructed open end of the device.	Obstruction of the device gives a false high reading
5. Have client blow out as hard and as fast as possible.	Maximal effort is required for an accurate reading.
6. Have client repeat steps 1 through 5 two more times, noting the highest number achieved.	Demonstrates the best effort.

STEP	RATIONALE

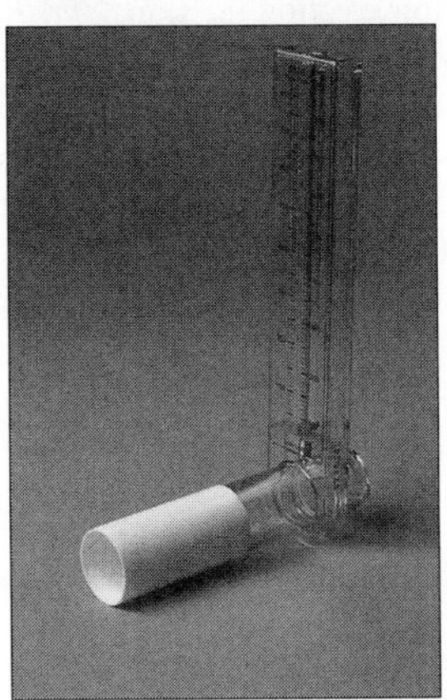

STEP 1 Peak flowmeter.

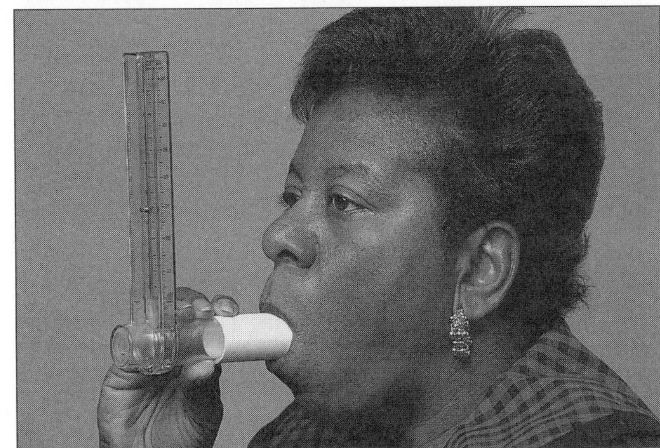

STEP 4 Correct use of peak flowmeter

EVALUATION

STEP	RATIONALE
1. Determine the client's PEFR and compare with the client's personal best.	Provides objective measure of client's symptoms. The personal best PEFR is obtained after the client is receiving effective therapy and has been determined to be maximally bronchodilated.
2. Reassess client for improvement in symptoms if bronchodilator therapy has been initiated.	PEFR is frequently measured following bronchodilator therapy to measure the client's response.
3. Observe client performing PEFR.	Documents learning and correct use of PEFR.

UNEXPECTED OUTCOMES AND RELATED INTERVENTIONS

- Client is unable to perform PEFR measurement
  - Indicates client is in distress and requires intervention such as bronchodilator therapy.
  - Client may need further demonstration on use of PEFR
  - Determine frequency of PEFR measurement if the client has experienced symptoms of airway obstruction.
- Client's PEFR measurement is less than 80% of personal best.
  - May indicate a poor effort by the client or severe airway obstruction.
  - Contact physician; client may need changes in bronchodilator or inhaled steroid therapy.

RECORDING AND REPORTING

- Record the PEFR measurement; in addition include:
  - The client's ability to use the peak flowmeter
  - Any symptoms the client may be experiencing
  - Any therapy the client may have received as a result of the PEFR measurement

TEACHING CONSIDERATIONS

- Begin teaching the client how to measure PEFR independently and record the measurements.
- Instruct the client in the care of the peak flowmeter.
- Teach the client how to recognize and record the best reading.
- Review the plan of action and when to notify the physician when there are changes in the PEFR to ensure understanding and ability to implement the plan.

HOME CARE CONSIDERATIONS

- Review the plan for notification of the physician when there are changes in the PEFR.
- Have the client demonstrate use of the peak expiratory flowmeter to demonstrate the client's ability to follow directions and use the flowmeter correctly.

Critical Thinking Exercises

1. Your client with asthma will be monitored with a peak expiratory flowmeter. What are the key concepts the client and family need to be taught?
2. The tidal volume level for your client on mechanical ventilation drops suddenly. What are the nursing interventions necessary to ensure that the client has adequate ventilation? What are the possible causes of the low tidal volume?
3. Your client is receiving oxygen therapy via nasal cannula at 3 L/min. He takes the cannula off because of discomfort at the nares and ears from the device. What are the causes of this discomfort? What are your interventions?

References

Gawlinski A, Dracup K: Effect of positioning on SvO2 in the critically ill patient with a low ejection fraction, *Nurs Res* 47(5):293, 1998.

Manning F and others: Effects of side lying on lung function in older individuals, *Phys Ther* 79(5):456, 1999.

Moody LE and others: Psychophysiologic predictors of weaning from mechanical ventilation in chronic bronchitis and emphysema, *Clin Nurs Res* 6(4):311, 1997.

Rice R: *Manual of home health nursing procedures,* ed 2, St. Louis, 2000, Mosby.

Weilitz PB: Respiratory system. In Leuckenotte AG: *Gerontologic Nursing,* ed 2, St. Louis, 2000, Mosby.

12

PERFORMING CHEST PHYSIOTHERAPY

Skills

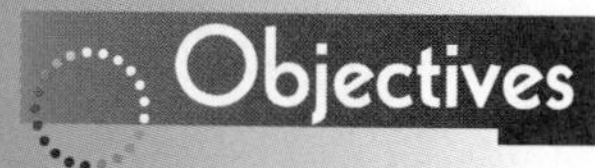

Objectives

Mastery of content in this chapter will enable the nurse to:

- Define the key terms listed.
- Assess the need to perform chest physiotherapy (CPT) maneuvers, including indications and physical assessment.
- Assess the need to modify or discontinue CPT maneuvers, including contraindications and individual variations.
- Explain how to prepare the client, the family, the nurse, and the therapist for the performance of each CPT maneuver.
- Identify goals for performing each CPT maneuver.
- Perform in a step-by-step method the outlined CPT maneuvers, including standard and modified versions.
- Describe expected and unexpected outcomes of each CPT maneuver.
- Describe discharge teaching and planning related to the use of each CPT maneuver in the home setting.

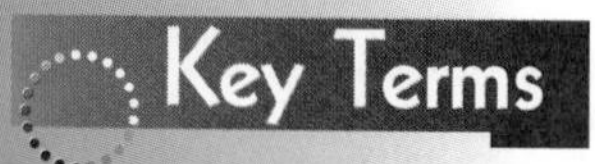

Key Terms

Chest physiotherapy
Cough
Mucociliary transport
Percussion
Postural drainage
Shaking
Vibration

Chest physiotherapy (CPT) consists of physical maneuvers such as cough, chest wall percussion, vibration and shaking, and postural drainage (PD). **Percussion** is a rhythmical force provided by clapping the caregiver's cupped hands against the client's thorax. Percussion assists in loosening retained secretions from the airway. Vibration and shaking are performed with the goal of moving secretions from the lung periphery to the larger airways. **Vibration** is performed by contracting all the muscles in the caregiver's upper extremities to cause vibration while applying pressure to the client's chest wall. **Shaking** is a stronger bouncing maneuver, which also supplies a concurrent, compressive force to the chest wall (Frownfelter and Dean, 1996). **Postural drainage** is achieved by positioning the client so that the position of the lung segment to be drained allows gravity to have its greatest effect (Frownfelter and Dean, 1996).

These maneuvers assist with airway clearance of mucus in clients with retained tracheobronchial secretions (Jones and Rowe, 1999). Examples of diseases associated with accumulation of excessive mucus in the tracheobronchial tree include atelectasis, bronchitis, asthma, cystic fibrosis, pneumonia, and bronchiectasis. Chest physiotherapy is often used with other therapeutic modalities, including antibiotic therapy, avoidance of specific airway irritants, smoking cessation, bronchodilator treatment, aerosol therapy, and systemic hydration and nebulization, to reduce mucus production and facilitate airway clearance. The goal is to improve respiratory gas exchange and to reduce and prevent further airway obstruction and ventilatory dysfunction. Research is inconclusive regarding the efficacy of CPT (Jones and Rowe, 1999).

The precise mechanism by which CPT maneuvers enhance clearance of airway secretions is not fully understood. The proposed mechanism of CPT is to facilitate movement of secretions from smaller peripheral airways into larger central airways, where coughing and suctioning are effective in removing them. Postural drainage involves placing the client in specific positions to use gravitational forces to assist in moving mucus from specific bronchi into the trachea. Exactly how externally applied forces of percussion, vibration and shaking are transmitted to the airways to move secretions toward the head is unclear. **Cough** is a natural lung clearance mechanism that aids in removal of mobilized secretions. Coughing forcefully exhales air, providing clearance of mucus primarily from the large central airways, including the trachea and mainstem bronchus.

When disease causes excessive sputum production, therapeutic interventions are needed to help natural airway clearance mechanisms (cough and mucociliary transport) clear the airways of obstructing mucus. In the normal lung the **mucociliary transport** system is able to keep the airways clear of excessive mucus and inhaled particles. This system lines the internal lumen of the entire tracheobronchial tree and consists of a thin layer of mucus that is constantly being propelled toward the larynx by cells that have hairlike projections called cilia. Inhaled particles are trapped on the mucus, and the cilia act as a conveyor belt to sweep the mucus toward the throat, where it can be swallowed or removed by coughing. In this way airways normally remain clear, and mucus is constantly being cleared almost as fast as it is made. Normal mucus remains thin, white, and watery.

In various disease states, mucus clearance slows down or the cilia are overwhelmed by production of excessively large quantities of mucus. The lung can no longer clear the mucus as fast as it is produced. Secretions stagnate in the airways, change color, and become thick and sticky. The cilia cannot remove large amounts of thick mucus from the lungs. In addition, many people with lung disease cannot cough effectively to clear airways. Therefore it becomes important to employ systemic hydration and other maneuvers to aid in clearing lung secretions as fast as they are made. These therapeutic modalities prevent mucus from stagnating and allow secretions to return to their normal thin, white, and watery consistency.

Fluids are an important part of a lung clearance program. They make the mucus thin and watery so that it can be mobilized, coughed up, and expectorated more easily. Unless contraindicated by other disease states, such as congestive heart failure or renal failure, fluids should be given along with CPT to make mucus thin and watery. During an acute exacerbation, it often takes three or four CPT treatments a day and 3 to 4 L of fluid a day to mobilize and thin secretions. During more stable states, one to two CPT treatments and 2 to 4 L of fluid a day can often keep secretions thin and watery, thereby preventing stagnation of mucus, which can lead to airway infection, airway obstruction, shortness of breath, increased work of breathing, and abnormal gas exchange.

This chapter presents two CPT skills as they are implemented in the clinical and home settings. Although they are separate skills, they must be thought of as different components of CPT. All must be mastered if treatment is to be effective.

Skill Performance Guidelines

The nurse plans the client's care and subsequent selection of CPT skills based on specific assessment findings. The following guidelines help the nurse in physical assessment and subsequent decision making:

1. Know the client's normal range of vital signs. Conditions such as atelectasis and pneumonia requiring CPT can affect a client's vital signs. The degree of change is related to the level of hypoxia, overall cardiopulmonary status, and tolerance to the procedure.
2. Know the client's present medications. Certain medications, particularly diuretics and antihypertensives, cause fluid and hemodynamic changes. These changes may decrease the client's tolerance of the positional changes of postural drainage. Steroid medications increase the client's risk of pathological rib fractures and often contraindicate rib shaking (Skill 12-2).
3. Know the client's medical and surgical history. Certain conditions, such as increased intracranial pressure, spinal cord injuries, or abdominal aneurysm resection, contraindicate the positional changes of postural drainage (Box 12-1). Thoracic trauma may contraindicate percussion, vibration and shaking.

Box 12-1 Contraindications for Postural Drainage

All Positions Are Contraindicated for the Following:

Intracranial pressure (ICP) >20 mm Hg
Head and neck injury until stabilized
Active hemorrhage with hemodynamic instability
Recent spinal surgery (e.g., laminectomy) or acute spinal injury
Active hemoptysis
Empyema
Bronchopleural fistula
Pulmonary edema associated with congestive heart failure (CHF)
Large pleural effusions
Pulmonary embolism
Aged, confused, or anxious patients
Rib fracture, with or without flail chest
Surgical wound or healing tissue

Trendelenburg Position Is Contraindicated for the Following:

Patients in whom increased ICP is to be avoided
Uncontrolled hypertension
Distended abdomen
Esophageal surgery
Recent gross hemoptysis related to recent lung carcinoma
Uncontrolled airway at risk for aspiration

Modified from AARC clinical practice guideline: postural drainage therapy, *Respir Care* 36(12):1418, 1991.

4. Know the client's level of cognitive function. Participation in controlled cough techniques requires the client to understand and to follow instructions. Congenital or acquired cognitive limitations may alter the client's ability to learn and to participate in these techniques.
5. Be aware of the client's exercise tolerance. Chest physiotherapy maneuvers are fatiguing. When the client is not used to physical activity, initial tolerance of the maneuvers may be decreased. However, with gradual increases in activity and planned CPT, the client's tolerance of the procedure improves.

Skill 12-1 Performing Postural Drainage

In health several factors provide for normal clearance of tracheobronchial secretions: normal functioning of the mucociliary escalator; adequate systemic hydration; absence of airway disease or infection; normal cough reflex; and normal ability to deep breathe, exercise moderately, and carry out activities of daily living. Loss of or alterations in one or several of these factors can interfere with normal clearance of tracheobronchial secretions. A good example is the client with severe bronchitis who gets an airway infection, becomes dehydrated because of anorexia, and stays in bed for several days. These circumstances can lead to stagnation of mucus in the airways. A postoperative client who is maintaining bed rest and cannot take deep breaths because of pain is also predisposed to abnormal clearance of tracheobronchial secretions.

Postural drainage achieves gravitational clearance of airway secretions from specific bronchial segments by using several different body positions. Each position drains a specific corresponding section of the tracheobronchial tree, either from the upper, middle, or lower lung field, into the trachea. Coughing or suctioning can then remove secretions from the trachea. Figure 12-1 shows the upper, middle, and lower lobe bronchi. The figures in Table 12-1 show the bronchial lobes and their corresponding body postures for drainage.

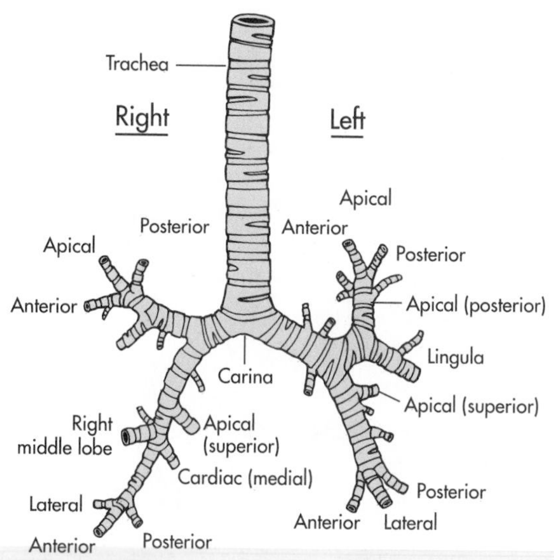

FIGURE **12-1** Tracheobronchial tree. (Modified from Frownfelter DL, Dean E: *Principles and practice of cardiopulmonary therapy*, ed 3, St. Louis, 1996, Mosby.)

Various pathophysiological conditions predispose the client to abnormal airway clearance and subsequent retention of lung secretions in peripheral airways. These retained secretions may be localized or diffuse. For example, clients with tuberculosis frequently have involvement of their upper lung fields, and posturing would be performed to drain only these specific upper lobe areas. In contrast, clients with bronchiectasis, asthma, bronchitis, or cystic fibrosis frequently have more diffuse involvement of many lung fields, which may require postural drainage of several areas. Clients maintaining bed rest who cannot turn may be placed in several or all drainage positions for several times throughout the day to prevent atelectasis and stasis of lung secretions. Areas are selected for drainage based on (1) knowledge of the client's condition and disease process, (2) physical assessment of the chest, (3) chest x-ray examination results, and (4) the extent of the pathologic condition and lobe involvement based on the physical examination and chest x-ray findings.

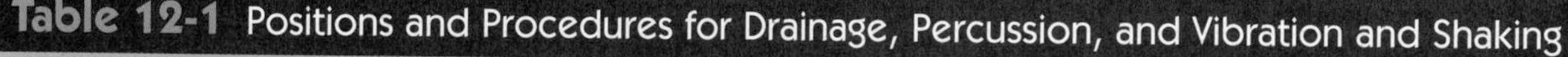

Table 12-1 Positions and Procedures for Drainage, Percussion, and Vibration and Shaking

Area and Procedure	Percussion	Vibration
Left and Right Upper Lobe Anterior Apical Bronchi		
Have client sit in chair, leaning back. Percuss and vibrate with heel of hands at shoulders and fingers over collarbones (clavicles) in front; can do both sides at same time. Note body posture and arm position of nurse. Nurse's back is kept straight, and elbows and knees are slightly flexed. 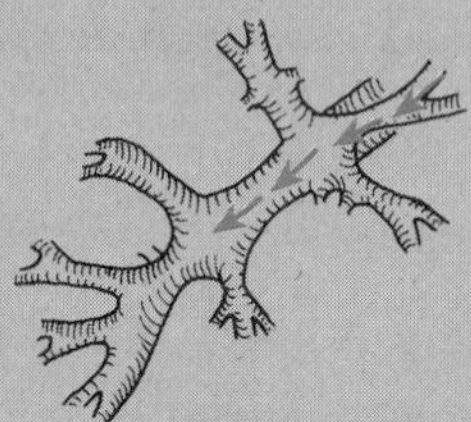	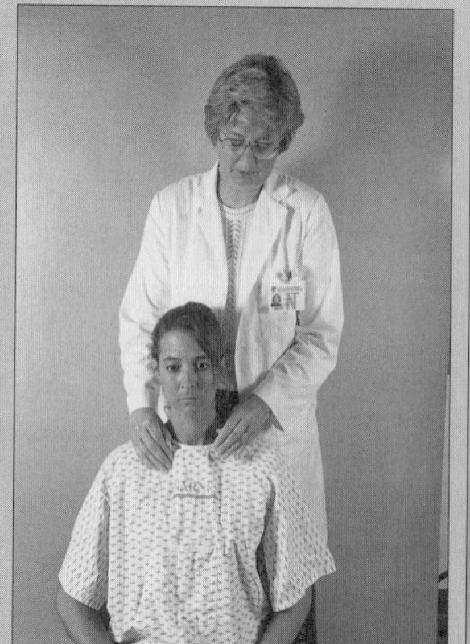	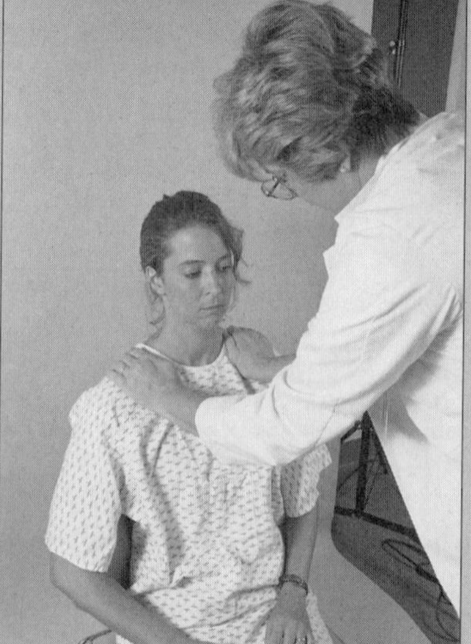
Direction of mucus flow through upper lobe anterior apical bronchi.	Position of hands for chest physiotherapy to left and right upper lobe anterior apical bronchi.	

Table 12-1 Positions and Procedures for Drainage, Percussion, and Vibration and Shaking—cont'd

Area and Procedure	Percussion	Vibration

Left and Right Upper Lobe Posterior Apical Bronchi

Have client sit in chair, leaning forward on pillow or table. Percuss and vibrate with hands on either side of upper spine. Can do both sides at same time.

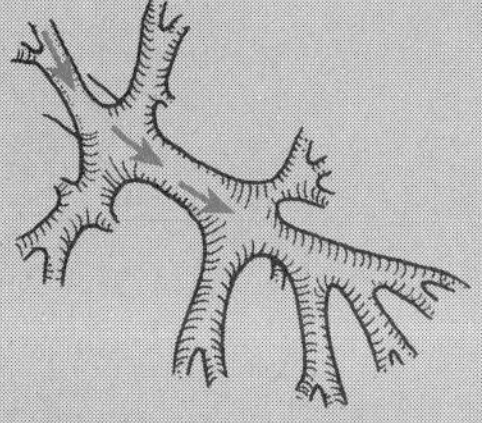

Direction of mucus flow through upper lobe posterior apical bronchi.

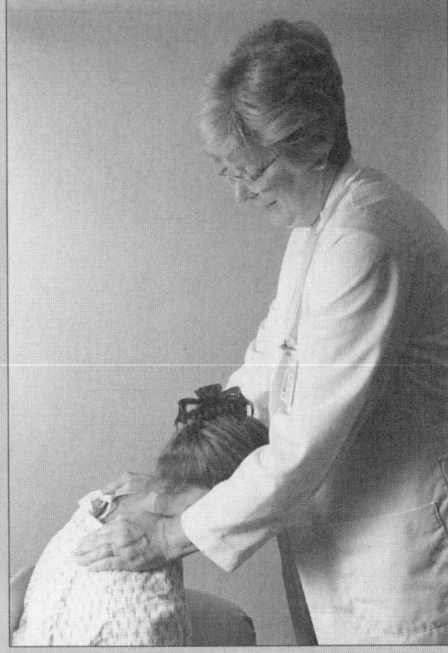

Position of hands for chest physiotherapy to left and right upper lobe posterior apical bronchi.

Right and Left Anterior Upper Lobe Bronchi

Have client lie flat on back with small pillow under knees. Percuss and vibrate just below clavicle on either side of sternum.

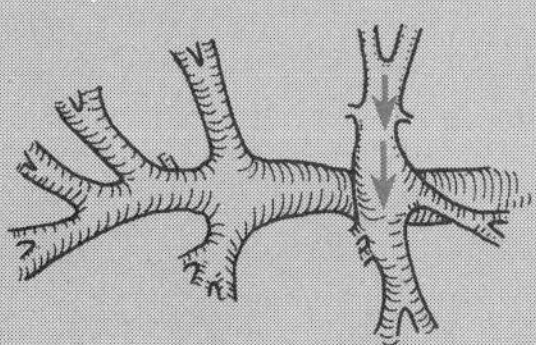

Direction of mucus flow through anterior upper bronchi.

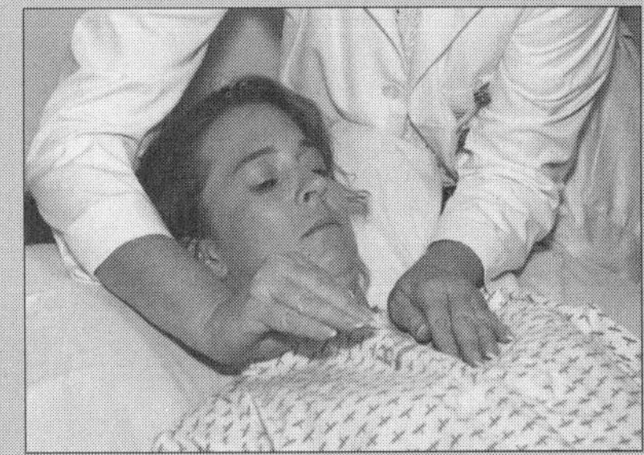

Position of hands for chest physiotherapy to right and left anterior upper lobe bronchi.

Left Upper Lobe Lingular Bronchus

Have client lie on right side with arm over head in Trendelenburg's position, with foot of bed raised 30 cm (12 in). Place pillow behind back, and roll client one-quarter turn onto pillow. Percuss and vibrate lateral to left nipple below axilla.

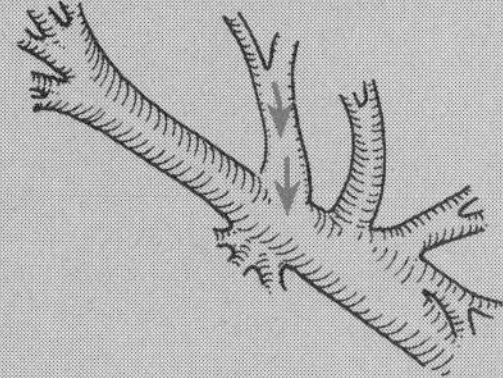

Direction of mucus flow through left upper lobe lingular bronchus.

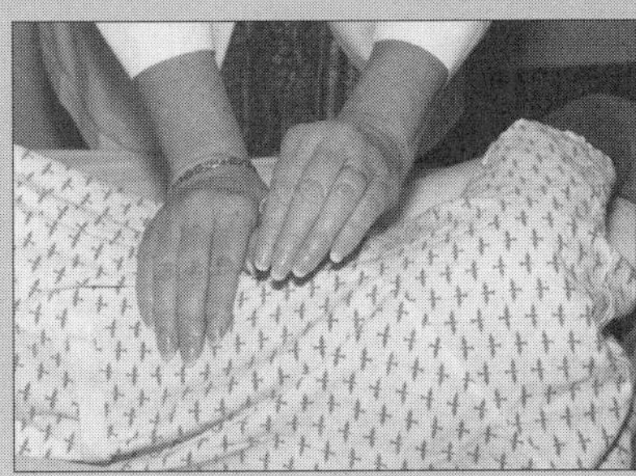

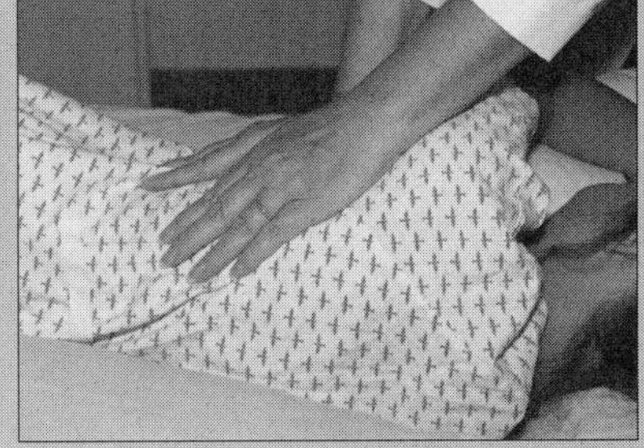

Position of hands for chest physiotherapy to left upper lobe lingular bronchus.

Continued

Table 12-1 Positions and Procedures for Drainage, Percussion, and Vibration and Shaking—cont'd

Area and Procedure	Percussion	Vibration
Right Middle Lobe Bronchus Have client lie on left side; raise foot of bed 30 cm (12 in). Place pillow behind back and roll client one-quarter turn onto pillow. Percuss and vibrate to right nipple below axilla. 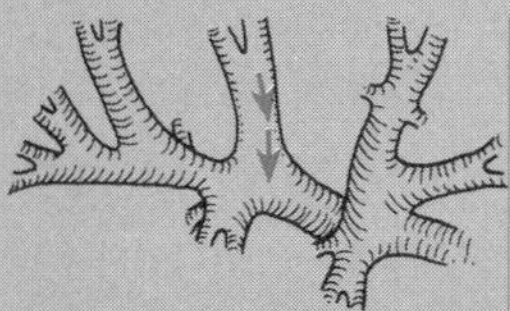 Direction of mucus flow through right middle lobe bronchus.	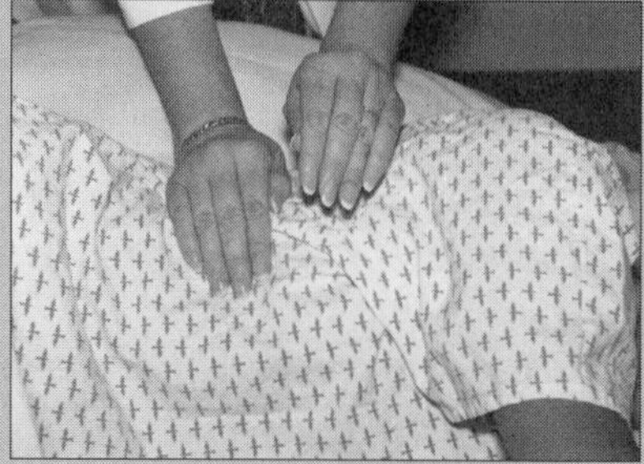 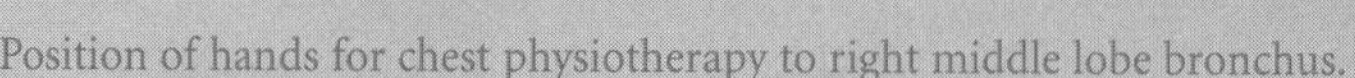 Position of hands for chest physiotherapy to right middle lobe bronchus.	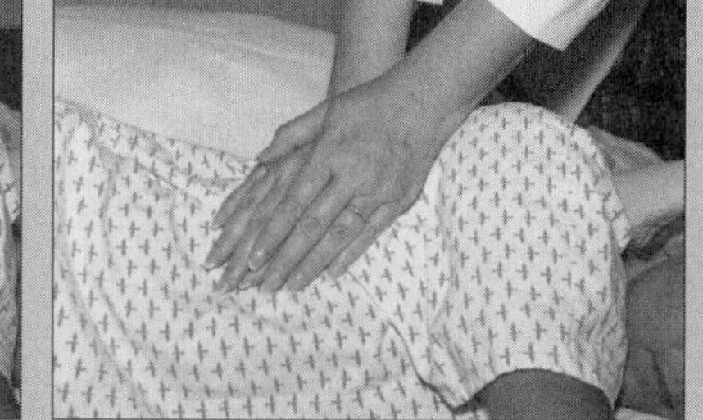
Left and Right Anterior Lower Lobe Bronchi Have client lie on back in Trendelenburg's position, with foot of bed elevated 45 to 50 cm (18 to 20 in). Have knees bent on pillow. Percuss and vibrate over lower anterior ribs on both sides. 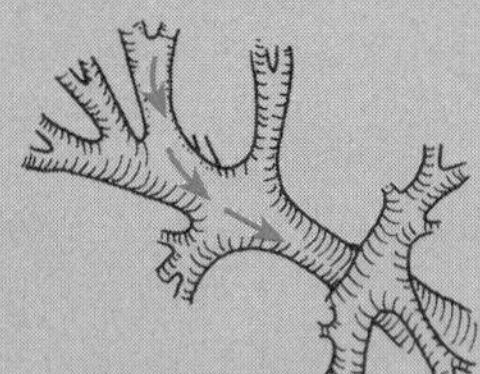 Direction of mucus flow through anterior lower lobe bronchi.	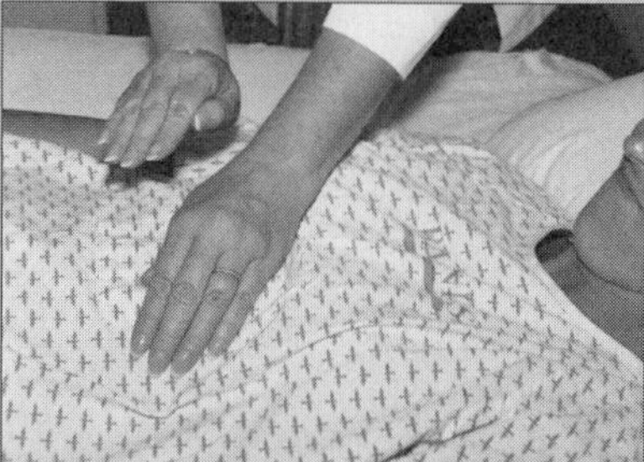 Position of hands for chest physiotherapy to left and right anterior lower lobe bronchi.	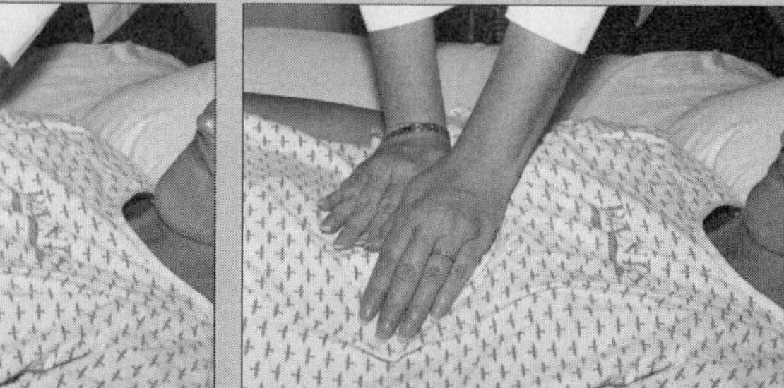
Right Lower Lobe Lateral Bronchus Have client lie on left side in Trendelenburg's position with foot of bed raised 45 to 50 cm (18 to 20 in). Percuss and vibrate on right side of chest below shoulder blades (scapulas) posterior to midaxillary line. 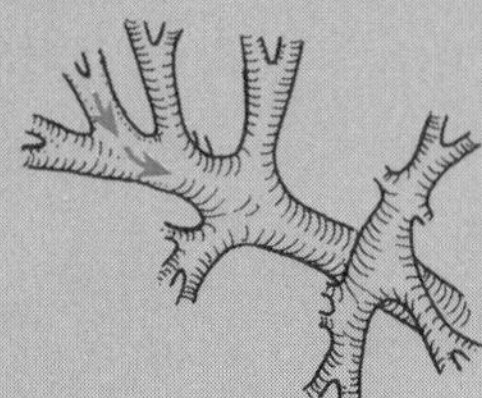 Direction of mucus flow through right lower lobe lateral bronchus.	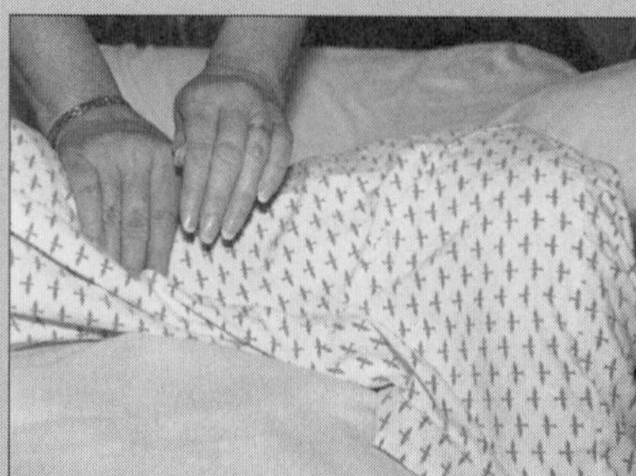 Position of hands for chest physiotherapy to right lower lobe lateral bronchus.	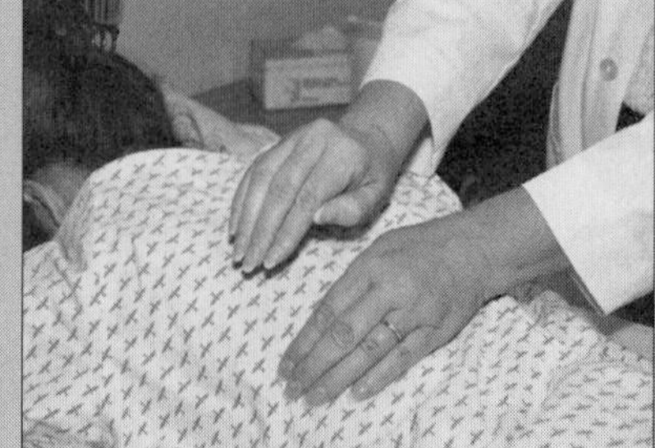

Table 12-1 Positions and Procedures for Drainage, Percussion, and Vibration and Shaking—cont'd

Area and Procedure	Percussion	Vibration
Left Lower Lobe Lateral Bronchus Have client lie on right side in Trendelenburg's position with foot of bed raised 45 to 50 cm (18 to 20 in). Percuss and vibrate on left side of chest below scapulas posterior to midaxillary line. 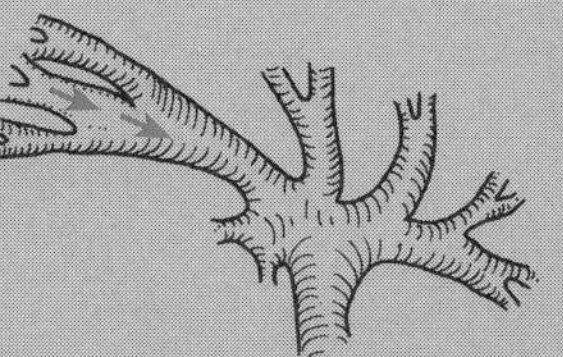 Direction of mucus flow through left lower lobe lateral bronchus.	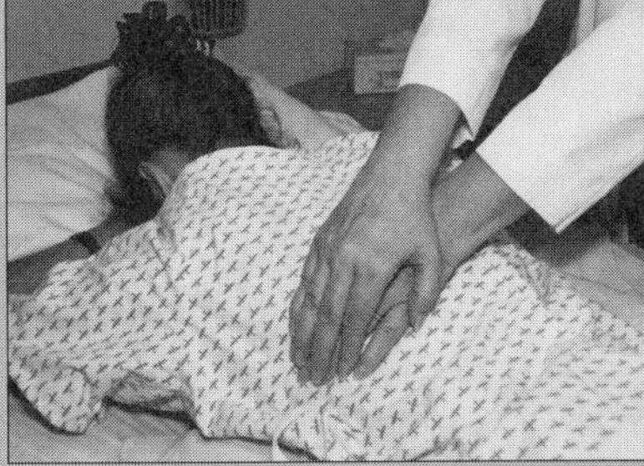	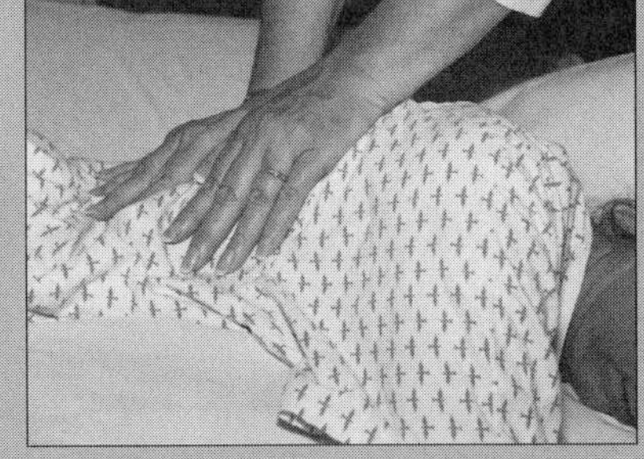
	Position of hands for chest physiotherapy to left lower lobe lateral bronchus.	
Right and Left Lower Lobe Superior Bronchi Have client lie flat on stomach with pillow under stomach. Percuss and vibrate below scapulas on either side of spine. 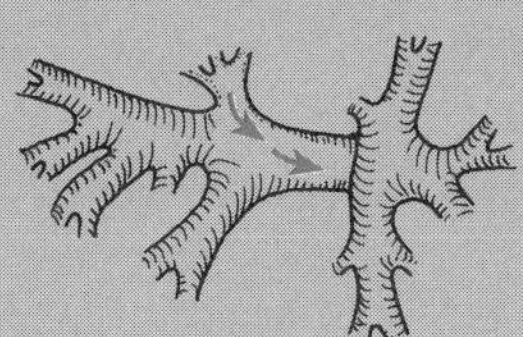 Direction of mucus flow through lower lobe superior bronchi.	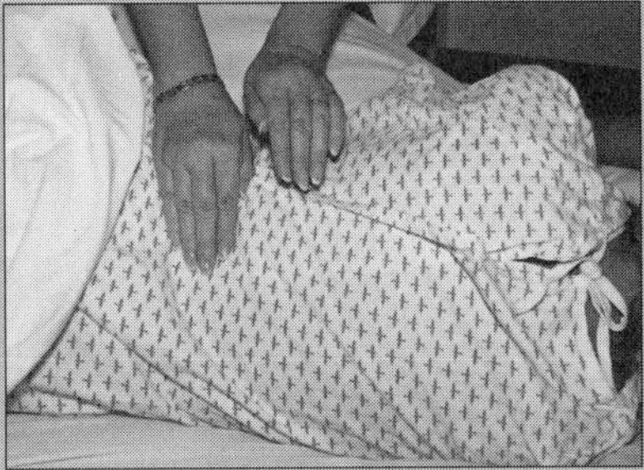	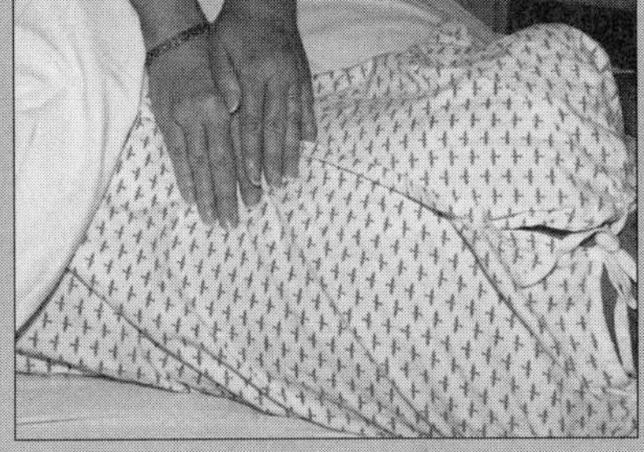
	Position of hands for chest physiotherapy to right and left lower lobe superior bronchi.	
Left and Right Posterior Basal Bronchi Have client lie on stomach in Trendelenburg's position with foot of bed elevated 45 to 50 cm (18 to 20 in). Percuss and vibrate over lower posterior ribs on either side of spine. 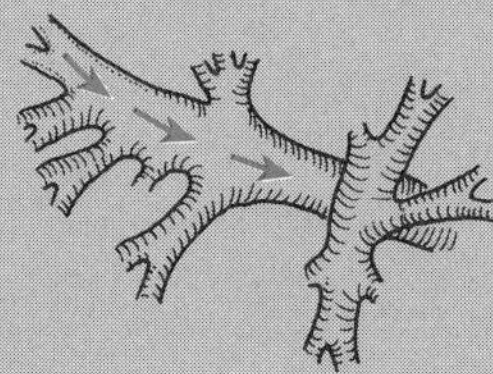 Direction of mucus flow through posterior basal bronchi.	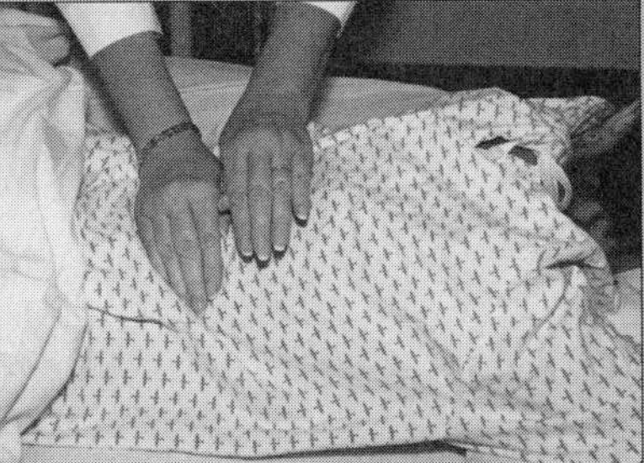	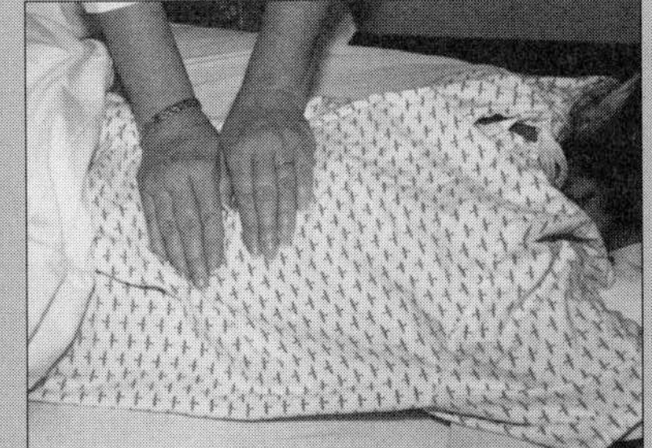
	Position of hands for chest physiotherapy to right and left posterior basal bronchi.	

Delegation Considerations

The skill of postural drainage can be delegated to appropriately trained assistive personnel. Before delegating this skill the client's chest x-ray films should be assessed and the client's chest should be examined to determine the proper positions to use. Assistive personnel should be warned to be alert for the client's tolerance of procedure and specific instruction regarding any client precautions related to disease or treatment.

Equipment

- Trendelenburg's hospital bed or tilt table
- Water pitcher and glass
- Chair (for draining upper lobes)
- One to four pillows
- Tissues and paper bag
- Clear graduated screw-top container

Step	Rationale
Assessment	
1. Assess for possible impairment of airway clearance.	Certain circumstances, disease processes, and conditions place client at risk for impaired airway clearance.

- ***Critical Decision Point***
  Contraindications to therapy may include use of contraindications to Trendelenburg's position or other postures that cause severe hypertension, severe hypoxemia, or severe shortness of breath. Procedure also contraindicated for head injuries, increased intracranial pressure, recent severe myocardial failure (see Box 12-1); lung hemorrhage; and certain surgical procedures, pain, or traction.

Step	Rationale
2. Identify signs and symptoms that indicate the need to perform postural drainage: x-ray film changes consistent with atelectasis, pneumonia, or bronchiectasis; ineffective coughing; thick, sticky, tenacious, and discolored secretions that are difficult to cough up; abnormal breath sounds, such as wheezing and crackling; palpable crepitus; increased vocal fremitus; complete loss or decrease in fremitus and breath sounds.	X-ray film data and signs and symptoms indicate accumulation of pulmonary secretions.
3. Identify which bronchial segments need to be drained by reviewing chest x-ray reports; auscultating over all lung fields for wheezes and crackles (Chapter 10); palpating over all lung fields for crepitus, fremitus, and chest expansion.	Areas of lung congestion and postures for drainage will vary, depending on disease process, client condition, and clinical problems. Areas most in need of and responsive to postural drainage usually can be easily identified by presence of early inspiratory crackles and palpable crepitus, which indicate secretions in the airways. If airway is completely plugged, breath sounds and chest excursion decrease.
4. Assess vital signs and pulse oximetry.	Provides baseline to evaluate client's response to therapy.
5. Determine client's understanding of and ability to perform home postural drainage.	Allows nurse to identify potential need for instruction. Home drainage is indicated in clients with chronic inability to clear lung secretions adequately, such as those with cystic fibrosis, chronic bronchitis, asthma, or bronchiectasis.

Nursing Diagnosis

Defining characteristics from the assessment data may reveal the following nursing diagnoses for clients requiring this skill:

- Ineffective airway clearance
- Ineffective breathing pattern
- Impaired gas exchange
- Deficient knowledge regarding the techniques of chest therapy

Related factors are individualized based on client's condition or needs.

Step	Rationale

Planning

Step	Rationale
1. **Expected outcomes** following completion of procedures:	
▪ Lung sounds improve or become clear. ▪ Sputum is more easily expectorated. ▪ Secretions appear more normal in color and consistency. ▪ Dyspnea is decreased.	Airways are clear of retained secretions.
▪ Results of pulmonary function and blood gas studies improve. ▪ Body temperature, white blood cell count, and chest x-ray films are normal.	No infectious process developing.
2. Prepare client:	
a. Explain purpose and rationale for procedure. Explain how it will be done, how long it will take, and any discomforts or side effects.	Helps promote cooperation. Well-prepared client is usually more relaxed and comfortable, which is essential for effective drainage.
b. Encourage high fluid intake program if not contraindicated by other diseases and if physician approves. Keep record of client's fluid intake.	Fluids thin secretions and make them easier to cough up. Clients need close monitoring and encouragement when first starting high fluid intake program.

• ***Critical Decision Point***

Contraindications to high fluid intake are congestive heart failure and renal failure. When forcing fluids, build up daily intake gradually and strive toward 8 to 12 8-oz glasses or until mucus is thin, white, and watery.

Step	Rationale
c. Plan treatments so they do not overlap with meals or tube feeding. Avoid postural drainage for 1 to 2 hours after meals or bolus tube feedings. Stop all continuous gastric tube feedings for 30 to 45 minutes before postural drainage. Check for residual feeding in client's stomach; if greater than 100 ml, hold treatment.	Postural drainage should be done when client's stomach is empty to avoid reflux or vomiting and aspiration of stomach contents.
d. Schedule treatments at appropriate times during day.	Postural drainage should be scheduled to obtain best results and should not conflict with other activities.
e. Have client remove any tight or restrictive clothing.	Helps client relax and allows deep breathing.

Implementation

Step	Rationale
1. Wash hands and apply gloves.	Reduces transmission of microorganisms.
2. Select congested areas to be drained based on assessment of all lung fields, clinical data, and chest x-ray data.	To be effective, treatment must be individualized to treat specific areas involved.
3. Place client in position to drain congested areas; first area selected may vary from client to client. (Refer to Table 12-1 for correct positioning to drain upper, middle, and lower lobe bronchi.) Help client assume position as needed. Teach client correct posture and arm and leg positioning. Place pillows for support and comfort. Drape client appropriately.	Specific positions are selected to drain each area involved.
4. Have client maintain posture for 10 to 15 minutes.	In adults, draining each area takes time.
5. During 10 to 15 minutes of drainage in each posture, perform chest percussion and vibration and shaking (Skill 12-2) over area being drained. Table 12-1 shows all postures and hand placement for percussion and vibration and shaking.	These maneuvers provide mechanical forces that aid in mobilization of airway secretions.
6. After 10 to 15 minutes of drainage in first posture, have client sit up and cough. Save expectorated secretions in a clear container. If client cannot cough, suctioning may need to be performed.	Any secretions mobilized into central airways should be removed by cough or suctioning before placing client into next drainage position. Coughing is most effective when client is sitting up and leaning forward.

STEP	RATIONALE
• ***Critical Decision Point*** *Sometimes client may experience transient dyspnea and fatigue because of irritation and bronchospasm from mobilizing secretions. Dyspnea usually subsides after sputum is coughed up.*	
7. Have client rest briefly if necessary.	Short rest periods between postures can prevent fatigue and help client better tolerate therapy.
8. Have client take sips of water.	Keeping mouth moist aids in expectoration of secretions.
9. Repeat Steps 3 through 8 until all congested areas selected have been drained. Each treatment should not exceed 30 to 60 minutes.	Postural drainage is used only to drain areas involved and is based on individual assessment.
10. Wash hands.	Reduces transmission of microorganisms.

EVALUATION

1. Ausculate lung fields.	Clearance of secretions usually relieves gurgling, early inspiratory crackles, and palpable crepitus.
2. Inspect character and amount of sputum.	Determines if secretions are adequately thinned.
3. Review diagnostic reports, including tests, chest x-ray films, and blood gas levels.	Provides objective data on improvements in lung function.
4. Obtain vital signs, pulse oximetry.	Procedure may result in dysrhythmias and decreases in oxygen saturation in some clients.
5. Have client explain purpose and procedure for postural drainage.	Evaluates client's understanding of procedure.

UNEXPECTED OUTCOMES AND RELATED INTERVENTIONS

- Client experiences severe dyspnea with bronchospasm, hypoxemia, and hypercarbia (hypercapnia).
  - Identify clients at risk for this unexpected outcome: (1) those with status asthmaticus and (2) those with severe exacerbation of bronchitis who are debilitated and tired and whose blood gas levels are consistent with severe hypoxemia and hypercarbia.
  - Chest therapy may have to be discontinued or modified for these clients. They may tolerate only 3 to 5 minutes of drainage per hour.
  - Bronchodilator inhalation should be scheduled 20 minutes before postural drainage.
- Hemoptysis occurs.
  - This may be caused by infection, erosion of blood vessels, or other causes.
  - In severe hemoptysis, stop therapy, call physician, remain calm, stay with client, request assistance, and keep client comfortable, calm, warm, and quiet.
- No secretions are obtained.
  - Continue therapy for several days to 1 week. There may be a lack of secretions, or secretions may be too thick to mobilize.
  - Secretions are not always mobilized and coughed up after each posture. If, after two or three coughs, nothing is expectorated, proceed with next posture. Often secretions are coughed up 30 to 60 minutes after postural drainage.
  - Improve hydration.
- There is no improvement in chest assessment: adventitious sounds are present, dyspnea occurs, there is poor chest excursion.
  - Increase frequency of therapy.
  - Consult physician for potential sputum culture and initiation of antibiotics.
  - Teach coughing exercises.
- Client's vital signs and oxygen saturation decline.
  - Notify physician.
  - Continue to monitor client's vital signs and oxygen saturation.
  - Modify type and frequency of postural drainage.
- Client unable to demonstrate or explain postural drainage.
  - Provide further instruction.

RECORDING AND REPORTING

- Record in nurses' notes pretherapy and posttherapy assessment of chest; frequency and duration of treatment; postures used and bronchial segments drained; cough effectiveness; need for suctioning; color, amount, and consistency of sputum; hemoptysis or other unexpected outcomes; client's tolerance and reactions.
- If client and family receive instruction in home care, chart instructions given, understanding of therapy, demonstration of skill, reactions to need for home care, barriers to learning and implementation, and referral for follow-up, that is, home care, rehabilitation, or pulmonary nurse specialist.
- Immediately report severe dyspnea, hemoptysis, severe bronchospasm, or hypotension to physician.

Teaching Considerations

- Best times for treatments are (1) in morning before breakfast, when client can clear secretions that accumulate overnight and (2) about 1 hour before bedtime, so that lungs are clear before sleeping and client has time after treatment to cough up any mobilized secretions. Frequency depends on need and client's tolerance and may vary from once daily to every 2 to 4 hours in an acute situation.
- If client is receiving inhaled bronchodilators or aerosol treatment, postural drainage should be done 20 minutes after such therapy. Plan for rest period after postural drainage.
- Do not schedule major activities (such as exercise or bath) right after chest therapy treatment, especially in clients with severe obstructive lung disease.
- Instruct client's family or primary caregiver to recognize when the client's respiratory status requires breathing exercises or postural drainage.
- Encourage primary caregiver or family member to encourage the client to participate in physical activities that will increase respiratory efficiency.
- Teach client and significant others how to assume postures at home. Some postures may need to be modified to meet individual needs; for example, side-lying Trendelenburg's position to drain lateral lower lobes may have to be done with client lying flat on side or in side-lying semi-Fowler's position if client is very short of breath.

Pediatric Considerations

- In the child with cystic fibrosis, chest physiotherapy is a cornerstone therapy and is usually performed at least twice daily, on rising in the morning and in the evening (Wong and others, 1999).
- Chest physiotherapy is not recommended during acute exacerbations of asthma (National Asthma Education and Prevention Program, 1997).

Gerontological Considerations

- Postural drainage in older adults should be done while taking extra care and assessment. Change positions more slowly, and closely assess for any changes in oxygen saturation or vital signs with position changes.
- Older adults with chronic cardiac and pulmonary conditions may not tolerate a supine or side-lying position for chest physiotherapy (CPT). In these positions clients experience decline in forced vital capacity (FVC) and subsequent decline in oxygen saturation (Manning and others, 1999).

Home Care Considerations

- Assess home environment for ventilation. Determine client's access to clean, fresh air. Assess the home for air conditioning and client's reaction to air conditioning.
- Discuss need for home postural drainage with family. Assess if they perceive need for home care and if any barriers exist to learning and implementing home program. If specialized home or outpatient follow-up is needed, refer client to pulmonary nurse specialist, pulmonary rehabilitation team, or home health care personnel.
- Obtain foam wedge or multiple pillows for correct positioning (Rice, 2000).
- In home setting, the Trendelenburg's position can be achieved in several ways. Select the most comfortable and practical method that best suits client:
  - Client can purchase slant board or make one out of old door or tabletop. Surface can be padded with foam or blankets.
  - Client's hips can be elevated with stack of old newspapers and pillows or foam wedge. These props tend to be uncomfortable and often flatten out because of client's body weight.
  - Wedge or stack of papers can be placed under bed board.

Skill 12-2 Performing Percussion and Vibration and Shaking

During postural drainage, physical maneuvers, such as percussion and vibration and shaking, can be performed on the rib cage over lung tissue by a trained nurse, therapist, or family member. The techniques are done on specific parts of the rib cage over each area being drained. Normally the mucociliary escalator and cough transport can effectively clear airway secretions. When airway clearance is impaired in certain disease states, however, these techniques are combined with postural drainage to help clear mucus. Exactly why these physical maneuvers enhance clearance of mucus is not known.

These techniques are defined and explained in detail in this skill. Percussion involves clapping the chest wall with cupped hands. If done correctly, it painlessly sets up vibrations in the chest to dislodge retained secretions. Vibration is a sustained contraction of the upper extremities of the caregiver to produce a downward vibrating pressure done only during exhalation with the flat part of the palm over the area being drained. Shaking is a more vigorous downward rocking motion on the rib cage done with the flat part of the hand during exhalation. These last two maneuvers are performed only during prolonged exhalation through pursed lips. They augment the natural movement of the rib cage during exhalation and assist with secretion clearance.

The natural expiratory movement of the chest wall involves (1) a decrease in the lateral and anteroposterior diameter of the lower ribs as they move downward and closer together and (2) a decrease in the anteroposterior diameter of the upper chest as the sternum, the clavicles, and the upper rib cage move downward. Pressure during vibration and shaking is always directed toward these natural expiratory movements of the rib cage. They become even more effective if the client can relax the rib cage muscles during exhalation and blow out using abdominal muscles. This relaxation during vibration and shaking enhances the rocking motion of the rib cage, makes vibration optimal, and assists in dislodging mucus plugs.

In diseases associated with mucus plugging, the rib cage frequently becomes hyperinflated because air is trapped behind obstructed airways. The ribs can become somewhat fixed in their upward and outward position and lose their excursion and flexibility; vibration and shaking can improve both. Vibration or shaking may be better tolerated than percussion in the immediate postsurgical client, providing no other contraindications exist.

Before attempting to master these techniques, the nurse must know that each posture is associated with a general area of the rib cage to be percussed and vibrated. These postures and the specific areas are shown in Table 12-1. Generally, for any given posture the area to be percussed and vibrated can be thought of as that portion of the rib cage at the greatest vertical height. Areas that are never percussed or vibrated regardless of their vertical height include the clavicles, breast tissue, sternum, spine, waist, and abdomen; the action must always stay over the ribs.

Delegation Considerations

The skill of percussion and vibration and shaking can be delegated to respiratory and physical therapists and appropriately trained assistive personnel. Before delegating this skill the client's chest x-ray films should be assessed and the client's chest should be examined for the proper positions to use. Assistive personnel should be warned to be alert for the client's tolerance of procedure and any client precautions related to disease or treatment.

Equipment

- Hospital bed or tilt table placed in Trendelenburg's position
- Chair (for upper lobes)
- One to four pillows
- Water pitcher and glass
- Tissues and paper bag
- Clear graduated screw-top container
- Mechanical vibrator or percussor (optional)
- Single layer of clothing

Step	Rationale
Assessment	
1. Assess breathing pattern, including muscles used for breathing, respiratory rate and depth, extent of excursion, and chest wall movement.	Certain disease states place client at risk for developing an ineffective breathing pattern. Rapid, shallow breathing with client using accessory muscles is seen in chronic obstructive lung disease, asthma, pain, hypoxemia, pneumonia, and atelectasis.

- ***Critical Decision Point***
  Percussion and vibration and shaking may be contraindicated in certain situations, including rib fracture, fracture of other rib cage structures such as clavicle or sternum, pain, severe dyspnea, and severe osteoporosis, so nurse should obtain physician's order. Thin, frail clients with osteoporosis are most susceptible to injury and should be taught other secretion control measures (e.g., forceful coughing, humidification).

Step	Rationale
2. Identify signs and symptoms and conditions that indicate need to perform these skills (Skill 12-1, Assessment).	When tolerated and not contraindicated, these techniques are done during postural drainage.
3. Identify and assess rib cage over bronchial segment being drained for pain, tenderness, abnormal configuration, abnormal excursion or chest wall movement during breathing, muscle tension.	Chest wall areas to be assessed and to receive percussion and vibration and shaking vary with each postural drainage position (Table 12-1).
4. Assess client's understanding and ability to cooperate with therapy, both in hospital and at home.	Assessment allows nurse to identify potential need for instruction of client, family, or significant others.

STEP	RATIONALE

Nursing Diagnosis

Defining characteristics from the assessment data may reveal the following nursing diagnoses for clients requiring this skill:

- Ineffective airway clearance
- Ineffective breathing pattern
- Impaired gas exchange
- Deficient knowledge regarding the techniques of chest therapy

Related factors are individualized based on client's condition or needs.

Planning

STEP	RATIONALE
1. **Expected outcomes** following completion of procedure:	
▪ Breathing pattern improves. ▪ Sputum is more easily expectorated. ▪ Secretions appear more normal in color and consistency. ▪ Dyspnea is decreased. ▪ Results of pulmonary function and blood gas studies improve.	Airways are clear of retained secretions.
▪ Body temperature, white blood cell count, and chest x-ray films are normal.	No infectious process developing.
2. Prepare client:	
a. Explain procedure in detail: how it will be done, how long it will take, and any discomforts or side effects.	Percussion and vibration and shaking cannot be done effectively without client's cooperation.
b. Encourage and help client to relax and deep breathe during procedure. Have client practice exhaling slowly through pursed lips while relaxing chest wall muscles. Client should blow out using abdominal muscles, not rib cage muscles.	Percussion and vibration and shaking are most effective if client breathes properly and works well with therapist. If done properly, these techniques should not cause pain or discomfort.

Implementation

STEP	RATIONALE
1. With client placed in appropriate drainage position (Skill 12-1, Implementation, Steps 1 through 3), assess and identify chest wall area to be percussed and vibrated (Table 12-1).	In general, for any given posture, rib cage area to be percussed and vibrated is in highest vertical position. Careful assessment of rib cage movement guides nurse in following natural movement during vibration and shaking.
2. Instruct client to relax by using one of these techniques: take slow, deep breaths, and exhale; use abdominal, diaphragmatic, or pursed-lip breathing.	Client should not lie passively but should relax and take deep breaths.
3. Use good body mechanics when clapping: elevate bed to comfortable working height, and stand close to bed with arms directly in front and knees slightly bent. Avoid bending over.	Use of good body mechanics avoids undue strain on therapist's back and legs.
4. Begin percussion on appropriate part of chest wall over draining area (Table 12-1). Perform percussion for 3 to 5 minutes in each posture as tolerated. Always ask if client is experiencing any discomfort, such as undue pressure or stinging of the skin.	Percussion helps clear mucus and should be painless, because air in hand acts as cushion.
a. Place hands side by side on chest wall over area to be drained. Hands should be cupped with fingers and thumbs held tightly together. Make sure that entire outer portion of hand makes contact with chest wall to avoid air leaks (Table 12-1).	This hand position creates an air pocket that sends vibrations through the chest wall but is not painful.

Step	Rationale
b. When clapping, most of arm movement should come from the elbow and wrist joint. Clapping can be done for 5 minutes without stopping or 2 to 3 minutes, alternating with vibration and shaking.	Using the larger muscles of the arms and shoulders improves endurance.
c. Alternately clap chest with cupped hands to create rhythmic popping sound resembling galloping horse. Clapping can be done at moderate or fast speed; whichever is most comfortable and effective.	The popping sound comes from the air pocket that is formed between the hand and the chest wall.
5. Perform chest wall vibration and shaking over each area being drained. See Table 12-1 for correct hand position to use in each posture. Vibrations are usually done in sets of three followed by coughing so that any mobilized mucus can be expectorated.	Vibration and shaking during slow exhalation and coughing help to clear mucus.
a. To perform vibration, gently place hands over area being drained, and have client take slow, deep breath through nose.	Slow inhalation helps relaxation.
b. Gently resist chest wall as it rises during inhalation.	Slight resistance on inhalation aids in expansion of rib cage.
c. Have client hold breath and then exhale through pursed lips, while contracting abdominal muscles and relaxing chest wall muscles. Chest wall should relax and fall.	Pursed-lip breathing makes exhalation easier. Relaxation of the chest wall makes vibrations more effective.
d. While client is exhaling, gently push down and vibrate with flat part of hand.	Vibrate only during exhalation so as to follow the natural downward movement of the rib cage.
e. Repeat vibration three times, then have client cascade cough by taking deep breath and doing series of small coughs until end of breath. Client should not inhale between coughs. Vibrate chest wall as client coughs. When applying pressure to ribs, always follow natural movement of rib cage. As client becomes comfortable and learns to relax rib cage during exhalation, chest wall movement and flexibility will increase. Allow client to sit up and cough as needed.	Coughing with vibrations aids in clearing mucus.
6. Assess client's tolerance of vibration and ability to relax chest wall and breathe properly as instructed.	Client's poor tolerance may necessitate discontinuing procedure.
7. Perform shaking with vibration.	Shaking helps to clear secretions from airway.
a. Place flat part of hand over area being drained (Table 12-1). Maintain good body mechanics: lower bed so client is about at nurse's hip level; work with arms directly in front; maintain good leverage; do not lean over or strain back.	Proper positioning of therapist prevents strain on back muscles.
b. Have client inhale slowly through nose.	
c. During inhalation, apply light pressure on ribs and stretch skin so it is tight.	
d. Have client hold breath for 2 seconds.	
e. As client exhales, increase pressure. Maintain pressure while applying intermittent rocking motion on ribs. Pressure is directed toward following natural expiratory rib cage movement.	This helps to dislodge mucus. It may be better tolerated than postural drainage in postoperative clients (Frownfelter and Dean, 1996).
f. Client must exhale through pursed lips and relax chest wall muscles as much as possible.	If rib cage is relaxed, ribs can be rocked more vigorously in direction they naturally move.
g. Repeat shaking three times, have client inhale deeply, and then do rib shaking during cascade cough.	Coughing helps to clear mobilized secretions.

Step	Rationale
h. Perform a total of three or four sets of three vibration and shaking and coughing in each posture as tolerated. Strength and frequency of vibration and shaking will vary: vibration requires all muscles in arm and shoulder to contract and tremble; shaking requires applying controlled pressure from shoulders and back while slightly leaning on chest; rocking motion is created by flexing and extending elbows using triceps.	
i. Suction if client is unable to cough up mucus (see Chapter 13).	
8. In each posture, complete vibration and shaking.	
9. If long-term therapy is needed, teach client and significant others the procedure for home use. If they cannot learn or use, refer for outpatient or home health follow-up.	Long-term use of these techniques can optimize airway clearance, reduce symptoms and infection, and improve chest mobility.

Evaluation

1. Evaluate changes in chest assessment following procedure.	These maneuvers usually relieve signs of congestion, slow respiratory rate, and improve chest mobility and expansion.
2. Inspect character of mucus.	Inspection determines if mucus is adequately thinned.
3. Review diagnostic test results for pulmonary function.	This determines airway clearance and oxygenation status.
4. Observe caregiver during percussion and vibration and shaking.	Return demonstration is an effective means to measure learning.

Unexpected Outcomes and Related Interventions

- Client experiences severe dyspnea with bronchospasm, hypoxemia, and hypercarbia (hypercapnia).
  - Identify clients at risk for this unexpected outcome: (1) those with status asthmaticus and (2) those with severe exacerbation of bronchitis who are debilitated and tired and whose blood gas levels are consistent with severe hypoxemia and hypercarbia.
  - Chest therapy may have to be discontinued or modified for these clients. They may tolerate only 3 to 5 minutes of drainage per hour.
  - Bronchodilator inhalation should be scheduled 20 minutes before postural drainage.
- Hemoptysis occurs.
  - This may be caused by infection, erosion of blood vessels, or other causes.
  - In severe hemoptysis, stop therapy, call physician, remain calm, stay with client, request assistance, and keep client comfortable, calm, warm, and quiet.
- No secretions are obtained.
  - Continue therapy for several days to 1 week. There may be a lack of secretions, or secretions may be too thick to mobilize.
  - Secretions are not always mobilized and coughed up after each posture. If, after two or three coughs, nothing is expectorated, proceed with next posture. Often secretions are coughed up 30 to 60 minutes after postural drainage.
  - Improve hydration.
- There is no improvement in chest assessment: adventitious sounds are present, dyspnea occurs, there is poor chest excursion.
  - Increase frequency of therapy.
  - Consult physician for potential sputum culture and initiation of antibiotics.
  - Teach coughing exercises.
- Client experiences rib fracture, rib pain, or tenderness of chest wall.
  - Notify physician.
  - Obtain chest x-ray examination.
  - Stop percussion, vibration, and shaking.

Recording and Reporting

- For treatment given along with postural drainage, record in nurses' notes pretherapy and posttherapy assessment of chest; assessment of chest mobility, client cooperation with and tolerance of procedure; client's ability to relax and breathe properly; duration of percussion; number of vibration and shaking series; cough effectiveness; suctioning.
- If client and family receive instruction in home care, chart instruction and skills given. Document demonstration of procedure, return demonstration, and follow-up activities.
- Immediately report severe dyspnea, hemoptysis, severe bronchospasm, or hypotension to physician.

Teaching Considerations

- Best times for treatments are (1) in morning before breakfast, when client can clear secretions that accumulate overnight and (2) about 1 hour before bedtime, so that lungs are clear before sleeping and client has time after treatment to cough up any mobilized secretions. Frequency depends on need and client's tolerance and may vary from once daily to every 2 to 4 hours in an acute situation.
- If client is receiving inhaled bronchodilators or aerosol treatment, postural drainage should be done 20 minutes after such therapy. Plan for rest period after postural drainage.
- Do not schedule major activities (such as exercise or bath) right after chest therapy treatment, especially in clients with severe obstructive lung disease.
- Instruct client's family or primary caregiver to recognize when the client's respiratory status requires breathing exercises or postural drainage.
- Encourage primary caregiver or family member to encourage the client to participate in physical activities that will increase respiratory efficiency.
- Teach client and significant others how to assume postures at home. Some postures may need to be modified to meet individual needs; for example, side-lying Trendelenburg's position to drain lateral lower lobes may have to be done with client lying flat on side or in side-lying semi-Fowler's position if client is very short of breath.

Pediatric Considerations

- Hand-held vibrators should be approved for use for a child in an oxygen-enriched environment (Wong and others, 1999).
- Larger children may benefit from a more powerful vibrator (Wong and others, 1999).

Gerontological Considerations

- Percussion and vibration and shaking usually have to be done more gently in the elderly.
- In the frail elderly use a mechanical vibrator on low speed instead of manual percussion and vibration and shaking.

Home Care Considerations

- Mechanical devices are sometimes used at home if (1) a trained therapist is not available or (2) client does not tolerate manual therapy. They are available through most home equipment companies.
- If home therapy is needed, instruct a family member in techniques of percussion and vibration and shaking. Assess willingness to learn and follow through in home setting.

Critical Thinking Exercises

1. What clinical situations may be responsible for development of ineffective airway clearance?
2. Describe how you would determine what position should be used on the chest wall for percussion and vibration and shaking.
3. You are caring for a client with a high spinal cord injury. However, he is able to breathe without a mechanical ventilator and his rehabilitation potential is quite good. How would you assess his ability to clear his airways?

References

AARC clinical practice guideline: postural drainage therapy, *Respir Care* 36(12):1418, 1991.

Frownfelter DL, Dean E: *Principles and practice of cardiopulmonary therapy,* ed 3, St. Louis, 1996, Mosby.

Jones AP, Rowe BH: Bronchopulmonary hygiene physical therapy in chronic obstructive pulmonary disease and bronchiectasis (Cochrane Review), *The Cochrane Library,* issue 3, Oxford, UK, 1999, Update Software.

Manning F, Dean E, Ross J, Abboud RT: Effects of side lying on lung function in older individuals. *Phys Ther* 79(5):456, 1999.

National Asthma Education and Prevention Program: *Expert Panel report H: guidelines for the diagnosis and management of asthma,* Bethesda, Md, 1997, National Heart Lung and Blood Institute, National Institutes of Health.

Rice R: *Manual of home health nursing procedures,* ed 2, St. Louis, 2000, Mosby.

Wong DL, and others: *Whaley and Wong's nursing care of infants and children,* ed 6, St. Louis, 1999, Mosby.

13

Airway Maintenance

Skills

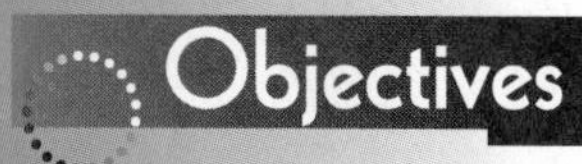

Objectives

Mastery of content in this chapter will enable the nurse to:

- Define the key terms listed.
- Identify guidelines used in managing the airway.
- Describe the methods of airway management for anatomical and artificial airways, respectively.
- Discuss the indications for airway suctioning.
- Discuss the indications for tracheostomy care.
- Suction the client's mouth of excess secretions.
- Suction the client's posterior pharynx or trachea through the nose.
- Suction the client's airway through an endotracheal tube.
- Suction the client's airway through a tracheostomy tube.
- Safely secure an endotracheal tube to the client's face.
- Safely secure a tracheostomy tube around the neck.
- Cleanse and dress the tracheostomy site.
- Correctly inflate the cuff on an endotracheal or tracheostomy tube.
- Change a tracheostomy tube.

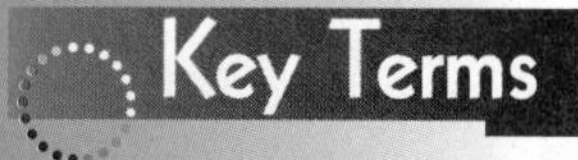

Key Terms

Artificial airway
Atelectasis
Bronchospasm
Bronchus
Closed system suction catheter
Cuff
Dead space
Endotracheal (ET) tubes
Fenestration
Hypercapnia
Hypoxemia
Hypoxia
In-line suction catheter
Intubation
Laryngospasm
Lower airway respiratory system
Nasal airway
Obturator
Oral airway
Outer cannula
Oxygen therapy
Patent
Pharynx
Respiratory distress
Sputum
Suction
Suction catheter
Tracheal stenosis
Tracheoesophageal fistula
Tracheomalacia
Tracheostomy
Upper airway
Yankauer suction

Many courses of action are available to promote an open or **patent** airway, which has the potential to become obstructed by mucus, mechanical obstruction (i.e., soft tissue in upper airway), or a foreign body. These actions may not require a physician's order, depending on the situation. The physician should be consulted if there is any concern about the appropriateness of the intervention or if the obstruction does not respond to treatment. The nurse must consider maintaining the patency of the nose and **upper airway,** as well as the trachea and **lower airway respiratory systems.** Based on continual assessment of the client, the nurse can include in the plan of care measures that aid in maintaining patency of the upper and lower airway. Hydration, nutrition, chest therapy airway clearance techniques, "flutter" mucous clearance device therapy, deep breathing, coughing, humidity, and aerosol therapy are noninvasive techniques that are helpful in maintaining a patent airway. For selected clients, medications such as antibiotics, bronchodilators, steroids, decongestants, antihistamines, and expectorants are adjuncts to these therapies.

In some clients use of the above techniques and medications is not sufficient to maintain a patent airway, and the client is at risk for development of **respiratory distress.** More invasive measures directed at maintaining airway patency may be necessary, especially in the critically ill client. This chapter focuses on nonemergent techniques designed to maintain patency of the anatomical and **artificial airways.** Techniques discussed include suctioning the anatomical and artificial airways (endotracheal tube, **tracheostomy** tube), caring for clients with an endotracheal tube or a tracheostomy tube, and properly inflating the **cuff** on an artificial airway.

Skill Performance Guidelines

1. Know the client's normal range of vital signs and oxygen saturation levels. Baseline vital signs serve as a means to identify individual abnormalities and to recognize the onset of illness or disease. Normal vital signs for one client may be abnormal for another client.
2. Know the client's medical history. Smoking alters normal mucocillary clearance. Certain disorders such as chronic obstructive pulmonary diseases (including asthma and cystic fibrosis, pneumonia, thoracic surgery, chest trauma, and abdominal surgery) place the client at increased risk for an obstructed airway. Other conditions that may increase the client's risk for aspiration of gastric contents into the lung and resulting airway obstruction include the presence of enteral feeding tubes or other nasal or oral gastric tubes, a decreased level of consciousness, and a decreased swallowing ability. Clients with a history of nasal problems, such as nasal trauma, nasal polyps, deviated nasal septum, or chronic sinus or allergy problems causing mucosal swelling, may have narrow nasal passages, which can affect the nurse's ability to easily pass a **suction catheter.**

3. Know the client's baseline respiratory assessment. Baseline assessment has two meanings. First, know what is historically normal for the client regarding pulmonary signs and symptoms, including chest assessment and **sputum** production. Second, know what the client's condition has been for the past 4, 8, 12, 16, or 24 hours. These are relative baseline measurements that assist the nurse in distinguishing between gradual and acute changes in the client's status.
4. Perform a systematic respiratory assessment of upper and lower airways, including identifying respiratory rate, respiratory pattern, respiratory muscles used, breath sounds, ability to cough effectively, integrity of the rib cage, and the characteristics of sputum production.
5. Determine the type and frequency of intervention, based on assessment findings. Care that is appropriate for one day or shift can change, resulting in an increase or decrease in frequency of care or alterations in the type of intervention.
6. Identify and become familiar with the application of equipment available at the institution. Many types of artificial airways, suction catheters, and suction machines are available. Knowing how to operate the equipment before it is needed benefits both the nurse and the client.
7. Test all equipment before use. Have adequate supplies on hand at the bedside. Equipment must work properly to provide safe nursing care. Determine that the suction machine is generating adequate negative suction pressure (Table 13-1) and that there are suction catheters at the bedside.
8. Know client's home care plan. Absence or interruption of certain therapies such as bronchodilators can place the client at risk for an obstructed airway during the hospitalization or after discharge from the hospital.
9. Know the side effects of medications and other therapies. Some medications such as beta-adrenergic blockers have the side effect of **bronchospasm.** An adverse effect of narcotics and sedatives is respiratory depression. Similarly, too much oxygen can reduce the drive to breathe in clients with **hypercapnia** (elevated arterial carbon dioxide tension). Position changes may affect the client adversely. For example, in clients with impaired spinal cord innervations of the respiratory muscles, supine positions place the diaphragm at a mechanical disadvantage and increase the risk of aspiration.

Table 13-1 Negative Pressure Settings for Suctioning

	Wall Suction	Portable Suction
Infants	40-60 mm Hg	3-5 mm Hg
Children	50-100 mm Hg	5-8 mm Hg
Adults	100-120 mm Hg	7-15 mm Hg

Skill 13-1 Performing Oral Pharyngeal Suctioning

Nurses use a Yankauer, or tonsillar tip, **suction** device to perform oral pharyngeal suctioning (Figure 13-1). A **Yankauer suction** catheter is made of rigid, minimally flexible plastic. The tip of this suction catheter usually has one large and several small eyelets through which the mucus enters with application of negative pressure. The Yankauer suction catheter is angled to facilitate removal of pharyngeal secretions through the mouth. This catheter is used instead of a standard suction catheter when oral secretions are extremely copious and thick because it can handle large volumes of secretions better than a standard suction catheter (Vanderberg, Lutz, and Vinson, 1999). The Yankauer suction catheter is not used to suction the nares because of its size.

The Yankauer suction device is useful in the removal of secretions from the mouth in clients after oral and maxillofacial surgery, trauma to the mouth, or neurovascular injury and cerebrovascular accident causing hemiparesis and drooling or impaired swallowing. Clients with artificial airways and impaired swallowing ability may require use of the Yankauer suction device to promote oral hygiene. Alert clients or assistive personnel can be easily taught how to use this apparatus and control the oral secretions.

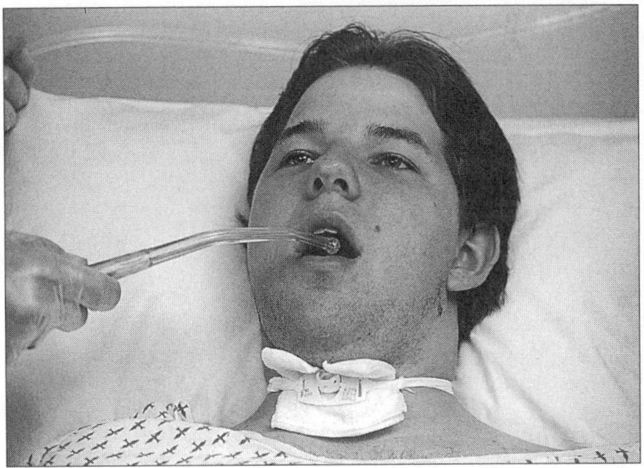

FIGURE 13-1 Oropharyngeal suctioning.

Delegation Considerations

The skill of performing oral pharyngeal (Yankauer) suctioning can be delegated to assistive personnel and sometimes to the client and family.

The client and care provider should be educated and assisted until competent in proper technique to apply, clean, and store Yankauer suction device.

The client and care provider must be taught appropriate suction limits for oral pharyngeal suctioning and the risks of applying excessive or inadequate suction pressure. Caution the client and care provider to avoid mouth sutures, avoid applying suction against sensitive tissues, and avoid dislodging tubings in the client's nose or mouth.

Equipment

- Towel, cloth, or disposable paper
- Nonsterile gloves
- Yankauer or tonsillar tip suction catheter
- Face shield or mask
- Disposable cup or nonsterile basin
- Tap water (about 100 ml)
- Portable or wall suction machine
- Connecting tubing (6 feet)
- Oral airway (if indicated)
- Washcloth (if indicated)

Step	Rationale

Assessment

Step	Rationale
1. Observe for signs and symptoms associated with upper airway secretions requiring oral pharyngeal suctioning: gurgling on inspiration or expiration, restlessness, obvious excess oral secretions, drooling, gastric secretions or vomitus in mouth, or coughing without clearing secretions from upper airway.	Physical signs and symptoms may indicate need to perform this procedure. Worsening status may result in total airway obstruction and hypoxia. The risk of aspiration of gastric contents and airway obstruction is increased in clients with vomiting, delayed gastric emptying, impaired esophageal sphincter control, hiatal hernia, impaired cough, impaired swallowing, or impaired gag reflex.

- ***Critical Decision Point***

  Signs and symptoms associated with ***hypoxia*** *(low oxygen utilization at the cellular or tissue level),* ***hypoxemia*** *(low oxygen tension in the blood), or hypercapnia (elevated carbon dioxide tension in the blood) may also be present: apprehension, anxiety, decreased ability to concentrate, lethargy, decreased level of consciousness (especially acute), increased fatigue and dizziness, behavioral changes (especially irritability), increased pulse rate, increased rate of breathing, decreased depth of breathing, elevated blood pressure, cardiac dysrhythmias, pallor, cyanosis, dyspnea, and use of accessory muscles for breathing.*

Step	Rationale
2. Determine client's knowledge about use of the catheter.	Reveals need for client instruction.
3. Identify risk factors such as impaired cough or gag reflex, weakened respiratory muscles, impaired swallowing, or decreased level of consciousness.	Risk factors may prevent client from protecting the airway from aspiration or from clearing secretions safely.

Nursing Diagnosis

Defining characteristics from the assessment data may reveal the following nursing diagnoses for clients requiring this skill:

- Ineffective airway clearance
- Risk for aspiration
- Ineffective breathing pattern
- Impaired gas exchange
- Risk for infection
- Deficient knowledge regarding airway clearance techniques and devices
- Impaired swallowing

Related factors are individualized based on client's condition or needs.

Planning

Step	Rationale
1. **Expected outcomes** following completion of procedure:	
▪ Upper airway (oral **pharynx**) is cleared of secretions.	Suctioning is effective.
▪ No gurgling is heard in pharynx on inspiration and expiration.	Presence of secretions in large upper airway produces noisy respirations.

STEP	RATIONALE
■ Drooling is diminished or absent.	Excessive drooling indicates that client is unable to handle oral secretions.
■ Vomitus or gastric secretions are absent from mouth.	Gastric secretions retained in oral cavity increase client's risk for aspiration pneumonia.
2. Explain to client how the procedure will help clear airway secretions and relieve some breathing problems. Explain that coughing, gagging, or (less commonly) sneezing is normal and lasts only a few seconds. Encourage client to cough out secretions during procedure. Practice, if able. Splint surgical incisions, if necessary.	Gagging or coughing will occur only when the posterior pharynx is deeply suctioned or as a result of excess secretions. Coughing secretions out of lower airway or posterior pharynx will decrease the amount of suctioning required. Encourages cooperation and minimizes risks and associated anxiety.
3. Position client and, if necessary, place towel across client's chest.	Promotes client comfort and removal of airway secretions. Towel protects client's gown and bed linen from contamination by secretions.

IMPLEMENTATION

STEP	RATIONALE
1. Wash hands and apply gloves. Apply mask or face shield.	Reduces transmission of microorganisms.
2. Fill cup or basin with approximately 100 ml of water.	For cleansing catheter after suctioning.
3. Turn suction device on; set regulator to appropriate negative pressure (see manufacturer's instructions).	Elevated pressure settings increase risk of trauma to the oral mucosa.
4. Connect one end of connecting tubing to suction machine and other to Yankauer suction catheter. Check that equipment is functioning properly by suctioning small amount of water from cup or basin.	Prepares suction apparatus. Ensures equipment function and lubricates catheter.
5. Remove client's oxygen mask, if present. Nasal cannula may remain in place. Keep oxygen mask near client's face. Try removing the straps from around the client's head that hold the mask in place and leaving the mask in place until ready to suction client.	Allows access to mouth. Reduces chance of hypoxia.

• ***Critical Decision Point***

Be prepared to quickly reapply supplemental oxygen if respiratory distress develops and at end of suctioning.

STEP	RATIONALE
6. Insert catheter into mouth along gum line to pharynx. Move catheter around mouth until secretions are cleared. Encourage client to cough. Replace oxygen mask.	Catheter provides continuous suction. Take care not to allow suction tip to invaginate oral mucosal surfaces. Coughing moves secretions from lower airway into mouth and upper airway.
7. Rinse catheter with water in cup or basin until connecting tubing is cleared of secretions. Turn off suction. May need to wash face if secretions are present on client's skin.	Rinses catheter and reduces probability of transmission of microorganisms. Clean suction tubing enhances delivery of set suction pressure. Prevents skin breakdown.
8. Reassess respiratory status. Repeat procedure, if indicated. May need to use standard suction catheter to reach into trachea if respiratory status not improved.	Directs nurse to continue or cease intervention or to choose another intervention.
9. Remove towel, and place in trash or in laundry if soiled. Reposition client; Sims' position encourages drainage and should be used if client has decreased level of consciousness.	Reduces transmission of microorganisms. Facilitates drainage of oral secretions.
10. Discard remainder of water into appropriate receptacle. Rinse basin in warm soapy water and dry with paper towels. Discard disposable cup into appropriate receptable. Place catheter in clean dry area.	Reduces transmission of microorganisms and maintains medical asepsis. Moist environment encourages microorganism growth.

• ***Critical Decision Point***

Catheter should be kept in nonairtight container such as brown paper or plastic bag attached to bed rail or in suction canister area. It should not be stored where it will come in contact with secretions or excretions or will contaminate clean supplies. Closure in an airtight container promotes bacterial growth.

STEP	RATIONALE
11. Remove gloves and mask or face shield and dispose in appropriate receptacle. Wash hands.	Reduces transmission of microorganisms to other clients. Clean equipment should not be handled with contaminated gloves.
12. Position client and provide oral hygiene as needed.	Promotes client's comfort.

EVALUATION

1. Compare assessment findings before and after procedure.	Identifies physiological response to the suction procedure.
2. Auscultate chest and airways for adventitious sounds.	Presence of lower airway adventitious sounds suggests a need for lower airway suctioning.
3. Observe client or family perform Yankauer suctioning.	Demonstrates learning.

UNEXPECTED OUTCOMES AND RELATED INTERVENTIONS

- Worsening respiratory distress
  - Implement nasal, oral pharyngeal, or tracheal suctioning.
  - Evaluate need for other means to protect airway (e.g., oral intubation, **oral airway,** positioning).
  - Provide supplemental oxygen.
  - Notify physician.
- Return of bloody secretions
  - Reduce the amount of suction pressure used.
  - Observe catheter tip for nicks, which can cause mucosal trauma.
  - Increase frequency of oral hygiene.

RECORDING AND REPORTING

- Record in nurses' notes respiratory assessments before and after suctioning; use of Yankauer suction catheter; duration of suctioning period (if unusual, as in nearly continuous secretions); secretions obtained—odor, amount, color, consistency; frequency of suctioning; client's tolerance of procedure; amount of negative suction pressure used (unless standardized in institution or deviation from usual).
- Record instruction to caregivers and ability to correctly perform procedure.
- Report any changes from client's baseline respiratory assessment.

TEACHING CONSIDERATIONS

- Instruct family or caregiver not to allow catheter to fall to the floor.
- Provide information regarding signs and symptoms of worsening respiratory status.
- Assess knowledge level of client, family, and primary caregiver to determine amount of instruction required and frequency of visits necessary to reach goals.

PEDIATRIC CONSIDERATIONS

- Maintain healthy infant in supine position (American Academy of Pediatrics, 1996).
- Position infants with breathing problems or excessive vomitus in prone position (Wong and others, 1999).
- Bulb syringe is used. Compress syringe before insertion to prevent forcing secretions into infant's bronchi (Wong and others, 1999).

GERONTOLOGICAL CONSIDERATIONS

- Clients with dysphagia may benefit from oral suctioning before, during, and after meals.
- Oral mucosa in older adults is fragile, and a lower suction pressure is needed.
- Older adults are prone to aspiration of oral secretions because of decreased cough and gag reflexes (Lueckenotte, 2000).

HOME CARE CONSIDERATIONS

- In the home the secretion collection container is cleaned and disinfected or changed every 24 hours according to home care or institutional protocol. In many institutions the disposable secretion collection canister is sealed and disposed of in its entirety as biohazardous material.
- Assess home for the presence of respiratory irritants, including cigarette smoke, dust, pollen, or chemicals.

Skill 13-2 Airway Management—Suctioning

The major differences between pharyngeal and tracheal suctioning are the depth suctioned and the potential for complications. Pharyngeal suctioning only removes secretions from the back of the throat and requires clean technique. Tracheal suctioning extends into the lower airway and necessitates aseptic technique. The nurse assesses the client to determine frequency and depth of suctioning. Some clients may require suctioning every hour or two, whereas others need to be suctioned only once or twice a day. How far to insert the suction catheter for tracheal suctioning depends on the size of the client, especially children.

Infants and young children can accept insertion of a catheter 8 to 14 cm (3 to 5.5 in), whereas the older child and adolescent can allow insertion of the catheter to a depth of 14 to 20 cm (5.5 to 8 in). These lengths vary with each child; children who are small for their age have shorter airways that require less deep suctioning. The nurse can estimate the correct catheter length by measuring the distance from nose (or mouth) to earlobe and nose (or mouth) to sternal notch for nasal (or oral) tracheal suctioning.

The nurse uses these techniques of suctioning primarily to remove accumulated nasal pharyngeal and tracheal secretions in the absence of an artificial airway. If the secretions are only in the nose and mouth, then only the pharynx requires suctioning, although in most instances the nurse will suction both the pharynx and the trachea. Secretions should be suctioned from the pharynx as often as necessary. Secretions that are not removed are more likely to be aspirated into the lungs, increasing the risk for potential infection and respiratory failure. In addition, the nurse may need to remove other body fluids, primarily blood and gastric contents, from the oral and posterior pharynx to prevent their aspiration as well.

The carina, located at the bifurcation of the mainstem bronchi, has many cough receptors. Many times the nurse will be able to stimulate a client's decreased cough reflex by passing a suction catheter to the carina. Once the client coughs, clearing of the lower airway is more effective.

Suctioning has many risks associated with performing the procedure. The most serious ones relate to hypoxemia, which may often result in cardiac dysrhythmias; laryngeal spasm; bradycardia, which is associated with stimulation of the vagus nerve; and nasal trauma and bleeding, which can develop from the suction catheter.

Performing Nasopharyngeal and Nasotracheal Suctioning

Nasopharyngeal and nasotracheal suctioning maintain a patent airway by removing secretions from the pharynx or throat and the trachea. This type of suctioning is used when suctioning with a Yankauer device is ineffective or inappropriate or when the lower airway requires removal of secretions. It involves inserting a small rubber or plastic tube into the naris to the pharynx or trachea and then applying negative pressure to withdraw mucus.

Performing Artificial Airway Suctioning

Endotracheal (ET) tubes and tracheostomy ("trach") tubes are artificial airways inserted to relieve mechanical airway obstruction, provide a route for mechanical ventilation, permit easy access for secretion removal, and protect the airway from gross aspiration in clients with impaired cough or gag reflexes (Figure 13-2).

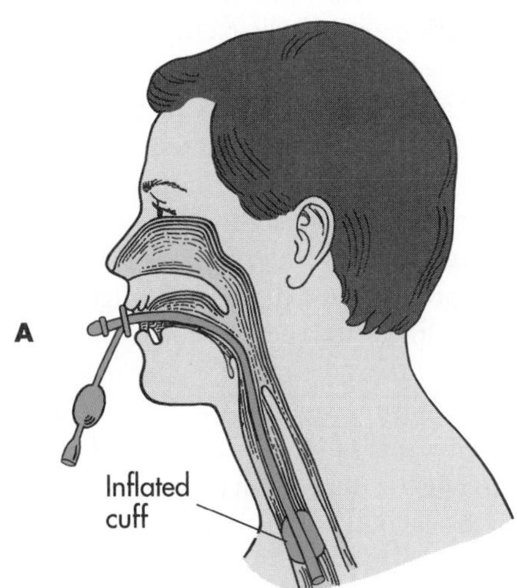

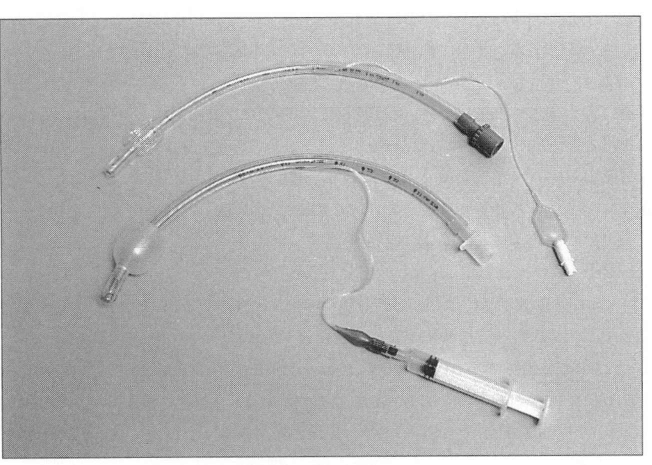

FIGURE **13-2** A, Endotracheal (ET) tube with inflated cuff. **B,** ET tubes with uninflated and inflated cuffs and syringe for inflation.

Endotracheal intubation is a procedure performed by a physician or specially trained personnel (e.g., nurse, respiratory therapist, or rescue personnel). An ET tube is inserted through the naris (nasal ET tube) or the mouth (oral ET tube) past the epiglottis and vocal cords into the trachea.

It remains somewhat controversial as to how long ET tubes are usually left in place; however, in most cases after 2 to 4 weeks a tracheostomy tube is inserted (St. John, 1999). A tracheostomy tube is inserted directly into the trachea through a small incision made in the client's neck by the surgeon. Although ET tubes are temporary, a tracheostomy tube can be temporary or permanent depending on the client's condition. One advantage of tracheostomy tubes in clients receiving mechanical ventilation is that they are shorter and decrease dead space ventilation. In selected clients decreasing **dead space** enhances the ability to wean from a mechanical ventilator, making the tracheostomy tube a temporary need. In other clients removal of critical airway structures with radical neck surgical procedures or uncorrectable airway obstructions dictate the need for a permanent tracheostomy tube.

ET tubes are usually made of plastic or rubber; tracheostomy tubes are made of several different materials, including various polyvinyl chloride– or silicone-based plastics and stainless steel or metallic compounds. Metal tracheostomy tubes are thermal sensitive and must be protected from extreme heat and cold to prevent tissue injury in the client. Most metal and plastic tracheostomy tubes contain an inner cannula that can be temporarily withdrawn for cleaning airway-occluding mucus without removing the entire tracheostomy tube.

Adult, but not pediatric, sizes of ET tubes have a cuff molded onto the tube to (1) prevent the aspiration of oral secretions or gastric contents into the lung or (2) obstruct the escape of air from mechanical ventilator breaths through the upper airway. Although pediatric tracheostomy tubes do not contain a cuff because of the small airway diameter of the child, adult sizes are available cuffed or noncuffed. A cuff on a tracheostomy tube serves the same purpose as one on an ET tube. Cuffs are made of a balloonlike inflatable plastic; usually they are manually inflated with air by the nurse or respiratory therapist. Plastic-covered foam cuffs are self–air inflating if the inflation port is left open to the atmosphere.

Tracheostomy tubes (see Skill 13-5) are available as either fenestrated or nonfenestrated. (A fenestration is a small hole.) In tracheostomy tubes the **fenestration** is usually on the outer, or greater, curve of the **outer cannula** of a tracheostomy tube; the inner cannula does not usually contain a fenestration. (ET tubes are not fenestrated primarily because of the risk of aspiration and also because of associated injury to the vocal cords with speech.) Fenestrated tubes are only indicated for clients who may be able to speak and do not need mechanical ventilation. When the cuff is deflated and the inner cannula is removed, a fenestrated tracheostomy tube permits the client to talk because exhaled air passes over the vocal cords. Phonation is optimized when the outer cannula is plugged, forcing all inhaled and exhaled air to travel by normal nasal and oral routes. A fenestrated tracheostomy tube usually allows the client to talk only in the absence of mechanical ventilation. (NOTE: Clients can also talk if there is no cuff or if the cuff is deflated when a nonfenestrated tracheostomy tube is used.) Newer types of cuffed tracheostomy tubes allow the client to talk during mechanical ventilation with the use of a narrow fenestrated catheter molded to the external surface of the outer cannula. This catheter is connected to an independent air source that blows air over the vocal cords, permitting phonation that ranges from an audible whisper to a clear voice. There are other tracheostomy tubes available that have valves to assist the client to speak (e.g., the Passey Muir tracheostomy tube).

Applying the laws of physics allows the nurse to understand the effects of secretions in the airway. Increasing the diameter of a tube (or artificial airway) decreases airway resistance. Decreasing the diameter of a tube increases airway resistance and therefore the work of breathing. Removing secretions from the artificial airway maintains patency, increases the diameter of the tube, and decreases the work of breathing. In addition, as stated before, a cough can be stimulated by suctioning; an effective cough reduces or eliminates the need for suctioning. The client helps maintain airway patency with facilitation of the natural cough reflex.

Usually suctioning is performed with the same kind of suction catheter as that used in nasal tracheal suctioning (see Table 13-2). However, this skill is easier to perform than nasal tracheal suctioning because there is already direct access to the lower airway. Systemic complications associated with ET or tracheostomy tube suctioning are similar to those related to nasal or oral tracheal tube suctioning, but the client who requires an artificial airway may have more physiologic compromise and may be at greater risk for development of complications. Some institutions use a **closed system suction catheter** or **in-line suction catheter** device, which assist in minimizing infections, especially in critically ill or highly contagious clients (see Skill 13-3).

Placement of an oral ET tube impedes performance of oral hygiene measures. Excessive manipulation of the tube can dislodge it; toothbrushing and mouth rinsing are difficult to perform because there is always the risk of fluid aspiration around the ET tube because the epiglottis is held open by the tube. The nurse promotes oral hygiene through the use of various techniques. One technique is to rotate the ET tube from one side of the mouth to the other on alternate days, thereby reducing pressure on the sides of the client's mouth and allowing improved visualization and cleaning of one side of the client's mouth. The use of a special toothbrush with a vacuum port also may be helpful in cleaning teeth and oral mucous membranes.

Table 13-2 Equipment Guidelines* for Intubation and Suctioning

Equipment	Infant (Premature Infant to 1 year)	Small Child (2-5 years)	School-Age Child (6-12 years)	Adolescent to Adult
Airway:				
Oral	00-2	2-3	3-4	4-5
Nasal (French)	12	10-20	20-24	24-36
Hand-held resuscitator size	Child	Child	Child/adult	Adult
Mask size	Premature infant/child	Child	Small adult	Adult
Laryngoscope blade size	0-1 (straight)	2 (straight)	2-3 (straight or curved)	4-5 (straight or curved)
Endotracheal tube size (mm)	2.5-4.0	4.0-5.0	5.0-6.5	7.0-9.0
Tracheostomy tube: Jackson size Inner	000-1	1-2	3-4	4-10
diameter (mm)	2.5-3.5	3.5-4.0	4.5-5.0	5.0-9.0
Suction catheter size (French)†	5-6	6-8	8-10	10-16

*These guidelines should be used as an estimate only: actual sizes depend on the size and individual needs of the patient.
†Catheter outer diameter should not exceed one half the internal diameter of the tube.
Data from St. John RE: Airway management, *Crit Care Nurse* 19(4):79, 1999.

Delegation Considerations

The skills of nasotracheal and endotracheal tube suctioning should not be delegated to assistive personnel. When the client is assessed by the nurse to be stable, the skill of performing tracheostomy tube suctioning can be delegated to assistive personnel and sometimes to the client in special situations. These situations include clients with permanent tracheostomy tubes after head and neck surgery and clients receiving mechanical ventilation at home. In these cases the client and care provider must be educated and assisted until competent in proper technique to suction, clean, and store catheter and suction machine. Client and care provider should be taught appropriate suction limits for suctioning tracheostomy tube and risks of applying excessive or inadequate suction pressure. Client and caregiver should also be taught signs and symptoms of hypoxemia and methods to prevent and treat hypoxemia and when to notify the physician.

Equipment

Oropharyngeal, Nasopharyngeal, and Nasotracheal Suctioning

- Appropriate-size suction catheter (smallest diameter that will remove secretions effectively) (see Table 13-2)
- Small Y-adapter (if catheter does not have a suction control port)
- Two sterile gloves or one sterile and one nonsterile glove
- Sterile basin
- Sterile normal saline solution or water (about 100 ml)
- Clean towel or paper drape
- Portable or wall suction
- Connecting tubing (6 feet)
- Nasal or oral airway (if indicated)
- Mask or face shield

Suctioning Artificial Airway

- Bedside table
- Suction catheter of appropriate size (see Table 13-2)
- Two sterile gloves or one sterile and one nonsterile glove
- Sterile setup
- Approximately 100 ml of sterile normal saline solution or water
- Clean towel or sterile drape
- Portable or wall suction apparatus
- 6 feet of connecting tubing
- Face shield

Step	Rationale
Assessment	
1. Assess signs and symptoms of upper and lower airway obstruction requiring nasal or oral tracheal suctioning, including: wheezes, crackles, or gurgling on inspiration or expiration; restlessness; ineffective coughing; unilateral, segmental, or lobar absent or diminished breath sounds (in absence of pneumonectomy or lobectomy); tachypnea; hypertension or hypotension; cyanosis; decreased level of consciousness, especially acutely; or excess nasal secretions, drooling, gastric secretions, or vomitus in mouth.	Physical signs and symptoms result from decreased oxygen to tissues, as well as pooling of secretions in upper and lower airways.
2. Determine the presence of apprehension, anxiety, decreased ability to concentrate, lethargy, decreased level of consciousness (especially acute), increased fatigue, dizziness, behavioral changes (especially irritability), decreased oxygen saturation (from pulse oximetry), increased pulse rate, increased rate of breathing, decreased depth of breathing, elevated blood pressure, cardiac dysrhythmias, pallor, cyanosis, dyspnea, or use of accessory muscles.	Signs and symptoms associated with hypoxia (low oxygen at the cellular or tissue level), hypoxemia (low oxygen tension in the blood), or hypercapnea (elevated carbon dioxide tension in the blood).
3. Assess for risk factors for upper or lower airway obstruction, including obstructive lung disease; pulmonary infections; impaired mobility; sedation; decreased level of consciousness; seizures; presence of feeding tube; decreased gag or cough reflex; decreased swallowing ability; allergies; sinus drainage; and head, neck, or chest tumors.	Presence of these risk factors may impair the client's ability to clear secretions from the airway and may necessitate nasopharyngeal or nasotracheal suctioning
4. Determine additional factors that normally influence upper or lower airway function; recent surgery, decreased level of consciousness, ineffective or absent cough, chemical neuromuscular blockade, neuromuscular diseases, congestive heart failure, pulmonary edema, adult respiratory distress syndrome, hyaline membrane disease, or diaphragmatic weakness or paralysis.	Allows nurse to identify clients at risk for airway obstruction needing ET or tracheostomy tube suctioning.
a. Fluid status	Fluid overload may increase amount of secretions. Dehydration promotes thicker secretions.
b. Lack of humidity	The environment influences secretion formation and gas exchange, necessitating airway suctioning when the client cannot clear secretions effectively.
c. Infection (e.g., pneumonia)	Clients with respiratory infections are prone to increased secretions that are thicker and sometimes more difficult to expectorate.
d. Anatomy	Abnormal anatomy can impair normal drainage of secretions. For example, nasal swelling, deviated septum, or facial fractures may impair nasal drainage. Tumors in or around the lower airway may impair secretion removal by occluding or externally compressing the lumen of the airway.
5. Examine sputum microbiology data.	Certain bacteria are more easily transmitted or require isolation because of virulence or antibiotic resistance.
6. Assess client's understanding of procedure.	Reveals need for client instruction and encourages cooperation.

STEP	RATIONALE

NURSING DIAGNOSIS

Defining characteristics from the assessment data may reveal the following nursing diagnoses for clients requiring this skill:

Ineffective airway clearance
Risk for aspiration
Ineffective breathing pattern
Impaired gas exchange
Risk for infection
Deficient knowledge regarding airway clearance techniques and devices
Impaired swallowing
Impaired spontaneous ventilation

Related factors are individualized based on client's condition or needs.

PLANNING

1. **Expected outcomes** following completion of procedure:
   - Lower and upper airways demonstrate absent or diminished crackles, wheezes, and gurgles on inspiration and expiration; return of absent or diminished breath sounds; normalization of heart rate, blood pressure, respiratory rate and effort; absence of drooling, gastric secretions, or vomitus in mouth, and nasal secretions.

     Airways are cleared of secretions. In the presence of infection more secretions are produced; as infection improves, the amount of secretions and the need for suctioning diminish.
   - Client verbalizes easier breathing, if able.

     Clear airway reduces work of breathing.
2. Explain to client how procedure will help clear airway and relieve breathing problems. Explain that temporary coughing, sneezing, gagging, or shortness of breath is normal during the procedure. Encourage client to cough out secretions. Practice coughing, if able. Splint surgical incisions, if necessary.

   Encourages cooperation and minimizes risks, anxiety, and pain of procedure.
3. Explain importance of and encourage coughing during procedure.

   Facilitates secretion removal and may reduce frequency and duration of future suctioning.
4. Assist client to assume position comfortable for nurse and client (usually semi-Fowler's or sitting upright with head hyperextended, unless contraindicated).

   Reduces stimulation of gag reflex, promotes client comfort and secretion drainage, prevents aspiration and nurse strain. Hyperextension facilitates insertion of catheter into trachea.
5. Place towel across client's chest, if needed.

   Reduces transmission of microorganisms by protecting gown from secretions.

IMPLEMENTATION

Performing Nasopharyngeal and Nasotracheal Suctioning

1. Wash hands and apply face shield if splashing is likely.

   Reduces transmission of microorganisms.
2. Connect one end of connecting tubing to suction machine, and place other end in convenient location near client. Turn suction device on and set vacuum regulator to appropriate negative pressure.

   Excessive negative pressure damages nasal pharyngeal and tracheal mucosa and can induce greater hypoxia.
3. If indicated, increase supplemental **oxygen therapy** to 100% or as ordered by physician. Encourage client deep breathing.

   These measures reduce suction-induced hypoxemia. Oxygen-sensitive clients include those with chronic heart and lung conditions and those with pneumonia.

   - ***Critical Decision Point***

     Oxygen must be readjusted as ordered by physician after procedure to avoid increased risk of oxygen toxicity and absorption, atelectasis from prolonged administration of high concentrations of oxygen, and increased carbon dioxide retention in clients with chronic obstructive lung diseases.

STEP	RATIONALE
4. Prepare suction catheter.	
a. Open suction kit or catheter with use of aseptic technique. If sterile drape is available, place it across client's chest or on the overbed table. Do not allow the suction catheter to touch any nonsterile surfaces.	Maintains asepsis and reduces transmission of microorganisms.
b. Unwrap or open sterile basin and place on bedside table. Be careful not to touch inside of basin. Fill with about 100 ml sterile normal saline solution or water (see illustration).	Saline or water is used to clean tubing after each suction pass.
c. Open lubricant. Squeeze small amount onto open sterile catheter package without touching package.	Prepares lubricant while maintaining sterility. Water-soluble lubricant is used to avoid lipoid aspiration pneumonia. Excessive lubricant can occlude catheter.
5. Apply sterile glove to each hand, or apply nonsterile glove to nondominant hand and sterile glove to dominant hand.	Reduces transmission of microorganisms and allows nurse to maintain sterility of suction catheter.
6. Pick up suction catheter with dominant hand without touching nonsterile surfaces. Pick up connecting tubing with nondominant hand. Secure catheter to tubing (see illustration).	Maintains catheter sterility. Connects catheter to suction.

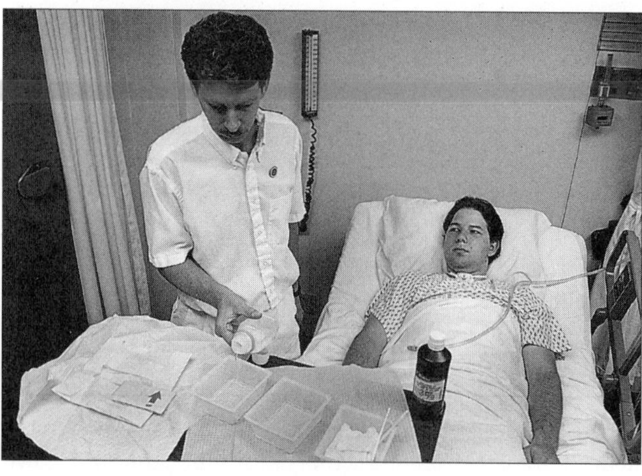

STEP **4b** Pouring sterile saline into tray.

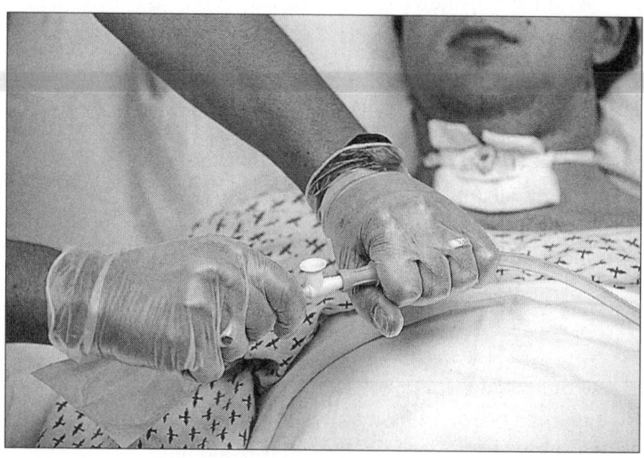

STEP **6** Attaching catheter to suction.

STEP	RATIONALE
7. Check that equipment is functioning properly by suctioning small amount of normal saline solution from basin.	Ensures equipment function. Lubricates internal catheter and tubing.
8. Lightly coat distal 6 to 8 cm (2 to 3 in) of catheter with water-soluble lubricant.	Lubricates catheter for easier insertion.
9. Remove oxygen delivery device, if applicable, with nondominant hand. Without applying suction and using dominant thumb and forefinger, gently but quickly insert catheter into naris during inhalation and following natural course of the naris, slightly slant the catheter downward or through mouth. Do not force through naris (see illustration).	Application of suction pressure while introducing catheter into trachea increases risk of damage to mucosa and increases risk of hypoxia because of removal of entrained oxygen present in airways.

- ***Critical Decision Point***

  Be sure to insert catheter during client inhalation, especially if inserting catheter into trachea, because epiglottis is open. Do not insert during swallowing or catheter will most likely enter esophagus. ***Never*** *apply suction during insertion. Client should cough. If client gags or becomes nauseated, catheter is most likely in esophagus and must be removed.*

STEP	RATIONALE

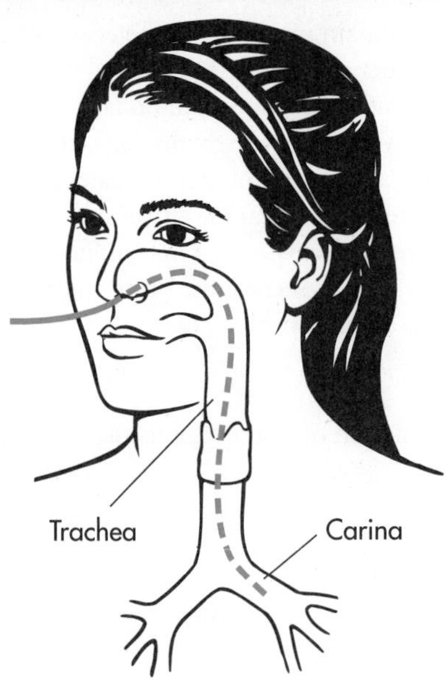

STEP 9 Pathway for nasotracheal catheter progression.

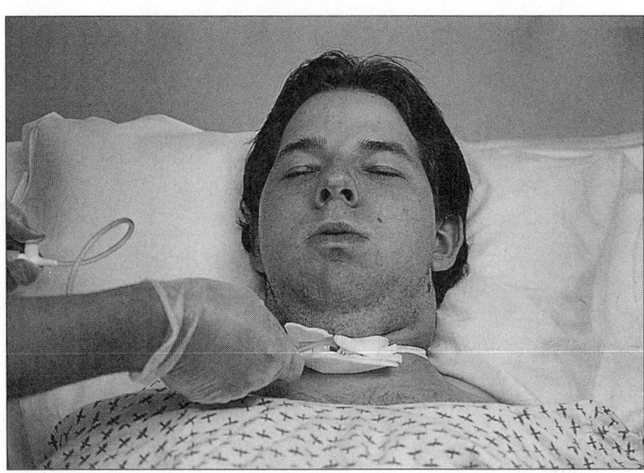

STEP 9b Suctioning tracheostomy.

a. Pharyngeal suctioning: In adults, insert catheter about 16 cm; in older children, 8 to 12 cm (3 to 5 in); in infants and young children, 4 to 8 cm (2 to 3 in). Rule of thumb is to insert catheter distance from tip of nose (or mouth) to base of ear lobe.
b. Tracheal suctioning: In adults, insert catheter about 20 cm; in older children, 14 to 20 cm (5.5 to 8 in); and in young children and infants, 8 to 14 cm (3 to 5.5 in) (see illustration).
c. Positioning: In some instances turning client's head to right helps nurse suction left mainstem bronchus; turning head to left helps nurse suction right mainstem bronchus. If resistance is felt after insertion of catheter for maximum recommended distance, catheter has probably hit carina. Pull catheter back 1 to 2 cm before applying suction.

- ***Critical Decision Point***
  Use the nasal approach and perform tracheal suctioning before pharyngeal suctioning whenever possible. The mouth and pharynx contain more bacteria than the trachea does. If copious oral secretions are present before beginning the procedure, suction mouth with oral suction device.

10. Apply intermittent suction for up to 10 seconds by placing and releasing nondominant thumb over vent of catheter and slowly withdrawing catheter while rotating it back and forth between dominant thumb and forefinger. Encourage client to cough. Replace oxygen device, if applicable.

Intermittent suction and rotation of catheter prevents injury to mucosa. If catheter "grabs" mucosa, remove thumb to release suction. Suctioning longer than 10 seconds can cause cardiopulmonary compromise, usually from hypoxemia or vagal overload.

- ***Critical Decision Point***
  Monitor client's vital signs and oxygen saturation using pulse oximetry throughout suction procedure. If the client's pulse drops more than 20 beats per minute or increases more than 40 beats per minute or if pulse oximetry falls below 90% or 5% from baseline, cease suctioning (Lewis and others, 2000).

STEP	RATIONALE
11. Rinse catheter and connecting tubing with normal saline or water until cleared.	Secretions that remain in suction catheter or connecting tubing decrease suctioning efficiency.
12. Assess for need to repeat suctioning procedure. When possible, allow adequate time (1 to 2 minutes) between suction passes for ventilation and oxygenation. Assist client to deep breathe and cough.	Observe for alterations in cardiopulmonary status. Suctioning can induce hypoxemia, dysrhythmias, laryngospasm, and bronchospasm. Deep breathing reventilates and reoxygenates alveoli. Repeated passes clear the airway of excessive secretions but can also remove oxygen and may induce **laryngospasm.**
13. When pharynx and trachea are sufficiently cleared of secretions, perform oral pharyngeal suctioning to clear mouth of secretions. Do not suction nose again after suctioning mouth.	Removes upper airway secretions. More microorganisms are generally present in mouth.
14. When suctioning is completed, roll catheter around fingers of dominant hand. Pull glove off inside out so that catheter remains coiled in glove. Pull off other glove over first glove in same way to seal in contaminants. Discard in appropriate receptacle. Turn off suction device.	Reduces transmission of microorganisms.
15. Remove towel, place in laundry or appropriate receptacle, and reposition client. (Nurse may need to wear clean gloves for personal care.)	Reduces transmission of microorganisms. Promotes comfort.
16. If indicated, readjust oxygen to original level because client's blood oxygen level should have returned to baseline.	Prevents absorption **atelectasis** and oxygen toxicity while allowing client time to reoxygenate blood.
17. Discard remainder of normal saline into appropriate receptacle. If basin is disposable, discard into appropriate receptacle. If basin is reusable, rinse it out and place it in soiled utility room.	Reduces transmission of microorganisms.
18. Remove face shield and discard into appropriate receptacle. Wash hands.	Reduces transmission of microorganisms.
19. Place unopened suction kit on suction machine table or at head of bed.	Provides immediate access to suction catheter for next procedure.
20. Assist client to a comfortable position and provide oral hygiene as needed.	
Performing Artificial Airway Suctioning	
1. Wash hands and apply face shield.	Reduces transmission of microorganisms.
2. Connect one end of connecting tubing to suction machine and place other end in convenient location. Turn suction device on and set vacuum regulator to appropriate negative pressure (see manufacturer's directions).	Excessive negative pressure damages tracheal mucosa and can induce greater hypoxia.
3. Prepare proper suction catheter (see Table 13-2):	Suction catheter's outer diameter should not exceed one-half of the internal diameter of the ET or tracheostomy tube (St. John, 1999).
4. Aseptically open suction catheter package. If sterile drape is available, place it across client's chest. Do not allow suction catheter to touch any nonsterile surface.	Prevents contamination of clothing and provides a sterile surface on which to lay suction catheter between passes, if needed. Prepares catheter and prevents transmission of microorganisms.
5. Unwrap or open sterile basin and place on bedside table. Be careful not to touch inside of basin. Fill with about 100 ml of sterile normal saline.	Normal saline is used to rinse catheter after suctioning.
6. Apply one sterile glove to each hand, or apply nonsterile glove to nondominant hand and sterile glove to dominant hand.	Reduces transmission of microorganisms and allows nurse to maintain sterility of suction catheter.
7. Pick up suction catheter with dominant hand without touching nonsterile surfaces. Pick up connecting tubing with nondominant hand. Secure catheter to tubing.	Maintains catheter sterility. Establishes suction.
8. Check that equipment is functioning properly by suctioning small amount of saline from basin.	Ensures equipment function; lubricates catheter and tubing.

Step	Rationale
9. Hyperinflate and/or hyperoxygenate client before suctioning, using manual resuscitation Ambu-bag connected to oxygen source (Chapter 11) or sigh mechanism on mechanical ventilator. Some mechanical ventilators have a button that when pushed delivers 100% oxygen for a few minutes and then resets to the previous value.	Hyperinflation decreases arterial oxygen desaturation and atelectasis caused by negative pressure of suctioning (St. John, 1999). Preoxygenation converts large proportion of resident lung gas to 100% oxygen to offset amount used in metabolic consumption while ventilator or oxygenation is interrupted, as well as to offset volume lost during suction procedure.
10. If client is receiving mechanical ventilation, open swivel adapter or if necessary remove oxygen or humidity delivery device with nondominant hand.	Exposes artificial airway.

- ***Critical Decision Point***

  Be careful not to allow client to remain on high fraction of inspired oxygen (FIO_2), such as 100%, too long. Atelectasis can develop.

Step	Rationale
11. Without applying suction, gently but quickly insert catheter using dominant thumb and forefinger into artificial airway until resistance is met or client coughs, then pull back 1 cm. (Best to time catheter insertion during client inspiration.)	Application of suction pressure while introducing catheter into trachea increases risk of damage to tracheal mucosa, as well as increased hypoxia related to removal of entrained oxygen present in airways. Pulling back stimulates cough and removes catheter from mucosal wall so that catheter is not resting against tracheal mucosa during suctioning.

- ***Critical Decision Point***

  If unable to insert catheter past the end of the ET tube, the catheter is probably caught in the Murphy eye (i.e., side hole at distal end of ET tube that allows for collateral air flow in event of mainstem ***intubation****). If this happens, rotate the catheter to reposition it away from the Murphy eye, or withdraw it slightly and reinsert with the next inhalation. Usually the catheter meets resistance at the carina. One indication that the catheter is at the carina is acute onset of coughing because the carina contains many cough receptors. The catheter should be pulled back.*

Step	Rationale
12. Apply intermittent suction by placing and releasing nondominant thumb over vent of catheter; slowly withdraw catheter while rotating it back and forth between dominant thumb and forefinger. Encourage client to cough. Watch for respiratory distress.	Intermittent suction and rotation of catheter reduces injury to tracheal mucosal lining. If catheter "grabs" mucosa, remove thumb to release suction (St. John, 1999).

- ***Critical Decision Point***

  If the client develops respiratory distress during the suction procedure, immediately withdraw the catheter and supply additional oxygen and breaths as needed. Oxygen can be administered directly through the catheter in an emergency. Disconnect suction and attach oxygen at prescribed flow rate through the catheter.

Step	Rationale
13. If client is receiving mechanical ventilation, close swivel adapter or replace oxygen delivery device.	Reestablishes artificial airway.
14. Encourage client to deep breathe, if able. Some clients respond well to several manual breaths from the mechanical ventilator or Ambu-bag.	Reoxygenates and reexpands alveoli. Suctioning can cause hypoxemia and atelectasis.
15. Rinse catheter and connecting tubing with normal saline until clear. Use continuous suction.	Removes catheter secretions. Secretions left in tubing decrease suction and provide environment for microorganism growth. Secretions left in connecting tube decrease suctioning efficiency.
16. Assess client's cardiopulmonary status (vital signs and oxygen saturation), secretion clearance, and complications. Repeat Steps 9 through 15 once or twice more to clear secretions. Allow adequate time (at least 1 full minute) between suction passes for ventilation and reoxygenation.	Suctioning can induce dysrhythmias, hypoxia, and bronchospasm and impair cerebral circulation or adversely affect hemodynamics (Kerr and others, 1999). Repeated passes with suction catheter clear airway of excessive secretions and promote improved oxygenation (Wood, 1998).
17. Perform nasal and oral pharyngeal suctioning. After naso- and oropharyngeal suctioning are performed, catheter is contaminated; do not reinsert into ET or tracheostomy tube.	Upper airway is considered "clean," and lower airway is considered "sterile." Therefore same catheter can be used to suction from sterile to clean areas, but not from clean to sterile areas.

Step	Rationale
18. Disconnect catheter from connecting tubing. Roll catheter around fingers of dominant hand. Pull glove off inside out so that catheter remains in glove. Pull off other glove over first glove in same way to contain contaminants. Discard into appropriate receptacle. Turn off suction device.	Reduces transmission of microorganisms. Clean equipment should not be touched with contaminated gloves.
19. Remove towel and place in laundry, or remove drape and discard in appropriate receptacle.	
20. Reposition client as indicated by condition. Nurse may need to reapply clean gloves for client's personal care.	Proper positioning based on client's condition promotes comfort and encourages secretion drainage and reduces risk of aspiration.
21. Discard remainder of normal saline into appropriate receptacle. If basin is disposable, discard into appropriate receptacle. If basin is reusable, rinse and place in soiled utility room.	Solution is contaminated.
22. Remove and discard face shield and wash hands.	Reduces transmission of microorganisms.
23. Place unopened suction kit on suction machine or at head of bed according to institution preference.	Provides immediate access to suction catheter for next procedure.

Evaluation

Step	Rationale
1. Compare client's respiratory assessments before and after suctioning.	Identifies physiological effects of suction procedure to restore airway patency.
2. Ask client if breathing is easier and if congestion is decreased.	Provides subjective confirmation that airway obstruction is relieved with suctioning procedure.
3. Observe airway secretions.	Provides data to document presence or absence of respiratory tract infection.

Unexpected Outcomes and Related Interventions

- Worsening respiratory assessment
  - Limit length of suctioning.
  - Determine need for more frequent suctioning, possibly of shorter duration.
  - Determine need for supplemental oxygen. Supply oxygen between suctioning passes.
  - Notify physician.
- Return of bloody secretions
  - Determine amount of suction pressure used. May need to be decreased.
  - Determine nurse's use of intermittent suction and catheter rotation.
  - Evaluate suctioning frequency.
  - Provide more frequent oral hygiene.
- Unable to pass suction catheter through first naris attempted
  - Try other naris or oral route.
  - Insert **nasal airway,** especially if suctioning through client naris frequently (St. John, 1999).
  - Follow naris floor to avoid turbinates.
  - If obstruction is mucus, apply suction to relieve obstruction, but do not apply suction to mucosa. If obstruction is felt to be a blood clot, consult with physician.
  - Increase lubrication.
- Paroxysms of coughing
  - Administer supplemental oxygen.
  - Allow client to rest between passes of suction catheter.
  - Consult with physician regarding need for inhaled bronchodilators or topical anesthetics.
- No secretions obtained
  - Evaluate client's fluid status.
  - Assess for signs of infection.
  - Determine need for chest physiotherapy (see Chapter 12).
  - Assess adequacy of humidification on oxygen delivery device.
- Unable to remove suction catheter (CRITICAL SITUATION).
  - Disconnect suction source from catheter, but leave catheter in trachea.
  - Connect oxygen source to catheter.
  - Notify physician immediately.
  - Anticipate physician's order for inhaled bronchodilator.
  - Prepare for emergency resuscitation.

Recording and Reporting

- Chart in nurses' notes respiratory assessments before and after suctioning; size of suction catheter used; duration of suctioning period, if unusual; route(s) used to suction; secretions obtained; odor, amount, color, and consistency of secretions; frequency of suctioning; client's tolerance of procedure; amount of negative suction pressure used (unless standardized in institution or deviation from usual).
- Report any change in client's respiratory status.

Teaching Considerations

- Instruct client that coughing may increase during the procedure.
- Explain why supplemental oxygen is given prior to suction.

Pediatric Considerations

- Small-diameter suction catheters required in pediatrics should be one half the diameter of the child's tracheostomy tube (Wong and others, 1999).
- Because of small diameter of suction catheter, thick secretions may be more difficult to remove.
- Vacuum pressure should range from 60 to 100 mm Hg for infants and children and 40 to 60 mm Hg for preterm infants (Wong and others, 1999).
- Distance suctioned should not be greater than 0.5 cm beyond the tip of the artificial airway. To determine distance, place catheter near a sample artificial airway (Wong and others, 1999).
- Infant airways have less cartilage and may collapse easily, especially in premature infants or those with reactive airways.
- Suctioning should require no more than 5 seconds (Chandre and Hazinski, 1997).

Gerontological Considerations

- Older adults have lost some properties of elastic recoil and gas exchange.
- Capillaries of older adults are often fragile, predisposing client to bleeding problems.
- Older clients may have coronary artery disease, which places them at increased risk for cardiopulmonary compromise. In addition, older adults may be taking blood-thinning medications such as aspirin for the prevention of coronary or cerebral artery occlusion.

Home Care Considerations

- Although most clients with airway clearance problems at home have a tracheostomy, some also require nasal pharyngeal suctioning. Catheters are often used for a 24-hour period and then cleaned and disinfected; or catheters are cleaned with soapy water after each use and discarded after 24 hours.
- In the home the secretion collection container is cleaned and disinfected or changed every 24 hours according to home care or institutional protocol.
- In the home setting stress the importance of brief intervals of applying suction pressure. Those performing suctioning should hold their breath during the application of negative suction pressure to help them remember to not suction too long.

Skill 13-3 Performing Endotracheal or Tracheostomy Tube Suctioning Using a Closed System (In-Line) Catheter

Use of a closed system catheter (in-line) allows quicker lower airway suctioning without applying gloves or a mask and does not interrupt ventilation and oxygenation in critically ill clients. In addition, the nurse is protected from contamination by the client's secretions (Noll, Hix, and Scott, 1990). With a closed-system method the client's artificial airway is not disconnected from the mechanical ventilator (Paul-Allen and Ostrow, 2000).

Delegation Considerations

The skill of endotracheal (ET) tube suctioning with a closed system (in-line) catheter should not be delegated to assistive personnel. The skill of performing tracheostomy tube suctioning with a closed system catheter can be delegated to assistive personnel or the client in special situations (e.g., when a client has a permanent tracheostomy tube and may be receiving mechanical ventilation in the home or extended care facility). The client and care provider must be educated and assisted until competent in proper technique to apply and care for closed system (in-line) catheter. Client and care provider should be taught appropriate suction limits for suctioning and risks of applying excessive or inadequate suction pressure.

Equipment

- Closed system or in-line suction catheter
- 10 ml or more of normal saline solution in syringe or vials
- Portable or wall suction apparatus
- 6 feet of connecting tubing
- Two clean gloves (optional)

STEP	RATIONALE

ASSESSMENT

1. Observe for signs and symptoms of lower airway obstruction possibly causing hypoxemia or hypercapnia requiring ET or tracheostomy tube suctioning:
   Secretions in artificial airway; coughing, wheezes, or crackles on inspiration and/or expiration; restlessness; ineffective cough; unilateral (in absence of lobectomy or pneumonectomy) or bilateral absent or diminished breath sounds; tachypnea; acute shallow respirations; acute tachycardia or bradycardia; acute hypotension or hypertension; cyanosis; decreased oxygen saturation by pulse oximetry; decreased level of consciousness, especially acute; or acute atelectasis or collapse of segment or lobe on chest x-ray films.

   Physical signs and symptoms result from lower airway obstruction and tissue hypoxia. Mucous plug obstructs airflow into the lung, resulting in atelectasis or collapse.

2. Determine factors that influence normal airway function: impaired cough or gag reflex, decreased level of consciousness, ineffective or absent cough reflex, heavy sedation, neuromuscular diseases affecting chest or abdominal muscles, pneumonia or bronchitis, chronic obstructive pulmonary disease (COPD), congestive heart failure, pulmonary edema, adult respiratory distress syndrome, hyaline membrane disease, or diaphragmatic paralysis.

   Allows nurse to accurately evaluate need to perform ET or tracheostomy tube suctioning. Client's inability to protect airway or clear secretions effectively indicates need for suctioning.

3. Examine sputum microbiology data.

   Certain bacteria are more easily transmitted or require isolation because of virulence or antibiotic resistance.

4. Assess client's understanding of procedure and feeling that lower airway congestion needs suctioning.

   Identifies need for client teaching and validates other assessments, indicating need to perform skill.

NURSING DIAGNOSIS

Defining characteristics from the assessment data may reveal the following nursing diagnoses for clients requiring this skill:

- Ineffective airway clearance
- Risk for aspiration
- Ineffective breathing pattern
- Impaired gas exchange
- Risk for infection
- Deficient knowledge regarding airway clearance techniques and devices
- Impaired swallowing
- Impaired spontaneous ventilation

Related factors are individualized based on client's condition or needs.

PLANNING

1. **Expected outcomes** following completion of procedure:
   - Client demonstrates absent or diminished crackles, wheezes, and gurgles on inspiration and expiration; return of absent or diminished breath sounds; normalization of heart rate, blood pressure, respiratory rate and effort; absence of drooling, gastric secretions or vomitus in mouth, and nasal secretions.

     Lower and upper airways are cleared of secretions, reducing risk of pulmonary infection. Containment of secretions reduces risk of droplet transmission to nurse or other client.

   - Client verbalizes easier breathing, if able.

     Clear airway reduces work of breathing.

2. Explain to client how procedure will help clear airway and relieve breathing problems. Explain that temporary coughing, sneezing, gagging, or shortness of breath is normal during the procedure. Encourage client to cough out secretions. Practice coughing, if able. Splint surgical incisions, if necessary.

   Encourages cooperation and minimizes risks, anxiety, and discomfort of procedure.

Step	Rationale
3. Explain importance of and encourage coughing during procedure with splinting.	Coughing facilitates secretion removal and may reduce frequency of future suctioning. Splinting reduces client pain and results in more effective cough effort.
4. Assist client to assume position comfortable for nurse and client (usually semi-Fowler's or sitting upright with head hyperextended, unless contraindicated).	Promotes client and nurse comfort, reducing nurse's back muscle strain. Promotes maximal lung expansion and deep breathing. Also reduces risk of aspiration.
5. Place towel across client's chest, if needed.	Reduces transmission of microorganisms by protecting client's gown from secretions.

Implementation

Step	Rationale
1. Wash hands and apply clean gloves.	Reduces transmission of microorganisms.
2. Attach suction	
a. In many institutions the catheter is attached to the mechanical ventilator circuit by a respiratory therapist. If catheter is not already in place, open suction catheter package using aseptic technique, attach closed suction catheter to ventilator circuit by removing swivel adapter and placing closed suction catheter apparatus on ET or tracheostomy tube, and connect Y on mechanical ventilator circuit to closed suction catheter with flex tubing (see illustrations).	The catheter becomes part of the circuit and is often changed by respiratory therapist with each circuit change or every 24 hours. Using a closed system maintains an aseptic environment (Paul-Allen and Ostrow, 2000).
b. Connect one end of connecting tubing to suction machine and connect other to end of closed system or in-line suction catheter, if not already done. Turn suction device on and set vacuum regulator to appropriate negative pressure (see manufacture's directions). Many closed system suction catheters require slightly higher suction pressures; consult manufacturer's guidelines (Connelly and Stone, 1991).	Prepares suction apparatus. Excessive negative pressure damages tracheal mucosa and can induce greater hypoxia. Inadequate suction pressure reduces effectiveness of suctioning, necessitating more passes or longer suctioning time.
3. Hyperinflate and/or hyperoxygenate client with Ambu-bag or manual breathing mechanism on mechanical ventilator according to institution protocol and clinical status (usually 100% oxygen).	Hyperoxygenation before and after suctioning decreases occurrence of arterial oxygen desaturation (St. John, 1999). Decreases atelectasis caused by negative pressure and increases oxygen available to tissues during suctioning (Paul-Allen and Ostrow, 2000).
4. Unlock suction control mechanism if required by manufacturer. Open saline port and attach saline syringe or vial.	Prepares suction apparatus.

A

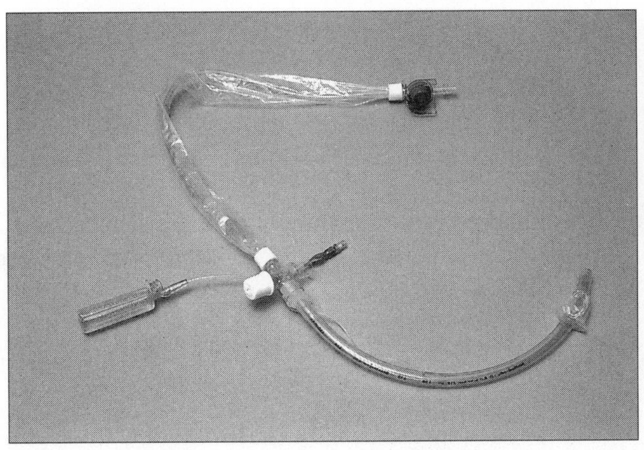

B

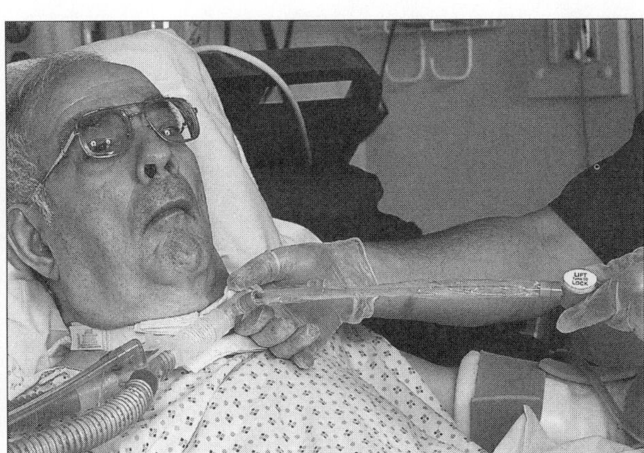

STEP **2a** **A**, Closed system suction catheter attached to endotracheal tube. **B**, Suctioning tracheostomy with closed-system suction catheter.

STEP	RATIONALE
5. Pick up suction catheter enclosed in plastic sleeve with dominant hand. If client requires normal saline, advance catheter 2 to 3 cm (1 to 1.5 in) and squeeze vial or push syringe with other hand to release 5 to 10 ml of normal saline during inspiratory cycle.	Saline travels down suction catheter and into airway. Timing delivery of the saline with inhalation allows saline to be delivered into the lung rather than blown into ventilator circuit.
6. Wait until client inhales normal saline or mechanical ventilator delivers a breath to disperse saline and then quickly but gently insert catheter on next inhalation. To insert catheter, use a repeating maneuver of pushing catheter and sliding (or pulling) plastic sleeve back between thumb and forefinger until resistance is felt or client coughs.	Catheter sterility and secretion containment are provided by plastic sheath. Mechanical ventilator breaths, oxygen, and positive end-expiratory pressure (PEEP) are not interrupted during suctioning. Catheter slides within the plastic sheath. Coughing occurs or resistance is felt when the catheter touches the carina.

- ***Critical Decision Point***
  Some catheters contain depth markings that are useful in positioning catheter.

STEP	RATIONALE
7. Encourage client to cough and apply suction by squeezing on suction control mechanism while withdrawing catheter. It is difficult to apply intermittent pulses of suction and nearly impossible to rotate the catheter compared with a standard catheter. Be sure to withdraw catheter completely into plastic sheath so it does not obstruct airflow.	Removes secretions from airway. Plastic sheath limits rotational movement of catheter. Catheter left in ET or tracheostomy tube limits airflow.
8. Reassess cardiopulmonary status, including pulse oximetry, to determine need for subsequent suctioning or complications. Repeat steps 5 through 8 one to two more times to clear secretions. Allow adequate time (at least 1 full minute) between suction passes for ventilation and reoxygenation.	Repeated passes clear airway of secretions to promote ventilation and oxygenation (Paul-Allen and Ostrow, 2000). Suctioning can cause complications such as dysrhythmias, hypoxia, and bronchospasm.
9. When airway is clear, withdraw catheter completely into sheath. Be sure that colored indicator line on catheter is visible in the sheath. Squeeze vial or push syringe while applying suction to rinse inner lumen of catheter. Use at least 5 to 10 ml of saline. Lock suction mechanism, if applicable, and turn off suction.	Black line is reference point to determine correct position of catheter when not in use. Inability to see black line suggests catheter is in airway and may be impeding airflow. Interior of catheter must be rinsed to prevent bacterial growth inside catheter. Failure to lock mechanism can result in inadvertent continuous suction and serious complications.
10. If client requires oral or nasal suctioning, perform Skill 13-1 or 13-2 with separate standard suction catheter.	Catheter is continuously connected to ET or tracheostomy tube and is considered sterile (Paul-Allen and Ostrow, 2000). Separate suction catheter is necessary for oral or nasal suctioning.
11. Reposition client.	Promotes comfort and drainage of secretions and prevents pressure areas.
12. Remove gloves and discard into appropriate receptacle and wash hands.	Reduces transmission of microorganisms.
13. Turn off suction device.	Clean equipment should not be touched with contaminated gloves or hands.

EVALUATION

STEP	RATIONALE
1. Compare client's respiratory assessments before and after suctioning.	Identifies objective measures to determine benefit of suctioning.
2. Observe airway secretions.	Documents presence or absence of respiratory tract infection.
3. Ask client if breathing is easier.	Provides subjective data about client's perception of effect of suctioning.

Unexpected Outcomes and Related Interventions

- Worsening respiratory status: see Unexpected Outcomes and Related Interventions for Skill 13-2
  - Evaluate size of suction catheter used to determine if it occluded lumen of tube by more than one half of tube diameter.
- Bloody secretions
  - Evaluate amount of suction pressure used. May need to be decreased.
  - Evaluate length of time between catheter insertion and removal of catheter.
  - Evaluate need for suctioning frequency.
- Paraoxysms of coughing
  - Consult physician about need for inhaled bronchodilators or topical anesthetic.
  - Allow client to rest between passes of suction catheter.
- No secretions were obtained (see Skill 13-2).
  - Consider using standard catheter once to determine if closed system catheter is ineffective.

Recording and Reporting

- Record in nurses' notes: respiratory assessments before and after suctioning; size of suction catheter used; amount of negative suction pressure used (unless standardized in institution or deviation from usual); duration of suctioning period, if unusual; route(s) used to suction; secretions obtained and odor, amount, color, consistency; frequency of suctioning; client's tolerance of procedure.
- Report changes in client's respiratory status.

Teaching Considerations

- Clients with permanent tracheostomies receiving mechanical ventilation at home will require family member to learn suction procedure and airway management.

Pediatric Considerations

- Closed system catheters are available only for older children and adult-size artificial airways.
- Weight of closed system catheters may displace ET tube more easily in child than adult because of short distance of trachea.
- Bronchospasm may develop more readily during suctioning in children with prematurity, underdeveloped airways, or reactive airways diseases (Wong and others, 1999).

Gerontological Considerations

- Older adults with ischemic cardiac or obstructive pulmonary disease may benefit from maintenance of oxygen supply during suctioning (Lueckenotte, 2000).

Skill 13-4 Performing Endotracheal Tube Care

After insertion of an endotracheal (ET) tube, the cuff is inflated. Preventing cuff-related problems is a critical component of nursing care and depends on securing the tube and inflating the cuff properly. In many institutions these functions are shared by nursing and respiratory therapy staff. An inadequately secured ET tube moves up and down the tracheobronchial tree. Allowing an ET tube to slip too far down into the lungs can prevent ventilation of a lung, usually the left lung (and sometimes the right upper lobe also) because of anatomical differences. Allowing an ET tube to slide too far up the tracheobronchial tree can allow air to escape through or damage the vocal cords and epiglottis or permit aspiration of upper airway secretions. Properly securing the ET tube prevents incidental extubation from coughing or pulling on the tube. In addition, movement of an ET tube can cause development of granulation tissue on the vocal cords, epiglottis, or trachea. Additional risks of movement of an artificial airway are **tracheal stenosis, tracheomalacia,** erosion of the innominate artery, and **tracheoesophageal fistula,** particularly when the cuff is overinflated. Risks for each of these complications can be reduced with proper nursing care.

After the tube is inserted and secured and the cuff is inflated (see Skill 13-6), the chief concern of the nurse is to maintain patency of the ET tube. In clients who cannot clear the airway of secretions, patency is achieved primarily through periodic suctioning of the artificial airway.

Delegation Considerations

This skill should not be delegated to assistive personnel.

Equipment

- Towel
- Endotracheal and oral pharyngeal suction equipment
- 1- or $1^1/_2$-inch wide adhesive or waterproof tape (do not use paper or silk tape) or commercial ET tube holder and mouthguard (follow manufacturer's instructions for securing)
- Nonsterile gloves (two pairs)
- Adhesive remover swab or acetone on cotton ball
- Mouthwash-soaked clean 4 × 4 inch gauze secured on tongue blade or sponge-tipped applicators
- Toothbrush, toothpaste (optional), and shaving supplies
- One wet and one soapy washcloth or paper towels
- Clean 2 × 2 inch gauze
- Tincture of benzoin, liquid adhesive, or skin prep pads
- Tongue blade (optional)
- Face shield, if indicated

Step	Rationale
Assessment	
1. Observe for signs and symptoms of need to perform ET tube care: soiled or loose tape; pressure sore on naris, lips, or corner of mouth; excess nasal or oral secretions; client moving tube with tongue, biting tube or tongue; tube repositioned by physician or other specially trained personnel; foul-smelling mouth.	Presence of ET tube impairs ability of client to swallow oral secretions. Client is also at increased risk for development of pressure areas from impaired circulation as tube is pulled or pressed against nasal or oral mucosa.
2. Observe for factors that increase risk of complications from ET tube: type and size of tube, movement of tube up and down trachea (in and out), duration of tube placement, cuff overinflation or underinflation, presence of facial trauma, malnutrition, and neck or thoracic radiation.	Nasal tube cannot be rotated from side to side like oral tube. Pressure sores are more likely. Tube moving up and down trachea predisposes client to develop tracheoesophageal fistula or tracheomalacia, tube can become dislodged from the lower airway (incidental extubation), or it can enter mainstem **bronchus.** Cuff underinflation may allow aspiration, whereas cuff overinflation may cause ischemia or necrosis of tracheal tissue from obstruction of capillary bed. Client can "tongue" oral tube easily and dislodge it. Longer duration of intubation is associated with increased risk of lower airway complications, as is facial trauma. Tissue is more prone to breakdown in presence of malnutrition and radiation.
3. Assess client's knowledge of procedure.	Encourages cooperation, minimizes risks and anxiety. Identifies teaching needs.

Nursing Diagnosis

Defining characteristics from the assessment data may reveal the following nursing diagnoses for clients requiring this skill:

- Ineffective airway clearance
- Risk for aspiration
- Ineffective breathing pattern
- Deficient knowledge regarding airway clearance techniques and devices
- Impaired skin integrity
- Impaired gas exchange
- Risk for infection
- Impaired swallowing
- Impaired spontaneous ventilation

Related factors are individualized based on client's condition or needs.

Planning

Step	Rationale
1. **Expected outcomes** following completion of procedure:	
▪ ET tube is maintained in correct position in client's trachea.	Complications of lower airway and vocal cords trauma prevented.

Step	Rationale
▪ Client's skin around mouth and oral mucous membranes does not have pressure areas or other injury from biting: tube is repositioned on opposite side of mouth or center of mouth at least every 24 to 48 hours according to institution protocol (oral ET tube only); oral airway, if used, is cleaned and reinserted to prevent biting of tongue or inner cheeks.	Endotracheal tube does not place undue pressure against corners of mouth causing pressure area. Client is not able to bite inner cheeks or tongue.
▪ Endotracheal tube is resecured at proper depth as evidenced by the following: clean tape is firmly secured to cheeks, upper lip or top of nose, and tube only; depth of tube is same as when started or as ordered (same centimeter marking at gums or lips); bilateral breath sounds are equal.	Endotracheal tube care prevents movement of tube out of airway or into mainstem bronchus.
2. Obtain another nurse's assistance in this procedure.	Reduces risk of incidental extubation of ET tube.
3. Explain procedure and client's participation, including importance of the following: not biting or moving ET tube with tongue; trying not to cough when tape is off ET tube; keeping hands down and not pulling on tubing; removal of tape from face can be uncomfortable.	Reduces anxiety, encourages cooperation, and reduces risks.
4. Assist client to assume position comfortable for both nurse and client (usually supine or semi-Fowler's).	Promotes client comfort; prevents nurse muscle strain.
5. Place towel across chest.	Reduces transmission of organisms and protects bed clothes and linens from contamination.

Implementation

Step	Rationale
1. Wash hands. Apply face shield if indicated.	Reduces transmission of microorganisms.
2. Administer endotracheal, nasopharyngeal, and oropharyngeal suction.	Removes secretions. Diminishes client's need to cough during procedure.
3. Connect oral suction catheter to suction source (see Skill 13-1).	Prepares client for oropharyngeal suctioning.
4. Prepare tape. Cut a piece of tape long enough to go completely around client's head from naris to naris plus 6 inches: adult 24 to 48 cm (1 to 2 feet). Lay tape adhesive side up on bedside table. Cut and lay 8 to 16 cm (3 to 6 inches) of tape, adhesive sides together, in center of long strip to prevent tape from sticking to hair. Smaller strip of tape should cover area between ears around back of head.	Preparing tape ahead allows nurse to have one hand positioned on ET tube throughout procedure. Adhesive tape must encircle head below ears with sufficient tape left to wrap around tube.
5. Apply gloves. Instruct helper to apply pair of gloves and hold ET tube firmly at client's lips or naris. Note the number marking on the ET tube at the gum line.	Reduces transmission of microorganisms. Maintains proper tube position and prevents incidental extubation.

• ***Critical Decision Point***

Do not allow helper to hold the tube away from the lips or naris. Doing so allows too much "play" in the tube and increases the risk of tube movement and incidental extubation. Never let go of the ET tube, even for a moment. Client could move or cough, and the tube could become dislodged.

Step	Rationale
6. Carefully remove tape from ET tube and client's face. If tape is difficult to remove, moisten with (soapy) wet washcloth, water, or adhesive tape remover. Discard type in appropriate receptacle if nearby.	Provides nurse with access to skin under tape for assessment and hygiene. Reduces transmission of microorganisms.
7. Use adhesive remover swab to remove excess adhesive left on face after tape removal. Wash adhesive remover from face.	Promotes hygiene. Unremoved adhesive can cause damage to skin and prevent poor adhesion of new tape.

STEP	RATIONALE
8. Remove oral airway or bite block, if present, and place on towel.	Provides access to and complete observation of client's oral cavity.

- ***Critical Decision Point***
  Do not remove oral airway if client is actively biting ET tube. Wait until tape is partially or completely secured to ET tube.

STEP	RATIONALE
9. Clean mouth, gums, and teeth opposite ET tube with non–alcohol-based mouthwash solution and 4 × 4 inch gauze, sponge-tipped applicators, or saline swabs. Brush teeth as indicated. If necessary, administer oropharyngeal suctioning with Yankauer suction catheter.	Promotes hygiene and reduces risk of infection to teeth and gums. Alcohol-based mouthwashes dry oral mucosa (Lewis and others, 2000).
10. *Oral ET tube only:* Remembering "cm" ET tube marking at lips or gums, with help of assistant move ET tube to opposite side or center of mouth. Do not change tube depth.	Prevents formation of pressure sores at sides of client's mouth. Ensures correct position of tube.
11. Repeat oral cleaning as in Step 9 on opposite side of mouth.	Removes secretions from mouth and oral pharynx.
12. Clean face and neck with soapy washcloth, rinse, and dry. Shave male client as necessary (see Chapter 6).	Moisture and beard growth prevent adhesive tape adherence.
13. Pour small amount of skin protectant or liquid adhesive on clean 2 × 2 inch gauze and dot on upper lip (oral ET tube) or across nose (nasal ET tube) and cheeks to ear. Allow to dry completely.	Protects skin from tape burns and makes more adherent.
14. Slip tape under client's head and neck, adhesive side up. Take care not to twist tape or catch hair. Do not allow tape to stick to itself. It helps to gently stick tape to tongue blade, which serves as a guide. Then slide tongue blade under client's neck. Center tape so that double-faced tape extends around back of neck from ear to ear.	Positions tape to secure ET tube in proper position.
15. On one side of face, secure tape from ear to naris (nasal ET tube) or over lip to ET tube (oral ET tube). Tear remaining tape in half lengthwise, forming two pieces that are $^1/_2$ to $^3/_4$ inches wide. Secure bottom half of tape across upper lip (oral ET tube) or across top of nose (nasal ET tube) to opposite ear (see illustration *A*). Wrap top half of tape around tube and up from bottom (see illustration *B*). Tape should encircle tube at least two times for security.	Secures tape to face. Using top tape to wrap prevents downward drag on ET tube.

A
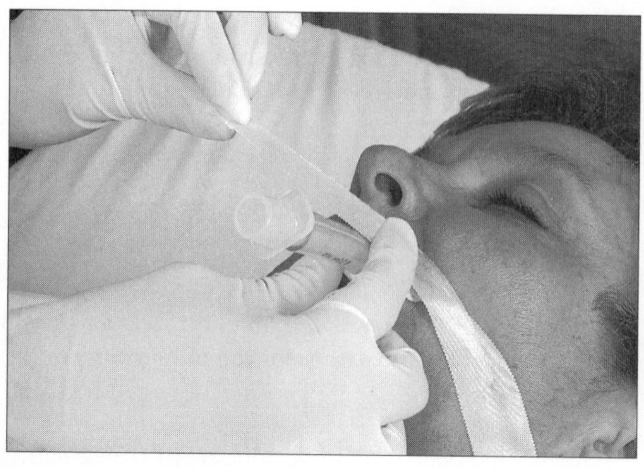

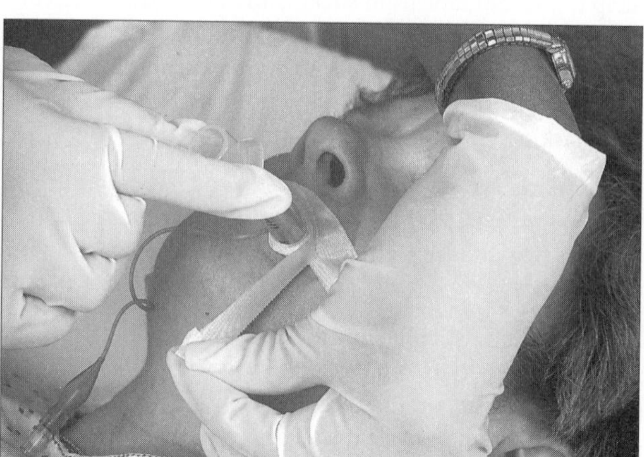
B

STEP **15** **A,** Securing bottom half of tape across client's upper lip. **B,** Securing top half of tape around tube.

STEP	RATIONALE
16. Gently pull other side of tape firmly to pick up slack and secure to opposite side of face and ET tube the same as the first piece. NOTE: ET tube is secured. Assistant can release hold (nurse may want assistant to help reinsert oral airway.)	Secures tape to face and tube. Endotracheal tube should be at same depth at the lips (see illustration). Check earlier assessment for verification of tube depth in centimeters.

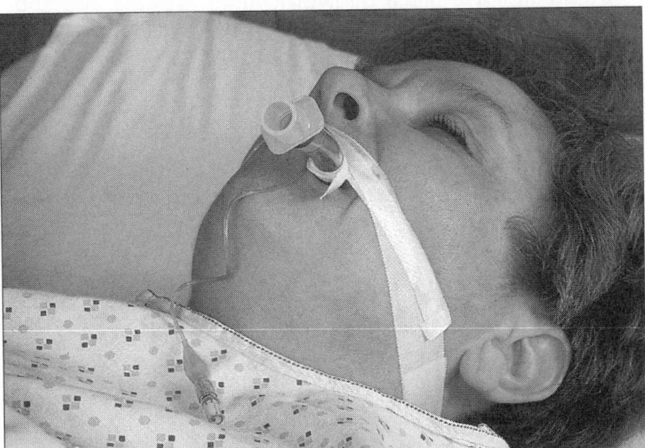

STEP **16** Tape securing endotracheal tube.

STEP	RATIONALE
17. If not already done, remove and clean oral airway in warm soapy water and rinse well. Hydrogen peroxide can aid in removal of crusted secretions. A mouthwash rinse will freshen client's mouth. Shake excess water from oral airway.	Promotes hygiene. Reduces transmission of microorganisms.
18. Reinsert oral airway without pushing tongue into oropharynx and secure with tape (Chapter 11).	Prevents client from biting ET tube and allows access for oral pharyngeal suctioning.
19. Discard soiled items in appropriate receptacle. Remove towel and place in laundry.	Reduces transmission of microorganisms.
20. Reposition client.	Promotes comfort.
21. Remove gloves and face shield, discard in receptacle, and wash hands. Assistant is also to remove gloves and wash hands before leaving client's room. Place clean items (e.g., tincture of benzoin, mouthwash, excess swabs) in place of storage.	Reduces transmission of microorganisms. Contaminated gloves and hands should not touch clean items.

EVALUATION

1. Compare respiratory assessments before and after ET tube care.	Identifies any changes in presence and quality of breath sounds after procedure.
2. Observe depth and position of ET tube according to physician recommendation.	Position of ET tube should not be altered.
3. Assess security of tape by gently tugging at tube.	Tape should remain attached to face. Client may cough.
4. Assess skin around mouth and oral mucous membranes for intactness and pressure areas.	Tape should not tear skin. Pressure areas should be absent.

UNEXPECTED OUTCOMES AND RELATED INTERVENTIONS

- Unexpected extubation
  - Remain with client.
  - Call for assistance.
  - Assess client for airway patency, spontaneous breathing, and vital signs.
  - Prepare for reintubation.
- Endotracheal tube is moving in and out.
  - Repeat taping procedure. If client is very active or if there are other reasons (e.g., excessive oral secretions or facial injury that impairs ability to apply tape effectively) and self-extubation is a concern, consider using a commercial mouth guard for holding ET tube. These devices generally secure with straps.

- In very active clients without facial injury who are at risk for self-extubation, consider applying a second piece of tape around the back of the head but going *over* the ears. This method of taping makes an X across the face and is more secure than a single piece of tape; however, the client may be at increased risk for skin injury with double the amount of tape.
- Unequal breath sounds
  - Evaluate ET tube for proper depth before and after ET tube care. If ET tube is deeper or shallower, reposition tube only if allowed by institution and nurse has received appropriate instructions
  - Notify physician, who may order chest x-ray film to verify placement, and then reposition ET tube.
  - Evaluate client for possible mucous plug.
- Pressure areas from tube
  - Increase frequency of ET tube care.
  - Apply antimicrobial ointment per institutional protocol. *Nasal ET tube only:* If tube is very painful for client, soak clean 2 × 2 inch gauze in anesthetic solution (e.g., xylocaine solution or xylocaine jelly). Open soaked 2 × 2 inch gauze and fold lengthwise one or two times (resulting in piece that is $^1/_2$ by 4 inches [1 cm by 10 cm]) and wrap around tube to center ET tube in naris and away from pressure area. Obtain physician's order if necessary.
  - Align oxygen and humidity supply tubings so that they do not pull ET tube, creating pressure areas.
  - Monitor for infection. If skin tear is present on cheeks or over nose or upper lip, apply protective barrier such as Stomadhesive patch or hydrocolloid dressing and apply tape to this. Change dressing according to institution protocol or manufacturer's recommendations.
- Air escaping around tube (see Skill 13-6)
  - Verify correct position of tube. If tube position is correct, assess proper cuff inflation. If tube position is incorrect, reposition according to protocol or notify physician (see Skill 13-6).

Recording and Reporting

- Note on Kardex with pencil: appropriate depth of ET tube, frequency of ET tube care, pressure sore care needed, and designated intervals. In some institutions this information is also placed on an index card and kept at the bedside for immediate referral.
- Record in nurses' notes: assessments before and after care, supplies used, client's tolerance of procedure, and frequency and extent of ET tube care.

Pediatric Considerations

- Neonatal and pediatric procedures for securing ET tubes and suctioning airways may vary (McLean and others, 1992; Warnock and Porpora, 1994).
- Infant skin may be more prone to tearing when tape is removed (Wong and others, 1999).

Gerontological Considerations

- Older adult skin may be more prone to tearing when tape is removed.
- Older adults with tendency toward inadequate nutrition may be more prone to complications (e.g., infection, breakdown of oral mucosa).

Skill 13-5 Performing Tracheostomy Care

A tracheostomy tube can cause development of granulation tissue on the vocal cords, epiglottis, or trachea. Additional risks of movement of an artificial airway are tracheal stenosis, tracheomalacia, erosion of the innominate artery, and tracheoesophageal fistula, particularly when the cuff is overinflated. Risks for each of these complications can be reduced with proper nursing care. (See additional material related to cuff inflation in Skill 13-6.)

Some clients with a tracheostomy tube are able to cough secretions out of the tracheostomy tube completely, whereas others are able only to cough secretions up into the tracheostomy tube. The latter clients may not require suctioning when an inner cannula is present because it can be safely removed, cleaned, and reinserted.

A comprehensive plan and execution of care include properly securing the tube, inflating the cuff, maintaining patency by suctioning and encouraging communication and oral hygiene. The intubated client is unable to speak because placement of the endotracheal (ET) and tracheostomy tube prevents normal airflow over and vibration of the vocal cords. When caring for an intubated client, the nurse is encouraged to use verbal and nonverbal communication skills to converse. Alphabet charts, pen and paper, slates or chalk boards, or magnetic pen doodle boards are some commonly used communication tools. There are many more simple to sophisticated communication devices that can be used. A speech therapist can assist the nurse in establishing effective communication.

Delegation Considerations

The skill of performing tracheostomy care can be delegated to assistive personnel and to the client under most situations. Clients with permanent tracheostomy tubes must learn this skill. In critically ill clients receiving mechanical ventilation, this skill usually should not be delegated to the client or family. The client and care provider must be educated and assisted until competent in proper technique to clean around the tracheostomy tube and to change the tracheostomy tube ties. The client and care provider must be taught emergency procedures in event tracheostomy tube inadvertently becomes dislodged when ties are changed.

Equipment

- Bedside table
- Towel
- Tracheostomy suction supplies
- Sterile tracheostomy care kit, if available (be sure to collect supplies listed that are not available in kit)
- Three sterile 4 × 4 inch gauze pads
- Hydrogen peroxide
- Normal saline solution
- Sterile cotton-tipped swabs
- Sterile tracheostomy dressing (precut and sewn surgical dressing)
- Sterile basin
- Small sterile brush
- Roll of twill tape, tracheostomy ties, or Velcro tracheostomy ties
- Scissors
- Sterile gloves (two)
- Face shield

Step	Rationale
Assessment	
1. Observe for signs and symptoms of need to perform tracheostomy care: excess peristomal secretions, excess intratracheal secretions, soiled or damp tracheostomy ties, soiled or damp tracheostomy dressing, diminished airflow through tracheostomy tube, or signs and symptoms of airway obstruction requiring suctioning (see Skill 13-2).	Signs and symptoms are related to presence of secretions at stoma site or within tracheostomy tube. The accompanying illustrations show a partially inflated cuff on an outer cannula, syringe used for cuff inflation, and an **obturator** that is used to insert outer cannula (see illustrations *A* and *B*).
2. Observe for factors (e.g., hydration, humidity, infection, nutrition, ability to cough) that normally influence tracheostomy airway functioning.	Allows nurse to accurately assess need to perform tracheostomy care.
3. Assess client's understanding of and ability to perform own tracheostomy care.	Allows nurse to identify potential need for instruction.
4. Check when tracheostomy care was last performed.	Tracheostomy care is provided at least every 8 to 12 hours and more often if indicated (e.g., increased airway secretions, infection [airway or stoma], increased secretions around stoma).

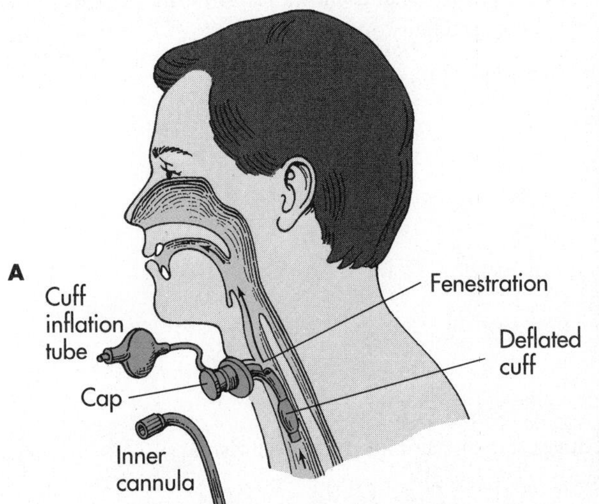

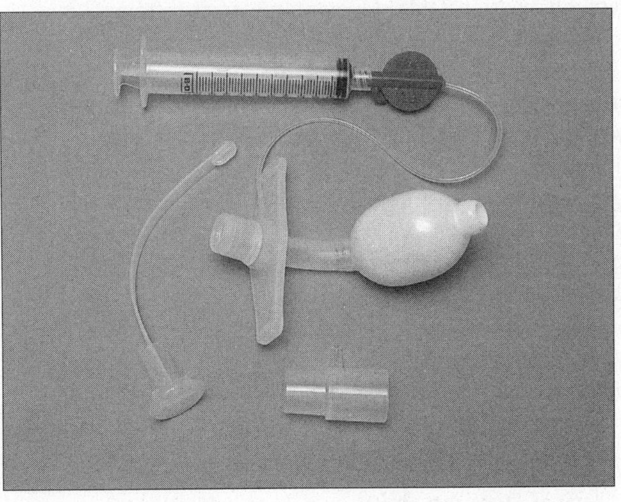

STEP 1 **A,** Tracheostomy tube (fenestrated) inserted with inner cannula removed, cuff deflated, and cap in place to allow speech (Lewis SL and others: *Medical surgical nursing: assessment and management of clinical problems,* ed 5, St. Louis, 2000, Mosby). **B,** Tracheostomy tube with obturator for insertion and syringe for inflation of cuff.

STEP	RATIONALE

NURSING DIAGNOSIS

Defining characteristics from the assessment data may reveal the following nursing diagnoses for clients requiring this skill:

- Ineffective airway clearance
- Risk for aspiration
- Ineffective breathing pattern
- Impaired gas exchange
- Risk for infection
- Deficient knowledge regarding airway clearance techniques and devices
- Impaired swallowing
- Impaired spontaneous ventilation

Related factors are individualized based on client's condition or needs.

PLANNING

STEP	RATIONALE
1. **Expected outcomes** following completion of procedure:	
▪ Inner cannula and outer cannula of trach tube are free of secretions; ties are clean, secured snugly, and tied in double square knot.	Trach tube is patent and secure. Tracheostomy tube that is clear and free of secretions optimizes the amount of oxygen delivered to client and limits risk of infection from retained secretions.
▪ Stoma site is pink, does not bleed, and is free of secretions.	Indicates absence of infection at stoma site. Dry, intact tracheostomy stoma reduces risk of subsequent systemic infection.
2. Have another nurse or family member assist in this procedure.	Prevents accidental extubation of tracheostomy tube.
3. Explain procedure and client's participation.	Encourages cooperation, minimizes risks, and reduces anxiety.
4. Assist client to position comfortable for both nurse and client (usually supine or semi-Fowler's).	Promotes client comfort and prevents nurse muscle strain.
5. Place towel across client's chest.	Reduces transmission of microorganisms.

IMPLEMENTATION

STEP	RATIONALE
1. Wash hands and apply gloves and face shield if applicable.	Reduces transmission of microorganisms.
2. Suction tracheostomy (see Skill 13-2 or 13-3). Before removing gloves, remove soiled tracheostomy dressing and discard in glove with coiled catheter.	Removes secretions to avoid occluding outer cannula while inner cannula is removed. Reduces need for client to cough.
3. While client is replenishing oxygen stores, prepare equipment on bedside table. Open sterile tracheostomy kit. Open three 4 × 4 inch gauze packages using aseptic technique and pour normal saline on one package and hydrogen peroxide on another. Leave third package dry. Open two cotton-tipped swab packages, and pour normal saline on one package and hydrogen peroxide on the other. Open sterile tracheostomy dressing package. Unwrap sterile basin and pour about 0.5 to 2 cm (½ inch) hydrogen peroxide into it. Open small sterile brush package and place aseptically into sterile basin. If using large roll of twill tape, cut appropriate length of tape (see Step 14) and lay aside in dry area. Do not recap hydrogen peroxide and normal saline.	Prepares equipment and allows for smooth, organized completion of tracheostomy care.
4. Apply gloves. Keep dominant hand sterile throughout procedure.	Reduces transmission of microorganisms.

• ***Critical Decision Point***

For tracheostomy tube with no inner cannula or Kistner button, complete Steps 10 through 22.

STEP	RATIONALE

TRACHEOSTOMY WITH INNER CANNULA CARE

Step	Rationale
5. Remove oxygen source and then inner cannula with nondominant hand. Drop inner cannula into hydrogen peroxide basin.	Removes inner cannula for cleaning. Hydrogen peroxide loosens secretions from inner cannula.
6. Place tracheostomy collar, T tube or ventilator oxygen source over outer cannula.	Maintains supply of oxygen to client.

- ***Critical Decision Point***
  T tube and ventilator oxygen devices cannot be attached to all outer cannulas when the inner cannula is removed.

Step	Rationale
7. To prevent oxygen desaturation in affected clients, quickly pick up inner cannula and use small brush to remove secretions inside and outside inner cannula.	Tracheostomy brush provides mechanical force to remove thick or dried secretions.
8. Hold inner cannula over basin and rinse with normal saline, using nondominant hand to pour normal saline.	Removes secretions and hydrogen peroxide from inner cannula.
9. Replace inner cannula and secure "locking" mechanism, if applicable. Reapply trach collar, T tube (Briggs), or ventilator oxygen source.	Secures inner cannula and reestablishes oxygen supply.

TRACHEOSTOMY STOMA AND FACE PLATE (includes tubes with no inner cannulas)

Step	Rationale
10. With hydrogen peroxide–saturated cotton-tipped swabs and 4 × 4 inch gauze, clean exposed outer cannula surfaces and stoma under faceplate extending 5 to 10 cm (2 to 4 inches) in all directions from stoma. Clean in circular motion from stoma site outward using dominant hand to handle sterile supplies.	Aseptically removes secretions from stoma site. Moving in outward circle pulls mucus and other contaminants from stoma to periphery.
11. With normal saline–saturated cotton-tipped swabs and 4 × 4 inch gauze, rinse hydrogen peroxide from tracheostomy tube and skin surfaces.	Rinses hydrogen peroxide from surfaces. If not removed from skin, hydrogen peroxide can promote tissue injury.
12. With dry 4 × 4 inch gauze, pat lightly at skin and exposed outer cannula surfaces.	Dry surfaces prohibit formation of moist environment for microorganism growth and skin excoriation.

TRACH TIES AND DRESSING CHANGE

Step	Rationale
13. Instruct assistant, if available, to apply gloves and securely hold tracheostomy tube in place. With assistant holding tracheostomy tube, cut ties. (Follow manufacturer's guidelines for Velcro ties. Be sure to cut off excess ties, if applicable.)	Promotes hygiene and reduces transmission of microorganisms. Secures trach tube. Reduces risk of incidental extubation.

- ***Critical Decision Point***
  Assistant must not release hold on tracheostomy tube until new ties are firmly tied. If working without an assistant, do not cut old ties until new ties are in place and securely tied.

Step	Rationale
14. Cut a length of twill tape long enough to go around client's neck two times (along 24 to 30 inches for an adult); cut ends on diagonal.	Cutting ends of tie on diagonal aids in inserting tie through eyelet.
15. Insert one end of tie through faceplate eyelet and pull ends even.	
16. Slide both ends of tie behind the head and around neck to other eyelet and insert one tie through second eyelet.	
17. Pull snugly.	Ensures tracheostomy will not come out.

Step	Rationale

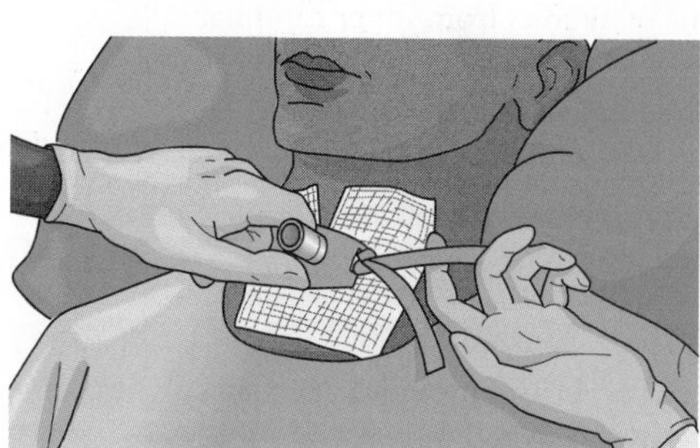

STEP **18** Tracheostomy ties properly placed.

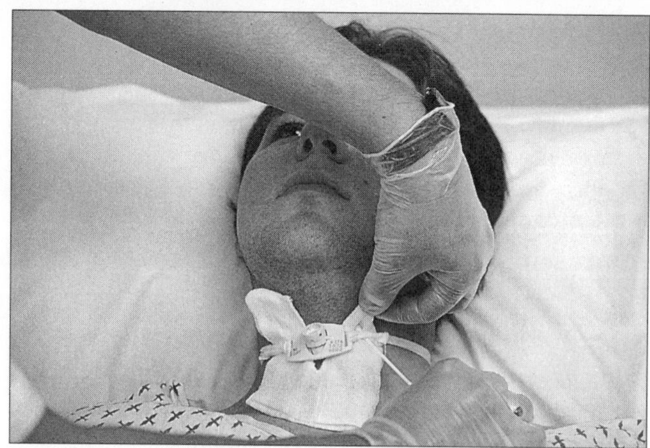

STEP **19** Applying tracheostomy dressing.

Step	Rationale
18. Tie ends securely in double square knot, allowing space for only one loose or two snug finger(s) in tie (see illustration).	One finger-length of slack prevents ties from being too tight when tracheostomy dressing is in place and also prevents movement of trach tube in lower airway.
19. Insert fresh tracheostomy dressing under clean ties and faceplate (see illustration).	Absorbs drainage. Dressing prevents pressure on clavicle heads.
20. Position client comfortably and assess respiratory status.	Promotes comfort. Some clients may require post–tracheostomy care suctioning.
21. Remove gloves and face shield and discard in appropriate receptacle.	Reduces transmission of microorganisms. Contaminated gloves should not touch clean supplies.
22. Replace cap on hydrogen peroxide and normal saline bottles. Store reusable liquids and unused supplies in appropriate place.	Once opened, normal saline can be considered free of bacteria for 24 hours, after which it should be discarded.
23. Wash hands.	Reduces transmission of microorganisms among clients.

Evaluation

Step	Rationale
1. Compare assessments before and after tracheostomy care.	Determines effectiveness of tracheostomy care.
2. Assess comfort of new tracheostomy ties.	Tracheostomy ties are uncomfortable and place client at risk for injury when they are too loose or too tight.
3. Inspect inner and outer cannulas for secretions.	Presence of secretions on cannulas indicates the need for more vigorous tracheostomy care.
4. Assess stoma for signs of infection or skin breakdown.	Broken skin places client at risk for infection. Stomal infection necessitates change in tracheostomy skin care plan.

Unexpected Outcomes and Related Interventions

- Excessively loose or tight tracheostomy ties
  - Adjust ties or apply new ties.
- Stomatitis
  - Increase frequency of tracheostomy care.
  - Consider intermittent application of heat to increase blood flow and promote healing.
  - Apply topical antibacterial solution, and allow it to dry and provide bacterial barrier.
  - Apply hydrocolloid or transparent dressing just under stoma to protect skin from breakdown. Consult with skin care specialist.
- Pressure area around tracheostomy tube
  - Increase frequency of tracheostomy care and keep dressing under faceplate at all times.
  - Consider using double dressing or applying hydrocolloid or Stomadhesive dressing around stoma.
- Accidental extubation
  - Call for assistance.
  - Replace old tracheostomy tube with new tube. Some experienced nurses or respiratory therapists may be able to quickly reinsert tracheostomy tube. Be sure to keep spare tracheostomy tube of same size and kind at bedside in event of emergency replacement. Same-size ET tube can be inserted in stoma in an emergency.

- Be prepared to manually ventilate clients in whom respiratory distress develops.
- Notify physician.
- Respiratory distress from mucous plug of cannula
  - Remove inner cannula, if applicable, for cleaning, or cannula can be suctioned.
  - Notify physician or specially trained personnel if tracheostomy tube requires replacement.

Recording and Reporting

- Chart in Kardex: type and size of tracheostomy tube, frequency of tracheostomy care, special care in event of stomatitis.
- Record in nurses' notes: assessments, supplies used, frequency and extent of tracheostomy care, client's tolerance of procedure.
- Report any change in client's respiratory status

Teaching Considerations

- Different types of tracheostomy tubes have different faceplates. Some are rigid, others are not. Instruct caregivers not to lift up on rigid faceplates or they may dislodge tube.
- Some commercial tracheostomy tube holders require removal of excess tie material to fit properly.
- If long-term placement of tracheostomy is anticipated, nurse should plan to teach client and family tracheostomy care.
- Clients with new tracheostomy frequently have blood secretions for 2 to 3 days after procedure or for 24 hours after each tracheostomy change.

Pediatric Considerations

- Children generally have shorter necks, so stoma may be more difficult to clean.
- Pediatric tracheostomy tubes (smaller than size 4) do not contain an inner cannula.
- Routine tracheostomy tube changes are carried out weekly after a tract has formed (Wong and others, 1999).

Gerontological Considerations

- Older adults may have more fragile skin and may be more prone to skin breakdown from secretions or pressure (Lueckenotte, 2000).
- Older adults with impaired nutrition may not heal well.

Skill 13-6 Inflating the Cuff on an Endotracheal or Tracheostomy Tube

The goals of correctly inflating the cuff on an artificial airway are to promote lung inflation for mechanical ventilation, to prevent aspiration of gastric contents, and at the same time to allow drainage of secretions that accumulate between the epiglottis and the cuff (Box 13-1). The amount of air inserted in the cuff is based on several factors; the two most important factors are the size of the client's trachea and the external diameter of the artificial airway. If two clients of approximately the same size are intubated—one with a size 6 and one with a size 8—the client with the larger tube (size 8) will require less air in the cuff. This is because the larger tube occludes more of the airway than the smaller tube does.

There is no recommendation on a preferred method for cuff inflation. The minimal leak technique and the minimal occlusive technique are both acceptable methods (St. John, 1999) (Table 13-3).

Box 13-1 Indications for Cuff Inflation

Mechanical Ventilation

- Continuous airway pressure
- Positive end-expiratory pressure (PEEP)
- Inability to meet ventilatory requirements with cuff down
- Inability to meet oxygen requirements with cuff down

Risk of Aspirating Gastric Contents

- Feeding tube, especially large bore, in stomach
- Gastroesophageal reflux disease
- Hiatal hernia
- During and after meals
- Impaired gastric emptying
- Decreased gag reflex
- Impaired swallowing

Delegation Considerations

The skill of inflating the cuff on an endotracheal or tracheostomy tube should not be delegated to assistive personnel.

Equipment

- Endotracheal/tracheostomy suction apparatus (Skill 13-2 or 13-3)
- Stethoscope
- 5- or 10-ml syringe
- Alcohol wipe
- Face shield, if indicated
- Gloves, if indicated

Table 13-3 Endotracheal and Tracheostomy Cuff Inflation Methods

INFLATION METHOD	PROCEDURE
Minimal occlusive volume	1. Inject air into the cuff until no airflow is auscultated over the trachea during the peak inflation pressure of a positive pressure breath 2. Record the cuff volume and pressure
Minimal leak technique	1. Inject air into the cuff until the air leak around the cuff is eliminated 2. Remove a small amount of air from the cuff until a slight leak occurs (50 to 100 ml tidal volume decrease) at peak inflation pressure during a positive pressure breath 3. Record the cuff volume and pressure

From St. John RE: Airway management, *Crit Care Nurse* 19(4):79, 1999.

STEP	RATIONALE

ASSESSMENT

1. Observe for signs and symptoms of need to perform care, including gurgling on expiration, decreased exhaled tidal volume (mechanically ventilated client), spasmodic coughing, tense test balloon on tube, flaccid test balloon on tube, and unexpected phonation.	Partially deflated cuff allows secretions to enter trachea and permits vocalization. High cuff pressure can result in necrosis, tracheomalacia, or tracheoesophageal fistula. Overinflated cuff may cause client to cough.
2. If client is discharged with a cuffed tracheostomy tube, determine caregiver's understanding of procedure.	Identifies teaching needs.

NURSING DIAGNOSIS

Defining characteristics from the assessment data may reveal the following nursing diagnoses for clients requiring this skill:

- Ineffective airway clearance
- Risk for aspiration
- Ineffective breathing pattern
- Impaired gas exchange
- Risk for infection
- Deficient knowledge regarding airway clearance techniques and devices
- Impaired swallowing
- Impaired spontaneous ventilation

Related factors are individualized based on client's condition or needs.

PLANNING

1. **Expected outcomes** following completion of procedure:	
▪ Mechanically ventilated clients receive prescribed tidal volume.	Proper inflation of cuff ensures client receives tidal volume.
▪ Minimal leak is auscultated at end inspiration.	Allows drainage of secretions during inhalation when airway is at widest but prevents gross aspiration during exhalation when airway is narrower. Prevents continuous contact of tracheal mucosa with cuff.
▪ No evidence of excessive phonation, aspiration of gastric or mouth contents, tracheoesophageal fistula, or tracheomalacia is found.	Proper level of cuff inflation is consistently maintained. Aspiration and phonation can occur when cuff is underinflated. Tracheoesophageal fistula and tracheomalacia can occur when the cuff is overinflated.
2. Explain procedure and client's participation. Explain that some coughing during procedure is normal.	Encourages cooperation, minimizes risks, and reduces anxiety.
3. Assist client to position comfortable for nurse and client (usually semi-Fowler's).	Promotes client comfort, prevents nurse muscle strain, and facilitates drainage.

STEP	RATIONALE

IMPLEMENTATION

Step	Rationale
1. Wash hands, and apply gloves and face shield, if indicated.	Reduces transmission of microorganisms.
2. Suction secretions through endotracheal (ET) or tracheostomy tube and also mouth.	Ensures patent airway and facilitates hearing airflow with stethoscope. Prevents aspiration of oral secretions when cuff is deflated.
3. Connect syringe to pilot balloon.	Allows immediate access to equipment for adjusting cuff pressure.
4. Place stethoscope in sternal notch or above tracheostomy tube and listen for minimal amount of air leak at end of inspiration (see illustration).	Assesses proper cuff inflation.

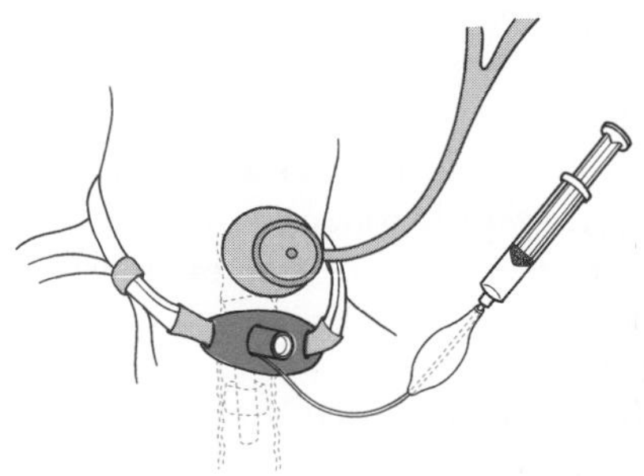

STEP **4** Inflating cuff on tracheostomy.

Step	Rationale
5. If no air leak is heard, remove all air from cuff.	Releases excessive cuff pressure, which reduces capillary blood flow and increases risk of tissue necrosis.
6. Inflate cuff according to agency policy (see Table 13-3).	Inflates cuff to minimal leak. If air leak is audible with ear, air leak is too large. If no air leak is heard, cuff is overinflated.
7. If excessive air leak is heard, slowly add air as in Step 6.	Air leak may prevent adequate lung expansion and increase risk of aspiration.
8. Remove stethoscope and wipe diaphragm with alcohol wipe.	Reduces transmission of microorganisms.
9. Remove syringe and discard into appropriate receptacle or store per policy. Do not leave attached to pilot balloon valve.	Reduces transmission of microorganisms.

- ***Critical Decision Point***
  Leaving syringe in pilot balloon can cause valve to break or "stick open." When syringe is removed, air is lost from cuff.

Step	Rationale
10. Reposition client.	Promotes comfort.
11. Remove gloves and face shield. Discard into appropriate receptacle. Wash hands.	Reduces transmission of microorganisms.

EVALUATION

Step	Rationale
1. Compare respiratory assessments before and after cuff care.	Determines effectiveness of cuff care procedure.
2. Observe exhaled tidal volume from mechanical ventilator.	Exhaled tidal volume should be not less than 50 ml of delivered tidal volume.
3. Auscultate for audible air leak.	Air leak should be heard only with stethoscope.
4. Observe for excessive phonation, presence of gastric secretions in airway secretions, or tracheoesophageal fistula.	Occurs with inadequate or excessive cuff inflation.

Unexpected Outcomes and Related Interventions

- Excessive cuff pressure
  - Remove air from cuff.
  - Reinflate with appropriate minimal leak technique.
- Excessive volume required to inflate cuff
  - Notify physician.
  - Consider client may need insertion of larger tube.
- Intratracheal bleeding
  - Notify physician.
  - Hyperinflate cuff with several additional milliliters of air to tamponade bleeding.
- Broken or open pilot balloon valve
  - Insert two- or three-way stopcock into valve, and turn off valve after cuff is properly inflated.
  - Clamp tubing between pilot balloon valve and ET tube or trach tube as close to balloon as possible.
  - Prepare for reinsertion of tube by trained personnel or physician.
- Excessive air leak
  - Reposition client or tubing.
  - Reinflate cuff if needed.
  - Prepare for insertion of new tube by physician or trained personnel if cuff ruptures.
  - Prepare to manually ventilate client if needed.
- Cuff requires increased amounts of air to maintain minimal leak.
  - Reassess position of tube.
  - Cuff of ET tube may be higher in trachea (where airway is wider) than previously.
  - Withdraw all air from cuff so pilot balloon is completely deflated (flat).
  - Remove syringe from pilot balloon. Watch to see if air reenters pilot balloon (cuff). If so, there is leak in cuff and tube requires replacement.
  - Fill cuff appropriately.
  - Apply gauze-padded clamps to pilot balloon tubing. (Do not use clamps with teeth, which will damage tubing.) If leak does not recur, pilot balloon valve may be broken. Institutional policy varies on how to correct this problem. Most tubes require replacement. Some institutions insert a blunt needle and stopcock in place of the broken valve. If leak recurs, cuff has a leak.
  - Tube must be replaced if client's cardiopulmonary status is compromised.

Recording and Reporting

- Record in nurses' notes: presence of minimal leak at end inspiration, volume of air injected into cuff, secretions obtained when suctioning, and frequency of cuff care. Documents safe cuff pressure levels.

Pediatric Considerations

- Pediatric tracheostomy tubes do not have cuffs.
- Neonatal and many pediatric ET tubes do not contain cuffs.

Critical Thinking Exercises

1. The Kardex indicates that correct placement for the ET tube is 24 cm at the lips. During assessment you observe that the loose tape is at 26.2 cm. What actions should you take?
2. The tracheostomy site is draining green purulent material, but you suction white material from the lungs. What actions are needed for this problem?
3. You are suctioning your client who has an endotracheal tube. You notice that the secretions are now thicker. What are your nursing actions with regard to client assessment and airway maintenance?

References

American Academy of Pediatrics Taskforce on Infant Positioning and SIDS: Positioning and sudden infant death syndrome (SIDS): update, *Pediatrics* 98(6):1216, 1996.

Chandre NC, Hazinski MF, editors: *Textbook of basic life support for health care providers,* Dallas, 1997, American Heart Association.

Connelly M, Stone K: Descriptive determination of negative airway pressure with closed system suctioning, *Heart Lung* 20(3):298, 1991.

DePew CL and others: Open vs closed-system endotracheal suctioning: a cost comparison, *Crit Care Nurse* 14(1):94, 1994.

Hagler DA, Traver GA: Endotracheal saline and suction catheters: sources of lower airway contamination, *Am J Crit Care* 3(6):444, 1994.

Kerr ME and others: Effect of endotracheal suctioning on cerebral oxygen in traumatic brain-injured patients, *Crit Care Med* 27(12):2776, 1999.

Lewis SL and others: *Medical-surgical nursing: assessment and management of clinical problems,* ed 5, St. Louis, 2000, Mosby.

Lueckenotte AG: *Gerontologic nursing,* ed 2, St. Louis, 2000, Mosby.

McLean S and others: Three methods of securing endotracheal tubes in neonates: a comparison, *Neonatal Network* 11(3):17, 1992.

Noll ML, Hix CD, Scott G: Closed tracheal suction systems: effectiveness and nursing implications, *AACN Clin Issues Crit Care Nurs* 1(2):318, 1990.

Paul-Allen J, Ostrow CL. Survey of nursing practices with closed-system suctioning, *Am J Crit Care* 9(1):9, 2000.

Raymond SJ: Normal saline instillation before suctioning: helpful or harmful? A review of the literature, *Am J Crit Care* 4(4):267, 1995.

Rudy EB and others: Endotracheal suctioning in adults with head injury, *Heart Lung* 20(6):667, 1991.

St. John RE: Airway management, *Crit Care Nurse* 19(4):79, 1999.

Vanderberg JT, Lutz RM, Vinson DR: Large-diameter suction system reduces oropharyngeal evacuation time, *J Emerg Med* 17(6):941, 1999.

Warnock C, Porpora K: A pediatric trach card: transforming research into practice . . . iatrogenic complications of deep suctioning are avoided, *Pediatr Nurs* 20(2):186, 1994.

Wong DL and others: *Whaley and Wong's Nursing Care of Infants and Children,* ed 6, St. Louis, 1999, Mosby.

Wood CJ: Endotracheal suctioning: a literature review, *Intensive Crit Care Nurs* 14(3):124, 1998.

14

Closed Chest Drainage Systems

Skills

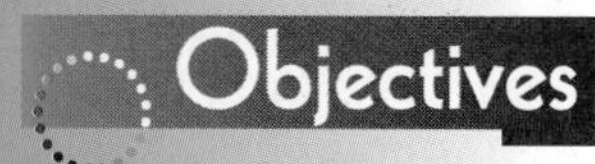

Mastery of content in this chapter will enable the nurse to:

- Define the key terms listed.
- Explain the physiology of normal respiration.
- List three common sites for chest tube placement.
- List three conditions requiring chest tube insertion.
- Describe two closed chest drainage systems: water-seal and waterless systems.
- Describe chest tube suction.
- Describe methods of troubleshooting chest tube systems.
- Discuss the care of clients with chest tubes.
- Describe autotransfusion.

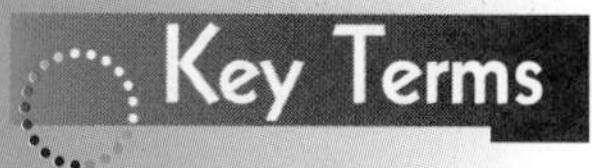

Air leak	Negative pressure
Atmospheric pressure	Parietal pleura
Chest tube	Pneumothorax
Hemothorax	Positive pressure
Intrapleural	Subcutaneous emphysema
Intrapulmonic	Tidaling
Mediastinal shift	Visceral pleura

The chest cavity is a closed structure bound by muscle, bone, connective tissue, vascular structures, and the diaphragm. This cavity has three distinct sections, each sealed from the others: one section for each lung and a third section for the mediastinum, which surrounds structures such as the heart, esophagus, trachea, and great vessels.

The lungs are covered with a membrane called the **visceral pleura.** The interior chest wall is lined with another membrane, called the **parietal pleura.** The potential space between the visceral and parietal pleura is filled with approximately 4 ml of lubricating fluid and is called the **intrapleural** space. To expand the lungs, negative intrapleural pressure must be maintained. During inspiration the intercostal muscles pull outward and the diaphragm contracts and pulls down, thereby increasing the size of the chest cavity. This increase in size causes an increase in the amount of **negative pressure** (vacuum effect) being exerted in the intrapleural space.

Inspiration occurs when the increased negative pressure pulls the lungs against the enlarged chest cavity, expanding their size. The expanding lungs cause the **intrapulmonic** pressure to fall lower than **atmospheric pressure.** This increase in negative pressure within the lungs causes air to rush into the lungs until the intrapulmonic pressure is equal to the pressure in the atmosphere. When the chest cavity stops expanding and the lungs are full of air, the respiratory muscles and diaphragm relax, returning the chest cavity to its resting stage. At this time the intrapulmonic pressure is the same as the atmospheric pressure. During expiration a passive relaxation of the respiratory muscles causes the chest cavity space to decrease. This decrease in space causes the intrapulmonic pressure to increase, which allows the air to leave the lungs.

Trauma, disease, or surgery can result in air, blood, or fluid leaking into the intrapleural space creating a **positive pressure** that collapses lung tissue. Small leaks may be absorbed spontaneously or may require interventions. Occasionally, in emergency situations and for some small pneumothoraxes, a catheter is inserted through the chest wall and a one-way valve (Heimlich valve) is attached to the catheter (Connor, 1987) (Figure 14-1). This one-way valve allows air and fluid to exit from the intrapleural space on expiration but prevents air from reentry during inspiration (Lewis, Collier, and Heitkemper, 2000). No drainage chamber is used with this simple device.

A pleural **chest tube** is inserted when air or fluid enters the intrapleural space, compromising oxygenation or ventilation (e.g., chest trauma, open chest surgery, or in the case of a large intrapleural leak). A closed chest drainage system with or without suction is attached to the chest tube to promote drainage of air and fluid. Lung reexpansion occurs as the fluid or air is removed from the intrapleural space.

The location of the chest tube indicates the type of drainage expected. Apical (second or third intercostal space) and anterior chest tube placement promotes removal of air, which is necessary in the case of a **pneumothorax** (collapsed lung caused by air in pleural space). Because air rises, these chest tubes are placed high, allowing evacuation of air from the intrapleural space and allowing the lung to reexpand (Figure 14-2). The air is discharged into the atmosphere, and there is little or no drainage in the collection chamber.

Chest tubes are placed low (usually in the fifth or sixth intercostal space) and posterior or lateral to drain fluid (Figures 14-2 and 14-3). Fluid in the intrapleural space is affected by gravity and localizes in the lower portion of the lung cavity when the client is sitting upright. Tubes placed in these posi-

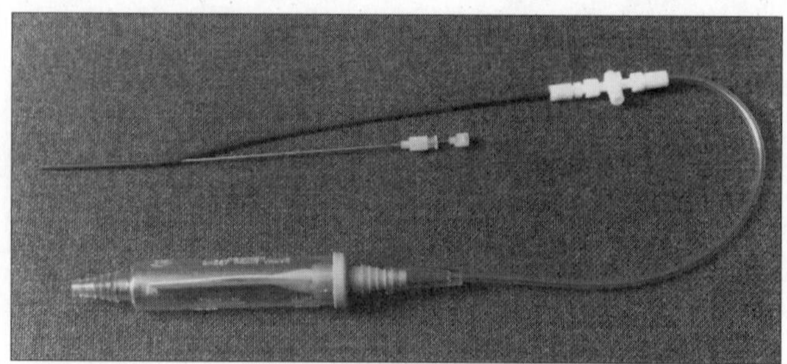

FIGURE 14-1 The one-way valve.

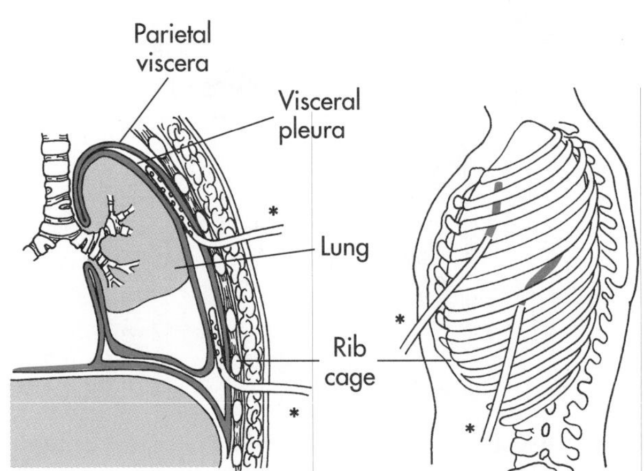

FIGURE 14-2 Diagram of sites for chest tube placement (sites indicated by *).

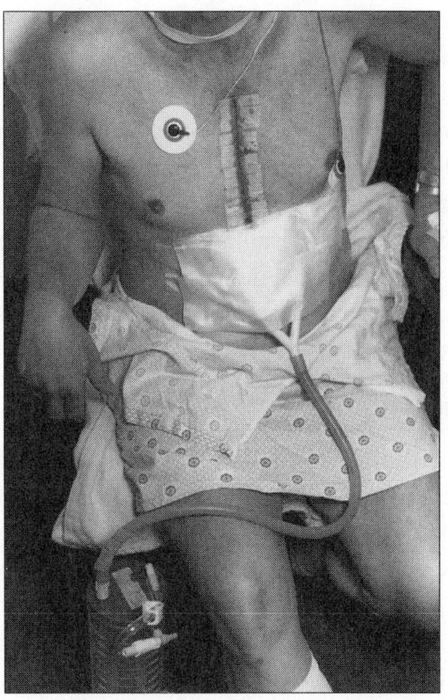

FIGURE 14-4 Mediastinal chest tube.

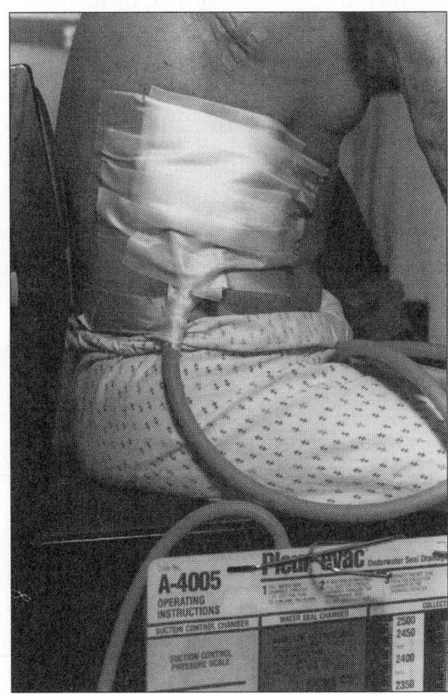

FIGURE 14-3 Pleural chest tube in place following open heart surgery.

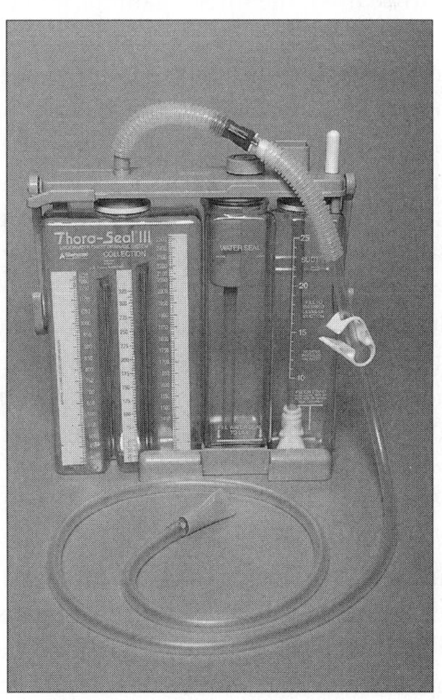

FIGURE 14-5 Disposable chest drainage system.

tions drain blood and fluid. Frequently applying suction assists this drainage. Fluid drainage is expected after open chest surgery and with some chest trauma.

A mediastinal chest tube is placed in the mediastinum, just below the sternum (Figure 14-4) and is connected to a drainage system. This tube drains blood or fluid, preventing its accumulation around the heart. A mediastinal tube is commonly used after open heart surgery. There is no **tidaling** (fluctuations or rocking) in mediastinal drainage because the tube is not placed in a lung cavity and therefore does not reflect intraplural pressure changes.

A variety of disposable commercial chest drainage systems are available. A one-bottle system allows air from the pneumothorax to bubble out of the water seal and escape through the air outlet while preventing air from reentering the intrapleural space. This system is not recommended for the evacuation of fluid because drainage would raise the level of the water-seal liquid. An increased height of fluid in the water seal increases the resistance to drainage on expiration and eventually stops the drainage entirely (Phipps and others, 1999).

A two- or three-chamber system drains both a **hemothorax** and a pneumothorax effectively (Figure 14-5). Water-seal or the newer waterless chest drainage systems can be purchased. Both systems are presented in this text. The two-chamber system permits liquid to flow into the collection chamber, and air flows into the water seal chamber. A three-chamber system promotes the drainage of fluid and air with controlled suction. In both systems the first chamber provides a compartment for fluid or blood drainage and a second compartment for either a water seal or a one-way valve. In the three-chamber system, the third compartment is for suction control, which may or may not be used.

Two-Chamber Water-Seal System

On expiration, fluid or air is forced out of the intrapleural space. Gravity pulls air or fluid through the chest tube into the drainage collection chamber. On entering the drainage collection chamber, this fluid or air displaces the air present in the chamber by pushing it through the water seal and out of the system into the atmosphere. The water-seal chamber must be left open to air in order to drain. If the tubing is clamped there is no mechanism for air to vent.

Three-Chamber Water-Seal System

If suction is to be used, the three-chamber water-seal system (see Figure 14-5) is set up with the suction control chamber added. A prescribed amount of sterile fluid (e.g., 20 cm of water) is poured into the suction control chamber, which is then attached to a suction source by tubing. The amount of sterile water added depends on the manufacturer's recommendations. The chamber is filled to the set volume for the prescribed amount of suction. Sterile water may need to be added several times a day because of evaporation. As the fluid level decreases the amount of suction also declines. The wall or portable suction device is turned up until the water in the suction control bottle exhibits a continuous, gentle bubbling. This provides the prescribed amount of suction (negative pressure).

If the suction source delivers more negative pressure than the suction control chamber water level allows, there is no danger because atmospheric air is pulled into the suction control chamber through an inlet, causing the excess suction to dissipate. The extra air pulled into the chamber causes vigorous bubbling. If this occurs, the suction source setting needs to be lowered to reduce noise and evaporation of the fluid. The absence of bubbling indicates that no suction is being exerted into the system. The suction setting should be raised to restore gentle bubbling.

Two-Chamber Waterless System

The waterless system's principles are similar to those of the water-seal system except that fluid is not required for setup. Since water is not used, accidentally tipping over the system does not compromise the client's condition.

The water seal is replaced by a one-way valve (Figure 14-6) located near the top of the system. Most of the container is the drainage chamber. The suction chamber does not depend on water. It contains a float ball, which is set by a suction control dial after the suction source is turned on. A diagnostic air-leak indicator is located on the face of the unit. It does require 15 ml of fluid for visualization. The indicator's function is to identify one of the following:

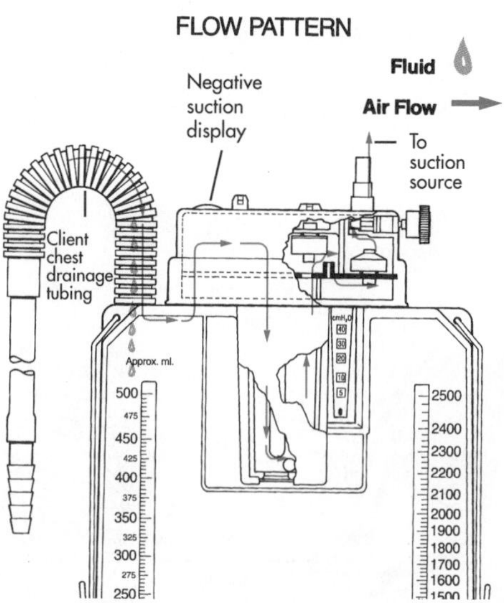

FIGURE 14-6 Disposable waterless chest drainage system with suction.

1. That the lung is expanding normally. This is indicated by a gentle tidaling of the fluid in the water seal or diagnostic indicator.
2. The lung is probably reexpanded if after 2 or 3 days the tidaling has stopped.
3. An air leak is in the system if, while facing the system, the observer sees the fluid bubbling left to right. The source of the air leak must be located and corrected.

Three-Chamber Waterless System

If suction is ordered, attach the suction chamber port to the suction source by tubing, turn the suction on, and set the float ball at the prescribed setting. If the float ball will not rise to the prescribed level, increase the suction source setting until it does. The system is now functioning with suction.

Both commercial systems have two suction settings: one at either the suction control chamber or at the float ball setting and the other at the suction source. The chamber or float ball setting is a safety factor to reduce the possibility that the intrapleural tissues will receive too much suction, causing injury.

Skill Performance Guidelines

1. Document client's baseline vital signs, lung sounds, and respiratory status. Changes in the vital signs or respiratory status can indicate a malfunction of the chest drainage system.
2. Observe the water seal for intermittent bubbling from its U tube or a rise and fall of fluid that is synchronous with res-

pirations. (For example, in a non–mechanically ventilated client during inspiration the fluid rises, and during expiration the fluid level falls. When a client is on a mechanical ventilator, the opposite occurs.)

a. Constant bubbling in the water seal or a sudden, unexpected stoppage of water-seal activity is considered abnormal and requires immediate attention.
b. Unexpected stoppage of activity may indicate a blockage. In these situations immediate attention and correction are indicated. After 2 to 3 days, tidaling or bubbling on expiration is expected to stop, indicating that the lung has reexpanded.

3. In the waterless system look for a rise and fall of fluid in the diagnostic air-leak indicator synchronous with respirations. Constant left-to-right bubbling (when facing the indicator) or violent rocking is considered abnormal and may indicate an air leak.
4. Know the amount of expected chest tube drainage.
   a. A sudden decrease in the amount of chest tube drainage can indicate a possible clot or obstruction in the chest tube.
   b. A sudden increase of more than 100 ml of drainage can indicate fresh bleeding from the thorax.
   c. Drainage from a pneumothorax is generally limited to the fluid caused by chest tube insertion trauma.
5. Know the expected color of the drainage. Drainage from recent open chest surgery is initially bright red and gradually becomes serous as the postoperative course continues. Pleural effusions usually drain straw-colored fluid. Empyema is a collection of pus in the pleural cavity, and the drainage is pus colored (Coote, 2000).
6. In the water system, observe for constant, gentle bubbling in the suction control chamber when it is connected to suction. In the waterless system a designated amount of suction is maintained by setting the suction source and dialing the prescribed suction level in the float ball column.
7. Assess both types of systems for air leaks. If an air leak exists, determine whether the air leak is within the client (client-centered **air leak**) or within the chest tube system (system-centered air leak). Remember that continuous bubbling in the water seal chamber with an absence of bubbles in the suction control chamber indicates that there is a leak in the system (Shuster, 1998). Ensure that all tubing connections are tight.
8. Note the color and amount of chest tube drainage on a regular basis (e.g., every hour initially and then every 4 hours). Make a mark to indicate the fluid level on the side of the drainage collection chamber at the end of the shift. Note the drainage amount as output.

Skill 14-1 Caring for Clients With Chest Tube Connected to Disposable Drainage Systems

There are two types of commercial drainage systems: the water-seal and the waterless systems.

Delegation Considerations

The skills in this chapter should not be delegated to assistive personnel. However, all staff should be informed about how to properly position clients with chest tubes in place. In addition, all staff should know expected client responses (e.g., normal fluctuation of fluid level, stable vital signs, expected type and amount of drainage). Finally, all staff should be instructed to immediately report problems such as disconnection of drainage tubing, sudden bleeding, or sudden shortness of breath.

Equipment

- Local anesthetic, if this is not an emergent procedure
- Prescribed drainage system
- Water suction system and: sterile water or normal saline (NS) solution to cover the lower 2.5 cm (1 inch) of water-seal U tube, sterile water or NS to pour into the suction control chamber if suction is to be used (see manufacturer's directions)
- Waterless system and vial of 30 ml injectable sodium chloride or water, 20-ml syringe, 21-gauge needle, and antiseptic swab
- Chest tube tray (all items are sterile): knife handle (1), chest tube clamp, small sponge forceps, needle holder, knife blade No. 10, 3-0 silk sutures, tray liner (sterile field), curved 8-inch Kelly clamps (2), 4 × 4 inch sponges (10), suture scissors, hand towels (3)
- Dressings: petrolatum gauze, split, chest-tube dressings, several 4 × 4 inch gauze dressings, large dressings (2), and 4-inch tape or elastic bandage (Elastoplast)
- Head cover
- Face mask/face shield
- Sterile gloves
- Rubber-tipped hemostats for each chest tube (2)
- 1-inch adhesive tape for taping connections

STEP	RATIONALE

ASSESSMENT

STEP	RATIONALE
1. Obtain baseline vital signs, oxygen saturation (SaO_2) and pulmonary assessment.	Baseline vital signs are essential for any invasive procedure. Clients requiring chest tube insertion frequently have respiratory distress, and vital signs are taken serially. Sharp stabbing chest pain with or without decreased blood pressure and increased heart rate may indicate a tension pneumothorax (Woodruff, 1999).
2. Observe for changes in heart rate, SaO_2, blood pressure, respiratory pattern, increased apprehension, and chest pain.	Changes in these parameters may indicate worsening of the initial condition.
3. Assess client for known allergies.	Povidone-iodine is an antiseptic used to cleanse the skin. Lidocaine is a local anesthetic administered to reduce pain. The chest tube will be held in place with tape. Iodine, lidocaine, and tape are common allergens.
4. Review client's medication record for anticoagulant therapy.	Anticoagulation therapy such as aspirin, warfarin, or heparin or platelet aggregation inhibitors such as ticlopidine can increase procedure-related blood loss.

NURSING DIAGNOSIS

Defining characteristics from the assessment data may reveal the following nursing diagnoses for clients requiring this skill:

Anxiety
Impaired gas exchange
Pain (acute)

Related factors are individualized based on client's condition or needs.

PLANNING

STEP	RATIONALE
1. **Expected outcomes** following completion of procedure:	
▪ Client is oriented and more relaxed.	Hypoxia relieved.
▪ Vital signs are stable.	Decreased hypoxia improves vital sign measure.
▪ Client reports no chest pain.	Reexpansion of the lung reduces chest pain.
▪ Breath sounds are auscultated in all lobes. Lung expansion is symmetrical, SaO_2 is stable or improved, and respirations are nonlabored.	Reexpansion of the lung promotes normal respirations.
▪ Chest tube remains in place and chest drainage system remains airtight.	Indicates correct placement and patency of the chest tube drainage system.
▪ Gentle tidaling (fluctuations or rocking) is evident in water seal or diagnostic indicator.	Indicates system is functioning normally. Reflects changes in intrapleural pressure.
2. Check agency policy and determine whether informed consent is needed.	In nonemergent situations most institutions require informed, written permission for chest tube insertion.
3. Review physician's role and responsibilities for chest tube placement (Table 14-1).	Helps differentiate physician and nurse roles so that the nurse can function more effectively.
4. Explain procedure to client.	Reduces anxiety and promotes client cooperation.
5. Wash hands.	Reduces transmission of microorganisms.
6. Set up the prescribed drainage system. Open system when physician is ready to insert chest tube.	Premature opening of the sterile chest drainage system increases risk of contamination of sterile equipment.
a. Water-seal system (check manufacturer's guidelines)	
(1) Obtain a chest drainage system. Remove wrappers and prepare to set up the system.	Maintains sterility of the system. The system is packaged in this manner so it can be used under sterile operating room conditions (Carroll, 1991).

Table 14-1 Physician's Role and Responsibility in Chest Tube Placement

ROLE	RESPONSIBILITY
Explain purpose, procedure, and possible complications to the client and have client sign consent form.	Provides informed consent.
Wash hands. Cleanse chest wall with antiseptic.	Reduces transmission of microorganisms.
Apply mask and gloves.	Maintains surgical asepsis.
Drape area of chest tube insertion with sterile towels.	Maintains surgical asepsis.
Inject local anesthetic and allow time to take effect.	Decreases pain during procedure.
Use blunt or sharp dissection to create incision in the skin and chest wall.	Opens chest for insertion of chest tube. A trocar is outdated and increases risk of tissue damage.
Thread a clamped chest tube through the incision. Physician clamps chest tube until system is connected to water seal.	Inserts chest tube into the intrapleural space. Clamping prevents entry of atmospheric air into the chest and worsening of the pneumothorax.
Suture chest tube in place, if suturing is policy or physician preference.	Secures chest tube in place.
Cover the chest insertion site with sterile petrolatum gauze, 4 × 4 inch gauze, and large dressing to form an occlusive dressing supported with an elastic bandage (Elastoplast).	Holds chest tube in place and occludes site around chest tube. Helps stabilize chest tube and holds dressing tightly in place. Helps prevent bacteria entry and air leak.
Water-seal system: Remove connector cover from client's end of chest drainage tubing with sterile technique. Secure drainage tubing to the chest tube and drainage system.	Physician is responsible for making certain that the system is set up properly, the proper amount of water is in the water seal, the dressing is secure, and the chest tube is securely connected to the drainage system.
Water-seal suction: Connect system to suction or supervise a nurse connecting it to suction, if suction is to be used.	The physician is responsible for determining and checking the amount of fluid that is to be added to the suction control chamber and prescribing the suction setting.
Waterless system: Remove connector cover from client's end of chest drainage tubing with sterile technique. Secure drainage tubing to the chest tube and drainage system.	Physician is responsible for making certain that the system is set up properly and the chest tube is securely connected to the drainage system.
Waterless suction: Turn on suction source. Set float ball level to prescribed setting.	Physician is responsible for prescribing level of float ball and prescribing the suction setting.
The physician or nurse adds sterile water or NS to diagnostic indicator.	Allows quick assurance that the system is functioning properly.
Unclamp the chest tube.	Connects chest tube to drainage.
In both systems the physician orders and reviews chest x-ray studies.	Verifies correct chest tube placement.

STEP	RATIONALE
(2) While maintaining sterility of the drainage tubing, stand the system upright and add sterile water or NS to the appropriate compartments.	Reduces possibility of contamination.
(a) For a two-chamber system (without suction), add sterile solution to the water-seal chamber (second chamber), bringing fluid to the required level as indicated.	Maintains water seal.
(b) For a three-chamber system (with suction), add sterile solution to the water-seal chamber (second chamber). Add amount of sterile solution prescribed by physician to the suction control (third chamber), usually 20 cm (8 inches). Connect tubing from suction control chamber to suction source.	Depth of fluid level dictates the highest amount of negative pressure that can be present within the system (Shuster, 1998). For example, 20 cm of water is approximately −20 cm of water pressure. Any additional negative pressure applied to the system is vented into the atmosphere through the suction control vent. This safety device prevents damage to pleural tissues from an unexpected surge of negative pressure from the suction source.
b. Waterless system (check manufacturer's guidelines)	
(1) Obtain a waterless system. Remove sterile wrappers and prepare to set up equipment.	Maintains sterility of the system. The system is packaged in this manner so it can be used under sterile operating room conditions.

Step	Rationale
(2) For a two-chamber system (without suction) nothing is added or needs to be done to the system.	The waterless two-chamber system is ready for connecting to the client's chest tube after opening the wrappers.
(3) For a three-chamber waterless system with suction: connect tubing from suction control chamber to the suction source.	The suction source provides additional negative pressure to the system.
(4) Instill 15 ml of sterile water or NS into the diagnostic indicator injection port located on top of the system.	This step is not necessary for mediastinal drainage because there will be no tidaling. Also, in an emergency it is not necessary because the system does not require water for setup.
7. Tape all connections in a double spiral fashion with 1-inch adhesive tape. Then:	Prevents atmospheric air from leaking into the system and the client's intrapleural space.
a. Check systems for proper functioning by:	
(1) Clamping the drainage tubing that will connect the client to the system.	
(2) Connecting tubing from the float ball chamber to the suction source.	
(3) Turning on the suction to the prescribed level.	Provides a chance to ensure an airtight system before connecting it to the client. Allows correction or replacement of system if it is defective before connecting it to the client. NOTE: Bubbling will be seen at first because there is air in the tubing and system initially. This should stop after a few minutes unless there are other sources of air entering the system.

• ***Critical Decision Point***

If bubbling continues, check connections and locate source of the air leak, as described in Table 14-2.

Step	Rationale
8. Turn off suction source and unclamp drainage tubing before connecting client to the system.	Having the client connected to suction when it is initiated could damage pleural tissues from sudden increase in negative pressure. The suction source is turned on again after the client is connected to the three-chamber system.
9. Position the client: During the chest tube insertion, the client will need to be positioned so the client's back or the side in which the tube will be placed is accessible to the physician. After the tube is placed, the client will be positioned in:	Permits optimal drainage of fluid and/or air.
a. Semi-Fowler's to high-Fowler's position to evacuate air (pneumothorax).	Air rises to the highest point in the chest. Pneumothorax tubes are usually placed on the anterior aspect at the midclavicular line, second or third intercostal space (Woodruff, 1999).
b. High-Fowler's position to drain fluid (hemothorax).	Permits optimal drainage of fluid. Posterior tubes are placed on the midaxillary line, fifth or sixth intercostal space.

Implementation

Step	Rationale
1. Wash hands and apply gloves.	Reduces transmission of microorganisms.
2. Administer parenteral premedications, such as sedatives or analgesics, as ordered.	Reduces client anxiety and pain during procedure.

• ***Critical Decision Point***

Many sedatives and analgesics suppress respirations and affect the blood pressure. Monitor the client closely to determine that the respiratory status is not worsened by the analgesics.

Step	Rationale
3. Assist physician in providing psychological support to the client. (See physician's responsibilities in Table 14-1.)	
a. Reinforce preprocedure explanation.	Reduces client anxiety and assists in efficient completion of procedure.
b. Instruct client throughout procedure.	

Table 14-2 Problem Solving With Chest Tubes

ASSESSMENT	INTERVENTION
Air leak can occur at insertion site, connection between tube and drainage, or within drainage device itself. Continuous bubbling is noted in water-seal chamber and water seal. Leaks are corrected when constant bubbling stops.	Locate leak by clamping tube at different intervals along the tube.
Assess for location of leak by clamping chest tube with 2 rubber shod or toothless clamps close to the chest wall. If bubbling stops, air leak is inside client's thorax or at chest insertions site.	NURSE ALERT: Unclamp tube, reinforce chest dressing, and notify physician immediately. **Rationale: Leaving chest tube clamped can cause collapse of lung, mediastinal shift, and eventual collapse of other lung from build up of air pressure within the pleural cavity.**
If bubbling continues with the clamps near the chest wall, gradually move one clamp at a time down drainage tubing away from client and toward suction control chamber. When bubbling stops, leak is in section of tubing or connection between the clamps.	Replace tubing or secure connection and release clamps.
If bubbling still continues, this indicates the leak is in the drainage system.	Change the drainage system.
Assess for tension pneumothorax: • Severe respiratory distress • Low oxygen saturation • Chest pain • Absence of breath sounds on affected side • Tracheal shift to unaffected side • Hypotension and signs of shock • Tachycardia	Make sure chest tubes are patent: remove clamps, eliminate kinks, or eliminate occlusion. **Rationale: Obstructed chest tubes trap air in intrapleural space when air leak originates within the thorax. Notify physician immediately and prepare for another chest tube insertion.** A flutter (Heimlich) valve or large-gauge needle may be used for short-term emergency release of pressure in the intrapleural space. Have emergency equipment, oxygen, and code cart available since condition is life-threatening.
Water seal tube is no longer submerged in sterile fluid due to evaporation.	Add sterile water to water-seal chamber until distal tip is 2 cm under surface level.

STEP	RATIONALE
4. Show local anesthetic to physician.	Allows physician to read label of drug before administering it to client.
5. Hold anesthetic solution bottle upside down with label facing physician. Physician will withdraw solution and inject into client's skin.	Allows physician to withdraw solution properly while maintaining surgical asepsis.
a. Physician places chest tube. (A standard procedure is detailed in Table 14-1.)	
6. Help physician attach drainage tube to chest tube.	Connects drainage system and suction (if ordered) to the chest tube.
7. Tape the tube connection between the chest and drainage tubes.	Secures chest tube to drainage system and reduces risk of air leaks causing breaks in the airtight system.
8. Check patency of air vents in system:	
a. Water-seal vent must not be occluded.	Permits the displaced air to pass into the atmosphere.
b. Suction control chamber vent must not be occluded when suction is used.	Provides safety factor of releasing excess negative pressure into the atmosphere.
c. Waterless systems have relief valves without caps.	
9. Coil excess tubing on mattress next to the client. Secure with a rubber band and safety pin or the system's clamp.	Prevents excess tubing from hanging over the edge of the mattress in a dependent loop. Drainage could collect in the loop and occlude the drainage system.
10. Adjust tubing to hang in a straight line from the chest tube to the drainage chamber.	Promotes drainage and prevents fluid or blood from accumulating in the pleural cavity.
11. If the chest tube is draining fluid, indicate the date and time (e.g., 0900) that drainage was begun on the drainage chamber's write-on surface.	Provides a baseline for continuous assessment of the type and quantity of drainage.

Step	Rationale
a. Assessment after chest-tube insertion is done every 15 minutes for the first 2 hours. This assessment interval then changes *on the basis of client's status.* Mark the time and level of drainage on the calibrated write-on strip periodically.	Permits timely and efficient account of the amount of drainage from the chest tube. Drainage is marked at specified periods of time and documented on the nurses' notes and intake and output (I&O) sheet. Ensures early detection of complications.
12. Strip or milk chest tube only if indicated (this means compressing the tube to encourage clots to press through the tube): Stripping—compression along length of the tubing beginning at client and continuing until drainage unit is reached. Milking—compressing and releasing the tube sequentially.	Stripping may cause complications because it creates excessive negative intrapleural pressure (over -100 cm H_2O pressure). Milking causes less of a pressure change.

• ***Critical Decision Point***

Check your institutional policy before stripping or milking chest tubes. This practice is being discontinued at most institutions because it is believed that stripping the tube greatly increases intrapleural pressure, which could damage the pleural tissue and cause or worsen an existing pneumothorax.

Step	Rationale
a. Postoperative mediastinal chest tubes are manipulated if nursing assessment indicates an obstruction of drainage resulting from clots or debris in the tubing.	Stripping is controversial and should be performed only if hospital policy permits and there is a physician's order (Phipps and others, 1999). Stripping creates a high degree of negative pressure and has potential of pulling lung tissue or pleura into drainage holes of the chest tube (Carroll, 1991).
13. Provide two rubber-tipped hemostats for each chest tube. Verify agency policy; rubber-tipped hemostats are usually attached to the bottom of the client's bed with adhesive tape or clamped to client's clothing during ambulation. a. Have the new system ready to be connected before clamping the tube, so that transfer can be rapid and the drainage system reestablished.	Chest tubes are double clamped under specific circumstances: To assess for an air leak (see Table 14-2). To empty or change the collection bottle or empty or change the collection bottle or chamber (Gross, 1993). To change disposable systems. To assess if client is ready to have chest tube removed. No bubbling occurs when the lung has fully expanded (Shuster, 1998).
14. Assist client to a comfortable position.	Reduces client anxiety and promotes cooperation.
15. Remove gloves and dispose of used soiled equipment.	Prevents accidents involving contaminated equipment.
16. Wash hands.	Reduces spread of microorganisms.

Evaluation

Step	Rationale
1. Monitor vital signs, oxygen saturation, pulmonary status, amount and type of drainage, and insertion site every 15 minutes for the first 2 hours.	Provides immediate information about procedure-related complications such as respiratory distress.
2. After first 2 hours, assess client's physical and psychological status at least every 4 hours or according to agency policy.	Detects early signs and symptoms of complications: Apprehension—increase in client anxiety, restlessness, and inability to concentrate. Respiratory distress—alteration in rate and/or depth of respirations, difficulty breathing, and breath sounds. **Subcutaneous emphysema**—air that is being trapped in the subcutaneous tissue.
3. Assess client for decreased respiratory distress and chest pain, breath sounds over affected lung area, and stable vital signs.	Increase in respiratory distress and/or chest pain, decrease in breath sounds over the affected and nonaffected lungs, marked cyanosis, asymmetrical chest movements, presence of subcutaneous emphysema around tube insertion site or neck, hypotension, tachycardia, and/or **mediastinal shift** are critical and indicate a severe change in client status, such as excessive blood loss or tension pneumothorax. Notify physician immediately (Godden, 1998).

STEP	RATIONALE
4. Observe: a. Chest tube dressing.	Ensure that dressing is occlusive and note any drainage.

• ***Critical Decision Point***
Check the dressing carefully. It can come loose from the skin, although this may not be readily apparent.

STEP	RATIONALE
b. Tubing should be free of kinks and dependent loops.	Straight and coiled drainage tube positions are optimal for pleural drainage. However, when dependent loop is unavoidable, periodic lifting and draining of the tube will also promote pleural drainage (Schmetz and others, 1999).
c. The chest drainage system should be upright and below level of tube insertion. Note presence of clots or debris in tubing.	System must be in this position to function and to facilitate proper drainage (Gordon and others, 1997).

• ***Critical Decision Point***
Monitor the position of the system relative to the chest tube carefully, especially during client transport.

STEP	RATIONALE
d. Water seal for fluctuations with client's inspiration and expiration.	
(1) Waterless system: diagnostic indicator for fluctuations with client's inspirations and expirations.	In the non–mechanically ventilated client, fluid should rise in the water seal or diagnostic indicator with inspiration and fall with expiration. The opposite occurs in the client who is mechanically ventilated. This indicates that the system is functioning properly (Lewis, Collier, and Heitkemper, 2000).
(2) Water-seal system: bubbling in the water-seal chamber (see Table 14-2).	When system is initially connected to the client, bubbles are expected from the chamber. These are from air that was present in the system and in the client's intrapleural space. After a short time, the bubbling stops. Fluid continues to fluctuate in the water seal on inspiration and expiration until the lung is reexpanded or the system becomes occluded.
e. Waterless system: bubbling in diagnostic indicator.	
f. Type and amount of fluid drainage: Nurse should note color and amount of drainage, client's vital signs, and skin color. What is the normal amount of drainage?	
(1) In the adult, less than 50 to 200 ml/hr immediately postoperative in a mediastinal chest tube (Johanson, Wells, Dungea, 1988); approximately 500 ml in the first 24 hours (Duncan and others, 1987). Dark-red drainage is expected only in the postoperative period, turning serous with time (Lewis, Collier, and Heitkemper, 2000).	
(2) Between 100 and 300 ml of fluid may drain in a pleural chest tube in an adult during the first 2 hours after insertion. This rate decreases after 2 hours; 500 to 1000 ml can be expected in the first 24 hours. Drainage is grossly bloody during the first several hours after surgery and then changes to serous (Lewis, Collier, and Heitkemper, 2000). Remember that a sudden gush of drainage may be retained blood and not active bleeding. This increase in drainage can result from client position change.	Reexpansion of lungs forces drainage into the tube. Coughing can also cause large gushes of drainage or air. Excessive amounts and/or the continued presence of frank bloody drainage the first several hours after surgery should be reported to the physician, along with client's vital signs and respiratory status.
g. Water-seal system: bubbling in the suction control chamber (when suction is being used) (see Table 14-2).	Suction control chamber has constant, gentle bubbling. Tubing to the suction source should be free of obstruction and the suction source should be turned to the appropriate setting.

STEP	RATIONALE
h. Waterless system: The suction control (float ball) indicates the amount of suction the client's intrapleural space is receiving.	The suction float ball dictates the amount of suction in the system. The float ball allows no more suction than dictated by its setting. If the suction source is set too low, the suction float ball cannot reach the prescribed setting. In this case the suction must be increased for the float ball to reach the prescribed setting.

UNEXPECTED OUTCOMES AND RELATED INTERVENTIONS

- Air leak unrelated to client's respirations
  - Locate source (see Table 14-2).
  - Notify physician.
- No chest tube drainage.
  - Observe for kink in chest drainage system.
  - Observe for possible clot in chest drainage system.
  - Observe for mediastinal shift or respiratory distress (medical emergency).
  - Notify physician.
- Chest tube is dislodged.
  - Immediately apply pressure over chest tube insertion site.
  - Have assistant apply gauze dressing and tape three sides.
  - Notify physician.
- Substantial increase in bright red drainage.
  - Obtain vital signs.
  - Monitor drainage.
  - Assess client's cardiopulmonary status.
  - Notify physician.
- Drainage system is damaged.
  - Observe for signs of increasing pneumothorax.
  - Obtain second sterile unit and reconnect system.

RECORDING AND REPORTING

- Record baseline vital signs, including SaO_2.
- Record vital signs and SaO_2 every 15 minutes for at least 2 hours postoperatively
- Record chest drainage output hourly for at least 2 hours and then record as client status indicates.
- Document time, type, and amount of drainage. Look at the fluid in the collection tubing, not just the fluid in the collection chamber. Is the drainage bright red, dark red, or pink? Is it opaque, or can you see through it?
- Record integrity of chest suction system (e.g., record the amount of bubbling in the water-seal suction control chamber, level of suction, intactness of system)
- Mediastinal drainage requires the following documentation: time, amount, and type of drainage every 15 minutes for 2 hours postoperatively, then as client status indicates.

TEACHING CONSIDERATIONS

- Instruct client and family regarding proper functioning of chest tube and drainage system.
- Instruct client to immediately report any changes in chest comfort.

PEDIATRIC CONSIDERATIONS

- If possible using pictures and special dolls, familiarize child and family with equipment before inserting chest drainage system (Wong and others, 1999).
- Allow child to play with equipment and special dolls before inserting chest drainage system.
- Chest tube drainage greater than 3 ml/kg/hr for more than 2 consecutive hours is excessive and may indicate postoperative hemorrhage (Wong and others, 1999).

GERONTOLOGICAL CONSIDERATIONS

- Fragility of the older adult's skin requires special care and planning for management of chest tube dressing. Frequently assess surrounding skin for signs of skin breakdown (Lueckenotte, 2000).

Skill 14-2 Assisting With Removal of Chest Tubes

Actual removal of a chest tube is the function of physicians and advanced practice nurses (APNs). An APN is a nurse with a master's degree in a specialized area of nursing. If nurses are to remove a chest tube, this procedure should be a written component of the agency's policy and procedure standards.

The nurse (1) prepares the client for chest tube removal by assessing the need for preremoval analgesia and obtaining the required medication orders (Houston and Jesurum, 1999) and (2) instructs the client about the process and what will be requested of the client (Mimnaugh and others, 1999). During removal of the chest tube, it is important that the client takes a deep breath and holds it until the physician has removed the tube. This maneuver prevents air from being sucked into the chest as the tube is pulled out and before an occlusive dressing is applied.

This skill details for the nurse the actual nursing responsibilities and physician action for chest tube removal.

Delegation Considerations

This skill should not be delegated to assistive personnel.

Equipment

- Suture set
- Sterile scissors
- Sterile forceps
- Clean gloves
- Sterile gloves
- Face mask/face shield
- Prepared sterile dressing: petrolatum-impregnated gauze, 4 × 4 inch gauze dressings, large dressings
- 4-inch adhesive tape or elastic bandage (Elastoplast) cut into strips

Step	Rationale
Assessment	
1. Assess status of lung reexpansion:	
a. Provide physician with results of chest x-ray film reveals total lung reexpansion.	Reveals position of lung tissue in chest cavity.
b. Note trend in water-seal fluctuation over last 24 hours.	Pleura of the expanded lung seal the holes on the internal tip of the chest tube, halting fluctuation in the water seal. A halt in fluctuation for 24 hours indicates lung is expanded.
c. Drainage decreases to less than 50 ml/day.	Drainage has been removed, allowing the lung to reexpand.
d. Percuss lung for resonance.	Normal percussion occurs with reexpansion.
e. Auscultate lung sounds.	Normal breath sounds are heard bilaterally with reexpansion.
2. Clamp chest tube before removal as ordered by the physician. Assess for changes in vital signs, chest pain, and level of apprehension.	Physician orders tube clamping before removal to assess client's tolerance.

- ***Critical Decision Point***
  If the client develops respiratory distress when the tube is clamped, assess the client, unclamp the tube, and call the physician.

Nursing Diagnosis

Defining characteristics from the assessment data may reveal the following nursing diagnoses for clients requiring this skill:

Risk for impaired gas exchange

Related factors are individualized based on client's condition or needs.

Step	Rationale
Planning	
1. **Expected outcomes** following completion of procedure:	
▪ Lung reexpansion is maintained.	Source of air or fluid loss is sealed or has healed.
▪ Client does not experience discomfort.	
▪ Spontaneous healing of chest tube insertion site occurs after removal of tube without infection or other complications.	Large nonporous occlusive dressing at puncture site promotes uncomplicated healing.
2. Explain procedure to client.	Reduces anxiety and promotes client cooperation (Mimnaugh and others, 1999).
Implementation	
1. Administer prescribed medication for pain relief about 30 minutes before procedure.	Reduces discomfort and relaxes client. Clients do report sensations ranging from pain to pulling when the chest tube is removed (Houston and Jesurum, 1999; Mimnaugh and others, 1999).
2. Wash hands and apply gloves and face shield if needed.	Reduces transmission of microorganisms.
3. Assist client in sitting on edge of bed or lying supine or on the side without chest tubes.	Physician prescribes client's position to facilitate tube removal.
4. Physician or APN prepares an occlusive dressing of petroleum gauze on a pressure dressing and sets it aside on a sterile field and applies sterile gloves.	Essential to prepare in advance for quick application to the wound on tube withdrawal.
5. Support client physically and emotionally while physician or APN removes dressing and clips sutures.	Clients state that when they know the tube is being pulled, they can mentally prepare themselves for the procedure. Support from the health care team reduces anxiety and promotes cooperation (Mimnaugh and others, 1999).
6. Physician or APN asks the client to take a deep breath and hold it or exhale completely and hold it.	Prevents air from being sucked into the chest as the tube is removed.
7. Physician or APN quickly pulls out the chest tube.	Prevents entry of air through the chest wound.
8. Aseptically apply sterile prepared dressing over the wound and firmly secure it in position with elastic bandage (Elastoplast) or wide tape. Sometimes skin clips or purse-string sutures are used to hold the wound together before dressing is applied.	Keeps wound aseptic. Prevents entry of air into the chest. Wound closure occurs spontaneously. Clips or sutures aid in skin closure.
9. Assist client to a comfortable position.	Assists in client's return to a comfortable status. Clients report that proper positioning and rest following chest tube removal assist in relief of procedure-related sensations of pain and pulling (Mimnaugh and others, 1999).
10. Remove used equipment from bedside. Place it in appropriate area for medical waste products.	Prevents spread of microorganisms.
11. Remove gloves and wash hands.	Reduces transmission of microorganisms.
Evaluation	
1. Assess lung sounds and observe client for subcutaneous emphysema or respiratory distress immediately after tube removal and during the first few hours after removal.	Provides for early notification of physician if adverse symptoms occur. Chest tubes may need reinsertion.
2. Assess client's vital signs, oxygen saturation, pulmonary status, and psychological status.	Detects early signs and symptoms of complications.
3. Review chest x-ray film.	Identifies early signs of incomplete lung expansion.
4. Ask about the client's level of pain or comfort. Observe for nonverbal cues of pain.	Could be signs that wound has not closed well. Determines client's tolerance of procedure.
5. Check chest dressing for drainage and patency. When changing dressing, note wound for signs of healing.	Ensures occlusion and proper healing of chest wound.

UNEXPECTED OUTCOMES AND RELATED INTERVENTIONS

- Client has dyspnea, chest pain, and labored respirations.
  - These are signs of recurrence of pneumothorax or hemothorax.
  - Notify physician.
  - Prepare for reinsertion of chest tube.

RECORDING AND REPORTING

- Record removal of tube, amount of drainage in the collection bottle, appearance of wound and dressing, and client's response. Client's response should also include vital signs and respiratory assessment.
- Report client's response to chest tube removal to next shift.

TEACHING CONSIDERATIONS

- Instruct client and family to immediately report signs of chest pain, shortness of breath, or sensations of chest discomfort.

PEDIATRIC CONSIDERATIONS

- Pediatric clients may usually require analgesia (e.g., morphine sulfate 0.1 mg/kg in combination with midazolam [Versed]) before the chest tube removal (Wong and others, 1999).
- EMLA (locally applied anesthetic patch) placed under the occlusive dressing at the chest tube insertion site 1 hour before tube removal reduces pain of procedure. However, child may still feel the "pulling" sensation of tube removal (Wong and others, 1999).

Skill 14-3 Reinfusion of Chest Tube Drainage

Reinfusion of chest tube drainage has become more widely used since the public has become aware of the risks associated with blood transfusions. When reinfusion is linked with chest drainage, it becomes a relatively risk-free, inexpensive, and easy method of replacing mediastinal blood previously lost during emergencies and open heart or thoracic surgery (see Chapter 20). Clients requiring this skill must also have an intravenous (IV) line in place (see Chapter 19).

DELEGATION CONSIDERATIONS

This skill should not be delegated to assistive personnel.

EQUIPMENT

- Adult/pediatric single-use chest drainage and autotransfusion unit
- Replacement bag (Figure 14-7)

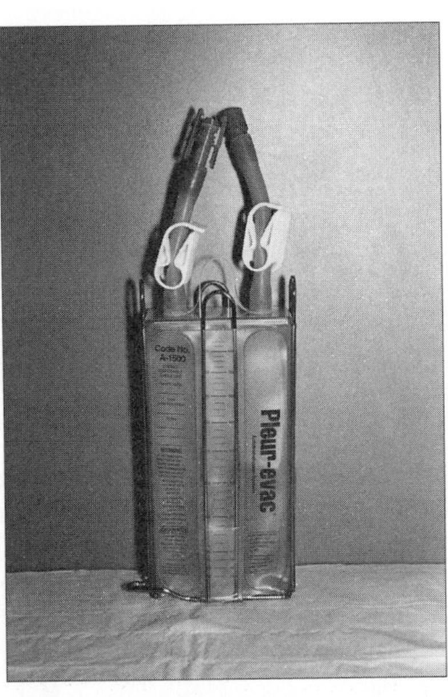

FIGURE 14-7 Example of reinfusion replacement bag.

STEP	RATIONALE

ASSESSMENT

STEP	RATIONALE
1. See Assessment for Skill 14-1. 2. Determine presence of active bleeding, at least 50 to 100 ml/hr through mediastinal tube.	Addition of the autotransfusion unit to the closed chest drainage unit requires no additional assessments.

NURSING DIAGNOSIS

Defining characteristics from the assessment data may reveal the following nursing diagnoses for clients requiring this skill:

Risk for infection

Risk for injury

Related factors are individualized based on client's condition or needs.

PLANNING

STEP	RATIONALE
1. **Expected outcomes** following completion of procedure:	
▪ Vital signs, hematocrit, and hemoglobin will stabilize.	Reinfusion prevents the loss of blood usually associated with closed chest drainage.
▪ The drainage system will function correctly, and the lung will reexpand in 48 to 72 hours.	Negative pressure will have been reestablished in the intrapleural space.
▪ The IV line will remain patent.	A patent IV is necessary for reinfusion of cleansed mediastinal tube drainage.
2. Explain procedure to client.	Reduces anxiety and promotes client cooperation.

IMPLEMENTATION

STEP	RATIONALE
1. System setup	
a. Set up the autotransfusion system according to technique that maintains the sterility of the unit and following the three steps printed on the front of the unit (see illustration).	Contamination of the unit provides a ready source of infection to client.

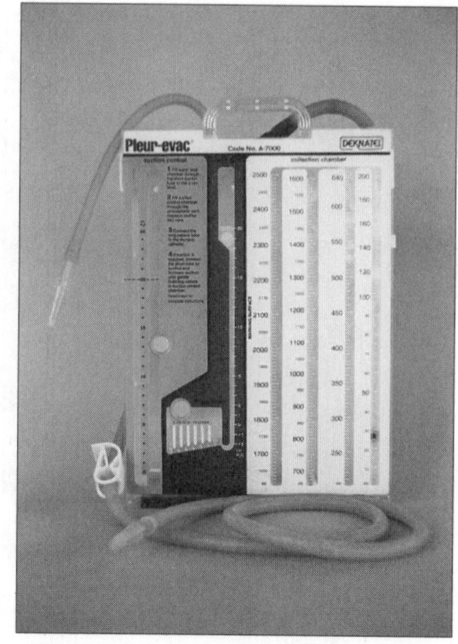

STEP **1a** Equipment needed for reinfusion of mediastinal chest tube drainage.

Step	Rationale
b. Make certain all connections are tight, and all clamps are open.	Tight connections ensure an airtight system, and open clamps allow chest drainage to enter the autotransfusion system (ATS) bag.
c. A 200 μm double-sided mesh filter is located in the ATS bag to filter the drainage.	Filtering the drainage removes extraneous materials and microemboli.
d. The ATS collection bag has a capacity of 1000 ml marked in increments of 25 ml and an area for marking times and amounts.	See Skill 14-1, Evaluation, Step 4f(1) for expected drainage amounts.
2. Wash hands and apply gloves.	Reduces transmission of microorganisms.
3. Continued collection:	
a. Open a replacement bag using proper technique, and close the two white clamps.	Contamination of the unit provides a ready source of contamination to the client. The closed clamps maintain a closed system during replacement.
b. Use the high-negativity relief valve to reduce excessive negativity.	This eases the removal of the initial collection bag from the metal support stand.
c. Bag transfer:	
(1) Close clamp on chest drainage tubing.	Prevents air from entering the chest cavity through the tube and collapsing the lung.
(2) Close the two white clamps on the top of the initial ATS collection bag.	Maintains a closed system for the reinfusion, preventing contamination of the blood.
(3) Connect the chest drainage tube to the new ATS bag with the red connectors.	Establishes a new autotransfusion system.
(4) Make certain that all connections are tight.	Ensures an airtight system.
(5) Open all clamps on chest drainage tube and replacement bag.	Reestablishes an autotransfusion collection system.
d. Connect the red and blue connectors on top of the initial collection bag and remove it by lifting it from the side hook and then from the foot hook.	Maintains a closed system within the bag and removes it for use in autotransfusion.
e. Secure the replacement bag by connecting the foot hook, replacing the metal frame into the side hook of the Pleur-evac unit, and pushing down to secure the frame onto the hook.	Provides safe attachment of the replacement bag to the Pleur-evac unit.
f. The replacement bag is removed by placing the thumbs on the top of the metal frame and pushing up with the fingers to slide the bag out.	
4. Reinfusion:	
a. Use a new microaggregate filter to reinfuse each autotransfusion bag.	Prevents the infusion of microemboli and provides maximal filtration for each bag.
b. Access the bag by inverting it and spiking the bag through the spike port with the microaggregate filter and twisting.	Connects the autotransfusion bag to the transfusion tubing.
c. With the bag upside down, gently squeeze the bag to remove the air and prime the filter with blood.	Gentle pressure is used to prevent hemolysis.
d. Hang the bag on an IV pole and continue to prime the tubing until all air is gone. Clamp the tubing, attach it to the client's IV access, and adjust the clamp to deliver the reinfusion at the appropriate rate.	Removes all air from the transfusion tubing. Reinfusion delivered either by gravity, application of a blood cuff (not to exceed 150 mm Hg pressure), or a blood-compatible IV pump (see Chapter 20).
e. If ordered, anticoagulants (citrate phosphate dextrose or heparin) can be added to the reinfusion through the self-sealing port in the autotransfusion connector.	Prevents clotting in the autotransfusion.
5. Discontinuing autotransfusion:	
a. Clamp the chest drainage tube and connect it directly to the Pleur-evac unit with the red and blue connectors.	Prevents air from entering the chest cavity through the tube and collapsing the lung.
b. Open the chest drainage tube clamp.	All drainage will be collected directly in the drainage unit and must be appropriately discarded.

Step	Rationale
6. Discard used supplies and wash hands.	Reduces transmission of microorganisms.

Evaluation

1. Monitor vital signs, hematocrit, and hemoglobin.	Helps determine the effects of the treatment.
2. Monitor chest drainage system and client's lung sounds.	Helps determine the proper functioning of the system and its effectiveness.
3. Assess the IV infusion site for infiltration and phlebitis.	A patent IV infusion site must be maintained.

Unexpected Outcomes and Related Interventions

- Chest tube becomes displaced.
  - Immediately apply pressure over chest tube insertion site.
  - Have assistant apply sterile petroleum occlusive dressing.
  - Notify physician.
- Client has dyspnea, chest pain, and labored respirations.
  - These are signs of recurrence of pneumothorax or hemothorax.
  - Notify physician.
  - Prepare for reinsertion of chest tube.
- Infection is evident.
  - Obtain wound cultures.
  - Obtain vital signs.

Recording and Reporting

- Record drainage, reinfusion with times, and amounts of each.
- Describe condition of IV infusion site.
- Report unusual findings and client responses to nurse in charge or physician.

Critical Thinking Exercises

1. Why is it important to check vital signs, check for air leaks, and note the amount of chest drainage every 15 to 30 minutes for at least 2 hours after the insertion of a chest tube?
2. You notice that your client's chest tube dressing is loose and away from his chest in several areas. What effect could this loose dressing have on the client's condition?
3. Your client is in respiratory distress. You notice that the water-seal chamber of the chest tube collection bottle is empty. What is the connection between the respiratory distress and the empty water-seal chamber?

References

Carroll PF: What's new in chest-tube management, *RN* 54(5):34, 1991.

Connor PA: When and how do you use a Heimlich flutter valve? *Am J Nurs* 87:288, 1987.

Coote N: Surgical versus non-surgical management of pleural empyema (Cochrane Review). *The Cochrane Library,* issue 2, 2000, Oxford, UK Update Software.

Duncan C, Erickson R, Weigel RM: Effect of chest tube management on drainage after cardiac surgery, *Heart-Lung* 16(1):1, 1987.

Godden J: Managing the patient with a chest drain: a review, *Nurs Stand* 12(32):35, 1998.

Gordon PA and others: Positioning of chest tubes: effects on pressure and drainage, *Am J Crit Care* 6:33, 1997.

Gross S: Current challenges, concepts, and controversies in chest-tube management, *AACN Clin Issues Crit Care Nurs* 4(2):260, 1993.

Houston S, Jesurum J: The quick relaxation technique: effect on pain associated with chest tube removal, *Appl Nurs Res* 12(4):196, 1999.

Johanson BC, Wells SJ, Dungea CU: *Standards for critical care,* ed 3, St. Louis, 1988, Mosby.

Lewis ML, Collier IC, Heitkemper M: *Medical-surgical nursing: assessment and management of clinical problems,* ed 5, St. Louis, 2000, Mosby.

Lueckenotte AG: *Gerontologic nursing,* ed 2, St. Louis, 2000, Mosby.

Mimnaugh L, and others: Sensations experienced during removal of tubes in acute postoperative patients, *Appl Nurs Res* 12(2):78, 1999.

Phipps WJ, and others, editors: *Medical-surgical nursing: concepts and clinical practice,* ed 6, St. Louis, 1999, Mosby.

Schmetz JO, and others: Effects of position of chest drainage tube on volume drained and pressure, *Am J Crit Care* 8(5):319, 1999.

Shuster PM: Chest tubes: to clamp or not to clamp, *Nurse Educ* 23(3):9, 1998.

Wong DL, and others: *Nursing care of infants and children,* ed 6, St. Louis, 1999, Mosby.

Woodruff DW: Pneumothorax, *RN* 62(9):62, 1999.

15

Emergency Measures for Life Support

Skills

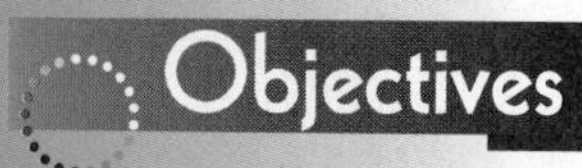

Objectives

Mastery of content in this chapter will enable the nurse to:

- Define the key terms listed.
- Describe the factors that place individuals at risk for foreign body airway obstruction.
- State signs and symptoms associated with foreign body airway obstruction.
- Discuss indications for a nasal airway.
- Discuss indications for an oral airway.
- Discuss indications for an Ambu-bag.
- State indications for cardiopulmonary resuscitation (CPR).
- State the goals for CPR.
- Demonstrate in a laboratory or clinical situation: removal of foreign body airway obstruction, insertion of a nasal airway and an oral airway, use of an Ambu-bag, and CPR.

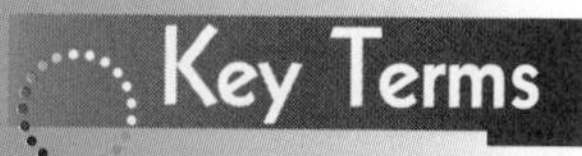

Key Terms

Airway obstruction
Ambu-bag
Aspiration
Cardiac output
Cardiopulmonary arrest
Cardiopulmonary resuscitation (CPR)
Foreign body airway obstruction maneuver (FBAOM)
Head tilt–chin lift
Heimlich maneuver
Minute ventilation
Nasal airway
Oral airway
Perfusion
Respiratory arrest
Ventilation

The oxygen transport system consists of the lungs and cardiovascular system. Adequacy of oxygen delivery depends on the amount of oxygen entering the lungs (**ventilation**), the blood flow to the lungs and to the body tissues (**perfusion**), the adequacy of diffusion of respiratory gases, the pumping ability of the heart, and the capacity of the blood to carry oxygen.

The blood's capacity to carry oxygen is influenced by the amount of dissolved oxygen in the plasma, the amount and type of hemoglobin, and the affinity of hemoglobin for oxygen. Also critical in the process of gas exchange is the ability of the heart to pump blood between the lungs and peripheral tissue.

Respiratory gases are exchanged in the alveoli and in the tissues. Oxygen is transferred from the lungs to the blood, and carbon dioxide is transferred from the blood to the lungs to be exhaled as a waste product. At the capillary level, oxygen is transferred from the blood to the tissues, and carbon dioxide is transferred from the tissues to the blood to return to the lungs and be exhaled. This transfer depends on the process of diffusion.

The hemoglobin molecule is the carrier for both oxygen and carbon dioxide; it combines with oxygen to form oxyhemoglobin. Whenever the concentration of inspired oxygen declines, there is less oxygen available for the tissues. Decreases in inspired oxygen concentration (F_IO_2) can be caused by an upper or lower airway obstruction, decreased environmental oxygen (as occurs at high altitudes), or absence of breathing, as in respiratory or cardiac arrest.

An acute **airway obstruction** reduces the amount of inspired oxygen delivered to the alveoli. As a result the amount of oxygen available for diffusion into the blood is decreased. A respiratory or cardiac arrest is an emergency situation that can occur at any time. Inability to exchange waste air for fresh air or lack of heart contraction to deliver blood to tissues impairs cellular oxygenation. Clients at risk for either type of arrest include those with airway obstruction, cardiopulmonary illnesses, severe fluid and electrolyte disturbances, and excessive ingestion of chemical substances.

Cardiopulmonary resuscitation should be performed only when true cessation of breathing and/or pulselessness has occurred. It is intended for clients who are expected to live. It should not be used in clients in the terminal stages of illness.

Skill Performance Guidelines

1. Maintenance of a safe environment for the child under 2 is essential. This age group is at greatest risk for foreign body **aspiration** of objects from their surroundings. Children frequently put coins, buttons, or small objects from the floor or tabletop into their mouths. This risk is increased due to the added mobility of this age group. Also, table foods that are not cut into an appropriate size pose a risk to the child's airway.
2. Older adults, especially those with primary neurological disorders should be observed for airway obstruction. These disorders result in a decreased gag reflex. Other causes of decreased gag reflex include alcohol, seizure, senile dementia, and strokes.
3. Counsel clients not to talk or laugh with food in their mouths. The inspiratory effort to initiate talking or laughing can cause aspiration of food and thus airway obstruction. Drinking liquids, especially alcohol, while chewing food can also cause choking and precipitate aspiration.
4. Know the client's baseline vital signs, noting any irregularities in cardiac rhythm. Dysrhythmias can precipitate a cardiopulmonary arrest. Cardiovascular conditions that place the client at risk for dysrhythmias include coronary artery disease, myocardial infarction, and open heart surgeries.

5. Know a client's most recent serum electrolyte values. Electrolyte imbalances (e.g., those involving potassium and calcium) can precipitate cardiopulmonary arrest.
6. When an overdose of a chemical substance is present, know the type and amount of the substance ingested. Certain chemicals, such as alcohol, tranquilizers, and depressants, depress the respiratory center and can result in a respiratory arrest. Overdoses of some drugs, such as heroin, can cause ventricular dysrhythmias and cardiopulmonary arrest.
7. Know the physician's orders and client's wishes regarding life-sustaining activities. Advance directives and living wills are a portion of the client's chart. Health care agencies have written policies and procedures for staff concerning the implementation of these decisions.

Skill 15-1 Removing a Foreign Body Airway Obstruction

An airway obstructed by a foreign body threatens life. In adults partially chewed food, especially meats and raw vegetables, and in children small toys or game pieces are the types of foreign bodies that most often result in partial or complete airway obstruction.

Inability to remove a foreign body impairs gas exchange and can result in unconsciousness and, possibly, cardiopulmonary arrest. Should arrest occur, cardiopulmonary resuscitation (CPR) must be initiated at once. However, CPR is ineffective if the foreign body remains in the airway. Efforts must continue to remove the obstruction. Often, full cardiac arrest can be prevented if the obstruction can be removed immediately. Prevention of foreign body aspiration is equally important.

In the adult and child, aspiration of a foreign body can be frequently prevented by (1) chewing pieces of food slowly and thoroughly, (2) avoiding excessive alcohol intake, especially at mealtime, (3) choosing age-appropriate toys and foods and restricting their use accordingly, (4) keeping children from placing small toys or game pieces in their mouths or noses, (5) avoiding excessive laughing, talking, and drinking during chewing and swallowing, (6) cutting food into small pieces, and (7) preventing children from walking, running, or playing with food in their mouth.

In the unconscious client the tongue is the most common cause of airway obstruction. Dentures and other nonpermanent dental work can become dislodged and obstruct the airway. In addition, it is not uncommon for an unconscious client or others with diminished or absent cough and gag reflexes (e.g., stroke victims) to vomit and then aspirate stomach contents, which may result in an airway obstruction. Excessive bleeding from head and facial injuries may also obstruct the airway.

In the unconscious client, aspiration of a foreign body can frequently be prevented by (1) removing all nonpermanent dental work, (2) inserting an oral airway (see Skill 15-3) to maintain tongue position, (3) inserting a nasogastric tube (see Chapter 25) to drain stomach contents, (4) placing the client in a side-lying position to prevent aspiration, and (5) when appropriate, inserting an endotracheal tube (this procedure is done by a physician or health care provider who is experienced and licensed to perform this skill) to maintain a patent airway and prevent aspiration (see Chapter 13).

The keys to successful management of foreign body airway obstruction (FBAO) are (1) early recognition that an obstructed airway exists and (2) recognition of the extent to which the airway is obstructed. If the client is able to breathe and/or speak without difficulty and cough forcefully, no immediate intervention is necessary. There may also be audible wheezing between coughs. Remain with the client until the obstruction is resolved.

The client who has difficulty breathing or is not breathing, is cyanotic, or is unable to speak, cough, or cough forcefully needs immediate assistance. In addition, a client may indicate complete airway obstruction by clutching the neck.

Delegation Considerations

The skill of removing a foreign body can be performed by trained assistive personnel. The care provider should be cautioned to allow clients experiencing foreign body obstruction to clear the airway themselves, if at all possible.

Equipment

Hospital Setting

- Emergency cart
- Suction equipment
- Face shield and gloves (if indicated and time permits)

Home Setting

- None; however, bulb syringe or kitchen baster may be useful in clearing oral secretions in an emergency. Any protective devices (e.g., mouth shield or gloves) should be utilized if they are available.

STEP	RATIONALE

ASSESSMENT

1. Identify signs and symptoms of foreign body airway obstruction needing immediate intervention:

   Clients at greater risk of foreign body aspiration include those with the following conditions: neuromuscular diseases such as myasthenia gravis and amyotrophic lateral sclerosis; cerebral vascular accident (stroke) with hemiparesis; cleft palate; lesions of head, neck, esophagus, or upper airway; seizure disorders; unconsciousness; heavy sedative or narcotic use; diminished or absent cough and gag reflexes.

   • ***Critical Decision Point***

   Do not leave clients who are experiencing a possible choking episode alone at any time. Intervention must be immediate if client's condition worsens.

   a. Cardiac: irregular pulse, rapid or slow pulse, cyanosis.
   b. Respiratory: irregular breathing pattern; choking; gagging; rapid or slow shallow breathing; apneic breathing periods; high-pitched inspiratory noises ("crowing" type); stridor; wheezing; inability to forcefully, effectively cough; inability to cough at all; inability to speak; use of accessory breathing muscles; possible cyanosis.
   c. Oral: blood or vomitus in mouth or on face, partially chewed food in mouth, freely floating dentures or nonpermanent dental work in mouth, tongue in posterior oropharynx.

      • ***Critical Decision Point***

      Postoperative oral surgery clients may experience more intense oral mucosal swelling or have their jaws wired together, thus requiring special attention to detailed assessment of their airway.

   d. Signs and symptoms of foreign body airway obstruction *that do not need immediate intervention* include ability to speak, cough forcefully, or breathe in and out; stable vital signs; alertness; and wheezing between coughs. If partial airway obstruction persists, seek help. Activate emergency medical system (EMS) if in community setting.
   e. The universal sign of obstructed airway is client clutching neck with thumb and fingers. Physical signs and symptoms may indicate need to perform **foreign body airway obstruction maneuver (FBAOM).**

2. If situation is not emergent assess for factors such as obesity or late stages of pregnancy and characteristics of foreign body.

   Such factors can influence outcome of FBAOM or require modification in intervention techniques.

3. Assess client's and family's understanding of FBAOMs and anticipated outcomes and ability to perform.

   Allows nurse to identify potential for teaching needs and determine if family is capable of assessment and intervention.

NURSING DIAGNOSIS

Defining characteristics from the assessment data may reveal the following nursing diagnoses for clients requiring this skill:

Ineffective airway clearance
Risk for aspiration
Ineffective breathing pattern
Impaired gas exchange
Ineffective cardiopulmonary tissue perfusion

Related factors are individualized based on client's condition or needs.

Step	Rationale
Planning	
1. **Expected outcomes** following completion of procedure:	
▪ Foreign body is dislodged and removed.	Airway cleared of obstruction.
▪ Nurse is able to identify clients and families needing instruction in FBAOM. If possible, explain FBAOMs to client and emphasize importance of relaxation during maneuvers.	Families need to know how to perform FBAOMs.
2. Help client assume a position that allows nurse to perform maneuvers easily. Unconscious clients should be placed on floor. Alert clients may be seated in chair or allowed to stand.	Protects client and nurse from injury.
3. Remove dentures or other nonpermanent dental work. Do not discard.	Prevents further airway obstruction.
4. Activate emergency medical services (EMS).	Additional help may be necessary. If available in the area, dial 911.

Implementation

Heimlich Maneuver

Heimlich maneuver is recommended for use in adults and children greater than 1 year old (American Heart Association [AHA], 2000). For clients who are in late stages of pregnancy or are markedly obese, chest thrusts should be administered. In infants under 1 year, back blows and chest thrusts should be used (AHA, 2000). **Always activate EMS immediately if outside a health care system.**

Conscious Client, Sitting or Standing

Step	Rationale
1. Stand behind client, and wrap arms around client's waist.	Allows access to client's chest and provides support.
2. Keep elbows bent.	Prevents squeezing client's ribs and ensures that force is applied directly under diaphragm.
3. Make a fist with one hand; place thumb side of fist against client's abdomen in midline slightly above navel and well below tip of xiphoid process.	Fist provides force without injury from fingers. While performing chest thrusts: if hands are too low, xiphoid process can be fractured. If hands are too high, intrathoracic pressure will not be sufficiently increased to expel foreign body. If client is supine, placing hands over xiphoid process or over ribs can cause fractures and internal injuries.
4. Grasp fist with other hand and press it into client's abdomen with a quick upward thrust (see illustration).	Subdiaphragmatic thrust elevates diaphragm, forcing air from lungs and possible expulsion of foreign body (AHA, 2000).

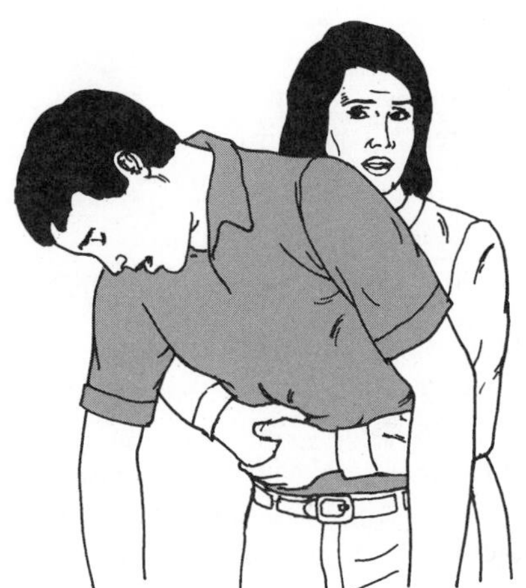

STEP 4 Heimlich maneuver.

STEP	RATIONALE
5. Repeat abdominal thrusts until object is expelled from airway or victim becomes unconscious. Each new thrust should be a separate and distinct movement (AHA, 2000).	Foreign body may not be removed on first attempt.
6. Periodically stop and assess the client for progress.	Partial dislodgement may have occurred.
7. Continue thrusts if client is still conscious and still obstructed.	Airway must be cleared to permit ventilation.

- ***Critical Decision Point***
  If client becomes unresponsive, position on floor.

Supine Client

STEP	RATIONALE
1. If client has become unconscious, position client face up and kneel astride or straddle victim's thighs. If rescuer is too short to reach across client, rescuer may straddle client.	Allows access to client's chest. This maneuver should only be used when client becomes unconscious.
2. Place heel of one hand against client's abdomen in midline slightly above navel and well below xiphoid process.	Correct hand position provides force for thrust without injury to internal body structures.
3. Perform finger sweep.	May facilitate removal of foreign body.
4. Open airway and try to ventilate victim's lungs.	Some obstructions may never come out until more extensive medical assistance can be provided. However, attempts to oxygenate client must still be attempted.

- ***Critical Decision Point***
  If client is obese or pregnant, apply chest thrusts.

STEP	RATIONALE
5. Place second hand directly on top of first, and lock fingers if desired.	Locking fingers prevents client injury and stabilizes heels of nurse's hands.
6. Press into client's abdomen with a quick upward thrust. Subdiaphragmatic thrust elevates diaphragm, forcing air from lungs.	
7. Repeat up to five times in unconscious client. Then open client's mouth and perform a finger sweep and attempt to ventilate (see Skill 15-5). If airway remains obstructed, repeat Steps 2-7 until object is dislodged and airway is patent or emergency personnel arrive and take over.	Foreign body may not be removed on first attempt.

- ***Critical Decision Point***
  If client resumes breathing, place client on side in recovery position. Remain with client.

Chest Thrusts

Sitting or Standing Client

- ***Critical Decision Point***
  In children, only abdominal thrusts are done.

STEP	RATIONALE
1. Stand behind client and encircle client's chest with both arms under client's armpits. Allow client's body to rest against nurse's (see illustration).	Allows easy access to client's chest and provides support for delivering thrusts.

- ***Critical Decision Point***
  If you cannot reach around victim, you can perform chest thrusts while victim is supine.

STEP	RATIONALE
2. Place thumb side of one fist on middle of client's breastbone, taking care to avoid xiphoid process and rib cage margin.	Correct hand position prevents injury to internal body structures.
3. Grab fist with other hand, and perform backward thrusts.	Provides force to increase intrathoracic pressure and possibly dislodge foreign body.
4. Repeat until foreign body is expelled or client becomes unresponsive (AHA, 2000).	Foreign body may not be removed on first attempt.

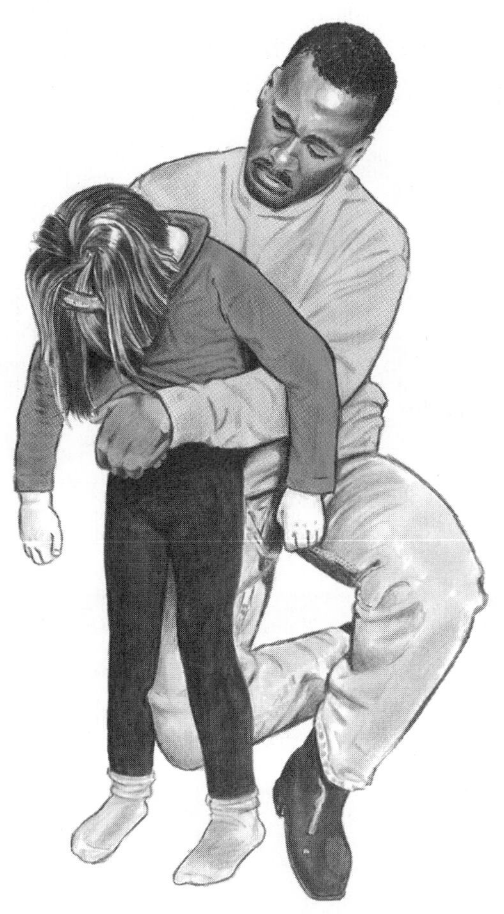

STEP 1 Abdominal thrusts for a responsive child with FBAO. (From American Heart Association: *Guidelines 2000 for cardiopulmonary resuscitation and emergency cardiovascular care: international consensus on science,* Dallas, 2000, The Association.)

STEP	RATIONALE
Supine Client	
1. Place client face up, and kneel close to client's side. If rescuer is too short to reach across client, rescuer may straddle client.	Allows easy access to client's chest. This position is also useful with pregnant or obese client that you cannot place your arms around.
2. Place heel of hand on lower half of sternum (similar to cardiac compressions).	Correct hand position prevents injury to internal body structures.
3. Press inward slowly and distinctly $1\frac{1}{2}$ to 2 inches in adults as for CPR (see Skill 15-5).	Increases intrathoracic pressure and forces exhalation to expel foreign body.
4. Repeat sequence until obstruction is relieved. Periodically open client's mouth, and perform a finger sweep and attempt to ventilate (see Skill 15-5). If airway remains obstructed, continue sequence until object is dislodged and airway is patent or emergency personnel arrive and take over.	Foreign body may not be removed with first attempt.
• ***Critical Decision Point*** *If foreign body not removed, resume chest thrust sequence.*	
Back Blows and Chest Thrusts for Infants	
1. Hold infant prone, resting on nurse's forearm, with infant's head lower than trunk, making certain to support head. (This can be performed standing or sitting. With larger infants, nurse should sit and rest forearm on thigh for support.) (See illustration, p. 416.)	Provides access to client's back and provides support for back blows. Head must be lower to encourage outward movement of foreign body and prevent reaspiration of foreign body.

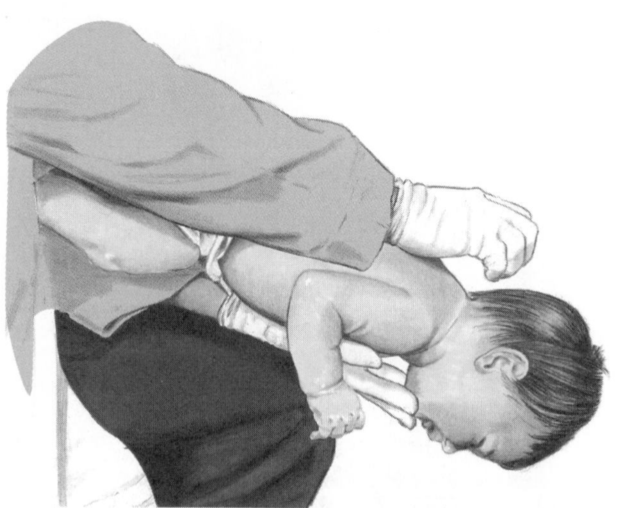

STEP 1 Infant back blows to relieve complete FBAO. (From American Heart Association: *Guidelines 2000 for cardiopulmonary resuscitation and emergency cardiovascular care: international consensus on science,* Dallas, 2000, The Association.)

STEP	RATIONALE
2. Using heel of hand, deliver up to five back blows forcefully between shoulder blades.	Increases intrathoracic pressure and forces exhalation to cough out foreign body. Careful placement of back blows is imperative because lower placement on back can result in internal organ damage.
3. Place free hand flat on infant's back, supporting head, and in such a way that infant is sandwiched between the two arms. Turn infant supine. Drape infant over thigh with infant's head lower than trunk, while continuing to support infant's head.	Repositions infant for chest thrusts.
4. Provide up to five downward thrusts over lower third of sternum (as in CPR, see Skill 15-5).	Increases intrathoracic pressure and forces exhalation to cough out foreign body.
5. Open airway and check for foreign object in back of client's throat. If visible, remove object, using finger sweep technique.	Object may have dislodged but not far enough to be ejected.
6. Attempt to ventilate.	Objects may never be completely ejected. Provision of oxygen needs to be attempted to assist client.
7. Repeat Steps 2 through 6 until foreign body is ejected.	

Finger Sweep

STEP	RATIONALE
1. Wash hands and apply gloves and face shield, if possible.	Reduces transmission of microorganisms.
2. Open client's mouth, grasping tongue and lower jaw with thumb and index finger and lift up.	Opens client's airway. Draws tongue away from back of throat.

- ***Critical Decision Point***
  Blind finger sweeps should not be performed in infants and children because foreign object may be forced back into airway.

- ***Critical Decision Point***
  In clients with a cervical spine injury pull tongue up and out of mouth and lower jaw slightly but do not move neck. If unable to open client's mouth easily, place thumb and index finger of one hand on upper and lower gum line and push teeth apart.

STEP	RATIONALE
3. Insert index finger of other hand along cheek to posterior pharynx and using a sweeping or hooking motion, dislodge foreign body and pull it up into and out of mouth (AHA, 2000).	Removes foreign body.

STEP	RATIONALE
4. When object is removed, assess airway and respiration and then obtain pulse. If pulse is absent, begin cardiopulmonary resuscitation (see Skill 15-5). If pulse is present but spontaneous respirations are absent, continue to ventilate client. In unconscious adults attempt rescue breathing (see Skill 15-5). In children, attempt ventilation; if unsuccessful, perform abdominal thrusts before attempting rescue breathing. In infants, perform back blows and chest thrusts.	Determines cardiopulmonary status. Inability to ventilate unconscious victim suggests presence of foreign body. Foreign body must be removed and airway patent before initiating chest compressions.
5. Repeat sequence of finger sweep and thrust maneuver as long as necessary.	Repeated attempts are often needed to clear foreign body.
6. Remove and dispose of gloves and face shield into appropriate receptacle. Wash hands.	Reduces transmission of microorganisms.

EVALUATION

1. Observe that foreign body is removed. Compare client's respiratory status before and after FBAOM, if possible. • ***Critical Decision Point*** *Presence of wheezing or rhonchi could indicate aspiration.*	Provides information concerning changes in client's vital signs.
2. If teaching caregivers, evaluate technique.	Practicing skills and demonstrating competence increases ability to perform in emergent situation.

UNEXPECTED OUTCOMES AND RELATED INTERVENTIONS

- Foreign body is not dislodged or is partially dislodged but not removed.
  - Call for immediate assistance.
- Client vomits.
  - Suction client's airway using oral catheter (see Chapter 13).
  - Position client on side to reduce risk for aspiration.
- Foreign body is dislodged but enters lung.
  - Repeat one or all maneuvers, and stay with client.
  - Obtain assistance.
  - Monitor pulse and respiratory status. Ventilate client if respirations are absent. Begin CPR if client suffers cardiac arrest (see Skill 15-5).
  - Prepare equipment for physician to perform intubation or tracheotomy.

RECORDING AND REPORTING

- Record and report nursing progress notes, including precipitating event, if known; maneuver(s) performed; and result of maneuver(s) performed.
- Record and report vital signs, if taken, and other assessments (skin color; ability to speak, breathe, and talk) before and after FBAOMs.

TEACHING CONSIDERATIONS

- Instruct client and family in how to avoid obstruction by avoiding talking while eating and removing, modifying, or avoiding offending agent; instruct client and family in maneuvers should obstruction occur again.
- Ask client and family to state signs and symptoms of foreign body obstruction.
- Have client and family perform techniques on manikins or become certified in CPR and airway techniques. Observe for correct technique.

PEDIATRIC CONSIDERATIONS

- Tachypnea places child at risk for aspiration.
- Meat is most common cause of obstruction in adults, whereas many foods, toys, coins, and other foreign bodies cause obstruction in children.
- Not every child who gags or coughs while eating is truly choking. A child in distress cannot speak, becomes cyanotic, and collapses (Wong and others, 1999). If distress is manifested by wheezing, difficulty breathing, drooling or a croupy cough, obstruction is most likely due to swelling in airway or epiglot-

tis and not a foreign body. This is an emergency situation, and infant or child needs immediate medical attention.

- In all children and infants (and occasionally adults) be careful when using finger sweep not to force foreign body deeper into throat. Blind finger sweep is not to be performed in infants and children (AHA, 2000).
- Back blows only are recommended for infants (from birth to 1 year old), according to the AHA (2000).
- Infant, up to 1 year of age, is placed over rescuer's arm with head lower than trunk. Children, usually ages 1 to 8, can be draped across rescuer's thighs with rescuer kneeling on floor, or child can be held from behind with nurse's arms wrapped around child's abdomen (Wong and others, 1999) or placed on floor with rescuer in straddle position (Wong and others, 1999).

GERONTOLOGICAL CONSIDERATIONS

- Chest walls of older adults are less compliant. Improper technique of FBAOM may result in fractured rib(s) or xiphoid process or internal injury.
- Older adults often cannot chew food as well. They may also have impaired swallowing because of illness, such as senile dementia, stroke, or Parkinson's disease, and as a result their risk for choking increases.

Skill 15-2 Inserting a Nasal Airway

A **nasal airway** is a flexible curved piece of rubber or plastic with one wide or trumpetlike end flange and one narrow end that, once inserted, extends from the nares (remains external to the nose) past the sinuses to the pharynx (Figure 15-1, *A*).

The nasal airway varies in length (measured in centimeters or inches) and diameter (measured in millimeters). Some companies indicate nasal airway size by number (e.g., 5, 6, 7, 8, 9, or 10), others by grouping two or more numerical sizes into one nasal airway (e.g., small, medium, or large). In general, a small nasal airway corresponds to a 5- or 6-mm diameter nasal airway, a medium nasal airway corresponds to a 7- or 8-mm diameter nasal airway, and a large nasal airway corresponds to a 9- or 10-mm diameter nasal airway.

The nurse chooses the size of a nasal airway based on the size (ideal body weight), nasal structure, sex, and age of the client. To determine the correct length, measure from the tragus of the ear to the nostril and add 1 inch. The largest airway possible should be utilized.

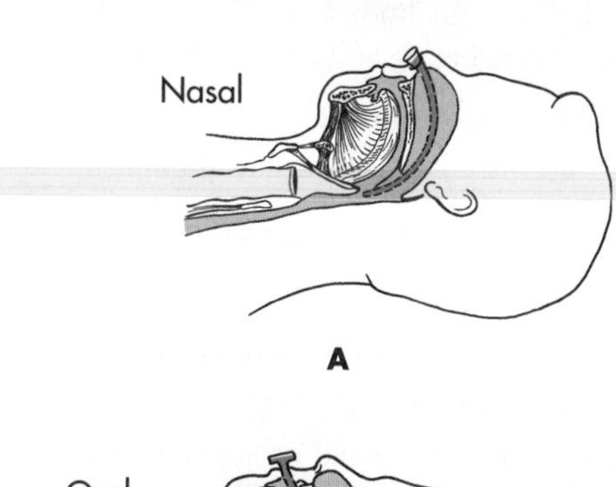

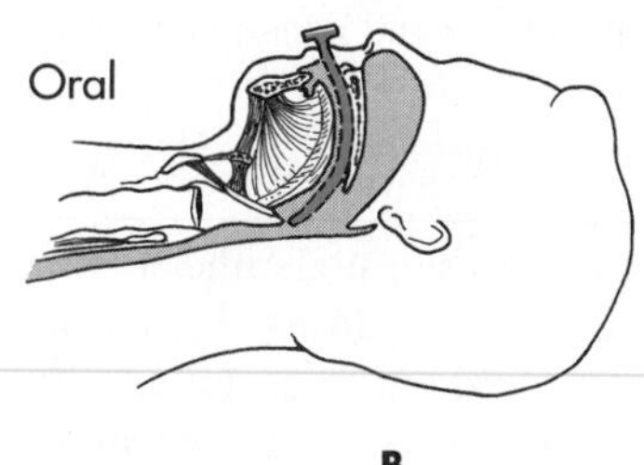

FIGURE 15-1 Placement of airways. **A,** Nasal. **B,** Oral.

DELEGATION CONSIDERATIONS

The skill of insertion of a nasal airway should not be delegated to assistive personnel.

EQUIPMENT

- Appropriate size nasal airway
- Nonsterile gloves
- Water-soluble lubricant
- Tissues
- Tape
- Appropriate suction equipment, if needed
- Face shield, if indicated

STEP	RATIONALE
ASSESSMENT	
1. Identify signs and symptoms of need to insert a nasal airway: frequent nasopharyngeal or nasotracheal suctioning, edematous nasal mucosa, and bleeding of nasal mucosa secondary to irritation from suctioning.	Clients with the following conditions are at greater risk for complication when nasal airway is inserted: chronic sinus infections or drainage, nasal fractures, spontaneous intranasal bleeding, deviated septum, and postoperative reconstructive nasal and facial surgery.

STEP	RATIONALE
2. Determine size of nasal airway to use:	Proper size ensures a patent airway and minimizes trauma to client.
a. Weight: (1) <100 lb: 5, 6, or small (20-24 French) (2) <100 to 150 lb: 7, 8, or medium (24-30 French) (3) >150 lb: 9, 10, or large (32-36 French)	
b. Gender: Males may use next larger size.	
3. Assess client's knowledge of procedure.	Identifies learning needs and can facilitate client's cooperation.

Nursing Diagnosis

Defining characteristics from the assessment data may reveal the following nursing diagnoses for clients requiring this skill:

- Ineffective airway clearance
- Impaired gas exchange
- Risk for infection
- Risk for impaired skin integrity
- Ineffective breathing pattern

Related factors are individualized based on client's condition or needs.

Planning

STEP	RATIONALE
1. **Expected outcomes** following completion of procedure:	
▪ Suctioning-induced nasal edema decreases, and bleeding diminishes immediately and ultimately stops.	Limited irritation results from insertion of nasal airway.
▪ Nasal air passage is patent.	Artificial airway maintains patency.
▪ Client is more cooperative to nasopharyngeal or nasotracheal suctioning.	Client is more comfortable because of decreased pain in nares from repeated suctioning; promotes ability to breathe more easily.
▪ No pressure area is evident on nares.	Prolonged use of nasal airway can result in pressure area around nares.
2. Explain reasons for insertion of airway and client's participation.	Relieves anxiety and encourages cooperation.
3. Help client assume comfortable position, usually semi-Fowler's.	Promotes client comfort.

Implementation

STEP	RATIONALE
1. Wash hands; put on gloves and face shield.	Reduces transmission of microorganisms.
2. Prepare nasal airway. Use principles of medical asepsis:	
a. Remove nasal airway from package; check for smooth edges.	Prevents insertion of damaged product that could produce further trauma.
b. Open water-soluble lubricant package; squeeze 10 to 15 ml of lubricant on nasal airway package or tissue.	Provides large surface area of lubricant with which to coat nasal airway.
c. Lubricate entire nasal airway, making sure narrow end is generously coated with lubricant.	Provides "slick" surface for insertion and prevents friction against dry mucous membranes, which causes trauma. Do not use a petroleum-based jelly. Non–water soluble lubricants can damage tissue lining of the nasal cavity and increase risk of infection.
3. Clean excess secretions from client's nares with tissues. Assess appropriate naris for insertion by alternately occluding each naris and asking client to inhale. If necessary, suction secretions (see Chapter 13).	Provides largest possible diameter airway for ease of insertion.

Step	Rationale
4. Holding nasal airway by wide end, insert it into naris using gentle inward and downward pressure until the trumpetlike end is at the naris.	Prevents trauma by following natural course of nasal structures.

- ***Critical Decision Point***
  Have client take slow deep breaths to ease insertion. If client gags, airway may be too large and different size should be selected.

Step	Rationale
5. Clean excess lubricant from client's face and nares.	Excess lubricant dries and acts as obstruction if not removed.
6. Secure airway if necessary (see Chapter 13 for taping endotracheal tube).	Prevents accidental removal and deeper penetration into nasal and pharyngeal structures.
7. Place client in comfortable position.	Promotes client comfort.
8. Remove gloves and face shield, and discard in appropriate receptacle. Wash hands.	Reduces transmission of microorganisms.
9. At least daily, remove nasal airway, clean in warm soapy water, and reinsert. Hydrogen peroxide can be used to remove crusts. Small brush is helpful to clean inner core of nasal airway. After cleansing, rinse nasal airway thoroughly.	Removes accumulated secretions and microorganisms. Nasal airway can obstruct drainage from sinuses; failure to remove and allow drainage can precipitate sinusitis.

- ***Critical Decision Point***
  Some institutions may require more frequent removal and alternating between nostrils.

Evaluation

1. Assess pressure points at end of flange.	Promotes early identification of impaired skin integrity.
2. Auscultate breath sounds.	Determines airway placement and effectiveness.
3. Observe nares over time to determine that previous edema and bleeding are diminished.	Airway reduces irritation from repeated NG or suction tube insertion.
4. Observe for patency of nasal airway.	Ensure airway is clear of mucous.
5. Assess client's respiratory status, and observe color, odor, consistency, and quantity of secretions.	Identifies client's response to insertion of nasal airway and/or removal of airway secretions.

Unexpected Outcomes and Related Interventions

- Nurse is unable to insert nasal airway.
  - Attempt to insert into other naris.
  - Use a smaller-size airway.
- Excessive edema or obstruction may be present.
  - Attempt to insert a smaller-size airway.
- Client begins to have nasal bleeding. Excessive epistaxis is dangerous in clients with hemophilia, active leukemia, aplastic anemia, or those on anticoagulant therapy.
  - Apply pressure over nasal pressure points for at least 5 to 10 minutes. Allows blood clotting system to form clot.
  - If bleeding continues, notify physician and follow instructions.
  - Monitor vital signs.
- Client complains of severe pain in ear and has fever.
  - Notify physician.
  - Assess external and internal ear.
- Client complains of headache (over sinuses) with or without fever. Nasal drainage becomes purulent.
  - Notify physician.
  - Palpate sinuses.

Recording and Reporting

- Record in nurses' progress notes:
  - Assessment finding for inserting nasal airway.
  - Size and site (right/left nares) of airway inserted.
  - Airway is in correct position; client's tolerance of procedure.
  - Secretions suctioned.
  - Method of securing (if done).
- Report the following in addition to what was recorded in progress notes:
  - Immediately report any respiratory distress.
  - Inability to remove secretions through airways.
  - Ear or headache pain.
  - Fever.

Pediatric Considerations

- Nasopharyngeal airways are more frequently used in young children and infants.

Gerontological Considerations

- In the older client mucosal membrane tissues are fragile and bleed easily. Gentle insertion is a must.

Skill 15-3 Inserting an Oropharyngeal Airway

An oropharyngeal airway is a semicircular-shaped, minimally flexible, curved piece of hard plastic (Figure 15-2). When inserted, it extends from just outside the lips, over the tongue, and to the pharynx (see Figure 15-1, *B*). **Oral airways** enable the nurse to suction through a central core or along the side of the airway, facilitate resuscitation, and maintain airway patency in the unconscious client. The airways facilitating resuscitation and maintaining airway patency in the unconscious client do not have a central core for suctioning.

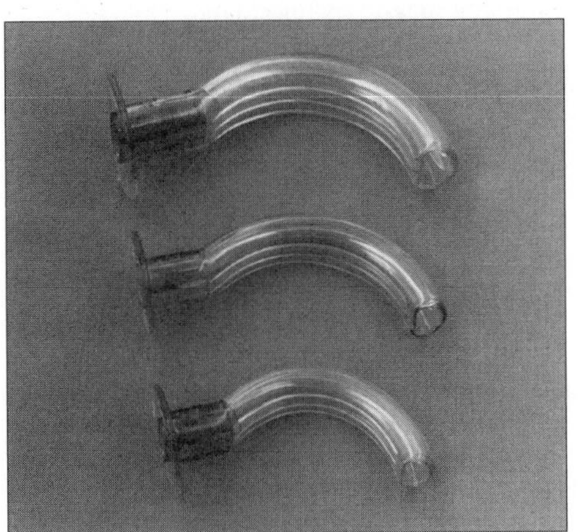

FIGURE **15-2** Oral airways.

The oral airway is sized for adults and children, varying in length and width. Pediatric sizes are 000, 00, 0, 1, 2, and 3. School-age children are usually size 3 or 4. Adult sizes are 4 through 10 or small, medium, and large. The nurse chooses the size of an oral airway based on the client's age and the width and length of the client's mouth. Size is correct if, when the flange is held parallel to the front teeth with the airway against the client's cheek, the end of the curve reaches the angle of the jaw. General size guidelines for choosing an oral airway for children are provided in Table 15-1.

Table 15-1 Oral Airway Guidelines for Size by Age

Size	Age
000	Premature neonates
00	Newborn
0	Newborn to 1 yr
1	1 to 2 yr
2	2 to 6 yr
3	6 to 18 yr
4 and larger	≥18 yr

Delegation Considerations

The skill of inserting an oropharyngeal airway should not be delegated to assistive personnel. When assistive personnel care for clients with an oropharyngeal airway, the care provider must be instructed to recognize and report signs of airway distress.

Equipment

- Appropriate-size oral airway
- Nonsterile gloves
- Tissues or washcloths
- Suction equipment, if indicated
- Tape (optional)
- Face shield, if indicated
- Tongue blade

Step	Rationale
Assessment	
1. Identify need to insert oral airway. Signs and symptoms include upper airway "gurgling" with respiratory cycle, no gag reflex, increased oral secretions or excretions, excessive drooling, grinding teeth, clenched teeth, biting of oral tracheal or gastric tubes, labored respirations, and increased respiratory rate.	These conditions place clients at risk for obstruction of upper airway. This airway is only used with unconscious client because in conscious client the gag reflex causes vomiting or retching when something is placed in pharynx.
2. Determine factors that normally influence upper airway functioning, such as age (children have a proportionally larger tongue), presence of nasal and oral airway, and drainage tubes (swallowing is more difficult with tubes in place).	Allows nurse to accurately assess need for oral airway. Clients at greater risk for upper airway obstruction are infants, children, and adults with cold and flu, loss of consciousness, seizure disorders, neuromuscular diseases, increased oral secretions or excretions, or facial trauma.

STEP	RATIONALE
3. Assess for presence of gag reflex; gently place tongue blade on back of client's tongue.	Provides guide as to when oral airway can be safely removed in postoperative client.

- ***Critical Decision Point***
  Never insert an oropharyngeal airway in a conscious client or a client with recent oral trauma, oral surgery, or loose teeth.

4. Assess client's and family's knowledge of procedure.	Identifies learning needs and facilitates client's cooperation with procedure.

NURSING DIAGNOSIS

Defining characteristics from the assessment data may reveal the following nursing diagnoses for clients requiring this skill:

Ineffective airway clearance
Risk for aspiration
Ineffective breathing pattern
Impaired gas exchange
Risk for infection

Related factors are individualized based on client's condition or needs.

PLANNING

1. **Expected outcomes** following completion of procedure:	
▪ Client's respiratory status improves, as evidenced by easier respirations with normal rate, easier removal of secretions, and lack of gurgling noise in throat with respirations.	Airway is cleared of secretions.
▪ Client is not able to grind teeth or bite tubes.	Oral airway prevents tooth contact with other teeth or with tubes.
▪ Client tongue does not relax back into pharynx and obstruct airway.	Oral airway keeps tongue in correct position to maintain patent airway.
2. Position client; semi-Fowler's position is preferred.	Promotes client comfort and provides easy access to oral cavity.

IMPLEMENTATION

1. Wash hands and apply nonsterile gloves and face shield (when possible).	Reduces transmission of microorganisms.
2. Whenever possible use padded tongue blade to open client's mouth; if necessary, use thumb and forefinger of nondominant hand to pry jaws and teeth apart.	Provides access to oral cavity.
3. Insert oral airway:	When inserting airway, take care not to push client's tongue into pharynx.
a. Hold oral airway with curved end up, insert distal end until airway reaches back of throat, then turn airway over 180 degrees and follow natural curve of tongue. Nurse may also hold airway sideways, insert halfway, and then rotate airway 90 degrees while gliding it over natural curvature of tongue. Outer flange should be just outside client's lips.	Provides patent airway and prevents displacement of client's tongue into posterior oropharynx.

- ***Critical Decision Point***
  In some clients it may be possible to depress tongue with tongue blade and inset airway with tip pointing down, sliding it over tongue.

STEP	RATIONALE
4. Secure with tape if client attempts to push out with tongue.	Prevents expulsion of airway. Taping an airway in place can limit client's ability to expel vomitus.
5. Suction secretions, as needed.	Removes secretions; maintains patent airway.
6. Reassess client's respiratory status.	Directs nurse to initiate intervention.
7. Clean client's face with soft tissue or washcloth.	Promotes hygiene.
8. Discard tissue into appropriate receptacle, place washcloth in dirty or soiled linen bag, remove gloves and face shield, and discard in appropriate receptacle; wash hands.	Reduces transmission of microorganisms.
9. Administer mouth care frequently.	Increases client comfort and removes debris. It also provides moisture to oral mucosal tissues.

- ***Critical Decision Point***

  Do not use lemon glycerin swabs for oral care because they are drying to mucosal tissues and promote bacterial growth. Oral airway may also need to be removed, cleaned, and reinserted in clients with a lot of oral mucous secretions. If secretions are left in place, they could occlude oral airway.

EVALUATION

1. Observe client's respiratory status, and compare respiratory assessments before and after insertion of oral airway.	Identifies client's response to insertion of airway.
2. Assess that airway is patent, that client does not occlude airway by biting tube, and that client's tongue does not obstruct airway.	Ensures oxygen delivery to client.

UNEXPECTED OUTCOMES AND RELATED INTERVENTIONS

- Client continually coughs and gags when airway is inserted.
  - Do not continue inserting airway if client begins to gag. Stimulation of gag reflex can cause vomiting and risk of aspiration.
  - Remove oral airway, and position client on side. Replace with smaller-size airway.
  - Assess need for airway.
- Airway obstruction not relieved.
  - Obtain immediate assistance.
  - Reinsert airway.
- Client pushes airway out of place or out of mouth.
  - Airway may not be properly secured.
  - Reassess client's need for oral airway.
- Nurse is unable to insert oral airway in client; client may be combative, or nurse may be unable to pry mouth open.
  - Obtain assistance.
  - Reassess client's need for oral airway.

RECORDING AND REPORTING

- Record in nurses' progress notes:
  - Assessment finding while inserting oral airway
  - Size of oral airway
  - Placement
  - Other procedures performed at same time, especially positioning, secretions obtained
  - Client's tolerance of procedure
- Report in addition to material recorded:
  - Respiratory distress
  - Vomiting
  - Pain

TEACHING CONSIDERATIONS

- Instruct family members in proper cleaning techniques. Observe their technique for adequacy.

PEDIATRIC CONSIDERATIONS

- Oral airways are seldom utilized in treatment of airway obstruction in children and infants. Due to narrowness of child's airway, oral airways are often more occlusive than beneficial (Wong and others, 1999).
- For infants and children the preferred method for inserting airway is with tip pointing to roof of mouth.

Skill 15-4 Using an Ambu-bag

"Ambu" stands for "air mask bag unit" (Figure 15-3). Many health professionals think of an **Ambu-bag** as being used only in emergency situations such as cardiopulmonary arrest, but it has many other uses. The Ambu-bag is important for providing manual hyperinflation of the lungs before and following suctioning secretions from the respiratory tract. Its use is also necessary in the transportation of ventilator-dependent clients between hospital areas.

An Ambu-bag has the following components: a mask, an endotracheal or tracheostomy tube adapter, a large reservoir or "bag," an oxygen adapter and sometimes reservoir tubing to increase oxygen concentration, and a valve or spring system to control air flow. Bags are available in infant, child, and adult models to deliver inhaled volumes of 240 to 2000 ml per breath, depending on the manufacturer.

Ambu-bags are not difficult to use. The mask is firmly placed over the client's nose and mouth to create a seal or is connected to the endotracheal or tracheostomy tube with the adapter. The reservoir is compressed with two hands, forcing air into the airways. Larger volumes are attained when using two hands, and as a result the client receives an adequate volume of air. When the bag is released, it self-inflates, ready for the next breath. It is usually necessary to attach the Ambu-bag to supplemental oxygen. Without this supplemental oxygen, the client receives ambient air.

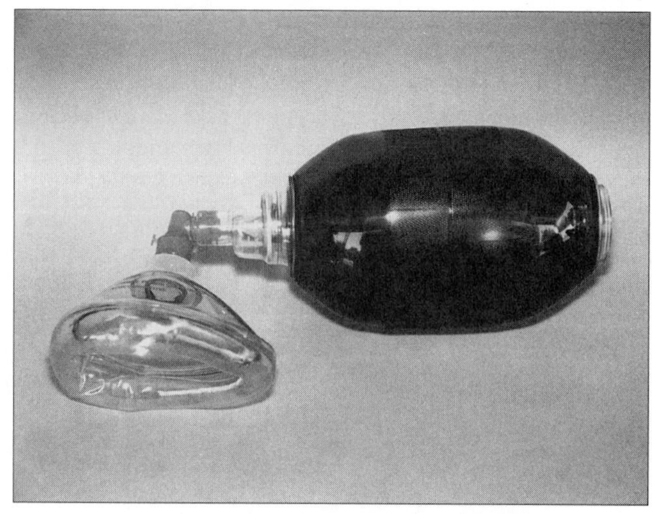

FIGURE **15-3** Ambu-bag.

Delegation Considerations

The skill of using an Ambu-bag should not be delegated to assistive personnel.

Equipment

- Two nonsterile gloves
- Ambu-bag with mask for nonintubated client or Ambu-bag with endotracheal (ET) or tracheal tube adapter for intubated clients; 15-mm Ambu-bag adapter must be obtained for most metal and silastic tracheostomy tubes
- Oxygen supply tubing and oxygen source, if needed
- Oral, nasotracheal, endotracheal, or tracheostomy suctioning apparatus
- Face shield, if indicated

Step	Rationale
Assessment	
1. Identify need to use Ambu-bag manual ventilator. Signs and symptoms of need for manual ventilatory assistance include diminished or absent respirations or pulse; apneic periods; cyanosis; acutely elevated $PaCO_2$; acutely decreased PaO_2, "bucking" or fighting mechanical ventilator; elevated intracranial pressure; thick, tenacious sputum; suctioning mucous plugs; and cardiopulmonary arrest.	Certain conditions place client at risk for needing Ambu-bag manual ventilatory assistance. Clients at greater risk of needing Ambu-bag are those with pneumonia, seizure or sleep apnea disorders, multiple trauma, cardiopulmonary arrest, sudden infant death syndrome, drug overdose, and neurological injury. Also at risk is ventilator-dependent client needing transportation to another hospital area.
2. Factors that affect respiratory drive include level of consciousness (LOC), neurological injury or central nervous system tumor, poor gas exchange (metabolic or respiratory alkalosis or acidosis), direct pulmonary injury, metabolic rate, and psychosocial factors.	Nurse is able to accurately assess need to provide Ambu-bag manual ventilation.

STEP	RATIONALE
3. In alert client, determine knowledge of procedure or determine caregiver knowledge of procedure (for home administration).	Identifies learning needs and opportunity for teaching.

NURSING DIAGNOSIS

Defining characteristics from the assessment data may reveal the following nursing diagnoses for clients requiring this skill:

- Ineffective airway clearance
- Ineffective breathing pattern
- Impaired gas exchange
- Impaired spontaneous ventilation

Related factors are individualized based on client's condition or needs.

PLANNING

STEP	RATIONALE
1. **Expected outcomes** following completion of procedure:	
▪ Improved vital signs and LOC and, when appropriate, intracranial pressure is decreased as evidenced by pressure waves and digital readout.	Ambu-bag manual ventilatory assistance was successful.
▪ Secretions are loosened and easier to remove as evidenced by improved respiratory rate, secretions or mucous plugs suctioned from large airways, clearing breath sounds, and decrease in restlessness.	Ambu-bag manual ventilatory assistance was successful.
▪ Arterial blood gas levels are improved in respiratory or cardiopulmonary arrest, during transportation, and after seizures and apneic episodes.	Ambu-bag manual ventilatory assistance restores more optimal oxygenation.
2. Explain procedure and client's participation.	Encourages cooperation and minimizes risks.
3. Position client comfortably.	Promotes client comfort, prevents strain on nurse.

IMPLEMENTATION

STEP	RATIONALE
1. If not emergency situation (e.g., cardiopulmonary arrest), wash hands and apply gloves and face shield.	Reduces transmission of microorganisms.
2. Prepare suction apparatus, if needed.	Readies equipment for use.
3. Connect oxygen supply tubing to Ambu-bag and oxygen flow meter. Adjust oxygen flow meter to ordered F_IO_2 or 100% F_IO_2, if indicated.	Provides supplemental oxygen. A high flow rate or "flush" position is necessary to meet **minute ventilation** needs of client.
4. If client is intubated and normal saline lavage is ordered to facilitate secretion removal:	
a. Remove oxygen delivery device.	Prepares artificial airway for hyperinflation with Ambu-bag.
b. Instill 5 to 10 ml sterile normal saline during inspiration.	Normal saline stimulates cough, which loosens secretions.
c. Connect Ambu-bag to artificial airway and administer one breath every 3 to 5 seconds to hyperventilate by compressing Ambu-bag with two hands.	Increases PaO_2 and decreases $PaCO_2$ before suctioning.
d. Suction client. Repeat the preceding step as needed.	Removes secretions. Normal saline instillation should not be routinely performed as part of suctioning. It does not liquefy secretions, may cause decreases in arterial oxygen saturation, and may also contribute to bacterial contamination of client's airway.
5. If client is unconscious and not intubated:	
a. Insert oropharyngeal airway.	Helps maintain airway patency.
b. If not contraindicated, tilt head using chin-lift maneuver.	Opens airway, facilitates ventilation, and reduces amount of air entering client's stomach.

Step	Rationale
c. Place Ambu-bag mask over client's nose and mouth. Maintain head in tilted position with last two fingers of nondominant hand. Apply pressure with remaining fingers and thumb to seal mask in place.	Correct placement of mask forms an occlusive seal for proper ventilation. Bag-mask ventilation requires two people. One person should provide a good seal with mask to face. Second provider ventilates, compressing Ambu-bag with two hands.
d. Second caregiver compresses bag. Administer breaths according to cardiopulmonary resuscitation (CPR) protocol.	Avoids hypocapnia (low $PaCO_2$) and hypercapnia (elevated $PaCO_2$). Provides adequate ventilation.

- ***Critical Decision Point***
  If chest fails to rise, reposition mask, make a firm seal, and compress bag again.

Step	Rationale
e. Be prepared to suction client as indicated. Client may need nasogastric tube insertion.	Pulmonary secretions may be loosened. Client may vomit if too much air is swallowed.
6. Assess client throughout procedure. Continue to "bag" client until assessment indicates it is no longer necessary, such as:	
a. Increased blood pressure; improved color, vital signs, and level consciousness; decreased coughing.	Provides supplemental ventilation and oxygenation. Assesses cardiopulmonary and neurological status.
b. Presence of spontaneous respirations	
c. Decreased intracranial pressure (ICP)	
7. Repeat Steps 4 through 6 as needed. Then remove bag, and replace oxygen delivery device.	Restores supplemental oxygen.
8. Turn off oxygen flow to Ambu-bag. Disconnect bag from oxygen tubing, if indicated. Some institutions leave bag connected to oxygen source at all times.	Discontinues oxygen supply to bag.
9. Reposition client.	Promotes comfort.
10. Remove "elbow" that connects bag to ET tube, tracheostomy tube, or mask, if able, and wash in warm soapy water. Shake off excess water and allow to dry. (Use of a towel to dry may leave unwanted particles.) When dry, reconnect mask or elbow to Ambu-bag.	Reduces transmission of microorganisms.
11. Remove gloves and face shield, and dispose of in proper receptacle. Wash hands.	Reduces transmission of microorganisms.

Evaluation

Step	Rationale
1. Monitor vital signs, oxygen saturation, and other physiological parameters, and compare assessments before and after Ambu-bag use.	Documents client's response to Ambu-bag procedure.
2. Observe that client's chest expands with each Ambu-bag ventilation.	Documents patent airway and that client is receiving ventilated breaths.
3. Observe the amount, quality, and consistency of suctioned secretions.	
4. If instructing caregivers, provide for return demonstration of technique.	Correctly performing technique independently is a reliable method of evaluating learning.

Unexpected Outcomes and Related Interventions

- Client becomes acidotic/hypercapnic:
  - Intubation and continuous ventilation needed.
  - Ventilator rate/tidal volume must be increased.
  - Client needs additional supplemental oxygen.
  - Inform physician.
- Client becomes alkalotic/hypocapnic:
  - Decrease volume/rate of bagging.
  - Observe for rebound hypoventilation.
  - Inform physician.

RECORDING AND REPORTING

- Chart in nurses' progress notes:
  - Assessments before and after bagging
  - Rate and volume of bagging
  - Amount of normal saline lavage, if used
  - Amount of supplemental oxygen used
  - Client's tolerance of procedure
  - Secretions suctioned (quality and quantity)
- Report the following in addition to material in nurses' notes:
  - Report any changes in client's vital signs and level of consciousness to physician or nurse in charge.

TEACHING CONSIDERATIONS

- Demonstrate techniques of bagging to caregivers. Allow time for practice on manikin.
- Assess for proper technique in administering procedure and cleaning equipment.

PEDIATRIC CONSIDERATIONS

- Infant and pediatric Ambu-bags are designed to provide tight seal and to deliver appropriate air volumes. Use of adult bag for infant or child is inappropriate.

GERONTOLOGICAL CONSIDERATIONS

- For older clients who are edentulous a tight seal may be difficult to obtain and sustain. For such clients the use of two caregivers, one to maintain seal and second to compress bag, is desirable.

Skill 15-5 Performing Cardiopulmonary Resuscitation

Cardiopulmonary arrest can occur at any time. It is characterized by an absence of pulse or respirations (**respiratory arrest** is the more common in children). If the nurse determines that the client has experienced cardiac arrest, **cardiopulmonary resuscitation (CPR)** must be initiated. Cardiopulmonary resuscitation is a basic emergency procedure for life support, consisting of artificial respiration and manual external cardiac massage. Cardiopulmonary resuscitation has three main goals, called the ABCs of cardiopulmonary resuscitation: establish an *A*irway, initiate *B*reathing, and maintain *C*irculation. When a cardiopulmonary arrest occurs, oxygen is not delivered to the tissues, carbon dioxide is not transported from the tissues, tissue metabolism becomes anaerobic, and metabolic and respiratory acidosis occurs. Tissue damage, including permanent heart and brain damage, occurs within 6 minutes. In a respiratory arrest, cessation of respiration occurs; the pulse often remains present for up to approximately 6 minutes.

Once it is determined that a respiratory or cardiac arrest has occurred, the nurse must quickly provide a patent airway by removing any obvious foreign body obstruction (see Skill 15-1), removing airway secretions (Chapter 13), inserting an oral airway (see Skill 15-3), and performing the jaw-thrust technique or hyperextending the neck as detailed in this skill.

The initiation of breathing is achieved by one of two methods. First, if immediately available, the nurse can use an Ambu-bag manual ventilator (see Skill 15-4). Second, the nurse can initiate mouth-to-mouth artificial ventilation as described in this skill. Cardiopulmonary mouth-to-mask devices are transparent masks with or without a one-way valve used to deliver artificial breaths via the mouth-to-mask technique (American Heart Association [AHA], 2000). These devices protect the nurse from the client's secretions during rescue breathing. These devices also promote more effective respirations by maintaining a better seal.

The maintenance of circulation is achieved by external cardiac compression. Three elements must be present to ensure safe and efficient cardiac massage. First, the client's spine must be supported during compression by placing the client on a hard surface such as a board or the floor. Second, sternal pressure must be forceful but not traumatic (Lewis and others, 2000). Third, to be safe and efficient, the nurse must have proper hand placement for compression.

DELEGATION CONSIDERATIONS

The skill of cardiopulmonary resuscitation can be performed by assistive personnel who are certified in basic life support techniques. The care provider should be cautioned to make certain the client is indeed pulseless before initiating chest compressions. The procedures for opening the airway should be reviewed with the care provider if the client has any risk for cervical neck trauma.

EQUIPMENT

- Ambu-bag, if available
- CPR mouth-to-mask device, if available
- Supplemental oxygen, if available
- Chest compression board, if available
- Gloves, if available
- Resuscitation cart, if available
- Face shield, if available

STEP	RATIONALE

ASSESSMENT

1. Determine if client is unconscious by shaking client and shouting "Are you OK?" — Confirms that client is unconscious as opposed to intoxicated, sleeping, or hearing impaired. Unconsciousness can be caused by substance abuse, hypoglycemia, ketoacidosis, and shock.

- ***Critical Decision Point***
  If unconscious person has adequate respirations and pulse, remain until further assistance is present. Place victim in recovery position. Continue to determine presence of respirations and pulse because respiratory or cardiopulmonary arrest is still possible.

2. Immediately activate emergency medical services (EMS) for adult client. If alone do CPR on infant or child for 1 minute, then activate EMS. — The majority of adult victims are in ventricular fibrillation and need defibrillation and dysrhythmic drugs as soon as possible.
3. Determine breathlessness and carotid or brachial (use with infants) pulse. — Presence of pulse and respirations contraindicates initiation of CPR.
   a. To determine breathlessness, open airway using head tilt–chin lift or jaw-thrust maneuver. Look, listen, and feel for exchange of air (AHA, 2000). — Tongue is most common cause of airway obstruction. Using these measures to open airway may alleviate cause of breathlessness.

NURSING DIAGNOSIS

Defining characteristics from the assessment data may reveal the following nursing diagnoses for clients requiring this skill:

Ineffective breathing pattern
Decreased cardiac output
Impaired gas exchange
Impaired spontaneous ventilation

Related factors are individualized based on client's condition or needs.

PLANNING

1. Call for assistance, seek help from passersby, or call for additional nurses. — One person cannot maintain CPR indefinitely. Without relief, rescuer fatigues, chest compressions are ineffective, and volume of air ventilated into victim's lungs decreases.
2. **Expected outcomes** following completion of procedure:
   - Client regains pulse and respirations. — CPR was successful.
   - Physician may terminate CPR. — Decision result of irreversible brain or cardiac damage or knowledge of advance directive.

IMPLEMENTATION

1. Place victim on hard surface such as floor, ground, or backboard. Victim must be flat. If necessary, logroll victim to flat, supine position using spine precautions. — External compression of heart is facilitated. Heart is compressed between sternum and spinal vertebrae, which must be on hard and firm surface.
2. Assume correct and comfortable position. — Nurse may be administering CPR for extended period, particularly in community setting. Correct, comfortable position decreases skeletal muscle fatigue and promotes more effective compressions.
   a. One-person rescuer:
      (1) Position to face victim, on knees, parallel to victim's sternum. — Allows rescuer to quickly move back and forth from victim's mouth to sternum.

STEP	RATIONALE
b. Two-person rescuer:	
(1) One person faces victim, kneeling parallel to victim's head. Second person moves to opposite side and faces victim, kneels parallel to victim's sternum.	Allows one rescuer to maintain breathing while other maintains circulation, without getting in each other's way.
3. If available, apply gloves and face shield.	Reduces transmission of microorganisms.
4. Open airway:	
a. If no head or neck trauma, use **head tilt–chin lift** method (AHA, 2000) (see illustration).	Spinal cord injury should be suspected with motor vehicle accident, falls, face or head injury or laceration, diving accident, or football or other contact sports injury. In these situations rescuer must use jaw-thrust maneuver. Tongue is most common cause of airway obstruction in unconscious client. Airway obstruction from tongue is relieved. If necessary, remove foreign body (see Skill 15-1).
b. Jaw-thrust maneuver (see illustration) can be used by health professionals but is not taught to general public. Grasp angles of victim's lower jaw and lift with both hands, displacing mandible forward while tilting head backward.	When head and/or neck trauma is suspected, this maneuver opens airway while maintaining proper head and neck alignment, thus reducing risk of further damage to neck.

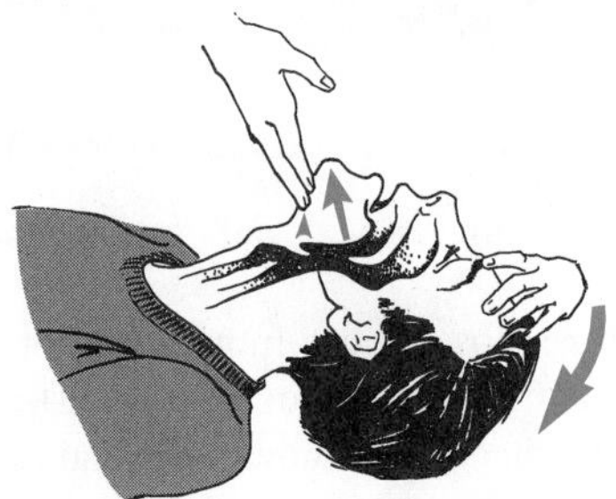

STEP **4a** Head tilt-chin lift.

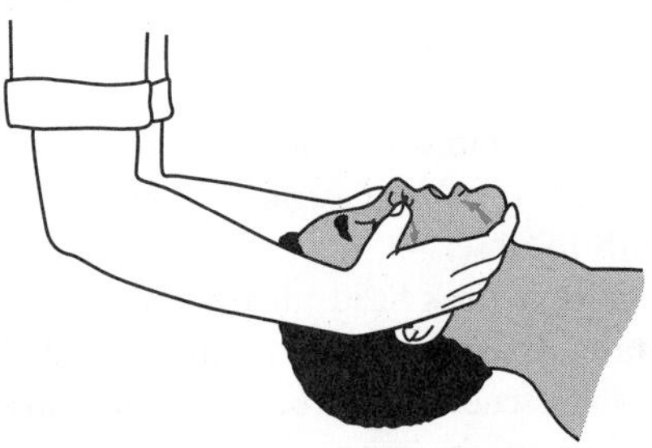

STEP **4b** Jaw thrust without head tilt.

STEP	RATIONALE
5. If readily available, insert oral airway (see Skill 15-3).	Maintains tongue on anterior floor of mouth and prevents obstruction of posterior airway by tongue.
6. If victim does not resume breathing, administer artificial respiration:	Airtight seal is formed, and air is prevented from escaping through nose.
a. Mouth-to-mouth:	

• ***Critical Decision Point***

Cardiopulmonary resuscitation pocket masks with one-way valves are available as required by Occupational Safety and Health Administration (OSHA) guidelines (Occupational Health and Safety Act, 1992). Oral airways are readily available in hospital and extended care and outpatient settings. However, they are not available in all community settings. Cardiopulmonary resuscitation can effectively be accomplished without oral airway or CPR pocket mask. However, rescuer must take appropriate measures to reduce transmission of infectious agents (e.g., hepatitis B, human immunodeficiency virus [HIV], herpes virus, tuberculosis) as proposed by Centers for Disease Control and Prevention (1989).

Adult

STEP	RATIONALE
(1) Pinch victim's nose with thumb and index fingers, and occlude mouth with nurse's mouth or use CPR pocket mask. Maintain head tilt–chin lift while administering breaths so air enters lungs and not stomach. Blow two slow full breaths into victim's mouth (each breath should take $1\frac{1}{2}$ to 2 seconds); allow victim to exhale between breaths. Continue giving 12 breaths per minute (AHA, 2000).	Hyperventilation is promoted and assists in maintaining adequate blood oxygen levels. In most adults this volume is 800 to 1200 ml and is sufficient to make chest rise. Rescuer should take a breath after each ventilation; this maximizes oxygen content and minimizes carbon dioxide concentration in delivered breaths (AHA, 2000).

STEP | RATIONALE

• ***Critical Decision Point***

An excess of air volume and fast inspiratory flow rates are likely to cause pharyngeal pressures that exceed esophageal opening pressures, allowing air to enter stomach and result in gastric distention, thereby increasing risk of vomiting and compromised respiration.

Child

(1) Place nurse's mouth over child's mouth (see illustration) or use CPR pocket mask. For mouth-to-mouth resuscitation of child, administer two slow breaths lasting 1 to 1½ seconds with a pause between. Continue giving 20 breaths per minute (AHA, 2000).

Airtight seal is formed, and air is prevented from escaping from nose.

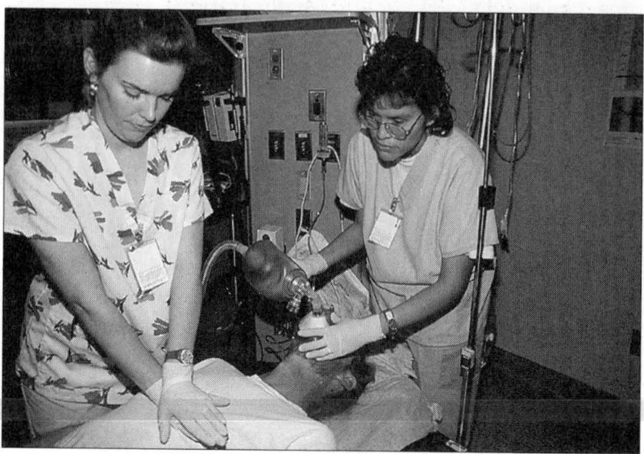

STEP **6c(1)** Two-rescuer breathing with Ambu-bag.

Infant

(1) Because infant's air passages are smaller and resistance to flow is quite high, making recommendations about force or volume of rescue breaths is difficult. Place nurse's mouth over infant's nose and mouth. However, three factors should be remembered: (1) rescue breaths are single most important maneuver in assisting nonbreathing child, (2) an appropriate volume is one that makes chest rise and fall, and (3) slow breaths provide an adequate volume at lowest possible pressure, thereby reducing risk of gastric distention.

b. Mouth-to-nose:

(1) Keep victim's head tilted with one hand on forehead. Use other hand to lift jaw and close mouth. Seal rescuer's lips around victim's nose and blow. Allow passive exhalation.

In some victims (those whose mouth cannot be opened or whose jaws or mouth is seriously injured) mouth to nose can be a more effective method of ventilation.

• ***Critical Decision Point***

It may be necessary to open victim's mouth on occasion to allow trapped exhaled air to escape.

c. Ambu-bag:

Adult and Child

(1) For Ambu-bag resuscitation use proper size face mask and apply it under chin, up and over victim's mouth and nose (see illustration).

Airtight seal is formed; as bag is compressed, oxygen enters client. Rescuer must squeeze bag fully to deliver 400 to 600 ml of air with supplemental oxygen or 700 ml of air without supplemental oxygen (AHA, 2000). This avoids overinflation and erroneous gastric inflation.

(2) Observe for rise and fall of chest wall with each respiration. Listen for air escaping during exhalation and feel for flow of air. If lungs do not inflate, reposition head and neck and check for visible airway obstruction, such as vomitus.

Repositioning ensures airway is properly opened and that artificial respirations are entering lungs.

7. Suction secretions if necessary, or turn victim's head to one side, unless contraindicated.

Suctioning prevents airway obstruction. Turning client's head to one side allows gravity to drain secretions.

8. Check for presence of carotid (adults/children) or brachial (infants) pulse after restoring breathing. Check pulse for 5 to 10 seconds.

Carotid artery pulse is most easily accessible and persists when other peripheral pulses are no longer palpable. Makes certain assessment is long enough to thoroughly assess absence of pulse. Following respiratory arrest pulse may be very slow and weak. Brachial pulse is most accessible and accurate pulse site in infant.

Performing external cardiac compressions on victim who has a pulse may result in serious medical complications.

STEP	RATIONALE

• ***Critical Decision Point***

In the nonintubated victim in acute care setting it may be possible to utilize two rescue breathers with Ambu-bag. In this case one rescuer maintains seal, and other utilizes two hands to compress bag, thus delivering greater volumes.

9. If pulse is absent, initiate chest compressions:

Places hands and fingers over heart in proper position. Prevents xiphoid process and rib fracture, which can further compromise cardiopulmonary status.

a. Assume correct hand position:

Adult

(1) Place hands over lower half of sternum, being careful to avoid xiphoid process on sternum. Keep hands parallel to chest and fingers above chest. Interlocking fingers is helpful. Keep fingers off chest wall. Extend arms and lock elbows. Maintain arms straight and shoulders directly over victim's sternum (see illustration).

It is critical to keep hands off xiphoid process by marking that area with two fingers of one hand and then placing heel of other hand next to them. Hand marking xiphoid process can then be moved and placed on top of other hand.

Child

(1) Place heel of one hand on lower half of sternum above xiphoid process (see illustration). Maintain head tilt with other hand, if possible.

Proper placement ensures heart compression, maintains patent airway.

Infant

(1) Place index and middle fingers of one hand on lower half of sternum above xiphoid process. Fingers should be 1 cm below nipple line and perpendicular to sternum and not slanted (see illustration).

Finger placement prevents abdominal injury.

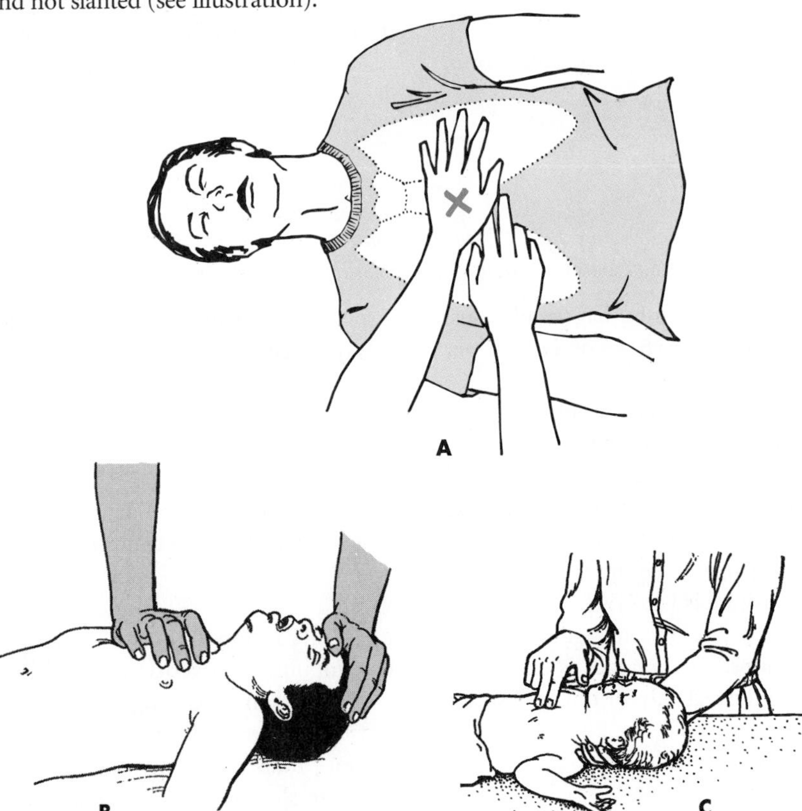

STEP **9a(1)** **A,** Proper hand position—adult. **B,** Proper hand position—child. **C,** Proper hand position—infant.

STEP	RATIONALE

(2) An alternative technique is to place both thumbs side by side over lower half of sternum about xiphoid process.

- ***Critical Decision Point***
  Ensure fingers are off ribs.

b. Compress sternum to proper depth from shoulders and then release pressure, maintaining contact with skin to ensure ongoing proper placement of hands. Do not rock, but transmit weight vertically down.

Compression occurs only on sternum and is meant to squeeze heart between sternum and spine. Pressure necessary for external compression is created by nurse's upper arm muscle strength and upper body. When compression is released, heart fills.

(1) Adult and adolescent: 4 to 5 cm ($1\frac{1}{2}$ to 2 inches) (see illustration)
(2) Older child: 3 to 4 cm (1 to $1\frac{1}{2}$ inches)
(3) Toddler and preschooler: 2 to 4 cm ($\frac{3}{4}$ to $1\frac{1}{2}$ inches)
(4) Infant: 1 to 2 cm ($\frac{1}{2}$ to 1 inch)

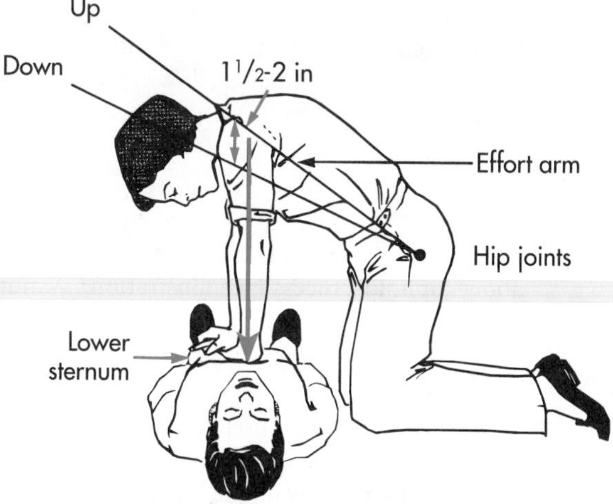

STEP **9b(1)** Compression occurs only on sternum. Pressure necessary for external compression is created by nurse's upper arm muscle strength.

c. Maintain proper rate of compression:
- Adult and adolescent: 80 to 100 per minute (count "one 1000; two 1000")
- Child: at least 100 per minute
- Infant: at least 100 per minute

Proper number of compressions per minute should be delivered to ensure adequate **cardiac output.**

- ***Critical Decision Point***
  Ratio of compressions to breaths in adult CPR for both one rescuer and two rescuers is 15 to 2. Infant and child CPR is performed at a ratio of 5 compressions to 1 breath.

d. Continue mouth-to-mouth or Ambu-bag ventilations:
- Adult and adolescent: every 5 seconds (12 per minute)
- Older child: every 4 seconds (15 per minute)
- Child: every 3 seconds (20 per minute)
- Infant and toddler: every 3 seconds (20 per minute)

Promotes adequate ventilations to excrete waste gas and supply oxygen.

10. Palpate for carotid or brachial pulse with each external chest compression for first full minute (two-person rescue). If carotid pulse is not palpable, compressions are not strong enough or hand position is incorrect.

Assessment of pulse validates that adequate stroke volume is achieved with each compression.

11. Continue CPR until relieved, until victim regains spontaneous pulse and respirations, until rescuer is exhausted and unable to perform CPR effectively, or until physician discontinues CPR.

Artificial cardiopulmonary function is maintained.
Cardiopulmonary resuscitation is interrupted when changing CPR personnel, during defibrillation, or when transporting victim. During intubation, CPR may be interrupted for more than 5 seconds but should not exceed 30 seconds. Nurse should remind rescue team of number of seconds elapsing during intubation.

STEP	RATIONALE
12. Remove and discard into appropriate receptacle: gloves, face shield, and pocket mask.	Reduces transmission of microorganisms.

EVALUATION

1. Palpate carotid pulse at least every 5 minutes after first minute of CPR.	Documents adequacy of external cardiac compressions.
2. Observe for spontaneous return of respirations or heart rate.	Performance of CPR on client with a pulse is dangerous.
3. Cardiopulmonary resuscitation is not interrupted for more than 5 seconds.	Maintains adequacy of oxygenation and circulation.

UNEXPECTED OUTCOMES AND RELATED INTERVENTIONS

- Client develops skeletal injury, such as fractured ribs or sternum, or internal organ injury, such as lacerated lung or liver.
  - Obtain appropriate diagnostic tests to document rib fracture.
  - Assess client's postarrest breathing for symmetry and pain.
  - Observe for hemoptysis or gastrointestinal bleeding.
  - Observe for distending abdomen.
- Client's CPR is unsuccessful.
  - Contact chaplain services.
  - Contact social worker.
  - Complete postmortem care on client (see Chapter 43).
  - Provide for privacy for client's family to say their good-byes to client.
- Rescuer is unassisted, tires, and is unable to continue.
  - Obtain assistance.

RECORDING AND REPORTING

- Immediately report arrest indicating exact location of victim.
  - In hospital setting, follow hospital policy. In community setting, dial 911 or other emergency number.
- Record in nurses' notes onset of arrest, medication given, procedures performed, and victim's response.

TEACHING CONSIDERATIONS

- If client is at risk for cardiopulmonary arrest, the family or caregivers should be instructed and certified in CPR by certified instructor from institution, American Red Cross, or American Heart Association.
- Client and family should keep emergency numbers taped to phone. These numbers may include fire department, ambulance, hospital, and physician. Instruct client and family whom to call. Family may also need to know what to do when client is found "deceased."
- It is extremely helpful if family has list of medications client is presently taking.

PEDIATRIC CONSIDERATIONS

- All persons involved in administering CPR must understand different breathing/compression ratios, hand (fingers) placement, and depth of compression in children and infants compared with adults.
- Infants and children experience only respiratory arrest much more frequently than full cardiopulmonary arrest.

GERONTOLOGICAL CONSIDERATIONS

- In older adult compressions often result in rib or cartilage fractures. Cardiopulmonary resuscitation should be continued.

HOME CARE CONSIDERATIONS

- In community setting, instruct someone to call for emergency medical service. Dial 0 or 911, depending on community resources. Tell operator or dispatcher exact location of victim; do not hang up (enhanced 911 can find location).
- Soft surface such as mattress, car seat, or grassy surface decreases efficiency of external cardiac compressions.

Critical Thinking Exercises

1. Your client keeps coughing out the oral airway. What assessments are needed to determine if the oral airway is still necessary?
2. You are the first person on the scene of a choking victim. The individual runs to the rest room. What should be your response?
3. How would you modify CPR or FBAOM for a pregnant client?

References

American Heart Association: *Guidelines 2000 for cardiopulmonary resuscitation and emergency cardiovascular care: international consensus on science,* Dallas, 2000, The Association.

Centers for Disease Control and Prevention: Guidelines for prevention of transmission of human immunodeficiency virus and hepatitis B virus to health-care and public safety workers, *MMWR Morbid Mortal Wkly Rep* 38(suppl 6):1, 1989.

Lewis SM and others: *Medical-surgical nursing,* ed 5, St. Louis, 2000, Mosby.

Occupational Health and Safety Act, 1992: *Occupational exposure to blood borne pathogens,* OSHA 3127, 1992.

Wong DL and others: *Whaley and Wong's nursing care of infants and children,* ed 6, St. Louis, 1999, Mosby.

16

Preparing for Medication Administration

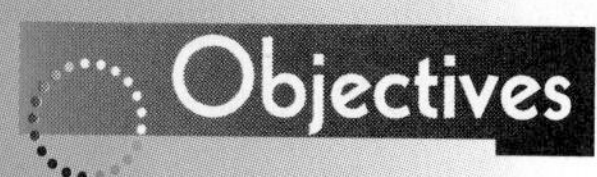

Mastery of content in this chapter will enable the nurse to:

- Define the key terms listed.
- Identify guidelines for safe administration of medications.
- Discuss common types of drug actions.
- Identify the system of measurement for a given prescribed drug.
- Calculate drug doses.
- Describe two methods for delivering medications to the nursing unit.
- Describe the five rights of drug administration.
- Explain cultural variations to consider in drug administration.
- Identify steps to take in reporting drug errors.

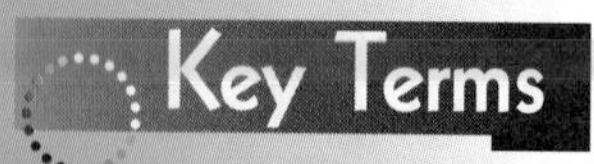

Adverse drug reactions (ADRs)
Anaphylaxis
Drug dependence
Drug plateau
Drug polymorphism
Drug tolerance
Duration of action
Floor stock
Idiosyncratic reaction
NPO
Onset of drug action
Over-the-counter (OTC) drug
Parenteral
Peak action
Peak level
Plateau
Polypharmacy
PRN
Side effect
Synergistic reaction
Telephone order
Toxic effects
Unit-dose system
Verbal order

Safe and accurate administration of medications is one of the nurse's most important responsibilities when caring for clients. The nurse's judgment is critical to confirm that the right drug is being given to a client, that it is administered properly, and that appropriate observations and measurements are made to evaluate the drug's effect and the client's response. The RN is empowered to administer medications under the direction of a licensed physician (Sullivan, 1998). Advanced practice nurses (APNs) have some prescriptive authority in almost every state, but the degree of required physician involvement varies. Medication administration, including the evaluation of client responses, cannot be delegated to assistive personnel. Assistive personnel should be instructed to report client complaints related to the signs and symptoms a drug may be intended to treat or control or any possible side effects.

Drug Forms

Drugs are available in a variety of forms or preparations. The form of the drug determines its route of administration. The composition of a drug is designed to enhance its absorption and metabolism within the body. Drugs are available in several forms (Table 16-1) such as solid, liquid, and powder.

Drug Actions

When administering medications, the nurse should be aware that a drug always has a desired or therapeutic effect. However, because of a drug's chemical makeup and physiological action, it can produce more than one effect. The different types of effects are summarized below.

Therapeutic Effects

The therapeutic effect is the intended or desired physiological response a drug causes. Each drug has a therapeutic effect for which it is prescribed. For example, the nurse administers morphine sulfate, an analgesic, to relieve a client's pain. A single medication may have many therapeutic effects. For example, acetaminophen creates analgesia, reduces inflammation, and reduces fever.

Adverse Drug Reactions

Drugs can react in the body to produce unpredictable and sometimes unexplainable responses (McKenry and Salerno, 1998). No drug is totally safe and absolutely free of nontherapeutic effects. The literature provides an array of definitions for **adverse drug reactions (ADRs)** (Table 16-2). Clinical recognition of ADRs is the important first step in identifying nontherapeutic effects of medications (Arnold, 1998). There are many drug-induced events that initially may seem trivial, expected, and not worth noting but later prove to be serious indicators of drug-induced injury. The nurse must understand that there is a continuum of ADRs, ranging from mild, expected side effects to life-threatening allergic and toxic effects. Prompt recognition and reporting of ADRs can prevent serious injury to clients. Box 16-1 highlights clients most at risk for ADRs. Although no client is totally risk free from having an ADR, clients falling into one or more risk categories require close monitoring (Arnold, 1998). Each health care agency has specific policies for reporting ADRs.

Side Effects. Typically drug side effects include those effects of drug therapy that are easily tolerated, not serious, and almost always expected (Arnold, 1998). The American Society of Health-System Pharmacists defines a side effect as an expected, well-known reaction resulting in little or no change in client management (Johnson and others, 1995). **Side effects** may be harmless or injurious. In the example of codeine phosphate, administered for analgesia, constipation is a common side effect. If the side effects are serious enough to outweigh

Table 16-1 Forms of Medication by Route of Administration

MEDICATION FORMS COMMONLY PREPARED FOR ADMINISTRATION BY ORAL ROUTE	
Solid Forms	
Capsule	Medication encased in a gelatin shell.
Tablet	Powdered medication compressed into hard disk or cylinder.
Liquid Forms	
Elixir	Clear fluid containing water and alcohol.
Extract	Concentrated drug form made by removing the active portion of a drug from its other components.
Solution	One or more substances dissolved in water.
Suspension	Finely dissolved particles in a liquid medium.
Syrup	Medication dissolved in a concentrated sugar solution.
Other Oral Forms and Terms Associated With Oral Preparations	
Troche (lozenge)	Medication that dissolves in mouth, not meant for ingestion.
Aerosol	Aqueous medication sprayed and absorbed in the mouth and upper airway, not meant for ingestion.
Enteric coated	Tablet that is coated so that it does not dissolve in stomach, meant for intestinal absorption.
Sustained release	Tablet or capsule that contains small particles of a drug coated with material that requires a varying amount of time to dissolve.
MEDICATION FORMS COMMONLY PREPARED FOR ADMINISTRATION BY TOPICAL ROUTE	
Aqueous	One or more substances dissolved in water.
Cream	Nongreasy, semisolid preparation.
Liniment	Oily liquid.
Lotion	Emollient liquid that can be clear solution, suspension, or emulsion.
Paste	Medication preparation that is thick and has poor skin penetration.
Transdermal patch	Disk or patch embedded with a drug that is absorbed through the skin over a designated period of time.
MEDICATION FORMS COMMONLY PREPARED FOR ADMINISTRATION BY PARENTERAL ROUTE	
Solution	Preparation that contains water with one or more dissolved compounds. The solution must be sterile.
Powder	Particles of drug that are reconstituted with water, dissolved, and administered parenterally. The solution must be sterile.
MEDICATION FORMS COMMONLY PREPARED FOR INSTILLATION INTO BODY CAVITIES	
Suppository	Drugs mixed with gelatin and shaped for insertion into a body cavity. The suppository is meant to dissolve, releasing the drug.
Intraocular disk	Disk (similar to a contact lens) embedded with a drug that is inserted into the client's eye. The drug is absorbed over a designated period of time.

Table 16-2 Definitions of Adverse Drug Reactions

DEFINING TERM	DESCRIPTORS	OUTCOME
Noxious	Excess therapeutic effect	Discontinue drug.
Unintended	Undesirable clinical effect	Change drug therapy.
Harmful	Abnormal sign	Serious injury or death.
Undesirable	Abnormal symptom	Results in disability.
Untoward	Abnormal laboratory result	Results in loss of work.
Unexpected	Creates illness/injury	Medical follow-up and/or treatment.
Iatrogenic	Illness resulting from medical intervention	Prolonged hospitalization.
Disabling	Unacceptable to client or MD.	Disciplinary measures, demand for compensation, regulatory measures, requires supportive treatment, negatively affects prognosis.

Modified from Arnold GJ: Clinical recognition of adverse drug reactions: obstacles and opportunities for the nursing profession, *J Nurs Care Qual* 13(2):45, 1998.

Box 16-1 Clients at Increased Risk for Adverse Drug Reactions

- Clients taking a drug for the first time
- Very young and elderly
- Women
- Clients taking more than four to five medications (polypharmacy)
- Clients extremely underweight or overweight
- Clients with renal and/or hepatic disease
- Clients with altered blood flow conditions
- Clients with a past history of an ADR
- Clients with depression or anxiety
- Clients with sensory deprivation or overload
- Clients who abuse alcohol, nicotine, or street drugs
- Clients who treat selves with over-the-counter drugs

Modified from Arnold GJ: Clinical recognition of adverse drug reactions: obstacles and opportunities for the nursing profession, *J Nurs Care Qual* 13(2):45, 1998.

Table 16-3 Mild Allergic Reactions

Symptom	Description
Urticaria (hives)	Raised, irregularly shaped skin eruptions with varying sizes and shapes; eruptions have reddened margins and pale centers.
Eczema (rash)	Small, raised vesicles that are usually reddened; often distributed over the entire body.
Pruritus	Itching of the skin; accompanies most rashes.
Rhinitis	Inflammation of mucous membranes lining the nose, causing swelling and a clear watery discharge.
Wheezing	Constriction of smooth muscles surrounding bronchioles that decreases diameter of airways; occurs primarily on inspiration because of severely narrowed airways; development of edema in pharynx and larynx further obstructs airflow.
Angioedema	An acute, painless, dermal, subcutaneous, or submucosal swelling of short duration involving the face, neck, lips, larynx, hands, feet, genitalia, or viscera.
Fever	Abnormal elevation of body temperature above 37° C (98.6° F)

the beneficial effects of a drug's therapeutic action, the prescriber may discontinue the drug. Clients may stop taking medications because of side effects. Any side effect should be reported to a physician and pharmacist to ensure that they are not incorrectly interpreted as a more serious adverse effect.

Toxic Effects. After prolonged intake of high doses of medication, ingestion of drugs intended for external application, or when a drug accumulates in the blood because of impaired metabolism or excretion, a toxic effect may develop. **Toxic effects** may be lethal, depending on the drug's action. For example, morphine acts on the central nervous system to relieve pain by producing a combination of depressing and stimulating effects. Toxic levels of morphine cause severe respiratory depression and death.

Idiosyncratic Reactions. Medications may cause unpredictable effects, such as an **idiosyncratic reaction,** in which a client overreacts or underreacts to a drug or has a reaction different from normal. Predicting which clients will have an idiosyncratic response is impossible. For example, Ativan, an antianxiety medication, when given to an older adult may cause agitation and delirium.

Allergic Reactions. Allergic reaction is another unpredictable response to a drug. Exposure to an initial dose of a medication may cause an immunologic response. The drug acts as an antigen, which causes antibodies to be produced. With repeated administration the client develops an allergic response to the drug, its chemical preservatives, or a metabolite of it.

An allergic reaction may be mild or severe. Allergic symptoms vary, depending on the client and the drug. Among the different classes of drugs, antibiotics cause a high incidence of allergic reactions. Common, mild allergy symptoms are summarized in Table 16-3. Severe or anaphylactic reactions are characterized by sudden constriction of bronchiolar muscles, edema of the pharynx and larynx, severe wheezing, and shortness of breath. The client may become severely hypotensive, necessitating emergency resuscitation measures. **Anaphylaxis** can be fatal.

It is common practice for clients who are hospitalized or in extended treatment facilities and who have a known drug allergy to have this information recorded in a clearly identifiable place to be easily seen by all those involved in the client's care. In many institutions this information is often recorded on the front of the client's medical record or on a specially designed label or sticker that is easy to see. Client allergies should always be recorded on the client's medication administration record (MAR). Clients cared for in other settings (e.g., home, community clinics) and who have a known history of an allergy to a medication or substance should be encouraged to wear an identification bracelet or medical alert medal, which alerts all health care providers to the allergies in case the client is found unconscious. A client should never be given a drug that has caused an allergic reaction in the past. It is impossible to know how sensitive an individual is to a medication and how severe an allergic reaction might be. Even though a client may have a mild allergy, continued exposure to a medication can cause the client to develop a more severe allergic response over time.

Drug Tolerance and Dependence. **Drug tolerance** exists when there is a decreased physiological response after repeated administration of a drug or a chemically related substance (McKenry and Salerno, 1998). It is usually noted clinically when clients receive the same drug for long periods of time and require higher doses to produce the same effect. Drugs known to produce tolerance include opium alkaloids, nitrites, barbiturates, and alcohol. Generally clients hospital-

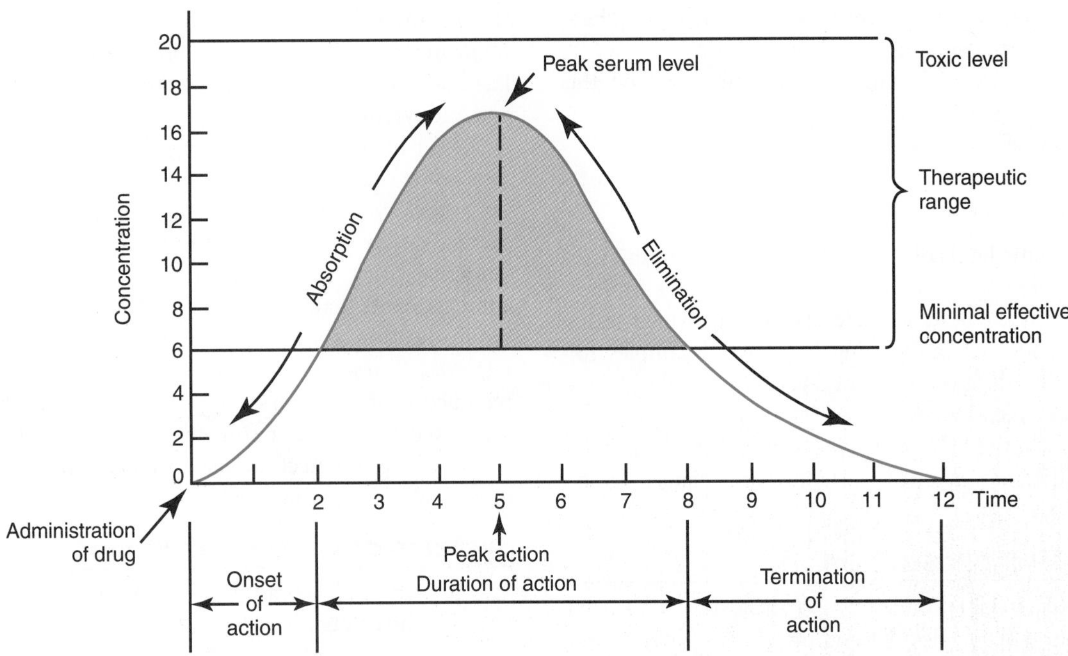

FIGURE **16-1** Plasma level profile of a drug. (From McKenry LM, Salerno E: *Mosby's pharmacology in nursing,* ed 20, St. Louis, 1998, Mosby.)

ized for acute episodes of illness do not develop tolerance. It may take a month or even longer for this phenomenon to occur (McCaffery and Pasero, 1999). Cross-tolerance may occur following tolerance to a drug. In cross-tolerance a client develops tolerance to other drugs with similar actions (Johnson, 1997).

Drug tolerance is not the same as drug dependence. Two types of **drug dependence** exist: psychological (or addiction) and physical, In psychological dependence the client desires the medication or drug for some benefit other than the intended effect. The individual believes a desirable effect will result when taking the medication. An example is the drug marijuana, which many individuals use thinking it causes relaxation. Physical dependence involves a physiological adaptation to a drug that manifests itself by intense physical disturbance when the drug is withdrawn. An example is the repeated use of codeine for reducing mild to moderate pain. When clients receive medications for a short term (such as for postoperative pain), dependence is rare (McCaffery and Pasero, 1999). If a client has dependence on and tolerance to alcohol, a higher-than-usual drug dose may be required for the desired effect of some medications.

Drug Interactions. When one drug modifies the action of another drug, a drug interaction occurs. Drug interactions are common in individuals taking many medications. A drug may potentiate or diminish the action of other drugs and may alter the way in which another drug is absorbed, metabolized, or eliminated from the body. This is a common problem in older adults, who tend to have multiple physicians prescribe a variety of medications without discontinuing any previous drugs.

When two drugs are given simultaneously, they can have a synergistic or additive effect. With a **synergistic reaction** the physiological action of the two drugs in combination is greater than the effect of the drugs when given separately. Alcohol is a central nervous system depressant that has a synergistic effect on antihistamines, antidepressants, and narcotic analgesics.

A drug interaction is sometimes desirable. Often a physician orders combination drug therapy to create a drug interaction for therapeutic benefit. For example, a client with moderate hypertension typically receives several drugs, such as diuretics and vasodilators, that act together to keep blood pressure at a desirable level.

Drug Dose Responses

After the nurse administers a drug, it undergoes absorption, distribution, metabolism, and excretion (Figure 16-1). These processes determine how much of the administered dose reaches the site of action. These processes are influenced by many things such as body surface area, body water content, body fat content, and protein stores.

When certain medications such as antibiotics are prescribed, the goal is to achieve a constant drug blood level within a safe therapeutic range. The client and nurse must follow regular dosage schedules and administer prescribed doses at correct intervals. Knowledge of the following time intervals of drug action also helps to anticipate a drug's effect:

1. **Onset of drug action**—Period of time it takes after a drug is administered for it to produce a therapeutic effect

2. **Peak action**—Time it takes for a drug to reach its highest effective concentration, or **peak level**
3. **Duration of action**—Length of time during which the drug is present in a concentration great enough to produce a therapeutic effect
4. **Plateau**—Blood serum concentration reached and maintained after repeated, fixed doses

The therapeutic levels of certain drugs, such as antibiotics, can be monitored by laboratory testing. A blood sample is drawn to identify the peak serum level of a drug, which varies according to the specific drug involved. Blood samples for trough levels, or the lowest serum levels, are usually drawn just before the next scheduled dose of medication. Precise coordination with the laboratory is essential for obtaining meaningful information. These data allow physicians to modify drug dosages.

Routes of Administration

The route chosen for administering a drug depends on its properties and desired effect and on the client's physical and mental condition. The nurse is often the best person to judge the route most desirable for a client. Table 16-4 summarizes the routes of drug administration. Table 16-5 summarizes the factors that influence the choice of administration routes.

Drug Distribution

Drug distribution is the responsibility of the institution or community pharmacy. In a hospital a variety of systems may be used to distribute medications to a nursing unit. The standard for drug distribution is the **unit-dose system.** In this system, each client on the nursing unit has a medication drawer (on a cart or in a predetermined cabinet) that contains enough of the client's current medications, usually, for a 24-hour period. The advantage to unit-dose dispensing of medications is that it reduces drug cost for institutions and also reduces medication errors.

Some drugs may be distributed as floor stock. **Floor stock** are medications that are distributed to the nursing unit in bulk (either individually wrapped or in bottles). Medications that are appropriate for floor stock are often those that are routinely prescribed or prescribed on an as-needed (PRN) basis. Examples of these medications are stool softeners, antacids, and antipyretics.

Newer medication dispensing systems, such as computer-assisted or electronic devices, are variations of unit-dose and floor stock systems. These systems are self-contained and can carry a variety of unit-dose and floor stock medications and stock narcotics. The medications are housed in individual compartments that are accessed by the nurse after requesting the medication from a computerized screen. All medications retrieved from these electronic medication stations are recorded in the system's computer. Frequently these systems are linked to computer software programs in the pharmacy that can help to detect dosage errors and incompatible drugs or send alerts regarding clients' drug allergies.

Table 16-4 Routes of Drug Administration

NONPARENTERAL	
Oral	By mouth
Sublingual	Under the tongue
Topical	On the skin (as a cream or patch) and eye/ear drops
Suppository	Into the rectum or vagina
PARENTERAL	
Intramuscular (IM)	Into a muscle
Subcutaneous (SQ)	Into the subcutaneous tissue of the skin
Intradermal (ID)	Into the dermis of the skin
Intravenous (IV)	Into a vein

Systems of Drug Measurement

The proper administration of medication depends on the nurse's ability to compute drug doses accurately and measure medications correctly. A careless mistake in placing a decimal point or adding a zero to a dose can lead to a fatal error. The prescriber and client depend on the nurse to check the dose before administering a drug. The most common system used in the measurement of medications is the metric system. The apothecary and household measures can also be used.

Metric System

As a decimal system, the metric system is the most logically organized of the measurement system. Metric units can be easily converted and computed through simple multiplication and division. Each basic unit of measure is organized into units of 10. Multiplying or dividing by 10 forms secondary units. In multiplication, the decimal point moves to the right; in division, the decimal moves to the left.

The basic units of measure in the metric system are the meter (length), the liter (volume), and the gram (weight). For drug calculations the nurse uses primarily volume and weight units. In the metric system small or large letters are used to designate the basic units:

Gram = g or Gm
Liter = l or L

Small letters are abbreviations for subdivisions of major units:

Milligram = mg
Milliliter = ml

A system of Latin prefixes designates subdivision of the basic units: deci- (1/10 or 0.1), centi- (1/100 or 0.01), and milli- (1/1000 or 0.001). Greek prefixes designate multiples of the basic units: deka- (10), hecto- (100), and kilo- (1000).

For example: 1 gram = 1000 milligrams (mg)

When writing drug dosages in metric units, physicians and nurses use either fractions or multiples of a unit. Fractions are always in decimal form, and a zero is placed in front of the decimal to prevent error. For example, Premarin .625 mg

Table 16-5 Factors Influencing Choice of Administration Routes

Advantages by Route	Disadvantages/Contraindications
Oral, Buccal, Sublingual	
Easy and comfortable to administer, convenient, economical; may produce local or systemic effects. Rarely causes anxiety for client.	Avoid giving to clients with alterations in gastrointestinal function (e.g., nausea and vomiting), reduced motility (after general anesthesia or inflammation of bowel), and surgical resection of portion of gastrointestinal tract. Some drugs are destroyed by gastric secretions. Oral administration is contraindicated in clients who are NPO and unable to swallow (e.g., clients with neuromuscular disorders, esophageal strictures, and lesions of the mouth). Oral medications cannot be given when client has gastric suction and are contraindicated in clients before some tests or surgery. An unconscious or confused client may be unable or unwilling to swallow or hold medication under the tongue. Oral medications may irritate the lining of the gastrointestinal tract, discolor teeth, or have an unpleasant taste.
Parenteral (SQ, IM, IV, Intradermal, Intrathecal, Epidural)	
Routes provide means of administration when oral drugs are contraindicated. More rapid absorption occurs than with topical or oral routes. IV infusion provides drug delivery when client is critically ill. If peripheral perfusion is poor, IV route is preferred over injections. Intrathecal route allows drugs that cannot pass through the blood-brain barrier to enter cerebrospinal fluid.	Risk of introducing infection, drugs are expensive, and these routes are avoided in clients with bleeding tendencies. Risk of tissue damage with SQ injections. IV and IM infusions are rapidly absorbed, requiring close monitoring. All parenteral routes cause considerable anxiety in many clients, especially children.
Epidural provides excellent pain control.	Limits mobility during administration. Risk of infection.
Skin	
Topical	
Topical skin applications provide primarily local effect. Route is painless. Limited side effects occur.	Extensive applications may require dressings that can be bulky for a client when maneuvering. Do not apply to skin if abrasions are present. Drugs can be absorbed by person applying it if gloves are not worn.
Transdermal	
Transdermal applications provide prolonged systemic effects, with limited side effects.	Application leaves oily or pasty substance on skin and may soil clothing. Client may have sensitivity to adhesive.
Mucous Membranes*	
Therapeutic effects are provided by local application to involved sites. Aqueous solutions are readily absorbed and capable of causing systemic effects. Mucous membranes provide route of administration when oral drugs are contraindicated.	Mucous membranes are highly sensitive to some drug concentrations. Insertion of rectal and vaginal medications often causes embarrassment. Rectal suppositories are contraindicated if clients have had rectal surgery or if active rectal bleeding is present. If eardrum is ruptured, otic medications may be contraindicated.
Inhalation	
Inhalation provides rapid relief for local respiratory problems. Route provides easy access for introduction of general anesthetic gases.	Some local agents can cause serious systemic effects. If clients unable to administer inhaler correctly drug will be ineffective. Difficult to learn for older adults and children.
Intraocular Disk	
Route is advantageous in that it does not require frequent administration like eye drops. The client can also wear disk when sleeping or swimming. Dry eyes do not affect drug delivery.	Local reactions can occur such as tearing, itchiness, or redness of the eyes. Client must be taught how to insert disk into and remove from the eye. Client may be anxious about doing this. Medication can be expensive. Medication is contraindicated in clients with infections of the eye.

*Includes eyes, ears, nose, and vaginal, rectal, buccal, and sublingual routes.

should be written 0.625 mg. Some institutions further recommend having a zero after a decimal point to reduce chance of error. For example, heparin 10,000 units should be written 10,000.0 units.

Apothecary System

The apothecary system of measurement is one of the oldest systems of measurement. It is seldom used; however, some drug companies still include apothecary measures in addition to metric. The basic units of measure in the apothecary system include weight (grains) and volume (minims, drams, and ounces). The measures used in this system are approximates, and a 10% variance has become acceptable in preparation and administration of most medications. The apothecary system often uses roman numerals and fractions. The symbol "ss" is used for the fraction $^1/_2$. Unlike the metric system, in the apothecary system the abbreviation or symbol for a unit of measure is written before the amount or quantity.

Household Measurements

Household measures are familiar to most people and are used when more accurate systems of measure are unnecessary. Included in household measures are drops, teaspoons, tablespoons, cups, and glasses for volume; and ounces and pounds for weight. Although pints and quarts are considered household measures, they are used in the apothecary system.

Medication Administration

Preparing and administering medications requires accuracy by the nurse. The nurse must pay full attention to the procedure and try not to do other tasks simultaneously. Accuracy is greatest when the nurse observes the five rights of drug administration.

1. The *right* drug
2. The *right* dose
3. The *right* client
4. The *right* route
5. The *right* time

Correct Transcription and Communication of Orders *(Right Drug)*

A medication order is required for any drug to be administered by a nurse. The nurse should be aware of the nurse practice act and institutional policies regarding which providers, other than physicians, may prescribe medications. The nurse or a designated unit secretary writes the prescriber's complete order on the appropriate MAR (Figure 16-2). The transcribed order includes the client's full name, room, and bed number (which is usually prestamped on the order form); date the order is written; date the drug order expires (if applicable); drug name, dose, and frequency, and route of administration. Each time a drug dose is prepared the nurse refers to the MAR. With unit-dose systems, only one transcription is necessary, limiting the opportunity for errors. When transcribing orders, the nurse should be sure names, dosages, and symbols are legible and not smudged. When the nurse is checking an order transcribed by the unit secretary, every element of the order is to be checked for accuracy and legibility. An RN is responsible for checking and initialing all transcribed orders against the original orders.

In some institutions a computer printout lists all currently ordered medications with dosage information. Orders are entered daily into the computer, preventing the need for transcription of orders. The same printout may be used to record medications given.

If a medication order seems incorrect or inappropriate, the nurse consults the prescriber. For example, if a prescribed drug name does not seem appropriate for the client's known condition the nurse should check. Similarly, if a dosage seems out of range of normal, the nurse should confirm the correct ordered dosage. The nurse who gives the wrong medication or an incorrect dosage is legally responsible for the error.

A **verbal order** is a medication or treatment order received by the nurse in the presence of the prescriber. Verbal orders should be limited to emergency situations when the prescriber has no time to write the order. Verbal orders are entered into the client's medical record by the nurse and transcribed the same was as if the prescriber wrote the order (Figure 16-3). The name of the prescriber is written next to that of the nurse.

Telephone orders are medication orders given over the phone, usually after the nurse updates the prescriber about a change in a client's condition. A telephone order is transcribed the same as a verbal order. Institutional and state regulations require verbal and telephone orders to be signed by the provider within 24 hours. Therefore it is important to limit its use as much as possible.

Accurate Dose Measurement *(Right Dose)*

When a medication must be prepared from a dose other than what is ordered, the chance of errors increases. After calculating the dose, have a second nurse check the calculation, especially if you are unsure, or if the drug is potentially toxic. After calculating doses, the nurse uses appropriate measuring devices to prepare the medication. Liquid preparations may be measured using a medicine cup marked in ml (cc) or a syringe for oral use (Figure 16-4). A syringe without a needle is used when the order is for less than 5 ml of liquid. Some pediatric medications come with a scaled dropper. Key principles for the nurse to observe when using measuring receptacles:

1. Drugs poured into medication cups should be done so at eye level. This allows the nurse to accurately see the desired amount. The amount of poured liquid should be even with the base of the meniscus (Figure 16-5).
2. Pour liquid medications away from a label to ensure that liquid will not run down a label, making it difficult to read.
3. Drugs drawn into syringes should be drawn slowly to prevent air bubbles from entering the syringe. Air displaces medications and may lead to inaccurate measurement of doses.

Room: 3700-03

Patient: PDM, Pharmacy
Birth: 11/30/79 Admit: 01/01/00
MRN: 2000403 Acct: 900015
A Doctor: Jim Smith

Age: 20 y Ht: 5 ft 2 in Wt: 125.2 lbs
Metric: Ht: 1 m 57 cm Wt: 56.79 kg

Saint Francis Medical Center

MEDICATION ADMINISTRATION RECORD

Date: 01/18/00 – 01/19/00

ADEs/Nondrug allergies: Latex – Zosyn – Amoxicillin – Insulins – Darvocet – Lugols soln. – Antihi +

Medication	0800	0900	1000	1100	1200	1300	1400	1500	1600	1700	1800	1900	2000	2100	2200	2300	2400	0100	0200	0300	0400	0500	0600	0700
P00014 Bacitracin ointment AKA: Bacitracin ointment Dose: Apply STRGH: 30 gm/tube TID Topical: Right lower leg For external use only Testing			RL 10																					
P00029 Insulin/human regular AKA: Humulin R Dose: 15 units Strgh: 1 ml = 100 units AC SQ	RL 0730																							
P00030 Fexofenadine 60 mg/psuedo 120 mg AKA: Allegra–D Sr Tab Dose: 1 tab STRGH: 60/120/tab BID Oral Auto Sub: 1 Allegra–D Tab bid For Claritin–D 12 hr and 24 hr Per P&T Comm			RL 10																					
P00036 Aspirin AKA: Aspirin 325 mg Tab Dose: 2 tab 650 mg STRGH: 325 mg/tab Q3–4h Oral Testing						RL 1315																		
P00039 Haloperidol tablet AKA: Haldol 0.5 mg tab Dose: 1 mg STRGH: 1 mg/tab QHS Oral																								
P00035 Zolpidem AKA: Ambien 5 mg tab Dose: 5 mg STRGH: 5/tab QHS PRN Oral MR × 1 Testing																								

Circle = Dose not given
Initials = Dose given
Deltoid = R.D., L.D.
Vastus Lateralis = R.V.L., L.V.L.
Lower Abdominal = R.L.A., L.L.A.
Anterior Gluteal = R.A.G., L.A.G.
Posterior Gluteal = R.P.G., L.P.G.

Page: 01 (continued)

Initials and signature	Initials and signature	Initials and signature
Rita Lassater RL		
Initials and signature	Initials and signature	Initials and signature
Initials and signature	Initials and signature	Initials and signature

FIGURE **16-2** Medication administration record (MAR). (Courtesy Saint Francis Medical Center.)

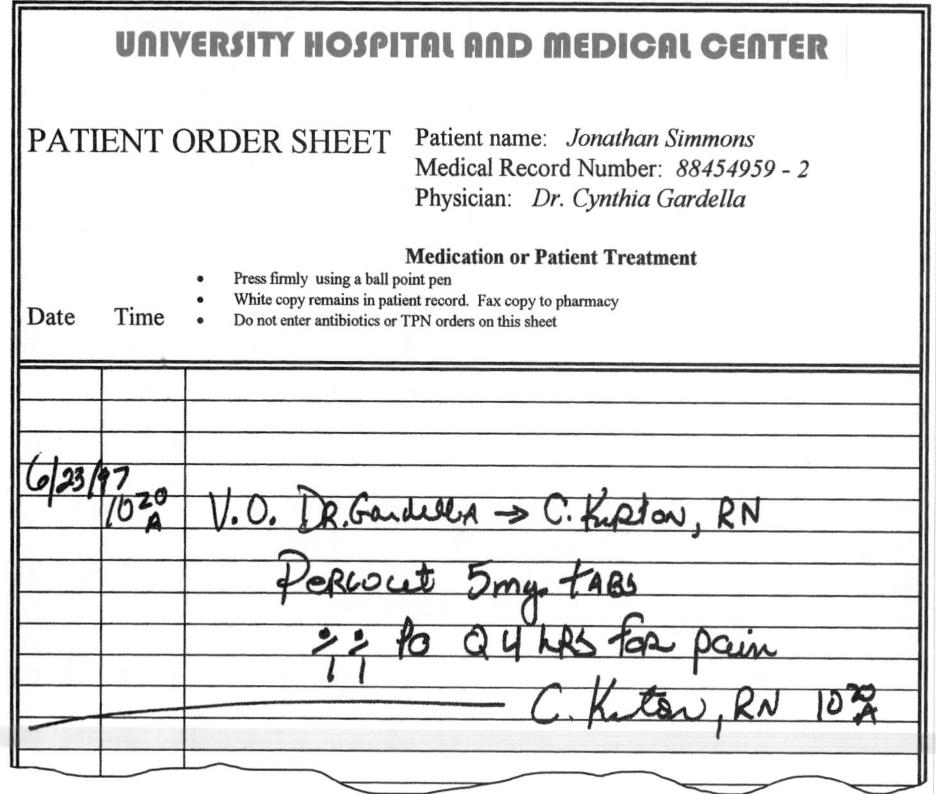

UNIVERSITY HOSPITAL AND MEDICAL CENTER

PATIENT ORDER SHEET

Patient name: *Jonathan Simmons*
Medical Record Number: *88454959 - 2*
Physician: *Dr. Cynthia Gardella*

Medication or Patient Treatment

- Press firmly using a ball point pen
- White copy remains in patient record. Fax copy to pharmacy
- Do not enter antibiotics or TPN orders on this sheet

Date	Time	Medication or Patient Treatment
6/23/97	10^20 A	V.O. Dr. Gardella → C. Kurton, RN
		Percocet 5mg tabs
		ii po Q 4 hrs for pain
		C. Kurton, RN 10^20 A

FIGURE **16-3** Example of a verbal order.

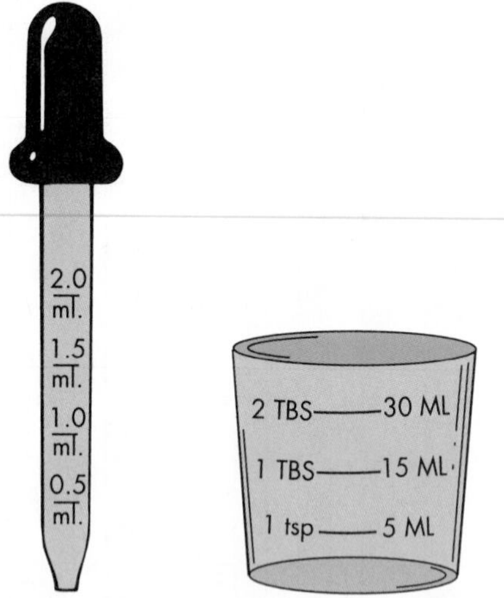

FIGURE **16-4** Scaled dropper and cup to measure oral liquids. (From Clayton BD, Stock YN: *Basic pharmacology for nurses,* ed 11, St. Louis, 1997, Mosby.)

Administration to the *Right Client*

Once a nurse is prepared to administer a drug, the client's identification band (ID bracelet) is checked against the MAR, and the client is asked to state his or her full name. "Please state your name," is the best question to ask for the client's name. Do not enter a room and state the client's name for him, "Mr. Miles, here is your medication." This assumes that the client, by acknowledging your presence, is indeed who you say he is. This procedure is most convenient when the nurse is able to bring a drug cart to the hall outside a client's room, refer to the MAR, and then enter the client's room.

There will be situations when clients are confused or unresponsive. The nurse then compares the medical record number on the MAR with the client's ID bracelet. If the client is a child, parents or legal guardians can be used to identify the child. The practice of checking clients' identification is invaluable in preventing errors, especially when caring for multiple clients. It is also essential even after caring for the same client for several days. If a client questions the practice of identification verification, explain that this is a routine practice for making sure clients receive the correct medication.

Administering by the *Right Route*

The prescriber's order must designate a route of administration. If the route of administration is missing or if the specified route is not the recommended route, the nurse must consult the prescriber immediately. When an injection is administered, the nurse must use only preparations intended for parenteral use. Injection of a liquid intended for oral use can produce local complications, such as sterile abscess, or fatal systemic ef-

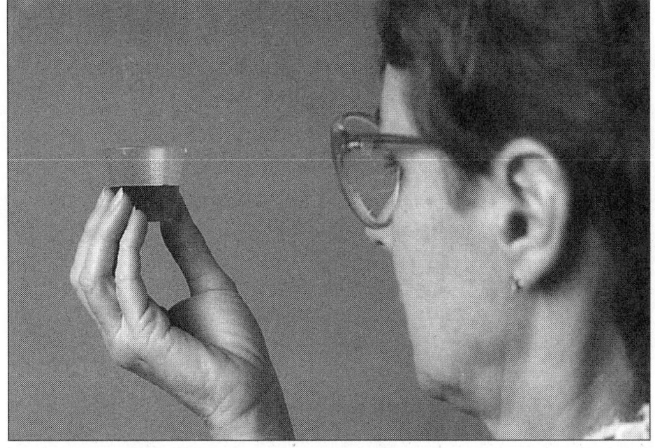

FIGURE 16-5 A, Pour the desired volume of liquid so that the base of the meniscus is level with line on scale. B, Nurse looks at base of meniscus to confirm volume poured.

fects. Medication companies label parenteral medication "for injectable use only."

Administering a Drug at the *Right Time*

Each agency has routine time schedules for medications ordered at standard intervals. For example, medications to be given tid (three times a day) may be routinely scheduled for 0800, 1400, and 2000, or 0900, 1300, and 1900, depending on agency policy. A drug may also be ordered q8h (every 8 hours), which is also three times a day, however, the medication ordered q8h needs to be given around the clock to maintain adequate therapeutic blood levels. *All routinely ordered medications should be given within 30 minutes before or after the scheduled time;* however, nursing judgment may allow some variance, depending on the medication involved.

A medication may also be ordered for special circumstances. A preoperative medication may be ordered "stat" (to be given immediately); "now," which means as soon as available, usually within an hour; or "on call," which means the operating room or treatment area will notify the nurse when it is the appropriate time. A drug may be ordered AC (before meals) or PC (after meals). Insulin and oral hypoglycemic agents should be given at a precise interval before a meal.

Some medications require the nurse's clinical judgment in determining the right administration time. A medication that is ordered **prn** (pro re nata) is intended to be given according to circumstances or when needed. For example, when a prn analgesic is ordered "q3-4h prn" the nurse needs to assess the characteristics and severity of the pain to determine when to administer within the 3- to 4-hour time span or longer. In the case of a stool softener, an order for sodium docusate "prn daily" requires the nurse to assess the character of a client's stool daily. In the case of acute pain, many experts recommend around-the-clock administration until the pain subsides. If the nurse waits to administer the drug until the client's pain is severe, the medication may not be effective.

Preparation of Medications

Before the actual administration of medications, the nurse may need to carry out several steps: interpreting drug labels, conversion of units within a system or between systems, and calculation of drug doses. It is important to remember. *Drugs ordered in units and milliequivalents are not convertible to metric, apothecary, or household measurements.*

Interpreting Drug Labels

Drug labels include seven basic pieces of information: the trade name of the drug in large letters, the generic name in smaller letters, the form of the drug, the dose, the expiration date, the lot number, and the name of the manufacturer (Figure 16-6). The trade name given by the manufacturer often suggests the action of the drug. The generic name is the chemical name.

Conversions

Drugs are not always dispensed in the unit of measure in which they are ordered. Drug companies package and bottle certain standard equivalents. The nurse often must convert available units of volume and weight to desired doses or vice versa. The nurse must know approximate equivalents in all of the measurement systems or make use of conversion tables (Box 16-2). An example follows:

The nurse receives an order: ceftazidine 1 g IV.
The pharmacy supplies ceftazidine in 500-mg vials.
Since the drug dose on the drug label is in milligrams, conversion should be from grams to milligrams.
To convert gram to milligrams, move the decimal point three spaces to the right.

$$1.0 \text{ g} = 1000 \text{ mg}$$

Once this information is known the nurse can move to the next step: dose calculations.

Dose Calculations

Dose calculations are necessary when the dose on the drug label differs from the dose ordered. There are several methods for calculating doses. The most common methods are ratio-proportion or use of a formula. Dimensional analysis is becoming a popular method for dose calculation because it involves simple multiplication and division and does not require algebra (Box 16-3).

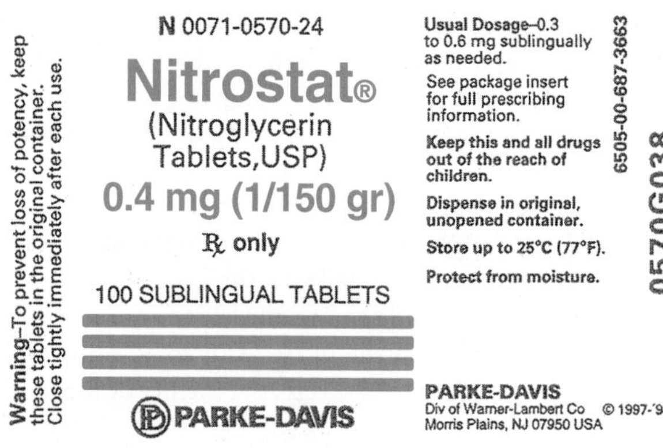

FIGURE **16-6** Interpreting a drug label. (Courtesy of Warner-Lambert Company.)

Box 16-2 Approximate Equivalents

1 gr* = 60 mg
1 g = 1000 mg = 16 gr*
1000 mcg (μg) = 1 mg
1000 g = 1 kg = 2.2 lb*
1 mL or ml (1 cc) = 15–16 minims* = 15 drops (gH)
4–5 ml = 1 tsp†
15 ml = 3 tsp = 1 tbs†
30 ml = 1 fluid oz†
240 ml = 8 fluid oz* = 1 cup†
1000 ml = 1L

*Apothecary measure.
†Household measure.

Box 16-3 Dimensional Analysis

Step 1. Identify the starting factor (amount ordered), which is the first item of the equation, and the answer label (tablets, capsules, or ml), which is the last item.

Step 2. Identify appropriate equivalents with a 1:1 ratio (e.g., 1 g = 1000 mg). Set up the equation so that labels can be canceled; for example, if mg is in the numerator, mg must be in the denominator to cancel.

Step 3. Solve the equation.

a. Cancel labels first; the answer label should not cancel.
b. Reduce numbers to lowest terms.
c. Multiply/divide to solve equation.
d. Reduce answer to lowest terms, convert to decimal, and round to a measurable quantity.

$$\text{Starting factor} \times \frac{\text{Equivalent}}{\text{Equivalent}} = \text{Answer label}$$

Pediatric Doses. Children vary in age, weight, and the ability to absorb, metabolize, and excrete medications. Children's doses are lower than those of adults, and caution is needed in preparing medications. In addition, a standard medication dose is nearly nonexistent in pediatrics (McKenry and Salerno, 1998). Drugs may or may not be prepared and packaged in doses appropriate for children. Preparing appropriate doses often requires calculation based on body weight or body surface area. A child's parents may be helpful in determining the best way to give a child medication. Sometimes it is more effective to have the parent give the drug as the nurse stands by.

Example 1
When the dose ordered has the same label as the dose available:
Dose ordered: 0.5 g
Tablets available: 0.25 g per tablet

Step 1. The starting factor is 0.5 g.
The answer label is tablets; that is, How many tablets should be given?

Step 2. Formulate the conversion equation:
The equivalent needed is 1 tablet = 0.25 g.

$$\frac{0.5\text{ g}}{1} \times \frac{1\text{ tab}}{0.25\text{ g}} = ?$$

Cancel labels (g)
NOTE: if properly written, all labels except the answer label will cancel.

Step 3. Solving the equation:
Reduce the numerical values and multiply the numerators and the denominators.

$$\frac{\overset{2}{\cancel{0.5\text{ g}}}}{1} \times \frac{1\text{ tab}}{\cancel{0.25\text{ g}}} = 2\text{ tabs}$$

Example 2
When the dose ordered has a different label than the dose available:
Dose ordered: 0.5 g
Tablets available: 250 mg per tablet

Step 1. The starting factor is 0.5 g.
The answer label is tablets; that is, How many tablets should be given?

Step 2. Formulate the conversion equation:
The equivalents needed are 1 g = 1000 mg and 1 tab = 250 mg.

$$\frac{0.5\text{ g}}{1} \times \frac{1000\text{ mg}}{1\text{ g}} \times \frac{1\text{ tab}}{250\text{ mg}} = ?$$

Cancel labels (g. mg).

Step 3. Solve the equation:
Reduce the values and multiply the numerators and the denominators

$$\frac{0.5\,\cancel{g}}{} \times \frac{\overset{4}{\cancel{1000\text{ mg}}}}{\underset{2}{\cancel{1\text{ g}}}} \times \frac{1\text{ tab}}{\cancel{250\text{ mg}}} = \frac{4}{2} = 2\text{ tabs}$$

Example 3
When the dose ordered is available in a liquid form:
Dose ordered: Keflex 250 mg PO
Available: 125 mg per 5 ml

Step 1. The starting factor is 250 mg.
The answer label is ml.

Step 2. Formulate the conversion equation:

$$\frac{250\text{ mg}}{1} \times \frac{5\text{ ml}}{125\text{ mg}} = \text{ml}$$

Cancel labels (mg).

Step 3. Solve the equation:
Reduce and multiply

$$\frac{\overset{2}{\cancel{250\text{ mg}}}}{1} \times \frac{5\text{ ml}}{\cancel{125\text{ mg}}} = 10\text{ ml}$$

Example 4
When dose is ordered based on body surface area (commonly done for pediatric doses). The body surface area is estimated on the basis of weight, using standard charts or nomogram. The formula is a ratio of the child's body surface area compared with the body surface area of an average adult (1.7 square meters, or 1.7 m^2).

$$\text{Child's dose} = \frac{\text{Surface area of child}}{1.7\text{ m}^2} \times \text{Normal adult dose}$$

Physician orders ampicillin for a child weighing 12 kg, and the nomogram chart shows that the body surface area is 0.54 m^2. The normal single dose is 250 mg.

1. Child's dose $= \frac{0.54\text{ m}^2}{1.7\text{ m}^2} \times 250\text{ mg}$
2. The m^2 units cancel out and can be ignored.
3. Child's dose $= \frac{0.54}{1.7} \times 250\text{ mg}$
   $0.3 \times 250\text{ mg} = 75\text{ mg}$
   Child's dose = 75 mg

Older Adult Dosages. In 1992 Kovach (1992) reported that older adults consume 31% of all prescription drugs and over 40% of **over-the-counter (OTC) drugs** in the United States. As the number of older adults continues to increase, it is important for nurses to understand age-related alterations in drug pharmacokinetics and the implications for safe drug administration (Box 16-4). A common problem for older adult clients is **polypharmacy,** the use of a number of different drugs (four or five) for one or more health problems (McKenry and Salerno, 1998). Polypharmacy increases the chances of drug interactions occurring. These interactions can be mistaken as drug toxicity, an increase in disease severity or suboptimal treatment, or an apparently unrelated event (Lueckenotte, 2000). The nurse, physician, and pharmacist share the responsibility of reducing or eliminating the adverse risk factors associated with various drug regimens older adults typically receive. The nurse must conduct a thorough assessment of the client's health status, current medication regimen, reason for existing and proposed medications, and any environmental factors that can influence accurate and safe medication administration by the client and caregivers. Although there are no stanardized dosages for older adults, the nurse can play an important role in recognizing physiologic changes in the client (e.g., reduction in renal function or change in gastric motility) that influence dosages prescribed. Frequently physicians will lower recommended adult dosages to treat older adult clients. The potent medications available to treat older adults often have a narrow index between effectiveness and toxicity (McKenry and Salerno, 1998). The drugs most commonly prescribed for older adults, which therefore commonly cause problems for older adults, are listed in Box 16-5.

Box 16-4 Altered Pharmacokinetics in Older Adults

Absorption	↑ Gastric pH
	↓ Intestinal blood flow
Distribution	↓ Lean body mass
	↑ Adipose (fat) stores
	↓ Total body water
	↓ Serum albumin
Metabolism	↓ Liver size
	↓ Liver blood flow
	↓ Liver functions (microsomal enzyme activity)
Excretion	↓ Kidney function

Box 16-5 Drugs Most Commonly Prescribed for Older Adults

- Diuretics
- Potassium salts
- H_2 antagonists
- Nitroglycerine
- Insulin
- Digitalis preparations
- Beta blockers
- Antianxiety agents
- Antihypertensives

From McKenry LM, Salerno E: *Mosby's Pharmacology in Nursing,* ed 20, Mosby, St. Louis, 1998.

Nursing Process in Medication Administration

Medication administration should be done in a safe and orderly manner. Application of the nursing process ensures that good clinical judgment is integrated into the client's care.

Assessment

Nursing assessment relating to drug therapy involves client assessment and medication review. The nurse determines if a client has a history of medication allergies. The hospitalized client's medical record should be clearly marked with a list of allergies, and the client should have an allergy band. A client should never be given a medication to which he or she is known to be allergic.

A careful assessment of the client's physiological status is also important. How is the client tolerating food or liquids by mouth? Does the client have abnormal laboratory values suggesting a change in renal or liver function? Does the client's blood pressure contraindicate administration of a drug? Is the client becoming less responsive at times, making him or her prone to aspiration of a liquid medication? These are just examples of conditions the nurse considers when helping to judge the appropriateness of a medication and/or the route for administration. Nursing assessment also reveals if it is necessary to withhold a prescribed medication. Any withheld medication should be reported to the prescriber.

Assessing the client's current medication history is useful when attempting to determine the reason for the client's presenting signs and symptoms. This is especially true in urgent situations. In clinic and medical office settings, nurses often ask clients to bring a list of their current medications for review. Review of current medications also allows the nurse to simultaneously assess the client's knowledge level necessary for safe self-administration of medications. Does the client know the drug's dosage schedule, purpose, common side effects, and actions to take when side effects develop?

In the home care setting, nursing assessment should also include a review of the environment where the client self-administers medications. Are medications stored safely away from children? Are there facilities to adequately prepare the medications? Is there a mechanism to dispose of biomedical equipment (e.g., needles and syringes)? The nurse also determines the family member's or significant other's ability to assist with medication administration.

A medication review requires the nurse to methodically consider what is known about each medication. A nurse should have an understanding of a drug's purpose, action, normal dosage and route, time interval for action, expected side effects, and the specific reason for why a client has the drug prescribed. Nursing implications for administering each drug safely will depend on the type of drug being given (e.g., all antihypertensives should require a blood pressure measurement before administration). When in doubt about drug information, the nurse checks available drug references or the pharmacy.

Planning

When administering medications, three basic goals should be met:

1. The drug's therapeutic effect is achieved.
2. There are no complications related to the prescribed medication and the method of administration.
3. Client and family will understand how to self-administer drug therapy safely.

Implementation

The principles of safe and effective drug preparation and administration must be followed for each client.

Preadministration Activities

1. Ensure that a medication order has not expired. Follow institutional policy for medication order renewal.
2. Follow guidelines described earlier for drug calculation.
3. Review any preadministration assessments (e.g., vital signs, review of laboratory results).
4. Use good medical aseptic technique, wash hands before preparing a dose of medication. Avoid touching tablets and capsules. Use sterile technique for **parenteral** medications (chapter 32).
5. To avoid common errors do not prepare medications from containers with labels that are unmarked or illegible; do not give medications that have changed from clear to cloudy or have changed color; discard a liquid medication if sediment can be seen in the bottom of its container, unless the medication is a suspension; and always check the drug expiration date.

Drug Administration

1. Follow the five rights of medication administration. *Never administer a drug prepared by another nurse.*
2. When entering the room, inform the client of each drug's name and its purpose. This is a good time to review any drug information that will be necessary for the client to know for self-administration.
3. Tablets and capsules should be kept in their wrappers and opened at the client's bedside. This allows you to review each drug with the client. Respect the client's right to refuse a medication. If a client refuses medication, never return unwrapped medication to a container; discard it. If the medication wrapper remains intact, the medication may be returned to the client's unit-dose drawer. When medication is refused, determine the reason for it, and take action accordingly. Refusal of medications must be documented and the physician notified within 24 hours.
4. Remain with the client as the client takes the medication. Provide assistance if necessary (e.g., for the client who is weak and unable to administer eye drops). Do not leave medications at a client's bedside without a prescriber's order to do so.

Postadminstration Activities

1. After administering a drug, record the following information on the MAR or other appropriate form (e.g., nurses' notes) required by the institution:
   - Drug name
   - Dose
   - Route of administration
   - Time of administration
   - Any unexpected client responses (see evaluation)
   - Pertinent data or assessment collected at time of administration
   - Signature and title of nurse administering drug
2. If the client refuses a medication, document the reason for refusal in the nurses' notes. The MAR may require a special symbol that indicates that the client refused the medication.

Evaluation

Once a medication is administered, the nurse is responsible for critically evaluating what is known about the client's condition, how the drug is expected to affect the client, and how the client actually responds. This means the nurse is looking for therapeutic effects as well as adverse outcomes. Should adverse outcomes develop, the nurse recognizes the clinical signs and responds quickly.

1. Monitor client's physical response to the drug (e.g., vital signs, urine output, relief of pain or other symptoms)
2. Monitor client's behavioral responses to the drug (e.g., level of anxiety, agitation, consciousness).
3. Observe injection sites for bruises, inflammation, localized pain, numbness, or bleeding.
4. Determine client's understanding of drug therapy and ability to self-administer medication.

Special Considerations When Administering Medications

Children

When the nurse is administering medications to a child, the parents can be a valuable resource. Nearly all parents have administered medications to their child and can describe the approaches that they have found to work. Parents can also offer information regarding the child's reaction to similar experiences if the child has been previously hospitalized or has been given medications in a practitioner's office (Wong and others, 1999). It may be less traumatic to the child if a parent gives the medication under the nurse's supervision. Typically children require extra psychological preparation and patience when parenteral medications are administered. Children rarely become accustomed to the discomfort of an injection.

Older Adults

McKenry and Salerno (1998) recommend that nurses make geriatric drug therapy as simple as possible. Conferring with the prescriber may help to limit the number of medications a client is taking. The nurse should also work closely with family caregivers to determine if drug schedules are best suited to the client's typical routine.

Nurses should suspect medications as a cause whenever they notice a change in an older adult client's behavior, particularly restlessness, irritability, and confusion. These symptoms are characteristic of drug toxicity (McKenry and Salerno, 1998). Instructing assistive personnel to alert the nurse to any changes in client behavior is prudent. What is frequently described as "senility" is often drug-induced lethargy or confusion.

Environmental, Genetic, and Cultural Factors

Recent studies suggest that ethnicity affects how individuals react to drugs (Kudzma, 1999). When individuals show a variation in response to a drug it is called **drug polymorphism.** Factors that contribute to polymorphism are environmental, genetic, and cultural. Environmental factors affect a drug's half-life and assimilation. For example, diet can affect drug absorption. If a client eats a high-fat diet, certain medications may work more effectively than others. The Japanese typically eat diets high in sodium chloride, which often makes antihypertensive medications less effective.

Genetic polymorphism affects drug efficacy because of genetic influence on liver metabolism, which in turn directs the secretion of liver enzymes. People with insufficient metabolism are slow or poor metabolizers, whereas those who metabolize at a faster rate are called rapid or extensive metabolizers. In the example of debrisoquin, an antihypertensive compound, extensive metabolizers oxidize the compound faster. However, about 3% to 9% of whites in the United States, Canada, Britain, Denmark, Sweden, and Switzerland are poor metabolizers of debrisoquin. Because many drugs are metabolized similarly to debrisoquin, this polymorphism is clinically significant (Kudzma, 1999).

Culturally, a client's values and beliefs affect drug response. Medication adherence is significantly influenced by a client's level of education, prior experience with drug therapy, and the family's influence on actions. In Japan, for example, nausea, vomiting, and bowel changes related to medication use are underreported because it is not acceptable to complain about gastrointestinal problems. Often a person's cultural background results in the use of herbal and homeopathic remedies that can alter response to a drug.

Although most practitioners do not consider ethnicity when prescribing medications, Kudzma (1999) predicts this will change. Other countries have responded. In Japan all clinical drug studies must be replicated on Japanese subjects, in recognition of the differences in medication response due to genetics.

Special Handling of Medications

Controlled Substances

Any medication that has the potential for abuse is handled in a manner differently than other drugs. These medications are called controlled substances and are often referred to as narcotics. Narcotics delivered to a nursing unit are kept in a locked cabinet. At the beginning of each shift, two registered nurses must count all of the narcotics in the locked cabinet and record the count on a narcotic administration record. Computerized or electronic distribution systems may make counting narcotics unnecessary by automatically counting and recording the nurse's electronic signature as the dose is dispensed. Any discrepancies found in a narcotic count are investigated by RNs. Any narcotics unaccounted for must be reported to the nurse manager or supervisor immediately.

When administering narcotics to a client, the nurse follows these general guidelines:

1. Before obtaining the narcotic, check the narcotic administration record for the number of narcotics left in stock. Compare this number with the actual supply available. If it is correct, obtain the desired dose of narcotic. If the count is incorrect, notify the nurse manager and follow institutional policy.
2. Count the remaining supply. The following information is often recorded on the narcotic administration sheet after removal of your dose:
   - Client's name
   - Prescribing physician
   - Client's medical record number
   - Dose of the drug ordered
   - Number of tablets (or injectables) remaining
   - Nurse's signature
3. Administer the narcotic according to policy.
4. If the narcotic cannot be given to the client (e.g., client refuses, medication is contaminated, vital signs change) or not all is used, the medication must be "wasted." Narcotic wasting often requires that another nurse witness the administering nurse discard the medication according to hospital policy. When narcotics are wasted, this information is recorded on the narcotic administration form or another designated form. The witnessing nurse records on that form a signature indicating the medication has been discarded properly. In electronic systems the information is recorded in the computer.

Medication Errors

A medication error is any preventable event that may cause or lead to inappropriate medication use or client harm while the medication is in the control of the health care professional, client, or consumer (United States Pharmacopeia Convention, Inc, 1997). For example, medication errors include administration of the wrong drug, route, and time interval, as well as administering extra doses or failing to administer a drug. Medication errors can be related to professional practice, health care product design, or procedures and systems such as product labeling and distribution. When an error occurs, the client's safety becomes the top priority. The nurse assesses and examines the client's condition and notifies the physician of the incident as soon as possible. Once the client is stable, the nurse reports the incident to the appropriate person in the institution (e.g., manager or supervisor).

Box 16-6 Steps to Take in Preventing Medication Errors

- Follow the five rights of medication administration.
- Be sure to read labels at least three times (comparing MAR with label): before, during, and after administering the drug.
- Do not allow any other activity to interrupt your administration of medication to a client.
- Double check all calculations.
- Document all medications as soon as they are given.
- When you have made an error, reflect on what went wrong, ask how you could have prevented the error.
- Evaluate the context for any medication error to determine if nurses have the necessary resources for safe medication administration.
- When repeated medication errors occur within a work area, identify and analyze the factors that may have caused the errors and take corrective action.
- Attend in-service programs that focus on the drugs you commonly administer.

The nurse is also responsible for reporting the incident. A written incident report usually must be filed within 24 hours of an incident. The report includes client identifying information, the location and time of the incident, an accurate, factual description of what occurred and what was done, and the signature of the nurse involved. The incident report is not a permanent part of the medical record and should not be referred to in the record. This is to legally protect the health care professional and institution. Institutions use incident reports to track incident patterns and to initiate quality improvement programs as needed. Depending on the circumstances and the severity of the outcome, the nurse or institution may be responsible for reporting the incident to the Joint Commission on Accreditation of Healthcare Organizations (JCAHO), MedWatch (FDA's Medical Products Reporting Program), or U.S. Pharmacopeia's Medication Errors reporting program (Morris, 1999).

It is good risk management to report all medication errors, including mistakes that do not cause obvious or immediate harm or near misses. When there has been no harm from a medication error, the institution can still learn why the mistake occurred and what can be done to avoid similar errors in the future. Prevention is the key. Box 16-6 lists steps to take in preventing medication errors.

Client and Family Teaching

A properly informed client is more likely to take medications correctly than one who is unsure about the purpose of a medication and how it will affect his or her daily lifestyle. The nurse provides information about the purpose of medications, their actions, side effects, dosage schedules, actions to take in case of side or toxic effects, and administration guidelines. It is never too early to begin instruction. When a client receives an order for a new medication, the nurse covers a comprehensive range of information about the drug. If a client has been receiving a medication, the nurse assesses the client's knowledge base and fills in where gaps or misunderstandings exist. When teaching clients it is best to include persons who may become involved in their care (e.g., family, friends, partners) or who are available should a client become ill at home.

Reinforcing Adherence

Taking prescribed medications routinely can become a challenge, depending on a person's lifestyle and the number of medications prescribed. When providing instruction, have the client or family member repeat the name and use for each medication plus the dosing instructions. Use of teaching pamphlets or drug information leaflets can help to reinforce important information. Determine if the client requires a compliance aid or memory cue. This is especially important in older adults. Drug dose containers, organized by the hours and days of the week, can be very useful. In the event clients miss a dose of medication, they need to know how to adjust their medication schedule safely.

Teaching Clients About Side Effects

All medications have side effects. The nurse teaches the client and family members about side effects associated with each medication prescribed, focusing on the side effects that are the *most likely* to occur early after administration. For example, some antibiotics cause hypersensitivity and should be used with caution for clients who have liver or kidney disease. Hypersensitivity reactions are likely to occur shortly after taking a few doses of an antibiotic. Other side effects tend to occur after long-term antibiotic administration. Teach clients about side effects in terms of things they can see, feel, touch, or hear. For example, thrombocytopenia, a reduction in the number of platelets in the blood, can be a side effect of a drug. The client cannot see, touch, or hear thrombocytopenia. However, thrombocytopenia can cause bleeding, and there are ways the client can look for evidence of bleeding in any part of the body (e.g., bruising of the skin, blood in urine or stool, nosebleeds). Be sure to teach the client what to do about side effects when they are discovered.

Teaching Drug Safety

Evaluating the effectiveness of teaching ensures that the client can administer drugs in a safe manner. Have clients describe their drug schedules and then have a discussion that allows them to ask questions and clarify their understanding:

- Why are you taking this medication?
- How often do you take this medication?
- How much do you take?
- What side effects can occur?
- What do you do when side effects occur?

Another method to evaluate client understanding of medications is to create medication cards with the name of the drug on the front of the card and all pertinent drug information on the back of the card. The nurse flashes the card in front of the client and asks the client to read the name of the medication. This also ensures that the client can read the name of the medication. If the client correctly identifies the name of the medication, further discussion about drug doses and side effects can be conducted.

It may be helpful to have actual medication bottles labeled with the drug name available at a teaching session. Drug bottles often have fine print and may not be easily read by the client with impaired visual acuity. This would be the time to discover visual limitations so that a larger print label can be provided.

The nurse also evaluates the client's sensory, motor, and cognitive functions, which, when impaired, may affect the client's ability to safely self-administer medications. This includes the ability to open medication containers, prepare a dose in a syringe, or read a label. When impairments are assessed, family members, friends, or home health aides may be available to assist with medication administration.

Critical Thinking Exercises

1. You have given Mrs. Vena her prescribed medications and cough elixir. She asks you, "Now you didn't give me any codeine, did you? I'm allergic to it." You reply that there is no codeine in her medications. After returning to the medication room, you think again and recheck the bottle of cough elixir and find that it contains codeine. What would you do?
2. Mr. Feit is 80 years old and suffers chronic renal disease. He is receiving an antihypertensive, a stool softener, an antianxiety agent, and a nonsteroidal antiinflammatory agent. When you go into Mr. Feit's room to administer nursing care in the evening, you assess him to be confused. When reporting this change to the nurse in charge, he tells you that Mr. Feit may be having a reaction to the antianxiety agent. What is the clinical problem, and why is Mr. Feit at risk?
3. You receive an order for Glucotrol (glipizide) 10.0 mg. PO daily, to be given in two equally divided doses, one dose before breakfast and one dose before dinner. The tablet is available in 2.5 mg. How many tablets does the client receive in each dose? Use dimensional analysis to compute your answer.
4. Cindi is a third-year nursing student. She is checking a transcription taken off by a secretary. Cindi is able to read the name of the medication clearly, but the dosage is smudged. Which of the five rights for medication administration is threatened? What should Cindi do?

References

Arnold GJ: Clinical recognition of adverse drug reactions: obstacles and opportunities for the nursing profession, *J Nurs Care Qual* 13(2):45, 1998.

Clayton BD, Stock YN: *Basic pharmacology for nurses,* ed 11, St. Louis, 1997, Mosby.

Johnson, DS: *Psychiatric-mental health nursing: adaptation and growth,* ed 4, Philadelphia, 1997, Lippincott.

Johnson PE and others: ASHP guidelines on adverse drug reaction monitoring and reporting, *Am J Health-System Pharm* 52:417, 1995.

Kovach LJ: Polypharmacy in the elderly, *Pharm Ther J* 17(11):1709, 1992.

Kudzma EC: Culturally competent drug administration, *Am J Nurs* 99(8):46, 1999.

Lueckenotte AG: *Gerontologic nursing,* ed 2, St. Louis, 2000, Mosby.

McCaffery M, Pasero C: *Pain,* ed 2, St. Louis, 1999, Mosby.

McKenry LM, Salerno E: *Mosby's pharmacology in nursing,* ed 20, St. Louis, 1998, Mosby.

Morris MR: Preventing med errors, *RN* 62(9):69, 1999.

Sullivan GH: When can RNs administer meds independently? *RN* 61(2);55, 1998.

United States Pharamcopeia Convention, Inc: Definition of medication errors, *USP Quality Rev,* no. 57, January 1997.

Wong D and others: *Whaley and Wong's nursing care of infants and children,* ed 6, St. Louis, 1999, Mosby.

17

ORAL AND TOPICAL MEDICATIONS

Skills

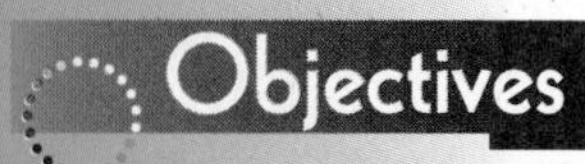

Mastery of content in this chapter will enable the nurse to:

- Define the key terms listed.
- Correctly administer a medication by oral, nasogastric, skin (topical), ophthalmic, otic, vaginal, and rectal routes.
- Correctly administer medications for irrigation and instillation.
- Identify guidelines for administering oral, nasogastric, skin (topical), ophthalmic, otic, vaginal, and rectal medications.
- Describe factors to assess before administering medications.
- Differentiate types of topical administrations that require sterile technique and those that require clean medical aseptic technique.
- Instruct clients in proper use of metered-dose inhalers (MDIs) and small-volume nebulizers.
- Identify conditions contraindicating the administration of medications.
- Prepare a teaching plan regarding medication use for a selected client.

Key Terms

A.D.
Adrenergic drug
Anaphylaxis
Anesthetics
Antianginal
A.S.
A.U.
Cerumen
Cycloplegic
Dermatitis
Dermatological
Eczema
Glaucoma
Lotion
Metered-dose inhalers (MDIs)
Mydriatics
Nares
Nasal
Nebulizer
Nitroglycerin
O.D.
Ointment
Ophthalmic
Orifice
O.S.
Otic
O.U.
Overdose
Pillating device
Pruritus
Suppository
Suspension
Sympathomimetic
Topical
Transdermal
Vertigo

The easiest and most desirable way to administer medications is by mouth. Clients usually are able to ingest or self-administer oral drugs with a minimum of problems. Situations, however, may arise that contraindicate the client's receiving medications by mouth, such as the presence of gastrointestinal alterations, the inability of a client to swallow food or fluids, and the use of gastric suction. An important precaution to take when administering any oral preparation is to protect clients from aspiration. Aspiration occurs when food, fluid, or medication intended for gastrointestinal administration inadvertently is administered into the respiratory tract. The nurse protects the client from aspiration by assessing the client's ability to safely swallow oral medications (Box 17-1). Properly positioning the client is also essential in preventing aspiration. Unless contraindicated, the nurse positions the client in a seated position when administering oral medications. The lateral position can also be used when the client's swallow, gag, and cough are intact. A client who has difficulty swallowing should be evaluated by appropriate personnel (e.g., speech therapist) before receiving oral preparations.

Topical administration of medications involves applying drugs locally to skin, mucous membranes, or tissue membranes. The nurse applies medications to the skin by painting, spraying, or spreading medication over an area, applying moist dressings, soaking body parts in solution, or

Box 17-1 Dysphagia

Dysphagia, or difficulty in swallowing, may lead to aspiration. A variety of signs and symptoms may be associated with dysphagia:

- Choking while eating or drinking
- Facial droop
- Drooling or leakage of food from the mouth
- Coughing during or after meals
- Holding pockets of food in the cheeks
- Absent or diminished gag reflex
- Gurgly voice quality
- Increased congestion or secretions after eating or drinking

The client's swallow, cough, and gag reflexes must be carefully assessed. Swallowing can be assessed at the bedside by placing the thumb and index finger on both sides of the client's Adam's apple and feeling for elevation of the larynx when the client tries to swallow. The elevation should be symmetrical. See Chapter 33 on proper techniques of coughing. If the client has intact swallow and cough reflexes, then assess the gag reflex by gently stroking the back of the throat on each side with a tongue blade.

If swallowing difficulties are suspected or detected, a referral to a speech pathologist is needed for definitive diagnosis. Dysphagia that is not recognized or managed may lead to aspiration pneumonia.

Data from Kayser-Jones J, Pengilly K: Dysphagia among nursing home residents, *Geriatr Nurs* 20(2):77, 1999; Mahan LK, Escott-Stump S: *Krause's food, nutrition, and diet therapy*, ed 10, Philadelphia, 2000, WB Saunders.

giving medicated baths. Adhesive-backed medicated disks can also be applied to the skin to provide a continuous release of medication over several hours or days. Systemic effects from topical agents can occur if the skin is thin, if the drug concentration is high, or if contact with the skin is prolonged.

Topical administration avoids puncturing skin and lessens the risk of infection and tissue injury that may occur with injections. Gastrointestinal disturbances are encountered less frequently than with oral administration. The risk of serious side effects is generally low, but serious systemic effects can occur.

Drugs applied to membranes such as the cornea of the eye or rectal mucosa are absorbed quickly because of the membrane's vascularity. When drug concentrations are high, systemic effects can occur. For example, bradycardia may occur following atropine instillation to the eye. Mucous and other tissue membranes differ in their sensitivity to medications. The cornea of the eye, for example, is extremely sensitive to chemicals. Clients commonly experience burning sensations during administration of eye and nose drops. Medications are generally less irritating to vaginal or rectal mucosa.

Medications for topical use can be administered in the following ways:

1. Direct application of liquid—eye drops, gargling, swabbing the throat.
2. Inserting drug into a body cavity—**suppository** insertion into rectum or vagina or creams and foams inserted into the vagina.
3. Instillation of fluid into body cavity (fluid is retained)—ear drops, nose drops, bladder and rectal instillation.
4. Irrigation of body cavity (fluid is not retained)—flushing eye, ear, vagina, bladder, or rectum with medicated fluid.
5. Spraying—instillation into nose or throat.
6. Inhalation of medicated aerosol spray—distributes medication throughout the **nasal** passages and tracheobronchial airway. There are two types of **nebulizers** designed for this purpose: **metered-dose inhalers (MDIs)** and small-volume nebulizers.
7. Direct application to skin or mucosa—**lotion, ointment,** cream, powder, spray, patch, and disk.

Skill Performance Guidelines

1. Assess client's sensory function, including sight, hearing, touch, and physical coordination. Sensory and coordination deficits may impair client ability to see medications, open prescription bottles, and read labels at home.
2. Clients often receive more than one oral medication at a time. The nurse evaluates each medication for potential drug-drug or drug-food interactions. Always consult with the pharmacist when in doubt.
3. Evaluate whether medication can be taken with food. Some drugs require an empty stomach to enhance absorption. Other drugs can irritate the stomach lining and should always be taken with food.
4. For all medications administered orally or topically, gather information pertinent to the drug(s) ordered: purpose, normal dosage and route, common side effects, time of onset and peak action, nursing implications.
5. For all medications administered orally or topically, review prescriber's order for client's name, name of drug, strength, time of administration, and site of application.
6. Administration of some medications require specific nursing actions. For example, the nurse should monitor the client's apical pulse and serum drug levels before administering digoxin.
7. Before applying topical medication, bathe any surface that may be contaminated with blood, body fluids, secretions, or excretions.
8. Use clean disposable gloves when applying topical medications to prevent absorption of the medication into the nurse's skin.
9. Some topical medications are poorly absorbed on peripheral extremities. Follow manufacturer's recommendation for proper application of medication.
10. Check for client allergies prior to administration, particularly to preservatives or fragrances in topical medications.
11. Know potential local and systemic effects of all topically applied medications.
12. If clients are mentally and physically able, prepare the clients for discharge by instructing them on self-administration techniques.
13. Check the expiration date for all medications.

Skill 17-1 Administering Oral Medications

The easiest and most desirable way to administer medications is by mouth. The majority of medications the nurse administers are given by this route. The nurse usually prepares the medications for the client to self-administer and prepares oral medications in an area designed for medication preparation or at the unit-dose cart.

Delegation Considerations

The skill of administering oral medications should not be delegated to assistive personnel. Assistive personnel should be instructed about potential side effects of medications and to report their occurrence.

Equipment

- Medication cart or tray
- Disposable medication cups
- Glass of water, juice, or preferred liquid
- Drinking straw
- Pill-crushing or pillating device (optional)
- Paper towels
- Medication administration record (MAR) or computer printout

Step	Rationale
Assessment	
1. Assess for any contraindications to client receiving oral medication: Is client able to swallow? Is client suffering from nausea/vomiting? Is client diagnosed as having bowel inflammation or reduced peristalsis? Has client had recent gastrointestinal surgery? Does client have gastric suction? Is the client restricted to nothing by mouth (NPO)? What is the client's level of consciousness?	Alterations in gastrointestinal function interfere with drug absorption, distribution, and excretion. Clients with gastrointestinal suction might not receive benefit from the medication because it may be suctioned from gastrointestinal tract before it can be absorbed. Clients with altered levels of consciousness may not be able to swallow oral medications.

- ***Critical Decision Point***
  Clients with neuromuscular disorders, esophageal strictures, lesions of the mouth, and those who are unresponsive or comatose and cannot swallow should not receive medications by the oral route. The nurse should request that the prescriber order the medication by an alternate route (e.g., intravenously).

Step	Rationale
2. Assess client's medical history, history of allergies, medication history, and diet history. Drug allergies should be listed on each page of the MAR and prominently displayed on the client's medical record.	These factors can influence how certain drugs act. Information also reflects client's need for medications.
3. Gather and review assessment and laboratory data that may influence drug administration, such as medication history, vital signs, and renal and liver function studies.	Physical examination or laboratory data may contraindicate drug administration. Medication history may reveal past problems with medication administration. Renal and liver function status will affect metabolism and excretion of the medication (Lilley and Aucker, 1999).

- ***Critical Decision Point***
  If contraindications exist, withhold medication and inform prescriber of your findings.

Step	Rationale
4. Assess clients knowledge regarding health and medication use. Consider drug use problems such as drug tolerance, noncompliance, abuse, addiction, or dependence.	Determines client's need for drug education. Also assists in identifying client's adherence to drug therapy at home.

- ***Critical Decision Point***
  If drug use problem is suspected, refer client to the appropriate health care professional.

Step	Rationale
5. Assess client's preferences for fluids.	Offering fluids during drug administration is an excellent way to increase client's fluid intake. Fluids ease swallowing and facilitate absorption from the gastrointestinal tract. However, fluid restrictions must be maintained if ordered.
6. Assess whether the medication can be administered with the preferred fluid.	Some fluids may interfere with absorption of the medication. For example, taking tetracyclines with milk products greatly reduces their absorption. (Lilley and Aucker, 1999)

STEP	RATIONALE

NURSING DIAGNOSIS

Defining characteristics from the assessment data may reveal the following nursing diagnoses for clients requiring this skill:

- Impaired swallowing
- Risk for aspiration
- Deficient knowledge regarding drug therapy
- Noncompliance regarding drug regimen

Related factors are individualized based on client's condition or needs.

PLANNING

Step	Rationale
1. **Expected outcomes** following completion of procedure:	
▪ Client experiences desired medication effect within period of onset of medication.	Drug has exerted its therapeutic action.
▪ Client denies any gastrointestinal discomfort or symptoms of alterations.	Oral medications can irritate gastrointestinal mucosa.
▪ Client explains purpose of medication and drug dose schedule.	Demonstrates understanding of drug therapy.
2. Check accuracy and completeness of each MAR or computer printout with prescriber's written medication order. Check client's name, drug name and dosage, route of administration, and time for administration. Compare MAR or computer printout with medication label.	The order sheet is the most reliable source and only legal record of drugs client is to receive. Ensures client receives correct medication.

• ***Critical Decision Point***
Incomplete or unclear orders should be clarified with the prescriber before implementation.

Step	Rationale
3. Recopy or reprint any portion of the MAR that is illegible.	Soiled or illegible MAR forms or computer printouts can be a source of drug error.
4. Check client's identification bracelet and ask name.	Ensures correct client receives medication.
5. Explain procedure to client. Be specific if client wishes to self-administer drug.	Makes client a participant in care and minimizes anxiety. Begins client teaching regarding medications. Enables client to self-administer drug if physically able.

IMPLEMENTATION

Step	Rationale
1. Prepare medications:	
a. Wash hands.	Reduces transfer of microorganisms.
b. Arrange medication tray and cups in medication preparation area or move medication cart to position outside client's room.	Organization of equipment saves time and reduces error.
c. Unlock medicine drawer or cart.	Medications are safeguarded when locked in cabinet or cart.
d. Prepare medications for one client at a time. Keep all pages of MARs or computer printouts for one client together.	Prevents preparation errors.
e. Select correct drug from stock supply or unit-dose drawer. Compare label of medication with MAR or computer printout (see illustration).	Reading label and comparing it against transcribed order reduces errors.
f. Calculate drug dose as necessary. Double-check calculation.	Double-checking reduces risk of error.

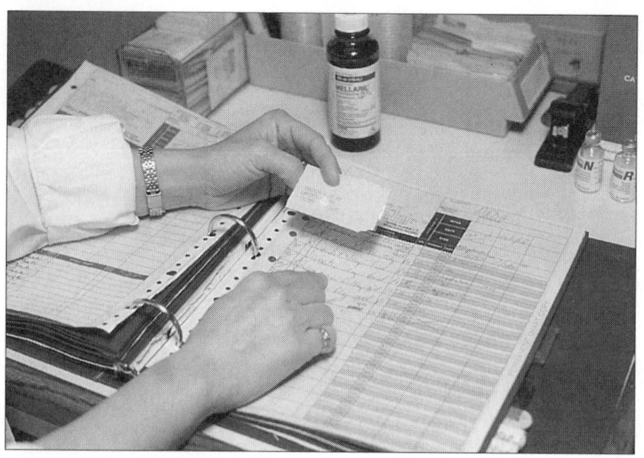

STEP **1e** The nurse checks the label of the medication with the transcribed medication order.

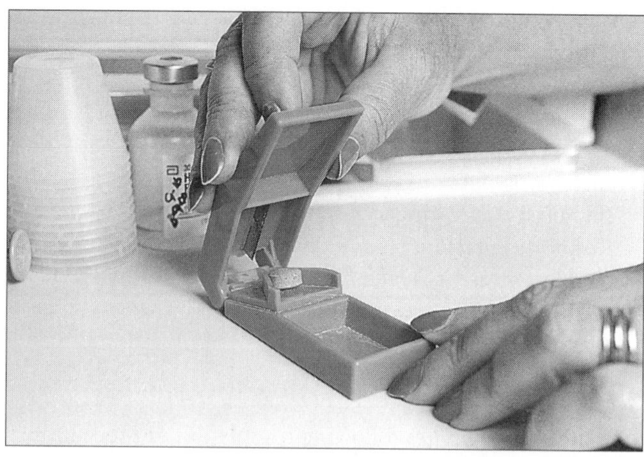

STEP **1g** Tablet is placed in pillating device and cut in half.

STEP	RATIONALE
g. To prepare tablets or capsules from a floor-stock bottle, pour required number into bottle cap and transfer medication to medication cup. Do not touch medication with fingers. Extra tablets or capsules may be returned to bottle. Medications that need to be broken to administer half the dosage can be broken, using a gloved hand, or cut with a **pillating device** (see illustration). Tablets that are to be broken in half must be prescored. Prescored tablets are identified by a manufactured line that transverses the center of the tablet.	Drugs are very expensive; avoid waste. Tablets that are not prescored cannot be broken into equal halves, and the result will be inaccurate dose.
h. To prepare unit-dose tablets or capsules, place packaged tablet or capsule directly into medicine cup. (Do not remove wrapper.)	Wrapper maintains cleanliness of medications and identifies drug name and dose.
i. All tablets or capsules to be given to client at same time may be placed in one medicine cup except for those requiring preadministration assessments (e.g., pulse rate or blood pressure).	Keeping medications that require preadministration assessments separate from others make it easier for the nurse to withhold drugs as necessary.
j. If client has difficulty swallowing, use pill-crushing device such as a mortar and pestle to crush pills (see illustration). If a pill-crushing device is not available, place tablet between two medication cups and grind with a blunt instrument. Mix ground tablet in small amount of soft food (custard or applesauce).	Large tablets can be difficult to swallow. Ground tablet mixed with palatable soft food is usually easier to swallow.

• ***Critical Decision Point***

Not all drugs can be crushed (e.g., capsules, enteric-coated, and long-acting/slow-release drugs). The coating of these drugs is designed to protect the stomach from irritation or protect the drug from destruction from stomach acids. Consult with pharmacist when in doubt (Miller and Miller, 2000).

STEP	RATIONALE
k. Prepare liquids:	
(1) Remove bottle cap from container and place cap upside down on work surface.	Prevents contamination of inside of cap.
(2) Hold bottle with label against palm of hand while pouring.	Spilled liquid will not drip and soil or fade label.
(3) Hold medication cup at eye level and fill to desired level on scale. Scale should be even with fluid level at its surface or base of meniscus, not edges (see illustration).	Ensures accuracy of measurement.

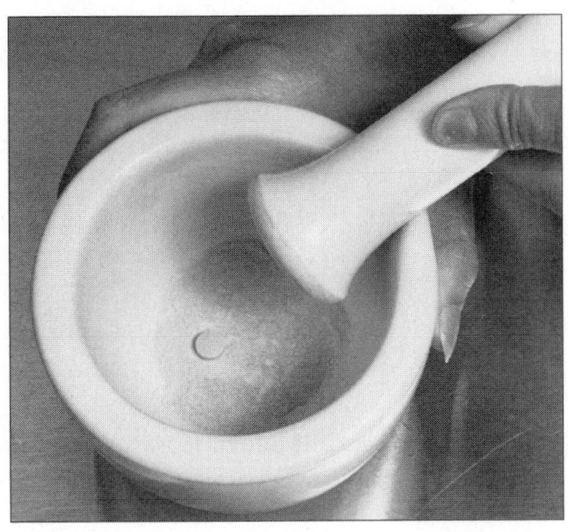

STEP **1j** Pill placed in mortar for crushing.

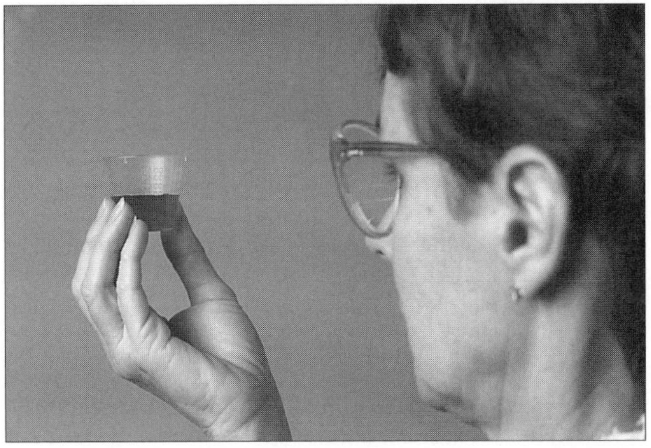

STEP **1k(3)** Pour the desired volume of liquid so that base of meniscus is level with line on scale.

STEP	RATIONALE
(4) Discard any excess liquid into sink. Wipe lip and neck of bottle with paper towel and recap the bottle.	Prevents contamination of bottle's contents and prevents bottle cap from sticking.
(5) Liquid medications packaged in single-dose cups need not be poured into medicine cups. They can be administered directly from the single-dose cup.	Avoids unnecessary manipulation of dose.
(6) For small doses of liquid medications, draw liquid into a calibrated oral syringe, with needle attached.	This technique is more accurate for measuring small doses of liquid medications.
l. Check expiration date on all medications.	Medications used past expiration date may be inactive or harmful to client.
m. When preparing narcotics, check narcotic record for previous drug count and compare with supply available.	Controlled substance laws require careful monitoring of dispensed narcotics.
n. Compare MAR or computer printout with prepared drug and container.	Reading label second time reduces error.
o. Return stock containers or unused unit-dose medications to shelf or drawer and read label again.	Third check of label reduces administration errors.
p. Do not leave drugs unattended.	Nurse is responsible for safekeeping of drugs.
2. Administer medications:	
a. Take medications to client at correct time.	Medications are administered within 30 minutes before or after prescribed time to ensure intended therapeutic effect. Stat or single-order medications should be given at time ordered.
b. Identify client by comparing name on MAR or computer printout with name on client's identification bracelet. Ask client to state name.	Identification bracelets are made at time of client's admission and are the most reliable source of identification. Replace any missing or faded identification bracelets.
c. Explain purpose of each medication and its action to client. Allow client to ask any questions about drugs.	Client has right to be informed, and client's understanding of purpose of each medication improves compliance with drug therapy.

- ***Critical Decision Point***
  If client refuses medication, withhold medication and notify prescriber.

d. Assist client to a seated or side-lying position if sitting is contraindicated by client's condition.	Decreases risk of aspiration during swallowing.

- ***Critical Decision Point***
  Check the client's swallow, cough, and gag reflexes (see Box 17-1) if in doubt about client's ability to manage oral medications. Withhold medication if swallow, cough, or gag is impaired and notify physician.

Step	Rationale
e. Administer drugs properly:	
(1) Client may wish to hold solid medications in hand or cup before placing in mouth.	Client can become familiar with medications by seeing each drug.
(2) Offer water or juice to help client swallow medications.	Choice of fluid promotes client's comfort and can improve fluid intake.
(3) For sublingual-administered drugs, have client place medication under tongue and allow it to dissolve completely. Caution client against swallowing tablet.	Drug is absorbed through blood vessels of undersurface of tongue. If swallowed, drug is destroyed by gastric juices or so rapidly detoxified by liver that therapeutic blood levels are not attained.
(4) For buccal-administered drugs, have client place medication in mouth against mucous membranes of the cheek until it dissolves.	Buccal medications act locally on mucosa or systemically as they are swallowed in saliva.

• ***Critical Decision Point***
Avoid administering liquids until buccal/sublingual medication has dissolved.

Step	Rationale
(5) Caution client against chewing or swallowing lozenges.	Drug acts through slow absorption through oral mucosa, not gastric mucosa.
(6) Mix powdered medications with liquids at bedside and give to client to drink.	When prepared in advance, powdered drugs may thicken and even harden, making swallowing difficult.
(7) Give effervescent powders and tablets immediately after dissolving.	Effervescence improves unpleasant taste of drug and often relieves gastrointestinal problems.
f. If client is unable to hold medications, place medication cup to the lips and gently introduce each drug into the mouth, one at a time. Do not rush.	Administering single tablet or capsule eases swallowing and decreases risk of aspiration.
g. If tablet or capsule falls to the floor, discard it and repeat preparation.	Drug is contaminated when it touches floor.
h. Stay until client has completely swallowed each medication. Ask client to open mouth if uncertain whether medication has been swallowed.	Nurse is responsible for ensuring that client receives ordered dosage. If left uanttended, client may not take dose or may save drugs, causing risk to health.
i. For highly acidic medications (e.g., aspirin), offer client nonfat snack (e.g., crackers) if not contraindicated by client's condition.	Reduces gastric irritation. The fat content of foods may delay absorption of the medication.
j. Assist client in returning to comfortable position.	Maintains client's comfort.
k. Dispose of soiled supplies and wash hands.	Reduces transmission of microorganisms.
l. Record administration of medication on MAR or computer printout. Return MAR or computer printouts to appropriate file for next administration time.	Timely recording reduces medication errors. Computer printouts or MAR are used as reference for when next dose is due. Loss can lead to administration error.
m. Replenish stock such as cups and straws, return cart to medicine room, and clean work area.	Clean working space assists other staff in completing duties efficiently.

Evaluation

Step	Rationale
1. Return within 30 minutes to evaluate client's response to medications.	Evaluates drug's therapeutic benefit and can detect onset of side effects or allergic reactions.
2. Ask client or family member to identify drug name and explain purpose, action, dose schedule, and potential side effects of drug.	Determines level of knowledge gained by client and family.

Unexpected Outcomes and Related Interventions

- Client exhibits adverse effects (side effect, toxic effect, allergic reaction).
  - Symptoms such as urticaria, rash, **pruritus,** rhinitis, and wheezing may indicate allergic reaction.
  - Always notify prescriber and pharmacy when the client exhibits adverse effects. Withhold further doses.
- Client is unable to explain drug information.
  - Further assess the client's or family member's knowledge of medications and guidelines for drug safety.
  - Further instruction is necessary.

Recording and Reporting

- Record actual time each drug was administered on MAR or computer printout immediately after administration. Include initials or signature. Do not chart medication administration until *after* it is given to client.
- If drug is withheld, record reason in nurses' notes. Circle time the drug normally would have been given on MAR or computer printout.
- Report adverse effects/client response and/or withheld drugs to nurse in charge or physician. Depending on medication, immediate prescriber notification may be required.

Teaching Considerations

- Instruct client on specific information pertaining to drug regimen (purpose, action, dose, dosage intervals, side effects, foods to avoid or take with drugs).
- All clients should learn the basic guidelines for drug safety (see Chapter 39).

Pediatric Considerations

- Liquid forms of medication are safer to swallow to avoid aspiration of small pills.
- Bitter or distasteful oral preparation will be rejected by the child. Mix the drug with a small amount (about 1 tsp) of a sweet-tasting substance, such as jam, applesauce, honey, or fruit puree. Do not use honey in infants because of the risk of botulism. The nurse can also offer the child juice or an ice pop after medication administration. Do not place medication in a favorite food; the child may refuse the food at a later time.
- Measure small amount of liquid medications using a plastic calibrated syringe. Amounts less than a teaspoon are impossible to measure accurately with a molded medicine cup (Wong and others, 1999).

Gerontological Considerations

- Physiologic changes of aging influence how oral medications are distributed, absorbed, and excreted. Common changes include loss of elasticity in oral mucosa; reduction in parotid gland secretion, causing dry mouth; delayed esophageal clearance, impaired swallowing; reduction in gastric acidity and stomach peristalsis, increased susceptibility to highly acidic drugs; and reduced colon motility, slowing drug excretion.
- Rinse client's oral cavity frequently with tepid water, floss daily, and brush gently.
- Administer a full glass of water (unless restricted) with medications to aid passage of the drug. Give client time to swallow.
- Older adults may have several health problems or chronic conditions that require the use of multiple drugs, often prescribed by different health care providers. This polypharmacy creates a high risk for drug interactions and adverse reactions.
- The most common adverse reactions that may occur in older adults are lethargy, sedation, falls, and confusion.
- When instructing about the medication regimen, include client's spouse or another family member. If possible, provide a written medication schedule for client to follow at home (Ebersole and Hess, 1998).

Home Care Considerations

- See Skill 39-3, Medication and Medical Device Safety, and Skill 40-4, Helping Clients With Self-Medication.

Skill 17-2 Administering Medications by Nasogastric Tube

Clients with nasogastric tubes often receive nothing by mouth. Oral medications that need to be administered to these clients can be given by nasogastric tube. Medications should not be administered into nasogastric/intestinal tubes that are inserted for decompression. To administer medications by a nasogastric tube, the nurse modifies the form of a tablet to be administered by crushing and dissolving it. Medications may also be available in liquid form. Generally, sustained-release, chewable, long-acting, or enteric-coated tablets and capsules are not administered by gastric tubes. Consult with the hospital pharmacy when in doubt.

Delegation Considerations

The skill of administering medications by nasogastric tube should not be delegated to assistive personnel. Assistive personnel should be instructed about potential side effects of medications and to report their occurrence.

Equipment

- 60-ml syringe: cone tip for large-bore tubes (Asepto syringe or Toomey syringe); Luer-lok tip for small-bore tubes
- Gastric pH test tape
- Graduated container
- Water
- Medication to be administered
- Pill crusher if medication in tablet form
- Medication administration record (MAR) or computer printout
- Disposable gloves

STEP	RATIONALE

ASSESSMENT

1. Assess for any contraindications to client receiving oral medication. Has the client been diagnosed as having bowel inflammation or reduced peristalsis? Has client had recent gastrointestinal surgery? Does client have gastric suction? Can the suction be temporarily turned off?

   Alterations in gastrointestinal function interfere with drug distribution, absorption, and excretion. Clients with gastrointestinal suction might not receive benefit from the medication because it may be suctioned from gastrointestinal tract before it can be absorbed.

   - ***Critical Decision Point***

     Always review client's postoperative orders for gastric tube care. Manipulation and irrigation of tube or instillation of medication may be contraindicated.

2. Assess client's medical history, history of allergies, medication history, and diet history.

   These factors can influence how certain drugs act. Information also reflects client's need for medications.

3. Gather and review assessment and laboratory data that may influence drug administration, such as medication history, vital signs, and renal and liver function studies.

   Physical examination or laboratory data may contraindicate drug administration. Medication history may reveal past problems with medication administration. Renal and liver function status will affect metabolism and excretion of the medication (Lilley and Aucker, 1999).

   - ***Critical Decision Point***

     If contraindications exist, withhold medication and inform the prescriber of your findings.

4. Before administration of medications verify placement of the gastric tube (see Skill 22-2).

   Reduces the risk of aspiration.

NURSING DIAGNOSIS

Defining characteristics from the assessment data may reveal the following nursing diagnoses for clients requiring this skill:

Impaired swallowing
Risk for aspiration
Feeding self-care deficit

Related factors are individualized based on client's condition or needs.

PLANNING

1. **Expected outcomes** following completion of procedure:
   - Client experiences desired medication effect within period of onset of medication.

     Drug has exerted its therapeutic action.

   - Client's feeding tube remains patent after administration of medication.

     A patent nasogastric tube indicates passage of medication into stomach, ensuring proper absorption. A blocked tube can later interfere with irrigation and fluid instillation.

2. Check accuracy and completeness of each MAR or computer printout with prescriber's written medication order. Check client's name, drug name and dosage, route of administration, and time for administration. Compare MAR or computer printout with medication label.

   The order sheet is the most reliable source and only legal record of drugs client is to receive. Ensures client receives correct medication.

3. Check client's identification bracelet and ask name.

   Ensures correct client receives medication.

4. Explain procedure to client, including description of medication to be instilled into nasogastric tube.

   Makes client a participant in care and minimizes anxiety. Begins client teaching regarding medications.

IMPLEMENTATION

1. Wash hands.

   Reduces transfer of microorganisms.

STEP	RATIONALE
2. Prepare medications for instillation into feeding tube. Prepare graduated container by pouring 50 to 100 ml of water into it.	Adequate preparation saves nursing time.

- ***Critical Decision Point***

  Whenever possible, liquid medications are preferred to crushed tablets, but if tablets must be crushed, the tubing must be flushed before and after the medication to prevent the drug from adhering to the inside of the tube (McKenry and Salerno, 1998). Concentrated medications need to be thoroughly diluted. Dilution is particularly important when the feeding tube extends beyond the pylorus, where residual volume is insufficient to dilute medications and avoid cramping (Klang, 1996).

STEP	RATIONALE
a. Crush tablets using a pill-crushing device such as a mortar and pestle to grind pills into a fine powder. If a pill-crushing device is not available, place tablet between two medication cups and grind with a blunt instrument. Dissolve in at least 30 ml of warm water.	
b. Capsules: Ensure that contents of capsule (granules or gelatin) can be expressed from its covering (consult with pharmacist). Open capsule or pierce gelcap with sterile needle and empty contents into 30 ml of warm water. Gelcaps can also be dissolved in warm water.	Ensures contents of tablets or capsules are a fine powder or solution so as not to occlude nasogastric tube.
3. Prepare client by placing the client in a high-Fowler's position (if not contraindicated by client's medical condition)	Reduces risk of aspiration.
4. Apply clean gloves.	Reduces transfer of microorganisms.
5. Aspirate stomach contents (see illustration). Note volume. Return aspirate to client by flushing tube with 30 ml of air and then pull back on syringe. More than one bolus of air may be necessary (Metheny and others, 1993).	

- ***Critical Decision Point***

  If large volume aspirate is found (e.g., 100 ml or more), return aspirate to client, withhold medication, and notify client's health care provider. Large volume aspirates (e.g., 100 to 150 ml) indicates delayed gastric emptying, which may contribute to gastric distention, esophageal reflux, and vomiting; all of which place the client at risk for aspiration (Mahan and Escott-Stump, 2000). Returning aspirate to client prevents excessive loss of electrolytes.

STEP	RATIONALE
6. Pinch nasogastric tube and remove syringe. Draw up 30 ml of water in syringe. Reinsert tip of syringe into nasogastric tube and flush tube.	Pinching nasogastric tube prevents leakage or spillage of stomach contents. Flushing ensures tube is patent.
7. Remove bulb or plunger of syringe.	Removal of bulb or plunger prepares syringe for delivery of medications.

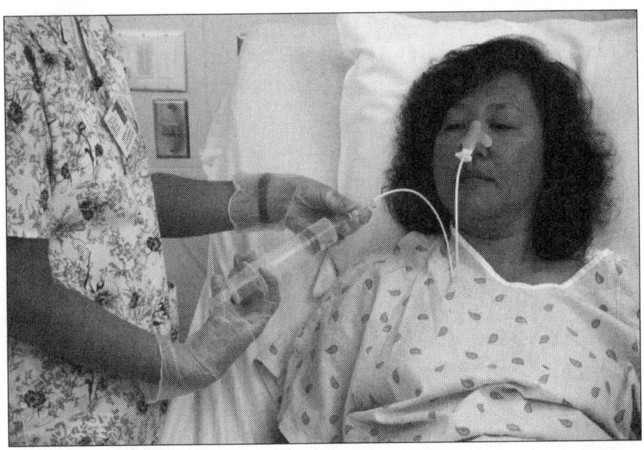

STEP 5 Nurse pulls back on syringe to aspirate stomach contents.

Step	Rationale
8. Administer first dose of medication by pouring into syringe. Follow medication with 30 ml of water, if only one dose of medication is administered.	Ensures instillation of each medication. Maintains patency of nasogastric tube (Simon and Fink, 1999).

- ***Critical Decision Point***
  If water or medication does not flow freely, a gentle push with bulb of Asepto syringe or plunger of Toomey syringe may facilitate flow of fluid.

Step	Rationale
9. Be sure to rinse tube thoroughly with warm water before and after giving medications.	Drugs in syrup form, such as iron elixirs, are acidic. Often these drugs clump, clogging feeding tubes when they come in contact with enteral formulas (Klang, 1996).
10. To administer more than one medication, give each separately with a 5-ml warm water rinse between doses (McConnell, 1998).	Keeping the medications separate allows for accurate identification of medication if a dose is spilled.
11. Follow last dose of medication with 30 to 60 ml of water.	Maintains patency of nasogastric tube. Ensures passage of medication into stomach (Simon and Fink, 1999).
12. When tube feeding is not being administered, clamp the proximal end of the feeding tube and cap end of tube.	Prevents air from entering the stomach between medication doses.
13. When continuous tube feeding is being administered by an infusion pump:	
a. Follow medication administration Steps 1-12, then stop the feeding for 1 hour (check agency policy).	Allows for adequate absorption of medication.
14. Remove gloves, dispose of soiled supplies, and rinse graduated container and syringe with tap water. Wash hands.	Reduces transmission of microorganisms.

Evaluation

1. Return within 30 minutes to evaluate client's response to medications.	By monitoring client's response, nurse assesses drug's therapeutic benefit and can detect onset of side effects or allergic reactions.

Unexpected Outcomes and Related Interventions

- Client does not receive medication as prescribed because of a blocked nasogastric tube
  - Requires interventions to unclog tube to ensure drug delivery (Box 17-2).

Box 17-2 Unclogging a Blocked Feeding Tube

- Prevent tube from becoming blocked by flushing it with 30 ml of warm water before and after administering each dose of medication and every 4 to 6 hours around the clock.
- Do not use cranberry juice or soda to flush or unblock the feeding tube. They only make the tube sticky.
- If tube is blocked, get an order for a pancrelipase tablet (such as Viokase Tablets) and a sodium bicarbonate tablet (to help balance the pH). Crush these tablets together and mix them to form a slurry. Instill into feeding tube. Keep the mixture in your client's feeding tube for 15 to 30 minutes and then irrigate.
- The tube may have to be removed and a new one reinserted if the medication is urgent.

Modified from: Klang M: Medicating tube-fed patients, *Nursing* 26:18, 1996.

- Client exhibits adverse effects (side effect, toxic effect, allergic reaction).
  - Symptoms such as urticaria, rash, pruritus, rhinitis, and wheezing may indicate allergic reaction.
  - Always notify prescriber, and pharmacy, when client exhibits adverse effects
  - Withhold further doses.

Recording and Reporting

- Record in nurses' notes method used to check placement of nasogastric tube, volume of stomach aspirate, and pH of stomach aspirate (see Chapter 22).
- Record actual time each drug was administered on MAR or computer printout immediately after administration. Include initials or signature. Do not chart medication administration until *after* it is given to client.
- Record total amount of fluid used for medication administration on proper intake/output sheet.
- If drug is withheld, record reason in nurses' notes. Circle time the drug normally would have been given on MAR or computer printout.
- Report adverse effects/client response and/or withheld drugs to nurse in charge or physician. Depending on medication, immediate prescriber notification may be required.

PEDIATRIC CONSIDERATIONS

- Volumes for instillation of medications or for irrigation of nasogastric tubes may be smaller. Check agency policy (Miller and Miller, 2000).

Skill 17-3 Administering Skin Applications

Many locally applied drugs such as lotions, patches, pastes, and ointments can create systemic and local effects if absorbed through the skin. To protect the nurse from accidental exposure, the nurse should apply these drugs using gloves and applicators. If the client's skin is intact, the nurse uses clean technique when applying lotions, patches, and ointments. If the client has an open wound, sterile technique is important.

Skin encrustations and dead tissue harbor microorganisms and block contact of medications with the tissues to be treated. Simply applying new medications over previously applied drugs does little to prevent infection or offer therapeutic benefit. The nurse cleans the skin thoroughly before applying medications by washing the area gently with soap and water, soaking an involved site, or locally debriding tissue.

Each type of medication, whether an ointment, lotion, powder, or patch, should be applied in a specific way to ensure proper penetration and absorption. For example, the nurse applies lotions and creams by spreading them lightly onto the skin's surface, whereas powders are dusted lightly over affected areas.

DELEGATION CONSIDERATIONS

The skill of administering skin (topical) medications should not be delegated to assistive personnel. Some institutions may permit assistive personnel to apply some forms of topical agents during morning care; check agency policies. Assistive personnel should be instructed about the expected therapeutic effects and potential side effects of medications and to report their occurrence.

EQUIPMENT

- Clean gloves (for intact skin) or sterile gloves (nonintact skin)
- Ordered agent (powder, cream, lotion, ointment, spray, patch)
- Cotton-tipped applicators or tongue blades (optional)
- Basin of warm water, washcloth, towel, nondrying soap
- Sterile dressing, tape
- Medication administration record (MAR) or computer printout

STEP	RATIONALE
ASSESSMENT	
1. Assess condition of client's skin. First wash site thoroughly with mild, nondrying soap and warm water, rinse, and dry. Be sure any previously applied medication or debris is removed. Assess for symptoms of skin irritation such as pruritus or burning.	Cleansing site thoroughly allows nurse to obtain a proper assessment of skin surface. Assessment provides baseline to determine change in condition of skin after therapy. Application of certain topical agents can lessen or aggravate these symptoms.
2. Further inspect the condition of the skin or membranes. Do not administer topical medications to skin whose integrity is altered, unless indicated.	
3. Determine whether client has known allergy to topical agent. Ask if client has had reaction to a cream or lotion applied to the skin.	Allergic contact **dermatitis** is relatively common and can worsen **dermatological** condition.
4. Determine amount of topical agent required for application by assessing affected area, reviewing prescriber's order, and reading application directions carefully (a thin, even layer is usually adequate).	An excessive amount of topical agent can cause chemical irritation of skin, negate drug's effectiveness, and/or cause adverse systemic effects, such as decreased white cell counts.

Step	Rationale
5. Assess client's knowledge of action and purpose of medication being given and interest in treating health problem.	Reveals client's level of understanding and whether instruction is necessary.
6. Determine if client is physically able to apply medication by assessing fine grasp, hand strength, reach, and coordination.	Necessary if client is to self-administer drug in the home.

Nursing Diagnosis

Defining characteristics from the assessment data may reveal the following nursing diagnoses for clients requiring this skill:

- Impaired skin integrity
- Ineffective therapeutic management regimen
- Deficient knowledge regarding medication application
- Pain (acute, chronic)
- Impaired physical mobility

Related factors are individualized based on client's condition or needs.

Planning

Step	Rationale
1. **Expected outcomes** following completion of procedure:	
▪ Client is able to identify drug and describe action, purpose, dose, side effects, and schedule of medication.	Demonstrates learning.
▪ Client is able to apply medication without assistance on prescribed schedule.	Demonstrates learning and compliance.
▪ With repeated applications, skin becomes clear, without inflammation or drainage from lesions.	Existing lesions heal and/or disappear as a result of medications' therapeutic action.
2. Check accuracy and completeness of each MAR or computer printout with prescriber's written medication order. Check client's name, drug name and dosage, route of administration, and time for administration. Compare MAR or computer printout with medication label.	The order sheet is the most reliable source and only legal record of drugs client is to receive. Ensures client receives correct medication.
3. Check client's identification bracelet and ask name.	Ensures correct client receives medication.
4. Explain procedure to client, including description of skin area to be treated.	Makes client a participant in care and minimizes anxiety.

Implementation

Step	Rationale
1. Wash hands and arrange supplies at bedside. If skin is broken (e.g., wound), use sterile gloves; otherwise apply clean gloves.	Reduces transmission of infection. Sterile gloves are used when applying agents to open noninfectious skin lesions. Topical agents are not usually premeasured in medication room.
2. Close room curtain or door and position client comfortably. Remove gown or bed linen so as to keep unaffected skin areas draped.	Provides client privacy and easy access to area being treated. Promotes client's comfort.
3. Apply topical agent.	
a. Technique for applying creams, ointments, and oil-based lotions:	
(1) Place approximately 1 to 2 teaspoons of medication in palm of gloved hand and soften by rubbing briskly between hands.	Softening of topical agent makes it easier to spread on skin.
(2) Once medication is thin and smooth, spread it evenly over skin surface, using long, even strokes that follow direction of hair growth.	Ensures even distribution of medication. Technique prevents irritation of hair follicles.
(3) Explain to client that skin may feel greasy after application.	Ointments often contain oils.

Step	Rationale
b. Technique for applying **nitroglycerin** (an **antianginal**) ointment:	
(1) Apply desired number of inches of ointment over paper measuring guide (see illustration).	Ensures correct dose of medication. Antianginal (nitroglycerin) ointments are usually ordered in inches and can be measured on small sheets of paper marked off in ½-inch markings. Unit-dose packages are available. (**Warning:** One package equals 1 inch; smaller amount should not be measured from this package.)
(2) Remove previous dose paper. Wipe off residual medication with tissue.	Prevents **overdose** that can occur with multiple dose papers left in place.
(3) Antianginal medication may be applied to the chest area, back, upper arm, or legs. Do not apply on hairy surfaces or over scar tissue.	If client complains of headaches, apply ointment farther from head. Application on hairy surfaces or scar tissue may interfere with absorption.
(4) Rotate site when applying nitroglycerin pastes.	Prevents skin irritation.
(5) Apply ointment to skin surface by holding edge or back of the paper measuring guide and placing ointment and wrapper directly on the skin (see illustration). Do not rub or massage ointment into skin.	Minimizes chance of ointment covering gloves and later touching nurse's hands. Medication is designed to absorb slowly over several hours; massaging may increase absorption rate.

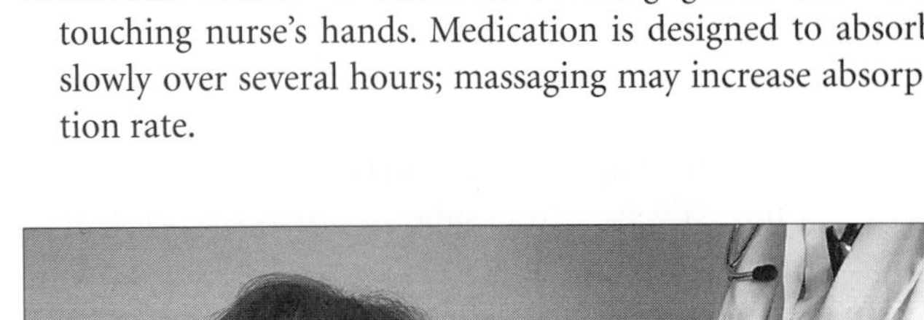

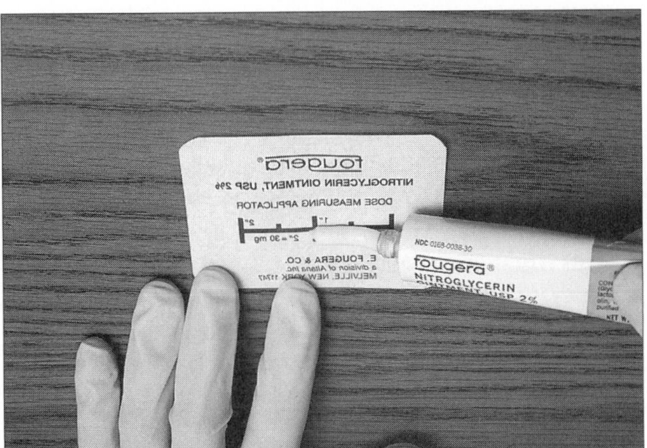

STEP **3b(1)** Ointment spread in inches over measuring guide.

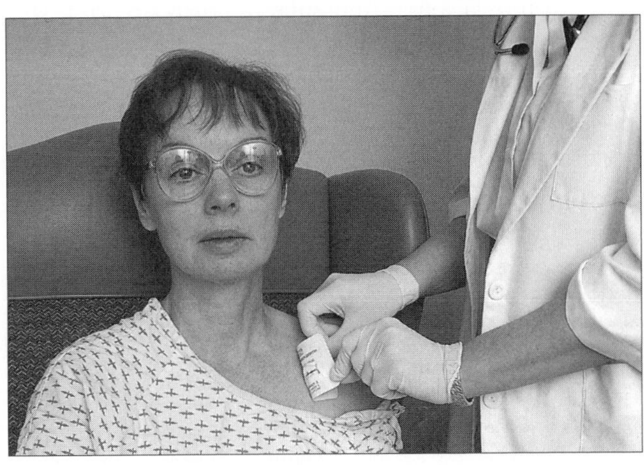

STEP **3b(5)** Nurse applies wrapper with medication on client's skin.

Step	Rationale
(6) Date and initial paper and note time.	Prevents missing doses.
(7) Secure ointment and paper with a strip of tape (optional). Plastic wrap may be used as an occlusive dressing.	Prevents staining of clothing or inadvertent removal of the medication (Lilley and Aucker, 1999).
c. Technique for applying a **transdermal** patch:	
(1) Choose a clean, dry area of the body that is free of hair.	Increases absorption.

• ***Critical Decision Point***

Do not attempt to apply the patch on skin that is oily, burned, broken out, cut, or irritated in any way.

Step	Rationale
(2) Carefully remove the patch from its protective covering. Hold the patch by the edge; do not touch the adhesive edges.	Touching only the edges assures that the patch will adhere and that the medication dose has not been changed.
(3) Immediately apply the patch, pressing firmly with the palm of one hand for 10 seconds. Make sure it sticks well, especially around the edges.	

Step	Rationale
(4) Date and initial patch and note time.	Visual reminder prevents missing or extra doses.
(5) When the next dose is due, remove the old patch and choose a different site. Do not apply to previously used sites for at least 1 week.	Rotation of sites reduces skin irritation from medication and adhesive.

• ***Critical Decision Point***

It is recommended that nitroglycerin transdermal patches be removed after 10 to 12 hours to allow for a nitrate-free interval and reduce the chance of tolerance to the medication. Check with the client's prescriber (Lilley and Aucker, 1999).

Step	Rationale
(6) Dispose of patches by folding in half with sticky sides together. Throw the patch in the trash away from children and pets.	Proper disposal protects others from accidental exposure to medication.
d. Technique for applying aerosolized medication (spray):	
(1) Shake container vigorously.	Mixes contents and propellant to ensure distribution of fine, even spray.
(2) Read container's label for distance recommended to hold spray away from area (usually 6 to 12 inches, 15 to 30 cm).	Proper distance ensures fine spray hits skin surface. Holding container too close results in thin, watery distribution.
(3) If neck or upper chest is to be sprayed, ask client to turn face away from spray or briefly cover face with towel.	Prevents inhalation of spray.
(4) Spray medication evenly over affected site (in some cases spray is timed for select period of seconds).	Entire affected area of skin should be covered with thin spray.
e. Technique for applying a **suspension**-based lotion:	
(1) Shake container vigorously.	Mixes powder throughout liquid to form well-mixed suspension.
(2) Apply small amount of lotion to small gauze dressing or pad and apply to skin by stroking evenly in direction of hair growth.	Method of application leaves protective film of powder on skin after water base of suspension dries. Technique prevents irritation to hair follicles.
(3) Explain to client that area will feel cool and dry.	Water evaporates to leave thin layer of powder.
f. Technique for applying a powder:	
(1) Be sure skin surface is thoroughly dry.	Minimizes caking and crusting of powder.
(2) Fully spread apart any skin folds such as between toes or under axilla and dry with a towel.	Fully exposes skin surface for application.
(3) Dust skin site lightly with dispenser so that area is covered with fine, thin layer of powder.	A thin layer of powder has slight lubricating properties to reduce friction and promote drying (Lilley and Aucker, 1999).
4. Cover skin area with dressing if ordered by physician.	May help prevent agent from being rubbed off skin. Protects clothing from being stained.
5. Assist client to comfortable position, reapply gown, and cover with bed linen as desired.	Provides for client's sense of well-being.
6. Remove gloves, dispose of soiled supplies in receptacle especially designated for such articles, and wash hands.	Keeps client's environment neat and reduces transmission of infection and/or residual medication to children, pets, or others.

Evaluation

Step	Rationale
1. Ask the client or significant other to name the medication and its action, purpose, dose, schedule, and side effects.	Evaluates learning.
2. Have client keep a diary of doses taken.	Confirm compliance with prescribed therapy.
3. Observe client apply lotion, ointment, or patch.	Return demonstration measures learning.
4. Inspect condition of skin between applications.	Determines if skin condition improves.

Unexpected Outcomes and Related Interventions

- Skin site may appear inflamed and edematous with blistering and oozing of fluid from lesions.
  - These signs are indicative of subacute inflammation or **eczema** that can develop from worsening of skin lesions.
  - Notify prescriber, alternate therapies may be needed.
- Client continues to complain of pruritus and tenderness.
  - Indicates slow or impaired healing.
  - Notify prescriber; alternate therapies may be needed.
- Client is unable to explain information about drug.
  - Reinstruction is necessary, or client is unable to learn.
  - Offer client or family member opportunity to apply topical agent during next application and to ask questions.
- Client fails to administer drug as ordered.
  - Indicates need to reexplore client's health beliefs and resources.

Recording and Reporting

- Describe condition of skin before topical agent application in nurses' notes.
- Record actual time each drug was administered, type of agent applied, strength, and site of application in nurses' notes and on MAR or computer printout immediately after administration. Include initials or signature. Do not chart medication administration until *after* it is given to client.
- If drug is withheld, record reason in nurses' notes. Circle time drug normally would have been given on MAR or computer printout.
- Report adverse effects/client response and/or withheld drugs to nurse in charge or physician. Depending on medication, immediate prescriber notification may be required.
- Report any abnormalities in condition of skin to nurse in charge or physician.

Teaching Considerations

- If skin is inflamed, use only warm water rinse without soap for cleansing.
- When applying creams or ointments do not pat or rub skin. This may cause irritation.
- When applying powders, take care that the client does not inhale the powdered medication.
- Include a family member or friend when possible during instruction about topical application of medications.
- When instructing client, be sure lighting is adequate and area to be treated is well exposed.
- Have client demonstrate the application technique to ensure effective therapy and compliance (Lilley and Aucker, 1999).

Gerontological Considerations

- Many changes occur in the skin of the older adult client. The nurse should be aware of these changes when applying topical medications so that proper application can occur. For example, the older adult client's skin is often subject to increased capillary fragility, which can lead to bruising. The nurse handles the skin gently when applying an ointment. Table 17-1 lists common age-related skin changes and assessment findings.

Home Care Considerations

- Instruct client to dispose of applicators, patches, and similar materials into cardboard or plastic disposable containers. Careful disposal is necessary to ensure the safety of client, other adults, pets, and children.

Table 17-1 Effect of Aging on the Integumentary System

Changes	Assessment Findings
Decreased subcutaneous fat, muscle laxity, degeneration of elastic fibers, collagen stiffening	Increased wrinkling, sagging breast and abdomen, redundant flesh around eyes, slowness of skin to flatten when pinched together (tenting)
Decreased extracellular water, surface lipids, and sebaceous gland activity	Dry, flaking skin with possible signs of excoriation caused by pruritus
Increased capillary fragility and permeability	Evidence of bruising
Increased melanocytes in basal layer with pigment accumulation	Senile lentingines on face and back of hands
Diminished blood supply	Decrease in rosy appearance of skin and mucous membranes; cool to touch; diminished awareness of pain, touch, temperature, and peripheral vibration
Decrease in skin cell proliferative capacity	Diminished rate of wound healing

Modified from Lewis SM and others: *Medical-surgical nursing: Assessment and management of clinical problems,* ed 5, St. Louis, 2000, Mosby.

Skill 17-4 Administering Eye Medications

Common eye **(ophthalmic)** medications used by clients are drops, and ointments, including over-the-counter preparations such as artificial tears and vasoconstrictors (e.g., *Visine* and *Murine*). However, many clients receive prescribed ophthalmic drugs for eye conditions such as **glaucoma** and infections and following cataract extraction. In addition, a third type of delivery system, the intraocular disk, is being used. Medications delivered this way resemble a contact lens. The disk is placed into the conjunctival sac, where it remains in place for up to 1 week.

The eye is the most sensitive organ to which the nurse applies medications. The cornea is richly supplied with sensitive nerve fibers. Care must be taken to prevent instilling medication directly onto the cornea. The conjunctival sac is much less sensitive and thus a more appropriate site for medication instillation.

Any client receiving topical eye medications should learn correct self-administration of the medication, especially clients with glaucoma, who must often undergo lifelong medication administration for control of their disease. Nurses can easily instruct clients while administering medications. At times it may become necessary for family members to learn how to administer eye medications. This is particularly true immediately after eye surgery, when a client's vision is so impaired that it is difficult to assemble needed supplies and handle applicators correctly.

Eye medications come in a variety of concentrations. Instilling the wrong concentration may cause local irritation of eyes, as well as systemic effects. Certain eye medications, such as **mydriatics** and **cycloplegics,** temporarily blur a client's vision. Use of the wrong drug concentration can prolong these undesirable effects.

Delegation Considerations

The skill of administering eye medications should not be delegated to assistive personnel. Assistive personnel should be instructed about potential side effects of medications and to report their occurrence. In addition, the care providers should be notified if vision impairment is possibility after administration of eye medications.

Equipment

- Medication bottle with sterile eye dropper or ointment tube
- Medicated intraocular disk
- Cotton ball or tissue
- Washbasin filled with warm water and washcloth
- Eye patch and tape (optional)
- Clean gloves
- Medication administration record (MAR) or computer printout

Step	Rationale
Assessment	
1. Review prescriber's medication order for number of drops (if a liquid) and eye (right, **O.D.;** left, **O.S.;** both, **O.U.**) to receive medication.	Ensures correct administration of medication.
2. Assess condition of external eye structures (may also be done just before drug instillation.)	Provides baseline to later determine if local response to medications occurs. Also indicates need to clean eye before drug application.
3. Determine whether client has any known allergies to eye medications. Also ask if client has allergy to latex.	Protects client from risk of allergic drug response. Latex allergy requires use of nonlatex gloves.
4. Determine whether client has any symptoms of visual alterations.	Certain eye medications act to either lessen or increase these symptoms. Nurse must be able to recognize change in client's condition.
5. Assess client's level of consciousness and ability to follow directions.	If client becomes restless or combative during procedure, a greater risk of accidental eye injury exists.
6. Assess client's knowledge regarding drug therapy and desire to self-administer medication.	Clients level of understanding may indicate need for health teaching. Motivation influences teaching approach.
7. Assess client's ability to manipulate and hold dropper.	Reflects client's ability to learn to self-administer drug.

STEP	RATIONALE

NURSING DIAGNOSIS

Defining characteristics from the assessment data may reveal the following nursing diagnoses for clients requiring this skill:

- Health-seeking behaviors (self-care)
- Risk for injury
- Impaired physical mobility
- Pain (acute, chronic)
- Deficient knowledge (regarding drug actions and purpose and self-administration)
- Disturbed sensory perception (visual)

Related factors are individualized based on client's condition or needs.

PLANNING

Step	Rationale
1. **Expected outcomes** following completion of procedure:	
▪ Client experiences desired effect of medication.	Drug is administered correctly without injury to client.
▪ Client denies discomfort.	Drug is administered correctly without injury to client.
▪ Client experiences no side effects and symptoms (e.g., irritation) are relieved.	Drug is distributed and absorbed properly.
▪ Client is able to discuss information about medication and technique correctly.	Demonstrates learning.
▪ Client demonstrates self-instillation of eye drops.	Demonstrates learning.
2. Check accuracy and completeness of each MAR or computer printout with prescriber's written medication order. Check client's name, drug name and dosage, route of administration, and time for administration. Compare MAR or computer printout with label of eye medication.	The order sheet is the most reliable source and only legal record of drugs client is to receive. Ensures right drug is administered.
3. Check client's identification bracelet and ask name.	Ensures correct client receives medication.
4. Explain procedure to client.	Relieves anxiety about medication being instilled into eye.

IMPLEMENTATION

Step	Rationale
1. Wash hands and arrange supplies at bedside; apply clean gloves.	Reduces transmission of microorganisms; ensures a smooth, orderly procedure.
a. If eye drops are stored in refrigerator, rewarm to room temperature before administering.	Reduces irritation to eye due to cold temperature of solution.
2. Ask client to lie supine or sit back in chair with head slightly hyperextended.	Position provides easy access to eye for medication instillation and minimizes drainage of medication through tear duct.

• ***Critical Decision Point***

Do not hyperextend the neck of a client with cervical spine injury.

Step	Rationale
3. If crusts or drainage are present along eyelid margins or inner canthus, gently wash away. Soak any crusts that are dried and difficult to remove by applying damp washcloth or cotton ball over eye for a few minutes. Always wipe clean from inner to outer canthus (see illustration).	Crusts or drainage harbor microorganisms. Soaking allows easy removal and prevents pressure from being applied directly over eye. Cleansing from inner to outer canthus avoids entrance of microorganisms into lacrimal duct.
4. Hold cotton ball or clean tissue in nondominant hand on client's cheekbone just below lower eyelid.	Cotton or tissue absorbs medication that escapes eye.
5. With tissue or cotton resting below lower lid, gently press downward with thumb or forefinger against bony orbit (see illustration). Never press directly against client's eyeball.	Technique exposes lower conjunctival sac. Retraction against bony orbit prevents pressure and trauma to eyeball and prevents fingers from touching eye. Pressure to the eyeball may cause damage.

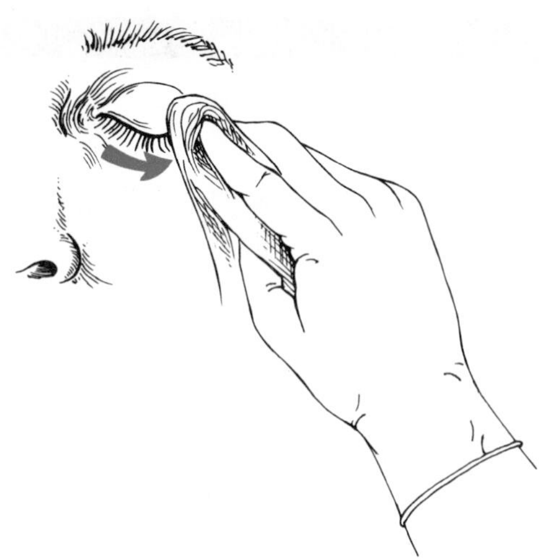

STEP **3** Cleanse eye, washing from inner to outer canthus before administering drops or ointment.

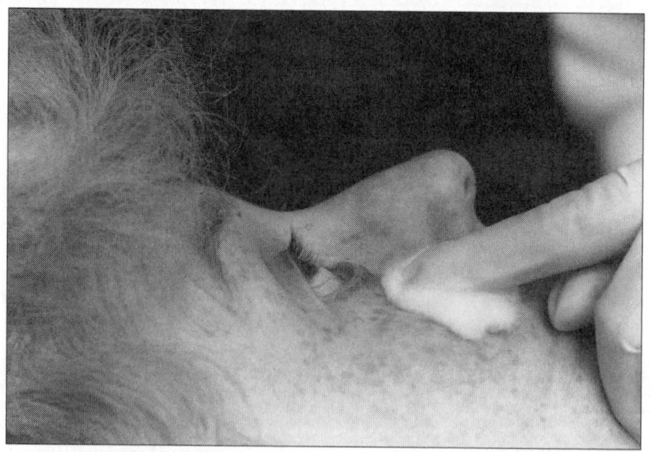

STEP **5** Nurse retracts lower conjunctival sac.

Step	Rationale
6. Ask client to look at ceiling.	Action moves sensitive cornea up and away from conjunctival sac and reduces stimulation of blink reflex.
7. Instill eye drops while explaining steps to client:	
a. With dominant hand resting on client's forehead, hold filled medication eye dropper approximately 1 to 2 cm ($\frac{1}{2}$ to $\frac{3}{4}$ inch) above conjunctival sac (see illustration).	Helps prevent accidental contact of eye dropper with eye structures, thus reducing risk of injury to eye and transfer of infection to dropper. Ophthalmic medications are sterile.
b. Drop prescribed number of medication drops into conjunctival sac.	Conjunctival sac normally holds 1 or 2 drops. Provides even distribution of medication across eye.
c. If client blinks or closes eye or if drops fall on outer lid margins, repeat procedure.	Therapeutic effect of drug is obtained only when drops enter conjunctival sac.
d. When administering drugs that cause systemic effects, with a clean tissue apply gentle pressure to client's nasolacrimal duct for 30 to 60 seconds.	Prevents overflow of medication into nasal and pharyngeal passages. Prevents absorption into systemic circulation.
e. After instilling drops, ask client to close eye gently.	Helps to distribute medication. Squinting or squeezing of eyelids forces medication from conjunctival sac.

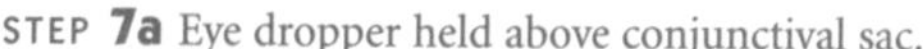

STEP **7a** Eye dropper held above conjunctival sac.

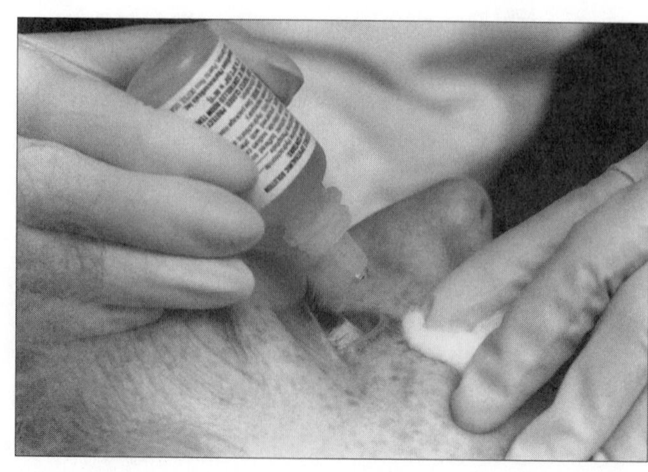

STEP	RATIONALE
8. Instill eye ointment:	
a. Ask client to look at ceiling.	Action moves sensitive cornea up and away from conjunctival sac and reduces stimulation of blink reflex.
b. Holding ointment applicator above lower lid margin, apply thin ribbon of ointment evenly along inner edge of lower eyelid on conjunctiva (see illustration) from the inner canthus to outer canthus.	Distributes medication evenly across eye and lid margin.
c. Have client close eye and rub lid lightly in circular motion with cotton ball, if rubbing is not contraindicated.	Further distributes medication without traumatizing eye.

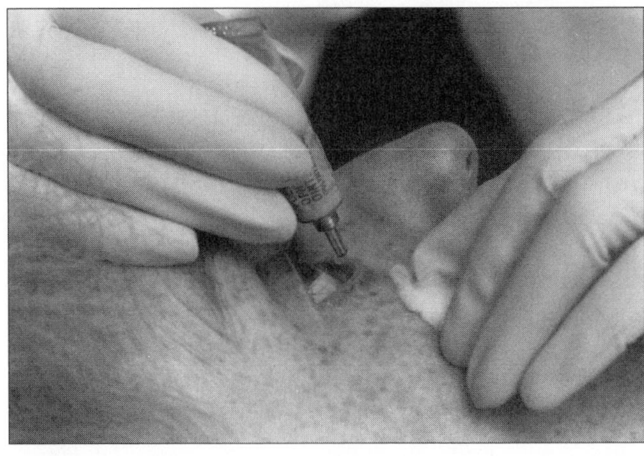

STEP **8b** Nurse applies ointment along lower eyelid.

STEP	RATIONALE
9. Intraocular disk	
a. Application:	
(1) Wash hands and apply gloves.	Reduces transmission of microorganisms.
(2) Open package containing the disk. Gently press your fingertip against the disk so that it adheres to your finger. (NOTE: It may be necessary to moisten gloved finger with sterile saline.) Position the convex side of the disk on your fingertip.	Allows nurse to inspect disk for damage or deformity. Prepares disk for proper administration.
(3) With your other hand, gently pull the client's lower eyelid away from his eye. Ask client to look up.	Prepares conjunctival sac for receiving medicated disk.
(4) Place the disk in the conjunctival sac, so that it floats on the sclera between the iris and lower eyelid.	Ensures delivery of medication.
(5) Pull the client's lower eyelid out and over the disk.	Ensures accurate medication delivery.

• ***Critical Decision Point***

You should not be able to see the disk at this time. Repeat Step (5) if you can see the disk.

STEP	RATIONALE
b. Removal:	
(1) Wash hands and apply gloves.	
(2) Explain procedure to client.	
(3) Gently pull on the client's lower eyelid to expose the disk.	
(4) Using your forefinger and thumb of your opposite hand, pinch the disk and lift it out of the client's eye.	
10. If excess medication is on eyelid, gently wipe it from inner to outer canthus.	Promotes comfort and prevents trauma to eye.
11. If client had eye patch, apply clean one by placing it over affected eye so entire eye is covered. Tape securely without applying pressure to eye.	Clean eye patch reduces chance of infection.

Step	Rationale
12. Remove gloves, dispose of soiled supplies in proper receptacle, and wash hands.	Maintains neat environment at bedside and reduces transmission of microorganisms.
13. Clients experienced in self-instillation may be allowed to give drops under nurse's supervision (check agency policy).	

Evaluation

1. Note client's response to instillation; ask if any discomfort was felt.	Determines if procedure was performed correctly and safely.
2. Observe response to medication by assessing visual changes and noting any side effects.	Evaluates effects of medication.
3. Ask client to discuss drug's purpose, action, side effects, and technique of administration.	Determines client's level of understanding.
4. Have client demonstrate self-administration of next dose.	Provides feedback regarding competency with skill.

Unexpected Outcomes and Related Interventions

- Client complains of burning or pain or experiences local side effects (e.g., headache, bloodshot eyes, local eye irritation).
  - Eye drops may have been instilled onto the cornea, or the dropper touched the surface of the eye.
  - The drug concentration and client's sensitivity both influence the chances of side effects developing.
  - Notify prescriber for a possible adjustment in medication type and dosage.
- Client experiences systemic effects from drops (e.g., increased heart rate and blood pressure from epinephrine, decreased heart rate and blood pressure from timolol).
  - Systemic absorption through tear duct can cause potentially dangerous effects.
  - Ophthalmic **anesthetics** and antibiotics may cause the same type of adverse reactions as systemically administered drugs (e.g., **anaphylaxis**).
  - Notify prescriber immediately
  - Remain with client
  - Withhold further doses.
- Client is unable to discuss information about medication correctly.
  - Reinstruction is needed, or client is unable to learn.
- Client is unable to instill eye drops.
  - Further practice is necessary.
  - Clients who will be administering drugs at home should demonstrate instillation until performed correctly. Otherwise instruct family member.

Recording and Reporting

- Record drug, concentration, number of drops, time of administration, and eye (left, right, or both) that received medication on MAR or computer printout immediately after administration. Include initials or signature. Do not chart medication administration until *after* it is given to the patient.
- If drug is withheld, record reason in nurses' notes. Circle time the drug normally would have been given on MAR or computer printout.
- Record appearance of eye in nurses' notes.
- Report adverse effects/client response and/or withheld drugs to nurse in charge or physician. Depending on medication, immediate prescriber notification may be required.

Teaching Considerations

- Warn clients receiving mydriatics that vision will be temporarily blurred. Wearing sunglasses will reduce photophobia.
- Clients who receive medications that paralyze the ciliary muscles of the eye (e.g., scopolamine, Isopto Hyoscine, Atropine, Isopto Atropine, and cycloplegics) should temporarily not drive or attempt to perform any activity that requires acute vision.
- Many clients lack confidence in their ability to instill drops without supervision. Others are unable to manipulate the dropper or are unable to see. The nurse teaches others, such as a family member, to instill drops into client's eye.

Pediatric Considerations

- When instilling drops in an infant or young child, have parent gently restrain child's head with child in parent's lap. Be sure that child's hands do not interfere with instillation.
- Infants often clench the eyes tightly to avoid eye drops. To administer drops in an uncooperative infant, with the head gently restrained, place the drops at the nasal corner where the lids meet. When the child opens the eye the medication will flow into the eye.
- Eye ointments are easily placed into the sleeping child's eye.

Gerontological Considerations

- Before discharging older adult client, nurse evaluates client's ability to perform all the necessary steps for the administration of eye drops and ointments.
- Nurse teaches family members of clients unable to perform the necessary skills. Clients without this type of assistance should be evaluated for home health nursing.

Home Care Considerations

- Clients with chronic health care problems should consult with their health care provider before using over-the-counter eye medications.
- When using over-the-counter eye drops, clients should not share medications with other family members. Risk of infection transmission is high.

Skill 17-5 Administering Ear Drops

When administering ear (**otic**) medications the nurse should be aware of certain safety precautions. Internal ear structures are very sensitive to temperature extremes. Failure to instill a solution at room temperature can cause **vertigo** (severe dizziness) or nausea and debilitate a client for several minutes. Although structures of the outer ear are not sterile, use sterile drops and solutions in case the eardrum is ruptured. Entrance of nonsterile solutions into the middle ear can cause serious infection. A final precaution is to avoid forcing any solution into the ear. The nurse must not occlude the ear canal with a medicine dropper, because this can cause pressure within the canal during instillation and subsequent injury to the eardrum. If these precautions are followed, instillation of ear drops is a safe and effective therapy.

Delegation Considerations

The skill of administering ear medications should not be delegated to assistive personnel. Assistive personnel should be instructed about potential side effects of medications and to report their occurrence.

Equipment

- Medication bottle with dropper
- Cotton-tipped applicator
- Cotton ball (optional)
- Clean gloves (optional, only if client has drainage)
- Medication administration record (MAR) or computer printout

Step	Rationale
Assessment	
1. Review prescriber's medication order for number of drops to instill, and ear (right, **A.D.**; left, **A.S.**; both, **A.U.**) to receive medication.	Ensures safe and correct administration of medication.
2. Assess condition of external ear structures and canal (see Chapter 10).	Provides baseline to later determine if local response to medication occurs, whether client's condition improves, or whether it will be necessary to clean ear before instilling medication.
3. Determine whether client has symptoms of discomfort and/or hearing impairment.	Disorders of external ear can be painful. Occlusion of external ear canal by swelling, drainage, or **cerumen** can impair hearing acuity. These conditions may change after drug instillation and require ongoing monitoring.
4. Assess client's level of consciousness and ability to follow instructions.	Client must lie still during drug administration. Sudden movements can cause injury from ear dropper.
5. Assess client's level of knowledge regarding drug therapy and motivation to self-administer medication.	Client's knowledge level determines whether health teaching is required. Motivation influences teaching approach.
6. Assess client's ability to grasp and manipulate dropper.	Determines client's ability to self-administer drug.

STEP	RATIONALE

NURSING DIAGNOSIS

Defining characteristics from the assessment data may reveal the following nursing diagnoses for clients requiring this skill:

Health-seeking behaviors (self-care)
Risk for injury
Impaired physical mobility
Deficient knowledge regarding drug actions and purpose
Pain (acute, chronic)
Disturbed sensory perception (auditory)

Related factors are individualized based on client's condition or needs.

PLANNING

Step	Rationale
1. **Expected outcomes** following completion of procedure:	
▪ Client denies discomfort during administration.	Procedure is performed correctly without injury to client.
▪ Ear canal becomes clear, without drainage, excess cerumen, or inflammation, as medication is repeatedly instilled.	Drug action is effective.
▪ Client's hearing acuity improves.	This response occurs only if hearing loss was caused by obstruction in external ear canal.
▪ Client is able to explain steps for instilling eardrops and demonstrates technique for administration.	Cognitive and psychomotor learning occurs.
2. Check accuracy and completeness of each MAR or computer printout with prescriber's written medication order. Check client's name, drug name and dosage, route of administration, and time for administration. Compare MAR or computer printout with label of ear medication.	The order sheet is the most reliable source and only legal record of drugs client is to receive. Ensures right drug is administered.
3. Check client's identification bracelet and ask name.	Ensures right client receives drug.
4. Explain each step of procedure to client, allowing for questions.	Reduces client anxiety; timing of instruction enhances learning.

IMPLEMENTATION

Step	Rationale
1. Wash hands and arrange supplies at bedside. Apply clean gloves (if drainage is present).	Reduces transmission of microorganisms; helps nurse perform procedure smoothly.
2. Warm medication by running warm water over the bottle (without damaging the label directions or allowing water to get into the bottle).	Prevents nausea and vertigo that may occur if the medication is too cold.
3. Have client assume side-lying position (if not contraindicated by client's condition) with ear to be treated facing up, or client may sit in chair or at the bedside. The nurse should stabilize the client's head with his or her hand.	Position provides easy access to ear for instillation of medication. Ear canal is in position to receive medication. Stabilizing the head promotes safety during instillation with a dropper.
4. For adults and children over age 3, gently pull the pinna up and back; in children age 3 or less, the pinna should be pulled down and back (Lilley and Aucker, 1999) (see illustrations).	Straightening of ear canal provides direct access to deeper external ear structures. Developmental differences in younger children and infants necessitate different methods of doing this.
5. If cerumen or drainage occludes outermost portion of ear canal, wipe out gently with cotton-tipped applicator (see illustration).	Cerumen and drainage harbor microorganisms and can block distribution of medication.

• ***Critical Decision Point***
Do not force wax inward to block or occlude canal.

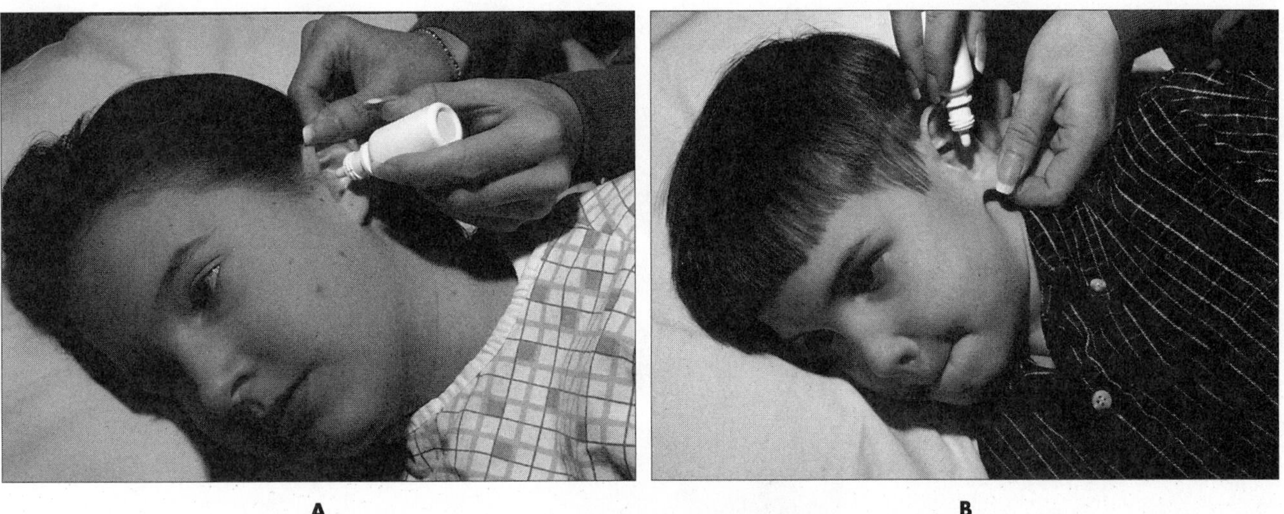

A B

STEP 4 **A,** Pull the pinna up and back for adults and children over age 3. **B,** Pull the pinna down and back for children age 3 or less. (From Lilley LL, Aucker RS: *Pharmacology and the nursing process,* ed 2, St. Louis, 1999, Mosby.)

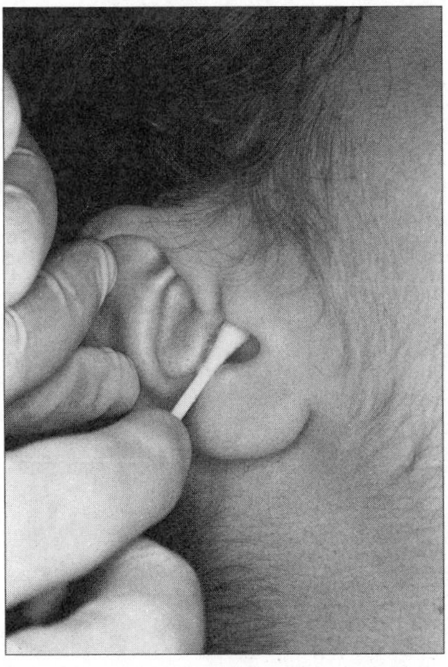

STEP 5 Always cleanse only outer canal. Do not push secretions into ear.

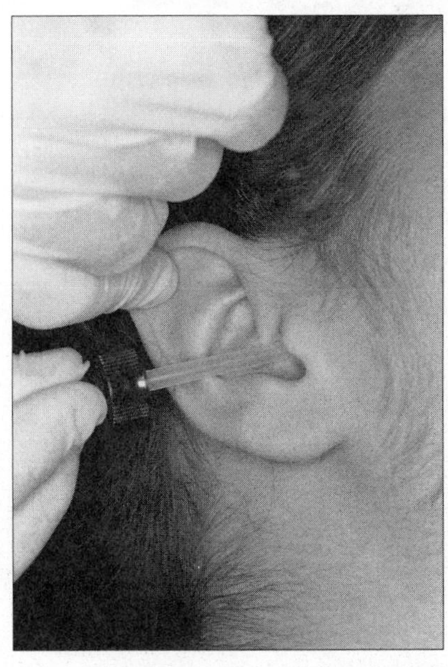

STEP 6 Nurse instills ear drops.

STEP	RATIONALE
6. Instill prescribed drops holding dropper 1 cm (½ inch) above ear canal (see illustration).	Forceful instillation of drops into occluded canal can cause injury to eardrum.
7. Remove gloves, dispose of soiled supplies, and wash hands.	Reduces transmission of microorganisms.
8. Ask client to remain in side-lying position for 5 to 10 minutes. Apply gentle massage or pressure to tragus of ear with finger (see illustration).	Allows complete distribution of medication. Pressure and massage moves medication inward.

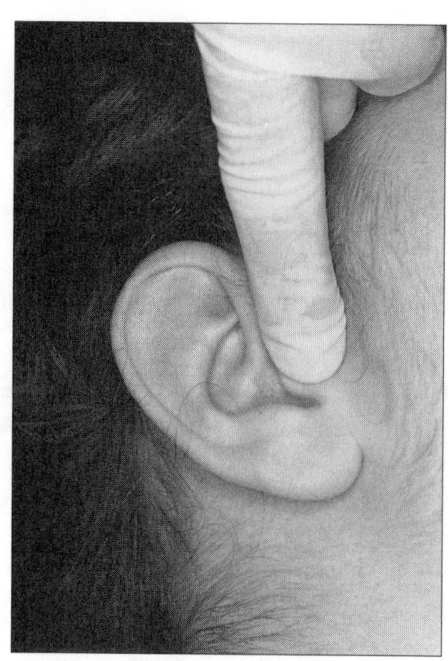

STEP **8** Nurse applies pressure to tragus of ear.

STEP	RATIONALE
9. At times, the prescriber orders insertion of portion of cotton ball into outermost part of canal. Do not press cotton into canal.	Inserting cotton into outer canal prevents escape of medication when client sits or stands. Cotton should not block canal to impair hearing.
10. Remove cotton after 15 minutes.	Time period promotes drug distribution and absorption.
11. Dispose of soiled supplies and wash hands.	Reduces transmission of microorganisms.
12. Assist client to comfortable position after drops are absorbed.	Restores comfort.

EVALUATION

1. Ask client if any discomfort is felt during instillation.	Determines if procedure is performed correctly and reveals severity of symptoms.
2. Evaluate condition of external ear between drug instillations.	Determines response to medication.
3. Evaluate client's hearing acuity.	Hearing may change after drug administration.
4. Ask client to explain technique for instilling ear drops and purpose of medication.	Evaluates degree of learning.
5. Have client demonstrate self-administration of next dose.	Provides feedback regarding competency with skill.

UNEXPECTED OUTCOMES AND RELATED INTERVENTIONS

- Ear canal is inflamed, swollen, tender to palpation. Drainage is present.
  - Symptoms of continuing ear infection are present; notify prescriber.
- Client's hearing acuity continues to be reduced.
  - Obstruction within ear canal is unrelieved. Notify prescriber.
- Ear canal is occluded by cerumen.
  - Wax has become impacted in canal. Ear irrigation may be necessary to remove wax impaction.
- Client is unable to explain drug information and steps for drug instillation.
  - Nurse must repeat instructions, or client is unable to learn.
- Client has difficulty self-administering ear drops.
  - Reinstruction is needed. Have client demonstrate instillation of ear drops until performed correctly.

RECORDING AND REPORTING

- Record drug, concentration, number of drops, time administered, and ear (left, right, or both) into which drops in-

stilled on MAR or computer printout immediately after administration. Include initials or signature. Do not chart medication administration until *after* it is given to client.
- If drug is withheld, record reason in nurses' notes. Circle time the drug normally would have been given on MAR or computer printout.
- Record condition of ear canal in nurses' notes.
- Report any sudden change in client's hearing acuity.
- Report adverse effects/client response and/or withheld drugs to nurse in charge or physician. Depending on medication, immediate prescriber notification may be required.

Teaching Considerations

- If client suffers hearing loss, use communication techniques such as enunciating words, getting client's attention, speaking in normal tone of voice, talking toward client's best ear.
- This procedure is simple to teach clients and family members.
- Instruct client in proper way to cleanse ears and to avoid use of sharp objects in ear canal.
- Teach the signs of hearing loss and the need for frequent follow-ups are to parents with children who have chronic otitis media.

Pediatric Considerations

- For children younger than 3 years of age gently pull the pinna of the ear downward and straight back. Ensure that parents and/or caregivers are aware of the proper method of administration.
- Infants or young children should be restrained in supine position with head turned to expose affected ear. Hold child in this position until the drug has time to be absorbed.
- Cotton pledgets may be used to prevent medication from flowing out of external canal. They should be inserted loose enough to allow any discharge to exit from ear. To prevent cotton from absorbing medication in ear, premoisten cotton with a few drops of medication (Wong and others, 1999).

Gerontological Considerations

- Some older adults experience excessive accumulation of cerumen in the ear. This should be removed before administration of medication.

Skill 17-6 Administering Ear Irrigations

Medications used to irrigate or wash out a body cavity such as the ear (otic) are delivered through a stream of solution. The common indications for irrigation of the external ear are presence of a foreign body, local inflammation of the canal, and accumulation of cerumen. Irrigations should be done with liquid warmed to body temperature to avoid vertigo (dizziness) or nausea in clients (McKenry and Salerno, 1998). The greatest danger during administration of ear irrigation is rupture of the tympanic membrane. Fluids must not be instilled under pressure or with the ear canal occluded by the irrigating device.

Delegation Considerations

The skill of ear irrigation should not be delegated to assistive personnel. Assistive personnel should be instructed about potential side effects of medications and to report their occurrence.

Equipment

- Clean disposable gloves
- Otoscope (optional)
- Irrigation syringe
- Basin
- Towel
- Cotton balls
- Prescribed irrigation solution warmed to body temperature or mineral oil, over-the-counter softener
- Medication administration record (MAR) or computer printout

Step	Rationale
Assessment	
1. Review prescriber's medication order, including solution to be instilled and the affected ear(s) (right, A.D.; left, A.S.; both, A.U.) to receive irrigation.	Ensures safe and correct administration of medication.
2. Review medical record for history of ruptured tympanic membrane, or visualize client's tympanic membrane using an otoscope.	Ruptured membrane contraindicates irrigation.

STEP	RATIONALE
3. Inspect the pinna and external auditory meatus for redness, swelling, drainage, abrasions, and presence of cerumen or foreign objects.	Findings provide baseline to monitor effects of medication or solution.
a. Always attempt to remove foreign objects in the ear by first simply straightening the ear canal.	This may cause the object to fall out.
b. If vegetable matter (such as a dried bean or pea) is occluded in the canal, do not perform an irrigation.	Children often place vegetable matter in the ear. The material can swell on contact with water, and cause further damage to the canal.
4. Ask if client is experiencing discomfort. Note client's ability to hear clearly.	Pain is symptomatic of external ear infection or inflammation. Occlusion of auditory canal by cerumen or foreign object can impair hearing.
5. Review client's knowledge of purpose for irrigation and of normal care of the ears.	May indicate need for instruction regarding hygiene.

Nursing Diagnosis

Defining characteristics from the assessment data may reveal the following nursing diagnoses for clients requiring this skill:

- Risk for injury
- Deficient knowledge regarding irrigation purpose
- Pain (acute, chronic)
- Disturbed sensory perception (auditory)
- Risk for infection

Related factors are individualized based on client's condition or needs.

Planning

STEP	RATIONALE
1. **Expected outcomes** following completion of procedure:	
▪ Client denies pain during instillation.	Fluid is properly instilled.
▪ Client hears conversation more clearly.	Obstruction in ear canal is resolved.
▪ Client is able to discuss purpose of irrigation and describe correct ear care techniques.	Feedback reflects client's learning.
▪ Skin overlying meatus and canal becomes clear, without redness, swelling, tenderness, or discharge. Canal is clear of cerumen and foreign material.	Inflammation, irritation, and occlusion of canal are relieved.
2. Check accuracy and completeness of each MAR or computer printout with prescriber's written medication or procedure order. Check client's name, drug name and dosage, route of administration, and time for administration. Compare MAR or computer printout with label of ear irrigation solution.	The order sheet is the most reliable source and only legal record of drugs or procedure the client is to receive. Ensures client receives correct medication.
3. Check client's identification by reading identification bracelet and asking name.	Ensures correct client receives irrigation.
4. If client is found to have impacted cerumen, instill 1 to 2 drops of mineral oil or over-the-counter softener into ear twice a day for 2 to 3 days before irrigation.	Loosens cerumen and ensures easier removal during irrigation.
5. Explain procedure. Warn that the irrigation may cause sensation of dizziness, ear fullness, and warmth.	Prepares client to anticipate effects of irrigation and promotes cooperation.

Implementation

STEP	RATIONALE
1. Wash hands, arrange supplies at bedside, and apply gloves.	Reduces transfer of microorganisms; helps nurse to perform procedure smoothly.
2. Close curtain or room door.	Maintains privacy.

Step	Rationale
3. Assist client to a sitting or lying position with head turned toward affected ear (see illustration). Place towel under client's head and shoulder and have client, if able, hold basin under affected ear.	Position minimizes leakage of fluids around neck and facial area. Solution will flow from ear canal to basin.
4. Pour irrigating solution into sterile round basin.	
5. Gently clean auricle and outer ear canal with moistened cotton applicator. Do *not* force drainage or cerumen into the ear canal.	Prevents infected material from reentering ear canal. Forceful instillation of solution into occluded canal can cause injury to eardrum
6. Fill irrigating syringe with solution (approximately 50 ml).	Enough fluid is needed to provide a steady irrigating stream.
7. For adults and children over age 3, gently pull pinna up and back; in children age 3 or less, pinna should be pulled down and back (Lilley and Aucker, 1999).	Straightening of ear canal provides direct access to deeper external ear structures. Developmental differences in younger children and infants necessitate different techniques. Allows fluid to flow through length of canal.
8. Slowly instill irrigating solution by holding tip of syringe 1 cm (½ inch) above opening to ear canal. The fluid should be directed toward the superior aspect of ear canal. Allow fluid to drain out during instillation. Continue until canal is cleansed or solution is used (see illustration).	Slow instillation prevents buildup of pressure in ear canal and ensures contact of solution with all canal surfaces.

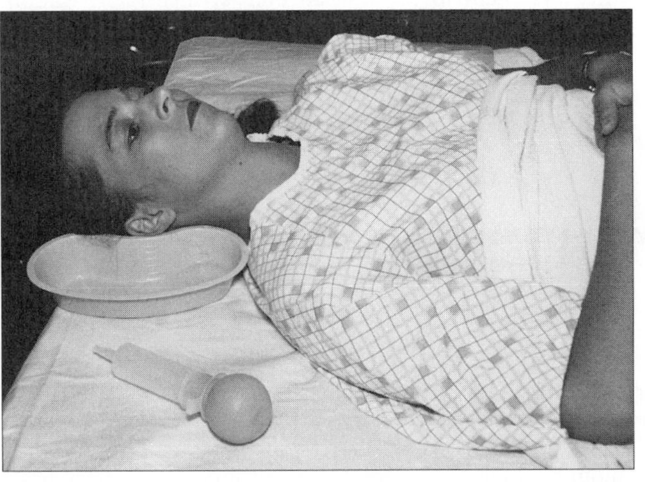

STEP 3 Irrigating basin is positioned under ear.

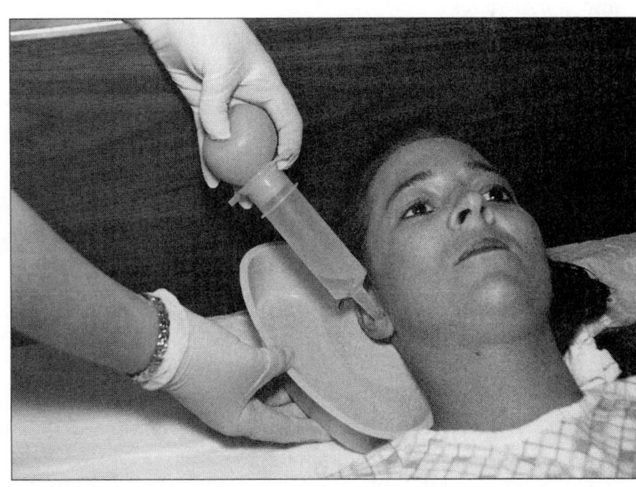

STEP 8 Tip of syringe does not occlude ear canal during irrigation.

Step	Rationale
9. Do *not* occlude ear canal with tip of syringe.	Buildup of fluid in ear canal under forced pressure could cause rupture of tympanic membrane.
10. Dry outer ear canal with cotton ball. Leave cotton loosely in place for 5 to 10 minutes.	Maintains comfort. Absorbs excess moisture in ear canal.
11. Assist client to a sitting position.	Maintains comfort.
12. Wash hands, remove gloves, and dispose of supplies.	Reduces transmission of infection.

Evaluation

Step	Rationale
1. Ask client if discomfort is noted during instillation of solution.	Fluid instilled improperly under pressure causes discomfort.
2. Reinspect condition of meatus and canal.	Determines if solution relieves symptoms and removes foreign materials.
3. Measure client's hearing acuity.	Determines if conduction deafness is relieved.
4. Ask client to describe purpose of irrigation and proper techniques for ear care.	Reflects client's understanding of procedure and proper hygiene.

Unexpected Outcomes and Related Interventions

- Client experiences increased ear pain.
  - Rupture of eardrum may have occurred. Notify prescriber immediately.
- Ear canal remains occluded with cerumen.
  - Repeat irrigation is required.
- Foreign body remains in ear canal.
  - Refer clients to an otolaryngologist if a foreign object remains after irrigation.
- Client is unable to explain ear care practices.
  - Reinstruction is necessary.

Recording and Reporting

- Record in nurses' notes and/or MAR or computer printout, the procedure, amount of solution instilled, time of administration, and ear receiving irrigation. Include initials or signature. Do not chart medication administration until *after* it is given to client.
- Record appearance of external ear and client's hearing acuity in nurses' notes.
- If drug is withheld, record reason in nurses' notes. Circle time the drug normally would have been given on MAR or computer printout.
- Report adverse effects/client response and/or withheld drugs to nurse in charge or physician. Depending on medication, immediate prescriber notification may be required.

Teaching Considerations

- Instruct client that cerumen has an antibacterial effect that maintains an acid pH in the auditory canal.
- Instruct clients to clean ears daily with a washcloth, soap, and warm water.
- Warn clients against placing objects (including cotton swabs) in ears.

Pediatric Considerations

- When cleansing the ear of a small child, be certain child's head is immobilized to prevent puncturing eardrum. It may be necessary to have child's parent participate in this procedure.

Home Care Considerations

- Instruct client to use a clean bulb syringe for irrigation. Mineral oil drops or over-the-counter otic preparations may be used to facilitate removal of cerumen, but client should be instructed to consult a health care provider if problems continue (McKenry and Salerno, 1998).

Skill 17-7 Administering Nasal Instillations

Clients with nasal sinus alterations may receive drugs by spray, drops, or tampons. The most commonly administered form of nasal instillation is a decongestant spray or drops used to relieve sinus congestion and cold symptoms. Many over-the-counter nose drops contain **sympathomimetic** drugs (such as Afrin or Neo-Synephrine). These drugs are relatively safe when administered nasally because only small doses are needed. However, the drugs can enter the systemic circulation by way of the nasal mucosa or gastrointestinal tract if an excess amount is swallowed. Repeated use of sprays can worsen nasal congestion because of a rebound effect. It is easy for a client to self-administer sprays. The client can be placed in a seated position with the head in a slightly hyperextended position.

Nasal drops (prescribed) often contain antibiotics for the treatment of sinus infections. Proper positioning of clients during instillation of drops is essential for medication to reach the affected sinus. The client should be instructed to lie in the supine position with head tilted back.

Delegation Considerations

The skill of administering nasal medications should not be delegated to assistive personnel. Assistive personnel should be instructed about potential side effects of medications and to report their occurrence.

Equipment

- Prepared medication with clean dropper or spray container
- Facial tissue
- Small pillow (optional)
- Washcloth (optional)
- Gloves (optional, only if client has extensive nasal drainage)
- Medication administration record (MAR) or computer printout

STEP	RATIONALE

ASSESSMENT

Step	Rationale
1. For nasal drops, determine which sinus is affected by referring to medical record.	Affects client's position during drug instillation.
2. Assess client's history of hypertension, heart disease, diabetes, and hyperthyroidism.	These conditions can contraindicate use of decongestants that stimulate the central nervous system. Side effects of transient hypertension, tachycardia, palpitations, and headache may occur.
3. Inspect condition of nose and sinuses. Palpate sinuses for tenderness. Note type of drainage, if present.	Provides baseline to monitor effects of medication. Presence of discharge interferes with drug absorption. Clear nasal discharge indicates sinus problem. Yellow or greenish discharge indicates infection.
4. Assess client's knowledge regarding use of nasal instillations and technique for instillation and willingness to learn self-administration.	May require health teaching regarding use of drugs. Motivation influences teaching approach.

NURSING DIAGNOSIS

Defining characteristics from the assessment data may reveal the following nursing diagnoses for clients requiring this skill:

- Health-seeking behaviors (self-care)
- Risk for injury
- Deficient knowledge regarding drug action and purpose
- Pain (acute, chronic)

Related factors are individualized based on client's condition or needs.

PLANNING

Step	Rationale
1. **Expected outcomes** following completion of procedure:	
■ Client is able to breathe with ease through nose.	Nasal congestion has been relieved.
■ Client's nasal sinuses become clear, moist, pink, without drainage after repeated instillations (applies to antiinfective medications).	Inflammation of mucosa has been relieved.
■ Client is able to explain medication's purpose and administers nasal instillations correctly.	Feedback reflects client's learning.
2. Check accuracy and completeness of each MAR or computer printout with prescriber's written medication order. Check client's name, drug name and dosage, route of administration, and time for administration. Compare MAR or computer printout with label of nasal medication.	The order sheet is the most reliable source and only legal record of drugs client is to receive. Ensures right drug is administered.
3. Check client's identification bracelet and ask name.	Ensures right client receives drug.
4. Explain procedure to client regarding positioning and sensations to expect, such as burning or stinging of mucosa or choking sensation as medication trickles into throat.	Helps client anticipate experience of procedure to reduce anxiety.

IMPLEMENTATION

Step	Rationale
1. Wash hands. Arrange supplies and medications at bedside.	Reduces transmission of microorganisms; ensures smooth, orderly procedure.
2. Instruct client to clear or blow nose gently unless contraindicated (e.g., risk of increased intracranial pressure or nosebleeds).	Removes mucus and secretions that can block distribution of medication.

STEP	RATIONALE
3. Administer nasal drops:	
a. Assist client to supine position.	Proper positioning provides access to specific nasal passages.
b. Position head properly:	
(1) For access to posterior pharynx, tilt client's head backward.	
(2) For access to ethmoid or sphenoid sinus, tilt head back over edge of bed or place small pillow under client's shoulder and tilt head back (see illustration).	
(3) For access to frontal and maxillary sinus, tilt head back over edge of bed or pillow with head turned toward side to be treated (see illustration).	Position allows medication to drain into affected sinus.

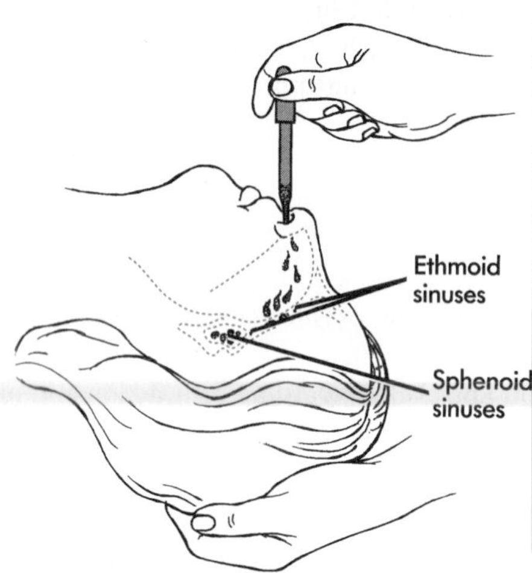

STEP 3b(2) Position for instilling nose drops into ethmoid or sphenoid sinus.

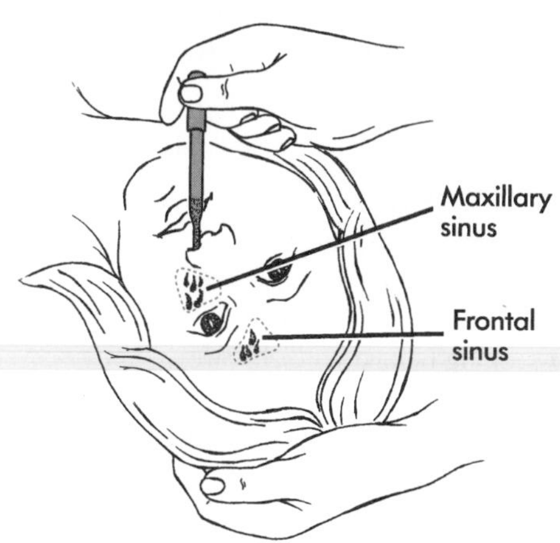

STEP 3b(3) Position for instilling nose drops into frontal and maxillary sinus.

STEP	RATIONALE
c. Support client's head with nondominant hand.	Prevents straining of neck muscles.
d. Instruct client to breathe through mouth.	Mouth breathing reduces chance of aspirating nasal drops into trachea and lungs.
e. Hold dropper 1 cm (½ inch) above **nares** and instill prescribed number of drops toward midline of ethmoid bone.	Avoids contamination of dropper. Instilling toward ethmoid bone facilitates distribution of medication over nasal mucosa.
f. Have client remain in supine position 5 minutes.	Prevents premature loss of medication through nares.
g. Offer facial tissue to blot runny nose, but caution client against blowing nose for several minutes.	Allows maximal amount of medication to be absorbed.
4. Assist client to a comfortable position after drug is absorbed.	Restores comfort.
5. Dispose of soiled supplies in proper container and wash hands.	Maintains neat, orderly environment. Reduces spread of microorganisms.

EVALUATION

1. Observe client for onset of side effects 15 to 30 minutes after administration.	Drugs absorbed through mucosa can cause systemic reaction.
2. Ask if client is able to breathe through nose after decongestant administration. May be necessary to have client occlude one nostril at a time and breathe deeply.	Determines effectiveness of decongestant medication.
3. Reinspect condition of nasal passages between instillations.	Condition of mucosa reveals response to medication.
4. Ask client to review risks of overuse of decongestants and methods for administration.	Feedback ensures that client can self-administer drugs properly.
5. Have client demonstrate self-medication.	Feedback demonstrates learning.

Unexpected Outcomes and Related Interventions

- Client is unable to breathe easily through nasal passages. Mucosa appears swollen and, congestion is unrelieved.
  - Client may be experiencing rebound effect. Stop medication use, and notify prescriber.
- Nasal mucosa remains inflamed and tender with discharge from nares.
  - Inflammatory or infectious process remains. May need to consider alternative therapy.
- Client complains of sinus headache. Sinuses remain congested.
  - May need to consider alternative therapy.
- Client is unable to explain technique and risks of drug therapy.
  - Further explanation is required.
- Client is unable to self-administer medication.
  - Reinstruction is necessary.

Recording and Reporting

- Record medication administration on MAR or computer printout immediately after administration, including drug name, concentration, number of drops; nostril into which drug was instilled; and time of administration. Include initials or signature. Do not chart medication administration until *after* it is given to client.
- If drug is withheld, record reason in nurses' notes. Circle time the drug normally would have been given on MAR or computer printout.
- Record client's response in nurses' notes.
- Report any unusual systemic effects or adverse effects/client response and/or withheld drugs to nurse in charge or physician. Depending on medication, immediate prescriber notification may be required.

Teaching Considerations

- Instruct clients that each family member should have a different dropper or spray applicator. Applicators should be washed or rinsed after each use.
- Use over-the-counter nasal sprays or nose drops for only one illness; bottles become easily contaminated with bacteria.
- Caution clients against overuse of nasal spray decongestants because they can cause rebound effect, worsening of mucosal swelling. Risk increases as more drug is used.

Pediatric Considerations

- Positioning child with head extended over edge of bed or pillow facilitates smooth instillation of nasal drops. Instruct child or parent to remain in this position for at least 1 minute to ensure that drops come into contact with affected tissue.
- Infants are nose breathers, and the possible congestion caused by nasal medications may inhibit their sucking. Nose drops, if ordered, should be administered 20 to 30 minutes before feedings (McKenry and Salerno, 1998).

Skill 17-8 Using Metered-Dose Inhalers

Inhaled medications are usually designed to produce local effects; for example, bronchodilators open narrowed bronchioles, and mucolytic agents liquefy thick mucous secretions. However, because these medications are absorbed rapidly through the pulmonary circulation, some have the potential for producing systemic side effects (e.g., isoproterenol [Isuprel] dilates bronchioles but can also cause cardiac dysrhythmias).

Clients who receive drugs by inhalation frequently suffer from chronic respiratory disease. Drugs administered by inhalation provide control of airway hyperactivity or constriction. Because clients depend on these medications for disease control, they must learn about the medications and how to administer them safely. Metered-dose inhalers (MDIs) and small-volume nebulizers (see Skill 17-9) are two devices that deliver medications.

Metered-dose inhalers (MDI) are handheld devices that disperse medications through an aerosol spray, mist, or fine powder to penetrate lung airways (Figure 17-1). The deeper passages of the respiratory tract provide a large surface area for drug absorption. The alveolar-capillary network absorbs medication rapidly.

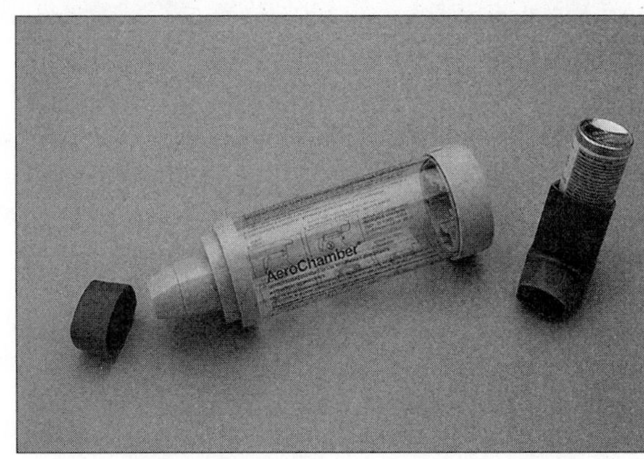

FIGURE 17-1 Example of a metered-dose inhaler (MDI) with spacer.

Drugs can be administered by MDIs in high concentrations with few side effects. An MDI delivers a measured dose of the drug with each push of a canister. Approximately 5 to 10 pounds of pressure must be used to activate the aerosol. This may be a problem for older age clients because hand strength diminishes with age. Because use of a metered-dose inhaler requires coordination during the breathing cycle, many client spray only the back of their throats and fail to receive a full dose. The inhaler must be depressed to expel medication just as the client inhales. This ensures the medication reaches the lower airways. Poor coordination can be solved by the use of spacer devices (Aerochamber, Inspirease) or the use of a breath-activated MDI (Maxair Autoinhaler) (Weilitz and Van Sciver, 1999). Box 17-3 summarizes common problems in using an inhaler.

Box 17-3 Common Problems in Using an Inhaler

1. Not taking the medication as *prescribed,* but taking either too much or too little.
2. Incorrect activation. This usually occurs through pressing the canister *before* taking a breath. Both should be done simultaneously so that the drug can be carried down to the lungs with the breath.
3. Forgetting to shake the inhaler. The drug is in a suspension, and therefore particles may settle. If the inhaler is not shaken, it may not deliver the correct dose of the drug.
4. Not waiting long enough between puffs. The whole process should be repeated to take the second puff, otherwise an incorrect dose may be delivered, or the drug may not penetrate into the lungs.
5. Failure to clean the valve. Particles may jam up the valve in the mouthpiece unless it is cleaned occasionally. This is a frequent cause of failure to get 200 puffs from one inhaler.
6. Failure to observe whether the inhaler is actually releasing a spray. If it is not, this should be checked with the pharmacist.

Delegation Considerations

The skill of administering MDI medications should not be delegated to assistive personnel. Assistive personnel should be instructed about potential side effects of medications and to report their occurrence. In addition, the care provider should report paroxysmal coughing, ineffective breathing patterns, and other respiratory difficulties.

Equipment

- Metered-dose inhaler with medication canister
- Stethoscope
- Spacer device, such as Aerochamber or Inspirease (optional)
- Facial tissues (optional)
- Wash basin or sink with warm water
- Paper towel
- Medication administration record (MAR) or computer printout

Step	Rationale
Assessment	
1. Assess respiratory pattern and auscultate breath sounds.	Establishes baseline of airway status.
2. Assess client's readiness to learn: client asks questions about medication, disease, or complications; requests education in use of inhaler; is mentally alert; participates in own care.	Affects client's ability to understand explanations and actively participate in teaching process.
3. Assess client's ability to learn: client should not be fatigued, in pain, or in respiratory distress; assess level of understanding of technical vocabulary terms.	Mental or physical limitations affect client's ability to learn and methods nurse uses for instruction.
4. Assess client's knowledge and understanding of disease and purpose and action of prescribed medications.	Knowledge of disease is essential for client to realistically understand use of inhaler.
5. Assess client's ability to hold, manipulate, and depress canister and inhaler.	Any impairment of grasp or presence of hand tremors interferes with client's ability to depress canister within inhaler.
6. Assess drug schedule and number of inhalations prescribed for each dose.	Influences explanations nurse provides for use of inhaler.
7. If previously instructed in self-administration of inhaled medicine, assess client's technique in using an inhaler.	Nurse's instruction may require only simple reinforcement, depending on client's level of dexterity.

STEP	RATIONALE

NURSING DIAGNOSIS

Defining characteristics from the assessment data may reveal the following nursing diagnoses for clients requiring this skill:

- Health-seeking behaviors (self-care)
- Risk for injury
- Ineffective breathing pattern
- Impaired gas exchange
- Ineffective therapeutic regimen management
- Deficient knowledge regarding use of MDI

Related factors are individualized based on client's condition or needs.

PLANNING

Step	Rationale
1. **Expected outcomes** following completion of procedure:	
■ Client describes techniques for use of MDI.	Ensures compliance with therapeutic regimen.
■ Client correctly self-administers metered dose.	Demonstrates learning.
■ Client's breathing pattern improves, and airways become less restricted.	Demonstrates proper administration and therapeutic effect of medication.
■ Client's gas exchange is adequate.	Demonstrates proper administration and therapeutic effect of medication.
2. Check accuracy and completeness of each MAR or computer printout with prescriber's written medication order. Check client's name, drug name and dosage, route of administration, and time for administration. Compare MAR or computer printout with medication label.	The order sheet is the most reliable source and only legal record of drugs client is to receive. Ensures client receives correct medication.
3. Check client's identification bracelet and ask name.	Ensures correct client receives medication.
4. Explain procedure to client. Be specific if client wishes to self-administer drug. Explain where and how to set up in the home.	Makes client a participant in care and minimizes anxiety.
5. Provide adequate time for teaching session.	Prevents interruptions. Instruction should occur when client is receptive.

IMPLEMENTATION

Step	Rationale
1. Wash hands and arrange equipment needed.	Reduces transfer of microorganisms and saves time.
2. Allow client opportunity to manipulate inhaler, canister, and spacer device (see Figure 17-1). Explain and demonstrate how canister fits into inhaler.	Client must be familiar with how to use equipment.
3. Explain what metered dose is, and warn client about overuse of inhaler, including drug side effects.	Client must not arbitrarily administer excessive inhalations because of risk of serious side effects and/or tolerance developing to medications. If drug is given in recommended doses, side effects are uncommon.
4. Explain steps for administering inhaled dose of medication (demonstrate steps when possible):	Use of simple, step-by-step explanations allows client to ask questions at any point during procedure.
a. Remove mouthpiece cover from inhaler.	
b. Shake inhaler well for 2 to 5 seconds.	Ensures mixing of medication in canister.
c. Hold inhaler upside down.	
d. Instruct client to position inhaler in one of two ways.	
(1) Place inhaler in mouth with opening toward back of throat closing lips tightly around it (see illustration).	
(2) Position the device 1 to 2 inches in front of widely opened mouth (see illustration).	Directs aerosol spray toward airway. Positioning the mouthpiece 1 to 2 inches from the mouth is considered the best way to deliver the medication without a spacer.
e. Have client take a deep breath and exhale completely.	Prepares client's airway to receive the medication.
f. With inhaler properly positioned, have client hold inhaler with thumb at the mouthpiece and the index finger and middle finger at the top (Lilley and Aucker, 1999).	Proper hand position ensures proper activation of metered-dose inhaler.

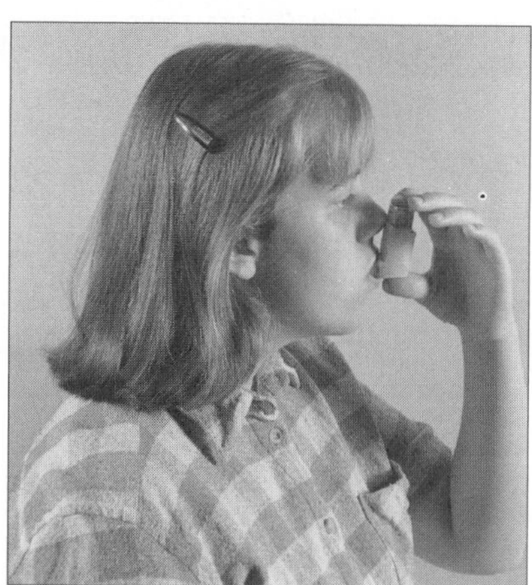

STEP **4d(1)** One technique for use of the inhaler. The client opens lips and places inhaler in mouth with opening toward back of throat.

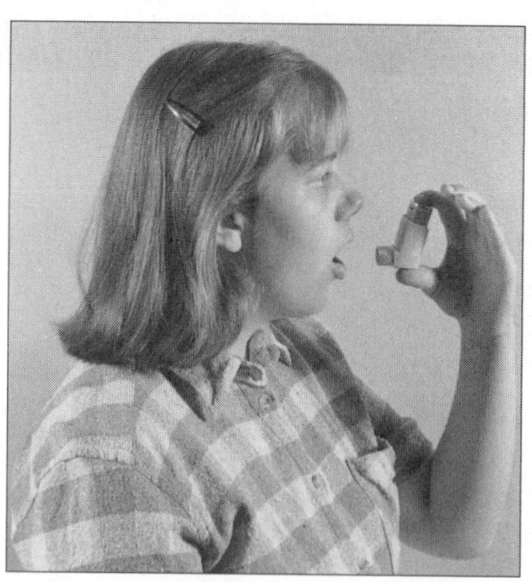

STEP **4d(2)** One technique for use of the inhaler. The client positions the mouthpiece 1 to 2 inches from the mouth. This is considered the best way to deliver the medication.

Step	Rationale
g. Instruct client to tilt head back slightly, inhale slowly and deeply through mouth, depress medication canister fully.	Medication is distributed to airways during inhalation. Inhalation through mouth rather than nose draws medication more effectively into airways.
h. Hold breath for approximately 10 seconds.	Allows tiny drops of aerosol spray to reach deeper branches of airways.
i. Exhale slowly through nose or pursed lips.	Keeps small airways open during exhalation.
5. Explain steps to administer inhaled dose of medication using a spacer device (demonstrate when possible):	
a. Remove mouthpiece cover from metered-dose inhaler and mouthpiece of spacer device.	Inhaler fits into end of spacer device.
b. Insert MDI into end of spacer device.	A spacer device traps medication released from MDI; client then inhales the drug from the device. These devices improve delivery of correct dose of inhaled medication (Wong and others, 1999).
c. Shake inhaler well for 2 to 5 seconds.	Ensures mixing of medication in canister.
d. Place spacer device mouthpiece in mouth and close lips. Do not insert beyond raised lip on mouthpiece. Avoid covering small exhalation slots with the lips.	Medication should not escape through mouth.
e. Breathe normally through spacer device mouthpiece (see illustration).	Allows client to relax before delivering medication.

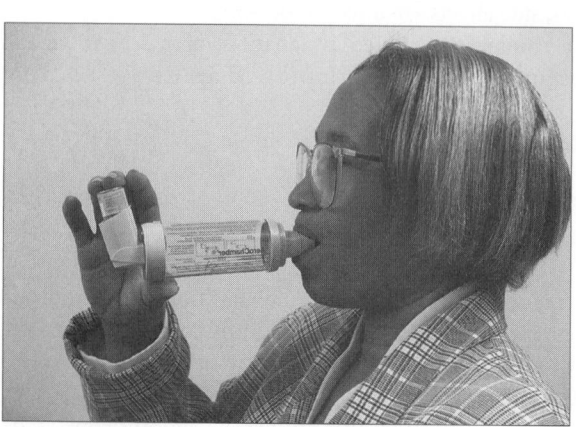

STEP **5e**

Step	Rationale
f. Depress medication canister, spraying one puff into spacer device.	Emits spray that allows finer particles to be inhaled. Large droplets are retained in spacer device.
g. Breathe in slowly and fully (for 5 seconds).	Ensures particles of medication are distributed to deeper airways.
h. Hold full breath for 5 to 10 seconds.	Ensures full drug distribution.
6. Instruct client to wait 2 to 5 minutes between inhalations or as ordered by prescriber.	Drugs must be inhaled sequentially. First inhalation opens airways and reduces inflammation. Second or third inhalations penetrate deeper airways.
7. Instruct client against repeating inhalations before next scheduled dose (see Box 17-3).	Drugs are prescribed at intervals during day to provide constant drug levels and minimize side effects. Beta-adrenergic MDIs are used either on an "as needed" basis or regularly every 4 to 6 hours.
8. Explain that client may feel gagging sensation in throat caused by droplets of medication on pharynx or tongue.	Results when inhalant is sprayed and inhaled incorrectly.
9. Instruct client in removing medication canister and cleaning inhaler in warm water.	Accumulation of spray around mouthpiece can interfere with proper distribution during use.
10. Ask if client has any questions.	Clarifies misconceptions or misunderstanding.

Evaluation

1. Have client explain and demonstrate steps in use of inhaler.	Return demonstration provides feedback for measuring client's learning.
2. Ask client to explain drug schedule.	Improves likelihood of compliance with therapy.
3. Ask client to describe side effects of medication and criteria for calling physician.	Allows client to recognize signs of overuse and need to seek medical support when drugs are ineffective.
4. After medication administration, assess client's respirations and assess breath sounds.	Determines status of breathing pattern and adequacy of ventilation.

Unexpected Outcomes and Related Interventions

- Client's respirations are rapid and shallow, breath sounds indicate wheezing.
  - May need to reassess type of medication or delivery method.
- Client experiences paraoxysms of coughing.
  - Aerosolized particles irritate posterior pharynx. Notify prescriber; may need to reassess type of medication or delivery method.
- Client needs a bronchodilator more than every 4 hours.
  - May indicate respiratory problems; reassessment of type of medication and delivery methods needed.
- Client experiences cardiac dysrhythmias, especially if receiving beta-adrenergics.
  - If client experiences symptoms with the dysrhythmias (e.g., light-headedness, syncope), withhold all further doses of medication. Discuss with prescriber.
- Client may not be able to self-administer medication properly.
  - Alternative delivery routes or methods may need to be explored.
- Client is unable to explain technique and risks of drug therapy.
  - Further teaching may be required.

Recording and Reporting

- Record actual time each drug was administered, dosage, and concentration on MAR or computer printout immediately after administration. Include initials or signature. Do not chart medication administration until *after* it is given to client.
- If drug is withheld, record reason in nurses' notes. Circle time the drug normally would have been given on MAR or computer printout.
- Record client's response to the medication, including pulse, respirations, breath sounds assessed, and any adverse effects.
- Document what skills were taught and client's ability to perform them.
- Report adverse effects/client response and/or withheld drugs to nurse in charge or physician. Depending on medication, immediate prescriber notification may be required.

Teaching Considerations

- Client may need supervised practice for several different steps of procedure before being able to perform each skill independently. Clients may have difficulty with timing inspiration with medication dispersal without proper instruction (Owen, 1999).
- Teach client how to determine fullness of canisters, using displacement in water technique (Figure 17-2).
- Do not try to teach client how to use an inhaler during an episode of shortness of breath. Client's attention span will be very poor.

Pediatric Considerations

- Because of difficulty coordinating actuation and inhalation, the use of a spacer device is recommended for young children (Wong and others, 1999).
- Bronchodilators are used often in children, but use with extreme caution and monitor for adverse effects such as tremors, restlessness, dizziness, gastrointestinal upset, and tachycardia (Lilley and Aucker, 1999).
- Educate child and parent about the need to use inhaler during school hours. Help family find resources within the school or day care facility. Keep in mind that many school systems do not permit self-administration of MDIs. Follow the school's policy regarding having the MDI available for use during school hours. A physician's order may be necessary.

Gerontological Considerations

- Older adult clients may be unable to depress medication canister because of weakened grasp or may be unable to coordinate actuation of the canister with inhalation. The use of a spacer device may be necessary.

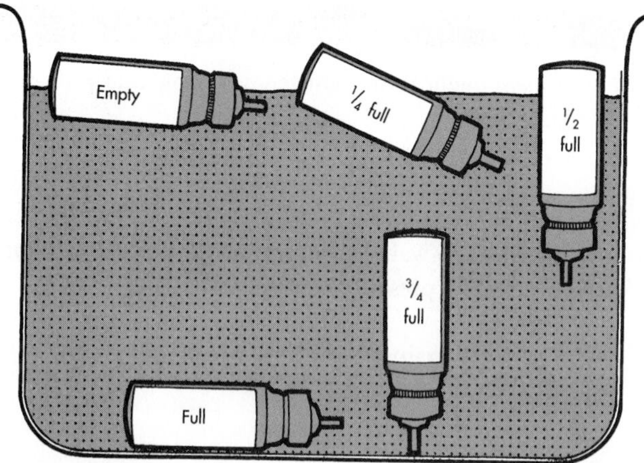

FIGURE 17-2 A simple method of estimating amount left in the inhalant canister is to place it in a container filled with water. The position the canister takes in the water determines the amount of inhalant remaining.

Home Care Considerations

- Remind clients to carry prescribed inhalers to use as immediate treatment in case of an acute asthma attack.

Skill 17-9 Using Small-Volume Nebulizers

Nebulization is a process of adding medications or moisture to inspired air by mixing particles of various sizes with air. Adding moisture to the respiratory system through nebulization may improve clearance of pulmonary secretions. Medications such as bronchodilators, mucolytics, and corticosteroids are often administered by nebulization.

Small-volume nebulizers provide medications in an aerosolized form that can be inhaled by the client into the tracheobronchial tree and possibly into the bloodstream through the alveoli. As a result, systemic effects from the medications may occur.

Clients who receive drugs by inhalation frequently suffer from chronic lung disease. Drugs administered by inhalation provide control of airway hyperactivity or constriction. Because clients depend on these medications for disease control, they must learn how they work and how to administer them safely.

Delegation Considerations

The skill of administering medications by nebulizer should not be delegated to assistive personnel. Assistive personnel should be instructed about potential side effects of medications and to report their occurrence. In addition, the care provider should report paroxysmal coughing, ineffective breathing patterns, and other respiratory difficulties.

Equipment

- Medication ordered
- Diluent (if needed)
- Nebulizer bottle and tubing assembly
- Small-volume nebulizer machine (often called handheld nebulizer or simply nebulizer)
- Stethoscope
- Medication administration record (MAR) or computer printout

Step	Rationale
Assessment	
1. Assess client's medical history, history of allergies, medication and diet history.	These factors can influence how certain drugs act. Information also reflects client's need for medications.
2. Assess client's ability to assemble, hold, and manipulate the nebulizer equipment.	Any impairment of grasp or presence of hand tremors interferes with client's ability to use the equipment.

• ***Critical Decision Point***
If client is unable to hold the nebulizer mouthpiece during the treatment, use an aerosol mask in place of the mouthpiece. Such masks are also used for children. This ensures proper deposition of medication.

Step	Rationale
3. Assess drug ordered, including amount, type and amount of diluent (if unit dose is not available), and frequency.	Legal order for medication therapy must be complete. Unit-dose medications do not require dilution; however, a diluent may be used along with a unit-dose medication if a different percentage of drug is desired.
4. Assess pulse, respirations, and breath sounds before beginning treatment.	Establishes a baseline for comparison during and after treatment.

Nursing Diagnosis

Defining characteristics from the assessment data may reveal the following nursing diagnoses for clients requiring this skill:

- Ineffective breathing pattern
- Impaired gas exchange
- Health-seeking behaviors (self-care)
- Risk for injury
- Ineffective therapeutic regimen management
- Deficient knowledge regarding use of small-volume nebulizers

Related factors are individualized based on client's condition or needs.

Planning

Step	Rationale
1. **Expected outcomes** following completion of procedure:	
▪ Client's breathing patterns are effective.	Demonstrates proper administration and therapeutic effect of medication.
▪ Client's gas exchange is adequate.	Demonstrates proper administration and therapeutic effect of medication.
▪ Client describes techniques for use of small-volume nebulizers.	Increases likelihood of compliance with therapeutic regimen.
▪ Client correctly self-administers medication using small-volume nebulizer.	Demonstrates learning.
2. Check accuracy and completeness of each MAR or computer printout with prescriber's written medication order. Check client's name, drug name and dosage, route of administration, and time for administration. Compare MAR or computer printout with medication label.	The order sheet is the most reliable source and only legal record of drugs client is to receive. Ensures client receives correct medication.
3. Check client's identification bracelet and ask name.	Ensures correct client receives medication.
4. Explain procedure to client. Be specific if client wishes to self-administer drug.	Makes client a participant in care and minimizes anxiety. Begins client teaching regarding medications. Enables client to self-administer drug if physically able and motivated.

Implementation

Step	Rationale
1. Wash hands and arrange equipment needed.	Reduces transfer of microorganisms and saves time.
2. Explain the use of the nebulizer, and warn client of possible drug side effects.	Helps to make client more knowledgeable about treatment and medication.

STEP	RATIONALE
3. Assemble nebulizer equipment per manufacturer's directions (see illustration).	Assembly may vary slightly with different manufacturers. Proper assembly ensures safe delivery of medication.
4. Add prescribed medication and diluent (if needed) to nebulizer.	Ensures proper dose and delivery of ordered medication.
5. Have client hold mouthpiece between lips with gentle pressure (see illustration).	
a. If client is a child or infant or an adult who is fatigued, who cannot follow instructions, or who is unable to follow instructions, use a face mask.	Use of a face mask does not require client to remember to hold mouthpiece correctly. Correct delivery ensures sufficient deposition of medication.
b. Use special adapters for clients with a tracheostomy.	

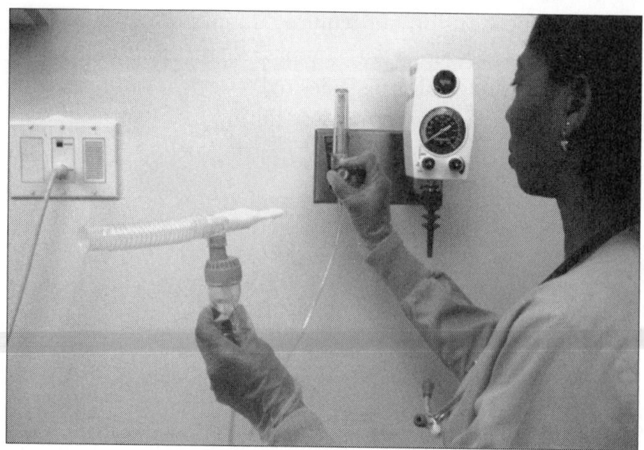

STEP 3 Nebulizer tubing, reservoir, and mouthpiece.

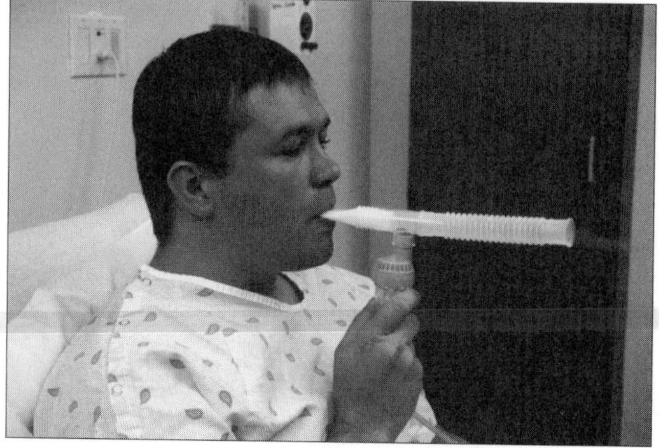

STEP 5 Nebulizer mouthpiece placed between client's lips.

STEP	RATIONALE
6. Have client take a deep breath, slowly, to a volume slightly greater than normal. Encourage a brief, end-inspiratory pause. Then have the client exhale passively.	Promotes greater deposition of medication in the airways.
a. If client is dyspneic, encourage client to hold every fourth or fifth breath for 5 to 10 seconds.	Improves effectiveness of medication.
7. Turn on the small-volume nebulizer machine, and ensure that a sufficient mist is formed.	Verifies that the equipment is working properly during delivery of medication.
a. Tap the nebulizer cup occasionally during treatment and toward the end of the treatment.	Releases droplets that may be clinging to the side of the cup, thus allowing for renebulization of the solution.
b. Remind client to repeat the breathing pattern described in Step 6 until the drug is completely nebulized.	Maximizes effectiveness of medication.
(1) Some practitioners set a timed limit as the length of the treatment rather than waiting for the medication to completely nebulize.	
c. Monitor client's pulse during procedure, especially if beta-adrenergic blockers are used.	Enables nurse to observe for potential side effects of medications.
8. When medication is completely nebulized, turn off machine, and store tubing assembly per institution policy.	Proper storage reduces transfer of microorganisms.
a. Shake the nebulizer bottle, attempting to remove all remaining solution. Never rinse with tap water.	Tap water may contain microorganisms.
9. If steroids are nebulized, encourage client to rinse mouth and gargle with warm water after nebulizer treatment.	Removes medication residue from oral cavity and helps to prevent thrust, a possible side effect of therapy with these drugs.

• ***Critical Decision Point***

Some respiratory medications can cause systemic effects such as restlessness, nervousness, and palpitations. Administer these medications with caution to clients with cardiac disease because of the possibility of hypertension, arrhythmias, or coronary insufficiency. If severe bronchospasm occurs during treatment, discontinue drug immediately and notify physician.

STEP	RATIONALE

EVALUATION

Step	Rationale
1. Assess client's pulse, respiratory rate, and breath sounds after procedure.	Allows comparison with baseline data and evaluation of effectiveness of procedure.
2. Have client explain and demonstrate steps in use of small-volume nebulizer.	Return demonstration provides feedback for measuring client's learning.
3. Ask client to explain drug schedule.	Improves likelihood of compliance with therapy.
4. Ask client to describe side effects of medication and criteria for calling physician.	Allows client to recognize signs of overuse and need to seek medical support when drugs are ineffective.

UNEXPECTED OUTCOMES AND RELATED INTERVENTIONS

- Client's breathing pattern is ineffective; respirations are rapid and shallow.
  - May need to reassess type of medication or delivery method.
- Client experiences paroxysms of coughing.
  - Aerosolized particles irritate posterior pharynx. Notify prescriber; may need to reassess type of medication or delivery method.
- Client experiences cardiac dysrhythmias as a side effect of medication. Notify prescriber.
- Client may not be able to self-administer medication properly.
  - Alternative delivery routes or methods may need to be explored.
- Client is unable to explain technique and risks of drug therapy.
  - Further teaching may be required.

RECORDING AND REPORTING

- Record drug used, dosage and concentration, and time and date of administration on MAR or computer printout immediately after administration. Include initials or signature. Do not chart medication administration until *after* it is given to client.
- Record client's response to the medication, including pulse, respirations, and breath sound assessed.
- If drug is withheld, record reason in nurses' notes. Circle time the drug normally would have been given on MAR or computer printout.
- Document what skills were taught and client's ability to perform them.
- Report adverse effects/client response and/or withheld drugs to nurse in charge or physician. Depending on medication, immediate prescriber notification may be required.

TEACHING CONSIDERATIONS

- When teaching self-administration, do not try to teach client how to use a nebulizer during an episode of shortness of breath. Client's attention span will be very poor.
- Teach client that length of treatment is usually 10 to 15 minutes, if equipment is working properly and correct medication and diluent are used. If treatment time is prolonged, check nebulizer or compressor function.
- Use all the medication in nebulizer cup for each treatment. Teach client not to store medication in nebulizer for later use (Ashwill and Droske, 1997).
- Review all steps of the procedure with client before discharge, and ask client to demonstrate the proper technique. Reinforce teaching as needed.
- Advise clients taking long-acting beta-agonists, which are used for long-term control of symptoms, about possible adverse effects: nervousness, restlessness, tremor, headache, nausea, rapid or pounding heart, and dizziness. Emphasize that the drug should only be taken as ordered so that a tolerance to the drug is not developed (Owen, 1999).
- Teach clients to use small handheld peak flowmeters to monitor response to therapy when bronchodilators or bronchospasm prevention drugs (steroids) are prescribed (Beare and Myers, 1998).

PEDIATRIC CONSIDERATIONS

- A mask may be used for the nebulizer treatment if child is too young to hold mouthpiece correctly for the duration of the treatment.
- Instruct child to breathe normally with mouth open to provide a direct route to the airways for the medication (Wong and others, 1999).
- Educate child and parent about the need to use nebulizer during school or day care hours. Help family find resources within the school or day care facility. Follow the school's policy regarding having the nebulizer and medication available for use during school hours. A physician's order may be necessary.

HOME CARE CONSIDERATIONS

- When at home, nebulizer parts should be rinsed after each use with clear water and air dried. In addition, parts should be cleaned daily with warm, soapy water, rinsed, and allowed to dry.
- Once a week, nebulizer parts should be soaked in a solution of vinegar and water (one part white vinegar to four parts water) for 30 minutes, rinsed thoroughly with clean water, and air dried. Nebulizer parts should never be stored until totally dried. Wet equipment encourages growth of bacteria and mold (Ashwill and Droske, 1997).
- Follow manufacturer's recommendations for maintenance of small-volume nebulizer machine, including changing the filters when they become discolored (grayish).

Skill 17-10 Administering Vaginal Instillations

Female clients can often develop vaginal infections that require topical application of antiinfective agents. Vaginal medications are available in foam, jelly, cream, or suppository form. Medicated irrigations or douches can also be given. However, their excessive use can lead to vaginal irritation.

Vaginal suppositories are oval shaped and come individually packaged in foil wrappers. They are larger and more oval than rectal suppositories. (Figure 17-3 provides a comparison with rectal suppositories.) Storage in a refrigerator prevents the solid suppositories from melting. A suppository is inserted into the vagina with an applicator or a gloved hand. After insertion, body temperature causes the suppository to melt, and the medication is then distributed. Foam, jellies, and creams are administered with an inserter or applicator. Clients often prefer administering their own vaginal medications and should be given privacy to do so. After instillation of the drug, a client may wish to wear a perineal pad to collect excess drainage. Because vaginal medications are frequently given to treat infection, any discharge may be foul smelling. Good aseptic technique should be followed, and the client should be offered frequent opportunities to maintain perineal hygiene (see Skill 6-2).

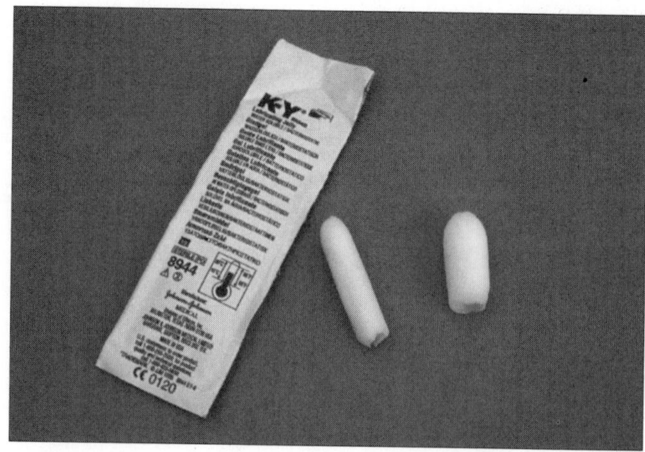

FIGURE 17-3 Vaginal suppositories are larger and more oval than rectal suppositories.

Delegation Considerations

The skill of vaginal instillations should not be delegated to assistive personnel. Assistive personnel should be instructed about potential side effects of medications and to report their occurrence.

Equipment

- Vaginal cream, foam, jelly, tablet, or suppository, or irrigating solution
- Applicators (if needed)
- Disposable gloves
- Tissues
- Paper towel
- Perineal pad
- Drape
- Water-soluble lubricants
- Bedpan
- Irrigation or douche container
- Medication administration record (MAR) or computer printout

Step	Rationale
Assessment	
1. Review prescriber's order, including client's name, drug name, form (foam, jelly, cream, tablet, or suppository), route, dosage, and time of administration.	Ensures safe and correct administration of medication.
2. Review pertinent information related to medication, including action, purpose, side effects, and nursing implications.	Allows nurse to administer drug properly and to monitor client's response.
3. Ask if client is experiencing any symptoms of pruritus, burning, or discomfort.	Assesses for symptoms of vaginal irritation.
4. Have client void.	Empties bladder and promotes comfort during insertion.
5. Assess client's ability to manipulate applicator or suppository and to properly position self to insert medication (may be done just before insertion).	Mobility restriction indicates level of assistance required from nurse.
6. Review client's knowledge of purpose of drug therapy and interest in self-administering medication.	May indicate need for health teaching. Understanding influences compliance with therapy.

STEP	RATIONALE

NURSING DIAGNOSIS

Defining characteristics from the assessment data may reveal the following nursing diagnoses for clients requiring this skill:

- Health-seeking behaviors (self-care)
- Noncompliance with drug therapy
- Impaired physical mobility
- Deficient knowledge regarding vaginal medication administration
- Pain (acute, chronic)
- Sexual dysfunction

Related factors are individualized based on client's condition or needs.

PLANNING

1. **Expected outcomes** following completion of procedure:
   - Vaginal tissues are pink and smooth. Genitalia are clear and without discharge. — Tissues take on normal characteristics.
   - Client denies symptoms of discomfort and expresses relief from symptoms of infection/inflammation. — Inflammation or infection has resolved.
   - A small amount of discharge may be seen that is the color of medication exiting from vaginal canal. — When suppository or cream becomes distributed, small amount may escape from the vaginal **orifice.**
   - Client is able to discuss information about prescribed drug. — Feedback reflects client's learning.
   - Client self-administers suppository or medication. — Demonstrates learning.
2. Check accuracy and completeness of each MAR or computer printout with prescriber's written medication order. Check client's name, drug name and dosage, route of administration, and time for administration. Compare MAR or computer printout with medication label. — The order sheet is the most reliable source and only legal record of drugs client is to receive. Ensures right medication is administered.
3. Check client's identification bracelet and ask name. — Ensures correct client receives medication.
4. Explain procedure to client. Be specific if client plans on self-administering medication. — Promotes client's understanding. Enables client to self-administer drug if physically able.

IMPLEMENTATION

1. Wash hands, arrange supplies at bedside, and apply clean gloves. — Reduces transfer of microorganisms; helps nurse perform procedure smoothly.
2. Close room curtain or door. — Provides privacy.
3. Assist client to lie in dorsal recumbent position. Clients with restricted mobility in knees or hips may lie supine with legs abducted. — Position provides easy access to and good exposure of vaginal canal. Dependent position also allows suppository to dissolve in vagina without escaping.
4. Keep abdomen and lower extremities draped. — Minimizes client's embarrassment by limiting exposure.
5. Be sure vaginal orifice is well-illuminated by room light. Otherwise position portable gooseneck lamp. — Proper insertion requires visualization of external genitalia if not self-administered.
6. Inspect condition of external genitalia and vaginal canal (Chapter 10). — Provides baseline to monitor effect of medication.
7. For suppository insertion:
   a. Remove suppository from wrapper and apply liberal amount of water-soluble lubricant to smooth or rounded end (see illustration). Be sure that suppository is at room temperature. Lubricate gloved index finger of dominant hand. — Lubrication reduces friction against mucosal surfaces during insertion. Use of petroleum jelly may leave a residue that harbors bacteria and yeast fungi.
   b. With nondominant gloved hand, gently separate labial folds, in the front-to-back direction. — Exposes vaginal orifice.

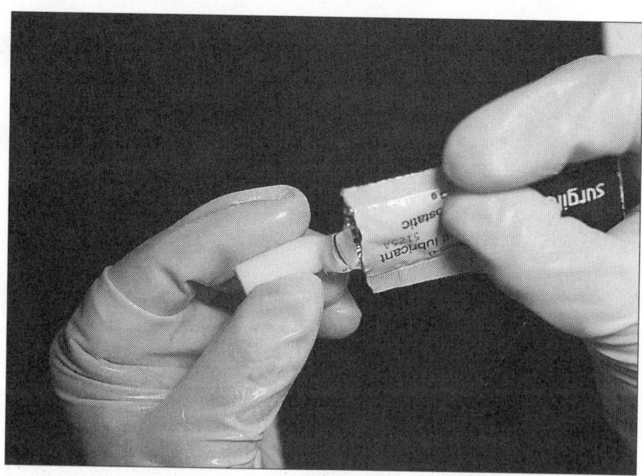

STEP **7a** Lubricate tip of suppository.

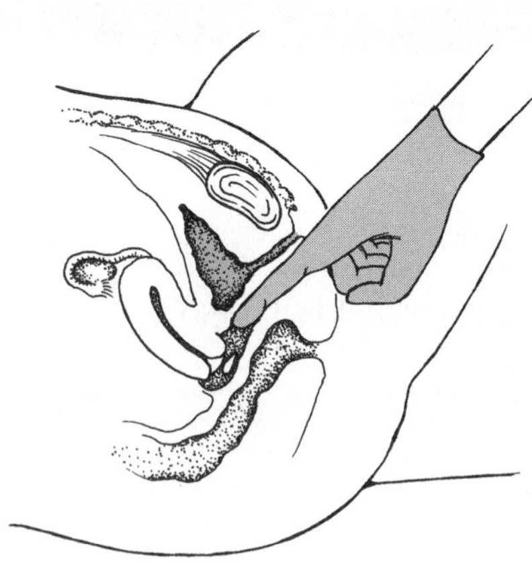

STEP **7c** Angle of suppository insertion.

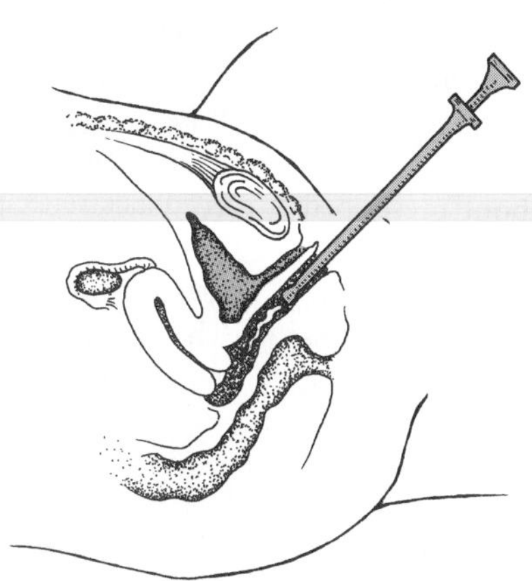

STEP **8c** Applicator inserted into vaginal canal. Plunger pushed to instill medication.

STEP	RATIONALE
c. Insert rounded end of suppository along posterior wall of vaginal canal entire length of finger (7.5 to 10 cm or 3 to 4 in) (see illustration).	Proper placement of suppository ensures equal distribution of medication along walls of vaginal cavity.
d. Withdraw finger and wipe away remaining lubricant from around orifice and labia.	Maintains comfort.
8. For application of cream or foam:	
a. Fill cream or foam applicator following package directions.	Dose is instilled based on volume in applicator.
b. With nondominant gloved hand, gently separate labial folds.	Exposes vaginal orifice.
c. With dominant gloved hand, insert applicator approximately 5 to 7.5 cm (2 to 3 inches). Push applicator plunger to deposit medication into vagina (see illustration).	Allows equal distribution of medication along vaginal walls.
d. Withdraw applicator and place on paper towel. Wipe off residual cream from labia or vaginal orifice.	Maintains client comfort. Residual cream on applicator may contain microorganisms.

Step	Rationale
9. For irrigation and douche:	
a. Place client on bedpan with absorbent pad underneath.	Allows hips to be higher than shoulders and solution reaches posterior wall of vagina. Bedpan collects solution.
b. Be sure fluid is at body temperature. Run fluid through container nozzle (priming the tubing).	Body temperature promotes client comfort. Priming tubing removes air and moistens the nozzle tip.
c. Gently separate labial folds and direct nozzle toward sacrum, following the floor of the vagina.	Correct angle allows nozzle access into the vagina.
d. Raise container approximately 30 to 50 cm (12 to 20 inches) above level of vagina. Insert nozzle 7 to 10 cm (3 to 4 inches). Allow solution to flow while rotating nozzle. Administer all the irrigating solution.	Rotating nozzle allows irrigation of all areas in vagina.
e. Withdraw nozzle and assist client to a comfortable sitting position.	Remaining solution drains by gravity.
f. Allow client to remain on bedpan for a few minutes. Cleanse perineum with soap and water.	Ensures all solution drains from vagina. Provides comfort for the client.
g. Assist client off bedpan. Dry perineal area.	
10. Instruct client who received suppository, cream, or tablet to remain on her back for at least 10 minutes.	Allows melting and spreading of the medication throughout vaginal cavity and prevents loss through the orifice.
11. If applicator is used, wash with soap and warm water, rinse, and store for future use.	Vaginal cavity is not sterile. Soap and water assist in removal of bacteria and residual cream from applicator.
12. Offer perineal pad when client resumes ambulation.	Provides client comfort.
13. Discard gloves by turning them inside out, and dispose of gloves and other soiled equipment in appropriate receptacle. Wash hands.	Reduces transmission of microorganisms.

Evaluation

1. Inspect condition of vaginal canal and external genitalia between applications.	Determines whether vaginal medication effectively reduced irritation or inflammation of tissues.
2. Question client regarding continued pruritus, burning, or discomfort.	Determines whether symptoms are relieved.
3. Ask client to discuss purpose, action, and side effects of medication.	Reflects client's understanding of drug therapy.
4. Have client demonstrate administration of next dose.	Reflects learning of technique.

Unexpected Outcomes and Related Interventions

- A thick, white, patchy, curdlike discharge is clinging to vaginal walls. Vaginal walls appear bright pink or inflamed.
  - Possible signs of yeast infection, a common female disorder. Continue medication administration, and report if symptoms continue or appear to get worse.
- Client reports localized pruritus and burning.
  - Result of infection or inflammation, but a possible side effect of some medications (such as miconazole).
  - Monitor symptoms, report if they are worse.
- Client is unable to discuss drug therapy correctly.
  - Requires repeated instruction, or client is unable to learn.
- Client is unable to self-administer medication.
  - Reinstruction is necessary.

Recording and Reporting

- Record appearance of vaginal canal and genitalia in nurses' notes, and report any unusual findings.
- Record actual time each drug (or solution if vaginal instillation) was administered on MAR or computer printout immediately after administration. Include initials or signature. Do not chart medication administration until *after* it is given to client.
- If drug is withheld, record reason in nurses' notes. Circle time the drug normally would have been given on MAR or computer printout.
- If symptoms do not disappear, or if they get worse, report to prescriber.
- Report adverse effects/client response and/or withheld drugs to nurse in charge or physician.

Teaching Considerations

- Teach client value of and technique for regular perineal hygiene.
- Encourage client to take *all* of the medication as prescribed, for the prescribed amount of time, to ensure effectiveness of the treatment.
- Women taking clotrimazole for the treatment of vaginal infection should be told to abstain from sexual intercourse until treatment is completed and the infection resolved (Lilley and Aucker, 1999).

Skill 17-11 Administering Rectal Suppositories

A variety of medications may be given rectally. Drugs administered rectally exert either a local effect on gastrointestinal mucosa, such as promoting defecation, or exert systemic effects, such as relieving nausea or providing analgesia. The rectal route is not as reliable as oral or parenteral routes in terms of drug absorption and distribution. However, the medications are relatively safe, since they rarely cause local irritation or side effects. Rectal medications are contraindicated in clients with rectal surgery or active rectal bleeding.

Rectal suppositories differ in shape from vaginal suppositories, being thinner and bullet shaped. (See Figure 17-3 for comparison with vaginal suppositories.) The rounded end prevents anal trauma during insertion. When the nurse administers the suppository, placing it past the internal anal sphincter and against the rectal mucosa is important. Improper placement can result in expulsion of the suppository before the medication dissolves and is absorbed into the mucosa. Never force a suppository into a mass of fecal material. It may be necessary to administer a small cleansing enema before a suppository can be inserted. If a client prefers to self-administer a suppository, the nurse should give specific instructions so that the medication is deposited correctly. Do not cut the suppository into sections to divide the dosage; the active drug may not be distributed evenly within the suppository, and the result may be an inaccurate dose (McKenry and Salerno, 1998).

Delegation Considerations

The skill of rectal medication administration should not be delegated to assistive personnel. Assistive personnel should be instructed about potential side effects of medications and to report their occurrence. The care provider should also report if the intended therapeutic response occurs (e.g., reduction of fever or bowel movement).

Equipment

- Rectal suppository
- Lubricating jelly (water soluble)
- Clean gloves
- Tissue
- Drape
- Medication administration record (MAR) or computer printout

Step	Rationale
Assessment	
1. Review prescriber's order, including client's name, drug name, dosage, form, route, and time of administration.	Ensures safe and correct administration of medication.
2. Review pertinent information related to medication, including action, purpose, side effects, and nursing implications.	Allows nurse to administer drug properly and to monitor client's response.
3. Review medical record for history of rectal surgery or bleeding.	Conditions contraindicate use of suppository.
4. Review any presenting signs and symptoms of gastrointestinal alterations (e.g., constipation or diarrhea).	Conditions may indicate use of suppository.
5. Assess client's ability to hold suppository and to position self to insert medication.	Mobility restriction indicates need for nurse to assist with drug administration.
6. Review client's knowledge of purpose of drug therapy and interest in self-administering suppository.	May indicate need for health teaching. Level of motivation influences teaching approach.

STEP	RATIONALE

NURSING DIAGNOSIS

Defining characteristics from the assessment data may reveal the following nursing diagnoses for clients requiring this skill:

Constipation
Health-seeking behaviors (self-care)
Impaired physical mobility
Deficient knowledge regarding suppository administration
Pain (acute, chronic)

Related factors are individualized based on client's condition or needs.

PLANNING

Step	Rationale
1. **Expected outcomes** following completion of the procedure:	
▪ Client reports relief or reduction in symptoms for which medication is prescribed.	Drug acts effectively.
▪ Client describes purpose of medication.	Feedback reflects client's learning.
▪ Client self-administers suppository.	Demonstrates learning.
2. Check accuracy and completeness of each MAR or computer printout with prescriber's written medication order. Check client's name, drug name and dosage, route of administration, and time for administration. Compare MAR or computer printout with medication label.	The order sheet is the most reliable source and only legal record of drugs client is to receive. Ensures right medication is administered.
3. Check client's identification bracelet and ask name.	Ensures correct client receives medication.
4. Explain procedure to client. Be specific if client wishes to self-administer drug.	Promotes client's understanding and cooperation. Enables client to self-administer drug safely if physically able and motivated.

IMPLEMENTATION

Step	Rationale
1. Wash hands, arrange supplies at bedside, and apply gloves.	Reduces transfer of microorganisms, helps nurse perform procedure smoothly.
2. Close room curtain or door.	Maintains privacy and minimizes embarrassment.
3. Assist client in assuming a left side-lying Sims' position with upper leg flexed upward.	Position exposes anus and helps client to relax external anal sphincter. Left side lessens the likelihood of the suppository or feces being expelled.

• ***Critical Decision Point***
If client has mobility impairment that prevents a left side-lying Sim's position, assist client to a left lateral position. Obtain assistance from another health care provider to help client turn, and use pillows under client's upper arm and leg for support and comfort.

Step	Rationale
4. Keep client draped with only anal area exposed.	Maintains privacy and facilitates relaxation.
5. Examine condition of anus externally and palpate rectal walls as needed (see Chapter 10). Dispose of gloves by turning them inside out and placing them in proper receptacle if they become soiled.	Determines presence of active rectal bleeding. Palpation determines whether rectum is filled with feces, which may interfere with suppository placement. Reduces transmission of infection.

• ***Critical Decision Point***
Do not palpate client's rectum if client has had rectal surgery. Generally, rectal suppository is contraindicated in the presence of active rectal bleeding, and diarrhea (McKenry and Salerno, 1998).

Step	Rationale
6. Apply new pair of disposable gloves (if previous gloves were soiled and discarded).	Minimizes contact with fecal material to reduce transmission of infection.
7. Remove suppository from foil wrapper and lubricate rounded end with water soluble lubricant. Lubricate gloved index finger of dominant hand. If client has hemorrhoids, use liberal amount of lubricant and handle area gently.	Lubrication reduces friction as suppository enters rectal canal.

STEP	RATIONALE
8. Ask client to take slow deep breaths through mouth and to relax anal sphincter.	Forcing suppository through constricted sphincter causes pain.
9. Retract client's buttocks with nondominant hand. With gloved index finger of dominant hand, insert suppository gently through anus, past internal sphincter, and against rectal wall, 10 cm (4 inches) (see illustration).	Suppository must be placed against rectal mucosa for eventual absorption and therapeutic action.

- ***Critical Decision Point***
  Suppository should not be inserted into a mass of fecal material; medication effectiveness will be reduced.

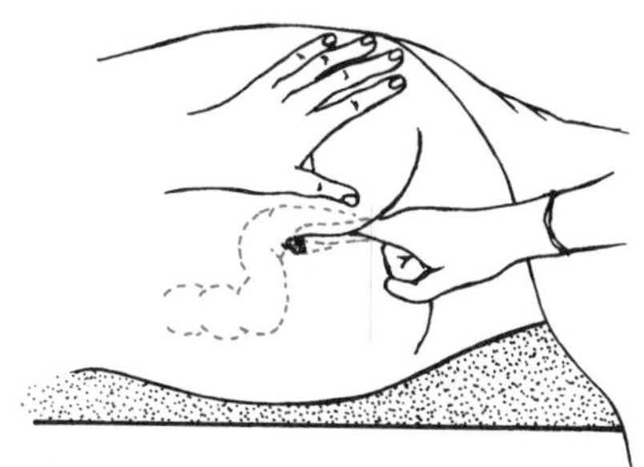

STEP 9 Insert rectal suppository past sphincter and against rectal wall.

STEP	RATIONALE
10. Withdraw finger and wipe client's anal area.	Provides comfort.
11. Discard gloves by turning them inside out, and dispose of in appropriate receptacle.	Reduces transfer of microorganisms.
12. Ask client to remain flat or on side for 5 minutes.	Prevents expulsion of suppository.
13. If suppository contains laxative or fecal softener, place call light within reach so client can obtain assistance to reach bedpan or toilet.	Ability to call for assistance provides client with sense of control over elimination.
14. Wash hands and dispose of gloves and other equipment.	Reduces risk of transfer of infection.

EVALUATION

STEP	RATIONALE
1. Return within 5 minutes to determine if suppository was expelled.	Determines if drug is properly distributed. Reinsertion may be necessary.
2. Ask if client experienced localized anal or rectal discomfort during insertion.	Determines whether insertion of suppository was irritating.
3. Evaluate client for relief of symptoms for which medication was prescribed to relieve or eliminate (within time expected action of drug occurs).	Determines medication's effectiveness.
4. Ask client to explain purpose of medication.	Reflects client's understanding of drug therapy.
5. Have client demonstrate administration of next dose of medication.	Demonstration measures learning.

UNEXPECTED OUTCOMES AND RELATED INTERVENTIONS

- Side effects of specific medication develop, depending on type of drug administered.
  - May require alternate therapy.
- Symptoms previously reported are unrelieved.
  - May require alternate therapy.
- Client reports rectal pain during insertion.
  - Suppository may need to be better lubricated, or rectal route may be contraindicated.
- Client is unable to explain purpose of drug therapy.
  - Reinstruction is necessary, or client is unwilling or unable to learn.
- Client is unable to self-administer medication.
  - Reinstruction is necessary.

RECORDING AND REPORTING

- Record actual time each drug was administered on MAR or computer printout immediately after administration. Include initials or signature. Do not chart medication administration until *after* it is given to client.

- If drug is withheld, record reason in nurses' notes. Circle time the drug normally would have been given on MAR or computer printout.
- Record client's response to medication, including any unusual reactions.
- Report adverse effects/client response and/or withheld drugs to nurse in charge or physician. Depending on medication, immediate prescriber notification may be required.

Teaching Considerations

- If client chooses to self-administer suppositories, teach principles and techniques of infection control to prevent contact with and spread of fecal material.
- Long-term use of laxatives often results in decreased bowel tone and may result in dependency. Client should be taught nonpharmacologic measures (fiber and fluid intake, dietary habits) to promote healthy bowel elimination (Lilley and Aucker, 1999).

Pediatric Considerations

- With children, it may be necessary to gently hold or tape the buttocks together for 5 to 10 minutes to relieve pressure on the anal sphincter until the urge to expel the suppository is gone (Wong and others, 1999).

Gerontological Considerations

- Older adult clients with loss of sphincter control may have difficulty retaining suppository.

Critical Thinking Exercises

1. Your client has the following medications ordered: digoxin, 0.125 mg qd; Slow-K, one tablet bid, furosemide, 40 mg qd; Nitro-Bid, 1 capsule q8h. This morning a nasogastric feeding tube was inserted, and all medications are to be given through the tube. How would you give these medications? (Check a pharmacology text to help you answer this question.)
2. A young mother has brought her 4-year-old child to the clinic because of an eye infection. The child's eyes are crusted with drainage. A prescription for antibiotic eye drops is given. What do you need to teach regarding this procedure?
3. You receive a phone call from the daughter of a 68-year-old client who is on home handheld nebulizer treatments. She states that the treatments are lasting almost 45 minutes even though she is using the same amount of medication and diluent. What could be the problem?
4. Your client has a partial-thickness burn, 20% body surface area on the lower abdomen and left thigh. He has been applying Silvadene q8h to the wound at home for the last 3 days. You discover upon your home visit that he has used almost 8 ounces of ointment, which should have lasted approximately 2 weeks, and that it is caked on the wound. How would you teach the client appropriate application of Silvadene to his burns?

References

Ashwill JW, Droske SC: *Nursing care of children,* Philadelphia, 1997, WB Saunders.

Beare PG, Myers JL: *Adult health nursing,* ed 3, St. Louis, 1998, Mosby.

Ebersole P, Hess P: *Toward healthy aging,* ed 5, St. Louis, 1998, Mosby.

Kayser-Jones J, Pengilly K: Dysphagia among nursing home residents, *Geriatr Nurs* 20(2):77, 1999.

Klang M: Medicating tube-fed patients, *Nursing* 26:18, 1996.

Lewis SM and others: *Medical-surgical nursing: assessment and management of clinical problems,* ed 5, St. Louis, 2000, Mosby.

Lilley LL, Aucker RS: *Pharmacology and the nursing process,* ed 2, St. Louis, 1999, Mosby.

Mahan LK, Escott-Stump S: *Krause's food, nutrition, and diet therapy,* ed 10, Philadelphia, 2000, WB Saunders.

McConnell EA: Clinical do's & don'ts: giving medications through an enteral feeding tube, *Nursing* 28(3), 66, 1998.

McKenry LM, Salerno E: *Pharmacology in nursing,* ed 20, St. Louis, 1998, Mosby.

Metheny N and others: Effectiveness of pH measurements in predicting feeding tube placement: an update, *Nurs Res* 42(6):324, 1993.

Miller D, Miller H: To crush or not to crush, *Nursing* 30(2):51, 2000.

Owen CL: New directions in asthma management, *Am J Nurs* 99(3):26, 1999.

Simon T, Fink O: Current management of endoscopic feeding tube dysfunction, *Surg Endosc* 13:403, 1999.

Weilitz PB, Van Sciver T: Obstructive pulmonary disease. In Lewis SM, Collier IC, Heitkemper MM, Dirksen SR, editors: *Medical surgical nursing: assessment and management of clinical problems,* ed 5, St. Louis, 1999, Mosby.

Wong D and others: *Whaley and Wong's nursing care of infants and children,* ed 6, St. Louis, 1999, Mosby.

18

Parenteral Medications

Skills

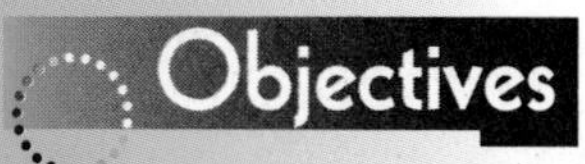

Objectives

Mastery of content in this chapter will enable the nurse to:

- Define the key terms listed.
- Correctly prepare injectable medications from a vial and an ampule.
- Identify advantages, disadvantages, and risks of administering medications by each injection route.
- Explain the importance of selecting the proper size syringe and needle for an injection.
- Discuss factors to consider when selecting injection sites.
- Discuss ways to promote client comfort while administering an injection.
- Correctly administer a subcutaneous, intramuscular, and intradermal injection.
- Correctly add medications to intravenous fluid containers.
- Compare the risks of three different intravenous routes.
- Correctly administer an intravenous infusion by intravenous piggyback, large-volume infusion, or bolus through a hanging intravenous line or a saline lock.
- Initiate, maintain, and discontinue a continuous subcutaneous medication.

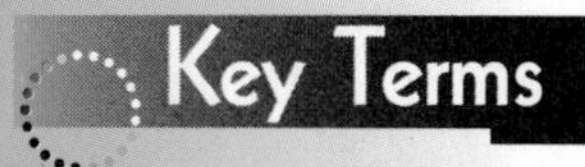

Key Terms

Air embolus
Ampules
Anaphylactic reaction
Aqueous
Aspirate
Bolus
Compatibility
Continuous subcutaneous infusion (CSQI or CSCI)
Diluent
Extravasation
Heparin lock
Hypodermoclysis
Incompatibility
Induration
Infiltration
Infusion
Injection
Intradermal (ID) injection
Intramuscular (IM) injection
Intravenous (IV) injection
Parenteral
Phlebitis
Piggyback infusion
Saline lock
Subcutaneous (SC, SQ) injection
Vial
Z-track method

Parenteral injections are used to instill medications into body tissues. The procedures for administering parenteral medications are invasive and thus pose greater risk than that associated with administering oral medications. Injected drugs act more quickly than oral medications because they reach the bloodstream either directly or by rapid absorption through the tissues. Thus the client's condition can change rapidly. The nurse must monitor the client's response closely and be aware of potential adverse or allergic reactions and the risk of infection that occurs once a needle pierces the skin or enters a port of the intravenous system. The nurse uses strict aseptic technique whenever preparing and administering injections. Infection can originate from a variety of sources (Table 18-1).

Parenteral drugs can be administered through four different routes:

1. **Subcutaneous (SC, SQ) injection**—injection into tissues just below the dermis of the skin
2. **Intramuscular (IM) injection**—injection into the body of a muscle
3. **Intradermal (ID) injection**—injection into the dermis just under the epidermis
4. **Intravenous (IV) injection**—injection into a vein

Each type of **injection** requires a certain set of skills to make certain that the medication reaches the proper location. Failure to inject a medication correctly can result in complications such as a drug response that is too rapid, nerve injury with associated pain, localized bleeding, tissue necrosis, and sterile abscess.

Parenteral medication is delivered to a client by using a needle and syringe. Needles and syringes come in a variety of sizes. The nurse determines the appropriate size of syringe and length of needle based on the type of medication to be delivered, the volume of solution to be delivered, and the medication route. A variety of electronic pumps also can be used to deliver parenteral medications. Electronic pumps ensure a constant delivery of medication. They are often used when vasoactive substances are delivered. Vasoactive medications can produce rapid, dramatic physiological changes, such as alterations in blood pressure or heart rate. Use of electronic pumps with these medications ensures a more controlled administration of set doses.

Syringes

A syringe consists of a cylindrical barrel, a tip designed to fit the hub of a hypodermic needle, and a close-fitting plunger (Figure 18-1). Syringes are single-use and disposable. They are packaged separately, with or without a sterile needle, in a paper wrapper or rigid plastic container. Syringes, in general, are classified as non–Luer-lok or Luer-lok. This nomenclature is based on the design of the syringe's tip. Non–Luer-lok syringes use needles that slip onto the tip. Luer-lok syringes (Figure 18-2, *A*) require special needles that are twisted onto the tip and lock themselves in place. The Luer-lok design prevents the inadvertent removal of the needle from the syringe.

Table 18-1 Preventing Infection During an Injection

PRINCIPLE	TECHNIQUE
Prevent contamination of solution.	Add date, time, and initials to vials when opened. A multi-dose vial, properly labeled, can be used up to 30 days. Swab top of opened or unopened multidose vials with alcohol before piercing.
Prevent needle contamination.	Avoid letting needle touch contaminated surface: outer edges of ampule or vial, outer surface of needle cap, nurse's hands, countertop, or table surface.
Prevent syringe contamination.	Avoid touching length of plunger or inner part of barrel. Keep tip of syringe covered with cap or needle.
Prepare skin.	Wash grossly contaminated sites with soap and water. Before giving an injection, use an alcohol swab to clean site; swab from center of site and move outward approximately 5 cm from center (2 inches).
Prior to handling any equipment, hand washing is essential to reduce the transfer of microorganisms.	Wash hands for a minimum of 15 seconds.

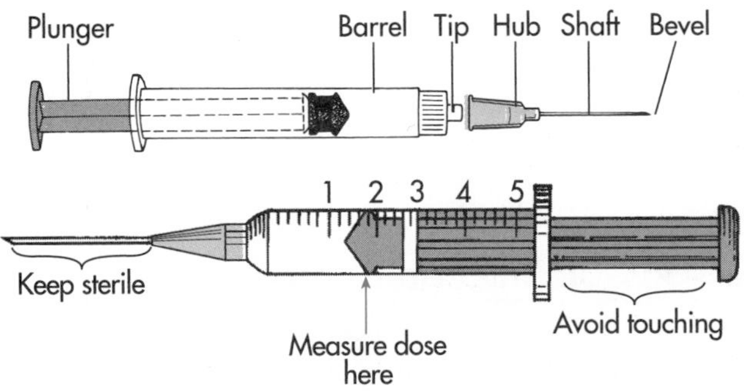

FIGURE **18-1** Parts of a syringe.

Syringes come in various sizes, ranging from 1 to 60 ml in capacity (Figure 18-2). The nurse, using knowledge about the types of syringes and the location of an injection, determines which is the most appropriate to use. The nurse uses large syringes to administer certain IV drugs and to add medications to IV solutions. It is unusual to use a syringe larger than 5 ml for an injection. A 2- to 3-ml syringe is adequate for IM and SC injections (Figure 18-2, *A*). Some syringes have two scales along the barrel. One scale is divided into minims and the other into tenths of a milliliter. Before use, the nurse carefully examines the syringe to ensure that the correct scale is being used. The tuberculin syringe (Figure 18-2, *B*) has a long, thin barrel with a preattached thin needle. The syringe, calibrated in sixteenths of a minim and hundredths of a milliliter, has a capacity of 1 ml. The nurse uses a tuberculin syringe to prepare small amounts of medication such as small, precise doses for infants or young children. Insulin syringes (Figure 18-2, *C* and *D*) hold 0.3 ml, 0.5 ml, or 1 ml and are calibrated in units. Insulin syringes that hold 0.3 ml and 0.5 ml are known as low-dose syringes (30 units per 0.3 ml or 50 units per 0.5 ml) and are easier to read. Insulin syringes in the United States and Canada are U-100s, designed for use with U-100–strength insulin. Each milliliter of solution contains 100 units of insulin.

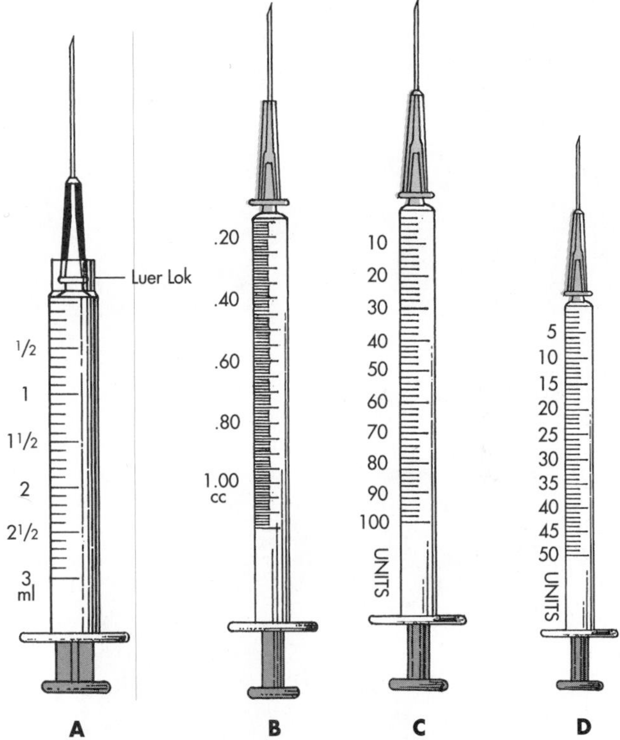

FIGURE **18-2** Types of syringes. **A,** Syringe with 3-ml capacity is marked in 0.1 (tenths). **B,** Tuberculin syringe is marked in 0.01 (hundredths) for doses of less than 1 ml. Insulin syringes marked in units in two sizes: **C,** 100 U; or **D,** 50 U (low-dose).

Needles

Needles come packaged in individual sheaths to allow flexibility in choosing the right needle for a client. Some needles are preattached to standard size syringes.

A needle has three parts: the hub, which fits onto the tip of a syringe; the shaft, which connects to the hub; and the bevel,

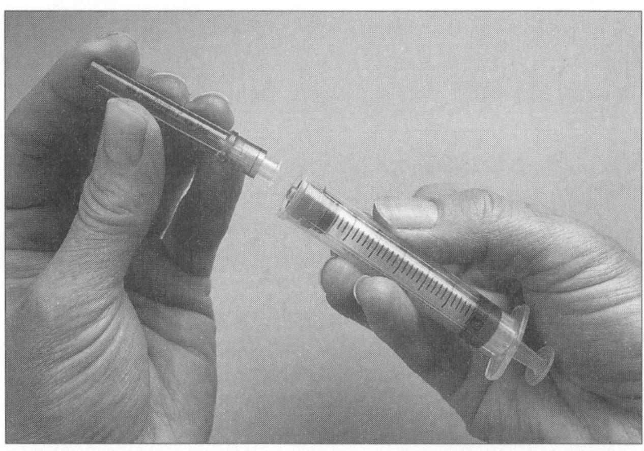

A

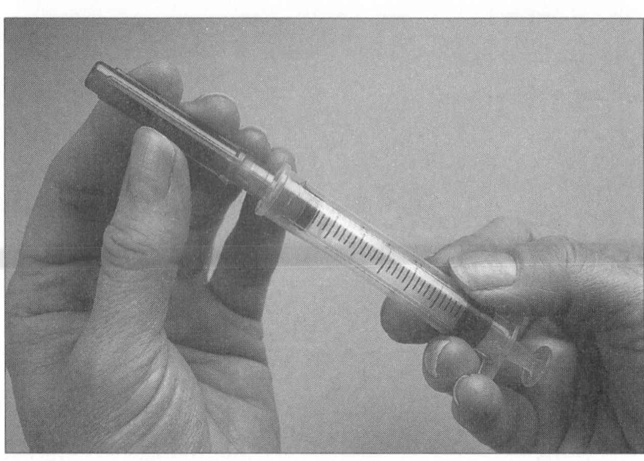

B

FIGURE **18-3** **A,** Cap placed on syringe tip. **B,** Cap secured.

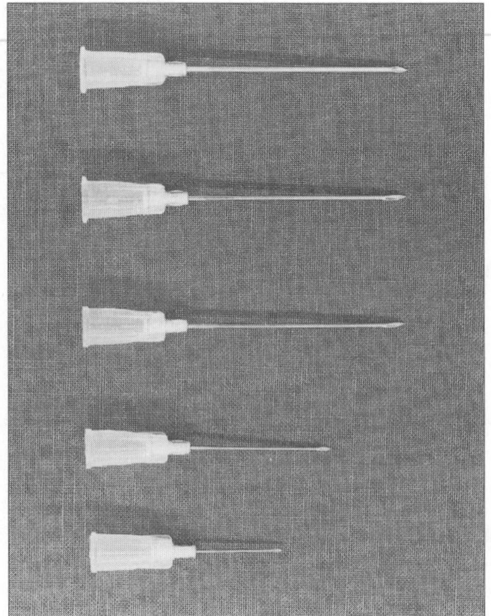

FIGURE **18-4** Hypodermic needles arranged in order of gauge. *Top to bottom:* 19 gauge, 20 gauge, 21 gauge, 23 gauge, and 25 gauge.

or slanted tip (see Figure 18-1). The needle hub, shaft, and bevel must remain sterile at all times. To prevent contamination, the nurse places the needle onto the syringe with the cap intact, using gentle force (Figure 18-3).

Needle Features

The tip of a needle, or the bevel, is always slanted. The bevel creates a narrow slit when injected into tissue; the slit quickly closes when the needle is removed to prevent leakage of medication, blood, or serum. A short beveled tip is best for IV injections because it is not easily occluded against the inside of a blood vessel wall. Long beveled tips are sharper and narrower, which minimizes discomfort when tissue is entered for an SC or IM injection.

Needles vary in length from $\frac{1}{4}$ inch to 3 inches (Figure 18-4). The nurse chooses the needle length according to the client's size and weight and the type of tissue into which the drug is to be injected. A child or slender adult generally requires a shorter needle. The nurse uses a longer needle (1 inch to $1\frac{1}{2}$ inches) for IM injections and a shorter needle ($\frac{3}{8}$ to $\frac{5}{8}$ inch) for SC or ID injections. As the needle gauge gets smaller, the needle diameter becomes larger. The selection of a gauge depends on the viscosity of fluid to be injected or infused. The rationale for needle selection is included in each skill.

Disposable Injection Units

Disposable single-dose prefilled syringes are available for some medications. With these syringes the nurse does not need to prepare medication doses, except perhaps to expel portions of unneeded medication.

The Tubex and Carpujet injection systems include reusable syringes that hold disposable, prefilled sterile-cartridge-needle units (Figure 18-5). The nurse slips the cartridge into the syringe, secures it (following package directions), and checks for air bubbles in the syringe. The nurse advances the plunger to expel air and excess medication, as with a regular syringe. Another type of injection system involves screwing a plunger-like device into the end of a prefilled vial containing a needle. After the medication is given, the entire unit is disposed of in a receptacle. This design reduces the risk of needle-stick injury.

Protecting Yourself From Needle-Stick Injury

The most frequent route of exposure to blood-borne disease is from needle-stick injuries (Rogers, 1997, American Nurses Association, 2000). To reduce the frequency of needle-stick injury, many institutions now supply "safety devices" for the nurse to use when handling needles or sharp cannulas. One example is the safety syringe, which is equipped with a plastic guard or shield that slips over the needle as it is withdrawn from the skin (Figure 18-6, *A, B*). Another example is needleless IV line connection systems (Figure 18-6, *C, D, E*). Box 18-1 lists recommendations for health care workers to use to decrease the risk of needle-stick injuries.

Skill Performance Guidelines

1. Use strict aseptic technique during all steps of preparation and administration.
2. To prepare medication for administration, fill a syringe by aspirating the fluid. Pull the plunger outward from the barrel while keeping the attached needle tip immersed in the medication solution. To prevent contamination and maintain sterility, hold only the outside of the syringe barrel and the handle on the plunger. Avoid touching the tip of the needle, the inside of the barrel, the shaft of the plunger, or the needle with an unsterile object.
3. Know the volume and characteristics of the medication to be administered. Injecting too large a volume of medication can cause extreme pain and local tissue damage.
4. Identify the bony prominences and anatomical structures that outline the chosen injection sites. Correct identification of the specific muscle mass will prevent injury to major nerves and blood vessels located near the injection site.
5. Insert the needle at the proper angle to deliver medication into the correct tissue (Figure 18-7).
6. Before injecting an intramuscular medication, aspirate by pulling back on the plunger to ensure that the needle has not pierced a vein or artery. Injection directly into a blood vessel can cause a rapid drug response. If blood is aspirated, remove the needle, dispose of the syringe and medication, and prepare a new dose of medication.
7. Attempt to minimize the client's discomfort when giving an injection by observing the following guidelines: Use sharp beveled needles in the shortest length and smallest gauge possible. Change the needle if liquid medication has coated the shaft of the needle. Position and flex client's limbs appropriately to reduce muscular tension. Divert the client's attention from the injection procedure. Insert the needle smoothly and quickly. Do not hesitate, and slowly push the needle into tissue. Inject the medication slowly but smoothly to reduce pain. Hold the syringe steady once the needle is in the tissue to prevent tissue damage. Withdraw the needle smoothly at the same angle used for insertion. Gently apply an antiseptic pad (e.g., alcohol) or a dry, sterile gauze pad to the site. Apply gentle pressure at the injection site. Rotate injection sites to prevent the formation of **indurations** and abscesses.
8. Use the guidelines for administering medications, including the five rights to medication administration, listed in Chapter 16.
9. Do not recap needles after administering injections, and dispose of all needles in an appropriate puncture-proof and leak-proof container (NIOSH, 1999).

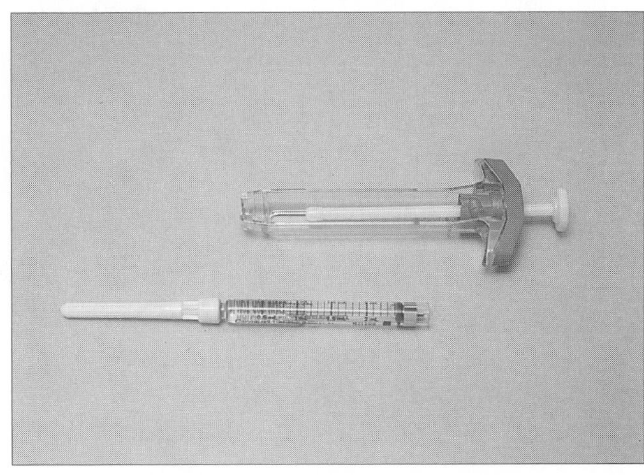

A

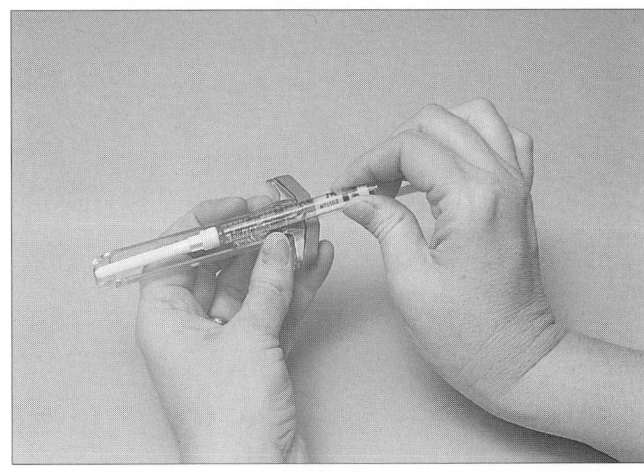

B

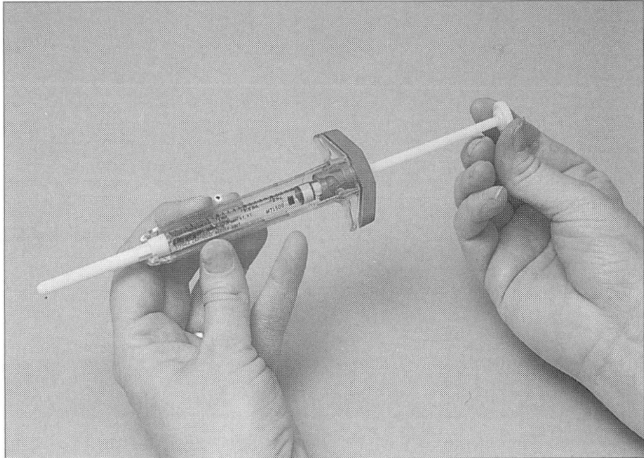

C

FIGURE **18-5** **A,** Carpujet syringe and prefilled sterile cartridge with needle. **B,** Assembling the Carpujet. **C,** The cartridge slides into the syringe barrel, turns, and locks at the needle end. The plunger then screws into the cartridge end.

A

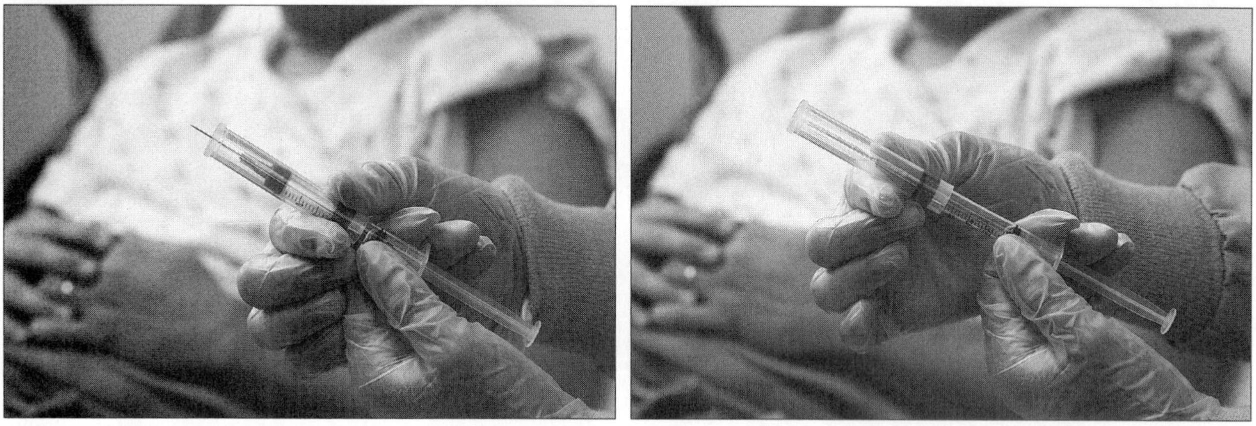

B

C

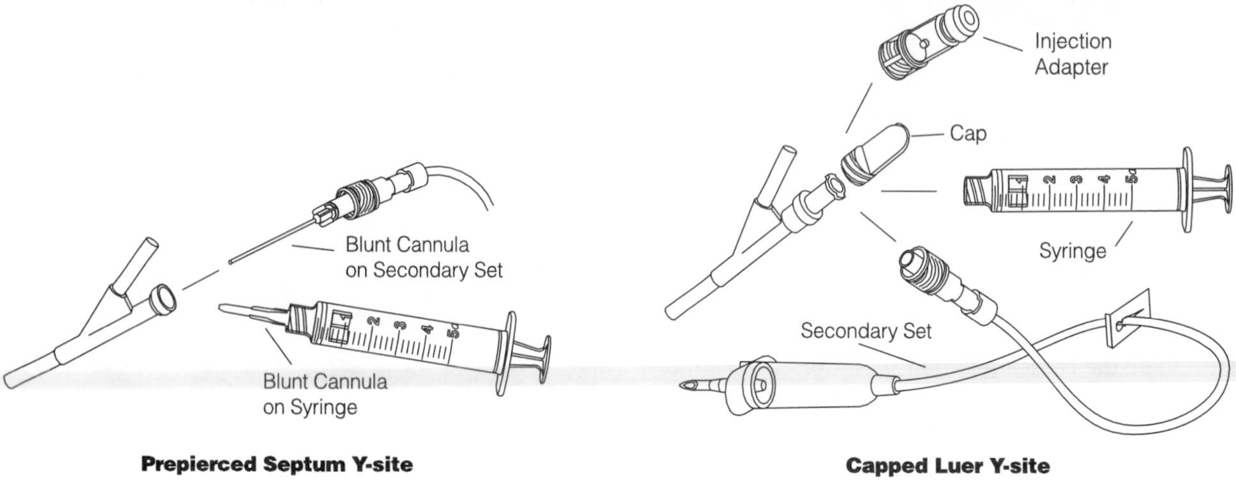

Blunt Cannula
on Secondary Set
Blunt Cannula
on Syringe
Prepierced Septum Y-site
Injection
Adapter
Cap
Syringe
Secondary Set
Capped Luer Y-site

D

E

Cap
Syringe
Secondary Set
Valved Connector Y-site
C441HN3B-01

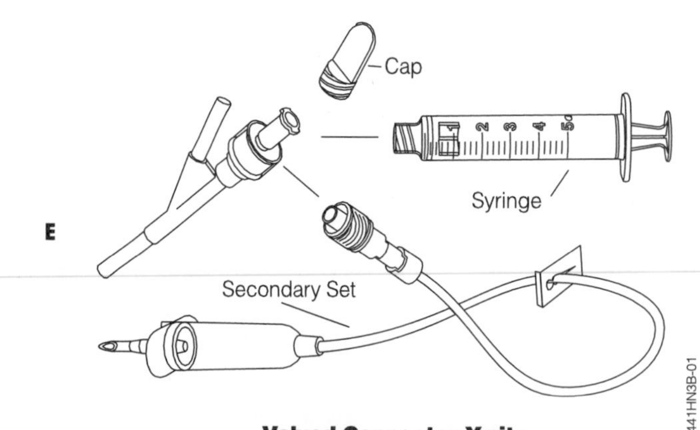

FIGURE **18-6** **A,** Protective syringe shown with sheath partially retracted. **B,** Sheath pulled and locked over needle. **C,** Prepierced Septum Y-site. **D,** Capped Luer Y-site. **E,** Valved Connector Y-site. (C, D, and E from Health Devices Needlestick-Prevention Device Selection Guide, Plymouth Meeting, Penn., 2000, ECRT.)

Box 18-1 Recommendations for the Prevention of Needle-Stick Injuries

1. Avoid using needles when effective needleless systems or devices with safety features are available.
2. Avoid recapping needles.
3. Plan safe handling and disposal of needles before beginning a procedure that requires the use of a needle.
4. Immediately dispose of used needles into puncture-proof and leak-proof sharps disposal containers.
5. Inform your employer of potential or actual hazards from needles in your work environment.
6. Participate in educational offerings regarding blood-borne pathogens, and follow recommendations for infection prevention, including receiving the hepatitis B vaccine.
7. Report all needle-stick and sharps-related injuries immediately, according to institutional policies to ensure the receipt of appropriate follow-up care.
8. Participate in the selection and evaluation of needleless systems and devices with safety features within your place of employment whenever possible.

Modified from National Institute for Occupational Safety and Health (NIOSH): NIOSH alert: preventing needlestick injuries in health care settings, NIOSH Publications Dissemination DHHS (NIOSH) Pub No. 2000-108, November 1999.

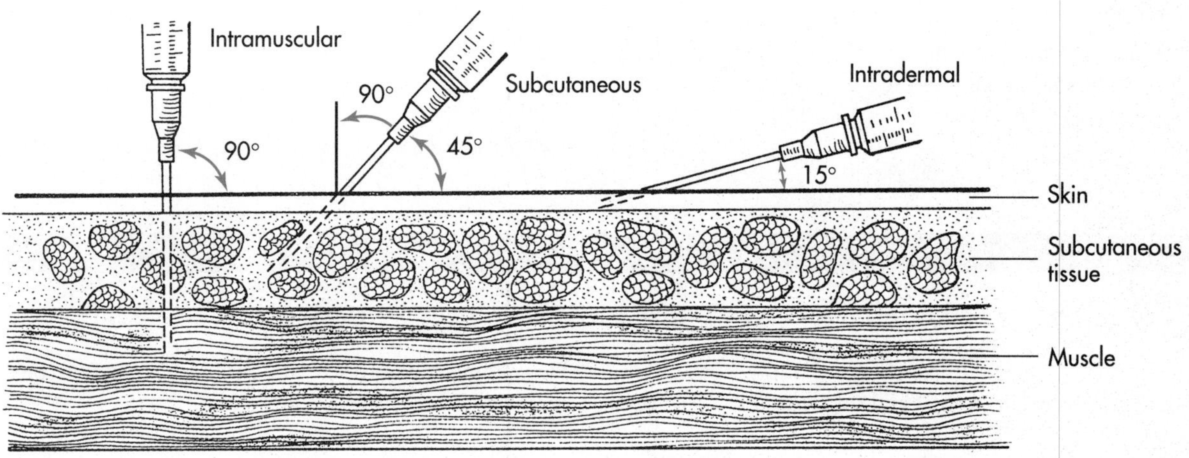

FIGURE **18-7** Comparison of the angles of insertion of IM (90 degrees), SQ (45 to 90 degrees) and ID (15 degrees) injections.

Skill 18-1 Preparing Injections From Ampules and Vials

Ampules contain single doses of injectable medication in a liquid form. They are available in sizes from 1 to 10 ml or more (Figure 18-8). An ampule is made of glass with a constricted neck that must be snapped off to allow access to the medication. A colored ring around the neck indicates where the ampule is prescored to be broken easily. Medications are easily withdrawn from the ampule by aspirating the fluid with a filter needle and syringe. Filter needles are used when preparing medications from glass ampules to prevent glass particles from being drawn into the syringe with the medication (Meister, 1998). The fluid enters the syringe because pulling on the plunger creates a vacuum in the syringe barrel.

A **vial** is a plastic or glass container with a rubber seal at the top (see Figure 18-8). A vial that is entered and then discarded, regardless of the amount of medication used, is called a single-dose vial. A vial that can be entered into several times and contains several doses of medication is called a multidose vial. The date that multidose vials are opened should be written on the label. Institutional policies vary on how long opened multidose vials can be used. Do not use and properly dispose of vials that have exceeded the time allowed by institutional policy.

A metal or plastic cap protects the vial's rubber seal. It is removed when the nurse is first preparing the vial for use. Vials contain liquid or dry forms of medications; drugs that are unstable in solution are packaged in a dry powder form. The vial label specifies the amount of diluent to be used to dissolve the powdered drug to prepare a desired drug concentration. Unlike the ampule, the vial is a closed system, and air must be injected into the container to permit easy withdrawal of the solution. Some medications, even when in a vial, may need to be drawn up with a filter needle because of the nature of the drug. Institutional policies will indicate which drugs should be prepared with a filter needle.

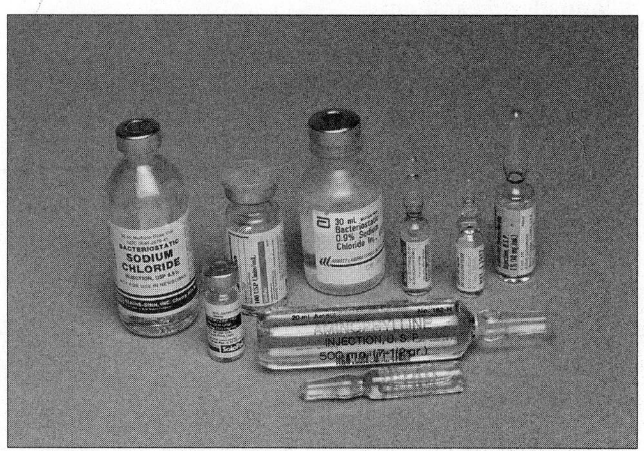

FIGURE **18-8** Assorted ampules and vials.

Delegation Considerations

The skill of preparing injections from ampules and vials should not be delegated to assistive personnel.

Equipment

Medication in an Ampule

- Syringe, needle, and filter needle
- Small gauze pad or alcohol swab

Medication in a Vial

- Syringe and two needles (filter needle if indicated) or syringe with vial adapter and needle
- Small gauze pad or alcohol swab
- Diluent, for example, normal saline or sterile water (if indicated)

Both

- Medication administration record or computer printout

Step	Rationale
Assessment	
1. If medication is to be injected, assess the client's body build, muscle size, and weight and the desired route of administration.	Determines type and size of syringe and needles to be used for injection.
2. Check medication's expiration date printed on vial or ampule.	Medications that have expired should not be used because the potency of medications change when the medications become outdated.
Planning	
1. **Expected outcomes** following completion of procedure:	
▪ Proper dose is prepared. No air bubbles are present within syringe barrel.	Air bubbles displace medication. Elimination of air ensures medication dose is accurate.
2. Check medication administration record or computer printout.	Verifies orders.
Implementation	
1. Wash hands.	Reduces transmission of microorganisms.
2. Assemble supplies at work area in medicine area.	Organization saves nursing time.
3. Check medication order, medication administration record, or printout against label on the ampule or vial.	Ensures right drug and dose are prepared.
4. **Ampule preparation:**	
a. Tap top of ampule lightly and quickly with finger until fluid moves from neck of ampule (see illustration).	Dislodges any fluid that collects above neck of ampule. All solution moves into lower chamber.

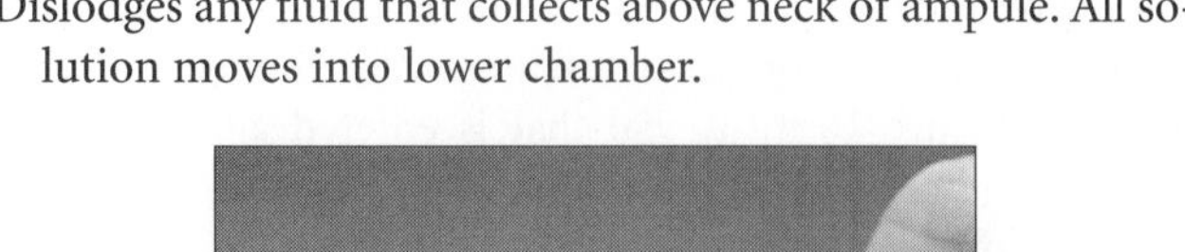

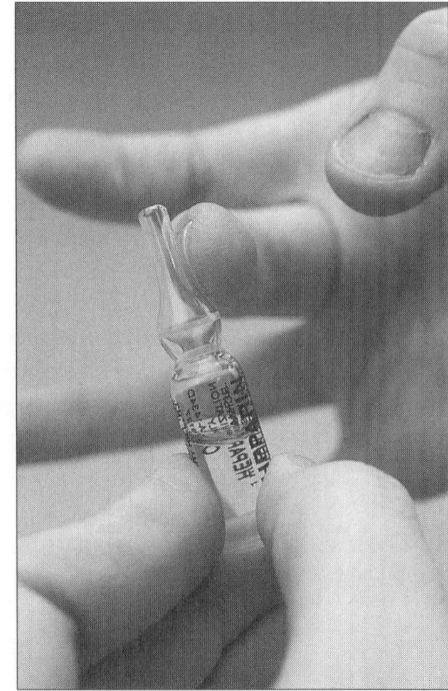

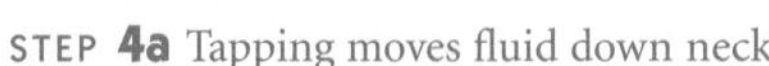

STEP **4a** Tapping moves fluid down neck.

STEP	RATIONALE
b. Place small gauze pad around neck of ampule (see illustration).	Placing pad around neck of ampule protects nurse's fingers from trauma as glass tip is broken off. *Do not use wet alcohol swab to wrap around top of ampule because alcohol may leak into ampule.*
c. Snap neck of ampule quickly and firmly away from hands (see illustration).	Protects nurse's fingers and face from being cut by glass.

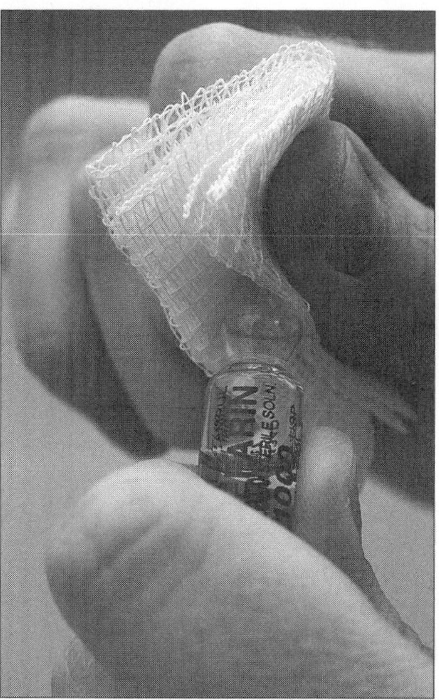

STEP **4b** Gauze pad placed around neck of ampule.

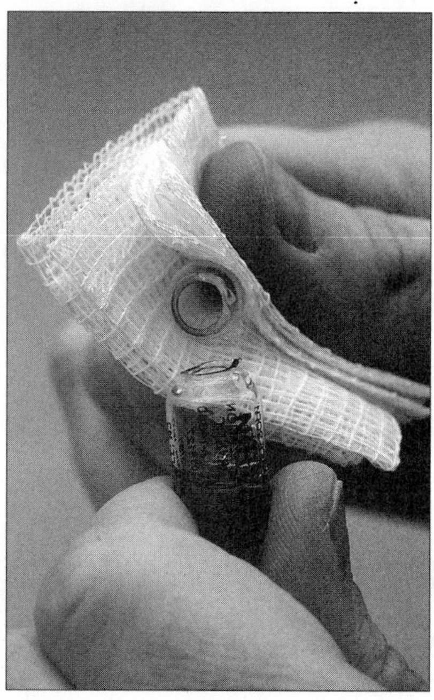

STEP **4c** Neck snapped away from hands.

STEP	RATIONALE
d. Draw up medication quickly, using a filter needle long enough to reach bottom of ampule.	System is open to airborne contaminants. Needle must be long enough to access medication in ampule so it can be drawn up.
e. Hold ampule upside down, or set it on a flat surface. Insert filter needle into center of ampule opening. Do not allow needle tip or shaft to touch rim of ampule.	Broken rim of ampule is considered contaminated. When ampule is inverted, solution dribbles out if needle tip or shaft touches rim of ampule.
f. Aspirate medication into syringe by gently pulling back on plunger (see illustrations).	Withdrawal of plunger creates negative pressure within syringe barrel, which pulls fluid into syringe.
g. Keep needle tip under surface of liquid. Tip ampule to bring all fluid within reach of the needle.	Prevents aspiration of air bubbles.
h. If air bubbles are aspirated, do not expel air into ampule.	Air pressure may force fluid out of ampule and medication will be lost.
i. To expel excess air bubbles, remove needle from ampule. Hold syringe with needle pointing up. Tap side of syringe to cause bubbles to rise toward needle. Draw back slightly on plunger, and then push plunger upward to eject air. • ***Critical Decision Point*** *When expelling air bubbles, do not eject fluid.*	Withdrawing plunger too far will remove it from barrel. Holding syringe vertically allows air bubbles to rise to top of barrel and fluid to settle in bottom of barrel. Pulling back on plunger allows fluid within needle to enter barrel so fluid is not expelled. Air at top of barrel and within needle is then expelled.
j. If syringe contains excess fluid, use sink for disposal. Hold syringe vertically with needle tip up and slanted slightly toward sink. Slowly eject excess fluid into sink. Recheck fluid level in syringe by holding it vertically.	Medication is safely dispersed into sink. Position of needle allows medication to be expelled without it flowing down needle shaft and onto nurse's hand. Rechecking fluid level ensures proper dose.
k. Cover needle with its safety sheath or cap. Change needle on syringe.	Prevents contamination of needle. Filter needles cannot be used for injection.

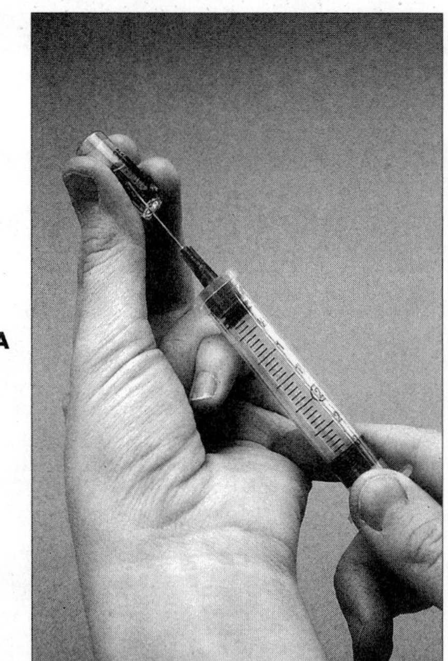

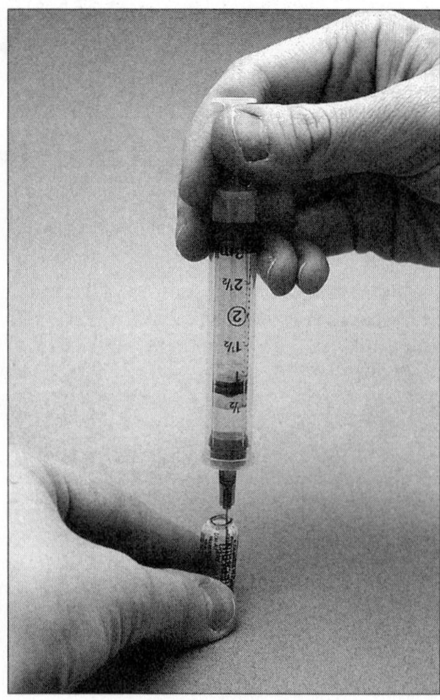

STEP **4f** **A,** Medication aspirated with vial inverted. **B,** Medication aspirated with vial on flat surface.

STEP	RATIONALE
5. Vial containing a solution:	
a. Remove cap covering top of unused vial to expose rubber seal. If using a multidose vial that has been opened, cap is already removed. Firmly and briskly wipe surface of rubber seal with alcohol swab and allow it to dry.	Vials come packaged with cap that cannot be replaced after removal. Not all drug manufacturers guarantee that caps of unused vials are sterile (Posey and Long, 1996). Therefore caps must be swabbed with alcohol before drawing up medication. Allowing alcohol to dry prevents alcohol from coating needle and mixing with medication.
b. Pick up syringe (with vial adapter or needle) and remove needle cap (see illustration). Pull back on plunger to draw amount of air into syringe equivalent to volume of medication to be aspirated from vial.	Air must first be injected into vial to prevent buildup of negative pressure in vial when aspirating medication.

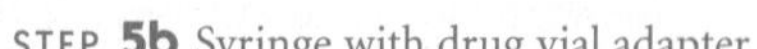
STEP **5b** Syringe with drug vial adapter.

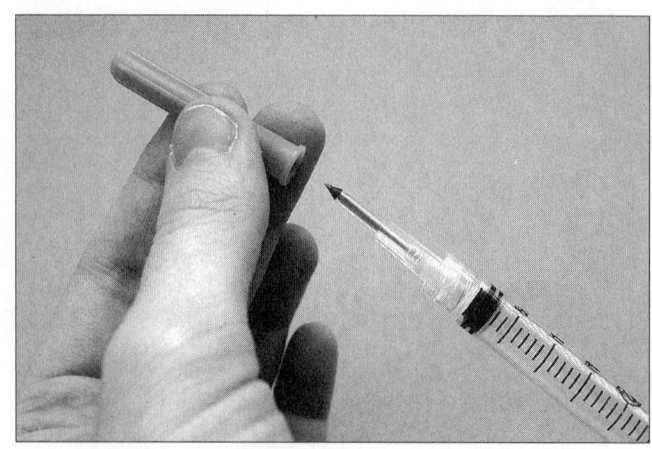

STEP	RATIONALE
c. With vial on flat surface, insert tip of needle through center of rubber seal (see illustration).	Center of seal is thinner and easier to penetrate. Firm pressure prevents coring of rubber seal, which could enter vial or needle.
d. Inject air into the vial's airspace, holding on to plunger.	Air must be injected before aspirating fluid. Injecting into vial's airspace prevents formation of bubbles and inaccuracy in dose.

• ***Critical Decision Point***
Hold plunger with firm pressure; plunger may be forced backward by air pressure within the vial.

STEP	RATIONALE
e. Invert vial while keeping firm hold on syringe and plunger (see illustration). Hold vial between thumb and middle fingers of nondominant hand. Grasp end of syringe barrel and plunger with thumb and forefinger of dominant hand to counteract pressure in vial.	Inverting vial allows fluid to settle in lower half of container. Position of hands prevents forceful movement of plunger and permits easy manipulation of syringe.

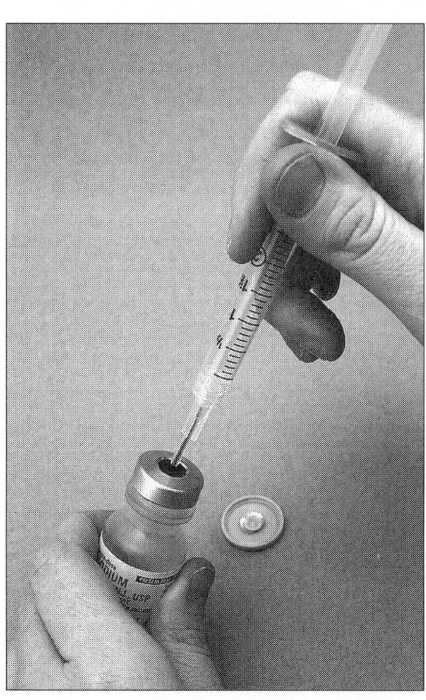

STEP **5c** Insert adapter through center of vial diaphragm.

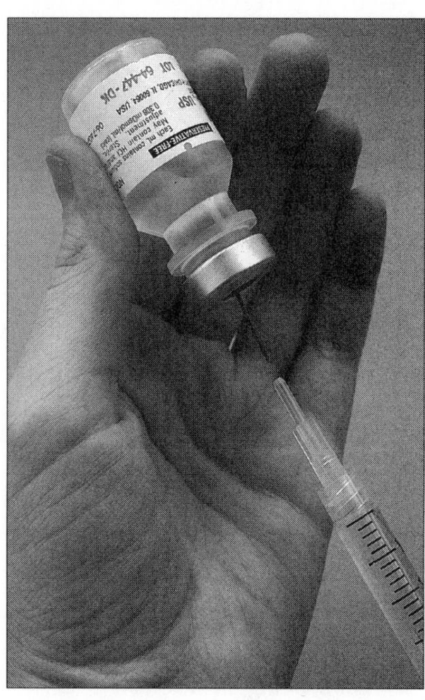

STEP **5e** Withdraw fluid with vial inverted.

STEP	RATIONALE
f. Keep tip of adapter/needle below fluid level.	Prevents aspiration of air.
g. Allow air pressure from the vial to fill syringe gradually with medication. If necessary, pull back slightly on plunger to obtain correct amount of medication.	Positive pressure within vial forces fluid into syringe. Pulling back too quickly or forcefully on the plunger will pull unwanted air into the syringe.
h. When desired volume has been obtained, position adapter/needle into vial's airspace; tap side of syringe barrel carefully to dislodge any air bubbles. Eject any air remaining at top of syringe into vial.	Forcefully striking barrel while needle is inserted in vial may bend needle. Accumulation of air displaces medication and causes dose errors.
i. Remove adapter/needle from vial by pulling back on barrel of syringe.	Pulling plunger rather than barrel causes plunger to separate from barrel, resulting in loss of medication.
j. Hold syringe at eye level, at 90-degree angle, to ensure correct volume and absence of air bubbles. Remove any remaining air by tapping barrel to dislodge any air bubbles. Draw back slightly on plunger; then push plunger upward to eject air. Do not eject fluid.	Holding syringe vertically allows air to rise to top of barrel and fluid to settle in bottom of barrel. Pulling back on plunger allows fluid within needle to enter barrel so fluid is not expelled. Air at top of barrel and within needle is then expelled.

Step	Rationale

- ***Critical Decision Point***

  When preparing medication from single-dose vial, do not assume that volume listed on label is total volume in vial. Some manufacturers provide small amount of extra liquid, expecting loss during preparation. Be sure to draw up only desired volume.

Step	Rationale
k. If medication is to be injected into client's tissue, change adapter/needle with a new needle of appropriate gauge and length according to route of medication.	Inserting needle through a rubber stopper may dull beveled tip. New needle is sharper. An adapter must be changed for a needle. Because no fluid is along shaft new needle will not track medication through tissues.
l. For multidose vial, make label that includes date of opening, mixing (if necessary), concentration of drug per milliliter, and nurse's initials.	Ensures that future doses will be prepared correctly. Some drugs must be discarded after certain number of days after opening or mixing of vial.
6. Vial containing a powder (reconstituting medications):	
a. Remove cap covering vial of powdered medication and cap covering vial of proper **diluent.** Firmly swab both caps with alcohol swab and allow alcohol to dry.	Vials come packaged with cap that cannot be replaced after removal. Not all drug manufacturers guarantee that caps of unused vials are sterile (Posey and Long, 1996). Therefore caps must be swabbed with alcohol before drawing up medication. Allowing alcohol to dry prevents alcohol from coating needle and mixing with medication.
b. Draw up diluent into syringe following Step 5b through j.	Prepares diluent for injection into vial containing powdered medication.
c. Insert tip of needle through center of rubber seal of vial of powdered medication. Inject diluent into vial. Remove needle from vial and cover with its safety sheath or cap.	Diluent begins to dissolve and reconstitute medication. Maintaining sterility of needle and syringe allows syringe to be used to draw up medication once it is reconstituted.
d. Mix medication thoroughly. Roll in palms. Do not shake.	Ensures proper dispersal of medication throughout solution.
e. Reconstituted medication in vial is ready to be drawn into syringe. Read label carefully to determine concentration after reconstitution.	Once diluent has been added, concentration of medication (mg/ml) determines amount to be given.
f. Draw up medication into syringe following Steps 5b through 1.	

- ***Critical Decision Point***

  Some institutions require that medications prepared for parenteral administration be verified for accuracy by another nurse (Zimmerman and Pierce, 1998). Check individual institution guidelines before administering medication.

Step	Rationale
7. Dispose of soiled supplies. Place broken ampule and/or used vials and used needle in puncture-proof and leak-proof container. Clean work area and wash hands.	Proper disposal of glass and needle prevents accidental injury to staff. Controls transmission of infection.

Evaluation

Step	Rationale
1. Compare dose in syringe with desired dose.	Ensures that accurate dose has been prepared.

Unexpected Outcomes and Related Interventions

- Air bubbles remain within syringe barrel.
  - Expel air from syringe, and add medication to syringe until correct dose is prepared.
- Excess or insufficient volume of medication is prepared.
  - Correct amount of medication in syringe before administering to ensure correct dose of medication is given.

Skill 18-2 Mixing Medications From Two Vials

Occasionally the nurse must mix medications from two vials or from a vial and an ampule. This avoids the need to give a client more than one injection at a time. It is essential that any medications to be mixed are compatible. When mixing medications, the nurse must remember the differences in how to aspirate fluid correctly from each type of container. When using multidose vials, the nurse must not contaminate the vial's contents with medication from another vial or ampule.

Mixing medications from a vial and an ampule is simple because adding air to withdraw medication from an ampule is unnecessary. The nurse prepares medications from the vial first and then, using the same syringe and needle, withdraws medication from the ampule. Mixing medications from two vials is somewhat more complicated because air must be added to both vials.

Special consideration must be given to the proper preparation of insulin, which comes in vials. Insulin is the hormone used to treat diabetes. Often clients with diabetes receive a combination of different types of insulin to control their blood sugar levels. Regular insulin is a clear solution that can be given subcutaneously, intravenously, or intramuscularly. The other types of insulin contain the addition of a protein that slows absorption. Cloudy insulin preparations cannot be given intravenously or intramuscularly.

Some insulins can be mixed in the same syringe. However, when insulins are mixed, chemical changes may occur either immediately or over time. This can result in a client response to insulin that is different than the response that would occur if the insulins had been given separately. Box 18-2 lists recommendations from the American Diabetes Association for mixing insulins.

Box 18-2 Recommendations for Mixing Insulins

- Clients whose blood sugar levels are well controlled on a mixed-insulin dose should maintain their individual routine when preparing and administering their insulin.
- Insulin should not be mixed with any other medications or diluent unless approved by the prescribing physician or advanced practice nurse.
- Commercially available premixed insulins may be used if the ratio of the insulins within the vial matches the client's current insulin requirements.
- Rapid-acting insulins that are mixed with NPH or Ultralente insulins should be injected within 15 minutes before a meal to promote consistent absorption of insulin.
- Short-acting and Lente insulins should not be mixed unless the client's blood sugar levels are currently under control with this mixture.
- Phosphate-buffered insulins (e.g., NPH) should not be mixed with Lente insulins. If they are mixed, a precipitate may form and the time of onset and peak action of the insulins will change.
- Consult manufacturers of insulins whenever their recommendations conflict with these recommendations.

Modified from American Diabetes Association: Insulin administration: clinical practice recommendations, *Diabetes Care* 20(suppl 1):46S, 1997.

Delegation Considerations

The skill of mixing medications from two vials should not be delegated to assistive personnel.

Equipment

- Single-dose or multidose vials and ampules containing medications
- Syringe with needle or syringe with vial adapter and syringe
- Extra needle for injection
- Alcohol swab
- Puncture-proof container for disposing of syringes, needles, and glass
- Medication administration record or computer printout

Step	Rationale
Assessment	
1. Check medication administration record or computer printout.	Verifies order.
2. Assess client's body build, muscle size, and weight and desired route of medication administration.	Determines type and size of syringe and needles for injection.
3. Consider medications to be mixed, compatibility of medications, and type of injection.	Determines if medications can be mixed, order of drawing up medications, and size of syringe.
4. Check medication's expiration date printed on vial or ampule.	Medications that have expired should not be used because the potency of medications change when the medications become outdated.

STEP	RATIONALE

PLANNING

1. **Expected outcomes** following completion of procedure:
   - Combined medications equal correct dose. No air bubbles are present in syringe barrel. — Indicates medication is prepared correctly.

IMPLEMENTATION

1. Wash hands. — Reduces transmission of microorganisms.
2. Assemble supplies at work area in medication preparation area. — Organization saves nursing time.
3. **Mixing medications from vials:**
   a. Take syringe (with vial adapter and needle) and **aspirate** volume of air equivalent to first dose of medication (vial A). — Air must be introduced into vial to create positive pressure needed to withdraw solution.
   b. Inject air into vial A, making sure needle does not touch solution (Figure 18-9, *A*). — Prevents cross contamination.
   c. Holding on to plunger, withdraw needle/adapter and syringe from vial A. Aspirate air equivalent to second dose of medication (vial B). — If plunger is not held in place, injected air may escape from vial A. Air is injected into vial B to create positive pressure needed to withdraw desired dose.
   d. Insert needle/adapter into vial B, inject air, and then fill syringe with proper volume of medication from vial (Figure 18-9, *B*). — First portion of dose has been prepared.
   e. Withdraw needle and syringe from vial B. Ensure that proper volume has been obtained. — Ensures correct dose is prepared.
   f. Determine at which point on syringe scale combined volume of medications should measure. — Prevents accidental withdrawal of too much medication from second vial.
   g. Insert needle/adapter into vial A, being careful not to push plunger and expel medication into vial. Invert vial and carefully withdraw desired amount of medication into syringe (Figure 18-9, *C*). — Positive pressure within vial A allows fluid to fill syringe without need to aspirate.
   h. Withdraw needle/adapter and expel any excess air or fluid from syringe. Check fluid level in syringe. — Air bubbles should not be injected into tissues. Excess fluid causes incorrect dose.

• ***Critical Decision Point***

If too much medication is withdrawn from second vial, discard syringe and start over. Do not push medication back into vial.

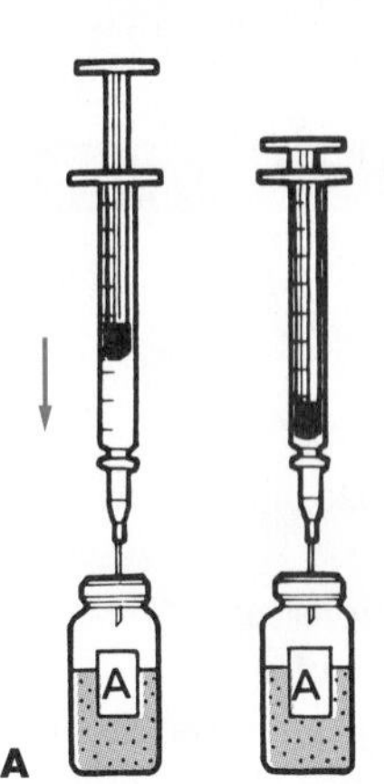

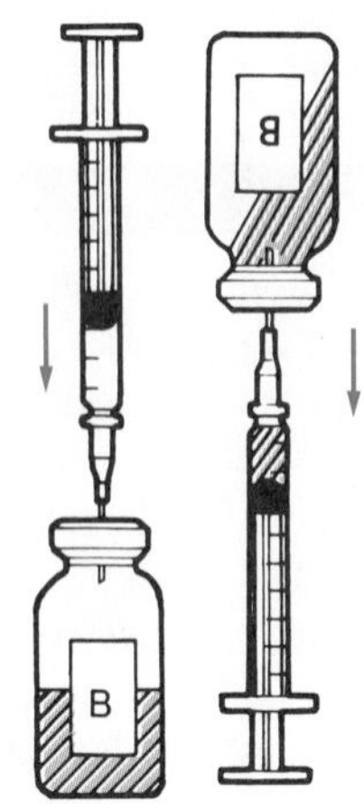

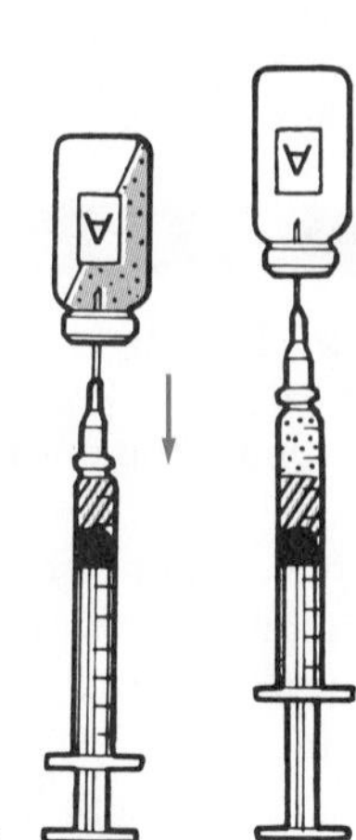

FIGURE **18-9** **A,** Injecting air into vial A. **B,** Injecting air into vial B and withdrawing dose. **C,** Withdrawing medication from vial A; medications are now mixed.

STEP	RATIONALE
i. Change needle/adapter to appropriate needle gauge and length according to route of medication. Keep needle sheathed or capped until administration time.	New needle prevents tracking of medication into tissues. Cover or cap maintains needle sterility.
j. Dispose of soiled needle/adapter and supplies in proper receptacles.	Controls spread of infection and prevents accidents.
k. Wash hands.	Reduces transmission of infection.
4. **Mixing insulin:**	
a. If mixing modified insulin (cloudy) and unmodified insulin (clear), take insulin syringe and aspirate volume of air equivalent to dose to be withdrawn from modified insulin first (see illustration). If two modified forms of insulin are mixed, it makes no difference which vial is prepared first.	Air must be introduced into vial to create pressure needed to withdraw solution.
b. Inject air into vial of modified insulin (cloudy vial). Be sure that needle/adapter does not touch solution.	Prevents cross contamination.
c. Withdraw needle/adapter and syringe from vial without aspirating medication. Aspirate air equivalent to dose to be withdrawn from unmodified regular insulin (clear vial).	Air is injected into vial to withdraw desired dose.
d. Insert needle/adapter into vial of unmodified regular insulin (clear vial), inject air, and then fill syringe with proper regular insulin dose (see illustration).	First portion of dose has been prepared. Always fill syringe with unmodified (regular) insulin first to prevent contamination of the regular insulin bottle with NPH or Lente insulin. The immediate effect required from short-acting regular insulin can be modified if contaminated by longer-acting insulin.

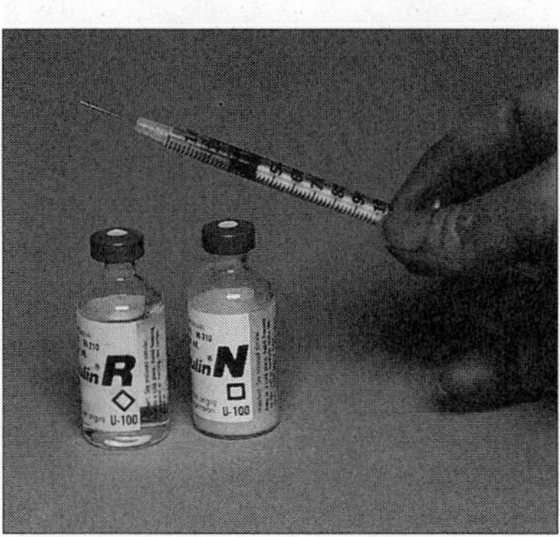

STEP **4a** Vials of insulin and syringe with air aspirated.

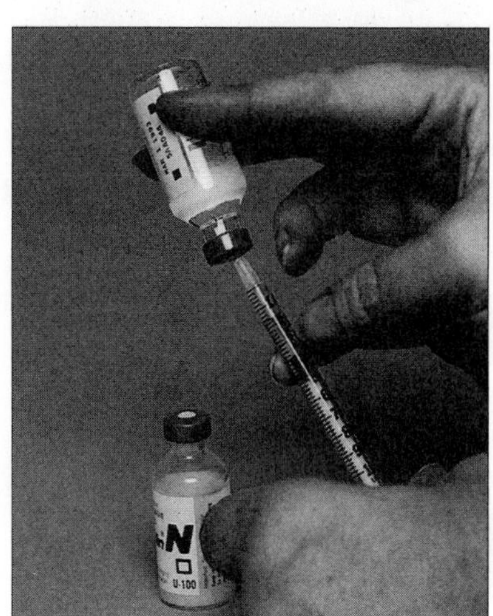

STEP **4d** Withdrawal of regular insulin.

STEP	RATIONALE
e. Withdraw needle/adapter and syringe from vial by pulling on barrel; check dose.	Prevents accidental pulling of plunger, which may cause loss of medication. Ensures correct dose prepared.

- ***Critical Decision Point***
  Some institutions require insulin doses to be verified by another nurse for accuracy (Zimmerman and Pierce, 1998). If indicated by institutional policy, have dose of regular insulin verified before proceeding with mixing of insulin at this time. Have dose verified after the medications are mixed as well.

STEP	RATIONALE
f. Determine at which point on syringe scale combined units of insulin should measure by adding the number of units of both insulins together (e.g., 5 U Regular + 12 U NPH = 17 U total).	Prevents accidental withdrawal of too much insulin from second vial.

STEP	RATIONALE
g. Insert needle/adapter into vial of modified insulin (cloudy vial). Be careful not to push plunger and expel medication into vial. Invert vial and carefully withdraw desired amount of insulin into syringe (see illustration).	Positive pressure within vial of modified insulin allows fluid to fill syringe without need to aspirate.
h. Withdraw needle/adapter and check fluid level in syringe. Change needle/adapter to appropriate gauge. Keep needle of prepared syringe sheathed or capped until administering medication.	Ensures accurate dose. Inaccurate doses of insulin can cause serious hypoglycemia or hyperglycemia. Keeping needle capped or sheathed keeps needle sterile for insulin administration.
i. Dispose of soiled supplies in proper receptacle.	Controls spread of infection.
j. Wash hands.	Reduces transmission of infection.

EVALUATION

1. Check syringe carefully for total combined dose of medications.	Accurate dose ensures safe medication administration.

- ***Critical Decision Point***

  Administer mixture of insulins within 5 to 15 minutes of preparation. Short-acting and regular insulins bind with intermediate and long-acting insulins, reducing the action of regular insulin.

STEP **4g** Withdrawal of modified insulin.

UNEXPECTED OUTCOMES AND RELATED INTERVENTIONS

- Air bubbles remain in syringe barrel.
  - Expel air from syringe and add medication to syringe until correct dose is prepared.
- Excess or insufficient volume of medication is prepared.
  - Be sure correct amount of medication is in syringe before administering to ensure correct dose of medication is given.

TEACHING CONSIDERATIONS

- Because insulin is essential to life, clients must be able to prepare and inject insulin as ordered (see Chapter 40).
- Assess client's ability to mix insulin by having client complete a return demonstration of insulin preparation. Insulin can be prescribed in premixed formulations. The nurse should communicate if the client is unable to mix insulin accurately and should discuss changing the client's insulin type to a premixed formula with the client's health care provider.

PEDIATRIC CONSIDERATIONS

- Children of about 8 or 9 years should be able to prepare and administer their own injections, including insulin.
- Children may need participation/supervision of a parent or legal guardian through adolescence.
- The nurse assesses the pediatric client's physical readiness, psychological readiness, and development in activities of daily living before teaching the client how to prepare and self-administer injections, such as insulin.

- Family education is essential to successful disease management and medication administration in the pediatric client, especially when the preparation and administration of medications in a syringe are required.

GERONTOLOGICAL CONSIDERATIONS

- Physiological changes in the older adult, such as decreased peripheral vision, presbyopia, and reduction in the power of skeletal and voluntary muscle contractions, may make it difficult for clients to prepare and self-administer injections.
- The nurse assesses the older client's physical readiness, psychological readiness, and development in activities of daily living before teaching a client how to prepare and self-administer injections, such as insulin.
- Clients unable to perform the task may be assisted by family members, a visiting nurse, or home health attendants.

HOME CARE CONSIDERATIONS

- Some clients may prefer to use their syringe more than once. Many studies have shown that it is both safe and practical for the syringe to be used more than once if the client desires as long as the syringe is not contaminated when used and is recapped after each use. For example, insulin preparations have bacteriostatic additives that inhibit growth of bacteria commonly found on the skin (American Diabetes Association, 1997).

Skill 18-3 Administering Intradermal Injections

The nurse typically gives intradermal injections for skin testing, for example, in tuberculin screening and allergy tests. Because these medications are potent, they are injected into the dermis, where blood supply is reduced and drug absorption occurs slowly. A client may have an **anaphylactic reaction** if the medications enter the client's circulation too rapidly. For clients with a history of numerous allergies, the physician often performs skin testing.

Skin testing often requires the nurse to visually inspect the test site; therefore intradermal sites should be free of lesions and relatively hairless. The inner forearm and upper back are ideal locations.

To administer an injection intradermally, the nurse uses a tuberculin or small syringe with a short (¼ to ½ inch), fine-gauge (26 or 27) needle. The angle of insertion for an intradermal injection is 5 to 15 degrees (see Figure 18-7). Only small amounts of medication (0.01 to 0.1 ml) are injected intradermally. If a bleb does not appear or if the site bleeds after needle withdrawal, the medication may have entered subcutaneous (SC) tissues. In this situation skin test results will not be valid.

DELEGATION CONSIDERATIONS

The skill of administering intradermal injections should not be delegated to assistive personnel. Assistive personnel should be instructed to report any unexpected drug reactions as soon as possible.

EQUIPMENT

- 1-ml tuberculin syringe with preattached 26- or 27-gauge needle
- Small gauze pad and/or alcohol swab
- Vial or ampule of skin test solution
- Disposable gloves
- Medication administration record (MAR) or computer printout
- Skin pencil

STEP	RATIONALE
ASSESSMENT	
1. Review physician's medication order for client's name, drug name, dose, time, and route of administration.	Ensures safe and correct administration of medication.
2. Collect drug reference information regarding expected reaction when testing skin with specific allergen or medication and appropriate time to read site.	Type of reaction depends on client's ability to mount a cell-mediated response. Knowledge of expected and adverse reactions to skin testing helps the nurse determine future assessment criteria, including what symptoms to monitor for and how frequently and when to reassess client.

Step	Rationale
3. Assess client's history of allergies, type of substance, and normal allergic reaction.	Nurse should not administer any substance to which client is known to be allergic.
4. Assess client's knowledge of purpose and reactions of skin testing.	Reveals need for client instruction.

Nursing Diagnosis

Defining characteristics from the assessment data may reveal the following nursing diagnoses for clients requiring this skill:

- Anxiety
- Fear
- Health-seeking behaviors regarding disease screening practices
- Knowledge deficit regarding skin testing

Related factors are individualized based on client's condition or needs.

Planning

Step	Rationale
1. **Expected outcomes** following completion of procedure:	
▪ Client experiences very mild burning sensation during injection but no discomfort after injection.	Normal reaction to medication deposited in dermis.
▪ Small light-colored bleb approximately 6 mm (¼ inch) in diameter forms at site and gradually disappears. Minimal bruising may be present.	Medication is in dermis and is eventually absorbed. Bruising is result of minor bleeding from capillaries.
▪ Client is able to identify signs of a skin reaction and their significance.	Demonstrates learning.
2. Wash hands thoroughly.	Reduces transfer of microorganisms.
3. Prepare correct dose from vial or ampule (see Skill 18-1). Check dose carefully.	Ensures that medication is sterile and dose is accurate.
4. Identify client by checking identification bracelet and asking client's name. Compare with medication administration record.	Ensures that correct client receives ordered drug.
5. Explain steps of procedure, and tell client that injection will cause a slight burning or sting.	Helps minimize client's anxiety.

Implementation

Step	Rationale
1. Close room curtain or door.	Provides privacy.
2. Select appropriate injection site. Inspect skin surface over sites for bruises, inflammation, or edema. Note lesions or discolorations of skin. If possible, select site three to four finger widths below antecubital space and one hand width above wrist. If forearm cannot be used, inspect the upper back. If necessary, sites appropriate for subcutaneous injections (see Figure 18-10, p. 523) can be used (Workman, 1999).	Injection sites should be free of abnormalities that may interfere with drug absorption. An intradermal site should be clear so that results of skin test can be seen and interpreted correctly.
3. Assist client to comfortable position. Extend and support elbow and forearm on flat surface if using arm.	Stabilizes injection site for easiest accessibility.
4. Wash hands and apply disposable gloves.	Follow Centers for Disease Control and Prevention recommendations to prevent accidental exposure to blood and body fluids (National Institute for Occupational Safety and Health, 1999).

STEP	RATIONALE
5. Cleanse site with an antiseptic swab. Apply swab at center of the site and rotate outward in a circular direction for about 5 cm (2 inches).	Mechanical action of swab removes secretions containing microorganisms.
6. Hold swab or square of sterile gauze between third and fourth fingers of nondominant hand.	Gauze or swab remains readily accessible when needle is withdrawn.
7. Remove needle cap or sheath from needle by pulling it straight off.	Keeping needle from touching sides of cap prevents contamination.
8. Hold syringe between thumb and forefinger of dominant hand with bevel of needle pointing up.	Smooth injection requires proper manipulation of syringe parts. With bevel up, medication is less likely to be deposited into tissues below dermis.
9. With nondominant hand, stretch skin over site with forefinger or thumb.	Needle pierces tight skin more easily.
10. With needle almost against client's skin, insert it slowly at 5- to 15-degree angle until resistance is felt. Then advance needle through epidermis to approximately 3 mm (⅛ inch) below skin surface. Needle tip can be seen through skin (see illustration).	Ensures that needle tip is in dermis.
11. Inject medication slowly. Normally resistance is felt. If not, needle is too deep; remove and begin again.	Slow injection minimizes discomfort at site. Dermal layer is tight and does not expand easily when solution is injected.

• ***Critical Decision Point***
It is not necessary to aspirate because dermis is relatively avascular.

STEP	RATIONALE
12. While injecting medication, notice that small bleb resembling mosquito bite appears on skin's surface (see illustration).	Bleb indicates that medication is deposited in dermis.
13. Withdraw needle while applying alcohol swab or gauze gently over site.	Support of tissue around injection site minimizes discomfort during needle withdrawal. Dry gauze may minimize client discomfort associated with alcohol on nonintact skin.
14. Do not massage site.	Massage may disperse medication into underlying tissue layers and alter test results.
15. Assist client to comfortable position.	Gives client sense of well-being.
16. Discard uncapped needle or needle enclosed in safety shield and attached syringe in puncture-proof and leak-proof receptacles.	Prevents injury to clients and health care personnel. Capping of needles places the health care worker at risk for a needle-stick injury. Safety shields protect against needle sticks.
17. Remove gloves and wash hands.	Reduces transmission of microorganisms.

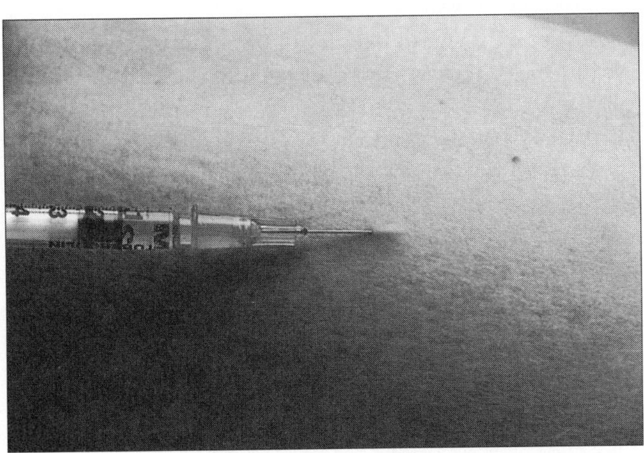

STEP **10** Intradermal needle tip inserted into dermis.

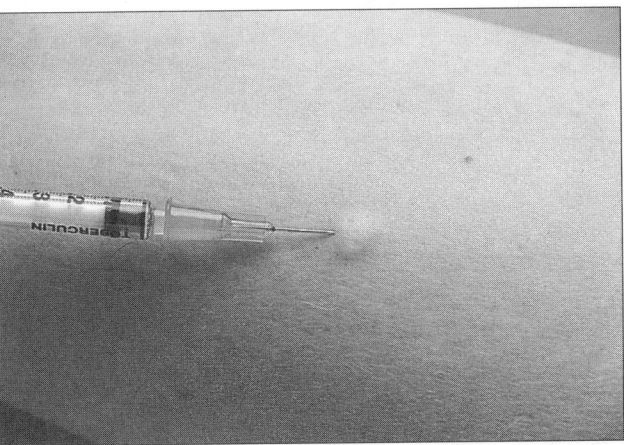

STEP **12** Injection creates small bleb.

STEP	RATIONALE
18. Read site within appropriate amount of time, designated by type of medication or skin test given.	The results of skin testing are determined at various times, based on the type of medication used or the type of skin testing. Refer to the manufacturer's directions to determine when to read the test's results.

- ***Critical Decision Point***

  Positive tuberculin reaction is indicated by induration (hardening) of skin around injection site of 10 mm or more in immunocompetent clients and 5 mm or more in immunocompromised clients. Read at 48 to 72 hours. Induration of 5 to 9 mm is doubtful unless known exposure has occurred. Explain that a positive tuberculin test indicates exposure, not active disease.

EVALUATION

Step	Rationale
1. Stay with client and observe for any allergic reactions.	Severe anaphylactic reaction is characterized by dyspnea, wheezing, and circulatory collapse and requires immediate attention.
2. Inspect bleb. Use skin pencil to draw circle around perimeter of injection site.	Site must be read at various intervals to determine test results. Pencil mark makes site easy to find.
3. Ask client to discuss implications of skin testing and signs of hypersensitivity.	Client's ability to recognize signs of skin testing helps to ensure timely reporting of results.

UNEXPECTED OUTCOMES AND RELATED INTERVENTIONS

- Raised, reddened, or hard zone forms around test site (induration), indicating sensitivity to injected allergen (positive test for tuberculin skin testing).
  - Document results, and notify client's health care provider.
- Onset of allergic reaction develops within minutes.
  - Follow institutional policy or guidelines for appropriate response to allergic reactions, and notify client's health care provider.
- Client is unable to explain purpose or signs of skin testing.
  - Provide further instruction, or recognize client is unable to learn at this time.

RECORDING AND REPORTING

- Record amount and type of testing substance and date and time on MAR.
- Record area of injection and appearance of skin in nurses' notes.
- Report any undesirable effects from medication to client's health care provider, and document adverse effects according to institutional policy.

TEACHING CONSIDERATIONS

- Teach clients that negative skin tests may not rule out allergies, especially when low concentrations of medication are used.
- Client should wear medical identification band listing all substances to which client is allergic.
- Caution client not to wash off markings around injection site.
- When clients are tested in a clinic or other outpatient setting, have them call in results of skin tests if a follow-up appointment is not made.
- Explain to client how to observe for skin reactions.

PEDIATRIC CONSIDERATIONS

- Only amounts up to 0.5 ml can be administered intradermally to small children (Wong and others, 1999).

GERONTOLOGICAL CONSIDERATIONS

- The skin becomes less elastic during physiological changes in the older adult. Therefore the skin must be held taught to ensure the intradermal injection is administered correctly.

Skill 18-4 Administering Subcutaneous Injections

A subcutaneous (SC) injection involves depositing medication into the loose connective tissue underlying the dermis. Subcutaneous tissue is not as richly supplied with blood vessels as muscles; thus drugs are not absorbed as quickly as those given intramuscularly (IM). One exception is heparin, which is absorbed quickly by both SC and IM routes. Anything affecting local blood flow to tissues, such as physical exercise or the local application of hot or cold compresses, influences the rate of drug absorption. Conditions such as circulatory shock or occlusive vascular disease impair client's blood flow and thus contraindicate SC injections.

Drugs given subcutaneously are isotonic, nonirritating, nonviscous, and water soluble. Examples of drugs given by this route are epinephrine, insulin, tetanus toxoid, allergy medications, narcotics, and heparin. Only small doses of medications (0.5 to 1 ml) should be given subcutaneously. The tissue is sensitive to irritating solutions and large volumes of medications. Medications collecting within the tissues can cause sterile abscesses, which appear as hardened, painful lumps.

The best sites for SC injections include vascular areas around the outer aspect of the upper arms, the abdomen from below the costal margins to the iliac crests, and the anterior aspect of the thighs (Figure 18-10). These areas are easily accessible, especially for clients who must self-administer subcutaneous injections, such as insulin. They also are large enough areas so that multiple injections may be rotated within each anatomical location.

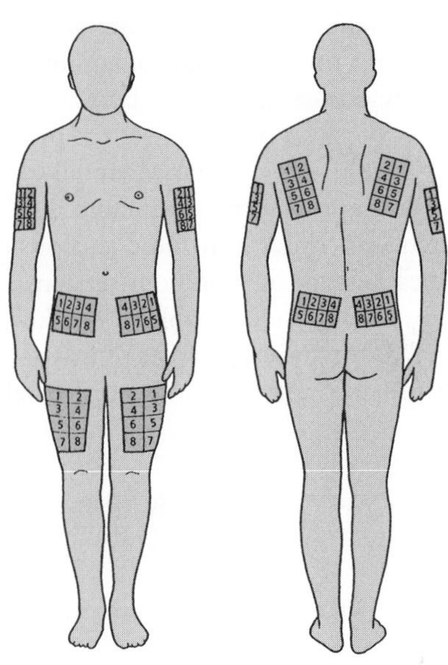

FIGURE 18-10 Common sites for subcutaneous injections.

The site most frequently recommended for insulin and heparin injections is the abdominal wall. Other sites include the scapular areas of the upper back and the upper ventral or dorsal gluteal areas. Injection sites should be free of infection, skin lesions, scars, bony prominences, and large underlying muscles or nerves. Rotation of injection from major site to major site (e.g., rotating from abdomen to upper arms to thighs from one injection to the next), once a common practice for clients who use insulin, is no longer recommended. Human insulins carry a much lower risk for hypertrophy and are almost exclusively prescribed for clients. Therefore clients can choose one anatomical area (e.g., the abdomen) and systematically rotate sites within that region. Once all potential sites within that area are used, the client may choose either to move to another anatomical site (e.g., the thigh) or to start the rotation pattern over in the same anatomical area. Rotating injection sites within one area decreases the variability in insulin absorption from one day to the next, helping clients maintain better control of their blood sugar levels (American Diabetes Association, 1997).

The amount of adipose tissue on the client's body influences the nurse's choice of needle length and angle of needle insertion. Generally a 25-gauge ⅝-inch needle with a medium bevel inserted at a 45- to 90-degree angle (see Figure 18-7) deposits medication into the SC tissue of a normal-size client. If a client is obese, the nurse often pinches the tissue and uses a needle long enough to insert through the fatty tissue at the base of the skinfold. The preferred needle length is one half the width of the skinfold. A ⅞-inch needle is the longest needle for SC use. For injection in obese clients, the angle of insertion is 90 degrees. Cachectic clients may have insufficient tissue for subcutaneous injections. Insulin is injected into the abdomen usually at a 90-degree angle. To ensure that the medication reaches SC tissue, follow this rule: if 2 inches of tissue can be grasped, the needle should be inserted at a 90-degree angle; if 1 inch of tissue can be grasped, the needle should be inserted at a 45-degree angle. The upper abdomen is the best injection site for clients with little peripheral subcutaneous tissue.

Delegation Considerations

The skill of administering subcutaneous injections should not be delegated to assistive personnel. Assistive personnel should be instructed to report any unexpected drug reactions or pain at injection site as soon as possible.

Equipment

- Syringe (1 to 3 ml)
- Needle (27 to 25 gauge, ⅜ to ⅝ inch)
- Alcohol swab
- Small gauze pad (optional)
- Medication ampule or vial
- Disposable gloves
- Medication administration record (MAR) or computer printout

STEP	RATIONALE

ASSESSMENT

Step	Rationale
1. Review physician's medication order for client's name, drug name, dose, time, and route of administration.	Ensures safe and correct administration of medication.
2. Gather drug reference information pertinent to drug(s) ordered: action, purpose, time of onset and peak action, normal dosage, side effects, and nursing implications.	Nurse must be able to anticipate drug's effects and observe client's response. Allows nurse to judge appropriateness of therapy as client's condition changes.
3. Assess for factors that may contraindicate SC injections, such as circulatory shock or reduced local tissue perfusion.	Reduced tissue perfusion interferes with drug absorption and distribution.
4. Assess indications for SC injections: unconscious or confused client; client who is unable to swallow or has gastrointestinal disturbances; presence of gastric suction.	Contraindicates use of oral medications; therefore parenteral route is more desirable. Some medications are not absorbed from the gastrointestinal tract.
5. Assess client's medical history, history of allergies, and medication history.	May influence how drug acts. Information also indicates client's need for medication or contraindications for medication use.
6. Assess adequacy of client's adipose tissue.	Physiological changes of aging or client illness may influence amount of SC tissue a client possesses. This influences methods for administering injections.
7. Assess client's knowledge regarding medication to be received.	Information may pose implications for client education. Assessment may also reveal drug use problems at home.
8. Observe client's verbal and nonverbal responses toward injection.	Injections can be painful. Clients may experience considerable anxiety, which can increase pain.

NURSING DIAGNOSIS

Defining characteristics from the assessment data may reveal the following nursing diagnoses for clients requiring this skill:

- Anxiety
- Fear
- Ineffective health maintenance
- Deficient knowledge regarding medication administration or drug therapy
- Pain (acute)

Related factors are individualized based on client's condition or needs.

PLANNING

Step	Rationale
1. **Expected outcomes** following completion of procedure:	
▪ Client experiences no pain or mild burning at injection site.	Subcutaneous medications are usually nonirritating to tissues, but displacement of tissues or medication may cause mild burning.
▪ Desired effect of medication achieved with no signs of allergies or undesired effects	Drug action is effective.
▪ Client explains purpose, dosage, and effects of medication.	Demonstrates learning.
2. Check medication administration record or computer printout.	Verifies order.
3. Prepare correct medication dose from ampule or vial (see Skill 18-1 or 18-2). Check dose carefully.	Ensures that medication is sterile and dose is accurate. Preparation techniques differ for ampule and vial.
4. Identify client by checking identification bracelet and asking client's name. Compare with medication administration record.	Ensures that correct client is receiving medication.
5. Explain procedure to client and proceed in calm, confident manner.	Helps client anticipate nurse's actions. Calm approach minimizes client's anxiety.

STEP	RATIONALE
IMPLEMENTATION	
1. Close room curtains or door.	Provides privacy.
2. Wash hands and apply disposable gloves.	Follows Centers for Disease Control and Prevention recommendations to prevent accidental exposure to blood and body fluids (National Institute for Occupational Safety and Health [NIOSH], 1999).
3. Keep sheet or gown draped over body parts not requiring exposure.	Respects client's dignity while area to be injected is exposed.
4. Select appropriate injection site. Inspect skin's surface over site for bruises, inflammation, or edema. Palpate site for masses, edema, or tenderness. NOTE: When administering heparin subcutaneously, use abdominal injection sites.	Injection site should be free of lesions that might interfere with drug absorption. NOTE: Anticoagulant may cause local bleeding and bruising when injected into areas such as arms and legs, which are involved in muscular activity.

- ***Critical Decision Point***
  If client is receiving heparin and is experiencing bruising with use of 1-ml or tuberculin syringe, try administering heparin injections with a 3-ml syringe. This may help reduce extent of bruising associated with heparin therapy (Hadley, Chang, and Rogers, 1996).

STEP	RATIONALE
5. Be sure that needle size is correct by grasping skinfold at site with thumb and forefinger. Measure skinfold from top to bottom; be sure that needle is approximately one half this length.	Subcutaneous injections can be inadvertently given in the muscle, especially in the abdomen and thigh sites (Peragallo-Dittko, 1997). Appropriate size of needle ensures that medication will be injected into SC tissue as ordered.
6. Assist client to comfortable position. Instruct client to relax arm, leg, or abdomen, depending on site chosen for injection. Talk with client about subject of interest.	Relaxation of area minimizes discomfort during injection. Promoting client's comfort through positioning and distraction helps reduce anxiety.
7. Re-locate site using anatomical landmarks.	Accurate injection of medication requires insertion in correct site to avoid injury to underlying nerves, bone, or blood vessels.
8. Cleanse site with antiseptic swab (see illustration). Apply swab at center of site and rotate outward in circular direction for about 5 cm (2 inches).	Mechanical action of swab removes secretions containing microorganisms.

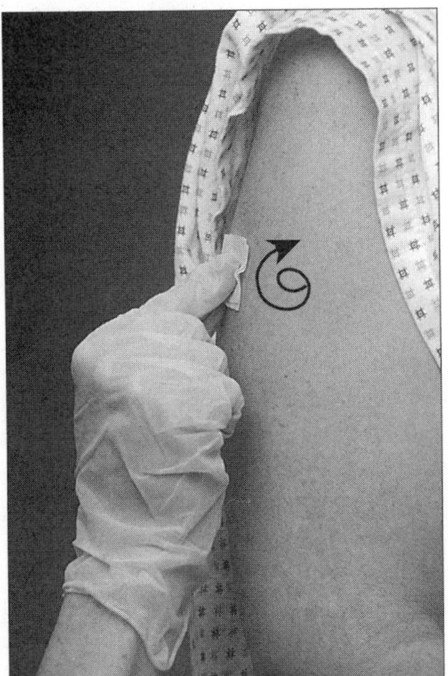

STEP **8** Cleansing site with circular motion.

Step	Rationale
9. Remove needle cap or sheath from needle by pulling it straight off.	Preventing needle from touching sides of cap prevents contamination.
10. Hold swab or square of sterile gauze between third and fourth fingers of nondominant hand.	Swab or gauze remains readily accessible for when needle is withdrawn.
11. Hold syringe between thumb and forefinger of dominant hand as if grasping a dart, holding syringe across tops of fingertips (see illustration).	Quick, smooth injection requires proper manipulation of syringe parts.

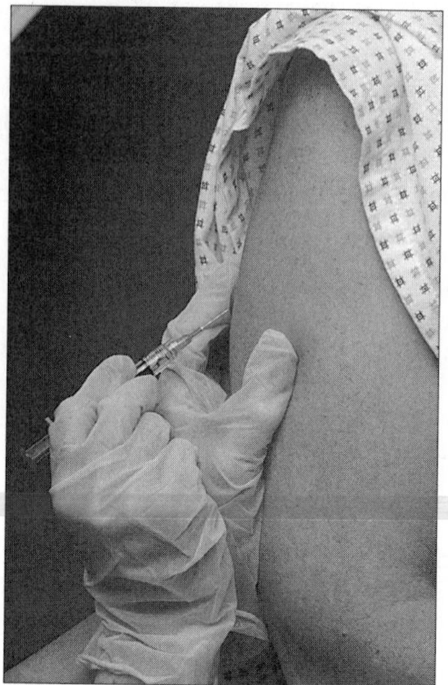

STEP **11** Holding syringe as if grasping a dart.

Step	Rationale
12. Administer injection:	
a. For average-size client, spread skin tightly across injection site or pinch skin with nondominant hand.	Needle penetrates tight skin easier than loose skin. Pinching skin elevates SC tissue.
b. Inject needle quickly and firmly at 45- to 90-degree angle. (Then release skin, if pinched.)	Quick, firm insertion minimizes discomfort. (Injecting medication into compressed tissue irritates nerve fibers.)
c. For obese client, pinch skin at site and inject needle at 90-degree angle below tissue fold.	Obese clients have fatty layer of tissue above SC layer.
13. After needle enters site, grasp lower end of syringe barrel with nondominant hand. Move dominant hand to end of plunger and slowly inject medication. Avoid moving syringe.	Properly performed injection requires smooth manipulation of syringe parts. Movement of syringe may displace needle and cause discomfort.

- ***Critical Decision Point***

  Aspiration after injecting a SC medication is not necessary. Piercing a blood vessel in an SC injection is very rare (Peragallo-Dittko, 1997). Aspiration after injecting heparin and insulin is not recommended (Ross & Soltes, 1995; ADA, 1997).

Step	Rationale
14. Withdraw needle quickly while placing antiseptic swab or sterile gauze gently above or over site.	Supporting tissues around injection site minimizes discomfort during needle withdrawal. Dry gauze may minimize client discomfort associated with alcohol on nonintact skin.
15. Apply gentle pressure to site. *Do not massage site.* (If heparin is given, press alcohol swab or gauze to site for 30 to 60 seconds.)	Aids absorption. Massage can damage underlying tissue.
16. Assist client to comfortable position.	Gives client sense of well-being.
17. Discard uncapped needle or needle enclosed in safety shield (see illustrations) and attached syringe in puncture-proof and leak-proof receptacle.	Prevents injury to client and health care personnel. Recapping needles increases risk of needle-stick injury (NIOSH, 1999).

A 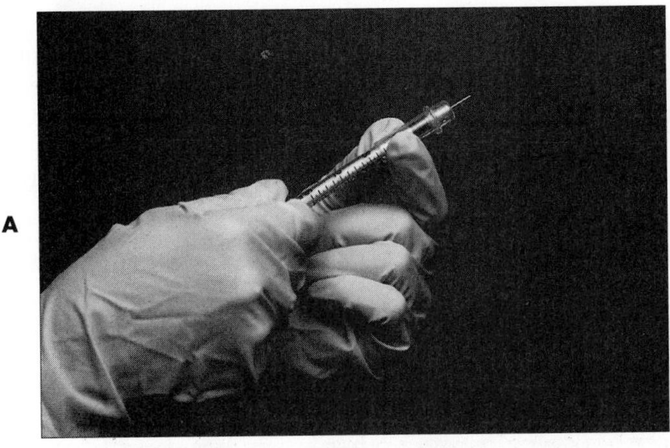 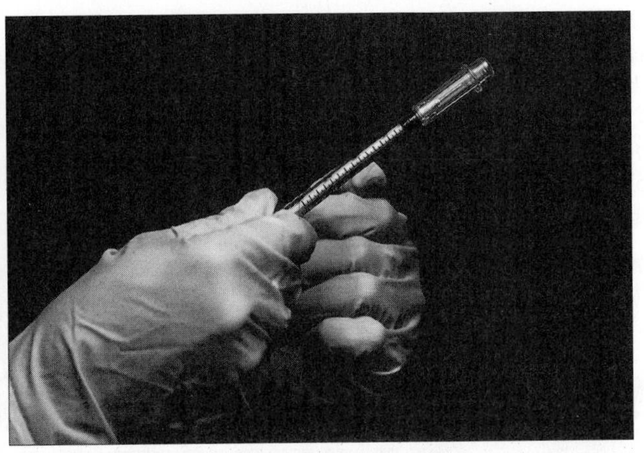 B

STEP **17** Needle with plastic guard to prevent needle sticks. **A,** Position of guard before injection. **B,** After injection the guard locks in place, covering the needle.

STEP	RATIONALE
18. Dispose of used supplies, remove gloves, and wash hands.	Reduces transmission of microorganisms.

EVALUATION

1. Return to room and ask if client feels any acute pain, burning, numbness, or tingling at injection site.	Continued discomfort may indicate injury to underlying bones or nerves.
2. Observe client's response to medication at times that correlate with the medication's onset, peak and duration.	Determines efficacy of drug and allows evaluation of undesirable side effects.
3. Ask client to explain purpose and effects of medication.	Evaluates client's understanding of information taught.

UNEXPECTED OUTCOMES AND RELATED INTERVENTIONS

- Client complains of localized pain or continued burning at injection site, indicating potential injury to nerve or tissues.
  - Assess injection site, and notify client's health care provider.
- Client displays signs of urticaria, eczema, pruritus, wheezing, and dyspnea.
  - Follow institutional policy or guidelines for appropriate response to allergic reactions, and notify client's health care provider immediately.

RECORDING AND REPORTING

- Immediately after administration, chart medication dose, route, site, time, and date given on MAR to record care provided and prevent future drug administration errors. Correctly sign MAR according to institutional policy.
- Record client's response to medication.
- Report any undesirable effects from medication to client's health care provider and document adverse effects according to institutional policy.

TEACHING CONSIDERATIONS

- Instruct client to wear medical identification bracelet indicating important medical information, including diseases client has (e.g., diabetes) and allergies.
- Clients who require daily injections will need to learn techniques of self-administration (see Skills 40-5 and 40-6). A family member or a significant other should also be taught injection techniques.
- Clients with hypertrophy of skin due to repeated insulin injections (common with beef or pork insulin formulations) should be taught to avoid site until problem resolves.

PEDIATRIC CONSIDERATIONS

- Only amounts up to 0.5 ml may be administered subcutaneously to small children (Wong and others, 1999).

GERONTOLOGICAL CONSIDERATIONS

- Aging clients have reduced subcutaneous skinfold thickness, and skin is less elastic than that of younger clients. The upper abdominal site is the best site to use when the client has little subcutaneous tissue.

HOME CARE CONSIDERATIONS

- Most insulin preparations have bacteriostatic properties that inhibit the growth of bacteria found on the skin. Therefore clients with diabetes may reuse their syringes at home if desired. Syringes should be discarded into a hard plastic container, such as a laundry detergent bottle, when the needles become dull, bent, or contact any surface other than the skin. Wiping the needle off with alcohol is not recommended, as that may remove the silicon coating on the needle that makes injections less painful. Clients with poor personal hygiene, an acute illness, and open wounds on hands or clients who are immunocompromised should not reuse syringes (American Diabetes Association, 1997).

Skill 18-5 Administering Intramuscular Injections

An injection given by the intramuscular (IM) route deposits medication into deep muscle tissue. The vascularity of muscle tissue results in fast drug absorption. An **aqueous** solution is absorbed in 10 to 30 minutes, as opposed to at least 30 minutes when given subcutaneously (McConnell, 1982). However, an increased risk of injecting drugs directly into blood vessels exists. As with subcutaneous (SC) injections, any factor that interferes with local tissue blood flow affects the rate and extent of drug absorption.

A nurse uses a longer and larger-gauge needle to pass through SC tissue and penetrate deep muscle tissue. Generally for the average adult a 21- to 25-gauge $1\frac{1}{2}$-inch needle inserted at a 90-degree angle will pass through SC tissue and enter deep muscle (see Figure 18-7, p. 509). Intramuscular injection sites should be rotated to decrease the risk of hypertrophy. An older adult or cachectic client may require a shorter, smaller-gauge needle because of muscle atrophy. For well-developed children a 1-inch needle will usually penetrate deep muscle. Emaciated muscles absorb medication poorly and should be avoided when possible.

The following guidelines are helpful in estimating the needle length necessary for IM injections into the vastus lateralis or deltoid muscle. If using the deltoid muscle, grasp the muscle between the thumb and index finger. Use a needle that is about half the distance between the two fingers. When using the vastus lateralis, grasp the subcutaneous tissue between the thumb and index finger and use a needle that is slightly greater than half the distance between the two fingers (Wong and others, 1999).

Muscle is less sensitive to irritating and viscous drugs. A normal, well-developed adult client can safely tolerate as much as 4 ml of medication in larger muscles such as the gluteus medius (Beyea and Nicoll, 1995). Older infants and small children (e.g., under the age of 2) receiving IM injections should receive no more than 1 ml of medication (Wong and others, 1999).

The **Z-track method** is recommended for IM injections. The Z-track technique, pulling the skin either downward or laterally before injection, reduces leakage of medication into subcutaneous tissue and minimizes pain (Beyea and Nicoll, 1995). The nurse applies a new needle to the syringe after preparing the drug so that no solution remains on the outside needle shaft. Then the nurse selects an IM site, preferably in a large, deep muscle such as the ventrogluteal. The overlying skin and SC tissues are pulled approximately 2.5 to 3.5 cm (1 to $1\frac{1}{2}$ inches) down or laterally to the side with the ulnar side of the nondominant hand (McConnell, 1999). The skin is held in this position until the injection has been administered. The area is cleansed with an antiseptic swab. Holding the syringe in the dominant hand, the nurse injects the needle quickly through the skin, deep into the muscle. The nurse slowly injects the drug if there is no blood return on aspiration. The needle remains inserted for 10 seconds to allow the medication to disperse evenly (McConnell, 1999). The nurse releases the skin after withdrawing the needle, which leaves a zigzag path that seals the needle track wherever tissue planes slide across each other (Figure 18-11). The drug is less likely to escape from the muscle tissue.

VENTROGLUTEAL MUSCLE

The ventrogluteal muscle involves the gluteus medius and minimus. It is situated deep and away from major nerves and blood vessels and is a safe site for all clients. Research has shown that injuries such as fibrosis, nerve damage, abscess, tissue necrosis, muscle contraction, gangrene, and pain have been associated with all the common IM sites except the ventrogluteal site. *The ventrogluteal site is the preferred injection site for adults and anyone over 7 months old* (Beecroft and Kongelbeck, 1994; Beyea and Nicoll, 1995). This site is also safe for children younger than 7 months (Wong and others, 1999).

The nurse locates the muscle by placing the heel of the hand over the greater trochanter of the client's hip with the wrist almost perpendicular to the femur. The right hand is used for the left hip, and the left hand is used for the right hip. The nurse points the thumb toward the client's groin and the fingers toward the client's head, points the index finger to the anterior superior iliac spine, and extends the middle finger back along the iliac crest toward the buttock. The index finger, the middle finger, and the iliac crest form a V-shaped triangle, and the injection site is the center of the triangle (Figure 18-12).

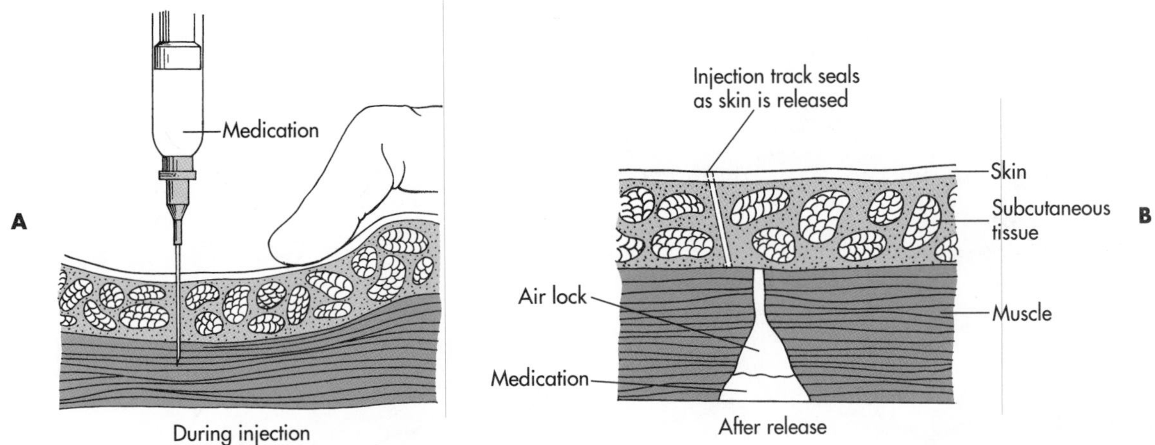

FIGURE **18-11** A, Pull on overlying skin before needle insertion and during IM injection moves tissues to prevent later tracking. **B,** The Z-track left after injection prevents the deposit of medication through sensitive tissue.

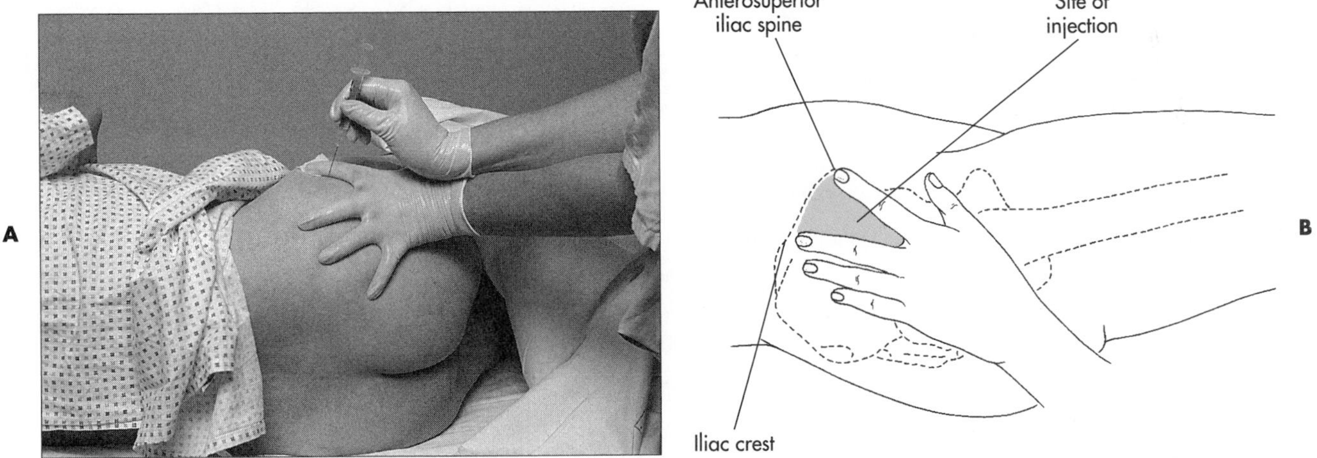

FIGURE **18-12** A, Injection site for ventrogluteal muscle avoids major nerves and blood vessels. **B,** Anatomical view of ventrogluteal muscle injection site.

Vastus Lateralis Muscle

The vastus lateralis muscle is another injection site used in the adult client and is the preferred site for infants under 7 months of age (Beyea and Nicoll, 1995; Wong and others, 1999). The muscle is thick and well developed. It is located on the anterior lateral aspect of the thigh; in an adult it extends from a handbreadth above the knee to a handbreadth below the greater trochanter of the femur (Figure 18-13). The middle third of the muscle is the suggested site for injection. The width of the muscle usually extends from the midline of the thigh to the midline of the thigh's outer side.

Deltoid Muscle

Although the deltoid site is easily accessible, the muscle is not well developed in many adults. The radial and ulnar nerves and the brachial artery lie within the upper arm along the humerus (Figure 18-14, *A*). The nurse should use this site only for small medication volumes (0.5 to 1.0 ml) and when other sites are inaccessible because of dressings or casts.

To locate the deltoid muscle the nurse fully exposes the client's upper arm and shoulder. A tight-fitting sleeve should not be rolled up. The nurse instructs the client to relax the arm at the side and flex the elbow by placing the hand on the hip or relaxing the lower arm across the abdomen or lap. The client may sit, stand, or lie down (Figure 18-14, *B*). The nurse palpates the lower edge of the acromion process, which forms the base of a triangle in line with the midpoint of the lateral aspect of the upper arm. The injection site is in the center of the triangle, about 2.5 to 5 cm (1 to 2 inches) below the acromion process (see Figure 18-14, *A*). The nurse may also locate the site by placing four fingers across the deltoid muscle, with the top finger along the acromion process. The injection site is then three finger widths below the acromion process.

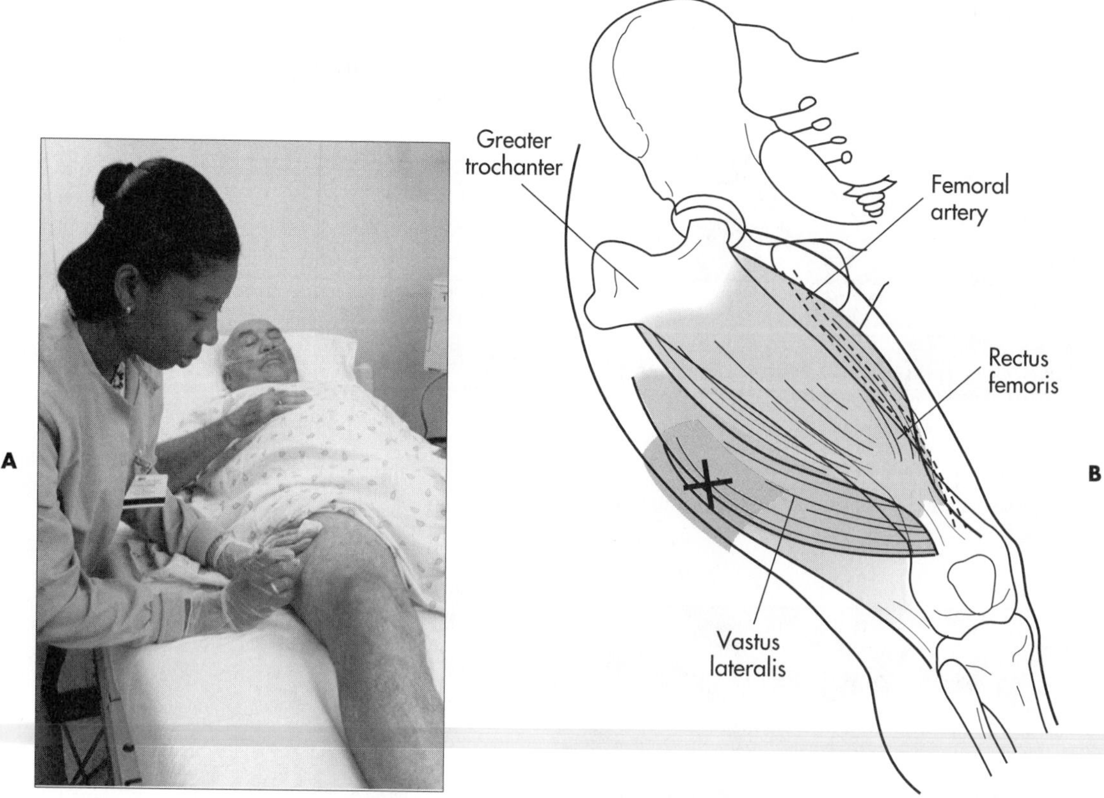

FIGURE **18-13** **A,** Giving IM injection in vastus lateralis site. **B,** Landmarks for vastus lateralis site.

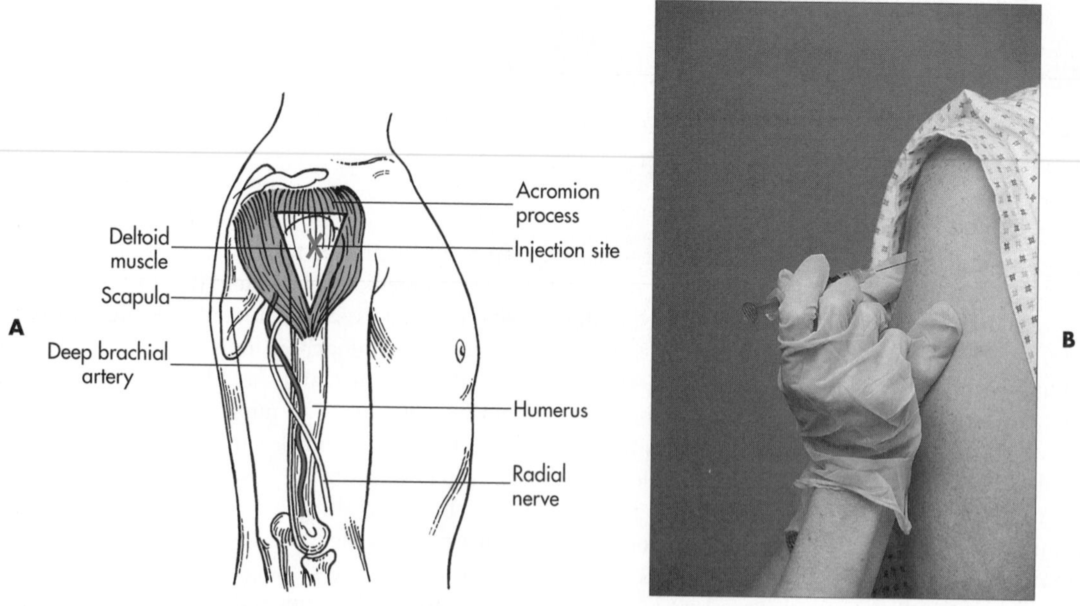

FIGURE **18-14** **A,** Landmarks for deltoid site. **B,** Giving IM injection in deltoid site.

Delegation Considerations

The skill of administering intramuscular medications should not be delegated to assistive personnel. Assistive personnel should be instructed to report any unexpected drug reactions or pain at injection site as soon as possible.

Equipment

- Syringe: 2 to 3 ml for adult; 0.5 to 1 ml for infants and small children
- Needles (2): 21 to 25 gauge, 1 to 1½ inches for adults; 1 inch for children
- Alcohol swab
- 2 × 2 gauze pad (optional)
- Medication ampule or vial
- Disposable gloves
- Medication administration record (MAR) or computer printout

Step	Rationale

Assessment

Step	Rationale
1. Review physician's medication order for client's name, drug name, dose, time, and route of administration.	Ensures safe and correct administration of medication.
2. Gather drug reference information pertinent to drug(s) ordered: action, purpose, time of onset and peak action, normal dose, common side effects, nursing implications.	Nurse must be able to anticipate drug's effects and observe client's response. Allows nurse to judge appropriateness of therapy as client's condition changes.
3. Consider factors that may contraindicate IM injection, for example, muscle atrophy, reduced blood flow, or circulatory shock.	Atrophied muscle absorbs medication poorly. Factors interfering with blood flow to muscles impair drug absorption.

- ***Critical Decision Point***
  Consider calling prescriber for alternate route of medication administration. Because of the documented adverse effects of IM injections, other routes of medication injection are safer (Beecroft and Kongelbeck, 1994).

Step	Rationale
4. Assess client's medical history, history of allergies, and medication history.	May influence action of certain drugs. Information also indicates client's need for medication.
5. Assess client's knowledge regarding medication and dosage schedule.	Information may pose implications for client education.
6. Observe client's verbal and nonverbal responses toward receiving injection.	Injections can be painful. Clients may experience considerable anxiety or fear, which can increase pain.

Nursing Diagnosis

Defining characteristics from the assessment data may reveal the following nursing diagnoses for clients requiring this skill:

- Anxiety
- Fear
- Deficient knowledge regarding medication administration or drug therapy
- Pain (acute)

Related factors are individualized based on client's condition or needs.

Planning

Step	Rationale
1. **Expected outcomes** following completion of procedure:	
▪ Client experiences temporary mild burning at injection site.	Insertion of needle and/or injection of medications into tissues may cause discomfort.
▪ No allergies or undesired effects occur.	Drug action is normal.
▪ Client explains purpose and effects of medication.	Demonstrates learning.
▪ Client demonstrates no behaviors reflecting anxiety.	Anticipatory guidance relieves anxiety.
2. Prepare correct dose from ampule or vial (see Skill 18-1 or 18-2). Check dose carefully.	Ensures that medication is sterile and dose is accurate.

Step	Rationale
3. Change needle on syringe.	Prevents tracking of irritating substances as needle passes into muscle.
4. For adults select a 1.5-inch, 21- to 25-gauge needle. For children select a 1-inch needle.	Needle must be long enough to reach muscle. Adipose tissue layer over the ventral gluteal muscle is less than 3.75 cm (1.47 inches) in depth (Beyea and Nicoll, 1995).
5. Identify client by checking identification bracelet and asking client's name. Compare with medication administration record.	Ensures that correct client is receiving medication.
6. Explain procedure, location of injection site, and how positioning lessens discomfort. Proceed in calm manner.	Allows client to anticipate injection so as to lessen anxiety.

Implementation

Step	Rationale
1. Close room curtains and/or door.	Provides client privacy.
2. Wash hands and apply gloves.	Follows Centers for Disease Control and Prevention recommendations to prevent accidental exposure to blood and body fluids (National Institute for Occupational Safety and Health [NIOSH], 1999).
3. Keep sheet or gown draped over body parts not requiring exposure.	Maintains client's dignity.
4. Select appropriate injection site by assessing size and integrity of muscle. Palpate for areas of tenderness or hardness. Note presence of bruising or area of infection.	The ventrogluteal site is the preferred site for children over 7 months and adults unless there are contraindications to this site. For example, the hepatitis-B vaccine should be administered in the deltoid in all clients greater than 7 months of age. In infants less than 7 months, the vastus lateralis should be used (Beyea and Nicoll, 1995).

- ***Critical Decision Point***
  When choosing an injection site, do not use an area that is bruised, has indurations, or has signs associated with infection.

Step	Rationale
5. Assist client to comfortable position, depending on site chosen: ventrogluteal—client lies on side or back, flexes knee and hip on side to be injected; vastus lateralis—client lies flat, supine, with knee slightly flexed; deltoid—client may sit or lie flat with hand on hip or lower arm flexed but relaxed across abdomen or lap (Box 18-3).	Position that reduces strain on muscle minimizes discomfort of injection.

- ***Critical Decision Point***
  Ensure that client's position for injection is not contraindicated by medical condition.

Step	Rationale
6. Re-locate site using anatomical landmarks.	Injection into correct anatomical site prevents injury to nerves, bones, and blood vessels.
7. Position nondominant hand just below site and pull the skin over with ulnar side of hand to administer in a Z-track.	Reduces discomfort and incidence of lesions.

Box 18-3 Positioning Client for Comfort With Intramuscular Injection

- Giving an injection to a client in the side-lying position: Have the client flex the knee, then pivot the leg forward from the hip approximately 20 degrees so it can rest on the bed.
- Giving an injection to a client in the supine position: Have the client flex the knee on the side where the injection is to be administered.
- Giving an injection to a client in the prone position: Have the client "toe in" to rotate the femur internally.

Modified from Beyea SC, Nicoll LH: Back to basics: administering IM injections the right way, *Am J Nurs* 96(1):34, 1996.

STEP	RATIONALE

- ***Critical Decision Point***
  If client's muscle mass is small, do not use the Z-track method. Instead, grasp body of muscle between thumb and fingers (Workman, 1999).

Step	Rationale
8. Cleanse site with antiseptic swab. Apply swab to center of site and rotate outward in circular direction for about 5 cm (2 inches).	Mechanical action of swab removes secretions containing microorganisms.
9. Hold swab or square of sterile gauze between third and fourth fingers of nondominant hand.	Swab or gauze remains readily accessible for when needle is withdrawn.
10. Place needle cap or sheath from needle in between thumb and index finger of nondominant hand. Hold barrel in dominant hand and pull cap straight off.	Preventing needle from touching sides of cap prevents contamination.
11. Hold syringe between thumb and forefinger of dominant hand as if holding a dart. Hold it with palm down at 90-degree angle to injection site.	Quick, smooth injection requires proper manipulation of syringe. Needle must be injected at 90-degree angle to enter muscle.
12. Administer injection:	
a. Inject needle quickly at 90-degree angle into muscle.	Smooth, quick injection lessens pain. Angle ensures that medication reaches muscle mass.
b. After needle enters site, grasp lower end of syringe barrel with nondominant hand to stabilize syringe. Continue to hold skin tightly with nondominant hand. Move dominant hand to end of plunger. Avoid moving syringe.	Smooth manipulation of syringe parts reduces discomfort from needle movement. Skin must remain pulled until after drug is injected to ensure Z-track administration.
c. Pull back on plunger 5 to 10 seconds. If no blood appears, inject medication slowly at a rate of 10 sec/ml.	Aspiration of blood into syringe indicates intravenous (IV) placement of needle. Intramuscular medications are not for IV use. Slow injection reduces pain and tissue trauma (Beyea and Nicoll, 1995).

- ***Critical Decision Point***
  If blood appears in syringe, remove needle and dispose of medication and syringe properly. Repeat preparation procedure.

Step	Rationale
d. Wait 10 seconds, then smoothly and steadily withdraw needle and release skin while placing antiseptic swab or dry gauze gently above or over injection.	Support of tissues around injection site minimizes discomfort during needle withdrawal. Dry gauze may minimize client discomfort associated with alcohol on nonintact skin.
13. Apply gentle pressure. *Do not massage site.*	Massage can damage underlying tissue.
14. For ventrogluteal and vastus lateralis sites, encourage leg exercises.	Promotes drug absorption.
15. Discard uncapped needle or needle enclosed in safety shield and attached syringe into puncture-proof and leak-proof receptacle.	Prevents injury to client and health care personnel. Recapping needles increases risk of needle-stick injury (NIOSH, 1999).
16. Dispose of soiled supplies, remove gloves, and wash hands.	Reduces transmission of microorganisms.

EVALUATION

Step	Rationale
1. Return to room and ask if client feels any acute pain, burning, numbness, or tingling at injection site.	Continued discomfort may indicate injury to underlying bones or nerves.
2. Inspect site, note any bruising or induration.	Bruising or induration indicates complication associated with injection. Document findings and notify health care provider. Apply warm compress to site.
3. Observe client's response to medication at times that correlate with the medication's onset, peak, and duration.	Intramuscular medications are absorbed quickly; undesired effects may also develop rapidly. Nurse's observations determine efficacy of drug action.
4. Ask client to explain purpose and effects of medication.	Evaluates client's understanding of information taught.

UNEXPECTED OUTCOMES AND RELATED INTERVENTIONS

- Client continues to complain of localized pain, numbness, or tingling, indicating potential injury to nerves or tissues.
  - Assess injection site and other involved areas, and notify client's health care provider.
- Client develops signs and symptoms of allergy or side effects.
  - Follow institutional policy or guidelines for the appropriate response and reporting of adverse drug reactions, and notify client's health care provider immediately.

RECORDING AND REPORTING

- Immediately chart medication, dose, route, site, time, and date given on MAR. Correctly sign according to institutional policy.
- Record client's response to medication if indicated (for example, response to pain medication).
- Document and report any undesirable effects from medication to client's health care provider. Be aware that possible allergic reactions may not appear for several hours after a medication is given, especially when the client is receiving the medication for the first time.

TEACHING CONSIDERATIONS

- Clients who require regular injections, for example, vitamin B_{12}, will need to learn techniques of self-administration (see Skills 39-1 and 40-4). A family member or significant other should also be taught injection techniques and the importance of rotating sites to decrease the risk for hypertrophy.
- Instruct client and family member or significant other to observe injection sites for complications and to report complications to a health care provider immediately.
- Instruct client and family member or significant other to observe for effectiveness of medication and adverse reactions. Client or caregiver should report ineffectiveness of medication and adverse reactions to the health care provider.
- Have client perform several return demonstrations of preparing medications from vial or ampule and on injection technique.

PEDIATRIC CONSIDERATIONS

- The deltoid muscle is no longer recommended as an injection site in children.
- Children may be extremely anxious or fearful of needles. Assistance with proper positioning and holding of the child may be necessary. Distraction can help alleviate the child's anxiety.
- If possible, apply EMLA cream to site 2½ hours before IM injection or a vapocoolant spray just before injection to decrease pain (Wong and others, 1999).

GERONTOLOGICAL CONSIDERATIONS

- Older clients are more likely to have muscle atrophy. Therefore the nurse must carefully assess the injection site and may need to grasp the muscle between the thumb and fingers.

HOME CARE CONSIDERATIONS

- Needles and equipment should be disposed of in a hard, plastic receptacle. If a red biohazardous sharps container is unavailable, a large detergent or fabric softener bottle may be used.
- See Skills 39-1 and 40-4.

Skill 18-6 Adding Medications to Intravenous Fluid Containers

Intravenous (IV) **infusion** medications enter the venous circulation directly and thus can cause rapid effects. The nurse must observe the client closely for symptoms of adverse reactions. Special attention is given to dose calculation and drug preparation. The nurse carefully checks the five rights of safe drug administration and is aware of the desired action and potential side effects of each medication.

Mixing drugs in large volumes of fluids is relatively safe and easy. The nurse or pharmacist dilutes IV medications in volumes of 50 to 1000 ml of compatible IV fluids such as normal saline, dextrose and water, or lactated Ringer's solution. In many hospital settings the pharmacy adds drugs to primary containers of IV solutions to ensure asepsis. The pharmacist may use special plastic caps to seal containers previously mixed. Because a drug in an IV solution is not in a concentrated form, the risk of side effects or fatal reactions is minimal. Vitamins and potassium chloride are two types of drugs commonly added to IV fluids.

Many parenteral medications are highly alkaline and irritating to muscle and subcutaneous (SC) tissue. Thus the IV route is best to minimize client discomfort. The nurse administers drugs intravenously by five methods:

1. As mixtures within large volumes of IV fluids
2. By **piggyback infusion** of a solution containing the prescribed medication and a small volume of fluid (50 ml, 100 ml) through an adjoining container or existing IV line (see Skill 18-7)
3. By volume-control administration device, in which a small container, holding 50 to 150 ml of fluid, is attached below the primary infusion bag (see Skill 18-7)

4. By various electronic infusion devices (see Skill 18-7)
5. By injection of a bolus or small volume of medication through an existing IV infusion line or heparin or saline IV lock (see Skill 18-8)

In all the methods the client has either an existing IV infusion line or an IV access site in the form of a **heparin lock** or a **saline lock.** In most institutions and settings there are policies that identify the medications that nurses are allowed to inject directly into a client's veins through venipuncture.

Delegation Considerations

The skill of adding medications to intravenous fluid containers should not be delegated to assistive personnel.

Equipment

- Vial or ampule of prescribed medication
- Syringe of appropriate size (1 to 20 ml)
- Sterile needle (1 to 1½ inch, 19 to 21 gauge) with special filters if indicated
- Correct diluent if indicated (e.g., sterile water, normal saline)
- Sterile IV fluid container (bag or bottle, 50 to 1000 ml in volume)
- Alcohol or antiseptic swab
- Label to attach to IV bag or bottle
- Medication administration record or computer printout

Step	Rationale
Assessment	
1. Check physician's order to verify the client's name, drug name, dose, time, route, and appropriate type and amount of IV solution to use.	Client's overall physical condition and compatibilities of ordered medication dictate type of IV solution used to ensure safe and accurate drug administration.
2. Collect medication reference information necessary to administer drug safely, including action, purpose, side effects, normal dose, rate of administration, time of peak onset, and nursing implications.	Allows nurse to give drug safely and to monitor client's response to therapy.
3. When more than one medication is to be added to IV solution, assess for **compatibility** of medications. Check institutional reference for drug compatibility list.	Drug **incompatibility** often becomes apparent when drugs are mixed together. Chemical reactions that occur result in clouding or crystallization of IV fluids.
4. Assess client's systemic fluid balance, as reflected by skin hydration and turgor, body weight, pulse, blood pressure, and electrolyte laboratory values.	Danger of continuous IV infusions, especially in older adults or children, is that fluids may infuse too rapidly, causing circulatory overload (Powers, 1999; Wong and others, 1999).
5. Assess client's history of drug allergies.	Intravenous administration of drugs causes rapid effects. Allergic response can be immediate.
6. Assess IV insertion site for signs of **infiltration** or **phlebitis** (see Chapter 19). Presence of complication will require IV to be restarted.	An intact, properly functioning site ensures that medication is given safely.

Nursing Diagnosis

Defining characteristics from the assessment data may reveal the following nursing diagnoses for clients requiring this skill:

Deficient knowledge regarding medication therapy
Risk for imbalanced fluid volume

Related factors are individualized based on client's condition or needs.

Planning

Step	Rationale
1. **Expected outcomes** following completion of procedure:	
▪ Proper medication dose and IV mixture is prepared.	
▪ Client experiences no medication side effects or adverse reactions.	Drugs were given safely.

Step	Rationale
▪ Client develops no signs or symptoms of fluid volume excess.	Intravenous rate is correctly maintained.
▪ Intravenous site remains free of swelling or inflammation.	Fluid was delivered without infusion site complications.
▪ Client will explain purpose and side effects of medication.	Demonstrates learning.
2. Assemble supplies in medication area.	Ensures orderly procedure with less chance of supply contamination.
3. Prepare prescribed medication from vial or ampule. (If filter needle is used, replace it with regular needle before injecting medication into IV fluid container.)	Different techniques are used for each type of container.
4. Identify client by reading identification band and asking name. Compare with medication administration record.	Ensures that correct client receives ordered medication.
5. Prepare client by explaining that medication is to be given through existing IV line or one to be started. Explain that no discomfort should be felt during drug infusion. Encourage client to report symptoms of discomfort.	Most IV medications do not cause discomfort when diluted. However, potassium chloride can be irritating. Pain at insertion site may be early indication of infiltration.

Implementation

Step	Rationale
1. Wash hands thoroughly.	Reduces transfer of microorganisms.
2. **To add medication to new container:**	
a. Solution in a bag: Locate medication injection port on plastic IV solution bag. Port has small rubber stopper at end. Do not select port for IV tubing insertion or air vent.	Medication injection port is self-sealing to prevent introduction of microorganisms after repeated use.
b. Solution in a bottle: Locate injection site on IV solution bottle, which is often covered by a metal or plastic cap.	Accidental injection of medication through main tubing port or air vent can alter pressure within bottle and cause fluid leaks through air vent. Cap seals bottle to maintain its sterility.
c. Wipe off port or injection site with alcohol or antiseptic swab.	Reduces risk of introducing microorganisms into bag during needle insertion.
d. Remove needle cap or sheath from syringe and insert needle or needleless adapter of syringe through center of injection port or site; inject medication.	Injection of needle into sides of port may produce leak and lead to fluid contamination.
e. Withdraw syringe from bag or bottle.	Open tubing port in bottle provides direct route for microorganisms to enter solution. Bags have self-sealing port.
f. Mix medication and IV solution by holding bag or bottle and turning it gently end to end.	Allows even distribution of medication.
g. Complete medication label with name and dose of medication, date, time, and nurse's initials. Stick it on bottle or bag. *Optional* (check institution's policy): Apply a flow strip that identifies the time that the solution was hung and intervals indicating fluid levels (see illustration).	Label can be easily read during infusion of solution. Informs nurses and physicians of contents of bag or bottle.

• ***Critical Decision Point***

Do not use felt-tip markers on plastic IV bag surface. The ink can penetrate the plastic and leak into the IV solution.

Step	Rationale
h. Spike bag or bottle with IV tubing and hang (see Chapter 19). Regulate infusion at ordered rate.	Ensures medication is given over appropriate amount of time.

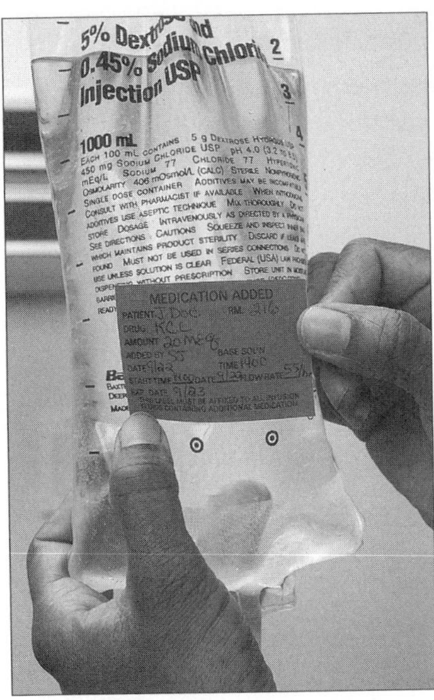

STEP **2g** Label affixed to IV bag.

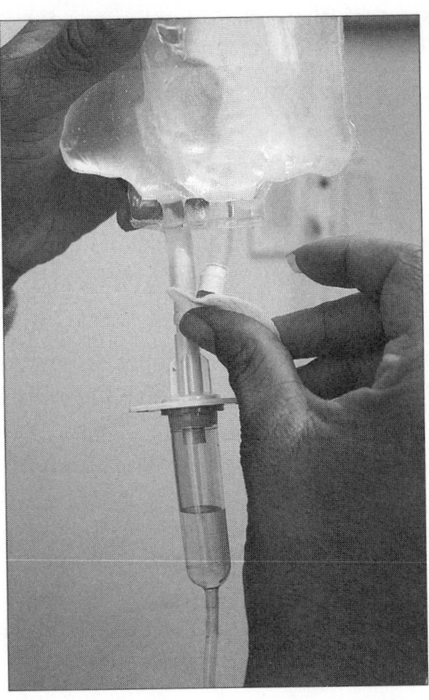

STEP **3a(3)** Injection port cleansed with alcohol.

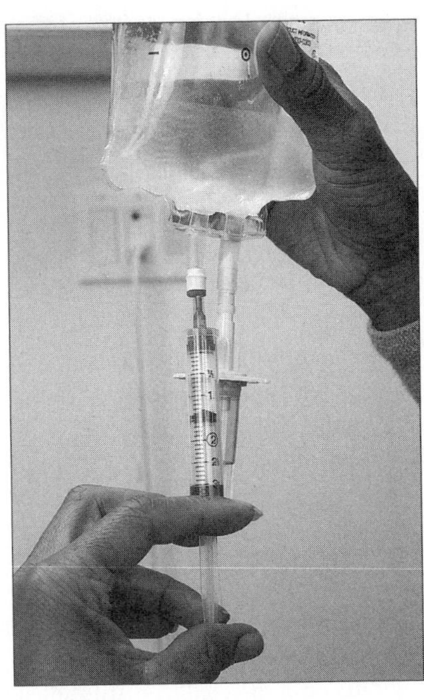

STEP **3a(4)** Medication injected through port.

STEP	RATIONALE
3. To add medication to existing container:	
• ***Critical Decision Point*** *Because there is no way to know exactly how much IV fluid is in an existing hanging IV container, there is no way for the nurse to determine the exact concentration of the medication in the IV solution. Therefore it is recommended that medications should be added to new containers whenever possible.*	
a. Prepare vented IV bottle or plastic bag:	
(1) Check volume of solution remaining in bottle or bag.	Proper minimal volume (see drug insert) is needed to dilute medication adequately.
(2) Close off IV infusion clamp.	Prevents medication from directly entering circulation as it is injected into bag or bottle.
(3) Wipe off medication port with an alcohol or antiseptic swab (see illustration).	Mechanically removes microorganisms that could enter container during needle insertion.
(4) Insert syringe needle through injection port and inject medication (see illustration).	Injection port is self-sealing and prevents fluid leaks.
(5) Lower bag or bottle from IV pole and gently mix. Rehang bag.	Ensures medication is evenly distributed.

Step	Rationale
b. Complete medication label and stick it to bag or bottle.	Informs nurses and physicians of contents of bag or bottle.
c. Regulate infusion to desired rate.	Ensures medication is given over the appropriate amount of time.

- ***Critical Decision Point***
  Some medications, for example, potassium chloride boluses, can cause serious adverse reactions, including cardiac dysrhythmias. These IV medications should be infused on an IV pump. Check institutional policies for which IV medications require administration on an IV pump.

Step	Rationale
4. Properly dispose of equipment and supplies. Do not cap needle of syringe. Specially sheathed needles are discarded as a unit with needle covered.	Proper disposal of needle prevents injury to nurse and client. Capping of needles increases risk of needle-stick injuries.
5. Wash hands.	Reduces transmission of microorganisms.

Evaluation

Step	Rationale
1. Observe client for signs or symptoms of drug reaction.	Intravenous medications can cause rapid effects.
2. Assess IV insertion site and rate of infusion every 1 to 2 hours or as directed by institutional policy.	Over time IV site may become infiltrated or needle may become malpositioned. Flow rate may change according to client's position or volume left in container.
3. Observe IV site for signs or symptoms of infiltration or phlebitis.	Infiltrated drugs can injure tissue. Phlebitis indicates need to restart IV.
4. Observe for signs and symptoms of fluid volume excess.	Rapid uncontrolled infusion can cause circulatory overload.
5. Have client explain purpose and effects of drug therapy.	Demonstrates learning.

Unexpected Outcomes and Related Interventions

- Client has adverse reaction to medication.
  - Follow institutional policy or guidelines for the appropriate response to and reporting of adverse drug reactions, and notify client's health care provider immediately.
- Client develops signs of fluid volume excess (e.g., abnormal breath sounds [crackles], blood pressure changes, jugular venous distention, edema, shortness of breath, intake greater than output).
  - Stop IV infusion, and notify client's health care provider immediately.
- Intravenous site becomes swollen, warm, reddened, and tender to touch (see Chapter 19), indicating phlebitis.
  - Stop IV infusion, and discontinue IV.
  - Treat IV site as indicated by institutional policy, and insert new IV site if continuation of IV therapy is indicated.
- Intravenous site becomes cool, pale, and swollen (see Chapter 19), indicating infiltration. Some IV medications are extremely harmful to subcutaneous tissue.
  - Stop IV infusion, and discontinue IV. For infiltration, keep affected area elevated.
  - Provide IV **extravasation** care (e.g., injecting phentolamine [Regitine] around the IV infiltration site) as indicated by institutional policy, or use a medication reference/manual or consult a pharmacist to determine appropriate follow-up care.

Recording and Reporting

- Record solution and medication added to parenteral fluid on appropriate form (Figure 18-15).
- Report any adverse effects to client's health care provider, and document adverse effects according to institutional policy.

Teaching Considerations

- Clients or caregivers who will be expected to perform this skill should be taught both how to prepare the medication in a syringe and how to mix the medication in the IV solution. Allow plenty of time for learning, reinforcement, and return demonstration to ensure the medication can be prepared accurately.

Home Care Considerations

- Clients or their caregivers should keep a record of medications that are mixed and when they are given at home. Records should include the name of the medications being mixed, the solution they are mixed in, and when they are infused.

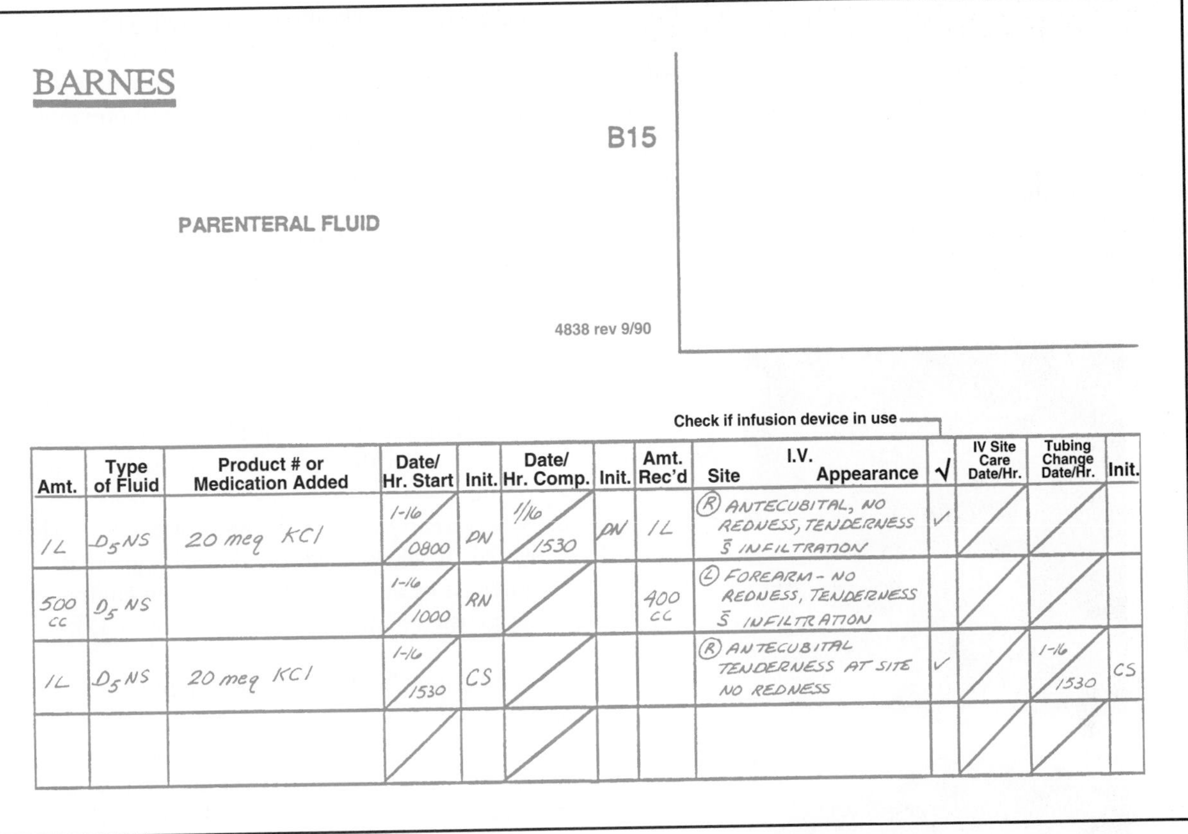

BARNES

B15

PARENTERAL FLUID

4838 rev 9/90

Check if infusion device in use

Amt.	Type of Fluid	Product # or Medication Added	Date/ Hr. Start	Init.	Date/ Hr. Comp.	Init.	Amt. Rec'd	I.V. Site Appearance	√	IV Site Care Date/Hr.	Tubing Change Date/Hr.	Init.
1L	D_5NS	20 meq KCl	1-16 / 0800	DN	1/16 / 1530	DN	1L	Ⓡ ANTECUBITAL, NO REDNESS, TENDERNESS $\bar{S}$ INFILTRATION	✓			
500 cc	D_5 NS		1-16 / 1000	RN			400 cc	Ⓛ FOREARM - NO REDNESS, TENDERNESS $\bar{S}$ INFILTRATION				
1L	D_5NS	20 meq KCl	1-16 / 1530	CS				Ⓡ ANTECUBITAL TENDERNESS AT SITE NO REDNESS	✓		1-16 / 1530	CS

FIGURE **18-15** Example of documentation form for parenteral fluids.

Skill 18-7 Administering Intravenous Medications by Intermittent Infusion Sets and Miniinfusion Pumps

Administering drugs by intermittent infusion is a method in which the nurse dilutes intravenous (IV) medications in small volumes of solution and administers them over a short period. Administering drugs by this method reduces the risk of rapid drug-dose infusion and provides greater comfort and independence for the client. Clients receiving drugs by intermittent infusion have an established IV line that is kept patent by intermittent flushes of normal saline.

Intermittent infusion of drugs can be administered in several ways:

1. *Tandem.* A tandem setup is a small (25 to 100 ml) IV bag or bottle connected to a short tubing line to the *lower* Y-port of a primary infusion line or to an intermittent venous access (Figure 18-16, *A*). The tandem set is placed at the same height as the primary infusion bag or bottle. In the tandem setup the tandem and the main line infuse simultaneously. The nurse must monitor the tandem setup closely. If the tandem setup is not immediately clamped when the medication is infused, the IV solution from the primary line will back up into the tandem line.

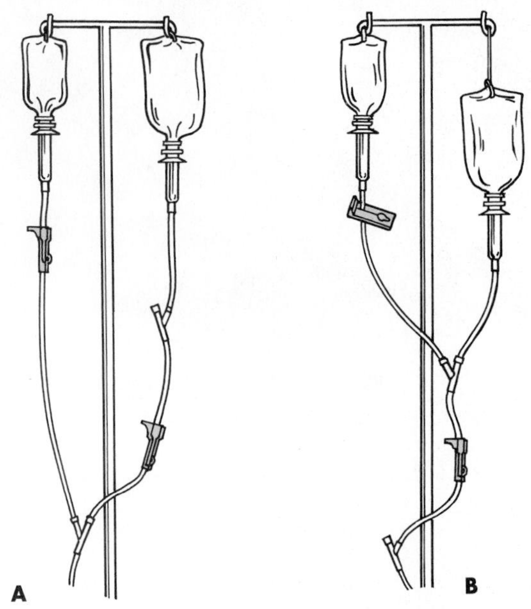

FIGURE **18-16** Intermittent infusion sets. **A,** Tandem set. **B,** Piggyback set.

2. *Piggyback.* A piggyback is a small (25 to 250 ml) IV bag or bottle connected to short tubing lines that connect to the *upper* Y-port of a primary infusion line or to an intermittent venous access (Figure 18-16, *B*). The piggyback tubing is a microdrip or macrodrip system (see Chapter 19). The set is called a "piggyback" because the small bag or bottle is set higher than the primary infusion bag or bottle. In the piggyback setup the main line does not infuse when the piggybacked medication is infusing. The port of the primary IV line contains a back check valve that automatically stops the flow of the primary infusion once the piggyback infusion flows. After the piggyback solution infuses and the solution within the tubing falls below the level of the primary infusion drip chamber, the back-check valve opens and the primary infusion again flows.
3. *Volume-control administration.* Volume-control administration (e.g., Volutrol, Buretrol, Pediatrol) sets are small (50 to 150 ml) containers that attach just below the primary infusion bag or bottle. The set is attached and filled in a manner similar to that used with a regular IV infusion. However, the priming filling of the set is different, depending on the type of filter (floating valve or membrane) within the set. Follow the package directions for priming sets.
4. *Miniinfusion pump.* The miniinfusion pump is battery operated. It allows medications to be given in very small amounts of fluid (5 to 60 ml) within controlled infusion times using standard syringes (Figure 18-17).

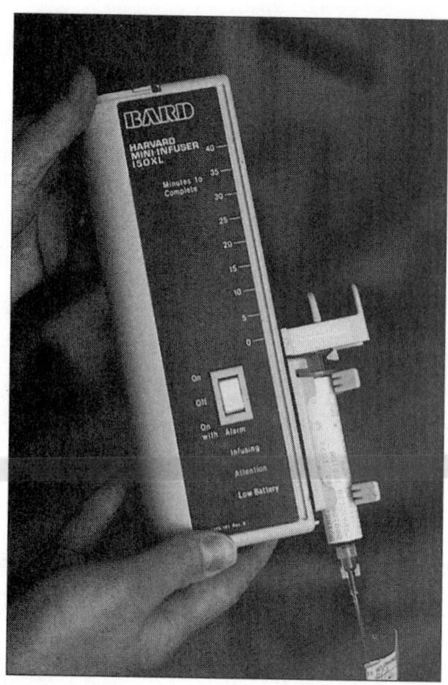

FIGURE **18-17** Subcutaneous infusion set.

The Centers for Disease Control and Prevention (CDC) and the Occupational Safety and Health Administration (OSHA) have made very strong recommendations that all intermittent infusion systems be needleless (National Institute for Occupational Safety and Health [NIOSH], 1999; OSHA, 2000). This can be achieved by using stopcocks or a needleless system (Figure 18-18) to attach medication tubings to the main line. Needleless infusion lines have blunt-ended cannulas or recessed connection ports, eliminating the risk of exposure to an IV needle.

A

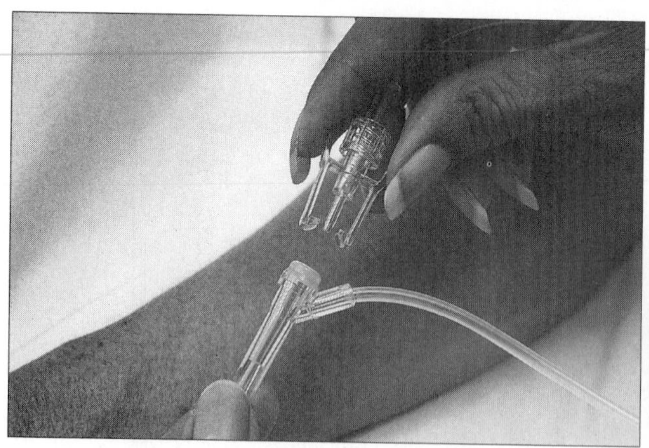

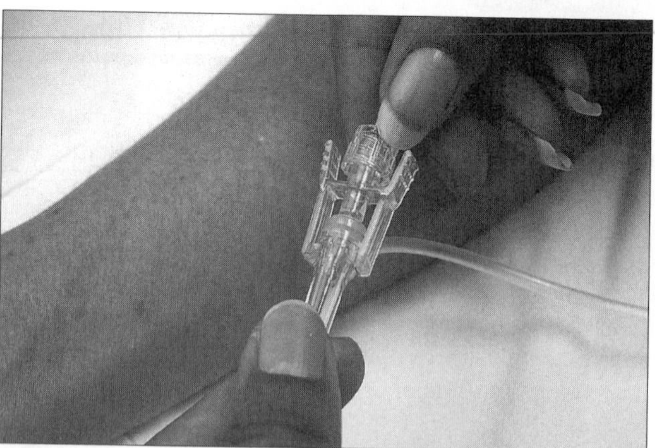

B

FIGURE **18-18** **A,** Needleless lever lock cannula system. **B,** Blunt-ended cannula inserts into port and locks.

Delegation Considerations

The skill of administering intravenous medications by intermittent infusion sets and miniinfusion pumps should not be delegated to assistive personnel. Assistive personnel should be instructed to report any unexpected drug reactions or reported discomfort at infusion site as soon as possible.

Equipment

- Antiseptic swab
- IV pole or rack
- Medication administration record (MAR) or computer printout
- Medication label

Piggyback, Tandem, or Miniinfuser Pump

- Medication prepared in 5- to 250-ml labeled infusion bag or syringe
- Short microdrip or macrodrip tubing set for piggyback (may have needleless system attachment)
- IV pump or miniinfusion pump, if indicated
- Adhesive tape (optional)

Volume-Control Administration Set

- Volutrol or Buretrol, Pediatrol
- Infusion tubing (may have needleless system attachment)
- Syringe (1 to 20 ml)
- Vial or ampule of ordered medication

Step	Rationale
Assessment	
1. Check physician's order to determine type of IV solution to be used, type of medication, dose, route, and time of administration.	Client's overall physical condition dictates type of IV solution used. Ensures safe and accurate drug administration.
2. Collect drug reference information necessary to administer drug safely, including how quickly to infuse the medication and its action, purpose, side effects, normal dose, time of peak onset, and nursing implications.	Allows nurse to give drug safely and to monitor client's response to therapy.
3. Assess compatibility of drug with existing IV solution.	Drugs that are incompatible with IV solutions may result in clouding or crystallization of solution in IV tubing, which may harm the client.

- ***Critical Decision Point***
  Never administer IV medications through tubing that is infusing blood, blood products, or parenteral nutrition solutions.

Step	Rationale
4. Assess patency of client's existing IV infusion line (see Chapter 19).	Intravenous line must be patent and fluids must infuse easily for medication to reach venous circulation effectively.

- ***Critical Decision Point***
  If the client's IV site is saline locked, cleanse the port with alcohol and assess the patency of the IV by flushing the IV with 2 to 3 ml of sterile normal saline. Attach appropriate IV tubing to the saline lock, and administer the medication via piggyback, tandem, miniinfuser, or volume-control administration set. When the infusion is completed, disconnect the tubing, cleanse the port with alcohol, and flush the IV with 2 to 3 ml sterile normal saline. Maintain sterility of IV tubing between intermittent infusions.

Step	Rationale
5. Assess IV insertion site for signs of infiltration or phlebitis: redness, pallor, swelling, and tenderness on palpation.	Confirmation of placement of IV needle or catheter and integrity of surrounding tissues ensures that medication is administered safely.
6. Assess client's history of drug allergies.	Effects of medications can develop rapidly after IV infusion. Nurse should be aware of clients at risk and not administer the medication if the client has an allergy to it.
7. Assess client's understanding of purpose of drug therapy.	May reveal need for education.

STEP | RATIONALE

NURSING DIAGNOSIS

Defining characteristics from the assessment data may reveal the following nursing diagnoses for clients requiring this skill:

Deficient knowledge regarding drug therapy
Risk for imbalanced fluid volume
Risk for ineffective health maintenance

Related factors are individualized based on client's condition or needs.

PLANNING

1. **Expected outcomes** following completion of procedure:
   - Drug infuses without adverse reactions. — Drug was given safely with desired therapeutic effect.
   - Medication infuses within desired period. — Intravenous line remains patent.
   - Intravenous site remains intact without signs of swelling or inflammation or symptoms of tenderness at site. — Fluid infuses into vein rather than tissues.
   - Client is able to explain drug purpose, action, side effects, and dosage. — Demonstrates learning.
2. Assemble supplies at bedside. — Drug preparation usually is not required. Nurse may assemble infusion tubing and bag of medication in medication area or client's room.

IMPLEMENTATION

1. Wash hands. — Reduces transmission of microorganisms.
2. Check client's identification by looking at arm bracelet and asking client's name. — Ensures drug is administered to correct client.
3. Explain purpose of medication and side effects to client. Explain that medication is to be given through existing IV line. Encourage client to report symptoms of discomfort at site. — Keeps client informed of treatment. Clients who can verbalize pain at the IV site can help detect IV infiltrations early, lessening damage to surrounding tissues.
4. **Piggyback or tandem infusion:**
   a. Connect infusion tubing to medication bag (see Chapter 19). Allow solution to fill tubing by opening regulator flow clamp. Re-cover end of tubing. — Infusion tubing should be filled with solution and free of air bubbles to prevent **air embolus.**

   - ***Critical Decision Point***

     An alternative method to priming the tubing is to clamp the infusion tubing, connect it to the medication bag, connect the medication tubing to the main IV tubing, lower the medication bag below the level of the main IV bag, unclamp the medication tubing, and allow the solution in the main IV bag to back up into the medication tubing. Clamp the medication tubing once the main IV bag has filled it, and hang medication bag on IV pole. This method prevents the loss of any medication during the priming of the medication tubing. It can also be used when clients are receiving more than one IV piggyback medication. To do this, lower the used medication bag and let it backflow until approximately 10 to 25 ml of the main IV solution enters the empty medication bag. Clamp the medication tubing, remove the used IV medication bag and connect the new IV medication bag. This clears out the tubing for the next IV medication, decreases the risk of contaminating the IV system, and saves money for the client because only one set of tubing is used for every IV medication ordered for the client.

   b. Hang piggyback medication bag above level of primary fluid bag. (Hook may be used to lower main bag.) Hang tandem infusion at same level as primary fluid bag. — Height of fluid bag affects rate of flow to client.

STEP	RATIONALE
c. Connect tubing of piggyback or tandem infusion to appropriate connector on primary infusion line:	
(1) *Stopcock:* Wipe off stopcock port with alcohol swab and connect tubing. Turn stopcock to open position.	Stopcock eliminates need for needle.
(2) *Needleless system:* Wipe off needleless port, and insert tip of piggyback or tandem infusion tubing. Lock into place as indicated by manufacturer of needleless system.	The CDC strongly recommends needleless connections to prevent accidental needle-stick injuries (National Institute for Occupational Safety and Health, 1999). Establishes route for IV medication to enter main IV line.
(3) *Tubing port:* Connect sterile 21- to 23-gauge needle to end of piggyback or tandem infusion tubing, remove cap, cleanse injection port on main IV line, and insert needle through center of port. Consider placing a piece of tape at the junction of where the needle enters the IV port to secure the medication line to the main IV line.	Prevents introduction of microorganisms during needle insertion.
d. Regulate flow rate of medication solution by adjusting regulator clamp or IV pump infusion rate. Rate of flow should be determined by institutional policy. If a policy does not exist, consult a pharmacist or a drug manual. (Usually medications are recommended to infuse within 20 to 90 minutes.)	Provides slow, safe, intermittent infusion of medication and maintains therapeutic blood levels.
e. After medication has infused, check flow regulator on primary infusion. Back-check valve on piggyback stops flow of the primary infusion until piggyback infuses. The tandem and primary infusions flow together until the tandem set empties. The primary infusion should automatically begin to flow after the piggyback or tandem solution is empty.	Valve prevents backup of medication into main infusion line. Checking flow rate ensures proper administration of IV fluids.
f. Regulate main infusion line to desired rate, if necessary.	Infusion of piggyback or tandem may interfere with main line infusion rate.
g. Leave IV piggyback bag and tubing in place for future drug administration, or discard in appropriate containers.	Establishment of IV piggyback or tandem line produces route for microorganisms to enter main line. Repeated changes in tubing increase risk of infection transmission (check agency policy).
5. Miniinfusion administration:	
a. Connect prefilled syringe to miniinfusion tubing.	Special tubing designed to fit syringe delivers medication to main IV line.
b. Carefully apply pressure to syringe plunger, allowing tubing to fill with medication.	Ensures that tubing is free of air bubbles to prevent air embolus.
c. Place syringe into miniinfusion pump (follow product directions). Be sure that syringe is secure.	
d. Connect miniinfusion tubing to main IV line.	
(1) *Stopcock:* Wipe off stopcock port with alcohol swab and connect tubing. Turn stopcock to open position.	Stopcock reduces risk of needle-stick injuries.
(2) *Needleless system:* Wipe off needleless port, and insert tip of miniinfuser tubing.	Needleless system reduces risk of needle-stick injuries.
(3) *Tubing port:* Connect sterile 21- to 23-gauge needle to miniinfuser tubing, remove cap, cleanse injection port on main IV line or saline lock, and insert needle through center of port. Consider placing tape where IV tubing enters port to keep connection secured.	Cleansing reduces transmission of microorganisms.

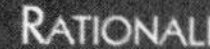

Step	Rationale
e. Hang infusion pump with syringe on IV pole alongside main IV bag. Set pump to deliver medication within time recommended by institutional policy, a pharmacist, or a medication reference manual. Press button on pump to begin infusion (see illustration). *Optional:* Set alarm.	Pump automatically delivers medication at safe, constant rate based on volume in syringe. (Alarm is used if medication is delivered into heparin/saline lock.)
f. After medication has infused, check flow regulator on primary infusion. Infusion should automatically begin to flow once pump stops. Regulate main infusion line to desired rate as needed. NOTE: If stopcock is used, turn off miniinfusion line.	Maintains patency of primary IV line.

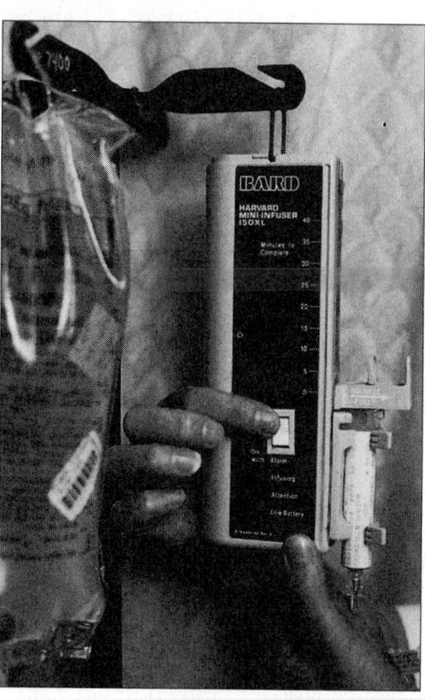

STEP **5e** Miniinfusion pump.

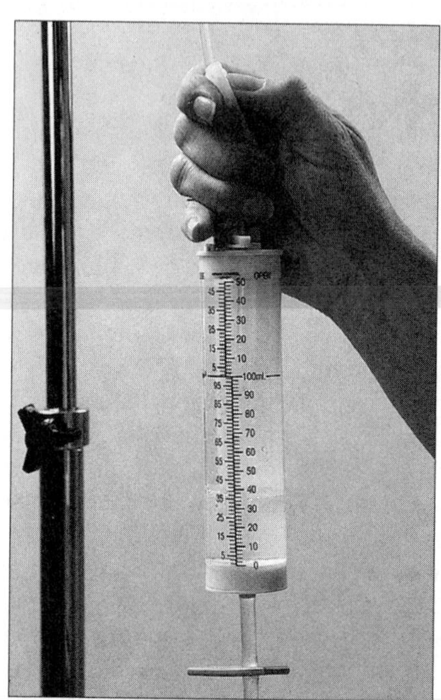

STEP **6b** Filling volume-control administration device.

Step	Rationale
6. **Volume-control administration set (e.g., Volutrol):**	
a. Prepare medication from vial or ampule (see Skill 18-1).	Ensures that medication is sterile.
b. Fill Volutrol with desired amount of fluid (usually 50 to 100 ml) by opening clamp between Volutrol and main IV bag (see illustration).	Small volume of fluid dilutes IV medication and reduces risk of too-rapid infusion.
c. Close clamp. Check to be sure clamp on air vent of Volutrol chamber is open.	Prevents additional leakage of fluid into Volutrol. Air vent allows fluid in Volutrol to exit at regulated rate.
d. Clean injection port on top of Volutrol with antiseptic swab.	Prevents introduction of microorganisms during needle insertion.
e. Remove needle cap or sheath, insert syringe needle adapter through port, and then inject medication (see illustrations). Gently rotate Volutrol between hands.	Rotating mixes medication with solution in Volutrol to ensure equal distribution.
f. Regulate IV infusion rate to allow medication to infuse in time recommended by institutional policy, a pharmacist, or a medication reference manual.	For optimal therapeutic effect, drug should infuse in prescribed time interval.
g. Label Volutrol with name of drug, dose, total volume (including diluent), and time of administration.	Alerts nurses to drug being infused. Prevents other medications from being added to Volutrol.

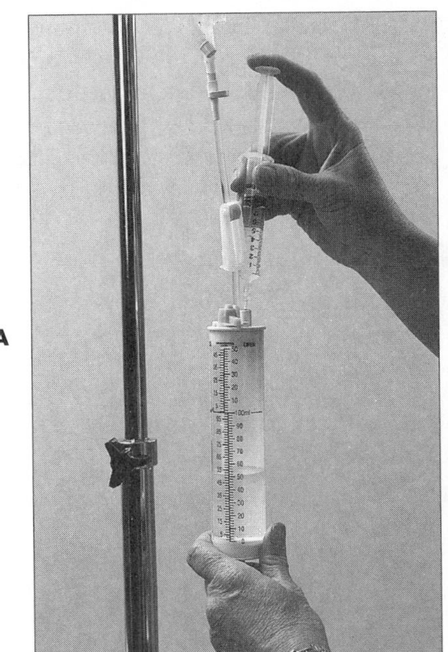
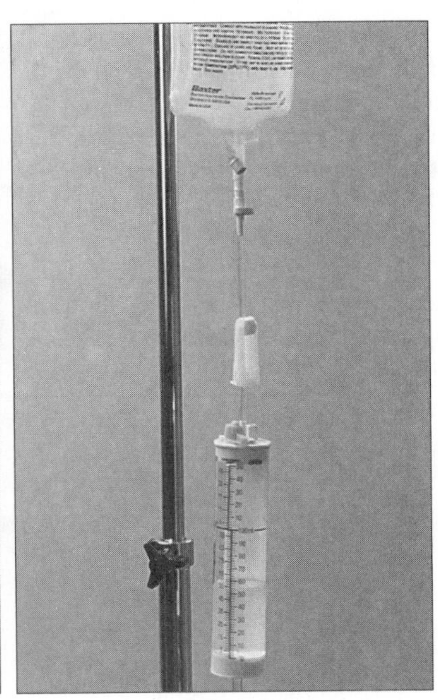

A B

STEP 6e A, Medication injected into device. B, Prepared device.

STEP	RATIONALE
h. Dispose of uncapped needle or needle enclosed in safety shield and syringe in proper container.	Prevents accidental needle sticks.
7. When medication has infused, be sure main IV solution is infusing as ordered or disconnect IV tubing from IV site and flush IV with either saline or heparin.	Assures continued patency of IV site.

EVALUATION

1. Observe client for signs of adverse reactions.	Intravenous medications act rapidly.
2. During the infusion, periodically check infusion rate and condition of IV site.	Intravenous line must remain patent for proper drug administration. Development of infiltration necessitates discontinuing infusion and possibly initiating IV extravasation care.
3. Ask client to explain purpose and side effects of medication.	Evaluates client's understanding of instruction.

UNEXPECTED OUTCOMES AND RELATED INTERVENTIONS

- Client develops adverse drug reaction.
  - Stop medication infusion immediately, and follow institutional policy or guidelines for appropriate response and reporting of adverse drug reactions.
  - Notify client's health care provider of adverse effects immediately.
- Medication does not infuse over desired period.
  - Can result from improper calculation of flow rate, malpositioning of IV needle at insertion site, or infiltration.
  - Determine reason, and take corrective action as indicated (e.g., correct flow rate, reposition IV, discontinue and restart IV).
- Intravenous site becomes swollen, warm, reddened, and tender to touch (see Chapter 19), indicating phlebitis.
  - Stop IV infusion, and discontinue IV.
  - Treat IV site as indicated by institutional policy and insert new IV site if continuation of IV therapy is indicated.
- Intravenous site becomes cool, pale, and swollen (see Chapter 19), indicating signs of infiltration.

- Some IV medications are extremely harmful to subcutaneous tissue. Provide IV extravasation care (e.g., injecting phentolamine [Regitine] around the IV infiltration site) as indicated by institutional policy, or use a medication reference or consult a pharmacist to determine appropriate follow-up care.

RECORDING AND REPORTING

- Immediately record drug, dose, route, and time administered on MAR or computer printout to record care provided and prevent future drug administration errors. Correctly sign MAR according to institutional policy.
- Record volume of fluid in medication bag or Volutrol on intake and output (I&O) form to monitor total fluid intake.
- Report any adverse reactions to client's health care provider. Client's response may indicate need for additional medical therapy.

HOME CARE CONSIDERATIONS

- See Skill 18-6, p. 534.

Skill 18-8 Administering Medications by Intravenous Bolus

An intravenous (IV) **bolus** involves introducing a concentrated dose of a drug directly into the systemic circulation. An IV bolus may be given directly into a vein, into an existing IV line through an injection port, or through a saline or heparin lock. A saline lock consists of an indwelling needle or catheter attached to a plastic tube with a sealed injection port on the end. Institutional policy dictates which medications the nurse may give by IV push.

The IV bolus allows no time to correct errors. Therefore nurses should be very careful in calculating the correct amount of the medication to give and may be required to have their calculations verified by another nurse. In addition, a bolus may cause direct irritation to the lining of blood vessels. Thus the nurse must be sure that the IV catheter or needle is correctly positioned in the client's vein. An IV bolus should never be given if the insertion site appears puffy or edematous or if the fluid from a connecting IV line cannot flow at the proper rate. Accidental injection of a medication into tissues surrounding a vein can cause pain, necrotic sloughing of tissues, and abscesses. The rate of administration of IV push drugs varies from drug to drug. Therefore the nurse must verify a medication's rate of administration with institutional guidelines before administering a drug. If institutional guidelines are not available, then use a medication manual to determine the appropriate rate of administration. The advantages and disadvantages to administering IV push medications are summarized in Box 18-4.

Box 18-4 Advantages and Disadvantages of the Intravenous Push Method

ADVANTAGES

- Rapid onset of medication's effects, which is especially helpful in clients experiencing critical or emergent alterations in health.
- Small amount of nursing time is required to prepare an IV push.
- Doses of medications are easily controlled. Therefore, dosages of short-acting medications can be titrated based on the client's individual requirements and responses to the drug therapy.
- IV push medications can be given one after another very quickly, avoiding the larger amounts of time that would be required if the medications had to be given by IV piggyback.

DISADVANTAGES

- Higher risk of side effects and adverse reactions; a temporary brief "toxicity" may occur since the medication peaks quickly with this route.
- If the medication is given very quickly (e.g., within 1 minute or less), there is little or no opportunity to stop the injection if an allergic reaction occurs.
- Increased risk of phlebitis, especially if a high concentrated medication is given or a small peripheral vein is used.

Modified from Keen JH: Slow down, *J Emerg Nurs* 21(4):323, 1995.

Delegation Considerations

The skill of administering medications by intravenous bolus should not be delegated to assistive personnel. Assistive personnel should be instructed to report any unexpected drug reactions or reported discomfort at infusion site as soon as possible.

Equipment

- Watch with second hand
- Medication administration record (MAR) or computer printout
- Disposable gloves
- Antiseptic swab

Intravenous Push (Existing Line)

- Medication in vial or ampule
- Syringe
- Needleless device or sterile needle (21 to 25 gauge)

Intravenous Push (Intravenous Lock)

- Medication in vial or ampule
- Syringe
- Vial of appropriate flush solution (saline most common, but heparin may also be used; if heparin is used, most common concentration is 10 to 100 units; check agency policy)
- Needleless device or sterile needle (21 to 25 gauge)

Step	Rationale
Assessment	
1. Check physician's order for type of medication, dose, time, and route of administration.	Ensures safe and accurate drug administration.
2. Collect drug reference information necessary to administer drug safely, including action, purpose, side effects, normal dose, time of peak onset, how slowly to give the medication, and nursing implications.	Allows nurse to give drug safely and to monitor client's response to therapy.

- ***Critical Decision Point***
  If a small amount of medication is given (e.g., less than 1 ml), dilute medication in 5 to 10 ml of normal saline or sterile water so that the medication does not collect in the "dead spaces" (e.g., Y-site injection port, IV cap) of the IV delivery system (Keen, 1995).

Step	Rationale
3. If drug is to be given through existing IV line, determine compatibility of medication with IV fluids and any additives within IV solution.	Intravenous medication may not be compatible with IV solution and/or additives.
4. Assess condition of IV needle insertion site for signs of infiltration or phlebitis.	Drug should not be administered if site is edematous or inflamed.
5. Check client's history of drug allergies.	Intravenous bolus delivers drug rapidly. Allergic reaction could prove fatal.
6. Assess client's understanding of purpose of drug therapy.	May reveal need for education.

Nursing Diagnosis

Defining characteristics from the assessment data may reveal the following nursing diagnoses for clients requiring this skill:

Deficient knowledge regarding medication therapy

Related factors are individualized based on client's condition or needs.

Planning

Step	Rationale
1. **Expected outcomes** following completion of procedure:	
▪ Drug infuses without adverse reactions occurring.	Drug is given safely.
▪ Intravenous site remains clear, without swelling.	Medication infuses without complications to IV site.
▪ Client will explain purpose and side effects of medication.	Demonstrates learning.
2. Assemble supplies in medication room.	Ensures sterile preparation of medications.
3. Prepare medication from vial or ampule (see Skill 18-1).	Ensures that medication is sterile and correctly prepared.

STEP	RATIONALE

IMPLEMENTATION

Step	Rationale
1. Wash hands.	Reduces transmission of microorganisms.
2. Check client's identification by looking at arm band and asking name. Compare with medication administration record.	Ensures that drug is administered to correct client.
3. Explain procedure to client. Encourage client to report symptoms of discomfort at IV site.	Informs client of planned therapies, keeps client involved in care, and helps identify possible infiltration early.
4. Put on disposable gloves.	Follows Centers for Disease Control and Prevention (CDC) recommendations to prevent accidental exposure to blood and body fluids (National Institute for Occupational Safety and Health [NIOSH], 1999).
5. **Intravenous push (existing line):**	
a. Select injection port of IV tubing closest to client. Whenever possible, injection port should be a stopcock or other needleless component.	The Occupational Safety and Health Administration (OSHA) and CDC strongly recommend that all IV injection sites be needleless to prevent needle-stick injuries (NIOSH, 1999).
b. Connect syringe to IV line: Clean port with antiseptic swab. Insert needleless tip of syringe or small-gauge needle containing drug through center of port.	Prevents introduction of microorganisms. Prevents damage to port diaphragm.
c. Occlude IV line by pinching tubing just above injection port (see illustration). Pull back gently on syringe's plunger to aspirate for blood return.	Final check ensures that medication is being delivered into bloodstream.

• ***Critical Decision Point***

In some cases, especially with a smaller gauge IV needle, blood return may not be aspirated, even if IV is patent. If IV site does not show signs of infiltration, and IV fluid is infusing without difficulty, proceed with IV push.

Step	Rationale
d. Release tubing and inject medication within amount of time recommended by institutional policy, pharmacist, or medication reference manual. Use a watch to time administrations (see illustration). Intravenous line may be pinched while pushing medication and released when not pushing medication. Allow IV fluids to infuse when not pushing medication.	Ensures safe drug infusion. Rapid injection of IV drug can be fatal. Allowing IV fluids to infuse while pushing IV drug will enable medication to be delivered to client at prescribed rate.

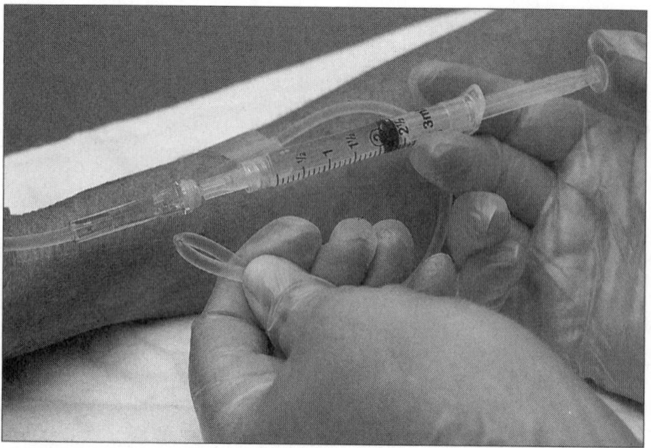

STEP **5c** Intravenous line pinched off for medication infusion.

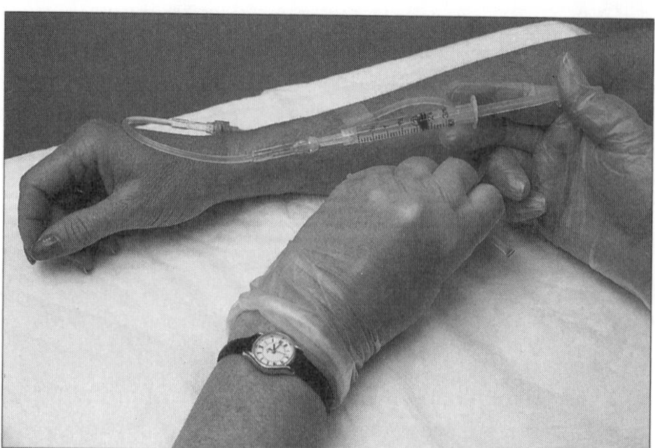

STEP **5d** Timing IV push administration.

STEP	RATIONALE

- ***Critical Decision Point***

If IV medication is incompatible with IV fluids, stop the IV fluids, clamp the IV line, flush with 10 ml of normal saline or sterile water, give the IV bolus over the appropriate amount of time, flush with another 10 ml of normal saline or sterile water at the same rate as the medication was administered, and then restart the IV fluids at the prescribed rate. If IV that is currently hanging is a medication (e.g., ranitidine), disconnect IV and administer IV push medication as outlined in Step 6 to avoid giving a sudden bolus of the medication in the existing IV line to the client. Allows nurse to give IV push medication through the existing line without creating potential risks associated with IV incompatibilities. Verify institutional policy regarding the stopping of IV fluids or continuous IV medications. If unable to stop IV infusion, start a new IV site (see Chapter 19) and administer medication using the IV push (IV lock) method.

e. After injecting medication, withdraw syringe, and recheck fluid infusion rate.

Injection of bolus may alter rate of fluid infusion. Rapid fluid infusion can cause circulatory fluid overload.

6. **Intravenous push (Intravenous lock):**
   a. Prepare flush solutions according to hospital policy.
      (1) Saline flush method (preferred method):
         - Prepare two syringes filled with 2 to 3 ml of normal saline (0.9%).

Normal saline has been found to be effective in keeping IV locks patent and is compatible with a wide range of medications.

      (2) Heparin flush method (traditional method):
         - Prepare one syringe with ordered amount of heparin flush solution.
         - Prepare two syringes with 2 to 3 ml of normal saline (0.9%).
   b. Administer drug:
      (1) Clean lock's injection port with antiseptic swab.

Cleaning prevents introduction of microorganisms during needle insertion.

      (2) Insert syringe with normal saline 0.9% through injection port of IV lock (see illustrations).
      (3) Pull back gently on syringe plunger and check for blood return.

Indicates if needle or catheter is in vein.

- ***Critical Decision Point***

In some cases, especially with a smaller gauge IV needle, blood return may not be aspirated, even if IV is patent. If IV site does not show signs of infiltration, and IV fluid is infusing without difficulty, proceed with IV push.

A
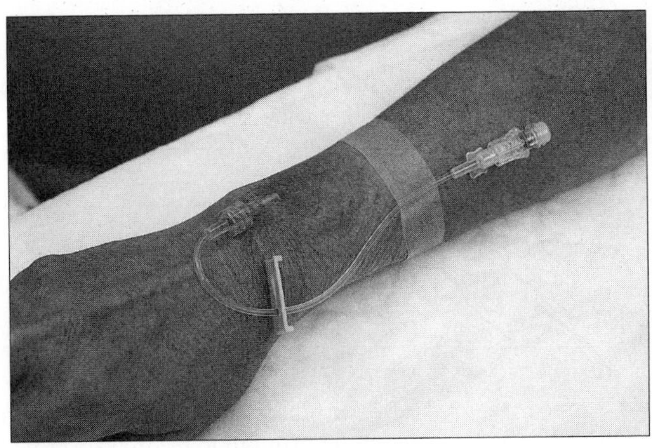
B
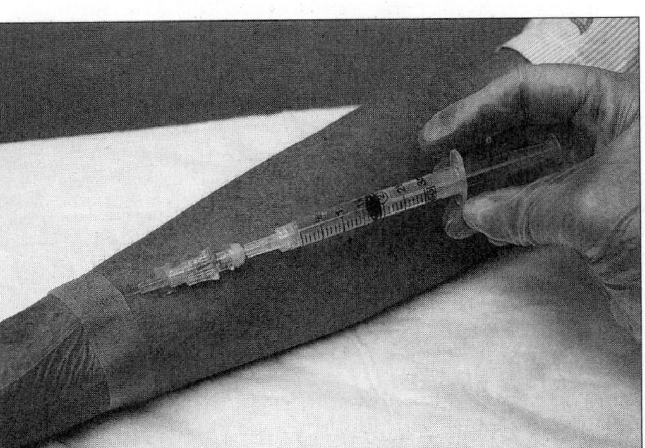

STEP **6b(2)** **A,** Intravenous catheter with saline lock adapter. **B,** Syringe inserted into injection port.

Step	Rationale
(4) Flush IV site with normal saline by pushing slowly on plunger.	Cleans needle and reservoir of blood. Flushing without difficulty indicates patent IV.

• ***Critical Decision Point***

Carefully observe the area of skin above the IV catheter. Note any puffiness or swelling as the IV site is flushed, which could indicate infiltration into the vein, requiring removal of catheter.

Step	Rationale
(5) Remove saline-filled syringe.	
(6) Clean lock's injection port with antiseptic swab.	Prevents transmission of infection.
(7) Insert syringe containing prepared medication through injection port of IV lock.	
(8) Inject medication within amount of time recommended by institutional policy, pharmacist, or medication reference manual. Use a watch to time administration.	Rapid injection of IV drug can cause death.
(9) After administering bolus, withdraw syringe.	
(10) Clean lock's injection site with antiseptic swab.	Prevents transmission of infection.
(11) Attach syringe with normal saline and inject normal saline flush at the same rate the medication was delivered.	Irrigation with saline prevents occlusion of IV access device and ensures all medication delivered (Keen, 1995). Flushing IV site at same rate as medication ensures that any medication remaining within IV needle is delivered at the correct rate.
(12) *Heparin flush option:* After instilling saline, attach syringe containing heparin flush. Inject heparin slowly and then remove syringe.	Maintains patency of IV needle by inhibiting clot formation. SASH method: Saline, Administration of medication, Saline, Heparin.
7. Dispose of uncapped needles and syringes in puncture-proof and leak-proof container.	Prevents accidental needle-stick injuries.
8. Wash hands.	Reduces transmission of microorganisms.

Evaluation

Step	Rationale
1. Observe client closely for adverse reactions during administration and for several minutes thereafter.	Intravenous medications act rapidly.
2. Observe IV site during injection for sudden swelling.	Determines development of infiltration into tissues surrounding vein.
3. Assess client's status after giving medication to evaluate the effectiveness of the medication.	Some IV bolus medications can cause rapid changes in the client's physiological status. Some drugs require careful monitoring and assessment and possibly future laboratory testing (e.g., vasopressors and antiarrhythmics require blood pressure and heart rate monitoring, whereas heparin requires laboratory studies after administration to determine if it is in a therapeutic level).
4. Ask client to explain drug's purpose and side effects.	Evaluates learning.

Unexpected Outcomes and Related Interventions

- Client develops adverse reaction to medication.
  - Stop delivering medication immediately, and follow institutional policy or guidelines for appropriate response and reporting of adverse drug reactions.
  - Notify client's health care provider of adverse effects immediately.
- Intravenous site becomes puffy.
  - Immediately discontinue administration of injection, and discontinue IV site.
  - Follow institutional guidelines on appropriate extravasation care.
- Client is unable to explain medication information.
  - Client requires reinstruction, or is unable to learn at this time.

Recording and Reporting

- Immediately record drug, dose, route, and time administered on MAR or computer printout to record care provided and prevent future drug administration errors. Correctly sign MAR according to institutional policy.
- Report any adverse reactions to client's health care provider. Client's response may indicate need for additional medical therapy.

PEDIATRIC CONSIDERATIONS

- Many practical problems exist when administering IV push medications to neonates, infants, and small children. The therapeutic dosage for these clients is often so small that it can be difficult to accurately prepare the prescribed dose, even with a tuberculin syringe. These drugs need to be infused very slowly and in small volumes because of the risk for fluid volume overload (Jew, Gordin, and Lengetti, 1997). Therefore, to maintain client safety, the nurse must carefully follow institutional policies when administering medications via IV bolus to this population.

Skill 18-9 Administering Continuous Subcutaneous Medications

The **continuous subcutaneous infusion (CSQI or CSCI)** route of medication administration is often used as an alternative to intravenous (IV) (e.g., IV bolus) or injection (e.g., intramuscular [IM], subcutaneous [SQ]) routes of medication administration. This route is mainly used for the administration of medications for pain management (e.g., opioids) and insulin. It has also been used with medications that stop preterm labor. No more than 1 to 2 ml/hr should be administered using CSQI. When the amount of fluid exceeds this amount, the absorption of the medication decreases (Poniatowski, 1991).

Continuous subcutaneous infusion is used in many settings, including the home, because it enables clients to manage their illness and/or pain without the risks and expenses involved with IV medication administration. When used for pain management, this route is also relatively easy to learn and understand. It has been associated with better pain control and less sleep disturbance related to pain when compared with intravenous pain medications (Dawson and others, 1999). Box 18-5 summarizes indications for the use of CSQI in clients requiring pain management. Selection criteria for clients considering an insulin pump as outlined by the American Association of Diabetes Educators' position statement (1997) are listed in Box 18-6.

The procedure to initiate and discontinue CSQI therapy is similar regardless of the type of medication that is being delivered. However, nursing assessment and interventions vary depending on the medication's classification and desired effect. For example, in pain management, the advanced practice nurse, physician, or pharmacist determines the drug dose based on how much pain medication the client uses in 24 hours. An equianalgesic chart is used to convert IV, IM, and oral (PO) medication doses to SQ doses. The nurse evaluates the effectiveness of the medication by assessing the client's pain. Alternatively, if the client is receiving insulin, the advanced practice nurse, physician, or pharmacist reviews how much insulin the client requires in a 24-hour period and the response to insulin in determining the appropriate basal (or continuous) rate and a sliding scale for the client to use before eating. The effectiveness of insulin therapy is evaluated by assessing the client's blood sugar levels and occurrences of hypoglycemia or hyperglycemia.

A small-gauge (25 to 27) winged or butterfly IV needle is used to deliver medications through CSQI (Figure 18-19). Alternatively, a special commercially prepared Teflon cannula may be used. Although Teflon needles are generally more expensive, they tend to be more comfortable for the client and

Box 18-5 Common Characteristics of Clients Receiving Pain Management by Continuous Subcutaneous Infusion

- Inability to tolerate oral medications (e.g., nausea and vomiting, dysphagia, malabsorption)
- Requires continuous or large amounts of medications to control pain
- Poor venous access
- Will require injections (e.g., SQ, IM) for more than 48 hours
- Is confused, drowsy, or has altered level of consciousness
- Inability to afford IV therapy

Box 18-6 Selection Criteria for Clients Using Insulin Pumps

- Requires or desires improved control of blood sugars levels
- Daily routine requires greater flexibility than allowed by traditional insulin injection schedules
- Strong motivation and commitment to use diabetes management skills
- Acceptance of responsibilities associated with the self-management of diabetes
- Ability to perform self–blood glucose monitoring and to operate the insulin pump
- Evidence of effective coping patterns
- Availability of support systems
- Availability of financial resources to cover costs associated with CSQI

Modified from American Association of Diabetes Educators: AADE position statement: education for continuous subcutaneous insulin infusion pump users, *Diabetes Educator* 23(4):397, 1997.

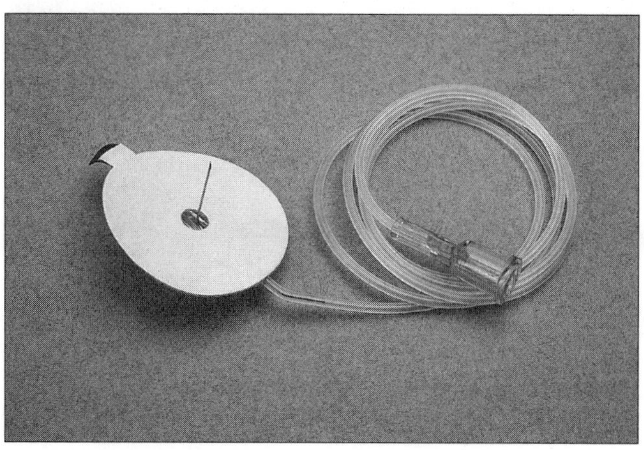

FIGURE **18-19** Small-gauge butterfly needle and tubing for CSQI therapy.

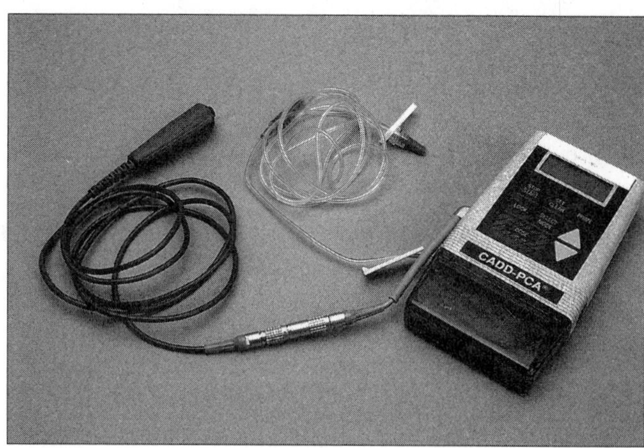

FIGURE **18-20** Medication pump.

have lower rates of complications when compared with winged IV needles (Macmillan and others, 1994). The choice of needle type is based on institutional guidelines or client preference. The needle used should be of the shortest length and the smallest gauge necessary to establish and maintain the infusion (Intravenous Nursing Society, 1998).

Anatomical sites for subcutaneous injections (see Figure 18-10) and the upper chest may be used for medication administration in this route. Site selection depends on the client's activity level and the type of medication delivered. For example, pain medications given to ambulatory clients are best delivered in the upper chest. This allows the client to move freely. Insulin is absorbed most consistently in the abdomen, thus a site in the abdomen away from the belt line is the preferred site for insulin administration. Sites should be free from irritation, away from bony prominences and the waistline, and rotated at least every 72 hours or whenever complications (e.g., infection, leaking) occur (Intravenous Nursing Society, 1998).

Medications given by the CSQI route require a computerized pump with safety features, including lockout intervals and warning alarms. A variety of medication pumps are currently available (Figure 18-20). If used at home, clients should be able to give themselves loading doses and boluses of the medication when needed. Ideally, medication pumps should be chosen for each individual, based on the medication being delivered and the client's needs. Other factors used in the selection process of the appropriate pump include the availability and cost of the pump and its supplies. When possible, clients using CSQI at home should be offered a selection of pumps and be allowed to choose the one that they find the easiest to use.

Delegation Considerations

The skill of administering continuous subcutaneous medications should not be delegated to assistive personnel. Assistive personnel should be instructed to report any unexpected drug reactions or leaking at insertion site as soon as possible.

Equipment

Initiation of CSQI Therapy

- Clean, nonsterile gloves
- Alcohol swab
- Povidone-iodine swab
- Small- (25- to 27-) gauge winged IV catheter with attached tubing or catheter designed especially for CSQI (e.g., Sof-set)
- Infusion pump
- Occlusive, transparent dressing
- Tape
- Medication in appropriate syringe or container

Discontinuing CSQI

- Clean, nonsterile gloves
- 2 × 2 gauze dressing and tape or adhesive bandage
- Alcohol swab and povidone-iodine swab (optional)

Step	Rationale
Assessment	
1. Check physician's order for type of medication, dosage, and route of administration.	Ensures safe and accurate drug administration.

STEP	RATIONALE
2. Collect drug reference information necessary to administer drug safely, including action, purpose, side effects, safe dosage range, and nursing implications. Verify that medication can be given through this route.	Allows nurse to give drug safely using this route and to monitor client's response to therapy.
3. Assess client's medical history, drug allergies, and medication history.	Indicates client's need for medication, contraindications for medication use, and risk for drug interactions.
4. Assess for factors that may contraindicate CSQI, such as circulatory shock or reduced local tissue perfusion.	Reduced tissue perfusion interferes with drug absorption and distribution.
5. Assess adequacy of client's adipose tissue to determine appropriate site.	Physiological changes of aging or client illness may influence amount of SQ tissue a client possesses. This influences choice of catheter insertion site.
6. Assess client's knowledge regarding medication to be received. (NOTE: Assess pain severity if analgesic to be given.)	Information may pose implications for client education.

NURSING DIAGNOSIS

Defining characteristics from the assessment data may reveal the following nursing diagnoses for clients requiring this skill:

- Anxiety
- Fear
- Ineffective health maintenance
- Risk for infection
- Risk for injury
- Deficient knowledge regarding CSQI therapy
- Pain (acute, chronic)

Related factors are individualized based on client's condition or needs.

PLANNING

STEP	RATIONALE
1. **Expected outcomes** following completion of procedure:	
▪ Needle insertion site remains free from infection.	Risk for infection at needle insertion site is a potential complication of CSQI therapy.
▪ Desired effect of medication achieved with no signs of allergies or undesired effects.	Medication is delivered effectively.
▪ Client explains purpose, dosage, and effects of medication and verbalizes understanding of CSQI therapy.	Demonstrates learning.
2. Check medication administration record, computer printout, or physician's order.	Ensures safe medication administration.
3. Prepare correct medication dose from vial or ampule (see Skill 18-1) or check dose on prefilled syringe and prime tubing with medication.	Ensures that medication is sterile and dose is accurate.
4. Obtain and program medication administration pump.	Needed for safe medication infusion.
5. Explain procedure to client and proceed in calm, confident manner.	Involves client in care and eases anxiety.

IMPLEMENTATION

STEP	RATIONALE
1. Provide for privacy.	Respects client's dignity.
2. Wash hands.	Reduces transmission of microorganisms.
3. **To initiate CSQI:**	
a. Select appropriate injection site. Most common sites used are subclavicular, abdominal, upper arms or thighs (Intravenous Nursing Society, 1998).	Site must be free from irritation and not over bony prominences.
b. Assist client to comfortable position.	Eases pain associated with insertion of needle.

Step	Rationale
c. Cleanse injection site with alcohol followed by povidone-iodine in a circular fashion. Allow both alcohol and povidone-iodine to dry.	Reduces risk of infection at insertion site.

- ***Critical Decision Point***
  Clients allergic to povidone-iodine or managing CSQI at home may use an antibacterial soap (e.g., Hibiclens, PhisoHex) instead of alcohol and povidone-iodine to cleanse insertion site (Frazzitta-Luerssen, 1997).

Step	Rationale
d. Put on clean, nonsterile gloves.	Follows Centers for Disease Control and Prevention (CDC) recommendations to prevent accidental exposure to blood and body fluids (National Institute for Occupational Safety and Health [NIOSH], 1999).
e. Hold needle in dominant hand, and remove needle guard.	Prepares needle for insertion.
f. Gently pinch or lift up skin with nondominant hand.	Ensures needle will enter subcutaneous tissue.
g. Gently and firmly insert needle at a 45- to 90-degree angle (see illustration).	Decreases pain related to insertion of needle.

- ***Critical Decision Point***
  Some prepackaged needles (e.g., Sof-Set, Sub-Q-Set) are inserted at a 90-degree angle. These needles are shorter than butterfly needles. Refer to manufacturer's directions.

Step	Rationale
h. Release skinfold and apply tape over "wings" of needle.	Secures needle.

- ***Critical Decision Point***
  Some cannulas have a sharp needle with a plastic catheter covering the needle. In this case, remove the needle and leave the plastic catheter in the skin.

Step	Rationale
i. Place occlusive, transparent dressing over insertion site (see illustration).	Protects site from infection and allows nurse to assess site during medication infusion.
j. Attach tubing from needle to tubing from infusion pump.	Allows medication to be administered.
k. Turn infusion pump on.	Initiates medication therapy.
l. Dispose of any sharps in appropriate leak-proof, puncture-resistant container. Discard used supplies and wash hands.	Prevents injury to client and health care personnel (NIOSH, 1999).
m. Assess site before leaving client, and instruct client to inform nurses if site becomes red or begins to leak.	A new site with a new needle must be initiated whenever erythema or leaking occurs (Intravenous Nursing Society, 1998).

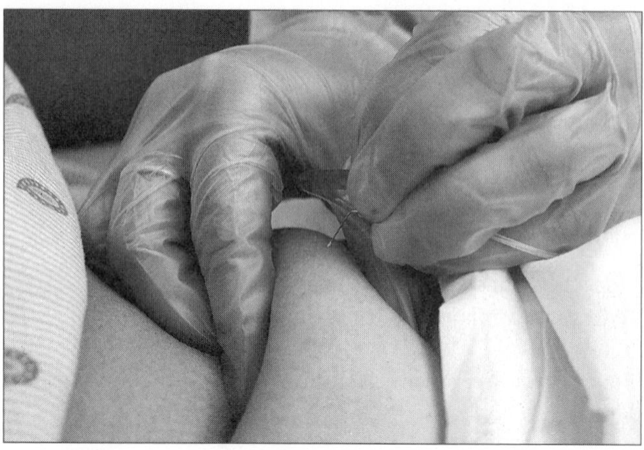

STEP **3g** Insertion of butterfly needle into subcutaneous tissue of abdomen.

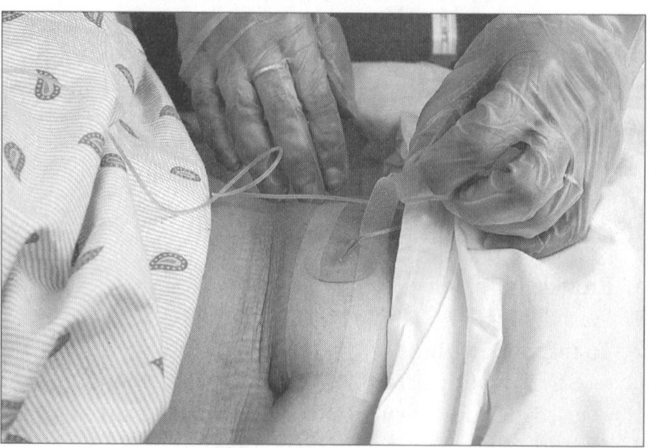

STEP **3i** Securing insertion site.

STEP	RATIONALE
4. To discontinue CSQI:	
a. Verify health care provider's order and establish alternative method for medication administration if applicable.	If medication will be required after discontinuing CSQI, a different medication and/or route may be necessary to continue to manage client's illness or pain.
b. Stop infusion pump.	Prevents spillage of medication.
c. Put on clean, nonsterile gloves.	Follows CDC recommendations to prevent accidental exposure to blood and body fluids (NIOSH, 1999).
d. Remove dressing without dislodging or removing the needle.	Exposes needle.

• ***Critical Decision Point***
If site is infected or if included in institutional guidelines, cleanse site with alcohol and then povidone-iodine swabs.

STEP	RATIONALE
e. Remove tape from the wings of needle and pull needle out at the same angle it was inserted.	Promotes comfort.
f. Apply pressure at site until no fluid leaks out of skin.	Dressing will stick to site if skin remains dry.
g. Apply 2 × 2 gauze dressing or adhesive bandage to site.	Prevents bacterial entry into puncture site.
h. Discard used supplies and wash hands.	Reduces transmission of microorganisms

EVALUATION

STEP	RATIONALE
1. Evaluate client's response to medication.	Indicates possible need to alter medication dosage based on client's response or presence of adverse effects. Decreased or absent response to medication may indicate client is not receiving medication into subcutaneous tissue (e.g., pump malfunction, medication leaking at site).
2. Observe site at least every 4 hours for redness, pain, drainage, or swelling.	Indicates infection at insertion site.

UNEXPECTED OUTCOMES AND RELATED INTERVENTIONS

- Client complains of localized pain or burning at needle's insertion site, or site appears red, swollen, or is leaking.
  - Symptoms indicate potential infection
  - Leakage at the site indicates needle is not securely in SQ tissue. Remove needle, and place new needle in a different site.
- Client displays signs of allergic reaction to medication.
  - Follow institutional policy or guidelines for appropriate response to allergic reactions, and notify client's health care provider immediately.
- Continuous subcutaneous infusion becomes dislodged.
  - Stop the infusion, apply pressure at the site until no fluid leaks out of skin, cover site with a 2 × 2 gauze dressing or adhesive bandage, and initiate a new site.
  - Assess client to determine effects of not receiving medication (e.g., assess pain level if client is receiving pain medication via CSQI).
  - Document dislodgement of CSQI, assessment findings, and nursing interventions in client's permanent record. Dislodgement of CSQI may necessitate notifying the client's primary care provider and/or documenting the event on an occurrence report per institutional policy.
- Desired effect of medication not achieved.
  - Follow established protocols for titration of medication, or notify client's health care provider for either change in dosage or medication.

RECORDING AND REPORTING

- Immediately after initiating CSQI, chart medication, dose, route, site, time, date, and type of medication pump in appropriate place in client's chart.
- Record client's response to medication and appearance of site every 4 hours or according to institutional policy.
- Report any adverse effects from medication or infection at insertion site to client's health care provider, and document according to institutional policy. Client's condition may indicate need for additional medical therapy.

TEACHING CONSIDERATIONS

- Instruct client to wear medical identification bracelet indicating important medical information, including disease client has (e.g., diabetes) and allergies.
- Clients receiving insulin require intensive diabetes management instruction (Box 18-7).

PEDIATRIC CONSIDERATIONS

- Despite the barriers to CSQI in adolescents with diabetes (e.g., frequent blood sugar testing, wearing tight clothing, transferring responsibility of diabetes management from parent to child), insulin pumps offer more flexibility, and insulin dosage can be quickly changed based on the client's current situation. To achieve successful diabetes management, intensive education is required both for the client and the family, especially during the first few weeks after starting CSQI. The nurse must ensure clients and their families have all the information and skills necessary to use CSQI. The nurse also plays an important role in follow-up care, education, and the enhancement of problem-solving skills (Boland, Ahern, and Grey, 1998).

GERONTOLOGICAL CONSIDERATIONS

- Continuous subcutaneous infusion can be used to deliver isotonic IV solutions to dehydrated older adults. This is called **hypodermoclysis** therapy. This method of providing hydration avoids the need to transfer the client from home or long-term care facility to an acute care hospital. Fluids should infuse slowly (e.g., 30 ml/hr) during the first hour of hypodermoclysis. If the client remains comfortable, the rate of infusion may be increased. Usually infusion rates do not exceed 80 ml/hr (Worobec and Brown, 1997). Fluids given through hypodermoclysis should only be administered for a short time. If long-term management is required, an IV access should be initiated.

HOME CARE CONSIDERATIONS

- When clients are going home using CSQI, the nurse should assess the client's readiness to learn before teaching how to administer medications using this route. A responsible caregiver should be included in the instructions. Clients and caregivers should understand the desired effect of the medication, side effects and adverse effects of the medication, operation of the pump, how to evaluate the effectiveness of the medication, when and how to assess and rotate injection sites, and when to call a health care provider for problems. They also need to determine where and how to obtain the required supplies (Poniatowski, 1991).

Box 18-7 Educational Topics Essential for Clients Receiving Insulin With Continuous Subcutaneous Infusion

- Blood sugar monitoring
- Meal planning and food choices
- Incorporating exercise into daily routine
- How to program and use the insulin pump
- Sick-day guidelines and management
- Treatment of hypoglycemia, including use of glucagon
- Treatment of hyperglycemia and prevention of diabetic ketoacidosis
- Prevention of infection, especially at site of infusion
- Problem-solving and decision-making skills
- Special considerations and precautions (e.g., what to do with pump when showering and sleeping)

Modified from American Association of Diabetes Educators: AADE position statement: Education for continuous subcutaneous insulin infusion pump users, *Diabetes Educator* 23(4):397, 1997.

Critical Thinking Exercises

1. You are administering an intravenous (IV) bolus of digoxin. During the administration of the medication, your client begins to complain of pain at the IV site. What steps would you take?
2. Your client has an order for 4 mg of dexamethasone (Decadron) to be given IV push now. You have never given this drug before. Describe the steps you should take before giving this medication. Give rationales for your answer.
3. Your client is receiving morphine through continuous subcutaneous infusion. He begins to complain of pain and rates it as an 8 on a 1 to 10 pain scale. What does this tell you about his level of pain control? Describe how you would manage his pain. What would you assess as his medication dosage is altered?
4. Your client is to receive 10 mg morphine sulfate intramuscularly for acute postoperative pain. The client is a 68-year-old woman who weighs about 120 lb and is 5 feet 5 inches. When you enter the room, the client asks you to give the injection in her arm. What would you do?

References

American Association of Diabetes Educators: AADE position statement: education for continuous subcutaneous insulin infusion pump users, *Diabetes Educator* 23(4):397, 1997.

American Diabetes Association: Insulin administration: clinical practice recommendations, *Diabetes Care* 20(suppl 1):46S, 1997.

American Nurses Association: Nursing facts about needlestick injuries, http://www.nursingworld.org/readroom/fsneedle.htm, January 31, 2000.

Beecroft PC, Kongelbeck RS: How safe are intramuscular injections? *AACN Clin Issues* 5(4):207, 1994.

Beyea SC, Nicoll LH: Administration of medications via the intramuscular route: an integrative review of the literature and research-based protocol for the procedure, *Appl Nurs Res* 8(1):23, 1995.

Beyea SC, Nicoll LH: Back to basics: administering IM injections the right way, *Am J Nurs* 96(1):34, 1996.

Boland E, Ahern J, Grey M: A primer on the use of insulin pumps in adolescents, *Diabetes Educator* 24(1):78, 1998.

Dawson L and others: Improving patients' postoperative sleep: a randomized control study comparing subcutaneous with intravenous patient-controlled analgesia, *J Adv Nurs* 30(4):875, 1999.

Frazzitta-Luerssen M.: Infusion site do's and don'ts, *Diabetes Forecast* 50(2):45, 1997.

Hadley SA, Chang M, Rogers K: Effect of syringe size on bruising following subcutaneous heparin injection, *Am J Crit Care* 5(4):271, 1996.

Intravenous Nursing Society: Standards for continuous subcutaneous medication administration, *J Intravenous Nurs* 21(suppl 1):S32, 1998.

Jew RK, Gordin P, Lengetti E: Clinical implications of IV drug administration in infants and children, *Crit Care Nurse* 17(4):62, 1997.

Keen JH: Slow down, *J Emerg Nurs* 21(4):323, 1995.

Macmillan K and others: A prospective comparison study between a butterfly needle and a Teflon cannula for subcutaneous narcotic administration, *J Pain Symptom Manage* 9(2):82: 1994.

McConnell EA: The subtle art of really good injections, *RN* 45:24, 1982.

McConnell EA: Administering a Z-track IM injection, *Nursing* 29(1):26, 1999.

Meister FL: Ask the experts, *Crit Care Nurse* 18(4):97, 1998.

National Institute for Occupational Safety and Health (NIOSH): NIOSH alert: preventing needlestick injuries in health care settings, NIOSH Publications Dissemination DHHS (NIOSH) Pub No. 2000-108, November 1999.

Occupational Safety and Health Administration (OSHA): OSHA instruction on enforcement procedures for the occupational exposure to bloodborne pathogens, http://www.osha-slc.gov/OshDoc/Directive data/CPL 2-2 44D.html, January 31, 2000.

Peragallo-Dittko V: Rethinking subcutaneous injection technique, *Am J Nurs* 97(5):71, 1997.

Poniatowski BC: Continuous subcutaneous infusions for pain control, *J Intravenous Nurs* 14(1):30, 1991.

Posey D, Long B: Always swab the stopper on vials before each use, *RN* 59(2):9, 1996.

Powers FA: Your elderly patient needs I.V. therapy . . . Can you keep her safe? *Nursing* 29(7), 1999.

Rogers B: Is health care a risky business? *Am Nurse,* 29(5):5, 1997.

Ross S, Soltes D: Heparin and haematoma: Does ice make a difference? *J Adv Nurs* 21, 434, 1995.

Wong DL and others: *Whaley and Wong's nursing care of infants and children,* ed 6, St. Louis, 1999, Mosby.

Workman B: Safe injection techniques, *Nurs. Stand* 13(39):47, 1999.

Worobec F, Brown MK: Hypodermoclysis therapy in a chronic care hospital setting, *J Gerontol Nurs* 23(6):23, 1997.

Zimmerman PG, Pierce B: Double-checking medications, *J Emerg Nurs* 24(6):586, 1998.

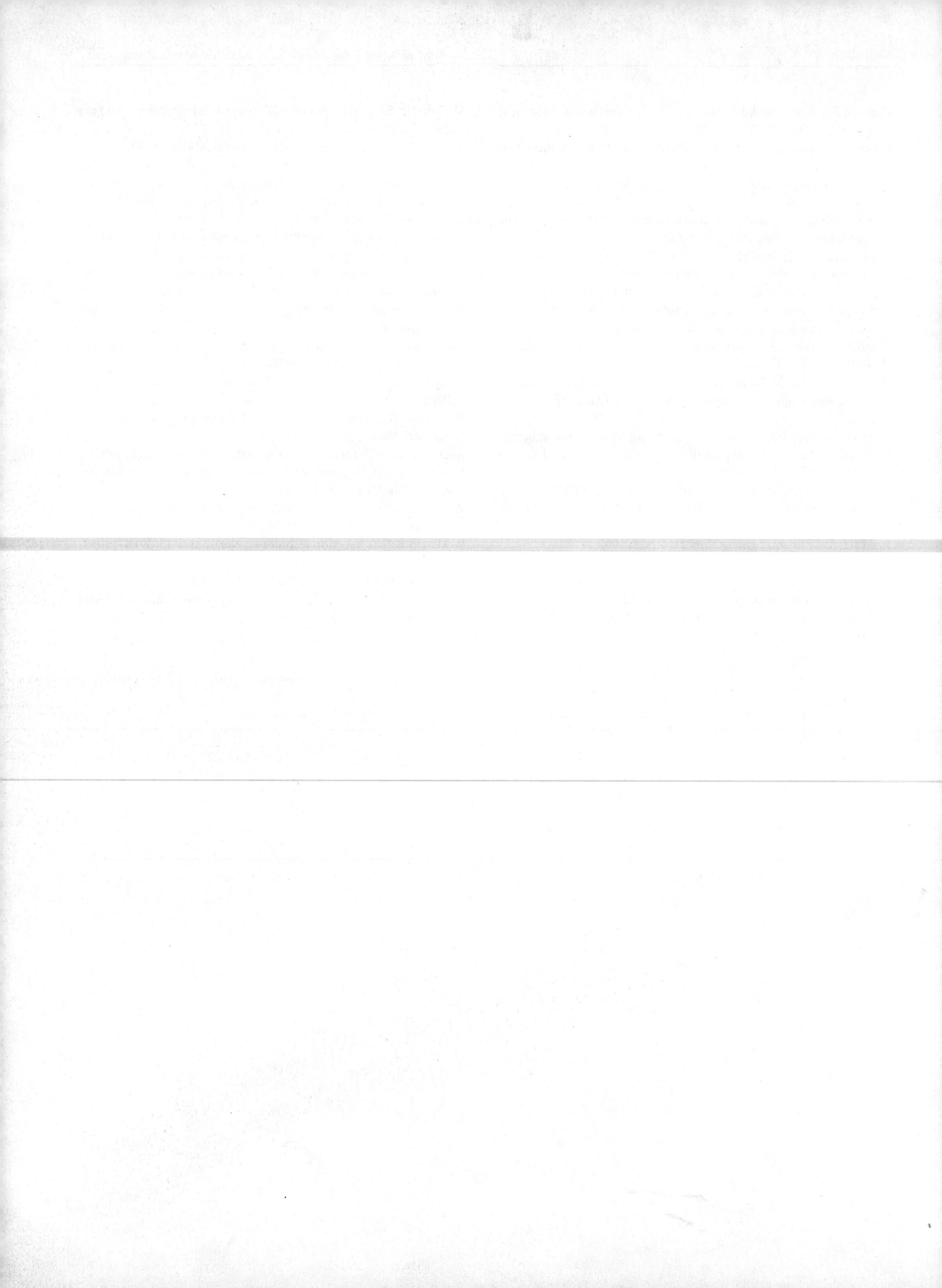

19

INTRAVENOUS AND VASCULAR ACCESS THERAPY

Skills

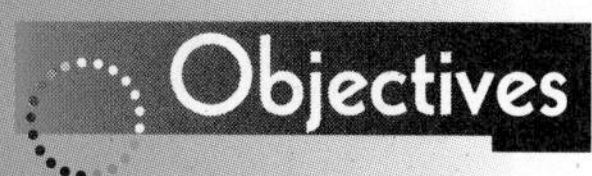

Mastery of content in this chapter will enable the nurse to:

- Define the key terms listed.
- Discuss conditions requiring intravenous (IV) therapy.
- Explain how to prepare the client and family for IV therapy.
- Discuss factors that increase the risk of complications from IV therapy.
- Identify individualized outcomes for clients requiring IV therapy.
- Explain techniques used to prevent transmission of infection for a client receiving IV therapy.
- Demonstrate initiation of IV therapy, regulation of IV flow rate, changing of IV solutions, changing of IV tubing, changing of IV dressings, and discontinuing a peripheral IV.
- Identify common types of vascular access devices (VADs) and describe their care and maintenance.
- Identify the educational needs of clients with VADs.

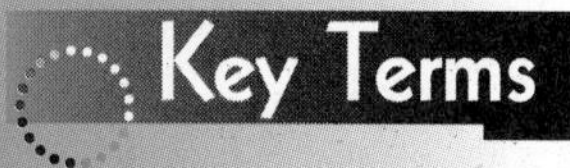

Cannula
Central venous catheter (CVC)
Drop factor
Electrolyte
Electronic infusion device (EID)
Embolus (Emboli)
Exit site
Fluid volume deficit (FVD)
Fluid volume excess (FVE)
Heparin lock
Hypertonic
Hypokalemia
Hypotonic
Implanted infusion port
Infiltration
Infusion pump
Injection cap
Isotonic
IV plug
Noncoring Huber needle
Over-the-needle catheter (ONC)
Percutaneous
Peripherally inserted central catheter (PICC)
Phlebitis
Saline lock
Sharps container
Subcutaneous tunnel
Thrombosis
Vascular access device (VAD)
Venipuncture

Parenteral Replacement of Fluids

Fluids may be infused directly into the circulating blood volume to supplement or replace body fluids. This form of therapy is common for clients requiring surgery and for clients too ill to tolerate oral or enteral nutrition. Parenteral fluid replacement includes intravenous (IV) fluid and electrolyte therapy, blood therapy (Chapter 20), total parenteral nutrition (TPN) and peripheral parenteral nutrition (PPN) (Chapter 23). The goal of IV fluid administration is to correct or prevent fluid and electrolyte imbalances, correct or prevent nutritional imbalances, or to provide IV medication therapy. When IV therapy is necessary, the nurse must know the correct solution and equipment needed and how to initiate an infusion, regulate the fluid infusion rate, care for and maintain the system, identify and correct problems, and discontinue the infusion.

Intravenous Solutions

Prepared IV solutions fall into three general categories: isotonic, hypotonic, and hypertonic (Table 19-1). An **isotonic** solution has a total electrolyte content of approximately 310 mEq/L. A **hypotonic** solution has a total electrolyte content of less than 250 mEq/L. A **hypertonic** solution has a total electrolyte content of 375 mEq/L or greater (Metheny, 2000). All IV fluids should be carefully given, especially hypertonic solutions, because these solutions pull fluid into the vascular space by osmosis, resulting in an increased vascular volume that can result in pulmonary edema, particularly in clients with cardiac or renal diseases. The type and amount of IV solution ordered by the physician are determined by the client's serum electrolyte values and fluid volume balance. The nurse must understand the rationale for IV fluid administration and the type of IV solution ordered. Because the names of IV solutions are often abbreviated or shortened, the nurse must be careful to give the correct solution (Box 19-1).

In addition to the specific IV fluid ordered, the physician often includes additives such as vitamins or potassium. Clients with properly functioning kidneys who are NPO (nothing by mouth) should have potassium added to the IV solution. Prepared bags of IV fluids with potassium already added should be used if available to decrease the chance of fluid contamination. If the physician's order does not include potassium, the nurse should double-check the order. Kidneys routinely excrete potassium, and if there is no potassium intake orally or parenterally, **hypokalemia** can develop.

Intravenous Catheters

The majority of peripheral venous catheters in the United States are made of silicone and polymers, including polyurethane and flexane (Orr, 1999). Metal needles, once the only type of intravenous device, are used infrequently because of the high degree of vein trauma and complication of IV infiltration. Many companies make a short catheter with a removable needle that looks just like a butterfly needle minus the needle. Despite advancements in catheter products, there is still risk of injury to blood vessel walls. Stiffer catheter materials, such as polyurethane, have been shown to result in more

Table 19-1 Composition and Use of Commonly Prescribed Crystalloid Solutions

Solution	Tonicity	mOsm/L (mmol/L)	Glucose (g/L)	Indications and Considerations
Dextrose in Water				
5%	Isotonic	278	50	Provides free water necessary for renal excretion of solutes Used to replace water losses and treat hypernatremia Provides 170 calories/L Does not provide any electrolytes
10%	Hypertonic	556	100	Provides free water only, no electrolytes Provides 340 calories/L
Saline				
0.45%	Hypotonic	154	0	Provides free water in addition to Na^+ and Cl^- Used to replace hypotonic fluid losses Used as maintenance solution although it does not replace daily losses of other electrolytes Provides no calories
0.9%	Isotonic	308	0	Used to expand intravascular volume and replace extracellular fluid losses Only solution that may be administered with blood products Contains Na^+ and Cl^- in excess of plasma levels Does not provide free water, calories, other electrolytes May cause intravascular overload or hyperchloremic acidosis
3.0%	Hypertonic	1026	0	Used to treat symptomatic hyponatremia Must be administered slowly and with extreme caution because it may cause dangerous intravascular volume overload and pulmonary edema
Dextrose in Saline				
5% in 0.225%	Isotonic	355	50	Provides Na^+, Cl^-, and free water Used to replace hypotonic losses and treat hypernatremia Provides 170 calories/L
5% in 0.45%	Hypertonic	432	50	Same as 0.45% NaCl except provides 170 calories/L
5% in 0.9%	Hypertonic	586	50	Same as 0.9% NaCl except provides 170 calories/L
Multiple Electrolyte Solutions				
Ringer's solution	Isotonic	309	0	Similar in composition to plasma except that it has excess Cl^-, no Mg^{2+}, and no HCO_3^- Does not provide free water or calories Used to expand the intravascular volume and replace extracellular fluid losses
Lactated Ringer's (Hartmann's) Solution	Isotonic	274	0	Similar in composition to normal plasma except does not contain Mg^{2+} Used to treat losses from burns and lower gastrointestinal tract May be used to treat mild metabolic acidosis but should not be used to treat lactic acidosis Does not provide free water or calories

Modified from Horne MM, Easterday Heitz U, Swearingen PL: *Pocket guide to fluid, electrolyte, and acid-base balance,* ed 3, St. Louis, 1997, Mosby.

Box 19-1 Common Names for Intravenous Solutions

SOLUTION	COMMON NAMES
0.9% sodium chloride	Normal saline
	0.9% NaCl
	0.9% NS
	NS
0.45% sodium chloride	One-half-strength normal saline
	0.45% NaCl
	0.45% NS
	½ NaCl
	½ NS
Dextrose 5% in 0.9% sodium chloride	D_5 normal saline
	D_5 0.9% NaCl
	D_5 0.9% NS
	D_5 NS
Dextrose 5% in 0.45% sodium chloride	D_5 One-half-strength normal saline
	D_5 0.45% NaCl
	D_5 0.45 NS
	D_5 ½ NaCl
	D_5 ½ NS
Lactated Ringer's	LR
Dextrose 5% in lactated Ringer's	D^3 LR

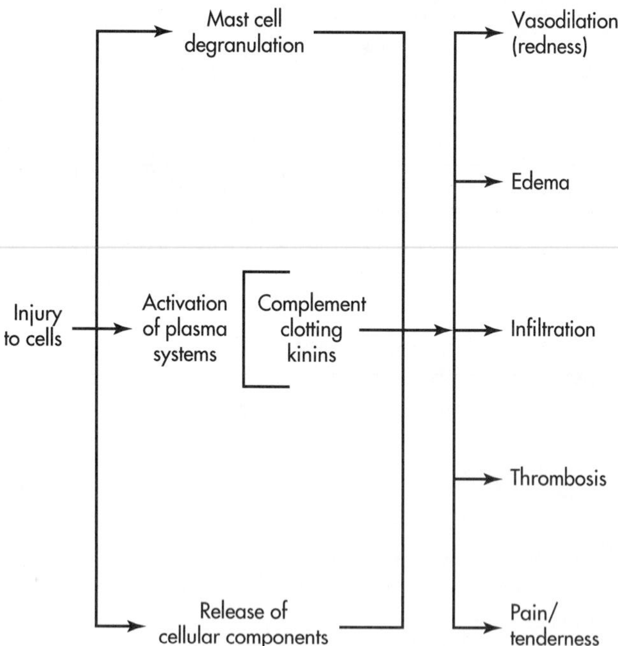

FIGURE **19-1** Response to injury to blood vessel walls by IV catheter. (Modified from Lawson T: Vein trauma during catheter advancement, *J Vasc Acces Device*, Sp 1998, p. 22.)

thrombosis of veins than silicone. Intravenous catheters that are stiff and have a rough surface result in thrombophlebitis, fibrin sheath formation, and congregation of platelets (Lawson, 1998). Various cellular processes come into play once an injury to a vein occurs, resulting in clinical signs of redness, edema, infiltration, **thrombosis,** and pain at a catheter entrance site (Figure 19-1).

Venous access poses significant risks to clients, however intravenous therapy is often critical to a client's proper clinical management and recovery. Commonly used **over-the-needle catheters (ONC)** comprise a metal stylet, which is used to pierce the skin, and a Teflon, polyurethane, or silicone catheter, which is threaded into a vein and remains there for the instillation of fluid. These flexible catheters do not dislodge from the vein as easily as butterfly needles. In addition, large volumes of fluids and medications can be quickly administered through the catheter without a high risk of infiltration. A 20- to 22-gauge flexible catheter is used in most situations for adults, whereas a 22- to 24-gauge catheter can be used for children and older adults or for any other client with small or fragile veins. In general, use the smallest catheter that will deliver the needed fluids at the appropriate rate. If the administration of large volumes of IV fluids or blood or blood products is anticipated, a size 20-gauge or 18-gauge angiocatheter is necessary to allow rapid infusion of IV fluids or viscous blood product solutions.

Health care workers are at high risk for accidental needle sticks and sharp injuries. Common causes of accidental needle-stick injuries include recapping incidents, assembling or accessing IV tubing devices, disposing of contaminated sharps, using alternative methods to cover used needles on IV needle assemblies, and intentionally detaching IV lines. IV catheters and butterfly or winged catheters are devices commonly associated with a high risk for injuries. To help prevent accidental injury, needles should not be recapped and are disposed of in puncture-proof containers, referred to as **sharps containers.** In emergencies a one-handed "scoop" technique may be used to cover needles (Occupational Safety and Health Administration, 1991) (Figure 19-2). The caregiver places the cap on a flat surface and *with one hand only,* will slide the needle into the cap. Most health care agencies now use needleless devices that eliminate the use of needles altogether. However, this chapter will address use of needle devices as an option. The needleless devices use protective covers and valvelike systems and come in a variety of needle, catheter, and tubing products.

Skill Performance Guidelines

1. Know the client's normal range of vital signs before instituting intravenous therapy. Altered fluid or electrolyte imbalances can affect vital signs. Dehydration can produce hypotension and tachycardia. Fluid overload can result in hypertension and a bounding pulse. Disturbances in serum potassium can result in an irregular pulse.
2. Know the client's developmental stage. The proportion of total body water to body mass changes from infancy to the older adult years.
3. Know the client's weight. Body size affects total body water. Fat contains no water; the obese client thus has proportionately less body water.

A

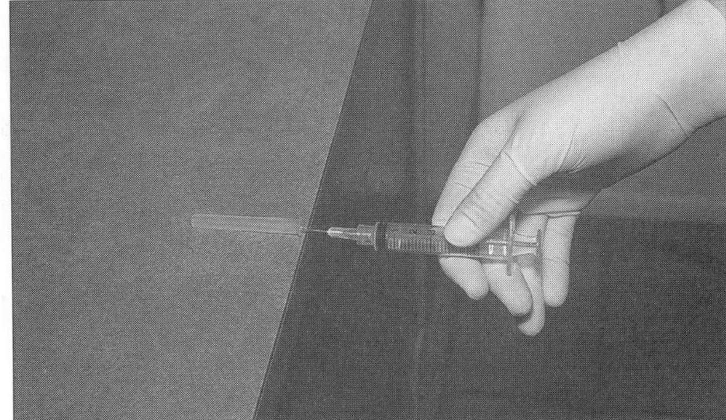

B

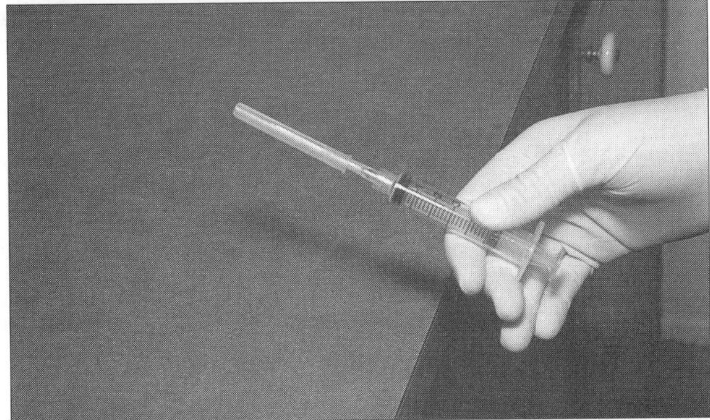

C

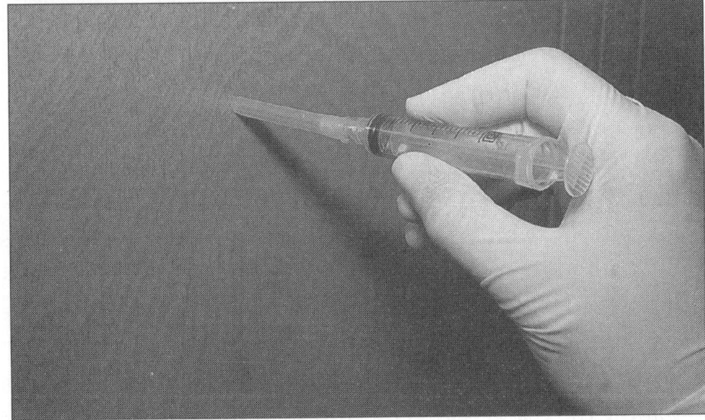

FIGURE **19-2** **A,** Insert contaminated needled into cap using one hand. **B,** Have cap slip fully over needle. **C,** Push cap against firm surface.

Box 19-2 CDC Guidelines to Decrease Intravascular Infection Related to IV Therapy

- Palpate catheter insertion site for tenderness daily through the intact dressing.
- Visually inspect a catheter site if client develops tenderness at site, fever without obvious source, or symptoms of local or bloodstream infection.
- Wash hands before and after palpating, inserting, replacing, or dressing any intravascular device.
- Cleanse skin site before venipuncture with an appropriate antiseptic, including 70% alcohol, 10% povidone-iodine.
- Do not palpate insertion site after skin has been cleansed with antiseptic.
- Use sterile gauze or transparent dressing to cover a catheter site.
- Replace IV tubing, including piggyback tubing and stopcocks, no more frequently than at 72-hour intervals unless clinically indicated.
- Replace tubing used to administer blood, blood products, or lipid emulsions within 24 hours of initiating infusion.
- There are no recommendations for the hang time of IV fluids.
- Replace dressing over peripheral venous catheters when catheter is replaced or when dressing becomes damp, loosened, or soiled.
- Clean injection ports with 70% alcohol or povidone-iodine before accessing system.
- Do not use in-line filters routinely for infection control.
- In adults, replace short, peripheral venous catheters and rotate sites every 48 to 72 hours.
- In adults, replace heparin locks every 96 hours.
- Do not routinely apply topical antimicrobial ointment to the insertion site of peripheral venous catheters or central venous catheter-insertion sites.
- No recommendation for the frequency of replacement of peripherally inserted central catheter (PICC).

Modified from Centers for Disease Control and Prevention: Guideline for prevention of intravascular device-related infections, *Infect Control Hosp Epidemiol* 17(7):438, 1996a.

4. Know the client's medical history and present medications or therapies. Certain drugs such as diuretics or steroids affect fluid and electrolyte balance. Likewise, a client may be on a specific diet, such as a low-sodium diet for water retention. Determine whether the client has had IV therapy before.
5. Beware of prolonged environmental conditions that can affect the client's fluid status. Prolonged exposure to hot, humid weather can lead to fluid and electrolyte imbalances, particularly in the infant, the older adult, and the chronically ill client.
6. Know if the client is right- or left-handed. When possible, place an IV into the nondominant arm.
7. Determine that the present IV system is intact. A system in which none of the connections have separated ensures that the sterility of the system has been maintained and that no fluid or medication has been lost. If the nurse suspects that the infusion tubing has separated from the IV catheter or needle, sterility is no longer assumed, and a new system, including sterile tubing, solution, and catheter or needle must be reestablished.
8. Note when the last IV tubing and dressing change occurred (Box 19-2).
9. Maintain sterility of a patent IV system using the Centers for Disease Control (CDC) (1996a) recommendations (see Box 19-2).
10. Know the standard precautions for infection control and the Occupational Safety and Health Administration (OSHA) standards for occupational exposure to bloodborne pathogens (Box 19-3).

Box 19-3 OSHA Standards for Reducing Occupational Exposure to Bloodborne Pathogens

1. Gloves must be worn when there is a reasonable expectation that the employee may contact blood, for example, during venipuncture or while changing IV administration sets.
2. Contaminated needles and other sharps must be placed in puncture-resistant containers properly labeled as a biohazard; when the containers are full, they are to be sealed and disposed of properly.
3. Contaminated needles should not be bent, sheared, recapped, or removed from the syringe after use.
4. Reports to OSHA of needle-stick injuries are required, and the health care agency must provide medical evaluation and follow-up.
5. Hepatitis B vaccination is to be made available to all employees who have occupational exposure.
6. Training and education must be offered to high-risk workers, such as nurses who initiate IV therapy, concerning precautions for prevention of exposure and use of personal protective equipment.
7. Each facility must have an infection control plan, including methods for reduction of the health care worker's exposure to biohazardous wastes.
8. Facilities must have engineering and work practice controls to eliminate or minimize employee exposure. Controls may include sharps disposal containers and self-sheathing needles.

From Occupational Safety and Health Act: Bloodborne pathogens, *Federal Register* 56(235):64, 175, Dec 6, 1991.

Skill 19-1 Initiating Intravenous Therapy

The goal of intravenous (IV) fluid administration is correction or prevention of fluid and electrolyte disturbances in clients who are or may become acutely ill. For example, a client with third-degree burns over 40% of the body is critically ill and has severe fluid and electrolyte imbalances. Fluid therapy must be continuously regulated in a burn client because of continual changes in fluid and electrolyte balance. A client who is NPO (nothing by mouth) after surgery receives IV fluid replacement to prevent fluid and electrolyte imbalances; the infusion is usually discontinued when the client resumes oral intake. Another reason to perform a venipuncture is to provide IV access for intermittent or emergency medication administration. This administration route is often accomplished through the use of a **heparin** or normal **saline lock,** which is an IV catheter attached to an injection cap to maintain a closed system. Sometimes a short piece of extension tubing is used. The heparin or saline lock is flushed with a heparin or normal saline solution every 8 hours or before and after each administration of medication to maintain patency of the IV catheter (see Chapter 18). Ideally, peripheral IV access should not be used for administration of medications that are irritants or vesicants (e.g., chemotherapy, total parenteral nutrition). These types of medications should be administered through a central venous access site whenever possible (see Chapter 23).

Concern for the personal safety of nurses who work with IV therapy products is very important because of the possibility of transmission of organisms such as hepatitis B virus (HBV) and human immunodeficiency virus (HIV). The most common cause of exposure of nurses to blood during IV therapy is by needle stick. To prevent this, there are products that decrease the chance of an accidental needle stick. Products that allow the connection of multiple tubings for IV solution or medication administration without the use of needles (needleless systems) are available. Other products with recessed needles or needle protectors can be used to prevent contact with exposed needles.

Delegation Considerations

The skill of initiating peripheral intravenous therapy should not be delegated to assistive personnel.

Equipment

- Correct IV solution (with time tape attached)
- Proper IV access devices for venipuncture (will vary with client's body size and reason for IV fluid administration) (Figure 19-3)
- IV start kit (available in some agencies): may contain a sterile drape to place under the client's arm, cleansing and antiseptic preparations, dressings, and a small roll of sterile tape.

For IV Fluid Infusion

- Administration set (choice depends on type of solution and rate of administration; infants and children require microdrip tubing, which provides 60 gtt/ml)
- 0.22 μmm filter (if required by agency policy or if particulate matter is likely)
- Extension tubing
- Alcohol and povidone-iodine cleansing swabs or sticks
- Disposable gloves
- Tourniquet (can be a source of contamination; use a single-use product)
- Arm board, if needed (used to maintain wrist or elbow joint position when catheter is placed close to or over a joint [Figure 19-4]; will help prevent infiltration of IV)

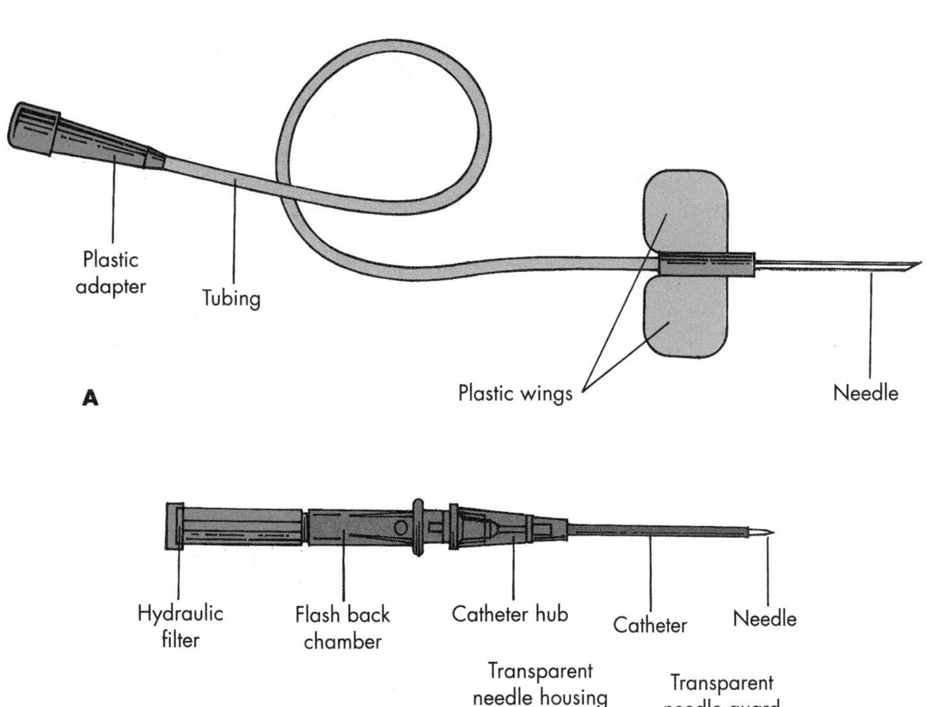

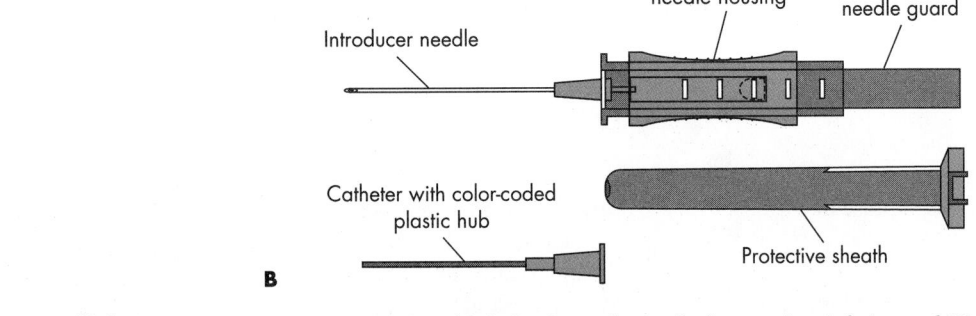

FIGURE **19-3** IV access device options. **A,** Winged infusion butterfly needle for one-time infusion and IV push only. **B,** Short over-the-needle catheter (ONC) for continuous and intermittent infusions (less than 1 week).

- Nonallergenic tape
- Towel (to place under client's hand or arm)
- IV pole, rolling or ceiling mounted
- Special gown with snaps at shoulder seams (makes removal with IV tubing easier), if available
- Needle disposal container (also called sharps container)

For Heparin or Normal Saline Lock

- Injection cap (also called **IV plug,** PRN adapter)
- IV loop or short piece of extension tubing, if necessary
- 1 to 3 ml of normal saline or heparin flush (10 U/ml as ordered)
- Syringes and 25-gauge needles

Gauze Dressing Only

- 2 × 2 or 4 × 4 sterile gauze sponge

Transparent Dressing Only

- Transparent dressing

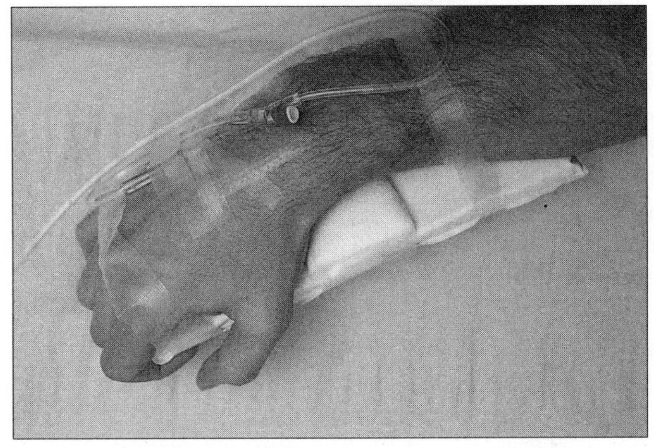

FIGURE **19-4** Arm positioned and taped on arm board.

STEP	RATIONALE

ASSESSMENT

Step	Rationale
1. Review physician's order for type and amount of IV fluid and rate of fluid administration. In addition, nurse follows five rights for administration of medications (see Chapter 16).	An order requesting the initiation of a peripheral IV access and administration of an IV solution must be made by a physician prior to the implementation of this procedure.

- ***Critical Decision Point***
  In most medical facilities, physicians do not write an order to "initiate peripheral access" or "perform venipuncture." "Start IV" may be written followed by the exact IV therapy order. The order to perform the venipuncture is implied. If the order is confusing or in question, clarify with the physician before proceeding.

Step	Rationale
2. Assess for clinical factors/conditions that will respond to or be affected by IV fluid administration:	Provides baseline to determine effect IV fluids have on client's fluid and electrolyte balance.
a. Peripheral edema—can be rated for severity by assessing pitting over bony prominences. 1+ indicates barely detectable edema to 4+ for deep persistent pitting (see Chapter 10).	Indicates expanded interstitial volume. This is usually most evident in dependent areas (i.e., feet and ankles). Fluid overload will worsen edema.
b. Greater than 2% increase or decrease in body weight.	Daily weights document fluid retention or loss. Change in body weight of 1 kg corresponds to 1 L of fluid retention or loss (Horne and Swearingen, 1997).
c. Dry skin and mucous membranes	May signal fluid volume deficit.
d. Distended neck veins	Suggests fluid volume excess.
e. Blood pressure changes	Elevated blood pressure may indicate volume excess due to increase in stroke volume. Decreased blood pressure may indicate fluid volume deficit due to a decrease in stroke volume.
f. Irregular pulse rhythm; increased pulse rate	Rhythm changes may occur with potassium, calcium, and/or magnesium abnormalities; rate change may occur with fluid volume deficit.
g. Auscultation of crackles or rhonchi in lungs	May signal fluid buildup in the lungs due to fluid volume excess.
h. Inelastic skin turgor (after pinching, fails to return to normal position within 3 seconds)	With fluid volume deficit, the pinched skin stays elevated for several seconds.

- ***Critical Decision Point***
  This is a less reliable indicator for older adults because their skin has lost elasticity naturally due to aging.

Step	Rationale
i. Anorexia, nausea, and vomiting	May occur with acute fluid volume deficit or fluid volume excess.
j. Thirst	Symptomatic of fluid volume deficit.
k. Decreased urine output	During dehydration, kidney attempts to restore fluid balance by reducing urine production. Average daily adult urine output is 1500 ml; urine output of less than 400 ml/24 hr (oliguria) signals the retention of metabolic wastes (Horne and Swearingen, 1997).
l. Behavioral changes (e.g., restlessness, confusion)	May occur with fluid volume deficit or acid-base imbalance.
3. Assess client's previous or perceived experience with IV therapy and arm placement preference.	Determines level of emotional support and instruction needed.
4. Obtain information from drug reference books or pharmacist about composition of IV fluids, purposes of administration, potential incompatibilities, and side effects to monitor for.	This allows detection of an inadvisable IV fluid order and helps to determine priority assessments.
5. Determine if client is to undergo any planned surgeries or is to receive blood infusion later.	Allows nurse to anticipate and place large gauge catheter (e.g., 18 or 16) for fluid infusion and avoids placement in area that will interfere with medical procedures.

STEP	RATIONALE
6. Assess for the following risk factors: child or older adult; presence of heart failure or renal failure, skin lesions, infection, low platelet count or receiving anticoagulants.	Persons at extremes in age develop fluid imbalances more rapidly because they have a proportionately larger extracellular fluid volume; persons with heart failure cannot adapt to sudden increases in vascular volume, and persons with renal failure cannot eliminate excess extracellular fluid. Skin lesions or infection may influence choice of access site. Low platelets or use of anticoagulants increase client's risk for bleeding from IV site.
7. Assess laboratory data and client's history of allergies.	May reveal information that affects insertion of devices, such as fluid volume deficit or allergy to iodine, adhesive, or latex.

Nursing Diagnosis

Defining characteristics from the assessment data may reveal the following nursing diagnoses for clients requiring this skill:

Risk for imbalanced fluid volume
Risk for deficient fluid volume
Risk for infection

Related factors are individualized based on client's condition or needs.

Planning

STEP	RATIONALE
1. **Expected outcomes** following completion of procedure:	
▪ Fluid and electrolyte balance returns to normal; vital signs and other abnormal assessment parameters stabilize and return to normal.	Indicates correction of fluid and electrolyte imbalances and circulatory system's response to fluid and electrolyte replacement.
▪ IV line is patent.	Ensures free instillation of IV fluids without infiltration.
▪ Infiltration is absent with no swelling and pallor at venipuncture site.	Infiltration results from dislodging of catheter or needle into subcutaneous space.
▪ Inflammation is absent.	Inflammation results from irritation of vein by catheter, IV solution, additives, or bacteria.
▪ Client will understand purpose and risks of IV therapy.	Increases likelihood of client and family adherence to IV treatment modalities.
2. Prepare client and family by explaining the procedure, its purpose, and what is expected of client. Also explain sensations client is to expect.	Cognitive and sensory information decrease anxiety and help to promote cooperation.
3. Assist client to comfortable sitting or supine position.	
4. Wash hands.	Reduces transmission of infection.
5. Organize equipment on clean, clutter-free bedside stand or overbed table.	Reduces risk of contamination and accidents.

Implementation

STEP	RATIONALE
1. Change client's gown to the more easily removed gown with snaps at the shoulder, if available.	Use of a special IV gown facilitates safe removal of the gown once IV has been inserted.
2. Open sterile packages using sterile aseptic technique (see Chapter 32).	Maintains sterility of equipment and reduces spread of microorganisms.
3. Prepare IV infusion tubing and solution.	
a. Check IV solution, using five rights of drug administration (see Chapter 16). Make sure prescribed additives, such as potassium and vitamins, have been added. Check solution for color, clarity, and expiration date. Check bag for leaks, which is best if done before reaching the bedside.	IV solutions are medications and should be carefully checked to reduce risk of error. Solutions that are discolored, contain particles, or are expired are not to be used. Leaky bags present an opportunity for infection and must not be used.

Step	Rationale
b. Open infusion set, maintaining sterility of both ends of tubing. Many sets allow for priming of tubing without removal of end cap.	Prevents bacteria from entering infusion equipment and bloodstream.
c. Place roller clamp (see illustration) about 2 to 5 cm (1 to 2 inches) below drip chamber and move roller clamp to "off" position (see illustration).	Close proximity of roller clamp to drip chamber allows more accurate regulation of flow rate. Moving clamp to "off" prevents accidental spillage of IV fluid on client, nurse, bed, or floor.
d. Remove protective sheath over IV tubing port on plastic IV solution bag (see illustration).	Provides access for insertion of infusion tubing into solution.
e. Insert infusion set into fluid bag or bottle: Remove protector cap from tubing insertion spike, not touching spike, and insert spike into opening of IV bag (see illustration). Cleanse rubber stopper on bottled solution with antiseptic and insert spike into black rubber stopper of IV bottle.	Flat surface on the top of bottled solution may contain contaminants, whereas opening to plastic bag is recessed. Prevents contamination of bottled solution during insertion of spike.

A

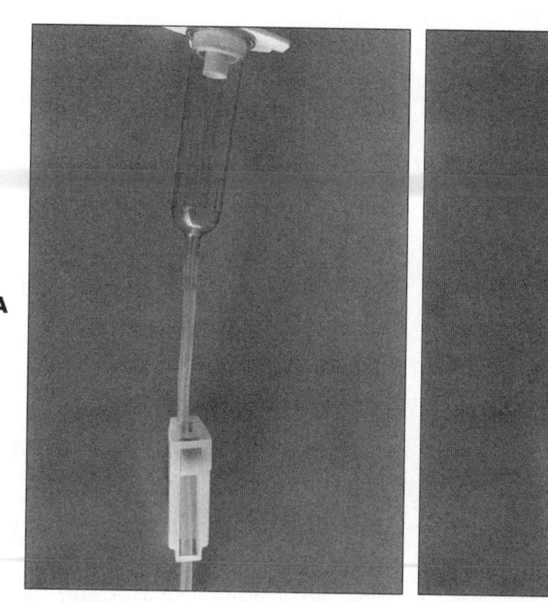

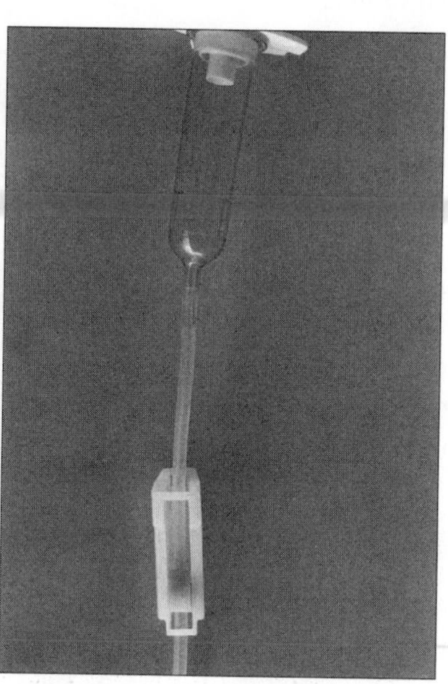

B

STEP 3c **A,** Roller clamp in open position. **B,** Roller clamp in closed position.

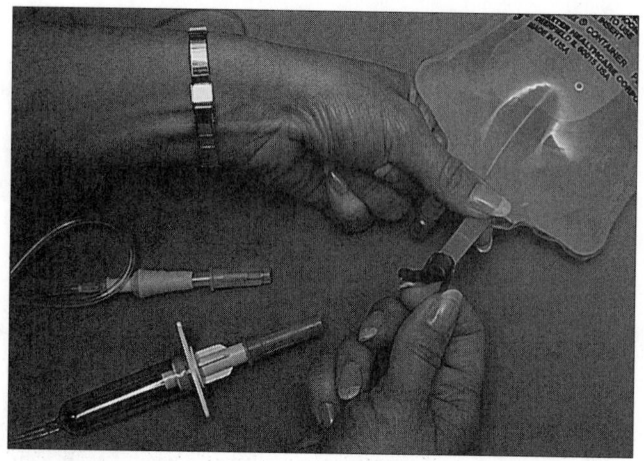

STEP 3d Removing protective sheath from IV bag port.

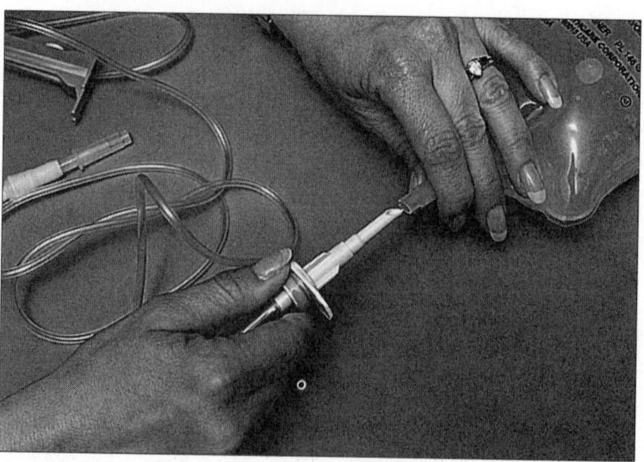

STEP 3e Inserting spike into IV bag.

STEP	RATIONALE

- ***Critical Decision Point***
  Do not touch spike because it is sterile. If contamination occurs (e.g., spike is accidently dropped on the floor), then discard that IV tubing and obtain a new one.

f. Prime infusion tubing by filling with IV solution: — Ensures tubing is cleared of air prior to connection with IV site.

(1) Compress drip chamber and release, allowing it to fill one-third to one-half full (see illustration). — Creates suction effect; fluid enters drip chamber to prevent air from entering tubing.

g. Remove protector cap on end of tubing (some tubing can be primed without removal) and slowly release roller clamp to allow fluid to travel from drip chamber through tubing to needle adapter. Return roller clamp to "off" position after tubing is primed (filled with IV fluid). — Slow fill of tubing decreases turbulence and chance of bubble formation. Removes air from tubing and permits tubing to fill with solution. Closing the clamp prevents accidental loss of fluid.

h. Be certain tubing is clear of air and air bubbles. To remove small air bubbles, firmly tap IV tubing where air bubbles are located. Check entire length of tubing to ensure that all air bubbles are removed (see illustration). If multiple port tubing is used, turn ports upside down and tap to fill and remove air. — Large air bubbles can act as **emboli.**

- ***Critical Decision Point***
  An extra extension tubing may be added to IV tubing to allow for more length, which will enable client to move more freely while still keeping IV line stable.

i. Replace cap protector on end of infusion tubing. — Maintains system sterility.

4. Prepare heparin or normal saline lock for infusion:

a. If a loop or short extension tubing is needed because of an awkward IV site placement, use sterile technique to connect the IV plug to the loop or short extension tubing. Inject 1 to 3 ml normal saline through the plug and through the loop or short extension tubing before connecting to IV site. — Removes air to prevent introduction into the vein. Do the same with the saline plug.

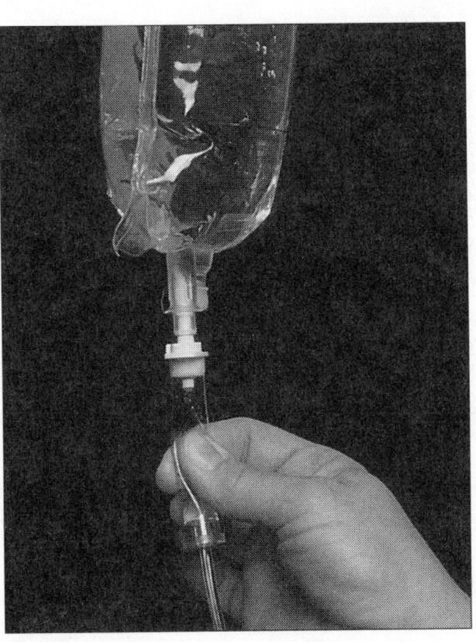

STEP **3f** Squeezing drip chamber to fill with fluid.

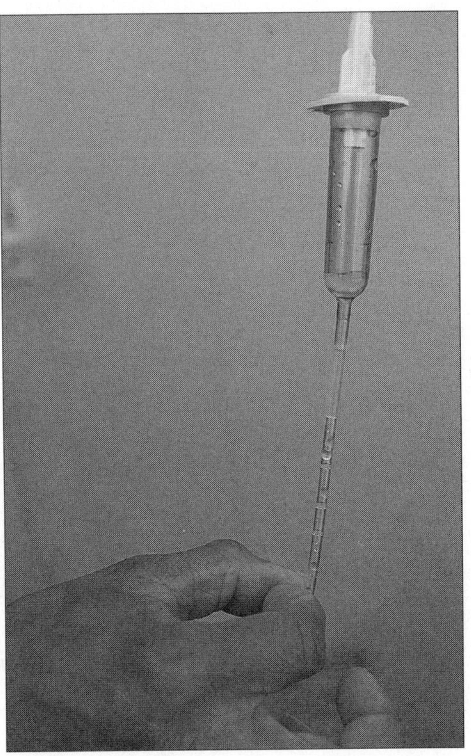

STEP **3h** Removing air bubbles from tubing.

STEP	RATIONALE
5. Apply disposable gloves. Eye protection and mask may be worn (see agency policy) if splash or spray of blood is possible.	Reduces transmission of microorganisms. Decreases exposure to HIV, hepatitis, and other blood-borne organisms (Centers for Disease Control and Prevention [CDC], 1996b) and prevents spraying of blood on nurse's mucous membranes.
6. Identify accessible vein for placement of IV catheter or needle. Apply flat tourniquet around arm, above antecubital fossa (see illustration) or 4 to 6 in (10 to 15 cm) above proposed insertion site. Do not apply tourniquet too tightly to avoid injury or bruising to skin. Check for presence of radial pulse. Try applying tourniquet on top of a thin layer of clothing such as a gown sleeve. It may become necessary to remove tourniquet and move lower down arm.	Tourniquet impedes venous return but should not occlude arterial flow. If vein cannot be found in antecubital fossa, move down along arm to locate vessel in lower arm or hand.
7. Select the vein for IV insertion. The cephalic, basilic, and median cubital are preferred in adults (see illustration).	
a. Use the most distal site in the nondominant arm, if possible. Clip arm hair with scissors if necessary.	Venipuncture should be performed distal to proximal, which increases the availability of other sites for future IV therapy. Hair impedes venipuncture or adherence of dressing.

- ***Critical Decision Point***

  Do not shave area. Shaving may cause microabrasions and predispose to infection.

b. Avoid areas that are painful to palpation.

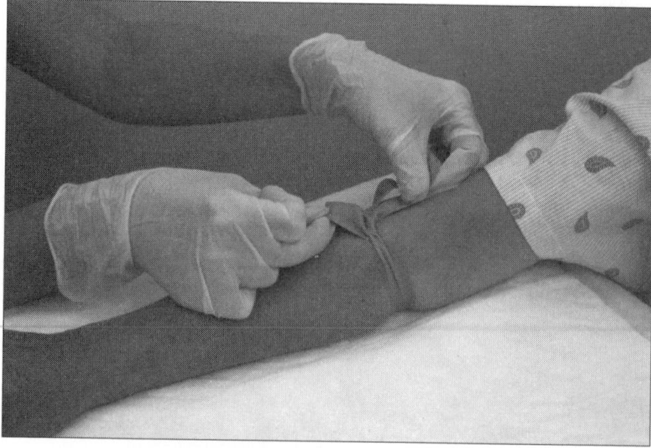

STEP **6** Tourniquet placed on arm for initial vein selection.

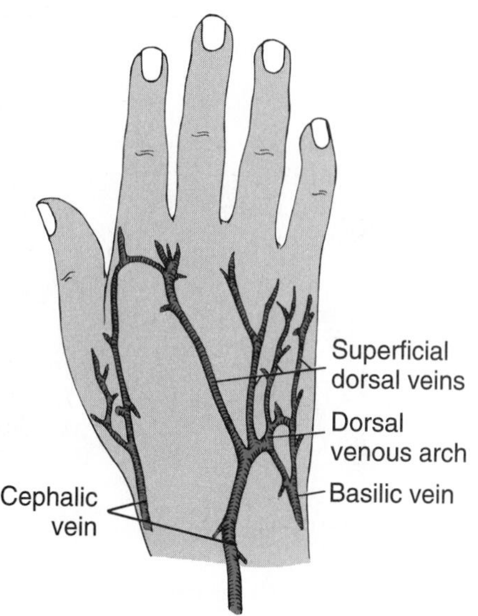

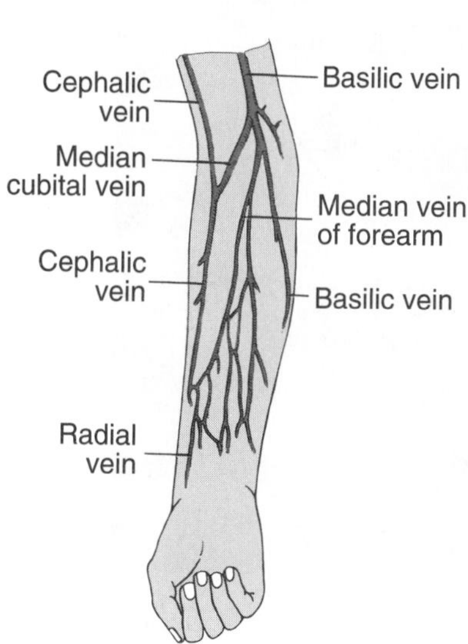

STEP **7** Cephalic, basilic, and median cubital veins are best for IV placement in adults.

STEP	RATIONALE
c. Select a vein large enough for catheter placement.	Prevents interruption of venous flow while allowing adequate blood flow around the catheter.
d. Choose a site that will not interfere with client's activities of daily living (ADLs) or planned procedures.	Keeps client as mobile as possible.
e. Palpate the vein by pressing downward and noting the resilient, soft, bouncy feeling as the pressure is released. Always use the same finger to palpate.	Use of the same finger causes a development of sensitivity to better assess the vein's condition (Perucca, Micek, 1993).
f. If possible, place extremity in dependent position.	Permits venous dilation and visibility.
g. Select well-dilated vein. Methods to foster venous distention include:	Increases the volume of blood in the vein at the venipuncture site.
(1) Stroking the extremity from distal to proximal below the proposed venipuncture site.	
(2) Having client alternately open and close the fist.	Muscle contraction increases the amount of blood in the extremity.
(3) Light tapping over a vein.	May help to foster venous dilation.
(4) Applying warmth to the extremity for several minutes, for example, with a warm washcloth.	Increases blood supply and fosters venous dilation.

• ***Critical Decision Point***

Vigorous friction and multiple tapping of the veins, especially in older adults, may cause hematoma and/or venous constriction (Whitson, 1996).

STEP	RATIONALE
h. Avoid sites distal to previous venipuncture site, sclerosed or hardened cordlike veins, infiltrate site or phlebotic vessels, bruised areas, and areas of venous valves or bifurcation.	Such sites can cause infiltration of newly placed IV catheter and excessive vessel damage.
i. Avoid fragile dorsal veins in older adult clients and vessels in an extremity with compromised circulation (e.g., in cases of mastectomy, dialysis graft, or paralysis).	Venous alterations can increase risk of complications (e.g., infiltration and decreased catheter dwell time).
8. Release tourniquet temporarily and carefully.	Restores blood flow while preparing for venipuncture.
9. Place needle adapter end of infusion set nearby on sterile gauze or sterile towel.	Permits smooth, quick connection of infusion to IV needle once vein is punctured.
10. Place tourniquet 10 to 12 cm (4 to 5 inches) above anticipated insertion site (see illustration). Check presence of distal pulse.	Diminished arterial flow prevents venous filling. The pressure of the tourniquet should cause the vein to dilate.
11. (If area of insertion appears to need cleansing, use soap and water first.) Then cleanse insertion site using firm, circular motion (middle to outward) with povidone-iodine or 70% alcohol solution; refrain from touching the cleansed site; allow the site to dry for at least 2 minutes (povidone) or 60 seconds (alcohol) (see illustration).	Touching the cleansed area would introduce organisms from the nurse's hand to the site. Drying prevents chemical reactions between agents and allows time for maximum microbicidal activity of agents (Baranowski, 1993).

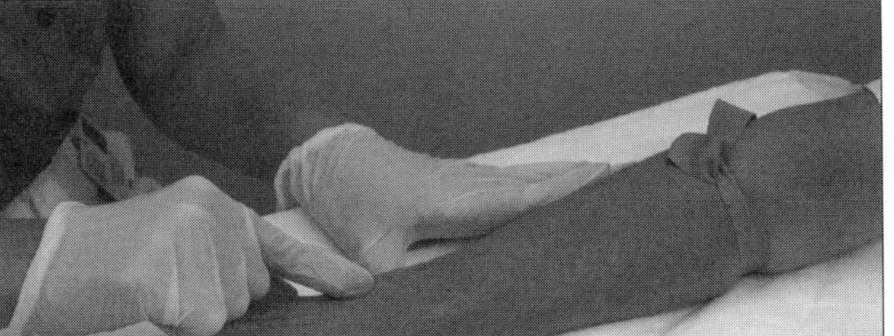

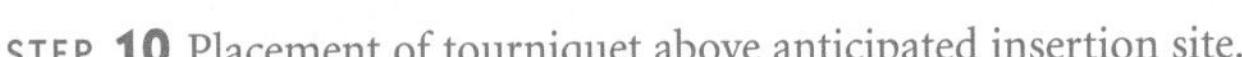

STEP **10** Placement of tourniquet above anticipated insertion site.

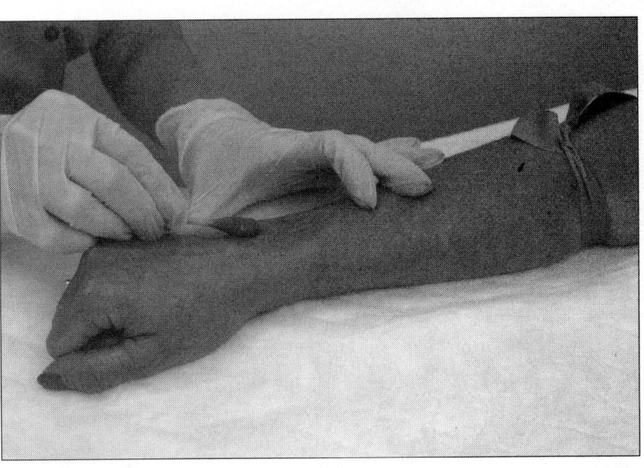

STEP **11** Cleanse insertion site with antiseptic prep.

STEP	RATIONALE
12. Perform **venipuncture.** Anchor vein by placing thumb over vein and by stretching the skin against the direction of insertion 2 to 3 inches (5 to 7.5 cm) distal to the site (see illustration). Warn client of a sharp, quick stick. a. *Over-the-needle catheter (ONC):* Insert with bevel up at 20- to 30-degree angle slightly distal to actual site of venipuncture in the direction of the vein. b. *IV catheter safety device:* Insert using same position as for ONC (see illustration). c. *Butterfly needle:* Hold needle at 20- to 30-degree angle with bevel up slightly distal to actual site of venipuncture.	Stabilizes vein for needle insertion. Places needle parallel to vein. When vein is punctured, risk of puncturing posterior vein wall is reduced.

- ***Critical Decision Point***

  Only one needle/catheter should be utilized for each attempt at insertion.

STEP	RATIONALE
13. Look for blood return through flashback chamber of catheter, or tubing of butterfly needle, indicating that needle has entered vein (see illustration). Lower needle until almost flush with skin. Advance catheter another $\frac{1}{4}$ inch into vein and then loosen stylet. Continue to hold skin taut and advance catheter into vein until hub rests at venipuncture site. *Do not reinsert the stylet once it is loosened.* (If available, advance the safety device by using push-off tab to thread the catheter; *see illustration.*) Advance butterfly needle until hub rests at venipuncture site.	Increased venous pressure from tourniquet increases backflow of blood into catheter or tubing. Reinsertion of the stylet can cause catheter breakage in the vein.

A
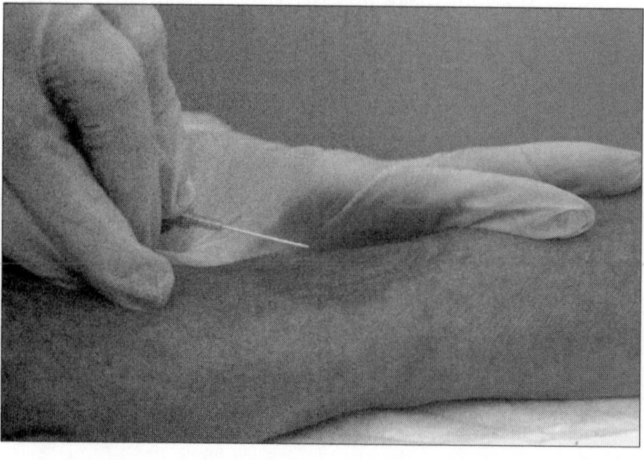
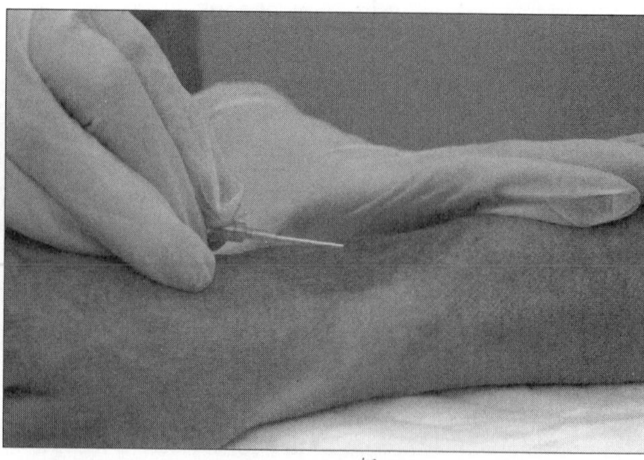
B

STEP **12** **A,** Illustration of ONC with bevel angled 20 to 30 degrees above vein. **B,** IV catheter tip enters vein.

A
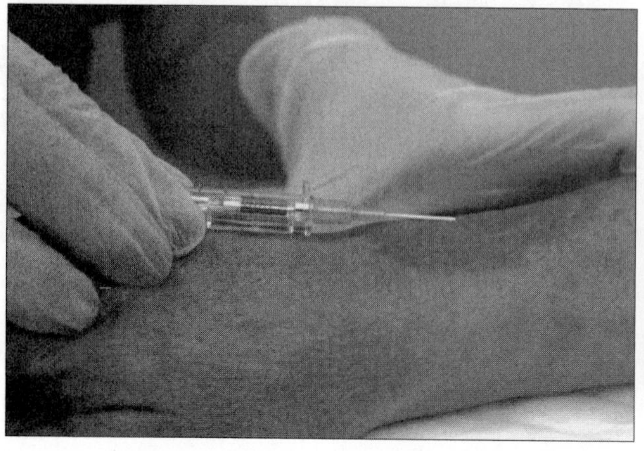
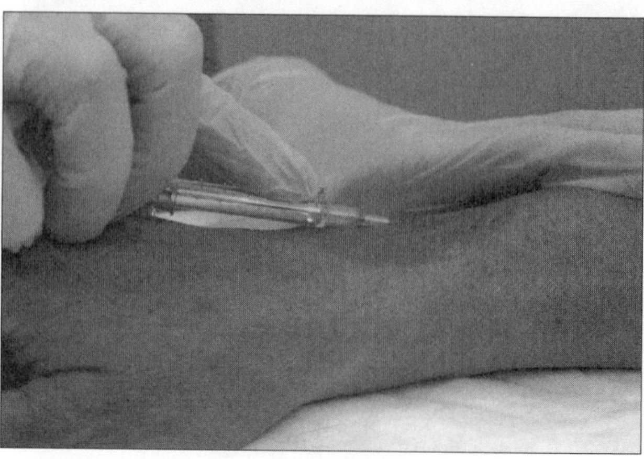
B

STEP **13** **A,** Blood return indicates catheter placed inside vein. **B,** Advance catheter into vein using one-handed technique.

STEP	RATIONALE

- ***Critical Decision Point***
  No more than three attempts at initiating the IV access should be made by a single nurse.

14. Stabilize catheter/needle with one hand and release tourniquet with other (see illustration). Apply gentle but firm pressure with index finger of nondominant hand 1 ¼ inches (3 cm) above the insertion site (see illustration). Keep a needle stable. Remove the stylet of ONC. Do not recap the stylet. For a safety device, slide the catheter off the stylet while gliding the protective guard over the stylet. A click indicates the device is locked over the stylet. (NOTE: techniques will vary with each IV device.)

    Permits venous flow, reduces backflow of blood, and allows connection with administration set with minimal blood loss.

15. Quickly connect needle adapter of infusion tubing set (see illustration) or the heparin/saline lock adapter to hub of catheter or butterfly tubing. Do not touch point of entry of needle adapter.

    Prompt connection of infusion set maintains patency of vein and prevents risk of exposure to blood. Maintains sterility.

16. *Intermittent infusion:* Hold the heparin/saline lock firmly with nondominant hand and clean with alcohol. Insert prefilled syringe containing flush solution into injection cap (see illustration). Flush injection cap slowly with flush solution. Withdraw the syringe while still flushing.

    "Positive pressure flushing" allows fluid to displace the removed needle, creates positive pressure in the catheter, and prevents reflux of blood during flushing. Stabilizing the cannula prevents accidental withdrawal or dislodgement.

A
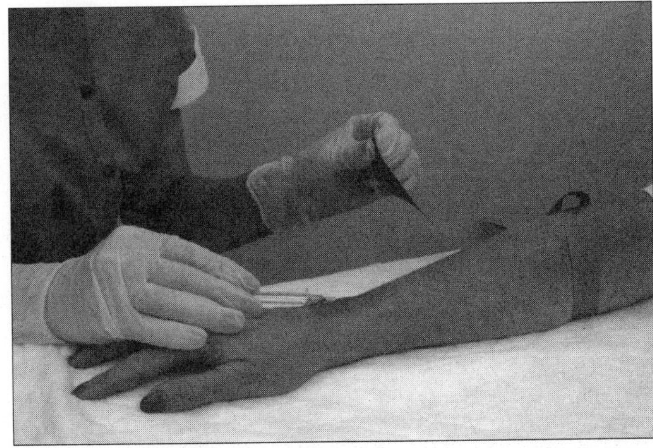

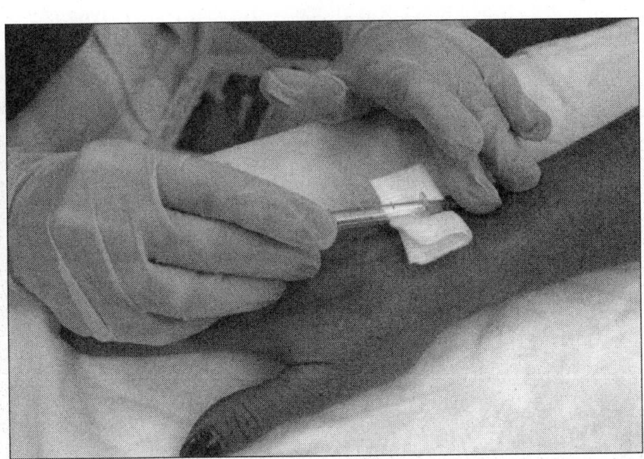
B

STEP **14** **A,** Stabilize catheter with one hand and release tourniquet with other. **B,** Apply pressure above insertion site while preparing to attach infusion tubing.

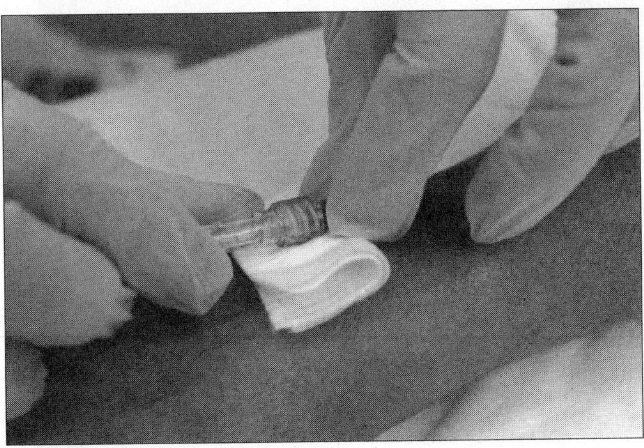

STEP **15** Connect IV tubing adaptor to ONC catheter hub.

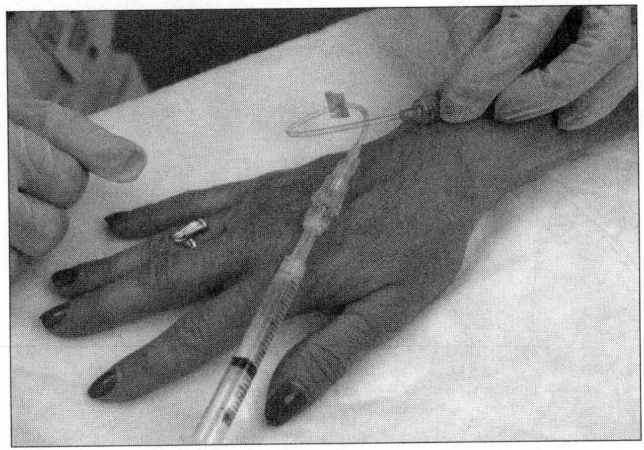

STEP **16** Syringe containing saline flush connected to heparin lock injection cap.

STEP	RATIONALE
17. *Continuous infusion:* Begin infusion by slowly opening the slide clamp or adjusting the roller clamp of the IV tubing.	Initiates flow of fluid through IV catheter, preventing clotting of device.

- ***Critical Decision Point***
  Be sure to calculate rate so as not to infuse IV solution too rapidly or too slowly.

STEP	RATIONALE
18. Tape or secure catheter/butterfly needle (procedures can differ; follow agency policy):	
a. Sterile gauze dressing: Place narrow piece ($\frac{1}{2}$ inch) of tape under catheter hub with sticky side up and cross tape over catheter hub (see illustrations). Place tape only on the catheter, *never* over the insertion site. Secure site to allow easy visual inspection. Avoid applying tape around the arm.	Prevents accidental removal of catheter from vein. Prevents back-and-forth motion, which can irritate the vein and introduce bacteria on the skin into the vein.
b. Transparent dressing: secure catheter/butterfly needle with nondominant hand while preparing to apply dressing.	Prevents accidental dislodgement of catheter.
19. Apply sterile dressing over site.	
a. Sterile gauze dressing.	
(1) Fold a 2 × 2 gauze in half and cover with a 1-inch–wide tape extending about an inch from each side. Place under the tubing/catheter hub junction. Curl a loop of tubing alongside the arm and place a second piece of tape directly over the tubing and padded 2 × 2, securing tubing in two places (see illustration).	Tape on top of gauze makes it easier to access hub/tubing junction. Gauze pad elevates hub off skin to prevent pressure area. Securing loop of tubing reduces risk of dislodging catheter.
(2) Place 2 × 2 gauze pad over insertion site and catheter hub. Secure all edges with tape. Do not cover connection between IV tubing and catheter hub.	
b. Transparent dressing:	
(1) Carefully remove adherent backing. Apply one edge of dressing and then gently smooth remaining dressing over IV site, leaving connection between IV tubing and catheter hub uncovered (see illustration)	Occlusive dressing protects site from bacterial contamination. Connection between administration set and hub needs to be uncovered to facilitate changing the tubing if necessary. CDC (1996a) no longer recommends application of antimicrobial ointment to catheter site.
(2) Follow step 19a(1).	

A

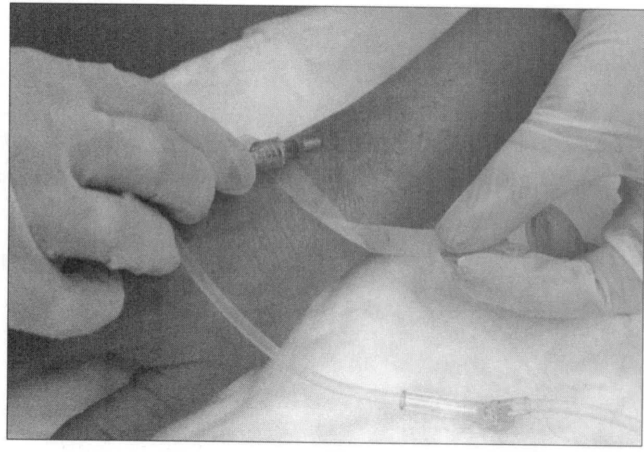

B

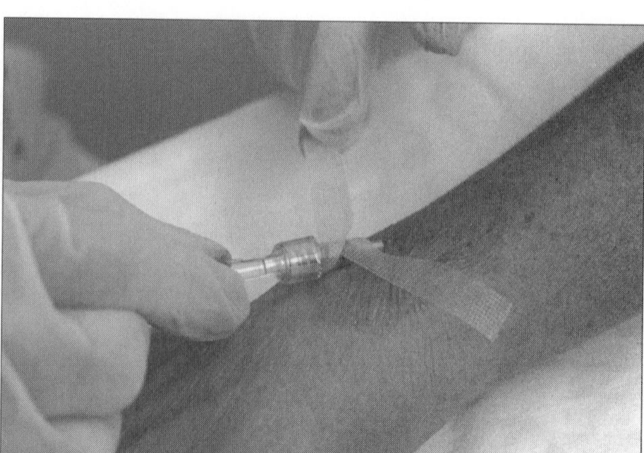

STEP **18a** **A,** Slide tape under ONC catheter hub. **B,** Cross tape ends over hub.

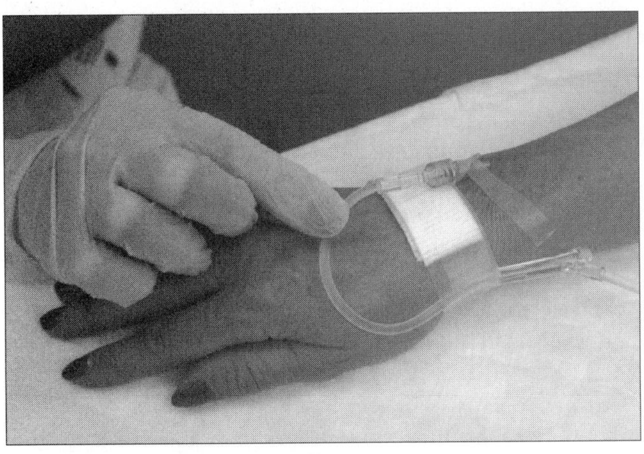

STEP **19a(1)** Place folded 2 × 2 gauze under catheter hub junction and secure loop of tubing with tape.

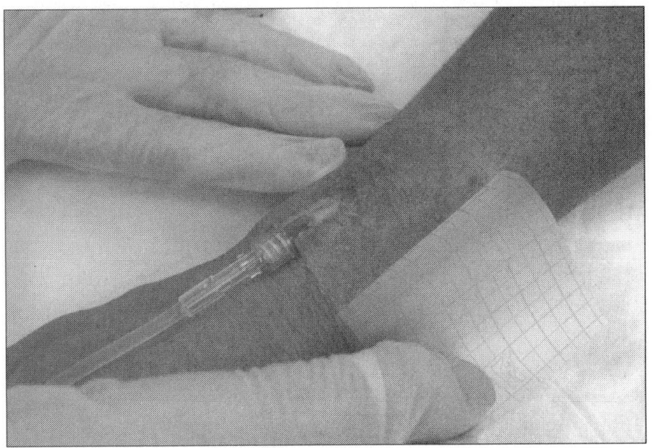

STEP **19b(1)** Apply transparent dressing over IV site and catheter.

STEP	RATIONALE
20. For IV fluid administration recheck flow rate to correct drops per minute (Skill 19-3).	Manipulation of catheter during dressing application may alter flow rate. Maintains correct rate of flow for IV solution. Flow can fluctuate so it must be checked at intervals for accuracy.
21. Write date and time of IV placement, catheter/needle gauge size on dressing.	Provides immediate access to data as to when IV was inserted and when subsequent dressing changes are needed.
22. Dispose of used stylet or other sharps in appropriate sharps container. Discard supplies. Remove gloves and wash hands.	Reduces transmission of microorganisms and protects staff from infection and injury.
23. Instruct client on how to move about in and out of bed without dislodging IV catheter.	
24. Peripheral IV access should be changed every 48 to 72 hours (CDC, 1996a) or per physician orders or more frequently if complications occur.	Incidence of complications may be higher when peripheral IV is allowed to remain in a vein over 72 hours. However, Homer and Holmes (1998) studied 722 clients with peripheral IV catheters and found that restarting catheters at 72 hours did not reduce the risk of complication when compared to simply continuing therapy with original catheter.
25. When solution has less than 100 ml remaining, present nursing shift should have new solution at client's bedside and slow flow rate.	This reduces risk of solution emptying during change-of-shift report.

EVALUATION

1. Observe client every 1 to 2 hours:	
a. Check if correct amount of IV solution has infused by looking at time tape on IV bag or by checking infusion pump record.	Correct administration of fluid volume prevents fluid imbalance.
b. Count drip rate (if gravity drip) or check rate on infusion pump.	Accurate monitoring of drip rate further ensures correct volume administration.
c. Check patency of IV catheter or needle: briefly compress cannulated vein proximal to site. Observe for slowing or momentary cessation of IV rate.	Compression results in mechanical obstruction of vein. When IV catheter is patent, compression results in slowing or cessation of flow rate. No change in flow rate may indicate infiltration.

• ***Critical Decision Point***

If IV is positional, fluid will run less slowly or stop depending on position of client's arm. Instruct client to position arm to maintain flow; if this continues, IV may have to be restarted.

STEP	RATIONALE
d. Observe client during compression of vessel for signs of discomfort.	Tenderness can be early sign of phlebitis.
e. Inspect insertion site, note color (e.g., redness or pallor). Inspect for presence of swelling. Palpate temperature of skin above dressing.	Redness or inflammation along with tenderness and warmth indicate vein inflammation or phlebitis. Swelling above insertion site and cool temperature may indicate infiltration of fluid into tissues.
2. Observe client every hour to determine response to therapy (e.g., I&O, weights, vital signs, postprocedure assessments).	IV fluids and additives are given to maintain or restore fluid and electrolyte balance. If I&O, weights, or vital signs change unexpectedly, fluid volume alterations can be serious.

Unexpected Outcomes and Related Interventions

- **Fluid volume deficit (FVD)** as manifested by decreased urine output, dry mucous membranes, hypotension, tachycardia.
  - Notify physician; may require readjustment of infusion rate.
- **Fluid volume excess (FVE)** as manifested by crackles in the lungs, shortness of breath, edema.
  - Reduce IV flow rate if symptoms appear, and notify physician.
- Electrolyte imbalances as manifested by abnormal serum electrolyte levels, changes in mental status, alterations in neuromuscular function, changes in vital signs, and other manifestations.
  - Notify physician. Additives in IV or type of IV fluid may be adjusted.
- **Infiltration** as indicated by swelling and possible pitting edema, pallor, coolness, pain at insertion site, possible decrease in flow rate (see Table 19-2).
  - Stop infusion and discontinue IV (see Skill 19-8). Elevate affected extremity. Restart new IV if continued therapy is necessary.
- **Phlebitis** is indicated by pain, increased skin temperature, erythema along path of vein (see Table 19-3).
  - Stop infusion and discontinue IV (see Skill 19-8). Restart new IV if continued therapy is necessary.
  - Place moist warm compress over area of phlebitis.
- Bleeding occurs at venipuncture site. Bleeding from vein is usually slow, continuous seepage. Common in clients who have received heparin, have a bleeding disorder, or the IV site is over bend in arm/hand.
  - If bleeding occurs around venipuncture site and catheter is within vein, gauze dressing may be applied over site. Be

Table 19-2 Infiltration Scale

Grade	Clinical Criteria
0	No symptoms
1	Skin blanched Edema <1 inch in any direction Cool to touch With or without pain
2	Skin blanched Edema 1–6 inches in any direction Cool to touch With or without pain
3	Skin blanched, translucent Gross edema >6 inches in any direction Cool to touch Mild-moderate pain Possible numbness
4	Skin blanched, translucent Skin tight, leaking Skin discolored, bruised, swollen Gross edema >6 inches in any direction Deep pitting tissue edema Circulatory impairment Moderate to severe pain Infiltration of any amount of blood product, irritant, or vesicant

From Intravenous Nurses Society: Infusion nursing standards of practice, *J Intraven Nurs* 23(65):557, 2000.

Table 19-3 Phlebitis Scale

Grade	Clinical Criteria
0	No symptoms
1	Erythema at access site with or without pain
2	Pain at access site with erythema and/or edema
3	Pain at access site with erythema and/or edema Streak formation Palpable venous cord
4	Pain at access site with erythema and/or edema Streak formation Palpable venous cord >1 inch in length Purulent drainage

From Intravenous Nurses Society: Infusion nursing standards of practice, *J Intraven Nurs* 23(65):556, 2000.

aware that if gauze dressing is used, it must be removed to accurately assess insertion site.
- Blood on the dressing can result when the administration set becomes disconnected from the catheter's hub. When blood appears on the dressing, verify that the system is intact and change the dressing.

Recording and Reporting

- Record in nurses' notes number of attempts at insertion, type of fluid, insertion site by vessel, flow rate, size and type catheter or needle, and when infusion was begun. A special parenteral therapy flow sheet may be used (Figure 19-5)
- If an electronic infusion device is used, document type and rate of infusion. Include the number on the pump.
- Record client's response to IV fluid, amount infused, and integrity and patency of system every 4 hours or according to agency policy.
- Report to oncoming nursing staff: type of fluid, flow rate, status of venipuncture site, amount of fluid remaining in present solution, expected time to hang next IV bag or bottle, and any side effects.
- Report to physician adverse reactions such as pulmonary congestion, shock, thrombophlebitis.

Teaching Considerations

- Instruct client about signs and symptoms of infiltration, phlebitis, and inflammation. Client can report early onset to nurse.
- Instruct client to inform nurse if flow slows or stops or blood is seen in the tubing or on the dressing.
- Instruct client how to ambulate with IV pole or stand.
- Instruct client to ask for assistance when bathing or when changing gown.

Pediatric Considerations

- Pediatric veins are very fragile. Avoid sites that are easily moved or bumped. Use commercial protective device to cover area.
- In addition to the usual venipuncture sites, the veins in the scalp or the foot are used in infants.
- If clients are older children, allowing them to select IV site may increase cooperation because they have some control over their treatment.
- Most IV infusions in pediatric clients require a 22- to 24-gauge catheter.
- When child is critically ill or long-term IV access is anticipated, PICC catheter, Broviac catheter, or implanted port may be used to access larger vein.
- Choosing age-appropriate activities compatible with the maintenance of the IV infusion is important to maintain normal growth and development.

Gerontological Considerations

- Apply good communication principles for communicating clearly to older adults when instruction is provided. Be sure client can hear you and is able to read any printed materials used.
- Gerontological veins are very fragile; there is less subcutaneous support tissue, and there is thinning of the skin. Take more time to select a site. Avoid sites that are easily moved or bumped. Sometimes dorsal metacarpal veins may not be the best choice. (Use commercial protective device to protect site.)
- In older clients, use the smallest gauge possible. For example, a 22-gauge needle is adequate for fluid and medication therapy; a 24-gauge is increasingly more popular in older adults (Whitson, 1996). This is less traumatizing to the vein and allows better blood flow to provide increased hemodilution of the IV fluids or medications (Coulter, 1992).
- If possible, avoid the back of the older adult's hand or the dominant arm for venipuncture because these sites greatly interfere with the older adult's independence.
- If the older adult has fragile skin and veins, use minimal tourniquet pressure or no tourniquet at all.
- When the older adult has lost subcutaneous tissue, the veins lose stability and roll away from the needle. To stabilize the vein, apply traction to the skin below the projected insertion point (Whitson, 1996).
- Use a lower angle of approach (e.g., 5 to 15 degrees on insertion) to accommodate more superficial veins (Whitson, 1996).
  - Use paper tape on fragile skin. Use just enough to secure the device to prevent an in-and-out motion of the device with movement (Whitson, 1996).
  - Older adults may not complain of pain at the insertion site. A large amount of fluid may infiltrate before a client experiences discomfort. Be vigilant in checking an older adult's IV site.

Home Care Considerations

- Ensure that the client is able and willing to self-administer IV therapy or that there is a reliable caregiver to provide IV therapy care at home.
- Determine the client's ability to obtain help, for example, availability of caregiver, presence of and ability to use telephone.
- Ensure that all needles and equipment contaminated by blood are disposed of in puncture-resistant containers with lids, for example, plastic milk cartons or coffee cans. Some suppliers will provide sharps containers for needle disposal (see Chapter 39).
- Instruct client and primary caregiver about procedures of IV therapy, including hand washing, sterile technique while manipulating syringes and other supplies.
- Teach client and primary caregiver to take tub bath but not to let IV tubing touch water and to unplug pump first if one is used. If showering is mandatory, the client must insert

ST. JOHN'S HOSPITAL
Springfield, Illinois

I.V. MAINTENANCE RECORD

I.V. FLUID & I.V. MEDICATION

Signature:

Site Code:
R.J. or L.J. – Right or Left Jugular
R.S.V. or L.S.V. – Right or Left Subclavian Vein
R.L.L. or L.L.L. – Right or Left Lower Leg
R.H. or L.H. – Right or Left Hand
R.F.A. or L.F.A. – Right or Left Forearm
R.U.A. or L.U.A. – Right or Left Upperarm
R.F. or L.F. – Right or Left Foot
R.S., L.S. or M.S. – Right, Left or Mid Scalp
R.F.V. or L.F.V. – Right or Left Femoral Vein
R.A.C. or L.A.C. – Right or Left Antecubital
R.W. or L.W. – Right or Left Wrist
K.V.O. – Keep Vein Open
H.L. – Heparin Lock
P.B. – Piggyback
P. – Push

Triple Lumen Catheter:
Proximal - 18 gauge (White) Draw blood, Blood Adm, Medications
Middle - 18 gauge (Blue) TPN, Medications
Distal - 16 gauge (Brown) Blood Adm., Colloids, Viscous Fluids, CVP Monitoring, Medications

Allergy:

No. of last I.V. ________ Letter of last expander ________

No. of last Blood/Component ________

DATE		
Night Nurse		
Day Nurse		
Evening Nurse		

Order Date		Amount, Solution, Infusing Time or Rate, Medication, Dose, Time	Site(s)			Pump	Time	Time
		One Time I.V. Meds.						
	No.	I.V. Fluids						

I.V. SITE ASSESSMENT

SITE CODE		TYPE CODE	
R.J. or L.J. – Right or Left Jugular	K.V.O. – Keep Vein Open	M.C. – Medicut	H.C. – Hickman Catheter
R.S.V. or L.S.V. – Right or Left Subclavian Vein	H.L. – Heparin Lock	A.C. – Angiocath	B.C. – Broviac Catheter
R.L.L. or L.L.L. – Right or Left Lower Leg	P.B. – Piggyback	S.V. – Scalpvein	M.L.C. – Multi-lumen Catheter
R.H. or L.H. – Right or Left Hand	P. – Push	A.S. – Angio-set	M.L.P. – Multi-lumen Proximal
R.F.A. or L.F.A. – Right or Left Forearm	Cath – Catheter	C.D. – Cutdown	M.L.M. – Multi-lumen Middle
R.U.A. or L.U.A. – Right or Left Upperarm		I.C. – Intracath	M.L.D. – Multi-lumen Distal
R.F. or L.F. – Right or Left Foot		I.P. – Infuse A Port	I. – Introducer
R.S., L.S. or M.S. – Right, Left or Mid Scalp			
R.F.V. or L.F.V. – Right or Left Femoral Vein			
R.A.C. or L.A.C. – Right or Left Antecubital			
R.W. or L.W. – Right or Left Wrist	NA – Not Applicable		

Document on each site once each shift & P.R.N. No space is to be left blank. Place "NA" in spaces which do not apply.

Date	Time	I.V. Site Start	I.V. Site d/c	Site Code	Cath Size	Type Code	Site Day	Cap Change	Dressing Change	I.V. Site: $\bar{s}$ tenderness redness, edema, drainage	Signature

FIGURE 19-5 IV maintenance record. (Courtesy St. John's Hospital, Springfield, Ill.)

hand and forearm into a plastic bag. Tape bag in place to ensure that IV site is completely covered.
- Instruct client to wear clothes with wide sleeves.
- Teach client about activity restrictions, for example, avoiding strenuous exercise of the arm with the IV.
- Teach client and family to monitor intake and output using household measuring devices.

Long-Term Care Considerations

- If a client is highly active or requires restraints at times, it may be wise to place the client's arm in an armboard to prevent the needle or catheter from becoming dislodged.

Skill 19-2 Inserting a Peripherally Inserted Central Catheter

Peripherally inserted central catheters (PICCs) provide alternate intravenous (IV) access when the client requires intermediate-length venous access (greater than 7 days to 3 months). PICC catheters are inserted through a vein in the antecubital fossa and advanced until the tip enters the central venous system (e.g., subclavian vein). In many states the PICC can be inserted only by an RN nurse who has received special training, consisting of didactic and practical instruction, and has demonstrated competency in PICC line insertion (Refer to Nurse Practice Act for your state.) In some institutions only IV therapy team members will insert PICC lines. Five primary methods of inserting PICC lines exist; thus extensive training is needed to know each method and the benefits and disadvantages to each (Thompson, 1999).

The staff nurse must still understand what a PICC line is and be aware of its appropriate care and maintenance. In comparison to centrally placed venous catheters, the PICC has less risk of pneumothorax, hemothorax, or air embolism and is more cost-effective. Compared to peripheral IV catheters, the PICC can be kept in place longer (more than 48 to 72 hours). In fact, PICC lines may remain in place as long as there are no signs of problems (e.g., infiltration, migration, infection). PICC lines are associated with less risk of infiltration and phlebitis because the IV fluids and medications are diluted in the greater volume of blood flow present in the larger veins (subclavian or superior vena cava) where the tip of the catheter is placed. However, other complications associated with PICC use include clotting, leaking, or breaking of the catheter. For successful catheter placement, the client must have a palpable cephalic or basilic vein located in the antecubital fossa.

PICCs vary in size from 16- to 24-gauge and in length from 40 to 65 cm (16 to 26 in). The length is chosen based on the distance from the client's antecubital fossa to the desired point of tip placement. Catheters can have a single or double lumen. A guide wire or stylet can be used when inserting a PICC to make the catheter stiffer and easier to advance. The catheter is made of soft materials, which cause minimal irritation to the vein.

PICCs can be used to infuse IV fluids, parenteral nutrition, blood and blood products, and medications such as antibiotics. The smaller-gauge catheters cannot be used for some types of infusions, especially those of blood, blood products, and parenteral nutrition. Not all PICCs can be used to draw blood. The nurse should be aware of product advantages and limitations of each device used.

Delegation Considerations

The skill of inserting a peripherally inserted central catheter should not be delegated to assistive personnel. If assistive personnel are involved in caring for clients with PICC lines, they should be instructed to report any client complaint regarding the IV device immediately. Assistive personnel should also be instructed in how to position and assist clients in moving when PICC lines are in place.

Equipment

Many manufacturers of PICCs provide an insertion kit that provides most of the required equipment, check how equipment is supplied in each agency. Not every kit contains the same supplies.

- Two pair of sterile gloves
- Two sterile drapes (1 fenestrated, 1 nonfenestrated)
- Sterile forceps (nontoothed)
- Sterile scissors
- Two sterile 4 × 4 gauze pads
- Tourniquet
- Three povidone-iodine swab sticks
- Three alcohol swab sticks
- Two sterile 2 × 2 gauze pads
- Transparent dressing
- Steri-strips
- Six 10-ml syringes with 1-inch, 21-gauge needles
- Short extension tubing (one for each lumen)
- Injection cap (one for each lumen) (Luer-lok)
- Two 10-ml vials of sterile normal saline for injection
- 10-ml vial of heparin (10 to 100 U/ml)
- PICC (size depends on size of client's vein and type of infusion ordered)
- Lidocaine (1% or 2% with or without epinephrine) or Enteric Mixture of Local Anesthetics (EMLA) lidocaine and prilocaine (topical lidocaine) for topical anesthesia
- Two tape measures (one sterile and one unsterile)
- Face mask, gown, goggles

STEP	RATIONALE

ASSESSMENT

1. Review physician's order for type of catheter, type of infusion, and desired placement of the catheter. An order requesting the insertion of a PICC line and administration of an IV solution must be made by a licensed physician prior to implementation of this procedure.
   - *Rationale:* Ensures safe and correct initiation of PICC. Catheter tip can be placed in either subclavian vein or in superior vena cava. (Superior vena cava is the most desired position.)
2. Know agency's policy concerning RN personnel who may start PICCs.
   - *Rationale:* Most agencies require special training and/or certification.
3. Review manufacturer's directions concerning the catheter and insertion technique. Each manufacturer publishes guidelines for a particular catheter. Five techniques exist for PICC insertion (Thompson, 1999):
   a. Break-away needle introducer (used for this procedure description)
   b. Over-the-needle
   c. Peel-away sheath
   d. Insertion through a standard over-the-needle IV cannula
   e. Modified or full Seldinger technique
   - *Rationale:* Adherence to guidelines facilitates safe insertion.
4. Assess client's understanding of length and type of therapy and management of PICC.
   - *Rationale:* Client or significant other should be assessed to assume management of PICC once discharged home. Dressing changes are often done by home care agency, in a clinic, or in a doctor's office.
5. Assess client's fluid, **electrolyte,** and nutritional status.
   - *Rationale:* Provides data to verify reason for IV therapy and to serve as a basis for evaluation.
6. Assess client's comfort, oxygenation, and elimination needs.
   - *Rationale:* Anticipation of these needs prevents interruption of sterile procedure.
7. Assess for drug allergies.
   - *Rationale:* Local lidocaine will be applied to skin for anesthetic purposes. Catheters may contain latex.

NURSING DIAGNOSIS

Defining characteristics from the assessment data may reveal the following nursing diagnoses for clients requiring this skill:

- Imbalanced nutrition: less than body requirements
- Deficient fluid volume
- Risk for imbalanced fluid volume
- Risk for infection
- Deficient knowledge regarding use of PICC

Related factors are individualized based on client's condition or needs.

PLANNING

1. **Expected outcomes** following completion of procedure:
   - Client tolerates positional changes during insertion of PICC line.
     - *Rationale:* Catheter insertion performed correctly with good sterile technique. In one study, phlebitis occurred in 7% of the clients after an average time of 19 days, clotting occurred in 5.6% of the clients, and broken catheters occurred 6.4% of the time (Loughran, Edwards, and McClure, 1992).
   - Client will have no complaint of pain or erythema at the insertion site; PICC remains patent; catheter should be intact without visible breakage.
   - Site is free of bleeding or hematoma.
     - *Rationale:* Catheter inserted into vein without trauma to tissues or vein wall.
   - Client is free of respiratory distress.
     - *Rationale:* No introduction of air embolus occurs.
   - Client's chest x-ray film shows proper placement of catheter tip.
     - *Rationale:* Tip must be located in superior vena cava or subclavian vein.
   - Fluid and electrolyte balance will be normal as measured by normal vital signs, serum electrolyte levels, intake and output.
     - *Rationale:* Reflects the correction or maintenance of normal fluid and electrolyte balance.

Step	Rationale
▪ Client will have normal body weight and other indicators of nutritional balance.	Body weight can be maintained or gained when the client receives parenteral nutrition.
▪ Client remains afebrile with normal white blood cell count (WBC).	Elevated body temperature is associated with catheter sepsis.
▪ Client explains purpose and type of PICC and discusses proper management skills for home care.	Improves likelihood of client's adherence to medical treatment plan.
▪ Client lists three signs and symptoms of infection, thrombosis, and air embolism and interventions for each.	Enables client to initiate corrective measures at home.
2. Explain procedure to client, including position that will be used and possible complications.	Decreases anxiety and promotes cooperation.
3. Verify that a consent form has been signed.	Many agencies require a consent form.
4. Measure circumference of client's upper arm and document in nurses' notes.	Provides a baseline for subsequent comparison to determine swelling, which can be associated with the advent of complications (e.g., venous **thrombosis**).

Implementation

Step	Rationale
1. Wash hands.	Reduces transmission of microorganisms.
2. Organize equipment on a clean, clutter-free bedside stand or clean overbed table.	Reduces risk of contamination and accidents.
3. Instruct client to wash arms thoroughly from fingertips to midbiceps using antibacterial soap and warm water. (Assist client as needed.) Then assist to comfortable position, supine.	Decreases bacteria prior to insertion.
4. Clip hair around insertion site if necessary.	Helps dressing and tape adhere to skin. Makes dressing removal less painful. Clipping prevents microabrasions, thus decreasing risk for infection.

• ***Critical Decision Point***
Do not shave area. Shaving causes microabrasions.

Step	Rationale
5. Identify an appropriate vein in antecubital fossa by placing a tourniquet around upper arm close to axilla and examining veins in antecubital fossa; release tourniquet, leaving it in place beneath arm.	Either basilic or cephalic vein may be used; basilic vein is preferred because it is less tortuous. Releasing tourniquet prevents venous engorgement.

• ***Critical Decision Point***
Veins that are sclerosed (often from frequent blood drawing) should be avoided because catheter will most likely be difficult to advance.

Step	Rationale
6. Position client in a supine position in bed with arm at a 45- to 90-degree angle (see agency policy) to client's trunk.	This provides a straighter course for advancing catheter to large veins in chest.
7. Measure distance from insertion site to proposed site for catheter tip using unsterile tape measure. For subclavian placement, measure from proposed insertion site up the arm to the shoulder and across to the midclavicular line. For superior vena cava placement, continue to the sternal notch and down to the third intercostal space on the right of the sternum.	Desired position of catheter may be indicated in physician's order or by type of therapy to be given. These landmarks correspond to the venous structures underneath (see illustration).

• ***Critical Decision Point***
Superior vena cava placement must always be confirmed by a chest x-ray examination.

Step	Rationale
8. Put on mask, gown, and goggles. Client may also wear mask.	Reduces transmission of microorganisms.

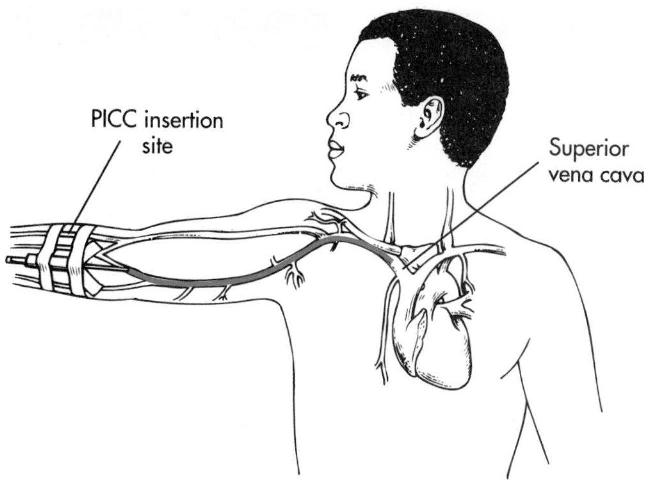

STEP 7 PICC line inserted at antecubital fossa, with tip advanced into superior vena cava.

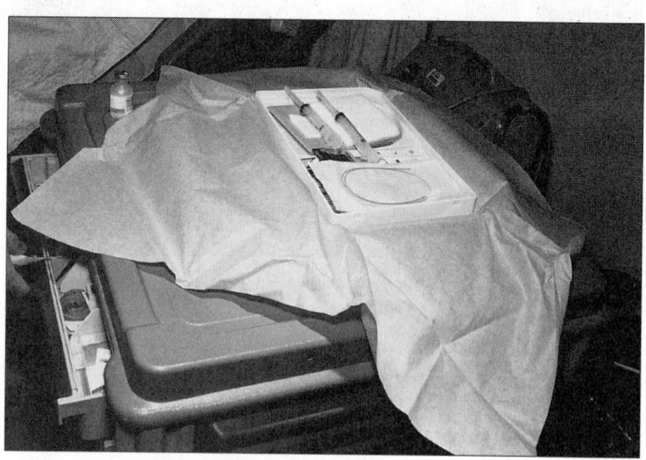

STEP 9 Equipment for PICC insertion.

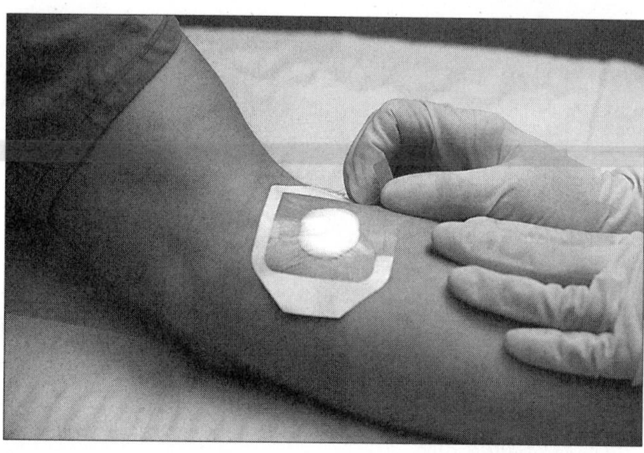

STEP 12 Application of topical lidocaine (EMLA) to site chosen for PICC insertion.

STEP	RATIONALE
9. Open sterile supplies or kit. Using kit's wrap as a sterile field, arrange supplies for efficient use; drop 4 × 4 gauze, extension tubings, and injection cap(s) onto field using sterile technique (see illustration). Cleanse top of normal saline, heparin, and lidocaine vials with alcohol and set aside on separate work surface.	Provides a sterile working surface. Facilitates efficient technique by having all supplies ready and accessible.
10. Put on sterile gloves.	Reduces transmission of microorganisms.
11. With another nurse or technician assisting, draw up lidocaine (optional), normal saline, and heparin for flushing.	Ensures sterile technique is observed.
12. If using EMLA for anesthetic, prepare by applying to insertion site ½ to 1 hour before venipuncture and cover with a layer of transparent dressing (see illustration).	Ensures skin is properly anesthetized.
13. Prepare catheter and tubing:	
a. Using sterile tape measure, measure catheter to length previously determined plus 1 inch.	Ensures that distal tip of catheter will be properly positioned. The extra length will extend out from venipuncture site.
b. Using sterile scissors, cut catheter tip at appropriate length (Optional step: check agency policy).	A straight cut may prevent catheter end from lying on intima and obstructing blood flow. A 45-degree bevel cut clearly identifies tip of catheter.

• ***Critical Decision Point***
Check agency policy. Not all catheters can be cut. Check product brochure.

STEP	RATIONALE
c. Attach injection cap to extension tubing (one set for each lumen). Using a 4 × 4 gauze to hold vial, draw up 5 ml of normal saline into a syringe for each lumen of catheter and flush each cap and tubing with 2 ml. Remove needle from syringe and flush catheter, leaving syringe in place.	Removes air from tubing and catheter, ensures patency of catheter, detects any leaks.
d. Inspect equipment for defects such as cracks or kinks. Verify patency of introducer.	Ensures proper function during and after insertion.
14. Prepare insertion site:	
a. Place sterile drape under access arm.	Reduces transmission of microorganisms.
b. Vigorously scrub insertion site using three alcohol swab sticks and allow to dry for 60 seconds. Follow by three povidone-iodine swab sticks (see illustration). A circular area from the middle of forearm to middle of upper arm should be cleaned with each swab stick, starting at venipuncture site and cleansing outward in a circular motion middle to outer edge. Cleansed area should be an approximate 6-inch concentric circular area from venipuncture site. Let povidone-iodine dry completely (at least 2 minutes).	Alcohol defats the skin; povidone-iodine is a topical antiinfective that reduces skin surface bacteria. Circular motion moves bacteria on skin away from insertion site. Use of separate swab sticks prevents bacteria from being reintroduced to venipuncture site. Povidone-iodine must dry to be effective in reducing microbial counts (Baranowski, 1993).

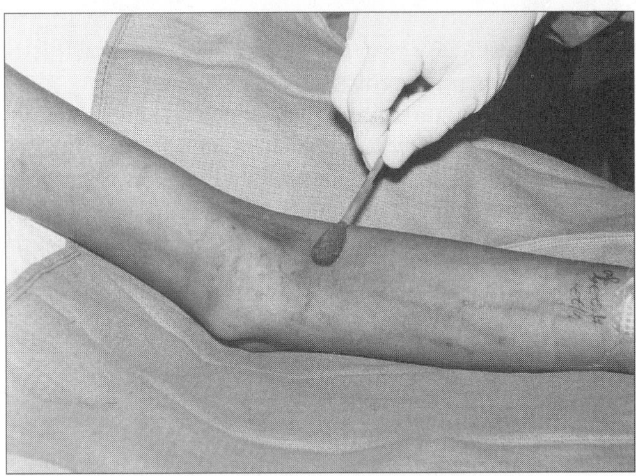

STEP **14b** Prepping PICC site.

STEP	RATIONALE
15. Remove gloves; reapply tourniquet if a single nonsterile tourniquet is used.	Tourniquet is not sterile; application of tourniquet impedes venous blood flow, resulting in an engorged vein to foster ease of venipuncture.
16. Put on a new pair of sterile gloves; use talc-free gloves or rinse gloves with sterile water.	Reduces the transmission of microorganisms; rinsing gloves prevents talc adherence to the catheter.
17. Place sterile 4 × 4 gauze over tourniquet or apply sterile tourniquet.	Allows removal of tourniquet without contaminating glove.
18. Place fenestrated drape over insertion site, being careful to avoid contamination of site.	Provides sterile field around venipuncture site.
19. If EMLA not applied, administer 0.1 to 0.2 ml of 1% lidocaine subcutaneously (SQ) at insertion site. Check agency policy and physician's order.	Local anesthetic reduces discomfort.

• ***Critical Decision Point***
Note lidocaine is used only when EMLA has not been used. ***Do not use both.***

STEP	RATIONALE
20. Insert introducer needle at a 20- to 30-degree angle, bevel up. Look for a brisk blood return through introducer (see illustration).	Angle lessens risk of puncture of posterior wall of vein. The introducer is large bore.

• ***Critical Decision Point***
Verify that blood return is venous, not arterial (arterial blood is pulsatile and bright red). Brachial vein is close to brachial artery and artery may be inadvertently cannulated.

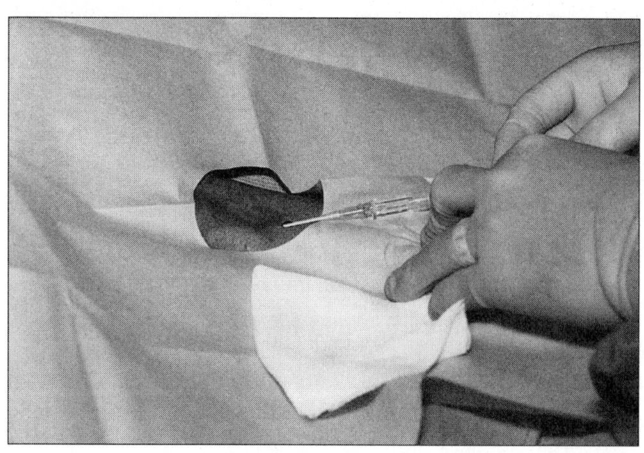

STEP **20** Introduction of PICC introducer needle into antecubital fossa.

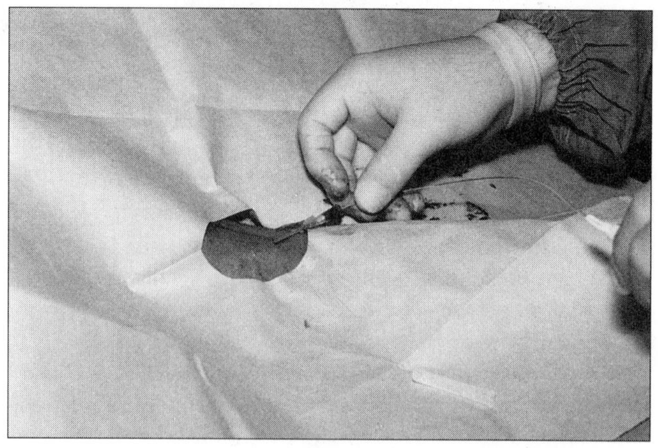

STEP **24** Advancing PICC line through vein.

STEP	RATIONALE
21. Lower introducer parallel to skin and advance (½ to 1 cm) further into vein.	Ensures that vein is securely cannulated.
22. Insert catheter through introducer needle, and advance it slowly approximately 2 to 3 inches (5 to 7.5 cm) using the nontoothed forceps. Agency policy differs concerning use of guide wire or stylet. If guide wire is used, ensure that it remains well within lumen of PICC during insertion. Take care that catheter remains on sterile field during insertion.	Allows catheter to travel through introducer into vein. Slow advancement prevents trauma to intima of vein (Loughran, Edwards, and McClure, 1992). Guide wire provides more rigidity to catheter to aid insertion. Otherwise, no significant difference was found between clients whose PICCs were begun with guide wires and those for whom guide wires were not used (Loughran, Edwards, and McClure, 1992).

- ***Critical Decision Point***
  If catheter leaves sterile field, it is considered contaminated and cannot be inserted. A new sterile catheter must be used.

STEP	RATIONALE
23. Release tourniquet, while stabilizing catheter, using sterile 4 × 4 gauze if a nonsterile tourniquet is used.	Allows further catheter advancement. Prevents contamination of glove.
24. Advance catheter an additional 6 inches (or more depending on client size) until tip of catheter is at the shoulder (see illustration). Catheter is marked at 10-cm intervals to facilitate identification of location of tip.	Ensures placement of catheter tip into central venous circulation.
25. Instruct client to turn head toward the side of the venous access and drop the chin to the chest.	This position closes the internal jugular vein, preventing accidental cannulation.
26. Continue to slowly advance catheter until predetermined length is reached.	Aids proper placement of tip of catheter.
27. Fully withdraw introducer needle. Either use forceps to maintain position of catheter or apply light pressure 2 inches above insertion site while introducer is withdrawn.	Introducer is removed to prevent accidental puncture of the vein. Pressure helps ensure that catheter will not be withdrawn with introducer. Pressure any closer to introducer may cause introducer to nick catheter.

- ***Critical Decision Point***
  Never withdraw the catheter through the introducer needle; *this may shear off the catheter, causing a catheter embolism.*

STEP	RATIONALE
28. When introducer is out, press wings together until they snap, then peel needle from around catheter.	Removes needle so that catheter cannot be inadvertently punctured.
a. Tell client that a snapping sound will be heard.	Prevents anxiety.
29. Remove guide wire using a gentle twisting motion.	Allows use of lumen, prevents damage to catheter and vein.
30. Attach a syringe filled with 3 ml of normal saline to lumen where guide wire had been, aspirate for a blood return, and flush catheter.	Verifies patency of distal lumen, prevents clotting.

Step	Rationale
31. Remove syringe from each lumen and attach extension tubing and cap to lumen.	Prevents blood loss, maintains closed system.
32. Cleanse insertion site with antiseptic swab if there has been oozing of blood. Allow to dry (see illustration).	Leakage around insertion site is not uncommon due to size of catheter gauge. Cleansing reduces risk of microorganism growth at site.
33. Anchor hub of catheter to skin with Steri-strips placed over catheter's hub (see illustration). Some agencies suggest that PICC should be sutured in place. Some state boards do not allow RNs to suture.	Helps to maintain catheter's position for long-term use.
34. Place 2 × 2 gauze pads directly over insertion site. Cover this with a transparent dressing (see illustration).	Provides pressure on insertion site for 24 hours to control oozing caused by large-gauge introducer. Later dressing replaced with transparent covering only.
35. Coil extension tubing and tape securely to client's arm. Do not pull or apply undue pressure to catheter when manipulating it. Label dressing with date and time of insertion, length and gauge of catheter.	Prevents inadvertent dislodgement. Prevents catheter breakage.
36. Flush each lumen with 3 ml of heparin solution.	Maintains patency of each lumen.
37. Dispose of equipment appropriately. Wash hands.	Reduces transmission of microorganisms.
38. Follow agency policy for x-ray verification of placement.	X-ray examination is usually done to verify placement in the superior vena cava before start of infusion therapy.

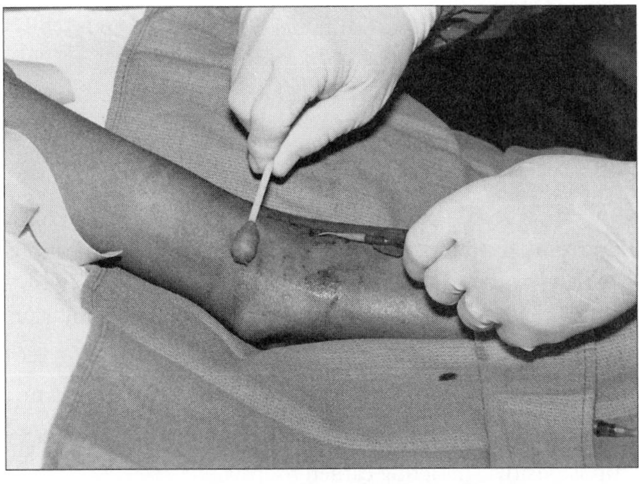

STEP **32** Cleanse site if there has been oozing of blood.

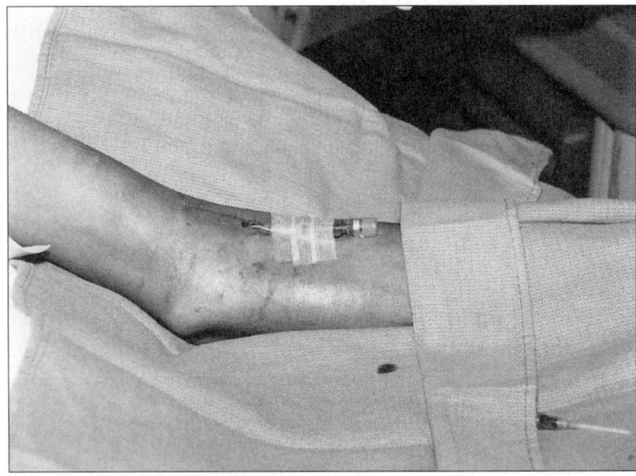

STEP **33** Anchor PICC catheter hub with Steri-strips.

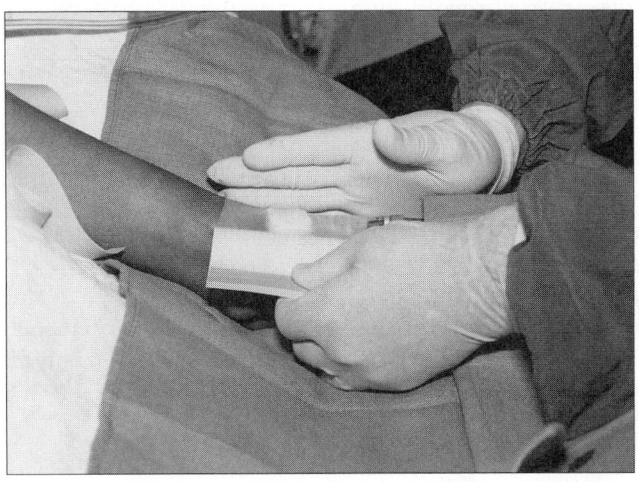

STEP **34** Apply transparent dressing over PICC catheter.

Step	Rationale
39. Regularly aspirate for blood return and flush the catheter with normal saline followed by heparin solution (10 to 100 U/ml) (according to agency policy).	Retains patency of catheter, preventing clotting.

Evaluation

1. Observe client and inquire about comfort level during insertion.	Procedure can be lengthy, causing client to become anxious.
2. Inspect and palpate PICC site immediately after insertion for bleeding or hematoma.	Bleeding will require new attempt with insertion of new catheter.
3. Note respiratory status.	PICC line insertion can result in air embolism.
4. Once PICC has been inserted, call for chest x-ray examination.	Determines that catheter is positioned in superior vena cava.

- ***Critical Decision Point***
  Chest x-ray examination is required for PICC lines placed in the superior vena cava.

5. Observe integrity of PICC routinely, according to agency policy.	Provides information concerning the most frequent complications associated with PICCs.
a. Assess insertion site for phlebitis, exudate, leaking, clotting, catheter breakage.	Ensures PICC line is functioning properly.
b. Verify that correct therapy is being delivered as ordered.	Ensures correct fluid is infusing.
c. Observe client for systemic complications such as air embolism, infection.	Timely identification of complications results in prompt treatment.
d. Measure amount of catheter that remains external with each dressing change.	Detects catheter migration.
6. Observe client to determine response to fluid and electrolyte therapy (see Skill 19-1).	PICCs provide a reliable method for delivering IV fluids and electrolytes.
7. Weigh client daily.	PICCs can provide parenteral nutrition.
8. Measure client's body temperature every 4 hours.	Elevated body temperature provides evidence of infection, which may be related to presence of PICC.
9. Review with client and ask to describe signs and symptoms of complications and steps for daily catheter maintenance.	Ensures client's ability to detect problems with PICC infusion and to adhere to daily care routines.

Unexpected Outcomes and Related Interventions

- There is blocked or difficult infusion of fluids through catheter, indicating occlusion that is either mechanical, nonthrombotic, or thrombotic (Bagnall-Reeb, 1998).
  - Assess tubing and catheter exit site to rule out external cause of obstruction. Tight sutures may need to be removed.
  - Chest x-ray examination may be ordered to determine internal compression.
  - Know drug incompatibilities to prevent precipitation of infused solution.
  - Assess change in ability to aspirate or withdraw from catheter. Look for clots visible in external portion of line. Physician or qualified RN may attempt aspiration of clot. Fibrinolytic therapy may be used (see agency policy).
- Client experiences pain and erythema at insertion site; blood or fluids leak from PICC insertion site.
  - Reinsertion in opposite arm with new sterile catheter may be necessary.
- Client develops a fever, elevated WBC, and culture of PICC tip is positive, indicting catheter sepsis.
  - PICC line is removed. Client may receive antibiotics.
- Client develops fluid volume deficit, fluid volume excess, or electrolyte imbalances.
  - Volume of fluid to be infused over 24 hours will be revised by prescriber. Additions or deletions may be made to additives in IV fluid.
- Client's body weight is less than ideal body weight. If parenteral nutrition is not administered accurately, client receives insufficient nutrients to support normal body weight.
  - Orders for parenteral nutrition will be revised to provide accurate caloric intake.
- Client develops sudden respiratory distress, which may indicate pulmonary embolus.
  - Notify physician immediately. Be prepared to obtain chest x-ray examination.

- Client develops irregular pulse.
  - May indicate catheter is in the right atrium, causing atrial irritation. Catheter may need to be withdrawn several centimeters.

Recording and Reporting

- Document date, time of PICC placement, length and size of PICC catheter, vein accessed, and arm circumference.
- Record PICC's gauge and length, insertion site, date and time of insertion, location of catheter tip, radiographic confirmation of location of catheter tip (if x-ray examination has been completed), presence or absence of signs and symptoms of complications.
- Report status of PICC, therapy being administered, and development of complications and their treatment.

Teaching Considerations

- Because PICC insertion and care may be unfamiliar to the client, careful and repeated verbal explanations with written follow-up are important.
- Instruct client and caregiver about signs and symptoms of the most common complications: phlebitis, clotting, leaking at catheter insertion site, or breaking of the catheter. Instruct client on how to respond to each of these complications.
- Because the dressing is the anchor for the PICC, client and caregiver need to notify nurse if dressing becomes loose. Nurse will perform a dressing change.
- If PICC becomes clotted, client should promptly seek care so that declotting measures can be instituted.
- Instruct clients about allowed activities:
  - The PICC dressing should not become wet, so bathing must be adapted to keep cannulated arm dry.
  - Client should avoid vigorous activities (e.g., weight lifting) because catheter may be damaged.
  - Client can move arm freely because there is less chance of infiltration and dislodgement than with a peripheral venipuncture using a short catheter. However, elbow flexion may be hampered by placement of dressing.

Pediatric Considerations

- An advantage of the use of PICCs for neonates is the longer duration of use compared with traditional peripheral catheters.
- In neonates the antecubital veins, long saphenous vein, superficial temporal vein, external jugular vein, popliteal vein, veins in the ankle, and axillary veins may be used.

Home Care Considerations

- Ensure that client is able and willing to care for PICC line and administer IV therapy or that there is a reliable caregiver or nursing support personnel at home to provide IV therapy care before insertion.
- The catheter can be inserted in the home, or client may have it inserted before discharge from the hospital.
- Common uses for PICCs in the home are long-term antibiotic/antiviral administration, pain control, parenteral nutrition, and hydration.
- Since client in the home setting may be more active, a secure dressing is required.
- Superior vena cava insertion is not practiced in the home setting because this requires an x-ray examination after insertion.

Skill 19-3 Regulating Intravenous Flow Rate

After an intravenous (IV) infusion is initiated and the line is patent, the nurse is responsible for regulating the rate of infusion according to the physician's orders. An infusion rate that is too slow can lead to further cardiovascular and circulatory collapse in a client who is dehydrated, in shock, or critically ill. In addition, if an infusion runs too slowly, the chances of the vein clotting off are greater. An infusion rate that is too rapid can result in fluid overload, which is particularly dangerous in certain cardiovascular, kidney, and neurological disorders and in the very young and very old.

The nurse calculates the infusion rate to prevent too-slow or too-rapid administration. Children, older adults, clients with severe head trauma, and clients susceptible to fluid volume excess (FVE) must be protected from sudden increases in infusion volumes. Sudden increases can occur accidentally. For example, a restless client may loosen the roller clamp with a sudden movement and thus increase the flow rate, or the flow rate may be accidentally increased if the client ambulates. A sudden increase in volume can make the client critically ill or even cause death in some cases. Two types of infusion devices, the electronic infusion pump and an IV volume-control device, assist the nurse in maintaining correct flow rates, maintaining catheter patency, and preventing runaway bolus IV infusions, and alert the nurse when an IV bag or bottle is empty or when an IV occlusion occurs. Many infusion pumps also record the volume of fluid infused.

An **infusion pump** is designed to deliver a measured amount of fluid over a period of time, that is, milliliters per hour. If the pump has a drop sensor, an alarm sounds if drops are not detected at the appropriate rate. The alarm will go off

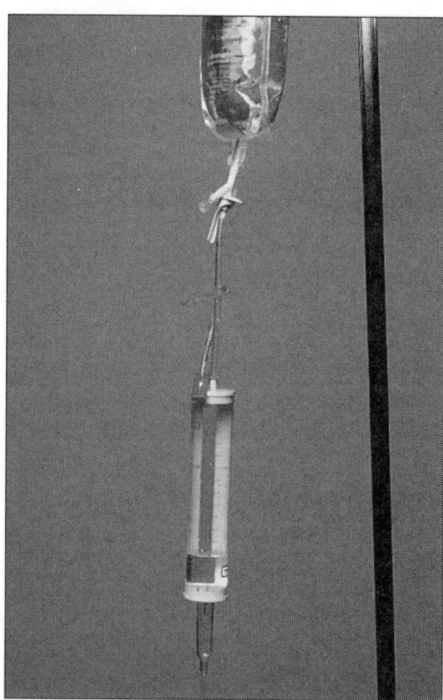

FIGURE **19-6** Volume control device.

when an IV bag or bottle becomes empty. An alarm also sounds if the pressure in the system increases. For example, when an infiltration of IV fluids forms within the subcutaneous tissue or if the client's arm position obstructs intravenous flow, pressure will build up and set off the alarm. Since the pump uses positive pressure, an infiltration may be extensive before the pump's alarm sounds. The nurse must use frequent inspection and palpation of the IV site to ensure timely detection of an infiltration. IV pumps have a high degree of accuracy and precision to ensure that IV fluid therapy is administered correctly.

An IV volume-control device delivers fluid with the aid of gravity. The IV container must be placed approximately 36 inches above the IV site to overcome venous resistance and operate properly. IV controllers deliver fluids based on a determination of drops per minute, which is in turn based on milliliters per hour. The nurse must monitor the volume delivered each hour to ensure that the calculated drops per minute deliver the actual volume desired. The actual volume delivered depends on the rate of infusion, the IV tubing size, and fluid viscosity. Because IV controllers cannot overcome increased resistance in the IV system, infiltrations can be more quickly detected by an IV controller than by a pump. This sensitivity also increases the number of nuisance alarms that occur when client movement is misinterpreted as increased resistance to flow. A volume-control device is a calibrated chamber placed between the IV bag or bottle and the insertion spike and drip chamber of the administration set (Figure 19-6). A small volume of IV fluid is placed in the chamber from the IV fluid container. This smaller volume is then delivered to the client. The advantage of this system is that only the smaller volume of fluid infuses if the rate of the IV is inadvertently increased. Volume-control devices are usually used when administering IV fluid to neonates and very young children.

Delegation Considerations

The skill of regulating intravenous flow rate should not be delegated to assistive personnel. Assistive personnel should be instructed to report if electronic infusion device alarm sounds.

Equipment

- Watch with second hand
- Paper and pencil
- IV infusion pump (optional)
- Volume-control device (optional)

Step	Rationale
Assessment	
1. Check client's medical record for correct solution and additives. Follow five rights of drug administration (Chapter 16). Usual order includes solution for 24 hours, usually divided into 2 or 3 L. Occasionally, IV order contains only 1 L to keep vein open (KVO). Record also shows time over which each liter is to infuse.	Five rights prevent medication administration error.
2. Observe for patency of IV line and catheter or needle:	For fluid to infuse at proper rate, IV line and needle must be free of kinks, knots, clots.
a. Open drip regulator and observe for rapid flow of fluid from solution into drip chamber, then close drip regulator to prescribed rate (see Implementation section).	Rapid flow of fluid into drip chamber indicates patency of IV line. Closing drip chamber to prescribed rate prevents fluid overload.
b. Compress cannulated vein slightly proximal to end of catheter and observe drip chamber.	Compression will temporarily cause cessation of drops from drip chamber, indicating catheter or needle is in vein. If fluid continues to drip, infiltration may be present and further assessment is needed.

STEP	RATIONALE
3. Check client's knowledge of how positioning of IV site affects flow rate.	Fosters client participation in maintaining most effective position of arm with IV equipment. Position or setting of control clamp or infusion device drip rate should be done only by health care provider.
4. Verify with client how venipuncture site feels; for example, determine if there is pain or burning.	Pain or burning may be early indication of phlebitis. Includes client in decision making.

NURSING DIAGNOSIS

Defining characteristics from the assessment data may reveal the following nursing diagnoses for clients requiring this skill:

- Deficient fluid volume
- Risk for imbalanced fluid volume
- Excess fluid volume

Related factors are individualized based on client's condition or needs.

PLANNING

1. **Expected outcomes** following completion of procedure:
   - Serum electrolytes remain within normal limits. — IV fluid assists in maintaining fluid and electrolyte levels.
   - Client receives prescribed volume of fluid over desired time interval. — When infusion rate remains within prescribed range, the therapeutic aim is achieved.
2. Have paper and pencil to calculate flow rate. — The beginning student is unfamiliar with IV fluid rates and should use mathematical calculations to obtain correct rate.
3. Know calibration (**drop factor**) in drops per milliliter (gtt/ml) of infusion set:
   Microdrip: 60 gtt/ml
   Macrodrip (Metheny, 2000):
   Abbott: 15 gtt/ml
   Travenol: 10 gtt/ml
   McGaw: 15 gtt/ml

   Microdrip tubing, also called pediatric tubing, universally delivers 60 gtt/ml and is used when small or very precise volumes are to be infused. However, there are different commercial parenteral administration sets for macrodrip tubing. Macrodrip tubing should be used when large quantities or fast rates are necessary.

   - ***Critical Decision Point***
     Know which company's infusion set an agency uses.
4. Select one of the following formulas to calculate flow rate after determining ml/hr.

   ml/hr = total infusion (ml)/hours of infusion

   (a) ml/hr/60 min = ml/min
   (b) Drop factor × ml/min = drops/min

   or

   (c) ml/hr × drop factor/60 min = drops/min

   Once hourly rate has been determined, these formulas give correct flow rate.

IMPLEMENTATION

STEP	RATIONALE
1. Read physician's orders, and follow five rights for correct solution and proper additives.	IV fluids are medications; following five rights decreases chance of medication error.
2. Intravenous fluids are usually ordered for 24-hour period, indicating how long each liter of fluid should run; for example, IV order for client is: *Bottle 1:* 1000 ml D_5W with 20 mEq KCl to run 8 hours *Bottle 2:* 1000 ml D_5W with 20 mEq KCl to run 8 hours *Bottle 3:* 1000 ml D_5W with 20 mEq KCl to run 8 hours *Total 24-hour IV intake:* 3000 ml	Determines volume of fluid that should infuse hourly.

STEP	RATIONALE

• ***Critical Decision Point***
It is common for physicians to write an abbreviated IV order such as: "D_5W with 20 mEq KCl 125 ml/hr continuous." This order implies that the IV should be maintained at this rate until order has been written for IV to be discontinued.

3. Determine hourly rate by dividing volume by hours, for example:

1000 ml/8 hr = 125 ml/hr

or if 3 L is ordered for 24 hours

3000 L/24 hr = 125 ml = 125 ml/hr

Provides even infusion of fluid over prescribed hourly rate.

4. Place marked adhesive tape or commercial fluid indicator tape on IV bottle or bag next to volume markings (see illustration)

Time taping IV bag gives nurse visual cue as to whether fluids are being administered over correct period of time. Time tapes should be used for all IV infusions, including those on therapies infused via **electronic infusion devices (EIDs).**

• ***Critical Decision Point***
Avoid drawing directly on IV bags with felt-tip pens or permanent markers because the ink could contaminate the solution (Millam, 1992).

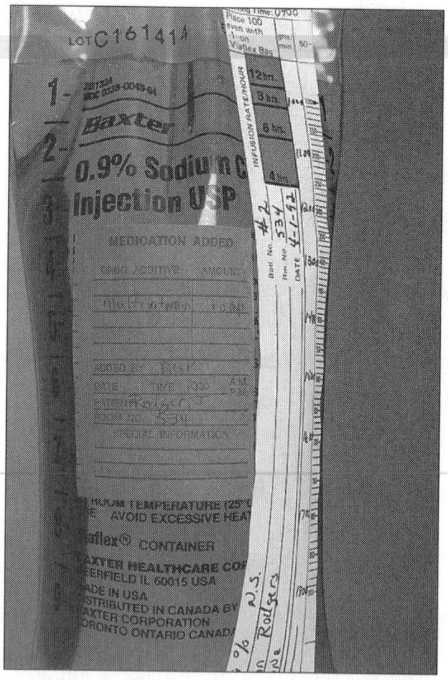

STEP **4** IV fluid bag with time tape.

5. After hourly rate has been determined, calculate minute rate based on drop factor of infusion set. Microdrip infusion set has a drop factor of 60 gtt/ml. Regular drip or macrodrip infusion set used in this example has drop factor of 15 gtt/ml. Using formula (see Planning, Step 4c), calculate minute flow rates: Bottle 1:1000 ml with 20 mEq KCl over 8 hours.

Allows nurse to calculate minute flow rate based on this formula:

Microdrip:

125 ml/hr × 60 gtt/ml = 7500 gtt/hr
7500 gtt ÷ 60 minutes = 125 gtt/min

When using microdrip, ml/hour always equals gtt/minute.

Macrodrip:

125 ml/hr × 15 gtt/ml = 1875 gtt/hr
1875 gtt ÷ 60 minutes = 31-32 gtt/min

Volume is multiplied by drop factor, and the product is divided by time (in minutes).

STEP	RATIONALE
6. Determine flow rate by counting drops in drip chamber for 1 minute by watch, then adjust roller clamp to increase or decrease rate of infusion (see illustration).	Determines if fluids are administered too slowly or too fast.
7. Follow this procedure for infusion controller or pump:	
a. Place electronic eye on drip chamber below origin of drop and above fluid level in chamber or consult manufacturer's directions for setup of the infusion (see illustration). If a controller is used, ensure that IV bag is 36 inches above IV site.	Electronic eye counts number of drops flowing from administration set to ensure that proper rate infuses. IV controller works by gravity.
b. IV infusion tubing is placed within ridges of control box in direction of flow (i.e., portion of tubing nearest IV bag at top and portion of tubing nearest client at bottom) or consult manufacturer's directions for use of pump (see illustration). Required drops per minute or volume per hour are selected, door to control chamber is closed, power button is turned on, and start button is pressed (see illustration).	Infusion pumps move fluid by compressing and milking IV tubing, thus propelling fluid through tubing.

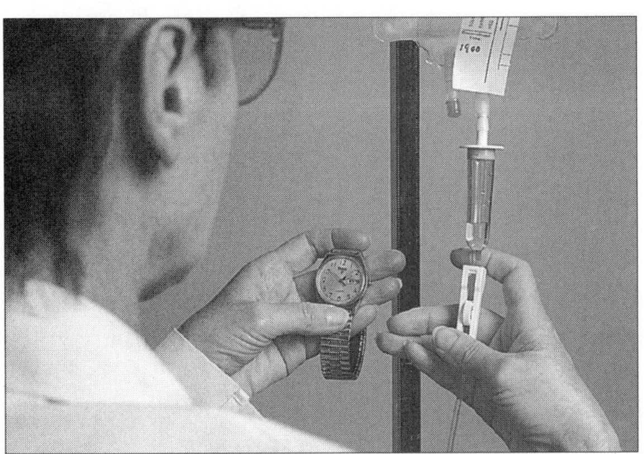

STEP **6** Counting IV drip rate.

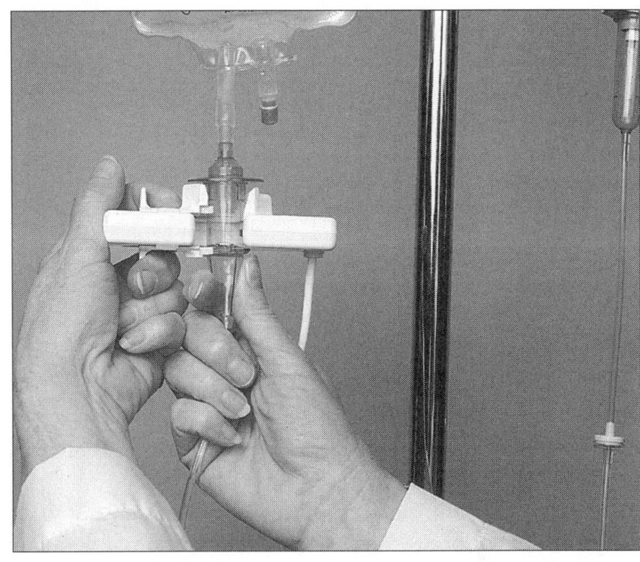

STEP **7a** Place electronic eye above fluid level in drip chamber.

A

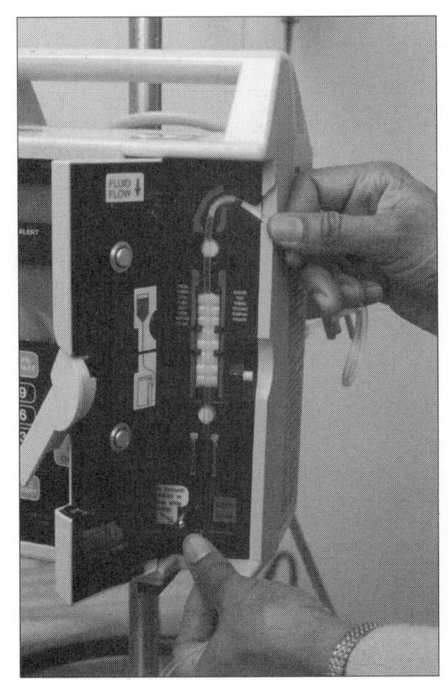

B

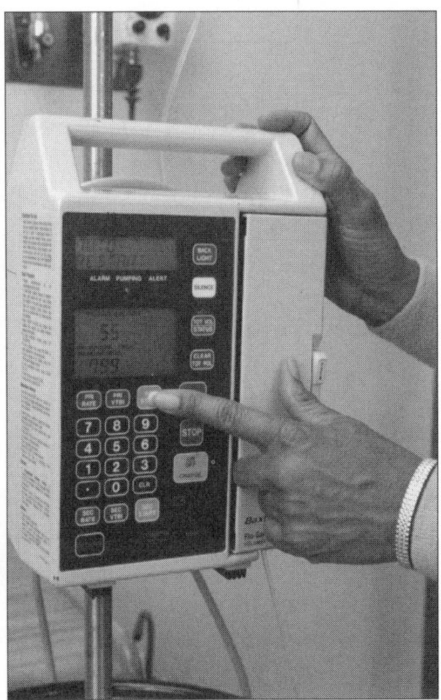

STEP **7b** **A,** Place infusing tubing within ridges of pump. **B,** Press start button to begin infusion.

STEP	RATIONALE
• ***Critical Decision Point*** *Special infusion tubing is required for some pumps. Check agency equipment and associated policies.*	
c. Open drip regulator completely while infusion controller or pump is in use.	Insures that pump freely regulates infusion rate.
d. Monitor infusion rates and IV site for infiltration according to agency policy. Rate of infusion should be checked by watch, even when infusion pump is used.	Infusion controllers or pumps are not infallible and do not replace frequent, accurate nursing evaluation. Infusion pumps may continue to infuse IV fluids after an infiltration has begun.
e. Assess patency of system when alarm sounds.	Alarm indicates that electronic eye has not noted precise number of drops from drip chamber. Alarm on infusion pump can be triggered by empty solution bag or bottle, kink in tubing, closed drip regulator, infiltrated or clotted needle, and/or air in the tubing.
8. Follow this procedure for volume-control device:	
a. Place volume-control device between IV bag and insertion spike of infusion set (see Figure 19-6).	Reduces risk of sudden increases in fluid volume.
b. Place 2 hours' allotment of fluid into device.	Prevents IV line from running dry if nurse does not return in exactly 60 minutes. In addition, if there is accidental increase in flow rate, client receives at most only a 2-hour allotment of fluid.
c. Assess system at least hourly; add fluid to volume control device. Regulate flow rate.	Maintains patency of system.

EVALUATION

STEP	RATIONALE
1. Monitor IV infusion at least every hour, noting volume of IV fluid infused and rate.	Ensures correct volume infuses over prescribed time period.
2. Observe client for signs of overhydration or dehydration to determine response to therapy and restoration of fluid and electrolyte balance.	Signs and symptoms of dehydration or overhydration warrant changing rate of fluid infused.
3. Evaluate for signs of infiltration: inflammation at site, clot in catheter, kink or knot in infusion tubing.	Prevents decrease or cessation of flow rate.

UNEXPECTED OUTCOMES AND RELATED INTERVENTIONS

- Sudden infusion of large volume of solution occurs with client having symptoms of dyspnea, crackles in the lung, and increased urine output, indicating fluid overload.
    - Slow infusion to KVO rate, and notify physician immediately. New IV orders will be required. Client may require diuretics.
- IV fluid bag runs empty with subsequent loss of IV line patency.
    - IV will be restarted.
- The IV infusion is slower than ordered.
    - Check client for positional change that might affect rate, height of IV bag, kinking of tubing.
    - An infiltration may be developing at IV site. Check condition of site.
    - If volume infused is deficient, consult physician for new order to provide necessary fluid volume

RECORDING AND REPORTING

- Record rate of infusion, drops/minute, and ml/hr in nurses' notes or parenteral fluid form every 4 hours or according to agency policy.
- Immediately record in nurses' notes any new IV fluid rates.
- Document use of any electronic infusion device or controlling device and number on that device.
- At change of shift or when leaving on break, report rate of infusion to nurse in charge or next nurse assigned to care for client.

TEACHING CONSIDERATIONS

- Client should know the prescribed hourly flow of IV fluids to provide an extra pair of eyes for observation.
- If an infusion pump is used, client should know its preset rate and the significance of alarms.

HOME CARE CONSIDERATIONS

- Ensure that client is able and willing to operate an infusion pump (if applicable) and administer IV therapy. If client is unable to provide self-care be sure that a reliable caregiver is available in the home.
- Make sure nurse is in the home when IV pump is delivered. This enables nurse to determine that equipment works properly.
- Teach client and primary caregiver to time drops per minute using watch with second hand.
- Ensure that client's electrical outlets are properly grounded.

Skill 19-4 Changing Intravenous Solutions

Clients receiving intravenous (IV) therapy may require frequent changing of IV solutions. The nurse must allow adequate time for this procedure and follow proper technique to prevent infection. Occasionally clients have an infusion only to deliver IV medication every 4, 6, or 8 hours (see Chapter 16). In this case an hourly infusion flow of about 10 to 25 ml/hr is used to keep the vein open (KVO) between doses, and usually a microdrip infusion set is used. Generally these clients do not use an entire IV solution bag. A new solution bag or bottle should be changed according to agency policy. The Centers for Disease Control and Prevention (CDC) (1996a) does not have a recommendation for hang time of IV fluids.

DELEGATION CONSIDERATIONS

The skill of changing intravenous solutions should not be delegated to assistive personnel.

EQUIPMENT

- Bottle/bag of IV solution as ordered by physician
- Time tape

STEP	RATIONALE
ASSESSMENT	
1. Check physician's orders for type of fluid and infusion rate.	Ensures that correct solution will be used.
2. If order is written for KVO or to keep open (TKO), note date and time when solution was last changed.	A hang time is no longer recommended by the Centers for Disease Control and Prevention (1996a) to ensure sterility of solutions in bag or bottle. Refer to agency policy.
3. Determine the compatibility of all IV fluids and additives by consulting appropriate literature or the pharmacy.	Incompatibilities can cause physical, chemical, and therapeutic client changes.
4. Determine client's understanding of need for continued IV therapy.	Reveals need for client instruction.
5. Determine if current IV access is patent.	If patency is not verified, a new IV access site may be needed. Notify physician.

NURSING DIAGNOSIS

Defining characteristics from the assessment data may reveal the following nursing diagnoses for clients requiring this skill:

Deficient fluid volume
Risk for imbalanced fluid volume
Risk for infection
Deficient knowledge related to purpose for IV therapy

Related factors are individualized based on client's condition or needs.

PLANNING

STEP	RATIONALE
1. **Expected outcomes** following completion of procedure:	
▪ Fluid infusion is correct.	Client receives correct fluid volume.
▪ IV line remains patent.	Ensures infusion of fluid into intravascular space.

Step	Rationale
2. Have next solution prepared at least 1 hour before needed. If prepared in pharmacy, be sure it has been delivered to client's hospital unit. Check that solution is correct and properly labeled. Check solution expiration date.	Adequate planning reduces risk of clot formation in vein caused by empty IV bag. Checking prevents medication error.
3. Check client's identification by checking arm bracelet and asking client to state name.	Ensures correct solution is administered to correct client.
4. Prepare to change solution when fluid remains only in neck of bottle or bag.	Prevents air from entering tubing and vein from clotting from lack of flow.
5. Prepare client and family by explaining the procedure, its purpose, and what is expected of client.	Decreases anxiety and promotes cooperation.
6. Be sure drip chamber is at least half full.	Provides fluid to vein while bag is changed.

IMPLEMENTATION

Step	Rationale
1. Wash hands.	Reduces transmission of microorganisms.
2. Prepare new solution for changing. If using plastic bag, remove protective cover from IV tubing port. If using glass bottle, remove metal cap and metal rubber disks.	Permits quick, smooth, and organized change from old to new solution.
3. Move roller clamp to stop flow rate.	Prevents solution remaining in drip chamber from emptying while changing solutions.
4. Remove old IV fluid container from IV pole.	Brings work to nurse's eye level.
5. Quickly remove spike from old solution bag or bottle and, without touching tip, insert spike into new bag or bottle.	Reduces risk of solution in drip chamber running dry and maintains sterility.

• ***Critical Decision Point***

If spike is contaminated, a new IV tubing set is required. Sterile IV tubing is good for 72 hours.

Step	Rationale
6. Hang new bag or bottle of solution.	Allows gravity to assist with delivery of fluid into drip chamber.
7. Check for air in tubing. If bubbles form, they can be removed by closing roller clamp, stretching tubing downward, and tapping tubing with finger (bubbles rise in fluid to drip chamber) (see illustration). For a larger amount of air, insert a needle and syringe into a port below the air, and aspirate the air into the syringe. Swab port with alcohol and allow to dry before inserting needle into port. Reduce air in tubing by priming slowly instead of allowing a wide-open flow.	Reduces risk of air embolus. Use of an air-eliminating filter also reduces this risk.

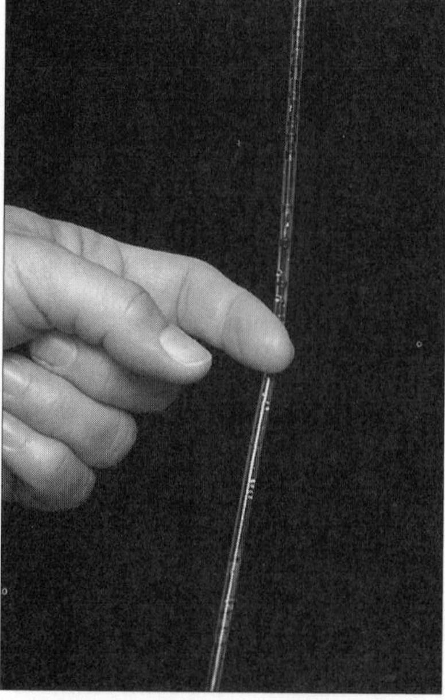

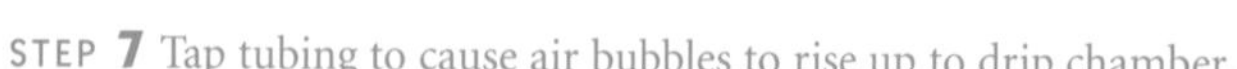
STEP 7 Tap tubing to cause air bubbles to rise up to drip chamber.

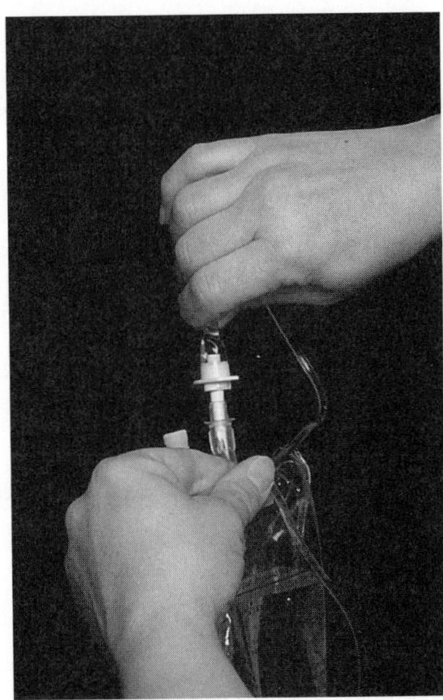

STEP 8 Squeeze drip chamber to remove a portion of fluid. Be sure to leave chamber one-third to one-half full.

STEP	RATIONALE
8. Make sure drip chamber is one-third to one-half full. If the drip chamber is too full, pinch off tubing below drip chamber, invert container, squeeze drip chamber (see illustration), hang up bottle, and release tubing.	Reduces risk of air entering tubing.
9. Regulate flow to prescribed rate.	Maintains measures to restore fluid balance and deliver IV fluid as ordered.

EVALUATION

1. Observe client for signs of overhydration or dehydration to determine response to IV fluid therapy.	Provides ongoing evaluation of client's fluid and electrolyte status.
2. Periodically check infusion rate.	Prevents improper fluid infusion.

UNEXPECTED OUTCOMES AND RELATED INTERVENTIONS

- Flow rate is incorrect; client receives too little or too much fluid.
  - Readjust infusion rate to ordered rate; evaluate client for adverse effects; notify physician.

RECORDING AND REPORTING

- Record amount and type of fluid infused and amount and type of new fluid according to agency policy. A special flow sheet may be used for parenteral fluids.

TEACHING CONSIDERATIONS

- Inform client of new solution, additives, flow rate, and potential side effects.

HOME CARE CONSIDERATIONS

- Ensure that client is able and willing to self-administer IV therapy (including changing IV solutions) and care for IV access site or that there is a reliable caregiver or nursing support person at home to provide this IV therapy care.
- If client or family must pick up antibiotics or other parenteral fluids from the hospital pharmacy, be sure physician's orders have been completed to avoid needless waiting by client or family at the hospital.
- Instruct client and primary caregiver how to perform an IV solution change.
- If medications are delivered to client's home, be sure to instruct client and/or caregiver on proper storage of these IV medications.

Skill 19-5 Changing Infusion Tubing

Changing intravenous (IV) infusion tubing is much simpler and more efficient if the nurse changes the tubing when preparing to hang a new bag or bottle. However, the Centers for Disease Control and Prevention (CDC) (1996a) recommends replacing tubing, including piggyback tubing and stopcocks, no more frequently than 72-hour intervals, assuming the system has not been contaminated. Situations arise when the nurse needs to change tubing without hanging a new bag. Such situations include accidental puncture of the tubing or after infusion of blood or a blood product (see Chapter 20).

Delegation Considerations

The skill of changing infusion tubing should not be delegated to assistive personnel.

Equipment

If a new IV dressing must be applied, assemble additional equipment (see Skill 19-6).

- Disposable nonsterile gloves

IV Infusion

- Infusion tubing
- 0.22 μmm filter and extension tubing (if necessary)

Heparin Flush

- Injection cap, loop, or short extension tubing (if necessary)

Normal Saline Flush

- Syringes
- Two sterile 2 × 2 gauze pads
- Tape

Step	Rationale
Assessment	
1. Determine when new infusion set is needed:	
a. Agency policy will indicate frequency of routine change for IV administration sets and heparin flushes OR	CDC (1996a) recommends tubing change no more often than 72-hour intervals.
b. Puncture of infusion tubing.	Punctured tubing results in fluid leakage and bacterial contamination.
c. Contamination of tubing.	Contamination of tubing allows entry of bacteria into client's bloodstream.
d. Occlusions in tubing. Such occlusions can occur after infusion of packed red cells, whole blood, albumin, other blood components, or administration of incompatible mixtures.	Whole blood or blood component products can occlude or partially occlude tubing because viscous solutions adhere to walls of tubing and decrease size of lumen.
2. Determine client's understanding of the need for continued IV infusions.	Reveals need for client instruction.

Nursing Diagnosis

Defining characteristics from the assessment data may reveal the following nursing diagnosis for clients requiring this skill:

Risk for infection

Related factors are individualized based on client's condition or needs.

Planning

Step	Rationale
1. **Expected outcomes** following completion of procedure:	
▪ Client's IV site will be free from redness, swelling, pain, or exudate.	Sterile IV tubing prevents bacterial growth.
▪ Client will experience no leakage of solution from tubing.	Intact system decreases risk of bacterial contamination.

STEP	RATIONALE
▪ Client's IV tubing will be patent.	Brief interruption of IV infusion will not result in clotting of catheter.
2. Prepare client and family by explaining the procedure, its purpose, and what is expected of client.	Decreases anxiety, promotes cooperation, and prevents sudden movement of extremity, which could dislodge IV needle or catheter.

IMPLEMENTATION

STEP	RATIONALE
1. Wash hands.	Reduces transmission of microorganisms.
2. Open new infusion set, keeping protective coverings over infusion spike and connector and connector site for butterfly needle or IV catheter.	Provides nurse with ready access to new infusion set and maintains sterility of infusion set.
3. Apply nonsterile, disposable gloves.	Reduces risk of exposure to human immunodeficiency virus (HIV), hepatitis, and other blood-borne bacteria (CDC, 1996a; Garner, 1996).
4. If needle or catheter hub is not visible, remove IV dressing as directed in Skill 19-6. Do not remove tape securing needle or catheter to skin.	Needle hub must be accessible to provide smooth transition when removing old and inserting new tubing.
5. **For IV infusion:**	
a. Move roller clamp on new IV tubing to "off" position.	Prevents spillage of solution after bag or bottle is spiked.
b. Slow rate of infusion by regulating drip rate on old tubing. Be sure rate is at keep vein open (KVO) rate.	Prevents complete infusion of solution remaining in tubing. Complete infusion of solution remaining in tubing increases risk of occlusion of IV catheter or needle.
c. With old tubing in place, compress drip chamber and fill chamber.	Provides surplus of fluid in drip chamber so there is enough fluid to maintain IV patency while changing tubing.
d. Remove old tubing from solution and hang or tape drip chamber on IV pole 36 inches above IV site.	Allows fluid to continue to flow through IV catheter while nurse is preparing new tubing.
e. Place insertion spike of new tubing into old solution bag opening and hang solution bag on IV pole.	Permits flow of fluid from solution into new infusion tubing.

• ***Critical Decision Point***
If spike becomes contaminated, a new IV tubing set is required.

STEP	RATIONALE
f. Compress and release drip chamber on new tubing; slowly fill drip chamber one-third to one-half full.	Allows drip chamber to fill and promotes rapid, smooth flow of solution through new tubing.
g. Slowly open roller clamp, remove protective cap from needle adapter (if necessary), and flush tubing with solution. Replace cap.	Removes air from tubing and replaces it with fluid.
h. Turn roller clamp on old tubing to "off" position.	Prevents spillage of fluid as tubing is removed from needle hub.
6. **For heparin lock:**	
a. If a new loop or short extension tubing is needed because of an awkward IV site placement, use sterile technique to connect a new **injection cap** to the loop or tubing.	
b. Swab injection cap with alcohol. Insert syringe with 1 to 3 ml saline, and inject through the injection cap into the loop or short extension tubing (see illustrations).	Removes air to prevent introduction into the vein.
7. Stabilize hub of catheter or needle, and apply pressure over vein just above insertion site. Gently pull out old tubing (see illustration *A*). Maintain stability of hub, and quickly insert needle adapter with new tubing and injection cap into hub (see illustrations *B* and *C*).	Prevents accidental displacement of catheter or needle. Prevents clot formation in catheter or needle and back flow of blood.
8. Open roller clamp on new tubing. Allow solution to run rapidly for 30 to 60 seconds.	Permits IV solution to enter catheter to prevent catheter occlusion.
9. Regulate IV drip (see Skill 19-3) according to physician's orders, and monitor rate hourly.	Maintains infusion flow at prescribed rate.

A 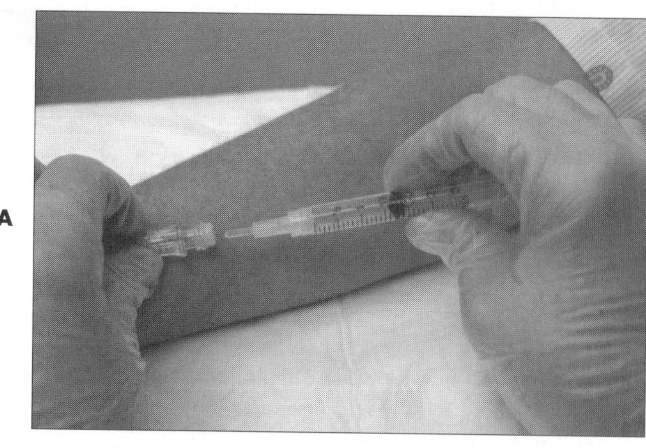 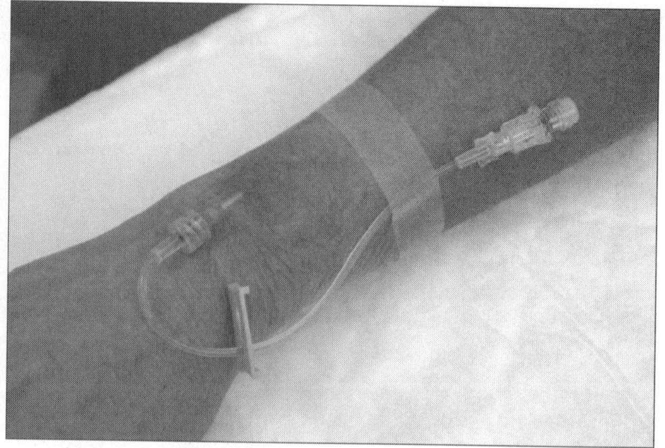 B

STEP 6b Inject saline into injection cap (**A**) connected to saline lock extension tube (**B**).

A 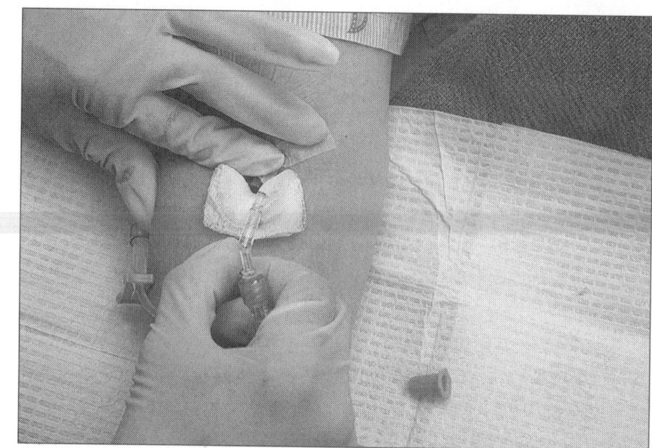 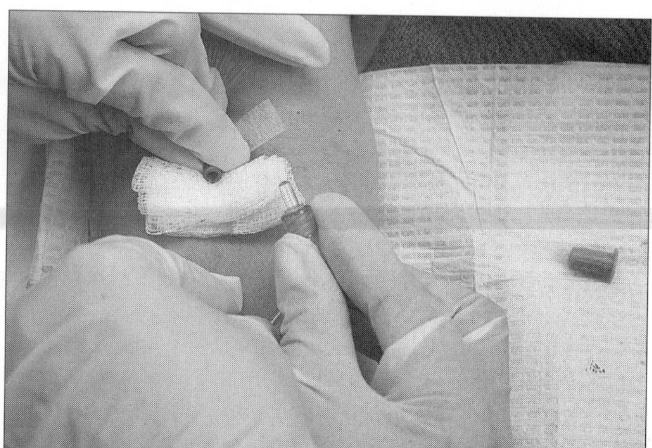 B

C 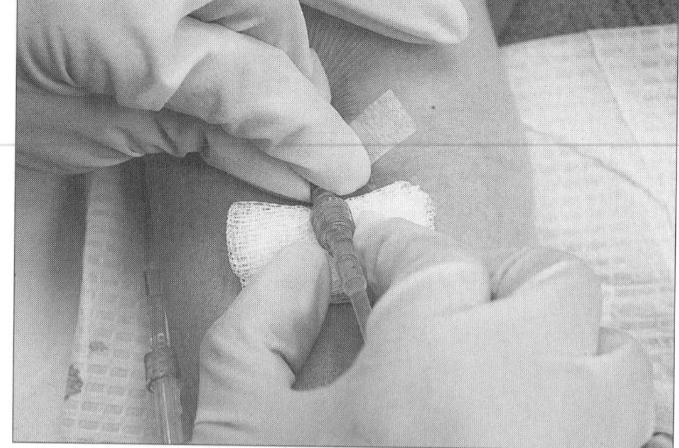

STEP 7 **A,** Maintain stability of catheter hub while removing old tubing. **B,** Connect new infusion tubing. **C,** Be sure connection at hub is secure.

Step	Rationale
10. If necessary, apply new dressing (see Skill 19-6).	Reduces risk of bacterial infection from skin.
11. Discard old tubing in proper container.	Reduces accidental transmission of microorganisms.
12. Remove and dispose of gloves. Wash hands.	Reduces transmission of microorganisms.

Evaluation

1. Evaluate flow rate, and observe connection site for leakage.	Maintains prescribed rate of flow of IV fluid and determines if fit is secure.

Unexpected Outcomes and Related Interventions

- Decreased or absent flow of IV fluid is indicated by decreased rate.
  - Assess IV infusion system for patency.
  - Recalibrate drip rate on new tubing.
  - Assess IV site for infiltration.

Recording and Reporting

- Record changing of tubing and solution on client's record. A special parenteral therapy flow sheet may be used.
- Mark a piece of tape or preprinted label with date and time of tubing change, and attach to tubing below the level of drip chamber.

Teaching Considerations

- Instruct client to notify nurse if fluid leaks around IV site or from the tubing itself or if tubing separates from catheter.

Home Care Considerations

- Instruct client or primary caregiver in procedure for performing a sterile IV tubing change.
- Ensure that client is able and willing to change infusion tubing and maintain IV access site or that there is a reliable person at home to provide this IV therapy care.

Skill 19-6 Changing a Peripheral Intravenous Dressing

Dressing applications are done for both intravenous (IV) infusion sites and heparin lock insertion sites at the time when the IV is inserted or when the IV site is changed. The IV site is usually changed every 72 hours, and the peripheral IV dressing is then applied. Otherwise, the peripheral IV dressing is not changed unless it becomes, wet, soiled, or loosened/removed (Centers for Disease Control and Prevention [CDC], 1996a). There is no difference in technique for the two. However a peripherally inserted central catheter (PICC) dressing change requires rigorous sterile technique.

The type of material used for the IV dressing depends on agency policy. The advantage of the transparent dressing is that the IV site can be inspected constantly without removal of the dressing. However, if there is significant drainage at the insertion site, a gauze dressing should be utilized. The dressings provide some protection and stability for the insertion site.

Using sterile technique during dressing changes reduces the risk of phlebitis and infection at the venipuncture site. Phlebitis is an inflammation of the vein and is associated with pain, redness, swelling, and a palpable venous cord (Intravenous Nurses Society, 1990). The occurrence of phlebitis increases the risk for developing a catheter-related infection.

A secure IV dressing is essential. Applying tape and a dressing that are not secure allows for IV catheter movement, which can result in infection or puncture of the vein by the catheter and flow of IV solution into the surrounding interstitial tissue. An infiltration is associated with slowed IV flow rate, tissue swelling around the IV site (especially proximal), and coolness. Changing a gauze dressing at routine intervals allows the visualization of the insertion site.

Delegation Considerations

The skill of changing a peripheral intravenous dressing should not be delegated to assistive personnel. Assistive personnel caring for clients with peripheral IVs should be instructed to report if a client complains of moistness or loosening of an IV dressing.

Equipment

- Povidone-iodine swab stick (three are needed for PICC dressing change)
- Alcohol swab stick (three are needed for PICC dressing change)
- Adhesive remover (if needed)
- Strips of sterile, precut tape
- Steri-strips (for PICC dressing)
- Disposable gloves
- Sterile gloves for PICC dressing change

For Gauze Dressing

- Sterile 2 × 2 gauze pad or
- Sterile 4 × 4 gauze pad

For Transparent Dressing

- Sterile transparent dressing

Step	Rationale

Assessment

Step	Rationale
1. Determine when dressing was last changed. Many institutions require nurse to write date and time on dressing and date the device was first placed.	Provides information regarding length of time that present dressing has been in place. In addition, nurse is able to plan for dressing change.
2. Observe present dressing for moisture and intactness.	Moisture is medium for bacterial growth and renders dressing contaminated. Nonadhering dressing increases risk of bacterial contamination to venipuncture site or displacement of IV catheter.
3. Observe IV system for proper functioning or complications: current flow rate, presence of kinks in infusion tubing or IV catheter. Palpate the catheter site through the intact dressing for subjective complaints of pain or burning.	Unexplained decrease in flow rate requires nurse to investigate placement and patency of IV catheter. Pain can be associated with both phlebitis and infiltration.
4. Inspect exposed catheter site for inflammation and swelling.	Inflammation indicates phlebitis. Swelling indicates infiltration, with fluid infusing into surrounding tissues. These signs require removal of IV catheter.
5. Monitor body temperature.	Elevated temperature may be related to infection at IV site.
6. Assess client's understanding of the need for continued IV infusion.	Reveals need for client instruction.

Nursing Diagnosis

Defining characteristics from the assessment data may reveal the following nursing diagnoses for clients requiring this skill:

Risk for infection

Pain (acute)

Related factors are individualized based on client's condition or needs.

Planning

Step	Rationale
1. **Expected outcomes** following completion of procedure:	
▪ Client will have patent IV as evidenced by absence of infiltration, phlebitis, or clot.	Maintains IV infusion as prescribed.
▪ Client's temperature remains normal.	
▪ IV insertion site is without pain, redness, swelling, or exudate.	Site remains uninfected.
2. Explain procedure and purpose to client and family. Explain that affected extremity must be held still and how long procedure will take.	Decreases anxiety, promotes cooperation, and gives client time frame around which personal activities can be planned.

Implementation

Step	Rationale
1. Wash hands. Apply disposable gloves.	Reduces transmission of microorganisms. Infections related to IV therapy are most often caused by catheter hub contamination, so careful technique must be used throughout the dressing change. Gloves reduce nurse's risk of exposure to human immunodeficiency virus (HIV), hepatitis, and other blood-borne viruses or bacteria.

STEP	RATIONALE
2. Remove tape, gauze, and/or transparent dressing from old dressing one layer at a time, leaving tape that secures IV needle or catheter in place. Be cautious if catheter tubing becomes tangled between two layers of dressing. When removing transparent dressing, hold catheter hub and tubing with nondominant hand.	Prevents accidental displacement of catheter or needle.
3. Observe insertion site for signs and/or symptoms of infection, namely redness, swelling, and exudate.	Presence of infection indicates need to discontinue IV at current site.
4. If infiltration, phlebitis, or clot occur or if ordered by physician, discontinue infusion (see Skill 19-8).	
5. If IV is infusing properly, gently remove tape securing needle or catheter. Stabilize needle or catheter with one hand. Use adhesive remover to cleanse skin and remove adhesive residue, if needed.	Exposes venipuncture site. Stabilization prevents accidental displacement of catheter or needle. Adhesive residue decreases ability of new tape to adhere tightly to skin.

- ***Critical Decision Point***
  Keep one finger over catheter at all times until tape is replaced for security. It may help to have another staff member assist.

STEP	RATIONALE
6. If changing dressing on PICC line, remove disposable gloves and apply sterile gloves.	
7. Using circular motion, cleanse peripheral IV insertion site with alcohol, then povidone-iodine solution (see illustration) starting at insertion site and working outwards, creating concentric circles. Allow each solution to dry for 2 minutes. For a PICC, cleanse with three alcohol swab sticks and allow to dry for 60 seconds (see illustration). Follow by three povidone-iodine sticks. Allow to dry for 2 minutes.	Circular motion prevents cross contamination from skin bacteria near venipuncture site. Povidone-iodine is a topical antiinfective that reduces skin surface bacteria; the solution must be dry to be effective in reducing microbial counts (Baranowski, 1993).
8. Tape or secure catheter.	
a. Applying gauze dressing: Place a narrow piece ($\frac{1}{2}$ inch) of tape under hub of catheter with adhesive side up and cross tape over hub. Place tape only on the catheter, *never over* the insertion site.	

A

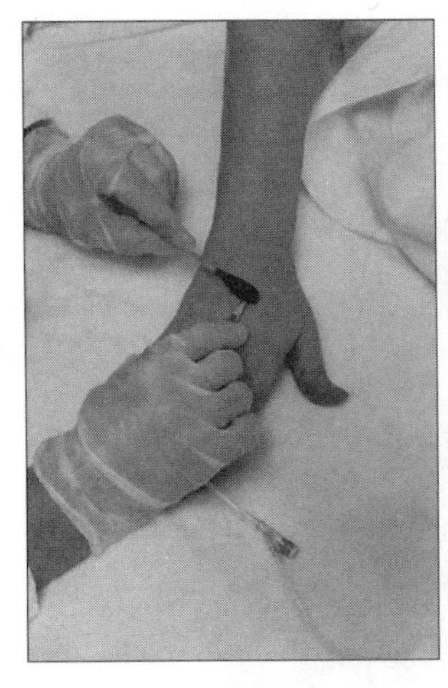

B

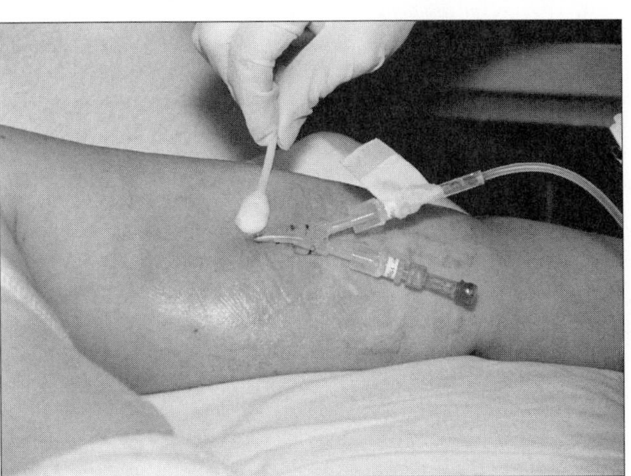

STEP **7** **A,** Cleanse IV site with antiseptic swab. **B,** Cleanse PICC site with alcohol.

STEP	RATIONALE
b. Applying transparent dressing: Secure catheter with nondominant hand while preparing to apply dressing.	

- ***Critical Decision Point***
  Do not tape over connection of access tubing or port to IV catheter.

STEP	RATIONALE
9. Apply sterile dressing over site:	
a. Sterile gauze dressing	
(1) Fold a 2 × 2 gauze in half and cover with a 1-inch-wide piece of tape extending about an inch from each side. Place gauze under the tubing/catheter hub junction (see illustration). Curl a loop of tubing alongside the arm and place a second piece of tape directly over the padded 2 × 2, securing tubing in two places (see illustration).	Gauze prevents pressure of catheter hub against skin. Securing loop of tubing reduces risk of dislodging catheter from accidental pull.
(2) For PICC catheter place several Steri-strips over catheter (see illustration).	Provides security to prevent catheter dislodgment. PICC lines are often sutured in place, preventing placement of gauze underneath.
(3) Place another 2 × 2 gauze pad over the venipuncture site and catheter hub. Secure all edges with tape. Do not cover connection between IV tubing and catheter hub.	Access to catheter hub is needed in times of emergency and when changing tubing.

A
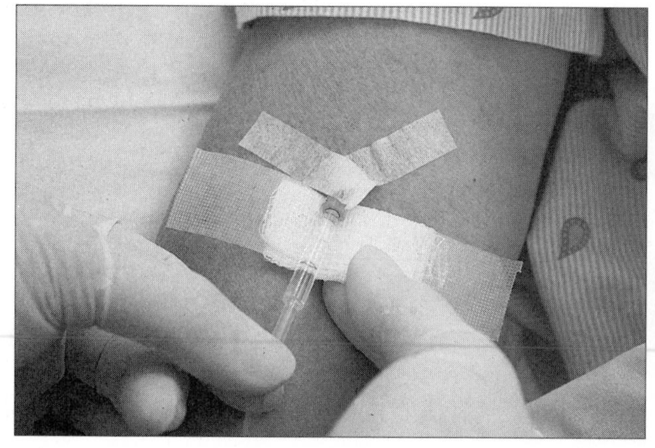
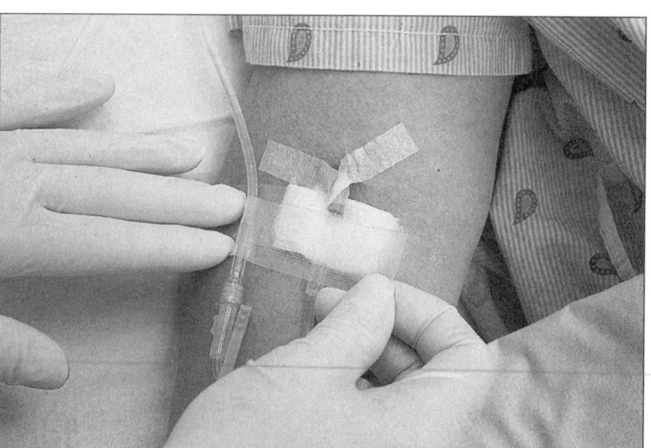
B

STEP **9a(1)** **A,** Place a folded 2 × 2 under catheter hub. **B,** Secure dressing and loop of IV tubing.

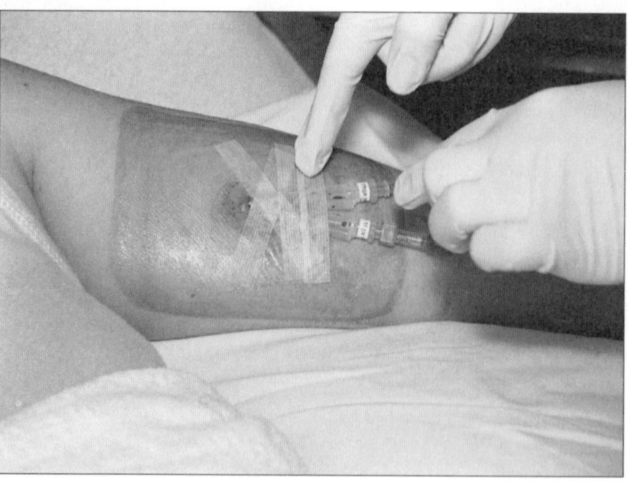

STEP **9a(2)** Taping PICC with Steri-strips.

STEP	RATIONALE
b. Transparent dressing	
(1) Carefully remove adherent backing. Apply one edge of dressing, and then gently smooth remaining dressing over IV site, leaving end of catheter hub uncovered.	Secures catheter and provides tight dressing seal.
10. Remove and discard gloves.	
11. Anchor IV tubing with additional pieces of tape if necessary. When using transparent dressing, avoid placing tape over dressing.	Prevents accidental displacement of IV needle or catheter or separation of IV tubing from needle adapter.
12. Place date and time of dressing change and size and gauge of catheter directly on dressing.	Documents dressing change.
13. Discard equipment and wash hands.	Reduces transmission of microorganisms.

EVALUATION

1. Observe IV flow rate and compare with rate at time dressing change began.	Validates that IV is patent and functioning correctly.
2. Monitor client's body temperature.	Elevated temperature indicates an infection that may be associated with bacterial contamination of the venipuncture site.

UNEXPECTED OUTCOMES AND RELATED INTERVENTIONS

- IV catheter or needle is infiltrated, as evidenced by decreased flow rate or edema, pallor, or decreased temperature around insertion site.
  - Stop infusion and discontinue IV (see Skill 19-8). Restart new IV in other extremity if continued therapy is necessary. Elevate affected extremity.
- Phlebitis is present, as evidenced by erythema and tenderness along vein pathway.
  - Stop infusion and discontinue IV (see Skill 19-8). Restart new IV in other extremity if continued therapy is necessary.
  - Apply warm moist compress to area of phlebitis
- IV catheter or needle is accidentally removed.
  - Restart IV if continued therapy is needed.
- Client has an elevated temperature.
  - Notify physician. IV may be removed and restarted. Client will be evaluated for source of infection.
- Insertion site is red and/or edematous and/or painful and/or has presence of exudate, indicating infection at venipuncture site.
  - IV is discontinued (see Skill 19-8). Antibiotic therapy may begin.
  - Apply warm moist compress to area of inflammation.

REPORTING AND RECORDING

- Record in nurses' notes time IV dressing was changed and type of dressing used. Include patency of system and description of venipuncture site.
- Report to nurse in charge or oncoming nursing shift that dressing was changed and any significant information about integrity of system.
- Report to physician any complications.

TEACHING CONSIDERATIONS

- Client should be instructed to notify nurse if skin under dressing or tape becomes reddened, itches, or burns or if dressing becomes loosened.

PEDIATRIC CONSIDERATIONS

- Pediatric clients may not be able to fully understand nurse's explanation. Presence of parent or security toy during procedure can help to decrease fear and increase cooperation.

GERONTOLOGICAL CONSIDERATIONS

- In the older adult with fragile skin, prevent skin tears by minimizing the use of tape directly on the skin.

HOME CARE CONSIDERATIONS

- Ensure that the client is able and willing to perform this procedure and care for IV access site or that there is a reliable caregiver or nursing support person at home to provide this IV therapy care.

Skill 19-7 Caring for Vascular Access Devices

Clients with chronic disease often need long-term intravenous (IV) therapy, which requires safe, repeated access to the venous system for administration of drugs, fluids, nutrition, and blood products. Frequent venipuncture and multiple IV lines pose problems and risks, including infection, pain, **and bruising.** Clients with chronic disease are generally more susceptible to infection and bleeding. Clients receiving multiple doses of chemotherapeutic drugs experience vein sclerosis or hardening. Eventually no suitable peripheral veins remain for drug administration.

The need for safe and convenient long-term IV therapy has led to the development of **vascular access devices (VADs),** which are catheters, **cannulas,** or infusion ports designed for long-term, repeated access to the venous or arterial systems. The nurse must be able to maintain the integrity of central venous catheters (CVCs) and implanted infusion ports and educate clients about the care of catheters for eventual home use.

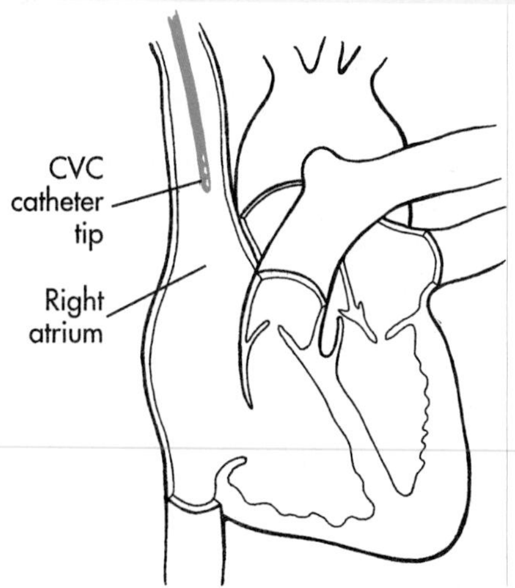

FIGURE **19-7** Catheter tip from CVC lies in right atrium.

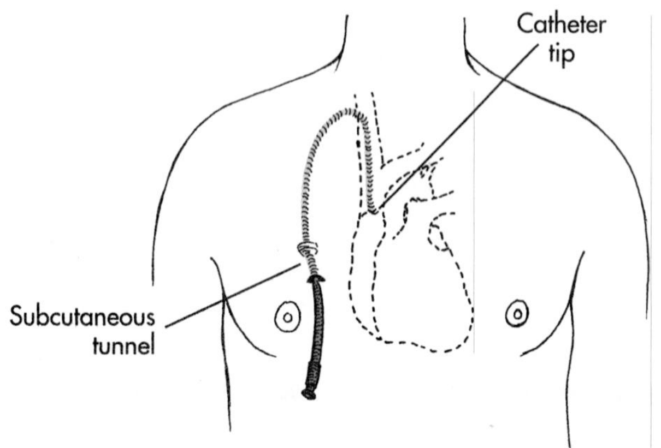

FIGURE **19-8** Small-gauge tunneled catheter is in place, threaded into right atrium.

To manage long-term IV therapy effectively the nurse must be familiar with the various types of VADs. Knowing the type of VAD can be confusing since catheters are often referred to by brand name instead of type and placement (e.g., Hickman, Groshong, Raaf, Port-a-Cath). Also, the literature does not indicate universal acceptance of one term to describe a particular catheter. For this skill VADs will be divided into two types: CVCs (tunneled and percutaneous) and implanted infusion ports. **Central venous catheters (CVCs)** are inserted into a large vein, typically the internal or external jugulars or the superior vena cava that leads to the right atrium of the heart (Figure 19-7). The large vessel lumen minimizes the risks of vessel irritation, inflammation, or sclerosis that commonly occur when smaller peripheral veins are used. These catheters are used to administer IV fluids, antibiotics, chemotherapy, and parenteral nutrition, to infuse medications and blood products, and to obtain blood samples.

Tunneled CVCs are surgically inserted with the client in the operating room under general or local anesthesia. First a tunnel is made through subcutaneous tissue, usually between the clavicle and nipple. The **subcutaneous tunnel** allows the catheter to remain in place longer because it creates space between the end of the catheter and the actual vein. The risk of infection is lower. Next, the catheter tip is inserted through the cephalic, internal or external jugular vein, or a similar large vein, and threaded into the right atrium (Figure 19-8). The catheter is held in place with a Dacron cuff that surrounds the catheter located on the chest wall. These catheters have single, double, or triple lumens, which are hollow tubes inside the catheter that allow simultaneous administration of several infusions.

The second type of CVC is the percutaneously placed catheter. The **percutaneous** catheter is inserted directly through the skin and into a large vein of the neck, usually the internal or external jugular (Figure 19-9), or subclavian (see

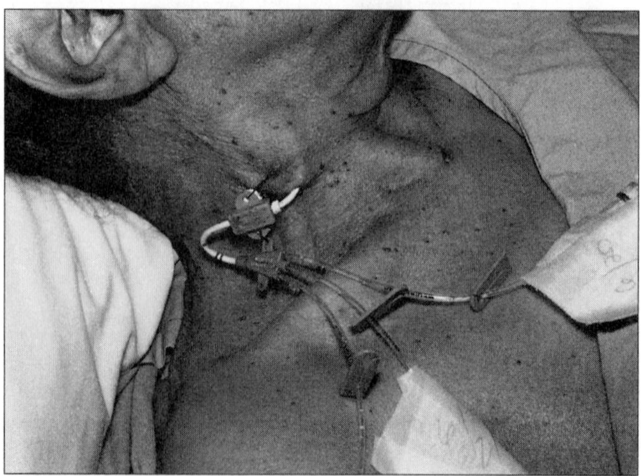

FIGURE **19-9** CVC placed in jugular vein.

A

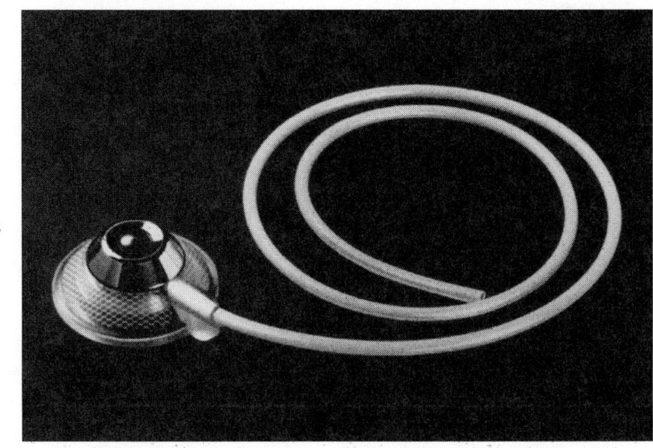

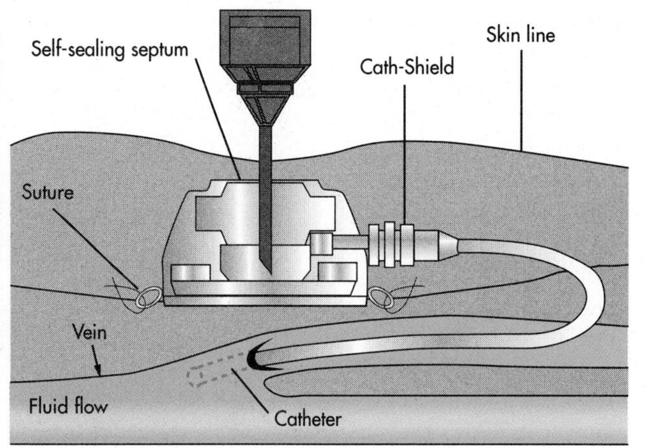

B

FIGURE **19-10** **A,** Implantable infusion port. **B,** Infusion port placed in subcutaneous pocket. (Courtesy SIMS Deltec, Inc., St. Paul, Minn.)

Chapter 23). If not inserted directly into a central vein, a CVC may also be inserted through large veins of the antecubital fossa and threaded into the tip of the right atrium (see Skill 19-2 for peripherally inserted central catheter (PICC) insertion). Various types of percutaneously placed central catheters are available. The length of time catheters are left in place depends on the type and the manufacturer's recommendations, the length of therapy, and the condition/functionality of the catheter.

The second type of VAD is the **implanted infusion port,** which consists of a self-sealing injection port housed in a plastic or metal case (Figure 19-10) and is connected most often to a silicone venous catheter. The port is also available with a double lumen catheter. The physician implants the infusion port under sterile conditions in an operating room with the client under local anesthesia. The infusion port usually rests in a subcutaneous pocket in the infraclavicular fossa, and the catheter is inserted into a large vein and threaded into the right atrium. The port can be easily palpated to determine placement. Specially designed **noncoring Huber needles** (straight or with 90-degree angles) are inserted through the skin to enter the port (Figure 19-11). Implanted infusion ports are used for administration of injections and for continuous infusions of all types: medications, chemotherapy, parenteral nutrition, and blood products. When not in use, no external catheter is present, and the port manufacturers recommend the port be heparinized every 4 weeks to maintain its patency. No other care is required for a port that is not being used.

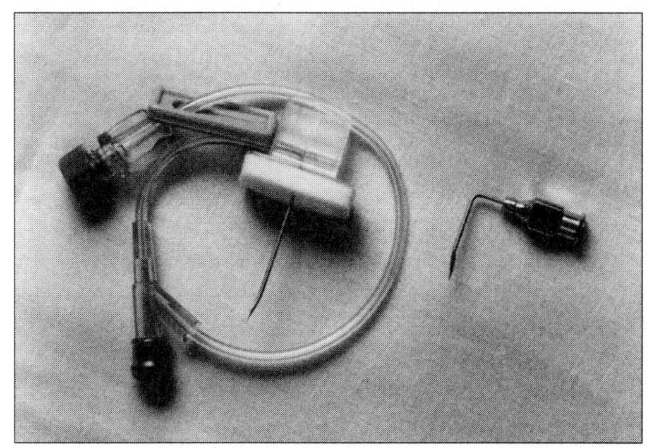

FIGURE **19-11** Assortment of Huber needles.

Care of VADs is simple as long as nurses and clients are aware of the purpose and function of the devices and the two most common complications, infection and clotting. In the home, most clients learn to use clean technique for dressing changes and catheter care. Within 2 to 3 weeks a transparent dressing is sufficient to cover catheter insertion sites. Clients can learn to initiate infusions, heparinize devices, and discontinue infusions.

Delegation Considerations

The skill of caring for a vascular access device in an acute care setting should not be delegated to assistive personnel. Assistive personnel should be instructed in the signs and symptoms of VAD complications to report.

Equipment

Blood Drawing

- Povidone-iodine and alcohol preparation swabs
- Four to five syringes (10 and 20 ml)
- Sterile drape
- Saline flush
- Heparin flush (100 U/ml)
- Plastic clamp
- Sterile Huber needle (20- to 22-gauge)
- Sterile needle (20- to 22-gauge)
- Blood tubes, labels, requisitions
- Gloves, gowns, masks

Administration of Drugs, Fluids, Blood Products

- Povidone-iodine and alcohol swabs
- Drug, fluid, blood product to be infused
- Sterile IV tubing

- IV pole, infusion pump, or blood pump
- Sterile drape
- Saline flush
- Sterile Huber needle (20- to 22-gauge)
- Sterile needle (20- to 22-gauge)
- Dressing supplies as indicated
- Gloves, gown, masks

Dressing Change

- Povidone-iodine and alcohol swabs
- Gloves
- Tape
- Sterile gauze 4 × 4 or 2 × 2 sponges (gauze dressing)
- Transparent occlusive dressing (transparent dressing)

Heparinization

- Povidone-iodine and alcohol preparation swabs
- Syringe (5 ml or 10 ml—see agency policy)
- Saline flush
- Heparin flush (100 U/ml)
- Plastic clamp
- Sterile needle (22-gauge)

Step	Rationale
Assessment	
1. Assess diagnosis of client's stage of disease and plan of therapy by review of medical record.	Allows nurse to understand need for vascular access in treatment of disease and in evaluation of response to therapy and to determine need to educate client about disease process and plan of therapy using VAD.
2. Review physician's order and assess treatment schedule: times for administration of fluids, drugs, blood products, nutrition, and blood sampling.	Allows nurse to schedule use of VAD for simultaneous administration of products, to educate client about schedule of administration, and to provide for comfort and reduction of anxiety about therapy.
3. Assess type of VAD in place.	Care and management depend on type and size of catheter, number of lumens, type of infusion port.
4. Assess need to use VAD for blood sampling.	Scheduling sampling needs allows nurse to minimize entering VAD system and allows for timely collection of specimens to evaluate therapy. Risk of infection increases with multiple entries into vascular system, especially in immunocompromised clients.

- ***Critical Decision Point***

In some situations, several tests can be run from one blood tube sample. For example, potassium, calcium, and magnesium test results can all be obtained from one full tube of blood versus three separate tubes. Always anticipate the need for a blood test (e.g., blood cultures if a client has developed an elevated temperature). If your next task was to draw blood for electrolyte results, you could eliminate reaccessing the VAD at a later time by asking the physician if blood cultures are to be drawn.

Step	Rationale
5. Assess VAD placement site for skin integrity and signs of infection: i.e., redness, swelling, tenderness, exudate, bleeding.	Clients requiring long-term IV therapy often have conditions placing them at risk for alterations in skin integrity and immune function.
6. Assess for proper function of VAD before therapy: integrity of port or catheter, ability to irrigate or infuse fluid, ability to aspirate blood.	Ensures proper function of VAD with minimal complications.
7. Assess need for irrigation and dressing change by referring to medical record, nurses' notes, and manufacturer's recommended guidelines for use.	Provides guidelines for maintaining catheter patency and preventing infection.
8. Assess client's reaction to VAD and knowledge of purpose, care, and maintenance. Ask client to discuss steps in care and to perform procedure (e.g., catheter site cleansing or dressing change).	Determines client's level of understanding. Allows nurse to educate client for home care of VAD.

STEP	RATIONALE

NURSING DIAGNOSIS

Defining characteristics from the assessment data may reveal the following nursing diagnoses for clients requiring this skill:

Risk for infection
Risk for injury
Impaired skin integrity
Deficient knowledge regarding use of VAD

Related factors are individualized based on client's condition or needs.

PLANNING

Step	Rationale
1. **Expected outcomes** following completion of procedure:	
▪ Site is intact, has normal color, and has no swelling.	Local signs of infection are absent.
▪ Systemic signs of infection (fever, malaise, increased white blood cell count [WBC]) are absent.	Catheter system remains sterile.
▪ Fluids, medications, blood products infuse without difficulty.	Patency of catheter is maintained.
▪ Blood can be aspirated from catheter.	Indicates patency.
▪ Catheter and connecting tube are intact.	Integrity of system is maintained.
▪ Catheter tip is correctly placed, as confirmed by x-ray examination.	Correct placement minimizes chances of displacement or occlusion.
▪ Client and family are able to explain the purpose of VAD therapy and perform dressing changes and skin care.	Demonstrates that client and family are learning.
2. Position client in supine position with head slightly elevated.	Stabilizes client and prevents accidental pulling or tugging at catheter. Location of infusion port requires palpation and examination in supine position.
3. Explain procedure and purpose to client and family. Instruct client to lie still.	Decreases anxiety and promotes cooperation.

IMPLEMENTATION

Administration of Infusions or Sampling of Blood From Implanted Infusion Port

Step	Rationale
1. Wash hands thoroughly. Mask self and client. Not all institutions require masking of the client. The client may, instead, be asked to turn head away from port site. Refer to agency policy.	Reduces transfer of microorganisms, prevents spread of airborne microorganisms while needle insertion site is exposed.
2. Prepare sterile field, and open sterile supplies.	Provides work space for use of sterile items.
3. Using alcohol, prepare client's skin overlying port septum, moving outward in concentric circles from insertion site out. Allow to dry for 60 seconds.	Rigorous skin preparation is necessary to prevent introducing bacteria into system.
4. In the same manner, use povidone-iodine swabs to cleanse skin overlying port septum. Allow to dry for 2 minutes.	Provides additional skin cleansing.
5. Apply sterile gloves.	Prevents transmission of microorganisms by nurse's hands.
6. As another nurse holds vial of saline, fill sterile syringe with saline solution.	Allows nurse filling syringe to not contaminate supplies.
7. Attach one end of sterile extension tubing to syringe and attach appropriate size Huber needle to other end. Fill tubing with saline solution.	Removes all air from tubing, reducing risk of air embolus.
8. Apply sterile drape to port site (may be optional in some agencies).	Provides sterile work area.

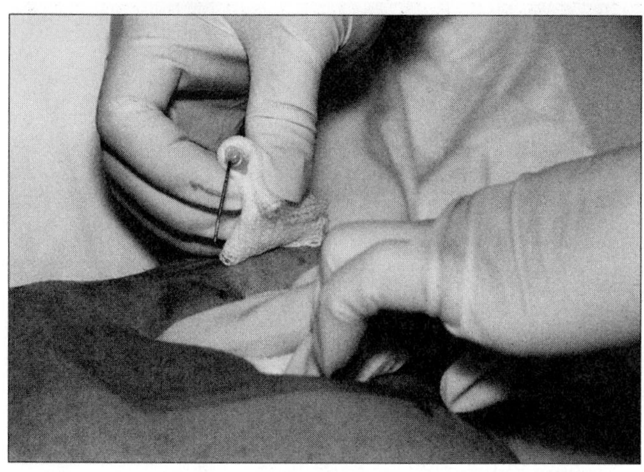

STEP **9** Palpate port septum before inserting Huber needle.

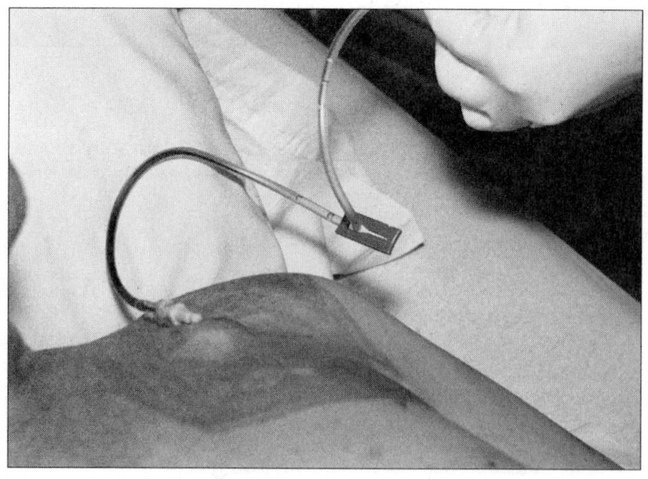

STEP **11** Aspirate blood return from port.

STEP	RATIONALE
9. Palpate port septum, observing strict aseptic technique (see illustration).	Entry site for needle insertion must be located to ensure proper needle entry.
10. While holding wings or needle hub, insert Huber needle through skin at a 90-degree angle and push firmly down until needle penetrates silicone septum and hits bottom of portal chamber.	Do not push too hard. If tip of the needle bends, septum can be damaged upon removal of needle.
11. Check for proper placement by attempting to withdraw blood by aspirating with the attached syringe (see illustration).	
12. If a good blood return is present, flush tubing with remaining saline in syringe. If a blood return is not obtained, fill another syringe, as in Step 6, and attempt to flush port with 10 ml normal saline.	Forceful irrigation against resistance may propel clotted blood into the client's muscular system.

- ***Critical Decision Point***

  Do not irrigate forcefully if resistance is felt. If unable to flush, reposition needle without completely withdrawing it from the skin or reprepping will be necessary. Never use a syringe less than 10 ml; exerts too high a psi pressure.

STEP	RATIONALE
13. Observe for swelling. If swelling occurs around needle insertion site, stop procedure and notify physician.	This may indicate that needle is not in port, but in surrounding subcutaneous tissue, or that there is a tear in the catheter.
14. To draw blood samples, first aspirate and discard 5 ml of fluid.	Avoids dilution of sample.
15. Withdraw necessary blood for each sample, using two 10-ml syringes equal to total volume withdrawn.	Eliminates repeated need to puncture infusion port for sampling.
16. Flush with 2 ml heparin (100 U/ml or institution policy).	Flush clears fibrin after blood draw.
17. Refill saline syringe and flush port with 20 ml normal saline.	Any fluid other than normal saline has potential for clotting blood or precipitating in catheter.
18. If continuous infusion is not indicated, heparinize port by flushing with 5 ml heparin (100 U/ml or institution policy) flush solution using positive pressure.	Prevents clot formation.
19. If IV fluid will be continuously administered, secure Huber needle with Steri-strips (see illustration). Cover the Huber needle and insertion site with a transparent dressing. If Huber needle does not sit flush on skin, place folded 2 × 2 gauze under hub and then cover with dressing.	Prevents accidental dislodging of needle at insertion site.

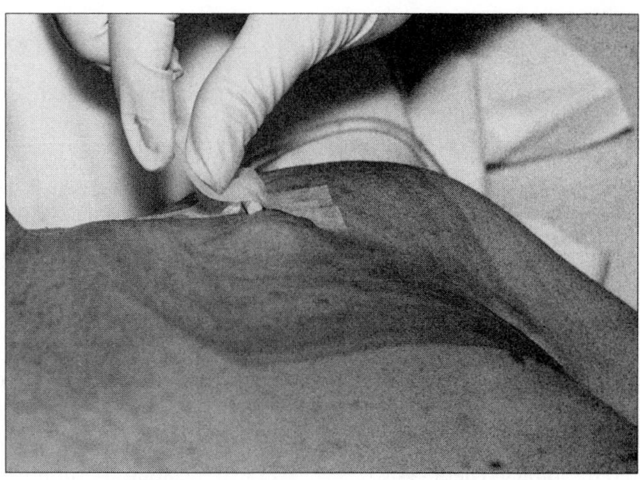

STEP **19** Secure Huber needle with Steri-strips.

STEP	RATIONALE
20. Connect IV infusion tubing with sterile tubing connected to Huber needle.	IV infusion system should be closed to maintain sterility.
21. Regulate IV infusion as ordered.	Maintains desired fluid intake and patency of catheter.
22. Dispose of all soiled supplies and used equipment. Send labeled specimens to laboratory. Remove gloves and wash hands.	Reduces spread of microorganisms.

Administration of Infusions or Sampling of Blood From Central Venous Catheter

STEP	RATIONALE
1. Wash hands thoroughly.	Reduces transmission of microorganisms.
2. Apply gloves. Apply gown and goggles (check agency policy) if blood sampling.	Prevents transfer of body fluids.
3. Use povidone-iodine and/or alcohol preparation swabs to cleanse injection cap or catheter hub according to agency policy.	Prevents introduction of microorganisms into catheter.
4. Prepare two syringes: one with 10 ml normal saline, the other with 20 ml saline.	Used to flush catheter.
5. If injection cap will be removed, clamp catheter.	Catheter must be clamped if injection cap is removed to prevent entrance of air.
6. If injection cap is in place, insert needle of syringe containing 10 ml normal saline and flush. If injection cap is removed, connect syringe tip to catheter hub, release clamp, flush with positive pressure, and reclamp.	Flushing ensures patency of catheter. Catheter must always be clamped during change of syringe or tubing to prevent exposure to air.

- ***Critical Decision Point***
  If catheter is occluded and resistance is felt, do not force flushing. Vigorous flushing may cause catheter rupture or embolization of catheter (Bagnall-Reeb, 1998). Notify physician.

STEP	RATIONALE
7. Connect syringe for blood sampling and release clamp. Aspirate 5 ml fluid, reclamp, and discard aspirate.	Avoids diluting sample.
8. Attach or insert syringe of size equal to volume of blood sample to withdraw to catheter. Release clamp. Withdraw necessary blood for samples and reclamp.	Samples should be collected at one time to minimize time needed to open catheter system.
9. Attach syringe filled with 2 ml heparin (100 U/ml) and flush.	Clears fibrin left after blood draw.

Step	Rationale
10. Attach or insert syringe filled with 20 ml normal saline to catheter. If clamp is present, release, flush vigorously, and reclamp.	Catheter should be cleared of all blood or medications that may clog catheter lumen or precipitate with additives in IV fluids.
11. If no continuous infusion is indicated, flush catheter with heparin or normal saline as appropriate. Connect syringe containing 5 ml heparin (100 U/ml) or normal saline flush solution. If clamp is present, release, flush with positive pressure, and reclamp.	A catheter not in use must be flushed to prevent clot formation. This is commonly done with heparin; however, Groshong catheters are flushed with normal saline only.
12. Replace new cap to end of catheter and remove clamp.	Maintains sterile seal to catheter.
13. If IV fluids will be administered, connect IV tubing to end of catheter, being sure both ends are sterile.	IV system should be closed to maintain sterility.
14. Regulate IV infusion as ordered.	Maintains ordered fluid intake and keeps catheter patent.
15. Tape all tubing connections, and pin tubing to client's gown.	Prevents accidental tubing disconnection and catheter displacement.
16. Dispose of soiled equipment and used supplies. Remove gloves and wash hands.	Reduces transmission of microorganisms.

Dressing Change

Step	Rationale
1. Wash hands and apply clean gloves.	Reduces transmission of microorganisms.
2. Mask self and client, if indicated (check agency policy).	Prevents exposure of catheter exit or placement site to airborne microorganisms.
3. Carefully remove old dressing in the direction the catheter was inserted, noting drainage and appearance of catheter or needle insertion site.	Remove tape carefully because clients frequently have alterations in skin integrity.
4. Inspect placement or exit site for signs of redness, swelling, inflammation, tenderness, or exudate.	This is a potential site of infection.
5. If catheter is tunneled, palpate Dacron cuff in subcutaneous tunnel.	Documenting position of cuff verifies proper placement.
6. Inspect catheter and hub for intactness, and remove clean gloves.	Catheter may become torn, cut, displaced, cracked, split.
7. Wash hands thoroughly and open dressing kit in a sterile manner. Most agencies have dressing kits that contain all needed dressing change supplies.	
8. Apply sterile gloves.	Prevents direct transmission of microorganisms to skin **exit site.**
9. Clean placement or exit site with alcohol swabs by starting from inside moving out in circular fashion, creating concentric circles. Maintain strict asepsis. Clean about a 3-cm area. Allow alcohol to remain on skin for at least 60 seconds (see illustration).	It is impossible to sterilize skin. Organisms that accumulate must be eliminated by mechanical and chemical means.

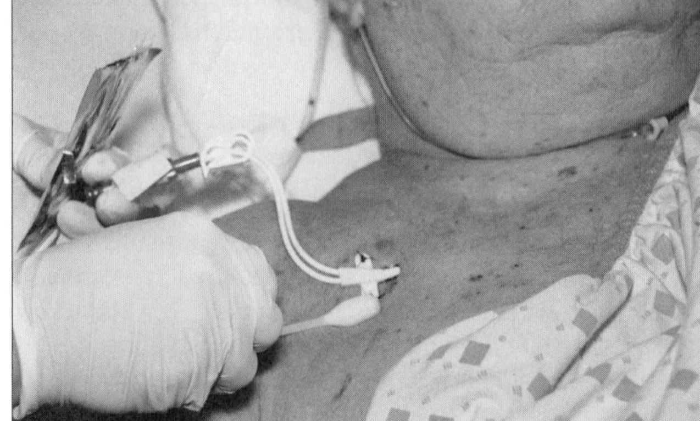

STEP 9 Cleanse central venous catheter site.

STEP	RATIONALE
10. Repeat Step 9 using povidone-iodine swabs. Allow to dry for 2 minutes.	Povidone-iodine must be dry to be effective in reducing microbial count (Baranowski, 1993).
11. Redress site using sterile gauze and tape or transparent dressing as indicated.	Prevents entrance of bacteria into exit or placement site.
12. Secure tubing or needle to client's gown. If catheter is not in use, loop catheter and tape to client's skin.	Prevents accidental pulling and displacement.
13. Label date, time of dressing change, and size of needle in place.	Documents dressing change. Provides guideline for time of next change.
14. Dispose of soiled supplies; remove gloves and wash hands.	Reduces transmission of microorganisms.

EVALUATION

1. When continuous infusions are administered, observe and calculate drip rate hourly. Note ease with which fluid rate can be increased.	To maintain proper fluid infusion, desired drip rate should be regulated continuously. A gradual slowing in rate or inability to increase rate may indicate catheter occlusion.
2. Routinely assess vital signs of client, noting changes symptomatic of infection.	Catheter-related sepsis can cause fever, chills, flushed skin, tachycardia.
3. Observe catheter or port exit or placement site when sites are exposed (Table 19-4).	Continual monitoring for signs of inflammation or infection is essential.
4. Observe all catheter connection points periodically.	An intact system prevents accidental blood loss or entrance of air.
5. Inspect condition of catheter and connecting tubing daily for leaks, holes, tears, splits, or cracked hubs.	Break in integrity of system predisposes client to hemorrhage or air embolus.
6. Consult x-ray examination reports for catheter placement.	A routine chest x-ray examination can locate position of catheter tip.
7. Evaluate ability of client and family to provide care and maintain catheter or infusion port through discussion and return demonstrations of dressing changes and skin care. Determine need for restrictions on daily activities.	Measures client's ability to care for self and any additional learning needs.

UNEXPECTED OUTCOMES AND RELATED INTERVENTIONS

- For catheter complications see Table 19-4.
- Client or family member is unable to explain or perform VAD care.
  - May indicate need for home health care referral or additional instruction.

RECORDING AND REPORTING

- Chart date and time of medications, blood products, parenteral nutrition given, and samples obtained, in nurses' notes or on medication administration record.
- Chart condition of exit site or port implantation site, including skin integrity, signs of infection, placement, integrity, and functionality of catheter.
- Chart dressing change procedure, label date, time, type, and size of needle in port.
- Chart patency of catheter, ability to draw blood, and difficulty with infusions.
- Chart measures taken to educate client in self-care and response to education.
- In emergency situations (damage to catheter, loss of patency, blood loss, air embolus, septic episode, local signs of infection), notify nursing or medical personnel immediately. Instruct client and family when to contact medical personnel.

TEACHING CONSIDERATIONS

- Discuss and provide written emergency measures and telephone numbers of health care personnel to be used in case of catheter damage; needle displacement; swelling, redness, or leakage at insertion site; occlusion of port or catheter; temperature above 100° F; and shaking chills.
- Provide written instruction for dressing changes, inspection of insertion site, irrigations, and tubing changes.
- Arrange for instruction and return demonstration of skills by client or caregiver.
- Have client or caregiver maintain a list of caregivers and telephone numbers (e.g., physician, nurse, social worker, pharmacist, dietitian).

Table 19-4 Complications of Vascular Access Devices

Complication	Assessment	Prevention	Intervention
Catheter damage, breakage	Observe for pinholes, leaks, tears, every shift Assess for drainage after flushing	Follow proper clamping procedure Avoid sharp objects near the catheter Avoid using needles longer than 1 inch through the injection cap Avoid inserting larger than 21-gauge needles through the injection cap	Use a catheter stylet for temporary repair Use permanent repair kit Remove catheter
Occlusion: thrombus, precipitation, malposition	Assess for blood return Assess for inability to infuse Assess equipment If port, reaccess and verify needle placement Assess with syringe directly on catheter Assess for discomfort or pain in shoulder, neck, or arm at insertion site Assess for neck or shoulder edema Assess sutures to ensure no restriction	Follow routine flushing with positive pressure Avoid tugging on VAD Administer low-dose oral anticoagulant therapy Avoid using excessive force Flush between drugs Flush vigorously after viscous solutions Avoid mixing incompatible drugs Avoid kinking catheter	Administer bolus of IV fluid Reposition client Have client cough and deep breathe Raise client's arm Obtain venogram Administer thrombolytics Remove catheter Obtain x-ray examination If precipitate, try hydrochloric acid or ethanol solution *Do not* use a 1-ml syringe to instill saline as pressures exceed 200 psi (Bagnall-Reeb, 1998)
Infection: exit site, tunnel, thrombus, port pocket	Assess exit site for redness, drainage, edema, or tenderness Assess vital signs Monitor laboratory findings	Use strict hand washing Use aseptic technique Adhere to dressing change technique Apply dressing over exit site Apply antibiotic or antimicrobial ointment at exit site	Administer antibiotic therapy Remove catheter Administer thrombolytic agent Replace catheter Obtain blood cultures peripheral and from VAD Do not use VAD if it has not been accessed
Dislodgement, twiddler's syndrome	Assess length of catheter daily Inform client of possible catheter dislodgement Identify edema at exit site or drainage Palpate exit site and tunnel for coiling Assess distended neck veins	Loop and tape the catheter securely Use occlusive dressing Use athletic sock for peripherally inserted central catheter Avoid pulling on VAD Handle with care Avoid manipulating catheter (port) by hand	Reinsert catheter Secure catheter with sutures Teach client not to manipulate catheter

Home Care Considerations

- Initiate early referral for discharge planning to social service, counselor, or home care coordinator for assessment of resources.
- Determine client and caregiver's acceptance of client's altered body image.
- Provide client with written list of providers for supplies and equipment.
- Assess willingness and ability of primary caregiver to assist in home management of device. Acceptance of altered body image influences primary caregiver's readiness to assist with care.

Table 19-4 Complications of Vascular Access Devices—cont'd

Complication	Assessment	Prevention	Intervention
Catheter migration, pinch-off syndrome, port separation	Assess for client complaints of gurgling sounds Assess for change in patency of catheter Obtain x-ray examination Assess edema of arm and hand on side of insertion Assess distended neck veins Assess for inability to infuse fluids Assess length of catheter daily	Avoid trauma Avoid placement near site of local disease	Reposition under fluoroscopy Remove catheter Stop all fluid administration
Skin erosion, hematomas, cuff extrusion, scar tissue formation over port	Assess for loss of viable tissue over implantation Assess for separation of exit site edges Assess for drainage at exit site Assess for redness Assess for edema, contusions Note if tunneled catheter is exposed	Maintain nutritional status Minimize edema with cold packs Avoid pressure or trauma Rotate site with each port access	Remove VAD Improve nutrition Provide appropriate skin care
Infiltration, extravasation	Assess for erythema Assess for edema Assess for spongy feeling Assess for labored breathing Assess for no blood return Assess for complaints of pain Assess for no free-flow IV drip	Do not administer vesicants Use own judgment to use without a blood return Use astute assessment skills Administer medications according to drug literature	Apply warm compress Provide emotional support Obtain x-ray examination Use antidotes Discontinue IV fluids
Pneumothorax, hemothorax, air emboli, hydrothorax	Use astute assessment skills Assess for subcutaneous emphysema Assess for chest pain Assess for dyspnea, apnea, hypoxia, tachycardia, hypotension, nausea, confusion	Use cap on distal end when not in use Do not leave catheter open to air	Insert chest tubes Elevate feet Administer oxygen Aspirate air, fluid Remove catheter If air emboli suspected, place client on left side with head elevated slightly
Incorrect placement	Cardiac dysrhythmias Assess for hypotension Assess for neck distention Assess for narrow pulse pressure Assess for inadequate blood withdrawal Assess for retrograde of blood	Obtain x-ray examination after placement Reposition catheter as warranted Use astute assessment skills	Obtain x-ray examination and electrocardiogram Stop all fluid administration Discontinue catheter Administer support medications

- Instruct client and caregiver in adaptations of hospital procedures that can be made at home (e.g., good hand washing instead of sterile gloves).
- Discuss troubleshooting and emergency care routines with caregiver in home.
- Assess home environment and determine suitable area for dressing changes, avoiding areas where contaminants are potential hazards.
- Determine ability of client to meet expenses of equipment involved in caring for VAD.

Skill 19-8 Discontinuing Peripheral Intravenous Access

The technique for discontinuing a peripheral intravenous (IV) line is relatively simple. The nurse follows infection control guidelines to minimize the chance of the client acquiring an injection. In addition, the nurse takes precautions to not cause discomfort or injury to the client.

Delegation Considerations

The skill of discontinuing a peripheral IV should not be delegated to assistive personnel. Assistive personnel should be instructed to observe the venipuncture site and to report any bleeding after the catheter/needle has been removed.

Equipment

- Disposable gloves
- Sterile 2 × 2 or 4 × 4 gauze sponge
- Tape

Step	Rationale
Assessment	
1. Observe IV site for signs and symptoms of infection, infiltration, or phlebitis.	Findings will determine if therapy is needed following catheter/needle removal.
2. Review physician's orders for discontinuation of IV.	Order required for procedure.
3. Assess client's understanding for the need for IV to be discontinued.	Determines need for instruction.

Nursing Diagnosis

Defining characteristics from the assessment data may reveal the following nursing diagnosis for clients requiring this skill:

Risk for infection

Related factors are individualized based on client's condition or needs.

Planning

Step	Rationale
1. **Expected outcomes** following completion of procedure:	
▪ IV will be removed with minimal trauma to client.	Hemostasis will be maintained.
▪ IV site will remain free of infection.	Venipuncture wound properly cleansed
2. Explain procedure to client, describing sensation (burning) to be felt when catheter is removed. Explain that affected extremity must be held still and how long procedure will take.	Prepares client to cooperate during procedure.

Implementation

Step	Rationale
1. Wash hands. Apply disposable gloves.	Reduces transmission of microorganisms.
2. Turn IV tubing roller clamp to "off" position.	Prevents spillage of IV fluid.
3. Remove IV site dressing, stabilizing IV device. Then remove tape securing needle or catheter.	Exposes needle or catheter with minimal discomfort.
4. Hold needle or catheter, and clean site with alcohol, then povidone iodine solution.	Removes secretions around skin puncture site.
5. Place clean sterile gauze over venipuncture site, apply light pressure, and remove catheter or needle by pulling straight away from insertion site in a slow, steady motion (see illustration). Inspect catheter for intactness after removal.	Prevents damage to client's vein; determines if catheter tip is intact.

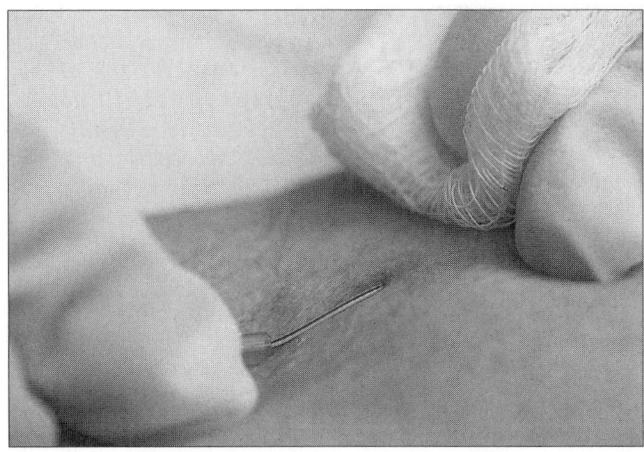

STEP **5** Remove IV catheter straight back.

STEP	RATIONALE

- ***Critical Decision Point***
  Do not raise or lift catheter before it is completely out of the vein to avoid trauma or hematoma formation.

6. Keep gauze in place and apply continuous pressure to site for 2 to 3 minutes. — Controls bleeding and hematoma formation.

- ***Critical Decision Point***
  If client has received anticoagulants (e.g., low-dose aspirin, coumadin, heparin), or has a low platelet count, apply steady pressure for 5 to 10 minutes and assess bleeding.

7. Apply clean folded gauze dressing over insertion site and secure with tape. — Maintains pressure to prevent bleeding and reduces bacterial entry into puncture site.
8. Discard used supplies, remove gloves, and wash hands. — Reduces transmission of microorganisms.

EVALUATION

1. Observe site for evidence of bleeding through dressing. — Additional pressure may be needed.
2. Observe site for redness, pain, drainage, or swelling. — May indicate infection or phlebitis at old IV site.

UNEXPECTED OUTCOMES AND RELATED INTERVENTIONS

- Venipuncture site is inflamed and/or has purulent drainage.
  - For treatment of phlebitis, apply moist, warm compress.
  - If area is infected, initiate appropriate wound care protocol (see Chapter 35).

RECORDING AND REPORTING

- Record in nurses' notes the time peripheral IV was discontinued. Include site assessment information and status of catheter.
- Report to nurse in charge or oncoming nursing shift that IV was discontinued and any significant complications.

TEACHING CONSIDERATIONS

- Instruct client to notify nurse if bleeding is noted at insertion site or if client experiences pain, tenderness, or drainage.

Critical Thinking Exercises

1. Mr. J. is visiting his daughter in the United States from Italy. He speaks no English. He is right-handed. While visiting, he develops pneumonia and requires intravenous (IV) antibiotics. He is found to have a rash on his left hand and wrist. What is the best place for his IV insertion site and why?
2. Mrs. C.'s IV order is 1000 ml normal saline (0.9% NS) with 20 mEq of KCl to run at 125 ml/hr. Which type of IV tubing should be used for this order (macrodrip = 10 gtt/ml; minidrip = 60 gtt/ml)? Calculate the drops per minute for this order. How long will a 1000 ml bag last?
3. Mr. K. has an IV infusion of 1000 ml D_5 0.45% NaCl infusing at 150 ml/hr into the right antecubital fossa. There was 700 ml left in the bag at the beginning of the shift. An hour later, you check the bag and note that there is 650 ml left in the bag. What are the possible causes for this? Describe how you should investigate to determine the actual cause.
4. Mrs. T. has had a peripheral catheter in place in the right arm for 3 days. She receives D_5 NS with 40 mEq potassium at 80 ml/hr. Your assessment of the IV site reveals tenderness around the site with localized redness. Mrs. T. tells you that her arm is painful. What might be the problem? What should you do?
5. Mrs. B. has heart failure. She is to receive 1000 ml 0.45% NS to run at 50 ml/hour. When you check the IV 2 hours later, you discover that 1000 ml 0.9% NS is infusing at 150 ml/hour. What is the highest priority action in this situation? For what complication is Mrs. B. at risk because of the IV fluids that were infusing? What assessments would indicate this complication?

References

Bagnall-Reeb J: Diagnosis of central venous access device occlusion, *J Intraven Nurs* 21(5S):S115, 1998.

Baranowski L: Central venous access device: current technologies, users, and management strategies, *J Intraven Nurs* 16(3):167, 1993.

Centers for Disease Control and Prevention: Guideline for prevention of intravascular device-related infections, *Infect Control Hosp Epidemiol* 17(7):438, 1996a.

Centers for Disease Control and Prevention, Hospital Infection Control Practice Advisory Committee: Guidelines for isolation precautions in hospitals, *Am J Infect Control* 24:24, 1996b.

Coulter K: Intravenous therapy for the elder client: implications for the intravenous nurse, *J Intraven Nurs* 15(suppl):S18, 1992.

Garner J: Guideline for isolation precautions in hospitals, *Infect Control Hosp Epidemiol* 17(1):53, 1996.

Homer LD, Holmes KR: Risks associated with 72- and 96-hour peripheral intravenous catheter dwell times, *J Intraven Nurs* 21(5):301, 1998.

Horne MM, Swearingen PL: *Pocket guide to fluid, electrolyte, and acid-base balance,* ed 3, St. Louis, 1997, Mosby.

Intravenous Nurses Society: Intravenous nursing standards of practice, *J Intraven Nurs* 13(suppl):S5, 1990.

Intravenous Nurses Society: Intravenous nursing standards of practice, *J Intraven Nurs* 21(15):535, 1998.

Intravenous Nurses Society: Infusion nursing standards of practice, *J Intraven Nurs* 23(65):556, 2000.

Lawson T: Vein trauma during catheter advancement, *J Vasc Access Device,* p 22, Spring 1998.

Lewis SM, Collier IC, Heitkemper MM: *Medical-surgical nursing,* ed 4, St. Louis, Mosby, 1996.

Loughran SC, Edwards S, McClure S: Peripherally inserted central catheters—guide wire versus non guide wire use: a comparative study, *J Intraven Nurs* 15(3):152, 1992.

Metheny N: *Fluid and electrolyte balance: nursing considerations,* ed 4, Philadelphia, 2000, Lippincott.

Millam DA: Starting IVs: how to develop your venipuncture experience, *Nursing* 22(9):33, 1992.

Occupational Safety and Health Act: Bloodborne pathogens, *Federal Register* 56(235):64, 175, Dec 6, 1991.

Orr ME: Vascular access device selection for parenteral nutrition. *Nutrition Clin Pract* 14:172-177, 1999.

Perucca R, Micek J: Treatment of infusion related phlebitis: review and nursing protocol. *J Intraven Nurs* 16:5, 286, 1993.

Thompson SE: Insertion of peripherally inserted central catheters for the administration of total parenteral nutrition, *Nutrition Clin Pract* 14:191, 1999.

Whitson M: Intravenous therapy in the older adult: special needs and considerations, *J Intraven Nurs* 19:251, 1996.

20

BLOOD THERAPY

Skills

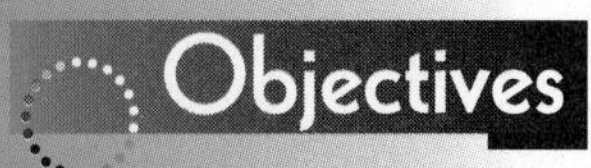

Objectives

Mastery of content in this chapter will enable the nurse to:

- Define the key terms listed.
- Discuss indications for blood therapy.
- Describe various transfusion reactions.
- Demonstrate the following skills on selected clients: initiating blood therapy, implementing autotransfusion, and monitoring for adverse reactions to transfusion.

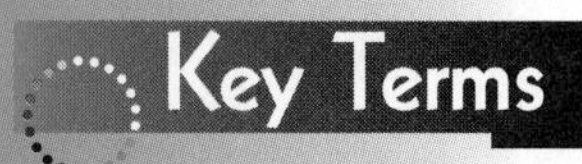

Key Terms

Agglutinate	Blood type
Allogeneic	Hemolysis
Autologous transfusion	Neutropenic
Autotransfusion	Reinfusion device
Blood group	Transfusion reaction
Blood transfusion	

Transfusion therapy is the intravenous (IV) administration of whole blood or blood components for therapeutic purposes. It may be used to restore intravascular volume with whole blood or albumin, to restore the oxygen-carrying capacity of blood by replacing red blood cells (RBCs), to replace clotting factors and/or platelets to reverse coagulopathy, or to replace white blood cells in **neutropenic** clients.

Despite precautions, blood component therapy is not without risk. Clerical errors, either in the collection or distribution of blood, may lead to the administration of incompatible units of blood. In addition, unforeseeable incompatibility and/or disease transmission remain a remote possibility. Fortunately, careful testing has reduced the aggregate per unit risk of transmitting hepatitis B, hepatitis C, human *T*-cell leukemia virus (HTLV), and human immunodeficiency virus (HIV) to less than 1:34,000. By comparison, the per unit risk of a transfused unit of RBCs being ABO incompatible is 1:33,000 (Shulman, Saxena, and Ramer, 1999).

To decrease some of the risks of transfusion, a client scheduled for major surgery in which a large volume of blood loss is anticipated (open heart, some orthopedic surgeries) may choose to donate 1 to 5 units of his or her own blood for perioperative or postoperative reinfusion (AuBuchon, 1997). Like **allogeneic** blood, autologous units are tested for HbsAg, HIV, hepatitis C, and syphilis. A biohazard label is applied to the autologous unit if the blood is reactive (American Association of Blood Banks, 1999). It is recommended that the client's donations cease more than 72 hours prior to surgery. A unit of RBCs can be stored for 5 to 6 weeks, or if frozen, for several years.

Another method used by clients as an alternative to anonymous allogeneic transfusion is the directed donation: a friend or relative donates blood specifically for a particular client's use. These donations must meet the same standards as any blood donation. Disadvantages include overt and covert pressure placed on the potential donor to donate blood. Directed donations are no safer than other allogeneic donations because potential donors may engage in behaviors that place them at high risk for hepatitis or HIV infection that they may be reluctant to admit.

Although the decision to transfuse is made by a physician, it is the nurse who must assess the client before, during, and after a transfusion. It is important that the nurse understand the rationale for transfusion of any component to be given, the expected outcomes, and the possible unanticipated outcomes so that the nurse may immediately identify any adverse effects of the therapy.

ABO System

Blood type in the ABO system is determined by the presence or absence of certain antigens on the surface of red blood cells. When the type A antigen is present, the **blood group** is called type A, and when the type B antigen is present, the blood group is type B. When both A and B antigens are present, the blood group is type AB, and when neither A nor B antigens are present, the blood group is type O.

Antibodies that react against the A and B antigens occur naturally in the plasma of people whose red blood cells do not carry them. These antibodies (agglutinins) react against the foreign antigens (agglutinogens), causing the incompatible red blood cells to **agglutinate** (clump together), resulting in a life-threatening hemolytic transfusion reaction. People with type A blood have anti-B antibodies, and people with type B blood have anti-A antibodies. People with type AB blood have neither antibody and therefore can receive all blood types, and people with type O blood have both, and therefore can receive only type O blood.

Rh System

Although six common types of Rh antigen may be present on the surface of red blood cells, the type D antigen is widely prevalent and is most likely to incite an immune response. It is the presence or absence of the D antigen that determines a person's Rh type (Mollison and Engelfriet, 1999). A person with the D antigen is considered Rh positive, and a person without the D antigen is considered Rh negative.

Unlike the ABO antigens, there are no naturally occurring antibodies to the Rh (D) antigen. A person with Rh-negative blood must first be exposed to Rh-positive blood before any Rh antibodies are formed. A person with Rh-negative blood who is exposed to a large amount (200 ml or more) of Rh-positive blood will develop enough antibodies to mount a severe transfusion reaction with repeat exposure. These antibodies take up to 2 weeks to form. Therefore, in the case of massive transfusion as used in trauma situations, Rh-positive blood may be used for a person with Rh-negative blood without adverse effect, provided that the person has not been exposed to Rh-positive blood in the past.

An Rh-negative mother previously exposed to Rh antigen can transfer Rh antibodies across the placenta to an Rh-positive fetus. This can result in severe fetal **hemolysis,** the breakdown of red blood cells, with resultant anemia and jaundice, and can be fatal to the infant.

Skill Performance Guidelines

1. Review hospital or agency policy and procedure regarding administration of blood or blood products, because it is designed to ensure safe administration of blood products.
2. Know the client's normal range of vital signs and medical history, including allergies. Administration of blood products increases intravascular volume and may elevate a client's blood pressure. This may be one of the desired effects of therapy. However, some clients cannot tolerate the volume load of a **blood transfusion** and may develop fluid volume excess, leading to markedly elevated blood pressure, tachycardia, pulmonary edema, or cardiac failure.
3. Monitor and document the client's vital signs immediately before initiation of therapy and closely during blood therapy as well. (Policies will differ between institutions regarding timing of vital sign monitoring throughout blood transfusions.) An elevation in temperature or heart rate may be one of the first signs that a person is having an adverse reaction to a transfusion. A client may also experience marked hypotension if a severe reaction occurs (see Table 20-2).
4. Understand the indications for and the goal of the transfusion therapy. This will allow the nurse to assist the physician in evaluating the outcome and assessing the need for any further therapy.
5. Assess the client's most recent serum electrolyte values. When blood is stored, there is continual destruction of RBCs, which releases potassium from the cells into the plasma. If blood is transfused rapidly, there may be transient hyperkalemia before the potassium is reabsorbed. Blood that is preserved with citrate phosphate dextrose (CPD) contains a high concentration of citrate ions. The excess citrate may combine with the ionized calcium in the recipient's blood, resulting in transient low ionized calcium levels (Simon and others, 1998). While ionized calcium deficiency resulting from blood transfusions is rare, it is more likely to occur in young children, older adults, or osteoporotic clients.
6. Verify the client's understanding of the procedure and its rationale. This may help to alleviate any anxiety the client may have over receiving blood products.

Skill 20-1 Initiating Blood Therapy

A variety of blood components exist, and their indications for use differ from one product to another (Table 20-1). It is the responsibility of the physician to determine which blood component should be administered to the client and the responsibility of the nurse to understand which components are appropriate in various situations. Before requesting a blood component for a client, the nurse must first ensure that a sample of the client's blood has been sent to the laboratory within the past 72 hours for blood typing and general compatibility screening. When sending a sample of a client's blood to the blood bank for crossmatching, the nurse must be meticulous in verifying the client's identifying information on the sample.

If a client is bleeding severely, requiring massive replacement of blood products, special infusion tubing may be obtained and hung through a pump that allows for rapid transfusion. A blood warmer may also be used, which warms the tubing and thus the infused product. Rapid transfusion of cold blood through a central line is discouraged because it is likely to cause dysrhythmias (Simon and others, 1998). Heating a unit of blood itself (in a microwave or under hot water) is inappropriate because these methods can cause destruction of the cells.

Delegation Considerations

Assistive personnel may obtain blood components from the blood bank in many institutions. Depending on the agency's policy, they may also assist in the verification procedure before the initiation of blood therapy. However, initiating blood therapy should not be delegated to assistive personnel. After the transfusion has been started and the client is stable, assistive personnel can monitor the client's vital signs. Assistive personnel should be taught the signs and symptoms of a transfusion reaction and the importance of immediately reporting if any of the signs or symptoms occur.

Equipment

- Blood administration set
- 0.9% NaCl (normal saline) intravenous (IV) solution
- Alcohol wipes
- Disposable, clean gloves
- Tape
- Blood pressure cuff and stethoscope
- Thermometer
- Signed transfusion consent form

If needed:

- Rapid infusion pump
- Leukocyte-depleting filter
- Blood warmer
- Pressure bag

Table 20-1 Blood and Blood Component Products*

Blood Product and Source	Volume and Infusion Time	Able to Transmit HIV/HBV†	ABO/Rh Testing Needed	Actions/Uses
Whole blood—single donor: allogeneic or autologous	300-550 ml < 4 hrs	Yes	Yes—Must be ABO identical Rh—Yes	Replaces red cell mass and plasma volume; expected to raise hemoglobin 1 g/100 ml and hematocrit by 3% in nonhemorrhaging adult (rarely used).
Packed red blood cells—single donor: allogeneic or directed	300-350 ml < 4 hrs	Yes	Yes/Yes	Preferred method of replacing red blood cell mass; expected to raise Hgb/HCT† level same as whole blood.
Leuko-poor RBCs—single donor: allogeneic or directed	200-250 ml < 4 hrs	Yes	Yes/Yes	Replaces RBCs while preventing febrile, nonhemolytic transfusion reactions; reduces risk of CMV transmission.
Irradiated RBCs—single donor: allogeneic or directed	250-350 ml < 4 hrs	Yes	Yes/Yes	Replaces RBCs while preventing transfusion-associated graft-versus-host disease; used in immunodeficient clients (any blood component can be irradiated).
Fresh frozen plasma (FFP)—single donor	200-250 ml < 4 hrs	Yes	Yes/No	Replaces plasma without RBCs or platelets; contains most coagulation factors and complement; used in the control of bleeding where replacement of coagulation factors is needed (e.g., DIC, TTP).
Cryoprecipitate—multiple donors, pooled	5-20 ml/unit; 1 unit/10 kg body weight 1-2 ml/min	Yes	No/No	Replaces factors VIII, XIII, von Willebrand's factor, and fibrinogen.
Platelets—multiple/random donor, pooled	40-70 ml/unit; 1 unit/10 kg body weight < 4 hrs.	Yes	Yes/Yes	Used in clients with thrombocytopenia. Certain microaggregate filters are not to be used with platelets—check manufacturer's instructions.
Platelets—single donor	200-500 ml < 4 hrs	Yes	Yes/Yes	Single-donor platelets are most useful in immunologically refractory clients when given as HLA matched with recipient. Each unit expected to raise platelet count by 5000-10,000/ml in a 70-kg client.
Colloid components—albumin 5% pooled	250-500 ml 1-10 ml/min	No	No/No	Oncotically equivalent to plasma, used to treat hypoproteinemia in burns and hypoalbuminemia in shock and ARDs; used to support blood pressure in dialysis and acute liver failure.
Colloid components—albumin 25% pooled	50-100 ml 0.2-0.4 ml/min	No	No/No	Increased circulating blood volume by increasing intravascular oncotic pressure.

*Other less commonly used blood components include factors VIII and IX concentrates, granulocytes, immunoglobulin, and saline-washed RBCs

†*HIV*, human immunodeficiency virus; *HBV*, hepatitis B virus, *Hgb*, hemoglobin; *HCT*, hematocrit; *RBC*, red blood cell; *CMV*, cytomegalovirus; *DIC*, disseminated intravascular coagulation; *TTP*, thrombotic thrombocytopenic purpura; *HLA*, human leukocyte antigen; *ARD*, acute respiratory disease.

Data from American Red Cross: Transfusion medicine update, *Blood Component Ther* 3(1), 1995; AuBuchon JP: Blood transfusion options: improving outcomes and reducing costs, *Arch Pathol Lab Med* 12(1):48, 1997; McKenry L, Salerno E: *Mosby's pharmacology in nursing*, ed 20, St. Louis, 1998, Mosby.

STEP	RATIONALE

ASSESSMENT

Step	Rationale
1. Verify that intravenous (IV) catheter to be used is patent (see Chapter 19). Catheters as small as 22 gauge and appropriate larger gauge (e.g. 19) may be used with pediatric or geriatric clients without damaging infused cells. (LaRocca, 1997)	Patent IV ensures that transfusion will be initiated and infused within time guidelines set forth. Large catheters promote optimal flow of blood components and guard against hemolysis. Use of a smaller catheter may require blood bank to divide the unit so that each half can be infused within the allotted time. Infiltration or signs of infection at IV site contraindicate use of that line.
2. Obtain client's transfusion history.	Identifies client's prior response(s) to transfusion of blood components. If client has experienced a reaction in the past, anticipate a similar reaction and be prepared to rapidly intervene.
3. Review physician's order for blood component transfusion. Check that transfusion consent has been properly completed.	A physician's order must be present before transfusing a blood product. Verifying order helps to ensure that appropriate blood component will be administered. Client consent must be obtained.
4. Know indication for blood product to be transfused (e.g., packed red blood cells [PRBCs] for a client with a low hematocrit from gastrointestinal bleeding).	Knowing rationale for product to be transfused facilitates evaluation of outcome of therapy.
5. Obtain and record vital signs immediately before initiation of transfusion.	Change from baseline vital signs will alert nurse to a potential transfusion reaction or adverse effect of therapy.

NURSING DIAGNOSIS

Defining characteristics from the assessment data may reveal the following nursing diagnoses for clients requiring this skill:

- Activity intolerance
- Ineffective peripheral tissue perfusion
- Decreased cardiac output
- Deficient fluid volume/excess fluid volume
- Deficient knowledge regarding purpose and risks of blood transfusions

Related factors are individualized based on client's condition or needs.

PLANNING

Step	Rationale
1. **Expected outcomes** following completion of the procedure:	
▪ Client will verbalize understanding of rationale for therapy.	Indicates learning has occurred.
▪ Client experiences improved activity tolerance.	Oxygenation is improved.
▪ Mucous membranes are pink, and client has brisk capillary refill.	Tissue perfusion is improved.
▪ Client's cardiac output returns to baseline.	Intravascular volume is restored.
▪ Client's systolic blood pressure improves, and urine output is ½ to 1 ml/kg/hr.	Parameters reflect optimal fluid status and adequate renal blood flow.
▪ Laboratory values will reflect improvement in targeted areas (hematocrit, coagulation values).	
2. Explain procedure to client and family. Have client sign any necessary consent forms.	Some agencies require clients to sign consent forms before receiving blood component therapy.

IMPLEMENTATION

1. **Preadministration**
   a. Obtain blood component from blood bank following agency protocol.

Step	Rationale
b. Correctly verify product and identify client with a person considered qualified by your agency.	Strict adherence to verification procedures before administration of blood or blood components reduces risk of administering the wrong blood to client. Most hemolytic transfusion reactions are caused by clerical errors (American Association of Blood Banks [AABB], 1999).
(1) Check client's first and last names by having client state name, if able. Also check client's identification number and date of birth on arm band and client record.	When a discrepancy is noted during verification procedure, do not administer the product. Notify blood bank and appropriate personnel as indicated by agency policy.
(2) Verify that component received from blood bank is component ordered by physician.	Ensures client receives correct therapy.
(3) Check that client's blood type and Rh type are compatible with donor blood type and Rh type. Be sure that transfusion is not discolored or has clots present.	Verifies accurate donor blood type. Air bubbles, clots, or discoloration may indicate bacterial contamination or inadequate anticoagulation of the stored component and would be contraindications for transfusion of that product.
(4) Check that unit number on unit of blood and on form from blood bank match.	Prevents accidental administration of wrong component.
(5) Check expiration date and time on unit of blood.	Expired blood should never be used, as the cell components deteriorate and may contain excess citrate ions.
(6) Record verification process as directed by agency policy.	
(7) Check appearance of blood product.	
c. Empty urine drainage collection container or have client void.	If a transfusion reaction occurs, a urine specimen containing urine produced after initiation of the transfusion will be sent to the laboratory.
2. Administration	
a. Wash hands, and apply clean, disposable gloves.	Utilizing standard precautions reduces risk for transmission of microorganisms.
b. Open blood administration set.	
c. For single-tubing administration, set roller clamp to "off" position.	Prevents accidental spillage of blood.
d. For Y tubing set all three roller clamps to off position.	Moving roller clamps to off position prevents accidental spilling and wasting of product.
e. Prepare blood component for administration.	
(1) For Single-Tubing Administration	
(a) Invert blood component bag gently, two to three times.	Equally distributes cells throughout preservative solution.
(b) Spike blood component unit. Squeeze drip chamber, allowing filter to fill halfway with blood. Open roller clamp slowly, and allow infusion tubing to fill with blood.	Priming tubing removes air from system.
(c) Close roller clamp when tubing is filled with blood.	Minimizes wasting any component.
(d) Set up a piggyback infusion of 0.9% saline IV solution to the single-tubing blood administration set, using a stopcock or needleless valve.	Saline should be readily available in case of a transfusion reaction.

- ***Critical Decision Point***
  Normal saline is used to prevent coagulation of the blood product. Solutions that contain dextrose will cause coagulation of donor blood.

- ***Critical Decision Point***
  Needle use should be minimized when infusing blood products because fragile blood cells can be damaged if forced through a needle. Also avoids risk of needle stick.

STEP	RATIONALE
(2) For Y tubing (see illustration)	Y tubing is used to facilitate maintenance of IV access in case a client will need more than 1 unit of blood. When utilizing Y tubing, normal saline can be easily infused following each transfusion (follow manufacturer's guidelines regarding the number of units that can be given before tubing must be changed).

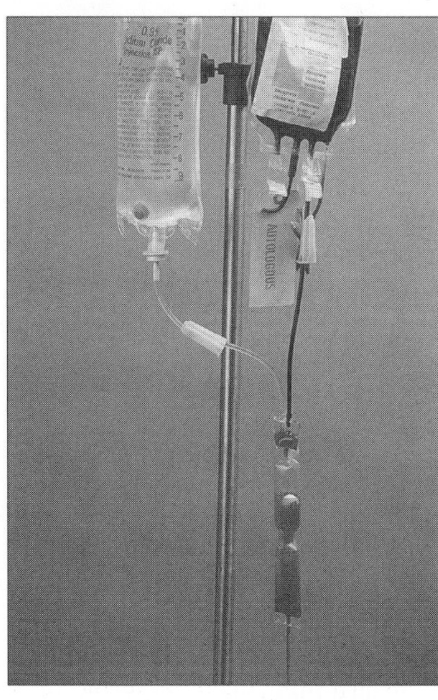

STEP **2e(2)** Blood administration setup with Y tubing.

STEP	RATIONALE
(a) Spike 0.9% normal saline IV bag.	
(b) Open roller clamp on tubing attached to saline bag. Squeeze drip chamber, allowing saline to cover the filter. Open roller clamp on common tubing.	Having both roller clamps open will prime the tubing with saline. Priming the tubing removes air from the system.
(c) Close lower roller clamp (clamp on the common tubing) after tubing is filled with saline.	This will prevent spilling or wasting of saline.
(d) Gently invert blood component bag two to three times.	This will equally distribute cells throughout preservative solution.
(e) Spike and hang blood component bag.	
(f) Close roller clamp leading from saline bag to drip chamber.	This will prevent blood from backing up into saline bag.
(g) Open roller clamp leading from blood component bag to drip chamber.	Primes tubing with blood component.
(h) Squeeze drip chamber, allowing blood to enter.	
f. Maintaining asepsis, attach primed tubing to IV catheter. Open lower clamp.	This initiates infusion of blood product into client's vein.
g. Remain with client during the first 5 to 15 minutes of a transfusion. Initial flow rate during this time should be 2 ml/min, or 20 gtts/min.	Most transfusion reactions occur within the first 5 to 15 minutes of a transfusion. Infusing a small amount of blood component initially minimizes the volume of blood to which the client is exposed, thereby minimizing the severity of a reaction.

- ***Critical Decision Point***
  The transfusion should be stopped and the physician notified immediately if signs of a transfusion reaction occur. (Refer to Skill 20-3 for signs and symptoms of a transfusion reaction.)

STEP	RATIONALE
h. Monitor client's vital signs 5 minutes after the blood product has begun infusing and per agency policy after that.	Frequent monitoring of vital signs will help to quickly alert nurse to a transfusion reaction.
i. Regulate rate of transfusion according to physician's orders. (Drop factor for blood tubing is 10 drops/ml.)	Maintaining the prescribed rate of flow decreases risk of fluid volume excess while restoring vascular volume.

STEP	RATIONALE

- ***Critical Decision Point***
  A unit of blood should not hang for more than 4 hours because of the danger of bacterial growth.

- ***Critical Decision Point***
  Medication should never be injected into an IV line with a blood component transfusing because of the risk of contaminating the blood product with bacteria.

STEP	RATIONALE
j. After blood has infused, clear IV tubing with 0.9% normal saline and discard blood bag according to agency policy.	Infusing IV saline solution infuses remainder of blood in IV tubing and keeps IV line patent for supportive measures in case of a transfusion reaction.
k. Appropriately dispose of all supplies. Remove gloves, and wash hands.	Standard precautions during a transfusion reduce transmission of microorganisms.

EVALUATION

STEP	RATIONALE
1. Monitor IV site and status of infusion each time vital signs are taken.	Detects presence of infiltration or phlebitis and verifies continuous and safe infusion of blood product.
2. Observe for any changes in vital signs and for chills, flushing, itching, dyspnea, rash, or other signs of transfusion reaction.	These may be early signs of a transfusion reaction (see Table 20-2).
3. Observe client and assess laboratory values to determine response to administration of blood component.	This aids in determining whether goals of therapy have been reached or if further blood component therapy will be required.

UNEXPECTED OUTCOMES AND RELATED INTERVENTIONS

- Client displays signs and symptoms of a transfusion reaction, which occurs when donor blood is incompatible with recipient's blood or when recipient has a sensitivity to a plasma protein in the transfused (donor's) blood
  - Stop transfusion.
  - Notify physician.
  - See Table 20-2 for interventions.
- Client develops infiltration or phlebitis at venipuncture site.
  - Remove IV and insert new catheter in different site.
  - The product may be restarted if remainder can be infused within 4 hours of initiation of transfusion.
  - Institute nursing measures to reduce discomfort at infiltrated or infected site.
- Rate of infusion slows in the absence of infiltration.
  - Gently flush IV line with normal saline or use a pressure bag to increase rate of flow of product.
- Fluid overload occurs, and/or client exhibits difficulty breathing or crackles upon auscultation.
  - Slow or stop transfusion, elevate head of bed, and inform physician of physical findings.
  - Administer diuretics, morphine, and/or oxygen as ordered by physician.
  - Continue frequent assessments, and closely monitor vital signs, intake and output.

RECORDING AND REPORTING

- Record type of blood component and amount administered, along with client's response to therapy. This may be documented on transfusion record itself, in nurses' notes, medication administration record, and/or intake and output sheet, depending on agency policy.
- Report signs and symptoms of a transfusion reaction immediately.

TEACHING CONSIDERATIONS

- Instruct client regarding rationale for transfusion and anticipated amount of time for completion of transfusion.
- Discuss with client and family the rationale for frequent vital sign monitoring throughout transfusion.
- Inform client and family to notify nurse in case of itching, swelling, dizziness, dyspnea, low back pain, or chest pain, because these may be indicative of a transfusion reaction.
- Instruct client to inform nurse if pain, swelling, or redness occurs at IV site, because these are indicative of infiltration.

PEDIATRIC CONSIDERATIONS

- The first 50 ml of a blood transfusion should be run very slowly in a pediatric client, and nurse should stay with child for that time.
- Smaller aliquots of blood are often available for use with pediatric clients (AABB, 1999).

GERONTOLOGICAL CONSIDERATIONS

- Older adults may have decreased cardiac function, thus requiring a slower infusion time. Half units may be obtained if a client is unable to tolerate the volume in a whole unit of blood or blood component.

HOME CARE CONSIDERATIONS

- Clients who have had prior transfusion reactions, acute angina, or congestive heart failure are not considered good candidates for home transfusion.
- If blood is given in the home setting, nurse must follow meticulous cross-check procedures to ensure proper administration of correct product.
- The transfusion must be initiated as soon as possible after component is obtained from blood bank. It should be transported in an insulated container with ice. Blood bank will determine appropriate temperature.
- The nurse must plan for client to have nursing personnel present during the entire transfusion process and for 30 to 60 minutes after transfusion.
- When blood sample is obtained for blood typing and crossmatching, identity band should be attached to client, with full name and identification number used by laboratory. This provides clear identification of client when blood component transfusion is initiated.
- Client and caregiver should be instructed regarding signs and symptoms of a delayed hemolytic transfusion reaction (unexplained fever, decrease in hemoglobin and hematocrit levels 2 to 14 days after transfusion) so that they can report them and receive treatment if necessary.

Skill 20-2 Autologous Transfusion

Autologous transfusion is the collection and reinfusion of a client's own blood. The blood for an autologous transfusion can be obtained by preoperative donation. Blood for an autologous transfusion can also be salvaged perioperatively, using machines that wash and filter the blood, removing anticoagulants and activated clotting factors, before returning it to the client's circulation (AuBuchon, 1997).

A client's blood can also be salvaged postoperatively (Figure 20-1). The client's blood is removed through tubes from the site of bleeding and filtered before reinfusion, and an anticoagulant such as heparin, acid citrate dextrose, or citrate phosphate dextrose (CPD) may be used to prevent clotting (AuBuchon, 1997; Simon and others, 1998). The blood must be reinfused within 6 hours of the beginning of collection. If more than 50% of the client's total blood volume is reinfused, replacement of clotting factors is necessary. This form of autologous transfusion is termed **autotransfusion.**

There are several advantages to autologous transfusions. They generally are safer for the client because they eliminate the risk of incompatibility reactions (except those due to cler-

A

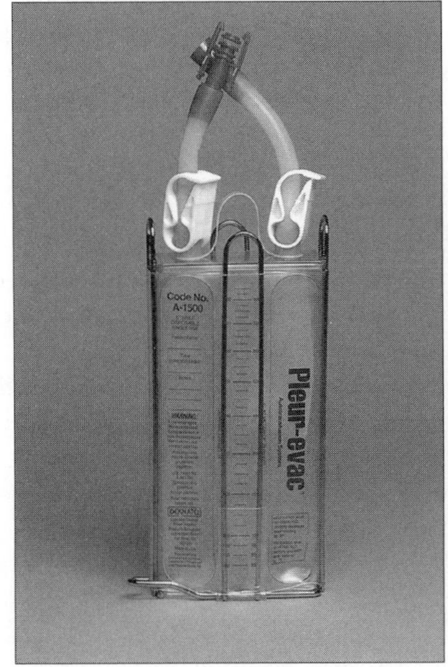

B

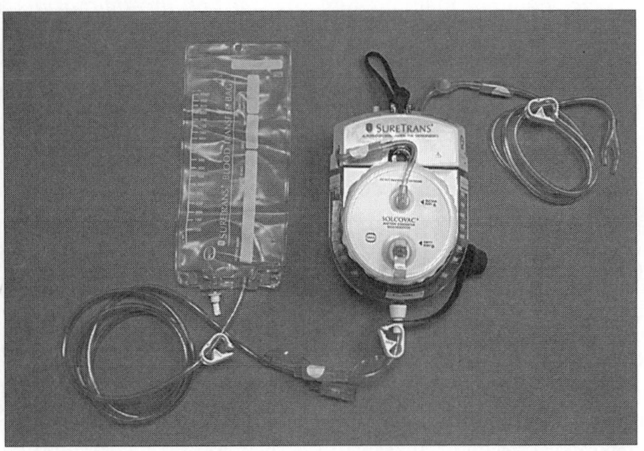

FIGURE **20-1** **A,** Pleur-evac thoracic autotransfusion device. **B,** SureTrans orthopedic autotransfusion device. (Courtesy Davol, Cranston, RI.)

ical errors) and exposure to blood-borne infectious agents (except for bacterial contamination). When preoperative donation is used, the need to carefully identify the blood unit and the client is as important as it is for an allogeneic transfusion, or the advantages are negated. The reinfused blood from perioperative blood salvage contains more viable red blood cells than does stored blood, its pH is normal, and there is a higher level of 2,3-diphosphoglycerate (2,3-DPG, a chemical that increases the oxygen-carrying capacity of hemoglobin). Another advantage of autologous transfusion is the conservation of the blood supply, especially if the client has a rare blood type (Mollison and Engelfriet, 1999).

Delegation Considerations

The skill of administering an autologous transfusion should not be delegated to assistive personnel. After the transfusion has been initiated and the client is stable, assistive personnel can monitor the client's vital signs and monitor the client for signs or symptoms of a transfusion reaction during the autologous transfusion.

Equipment

- Stethoscope and sphygmomanometer
- Pulse oximeter

For Perioperative Blood Salvage

- Cell saver or continuous collection container and appropriate tubing

For Postoperative Salvage via Drainage Tubes:

- Drainage collection and **reinfusion device**
- 0.9% normal saline intravenous (IV) solution
- Anticoagulant, if needed
- Transfer bag and tubing
- Label
- Disposable gloves

For blood donated preoperatively, follow steps in Skill 20-1

Step	Rationale
Assessment	
1. Verify that IV catheter to be used is patent and is a proper-size gauge.	Larger catheters promote optimal flow of blood components and guard against hemolysis. Infiltration or signs of infection at site contraindicates use of that line. Another IV access must be initiated, and infected or infiltrated line discontinued.
2. Obtain and record vital signs immediately before initiation of the transfusion.	Clients requiring autotransfusion are usually experiencing excessive blood loss, and hemodynamic status may be labile. It is important to be aware of baseline vital signs so that any deterioration in status may be quickly treated.

- ***Critical Decision Point***
  Although the threat of adverse reaction is decreased with autologous transfusion, client's baseline and serial vital signs should be monitored and recorded on the appropriate form.

Step	Rationale
3. Assess client's level of comfort before initiating autotransfusion.	Pain increases oxygen demand. When red blood cells (RBCs) are depleted, the body's ability to meet that demand is reduced. Client may need to be medicated for comfort to decrease metabolic demand.
4. Assess client's understanding of procedure and rationale.	Clarifying client's need for and associated benefits of therapy may alleviate some of the anxiety client may have regarding this procedure.

Nursing Diagnosis

Defining characteristics from the assessment data may reveal the following nursing diagnoses for clients requiring this skill:

- Ineffective peripheral tissue perfusion
- Deficient knowledge regarding benefits and risks of autotransfusion
- Decreased cardiac output
- Deficient fluid volume

Related factors are individualized based on client's condition or needs.

STEP	RATIONALE

PLANNING

1. **Expected outcomes** following completion of the procedure:
   - Cardiac output returns to baseline. — Intravascular volume is restored.
   - Mucous membranes are pink and moist. — Tissue perfusion is adequate. Intravascular volume is restored.
   - Capillary refill is brisk. — Peripheral tissue perfusion is adequate.
   - Urine output is ½ to 1 ml/kg/hr. — Parameters reflect optimal fluid balance.
   - Client will verbalize understanding of rationale for therapy. — Instruction is focused on purpose, benefits, and risks.
2. Explain procedure to client and family. Have client sign necessary consent forms. — Informed consent is necessary before a transfusion because of its inherent risks.

IMPLEMENTATION

1. Wash hands and put on appropriate attire: — Reduces transmission of microorganisms and prevents exposure from splashes of blood.
   a. Perioperative: surgical garb as appropriate (see Chapter 34).
   b. Postoperative: disposable gloves; gown and goggles if necessary.
2. Connect drainage tubes to collection container or cell-processing system. Minimize air bubbles by establishing secure connections. Follow agency and manufacturer's procedure for setup and maintenance of system. — Allows collection of client's blood for reinfusion, storage (no longer than 6 hours), or washing and spinning.
3. Follow manufacturer and institutional guidelines regarding reinfusion of drainage/blood.

EVALUATION

1. Observe client, and monitor vital signs and laboratory values. — Improvement in client's vital signs, cardiac output, tissue perfusion, fluid balance, and hemoglobin and hematocrit levels are expected.
2. Monitor IV site and status of infusion each time vital signs are measured. — Detects infiltration or phlebitis, verifies maintenance of constant infusion.

UNEXPECTED OUTCOMES AND RELATED INTERVENTIONS

- Client displays signs and symptoms associated with decreased cardiac output: hypotension, tachycardia, cold skin, decreased urine output.
  - Insure that transfusion is infusing at ordered rate, so that rate of volume replacement is sufficient. If blood loss is too rapid, allogeneic transfusion may be necessary.
- Infiltration or phlebitis at venipuncture site is present.
  - Remove IV, and insert new IV catheter in a different site.
  - Institute nursing measures to decrease discomfort at previous site.
- Rate of infusion slows in the absence of infiltration.
  - Gently flush line with normal saline.

RECORDING AND REPORTING

- Record amount of blood received by autotransfusion and client's response to therapy.
- Report to physician any deterioration in cardiac status.

TEACHING CONSIDERATIONS

- As with allogeneic transfusions, client receiving autologous transfusion should be instructed regarding rationale for transfusion and anticipated amount of time until completion.
- Instruct client to inform nurse if signs or symptoms of infiltration are present or if any symptoms of a transfusion reaction occur (see Table 20-2).

PEDIATRIC CONSIDERATIONS

- Autologous transfusion is not typically used in pediatric clients.

GERONTOLOGICAL CONSIDERATIONS

- Older adults may have decreased cardiac functioning, thus requiring careful monitoring of infusion time, as well as monitoring client for signs or symptoms of fluid overload.

HOME CARE CONSIDERATIONS

- Autologous transfusion is not typically used in the home setting.

Skill 20-3 Adverse Reactions to Transfusion

During the transfusion of blood products, a client is at risk for adverse reactions, particularly during the first 15 minutes. The nurse should remain with the client for that period to assess vital signs and the client's physiological response. Selected transfusion reactions are described in Table 20-2.

A **transfusion reaction** is a systemic response to the administration of a blood product that is either incompatible with that of the recipient, contains allergens to which the recipient is sensitive or allergic, or is contaminated with bacteria. Some clients with sensitivities to blood products as a result of frequent transfusions may require premedication with diphenhydramine.

Several types of adverse reactions may result from a blood transfusion. General adverse reactions (see Table 20-2) may have symptoms ranging from fever, chills, and skin rash to hypotension and cardiac arrest. A client may also experience a delayed transfusion reaction, which will not manifest itself for days or weeks. The primary risk for transfusion-associated death is the erroneous transfusion of ABO-incompatible allogeneic units (Linden and Tourault, 1997). Fatalities that occur as the result of a transfusion reaction must be reported to the Food and Drug Administration by the agency.

Other possible adverse outcomes that may result from transfusion therapy include circulatory overload and transmission of diseases such as hepatitis, cytomegalovirus, or human immunodeficiency virus (HIV). Currently all units of blood undergo extensive serological testing, thereby minimizing the risk of acquiring a blood-borne disease.

DELEGATION CONSIDERATIONS

Assistive personnel should be instructed regarding the signs and symptoms of a transfusion reaction and should immediately report if any of these occur.

STEP	RATIONALE
ASSESSMENT	
1. Observe for fever with or without chills.	Fever may be indicative of onset of an acute hemolytic reaction, febrile nonhemolytic reaction, or bacterial sepsis.
2. Observe client for tachycardia and/or tachypnea and dyspnea.	May indicate acute hemolytic reaction or circulatory overload. These symptoms may be accompanied by a cough in the case of circulatory overload.
3. Observe client for hives or skin rash.	These may be early indications of an allergic reaction, anaphylaxis, or graft-versus-host disease, which occurs after transfusion.
4. Observe client for flushing.	Flushing may be present in an acute hemolytic reaction or a febrile nonhemolytic reaction. Localized flushing may be present with an allergic reaction.
5. Observe client for gastrointestinal symptoms.	Nausea and vomiting may be present in acute hemolytic transfusion reactions, anaphylactic reactions, or sepsis. Diarrhea may be present in graft-versus-host disease or sepsis.

STEP	RATIONALE
6. Observe client for a fall in blood pressure.	Hypotension may be indicative of an acute hemolytic reaction, anaphylaxis, or sepsis.

- ***Critical Decision Point***
  Sepsis and other infections due to blood transfusion should be reported to your agency's infection control department, which will then communicate that information to the state health department and the Centers for Disease Control and Prevention.

STEP	RATIONALE
7. Observe the client for wheezing, chest pain, and (ultimately) cardiac arrest.	These are all indications of an anaphylactic reaction.
8. Be alert to client complaints of headache or muscle pain in the presence of a fever.	Both may be indicative of a febrile nonhemolytic reaction.
9. Monitor client for disseminated intravascular coagulation, renal failure, and hemoglobinemia/hemoglobinuria.	All are late signs of an acute hemolytic reaction.
10. Auscultate client's lungs, and monitor central venous pressure, if possible.	Crackles in bases of lungs and a rising central venous pressure (CVP) are indications of circulatory overload.
11. Observe client for jaundice and signs of liver failure and bone marrow suppression.	These are indicative of graft-versus-host disease and would occur following transfusion.
12. Monitor client's laboratory values for anemia refractory to transfusion therapy.	This could signify a delayed hemolytic reaction.
13. In client receiving massive transfusions, observe client for mild hypothermia, cardiac dysrhythmias, hypotension, and hypocalcemia.	Cold blood products can affect the cardiac conduction system, resulting in ventricular dysrhythmias. Other cardiac dysrhythmias, hypotension, and tingling may indicate hypocalcemia, which occurs when citrate (used as a preservative for some blood products) combines with client's calcium.

NURSING DIAGNOSIS

Defining characteristics from the assessment data may reveal the following nursing diagnoses for clients requiring this skill:

Anxiety
Decreased cardiac output
Excess fluid volume
Hyperthermia
Hypothermia
Impaired gas exchange
Pain (acute)

Related factors are individualized based on client's condition or needs.

PLANNING

STEP	RATIONALE
1. **Expected outcomes** following completion of the procedure:	
▪ Client will have pink mucous membranes and brisk capillary refill.	Tissue perfusion is improved.
▪ Client's cardiac output will return to baseline.	Intravascular volume is restored.
▪ Client will maintain core body temperature of 97° to 99° F.	Helps to confirm absence of transfusion reaction.
▪ Client will have urine output of 0.5 to 1 ml/kg/hr.	Reflects optimal fluid status.
▪ Client will maintain stable blood pressure.	Intravascular volume is restored. Absence of transfusion reaction.
▪ Client will maintain oxygen saturation of greater than 95%.	Improved tissue perfusion.
▪ Client will be comfortable and calm.	Absence of transfusion reaction. Appropriate nursing measures applied to keep patient at ease.
2. Explain treatment of a reaction to client and family.	

Table 20-2 Adverse Reactions to Blood Transfusions

Reaction	Mechanism	Onset	Signs and Symptoms
Acute hemolytic transfusion reaction	ABO, Rh incompatibility; causes intravascular destruction of transfused RBCs* as antibodies in recipient's plasma attach to antigens on donor RBCs	Within 5-15 min of initiation of transfusion	Characteristically begins with increase in temperature and heart rate; sensation of heat and pain along vein in which blood is being infused; chills, low back pain, headache, nausea, chest or back pain, dyspnea, hypotension, hemoglobinemia, hemoglobinuria (Hgb* molecules from hemolysis of RBCs is released into the plasma. This free Hgb, when filtered by the kidneys, may obstruct the renal tubules, leading to renal failure), disseminated intravascular coagulation, possibly death Can be life threatening
Delayed hemolytic transfusion reaction	Immune response mounted by recipient against non-ABO donor antigens; usually the result of destruction of transfused RBCs by alloantibodies not detected during the crossmatch	2-14 days	Unexplained fever, unexplained decrease in Hgb/HCT,* positive Coombs' test
Febrile, nonhemolytic	Accompanies ~1% of transfusions; possible sensitivity of recipient to the leukocytes or platelets in donor's blood	30 min after initiation to 6 hr after completion of transfusion	Fever greater than 1° C above baseline, flushing, chills, headache, muscle pain; occurs most frequently in immunosuppressed clients
Allergic reaction (mild to moderate)	Caused by recipient allergy to a plasma protein in donor's blood	During transfusion to 1 hr after transfusion	Local erythema, hives, and urticaria
Allergic reaction (severe)	Caused by recipient allergy to a donor antigen (usually IgA) Agglutination of RBCs obstructing capillaries and blocking blood flow, causing symptoms to all major organ systems.	Within 5-15 min of initiation of transfusion	Coughing, nausea, vomiting, respiratory distress, hypotension, loss of consciousness, possible cardiac arrest
Graft-versus-host disease	Reproduction of donor lymphocytes, usually in an immunocompromised recipient, which attack recipient's RBCs as if they were foreign proteins	Days to weeks	Skin rash, fever, jaundice due to liver dysfunction, bone marrow suppression
Circulatory overload	Can lead to pulmonary edema Occurs with transfusion of excessive volume or excessively rapid rate	Any time during or within 1-2 hr after completion of transfusion	Dyspnea, cough, crackles at lung bases, tachypnea, tachycardia, increased central venous pressure
Bacterial sepsis	Bacterial contamination of infused product	During transfusion to 2 hr after transfusion	High fever, chills, abdominal cramping, vomiting, diarrhea, profound hypotension

*RBC, red blood cell; Hgb, hemoglobin; IV, intravenous; HCT, hematocrit; PRBCs, packed red blood cells.

Data from LaRocca J, Otto S: *Mosby's pocket guide to intravenous therapy,* ed 3, St. Louis, 1997, Mosby; National Blood Resource Education Program Nursing Education Working Group: Transfusion nursing: trends and practices for the '90s, *Am J Nurs* 91(6):42, 1991; American Association of Blood Banks: *Circular of information for the use of human blood and blood components,* ARC 1751, January 1999.

Prevention	Management
Careful identification of client when blood sample is obtained for blood typing and compatibility screening, and when blood is released from blood bank; careful verification procedure at bedside prior to transfusion	Stop transfusion. Maintain IV* access. Notify physician. Monitor vital signs at least every 15 min. Correct arterial blood pressure, correct coagulopathy if present. Monitor intake and output hourly. (Attempts may be made to alkalinize the urine and initiate diuresis because this may prevent precipitation of hemoglobin within the renal tubules.) Dialysis may be required. Obtain blood and urine samples and send to laboratory with unused portion of unit of blood. Document reaction according to agency policy.
Careful crossmatching of donor and recipient blood Potential to be missed because it may occur several days after transfusion	Monitor laboratory values for anemia. (Recognition is important because subsequent transfusions may cause an acute hemolytic reaction.) If detected, notify physician and blood bank. Most delayed hemolytic reactions require no treatment.
Utilizing leukocyte-reduced blood products in clients who have experienced febrile nonhemolytic reactions in the past.	Stop transfusion. Administer antipyretics as ordered. Monitor temperature every 4 hr.
May administer antihistamines before transfusion if ordered	Stop transfusion. Notify physician and blood bank. Administer antihistamines as ordered. Monitor and document vital signs every 15 min. Transfusion may be restarted if fever, dyspnea, and wheezing are not present.
Transfusion of saline-washed or leukocyte-depleted RBCs	This is a life-threatening reaction. Stop transfusion. Maintain IV access. Notify physician and blood bank. Administer antihistamines, corticosteroids, epinephrine, and antipyretics as ordered. Measure and document vital signs every 5-15 min. Initiate cardiopulmonary resuscitation if necessary.
Administration of irradiated blood products as ordered	Administer methotrexate, corticosteroids as ordered.
Administering blood or component at rate prescribed by physician, usually no greater than 2-4 ml/kg/hr; paying particular attention to rate and volume in older adults, administering PRBCs* instead of whole blood; minimizing amount of saline infused with a transfusion	Slow or stop transfusion as ordered. Elevate client's head. Notify physician. Administer diuretics, oxygen, and morphine as ordered.
Proper care of blood or blood product from time of procurement through end of administration	Stop transfusion. Maintain IV access. Notify physician. Monitor and document vital signs. Obtain samples for blood culture and Gram's stain from recipient. Administer IV fluids, broad-spectrum antimicrobials, vasopressors, and steroids as ordered.

STEP	RATIONALE

IMPLEMENTATION

In the Event of Transfusion Reaction:

Step	Rationale
1. Stop the transfusion.	Severity of reaction is related to amount of component infused.
2. Remove tubing containing blood product and replace it with new tubing (see Chapter 19), except as noted below, in the case of mild allergic reaction.	Prevents additional blood in tubing from being infused.
3. Notify physician.	Transfusion reactions require immediate medical intervention. In the event of a mild allergic reaction, transfusion should be stopped and antihistamine administered per physician's order. Transfusion may then be restarted per physician's order.
4. Maintain patent intravenous (IV) line using 0.9% normal saline.	Medications and fluids will need to be administered for certain reactions.
5. Notify blood bank.	Blood bank will have a procedure to follow when notified of a transfusion reaction.
6. Obtain blood samples (if needed) from arm opposite transfusion. Check agency policy regarding number and type of tubes to be used.	Typically, one tube of blood will be crossmatched to pretransfusion sample to ensure that correct blood was given to recipient, and the blood will be checked for antibodies to determine the type of reaction. A second blood sample will be checked for free hemoglobin in the serum, indicating hemolysis, and a bilirubin level should be obtained.
7. Return remainder of blood component and attached blood tubing to the blood bank according to agency policy. (Blood will not usually need to be returned in the case of circulatory overload or an allergic reaction.)	A sample of this blood will be crossmatched to client's pretransfusion and posttransfusion samples to determine if error in crossmatching occurred.
8. Monitor and document client's vital signs every 15 minutes or more frequently if needed.	Maintains ongoing assessment of client's cardiopulmonary status.
9. Administer prescribed medications according to type and severity of transfusion reaction.	
a. Epinephrine	Stimulates sympathetic nervous system to relieve respiratory distress and combat vasodilation in anaphylaxis.
b. Antihistamine	Parenteral antihistamine diminishes some aspects of allergic response by blocking histamine receptors. May also be ordered pretransfusion in some cases.
c. Antibiotics	Administered when bacterial contamination/sepsis is suspected.
d. Antipyretics/analgesics	Administered to relieve fever and discomfort in acute hemolytic reactions, febrile nonhemolytic reactions, graft-versus-host disease, and bacterial sepsis.
e. Diuretics/morphine	May be administered in circulatory overload to reduce intravascular volume and decrease vascular tone.
f. Corticosteroids	Stabilizes cell membranes, decreasing histamine release. Administered in severe allergic reactions.
10. IV fluids	Rapid administration of IV fluids may help to counteract some of symptoms of anaphylactic shock.
11. In the event of cardiac arrest, initiate cardiopulmonary resuscitation (see Chapter 15).	Anaphylaxis can quickly lead to cardiopulmonary arrest. Prompt resuscitation may prevent further complications.

STEP	RATIONALE
12. Obtain first voided urine sample and send to laboratory. A catheter may need to be inserted to obtain the urine (see Chapter 24).	Hemoglobinuria occurs with acute hemolytic reactions. Degree of damage to kidneys is influenced by pH of urine and rate of urinary excretion. Attempts will be made to initiate diuresis and alkalinize the urine. If kidney damage is severe, dialysis may be required.

EVALUATION

1. Observe client to determine response to discontinuing transfusion or instituting measures to reduce transfusion reaction.	Provides continued monitoring of client's cardiopulmonary status and physiological response.

UNEXPECTED OUTCOMES AND RELATED INTERVENTIONS

- Client's physiological status worsens.
  - Appropriate interventions will be dictated by nature of crisis. Table 20-2 provides general guidelines.

RECORDING AND REPORTING

- Immediately report presence of transfusion reaction and client's physical assessment findings to nurse in charge and physician.
- Record exact time of transfusion reaction, assessment findings, and nursing and medical actions taken.

TEACHING CONSIDERATIONS

- Clients and caregivers should be taught signs and symptoms of transfusion reactions and steps to be taken should they occur.

PEDIATRIC CONSIDERATIONS

- Irradiated red blood cells and platelets are preferable in children under 6 years of age because of their immature immune systems and to avoid graft-versus-host disease (Lumadue and Ness, 1996).

GERONTOLOGICAL CONSIDERATIONS

- It is important to remember to administer blood components cautiously to older adults, considering both rate and amount of infusion, because they are more likely to develop circulatory overload than younger clients.

HOME CARE CONSIDERATIONS

- Certain adverse outcomes (development of hepatitis) or transfusion reactions (delayed hemolysis) occur days to weeks after client has received transfusion and may become evident in the home setting. It is important that client, family, and home health care workers are aware of signs and symptoms of these adverse occurrences and steps to be taken should they occur.

Critical Thinking Exercises

1. A 38-year-old client in room 428, Mr. Wagner, admitted with gastrointestinal bleeding, is awaiting a transfusion of packed red blood cells (PRBCs) for a hemoglobin level of 7.6 mg/100 ml. His blood pressure is 86/46 mmHg, and his mucous membranes are pale. You and another nurse check the information on the bag of blood obtained from the blood bank with the information on the client's record and find the information below. What should you do?

   Name: Will Warner
   Room number: 428
   ID number: 123-45-67
   Blood type: A-Pos.

2. Ten minutes after a transfusion of PRBCs began infusing, your formerly afebrile 26-year-old female client has a temperature of 101.6° F and feels tightness in her chest. What is the first thing you should do?
3. A 79-year-old client receiving fresh frozen plasma states she is having difficulty breathing, as you check on her 1 hour into the transfusion. What steps will you take?

References

American Association of Blood Banks: *Circular of information for the use of human blood and blood components,* ARC 1751, January 1999.

American Red Cross: Transfusion medicine update, *Blood Component Ther* 3(1), 1995.

AuBuchon JP: Blood transfusion options: improving outcomes and reducing costs, *Arch Pathol Lab Med* 121(1):40, 1997.

LaRocca J, Otto S: *Mosby's pocket guide to intravenous therapy,* ed 3, St. Louis, 1997, Mosby.

Linden JV, Tourault MA, Scribner CL: Decrease in frequency of transfusion reactions, *Transfusion* 37(2):243, 1997.

Lumadue JA, Ness PM: Current approaches to red cell transfusion, *Semin Hematol* 33(4):277, 1996.

McKenry L, Salerno E: *Mosby's pharmacology in nursing,* ed 20, St. Louis, 1998, Mosby.

Mollison PL, Engelfriet P: Blood transfusion, *Semin hematol* 36(4)(suppl 7):48, 1999.

National Blood Resource Education Program Nursing Education Working Group: Transfusion nursing: trends and practices for the '90s, *Am J Nurs* 91(6):42, 1991.

Shulman IA, Saxena S, Ramer L: Assessing blood administration practices, *Arch Pathol Lab Med* 123(7):595, 1999.

Simon TL and others: Practice parameter for the use of red blood cell transfusions, *Arch Pathol Lab Med* 122(2):130, 1998.

21

Oral Nutrition

Skills

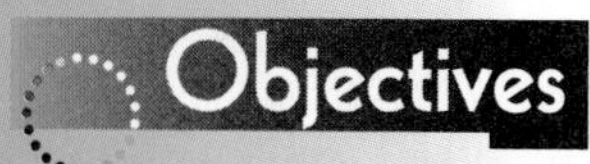

Objectives

Mastery of content in this chapter will enable the nurse to:

- Define the key terms listed.
- Perform accurate nutritional assessment.
- Identify clients appropriate for nutritional assessment.
- Assess client's ability to swallow.
- Provide mouth care after feeding a client.
- Demonstrate how to properly feed the client who cannot self-feed.
- Prepare the client to receive appropriate meals.
- Evaluate the client's tolerance of oral nutrition.
- Identify the client at risk for aspiration related to dysphagia.

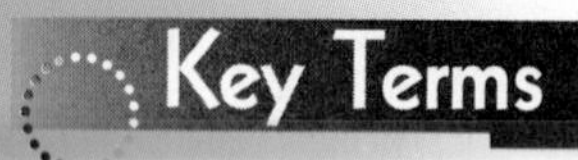

Key Terms

Anthropometrics
Aspiration
Basal energy expenditure (BEE)
Bolus
Dysphagia
Full liquid diet
Gag reflex
Kilograms
Malnutrition
Midarm circumference (MAC)
Nutritional risk
Prealbumin
Registered dietitian
Triceps skinfold (TSF)

Box 21-1 Components of a Nutritional Assessment (ABCD Approach)

Anthropometrics
- Triceps skinfold
- Midarm circumference
- Midarm muscle circumference

Biochemical Tests
- Protein status: albumin, **prealbumin**
- Nitrogen balance; 24-hour urinary nitrogen
- Immune function: total lymphocyte count
- Iron status

Clinical Observations

History
- Swallowing, GI, and elimination symptoms
- Functional status
- Social support
- Psychological status
- Ability to purchase food
- Religious and cultural food preferences

Physical Assessment
- Height
- Weight
- Usual height
- Ideal body weight
- Abdominal assessment
- Frame size

Dietary Evaluation
- 24-hour food recall
- Food frequency
- Food preferences
- Food allergies

Nutritional status for clients of any age reflects general health and can affect rate of recovery from procedures, surgery, or illness. When a client with a functional gastrointestinal (GI) tract is unable to obtain adequate oral nutrition, nutritional status can be compromised. A nurse's role may include performing nutritional assessment to determine if the client is already malnourished or at risk of becoming malnourished, feeding an adult client who cannot self-feed, and identifying a client who is at risk of aspiration during oral feeding. **Nutritional risk** is the potential to become malnourished because of factors that are primary, such as inadequate intake, or secondary, such as disease.

A comprehensive nutritional assessment is a procedure conducted to determine appropriate nutritional therapy based on the needs of the client (Grodner, Anderson, and DeYoung, 2000). Nutritional assessment includes collection of objective and subjective data that relate to nutritional status. This nutritional assessment may include an ABCD approach: Anthropometrics, Biochemical tests, Clinical observations, and Dietary evaluation (Box 21-1). No single biochemical test, such as serum albumin, can accurately indicate poor nutrition, but collectively biochemical tests, measurements of height and weight, and dietary histories can accurately reflect the client's nutritional status. Nurses can work with the **registered dietitian** to complete a nutritional assessment. Because nursing care involves frequent client contact, nurses who understand nutritional assessment can readily assess nutritional problems and evaluate the adequacy of the nutritional plan of care.

Adults usually eat independently, but they may need to be fed in the presence of physical or cognitive limitations. For example, neurological, neuromuscular, or orthopedic problems can impair a client's ability to manipulate feeding utensils. Clients' loss of independence and control when fed by another person can lead to psychological problems and depression. It is important for the nurse to understand the psychological and social impact of altered ability to self-feed and to give the client as much choice, time, and independence as possible.

Dysphagia (difficulty swallowing) is the most common cause of aspiration in adults during oral feeding. Dysphagia can be caused by neurological and neuromuscular diseases and by trauma to or surgical procedures of the oral cavity or throat. The nurse should suspect the presence of dysphagia when the client coughs or gags during eating, exhibits multiple attempts at swallowing, complains of food "getting stuck" in the throat, or has poor lip and tongue control. **Aspiration** of food can lead to pneumonia and death. Nursing interventions for the dysphagic client can help to avoid aspiration, such as placing a "dysphagia" sticker on each client's chart or at the top of the client's bed.

Skill Performance Guidelines

1. Identify who are at risk for **malnutrition.** The nurse can provide preventive care and seek appropriate resources for intervention, for example, dietitian, nutritionist.
2. Be aware of the signs and symptoms of malnutrition (Table 21-1). Clients who are not thin and visibly malnourished may still have nutritional problems (e.g., the obese client with adequate fat reserves but depleted circulating protein reserves). Nutritional care should be provided for all clients.
3. Use a systematic and organized approach to nutritional assessment. This allows the nurse to obtain complete, essential information without being repetitive.
4. Be aware of the client's social history. Clients may be interested in healthy nutritional practices but may be unable to implement them (e.g., no refrigeration at home, lack of money to buy food or infant formula). The nurse needs to be aware of limitations and work with the client toward realistic goals.
5. Review the client's medical history. Certain diseases, medications, and medical problems can influence nutritional status. Clients with some medical problems or nonfunctioning GI tracts cannot be treated with oral nutrition. Parenteral therapies may be necessary (American Society for Parenteral and Enteral Nutrition [ASPEN], 1995).
6. Verify that the type of feeding ordered is what has been provided to the client at the proper temperature. Knowledge of the different types of oral diets (e.g., diabetic diet, lactose intolerant diet) helps the nurse properly plan and recommend changes to meet client needs.
7. Promote factors that improve client's appetite, such as encouraging client to select foods, providing small, frequent meals, and arranging pleasant and comfortable surroundings.
8. An organized approach when feeding a client of any age helps the client feel more at ease, and appetite may increase in an unhurried atmosphere.
9. Be aware of the psychological impact on the adult client who cannot self-feed. Feeding in a timely, well paced, and understanding manner that allows maximal client independence can lessen the negative aspects of being fed by someone else. Instruct family members to provide a relaxed, social atmosphere when feeding the client and to allow the client to be as independent in feeding as possible. Assistive devices may enable the client to perform self-care.
10. Recognize symptoms such as coughing, gagging, multiple swallow attempts, or complaints of difficulty swallowing that may indicate dysphagia with aspiration.
11. Encourage clients and family members to keep menus from the hospital meal tray to use as a guide for preparing meals at home.

Table 21-1 Clinical Signs of Nutritional Status

Body Area	Signs of Good Nutrition	Signs of Poor Nutrition
General appearance	Alert: responsive	Listless, apathetic, cachexia, cachectic appearance
Weight	Weight normal for height, age, body build	Obesity or underweight appearance (special concern for underweight)
Posture	Erect posture; straight arms and legs	Sagging shoulders; sunken chest; humped back
Muscles	Well-developed, firm muscles; good tone; some fat under skin	Flaccid appearance, poor tone, underdeveloped tone; tenderness; edema; wasted appearance; inability to walk properly
Nervous system control	Good attention span; lack of irritability or restlessness; normal reflexes; psychological stability	Inattention; irritability; confusion; burning and tingling of hands and feet (paresthesia); loss of position and vibratory sense; weakness and tenderness of muscles (may result in inability to walk); decrease or loss of ankle and knee reflexes; absent vibratory sense
Gastrointestinal function	Good appetite and digestion; normal regular elimination; no palpable organs or masses	Anorexia; indigestion; constipation or diarrhea; liver or spleen enlargement

From Williams SR: *Nutrition and diet therapy,* ed 8, St. Louis, 1998, Mosby.

Continued

Table 21-1 Clinical Signs of Nutritional Status—cont'd

Body Area	Signs of Good Nutrition	Signs of Poor Nutrition
Cardiovascular function	Normal heart rate and rhythm; lack of murmurs; normal blood pressure for age	Rapid heart rate (above 100 beats/min); enlarged heart; abnormal rhythm; elevated blood pressure
General vitality	Endurance; energy, good sleep habits; vigorous appearance	Easily fatigued; lack of energy; falling asleep easily, tired and apathetic appearance
Hair	Shiny, lustrous appearance; firmness; strands not easily plucked, healthy scalp	Stringy, dull, brittle, dry, thin, and sparse, depigmented appearance; strands that can be easily plucked
Skin (general)	Smooth and slightly moist skin with good color	Rough, dry, scaly, pale, pigmented, irritated appearance; bruises; petechiae; subcutaneous fat loss
Face and neck	Uniform color; smooth, pink, healthy appearance; lack of swelling	Greasy, discolored, scaly, swollen appearance; dark skin over cheeks and under eyes; lumpiness or flakiness of skin around nose and mouth
Lips	Smoothness; good color; moist (not chapped or swollen) appearance	Dry, scaly, swollen appearance; redness and swelling (cheilosis); angular lesions at corners of mouth; fissures or scars (stomatitis)
Mouth, oral membranes	Reddish pink mucous membranes in oral cavity	Swollen, boggy oral mucous membranes
Gums	Good pink color; healthy and red appearance; lack of swelling or bleeding	Spongy gums that bleed easily; marginal redness, inflammation; receding gums
Tongue	Good pink or deep reddish color; lack of swelling; smoothness, presence of surface papillae; lack of lesions	Swelling, scarlet and raw appearance; magenta color, beefiness (glossitis); hyperemic and hypertrophic papillae; atrophic papillae
Teeth	Lack of cavities and pain; bright, straight appearance; lack of crowding; well-shaped jaw; clean appearance with no discoloration	Unfilled caries; absent teeth; worn surfaces; mottled (fluorosis), malpositioned appearance
Eyes	Bright, clear, shiny appearance; lack of sores at corner of membranes; eyelids moist and healthy pink color; lack of fatigue circles beneath eyes	Pale eye membranes (pale conjunctivas); redness of membrane (conjunctival infection); dryness; signs of infection; Bitot's spots, redness and fissuring of eyelid corners (angular palpebritis); dryness of eye membrane (conjunctival xerosis); dull appearance of cornea (corneal xerosis); soft cornea (keratomalacia)
Neck (glands)	Lack of enlargement	Thyroid enlargement
Nails	Firm, pink appearance	Spoon shape (koilonychia); brittleness; ridges
Legs, feet	Lack of tenderness, weakness, or swelling; good color	Edema; tender calf; tingling; weakness
Skeleton	Lack of malformations	Bowlegs; knock-knees; chest deformity at diaphragm; prominent scapulae and ribs

From Williams SR: *Nutrition and diet therapy*, ed 8, St. Louis, 1998, Mosby.

Skill 21-1 Performing Nutritional Assessment

Surveys have shown that malnutrition was present in approximately 50% of all hospitalized clients (Hall, 1999). The continuing decrease in length of stay in acute care facilities makes nutritional screening and assessment an essential component of care. Nutritional assessment is a specific, measurable means of identifying clients who may be malnourished. Clients may be assessed for a variety of reasons, including having diagnoses associated with nutritional problems (such as GI problems, trauma, burns, sepsis, or malabsorption), recent rapid weight loss, or history of poor dietary intake. The Joint Commission on Accreditation of Healthcare Organizations (JCAHO) standards now require the identification of clients who are nutritionally at risk by means of an initial screening mechanism (JCAHO, 2000). Clients who are identified to be at risk should have a nutritional assessment.

Four components of nutritional assessment are evaluated: (1) client history (medical, psychological, and social); (2) physical examination, which includes anthropometrics and clinical observations; (3) biochemical parameters; and (4) dietary history and evaluation (Grodner, Anderson, and DeYoung, 2000). Elements of the client history give background to factors influencing current nutritional status. The medical history indicates medications, surgery, and coexisting medical conditions compromising nutrition. Depression or abnormal psychiatric behavior leading to decreased food intake can be identified in the psychological history. A social history can give important insight into beliefs, the financial ability to obtain food, and food customs influencing nutrition. Assessment of dietary intake by sample menus, eating habits, or 24-hour recall can indicate food practices or avoidance of food groups that may impair nutritional status. A physical examination can also indicate impaired nutrition. Evaluation of body size, weight, and muscle wasting is accomplished through the use of **anthropometrics.** These can include measurements such as wrist circumference for body frame size, **midarm circumference** (MAC), and **triceps skinfold** (TSF) to measure muscle and fat reserves. Finally, biochemical parameters are evaluated that reflect the status of circulating proteins.

Nutritional assessment goals as outlined by ASPEN (1995) include the following:

1. Establish baseline subjective nutritional parameters.
2. Identify specific nutritional deficits.
3. Determine nutritional risk factors for individual clients.
4. Establish nutritional needs for individual clients.
5. Identify medical and psychosocial factors that may influence the prescription and administration of nutritional support.

Delegation Considerations

The interpretation of data collected during a nutritional assessment should not be delegated to assistive personnel. Delegation of steps in data collection, such as obtaining height and weight or helping the client to complete a 24-hour recall, may be appropriate.

Equipment

- Assessment sheet and pen
- Tongue blade, stethoscope, penlight
- Scale
- Tape measure
- Lange, Harpenden, or Holtain skin calipers (optional—if anthropometric measurements are obtained)

Step	Rationale
Assessment	
1. Determine need to perform nutritional assessment based on diagnosis and history.	Certain conditions place adult client at risk for malnutrition (Box 21-2).
2. Assess client for usual body weight, noting recent changes (see Chapter 10).	Sudden change in body weight unrelated to diet changes can indicate illness.
3. Review results of relevant laboratory tests (Table 21-2).	These biochemical parameters (tests ordered by physician) measure visceral and circulating protein status. Albumin and transferrin indicate visceral protein status. Total lymphocyte count (TLC) can reflect immunocompetence.
4. Determine what medications client is taking (over-the-counter and prescribed).	Certain medications can inhibit or potentiate action of other medications. Also, medications and nutrients may interact to either decrease medication function (e.g., foods rich in vitamin K, such as dark green vegetables and coumarin anticoagulants) or impair nutrient use (mineral oil laxatives). Nurses are expected to be aware of drug-drug and drug-nutrient interactions that may impair client care.
5. Determine clients ability to manipulate eating utensils and self-feed.	Difficulty in self-feeding creates significant risk for malnutrition.

Box 21-2 Adults at Nutritional Risk

Actual or potential for developing malnutrition:

- Involuntary weight loss or gain of >10% of usual body weight within 6 months or >5% of usual body weight within 1 month
- >20% over or under ideal body weight
- Presence of chronic disease
- Increased metabolic requirements

Altered diets or diet schedules:

- Receiving parenteral or enteral nutrition
- Recent illness, surgery, or trauma

Inadequate nutrition intake including not receiving food or nutrition products for >7 days

From American Society for Parenteral and Enteral Nutrition: The 1995 ASPEN standards for nutrition support: hospitalized patients, *Nurs Care Pract* 10(6):208, 1995.

Table 21-2 Selected Biochemical Tests for Nutritional Assessment

Biochemical Parameter	Laboratory Test	Normal Range	Implications for Abnormal Value
Visceral protein status	Serum albumin	3.5-5.0 mg/dl	Reflects liver's ability to synthesize plasma proteins; changes slowly
	Prealbumin	25-50 mg/dl	Sensitive to protein changes; useful in measuring short-term changes
Evaluation of protein intake	24-hour urinary nitrogen	Positive balance when compared with nitrogen intake	May indicate inadequate protein intake Nitrogen balance = (Protein intake/6.25) − 4 A positive nitrogen intake indicates that nitrogen can be stored instead of broken down for energy
Immune function	Total lymphocyte count (TLC)	>1500 cells/mm^3	May indicate poor dietary intake, possible immunocompromised status; is used more for nutritional screening with other biochemical parameters
Iron status	Hemoglobin	12-15 mg/dl	Decreased value indicates anemia; further testing is needed to determine if anemia is nutrition related

From Pagana KD, Pagana TJ: *Mosby's diagnostic and laboratory test reference*, ed 4, St. Louis, 1999, Mosby.

Step	Rationale

Nursing Diagnosis

Defining characteristics from the assessment data may reveal the following nursing diagnoses for clients requiring this skill:

- Risk for aspiration
- Risk for deficient fluid volume
- Imbalanced nutrition: more than body requirements
- Imbalanced nutrition: less than body requirements
- Risk for imbalanced nutrition: more than body requirements
- Feeding self-care deficit
- Deficient knowledge regarding nutritionally balanced diet
- Disturbed sensory perception (gustatory)
- Impaired swallowing

Related factors are individualized based on client's condition or needs.

Planning

1. **Expected outcomes** following completion of procedure:
   - Client denies any gastric, swallowing, or chewing problems or food intolerances. — Indicates absence of gastric disturbance or food intolerance.
   - Physical assessment and laboratory data are consistent with adequate nutritional status. — Indicates that client's nutritional intake is adequate to produce normal nutritional status.
2. Prepare equipment and supplies.
3. Explain to client purpose for nutritional assessment. — Ensures client's participation in care.
4. Prepare environment: quiet, undistracting. — Helps nurse to better obtain information.

Implementation

1. Obtain complete and thorough nursing history, including social, economic, and psychological information. — Allows nurse to identify those clients who have poor nutritional conditions or are at risk of developing nutritional deficiencies; is of significant importance in the care of acute and chronically ill clients (Correia, 1999).

STEP	RATIONALE
2. Either initiate diet diary or perform 24-hour recall interview. The use of food models may assist client to recall portions more accurately.	Both diet and 24-hour recall are effective methods for taking diet history. Diet diary is obtained over longer period and helps to determine food likes and dislikes, as well as allergies. The 24-hour recall is an account of everything client has consumed over that period of time; it is less time consuming but not as accurate. Both evaluate food consumption and eating habits (Grodner, Anderson, and DeYoung, 2000).
3. Document findings of diary on nutritional assessment sheet.	Prompt documentation of nutritional assessment is needed to plan, provide, and monitor client's nutritional status (Lyne, Prowse, 1999).
4. Assist client into bed.	Having client in bed facilitates physical assessment.
5. Perform physical assessment.	Through use of physical assessment, nurse will be able to detect signs and symptoms of malnutrition (see Table 21-1).
6. Help client to standing position, and be sure client is free of restrictive clothing.	Clients must be standing for anthropometric measurements.
7. Have client stand on scale, or if client is unable to stand, use chair, bed, or sling-type scale. Record weight; convert to **kilograms** (Weight ÷ 2.2 = kg).	Weight is a useful index of client's state of nutrition. Ideally, client should be weighed with same scale at same time of day with same amount of clothing for comparison of weight changes over time.
8. Measure client's height. If client is unable to stand, measure from heel to top of head while client is lying flat on bed and record.	Correct height measurement assists in calculating ideal body weight.
9. Calculate, or determine via standard height and weight chart, ideal body weight (IBW) with a range for normal of 10% above and 10% below IBW. Calculation of IBW can be accomplished using the following formula: ▪ Male: 106 pounds (47.7 kg) for the first 5 feet, then add 6 pounds per additional inch (2.25 kg per 2.5 cm). ▪ Female: 100 pounds (45 kg) for the first 5 feet, then add 5 pounds per additional inch (2.25 kg per 2.5 cm).	Determination of IBW using a standard chart may require the calculation of frame size.
10. Using measuring tape, measure the smallest portion of wrist distal to styloid process (bony prominence at wrist) (see illustration).	Wrist circumference and height are used to calculate body frame size (Table 21-3).

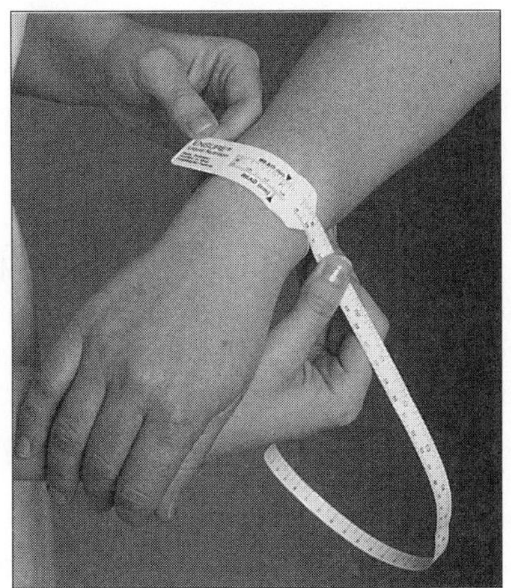

STEP **10** Wrist circumference.

Table 21-3 Calculation of Body Frame Size

$$\text{Ratio} = \frac{\text{Height (cm)}}{\text{Wrist circumference (cm)}}$$

FRAME SIZE	VALUES FOR MEN	VALUES FOR WOMEN
Small	10.4	11.0
Medium	9.6-10.4	10.1-11.0
Large	9.6	10.3

STEP	RATIONALE
11. With client's nondominant arm relaxed, measure circumference at midpoint of arm in centimeters (between tip of acromial process of scapula and olecranon process of ulna) and record (see illustration). If client is bedridden, measurements may be taken with arm bent and placed across chest.	Mid-upper arm circumference (MAC) estimates muscle wasting.

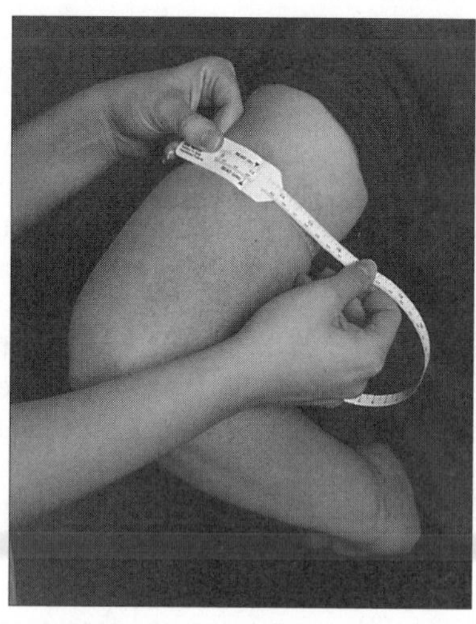

STEP **11** Measurement of mid-upper arm circumference (MAC).

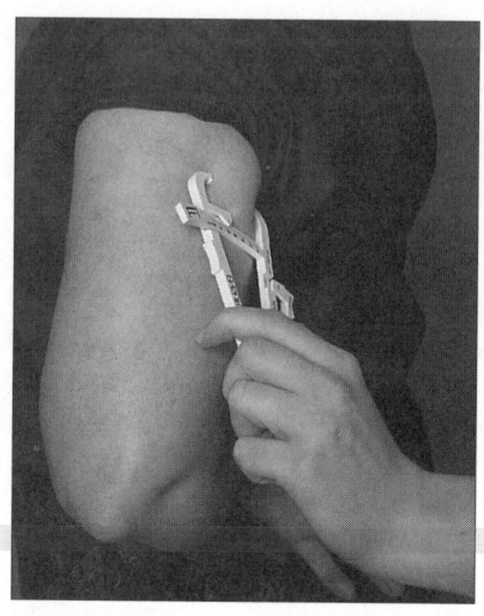

STEP **12** Triceps skinfold.

STEP	RATIONALE
12. With thumb and forefinger, pinch a double fold of fat lengthwise about 1 cm above midpoint of MAC. With other hand, place teeth of calipers on either side of fat fold. Calipers are placed below fingers so pressure is exerted from calipers rather than fingers. Record three separate readings in millimeters and document (see illustration).	Skinfold measurements are used to estimate fat content of subcutaneous tissue (e.g., biceps, scapula, abdominal muscles). TSF is most common and easiest to measure. Average the three readings of TSF.
13. Help client to comfortable position.	Remainder of assessment is composed of calculations and review of laboratory work.
14. Calculate and record midarm muscle circumference (MAMC). MAMC = MAC (cm) − [TSF (cm) × 3.14]	MAMC is estimation of skeletal muscle mass.
15. Wash hands.	Reduces transmission of microorganisms.
16. Explain to client that nutritional assessment is complete.	Allows time for clients to ask questions about assessment.

EVALUATION

STEP	RATIONALE
1. Review history and physical findings. Note abnormalities or areas of concern.	Completeness of data obtained from history and physical findings permits prompt interventions for nutritional alterations.
2. Discuss findings of diet history and 24-hour recall with client.	Reviewing findings with client determines status of dietary habits and client's knowledge.

Step	Rationale
3. Compare client's weight for height with ideal and usual weight.	Significant weight fluctuations or weight outside of normal range may indicate nutritional risk.
4. Compare anthropometric data against normal measurements.	Abnormal measurements indicate nutritional risk.
5. Compare biochemical test levels with client's levels.	Abnormal values, when considered with other nutritional parameters, may indicate malnutrition. Albumin is major protein produced by liver. It is a useful indicator for chronically malnourished clients. In an acute client, greater number of factors influence albumin (e.g., stress, hydration, surgery). Transferrin is more specific indicator of protein and calorie malnutrition than albumin.

Unexpected Outcomes and Related Interventions

- Body weight is below or above ideal body weight.
  - Check weight weekly and assess for change. Report significant changes to physician.
  - Document significant changes in intake, especially if client is at risk of malnutrition.
  - If client has lost more than 10% of body weight in a short time, weight-gain program is begun. A 500-kcal daily increase in calories provides 1-pound weight gain over 1 week.
  - Consult a dietitian to calculate client's caloric needs. A variety of formulas are available. Most commonly used formula is the Harris-Benedict equation for **basal energy expenditure (BEE).** Dietitian will:
    - Determine amount of protein client requires.
    - Determine route of nutrition (enteral [oral or tube] or parenteral). For parenteral nutrition (PN): the physician and dietitian will choose either peripheral or central PN and determine whether fat is needed (see Chapter 22).
- Laboratory tests are not within normal limits.
  - Inform physician.
  - Obtain serial laboratory parameters as ordered by physician or dietitian.

Recording and Reporting

- Record results on nutritional assessment form, making recommendations to the dietitian and documenting any significant differences from the norm (Figure 21-1).
- Report unusual findings to nurse in charge or physician.

Pediatric Considerations

- Anthropometric data includes measurement of length, weight, head circumference in young children, proportions, skinfold thickness, and arm circumference. These measurements are compared with standard growth charts to determine percentiles. The height and weight of children age 2 to 18 years is compared with standard growth charts for interpretation (Wong and others, 1999).
- Head circumference is measured in children up to 36 months of age and in any child whose head size is questionable. The head circumference is compared with standard growth charts for interpretation (Wong and others, 1999).

Gerontological Considerations

- The "normal" anthropometric standards were developed based on a healthy middle-age population and may not accurately reflect muscle wasting, decreased subcutaneous fat, or decreased skin elasticity in the older adult (Lueckenotte, 2000).
- Tools available for anthropometric measures for the older adult population have been published (*Nutritional Assessment of the Elderly Through Anthropometry,* 1988).
- Tools available in the Nutrition Screening Initiative (NSI, 1995) have been designed specifically for nutrition screening of older adults (Figure 21-2).

Nutritional Assessment

Date 12/11 Admit Date 12/7

Unit No.
Name
Address
DOB

Medical RADIATION ENTERITIS - CA
12/9 EXPLORATORY SURGERY
Social/Psych MILD DEPRESSION 2° DISEASE STATE
Diagnosis SMALL BOWEL OBSTRUCTION
Ht 183 cm Wt 71 Kg Usual Wt 82 Kg
% Change 13 IBW 80.9 (72.7 - 89)
Age 48 Sex (M) F

Drug Therapy ______ Insulin ______ Steroids
______ Narcotics (Other:) ______
PROCHLORPERAZINE, FENTANYL

Contributing Factors:
✓ Fever ___ Infection/Sepsis
___ Dysphagia ✓ Emesis
___ Chewing Probs.
___ Polytrauma ___ Diarrhea
✓ Chemo/(Radiation)
✓ Surgery
___ Other ______

Anthropometrics:
Wrist Circum. 6 1/2"
MAC 28.5
TSF
1 11.8
2 11.4
3 11.6
Ave. 11.6

Estimation of Intake:
Less than requirements ✓
Meeting requirements ______
More than requirements ______
Gastrointestinal Tract functional?
Yes ______ No ✓

Clinical/Lab Data:

	Normal		Mild		Moderate		Severe	
Albumin	>3.5		3.4-2.8		2.7-2.1	2.3	<2.1	
Total Lymph Count (TLC)	>1500		1499-1200		1199-800	1100	<800	
Transferrin	>200		199-150		149-100	138	<100	
% Usual Body Wt.	>95%		94-85%	86.5	84-75%		<74%	
% Ideal Body Wt.	>90%		89-80%	87.7	79-70%		<70%	
Skin Tests (# react./# placed)	4/4				1-2/4 (weak)	1/4	0/4 (anergic)	

Other ______

Recommendations:

______ Calories/day ______ gm protein/day

Route: ______ enteral-oral ______ enteral-tube feeding ______ parenteral

______

Signature

FIGURE 21-1 Nutritional assessment form.

The Warning Signs of poor nutritional health are often overlooked. Use this checklist to find out if you or someone you know is at nutritional risk.

DETERMINE YOUR NUTRITIONAL HEALTH

Read the statements below. Circle the number in the yes column for those that apply to you or someone you know. For each yes answer, score the number in the box. Total your nutritional score.

	YES
I have an illness or condition that made me change the kind and/or amount of food I eat.	2
I eat fewer than 2 meals per day.	3
I eat few fruits or vegetables, or milk products.	2
I have 3 or more drinks of beer, liquor or wine almost every day.	2
I have tooth or mouth problems that make it hard for me to eat.	2
I don't always have enough money to buy the food I need.	4
I eat alone most of the time.	1
I take 3 or more different prescribed or over-the-counter drugs a day.	1
Without wanting to, I have lost or gained 10 pounds in the last 6 months.	2
I am not always physically able to shop, cook and/or feed myself.	2
TOTAL	

Total Your Nutritional Score. If it's —

0-2 **Good!** Recheck your nutritional score in 6 months.

3-5 **You are at moderate nutritional risk.** See what can be done to improve your eating habits and lifestyle. Your office on aging, senior nutrition program, senior citizens center or health department can help. Recheck your nutritional score in 3 months.

6 or more **You are at high nutritional risk.** Bring this checklist the next time you see your doctor, dietitian or other qualified health or social service professional. Talk with them about any problems you may have. Ask for help to improve your nutritional health.

These materials developed and distributed by the Nutrition Screening Initiative, a project of:

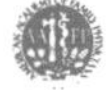
AMERICAN ACADEMY OF FAMILY PHYSICIANS

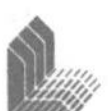
THE AMERICAN DIETETIC ASSOCIATION

NATIONAL COUNCIL ON THE AGING

Remember that warning signs suggest risk, but do not represent diagnosis of any condition. Turn the page to learn more about the Warning Signs of poor nutritional health.

FIGURE **21-2** Tool for nutrition screening of older adults. (Courtesy Nutrition Screening Initiative, Washington, DC.)

The Nutrition Checklist is based on the Warning Signs described below.
Use the word DETERMINE to remind you of the Warning Signs.

DISEASE

Any disease, illness or chronic condition which causes you to change the way you eat, or makes it hard for you to eat, puts your nutritional health at risk. Four out of five adults have chronic diseases that are affected by diet. Confusion or memory loss that keeps getting worse is estimated to affect one out of five or more of older adults. This can make it hard to remember what, when or if you've eaten. Feeling sad or depressed, which happens to about one in eight older adults, can cause big changes in appetite, digestion, energy level, weight and well-being.

EATING POORLY

Eating too little and eating too much both lead to poor health. Eating the same foods day after day or not eating fruit, vegetables, and milk products daily will also cause poor nutritional health. One in five adults skip meals daily. Only 13% of adults eat the minimum amount of fruit and vegetables needed. One in four older adults drink too much alcohol. Many health problems become worse if you drink more than one or two alcoholic beverages per day.

TOOTH LOSS/ MOUTH PAIN

A healthy mouth, teeth and gums are needed to eat. Missing, loose or rotten teeth or dentures which don't fit well or cause mouth sores make it hard to eat.

ECONOMIC HARDSHIP

As many as 40% of older Americans have incomes of less than $6,000 per year. Having less--or choosing to spend less--than $25-30 per week for food makes it very hard to get the foods you need to stay healthy.

REDUCED SOCIAL CONTACT

One-third of all older people live alone. Being with people daily has a positive effect on morale, well-being and eating.

MULTIPLE MEDICINES

Many older Americans must take medicines for health problems. Almost half of older Americans take multiple medicines daily. Growing old may change the way we respond to drugs. The more medicines you take, the greater the chance for side effects such as increased or decreased appetite, change in taste, constipation, weakness, drowsiness, diarrhea, nausea, and others. Vitamins or minerals when taken in large doses act like drugs and can cause harm. Alert your doctor to everything you take.

INVOLUNTARY WEIGHT LOSS/GAIN

Losing or gaining a lot of weight when you are not trying to do so is an important warning sign that must not be ignored. Being overweight or underweight also increases your chance of poor health.

NEEDS ASSISTANCE IN SELF CARE

Although most older people are able to eat, one of every five have trouble walking, shopping, and buying and cooking food, especially as they get older.

ELDER YEARS ABOVE AGE 80

Most older people lead full and productive lives. But as age increases, risk of frailty and health problems increase. Checking your nutritional health regularly makes good sense.

The Nutrition Screening Initiative, 2626 Pennsylvania Avenue, NW, Suite 301, Washington, DC 20037

© The Nutrition Screening Initiative is funded in part by a grant from Ross Laboratories, a division of Abbott Laboratories.

A5944(1.00)/DECEMBER 1995

FIGURE **21-2, cont'd** Tool for nutrition screening of older adults. (Courtesy Nutrition Screening Initiative, Washington, D.C.)

Skill 21-2 Assisting the Adult Client With Oral Nutrition

Assisting the adult with oral nutrition requires time, patience, knowledge, and understanding. Most people eat without assistance. However, with illness or trauma, the client may be physically unable to eat without assistance. Physical impairments that limit self-feeding include hemiplegia, fractured arm, quadriplegia, debilitating illness, or generalized weakness. The presence of intravenous (IV) catheters or tubings, dressings, and bandages can also limit self-feeding. In addition, some older adults tire quickly and may need to be assisted even though they can eat independently. Although adult feeding needs and techniques differ from those for infants, the adult who needs help to eat still needs compassion and understanding. Merely feeding the adult can be accomplished with common sense, but providing a socially meaningful mealtime requires education and experience on the part of the nurse.

Delegation Considerations

The skill of assisting the client with oral nutrition can be delegated to assistive personnel. Have care provider report incidence of coughing, gagging, or difficulty swallowing, immediately to nurse.

Equipment

- Two-handled cup with lid
- Plate with plate guard
- Utensils with splints
- Utensils with enlarged handles
- Towels

Step	Rationale
Assessment	
1. Assess that GI tract is functional, and determine what type of diet client can tolerate (Box 21-3).	Nurse's awareness of specific diet order provides appropriate nutrition.
2. Assess client's ability to swallow. In clients with neurological condition, assess **gag reflex.**	Some clients (those who have neurological diseases or are handicapped) may be at risk for dysphagia and aspiration and may not be able to tolerate a regular diet. Change in consistency of diet (thickened liquids, pureed, soft), swallow training, or alternative means of nutrition may be needed.
3. Place a tongue blade or an oral suction catheter tip on the back of client's tongue.	Clients who do not gag are at risk for aspiration (see Skill 21-3).
4. Determine to what extent client is able to self-feed. Assess physical motor skills, level of consciousness, visual acuity and peripheral vision, and mood.	Clients with any level of independence should not be totally fed by hospital staff. Thorough understanding of client's physical and cognitive limitations alerts the nurse to client's needs.
5. Assess client's appetite, tolerance of foods, cultural and religious preferences, and food likes and dislikes.	Awareness of client's needs before meals prevents misunderstanding and frustration for both nurse and client.
6. Assess whether client has food allergies.	Knowledge of client's food allergies prevents allergic reaction to food groups.

Nursing Diagnosis

Defining characteristics from the assessment data may reveal the following nursing diagnoses for clients requiring this skill:

- Risk for aspiration
- Risk for deficient fluid volume
- Feeding self-care deficit
- Disturbed sensory perception (gustatory)
- Impaired swallowing

Related factors are individualized based on client's condition or needs.

Planning

Step	Rationale
1. **Expected outcomes** following completion of procedure:	
■ Client denies any gastric, swallowing, or chewing problems or food intolerances.	Indicates absence of gastric disturbance or food intolerance.

Box 21-3 Diet Progression of Hospitalized Clients

Clear Liquid
Broth, bouillon, coffee, tea, carbonated beverages, clear fruit juices, gelatin, popsicles

Full Liquid
As above with addition of smooth textured dairy products, custards, refined cooked cereals, vegetable juice, pureed vegetables, all fruit juices

Pureed
All of above with addition of scrambled eggs, pureed meats, vegetables, fruits, mashed potatoes and gravy

Mechanical Soft
All of above with addition of ground or finely diced meats, flaked fish, cottage cheese, cheese, rice, potatoes, pancakes, light breads, cooked vegetables, cooked or canned fruits, bananas, soups, peanut butter

Soft
All of above with addition of moist tender meat, poultry, fish, soft casseroles, lettuce, tomatoes, soft fresh fruit, cake, cookies without nuts or coconut

From Grodner M, Anderson SL, DeYoung S: *Foundations and clinical applications of nutrition: a nursing approach,* ed 2, St. Louis, 2000, Mosby.

Step	Rationale
▪ Client's weight increases or remains the same over the time diet therapy is provided.	Nutritional intake exceeds or meets daily requirements.
▪ Client completes meal.	Prescribed dietary intake has been eaten; decreases risk of nutritional imbalances.
▪ Client is able to participate in independent feeding.	Enables client to be as independent as possible; provide assistive devices as needed to promote independence; involve family in mealtime if possible.
2. Prepare client's room for mealtime:	
a. Remove any unpleasant odors and sights (e.g., remove bedpans, bedside urinals, used dressings, trash).	Unsightly, odor-filled room can decrease client's appetite.
b. Clear overbed table.	
c. Set up chair for client and for nurse. Place bed in upright back position if client is unable to be up in the chair. Certain conditions, such as pressure ulcer, traction, or spinal surgery, may prevent positioning with head elevated.	Upright position assists client to keep food toward front of mouth prior to swallowing, reducing aspiration.
3. Prepare client for meal:	
a. Assist client with elimination needs.	Increases client's comfort and enjoyment of meal, and as a result client's nutritional intake may increase.
b. Help client wash hands.	Reduces spread of microorganisms.
c. Assist client with mouth care. Clients with dysphagia or dry mouth may benefit from clear water rinsing or swabbing.	Oral hygiene improves taste and increases appetite.
d. Clients with stomatitis (irritation of oral mucosa) may benefit from rinsing with a solution containing ½ to 1 teaspoon of salt to 1 pint of water.	Clients may avoid foods because of pain from mouth sores or esophagitis.
e. Help client to put in dentures and put on eyeglasses or insert contact lenses if used. Check that dentures are not too loose.	Enhances client's ability to chew and see food. Loose dentures inhibit normal chewing and pose a safety risk.

STEP	RATIONALE
f. Help client to comfortable sitting position. If client is unable to sit, turn client on side with the head of the bed elevated.	Minimizes risk of aspiration.
g. Obtain special devices and needed supplies to facilitate feeding (two-handled cup with lid, plate with plate guard, utensils with splints, utensils with enlarged handles, towels) before meal (see illustration).	Ensures organized, unhurried atmosphere.

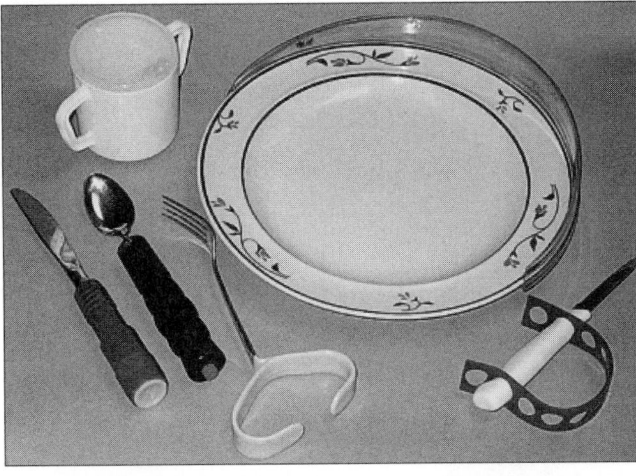

STEP 3g Mealtime equipment. *Clockwise from upper left:* two-handled cup with lid, plate with plate guard, utensils with splints, and utensils with enlarged handles. (From Elkin MK: *Nursing interventions and clinical skills,* ed 2, St. Louis, 1999, Mosby.)

IMPLEMENTATION

STEP	RATIONALE
1. Wash hands before preparing client's tray.	Reduces spread of microorganisms.
2. Assess tray for completeness and correct diet.	Prevents ingestion of incorrect or incomplete meal.
3. Prepare tray to meet client's needs: open cartons, remove lids, cut food, season food after asking client's preferences.	Clients with cognitive or physical impairments may not have the fine motor coordination needed to prepare tray for eating.
4. If client is able to eat independently, stop here. Return after 10 to 20 minutes.	Determines how well client is tolerating diet.
5. For client who cannot eat independently, begin feeding by assisting. ▪ Put yourself in a comfortable position. ▪ Ask client about any religious or cultural preferences before beginning feeding.	Sitting or standing close to client during feeding promotes psychologically comforting and caring environment, which may increase appetite. It is important that the caregiver be comfortable when feeding client, so as not to rush him or her through the meal.
6. Ask in what order client would like to eat, and cut food into bite-size pieces (see illustration). a. It may be helpful for slightly confused, visually impaired, or easily fatigued clients to have food identified by location on plate as if the plate were a clock (see illustration).	Allows client more independence and control. Small pieces are easier to chew and minimize risk of aspiration.
7. Feed client in a manner that facilitates chewing and swallowing.	
a. Older adult: feed small amounts at a time, assessing chewing, swallowing, and fatigue.	Decreased saliva production can impair swallowing in the older adult. Aspiration can result because of a decreased or absent gag reflex and relaxation of the lower esophageal sphincter (Williams, Hooper, 1999). Chewing and sitting up for feeding may accelerate onset of fatigue. Frequent rests may be helpful (White and others, 1991; Whitehouse, 1992).

STEP	RATIONALE

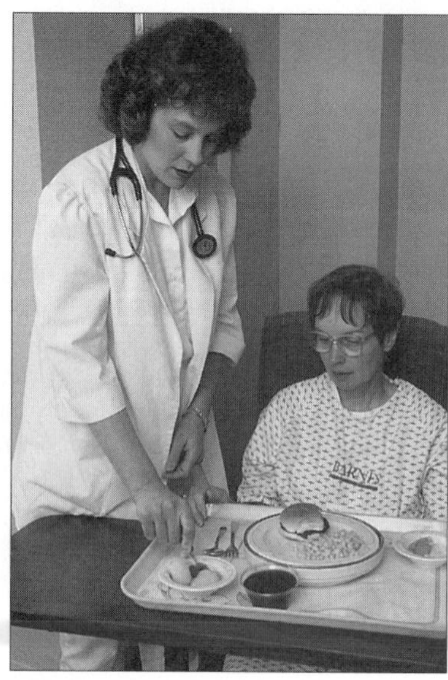
STEP 6 Nurse assisting client at mealtime.

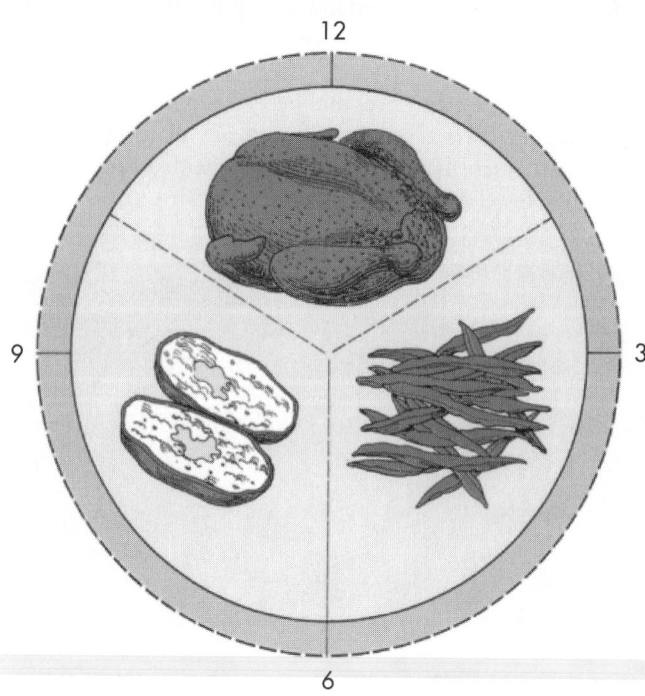

STEP 6a For the visually impaired client: "The potatoes are at 9 o'clock." (From Elkin MK: *Nursing interventions and clinical skills,* ed 2, St. Louis, 1999, Mosby.)

STEP	RATIONALE
b. Neurologically impaired client: feed small amounts at a time and assess for ability to chew, manipulate tongue to form a **bolus,** and swallow. Give small amounts of thin liquids (soup, beverages) and assess for swallowing.	Clients with limited tongue strength and control may be unable to move bolus to back of mouth for swallowing. Checking for "pocketed" food in mouth prevents aspiration.

• ***Critical Decision Point***
Clients with dysphagia who aspirate thin liquids may benefit from liquids thickened with commercial thickening products or from change in consistency of diet.

STEP	RATIONALE
c. Cancer client: check for food aversions before and during the meal.	May have strong, abnormal sense of taste and smell because of medications.
8. Provide fluids as requested. Do not allow client to drink all liquids at beginning of meal.	Assists with swallowing. Prevents client from filling up on liquids.
9. Talk with client during meal.	Meal should be a pleasant event. Conversation promotes socialization. Involve family if possible.
10. Use meal as an opportunity to educate client (e.g., topics related to nutrition, postoperative exercises, discharge plans).	Education can occur whenever nurse and client are together.
11. Assist client with hand washing and performing mouth care.	Mouth care after meals helps prevent dental caries.
12. Help client to resting position.	Client may feel tired after full meal. If client is prone to aspiration, leave head elevated 45 degrees for 30 minutes after meal.
13. Return client's tray to appropriate place and wash hands.	Reduces spread of microorganisms.

EVALUATION

STEP	RATIONALE
1. Observe client's ability to swallow.	Determines if client develops dysphagia and becomes prone to aspiration.
2. Weigh client daily (if nutrition has been inadequate).	Gradual weight gain reflects improved nutritional status.

STEP	RATIONALE
3. Determine client's tolerance to diet.	Overfeeding may cause nausea and vomiting. Underfeeding may leave client feeling hungry.
4. Monitor client's fluid and food intake.	Helps to determine whether client's nutritional and fluid needs are being met.
5. Observe client's ability to feed self.	Determines if client is gaining independence in feeding.

Unexpected Outcomes and Related Interventions

- Client is unable to complete meal.
  - Determine why client is unable to finish meal (e.g., inadequate personnel for feeding assistance, ingestion of large volume of liquids immediately before meal, improper diet).
  - Determine if client's food preferences are met.
  - Determine if client is in pain or uncomfortable.
  - Assess for constipation.
- Client chokes on food.
  - Suction food and secretions from mouth and airway.
  - If choking occurs often, contact physician.
  - Make appropriate referrals (e.g., speech therapy).

Recording and Reporting

- Document in client's chart: client's tolerance of diet, amount eaten, and intake and output.
- If client is on calorie counts, record caloric intake on appropriate form; if intake and output are being evaluated, record fluid intake on appropriate form.
- If clients are receiving oral nutritional supplements (special foods or medical nutritionals such as Ensure, Isocal, and Resource), record the amount taken and communicate client tolerance (likes or dislikes, supplements to fill or replace meals) to the health care team to evaluate supplement effectiveness.
- Report any swallowing difficulties, food dislikes, refusal to eat to nurse in charge.

Teaching Considerations

- Instruct client and family in required diet, including elimination of certain foods. Provide written instructions.
- Instruct client and family to maintain a nutritional balance of foods and to monitor intake of fluids, calories, fats, and salt.
- Teach family members to assist client in feeding self. Help client do as much as possible in feeding self.
- Instruct client and primary caregiver on importance of providing frequent mouth care.

Pediatric Considerations

- Infant feeding includes bottle or breast-feeding and the introduction of semisolid foods such as cereals at around 6 months; strained vegetables, meats, and fruits at around 8 months; and bite-size table foods at around 1 year. Cup feeding and finger foods are introduced as the child's fine motor skills develop (Wong and others, 1999).

Gerontological Considerations

- Older adult clients may have diminished appetite because of loss of taste and smell and decreased number of taste buds.
- Interactions between nutrients and medicines may affect taste of foods or metabolism, absorption, digestion, or excretion of drugs (Lueckenotte, 2000).

Home Care Considerations

- Assess familiarity of client and primary caregiver with proper nutritional standards.
- Assess financial resources of client and family to determine if they are able to purchase proper foods for client.
- Assess priority given by client and family to provision of a balanced nutritional plan.
- Help client, family, and primary caregiver to make eating an enjoyable experience.

Long-Term Care Considerations

- Meals are part of the resident's social interaction with other residents and staff, and, as a result, residents rarely eat meals in their rooms.
- Meals in long-term care settings may be in a social dining program, where residents eat in a dining room and food is served as in a restaurant; family dining, in which residents serve themselves from a common serving bowl; or in an assistive dining program, in which residents can receive assistance with meals (Sorrentino and Gorek, 1999).

Skill 21-3 Aspiration Precautions

Aspiration in the adult client usually occurs as a result of difficulties in swallowing (dysphagia). Dysphagia can result from neurological or neuromuscular diseases (stroke, amyotrophic lateral sclerosis, tremors, myasthenia gravis) and from trauma to or surgical procedures of the oral cavity or throat (cancer therapy, ingestion of caustic substances).

Symptoms (Figure 21-3) that suggest dysphagia include coughing and gagging while eating, multiple swallow attempts, choking, drooling, pockets of food in the mouth, a gargly sounding voice, and a sensation of food "getting stuck" in one's throat (Dangerfield and Sullivan, 1999). Clients who exhibit these symptoms should be evaluated for dysphagia. For clients with altered consciousness who ingest food orally, episodes of pneumonia may indicate aspiration of food or oral secretions.

A speech therapist or radiologist may conduct swallowing assessments. The speech therapist assesses the client's ability to swallow foods of various thicknesses. Thin liquids are typically the most difficult substances for a client with dysphagia. Radiological studies using radiopaque dyes that are swallowed are also used to diagnose dysphagia with aspiration.

Delegation Considerations

The assessment of client's role for aspiration and determination of positioning should not be delegated to assistive personnel. However, assistive personnel may feed clients after receiving instruction on aspiration precautions. Have staff report to the nurse in charge, as soon as possible, any onset of coughing, gagging, or pocketing of food.

Equipment

- Chair or electric bed (to allow client to sit upright)
- Thickening agents as needed (rice, cereal, yogurt, gelatin, commercial thickening agent)
- Tongue blade
- Penlight

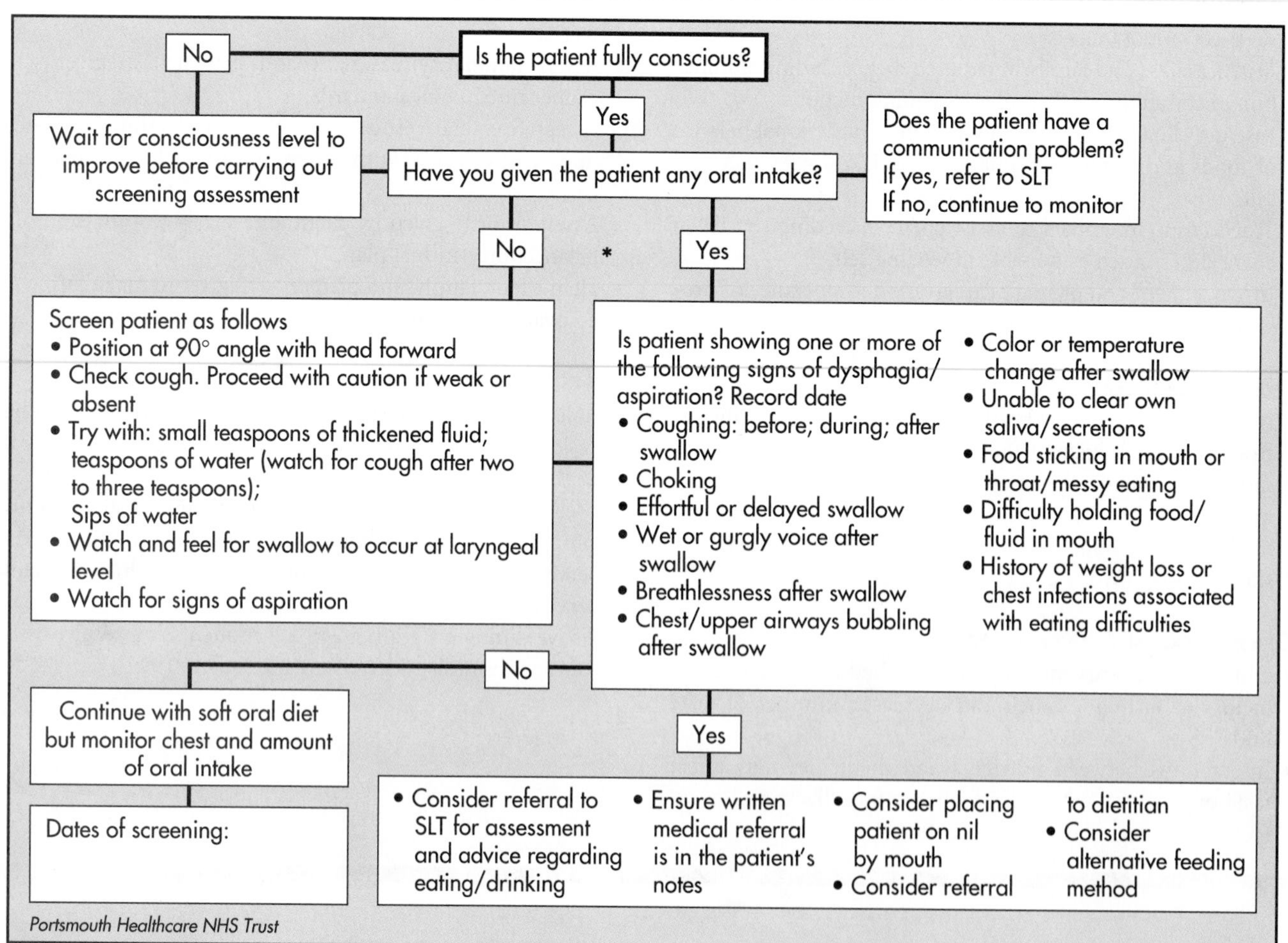

FIGURE **21-3** Screening assessment for dysphagic patients. (From Dangerfield L, Sullivan R: Screening for and managing dysphagia after stroke, *Nurs Times*, 95[19]:44, 1999.)

STEP	RATIONALE

ASSESSMENT

Step	Rationale
1. Perform nutritional assessment (see Skill 21-2).	Clients with aspiration from dysphagia may alter their eating patterns or choose foods that do not provide adequate nutrition.
2. Assess clients who are at increased risk of aspiration for signs and symptoms of dysphagia.	Client may exhibit symptoms or demonstrate poor lip and tongue control. Clients at risk include those who have neurological or neuromuscular diseases and those who have had trauma to or surgical procedures of the oral cavity or throat (Dangerfield and Sullivan, 1999).
3. Report signs and symptoms of dysphagia to the physician.	Client may need to have an evaluation performed by a radiologist or speech therapist.
4. Place an identification on client's chart or Kardex indicating that dysphagia is present.	Identifying client as dysphagic reduces risk of his or her receiving oral nutrients without supervision (Dangerfield and Sullivan, 1999).

NURSING DIAGNOSIS

Defining characteristics from the assessment data may reveal the following nursing diagnoses for clients requiring this skill:

Risk for aspiration
Disturbed sensory perception (gustatory)
Impaired swallowing

Related factors are individualized based on client's condition or needs.

PLANNING

Step	Rationale
1. **Expected outcome** following completion of procedure: ■ Client will not exhibit signs or symptoms that suggest aspiration is occurring.	Signs or symptoms associated with aspiration may indicate the need for further evaluation of swallowing, such as a fluoroscopic swallow study.

IMPLEMENTATION

Step	Rationale
1. Ask client about any difficulties with swallowing or chewing various textures of food.	Be alert for symptoms such as coughing, dyspnea, or drooling that suggest difficulty handling food, especially thin liquids.
2. Using penlight and tongue blade, gently inspect mouth for pockets of food.	Pockets of food in the mouth can indicate difficulty swallowing.
3. Elevate head of client's bed so that hips are flexed at a 90-degree angle and head is flexed slightly forward, or help client to same position in a chair.	Reduces risk of aspiration.
4. Offer client thicker foods, such as those that have been mixed in a blender, yogurt, creamed soups, gelatin, custard, or mashed potatoes, and assess client for signs or symptoms of difficulty swallowing.	Thicker foods are less likely to cause difficulty with swallowing.
5. If client manages thicker foods without difficulty, proceed gradually with foods of thinner consistency. Observe client closely for signs of dysphagia.	Thin liquids, such as coffee, tea, or sodas, are the most difficult foods for client with dysphagia to swallow (Dangerfield and Sullivan, 1999).
6. If no signs or symptoms of dysphagia are evident, assist client in completing the meal or place the meal within reach of client for self-feeding.	Client may not require adaptation of meal consistency but may still require appropriate positioning to reduce the risk of aspiration.
7. Ask client to remain sitting upright for at least 30 minutes after the meal.	Reduces the risk of gastroesophageal reflux, which can cause aspiration.

Step	Rationale
8. Help client to wash hands and perform mouth care.	Mouth care after meals helps prevent dental caries.
9. Return client's tray to appropriate place and wash hands.	Reduces spread of microorganisms.

Evaluation

1. Observe client's ability to ingest foods of various textures and thicknesses.	Indicates whether aspiration risk is increased with thin liquids.
2. Monitor client's food and fluid intake.	Client may avoid certain types and textures of food that are difficult to swallow.
3. Weigh client weekly.	Determines if weight is stable and reflects adequate caloric level.
4. Observe client's oral cavity after meal to detect pockets of food.	Determines presence of pockets of food when meal has included foods of various textures.

Unexpected Outcomes and Related Interventions

- Client coughs, gags, complains of food "stuck in throat," or has pockets of food in mouth.
  - Client may require a swallowing evaluation (Box 21-4).
  - Consider consultation with a speech therapist for swallowing exercises and techniques to improve swallowing and reduce risk of aspiration.
  - Notify physician of any symptoms that occurred during meal and which foods caused the symptoms.
- Client avoids certain textures of food.
  - Change consistency and texture of food.
- Client experiences weight loss.
  - Discuss findings with physician and/or dietitian.

Recording and Reporting

- Document the following in client's chart: client's tolerance of various food textures, amount of assistance required, position during meal, absence or presence of any symptoms of dysphagia, and amount eaten.
- Report any coughing, gagging, choking, or swallowing difficulties to nurse in charge or physician.

Box 21-4 Criteria for Dysphagia Referral

Before referral:

If the answer is yes to either of the following two questions the referral at this time is not appropriate.

- Is the patient unconscious or drowsy?
- Is the patient unable to sit in an upright position for a reasonable length of time?

Please consider the next two questions before making the referral:

- Is the patient dying?
- Does the patient have an esophageal problem which will require surgical intervention?

When observing the patient or giving mouth care look for:

- Open mouth (weak lip closure)
- Drooling
- Poor oral hygiene/thrush
- Weak tongue movements
- Slurred, indistinct speech
- Weak voice
- Weak involuntary cough
- Delayed cough (up to two minutes after swallow)
- General frailty
- Confusion/dementia
- No spontaneous swallowing movements

If any of the above are present the patient may have swallowing problems and may need referral to speech and language therapy.

From Dangerfield L, Sullivan R: Screening for and managing dysphagia after stroke, *Nurs Times,* 95(19):44, 1999.

Teaching Considerations

- Instruct caregivers regarding signs of aspiration and dysphagia.
- Instruct caregivers regarding specifics for foods and client positioning to reduce risk of aspiration.
- Teach family to use oral suction as needed.

Gerontological Considerations

- Older adults who have had a stroke or have Parkinson's disease are at risk for aspiration.
- If dysphagia is severe, an enteral feeding tube may be necessary (Lueckenotte, 2000) (see Chapter 22).

Critical Thinking Exercises

1. A client is 85% of normal body weight for height. What nutritional assessment parameters would help the nurse to determine if the client is malnourished?
2. An older adult client who has many medications complains of a loss of appetite and taste. What assessments are important to make for this client? How does the knowledge of pharmacology affect this client?
3. The nurse has performed a nutritional assessment for a client with a neurological condition that results in intermittent dysphasia. The client has lost 20 pounds over the last 6 months and has a serum albumin of 2.9 mg/dl. What are possible nursing interventions to assist the client in the management of the nutritional effects of dysphasia?

References

American Society for Parenteral and Enteral Nutrition: The 1995 ASPEN standards for nutrition support: hospitalized patients, *Nurs Care Pract* 10(6):208, 1995.

Correia MI: Assessing the nutritional assessment, *Nutr Clin Pract* 14:142, 1999.

Dangerfield L, Sullivan R: Screening for and managing dysphagia after stroke, *Nurs Times,* 95(19):44, 1999.

Elkin MK: *Nursing interventions and clinical skills,* ed 2, St. Louis, 1999, Mosby.

Grodner M, Anderson SL, DeYoung S: *Foundations and clinical applications of nutrition: a nursing approach,* ed 2, St. Louis, 2000, Mosby.

Hall J: Choosing nutrition support: how and when to initiate, *Nurs Case Manage* 4(5):212, 1999.

Joint Commission on Accreditation of Healthcare Organizations, *Comprehensive accreditation manual for hospitals,* Oakbrook, Ill, 2000, The Commission.

Lueckenotte AG: *Gerontologic nursing,* ed 2, St. Louis, 2000, Mosby.

Lyne P, Prowse MA: Methodological issues in the development and use of instruments to assess patient nutritional status or the level of risk of nutritional compromise, *J Adv Nurs* 30(4):835, 1999.

Nutrition Screening Initiative, 1010 Wisconsin Ave., Suite 800, Washington DC, 20007, 1995.

Nutritional assessment of the elderly through anthropometry, Columbus, Ohio, 1988, Ross Laboratories.

Pagana KD, Pagana TJ: *Mosby's diagnostic and laboratory test reference,* ed 4, St. Louis, 1999, Mosby.

Sorrentino SA, Gorek B: *Long-term care assistants,* ed 3, St. Louis, 1999, Mosby.

White JV and others: Consensus of the Nutrition Screening Initiative: risk factors and indications of poor nutritional status in older Americans, *J Am Diet Assoc* 91(7):783, 1991.

Whitehouse MJ: Nursing assessment of the elderly patient, *J Intr Nurs* 15:S14, 1992.

Williams LS, Hooper PD: *Understanding medical-surgical nursing,* Philadelphia, 1999, FA Davis.

Williams SR: *Nutrition and diet therapy,* ed 8, St. Louis, 1998, Mosby.

Wong DL and others: *Whaley & Wong's nursing care of infants and children,* ed 6, St. Louis, 1999, Mosby.

22

ENTERAL NUTRITION

Skills

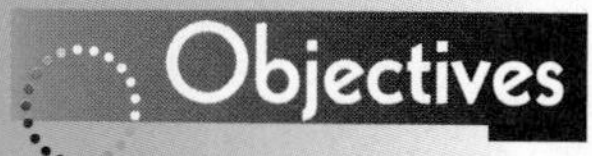

Objectives

Mastery of content in this chapter will enable the nurse to:

- Define the key terms listed.
- Assess the client who is to receive enteral tube feedings.
- Determine the appropriate route of intubation for the client.
- Demonstrate ability to correctly insert a small-bore feeding tube.
- Discuss the rationale for measuring pH to determine feeding tube placement.
- Demonstrate the appropriate technique for irrigating a small-bore feeding tube.
- Demonstrate the appropriate technique for administering syringe tube feedings.
- Demonstrate the appropriate technique for administering continuous tube feedings.
- Discuss the risk of aspiration for a client receiving nasoenteric versus jejunostomy tube feeding.
- Evaluate the client's tolerance of enteral feeding.

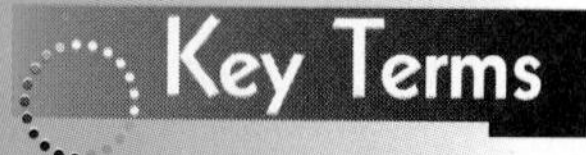

Key Terms

Enteral nutrition
Enteral tube feeding
Gastrostomy feeding tube
Jejunostomy feeding tube
Nasogastric (NG) feeding tube
Nasointestinal (NI) feeding tube

Enteral nutrition is the administration of nutrients directly into the gastrointestinal (GI) tract. The most desirable and appropriate method of providing nutrition is the oral route; unfortunately, this is not always possible. There are clients with a functional GI tract who are unable or unwilling to ingest oral nutrients. In this case **enteral tube feedings** are an alternative. A variety of enteral feeding formulas are available in whole protein or partially digested form. Special enteral formulas for renal disease, hepatic disease, pulmonary disease, or diabetes are also available. Adult and pediatric formulas can be chosen.

The skills presented in this chapter focus on the administration of nutritional feedings directly into the gastrointestinal tract with the goal of restoring the client's nutritional status. The nurse bases care on specific assessment findings in regard to clients' nutritional needs, gastrointestinal function, and the ability to tolerate enteral feedings.

Skill Performance Guidelines

1. Be aware of the purpose for the feeding and which clients are appropriate candidates. A feeding tube may not be appropriate for the client, and harm could occur at the time of insertion (e.g., upper GI bleeding, inadvertent placement of nasoenteral tube in the respiratory tract) or during the feeding (e.g., aspiration, electrolyte imbalance, fluid imbalance).
2. Be aware of the psychological implications associated with the insertion of a feeding tube. The client may become frightened and will need reassurance and encouragement throughout the insertion procedure.
3. Be aware of safety measures to prevent dislodgment of the feeding tube and aspiration of gastric contents by the client. Keep the head of the bed elevated 45 degrees for a client receiving tube feedings. Clients who are disoriented or comatose are at greater risk for aspiration than those who are alert and oriented.
4. Consider the client's medications and their route of delivery. Mixing medications with tube feeding formula should be avoided when possible. Some medications, particularly antibiotics and syrups, may lose their therapeutic effectiveness and disrupt emulsion of the feeding formula, resulting in a formula that resembles undigested milk. Tablets and pills, even when finely crushed, can clog a small-bore feeding tube. Certain medications should not be crushed because of an enteric coating that protects the stomach mucosa from irritation, because they are time-released, or because they should not be delivered directly into the intestine (see Chapter 17).
5. Know the client's activity pattern. Clients requiring physical or occupational therapy should have their tube feedings completed at least 1 hour before activity to decrease the risk of vomiting or abdominal discomfort.

Skill 22-1 Intubating the Client With a Small-Bore Nasogastric or Nasointestinal Feeding Tube

Large-bore nasogastric tubes are contraindicated when used primarily for enteral feedings, because they carry an increased risk of aspiration and are more irritating to the nasopharyngeal and esophageal mucosa (Lehmann, 1992). Occasionally, large-bore gastrointestinal tubes that were inserted for gastric decompression will be used to initiate enteral feeding because they are already in place. If the feeding continues for more than a few days, the nurse should consult with the physician about placement of a small-bore enteral feeding tube (Figure 22-1). Small-bore feeding tubes are available in weighted (tungsten) or unweighted designs. Weighted tubes were thought to pass more easily into the duodenum or jejunum via peristalsis; however, research has not demonstrated an advantage of the weight in promoting intestinal passage (Lord and others, 1993). Nonetheless, weighted tubes are used more frequently than nonweighted tubes for nasoduodenal and nasojejunal feedings because they are believed to remain in correct position longer than nonweighted tubes; however, research data regarding this belief are conflicting. Because the tubes are flexible, a guide wire or stylet is used to provide rigidity and to facilitate positioning and then removed once correct placement is verified. Small-bore tubes can be left in place for an extended period with less irritation to the nasopharyngeal, esophageal, and gastric mucosa.

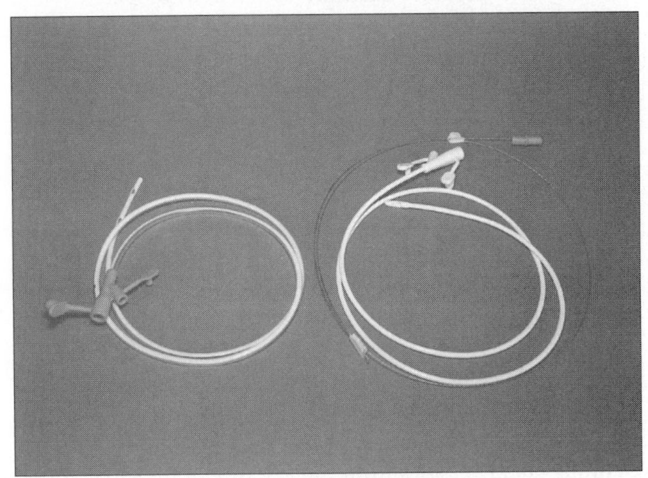

FIGURE **22-1** Small-bore feeding tube.

Placing a **nasogastric (NG)** or **nasointestinal (NI) feeding tube** requires a physician's order. Placement of a small-bore feeding tube needs to be verified by radiograph to determine that the tube is in the stomach or intestine rather than in the airways (Levy, 1998; Metheny and others, 1990a; Metheny and others, 1990b). Complications of prolonged intubation may include nasal erosion, sinusitis, esophagitis, gastric ulceration, and pulmonary aspiration.

Delegation Considerations

This skill should not be delegated to assistive personnel.

Equipment

- Nasogastric or nasointestinal tube (8 to 12 Fr) with guide wire or stylet
- 60-ml or larger Luer-lok or catheter-tip syringe
- Stethoscope
- Hypoallergenic tape and tincture of benzoin or tube fixation device
- pH indicator strip (scale 0.0 to 14.0)
- Glass of water and straw
- Emesis basin
- Safety pin
- Rubber band
- Towel
- Facial tissues
- Clean gloves
- Suction equipment in case of aspiration
- Penlight to check placement in nasopharynx
- Tongue blade

Step	Rationale
Assessment	
1. Assess client's need for enteral tube feedings and intubation: impaired swallowing, head or neck surgery, decreased level of consciousness, surgeries involving upper alimentary tract, or facial trauma; also assess weight for client's height, hydration status, electrolyte balance, and organ function.	Identifying clients who need tube feedings before they become nutritionally depleted facilitates preparation of nursing care plan and promotes client education. Enteral feeding preserves the function and mass of the gut, promotes wound healing, diminishes hypermetabolism in burn injuries, and may decrease the incidence of infection in critically ill clients (Zaloga, 1994).

STEP	RATIONALE
2. Assess patency of nares. Have client close each nostril alternately and breathe. Examine each naris for patency and skin breakdown.	Nares may be obstructed or irritated, or septal defect or facial fractures may be present. Assessment determines most patent naris.
3. Assess client's medical history: nosebleeds; nasal surgery; deviated septum; anticoagulant therapy, coagulopathy.	History of these problems may require nurse to seek physician's order to change route of nutritional support.
4. Assess client for gag reflex. Place tongue blade in client's mouth, touching uvula.	Assists nurse in identifying client's ability to swallow and determines if risk of aspiration exists.
5. Assess client's mental status.	Alert client is better able to cooperate with procedure. If vomiting should occur, an alert client can usually expectorate vomitus, which can help to reduce the risk of aspiration.
6. Assess for bowel sounds. Consult physician if bowel sounds are absent.	Absence of bowel sounds may indicate decreased or absent peristalsis and increased risk of aspiration or abdominal distention.

NURSING DIAGNOSIS

Defining characteristics from the assessment data may reveal the following nursing diagnoses for clients requiring this skill:

Imbalanced nutrition: less than body requirements
Impaired swallowing
Risk for aspiration

Related factors are individualized based on client's condition or needs.

PLANNING

STEP	RATIONALE
1. **Expected outcomes** following completion of procedure:	
▪ Tube is in stomach or intestine.	Correct placement.
▪ Feeding tube will remain patent.	Feeding tubes can become occluded with formula or medications; occlusion of feeding tube can result in need to insert new feeding tube.
▪ Client has no complaints or signs of discomfort or nasal trauma.	Tube correctly secured minimizes irritation to nares.
2. Explain procedure to client.	Increases client's cooperation with intubation procedure.
3. Explain to client how to communicate during intubation by raising index finger to indicate gagging or discomfort.	It is important for client to have a way of communicating to alleviate stress.

- ***Critical Decision Point***
  NG or NI feeding tubes may be inserted in clients with decreased level of consciousness, but risk of inadvertent respiratory placement is increased if there is an impaired gag reflex.

STEP	RATIONALE
4. Position client in sitting or high-Fowler's position. If client is comatose, place in semi-Fowler's position.	Reduces risk of pulmonary aspiration in event client should vomit.
5. Examine feeding tube for flaws: rough or sharp edges on distal end and closed or clogged outlet holes.	Flaws in feeding tube hamper tube intubation and can injure client.
6. Determine length of tube to be inserted and mark with tape or indelible ink (see illustration).	Being aware of proper length to intubate determines approximate depth of insertion.

- ***Critical Decision Point***
  Tip of tube must reach stomach. Measure distance from tip of nose to earlobe to xyphoid process of sternum (see illustration). Add additional 20 to 30 cm (8 to 12 inches) for nasointestinal tube (Welch, 1996; Lord and others, 1993; Hanson, 1979).

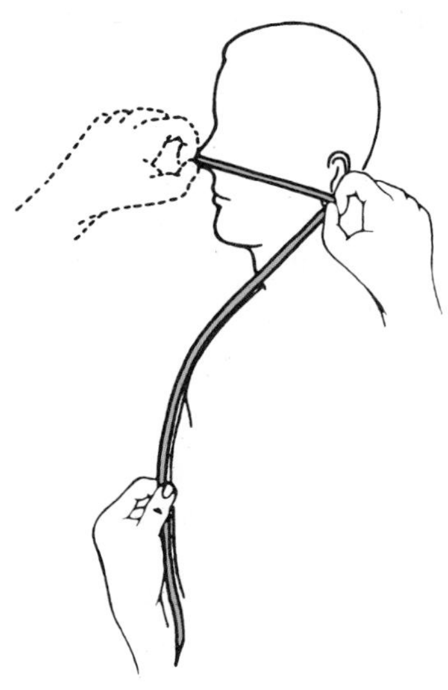

STEP 6 Determine length of tube to be inserted.

STEP	RATIONALE
7. Prepare NG or NI tube for intubation:	
a. Plastic tubes should *not* be iced.	Tubes will become stiff and inflexible, causing trauma to mucous membranes.
b. Wash hands.	Reduces spread of microorganisms.
c. Inject 10 ml of water from 30-ml or larger Luer-Lok or catheter-tip syringe into the tube.	Aids in guide wire or stylet insertion.
d. Make certain that guide wire is securely positioned against weighted tip and that both Luer-Lok connections are snugly fitted together.	Promotes smooth passage of tube into gastrointestinal (GI) tract. Improperly positioned stylet can induce serious trauma.
8. Cut adhesive tape 10 cm (4 inches) long, or prepare tube fixation device.	

IMPLEMENTATION

STEP	RATIONALE
1. Put on clean gloves.	Reduces transmission of microorganisms.
2. Inspect nares for any irritation or obstruction.	Avoid placement of tube in naris that is irritated.
3. Dip tube with surface lubricant into glass of water.	Activates lubricant to facilitate passage of tube into naris to GI tract.
4. Hand client a glass of water with straw or glass with crushed ice (if able to swallow).	Client will be asked to swallow water to facilitate tube passage.
5. Gently insert tube through nostril to back of throat (posterior nasopharynx). May cause client to gag. Aim back and down toward ear (see illustration).	Natural contours facilitate passage of tube into GI tract.
6. Have client flex head toward chest after tube has passed through nasopharynx.	Closes off glottis and reduces risk of tube entering trachea.

• ***Critical Decision Point***

Encourage client to swallow by giving small sips of water or ice chips when possible. Advance tube as client swallows. Rotate tube 180 degrees while inserting. Swallowing facilitates passage of tube past oropharynx. Rotating tube decreases friction.

STEP	RATIONALE
7. Emphasize need to mouth breathe and swallow during the procedure.	Helps facilitate passage of tube and alleviates client's fears during the procedure.

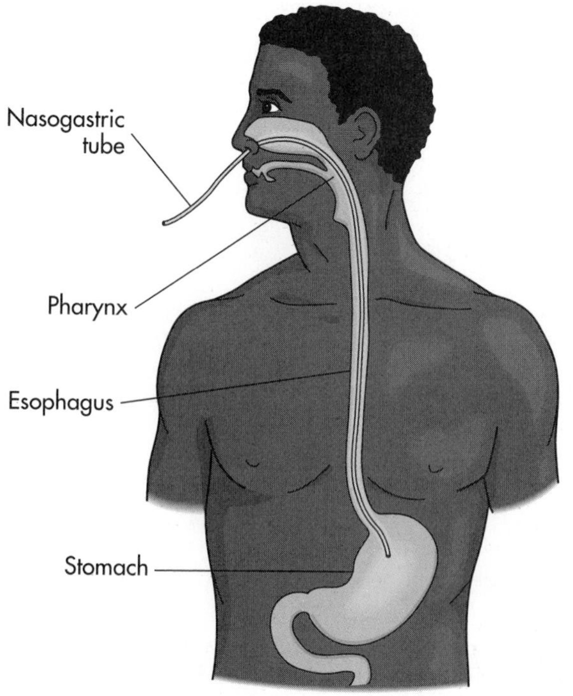

STEP **5** Nasogastric tube inserted through nose and esophagus into stomach.

STEP	RATIONALE
8. When tip of tube reaches the carina (about 25 cm [10 inches] in an adult), stop and listen for air exchange from the distal portion of the tube.	If air can be heard, tube could be in respiratory tract; remove tube and start over (Metheny, 2000).
9. Advance tube each time client swallows until desired length has been passed.	Reduces discomfort and trauma to client.

• ***Critical Decision Point***
Do not force tube. If resistance is met or client starts to cough, choke, or become cyanotic, stop advancing the tube and pull tube back.

STEP	RATIONALE
10. Check for position of tube in back of throat with penlight and tongue blade.	Tube may be coiled, kinked, or entering trachea.
11. Check placement of tube (see Skill 22-2).	Proper position is essential before initiating feedings.
12. After gastric aspirates are obtained, anchor tube to nose and avoid pressure on nares. Mark exit site with indelible ink. Use one of following options for anchoring:	A properly secured tube allows the client more mobility and prevents trauma to nasal mucosa.
a. **Apply tape:**	
(1) Apply tincture of benzoin or other skin adhesive on tip of client's nose and allow it to become "tacky."	Helps tape adhere better. Protects skin.
(2) Remove gloves and split one end of the adhesive tape strip lengthwise 5 cm (2 inches).	
(3) Wrap each of the 5-cm strips around tube as it exits nose (see illustration).	
b. **Apply tube fixation device** using shaped adhesive patch:	
(1) Apply wide end of patch to bridge of nose (see illustration).	
(2) Slip connector around feeding tube as it exits nose (see illustration).	

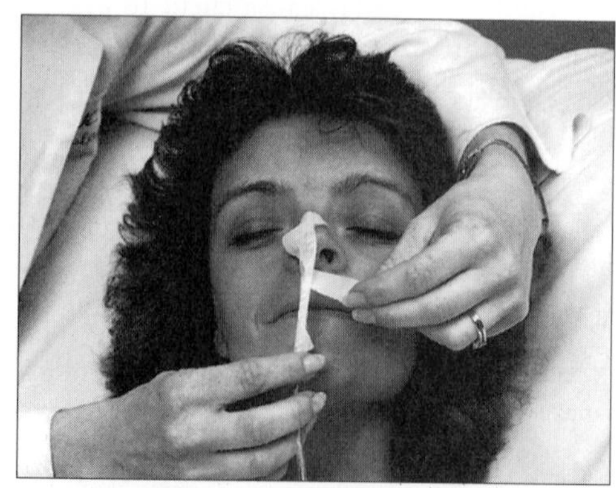

STEP **12a(3)** Wrapping tape to anchor nasoenteral tube.

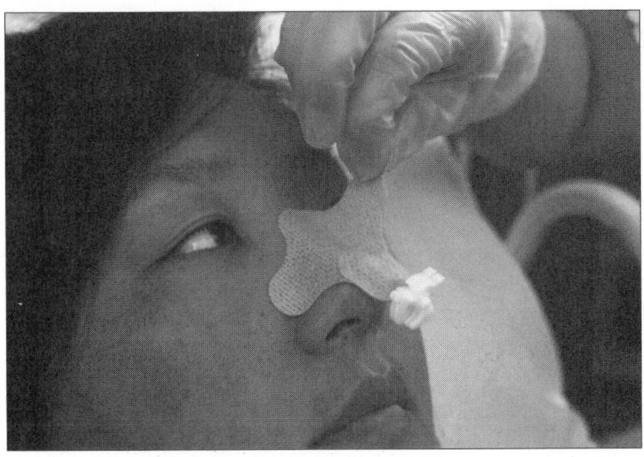

STEP **12b(1)** Applying patch to bridge of nose.

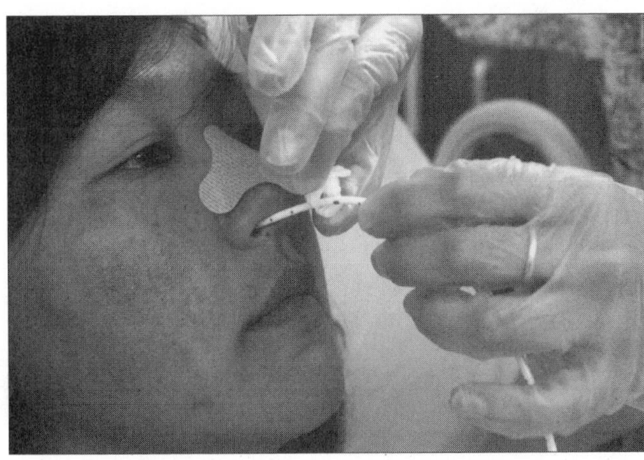

STEP **12b(2)** Slip connector around feeding tube.

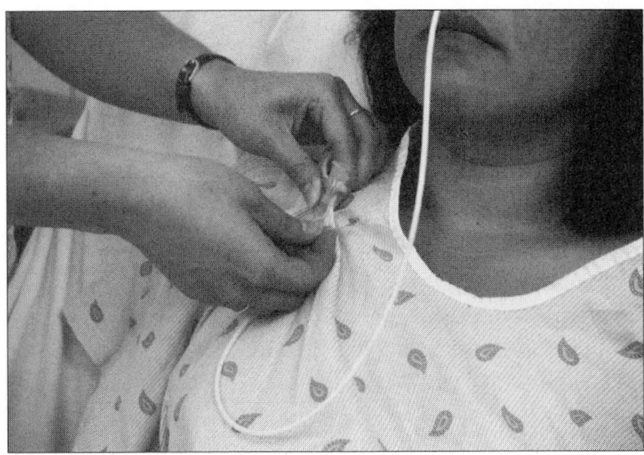

STEP **13** Fastening feeding tube to client's gown.

STEP	RATIONALE
13. Fasten end of nasogastric tube to client's gown by looping rubber band around tube in slip knot. Pin rubber band to gown (see illustration).	Reduces traction on the naris if tube moves.
14. For intestinal placement, position client on right side when possible until radiological confirmation of correct placement has been verified. Otherwise, assist client to a comfortable position.	Promotes passage of the tube into the small intestine (duodenum or jejunum).

- ***Critical Decision Point***

  Leave guide wire or stylet in place until correct position is ensured by x-ray film. Never attempt to reinsert partially or fully removed guide wire or stylet while feeding tube is in place.

STEP	RATIONALE
15. Obtain x-ray film of chest/abdomen.	Placement of tube is verified by x-ray examination (Metheny, 1988).
16. Apply gloves and administer oral hygiene (see Chapter 6). Cleanse tubing at nostril with washcloth dampened in soap and water.	Promotes client comfort and integrity of oral mucous membranes.
17. Remove gloves, dispose of equipment, and wash hands.	Reduces transmission of microorganisms.

STEP	RATIONALE

EVALUATION

1. Observe client to determine response to NG or NI tube intubation:
   a. Persistent gagging — Indicates prolonged irritation and stimulation of client's gag reflex. Can result in vomiting and increased risk of aspiration.
   b. Paroxysms of coughing — May indicate presence of NG or NI tube in client's airway.
2. Confirm x-ray results. — Verifies tube position.
3. Routinely note location of external exit site marking on the tube. — Can reveal if end of tube has migrated position.

UNEXPECTED OUTCOMES AND RELATED INTERVENTIONS

- Aspiration of stomach contents into respiratory tract (immediate response), evidenced by coughing, dyspnea, cyanosis, auscultation of crackles or wheezes.
  - Position client on side.
  - Suction nasotracheally or orotracheally.
  - Consult physician immediately to order a chest x-ray examination for confirming aspiration.
- Aspiration of stomach contents into respiratory tract (delayed response), evidenced by auscultation of crackles or wheezes, dyspnea, fever.
  - Consult physician to obtain order for chest x-ray examination.
  - Prepare for possible initiation of antibiotics.
- Displacement of feeding tube to another site (i.e., from duodenum to stomach), may occur when client coughs or vomits.
  - Aspirate GI contents and measure pH (Metheny and others, 1993a).
  - Remove displaced tube, and insert new tube.
- Clogging of feeding tube.
  - Assess patency of tube by aspirating.
  - Irrigate as needed.
- Nasal mucosa becomes inflamed, tender, and/or eroded.
  - Retape tube to relieve pressure on mucosa.
  - Consider removal of tube and reinsertion in opposite naris (physician's order required).

RECORDING AND REPORTING

- Record and report type and size of tube placed, location of distal tip of tube, client's tolerance of procedure, and confirmation of tube position by x-ray examination.

TEACHING CONSIDERATIONS

- Instruct family caregiver to offer oral hygiene frequently and to keep client's lips moistened.
- Teach family caregiver to report tension on feeding tube or displacement of tape, fixation device. Instruct caregiver to hold tube in place at nose while help is called.

PEDIATRIC CONSIDERATIONS

- Premature infant and neonate: Measure from bridge of nose to just beyond tip of sternum. Older child: Measure from tip of nose to earlobe to tip of sternum.
- In infant, observe for vagal stimulation during insertion of feeding tube, resulting in decreased heart rate.

GERONTOLOGICAL CONSIDERATIONS

- Ensure adequate lubrication of tube to decrease discomfort for the older adult, who may have decreased oral or nasopharyngeal secretions.

HOME CARE CONSIDERATIONS

- Assess client or primary caregiver's ability to maintain tube and feeding program.
- Assess environmental safety and sanitation of client's home to determine potential for infection or injury.
- Teach client or primary caregiver method of GI fluid pH measurement and expected range (see Skill 22-2).
- Teach family caregiver correct method for securing feeding tube to nares to eliminate pressure on nares and face and to allow enough tubing for movement.

Skill 22-2 Verifying Tube Placement for a Large-Bore or Small-Bore Feeding Tube

Small-bore feeding tubes can be inserted into the stomach for either intermittent or continuous feedings; they can also be inserted into the small intestine (duodenum or proximal jejunum) for continuous feedings. However, large-bore tubes are not suitable for small bowel feedings; further intermittent feedings are not administered into the small bowel. Testing placement of a small-bore or a large-bore feeding tube is a responsibility of the nurse. First, nurses must assess for gastrointestinal (GI) versus respiratory placement when tubes are initially blindly inserted. Failure to detect pulmonary placement of a feeding tube can lead to serious complications, especially if formula or medications are instilled through the tube. Documentation of nonrespiratory placement by x-ray examination is standard practice when a small-bore tube is initially inserted because such a tube can enter the airway without causing obvious respiratory symptoms. Even a large-bore tube may not produce obvious respiratory symptoms when accidentally inserted into the airway of a semiconscious or unconscious client.

Following verification that a tube is positioned in the desired site (either the stomach or small intestine), the nurse is responsible for ensuring that the tube has remained in the intended position before administering formula or medications through the tube. Therefore verification of correct tube placement is performed before each intermittent feeding, at least once every 12 hours when continuous feedings are given, and before medications are administered through the tube.

The risk for aspiration of regurgitated gastric contents into the respiratory tract is increased when the tip of a nasointestinal tube accidentally dislocates upward into the stomach or when the tip of either a nasogastric or nasointestinal tube dislocates upward into the esophagus.

Delegation Considerations

The verification of tube placement should not be delegated to assistive personnel.

Equipment

- 30-ml or larger Luer-lok or catheter-tip syringe
- Stethoscope
- Clean gloves
- pH indicator strip (scale 0.0 to 14.0)

Step	Rationale
Assessment	
1. Identify signs and symptoms of inadvertent respiratory migration of feeding tube: coughing, choking, or cyanosis.	Signs and symptoms indicate accidental insertion into airway. However, their absence does not ensure nonrespiratory placement, especially in a client with a decreased level of consciousness and/or altered cough and gag reflexes.
2. Identify conditions that increase the risk for spontaneous tube dislocation from the intended position: a. Retching/vomiting b. Nasotracheal suctioning c. Severe bouts of coughing.	Feeding tubes may become dislocated (e.g., stomach to esophagus, intestine to stomach).
3. Following a previous verification of correct position, make a mark on the tube where it extends from the naris with an indelible pen. Observe the external portion of the tube for movement of this mark away from the naris.	Increased external length of a tube may indicate that the distal tip is no longer in the correct position.
4. Review client's medication record—is client receiving a gastric acid inhibitor (e.g., cimetidine, ranitidine, famotidine, nizatidine) or a proton pump inhibitor (e.g., omeprazole)?	H_2 receptor antagonists reduce volume of gastric acid secretion and the concentration (acid content) of secretions (McKenry and Salerno, 1998).
5. Review client's record for history of prior tube displacement.	Clients who have a history of tube displacement are at increased risk.

STEP	RATIONALE

NURSING DIAGNOSIS

Defining characteristics from the assessment data may reveal the following nursing diagnoses for clients requiring this skill:

Risk for aspiration
Impaired gas exchange

Related factors are individualized based on client's condition or needs.

PLANNING

1. **Expected outcomes** following completion of procedure:
   - Tube feeding formula infuses smoothly into client's GI tract. — Feeding tube is patent and properly positioned.
   - Client does not experience respiratory distress (e.g., increased respiratory rate, coughing, poor color). — Client will develop respiratory distress if tube feedings or medications are administered through a tube inadvertently positioned in respiratory tract. Serious or even fatal results may follow such an event.
2. Explain procedure to client. — Increases client's cooperation. Well-informed client is more cooperative and relaxed.

IMPLEMENTATION

1. Wash hands and apply gloves. — Reduces transmission of microorganisms.
2. Perform measures to verify placement of tube:
   a. For intermittently fed clients, test placement immediately before feeding (usually a period of at least 4 hours will have elapsed since previous feeding).
   b. For continuously tube-fed clients, test placement at least once every 12 hours. — More frequent checking has been associated with increased clogging of small-bore tubes (Powell and others, 1993). To avoid this problem flush tube with water after checking the residual volume (Edwards and Metheny, 2000).
   c. Wait at least 1 hour after medication administration by tube or mouth. — Premature aspiration of contents will remove medication, reducing dose delivered to client. Approximately 1 hour is needed for medication to be absorbed or passed through stomach. Medication can also interfere with pH testing.
3. Draw up 30 ml of air into syringe, then attach to end of feeding tube. Flush tube with 30 ml of air prior to attempting to aspirate fluid. It will likely be more difficult to aspirate fluid from the small intestine than from the stomach. Repositioning the client from side to side may be helpful. More than one bolus of air through the tube may be needed in some cases. — Burst of air aids in aspirating fluid more easily (Metheny and others, 1993b).
4. Draw back on syringe and obtain 5 to 10 ml of gastric aspirate (see illustration). Observe appearance of aspirate. — Aspirates from nasogastric tubes of continuously tube-fed clients often have appearance of curdled enteral formula. In contrast, aspirates from nasointestinal tubes are often bile stained.
5. Gently mix aspirate in syringe. Measure pH of aspirated GI contents by dipping the pH strip into the fluid or by applying a few drops of the fluid to the strip (see illustration). Compare the color of the strip with the color on the chart provided by the manufacturer (see illustration) (Metheny and others, 1998b). — Quantity is sufficient for pH testing. Mixing ensures equal distribution of contents for testing. pH paper covering a range from 0 to 14 provides most accurate readings of gastric pH levels (Metheny and others, 1994).
   a. Gastric fluid from client who has fasted for at least 4 hours usually has pH range of 1 to 4. — Range of 1 to 4 is reliable indicator of stomach placement, especially when a gastric acid inhibitor is *not* being used.
   b. Fluid from nasointestinal tube of fasting client usually has pH greater than 6 (Metheny and others, 1989). — Intestinal contents are less acidic than stomach.

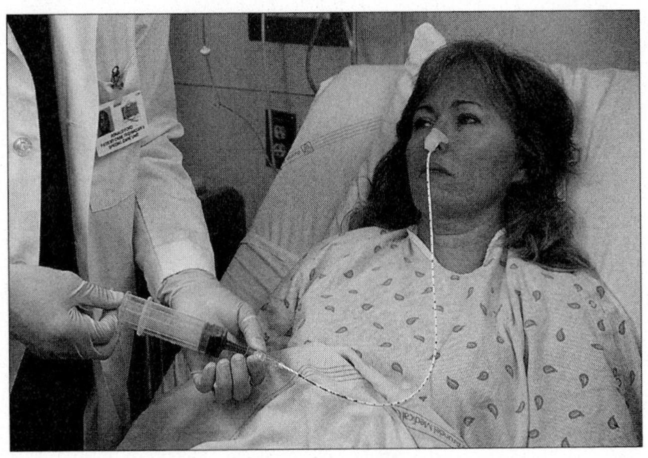

STEP 4 Obtaining gastric aspirate.

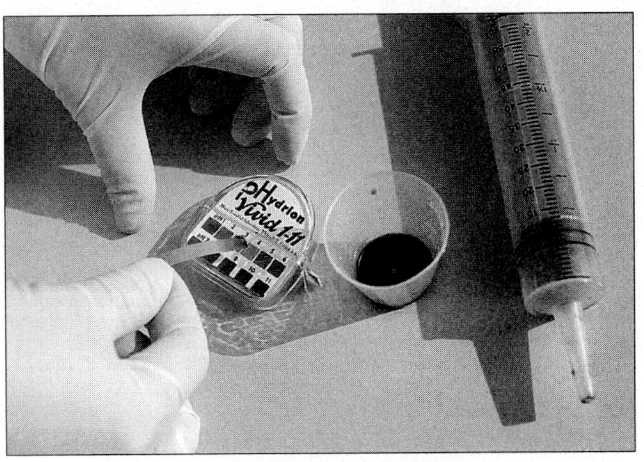

STEP 5 Compare color on test strip with color on pH chart.

STEP	RATIONALE
c. Client with continuous tube feeding may have pH of 5 or higher.	Formulas contain solutions that are basic.
d. pH of pleural fluid from the tracheobronchial tree is generally greater than 6.	The pH of pleural fluid makes it difficult to differentiate between respiratory and intestinal placement (Metheny and others, 1999a).

- ***Critical Decision Point***
  Auscultation is no longer considered a reliable method for verification of tube placement because a tube inadvertently placed in the lungs, pharynx, or esophagus can transmit a sound similar to that of air entering the stomach (El-Gamel and Watson, 1993; Ghahremani and Gould, 1986; Metheny and others, 1998a; Metheny and others 1998c).

STEP	RATIONALE
6. If after repeated attempts, it is not possible to aspirate fluid from a tube that was originally established by x-ray examination to be in desired position, and (a) there are no risk factors for tube dislocation, (b) tube has remained in original taped position, and (c) client is not experiencing difficulty, assume tube is correctly placed (Metheny and others, 1993a).	It is reasonable to assume tube is correctly placed. When abdominal x-ray films are obtained for clinical reasons, the nurse can take advantage of reports to monitor tube location.
7. Remove and dispose of gloves. Wash hands.	Reduces transmission of microorganisms.

EVALUATION

1. Observe client for respiratory distress:	
a. Persistent gagging	May indicate prolonged irritation; stimulation of client's gag reflex can result in vomiting and increased risk of aspiration.
b. Paroxysms of coughing	May indicate presence of nasogastric tube in client's airway.
c. Respiratory patterns (e.g., rate) that are inconsistent with baseline parameters	May indicate aspiration of contents, leading to aspiration pneumonia.
2. Observe flow rate of enteral formula:	
a. Slower rate than what is ordered	May indicate kink or clog within feeding tube, inaccurate setting on feeding pump, or malfunction of pump itself.
b. Excessive flow	May indicate inaccurate setting on feeding pump or malfunction of pump itself.

Unexpected Outcomes and Related Interventions

- Client develops severe respiratory distress evidenced by dyspnea and changes in arterial blood gas or oxygen saturation values, resulting from aspiration of large volume of fluid from distended stomach or from a tube accidentally displaced into esophagus.
  - Contact physician immediately.
  - Be prepared to obtain chest x-ray examination, initiate oxygen therapy.
  - Turn off feeding pump.

Recording and Reporting

- Record and report type of tube, length of tube inserted, pH, appearance of aspirate, and client's tolerance to tube feeding.

Teaching Considerations

- Instruct client to not pull or alter position of nasoenteral tube.

Pediatric Considerations

- In infant only, inject 0.5 to 1.0 ml of air during auscultation and before aspiration of gastric secretions for pH measurement.

Gerontological Considerations

- Assess client for use of medications that may affect the pH of gastric secretions, such as histamine-receptor antagonists, proton pump inhibitors or antacids.

Home Care Considerations

- Instruct client or family caregiver to check that tube is in correct position before administering formula or medications.
- Instruct client or primary caregiver not to proceed with feedings if there is any doubt as to proper placement of tube.
- For client who will require tube feedings at home, instruct client or family caregiver in method of gastric fluid pH measurement, expected range, and expected appearance of aspirate.

Skill 22-3 Irrigating a Small-Bore Feeding Tube

The skill of irrigating a small-bore feeding tube maintains patency of the tube. Patency of a tube may be questioned when air or fluid cannot be instilled through the tube. There are various factors that can cause tube occlusion. Certain tube-feeding formulas have properties that predispose to tube clogging (Simon and Fink, 1999). The frequency of tube obstruction increases when residuals are checked more often (Powell and others, 1993). There is a lower incidence of feeding-tube obstruction with intermittent than with continuous tube feeding, which is likely due to the delivery of a greater formula volume at a higher pressure with intermittent feedings (Ciocon, 1992). In addition, the administration of incompletely crushed tablets can easily occlude a tube.

Adequacy of nutritional support is essential in client care, and for this reason tubes must remain patent. Research suggests that unless effort is made to monitor and irrigate feeding tubes routinely, the amount of feeding a client receives is likely 15% to 20% below the amount ordered and 25% to 30% less than the goal (McClave and others, 1999).

There are variations in practice in regard to solutions used to irrigate feeding tubes. Research has shown that cranberry juice is far less effective than water in preventing tubes from clogging (Metheny 1988; Wilson, Haynes-Johnson, 1987). This skill discusses use of normal saline and tap water for irrigation.

Delegation Considerations

The skill of irrigating a small-bore feeding tube should not be delegated to assistive personnel. Assistive personnel should be instructed to report whenever a continuous tube feeding stops infusing.

Equipment

- 60-ml catheter-tip syringe
- Normal saline or tap water
- Towel
- Disposable gloves

STEP	RATIONALE

ASSESSMENT

Step	Rationale
1. Inspect the volume, color, and character of gastric aspirates (if obtainable).	Thick secretions and a reduced volume of secretions may indicate need to irrigate tube. Excess volume of secretions may indicate delayed gastric emptying.
2. Note ease with which tube feeding infuses through tubing.	Failure of formula to infuse as desired may indicate developing obstruction.
3. Monitor volume of tube-feeding formula administered during a shift and compare with ordered amount.	Indicates whether sufficient volume of feeding is infusing.
4. Refer to agency policies regarding routine irrigations (e.g., before medication administration).	Determines frequency of irrigations.

NURSING DIAGNOSIS

Defining characteristics from the assessment data may reveal the following nursing diagnosis for clients requiring this skill:

Risk for imbalanced nutrition: less than body requirements.

Related factors are individualized based on client's condition or needs.

PLANNING

Step	Rationale
1. **Expected outcomes** following completion of procedure:	
▪ Feeding tube remains patent.	Irrigation fluid clears inner lumen of feeding tube of accumulated solids and secretions.
▪ Client receives prescribed caloric intake.	Feeding infuses without interruption.
2. Explain procedure to client.	Minimizes anxiety during manipulation of tube.
3. Position client in high-Fowler's (if tolerated) or semi-Fowler's position.	Reduces risk of aspiration during irrigation.

IMPLEMENTATION

Step	Rationale
1. Wash hands.	Reduces transmission of microorganisms.
2. Prepare equipment at client's bedside and apply gloves.	
3. Determine that feeding tube is properly placed by checking pH (Skill 22-2), if fluid can be aspirated.	With tip of tube correctly placed in stomach, irrigation will not create risk of aspiration.
4. Draw up 30 ml of normal saline or tap water in syringe (see illustration).	This amount of solution will flush length of tube.
5. Kink feeding tube while disconnecting it from feeding-bag tubing or while removing plug at end of tube (see illustration). Place end of feeding bag tubing on towel.	Prevents leakage of gastric secretions.
6. Insert tip of catheter into end of feeding tube. Release kink and slowly instill irrigating solution (see illustration).	Infusion of fluid clears tubing.
7. If unable to instill fluid, reposition client on left side and try again.	Tip of tube may be against stomach wall. Changing clients' position may move tip away from stomach wall. Notify physician if unable to instill fluid.
8. When saline or tap water has been instilled, remove syringe. Reinstitute tube feeding, or administer medication as ordered.	Tubing is clear and patent.
9. Remove and discard gloves, dispose of supplies. Wash hands.	Reduces transmission of microorganisms.

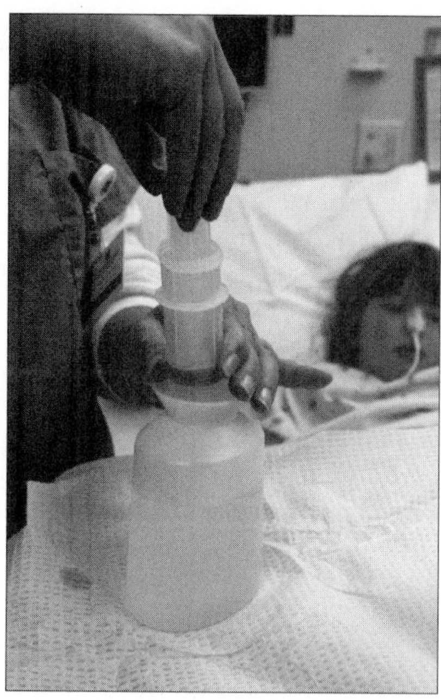

STEP 4 Draw up 30 ml normal saline into syringe.

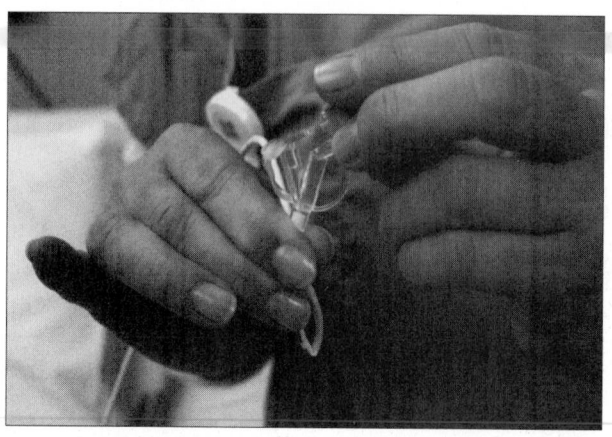

STEP 5 Kink tubing while unplugging feeding tube.

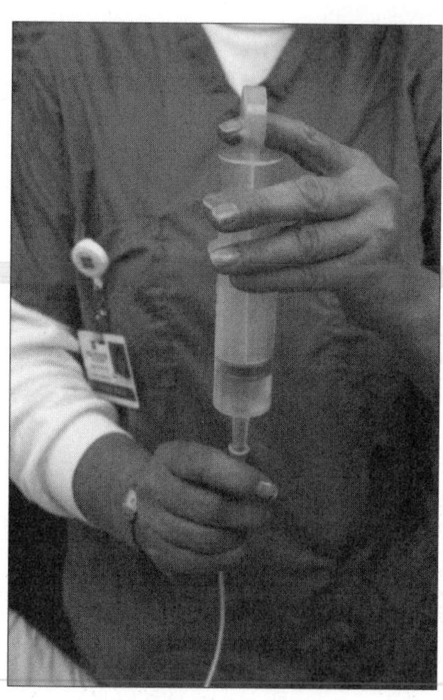

STEP 6 Irrigate feeding tube.

STEP	RATIONALE
EVALUATION	
1. Observe ease with which tube feeding instills through tubing.	A successfully irrigated tube is patent, allowing for free flow of tube-feeding solution.

Unexpected Outcomes and Related Interventions

- Tube remains obstructed.
  - Retry irrigation. If unsuccessful, notify physician. Tube may need to be removed and then reinserted.

Recording and Reporting

- Record time of irrigation, amount and type of fluid instilled, and results in progress notes or appropriate flow sheet.
- If client's intake and output are being monitored, record amount and type of fluid instilled.

Pediatric Considerations

- Irrigation of a tube requires a smaller volume of solution in children: 1 or 2 ml for small tubes to 5 to 15 ml or more for large ones (Wong and others, 1999).

Skill 22-4 Administering Enteral Feedings via Nasoenteric Tubes

Enteral nutrition refers to nutrients given via the gastrointestinal (GI) tract. Enteral feeding is preferred over parenteral nutrition (Chapter 23) because it improves utilization of nutrients, is generally safer for clients, maintains structure and function of the gut, and is less expensive. Not all clients are able to be fed enterally, but if the bowel can handle nutrients, this method should be used. The indications for enteral feeding include the following:

1. Clients who cannot eat (comatose clients with a functional gastrointestinal system; clients receiving mechanical ventilation; clients recovering from oral, head, and neck surgeries; clients with difficulty chewing or swallowing)
2. Clients who will not eat (older adults, confused clients, clients with eating disorders)
3. Clients who have increased energy requirements (clients with cancer, sepsis, infection, burns, trauma, or head injury)
4. Clients requiring bowel rest (mild inflammatory bowel disease, pancreatitis)

Enteral feedings are most commonly given via small-bore tubes, inserted through the nose and advanced to either the stomach or small intestine. Nasogastric feedings are the most common, allowing tube-feeding formulas to enter the stomach and then pass more gradually through the intestinal tract to ensure absorption. However, gastric ileus (decreased or absent peristalsis affecting the stomach but not the intestines), delayed gastric emptying, or gastric resections, contraindicate nasogastric feedings. Nasointestinal tubes allow for successful postpyloric feeding, in which formula is placed directly into the small intestine beyond the pyloric sphincter of the stomach (Kudsk, 1994). The advantage of nasointestinal feedings is decreased gastric reflux, which reduces the risk of aspiration.

Delegation Considerations

Administration of enteral tube feeding is a procedure that can be delegated to assistive personnel. The presence of peristalsis and tube placement should be verified before the feeding, and patency of the tube should be established by flushing it with water.

Also, the client should be sitting upright in a chair or in bed, and assistive personnel should be instructed to infuse the feeding slowly. In addition, assistive personnel should be instructed to report any difficulty infusing the feeding or any discomfort voiced by the client.

Equipment

- Disposable feeding bag and tubing or ready-to-hang system
- 30-ml or larger Luer-lok or catheter-tip syringe
- Stethoscope
- pH indicator strip (scale 0.0 to 14.0)
- Infusion pump (required for intestinal feedings): Use pump designed for tube feedings
- Prescribed enteral feeding
- Gloves
- Equipment to obtain blood glucose by finger stick

Step	Rationale
Assessment	
1. Assess client's need for enteral tube feedings: see indications above.	Identify clients who need tube feedings before they become nutritionally depleted.
2. Assess for signs and symptoms of malnutrition (see Chapter 21).	Certain conditions, such as gastrointestinal diseases, cancer, severe infections, head injury, trauma, and metabolic diseases, make clients candidates for enteral nutrition.
3. Assess client for food allergies.	Prevents client from developing localized or systemic allergic responses.
4. Auscultate for bowel sounds before feeding.	Absent bowel sounds may indicate decreased ability of GI tract to digest or absorb nutrients.
5. Obtain baseline weight and laboratory values. Assess client for fluid volume excess or deficit, electrolyte abnormalities, and metabolic abnormalities such as hyperglycemia.	Enteral feedings are to restore or maintain a client's nutritional status. Provides objective data to measure effectiveness of feedings.
6. Verify physician's order for formula, rate, route, and frequency. Laboratory data and bedside assessments, such as finger-stick blood-glucose measurement, are also ordered by physician.	Ensures correct formula will be administered in appropriate volume.

STEP	RATIONALE

NURSING DIAGNOSIS

Defining characteristics from the assessment data may reveal the following nursing diagnoses for clients requiring this skill:

Imbalanced nutrition: less than body requirements

Impaired swallowing

Related factors are individualized based on client's condition or needs.

PLANNING

Step	Rationale
1. **Expected outcomes** following completion of procedure:	
▪ Nutritional status is improved, as evidenced by increasing weight, improving laboratory values, and improved intake and output.	Indicates that client's nutritional needs are being met.
▪ Client has no signs of respiratory distress (e.g., increased respiratory rate, coughing, poor color), discomfort.	Entry of feeding tube into airways or aspiration of feeding causes respiratory distress.
2. Explain procedure to client.	Well-informed client is more cooperative and at ease.
3. Wash hands.	Reduces transmission of microorganisms.
4. Prepare feeding container to administer formula continuously:	
a. Check expiration date on formula and integrity of container.	Ensures GI tolerance of formula. Prevents leakage of tube feeding.
b. Have tube feeding at room temperature.	Cold formula may cause gastric cramping and discomfort because the liquid is not warmed by mouth and esophagus.
c. Connect tubing to container as needed or prepare ready-to-hang container.	Tubing must be free of contamination to prevent bacterial growth.
d. Shake formula container well, and fill container with formula (see illustration). Open stopcock on tubing, and fill tubing with formula to remove air. Hang on intravenous (IV) pole.	Filling the tubing with formula prevents excess air from entering gastrointestinal tract once infusion begins.
5. For intermittent feeding have syringe ready and be sure formula is at room temperature.	Cold formula causes gastric cramping.
6. Place client in high-Fowler's position or elevate head of bed at least 30 degrees.	Elevated head helps prevent aspiration.

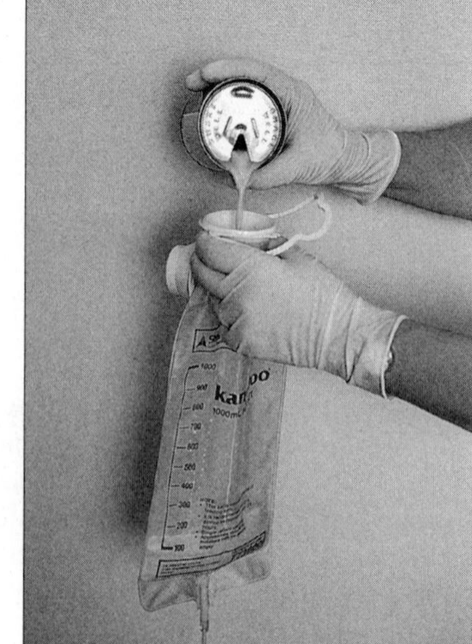

STEP **4d** Pour formula into feeding container.

Implementation

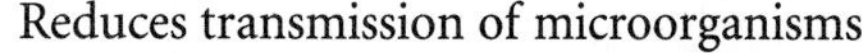

Step	Rationale
1. Apply gloves.	Reduces transmission of microorganisms.
2. Determine tube placement (see Skill 22-2). Consider together the results from pH testing and the aspirate's appearance.	On occasion, color alone may differentiate gastric from intestinal placement. Because most intestinal aspirates are stained by bile to a distinct yellow color, and most gastric aspirates are not, the difference can often distinguish the sites (Metheny and others, 1999). The pH of an aspirate offers valuable data as well in tracking advancement of a feeding tube (Metheny and others, 1998b).
3. Check for gastric residual (see illustration). a. Connect syringe to end of feeding tube, pull back evenly to aspirate gastric contents. b. Return aspirated contents to stomach unless the volume exceeds 100 ml (check agency policy).	Residual volume indicates if gastric emptying is delayed. Delayed gastric emptying may be reflected by 100 ml or more remaining in the client's stomach (McClave and others, 1992). Return of aspirate prevents fluid and electrolyte imbalance.

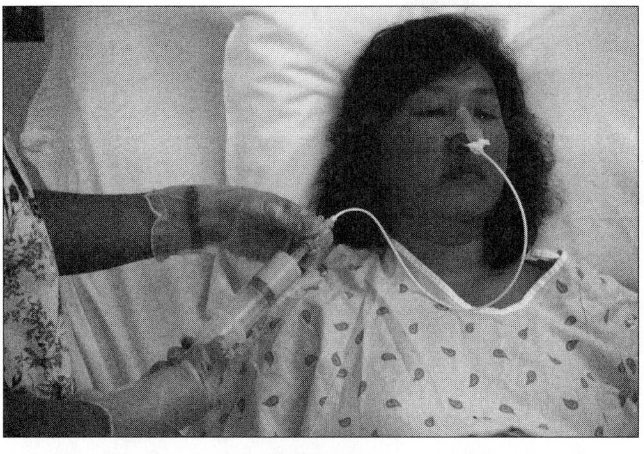

STEP 3 Check for gastric residual (small-bore tube).

Step	Rationale
4. Flush tubing with 30 ml water.	Ensures tube is clear and patent.
5. Initiate feeding:	
a. **Syringe or intermittent feeding**	
(1) Pinch proximal end of feeding tube.	Prevents air from entering client's stomach.
(2) Remove plunger from syringe and attach barrel of syringe to end of tube.	Barrel receives formula for instillation.
(3) Fill syringe with measured amount of formula (see illustration). Release tube, and elevate syringe to no more than 18 inches (45 cm) above insertion site and allow it to empty gradually by gravity. Refill until prescribed amount has been delivered to client.	Height of syringe allows for safe, slow, gravity drainage of formula.
(4) If feeding bag is used, attach gavage tubing to end of feeding tube. Set rate by adjusting roller clamp on tubing. Allow bag to empty gradually over 30 to 60 minutes (see illustration). Label bag with tube-feeding type, strength, and amount. Include date, time, and initials.	Gradual emptying of tube feeding by gravity from syringe or feeding bag reduces risk of abdominal discomfort, vomiting, or diarrhea induced by bolus or too-rapid infusion of tube feedings.
b. **Continuous-drip method**	
(1) Hang feeding bag and tubing on IV pole.	Continuous feeding method is designed to deliver prescribed hourly rate of feeding. This method reduces risk of abdominal discomfort. Clients who receive continuous drip feedings should have residuals checked every 8 to 12 hours and tube placement verified.

STEP	RATIONALE
(2) Connect distal end of tubing to proximal end of feeding tube.	
(3) Connect tubing through infusion pump and set rate (see manufacturer's directions) (see illustration).	Delivers continuous drip feeding.

- ***Critical Decision Point***
  Maximum hang time for formula is 8 hours in an open system, 24 hours in closed, ready-to-hang system.

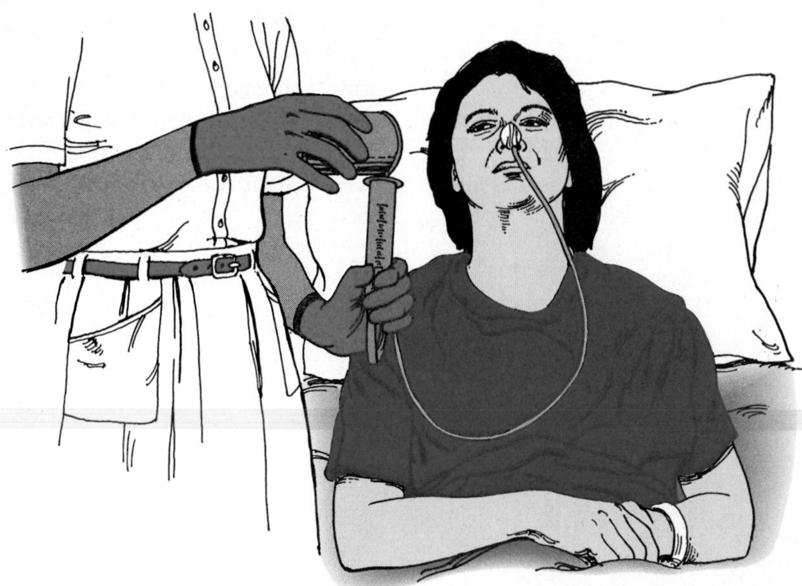

STEP **5a(3)** Fill syringe with formula.

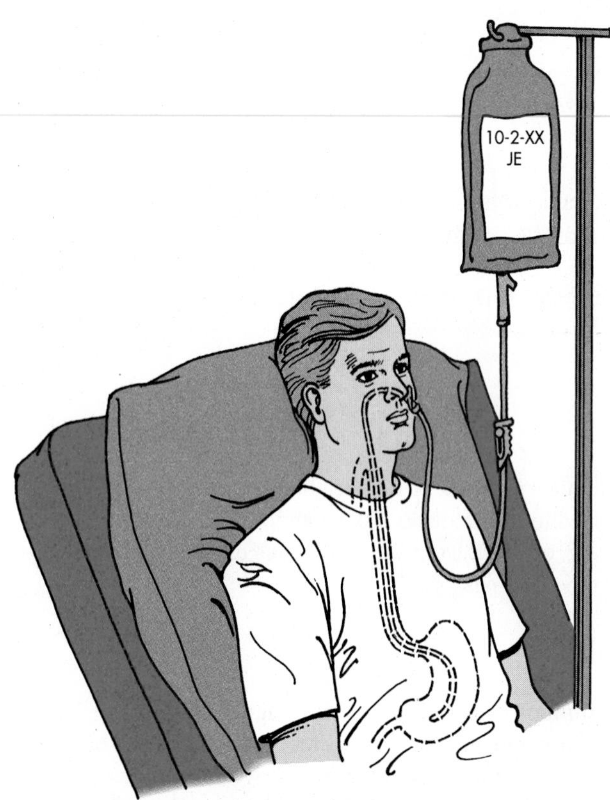

STEP **5a(4)** Administer feeding.

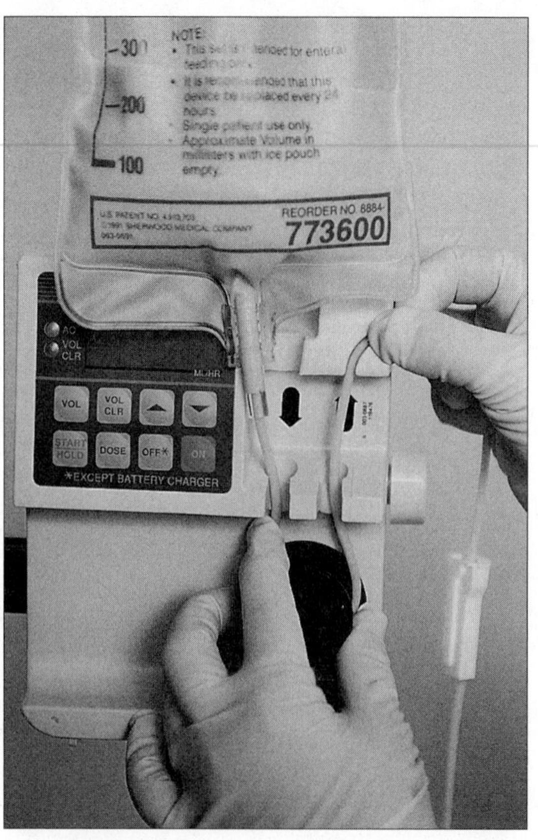

STEP **5b(3)** Connect tubing through infusion pump.

Step	Rationale
6. Advance rate of concentration of tube feeding gradually (see Box 22-1).	Prevents diarrhea and gastric intolerance to formula.
7. Following intermittent infusion or at end of continuous infusion, flush nasoenteral tubing with 30 ml of water, using irrigating syringe. Repeat every 4 to 6 hours around the clock (Simon and Fink, 1999). Have registered dietician recommend total free water requirement per day.	Provides client with source of water to help maintain fluid and electrolyte balance. Clears tubing of formula.
8. When tube feedings are not being administered, cap or clamp the proximal end of the feeding tube.	Prevents air from entering stomach between feedings.
9. Rinse bag and tubing with warm water whenever feedings are interrupted.	Rinsing bag and tubing with warm water clears old tube feedings and reduces bacterial growth.
10. Change bag and tubing every 24 hours.	Reduces incidences of bacterial growth.

Evaluation

Step	Rationale
1. Measure amount of aspirate (residual) every 8 to 12 hours.	Evaluates tolerance of tube feeding.
2. Monitor finger-stick blood glucose every 6 hours until maximum administration rate is reached and maintained for 24 hours.	Alerts nurse to client's tolerance of glucose. May require physician to revise type of formula administered.
3. Monitor intake and output every 8 hours (Metheny, 2000).	Intake and output are indications of fluid balance or fluid volume excess or deficit.
4. Weigh client daily until maximum administration rate is reached and maintained for 24 hours, then weigh client three times per week.	Weight gain is indicator of improved nutritional status; however, sudden gain of more than 2 lb in 24 hours usually indicates fluid retention.
5. Observe return of normal laboratory values.	Improving laboratory values (i.e., albumin, transferrin, and prealbumin) indicate an improved nutritional status.
6. Observe client's respiratory status.	Change in respiratory status can indicate aspiration of tube feeding.
7. Observe client's level of comfort.	Reduced gastric emptying can lead to abdominal discomfort.
8. Auscultate bowel sounds.	Confirms normal peristalsis is present.

Unexpected Outcomes and Related Interventions

- Gastric residual exceeds 100 ml. (See agency policy.)
  - Hold feeding.
  - Notify physician.
  - Maintain client in semi-Fowler's or at least have head of bed elevated 30 degrees.
  - Recheck residual in 1 hour.
- Client aspirates formula when tube inappropriately placed or client is positioned flat in bed.
  - Position client in Fowler's position, suction, and notify physician immediately.
  - Prepare for chest x-ray examination.
- Client develops diarrhea three times or more in 24 hours, indicating intolerance.
  - Notify physician and confer with dietitian to determine need to modify type of formula, concentration, or rate of infusion.
  - Determine if antibiotics and medications contain sorbitol, which can induce diarrhea (Guenther and others, 1991; Benya, Layden and Morhan, 1991).
- Client develops nausea and vomiting.
  - May indicate gastric ileus. Withhold tube feeding, and notify physician.
  - Be sure tubing is patent, aspirate for residual.

Recording and Reporting

- Record amount and type of feeding, client's response to tube feeding, patency of tube, and any side effects.
- Record volume of formula and any additional water on intake and output form.
- Report type of feeding, status of feeding tube, client's tolerance, and adverse effects.

Teaching Considerations

- Instruct client or family caregiver to keep formula refrigerated between feedings.
- Instruct client or family caregiver to administer feedings at room temperature.
- Teach client and family caregiver to check for secure attachment of feeding tube to nose. Explain that black marking should remain visible. Advise on method for hygiene for nares and face.
- Teach client and family caregiver to keep feeding tube capped or clamped between feedings and to give feedings with client in sitting position. If tolerated, client should remain upright for 1 hour after feedings.
- Instruct client or family caregiver to keep air from entering tubing via irrigating syringe and to irrigate with 30 to 60 ml of water before and after feedings, before and after medications, and before and after residual checks.
- Instruct client or family caregiver that client may complain of feelings of fullness, increased gas, belching, or diarrhea.
- Teach client or family caregiver method of GI fluid pH measurement, and expected range, and expected appearance of aspirates.

Pediatric Considerations

- Intermittent feeding is preferred in infants because of possible perforation of the stomach, nasal airway obstruction, ulceration, and irritation to mucous membranes with continuous feedings.

Gerontological Considerations

- Older adult clients may be more susceptible to hyperglycemia related to the glucose concentration in enteral formulas.

Home Care Considerations

- Instruct primary caregiver and client to monitor intake and output using household measuring devices.
- Ask client or care provider about any symptoms or discomfort during enteral feedings. Reinforce instruction to contact nurse if symptoms of discomfort occur.
- If enteral feeding is to be used at home for longer than 1 to 2 weeks, confirm with physician about gastrostomy placement.

Skill 22-5 Administering Enteral Feedings via Gastrostomy or Jejunostomy Tube

When clients cannot tolerate nasoenteral feeding tubes, there are options. Gastric feeding takes advantage of the stomach's capacity as a natural reservoir, permitting delivery of partially digested nutrients to the bowel at a normal physiologic rate. Gastric feedings via a **gastrostomy feeding tube** are relatively safe to administer, provided gastric emptying is normal. However, research has shown that aspiration rates are about the same in clients with gastrostomy as in those with nasogastric tubes (Metheny, 2000). A gastrostomy tube is inserted in the operating room or endoscopy suite by a surgeon or gastroenterologist. A large tube is surgically placed in the stomach and exits through an incision in the upper left quadrant of the abdomen where it is sutured in place. An alternative is a percutaneous endoscopic gastrostomy (PEG) tube, which is inserted with endoscopic visualization of the stomach. This tube also exits through a puncture wound in the upper left quadrant of the abdomen, but it is held securely in place by virtue of its design (Figure 22-2).

A

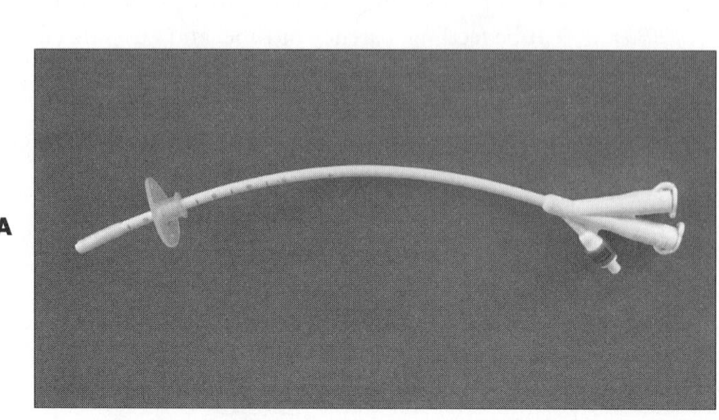

B

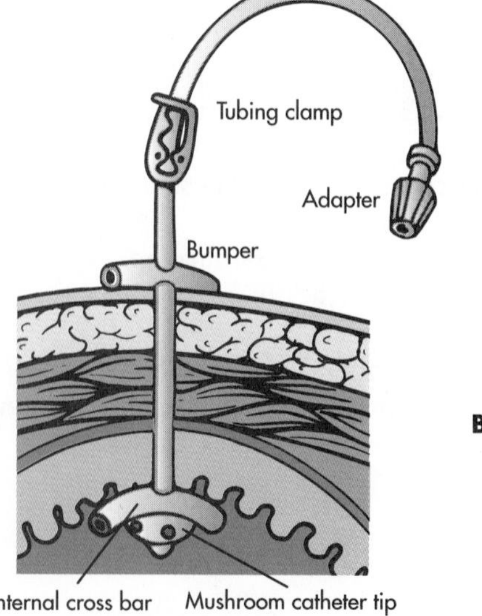

FIGURE 22-2 **A,** Percutaneous endoscopic gastrostomy (PEG) tube. **B,** Placement of PEG tube into stomach.

When clients have gastric ileus (decreased or absent peristalsis that affects the stomach but not the intestines), delayed gastric emptying, gastric resections, or neurological impairments that place them at greater risk of aspiration, enteral nutrition may be delivered via a jejunostomy tube. **Jejunostomy feeding tubes,** like gastrostomy tubes, can be inserted during surgery or endoscopy. Endoscopic insertion of a jejunostomy tube may be done through a PEG tube. After insertion of the large-bore PEG tube, the percutaneous endoscopic jejunostomy (PEJ) tube is passed through the PEG and advanced into the jejunum (Figure 22-3). A Y connector attached to the jejunostomy tube caps the PEG tube and closes the system. This Y connector labels the gastrostomy tube and designates the jejunostomy tube for feeding. The nurse must know which tube is gastric and which tube is jejunal.

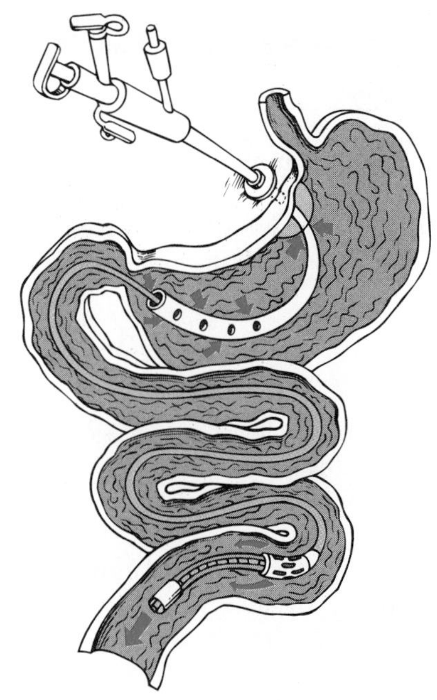

FIGURE **22-3** Endoscopic insertion of jejunostomy tube.

Delegation Considerations

Administration of enteral tube feeding via a gastrostomy or jejunostomy tube is a procedure that can be delegated to assistive personnel. Tube patency should be verified. Assistive personnel should be instructed to infuse the feeding slowly and to report any difficulty infusing the feeding or any discomfort voiced by the client.

Equipment

- Disposable feeding container or ready-to-hang bag
- 30-ml or larger Luer-lok or catheter-tip syringe
- Stethoscope
- Formula
- Infusion pump: use pump designed for tube feedings
- pH indicator strip (scale 0.0 to 14.0)
- Disposable gloves
- Equipment to obtain blood glucose by finger stick

Step	Rationale
Assessment	
1. Assess client's need for enteral feedings: impaired swallowing, decreased level of consciousness, surgeries of upper gastrointestinal tract, or need for long-term enteral nutrition.	Identifies clients who need tube feedings before they become nutritionally depleted. Enteral feeding preserves the function and mass of the gut, promotes wound healing, and may decrease infection in critically ill clients (Zaloga, 1994).
2. Assess client for food allergies.	Prevents client from developing localized or systemic allergic responses.
3. Auscultate for bowel sounds before feeding. Consult physician if bowel sounds are absent.	Bowel sounds indicate presence of peristalsis and ability of gastrointestinal tract to digest nutrients. Absent bowel sounds may indicate increased risk for abdominal distention and possibly aspiration.
4. Obtain baseline weight and laboratory values.	Enteral feedings are designed to restore or maintain nutritional status. Objective data measure effectiveness of feedings.
5. Verify physician's order for formula, rate, route, and frequency.	Tube feedings must be ordered by physician.
6. Assess gastrostomy/jejunostomy site for breakdown, irritation, or drainage.	Infection, pressure from gastrostomy tube, or drainage of gastric secretions can cause skin breakdown.

STEP	RATIONALE

NURSING DIAGNOSIS

Defining characteristics from the assessment data may reveal the following nursing diagnosis for clients requiring this skill:

Imbalanced nutrition: less than body requirements

Related factors are individualized based on client's condition or needs.

PLANNING

Step	Rationale
1. **Expected outcomes** following completion of procedure:	
▪ Nutritional status is improved, as evidenced by increasing weight, improving laboratory values, and improving intake and output.	Indicates that client's nutritional needs are being met.
▪ There are no signs of respiratory distress (e.g., increased respiratory rate, coughing, poor color).	Signs occur if vomitus or regurgitated feeding enters the respiratory tract.
▪ Skin surrounding stoma site is dry and intact.	Skin breakdown around gastrostomy site occurs from pressure of feeding tube or seepage of gastric contents around tube.
2. Explain procedure to client.	Well-informed client is more cooperative and feels more at ease.
3. Wash hands.	Reduces transmission of microorganisms.
4. Prepare feeding container to administer formula continuously:	
a. Have tube feeding at room temperature.	Cold formula may cause gastric cramping and discomfort because the liquid is not warmed by mouth and esophagus.
b. Connect tubing to container as needed or prepare ready-to-hang container.	Tubing must be free of contamination to prevent bacterial growth.
c. Shake formula container well. Fill container and tubing with formula.	Filling tubing with formula prevents excess air from entering gastrointestinal tract.
5. For intermittent feeding have syringe ready and be sure formula is at room temperature.	Cold formula causes gastric cramping.
6. Elevate head of bed 30 to 45 degrees.	Elevating client's head helps prevent chance of aspiration.

IMPLEMENTATION

Step	Rationale
1. Apply gloves and verify tube placement:	
a. **Gastrostomy tube:** Attach syringe and aspirate gastric secretions, observe their appearance, and check pH. Return aspirated contents to stomach unless the volume exceeds 100 ml. If the volume is greater than 100 ml on several consecutive occasions, hold feeding and notify physician (McClave and others, 1992).	Fluid from gastric tube of client who has fasted for at least 4 hours usually has pH range of 1 to 4, especially when client is not receiving a gastric-acid inhibitor. Continuous administration of tube feedings may elevate the pH (Metheny and others, 1999a). Gastric residual determines if gastric emptying is delayed. Delayed gastric emptying may be indicated by 100 ml or more remaining in client's stomach from previous feeding.
b. **Jejunostomy tube:** Aspirate intestinal secretions, observe their appearance and check pH.	
2. Flush with 30 ml water.	Ensures tube is clear and patent.
3. Initiate feedings:	
a. **Syringe feedings**	Gastrostomy and jejunostomy feedings are given continuously to ensure proper absorption. However, initial feedings may be given by bolus to assess client's tolerance (see Box 22-1).
(1) Pinch proximal end of the gastrostomy/jejunostomy tube.	Prevents excessive air from entering the client's stomach or leaking of gastric contents.

STEP	RATIONALE
(2) Remove plunger and attach barrel of syringe to end of tube, then fill syringe with formula.	
(3) Release tube and elevate syringe. Allow syringe to empty gradually by gravity, refilling until prescribed amount has been delivered to the client.	Gradual emptying of tube feeding by gravity reduces the risk of diarrhea induced by bolus tube feedings.
b. **Continuous drip method**	
(1) Fill feeding container with enough prescribed formula for 4 hours of feeding.	
(2) Hang container on IV pole, and clear tubing of air.	Allows for gravity flow of formula. Prevents accumulation of air in stomach.
(3) Thread tubing into feeding pump according to manufacturer's directions.	
(4) Connect end of feeding tubing to proximal end of gastrostomy/jejunostomy tube.	
(5) Begin infusion at prescribed rate.	Continuous feeding method is designed to deliver a prescribed hourly rate of feeding. This method reduces the risk of diarrhea. Clients who receive continuous-drip feedings should have residuals checked every 8 to 12 hours.
4. Administer water via feeding tube as ordered with or between feedings.	Provides client with source of water to help maintain fluid and electrolyte balance.
5. Flush tube with 30 ml of water every 4 to 6 hours around the clock and before and after administering medications via the tube (Simon and Fink, 1999).	Maintains patency of tube and provides client with some free water. Small jejunal tubes are very prone to clogging and are difficult to replace.
6. When tube feedings are not being administered, cap or clamp the proximal end of the gastrostomy/jejunostomy tube.	Prevents excess air from entering the gastrointestinal tract between feedings and prevents leakage of gastric contents.
7. Rinse container and tubing with warm water after all intermittent feedings.	Rinsing container and tube with warm water clears old tube feedings and prevents bacterial growth.

• ***Critical Decision Point***

Advance tube feeding rate gradually (Box 22-1). Tube feedings should be advanced gradually to prevent diarrhea and gastric intolerance of formula.

STEP	RATIONALE
8. The gastrostomy/jejunostomy exit site is usually left open to air. However, if a dressing is needed because of drainage, change dressing daily or as needed and report the drainage to the physician; inspect exit site every shift.	Leakage of gastric drainage may cause irritation and excoriation. Skin around feeding tube should be cleansed daily with warm water and mild soap; a small precut gauze dressing may be applied to exit site.
9. Dispose of supplies and wash hands.	Reduces transmission of microorganisms.

Box 22-1 Advancing the Rate of Tube Feeding

INTERMITTENT

1. Start formula at full strength for isotonic formulas (300 to 400 mOsm) or at ordered concentration.
2. Infuse formula over at least 20 to 30 minutes via syringe or feeding container.
3. Begin feedings with no more than 150 to 250 ml at one time. Increase by 50 ml per feeding per day to achieve needed volume and calories in six to eight feedings. (NOTE: Concentrated formulas at full strength may be infused at slower rate until tolerance is achieved.)

CONTINUOUS

1. Start formula at full strength for isotonic formulas (300 to 400 mOsm) or at ordered concentration. Usually hypertonic formulas are also started at full strength but at a slower rate.
2. Begin infusion rate at designated rate.
3. Advance rate slowly (e.g., 10 to 20 ml/hr) per day to target rate if tolerated (tolerance indicated by absence of nausea and diarrhea, and low gastric residuals).

STEP	RATIONALE
EVALUATION	
1. Evaluate client's tolerance of tube feeding. Check amount of aspirate (residual) every 8 to 12 hours.	Tolerance of tube feeding is evaluated by checking.
2. Monitor finger-stick blood glucose every 6 hours until maximum rate of administration is reached and maintained for 24 hours.	Alerts nurse to client's tolerance of glucose or fluid volume excess.
3. Monitor intake and output every 8 hours.	Intake and output are indications of fluid balance.
4. Weigh client daily until maximum administration rate is reached and maintained for 24 hours, then weigh client three times per week.	Weight gain is indicator of improved nutritional status; however, a sudden gain of more than 2 lb in 24 hours usually indicates fluid retention.
5. Observe return of normal laboratory values.	Improving laboratory values (i.e., albumin, transferrin, prealbumin) indicate return to normal nutritional status.
6. Observe stoma site for skin integrity.	Gastric secretions can cause injury and necrosis at stoma site.

UNEXPECTED OUTCOMES AND RELATED INTERVENTIONS

- Client aspirates formula when gastric emptying is delayed or formula is administered too rapidly and produces vomiting.
  - Position client in side-lying position, and suction airway to keep it clear. Do not initiate gagging during suctioning.
  - Notify physician; obtain chest x-ray film.
- Client develops diarrhea: diarrhea or liquid stools (three times or more in 24 hours) indicate intolerance. Antibiotics and medications containing sorbitol may also induce diarrhea.
  - Decrease rate of feeding, review medications, and notify physician.
  - Type of formula may be altered and antidiarrheal agents may be ordered.
- Client develops nausea and vomiting.
  - Palpate abdomen for distention, and check for bowel sounds to determine presence of gastric ileus.
  - Withhold feeding, and notify physician.
- Skin surrounding gastrostomy site breaks down.
  - Provide appropriate wound care (see Chapter 35).

RECORDING AND REPORTING

- Record amount and type of feeding, client's response to feeding, patency of tube, any untoward effects, and condition of gastrostomy/jejunostomy site in nurses' notes.
- Record amount of feeding on intake and output form.
- Report to oncoming nursing staff: type of feeding, status of gastrostomy tube, client's tolerance, and adverse effects.

TEACHING CONSIDERATIONS

- Teach client or primary caregiver to clean around tube with warm water and mild soap.
- Hydrogen peroxide diluted with water (50:50) can be used for the first few days after insertion of the tube to remove any crusting around exit site. A dressing is usually not necessary or recommended.
- If client has a large-bore tube, instruct client or primary caregiver to crush all pills completely and mix with water before administration through tube. If client has a small-bore tube, medications in liquid form are less likely to clog tube.
- Instruct client or primary caregiver to keep air from entering tubing via irrigating syringe and to irrigate with 30 to 60 ml of water before and after feedings, before and after residual checks, and before and after medications.

PEDIATRIC CONSIDERATIONS

- A low-profile gastrostomy tube (gastrostomy button) may be used for pediatric clients to decrease the chance of child pulling out or dislodging tube and for increased comfort. Low-profile tube has an adapter to allow syringe feeding or connection to a feeding container.
- Intermittent feeding is preferred in infants because of possible perforation of stomach and irritation to mucous membranes with continuous feedings.

GERONTOLOGICAL CONSIDERATIONS

- Older adults may have decreased gastric transit time so that formula remains in the stomach longer than for younger clients. Gastric residual checks are of special importance to decrease the risk of vomiting and aspiration during gastric feeding.

HOME CARE CONSIDERATIONS

- Instruct primary caregiver to maintain records of intake and output using household measuring devices.
- Flushing with 30 ml of tap water every 4 hours during continuous feeding, after residual checks, and before and after medication administration will help to increase absorption of medication and ensure patency and continued smooth infusion of feeding formula into client's gastrointestinal tract. Clients with fluid restriction should have a 10- to 30-ml flush.

Critical Thinking Exercises

1. Sylvia's client has been on intermittent tube feedings administered through a small-bore nasoenteric tube for 2 days. When the tube was first inserted 2 days ago, an x-ray film showed that the tube's distal tip was positioned in the gastric fundus. At 10 AM today, before giving an intermittent feeding, Sylvia found that fluid withdrawn from the feeding tube had a pH of 4 and looked like watery milk. At 4 PM today, before starting the next feeding, Sylvia found that fluid withdrawn from the tube had a pH of 6 and had a yellowish brown color. The client had a normal respiratory rate and was breathing without difficulty. What does this information reveal to Sylvia and what should she do?
2. Mr. Nielson has been on continuous tube feedings for 24 hours. He has had a gastric residual from his gastrostomy tube of 250 ml during the past three checks of his residual volume. What should you as the nurse be concerned about?
3. At 10:00 AM Todd administered medication via Ms. Lee's nasointestinal tube. He notices at approximately 11:30 AM that her continuous tube feeding is about an hour behind schedule. What should Todd do?
4. What unique aspect of nursing care is required when a client has a gastrostomy tube versus a nasogastric feeding tube?

References

Benya R, Layden T, Morhan S: Diarrhea associated with tube feeding: the importance of objective criteria: *J Clin Gastroenterol* 13(2):167, 1991.

Ciocon JO and others: Continuous compared with intermittent tube feeding in the elderly, *JPEN* 16:525, 1992.

Edwards S, Metheny N: Measurement of gastric residual volume: state of the science, *MedSurg Nurs* 9(3)125, 2000.

El-Gamel A, Watson D: Transbronchial intubation of the right pleural space: a rare complication of nasogastric intubation with a polyvinylchloride tube—a case study, *Heart Lung* 22:223, 1993.

Ghahremani GG, Gould RJ: Nasoenteric feeding tubes: radiographic detection of complications, *Dig Dis Sci* 31:574, 1986.

Guenther P and others: Tube feeding related diarrhea in acutely ill patients, *JPEN* 15(3):277, 1991.

Hanson RL: Predictive criteria for length of nasogastric tube insertion for tube feeding, *JPEN* 3:160, 1979.

Kudsk K: Clinical applications of enteral nutrition, *Nutr Clin Pract* 12(1):20, 1994.

Lehmann S: Parenteral and enteral access devices. In Teasley-Strausberg KM, editor: *Nutrition support handbook,* Cincinnati, 1992, Harvey Whitney Books.

Levy H: Nasogastric and nasoenteric feeding tubes, *Gastrointest Endosc Clin North Am* 8(3)529, 1998.

Lord L and others: Comparison of weighted vs unweighted enteral feeding tubes for efficacy of transpyloric intubation, *JPEN* 17(3):271, 1993.

McClave SA and others: Use of residual volume as a marker for enteral feeding intolerance: prospective blinded comparison with physical examination and radiographic findings, *JPEN* 16(2):99, 1992.

McClave SA and others: Enteral tube feeding in the intensive care unit: factors impeding adequate delivery, *Crit Care Med* 27(7):1252, 1999.

McKenry LM, Salerno E: *Mosby's pharmacology in nursing,* ed 20, St. Louis, 1998, Mosby.

Metheny N, Measures to test placement of nasogastric and nasoenteral feeding tubes: a review, *Nurs Res* 37(6):323, 1988.

Metheny N: Personal correspondence, 2000.

Metheny N and others: Effectiveness of pH measurements in predicting feeding tube placement, *Nurs Res* 38(5):285, 1989.

Metheny N and others: Detection of inadvertent respiratory placement of small-bore feeding tubes: a report of 10 cases, *Heart Lung* 19(6):631, 1990a.

Metheny N and others: Effectiveness of the auscultatory method in predicting feeding tube location, *Nurs Res* 39(5):262, 1990b.

Metheny N and others: Effectiveness of pH measurements in predicting feeding tube placement: an update, *Nurs Res* 42(6):323, 1993a.

Metheny N and others: How to aspirate fluid from small-bore feeding tubes, *Am J Nurs* 93(5):86, 1993b.

Metheny N and others: Characteristics of aspirates from feeding tubes as a method for predicting tube location, *Nurs Res* 43(5):282, 1994.

Metheny N and others: Detection of improperly positioned feeding tubes, *J Healthc Risk Manage* 18(3):37, 1998a.

Metheny N and others: pH, color, and feeding tubes, *RN* 61(1):227, 1998b.

Metheny N and others: Testing feeding tube placement: auscultation vs pH method, *Am J Nurs* 98(5):37, 1998c.

Metheny N and others: Indicators of feeding tube placement in neonates, *Nutr Clin Pract* 14(6):307, 1999a.

Metheny N and others: pH and concentration of bilirubin in feeding tube aspirates as predictors of tube placement, *Nurs Res* 48:189, 1999b.

Powell KS and others: Aspirating gastric residuals causes occlusion of small bore feeding tubes, *JPEN* 17:243, 1993.

Simon T, Fink AS: Current management of endoscopic feeding tube dysfunction, *Surgical Endoscopy* 13:403, 1999.

Welch SK: Certification of staff nurses to insert enteral feeding tubes using a research-based procedure, *NCP* 11(1):21, 1996.

Wilson M, Haynes-Johnson V: Cranberry juice or water? a comparison of feeding tube irrigants. *Nutr Support Serv* 7(7):23, 1987.

Wong D and others: *Whaley and Wong's nursing care of infants and children,* ed 6, St. Louis, 1999, Mosby.

Zaloga G: Timing and route of nutritional support. In Zaloga G, editor: *Nutrition in critical care,* St. Louis, 1994, Mosby.

23

Parenteral Nutrition

Skills

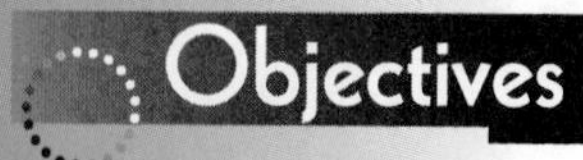

Objectives

Mastery of content in this chapter will enable the nurse to:

- Define the key terms listed.
- Identify clients who are candidates for parenteral nutrition.
- Describe factors influencing selection of appropriate sites for administering parenteral nutrition.
- Identify measures used to prevent complications of central parenteral nutrition.
- Demonstrate appropriate nursing care of the client receiving parenteral nutrition.
- Assist the physician with placement of a central vein catheter.
- Demonstrate a central line dressing change application.

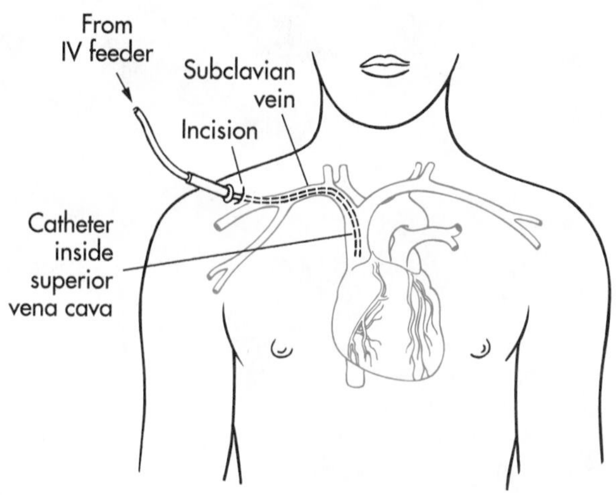

FIGURE **23-1** Placement of central venous catheter inserted into subclavian vein.

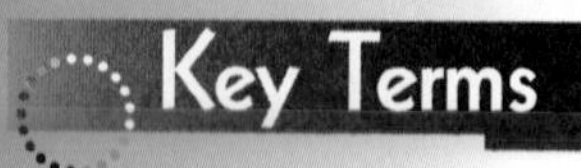

Key Terms

Amino acid
Dextrose
Enteral nutrition
Iso-osmotic solutions
Lipid emulsion
Nutritional support nursing
Osmolality
Parenteral nutrition (PN)
Peripherally inserted central catheter (PICC)
Pneumothorax
Trendelenburg position
Valsalva maneuver

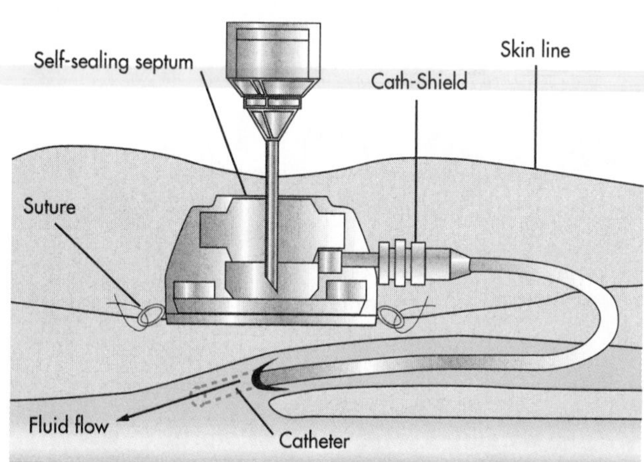

FIGURE **23-2** Cross section of implantable port displaying access of the port with a Huber needle. (Courtesy SIMS Deltec, Inc, St. Paul, Minn.)

Parenteral nutrition (PN) is the intravenous (IV) infusion of nutrients, including **amino acids** (protein/nitrogen), dextrose (carbohydrate/glucose), fat emulsions (fatty acids), vitamins, electrolytes, minerals, and trace elements. Nutrition through the gastrointestinal tract (**enteral nutrition**) is best and should be used when the client's gastrointestinal tract is functional before initiating parenteral nutrition. However, certain disease states that seriously impair gastrointestinal function or limit a client's ability to use enteral nutrition indicate the need for PN.

Parenteral nutrition cannot be administered without an appropriately placed vascular access device (Orr, 1999). PN solutions are usually hyperosmolar and must be administered into a large-diameter vein to prevent sclerosis of vein tissue. Administration into the central vascular system is indicated. Central vascular access devices currently used for PN administration include percutaneous central vein catheters (Figure 23-1), tunneled catheters, implanted subcutaneous ports (Figure 23-2), and **peripherally inserted central catheters (PICCs)** (Figure 23-3) (see Chapter 19). This chapter will discuss the administration of PN, using central venous access catheters. The ideal device used for PN is durable, reliable, and user-friendly, because most clients receiving PN will continue to receive the nutritional therapy in the home or long-term care setting.

The nurse plays an important role in assessing and identifying a client's need for parenteral nutrition. The first sign of a developing problem may be a pattern of declining oral food intake and reduced appetite. Frequently the nurse will be the first to identify risk factors, such as progressive weight loss, restricted or limited fluid intake, intolerance to enteral feedings, increased energy need (burns, sepsis, and trauma), or

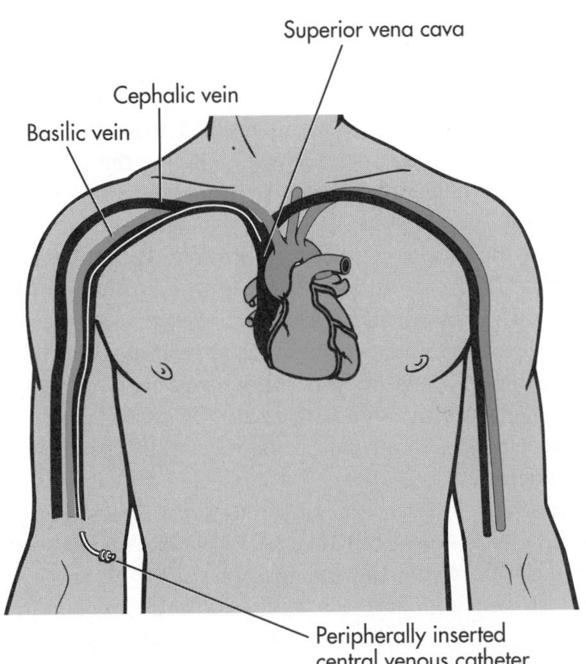

FIGURE **23-3** Placement of peripherally inserted central catheter (PICC) through antecubital fossa. (Modified from Lewis SM, Collier IC, Heitkemper MM, Dirksen SR: *Medical-surgical nursing: assessment and management of clinical problems,* ed 5, St. Louis, 2000, Mosby.)

being NPO (nothing by mouth) for 3 or more days. The nurse's assessment provides information for ultimately consulting with a dietitian and physician in an effort to initiate appropriate parenteral nutrition. The nurse also plays a role in the selection of the best vascular access site for PN administration (Table 23-1). Selection of an ideal vascular access device depends on several factors: client factors, device characteristics, therapeutic issues, and duration of therapy (Orr, 1999). For example, implanted ports and PICCs require the highest level of manual dexterity for home care clients to manage dressing changes and tubing manipulation. If possible, a port or PICC should be placed on the side opposite the client's dominant hand. When a client has a PICC, a willing and able caregiver is needed to assist with dressing changes to avoid the risk of catheter displacement and dressing contamination. Table 23-1 summarizes the factors to consider in device selection.

Parenteral nutrition can be administered as peripheral parenteral nutrition (PPN) or central parenteral nutrition (CPN). A parenteral nutrition solution with a final dextrose concentration of more than 10% must be delivered into the central venous system because of the hypertonicity of the solution (Orr, 1999). PPN is a solution that contains 10% or less dextrose and is a lower osmolality; 5% dextrose is actually an **iso-osmotic solution** (of similar **osmolality** as blood). PPN

Table 23-1 Factors in Determining Vascular Access Device Selection for Parenteral Nutrition

Client Factors	Device Characteristics	Therapeutic Factors	Duration of Therapy
Physiological	Design	Characteristics of solutions or emulsions:	PICCs can be placed for duration of 1 year.
Condition of veins	Low risk for infection	Dextrose concentration >10% requires central vein access	Implanted ports may remain in place for life of need or until portal head does not hold needle. Manufacturers recommend 1500 needle sticks with 20-gauge needle.
Hypercoagulability state	Antibacterial coatings	Solutions with osmolarity >600 mOsm/L requires central vein access	Hickman or Broviac catheter remains in place for life of need unless catheter becomes clotted, infected, or there is breakdown of catheter material.
Diabetes	Number of lumens	Disease or condition treated	Triple-lumen subclavian catheters used only for duration of acute care.
Skin disorders	Durability		
Previous surgery involving thorax or vascular system			
Known allergies to catheter materials			
Functional			
Poor vision			
Altered dexterity			
Developmental disabilities			
Frailty			
Psychological			
Needle phobia			
Body image impairment			
Previous experience with vascular access device			
Social Support			
Care provider availability			
Financial resources			

was meant to be administered through a short intravenous cannula into veins of the forearm or hand. However, PPN is often associated with an increased incidence of phlebitis and thrombosis of veins (Shuster, 1996; Shizgal and Knowles, 1991). Midline catheters have been argued to be appropriate devices for PPN administration; however, the catheters are only threaded to the upper arm, and the diameter and flow characteristics are not dramatically different from peripheral veins (Orr, 1999). Standards of care recommend midline catheters not be used for solutions or emulsions with a pH greater than 5 or an osmolarity greater than 500 mOsm (Intravenous Nurses Society, 1998). **Dextrose** concentration is the main factor in determining the osmolarity of PN. To calculate osmolarity:

$$\text{Total grams of CHO (carbohydrate)/L} \times 5 + \\ \text{Total grams of AA (amino acids)/L} \times 10 + \\ \text{Total number of cations (Na, K, Ca, Mg in mEq/L)} \times 2 = \text{Osmolarity}$$

Lipid emulsions were previously most often given as a separate infusion that was piggybacked into the PN solution. Today total nutrient admixture or three-in-one emulsions are used to provide nutritionally complete PN. Fats provide significant calories in the American diet and supply essential and nonessential fatty acids that are used as energy. The essential fatty acid present in **lipid emulsion** is linoleic acid; this acid cannot be made from other fats in human metabolism and therefore must be supplied. Linoleic acid is an omega-6 fatty acid. A client who is deficient in linoleic acid will be immunosuppressed and thus at risk for infection. A nutritional regimen that does not provide adequate fatty acids can lead to essential fatty acid deficiency (EFAD). Signs and symptoms of EFAD include dry scaly skin, sparse hair growth, impaired wound healing, decreased resistance to stress, increased susceptibility to respiratory tract infections, anemia, thrombocytopenia, and liver function abnormalities. EFAD is prevented by administering a minimum of 500 ml of 10% lipid emulsion two times per week (Abbot Labs, 1990).

Fat emulsion is a soybean or safflower oil base that is isotonic and may be infused with an amino acid and dextrose solution through a central or peripheral vein. Fats may be administered through a separate IV; given piggyback through a Y connector near the port of entry (Chapter 19); or given through admixing the amino acid, dextrose, and fat emulsion solution in one container (three-in-one system) to infuse over 24 hours. When administering fat (lipid) emulsions via piggyback infusion, the solution must be added below the infusion filter and inserted in the port nearest to the venipuncture site. The fat particles are large and cannot pass through the infusion filter. Not all clients should receive fat emulsion. Individuals for whom fat emulsions are contraindicated include those who have a disturbance of normal fat metabolism, such as pathological hyperlipemia.

Parenteral nutrition has significant physiological and psychological implications. Clients who are unable to eat may become socially isolated, suffer hunger pangs, have food cravings, or even hallucinate about food. A majority of social events focus around food, thereby excluding the client from complete participation. The nurse promotes the client's psychological well-being by discussing possible feelings and sensations with the client; describing possible alternatives to satisfy oral cravings, such as chewing gum or sucking on hard candies (if allowed); and offering activities that can help distract a client from hunger cravings and promote participation in social interactions. Many clients who receive parenteral nutrition are capable of some oral intake. Client and family education helps to alleviate many of the client's and family's fears and concerns.

The nursing committee of the American Society of Parenteral and Enteral Nutrition (ASPEN) has defined **nutritional support nursing** practice, the scope of nutritional support nursing, and the goals of nutritional support (ASPEN, 1996): Nutritional support nursing practice is the care of individuals with potential or known nutrition alterations. The goal of nutritional support nursing is to assist individuals in restoring and maintaining optimal nutritional health.

Skill Performance Guidelines

1. Identify clients who are candidates for PN. Clients unable to take nutrition orally or enterally and who are at risk of malnutrition because of actual or anticipated prolonged inability to ingest, digest, or absorb nutrients should be considered for PN. In addition, clients who are severely injured may receive PN and enteral nutrition.
2. Know when peripheral vein access can be used instead of central vein access. Clients who require short-term nutrition support, for whom central access placement is contraindicated or not feasible, who have adequate peripheral access, and who can tolerate larger volumes of fluid are candidates for peripheral parenteral nutrition.
3. Know the limits of solutions used for peripheral vein versus central vein access. Solutions with a final dextrose concentration of greater than 10% must be given via a central vein.
4. Be aware of complications associated with PN, including metabolic disturbances, fluid imbalance, technical management of catheter system, and infections.
5. Establish the client's normal range of vital signs, electrolyte balance, triglyceride levels, weight, and fluid status. Clients who receive PN may have rapid changes in these values.
6. Know the client's recent temperature range. Clients with peripheral or central IV lines are susceptible to septicemia; an elevated temperature can be an early indicator of a bacterial process.

Skill 23-1 Caring for the Client Receiving Central Venous Placement for Central Parenteral Nutrition

Central parenteral nutrition (CPN) is a form of nutritional support administered through central vein cannulation. A catheter is usually placed in the subclavian vein through infraclavicular venipuncture (see Figure 23-1). This site is preferred because it provides a flat, relatively immobile area on the chest and blood flows at a high rate, decreasing the risk of phlebitis or displacement. The nurse has an important role when assisting the physician in placing a CPN line. Attention to asepsis and positioning, being available to reassure the client during the procedure, and ensuring that the right equipment is available are critical to the success of the procedure. Because CPN is associated with numerous complications (Table 23-2), it is

Table 23-2 Complications of Central Parenteral Nutrition

PROBLEM	CAUSE	SYMPTOMS	IMMEDIATE ACTION	PREVENTION
Air embolism	IV tubing disconnected; part of catheter system open or removed without clamp on	Sudden respiratory distress; shortness of breath, coughing, chest pain, decreased blood pressure	Clamp catheter; position client in left Trendelenburg position; call physician; administer oxygen as needed.	Make sure all catheter connections are secure; clamp catheter when not in use.
Infection				
Localized infection (exit site, tunnel)	Poor aseptic technique in removal of skin flora during site preparation and dressing care	Exit site: erythema, tenderness, induration or purulence within 2 cm of skin at exit site Tunnel: same as above but extends beyond 2 cm from exit site	Call physician. Exit: warm compress, daily site care, oral antibiotics. Tunnel: remove catheter.	Use proper aseptic technique. Cleanse site with iodophor a minimum of 3 to 5 min.* Routine use of antibiotic ointment not recommended.
Systemic infection (catheter sepsis or bacteremia)	Catheter hub contamination; contamination of infusate; spread of bacteria through bloodstream from distant site	Systemic: isolation of same microorganism from blood culture and catheter segment, with client showing fever, chills, malaise, elevated white blood cell count	Systemic: antibiotics intravenously, remove catheter.	Do not disconnect tubing unnecessarily.
Hyperglycemia	Client receiving solution too quickly; too little insulin in solution; infection	Excessive thirst, urination, blood sugar >160 mg/100 ml, confusion	Call physician; may need to slow infusion rate (physician order).	Review medical history for glucose intolerance or diabetes; keep rate as ordered, never increase to "catch up." Use aseptic technique and routine blood glucose monitoring.
Hypoglycemia	CPN abruptly discontinued; too much insulin	Client is shaky, dizzy, nervous, anxious, senses hunger, blood sugar level <80 mg/100 ml	Call physician; if CPN discontinued abruptly, may need to restart D_{10} NS at previous CPN rate. If client has oral intake, give ½ cup fruit juice. Perform blood glucose monitoring; retest in 15 to 30 min.	Decrease CPN, "tapering" gradually until discontinued; blood glucose monitoring is used to ensure adequate insulin.

Data from Davis CL: Nursing care of total parenteral and enteral nutrition. In Fischer JE, editor: *Total parenteral nutrition,* ed 2, Boston, 1991, Little, Brown; Hickey MS: *Handbook of enteral, parenteral, and ARC/AIDS nutritional therapy,* St. Louis, 1992, Mosby; Pennington CR: Toward safer parenteral nutrition, *Aliment Pharmacol Ther* 4(5):427, 1990 (review article); Krzywda EA and others: Catheter infections: diagnosis, etiology, treatment, and prevention, *Nutr Clin Pract* 14:178, 1999; Mermel LA: Prevention of intravascular catheter-related infections, *Infect Dis Clin Pract* 3:391, 1994.

also vital that the nurse carefully monitor the CPN site and notify the physician of any symptoms or developing problems (Krzywda and others, 1999). Clients receiving CPN are at high risk for infection. Catheter-related bloodstream infections (CR-BSI) rank as the third most common nosocomial infection in intensive care units (CDC NNIS System, 1997).

Delegation Considerations

The skill of caring for a client receiving central venous placement for parenteral nutrition (PN) should not be delegated to assistive personnel. Assistive personnel should be instructed to report immediately if client's dressing becomes damp or soiled, catheter line appears to be pulled out farther than original insertion position, intravenous line becomes disconnected, client has a fever, or client complains of pain at the site.

Equipment

- Subclavian insertion tray *or* the following:
- Caps
- Sterile gowns
- Masks and protective eyewear
- Nonsterile gloves
- Sterile gloves
- Gauze pads
- Bottle of alcohol
- Alcohol swabs
- Surgical towels
- Povidone-iodine scrub
- Povidone-iodine swabs
- 1% lidocaine (Xylocaine)
- Central line catheter kit
- Sterile drapes
- Bath blanket or towel and protective pad
- 500-ml bottle 5% Dextrose in water
- Transparent dressing or gauze dressing for catheter insertion site
- Tape
- Intravenous infusion pump
- Tincture of benzoin (optional)

Step	Rationale
Assessment	
1. Assess need for CPN and determine client's current nutritional status and energy needs.	Provides baseline to compare changes after CPN is started.
a. Weight loss of 10% or more of usual body weight	Indicates malnourishment, a criteria for parenteral nutrition when GI function is altered.
b. Reduction in values for prealbumin, serum albumin, and total lymphocyte count, total iron-binding capacity	Serve as markers for nutritional risk but do not provide clinical measure for efficacy of parenteral nutrition. (Bozzetti and others, 2000).
c. Prolonged alteration in gastrointestinal function (malabsorption, recent gastrointestinal surgery, or paralytic ileus)	Rules out use of enteral nutrition to restore weight loss.
d. Reduced intake of calories	May result from factors such as loss of appetite, problems with chewing/swallowing, debilitating conditions causing fatigue or shortness of breath.
e. Intolerance to food/enteral feedings	Rules out use of enteral nutrition as a therapy.
2. Check physician's order for insertion of central vein catheter and for size and type of catheter.	Invasive procedure requires a consent. Physician may request a certain type or size of catheter.
3. Assess client's hydration status: skin turgor, texture, and fluid intake and output.	Dehydration depletes fluid volume and may make insertion of a central vein catheter more difficult.
4. Assess client for any surgical procedures of the upper chest or anatomical irregularities.	Previous surgical procedures or central vein catheterizations may indicate that a particular site should not be used. Scoliosis or other spine deformities may make positioning difficult.
5. Consider catheter material to be used, (e.g., silicone, polymers), and determine if client has allergy to material.	Prevents onset of hypersensitivity or allergic reaction from use of catheter.
6. Inspect condition of skin overlying supraclavicular and infraclavicular area.	Certain skin conditions where skin integrity is broken may contraindicate catheter insertion.
7. Assess client for allergy to iodine or lidocaine.	Solutions used during catheter insertion procedure. Allergic response could be fatal.

STEP	RATIONALE

NURSING DIAGNOSIS

Defining characteristics from the assessment data may reveal the following nursing diagnoses for clients requiring this skill:

Imbalanced nutrition: less than body requirements
Risk for infection
Deficient fluid volume
Excess fluid volume

Related factors are individualized based on client's condition or needs.

PLANNING

Step	Rationale
1. **Expected outcomes** following completion of procedure:	
■ Insertion occurs without complication.	Placement of a central vein catheter carries risks.
■ Insertion site is free of inflammation or breakdown.	Denotes absence of infection and skin changes at central venous site.
2. Explain to client steps for central line placement, the Valsalva maneuver, the need for CPN, and follow-up care. Provide time for client to ask questions.	Allows client to anticipate steps of procedure to minimize anxiety and to ensure client participation as needed.
3. Verify that consent was signed.	Consent document is required, because central line placement is considered an invasive procedure.

IMPLEMENTATION

Catheter Insertion

Step	Rationale
1. Nurse and physician wash hands.	Reduces transmission of microorganisms.
2. Physician, with assistance of nurse, positions client flat in bed, lying supine. Place rolled towel or bath blanket between client's scapulae and place protective pad under shoulder area.	Opens angle between clavicle and first rib; dilates veins to facilitate eventual catheter insertion.
3. Nurse puts on cap, mask, eyewear, and clean gloves. Physician should put on cap, gown, mask, eyewear, and sterile gloves.	Prevents transmission of infection.
4. Nurse opens central vein kit and adds any sterile equipment to kit for use during insertion (see Chapter 32).	Maintains sterile field
5. Nurse saturates 4 × 4 gauze pads with alcohol, and physician scrubs area using circular motion from shoulder to ear to chin to nipple for approximately 1 minute.	Alcohol cleans and defats skin.

• ***Critical Decision Point***
Do not use acetone to defat the skin. Acetone may cause inflammation of skin, client discomfort, and offers no antimicrobial benefit over alcohol (Maki and McCormack, 1987).

Step	Rationale
6. With povidone-iodine scrub, physician cleans same area for 1 minute.	Removes surface skin bacteria.
7. Physician wipes away excess scrub solution with sterile 4 × 4 gauze pad.	Avoids introduction of solution into skin during catheter insertion.
8. Physician changes sterile gloves.	Gloves become contaminated from surface bacteria picked up in solution.
9. Physician uses large sterile drape and sterile towels to create a sterile field. Physician finds anatomical landmarks and places fenestrated drape appropriately.	Provides sterile work space for catheter insertion. Clients whose catheters were placed using a mask, cap, sterile gloves, gown and large drape had lower colonization rate of bacteria than clients where sterile gloves and a small drape were used (Raad and others, 1994).

Step	Rationale
10. Physician prepares equipment in kit.	
11. Nurse sets up intravenous (IV) bag, fills tubing, and covers end of tubing with a sterile cap (see Chapter 19).	IV tubing is ready to be connected to IV catheter.
12. Nurse places client in **Trendelenburg position** and turns client's head away from site of insertion (see illustration).	With head down, below heart, position promotes maximal filling and distention of subclavicular vein.

STEP **12** Client positioned in Trendelenberg position in preparation for central venous catheter insertion.

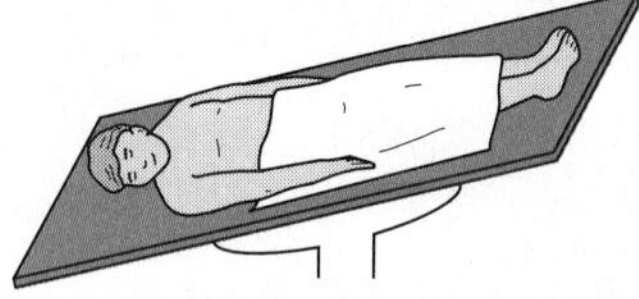

- ***Critical Decision Point***

  Trendelenburg position is contraindicated in clients with head injuries, increased intracranial pressure, and spinal cord injuries.

Step	Rationale
13. Nurse wipes off top of 1% lidocaine bottle with alcohol swabs and holds bottle upside down.	Removes surface bacteria; allows physician to withdraw lidocaine while maintaining asepsis.
14. Physician injects needle into bottle and withdraws approximately 3 to 4 ml lidocaine. Physician injects needle into site for subclavian puncture and anesthetizes venipuncture site, waiting 1 to 2 minutes for effect to take place.	Minimizes discomfort client feels during venipuncture.
15. Physician inserts IV catheter into subclavian vein. Usually this is done by locating the vein with a large-bore cannula, removing the needle from the cannula, threading a wire into the cannula and vein, removing the cannula over the wire, and threading the central vein catheter over the wire to the appropriate location (Seldinger technique) (Nussbaum and Fischer, 1994).	Large vein is less irritated by CPN solution.

- ***Critical Decision Point***

  *At time of insertion, nurse asks client to perform **Valsalva maneuver** (holding breath and straining). Maneuver is also performed whenever the catheter will be open to air. Valsalva maneuver increases intrathoracic pressure and prevents entry of air into the catheter. If client is unable to perform Valsalva maneuver, compress client's abdomen gently.*

Step	Rationale
16. When blood return is evident and catheter placement is appropriate, physician connects IV tubing to intravenous catheter.	Prevents air from entering venous system.
17. Nurse runs the IV fluid in at a rapid rate (macrodrip 20 to 30 gtt/min, microdrip 60 gtt/min) for 5 to 10 minutes.	Assesses whether fluid is infusing easily.
18. Nurse lowers IV bag below heart level.	Provides blood return to determine presence of catheter in venous system.
19. Nurse raises IV bag and slows rate to 30 to 40 ml/hr via infusion pump until chest x-ray study is obtained.	Central line cannulations increase risk of **pneumothorax** (entrance of air into pleural space). Chest x-ray examination verifies absence of pneumothorax and confirms location before fluids are administered at a rapid flow.
20. Physician sutures central venous catheter in place.	Suturing catheter to skin at insertion site assists in preventing accidental dislodgement.
21. Physician removes sterile drapes and completes procedure.	Occurs only if physician is not applying occlusive dressing to IV site.

Applying Occlusive Dressing

Step	Rationale
1. Nurse applies sterile gloves.	Maintains surgical asepsis.
2. With alcohol swab, start at catheter exit site and cleanse skin, working in a circular motion outward approximately 2 to 3 inches. (Do three times.) Allow to dry.	Removes blood and defats skin.

STEP	RATIONALE
3. With povidone-iodine swabs, repeat above step. Allow area to dry.	Disinfects skin. (Do not blow or fan dry.)

- ***Critical Decision Point***
  It is no longer recommended to routinely apply antimicrobial ointment to catheter insertion site at time of insertion or during routine dressing changes (see Chapter 19) (Pearson, 1996).

STEP	RATIONALE
4. Apply transparent or occlusive gauze dressing over site (see Chapter 36).	Reduces transmission of microorganisms to venipuncture site. Transparent dressing is less bulky, allows easy visualization of the site, and has waterproof and extended-wear properties (Krzywda and others, 1999).
5. Remove and dispose of gloves. Loop and tape tubing securely to client's shoulder. Do not kink tubing or apply tape over transparent dressing. Label dressing with date of insertion and catheter size.	Helps to reduce chance of accidentally pulling on catheter and causing dislodgement. Label provides reference for dressing change schedule.
6. Assist with chest x-ray examination.	Documents line position or presence of pneumothorax or other complications.
7. Reposition client.	Maintains comfort.
8. When position of central vein catheter is confirmed, prepare parenteral nutrition solution obtained from pharmacy for infusion via infusion pump (Skill 23-2).	Infusion pump will ensure regular infusion of prescribed volume of PN.
9. Dispose of supplies and wash hands.	Reduces transmission of microorganisms.

EVALUATION

STEP	RATIONALE
1. Observe client for shortness of breath, pain in the chest or shoulder within 23 to 48 hours after insertion of catheter.	Symptoms indicate delayed complication of pneumothorax.
2. Observe client for bleeding or swelling at the insertion site and occlusiveness of the dressing.	Symptoms may indicate infiltration of intravenous fluids into subcutaneous tissues or damage to vessel lumen. Dressing must remain occlusive to effectively protect against entrance of microorganisms.
3. Observe insertion site over time for erythema, warmth, tenderness, edema, or drainage.	Symptoms may indicate infection at line insertion site.
4. Measure client's body temperature routinely.	Fever can be early warning sign of systemic infection resulting from entrance of microorganisms into bloodstream.

UNEXPECTED OUTCOMES AND RELATED INTERVENTIONS (SEE TABLE 23-2)

- Displacement of the central vein catheter into veins of the neck or chest.
  - Physician will withdraw catheter and insert new catheter into different site.
- Pneumothorax resulting from insertion of catheter into pleural space.
  - Call physician immediately. Chest x-ray film will be obtained to confirm diagnosis.
  - Prepare for removal of catheter.
- Bleeding at the insertion site or into the pleural cavity.
  - Call physician.
  - Prepare for removal of catheter.
- Inability to place central vein catheter despite attempts.
  - Insertion of peripherally inserted central catheter line provides viable option for parenteral therapy if client has intact peripheral veins (Chapter 19).

RECORDING AND REPORTING

- Record condition of client before, during, and after procedure.
- Document size, type, and location of central catheter, presence or absence of blood return after placement of central vein catheter, type of dressing, and type and rate of PN infused.
- Document confirmation of appropriate position of central vein catheter following x-ray examination.

Teaching Considerations

- Instruct client to report discomfort around the site; in either arm, shoulder, or side of the neck; or any shortness of breath.

Pediatric Considerations

- Central vein catheters that are of a smaller diameter and shorter length are available for children and infants.

Gerontological Considerations

- Older adults may have difficulty with lying flat in bed, and a modification of the totally supine position during insertion may be necessary.

Home Care Considerations

- Clients or family members may need to learn to perform catheter site care and dressing changes for long-term central venous catheters.

Skill 23-2 Caring for the Client Receiving Central Parenteral Nutrition

Caring for clients receiving central parenteral nutrition (CPN) requires the use of strict aseptic technique and the nurse's application of critical thinking. Because of the composition of CPN fluids, clients can experience metabolic and fluid balance changes quickly. In addition, the clinical condition of clients receiving CPN is usually poor, with clients experiencing alterations in host defenses, severe underlying illnesses, and extremes of age. The nurse must be prepared to anticipate changes in the client's condition that may signal complications developing. Similarly, the nurse must use good judgment in maintaining the intravenous (IV) system and to ensure it is in proper working order.

Intravenous catheters used to provide parenteral nutrition are at an increased risk for infection compared with catheters used for other therapies such as antibiotics or chemotherapy (Krzywda and others, 1999). At one time it was assumed that the high concentration of dextrose supported bacterial growth. Dextrose, however, is highly acidic and not a good growth medium for many common bacteria and fungi (Orr, 1999). Nonetheless, preventing infection is a nursing priority when preparing and administering fluids and monitoring the infusion system.

Delegation Considerations

Caring for clients receiving CPN should not be delegated to assistive personnel. Assistive personnel should be instructed to report immediately if CPN infusion pump alarm sounds or if client complains of moist or leaking dressing/tubing.

Equipment

- IV infusion tubing
- CPN solution (IV) (Figure 23-4)
- IV filter (optional—0.22 μmm for dextrose/amino acids, 1.2 μm for three-in-one solutions)
- Intravenous infusion pump

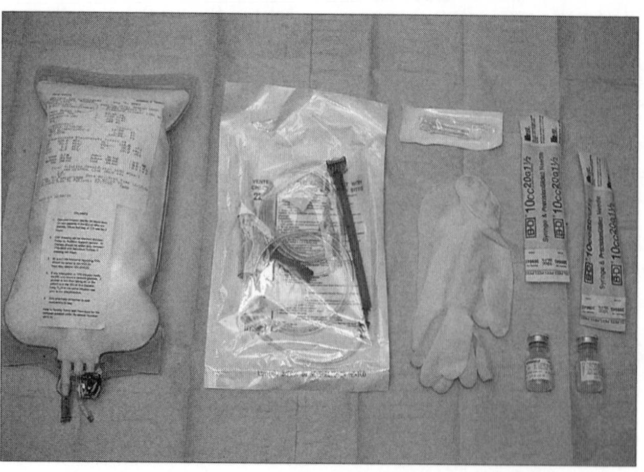

FIGURE 23-4 Parenteral nutrition solution and tubing.

STEP	RATIONALE

ASSESSMENT

STEP	RATIONALE
1. Assess client's nutritional status (see Skill 23-1), caloric intake, and weight.	Nurse needs to be aware of client's nutritional parameters to monitor and judge response to therapy.
2. Inspect condition of central vein access or peripherally inserted central catheter (PICC) access for presence of inflammation, edema, tenderness at site, and whether tubing is patent and not kinked.	Nurse monitors site to identify early signs of infection, infiltration, or disruption in system integrity. Development of complication may contraindicate infusion of fluids.
3. Assess client's blood glucose level (finger stick—see Chapter 41).	Provides baseline for measuring tolerance to high concentration of glucose infusion.
4. Assess factors influencing CPN administration.	Clients who have electrolyte disturbances, elevated blood glucose level, renal dysfunction, or hepatic dysfunction may require their CPN therapy to be adapted by composition or volume (requires physician order).
5. Assess vital signs and auscultate client's lung sounds.	Provides baseline for monitoring client's response to fluid infusion. Crackles in lungs are early indication of fluid volume excess.
6. Verify physician's order for nutrients, minerals, vitamins, trace elements, and electrolytes, as well as flow rate.	CPN must be ordered by physician and is often ordered daily in the hospital setting after review of laboratory values. In the home setting, orders may be obtained less frequently (e.g., weekly).

NURSING DIAGNOSIS

Defining characteristics from the assessment data may reveal the following nursing diagnoses for clients requiring this skill:

Imbalanced nutrition: less than body requirements

Risk for infection

Related factors are individualized based on client's condition or needs.

PLANNING

STEP	RATIONALE
1. **Expected outcomes** following completion of procedure:	
▪ Client's ideal weight gain is usually between 1 and 2 lb/week.	Weight is an indicator of how well the client is doing nutritionally and determines fluid volume. Weight gain greater than 1 lb/day indicates fluid retention.
▪ Serum glucose levels are less than 200 mg/100 ml.	A serum glucose level less than 200 mg/100 ml will reflect a metabolic tolerance to the concentrated glucose solution in PN.
▪ Central access catheter or PICC device is patent and site is free of pain, swelling, redness or inflammation. PICC site is free of phlebitis.	Ensures that CPN is infusing into the vein rather than into surrounding tissues and that there are no signs of an access device infection.
2. Explain purposes of CPN.	Promotes understanding and reduces anxiety.

IMPLEMENTATION

STEP	RATIONALE
1. Wash hands and put on gloves.	Reduces transmission of microorganisms.
2. Check that ordered parenteral nutrition (PN) solution is correct with correct additives and properly labeled. Check solution expiration date.	Prevents medication error.

STEP	RATIONALE
3. Inspect PN solution for particulate matter or, if it is a three-in-one solution, inspect emulsion for a cream layer or separation of the fat into a layer. If there is a thin layer of aggregated fat droplets about 1 to 2 cm in thickness, agitate bag (Driscoll and Baron, 2000).	Deterioration of a three-in-one solution results in breakdown of the emulsion.

- ***Critical Decision Point***
  Do not use PN solution if it has coalesced (thick, dense layer of fat droplets at surface, appearing 10 cm in thickness) or oiled out (fat droplets separate from solution and appear as a clear layer at surface). Notify the pharmacy, and request a new solution. (Driscoll and Baron, 2000).

STEP	RATIONALE
4. Check client's identification band and ask client to state name.	Ensures correct client receives correct intravenous solution.
5. Connect PN solution to appropriate intravenous tubing, prime tubing being sure no air bubbles remain, and turn off flow with roller clamp. Connect end of tubing to central or peripheral catheter line and open roller clamp to rate that maintains patency of line.	Air introduced into central circulation can result in an air embolus, a fatal complication. PN solutions need to be connected to new, sterile intravenous tubing every 23 hours.
6. Place IV tubing into an intravenous infusion pump, open roller clamp completely and regulate flow rate on pump as ordered (see Chapter 19) (see illustration).	CPN flow rates are ordered to meet client's metabolic and electrolyte needs. Rate must be maintained to prevent electrolyte imbalances. Typically the initial administration rate is 40 to 60 ml/hr. The rate is advanced each day toward the target rate to provide adequate calories and protein.

- ***Critical Decision Point***
  Rate of infusion may be increased gradually to prevent metabolic and electrolyte abnormalities. CPN is hyperosmolar and is usually tolerated when increased in stepwise fashion. Do not abruptly discontinue CPN, because this may lead to hypoglycemia. If discontinued suddenly, hang infusion of 5% Dextrose in water at same infusion rate (American Society for Parenteral and Enteral Nutrition [ASPEN], 1993).

STEP	RATIONALE
7. Discard used supplies and wash hands.	Reduces transmission of infection.

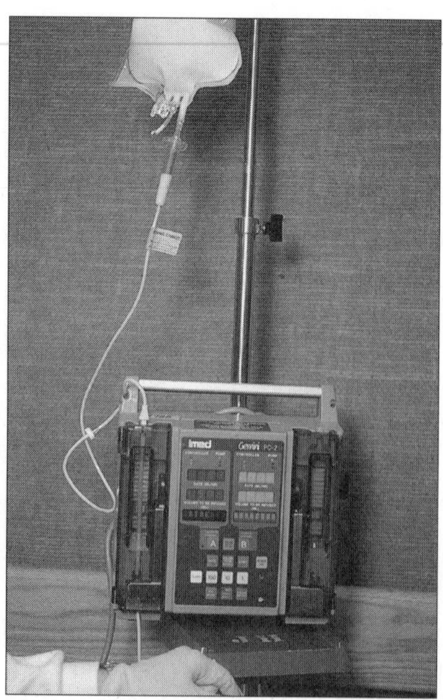

STEP **6** Parenteral nutrition solution infusing via infusion pump.

STEP	RATIONALE
EVALUATION	
1. Monitor flow rate routinely, at least hourly.	Too rapid or slow infusion could result in metabolic disturbances.
2. Obtain daily weights.	Over time, daily weights will reflect weight gain/loss resulting either from caloric intake or fluid retention.
3. Assess for fluid retention.	Weight gain in excess of 1 lb/day, dependent edema, lung crackles, and intake greater than output per each 24-hour period indicate fluid retention.
4. Monitor client's glucose and laboratory parameters to determine response to CPN.	Adequate tolerance is demonstrated by maintenance of normal electrolyte levels, satisfactory fluid balance, acceptable serum glucose levels, gradual increase in weight, and improvement in serum proteins.
5. Inspect central venous access site.	Determines presence of patency and absence of infection, infiltration, or phlebitis.

Unexpected Outcomes and Related Interventions

- There is redness, swelling, and tenderness around the venous access site, indicating possible exit site infection.
  - Notify physician. Apply warm compress, and initiate daily site care as ordered. Antibiotic therapy may begin.
- Client develops fever, malaise, and chills, indicating systemic infection.
  - Signs of exit site infection also may be present. Notify physician and consult about the need to obtain cultures of exit site or blood. Antibiotic therapy may begin.
- Infusion stops flowing or flows at a rate slower than ordered.
  - Venous access device may have become occluded with fibrin or particulate matter. Report the occlusion to the physician.
  - If the device is a surgically placed device or PICC (see Chapter 19), a thrombolytic agent may be ordered.
- Client experiences weight gain greater than 1 lb/day. Taut skin turgor may also be present. Crackles auscultated over lung fields.
  - Symptoms indicate fluid retention rather than restoration of body proteins.
- Serum glucose is greater than 200 mg/100 ml.
  - Indicates client's intolerance to glucose load in the CPN solution.
  - May document need for addition of insulin to the CPN, modification of CPN solution, or sliding-scale insulin coverage.
- Serum electrolytes are out of normal range.
  - May indicate movement of electrolytes in response to infusion of fluids and glucose.
  - The electrolyte levels in the solution may need to be adjusted.

Recording and Reporting

- Record condition of central venous access device, rate and type of infusion, intake and output each shift, vital signs, and weights.
- If signs of infection, occlusion, fluid retention, or infiltration occur, notify the physician.

Teaching Considerations

- Instruct client and family about the purpose and goals of CPN.
- Teach client and primary caregiver to monitor client's weight, calorie count, intake and output, and serum glucose.
- Teach client and primary caregiver about actions to take in case of emergency or unexpected outcomes.

Pediatric Considerations

- Indications for parenteral nutrition for infants include gastroschisis, congenital anomalies of the gastrointestinal system, and short-bowel syndrome.
- CPN can cause hepatobiliary dysfunction in infants.
- Catheter-related sepsis and thrombosis of central veins is more prevalent in the pediatric population (Chwals, 1994).

Gerontological Considerations

- Older adults may have impaired ability to manage higher fluid volumes, lipid intolerance, or an increased incidence of hyperglycemia.

Home Care Considerations

- Observe client and primary caregiver perform procedure in hospital before discharge (see Chapter 40).

Skill 23-3 Caring for the Client Receiving Peripheral Parenteral Nutrition With Lipid (Fat) Emulsion

The administration of parenteral nutrition via peripheral veins requires the use of lower concentrations of dextrose and amino acids to lower tonicity and lessen the risk of vein damage (Table 23-3). For example, 2 L of peripheral parenteral nutrition (PPN) consisting of 10% dextrose and 10% amino acids supplemented by 500 ml of 1% intravenous (IV) fat emulsion provide 2000 kcal/day. PPN is usually administered in conjunction with fat emulsion. Unfortunately, PPN is often difficult to maintain because of frequent episodes of phlebitis in superficial arm veins and infiltrations of solutions into subcutaneous tissue. Therefore the final dextrose concentration must be no greater than 10%, because the peripheral vein will sclerose at higher concentrations. However, solutions of lower concentration make it difficult to supply adequate calories and amino acids through a peripheral vein. This problem, in addition to the scarcity of adequate access sites, is the reason many experts recommend PPN for only short periods of time. Nutrients given through central veins may be very concentrated (e.g., 1800 mOsm). However, concentrations this great are not tolerated in peripheral veins because of their relatively low blood flow. Indications for PPN include the following:

1. Short-term need for parenteral nutrition: NPO (nothing by mouth) for more than 5 days but anticipation that the client will tolerate enteral or oral nutrition within 7 to 10 days.
2. History of problems with central vein access or inability to establish central vein access. Clients with a history of multiple central venous catheter infections or occlusions have increased risks associated with catheter placement. Multiple catheter placements may deplete access sites.
3. Adequate peripheral access. Despite its lower osmolality, PPN tends to cause phlebitis and may require frequent changes in the access location.
4. Ability to tolerate larger volumes of fluid. Because of the lower concentration of dextrose in PPN, a larger volume of fluid is required to attain adequate calories. Clients with impaired renal or cardiac function may not tolerate PPN.
5. Ability to tolerate lipid emulsions. Lipid is the most calorically dense nutrient, and PPN without lipid would not provide adequate calories unless very large volumes of fluid were provided. One liter of 10% dextrose provides only 340 kcal. Five hundred milliliters of 10% lipid provides 550 kcal.

Table 23-3 Comparison of Central Parenteral Nutrition (CPN) and Peripheral Parenteral Nutrition (PPN)

	CPN	PPN
Osmolality	1800 to 2000 mOsm	600 to 700 mOsm
Route of administration	Central venous catheter	Small peripheral vein
Usual daily caloric intake	2000 to 4000	700 to 2000
Fat emulsion	Minor caloric source; provides essential fatty acid	Major caloric source; provides essential fatty acid
Objectives	Weight maintenance; weight gain	Weight maintenance
Duration of therapy	6 days or longer	3 to 7 days

Delegation Considerations

The skill of caring for a client receiving peripheral parenteral nutrition with lipid emulsion should not be delegated to assistive personnel. Assistive personnel should be instructed to report if infusion pump alarm sounds.

Equipment

- PPN solution
- Lipid emulsion
- Two sets of IV tubing (filter optional—0.22 μm for amino acid/dextrose solution)
- Needle (19 gauge), Y connector, or stopcock
- Alcohol swab
- Infusion pump

Step	Rationale
Assessment	
1. Assess client for potential lipid intolerance. Assess serum triglyceride level. Serum triglyceride should be drawn before initiation of fat therapy (baseline) and 6 hours after fat has infused.	Determines client's ability to metabolize lipid.

STEP	RATIONALE
2. Select or initiate appropriate functional IV site to administer PPN and lipid emulsion. Assess its patency and function (Chapter 19).	Fat emulsions may be given through separate IV, piggybacked through peripheral line, or admixed in solution bag.
3. Check administration time for fat emulsion.	Fat emulsions may cause adverse symptoms if infused too rapidly as a separate infusion. The infusion time should be at least 4 hours. Fat emulsions should hang no longer than 10 hours as a separate infusion. When admixed with the PPN, fats are administered over 23 hours.
4. Check physician's order for volume of fat emulsion and PPN solution.	Fat emulsions and PPN must be ordered by physician.

NURSING DIAGNOSIS

Defining characteristics from the assessment data may reveal the following nursing diagnoses for clients requiring this skill:

Imbalanced nutrition: less than body requirements

Risk for infection

Related factors are individualized based on client's condition or needs.

PLANNING

1. **Expected outcomes** following completion of procedure:	
▪ Triglyceride level is stable.	Indicates physical tolerance to fat.
▪ Venipuncture site is free of phlebitis, pain, swelling, redness, and inflammation.	Ensures proper administration of PPN with lipids.
▪ Client does not show signs of systemic infection (e.g., elevated temperature).	Temperature is an indication of possible systemic infection related to parenteral nutrition.
2. Explain purposes of PPN.	Promotes understanding and reduces anxiety.
3. Place client in a comfortable position for IV insertion or initiation of infusion.	When clients are comfortable, they tolerate procedures more readily.
4. Check that ordered parenteral nutrition (PN) solution is correct with correct additives and properly labeled. Check solution expiration date. Inspect bottle for opacity and consistency in texture and color.	Prevents medication error.
5. Warm solution to room temperature if refrigerated.	Prevents change in body temperature from instillation of cold solution.

IMPLEMENTATION

1. Wash hands and put on gloves.	Reduces transmission of microorganisms.
2. Check client's identification band and ask client to state name.	Ensures correct client receives correct intravenous solution.
3. Connect tubing to PPN solution, run fat emulsion into IV tubing, and remove excess air. Turn roller clamp to off position.	To prevent air from entering vascular system, all tubing must be purged.
4. Clean peripheral line tubing injection port of primary IV with alcohol swab (Optional: use Y connector).	Removes surface organisms at injection site and prevents organisms from entering blood system.
5. Insert end of fat emulsion infusion tubing into injection port of main IV, proximal to the venipuncture site, below the infusion filter on the main parenteral nutrition line.	Fat emulsions cannot infuse through a 0.22 μm micron IV filter—the emulsion would separate.

Step	Rationale
6. Open roller clamp completely on fat emulsion infusion, and then set flow rate on infusion pump.	Up to 2.5 g fat per kilogram per day may be infused, but fat emulsion should not exceed 60% of total calories. Recommended daily fat percentage is 30% or less of total calories.
7. Begin PPN at ordered rate—10% fat emulsions are infused over at least 4 hours, and 20% fats are infused over at least 6 hours. All fats can hang for 10 hours; admixing fats can hang for 23 hours.	The rate of PPN administration does not need to be gradually increased. The lower concentration of dextrose allows most clients to tolerate the full administration rate without difficulty.
8. Discard supplies and wash hands.	Reduces transmission of infection.

Evaluation

Step	Rationale
1. Measure vital signs and client's general comfort level every 10 minutes for first 30 minutes.	Monitors client for fat emulsion intolerance.
2. Measure client's laboratory values daily.	Provides objective data to measure the response to therapy.
3. Monitor temperature every 4 hours, and regularly inspect venipuncture site for signs of phlebitis or infiltration.	Determines onset of fever, a complication of intolerance to fat emulsion or sepsis. Determines integrity of IV system.
4. Assess client's weight, intake and output (I&O), condition of peripheral extremities (for edema), and breath sounds.	Weight gain, I&O imbalance, peripheral edema, and crackles in lungs can indicate fluid retention.

Unexpected Outcomes and Related Interventions

- There is intolerance to fat emulsion, as evidenced by increased triglyceride levels, increased temperature (3° to 4° F), chills, headache, nausea and vomiting, muscle ache, backache, chest pain.
  - Confer with physician, and determine if fat emulsion should be discontinued.
- See Unexpected Outcomes and Related Interventions for Skill 23-2.

Recording and Reporting

- Record intake and output every shift on flow sheet.
- Record temperature every 4 hours.
- Record condition of IV site, type of PPN, and rate and status of infusion.

Teaching Considerations

- Teach client and primary caregiver to monitor client's weight, calorie count, intake and output, and IV site.

Pediatric Considerations

- Indications for parenteral nutrition for infants include gastroschisis, congenital anomalies of the gastrointestinal system, and short-bowel syndrome.
- Central parenteral nutrition (CPN) can cause hepatobiliary dysfunction in infants.
- Catheter-related sepsis and thrombosis of central veins is more prevalent in the pediatric population (Chwals, 1994).

Gerontological Considerations

- Older adults may have impaired ability to manage higher fluid volumes, lipid intolerance, or an increased incidence of hyperglycemia.

Home Care Considerations

- Observe client and primary caregiver perform procedure in hospital before discharge (see Chapter 40).

Critical Thinking Exercises

1. Mrs. Lester is a 70-year-old client with bilateral cataracts, high blood pressure, and osteoarthritis. She has been hospitalized for over 6 days following a resection of a tumor in her colon. Her inability to tolerate oral or enteral feedings has led her physician to order parenteral nutrition. It is possible that Mrs. Lester will be discharged home with parenteral nutrition. Mrs. Lester is widowed, but her sister lives a block away. What factors might influence the physician's choice of the type of vascular access device for Mrs. Lester?
2. The nurse assists the physician to place a central vein catheter. About 1 hour after the procedure, the client complains of pain and shortness of breath. The results of the chest x-ray examination are not yet available. What complication of central catheter placement might these symptoms indicate?
3. Before preparing to hang the first intravenous (IV) fluid bag of total parenteral nutrition (TPN), the nurse on the morning shift checks the client's weight and blood glucose level (finger stick). For what reason are these measures taken?

References

American Society for Parenteral and Enteral Nutrition: Guidelines for the use of parenteral and enteral nutrition in adult and pediatric patients, *JPEN* 17(4)(suppl):1SA, 1993.

American Society for Parenteral and Enteral Nutrition: Standards of practice: nutrition support nurses, *Nutr Clin Pract* 11(3):127, 1996.

Bozzetti F and others: Perioperative total parenteral nutrition in malnourished gastrointestinal cancer patients: a randomized clinical trial, *JPEN* 24(1):7, 2000.

CDC NNIS System: National Nosocomial Infections Surveillance (NNIS) report, data summary from October, 1986-April 1997, issued May 1997, *Am J Infect Control* 25:477, 1997.

Chwals WJ: Infant and pediatric nutrition. In Zaloga GP, editor: *Nutrition in critical care,* St. Louis, 1994, Mosby.

Davis CL: Nursing care of total parenteral and enteral nutrition. In Fischer JE, editor: *Total parenteral nutrition,* ed 2, Boston, 1991, Little, Brown.

Driscoll DF, Baron MN: Physiochemical stability of two types of intravenous lipid emulsions as total nutrient admixture, *JPEN* 24(1):15, 2000.

Hickey MS: *Handbook of enteral, parenteral, and ARC/AIDS nutritional therapy,* St. Louis, 1992, Mosby.

Intravenous Nurses Society: Revised intravenous nursing standards of practice, *J Intraven Nurs* 21:S49, 1998.

Krzywda EA and others: Catheter infections: diagnosis, etiology, treatment, and prevention, *Nutr Clin Pract* 14:178, 1999.

Lewis SM and others: *Medical-surgical nursing: assessment and management of clinical problems,* ed 5, St. Louis, 2000, Mosby.

Maki DG, McCormack KN: Defatting catheter insertion sites in TPN is of no value as an infection control measure, *Am J Med* 83:833, 1987.

Mermel LA: Prevention of intravascular catheter-related infections, *Infect Dis Clin Pract* 3:391, 1994.

Nussbaum MS, Fischer JE: Parenteral nutrition. In Zaloga GP, editor: *Nutrition in critical care,* St. Louis, 1994, Mosby.

Orr ME: Vascular access device selection for parenteral nutrition, *Nutr Clin Pract* 14:172, 1999.

Pearson ML (Hospital Infection Control Practices Advisory Committee): Guidelines for prevention of intravascular-device–related infections, *Infect Control Hosp Epidemiol* 17(7):438, 1996.

Pennington CR: Toward safer parenteral nutrition, *Aliment Pharmacol Ther* 4(5):427, 1990 (review article).

Raad II and others: Prevention of central venous catheter-related infections by using maximal sterile barrier precautions during insertion, *Infect Control Hosp Epidemiol* 15:231, 1994.

Shizgal HM, Knowles JB: Peripheral amino acids. In Fischer JE, editor: *TPN,* ed 2, Boston, 1991, Little, Brown.

Shuster MH: Parenteral nutrition. In Hennesy KA, Orr ME, editors: *Core curriculum for nutrition support nursing,* ed 3, Silver Spring Md, 1996, American Society for Parenteral and Enteral Nutrition.

24

Urinary Elimination

Skills

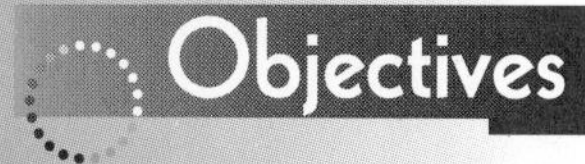

Mastery of content in this chapter will enable the nurse to:

- Define the key terms listed.
- Identify factors that alter normal voiding.
- Describe devices used to promote urinary drainage.
- Perform the following skills: place and remove urinal, insert urinary catheter, care for an indwelling urinary catheter, obtain residual urine, irrigate a catheter, remove a retention catheter, apply a condom catheter, and administer intermittent peritoneal and continuous ambulatory peritoneal dialysis.

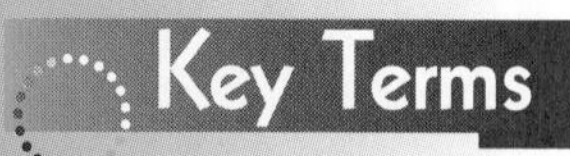

Catheterization
Dialysis
External urethral sphincter
Incontinence
Intake
Micturition
Nosocomial (hospital-acquired) infections
Output
Residual urine
Urinary retention
Urinary tract infections
Urine
Urine specific gravity
Void

Urinary elimination is a natural and often private process individuals take for granted until it is altered by some uncontrollable physiological factor. Clients needing assistance with urinary elimination may require physiological and psychological assistance from the nurse. Physiological support may require use of an invasive procedure such as the insertion of a catheter into the bladder. Psychological assistance may be needed to help the client adjust to an alteration in urinary elimination. Therefore the nurse must be competent in performing technical skills and sensitive to a client's psychological needs.

The urinary tract is susceptible to infections, particularly when invaded, as is the case when a sterile catheter is inserted. Therefore the nurse must be able to apply the principles of sterile asepsis when inserting a catheter. In addition, when caring for clients with catheters, nurses must follow medical asepsis guidelines such as hand washing to prevent cross contamination between clients and from objects to clients (Asci and Beyea, 1996).

Certain disease processes, medications, and stages of growth and development influence fluid and electrolyte status. Physical assessment findings can indicate that a fluid or electrolyte imbalance exists. The nurse must know the factors influencing fluid and electrolyte balance and the signs and symptoms of fluid imbalances. A client's hydration status is an important physiological indicator that is closely monitored, especially when the urinary system is altered. When clients have altered or impaired elimination, their **intake** (fluids ingested) and **output** (fluids excreted) (I&O) are often measured to help monitor fluid and electrolyte balance (see Chapter 10).

Skill Performance Guidelines

1. Know the client's usual fluid intake pattern, including the types and amounts of fluids and when they are ingested, and assess the client's fluid preferences regarding types, temperature, and amount of fluids preferred at one time.
2. Know the client's normal range of vital signs. Abnormal fluid and electrolyte balances can affect the amount of circulating blood volume. During dehydration, the blood pressure may be decreased and the pulse and body temperature may be elevated. Overhydration usually produces a bounding pulse; the rate may be either increased or decreased. Blood pressure may rise slightly, but body temperature remains unchanged.
3. Know the client's medical history, including diseases and any therapies the client is receiving that may affect bladder function. Clients with injuries from burns or trauma or cardiopulmonary or renal disease frequently have fluid imbalances. Medications may affect fluid and electrolyte balance. Diuretics are successfully used to regulate fluid balance; however, side effects can further potentiate fluid and electrolyte imbalances. Steroids are frequently used to treat severe inflammatory conditions, but they may cause the retention of sodium and water and increase excretion of potassium.
4. Be aware of environmental conditions that can affect fluid balance. Prolonged exposure to extreme environmental temperatures can cause increased loss of body fluids.
5. Know the signs of dehydration and fluid overload (Table 24-1).
6. Institute measurement of I&O when there is an anticipated or suspicious change in fluid balance. The nurse is responsible for the maintenance of accurate records. Measurements are kept throughout the day and totaled every 8 hours, but the nurse may determine that more frequent measurements are required (see Chapter 10).
7. Know the average output range for the clients for whom you are caring. Adult urinary output averages 1000 to 2400 ml in 24 hours. Minimum average hourly output is 30 ml; output is frequently monitored in acutely ill clients on an hourly or bihourly schedule.
8. It may be necessary to weigh the client to help assess fluid status. Remember to obtain weights with the same scale, same time of day, and with comparable articles of clothing, including bed linen if bed weights are necessary.
9. Consider the client's age when assessing micturition habits. Toilet training and enuresis are concerns that

Table 24-1 Signs of Dehydration and Fluid Overload

Eyes	*Dehydration:* sunken eyes, dry conjunctivae, decrease or absence of tearing *Fluid overload:* periorbital edema, blurred vision, papilledema
Mouth	*Dehydration:* sticky, dry mucous membrane; dry, cracked lips; decreased saliva; increased viscosity of saliva; furrowed, shrunken tongue *Fluid overload:* excessive salivation
Skin	*Dehydration:* increased skin temperature; dry, scaly skin; poor turgor *Fluid overload:* edema
Cardiovascular	*Dehydration:* increased pulse rate, weak pulse, hypotension, decreased capillary filling, increased hematocrit *Fluid overload:* bounding pulse rate, blood pressure normal with or without orthostatic changes, third heart sound (S_3), distended neck veins
Gastrointestinal	*Dehydration:* sunken abdomen *Dehydration or fluid overload:* vomiting, diarrhea, abdominal cramps
Renal	*Dehydration:* oliguria or anuria, **urine-specific gravity** increased (normal, 1.010 to 1.030) *Fluid overload:* decreased specific gravity, diuresis (if kidneys are normal)

arise in the toddler and preschooler. In the adult, increasing age may bring disease and physiological changes that predispose to **incontinence,** or the inability to control urination.

10. Encouraging fluids is a nursing responsibility. Any client not restricted in total fluid intake should be assessed; if oral intake is not minimally 1500 ml/day, a plan of care should be developed with the client to increase fluids. Clients with urinary problems may be hesitant to take fluids in fear of incontinence and/or increased urinary frequency. Education on the importance of fluid intake in maintaining urinary and overall health is vital.
11. Know the client's most recent serum electrolyte measurements. Abnormal electrolyte values can affect fluid balance and, if uncorrected, can lead to deterioration of the client's health status or even death.
12. Practice asepsis conscientiously. Because **urinary tract infections** are the most prevalent **nosocomial (hospital-acquired) infections,** it is imperative that the nurse adhere to standard precautions guidelines. Glove changes and hand washing between care of different clients is critically important. The nurse should teach clients, particularly girls and women, proper perineal hygiene habits (see Chapter 6).
13. Know the client's level of comfort. A client uncomfortable physically or psychologically may be unable to relax the **external urethral sphincter** (voluntary muscle at the neck of the bladder) and therefore not be able to urinate (**void**) or completely empty the bladder. The nurse can promote comfort measures by providing privacy, offering the client a warm bedpan, assisting the client into a normal voiding position (standing for a man, squatting for a woman), or reducing pain by administering a prescribed analgesic before helping the client walk to the bathroom. Distraction measures, such as turning on a sink faucet so the client can hear water running, may help the client to void.
14. Identify conditions that weaken abdominal or pelvic muscles such as multiple abdominal or gynecological surgeries or pregnancies. Clients with weak abdominal or pelvic floor muscles can be taught exercises to strengthen these muscles and increase the ability of the bladder to contract and promote better control of the external urethral sphincter.
15. Know the client's normal patterns of urination or **micturition.** The client should be taught not to ignore the urge to void. The nurse can assist by responding readily to the client's request to use a bedpan, urinal, bathroom, or commode. The nurse can also offer the client the opportunity to void after meals, at regular intervals throughout the day, and before bedtime. Clients taking diuretic medications should receive them early in the morning so they do not need to void during the night.
16. Consider the client's functional status. Mobility and sensory problems may influence access to toileting facilities. Assessments that should be made include use of walking aids, distance to the toilet, ability to remove clothing or to get in and out of the bathroom, and lighting.

Skill 24-1 Assisting a Client in Using a Urinal

The client's ability to void depends on feeling the urge to urinate and on being able to control the urethral sphincter. One factor that can interfere with micturition is bed rest or immobility, which does not allow the client to assume the normal position for emptying the bladder. The female client is accustomed to squatting, which promotes contraction of the pelvic and abdominal muscles that assist in sphincter control and bladder contraction. The nurse assists the bedridden woman in using a bedpan for voiding (see Chapter 25). A man voids more easily in the standing position. If a man cannot walk to the toilet facilities, he may stand at the bedside and void into a urinal (a plastic or metal receptacle for **urine**). If he is unable to stand at the bedside, the nurse needs to assist him in using the urinal in bed.

Delegation Considerations

The skill of assisting a client to use a urinal is often delegated to assistive personnel. The care provider should know standard precautions guidelines relating to body fluids, should be cautioned to be sensitive to the privacy needs of the client, and should be instructed to report information about urine such as changes in color, amount, or odor and the presence of incontinence. The care provider should be informed about the amount of assistance the client requires to use the urinal and if standing is permitted. In addition, the care provider should be reminded to teach the client and family about the procedure, so they can more fully understand and participate in care.

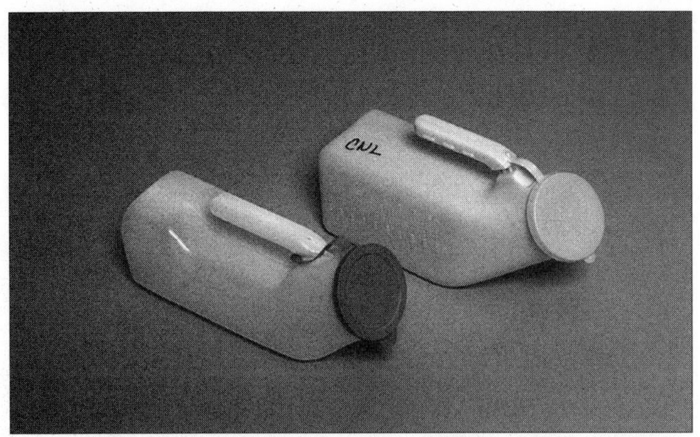

FIGURE 24-1 Types of male urinals.

Equipment

- Urinal (Figure 24-1)
- Disposable gloves
- Graduated cylinder (used for measuring volume if urinal is not marked)
- Supplies for diagnostic urine tests specimen collection

Step	Rationale
Assessment	
1. Assess client's normal urinary elimination habits.	Identifies normal pattern of urination; helps nurse to recognize when client may require use of urinal.
2. Assess for periods of incontinence.	May assist in planning when to offer urinal.
3. Palpate for distended bladder.	Indicates if bladder is full and client needs to void.
4. Assess client's cognitive and physical status.	Provides nurse with information about how much assistance is required to use urinal.
5. Assess client's knowledge regarding urinal use.	Reveals need for client instruction.

Nursing Diagnosis

Defining characteristics from the assessment data may reveal the following nursing diagnoses for clients requiring this skill:

Impaired urinary elimination
Impaired physical mobility
Deficient knowledge regarding use of urinal
Toileting self-care deficit

Related factors are individualized based on client's condition or needs.

Step	Rationale
Planning	
1. **Expected outcomes** following completion of procedure:	
■ Client is able to assist self with urinal. ■ Client remains continent.	Promotes self-care for toileting needs, decreases incontinence and its complications.
Implementation	
1. Wash hands and apply gloves.	Reduces transmission of microorganisms.
2. Provide privacy by closing bedside curtain or room door.	Promotes relaxation.
3. Assist client into appropriate position: position on side, back, or sitting with head of bed elevated or assist to standing position.	Men find it easier to void and empty bladder while standing.

STEP	RATIONALE
• ***Critical Decision Point*** *Always determine mobility status before having a client stand to void.*	
4. If possible, client should hold urinal and position penis in urinal. If client needs assistance, position penis completely within urinal and hold urinal in place or assist client to hold urinal.	Penis is placed completely within urinal to avoid urine spills.
5. Once client has finished voiding, remove urinal and wash and dry penis.	Prevents growth of microorganisms. Prevents skin breakdown.
6. Observe urine, empty and cleanse urinal, and return it to client for future use.	Avoids spilling and reduces odors.
7. Allow client to wash hands after voiding.	Reduces spread of microorganisms.
8. Remove and dispose of gloves; wash hands.	Reduces spread of microorganisms.

EVALUATION

1. Observe client for ability to use urinal and periods of incontinence.	Promotes modification of nursing care plan to include more assistance or increased frequency to assist client in using urinal.
2. Note amount, appearance, and odor of urine.	Indicates abnormalities.

UNEXPECTED OUTCOMES AND RELATED INTERVENTIONS

- Client is incontinent.
  - Increase frequency of prompted voidings.
  - Ensure client can reach urinal.
  - Monitor skin integrity.
  - Determine type of incontinence.
- Client unable to void using a urinal.
  - Attempt to place client in standing position and provide privacy (see Skill Performance Guidelines).
- Client experiences persistent urge, stress, or overflow incontinence.
  - Refer for urological evaluation.

RECORDING AND REPORTING

- Record and report client's ability to use urinal and characteristics of urinary output in nurses' notes.
- If I&O measurement is being monitored in client, include output data on flow sheet (see Chapter 10).
- Record client's voiding patterns, and report problems with voiding to physician.

TEACHING CONSIDERATIONS

- Clients should be taught not to ignore the urge to void. Poor habits may contribute to **urinary retention** (incomplete emptying of the bladder) problems.
- Hand washing is the best method for preventing infection. Clients may need this basic hygienic tip reinforced.
- Clients who are having difficulty with incontinence at night should be instructed to avoid tea, coffee, and other caffeine drinks during the evening hours.

PEDIATRIC CONSIDERATIONS

- Children who have been continent may become incontinent as a result of the stress from being ill and from separation from parents and home.
- Privacy norms will vary from household to household and with child's age. If child prefers privacy, nurse tries to prevent interruptions as child voids.
- Physiologically children can control their sphincters between the ages of 18 and 24 months (Wong and others, 1999).

GERONTOLOGICAL CONSIDERATIONS

- Aging process may impair micturition; elderly men may require urinal use more frequently to avoid urinary incontinence.
- The older man who is accustomed to standing to void may empty his bladder more readily if allowed to stand when using the urinal.
- Nocturia is common in older adults; use of urinal at night may help to prevent falls in an unfamiliar setting such as a hospital (Lueckenotte, 2000).

HOME CARE CONSIDERATIONS

- Incontinence is a major problem for homebound clients receiving Medicare reimbursement and nursing services. Often, however, clients will not report incontinence because of embarrassment (Hiser, 1999).
- Assess level of assistance required by client to determine if additional medical equipment (e.g., overbed trapeze, bedside commode) is necessary for the client to maintain continence.

- Before hospital discharge consider referral to home care agency to follow up and reinforce teaching concepts.

LONG-TERM CARE CONSIDERATIONS

- Urinary incontinence is a frequent problem in long-term care, but all residents should have a baseline assessment of any urinary problem. The assessment should include a history and physical examination, a voiding diary, a urinalysis, and postvoid residual urine determination. These guidelines were developed by the Omnibus Budget Reconciliation Act (OBRA) of 1987 (Ouslander and Schnelle, 1995).
- Urinary incontinence in nursing homes may be as high as 50% in some nursing facilities and is correlated with increased morbidity and health care costs (Ouslander and Schnelle, 1995).

Skill 24-2 Inserting a Straight or Indwelling Catheter

Catheterization of the bladder involves introducing a rubber or plastic tube through the urethra and into the bladder. The catheter provides for a continuous flow of urine in clients unable to control micturition or in those with obstruction to urine outflow. Because bladder catheterization carries the risk of the development of urinary tract infection (UTI), it is preferable to rely on less invasive measures to promote bladder emptying.

An indwelling or Foley catheter may remain in place for an extended period. It may be necessary to change indwelling catheters periodically. The nurse uses sterile asepsis when inserting an indwelling or straight catheter to reduce the risk of bladder infections. Intermittent catheterization, in which a straight catheter is used, can be repeated as necessary. Intermittent catheterization is a proven alternative for management of incontinence in many clients with spinal cord disease (Binard and others, 1996).

DELEGATION CONSIDERATIONS

The skill of urinary catheterization is not usually delegated to assistive personnel. The use of assistive personnel for inserting urinary catheters may occur in some settings, but it has not become routine practice. However, assistive personnel may assist with positioning the client, focusing lighting for the procedure, and aiding in the client's comfort during the procedure by measures such as holding the client's hand or keeping the client warm.

EQUIPMENT

- Catheterization kit (Figure 24-2) containing the following sterile items: gloves (extra pair optional); drapes, one fenestrated; lubricant; antiseptic cleansing solution; cotton balls; forceps; prefilled syringe with sterile water to inflate balloon of indwelling catheter; catheter of correct size and type for procedure (i.e., intermittent or indwelling); sterile drainage tubing with collection bag and multipurpose tube holder or tape, safety pin, and elastic band for securing tubing to bed if client is bedridden (for indwelling catheter); receptacle or basin (usually bottom of catheterization tray); and specimen container
- Blanket
- Waterproof absorbent pad
- Disposable gloves, basin with warm water, soap, face cloth, and towel
- Flashlight or other appropriate additional light as needed

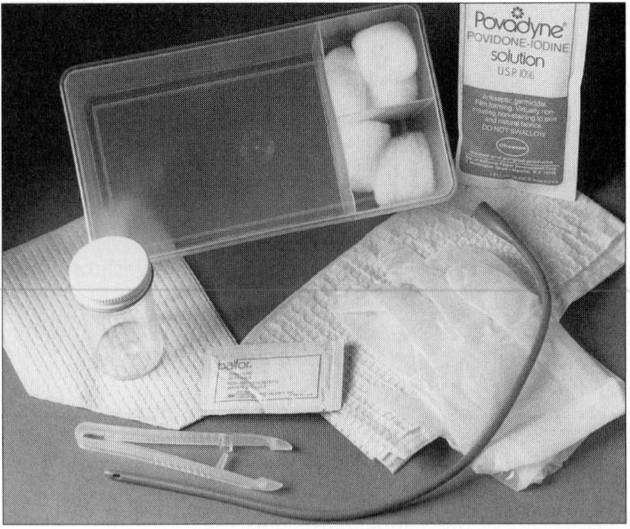

FIGURE 24-2 Catheterization kit.

Step	Rationale
Assessment	
1. Assess status of client:	
a. Time of last urination by asking client, checking intake and output (I&O) flow sheet.	Indicates likelihood of bladder fullness.
b. Level of awareness or developmental stage	Reveals client's ability to cooperate and level of explanation needed.
c. Mobility and physical limitations of client	Affect way that nurse positions client. Nurse can request additional nursing personnel to assist with this procedure if necessary.
d. Client's gender and age	Determines catheter size: 8 to 10 Fr is generally used for children, 14 to 16 Fr is indicated for women, 12 Fr may be considered for young girls, and 16 to 18 Fr is used for male clients unless larger size is ordered by physician.
2. Determine if client has distended bladder: bladder palpable above symphysis pubis; palpation causes urge.	Causes pain. Can indicate need to insert catheter if client is unable to void independently.
3. Assess for perineal anatomical landmarks, erythema, drainage, and odor.	Determines condition of perineum.
4. Assess for any pathological condition that may impair passage of catheter (e.g., enlarged prostate gland in men).	Obstruction prevents passage of catheter through urethra into bladder.

• ***Critical Decision Point***
Determine allergy to antiseptic, tape, latex, and lubricant. Betadine allergies are common; if the client is unaware of allergy, ask if allergic to shellfish.

Step	Rationale
5. Review client's medical record, including physician's order and nurses' notes.	Determine purpose of inserting catheter: preparation for surgery, urinary irrigations, collection of sterile urine specimen, or measurement of residual urine. Assess for previous catheterization, including catheter size, response of client, and time of last catheterization. Catheters may range in size from 6 Fr to 30 Fr (Evans, 1999).
6. Assess client's knowledge of the purpose for catheterization.	Reveals need for client instruction.

Nursing Diagnosis

Defining characteristics from the assessment data may reveal the following nursing diagnoses for clients requiring this skill:

- Acute pain
- Risk for infection
- Urinary retention

Related factors are individualized based on client's condition or needs.

Planning

Step	Rationale
1. **Expected outcomes** following completion of procedure:	
▪ Bladder distention relieved.	Removal of urine from bladder relieves sensation of fullness.
▪ Client will verbalize relief of discomfort in bladder within 24 hours of catheter insertion.	Patent catheter system keeps bladder empty and client comfortable.
▪ Minimum of 30 ml of urine is present in urinary collection bag every hour (see Chapter 10).	Verifies presence of catheter in bladder, catheter patency, and adequate perfusion to kidneys.
▪ Client verbalizes minimal pain during procedure.	Localized trauma may result from catheterization.
▪ Client verbalizes the purpose and expectations about the procedure.	Promotes cooperation.

Step	Rationale
Implementation	
1. Wash hands.	Reduces transmission of microorganisms. Infection is common after catheterization. Foley catheter systems are often colonized with bacteria within 48 hours of catheterization (Suchinski and others, 1999).
2. Close curtain or door.	Offers privacy, reduces embarrassment, and aids in relaxation during procedure.
3. Raise bed to appropriate working height.	Promotes use of proper body mechanics.
4. Facing client, stand on left side of bed if right-handed (on right side if left-handed). Clear bedside table and arrange equipment.	Successful catheter insertion requires nurse to assume comfortable position with all equipment easily accessible.
5. Raise side rail on opposite side of bed, and put side rail down on working side.	Promotes client safety.
6. Place waterproof pad under client.	Prevents soiling of bed linen.

- ***Critical Decision Point***
  Get assistance to position and to support weak or frail clients.

Step	Rationale
7. Position client:	Provides good visualization of perineal structures.
a. Female client:	
(1) Assist to dorsal recumbent position (supine with knees flexed). Ask client to relax thighs so the hip joints can be externally rotated.	Legs may be supported with pillows to reduce muscle tension and promote comfort.
(2) Position female client in side-lying (Sims') position with upper leg flexed at knee and hip if unable to be supine. If this position is used, nurse must take extra precautions to cover rectal area with drape during procedure to reduce chance of cross contamination.	This alternate position is used if client cannot abduct leg at hip joint (e.g., if client has arthritic joints). Also, this position may be more comfortable for client. Support client with pillows if necessary to maintain position.
b. Male client:	
(1) Assist to supine position with thighs slightly abducted.	Comfortable position for client that aids in visualization.
8. Drape client:	Avoids unnecessary exposure of body parts and maintains client's comfort.
a. Female client:	
(1) Drape with bath blanket. Place blanket diamond fashion over client, with one corner at client's neck, side corners over each arm and side, and last corner over perineum.	
b. Male client:	
(1) Drape upper trunk with bath blanket and cover lower extremities with bed sheets, exposing only genitalia.	
9. Wearing disposable gloves, wash perineal area with soap and water as needed; dry (see Chapter 6).	Reduces microorganisms near urethral meatus and allows further opportunity to visualize perineum and landmarks.
10. Position lamp to illuminate perineal area. (When using flashlight, have assistant hold it.)	Permits accurate identification and good visualization of urethral meatus.
11. Open package containing drainage system; place drainage bag over edge of bottom bed frame and bring drainage tube up between side rail and mattress.	Prepares bag for attachment to catheter.

- ***Critical Decision Point***
  This step is necessary only if indwelling catheter is to be inserted and drainage system is not part of the catheterization kit.

Step	Rationale
12. Open catheterization kit according to directions, keeping bottom of container sterile.	Prevents transmission of microorganisms from table or work area to sterile supplies. The materials in the kit are ordered in sequence of use.

STEP	RATIONALE
13. Place plastic bag that contains kit within reach of work area to use as waterproof bag to dispose of used supplies.	
14. Apply sterile gloves (see Chapter 32).	Allows nurse to handle sterile supplies without contamination.

- ***Critical Decision Point***
  If underpad is first item in kit, place the pad plastic side down under the client, touching only the edges so as to maintain sterility. Then apply sterile gloves (see Chapter 32 sterile fields).

STEP	RATIONALE
15. Organize supplies on sterile field. Open inner sterile package containing catheter. Pour sterile antiseptic solution into correct compartment containing sterile cotton balls. Open packet containing lubricant. Remove specimen container (lid should be loosely placed on top) and prefilled syringe from collection compartment of tray and set them aside on sterile field if needed.	Maintains principles of surgical asepsis and organizes work area.
16. Before inserting indwelling catheter, a common practice is to test balloon by injecting fluid from prefilled syringe into balloon port (see illustrations).	Checks integrity of balloon. Do not use the catheter if the balloon does not inflate or leaks. This is a controversial step. Follow manufacturer's recommendations. Checking the balloon in this way may stretch the balloon and cause increased trauma on insertion.
17. Lubricate catheter 2.5 to 5 cm (1 to 2 inches) for women and 12.5 to 17.5 cm (5 to 7 inches) for men. NOTE: Some catheter kits will have a plastic sheath over the catheter that must be removed prior to lubrication. (*Option:* physician may order use of lubricant containing local anesthetic.)	Eases insertion of catheter through urethral canal.
18. Apply sterile drape, keeping gloves sterile:	
a. Female client:	
(1) Allow top edge of drape to form cuff over both hands. Place drape down on bed between client's thighs. Slip cuffed edge just under buttocks, taking care not to touch contaminated surface with gloves.	Outer surface of drape covering hands remains sterile. Sterile drape against sterile gloves is sterile.
(2) Pick up fenestrated sterile drape and allow it to unfold without touching an unsterile object. Apply drape over perineum, exposing labia and being sure not to touch contaminated surface.	Maintains sterility of work surface.

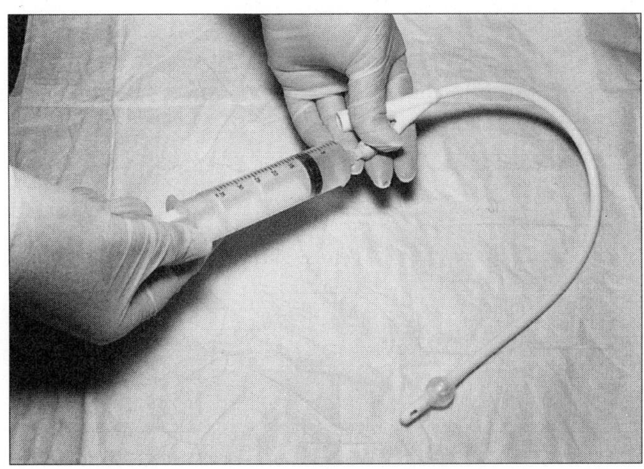

A

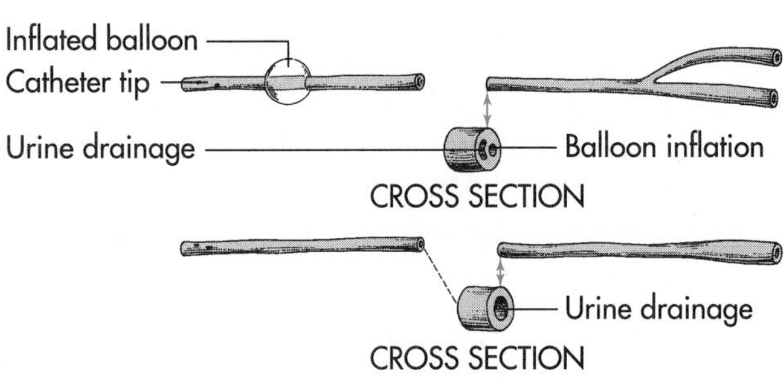

B

STEP **16** Types of urinary catheters. **A,** Indwelling (Foley) catheter. **B,** Straight catheter.

STEP	RATIONALE
b. Male client: Two methods are used for draping, depending on preference.	Maintains sterility of work surface.
(1) First method: Apply drape over thighs and under penis without completely opening fenestrated drape.	
(2) Second method: Apply drape over thighs just below penis. Pick up fenestrated sterile drape, allow it to unfold, and drape it over penis with fenestrated slit resting over penis.	
19. Place sterile tray and contents on sterile drape between legs. Open specimen container. NOTE: Client's size and positioning will dictate exact placement. This method works best with flexible, average-size clients.	Provides easy access to supplies during catheter insertion. Maintains aseptic technique during procedure.
20. Cleanse urethral meatus.	
a. Female client:	
(1) With nondominant hand, carefully retract labia to fully expose urethral meatus. Maintain position of nondominant hand throughout procedure.	Full visualization of urethral meatus is provided. Full retraction prevents contamination of urethral meatus during cleansing.

- ***Critical Decision Point***

  Closure of labia during cleansing requires that the procedure be repeated because the area has become contaminated.

STEP	RATIONALE
(2) Using forceps in sterile dominant hand, pick up cotton ball saturated with antiseptic solution and clean perineal area, wiping front to back from clitoris toward anus. Using a new cotton ball for each area, wipe along the far labial fold, near labial fold, and directly over center of urethral meatus.	Cleansing reduces number of microorganisms at urethral meatus (Asci and Beyea, 1996). Use of single cotton ball for each wipe prevents transfer of microorganisms. Preparation moves from area of least contamination to that of most contamination. Dominant hand remains sterile.
b. Male client:	
(1) If client is not circumcised, retract foreskin with nondominant hand. Grasp penis at shaft just below glans. Retract urethral meatus between thumb and forefinger. Maintain nondominant hand in this position throughout procedure.	Accidental release of foreskin or dropping of penis during cleansing requires process to be repeated because area has become contaminated.

- ***Critical Decision Point***

  If the foreskin does not remain retracted during insertion, then the cleansing procedure must be repeated because the area has become contaminated.

STEP	RATIONALE
(2) With dominant hand, pick up cotton ball with forceps and clean penis. Move it in circular motion from urethral meatus down to base of glans. Repeat cleansing three more times, using clean cotton ball each time.	Reduces number of microorganisms at urethral meatus and moves from areas of least to most contamination. Dominant hand remains sterile.
21. Pick up catheter with gloved dominant hand 7.5 to 10 cm (3 to 4 inches) from catheter tip. Hold end of catheter loosely coiled in palm of dominant hand (Optional: may grasp catheter with forceps). Place distal end of catheter in urine tray receptacle if straight catheterization is being done.	

- ***Critical Decision Point***

  Hold catheter near tip because it allows easier manipulation during insertion into urethral meatus and prevents distal end from striking contaminated surface.

STEP	RATIONALE
22. Insert catheter:	
a. Female client:	
(1) Ask client to bear down gently as if to void and slowly insert catheter through urethral meatus (see illustration).	Relaxation of external sphincter aids in insertion of catheter.
(2) Advance catheter a total of 5 to 7.5 cm (2 to 3 inches) in adult or until urine flows out catheter's end. When urine appears, advance catheter another 2.5 to 5 cm (1 to 2 inches). Do not force against resistance. Place end of catheter in urine tray receptacle.	Female urethra is short. Appearance of urine indicates that catheter tip is in bladder or lower urethra. Advancement of catheter ensures bladder placement.

• ***Critical Decision Point***

If no urine appears, check if catheter is in vagina. If misplaced, leave catheter in vagina as landmark indicating where not to insert, and insert another.

STEP	RATIONALE
(3) Release labia and hold catheter securely with nondominant hand. Inflate balloon if retention catheter is used (Box 24-1).	Bladder or sphincter contraction may cause accidental expulsion of catheter.
b. Male client:	
(1) Lift penis to position perpendicular to client's body and apply light traction (see illustration).	Straightens urethral canal to ease catheter insertion.
(2) Ask client to bear down as if to void and slowly insert catheter through urethral meatus.	Relaxation of external sphincter aids in insertion of catheter.

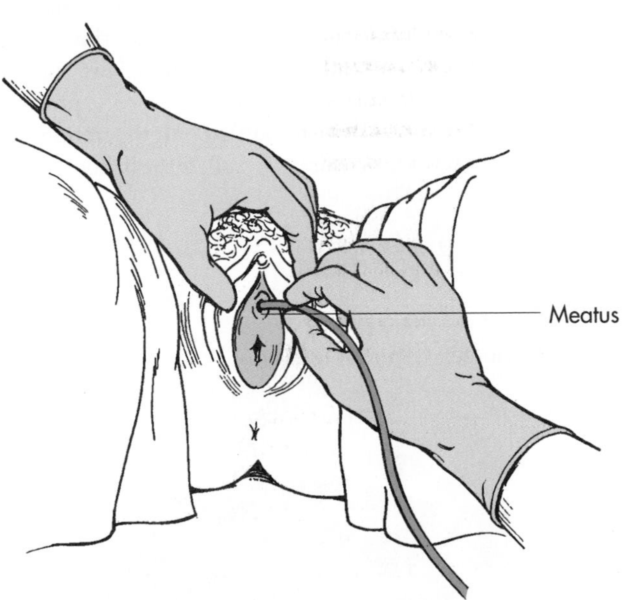

STEP **22a(1)** Inserting the catheter.

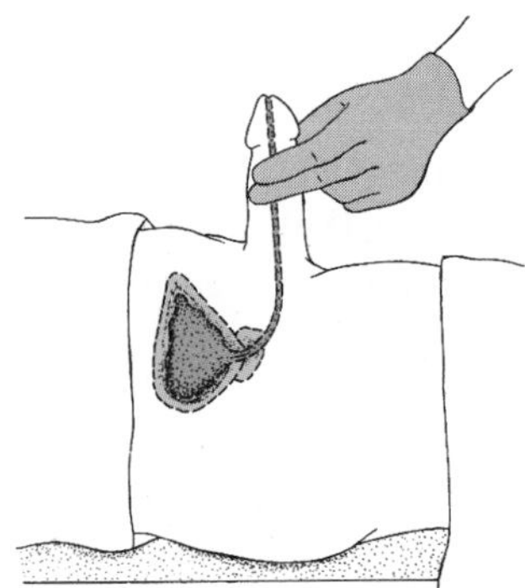

STEP **22b(1)** Structures of the male genitourinary system.

Box 24-1 Inflation of Balloon for Indwelling Catheter

Inflate balloon of indwelling catheter with amount of fluid recommended by the manufacturer.

a. While holding catheter with nondominant hand at urethral meatus, take end of catheter and place it between first two fingers of nondominant hand.
b. With free dominant hand, attach syringe to injection port at end of catheter.
c. Slowly inject total amount of solution. If client complains of sudden pain, aspirate solution and advance catheter farther.
d. After advancing catheter and inflating the balloon, release catheter and pull gently to feel resistance. Then move catheter slightly back into bladder.

STEP	RATIONALE
(3) Advance catheter 17 to 22.5 cm (7 to 9 inches) in adult or until urine flows out catheter's end. If resistance is felt, withdraw catheter; do not force it through urethra. When urine appears, advance catheter another 2.5 to 5 cm (1 to 2 inches). **Do not use force to insert a catheter.**	The adult male urethra is long. It is normal to meet resistance at the prostatic sphincter. When resistance is met, nurse should hold catheter firmly against sphincter without forcing catheter. After few seconds, sphincter relaxes and catheter is advanced. Appearance of urine indicates catheter tip is in bladder or urethra. Further advancement of catheter ensures proper placement.
(4) Lower penis and hold catheter securely in nondominant hand. Place end of catheter in urine tray receptacle. Inflate balloon if retention catheter is used (see Box 24-1).	Catheter may be accidentally expelled by bladder or urethral contraction. Collection of urine prevents soiling and provides output measurement.
(5) Reduce (or reposition) the foreskin.	Paraphimosis (retraction and constriction of the foreskin behind the glans penis), secondary to catheterization may occur if foreskin is not reduced.
23. Collect urine specimen as needed. Fill specimen cup or jar to desired level (20 to 30 ml) by holding end of catheter in dominant hand over cup.	Allows sterile specimen to be obtained for culture analysis.
24. Allow bladder to empty fully unless institution policy restricts maximal volume of urine drained with each catheterization (about 800 to 1000 ml).	Retained urine may serve as reservoir for growth of microorganisms (see Unexpected Outcomes and Related Interventions).

• ***Critical Decision Point***
If a straight, single-use catheter was inserted, withdraw catheter slowly but smoothly until removed.

STEP	RATIONALE
25. Inflate balloon fully per manufacturer's recommendations, and then release catheter with nondominant hand and pull gently to feel resistance.	Inflation of balloon anchors catheter tip in place above bladder outlet to prevent removal of catheter (see illustration). Note the size of balloon on the catheter. Most commonly a 5-ml balloon is used, but a 30-ml balloon may be ordered. A prefilled syringe may be included with the kit; use only the amount included. Do not overinflate or underinflate the balloon.

• ***Critical Decision Point***
If resistance is noted to inflation or the client complains of pain, the balloon may not be entirely within the bladder. Stop inflation; aspirate any fluid injected into the balloon and advance the catheter a little more before reattempting to inflate.

STEP	RATIONALE
26. Attach end of catheter to collecting tube of drainage system (see illustration). Drainage bag must be below level of bladder; do not place bag on side rails of bed.	Establishes closed system for urine drainage.

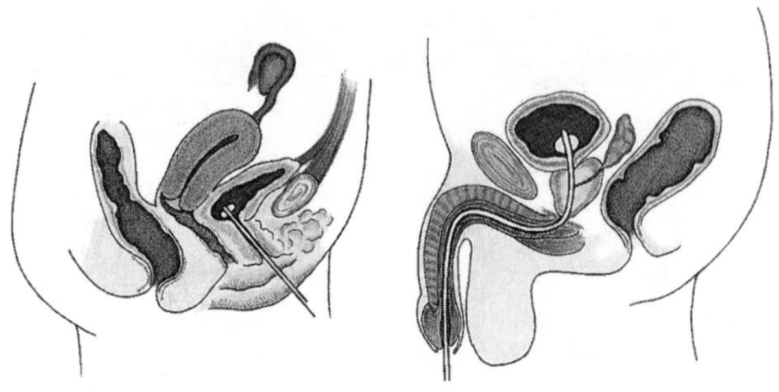

STEP **25** Inflation of balloon.

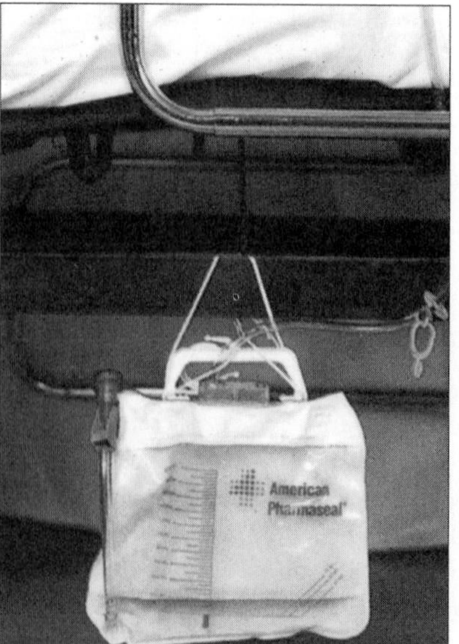

STEP **26** Drainage bag below level of bladder.

STEP	RATIONALE
27. Anchor catheter:	
a. Female client:	
(1) Secure catheter tubing to inner thigh with strip of nonallergenic tape (commercial multipurpose tube holders with a Velcro strap are available). Allow for slack so movement of thigh does not create tension on catheter (see illustration).	Anchoring catheter to inner thigh reduces pressure on urethra, thus reducing possibility of tissue injury in this area (Evans, 1999).
b. Male client:	
(1) Secure catheter tubing to top of thigh or lower abdomen (with penis directed toward chest). Allow slack in catheter so movement does not create tension on catheter (see illustration).	Anchoring catheter to lower abdomen reduces pressure on urethra at junction of penis and scrotum, thus reducing possibility of tissue injury in this area.

- ***Critical Decision Point***
  Be sure there are no obstructions in tubing. Coil excess tubing on bed and fasten it to bottom sheet with clip from kit or with rubber band and safety pin.

STEP	RATIONALE
28. Assist client to comfortable position. Wash and dry perineal area as needed.	Maintains comfort and security.
29. Remove gloves and dispose of equipment, drapes, and urine in proper receptacles.	Reduces transmission of microorganisms.
30. Wash hands.	Reduces spread of microorganisms.

EVALUATION

STEP	RATIONALE
1. Palpate bladder.	Determines if distention is relieved.
2. Ask about client's comfort.	Determines if client's sensation of discomfort or fullness has been relieved.
3. Observe character and amount of urine in drainage system.	Determines if urine is flowing adequately.
4. Determine that there is no urine leaking from catheter or tubing connections.	Prevents injury to client's skin and ensures a closed sterile system.

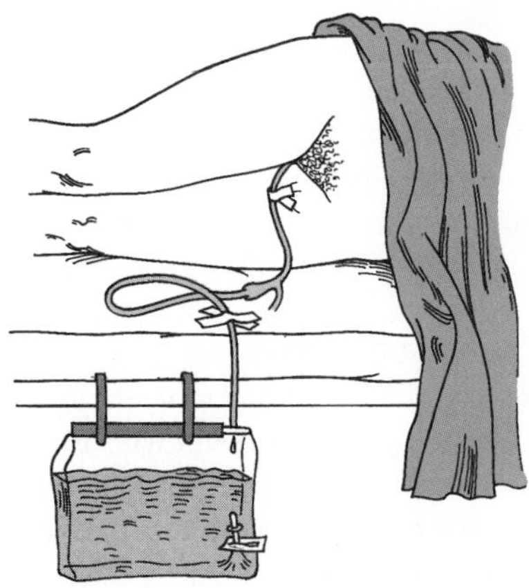

STEP **27a(1)** Securing the female indwelling catheter.

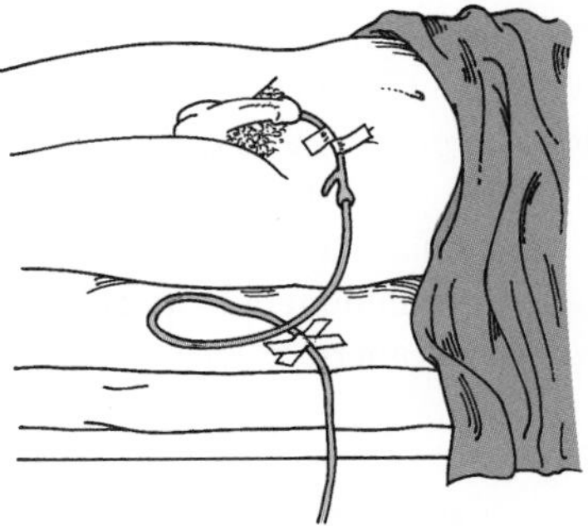

STEP **27b(1)** Securing the male indwelling catheter.

UNEXPECTED OUTCOMES AND RELATED INTERVENTIONS

- No urine is present.
  - *Female:* Catheter may be in vaginal opening. *Male:* Catheter may not be advanced far enough through prostatic urethra. Urine should drain freely. If not, nurse must further assess catheter placement and hydration status.
  - Assess the client for discomfort and check intake record. If catheter is in the bladder and no urine is produced within an hour, absence of urine should immediately be reported to physician.
- Catheter cannot be advanced.
  - Retry unless client is experiencing discomfort.
  - If catheter cannot be advanced, notify physician.

- Bladder discomfort persists despite catheter patency.
  - This may indicate urethral spasm or bladder infection. Notify physician.
- Leakage of urine from catheter.
  - Indicates improper catheter placement, possible balloon deflation, or too small a catheter. Reinflate balloon or replace catheter.
- More than 500 ml of urine drains from the catheter.
  - Check institution policy before beginning catheterization; some agencies restrict maximal amount of urine that can be drained at one time. This amount may vary from 800 to 1000 ml. Research has not shown that there is a limit to the amount of urine that can be drained (Williams, Wallhagen, and Dowling, 1993).
- Client with a spinal cord transection experiences the following symptoms: blood pressure (BP) elevated to 200 mm Hg systolic, bradycardia, headache, flushing and sweating above the spinal level of the injury. Spinal cord–injured (SCI) clients run the risk of autonomic dysreflexia (hyperreflexia) when exposed to a noxious stimulus such as a full bladder. Hyperreflexia is an autonomic response of the sympathetic system that results in dangerously high blood pressure. SCI clients who require intermittent catheterization are especially susceptible to dysreflexia.
  - Immediately elevate head of bed.
  - Empty a full bladder by unkinking tubing or removing any blockage in the catheter tubing.
  - Notify physician (Lombardo and Hartwig, 1997).

Recording and Reporting

- Report and record type and size of catheter inserted, amount of fluid used to inflate balloon, characteristics of urine, amount of urine, reasons for catheterization, specimen collection, and, if appropriate, client's response to procedure and teaching concepts. Identifies for other care providers pertinent information about the catheter and client's response to catheterization.
- Empty drainage bag and record amounts at least every 8 hours. Initiate I&O records (see Chapter 10). Bag should be emptied before it gets full (Evans, 1999).

Teaching Considerations

- Explain how the client can cooperate during the procedure.
- Explain to client that a burning and/or pressure sensation may be experienced during catheter insertion.
- Instruct client in ways to lie in bed with catheter. In the side-lying position facing the catheter, the tubing should drape over the thigh. In the side-lying position facing away from the catheter, the tubing should extend between the legs.
- Caution client against lying on tubing and against raising catheter bag and tubing above hips.
- Explain what is involved in the care of the catheter and drainage system.

Pediatric Considerations

- Children require smaller catheters than adults; an 8 to 10 Fr catheter with a 3-ml balloon is generally used for children.
- For an infant or young child, nurse must explain procedures to parent. Describe procedure to child at level they are able to understand (Wong and others, 1999).
- Catheterization in infants and children can be made easier by use of an adequate amount of lubricant that contains 2% lidocaine (Wong and others, 1999).

Gerontological Considerations

- A client with a catheter is especially vulnerable to UTI. The frail older adult client who is physically compromised runs the additional risk of developing septicemia, an infection that has spread to the blood. Septicemia is a potentially life-threatening complication. Therefore the client who is incontinent should not be routinely catheterized (Asci and Beyea, 1996).
- Ensuring adequate oral fluid intake of 2000 ml/day and assisting the older adult to toilet on a regular timed basis will help bladder retraining and minimize the need for excessive catheterization.
- Attached equipment such as a catheter may make it more likely that the older adult will not be fully ambulatory, thereby increasing the risks associated with decreased mobility. When catheters are required, they should be removed as soon as the client's condition allows.

Home Care Considerations

- Clients who are at home may use a leg bag during the day and switch to a large-volume bag at night so that sleep can remain uninterrupted.
- Clients may catheterize themselves at home on an intermittent basis using clean technique. Self-catheterization may be successful in maintaining continence and can result in fewer infections than the use of indwelling catheters.

Long-Term Care Considerations

- Appropriate use of indwelling catheters in long-term care may include incontinent residents who have wounds that are contaminated by urine and other means of control have been attempted and documented and in clients who are terminally ill (Ouslander and Schnelle, 1995).
- Urinary tract infection rates are high in nursing homes. This is thought to be due to lack of infection control knowledge and the skill level of some caregivers (Asci and Beyea, 1996).

Skill 24-3 Care and Removal of the Indwelling Catheter

Clients with indwelling catheters require specific perineal hygiene care to reduce the risk of urinary tract infection (UTI). Any secretions or encrustation at the catheter insertion site must be completely removed. Perineal care and the cleansing of the first 2 inches of the exposed catheter every 8 hours is minimally expected. This is often referred to as catheter care. The use of powders or lotions on the perineum is contraindicated because of the risk of growth of microorganisms, which may ascend the urinary tract.

Removal of a retention catheter is a skill requiring clean technique. When removing a retention catheter, the nurse must prevent trauma to the urethra. If the retention catheter balloon is not fully deflated, its removal can result in trauma and subsequent swelling of urethral meatus, and urinary retention can occur.

If the catheter was in place for more than several days, the client may experience dysuria resulting from inflammation of the urethral canal. Because of decreased bladder muscle tone, the client may urinate frequently.

Delegation Considerations

The skill of performing routine catheter care and removing a catheter can be delegated to assistive personnel. Instruct assistive personnel to report catheter drainage (color, odor, amount), catheter tubing (leaks, discharge, encrustation), and perineum (color, discharge, contamination from fecal incontinence) and amount of assistance client requires with positioning and understanding. Care provider should check size of balloon and size of syringe needed to deflate balloon and report if balloon does not deflate and/or if there is excessive burning or bleeding. Instruct care provider to not use force when removing catheter, and to monitor frequency and amount of urine voided.

Equipment

- Disposable gloves (needed for care and removal)
- Bed protector
- Bath blanket

For Catheter Care

- Soap, washcloth, basin, and water (to cleanse perineum before catheter care)
- Graduated cylinder (used if urine collection bag will be emptied)

For Removing a Catheter

- Syringe (same size as volume of solution used to inflate balloon) (information on balloon size can be obtained directly from balloon inflation valve on catheter)
- Waterproof pad
- Alcohol swab
- Correctly labeled sterile specimen container and 25-gauge ½-inch needle (if culture and sensitivity are to be obtained before catheter removal)

Step	Rationale
Assessment	
1. Determine how long catheter has been in place. Check agency policy to determine how often indwelling catheter must be changed.	Catheters in place for more than a few days are more likely to cause urethral irritation and buildup of encrustation.
2. Observe any discharge or encrustation around urethral meatus.	May indicate inflammatory process and may harbor bacteria.
3. Assess for complaints of pain or discomfort; determine location and type of pain client is experiencing; assess for presence of allergies (e.g., to antiseptic solution).	Indicates potential UTI.
4. Monitor client's temperature.	Possible symptom of UTI.
5. Determine client's fluid intake.	Lack of fluid intake reduces natural flushing of urinary system and increases chance of bacterial growth.
6. Assess urine color, clarity, odor, and amount.	Possible symptom of UTI, possible indicator of client's volume status.
7. Assess client's knowledge of catheter care or removal procedure.	Reveals need for client instruction.

Step	Rationale
8. Assess need or order for catheter removal.	Physician may have ordered catheter to be removed, enabling client to void after removal. Nurse may determine catheter needs to be removed to be replaced with another indwelling catheter.

Nursing Diagnosis

Defining characteristics from the assessment data may reveal the following nursing diagnoses for clients requiring this skill:

Impaired urinary elimination
Deficient knowledge regarding perineal care
Acute pain
Risk for infection
Toileting self-care deficit

Related factors are individualized based on client's condition or needs.

Planning

Step	Rationale
1. **Expected outcomes** following completion of procedure:	
▪ Urethral meatus is free of secretions and encrustation.	Indicates absence of irritation.
▪ Urine is clear, and volume is sufficient.	Indicates absence of UTI and adequate output.
▪ Client is afebrile.	Indicates absence of infection.
▪ Skin under tape site is intact and not abraded, open, or reddened.	
▪ Client will verbalize feeling of comfort after procedure is completed.	Cleansing relieves local discomfort.
▪ After catheter is removed the client voids without discomfort and voids a minimum of 250 ml of urine with each voiding within 6 to 8 hours of catheter removal.	Indicates return of voluntary bladder function.

Implementation

Step	Rationale
1. Wash hands and apply gloves.	Reduces transmission of microorganisms.
2. Close curtain or close door.	Provides privacy and reduces embarrassment to client, thus promoting relaxation.
3. Raise bed to appropriate working height. If side rails are raised lower side rail on working side.	Promotes use of proper body mechanics.
4. Organize equipment for perineal care or removal of catheter.	Increases efficiency of procedure.

• ***Critical Decision Point***
Get assistance for positioning the weak or frail client as necessary.

Step	Rationale
5. Position client and cover with bath blanket, exposing only perineal area. a. Female in dorsal recumbent position. b. Male in supine position.	Reduces client's embarrassment. Ensures easy access to perineal tissues.

Catheter Care

Step	Rationale
6. Place waterproof pad under client.	Protects bed from soiling.
7. Provide routine perineal care as outlined in Chapter 6.	Do not use powder after providing perineal care (Evans, 1999).
8. Assess urethral meatus and surrounding tissues for inflammation, swelling, and discharge, and ask client if burning or discomfort is felt.	Determines local infection and status of hygiene.

STEP	RATIONALE
9. Using a clean washcloth, wipe in circular motion along length of catheter for about 10 cm (4 inches).	Reduces presence of secretions or drainage on outside catheter surface.
• ***Critical Decision Point*** *Note the presence of any encrustation, and clean thoroughly.*	
10. Replace as necessary the adhesive tape or multipurpose tube holder that anchors catheter to client's leg or abdomen. Remove adhesive residue from skin.	Secures catheter, thus reducing risk of catheter being pulled and exposing portion of catheter that was in urethra. Also prevents drag on catheter and avoids creating pressure from balloon on bladder floor.
11. Avoid placing tension on the catheter.	Tension causes urethral trauma.
12. Replace tubing and collection bag as necessary and/or according to agency policy, adhering to principles of surgical asepsis.	Urinary tubing and collection bag should be changed if there are signs of leakage, odor, or sediment buildup. The catheterization system including the catheter may need to be replaced if leaking or blockage occurs.
13. Check drainage tubing and bag to ensure that:	
a. Tubing is not looped or positioned above level of bladder.	Prevents pooling of urine and reflux of urine into bladder.
b. Tubing is coiled and secured onto bed linen.	Prevents looping of tubing and subsequent pooling of urine.
c. Tube is not kinked or clamped.	Prevents stasis of urine in bladder. Also ensures that client is not lying on tubing, causing pressure on skin and increasing risk of pressure ulcer.
d. Collection bag is positioned appropriately on the bed frame.	Ensures appropriate drainage of urine.
14. Collection bag should be emptied as necessary but at least every 8 hours.	Urine in collection bag is excellent medium for growth of microorganisms.
Catheter Removal	
Refer to Steps 1 through 5 as necessary.	
15. Place waterproof pad:	Prevents soiling of bed linen. Provides wrapper to cover contaminated catheter after removal, thus eliminating possibility of urine contaminating nurse's gloved hand.
a. Between female's thighs (if in supine position)	
b. Over male's thighs	
16. Obtain sterile urine specimen if required (see Chapter 41).	Determines if bacteria are present in urine.
17. Remove adhesive tape or Velcro tube used to secure and anchor catheter. Cleanse any residue from skin.	Removes source of irritant on skin. Allows for positioning of catheter for removal.
18. Insert hub of syringe into inflation valve (balloon port). Aspirate entire amount of fluid used to inflate balloon (see illustration).	Deflates balloon to allow for removal. If solution is not completely aspirated, partially inflated balloon causes trauma to urethral wall as catheter is removed.
• ***Critical Decision Point*** *Do not use force to make the syringe fit into the valve.*	
19. Pull catheter out smoothly and slowly.	Prevents trauma to urethral mucosa.

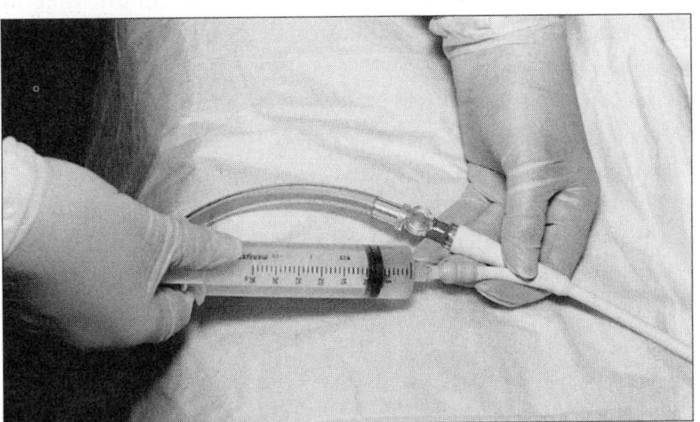

STEP **18** Aspirating fluid to deflate balloon.

STEP	RATIONALE
• ***Critical Decision Point*** *Stop pulling catheter if resistance is met; balloon is probably still inflated. Aspirate again to ensure all fluid has been removed. If still meet resistance, notify physician.*	
20. Wrap contaminated catheter in waterproof pad. Unhook collection bag and drainage tubing from bed.	Prevents contamination of nurse's hands.
21. When catheter care and/or removal is completed:	
a. Reposition client as necessary. Cleanse perineum as necessary. Lower level of bed, and position side rails accordingly.	Promotes client comfort and safety.
b. Measure and empty contents of collection bag.	Provides accurate recording of urinary output.
c. Dispose of all contaminated supplies correctly, remove gloves, and wash hands.	Reduces spread of microorganisms.

EVALUATION

1. Inspect the condition of the urethra and surrounding tissue, and ask client about discomfort.	Determines if area is cleansed properly and/or if client has any irritation.
2. Note character and amount of urine.	Helps indicate if infection is present and output is adequate before and after catheter removed.
3. Observe time and amount of first voided specimen.	Indicates return of bladder function.

UNEXPECTED OUTCOMES AND RELATED INTERVENTIONS

- Urethral or perineal irritation is present.
  - Observe for leaking, and replace catheter if necessary.
  - If catheter is present, ensure that indwelling catheter is anchored as outlined in Skill 24-2.
  - If securing catheter does not help or if catheter has been removed, notify physician of urethral irritation.
- Client has fever and/or odor is present, or client experiences small, frequent voidings or any burning or bleeding.
  - Monitor vital signs and urine, but report findings to physician because any of these symptoms/signs may indicate a UTI.
- Client experiences urinary retention and is unable to void after catheter removal.
  - Ensure adequate intake and privacy, and facilitate urination by relaxation (see Skill Performance Guidelines).
  - If client unable to void within 6 to 8 hours of catheter removal, notify physician.

RECORDING AND REPORTING

- Ensure that times for catheter care are set in the care plan. Clients with indwelling catheters should receive perineal and catheter care every 8 hours and after bowel movements.
- Record in nurses' notes when catheter care was given, removal of catheter and assessment of urethral meatus, and character of urine.

TEACHING CONSIDERATIONS

- Unless contraindicated, clients with a catheter should drink at least 2000 ml of fluid per day to promote continuous flushing of the bladder, preventing sediment from collecting in the catheter tubing.
- Instruct client to hold collection bag below the level of the bladder when ambulating.
- Instruct client to keep the collection bag off the floor, where microorganisms are abundant.
- Instruct client not to disconnect the catheter from the collection tubing and bag.

GERONTOLOGICAL CONSIDERATIONS

- The older adult client may exhibit atypical signs and symptoms of UTI. Although the usual symptoms of dysuria, urgency, frequency, odor, and hematuria should be assessed, they may not be present. The assessment must also include assessing for less specific signs such as fever and/or mental status changes including agitation, lethargy, and confusion.

HOME CARE CONSIDERATIONS

- Assess client and primary caregiver for ability and motivation to participate in routine catheter care.
- Silicone catheters may be a better choice for client in the home, where catheterization for longer periods of time may be done, because the silicone is less likely to become encrusted. Encrustation harbors microorganisms and increases irritation.

Skill 24-4 Obtaining Catheterized Specimens for Residual Urine

Residual urine is the volume of urine in the bladder after a normal voiding. Clients suspected of retaining urine are assessed for residual urine. Urinary retention is the inability of the bladder to fully empty.

Clients at risk for large residual volumes include those receiving bladder training exercises, such as those with spinal cord injuries, those who have suffered a cerebrovascular accident, and those who have had bladder surgery.

Delegation Considerations

The skill of obtaining catheterized specimens for residual urine should not be delegated to assistive personnel.

Equipment

- Equipment listed in Skill 24-3
- Straight catheter

Step	Rationale
Assessment	
1. Review prior intake and output (I&O) record.	Identifies usual amount of urine client voids during each voiding.
2. Determine if client experiences pain or discomfort when voiding.	Pain may be associated with bladder spasms.
3. Review physician's order to determine how often residual urine must be checked.	Order must be obtained from physician before nurse can catheterize client. Physician's order indicates when this procedure is no longer necessary (e.g., check residual urine twice a day until amount obtained is less than 100 ml).
4. Check time of last voiding before catheterization.	Residual urine determinations should be performed immediately after voiding to obtain accurate information about amount of urine remaining in bladder.
5. Assess client's knowledge regarding urinary retention.	Reveals need for client education.

Nursing Diagnosis

Defining characteristics from the assessment data may reveal the following nursing diagnoses for clients requiring this skill:

Impaired urinary elimination
Deficient fluid volume
Risk for deficient volume
Excess fluid volume
Deficient knowledge regarding residual urine
Acute pain
Risk for infection
Urinary retention

Related factors are individualized based on client's condition or needs.

Planning

Step	Rationale
1. **Expected outcomes** following completion of procedure:	
▪ Successive catheterizations result in decreasing amount of residual urine.	Client gains improved bladder control.
▪ Urine remains clear and dilute, without foul odor.	Removal of retained urine reduces medium for bacterial growth.
▪ Client will verbalize decrease in pain or discomfort with voiding.	Voiding at regularly scheduled times decreases residual volumes.
▪ The client explains the purpose of the procedure and what is expected.	Helps to minimize anxiety.

Step	Rationale

Implementation

1. Ask client to void completely, and measure volume of urine. — Determines how much client is able to void compared to how much urine remains in bladder which will be measured by catheterization.

- ***Critical Decision Point***
  Remind ambulatory clients not to dispose of urine and that it must be measured.

2. Wash hands. — Reduces transmission of infection.
3. Proceed as for inserting straight catheter (see Skill 24-2). — Insertion of straight catheter drains residual urine.
4. Accurately measure urine obtained. — Allows amount retained (catheterized amount) to be compared to amount voided.

Evaluation

1. Compare amount of urine voided and amount obtained on catheterization. — Difference indicates whether procedure should be repeated. Volume should be less than 100 ml.

Unexpected Outcomes and Related Interventions

- Residual volume is greater than 100 ml of urine.
  - Indicates inadequate bladder emptying; physician should be notified.
- Urinary incontinence of small amount of urine occurs.
  - Results from overflow incontinence from bladder distension. Physician should be notified.
- Client has signs and symptoms associated with bladder infection.
  - Monitor vital signs, and notify physician.

Recording and Reporting

- Report and record amount of urine voided, amount obtained from catheterization, and client's response. Communicates information to all members of health care team, indicating progress of therapy.
- Report presence of unexpected outcomes to physician and other team members as appropriate.
- Initiate a voiding diary if frequency or incontinence present.

Teaching Considerations

- Although straight catheters are used to drain residual urine, the physician may order an indwelling Foley catheter insertion if residual urine volumes exceed a certain volume. If physician's order is written in such a manner, nurse may elect to perform residual catheterization with Foley catheter. This procedure will need to be clarified and explained to the client, who may be anxious about urinary problems.
- Clients need to be informed about symptoms of UTI. Infections can increase bladder spasms and lead to worsening of urine retention.
- Urine retention predisposes the client to UTI and urinary calculi. Signs and symptoms of UTI are a change in urinary elimination such as frequency or nocturia; pain in back or on urination (dysuria); changes in urine including odor, blood, or sediment in urine and color changes to dark yellow or pink; and systemic symptoms as fever and chills. The major symptom of urinary calculi is pain that is described as dull and aching to intense, and the pain can be localized in the flank, back, lower abdomen, or groin. In addition, the client may present with fever, chills, nausea, and vomiting.

Pediatric Considerations

- Children require smaller catheters than adults; an 8 to 10 Fr catheter is generally used for children.
- For infant or child, nurse must explain procedures to parent. Describe procedure to child at the level he or she is able to understand.

Gerontological Considerations

- Urine retention is not considered a normal part of aging and therefore should not be dismissed.
- UTI that occurs as a result of residual urine can be devastating to the frail older adult. Septicemia, an infection that spreads into the circulation, may be life threatening.

Home Care Considerations

- Clients may need to be taught how to perform self-catheterization at home.
- Clients at home may use a double-voiding technique to help decrease the amount of residual urine. The client is instructed to void, wait about 5 minutes, and then void again. The relaxation between voidings may be helpful in cases of bladder outlet obstruction or weak contractility of the detrusor muscle (Gray, 1992).

Skill 24-5 Performing Catheter Irrigation

Catheter irrigations are performed on an intermittent or continuous basis to maintain catheter patency. There are two types of irrigation systems: closed bladder irrigation systems and open irrigation systems using disposable trays. A closed bladder irrigation system provides intermittent or continuous irrigation of the system without disrupting the sterile alignment of the catheter and drainage system (Figure 24-3), thus decreasing the risk of bacteria entering the urinary tract. The closed system is used most frequently in clients who have had genitourinary surgery. These clients are at risk for occlusion of the Foley catheter by small blood clots and mucous fragments; they are also at risk for UTI.

The open irrigation system is also used to maintain catheter patency. However, this system is used when bladder irrigations are required less frequently (e.g., every 8 hours) and there are no blood clots or large mucous shreds in the urinary drainage. This type of irrigation requires the nurse to aseptically break the closed drainage system and maintain surgical asepsis throughout the procedure. Both systems can be used to irrigate the bladder with a medication to treat an infection or local bladder irritation.

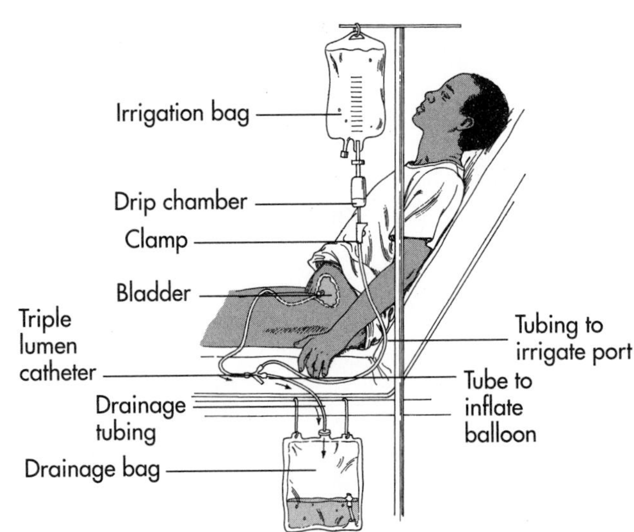

FIGURE 24-3 Closed continuous irrigation.

Delegation Considerations

The skill of catheter irrigation should not be delegated to assistive personnel.

Equipment

Closed Continuous Method

- Sterile irrigating solution (unless otherwise specified in order) at room temperature
- Irrigation tubing with clamp (with or without Y connector) (clamp regulates irrigation flow rate; Y connector allows IV bags to be connected to tubing)
- IV pole
- Y connector (optional) (used to connect irrigation tubing to double-lumen catheter)

Closed Intermittent Method

- Sterile irrigating solution at room temperature
- Sterile graduate container
- Sterile 30- to 50-ml syringe (used to instill irrigant into catheter)
- Sterile 19- to 22-gauge 1-inch needle
- Antiseptic swab
- Screw clamp (used to temporarily occlude catheter as irrigant is instilled)

Open Intermittent Method

- Sterile irrigating solution at room temperature
- Disposable sterile irrigation tray and set
- Bulb syringe or 60-ml piston type of syringe
- Sterile collection basin
- Waterproof drape
- Sterile solution container
- Antiseptic swabs
- Gloves
- Tape

Step	Rationale
Assessment	
1. Check client's record to determine:	
a. Purpose of closed bladder irrigation	Allows nurse to anticipate observations to make (e.g., blood or mucus in urine).

Step	Rationale
b. Physician's order for type and amount of irrigant	Order required to initiate therapy. Ensures that correct medication or solution and amount will be administered. Amount of solution used to flush system may be a nurse judgment or indicated by physician or institutional policy. Frequency of irrigation is based on need of client (e.g., client who has just had prostate gland surgery may require irrigations every 5 to 10 minutes in first hour, which are then tapered to every 4 hours).
c. Type of irrigation: continuous or intermittent	Allows nurse to select proper equipment. In continuous irrigation, clamp regulates slow, steady flow into bladder. Because outflow should correspond to regulated irrigation drip, patency of catheter must be checked frequently to prevent distention of bladder. For intermittent irrigation, flow from irrigating solution is clamped for specified time and then opened, and designated amount of irrigating solution is allowed to flush into bladder. Intermittent irrigation requires close observation of catheter patency between irrigations.
d. Type of catheter used:	Indicates if it is necessary to break system for irrigation.
(1) Triple lumen (one lumen to inflate balloon, one to instill irrigant solution, and one to allow outflow of urine (see Figure 24-3)	
(2) Double lumen (one lumen to inflate balloon, one to allow outflow of urine)	
2. Assess the following:	
a. Color of urine and presence of mucus, clots, or sediment	Indicates if client is bleeding or sloughing tissue and determines necessity for increasing irrigation rates with continuous irrigations or increasing irrigation frequency with intermittent irrigations.
b. Palpate bladder	
c. Existing closed system:	
(1) Note if fluid entering bladder and fluid draining from bladder are in appropriate proportions.	Determines presence of distention.
(2) Determine that drainage tubing is not kinked, clamped off incorrectly, or looped below bladder level.	Determines if system is obstructed. One would expect more output than fluid instilled because of urine production.
(3) Note amount of fluid remaining in existing irrigating solution container.	

• ***Critical Decision Point***

If fluid cannot enter or if fluid draining is less than amounts going in, stop the irrigation, assess, and notify the physician.

Step	Rationale
3. Review input and output (I&O) record.	Determines baseline for prior output measures. All clients with continuous bladder irrigations should have I&O measurements (see Chapter 10).
4. Assess client for presence of bladder spasms and discomfort.	Reveals need for bladder irrigation.
5. Assess client's knowledge regarding purpose of performing catheter irrigation.	Reveals need for client instruction.

Nursing Diagnosis

Defining characteristics from the assessment data may reveal the following nursing diagnoses for clients requiring this skill:

- Impaired urinary elimination
- Deficient knowledge regarding the need for bladder irrigation
- Acute pain
- Risk for infection

Related factors are individualized based on client's condition or needs.

STEP	RATIONALE

PLANNING

1. **Expected outcomes** following completion of this procedure:

Step	Rationale
▪ Output is greater than volume of irrigating solution used.	Indicates patency of drainage system. Patency promotes drainage of clots and mucus, which if trapped cause bladder spasms.
▪ Absence of pain or discomfort.	Surgery involving bladder and urethral structures results in discomfort.
▪ Absence of fever; urine is not concentrated or foul smelling.	Indicates infection not likely present.
▪ Client can explain purpose of procedure and what to expect.	Helps client relax and promotes cooperation.

IMPLEMENTATION

Step	Rationale
1. Wash hands.	Reduces transmission of microorganisms.
2. Provide privacy: Pull curtains around bed, and fold back covers so catheter is exposed at junction where it connects to drainage tubing. Cover client's chest with bath blanket.	Promotes client's self-esteem; shows respect for client while exposing only area nurse must see.
3. Position client in supine position, and remove tape or Velcro tube holder that is anchoring catheter to client. Be careful not to pull on catheter.	Allows for client comfort. Removing tape enables nurse to manipulate catheter.
4. Assess lower abdomen for signs of bladder distention.	Detects if catheter or closed irrigation system is malfunctioning, blocking urinary drainage.

Closed Intermittent Irrigation

Step	Rationale
5. Pour prescribed room-temperature sterile irrigating solution in sterile container.	
6. Draw sterile solution into syringe using aseptic technique.	Ensures sterility of irrigating fluid.

• ***Critical Decision Point***
Avoid cold solution as irrigation because it may cause bladder spasm.

Step	Rationale
7. Clamp indwelling retention catheter below soft injection port or on drainage tubing.	Occlusion of catheter provides resistance against which irrigant can be forcefully instilled into catheter.
8. Apply gloves.	Reduces risk of exposure to body fluids.
9. Cleanse catheter injection port with antiseptic swab (this same port is used for specimen collections).	Reduces transmission of infection.
10. Insert needle of syringe through port at 30-degree angle. (See manufacturer's instructions for possible variation).	Ensures needle tip enters lumen of catheter and that needle does not puncture tubing.
11. Inject fluid into catheter and bladder.	The injection dislodges clots and sediment.

• ***Critical Decision Point***
If catheter does not irrigate, tip may incorrectly be lodged in the urethra and not in the bladder. Use slow, even pressure when injecting fluid. Too much pressure may traumatize the bladder wall.

Step	Rationale
12. Withdraw syringe and remove clamp; allow solution to drain into urinary drainage bag. (Tubing clamped temporarily to allow instilled fluid to remain in bladder, especially if irrigant is medicated.)	Allows drainage to flow via gravity.

Closed Continuous Irrigation

NOTE: Supplies for closed irrigation system may be kept at bedside. Irrigating solution should be at room temperature. This practice is similar to that when bag of IV fluid is added to IV infusion. Check that solution, volume, client, route, and time are correct. Discard any sterile solution not used within 24 hours of opening. Check institutional policy. When irrigant is opened, it should be marked with the date and time.

Step	Rationale
13. Apply gloves and using aseptic technique, insert (spike) tip of sterile irrigation tubing into bag containing irrigation solution.	Reduces transmission of microorganisms.
14. Close clamp on tubing and hang bag of solution on IV pole.	Prevents loss of irrigating solution.
15. Open clamp and allow solution to flow through tubing, keeping end of tubing sterile; close clamp.	Removes air from tubing.

- ***Critical Decision Point***
  Be sure drainage bag and tubing are securely connected to drainage port of Y connector when using double-lumen catheter.

Step	Rationale
16. For continuous irrigation, calculate drip rate and adjust clamp on irrigation tubing accordingly; be sure clamp on drainage tubing is open, and check volume of drainage in drainage bag.	Ensures continuous, even irrigation of catheter system. Prevents accumulation of solution in bladder, which may cause bladder distention and possible injury.
17. For intermittent flow, clamp tubing on drainage system, open clamp on irrigation tubing, and allow prescribed amount of fluid to enter bladder (100 ml is normal for adult); close irrigation tubing clamp and then open drainage tubing clamp.	Fluid is instilled through catheter into bladder, flushing system. Fluid drains out after irrigation is complete.

- ***Critical Decision Point***
  Do not leave a clamped drainage bag unattended. Check frequently, at least every hour.

Open Irrigation

Step	Rationale
18. Apply gloves.	Reduces transmission of infection. Irrigation is a sterile procedure, but only parts of the system coming in contact with the inside of the catheter must remain sterile. The tip of the syringe, end of the catheter, end of the catheter tubing, and irrigant must remain sterile. Therefore the use of sterile gloves is optional.
19. Open sterile irrigation tray; establish sterile field, and pour required amount of sterile solution into sterile solution container. Replace cap on large container of solution.	Adheres to principles of surgical asepsis.
20. Position waterproof drape under catheter.	Prevents soiling of bed linen.
21. Aspirate 30 ml of solution into irrigating syringe.	Prepares irrigant for instillation into catheter.
22. Move sterile collection basin close to client's thigh.	Prevents soiling of bed linen and prohibits reaching over sterile area.
23. Wipe connection point between catheter and tubing with antiseptic wipe before disconnecting.	Reduces transmission of microorganisms.
24. Disconnect catheter from drainage tubing, allowing urine to flow into sterile collection basin; cover open end of drainage tubing with sterile protective cap and position tubing so it stays coiled on top of bed.	Maintains sterility of inner aspect of catheter lumen and drainage tubing; reduces potential of introducing pathogens into bladder.
25. Insert tip of syringe into lumen of catheter and gently instill solution.	Reduces incidence of bladder spasm but clears catheter of obstruction.

- ***Critical Decision Point***
  If strong resistance is noted, do not force the irrigation.

Step	Rationale
26. Withdraw syringe, lower catheter, and allow solution to drain into basin. Repeat, instilling solution and draining several times until drainage is clear of clots and sediment.	Allows drainage to flow by gravity. Provides for adequate flushing of catheter.
27. If solution does not return, have client turn onto side facing nurse; if changing position does not help, reinsert syringe and gently aspirate solution.	Change in position may move tip of catheter in bladder, increasing likelihood that fluid instilled will flow out.

STEP	RATIONALE
• ***Critical Decision Point*** *Observe client for indications of pain or discomfort.*	
28. After irrigation is complete, remove protector cap from drainage tubing adapter, cleanse adapter with alcohol swab, and reinsert adapter into lumen of catheter.	Reestablishes closed drainage system.
29. Anchor catheter to client's leg or thigh with tape or Velcro multipurpose tube holder (see Skill 24-2).	Prevents trauma to urethral tissue.
30. Assist client into comfortable position.	Promotes relaxation and rest.
31. Lower bed to lowest position, and position side rails accordingly.	Promotes client safety.
32. Dispose of contaminated supplies, remove gloves, and wash hands.	Reduces spread of microorganisms.

EVALUATION

1. Calculate fluid used to irrigate bladder and catheter, and subtract from volume drained.	Determines accurate urinary output.
2. Assess characteristics of output: viscosity, color, and presence of clots.	Data serve as baseline to judge response to therapy.
3. Observe for catheter patency.	Ensures bladder emptying freely.
4. Observe client for signs of pain and fever.	Evaluates for presence of infection.
5. Observe urine to determine clarity, concentration, and odor.	Determines presence of bacteria in urine.

UNEXPECTED OUTCOMES AND RELATED INTERVENTIONS

- Irrigating solution is not returned or is not flowing at prescribed rate, which indicates possible occlusion of Foley catheter.
  - Examine tubing for clots, sediment, and kinks.
  - Notify physician if irrigant is retained, client complains of pain, or bladder is distended.
- Signs of fever or cloudy, foul urine.
  - May indicate infection; physician should be notified.
  - Monitor vital signs and urine.
- Increase in bladder spasms. May indicate occlusion of catheter with foreign object (e.g., blood clot).
  - Notify physician if large clots or sediment is returned or if spasms increase or are unrelieved. May need to change from intermittent to continuous irrigation.

RECORDING AND REPORTING

- Record amount of solution used as irrigant, amount returned as drainage, characteristics of output, and urine output of drainage in nurses' notes and I&O sheet. Documents procedure and client's tolerance of it.
- Report catheter occlusion, sudden bleeding, infection, or increased pain to physician. May require more aggressive therapy. Reduces risk of urinary retention.

TEACHING CONSIDERATIONS

- Instruct client and primary caregiver to observe urine daily for changes in color, presence of mucus or blood, and changes in consistency and odor.
- Clients should be taught that bleeding is common after transurethral prostatectomy and that bright red-tinged urine during first 48 hours postoperatively followed by pink-tinged to clear urine by fifth postoperative day is expected.
- Instruct client to maintain adequate oral intake of 2 L/day (unless contraindicated).

GERONTOLOGICAL CONSIDERATIONS

- Benign prostatic hypertrophy is common as men age, and surgical intervention on the prostate gland may be required.

After surgery, continuous and rapid irrigation of the bladder with a three-way Foley catheter is often necessary to prevent clotting and obstruction of the catheter. Often irrigant is adjusted to keep urine pink rather than a set rate.

HOME CARE CONSIDERATIONS

- Assess the client and primary caregiver for ability and motivation to perform catheter irrigation.
- Assess client's environment for appropriate storage space for materials needed for procedure.
- Observe client and primary caregiver while they perform procedure.
- Refer client to home care agency for in-home follow-up.

Skill 24-6 Applying a Condom Catheter

The external application of a urinary drainage device is a convenient, safe method of draining urine in male clients. The condom catheter is suitable for incontinent or comatose clients who still have complete and spontaneous bladder emptying. The condom is a soft, pliable rubber sheath that slips over the penis and is kept in place with the use of an elastic adhesive strip (Figure 24-4). The catheter may be attached to a leg drainage bag or a standard urinary drainage bag. Often this is a nursing-instituted procedure, but check policies to determine if a physician's order is required.

The often advised frequency for changing a condom catheter is every 24 hours, but there is debate on this topic (Stelling and Hale, 1996). Close monitoring every 4 hours to detect potential problems is necessary, however. With each catheter change, the nurse cleanses the urethral meatus and penis thoroughly and looks for signs of skin irritation.

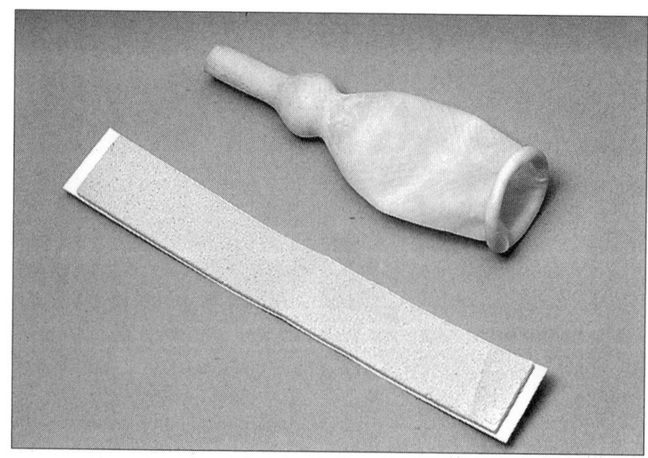

FIGURE **24-4** Condom catheter.

Delegation Considerations

The skills of applying a condom catheter can be delegated to assistive personnel. Consult policy, as delegation may vary with agencies. It is important that care provider knows standard precautions guidelines relating to body fluids and asks whether the client has a latex allergy. Before delegating the task, clarify that skin of penile shaft is intact and free from swelling, redness, or open lesions. The methods for applying the catheter differ from manufacturer to manufacturer so it is vital that the care provider understands how to apply the adhesive strip that secures the condom catheter.

Equipment

- Condom catheter kit (rubber condom sheath of appropriate size, strip of elastic adhesive, skin preparation)
- Urinary collection bag with drainage tubing or leg bag and straps
- Basin with warm water and soap
- Towels and washcloth(s)
- Bath blanket
- Nonsterile disposable gloves
- Scissors and/or safety razor

Step	Rationale
Assessment	
1. Assess urinary elimination pattern, client's ability to voluntarily urinate, and continence.	Clients who are incontinent are at risk for skin breakdown.
2. Assess mental status of client so appropriate teaching related to condom catheter can be implemented.	Some male clients may be incontinent only at night. Teaching can be implemented to instruct client on self-application.
3. Assess condition of penis.	Provides baseline to compare changes in condition of skin after condom catheter application.
4. Assess client's knowledge of the purpose of a condom catheter.	Reveals need for client instruction.

Nursing Diagnosis

Defining characteristics from the assessment data may reveal the following nursing diagnoses for clients requiring this skill:

- Risk for impaired skin integrity
- Deficient knowledge regarding application of condom catheter
- Toileting self-care deficit
- Total urinary incontinence

Related factors are individualized based on client's condition or needs.

STEP	RATIONALE

PLANNING

Step	Rationale
1. **Expected outcomes** following completion of procedure:	
▪ Client is continent with condom catheter intact.	Catheter is secure; normal voiding occurs. Application of the adhesive strip before or after the condom is applied varies with brand.
▪ Penile shaft is free of skin irritation or breakdown.	Indicates absence or irritation.
▪ Client can explain the purpose of the procedure and what to expect.	Reduces anxiety and promotes cooperation.

IMPLEMENTATION

Step	Rationale
1. Wash hands.	Reduces transmission of microorganisms.
2. Provide privacy by closing room door or bedside curtain.	Maintains client's self-esteem.
3. Raise bed to appropriate working height. If side rails raised, lower side rail on working side.	Promotes use of good body mechanics.
4. Assist client into supine position. Place bath blanket over upper torso. Fold sheets so lower extremities are covered; only genitalia should be exposed.	Promotes comfort; draping prevents unnecessary exposure of body parts.
5. Prepare urinary drainage collection bag and tubing. Clamp off drainage bag port. Secure collection bag to bed frame; bring drainage tubing up through side rails onto bed. Prepare leg bag for connection to condom if necessary.	Provides easy access to drainage equipment after condom catheter is in place.
6. Apply disposable gloves. Provide perineal care (see Chapter 6), and dry thoroughly.	Removes irritating secretions. Rubber sheath of condom rolls onto dry skin more easily.

• ***Critical Decision Point***

Clip hair at base of penis. In some cases shaving the hair at the base of the penis may be necessary. Hair adheres to condom and is pulled during condom removal or may get caught in rubber as condom catheter is applied.

Step	Rationale
7. Apply skin preparation to penis, and allow to dry. If client is uncircumcised, return foreskin to normal position.	Skin preparation has an alcohol base. Evaporation is necessary to prevent irritation.
8. With nondominant hand, grasp penis along shaft. With dominant hand, hold condom sheath at tip of penis and smoothly roll sheath onto penis.	Prepares penis for easy condom placement.

• ***Critical Decision Point***

Allow 2.5 to 5 cm (1 to 2 inches) of space between tip of glans penis and end of condom catheter (see illustration).

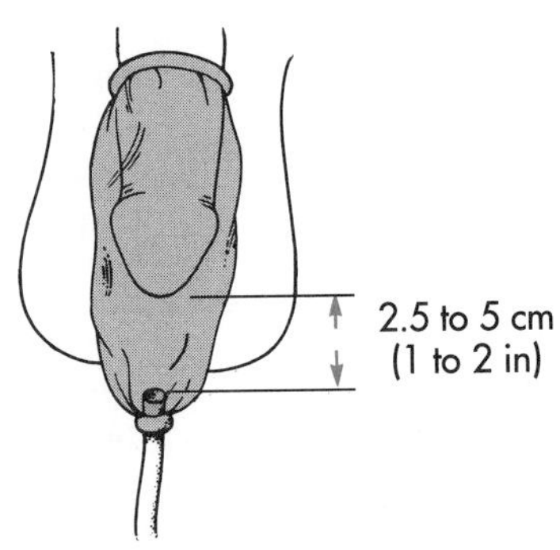

STEP **8** Distance between end of penis and tip of condom.

Step	Rationale
9. Spiral wrap penile shaft with strip of elastic adhesive. Strip should be spiral wrapped and not overlap itself. Do not use any tape except that provided by the manufacturer. Other tapes will not provide the flexibility needed for spiral wrap and may impair circulation to the penis. Never use adhesive tape in the application of the condom catheter because it may impede circulation.	Condom must be secured firmly so it is snug and stays on but not tight enough to cause constriction of blood flow. With some brands of catheters the adhesive strip is applied before the condom is applied.

- ***Critical Decision Point***

  Newer condom catheters are self-adhesive. When using a self-adhesive condom catheter, apply catheter as in Steps 7 and 8. Then apply gentle pressure on penile shaft for 10 to 15 seconds to secure catheter.

Step	Rationale
10. Connect drainage tubing to end of condom catheter. Be sure condom is not twisted. Catheter can be connected to large-volume bag or leg bag (see illustration).	Allows urine to be collected and measured. Keeps client dry. Twisted condom obstructs urine flow.

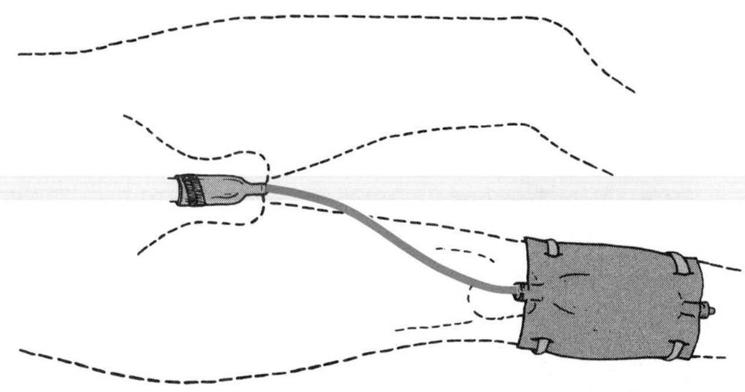

STEP **10** Leg bag.

Step	Rationale
11. Place excess coiling of tubing on bed and secure to bottom sheet.	Prevents looping of tubing and promotes free drainage of urine.
12. Place client in safe, comfortable position. Lower bed, and place side rails accordingly.	Promotes safety and comfort.
13. Dispose of contaminated supplies, and wash hands.	Reduces spread of microorganisms.

Evaluation

Step	Rationale
1. Observe urinary drainage.	Determines if normal voiding is occurring.
2. Inspect penis with condom catheter in place within 30 minutes after application. Look for swelling and discoloration, and ask client if there is any discomfort.	Determines if catheter has been applied incorrectly.
3. Remove and change condom, and inspect skin on penile shaft for signs of breakdown or irritation at least daily when hygiene is performed and when condom is reapplied.	Indicates if condom or urine is causing irritation or if adhesive is too restrictive. Frequent assessment of circulation of glans penis is important to determine if condom has been applied too tightly.

Unexpected Outcomes and Related Interventions

- Skin around penis is reddened and excoriated. Results from pressure of adhesive or contact with urine.
  - Check for allergy.
  - Remove condom, and notify physician.
  - Do not reapply until penis and surrounding tissue are free from irritation.
  - Some institutions apply a thin layer of plasticized skin spray to skin of penile shaft to protect skin from ulceration and irritation caused by rubber condom and adhesive holding it in place.
- Urination is reduced in amount and frequency.
  - Assess for kink in tubing.

- Assess condom application 30 minutes after applying, and inspect every 4 hours to determine if the penis circulation is adequate.
- Observe whether urine is pooling at tip of condom, bathing the penis in urine; reapply.

- Penile swelling or discoloration occurs.
  - Catheter has been improperly applied, or adhesive has been applied too snugly, resulting in impaired circulation. Remove catheter.
- Condom does not stay on.
  - Reapply as necessary. Reassess current condom size. See manufacturer's size chart.
- Venous circulation in leg impaired from leg bag strap.
  - Assess leg every 8 hours for circulatory impairment.
  - Apply a large Foley bag at night or continuous for a bedridden client.

Recording and Reporting

- Report and record pertinent information: condom application, condition of penis skin and scrotum, and voiding pattern.
- Monitor I&O as indicated.

Teaching Considerations

- Teach client to keep condom and catheter kink free and positioned below the level of the bladder.
- Teach client with leg bag to periodically assess leg straps for tightness and to report pain in leg.
- Teach client a collection bag that fills completely may put unnecessary tension on the catheter and contribute to problems keeping the catheter intact.

Gerontological Considerations

- Condom catheters are not recommended in clients with chronic urinary obstruction such as benign prostatic hypertrophy (Urinary Incontinence Guideline Panel, 1996).
- Clients with neuropathy should be carefully evaluated before application of the condom catheter.

Home Care Considerations

- Caregivers should be taught assessments to be made and what to report.
- Teach client to switch from leg bag to drainage bag at night.
- Modifications may need to be made in clothing to promote optimal drainage.

Skill 24-7 Care of a Suprapubic Catheter

Suprapubic catheters are inserted surgically into the bladder through the lower abdomen above the symphysis pubis (Figure 24-5). Although most successfully used for short periods with clients who have had gynecological and bladder surgery, the suprapubic catheter may be used for long-term care (Peate, 1997).

As with the indwelling urinary catheter, the suprapubic catheter predisposes the client to urinary tract infection (UTI), but the incidence may be lower than that with the indwelling catheter. The advantages of the suprapubic catheter for the client are that the client may void naturally when the catheter is clamped and it is more comfortable than the indwelling catheter. The procedure can be performed at the bedside with the client under local anesthesia, or it may be performed in surgery.

The nurse is responsible for maintaining the catheter while the client is in the nursing home or hospital and for teaching the client or caregiver about routine care. Daily care will depend on the institution's policy, but the cleaning and dressing of the catheter site is similar to that for any surgical drain.

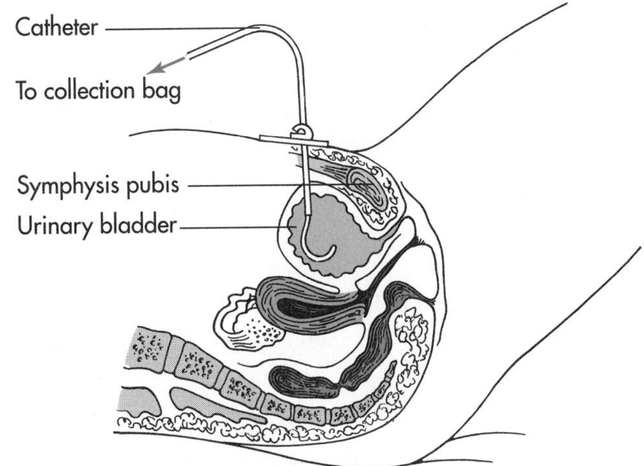

FIGURE 24-5 Suprapubic catheter in place.

Delegation Considerations

The skill of caring for a newly established suprapubic catheter should not be delegated to assistive personnel. However, assistive personnel may care for established suprapubic catheters. Have care provider report any change in client's comfort from tube or appearance of foul-smelling or discolored urine.

Equipment

- Gloves, sterile and clean
- Cleansing agent
- Sterile gauze for cleaning
- Sterile drain sponge (split gauze)
- Tape
- Dressing bag

Step	Rationale
Assessment	
1. Assess urine in bag for amount, clarity, color, odor, and sediment.	Abnormal findings may indicate potential complications such as UTI, decreased urinary output, and blockage.
2. Assess dressing for drainage and intactness.	Drainage indicates potential complication such as infection. Dressing coming off may be caused by tape choice or client picking at dressing.
3. Assess catheter insertion site for signs of inflammation such as redness, swelling, and discharge. Ask client if there is any pain at site.	If insertion is new, slight inflammation may be expected as part of wound healing. May indicate potential infection.
4. Assess how catheter is held in place.	The catheter may be sutured or may be retained by a manufactured seal or a water-filled balloon (much like an indwelling catheter in this latter example) (Peate, 1997).
5. Assess tape site for signs of irritation.	Taping over the same area over a prolonged period may lead to skin irritation and breakdown.
6. Assess for fever.	An increased temperature may indicate infection.
7. Check for allergies.	Client may be sensitive to tape or to antiseptic solution.
8. Assess client's knowledge of purpose of catheter and its care.	Determines level of instruction required.

Nursing Diagnosis

Defining characteristics from the assessment data may reveal the following nursing diagnoses for clients requiring this skill:

- Impaired urinary elimination
- Impaired skin integrity
- Functional urinary incontinence
- Deficient knowledge regarding care of suprapubic catheter
- Acute pain
- Risk for infection
- Total urinary incontinence
- Urge urinary incontinence
- Urinary retention

Related factors are individualized based on client's condition or needs.

Planning

Step	Rationale
1. **Expected outcomes** following completion of procedure:	
▪ Client will verbalize no pain or discomfort at insertion site.	Patent catheter system keeps bladder empty and client comfortable and without signs of infection.
▪ Minimum of 30 ml of urine is present in urinary collection bag every hour.	Verifies that there is adequate perfusion to kidneys and that catheter is not blocked.
▪ Urine remains clear and dilute without foul odor.	Removal of retained urine reduces medium for bacterial growth.
▪ Site remains dry, clean, and intact.	No indication of infection or breakdown develops.
▪ Client remains afebrile.	Indicates that no infection is developing.
▪ Client can explain the purpose and expected outcome.	Helps to minimize anxiety.

STEP	RATIONALE

IMPLEMENTATION

1. Wash hands. — Reduces transmission of infection.
2. Close curtain or door. — Provides privacy, reduces embarrassment, and relaxes client.
3. Prepare supplies and cleansing agent as for applying a dry dressing (see Chapter 36). — The catheter site is surgically made and therefore is treated similarly to other dressings (Peate, 1997).
4. Use nondominant sterile gloved hand to hold catheter erect while cleaning. Use gauze moistened with cleansing agent to clean site by swabbing in circular motion starting closest to the drain and continuing in outward widening circles for approximately 2 inches (5 cm) (see illustration). — Follows principle of sterile technique to move from area of least contamination to most. Cleanses microorganisms that could migrate to site.

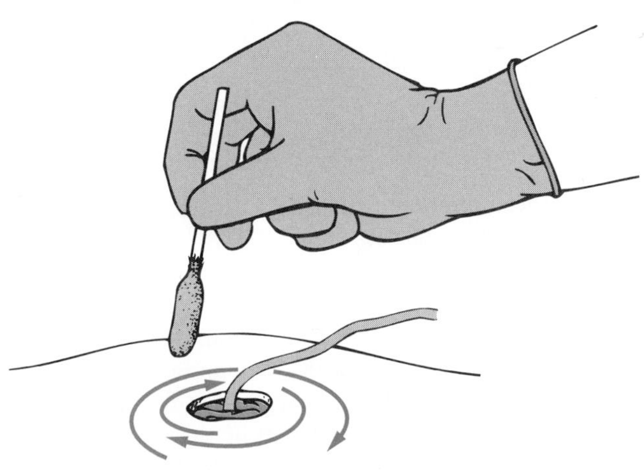

STEP 4 Clean in a circular pattern.

5. Use a new piece of moistened gauze to gently clean the base of the catheter, moving up and away from site of insertion. Do not pull catheter. — Removes microorganisms that reside on any drainage that adheres to tubing.
6. With dominant sterile gloved hand, apply split gauze around catheter and tape in place. — Serves to collect secretions.
7. Secure catheter to abdomen with tape or Velcro multipurpose tube holder to reduce tension on insertion site. — This technique is similar to that used for indwelling urinary catheter. Secures catheter and reduces risk of excessive tension on suture and/or body seal.
8. Check bag and tubing placement.
   - ***Critical Decision Point***
     Be sure there are no obstructions in tubing. Coil excess tubing on bed and fasten it to bottom sheet with clip from kit or with rubber band and safety pin.

EVALUATION

1. Ask client whether there is any pain or discomfort from suprapubic catheter. — Determines if bladder is draining and client is free of infection.
2. Observe client's urine for sediment, odor, or discoloration. — Possible signs of infection when present.
3. Inspect dressing at least every shift. — Dressings do not need to be changed daily unless there are indicators such as pain or discharge (Peate, 1997).
4. Monitor for signs of infection: elevated white blood cell count (WBC), positive urine culture, or elevated temperature.

Unexpected Outcomes and Related Interventions

- Catheter becomes dislodged.
  - Catheter is blocked by clots, accumulation of sediment, or position of catheter in bladder. The suprapubic catheter is often small bore and is easily blocked. Encourage client to drink at least 1500 ml of fluids per day if no restrictions.
  - Notify physician if blockage is persistent.
- Site continues to bleed after removal of old dressing.
  - Notify physician.
  - Monitor site, and assess vital signs.
- Client develops a UTI.
  - Encourage fluids, and notify physician.
  - Observe urine for color, consistency.
  - Monitor intake and output (I&O).
- Leakage of urine at site and skin breakdown.
  - Inspection and dressing changes are important in monitoring for these problems.
  - Notify physician.

Recording and Reporting

- Report and record dressing replacement, including assessments of wound and tolerance of client to dressing.
- Clients may have both an indwelling and a suprapubic catheter after gynecological or bladder surgery. Urine must be assessed in both drainage systems. (Most urine will be found in the suprapubic drainage system.) Record both outputs.
- Residual urine can be assessed by having client void while suprapubic drainage tubing is clamped; the residual urine is then measured by releasing the clamp. Residual urine amounts of less than 50 ml may indicate that bladder function has returned postoperatively.

Teaching Considerations

- Encourage clients to consume a minimum of 1500 ml of fluids daily.
- Clients should be taught to keep the drainage bag lower than the bladder and to keep tubing free of kinks.
- Clients should be informed that they may experience bladder spasms. The diameter of the suprapubic catheter is small and is easily occluded with clots, mucus, or sediment. Occlusion can lead to bladder irritation and spasms.
- Clients with both suprapubic and indwelling catheters should be informed that they will have the indwelling urinary catheter removed first, usually between the second and fourth postoperative day.

Home Care Considerations

- With shortened hospital stays it is common for the post-surgery client to go home with a suprapubic catheter.
- Client or caregiver needs to be taught how to clean and dress the suprapubic site and assess signs of infection at the site.
- Client or caregiver needs to be taught how to empty a catheter bag and assess urine for color, odor, clarity, and amount.

Skill 24-8 Peritoneal Dialysis and Continuous Ambulatory Peritoneal Dialysis

The kidneys are organs that filter and excrete excess fluid and solute wastes. When the kidneys fail, little to no urine is produced, electrolyte imbalances occur, and toxins accumulate in the blood. If excess fluid and toxins are not removed, death results.

Dialysis is a process that removes fluid and solute wastes from the blood or lymph. There are two major types of dialysis: hemodialysis and peritoneal dialysis. Hemodialysis nursing is a specialty practice that involves the shunting of the client's blood through a machine. Peritoneal dialysis is a procedure that infuses a hypertonic solution into the peritoneal cavity. The solution is left for a specified period of time and then drained. The semipermeable peritoneum membrane serves as a filter to remove excess water, electrolytes, and toxins from the blood. Peritoneal dialysis has three steps, each of which varies in length: (1) infusing the dialysate into the cavity, (2) allowing the fluid to dwell in the cavity, and (3) draining the dialysate from the cavity. These are sometimes referred to as "fill, dwell, and drain times."

Peritoneal dialysis can be performed for the acutely ill client or for the client with chronic renal failure. Acute intermittent peritoneal dialysis (IPD) is used within the hospital setting and involves the surgical insertion of a temporary catheter into the peritoneal cavity (Figure 24-6). An exchange or dialysis cycle in acute peritoneal dialysis ranges from ½ hour to 2 hours (Lancaster, 1995).

A second form of peritoneal dialysis is used with clients who need ongoing dialysis. Clients who require dialysis because of a chronic condition have long-term peritoneal catheters inserted and, based on need, may receive their dialysis in a variety of settings, including their homes. Therapy can be intermittent or continuous depending on the need.

Continuous ambulatory peritoneal dialysis (CAPD) is a type of therapy that has made home peritoneal dialysis feasible for the client with end-stage renal disease. With this type of dialysis, a permanent catheter is surgically implanted into the peritoneal cavity, and the processes of osmosis and diffusion remove fluid, excess electrolytes, and toxins from the blood. CAPD has the same three phases as acute peritoneal dialysis; however, the time cycle differs. Exchanges during the day are 3 to 6 hours long, and nighttime exchanges last 8 to 12 hours. During the "dwell time" an empty bag and drainage tubing are folded and concealed under the client's clothes (unless a bagless system is used). Afterward, the client drains the abdominal cavity, which is followed by reinstillation of fresh dialysate into the peritoneal cavity. The dialysate must be changed three to five times a day. One major advantage of CAPD is that it allows the client to be out of the hospital, maintain the system at home, and continue with daily activities.

A variation of the CAPD is continuous cyclic peritoneal dialysis (CCPD), which uses a cycler that automates the infusion of the dialysate. CCPD is often used to automate nighttime exchanges for clients in the home, or it may be used by hospital staff to automate the cycling process. When used for the client at night in the home, this process is referred to as nightly intermittent peritoneal dialysis.

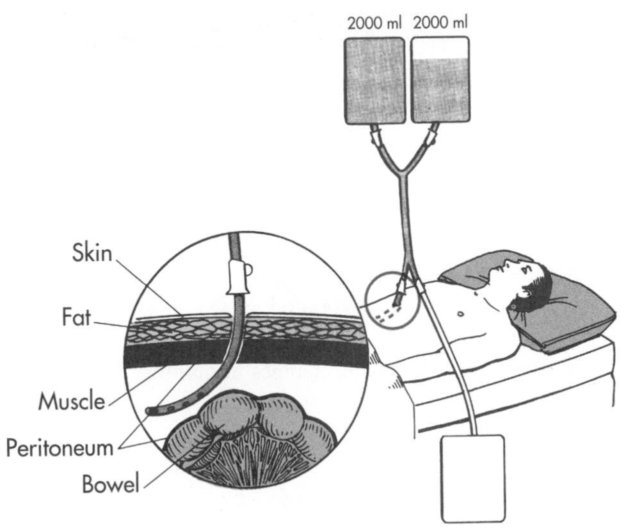

FIGURE **24-6** Patient receiving peritoneal dialysis. Dialysis fluid is being inserted into peritoneal cavity. (From Phipps WJ and others: *Medical-surgical nursing,* ed 6, St. Louis, 1999, Mosby.)

Delegation Considerations

The skills of peritoneal and continuous ambulatory dialysis should not be delegated to assistive personnel.

Equipment

- Ordered dialysate at 37° C (98° F)
- Sterile on-off pack containing titanium or plastic adapter and catheter cap
- Hydrogen peroxide
- Povidone-iodine solution
- Povidone-iodine ointment
- Mask, sterile gloves, goggles
- Intravenous (IV) pole
- Connector tubing (CAPD clients may not need)
- Sterile drainage bag
- IV bag label (IPD only)
- Peritoneal dialysis flow sheet (see Figure 24-7)

Step	Rationale
Assessment	
1. Obtain client's weight.	Provides baseline information about weight attributed to fluid retention. A daily weight gain of 1 kg is equivalent to 1 L of fluid.
2. Obtain vital signs.	Fluid volume changes associated with dialysis increase risk for hemodynamic blood pressure changes. In clients undergoing IPD, increased abdominal pressure may lead to bradycardia subsequent to vagal nerve stimulation (Lancaster, 1995).
3. Assess respiratory rate and auscultate lungs.	Pressure from fluid that is cycled into the peritoneal cavity may cause difficulty with breathing. Fluid volume changes may lead to fluid volume overload.
4. Measure abdominal girth.	Mark midpoint of client's abdomen. Keep mark as reference for future measurements. Provides baseline data regarding amount of fluid in peritoneal cavity.
5. Monitor for fluid and electrolyte balance.	Clients may experience hypervolemia or hypovolemia. Signs of hypervolemia include increased blood pressure, difficulty breathing, edema, and neck vein distention. Signs of hypovolemia include tachycardia, hypotension, poor skin turgor, and dry mucous membranes. With potassium imbalance, either hypokalemia or hyperkalemia may occur. Laboratory work must be performed to monitor for a potassium level alteration.

Step	Rationale
6. Inspect catheter site for erythema, tenderness, drainage, and swelling.	Indicates infection at catheter entry site, which increases risk for peritonitis.
7. Measure body temperature.	Provides baseline data about client's febrile status.
8. Review hospital or dialysis unit's procedure for IPD or CAPD.	There may be institutional variations regarding ordering of supplies; fill, dwell, and drain times; catheter care; and discharge teaching plan.
9. Review physician's orders:	
a. Verify dialysis solution and any medications added to solution.	IPD and CAPD require specific orders individualized to client's fluid needs and disease process.
b. Verify number of exchanges and infusion and dwell and drain times.	
10. Obtain laboratory data as ordered:	Documents fluid and electrolyte status and changes that occur from IPD or CAPD.
a. IPD: every 12 to 24 hours.	
b. CAPD: can vary depending on individual needs.	
11. Assess client's and family members' knowledge regarding the purpose of dialysis.	Reveals need for client instruction.

Nursing Diagnosis

Defining characteristics from the assessment data may reveal the following nursing diagnoses for clients requiring this skill:

- Deficient fluid volume
- Risk for deficient fluid volume
- Excess fluid volume
- Impaired home maintenance management
- Deficient knowledge regarding peritoneal dialysis
- Acute pain
- Risk for infection

Related factors are individualized based on client's condition or needs.

Planning

Step	Rationale
1. Expected outcomes following completion of procedure:	
▪ Decreased weight.	Indicates that excess fluid was removed. Indicates that more dialysate was removed than was instilled.
▪ Stable vital signs.	Indicates that there are no adverse hemodynamic responses.
▪ Decreased abdominal girth with IPD.	Indicates that no fluid was retained in peritoneal cavity.
▪ No erythema, tenderness, or drainage at catheter site.	Indicates absence of local inflammation at catheter site.
▪ No fever.	Indicates that no systemic infection is present.
▪ Dialysate return is clear or slightly light yellow.	Expected color of returned fluid; indicates absence of blood or bacteria in peritoneal cavity.
▪ Client is able to discuss principles of asepsis and peritoneal dialysis.	Discussing principles allows nurse to document cognitive learning.
▪ Client or caregiver will perform CAPD.	Demonstration is an effective measure to evaluate psychomotor learning.

Implementation

Step	Rationale
1. Wash hands and put on mask.	Reduces transmission of microorganisms.

- ***Critical Decision Point***

  When client is performing peritoneal dialysis in the home, client must wear mask.

Step	Rationale
2. Place client in semi-Fowler's or high-Fowler's position.	Instilling fluid into peritoneal cavity decreases diaphragmatic excursion. The semi-Fowler's or high-Fowler's position promotes optimal lung expansion.

Step	Rationale
3. Add medications aseptically immediately before beginning instillation of dialysate. Disinfect multiple-dose vials and injection ports of plastic bags. Label and record all medications added (Lancaster, 1995).	Reduces transmission of microorganisms into dialysate.

- ***Critical Decision Point***
  Maintain strict asepsis when adding medications to dialysate.

Step	Rationale
a. Heparin	Reduces accumulation of fibrin around catheter tip.
b. Prophylactic antibiotics	Reduce risk of peritonitis.
c. Insulin	Regular insulin is added to control serum glucose (Lancaster, 1995).
4. Attach two warmed dialysate bags to inflow tubing and attach to IV pole. Bags are punctured exactly as IV solution bags (see Chapter 19) or with special spiking devices.	Dialysate is warmed by dry heat through the use of warming pad, incubator, or microwave warming device. Hanging two bags promotes timely, organized follow-up exchanges. Standard IPD usually includes 24 exchanges in 24 hours. CAPD clients are instructed to hang only one bag because these clients have three to five exchanges daily.

- ***Critical Decision Point***
  Immersing dialysate in warm water is not recommended because of the chance of contamination (Lancaster, 1995). Dialysate that is too cold results in intolerance, cramps, and hypothermia.

Step	Rationale
5. Apply sterile gloves.	
6. Disinfect catheter cap and end of catheter; remove cap and disinfect adapter. Connect tubing, maintaining sepsis.	
7. With the CAPD system a Y connector that attaches on one side to the dialysate and the other side to the drainage bag may be used. The Y connector is attached aseptically.	This connection allows for flushing about 100 ml of dialysate into the drainage bag and then draining dialysate from the peritoneum. Research has shown this procedure, called the "flush before fill," to be effective in reducing the incidence of peritonitis (Lancaster, 1995).
8. Open clamp on first dialysate bag, and clamp on client line. Infuse solution over prescribed time (usually 2 L/10-15 min).	Permits instillation of dialysate into peritoneal cavity.
9. Clamp inflow tubing for prescribed dwell time:	
a. IPD: usually 30 minutes.	Prevents air from entering peritoneal cavity. Dwell time permits peritoneal membrane to exchange fluid, electrolytes, toxins from blood.
b. CAPD: 3 to 5 hours (CAPD client folds tubing and infusion bag on abdomen, which is concealed by clothing, and uses same bag and tubing for drain cycle).	

- ***Critical Decision Point***
  Monitor infusion and dwell time carefully. A timer may be used to signal the scheduled interval for each phase.

Step	Rationale
10. Remove first dialysate bag from IV pole. Place third warmed bag on pole.	Promotes organized procedure. When multiple exchanges are ordered, nurse should have two dialysate bags on IV pole.
11. Unclamp outflow tubing and drain (usually for 20 minutes). Evaluate drainage for clarity and color.	Permits drainage of dialysate and wastes from peritoneal cavity. During first two or three exchanges, it is common for dialysate to remain in cavity; excess should drain with later exchanges. The used dialysate should be clear (Scott, 1999).
12. Clamp outflow tubing.	Prevents untimed drain during subsequent exchange.
13. Empty and measure fluid in drainage bag.	Provides assessment of fluid balance of dialysate solution. If volume of fluid infused is more than amount drained, balance is positive (e.g., if 2000 ml of dialysate was infused and 1800 ml was drained, balance is positive 200 ml [+200 ml], meaning the client is retaining the fluid).

- ***Critical Decision Point***
  Wear gloves, mask, eye protection (or face shield), and gown when emptying because splashes may occur.

Step	Rationale
14. Remove contaminated items. Wash hands.	
15. Repeat steps until all exchanges are complete.	
16. During first exchanges, monitor client's vital signs every 15 minutes.	Promotes timely documentation of hemodynamic effects of IPD.
17. When all exchanges are complete:	
a. Acute-use catheter (short-term use): Disinfect, disconnect connections, and discard tubing. Disinfect catheter rim, and securely place sterile cap on end.	Keeps sterile catheter secure and closed to entrance of microorganisms.
b. Chronic-use catheter (long-term use): See guidelines made specifically for catheter.	Maintains patency of catheter insertion site.
18. Inspect catheter site; if dressing is reapplied, apply a clear transparent occlusive dressing (see Chapter 36).	Intact, dry dressing reduces risk of infection. If encrustations have developed, clean gently. Removal of crusts may cause further injury and may increase chance of infection (Scott, 1999).
19. Wash hands, and dispose of contaminated supplies according to agency policy.	Reduces transmission of microorganisms and blood-borne pathogens.

Evaluation

Step	Rationale
1. Obtain weight.	Decrease indicates removal of excess fluid; increase indicates retention of fluid.
2. Obtain dialysis fluid balance measurements.	Determines adequacy of fluid removal.
3. Obtain vital signs.	Documents tolerance to IPD.
4. Obtain body temperature.	Denotes presence or absence of infection.
5. Measure abdominal girth.	Provides an indirect measurement of fluid retention in peritoneal cavity.
6. Inspect catheter site for erythema, tenderness, drainage, and swelling.	Documents symptoms of infection.
7. Auscultate lungs for crackles.	Provides a measurement of fluid overload. As intravascular fluid increases, crackles are auscultated in bases of lungs.
8. Inspect returned dialysate solution.	Note blood, purulent discharge, fecal contents, or urine that may indicate infection, or perforation or fistula development.
9. Observe client performing CAPD.	Documents learning of skill.
10. Assess client's comfort level.	Clients may have incisional pain after access insertion. Clients undergoing peritoneal dialysis may also describe a feeling of fullness following instillation of a large volume of dialysate in the abdominal cavity.
11. Monitor laboratory work.	Imbalances in potassium may occur. A relative increase or decrease in hematocrit may indicate hypovolemia or hypervolemia, respectively.

Unexpected Outcomes and Related Interventions

- Increased weight or no weight change. Indicates fluid retained in peritoneal cavity.
  - Report to physician.
- Positive fluid balance. Indicates excess fluid retained.
  - Report to physician.
- Decreased blood pressure and tachycardia. Client unable to tolerate fluid volume, or catheter may have perforated bowel.
  - Report to physician.
  - Monitor client frequently.
- Increased abdominal girth. Indicates retained fluid.
  - Report to physician.
  - Assess for kinking in dialysis tubing.
- Erythema, tenderness, and drainage at catheter site. Indicates local inflammatory response.
  - Report to physician.
- Fever. Indicates systemic infection.
  - Report to physician.
- Dialysate drainage is abnormal.
  - Report to physician.

- Cramps. Indicates that dialysate is too cold, infusion is too rapid, volume is too much for client to tolerate, or electrolyte imbalances have occurred.
    - Check temperature of dialysate, check electrolyte levels, and compare volume to previous records.
    - Report to physician.
- Sudden respiratory distress. Indicates that volume is too excessive for client to tolerate.
    - Report to physician.
- Poor instillation flow or poor drainage.
    - Check for kink in inflow/outflow tubing or catheter.
- Leaking of dialysate from peritoneum.
    - Look for edema in abdominal wall, perineum, or penis (Lancaster, 1995).
    - Notify physician.
- Leak at catheter site. Indicates catheter displacement toward abdominal surface.
    - Notify physician.

Recording and Reporting

- Document client's weight, abdominal girth, and dialysis fluid balance before and after IPD. Notes presence or absence of retained fluid in peritoneal cavity.
- Document client's vital signs and respiratory status before, during, and after dialysis. Notes hemodynamic response.
- Document client's temperature and status of catheter site. Notes presence or absence of local or systemic infection.
- Record presence of pain or discomfort. Identify location, quality, and duration of pain. Report pain that is severe or unexpected.
- Record color of dialysate drainage. Notes abnormalities in drainage color.
- Record condition of catheter dressing or if new dressing is applied. Records status of dressing's condition and most recent dressing change.
- Note any unexpected outcomes and actions taken by nurse and physician. Records continuing care of client and possible future complications.
- Individual hospitals have individual flow sheets to record IPD fluids (Figure 24-7).
- When charting, it is important to note that if client is losing fluid weight, a negative balance is achieved. A positive balance means client is *retaining* instilled fluid.

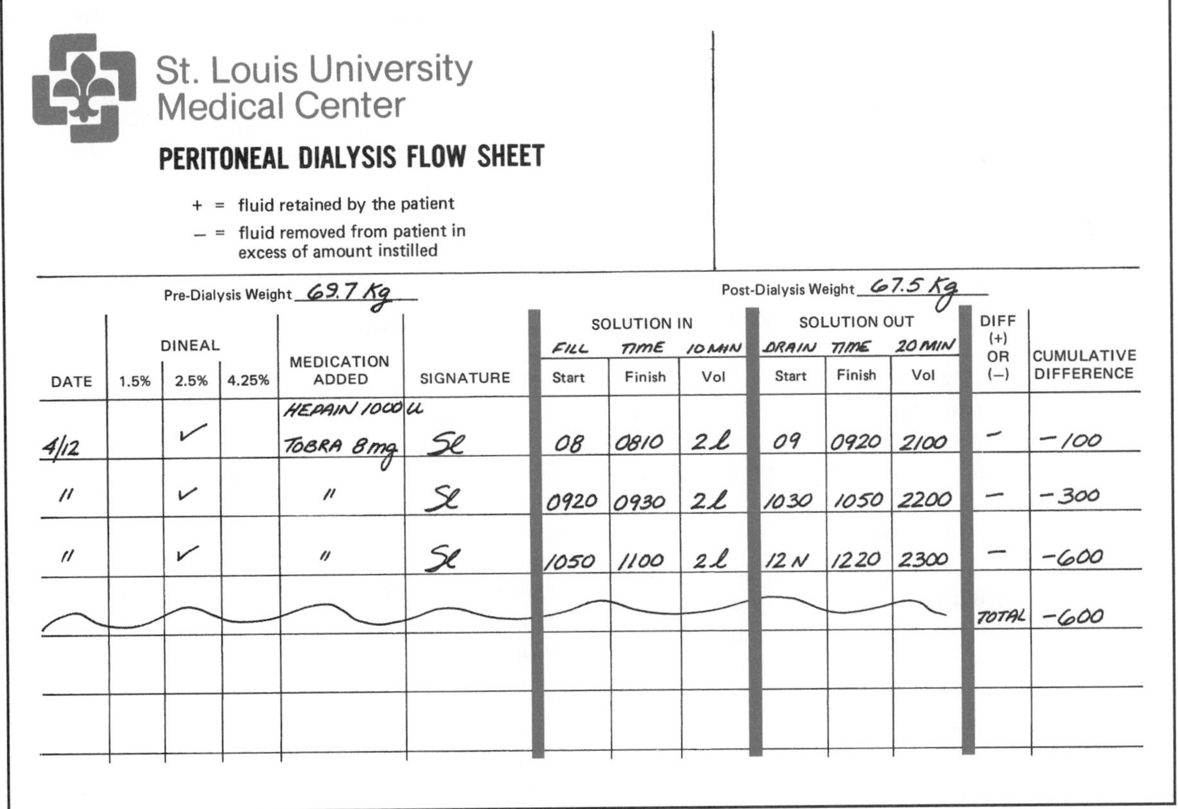

St. Louis University Medical Center

PERITONEAL DIALYSIS FLOW SHEET

\+ = fluid retained by the patient

– = fluid removed from patient in excess of amount instilled

Pre-Dialysis Weight 69.7 Kg

Post-Dialysis Weight 67.5 Kg

DATE	DINEAL 1.5%	DINEAL 2.5%	DINEAL 4.25%	MEDICATION ADDED	SIGNATURE	SOLUTION IN Start (FILL)	SOLUTION IN Finish (TIME)	SOLUTION IN Vol (10 MIN)	SOLUTION OUT Start (DRAIN)	SOLUTION OUT Finish (TIME)	SOLUTION OUT Vol (20 MIN)	DIFF (+) OR (–)	CUMULATIVE DIFFERENCE
4/12		✓		HEPAIN 1000 u TOBRA 8mg	Sl	08	0810	2 l	09	0920	2100	–	–100
//		✓		//	Sl	0920	0930	2 l	1030	1050	2200	–	–300
//		✓		//	Sl	1050	1100	2 l	12 N	1220	2300	–	–600
												TOTAL	–600

FIGURE **24-7** Peritoneal dialysis flow sheet. (Courtesy Saint Louis University Medical Center, St. Louis.)

Teaching Considerations

- Teach IPD clients what to expect during and after procedure.
- Teach scrub and exchange procedures to CAPD clients and/or caregivers according to policy and ask client to correctly demonstrate scrub and exchange procedure.
- Instruct client and/or caregivers in the common symptoms of fluid excess and deficit.
- Review teaching plan with client before discharge and during each clinic visit.
- Periodically review potential complications and signs and symptoms.
- Review medications and dietary and fluid restrictions.
- Instruct client when and whom to contact in emergency.
- Instruct client and/or caregivers how to take blood pressure correctly.
- Instruct client to weigh self correctly.
- Instruct client and/or caregiver about common symptoms associated with peritonitis.
- Client receiving IPD should be encouraged to move around in bed. However, movements should avoid stressing catheter or tubing. CAPD clients who are ambulatory should be encouraged to ambulate in between exchanges.
- Teach the client to check labels carefully. Peritoneal dialysis solutions are available in four dextrose concentrations (1.5%, 2.5%, 3.5%, and 4.25%), each with increasing osmolality to enhance fluid removal by osmosis (Scott, 1999).

Gerontological Considerations

- A major risk factor for death with CAPD is age greater than 65 years (Lancaster, 1995).
- The older adult client may be at risk for malnutrition related to loss of protein during dialysis, dietary restrictions, and loss of appetite.
- Clients on dialysis often suffer many complications; older adults are no exception. However, older adult client may be taking medications for other chronic health problems. Monitoring and assessment of medication therapy are ongoing.

Home Care Considerations

- CAPD clients must do the following correctly to complete CAPD exchanges:
  - Achieve expected outcomes under Planning.
  - Demonstrate CAPD scrub and aseptic exchange procedure.
  - State signs of infection.
  - Adhere to fluid, dietary, and medication therapies.
  - Perform activities of daily living. CAPD is designed so client can maintain normal daily activities.
  - The training interval for client undergoing CAPD is individualized to the client and family.
  - Centers for Disease Control and Prevention (CDC) recommendations require proper disposal of any used dialysate fluid.

Critical Thinking Exercises

1. Your are caring for a 63-year-old man who has dementia and is admitted from a nursing home with septicemia (systemic infection) secondary to a urinary tract infection (UTI). How will you care for the indwelling catheter that has been inserted?
2. You are caring for a 49-year-old woman who complains of moderate suprapubic pain (grade 5 on scale of 10). She has an order for a straight catheterization as needed (prn). What assessments would you make? Would you insert the straight catheter?
3. You are caring for an 85-year-old woman who has a Foley catheter in place. You are changing the bed when you notice a wet spot under her buttocks. What assessments do you need to make to determine if the catheter may be leaking?

References

Asci J, Beyea S: Urologic update: indwelling urinary catheters—an integrative review of the literature, *Online J Knowledge Synthesis Nurs* 3(2):1, 1996.

Binard J and others: Intermittent catheterization the right way! (volume vs time-directed), *J Spinal Cord Med* 19(3):194, 1996.

Evans E: Indwelling catheter care: dispelling the misconceptions, *Geriatr Nurs* 20(2):85, 1999.

Gray M: *Genitourinary disorders,* St. Louis, 1992, Mosby.

Hiser V: Nursing Interventions for urinary incontinence in home health, *J Wound Ostomy Continence Nurs* 26(3):142, 1999.

Lancaster L: *ANNA: curriculum for nephrology nursing,* ed 3, Pitman, NJ, 1995, Anthony J. Janetti.

Lombardo M, Hartwig M: Central nervous system injury. In Price S, Wilson L: *Pathophysiology: clinical concepts of disease,* ed 5, St. Louis, 1997, Mosby.

Lueckenotte A: *Gerontological nursing,* ed 2, 2000, Mosby.

Ouslander G, Schnelle J: Incontinence in the nursing home, *Am Coll Physicians* 122(6):438, 1995.

Peate I: Patient management following suprapubic catheterization, *Br J Nurs* 6(10):555, 1997.

Phipps WJ and others: *Medical-surgical nursing,* ed 6, St. Louis, 1999, Mosby.

Scott M: Caring for the orthopaedic patient receiving continuous ambulatory peritoneal dialysis, *Orthop Nurs* 18(4):59, 1999.

Stelling J, Hale A: Protocol for changing condom catheters in males with spinal cord injury, *SCI Nurs* 13(2):28, 1996.

Suchinski G and others: Treating urinary infections in the elderly, *Dimens Crit Care Nurs* 18(1):21, 1999.

Urinary Incontinence Guideline Panel: *Urinary incontinence in adults—clinical practice guidelines.* AHCPR Pub No 92-0686. Rockville, Md, 1996, Agency for Health Care Policy and Research, Public Health Services, U.S. Department of Health and Human Services.

Williams M, Wallhagen M, Dowling G: Urinary retention in hospitalized elderly women, *J Gerontol Nurs* 19(2):7, 1993.

Wong D and others: *Whaley & Wong's nursing care of infants and children,* ed 6, 1999, Mosby.

25

Bowel Elimination and Gastric Intubation

Skills

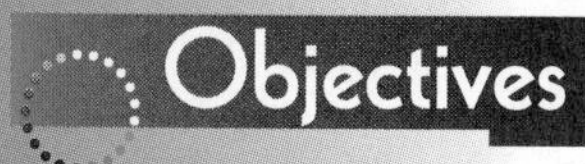

Objectives

Mastery of content in this chapter will enable the nurse to:

- Define the key terms listed.
- Describe factors that promote and impede normal bowel elimination.
- Discuss methods to relieve constipation or impaction.
- Describe approaches for managing a client's comfort during nasogastric tube insertion.
- Implement the following skills: assisting client in using a bedpan, digital removal of stool, enema administration, and insertion of a nasogastric tube.

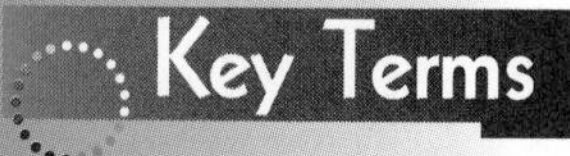

Key Terms

Cathartic
Cleansing enema
Colon
Constipation
Decompression
Defecation
Enema
Fracture pan
Hemorrhoids
Impaction
Medicated enema
Obstipation
Occult blood
Oil-retention enema

Regular elimination of bowel waste products is essential for normal body functioning and a sense of well-being. Because bowel function depends on the balance of several factors, physical and psychological, elimination patterns and habits vary among individuals. When ill at home or in a health care setting, people may not be able to maintain normal elimination habits and therefore might require a nurse's assistance to help with this body process. It is important for the nurse to always show respect for a client's privacy, provide necessary comfort measures, and attend to the client's emotional needs when performing required skills.

To assist clients with bowel elimination by performing skills competently, the nurse must have a clear understanding of normal elimination and factors that contribute to alterations. The nurse must be able to assist immobilized clients with the elimination process by helping them on and off bedpans. Often a nurse may be responsible for collecting stool specimens and ensuring that they are properly handled (see Chapter 41). If a client is constipated, the nurse may be expected to competently administer enemas or to digitally remove impacted stool. When clients undergo surgery or experience an alteration in gastrointestinal peristalsis, the insertion of a nasogastric tube may become necessary.

Skill Performance Guidelines

1. Determine a client's normal pattern of bowel elimination and try to accommodate that pattern while the client is in a health care setting. Determine the time the client normally has a bowel movement and the amount of assistance needed.
2. Provide privacy and try to reduce the client's embarrassment. If possible, the client should be encouraged to use the bathroom. However, if the nature of the illness limits physical activity, ensure as much privacy as possible during use of the bedpan or bedside commode.
3. Be aware of foods that promote normal peristaltic movement, including high-fiber foods such as raw fruit, whole grains, and green leafy vegetables, that are consistent with the client's prescribed diet. Immobilized clients should receive foods that promote peristalsis but not those that adversely affect bowel routine.
4. Unless contraindicated, encourage adequate hydration. Normally a person should drink 6 to 8 glasses of water per day. Warm fluids are especially effective in increasing peristalsis.
5. Encourage clients to be as active as physically possible. Physical activity promotes peristalsis, whereas immobilization decreases it.
6. Promote client comfort. The procedures designed to promote normal elimination or bowel **decompression** can create discomfort if not performed correctly.
7. Be aware of the side effects of medications the client receives. Some drugs may impair the normal elimination pattern by causing diarrhea or **constipation.** Also, general anesthetic agents used during surgery cause temporary cessation of peristalsis, which can affect the normal elimination pattern after surgery.
8. Consider the developmental changes that affect bowel functioning throughout the life span. For example, an older adult might become less active, muscle tone might be decreased, and eating patterns might change. These factors could result in constipation.
9. When handling or coming in contact with fecal matter always use standard precautions to prevent infection transmission.

Skill 25-1 Assisting the Client in Using a Bedpan

A client restricted to bed must use a bedpan for **defecation.** Women use bedpans to pass urine and feces, whereas men use bedpans only for defecation. Sitting on a bedpan can be extremely uncomfortable. The nurse should help the client assume a position similar to the natural squatting position.

Two types of bedpans are available (Figure 25-1). The regular bedpan, made of metal or hard plastic, has a curved, smooth upper end and a tapered lower end. The pan is approximately 5 cm (2 inches) deep. A **fracture pan,** designed for clients with body or leg casts or clients restricted from raising their hips (e.g., following total joint replacement), has a shallow upper end approximately 1.3 cm (½ inch) deep that slips easily under a client. The upper end of either pan fits under the client's buttocks toward the sacrum, with the lower end just under the upper thighs.

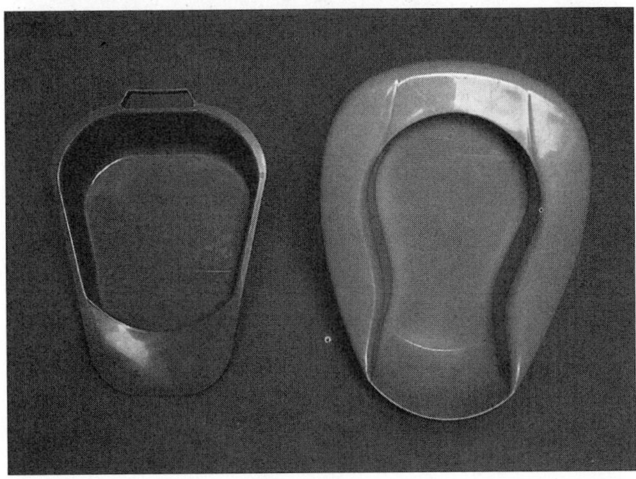

FIGURE **25-1** Types of bedpans. *Left,* Fracture bedpan. *Right,* Regular bedpan.

Delegation Considerations

The skill of assisting a client onto a bedpan can be delegated to assistive personnel. Be sure to inform and assist care provider in proper way to position clients who have mobility restrictions. Also instruct care provider about how to position clients who also have therapeutic equipment present, such as drains, intravenous catheters, or traction.

Equipment

- Disposable gloves
- Appropriate type of clean bedpan
- Bedpan cover
- Toilet tissue
- Specimen container (if necessary), plastic bag, clearly labeled with date, client's name, and identification number
- Washbasin, washcloths, towels, and soap
- Waterproof, absorbent pads
- Clean draw sheet (optional)

Step	Rationale
Assessment	
1. Assess client's normal bowel elimination habits: routine pattern, effect of certain foods/fluids and eating habits on bowel elimination, effect of stress and level of activity on normal bowel elimination patterns, current medications, normal fluid intake.	Managing a client's elimination problems depends on a thorough understanding of normal elimination and factors that may create alterations. Mass peristalsis is strongest during the hour after first meal of the day. Nurse should anticipate when to offer bedpan.
2. Auscultate abdomen for bowel sounds, and palpate for abdominal distention.	Normal bowel sounds occur irregularly at the rate of 5 to 35 per minute (Doughty and Jackson, 1993). A fecal-filled colon is palpated as a firm rounded mass. A distended bladder can be palpated as a smooth, round mass above the symphysis pubis.
3. Assess client to determine level of mobility and amount of assistance required.	Determines if client can assist in positioning on bedpan or if totally dependent on nurse's help. Older adult, obese clients who have had hip or knee surgery, and debilitated clients may require assistance of two or more nurses to help them onto or off of the bedpan. Assistance from additional personnel promotes safety for client and nurses.
4. Assess if client is allowed to sit up or must lie flat when using bedpan.	Determines most appropriate type of bedpan.

STEP	RATIONALE
5. Assess client's level of comfort. Especially note presence of rectal or abdominal pain or presence of hemorrhoids or irritation of skin surrounding anus.	Pain can limit client's ability to assist with positioning. Rectal or abdominal pain can reduce client's ability to bear down during defecation. Unexplained abdominal pain should be assessed by a physician before enema administration.
6. Determine if a stool specimen is needed.	Provides ample opportunity to obtain specimen container before placing the client on the bedpan.

NURSING DIAGNOSIS

Defining characteristics from the assessment data may reveal the following nursing diagnoses for clients requiring this skill:

- Bowel incontinence
- Risk for constipation
- Diarrhea
- Impaired physical mobility
- Acute pain

Related factors are individualized based on a client's condition or needs.

PLANNING

STEP	RATIONALE
1. **Expected outcomes** following completion of procedure:	
▪ Client is able to successfully defecate in bedpan.	Indicates normal elimination.
▪ Perianal skin is clear and intact.	No irritation has occurred; perianal skin is cleaned appropriately.
▪ Client eliminates without pain.	Client is positioned comfortably on bedpan.
2. Explain procedure to client, including self-help tips.	Information promotes client's independence, reduces anxiety, and helps client to better assist nurse during procedure.
3. Obtain assistance from additional nursing personnel as warranted.	Adequate personnel resources minimize muscle strain for client and nurse. Reduces client's discomfort.

IMPLEMENTATION

STEP	RATIONALE
1. Wash hands and apply gloves.	Reduces transmission of microorganisms.
2. Provide privacy by closing curtains around bed or door of room.	Reduces embarrassment and promotes bowel elimination.
3. Place bedpan under warm, running water for few seconds, then dry. Be careful that pan is not too hot.	Metal bedpans are very cold. Warm pan helps client to relax anal sphincter. Although plastic bedpans may not be as cold to touch as metal, warming them before use is still wise.
4. Put side rail up on opposite side of bed.	Protects client from falling out of bed. Client can use side rail to grasp onto and assist self to move about in bed.
5. Raise bed horizontally according to nurse's height.	Promotes use of good body mechanics and prevents muscle strain for nurse and client.
6. Have client assume supine position.	

• ***Critical Decision Point***

Observe for the presence of drains, dressings, intravenous fluids, traction. These devices may impede a client from assisting with the procedure and may also necessitate more personnel to assist in placing the client on a bedpan.

STEP	RATIONALE
7. Place client who is mobile in bed and can assist with procedure on bedpan.	
a. Raise client's head 30 to 60 degrees.	Prevents hyperextension of back and provides support to upper torso when client raises hips. Sitting position promotes defecation.
b. Remove upper bed linens just enough so they are out of the way, but do not unduly expose client.	Prevents embarrassment to client; demonstrates respect for client's sense of dignity.

Step	Rationale
c. Remove bedpan cover and place in accessible location.	
d. Instruct client on how to flex knees and lift hips upward.	Little effort should be required of client, whose body weight is supported by lower legs and feet and upper torso and arms.
e. Place hand closest to the client palm up, under client's sacrum, to assist lifting. As the client raises the hips, use other hand to slip bedpan under client (see illustration). Be sure open rim of bedpan is facing toward foot of bed. **Do not shove pan under client's hips.** (Option: Have client use overhead trapeze frame to raise hips.)	Nurse must ensure that bedpan is placed high enough under buttocks so feces enters pan. Incorrect placement of bedpan can cause discomfort for client and spillage of contents.
f. Option: If using a fracture pan, simply slip it under the client as the hips are raised (see illustration).	Requires less maneuvering by client.

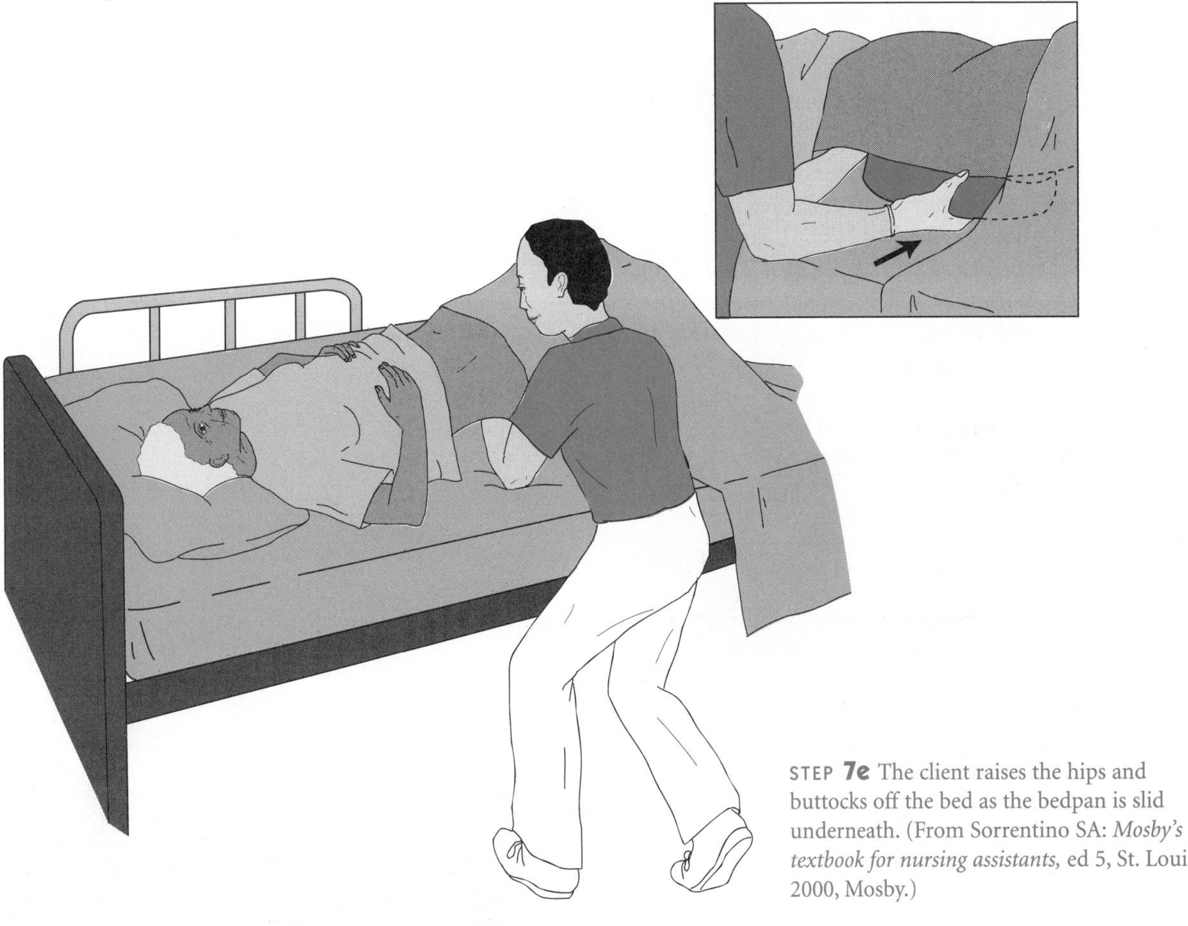

STEP **7e** The client raises the hips and buttocks off the bed as the bedpan is slid underneath. (From Sorrentino SA: *Mosby's textbook for nursing assistants,* ed 5, St. Louis, 2000, Mosby.)

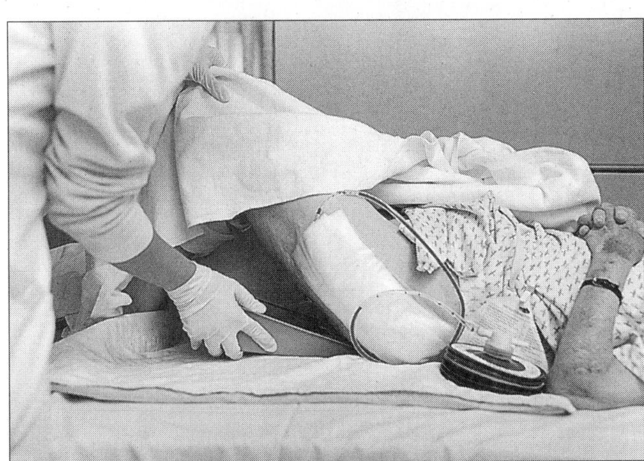

STEP **7f** Client lifts hips as fracture pan is positioned.

Step	Rationale
8. Place client who is immobile or has restrictions in mobility on bedpan.	
a. Lower the head of the bed flat (if tolerated by medical condition).	Assists client for whom it is unsafe to exert effort when lifting hips, who must remain flat, or who is unable to lift hips to roll onto bedpan.
b. Remove top linens as necessary to turn client while minimizing exposure.	Prevents embarrassment to client; demonstrates respect for client's sense of dignity.
c. Remove bedpan cover and place in accessible location.	
d. Assist the client to roll onto one side, backside towards you or turn client into side-lying position. Place bedpan firmly against client's buttocks and down into mattress. Be sure that open rim of bedpan is facing toward foot of bed (see illustrations).	Incorrect placement can cause discomfort to client and spillage of contents.

- ***Critical Decision Point***

  If client has had total hip replacement, the abduction pillow placed between the legs to prevent dislocation of the new joint must remain in place. Use a fracture pan.

Step	Rationale
e. Keeping one hand against the bedpan, place the other around the client's far hip. Ask the client to roll back onto the bedpan, flat in bed.	Positions client squarely on pan with minimal exertion.
f. Raise client's head 30 degrees to a comfortable level, unless contraindicated. Raise knee gatch (unless contraindicated) or ask client to bend the knees.	Client can assume sitting position unless the condition necessitates maintaining flat position. Sitting position promotes defecation.

A

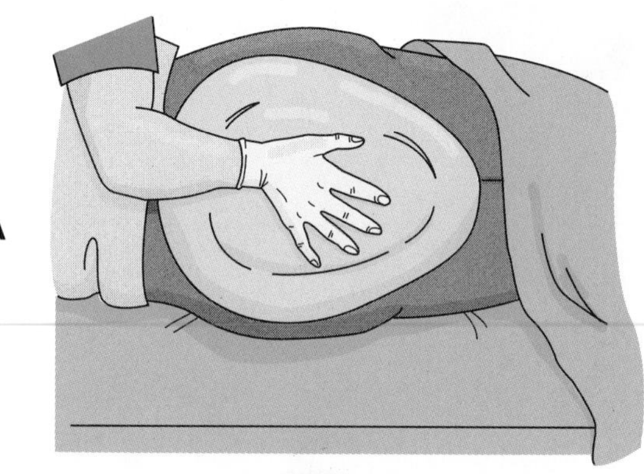

B

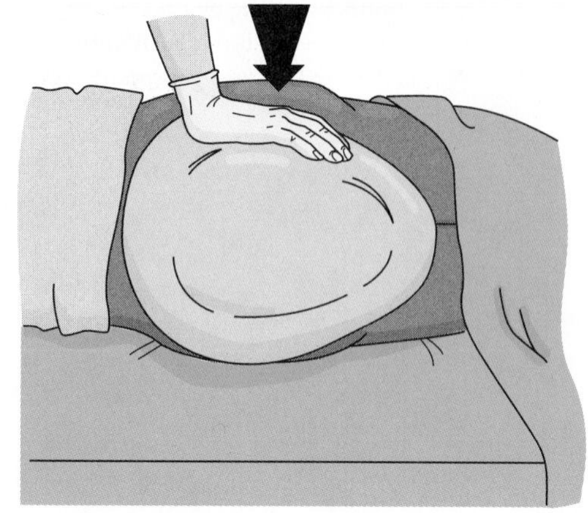

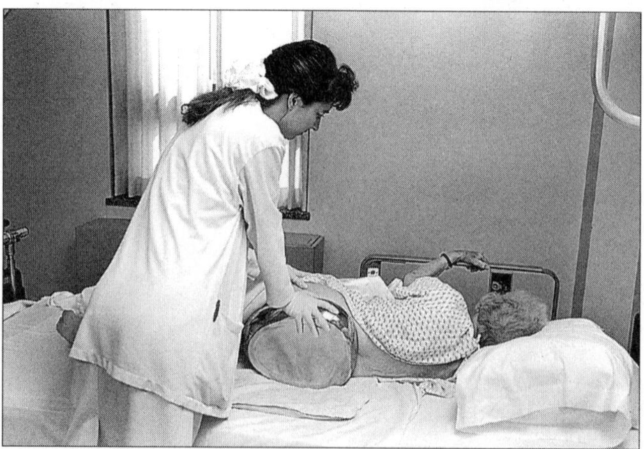

C

STEP **8d** **A,** Position the client on one side, and place the bedpan firmly against the buttocks. **B,** Push downward on the bedpan and toward the client. **C,** Nurse places bedpan in position. (*A* and *B* from Sorrentino SA: *Mosby's textbook for nursing assistants,* ed 5, St. Louis, 2000, Mosby.)

STEP	RATIONALE
9. Ensure that client is comfortable; cover client for warmth. Place small pillow or rolled towel under lumbar curve of back.	Provides added comfort. Pain reduces or eliminates urge to defecate, which can result in bowel elimination problems.
10. Ensure that call bell and toilet tissue are within easy reach for client.	Promotes safety by preventing client from reaching over edge of bed for objects out of reach.
11. Ensure that bed is in lowest position and upper side rails are up.	Promotes client safety.
12. Remove gloves and wash hands.	Reduces transmission of microorganisms.
13. Allow client to be alone, but monitor status and respond promptly to call signal.	Reassures client that nurse has not forgotten. Client may not be able to call nurse; the nurse is responsible for assessing client's status while on bedpan.
14. Apply new pair of gloves.	Reduces transmission of microorganisms.
15. Position client's bedside chair close to working side of bed.	Provides area to place bedpan and contents on chair after removal from client. Prevents spillage that could occur if full bedpan placed on bed surface.
16. Collect basin of warm water.	Allows client to wash hands after wiping perineal area (if appropriate); also allows nurse, wearing gloves, to use water to wash client's perineal area if client is unable to wipe thoroughly.
17. Move aside upper linens, keep client covered with towel.	Prevents undue embarrassment; maintains privacy.
18. Determine if client is able to wipe own perineal area. If not, using several layers of toilet tissue, wipe from mons pubis toward rectal area (for female client only); dispose of contaminated tissue in bedpan.	Cleansing from area of lesser contamination to greater contamination reduces spread of microorganisms.
19. Remove bedpan of mobile client.	
a. Ask client to flex knees, placing body weight on lower legs, feet, and upper torso; lift buttocks up from bedpan. At same time, place hand farthest from client on side of bedpan to support it (prevent spillage) and place other hand (closest to client) under sacrum to assist in lifting. After client is completely lifted off bedpan, remove pan and place it on bedside chair.	Nurse should avoid pulling or shoving pan from under hips because this action can pull skin and cause tissue injury.
b. Offer client opportunity to wash hands after having wiped perineal area (if appropriate).	Reduces spread of microorganisms.
20. Remove bedpan of immobile client.	
a. Lower head of bed.	Facilitates turning of client.
b. Assist client to roll onto side and off bedpan. Hold bedpan flat and steady while client is rolling off it; otherwise spillage will occur. Place bedpan and contents on bedside chair.	
c. Wipe client's anal area with tissue, depositing contaminated tissue in bedpan. If necessary, wash perineal area with warm, soapy water, drying area thoroughly.	Cleansing from area of lesser contamination to greater contamination reduces spread of microorganisms. Prevents excoriation and skin breakdown. Promotes personal hygiene. This is an excellent time to perform perineal hygiene (see Chapter 6).
21. Cover bedpan and contents with bedpan cover as soon as possible.	Reduces spread of offensive odors.
22. Return client to comfortable position, ensuring that bottom linens are clean and as wrinkle-free as possible. Soiled linens must be changed.	Reduces chance of skin breakdown when bedridden client lies on dry, wrinkle-free linens.
23. Position bed in its lowest position. Ensure that call bell, phone, drinking water, and desired personal items (e.g., books) are within easy access.	Promotes comfort and prevents injury to client.

Step	Rationale
24. If stool specimen is to be obtained, this is appropriate time to collect it. Wearing gloves, empty contents of bedpan into toilet or in special receptacle in appropriate utility room. Spray faucet attached to most institution toilets allows bedpan to be rinsed thoroughly. Use disinfectant if required by institution.	This should be done as soon as possible to prevent spread of offensive odor. Client uses same bedpan each time. (If it becomes very soiled, it could be replaced with clean one and soiled one sent for resterilization).
25. Replace all used equipment in appropriate location for subsequent use when required. Dispose of soiled linens correctly.	
26. Remove gloves and wash hands.	Reduces spread of microorganisms.

Evaluation

Step	Rationale
1. Assess characteristics of stool. Note color, odor, consistency, frequency, amount, shape, and constituents. Also assess characteristics of urine, if client voided in bedpan.	Identifies significant changes or findings.
2. Evaluate client's ability to use bedpan.	Provides continual assessment of ability to use bedpan.
3. Inspect client's perianal area and surrounding skin while removing bedpan.	Liquid stool predisposes client to skin breakdown.
4. Evaluate client's overall activity tolerance and comfort.	Defecation and use of the bedpan can be energy consuming.

Unexpected Outcomes and Related Interventions

- Client is unable to use bedpan.
  - If client's mobility allows, obtain order for use of a bedside commode.
- Client is incontinent of stool, resulting from client's embarrassment in using bedpan or nursing staff's delay in offering bedpan.
  - Talk to client about ways to make the procedure more comfortable.
  - Establish a regular schedule of offering pan or improve responsiveness when client calls for assistance.
- Client becomes constipated, resulting from pain of defecation, immobility, or unnatural position for defecation.
  - Consult with physician regarding administration of a stool softener.
  - Try offering dietary foods high in fiber.
  - Increase fluid intake if appropriate for client's medical condition.
- Client develops irritation and breakdown of skin around perianal area.
  - Administer regular perineal care (see Chapter 6).
- Blood in stool or black stool.
  - This diagnostic finding requires further testing for **occult blood** (see Chapter 41).

Recording and Reporting

- Record and report character and amount of stool in nurses' notes. Record urine output if client also voids.
- Complete laboratory requisition if stool or urine specimen was collected, and send to laboratory.

Teaching Considerations

- Some bedridden clients have overhead trapeze frame connected to bed to help lift themselves on and off bedpan. Teaching this activity can help to maintain strength of client's arms.
- Teach female clients to cleanse from area of lesser contamination to greater contamination (i.e., wiping from front to back). This reduces transmission of anal bacteria to urinary meatus and reduces risk of urinary tract infections.

Gerontological Considerations

- Older adults have some loss of sphincter control and often will require a quick response in providing a bedpan.
- Older adults may have limited movement in hips, requiring modification in pan placement.
- Incidence of constipation is greater because of changes in the nerves impulses. With aging these impulses may be dulled, and as a result the older adult does not perceive the need to defecate.
- Reinforce with older adult clients that as long as the consistency of the stool remains normal and that the bowel movements occur with regularity, they have no reason for concern (Lueckenotte, 2000).
- With increased age, transit time through the bowel increases, causing a normal lengthening of the time between bowel movements (Lueckenotte, 2000).

Home Care Considerations

- Assess client's home environment, routines, and activity of family members. When a bedpan must be used, determine availability of privacy and adequate time to use bedpan.

Skill 25-2 Removing Fecal Impaction Digitally

Constipation is a relatively common health problem for many adults who believe that a regular bowel habit requires having a daily bowel movement or a bowel movement at the same time each day (or both) (Prather and Ortiz-Camacho, 1998). Constipation is usually defined medically as infrequent stools. However, a consensus definition of functional constipation includes two or more of the following factors noted for at least 3 months: (1) straining with defecation at least one fourth of the time; (2) lumpy or hard stools (or both) at least one fourth of the time; (3) sensation of incomplete evacuation at least one fourth of the time; or (4) two or fewer bowel movements in a week (Thompson and others, 1992). There are a variety of interventions that can successfully relieve constipation. However, there are clients who develop **obstipation,** the absolute inability to pass stool.

Fecal **impaction,** the inability to pass a hard collection of stool, occurs in all age groups. Physically and mentally incapacitated persons and institutionalized older adult clients are at greatest risk (Prather and Ortiz-Camacho, 1998). Symptoms of fecal impaction include constipation, rectal discomfort, anorexia, nausea, vomiting, abdominal pain, diarrhea (around the impacted stool), and urinary frequency. When severe, fecal impaction can compromise a person's ventilation. The treatment for fecal impaction is prevention, but once it occurs digital removal of stool is the only alternative. This procedure can be very uncomfortable and embarrassing for the client. Excessive rectal manipulation may cause irritation to the mucosa, bleeding, and stimulation of the vagus nerve, which can cause a reflex slowing of the heart rate.

Delegation Considerations

This skill should not be delegated to assistive personnel. In some institutions only physicians perform this procedure.

Equipment

- Disposable gloves
- Water-soluble local anesthetic lubricant (NOTE: Some institutions require use of water-soluble lubricant without anesthetic when nurse performs procedure)
- Waterproof, absorbent pads
- Bedpan
- Bedpan cover
- Bath blanket
- Washbasin, washcloths, towels, and soap

Step	Rationale
Assessment	
1. Assess client to determine:	
a. Medical history of fecal impaction.	Can be a recurrent problem for institutionalized or disabled clients.
b. Last bowel movement.	Infrequent defecation increases chances of hard stool forming in rectum.
c. Consistency of stool, seepage of liquid stool. This situation may occur particularly in immobilized client. Client seems to continually or frequently be incontinent of liquid stool.	Symptomatic of an impaction high in colon. Client may be able to pass small pieces of hard stool or have episodes of passing small amounts of liquid stool (Prather and Ortiz-Camacho, 1998).
d. Expression of desire to defecate but inability to do so.	Large fecal mass causes rectal distention.
e. Complaints of pain when trying to defecate.	Pain often suppresses urge to defecate and compounds problem.
f. Normal bowel patterns, eating habits, exercise pattern or level of mobility, medications, especially narcotic analgesics.	Nurse must determine if these are contributing factors and attempt to include nursing actions in care plan that may help to prevent situation from recurring.
g. Client's normal vital signs.	Provides baseline measure. Vagus nerve stimulation during digital stimulation may result in reflex slowing of heart rate.

- ***Critical Decision Point***
  Clients with a history of dysrhythmia or heart disease have a greater risk of changes in heart rhythm. Be sure to monitor client's pulse before and during procedure. This procedure may be contraindicated in cardiac clients; if in doubt, verify with physician.

STEP	RATIONALE
h. Bowel sounds and abdominal distention.	Indicates presence of peristalsis but does not conclusively confirm gastrointestinal patency. Distention can contribute to constipation.
2. Check client's record to determine if physician's order exists to remove stool manually.	Because this procedure may involve excessive stimulation of vagus nerve, physician's order must be written in client's record before nurse can perform procedure.

NURSING DIAGNOSIS

Defining characteristics from the assessment data may reveal the following nursing diagnoses for clients requiring this skill:

Constipation
Diarrhea
Acute pain

Related factors are individualized based on client's condition or needs.

PLANNING

STEP	RATIONALE
1. **Expected outcomes** following completion of procedure:	
▪ Impacted stool is successfully removed.	Indicates rectum is clear of stool.
▪ Client is free of abdominal or rectal discomfort.	Fecal impaction causes direct pain to rectum and indirect abdominal discomfort through abdominal distention.
▪ Vital signs remain within client's baseline.	Indicates absence of vagal stimulation.
2. Explain procedure to client.	Information reduces anxiety and encourages client participation in a therapeutic elimination protocol.

IMPLEMENTATION

STEP	RATIONALE
1. Wash hands and apply gloves.	Prevents transmission of microorganisms.
2. Obtain assistance to help change client's position, if necessary. Raise bed horizontally to comfortable working height.	Promotes client safety and use of good body mechanics by nurse.
3. Keeping the far siderail raised, assist client to left side-lying position with knees flexed. Then raise near side rail.	Promotes client safety. Provides access to rectum.
4. Provide for privacy: pull curtains around bed or close door to room, drape bath blanket over client so client is minimally exposed.	Maintains client's dignity.
5. Drape client's trunk and lower extremities with bath blanket.	Prevents unnecessary exposure of body parts.
6. Place waterproof pad under buttocks.	Prevents soiling of bed linen.
7. Place bedpan next to client.	Bedpan is receptacle for stool.
8. Lubricate gloved index finger and middle finger of dominant hand with anesthetic lubricant.	Permits smooth insertion of finger into anus and rectum.

• ***Critical Decision Point***

Observe for the presence of perianal skin irritation. Presence of such indicates the need for postprocedure skin care to the perianal region to reduce pain during subsequent bowel elimination.

STEP	RATIONALE
9. Gradually insert the index finger and feel the anus relax around the finger. Then insert the middle finger (Prather and Ortiz-Camacho, 1998).	Maneuver helps to dilate the anal sphincter.
10. Gradually advance fingers slowly along rectal wall toward umbilicus.	Allows nurse to reach impacted stool high in rectum.

STEP	RATIONALE
11. Gently loosen fecal mass by moving fingers in a scissors motion to fragment the fecal mass (Prather and Ortiz-Camacho, 1998). Work fingers into hardened mass.	Loosening and penetrating mass allows nurse to remove it in small pieces, resulting in less discomfort to client.
12. Work stool downward toward end of rectum. Remove small sections of feces.	Prevents need to force finger up into rectum and minimizes trauma to mucosa.
13. Periodically assess heart rate and look for signs of fatigue.	Vagal stimulation slows heart rate and may cause dysrhythmia. Procedure may exhaust client.

- ***Critical Decision Point***
  Stop procedure if heart rate drops or rhythm changes from the client's baseline.

STEP	RATIONALE
14. Continue to clear rectum of feces, and allow client to rest at intervals.	Rest improves client's tolerance of procedure, allowing heart rate to slow.
15. After removal of impaction, provide washcloth and towel to wash buttocks and anal area.	Promotes client's sense of comfort and cleanliness.
16. Remove bedpan and inspect feces for color, consistency. Dispose of feces. Remove gloves by turning inside out and discarding in proper receptacle.	Reduces transmission of microorganisms.
17. Assist client to toilet or clean bedpan. (Procedure may be followed by enema or **cathartic.**)	Disimpaction may stimulate defecation reflex.
18. Wash hands.	Reduces transmission of microorganisms.

EVALUATION

1. Perform rectal examination for stool.	Determines if rectum is clear.
2. Reassess vital signs and compare to baseline values. Continue to monitor the client for 1 hour for bradycardia.	Determines extent of vagal stimulation.
3. Assess bowel sounds.	Determines peristaltic activity.
4. Palpate abdomen to determine if it is soft and nontender.	Discomfort is relieved.

UNEXPECTED OUTCOMES AND RELATED INTERVENTIONS

- Bleeding from rectum can occur if stool is large and hard.
  - Stop removal if bleeding becomes excessive.
  - Institute regimen of fecal softener and appropriate diet with fiber.
- Client experiences bradycardia and decreased blood pressure resulting from vagal stimulation.
  - Stop digital removal until vital signs stabilize.
  - Notify prescriber to determine if procedure should proceed.
- Client develops diarrheal stool following digital removal of hardened stool. Indicates hard stool remains in upper colon, with diarrheal stool leaking around area of impaction.
  - Institute cleansing enema or suppositories as ordered.
  - Increase client's intake of fluids and bulk in diet.

RECORDING AND REPORTING

- Record client's tolerance to procedure, amount and consistency of stool removed, and adverse effects.
- Report any adverse effects to nurse in charge or physician.

TEACHING CONSIDERATIONS

- If constipation and subsequent impaction are diet related, teach client about high-fiber nutritional products to increase bulk and the need for adequate fluid intake.
- If necessary, teach family caregivers about the effects of immobility, hydration, and nutrition on normal bowel elimination.

GERONTOLOGICAL CONSIDERATIONS

- Many older adult clients are especially prone to dysrhythmia and other problems related to vagal stimulation; monitor heart rate and rhythm closely.
- At least 28% of elderly clients are constipated as a result of insufficient dietary bulk, inadequate fluid intake, laxative abuse, diminished muscle tone and motor function, decreased defecation reflex, mental or physical illness, and presence of tumors or structures (Ebersole and Hess, 1998).
- For the elderly, instituting a diet adequate in dietary fiber (6 to 10 g per day) adds bulk, weight, and form to stool and improves defecation (Ebersole and Hess, 1998).
- Consider development of a regular toiling routine that includes responding to the urge to defecate (Lueckenotte, 2000).

Skill 25-3 Administering an Enema

An **enema** is the instillation of a solution into the rectum and sigmoid colon. Typically an enema is given to treat constipation or to empty the bowel prior to diagnostic procedures or certain types of abdominal surgery. Mosimann and Cornu (1998) suggest that clients who do not receive an enema prior to noncolonic abdominal operations have a return of peristalsis before those clients who have had enemas. Nevertheless, preoperative enemas are still very common for a number of surgeries.

Cleansing enemas promote complete evacuation of feces from the **colon.** They act by stimulating peristalsis through infusion of large volumes of solution. **Oil-retention enemas** act by lubricating the rectum and colon. Feces absorb oil and become softer and easier to pass. **Medicated enemas** contain pharmacological therapeutic agents and may be prescribed to reduce dangerously high serum potassium levels, as with use of a sodium polystyrene sulfonate *(Kayexalate)* enema, or to reduce bacteria in the colon before bowel surgery, as with use of a neomycin enema.

The primary reason for an enema is promotion of defecation. The fluid, depending on volume and type, breaks up the fecal mass, stretches the rectal wall, and initiates the defecation reflex. Clients should not rely on enemas to maintain bowel regularity because enemas do not treat the cause of irregularity or constipation. Frequent enemas disrupt normal defecation reflexes, resulting in dependence on enemas for elimination. Types of enemas:

Tap water (hypotonic) enema should not be repeated after first installation because water toxicity or circulatory overload can develop.

Physiological normal saline is safest. Infants and children can tolerate only this type because of their predisposition to fluid imbalance. If solution is prepared at home, mix 500 ml (1 pt) of tap water with 1 teaspoon table salt.

Hypertonic solution is useful for clients who cannot tolerate large volumes of fluid. Only 120 to 180 ml (4 to 6 oz) is usually effective (e.g., commercially prepared Fleet enema).

Soapsuds solution is pure soap added to either tap water or normal saline, depending on client's condition and frequency of administration. Use only castile pure soap. Recommended ratio of pure soap to solution is 5 ml (1 teaspoon) to 1000 ml (1 qt) warm water or saline. Soap should be added to enema bag after water is in place.

Oil retention enema uses an oil-based solution. Permits administration of a small volume, which is absorbed by the stool. The absorption of the oil softens stool for easier evacuation.

Carminative solution provides relief from gaseous distention. An example is MGW solution, which contains 30 ml of magnesium, 60 ml of glycerin, and 90 ml of water.

Delegation Considerations

The skill of administering an enema can be delegated to assistive personnel. Inform and assist care provider in proper way to position clients who have mobility restrictions. Instruct care provider about how to position clients who also have therapeutic equipment present, such as drains, intravenous catheters, or traction. Also be sure to teach care provider regarding signs and symptoms of client not tolerating the procedure, and when it must be stopped.

Equipment

Enema Bag Administration

- Disposable gloves
- Enema container (Figure 25-2)
- Tubing and clamp (if not already attached to container)
- Appropriate-size rectal tube (adult: 22 to 30 Fr; child: 12 to 18 Fr)
- Correct volume of warmed solution (adult: 750 to 1000 ml; child: 150 to 250 ml—infant, 250 to 350 ml—toddler, 300 to 500 ml—school-age child, 500 to 700 ml—adolescent)
- Water-soluble lubricant
- Waterproof, absorbent pads
- Bath blanket
- Toilet tissue
- Bedpan, bedside commode, or access to toilet

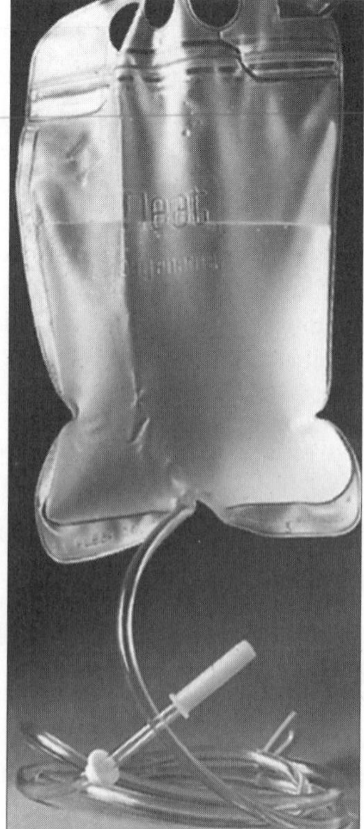

FIGURE 25-2 High-volume enema bag with tubing.

- Wash basin, washcloths, towel, and soap
- Intravenous (IV) pole

Prepackaged Enema

- Disposable gloves
- Prepackaged enema container with rectal tip (Figure 25-3)
- Water-soluble lubricant
- Waterproof, absorbent pads
- Bath blanket
- Toilet paper
- Bedpan, bedside commode, or access to toilet
- Washbasin, washcloths, towel, and soap

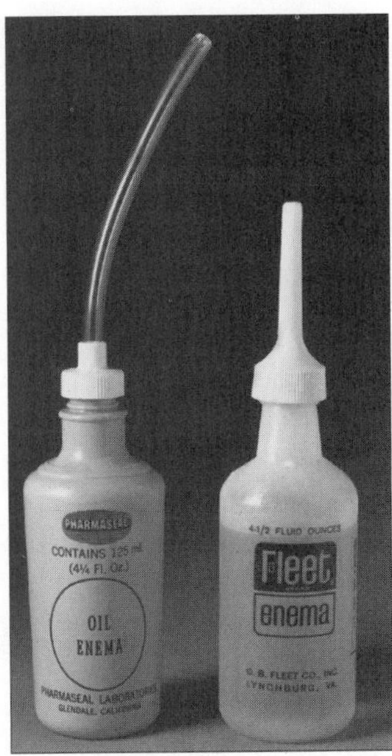

FIGURE **25-3** Prepackaged enema container with rectal tip(s).

STEP	RATIONALE
ASSESSMENT	
1. Assess status of client: last bowel movement, normal versus most recent bowel pattern, presence of hemorrhoids, mobility, bowel sounds, presence of abdominal pain.	Determines factors indicating need for enema and influencing the type of enema used. Also establishes baseline for bowel function.
2. Assess medical record for presence of increased intracranial pressure, glaucoma, or recent rectal or prostate surgery.	Conditions contraindicate use of enemas.
3. Inspect abdomen for presence of distention.	Establishes a baseline for determining effectiveness of enema.
4. Determine client's level of understanding of purpose of enema.	Allows nurse to plan for appropriate teaching measures.
5. Check client's medical record to clarify rationale for enema.	Determines purpose of enema administration: preparation for special procedure or relief of constipation.
6. Review physician's order for enema.	Order by physician is usually required for hospitalized client. Used to determine how many enemas client will require, type of enema to be given.

- ***Critical Decision Point***
  "Enemas until clear" order means that enemas are repeated until client passes fluid that is clear of fecal matter. Check agency policy, but usually client should receive only three consecutive enemas to avoid disruption of fluid and electrolyte balance.

NURSING DIAGNOSIS

Defining characteristics from the assessment data may reveal the following nursing diagnoses for clients requiring this skill:

Constipation
Acute pain
Risk for constipation

Related factors are individualized based on client's condition or needs.

STEP	RATIONALE

PLANNING

1. **Expected outcomes** following completion of procedure:
   - Stool is evacuated. — Solution clears rectum and lower colon of stool.
   - Enema return is clear. — All feces in colon have passed.
   - Abdominal distention is absent; client's discomfort is relieved. — Gas and feces have been expelled.
2. Collect appropriate equipment and arrange at bedside. — Ensures smooth procedure.
3. Correctly identify client and explain procedure. — Information promotes client cooperation and reduces anxiety.

IMPLEMENTATION

1. Wash hands and apply gloves. — Reduces transmission of microorganisms.
2. Provide privacy by closing curtains around bed or closing door. — Reduces embarrassment for client.
3. Raise bed to appropriate working height for nurse; raise side rail on opposite side. — Promotes good body mechanics and client safety.
4. Assist client into left side-lying (Sims') position with right knee flexed. Children may also be placed in dorsal recumbent position. — Allows enema solution to flow downward by gravity along natural curve of sigmoid colon and rectum, thus improving retention of solution.

   - ***Critical Decision Point***
     If client is suspected of having poor sphincter control, position the client on the bedpan in comfortable dorsal recumbent position. Clients with poor sphincter control cannot retain all of enema solution. Administering enema with client sitting on toilet is unsafe because curved rectal tubing can abrade rectal wall.

5. Place waterproof pad under hips and buttocks. — Prevents soiling of linen.
6. Cover client with bath blanket, exposing only rectal area, clearly visualizing anus. — Provides warmth, reduces exposure of body parts, allows client to feel more relaxed and comfortable.
7. Separate buttocks and examine perianal region for abnormalities including **hemorrhoids,** anal fissure, rectal prolapse (Moppett, 1999). — Findings will influence nurse's approach to insertion of enema tip. Prolapse contraindicates enema.
8. Place bedpan or commode in easily accessible position. If client will be expelling contents in toilet, ensure that toilet is free. (If client will be getting up to bathroom to expel enema, place client's slippers and bathrobe in easily accessible position.) — Used in case client is unable to retain enema solution.
9. Administer prepackaged disposable commercial Fleet enema.
   a. Remove plastic cap from tip of container. Tip of nozzle is already lubricated, but more water-soluble jelly can be applied as needed. — Lubrication provides for smooth insertion of rectal tube without causing rectal irritation or trauma (Saltzstein, Quebbeman, and Melvin, 1988).
   b. Gently separate buttocks and locate rectum. Instruct client to relax by breathing out slowly through mouth. — Breathing out promotes relaxation of external rectal sphincter.
   c. Expel any air from the enema container. — Introducing air into colon can cause further distention and discomfort (Moppett, 1999).
   d. Insert nozzle of container gently into anal canal, angling towards the umbilicus. — Gentle insertion prevents trauma to rectal mucosa (Saltzstein, Quebbeman, and Melvin, 1988).
      Adult: 7.5 to 10 cm (3 to 4 inches) (see illustration)
      Child: 5 to 7.5 cm (2 to 3 inches)
      Infant: 2.5 to 3.75 cm (1 to 1 ½ inches)

      - ***Critical Decision Point***
        If pain occurs or resistance is felt at any time during procedure, stop and confer with physician.

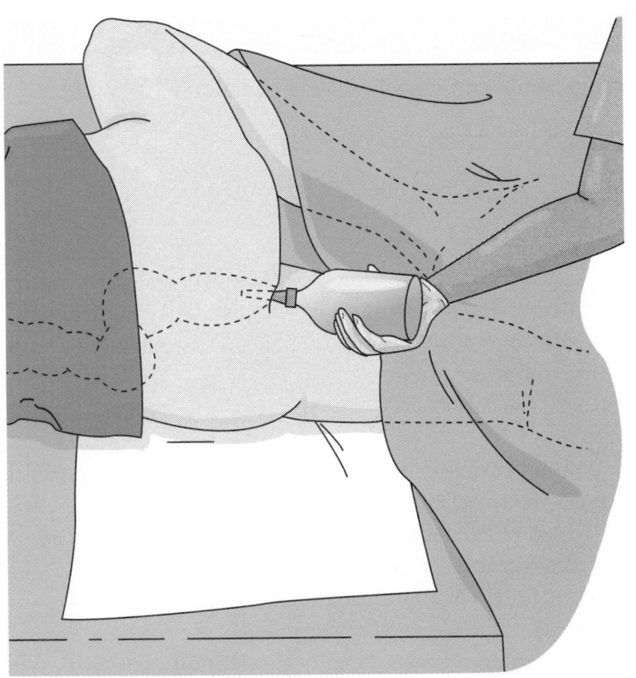

STEP **9d** The tip of the commercial enema is inserted into the rectum. (From Sorrentino SA: *Mosby's textbook for nursing assistants*, ed 5, St. Louis, 2000, Mosby.)

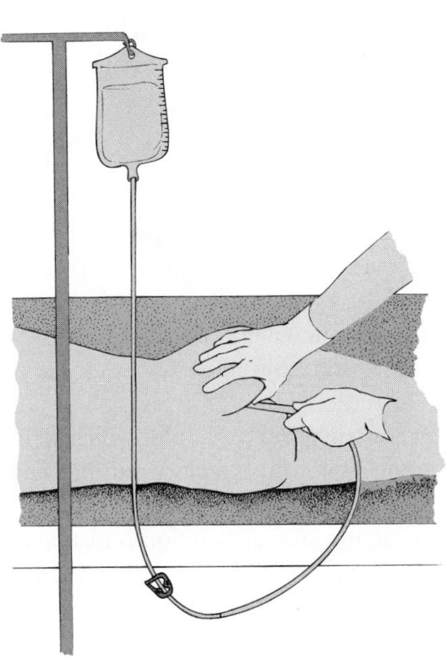

STEP **10f** Insertion of rectal tube into rectum.

STEP	RATIONALE
e. Squeeze bottle until all of solution has entered rectum and colon. (Most bottles contain approximately 250 ml of solution.) Instruct client to retain solution until the urge to defecate occurs, usually 2 to 5 minutes.	Hypertonic solutions require only small volumes to stimulate defecation.
10. Administer enema using enema bag:	
a. Add warmed solution to enema bag: warm tap water as it flows from faucet, place saline container in basin of hot water before adding saline to enema bag, and check temperature of solution by pouring small amount of solution over inner wrist.	Hot water can burn intestinal mucosa. Cold water can cause abdominal cramping and is difficult to retain.
b. Raise container, release clamp, and allow solution to flow long enough to fill tubing.	Removes air from tubing.
c. Reclamp tubing.	Prevents further loss of solution.
d. Lubricate 6 to 8 cm (3 to 4 inches) of tip of rectal tube with lubricating jelly.	Allows smooth insertion of rectal tube without risk of irritation or trauma to mucosa.
e. Gently separate buttocks and locate anus. Instruct client to relax by breathing out slowly through mouth.	Breathing out promotes relaxation of external anal sphincter.
f. Insert tip of rectal tube slowly by pointing tip in direction of client's umbilicus (see illustration). Length of insertion varies: Adult: 7.5 to 10 cm (3 to 4 inches) Child: 5 to 7.5 cm (2 to 3 inches) Infant: 2.5 to 3.75 cm (1 to 1 ½ inches)	Careful insertion prevents trauma to rectal mucosa from accidental lodging of tube against rectal wall. Insertion beyond proper limit can cause bowel perforation.
g. Hold tubing in rectum constantly until end of fluid instillation.	Bowel contraction can cause expulsion of rectal tube.

STEP	RATIONALE
h. Open regulating clamp, and allow solution to enter slowly with container at client's hip level.	Rapid instillation can stimulate evacuation of rectal tube.

- ***Critical Decision Point***
  If tube does not pass easily, do not force. Consider allowing a small amount of fluid to infuse and then try reinserting tube slowly.

STEP	RATIONALE
i. Raise height of enema container slowly to appropriate level above anus: 30 to 45 cm (12 to 18 inches) for high enema, 30 cm (12 inches) for regular enema, 7.5 cm (3 inches) for low enema. Instillation time varies with volume of solution administered (e.g., 1 L/10 min) (see illustration).	Allows for continuous, slow instillation of solution, raising container too high causes rapid instillation and possible painful distention of colon. High pressure can cause rupture of bowel in infant.
j. Lower container or clamp tubing if client complains of cramping or if fluid escapes around rectal tube.	Temporary cessation of instillation prevents cramping, which may prevent client from retaining all fluid, altering effectiveness of enema.
k. Clamp tubing after all solution is instilled.	Prevents entrance of air into rectum.
11. Place layers of toilet tissue around tube at anus and gently withdraw rectal tube.	Provides for client's comfort and cleanliness.
12. Explain to client that feeling of distention is normal, as well as some abdominal cramping. Ask client to retain solution as long as possible while lying quietly in bed. (For infant or young child, gently hold buttocks together for few minutes.)	Solution distends bowel. Length of retention varies with type of enema and client's ability to contract rectal sphincter. Longer retention promotes more effective stimulation of peristalsis and defecation.
13. Discard enema container and tubing in proper receptacle, or rinse out thoroughly with warm soap and water if container is to be reused.	Reduces transmission and growth of microorganisms.
14. Assist client to bathroom or help to position client on bedpan.	Normal squatting position promotes defecation.
15. Observe character of feces and solution (caution client against flushing toilet before inspection).	

- ***Critical Decision Point***
  When enemas are ordered "until clear," it is essential to observe contents of solution passed. The enema return is considered "clear" when no solid fecal material exists, but the solution may be colored.

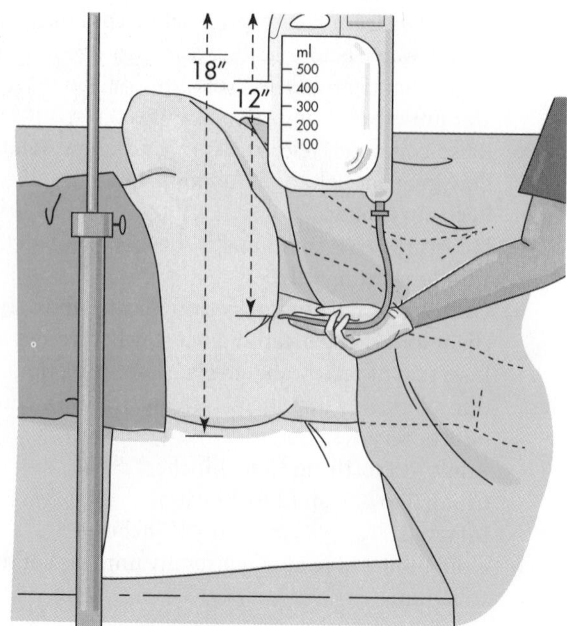

STEP **10i** An enema is given in the Sims' position. The IV pole is positioned so that the enema bag is 12 inches above the anus and approximately 18 inches above the mattress (depending on client's size). (From Sorrentino SA: *Mosby's textbook for nursing assistants,* ed 5, St. Louis, 2000, Mosby.)

STEP	RATIONALE
16. Assist client as needed to wash anal area with warm soap and water (if nurse administers perineal care, use gloves).	Fecal contents can irritate skin. Hygiene promotes client's comfort.
17. Remove and discard gloves and wash hands.	Reduces transmission of microorganisms.

EVALUATION

1. Inspect color, consistency, and amount of stool and fluid passed.	Determines if stool is evacuated or fluid is retained. Note abnormalities such as presence of blood or mucus.
2. Assess condition of abdomen.	Determines if distention is relieved.

UNEXPECTED OUTCOMES AND RELATED INTERVENTIONS

- Abdomen becomes rigid and distended due to perforation of bowel.
  - Stop enema if fluid is still instilling.
  - Notify physician immediately.
- Abdominal cramping or pain occurs from excess volume or cold temperature.
  - Slow rate of instillation of fluid.
- Bleeding develops.
  - Notify physician immediately.

RECORDING AND REPORTING

- Record type and volume of enema given, time administered, and characteristics of results.
- Report failure of client to defecate and any adverse effects to physician.

TEACHING CONSIDERATIONS

- Client should be instructed that enemas should not be given to treat cause of constipation.
- For self-administration, client should be instructed to lie in dorsal recumbent position with knees and hips flexed toward chest.
- Caution client against flushing toilet before nurse has inspected contents.

PEDIATRIC CONSIDERATIONS

- For infant or child, nurse may wish to involve parent in procedure.
- Children and infants usually do not receive prepackaged hypertonic enemas.

GERONTOLOGICAL CONSIDERATIONS

- Caution is needed when enemas are ordered "until clear" in the older adult population. Older adults may become fatigued, are at risk for fluid and electrolyte imbalances, and may experience changes in vital signs.
- Instruct older adults and their caregivers in how to modify diet to avoid constipation.
- Older adult may have difficulty retaining fluid. The nurse may gently hold buttocks together to assist.

HOME CARE CONSIDERATIONS

- Assess client's and primary caregiver's ability and motivation to administer enema and provide instruction as needed.
- Assess client's ability to administer enema if enema ordered is self-administrative type.
- Assess client's environment to identify location where enema may be administered with privacy.
- Teach skill; observe to determine level of understanding. Review possible complications and what action to take.

Skill 25-4 Inserting and Maintaining a Nasogastric Tube

There are times following major surgery or as a result of conditions affecting the gastrointestinal tract when normal peristalsis temporarily becomes altered. Because peristalsis is slowed or absent, a client cannot eat or drink fluids without causing abdominal distention. The temporary insertion of a nasogastric tube into the stomach serves to decompress the stomach, keeping it empty until normal peristalsis returns.

A nasogastric (NG) tube is a pliable tube that is inserted through the client's nasopharynx into the stomach. The tube has a hollow lumen that allows the removal of gastric secretions and the introduction of solutions into the stomach. There are times when a nasogastric tube can be used for enteral feedings, but a softer small-bore feeding tube is preferred for feeding purposes (see Chapter 22). The Levin and Salem sump tubes are the most common for stomach decompression. The Levin tube is a single lumen tube with holes near the tip. It may be connected to a drainage bag or an intermittent suction device to drain stomach secretions. The Salem sump tube is preferable for stomach decompression. The tube has two lumina: one for removal of gastric contents and one to provide an air vent. A blue "pigtail" is the air vent that connects with the second lumen. When the sump tube's main lumen is connected to suction, the air vent permits free, continuous drainage of secretions. The air vent should never be clamped off, connected to suction, or used for irrigation.

Nasogastric tube insertion does not require sterile technique. Clean technique is adequate. The procedure is uncomfortable, with clients experiencing a burning sensation as the tube passes through the sensitive nasal mucosa. One of the greatest nursing care challenges is keeping the client comfortable because the tube is a constant irritation to mucosa. The nurse routinely assesses the condition of the nares and mucosa for inflammation and excoriation. Supportive care includes changing soiled tape or fixation devices when they become soiled, keeping the nares lubricated and clean, and providing frequent mouth care to minimize the dehydration from mouth breathing.

Delegation Considerations

The skill of inserting and maintaining an NG tube should not be delegated. Assistive personnel may measure and record the drainage from an NG tube and provide oral and nasal hygiene measures. Caution personnel to anchor a tube during routine care to prevent accidental displacement.

Equipment

- 14 or 16 Fr NG tube (smaller-lumen catheters are not used for decompression in adults because they must be able to remove thick secretions).
- Water-soluble lubricating jelly
- pH test strips (measure gastric aspirate acidity)
- Tongue blade
- Flashlight
- Asepto bulb or catheter-tipped syringe
- 1-inch (2.5-cm) wide hypoallergenic tape or commercial fixation device
- Safety pin and rubber band
- Clamp, drainage bag, or suction machine or pressure gauge if wall suction is to be used
- Bath towel
- Glass of water with straw
- Facial tissues
- Normal saline
- Tincture of benzoin (optional)
- Disposable gloves

Step	Rationale
Assessment	
1. Inspect condition of client's nasal and oral cavity.	Baseline condition of nasal and oral cavity determines need for special nursing hygiene measures after tube placement.
2. Ask if client has had history of nasal surgery, and note if deviated nasal septum is present.	Nurse should insert tube into uninvolved nasal passage. Procedure may be contraindicated if surgery is recent.
3. Palpate client's abdomen for distention, pain, and rigidity. Auscultate for bowel sounds.	Baseline determination of level of abdominal distention and function later serves as comparison once tube is inserted.
4. Assess client's level of consciousness and ability to follow instructions.	Determines client's ability to assist in procedure.
5. Determine if client has had an NG tube insertion in the past.	Procedure is uncomfortable and requires thorough explanation. Client's previous experience will complement any explanations.

Step	Rationale
• ***Critical Decision Point*** *If client is confused, disoriented, or unable to follow commands, obtain assistance from another staff member to insert the tube.*	
6. Check medical record for physician's order, type of NG tube to be placed, and whether tube is to be attached to suction or drainage bag.	Procedure requires physician's order. Adequate decompression depends on NG suction.

Nursing Diagnosis

Defining characteristics from the assessment data may reveal the following nursing diagnoses for clients requiring this skill:

- Acute pain
- Impaired oral mucous membrane
- Deficient knowledge regarding purpose of gastric decompression
- Risk for impaired skin integrity

Related factors are individualized based on client's condition or needs.

Planning

Step	Rationale
1. **Expected outcomes** following completion of procedure:	
▪ Stomach will remain soft without distention.	NG tube is positioned in stomach, remains patent, and drains gastric secretions.
▪ Client nares and surface of nose remain clear, without abrasions or excoriation.	Absence of irritation from NG tube.
▪ Client's nasal mucosa will remain moist and intact.	Reduces risk of erosion developing.
2. Prepare equipment at the bedside. Have a 4-inch (10-cm) piece of tape ready with one end split in half.	Ensures well-organized procedure. Tape will be used to initially hold tube in place after insertion.
3. Identify client, and explain procedure. Let client know there will be a burning sensation in nasopharynx as tube is passed.	Identification prevents error of placing tube in wrong client. Explanation gains client's cooperation and ability to anticipate nurse's action.

Implementation

Step	Rationale
1. Wash hands and apply disposable gloves.	Reduces transmission of microorganisms.
2. Position client in high-Fowler's position with pillows behind head and shoulders. Raise bed to a horizontal level comfortable for the nurse.	Promotes client's ability to swallow during procedure. Good body mechanics prevents injury to nurse or client.
3. Pull curtain around the bed or close room door.	Provides privacy.
4. Stand on client's right side if right-handed, left side if left-handed.	Allows easiest manipulation of tubing.
5. Place bath towel over client's chest; give facial tissues to client.	Prevents soiling of client's gown. Tube insertion through nasal passages may cause tearing and coughing with increased salivation.
6. Instruct client to relax and breathe normally while occluding one naris. Then repeat this action for other naris. Select nostril with greater air flow.	Tube passes more easily through naris that is more patent.
7. Measure distance to insert tube:	
a. *Traditional method:* Measure distance from tip of nose to earlobe to xiphoid process (see illustration).	Tube should extend from nares to stomach; distance varies with each client.

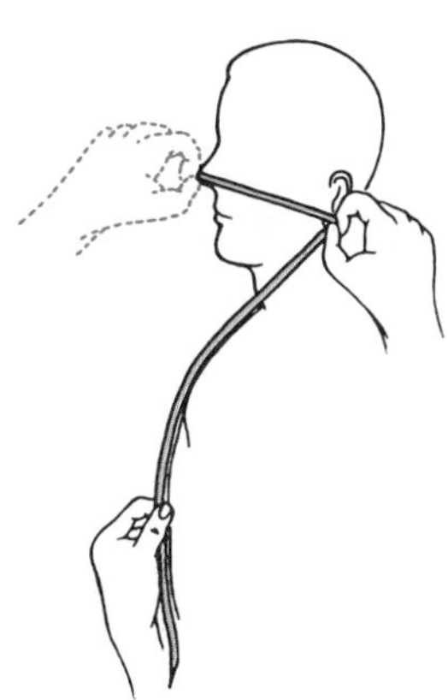

STEP **7a** Technique for measuring distance to insert NG tube.

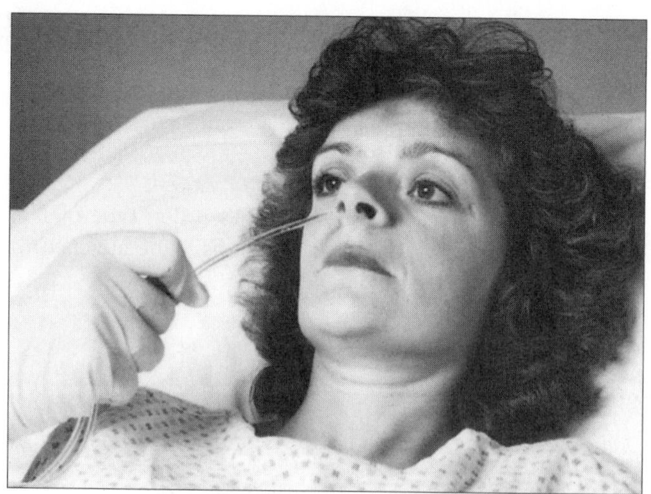

STEP **12** Insert NG tube with curved end pointing downward.

Step	Rationale
b. *Hanson method:* First mark 50-cm point on tube, then do traditional measurement. Tube insertion should be to midway point between 50 cm (20 inches) and traditional mark.	
8. Mark length of tube to be inserted with small piece of tape placed around tube so it can be easily removed.	Marks amount of tube to be inserted from naris to stomach.
9. Curve 10 to 15 cm (4 to 6 inches) of end of tube tightly around index finger, then release.	Curving tube tip aids insertion and decreases stiffness of tube.
10. Lubricate 7.5 to 10 cm (3 to 4 inches) of end of tube with water-soluble lubricating jelly.	Minimizes friction against nasal mucosa and aids insertion of tube.
11. Alert client that procedure is to begin.	Decreases client anxiety and increases client cooperation.
12. Initially instruct client to extend neck back against pillow; insert tube slowly through naris with curved end pointing downward (see illustration).	Facilitates initial passage of tube through naris and maintains clear airway for open naris.
13. Continue to pass tube along floor of nasal passage, aiming down toward ear. When resistance is felt, apply gentle downward pressure to advance tube (do not force past resistance).	Minimizes discomfort of tube rubbing against upper nasal turbinates. Resistance is caused by posterior nasopharynx. Downward pressure helps tube curl around corner of nasopharynx.
14. If resistance is met, try to rotate the tube and see if it advances. If still resistant, withdraw tube, allow client to rest, relubricate tube, and insert into other naris.	Forcing against resistance can cause trauma to mucosa. Helps relieve client's anxiety.

• ***Critical Decision Point***
If unable to insert tube in either naris, stop procedure and notify physician.

Step	Rationale
15. Continue insertion of tube until just past nasopharynx by gently rotating tube toward opposite naris.	
a. Stop tube advancement, allow client to relax, and provide tissues.	Relieves client's anxiety; tearing is natural response to mucosal irritation, and excessive salivation may occur because of oral stimulation.
b. Explain to client that next step requires that client swallow. Give client glass of water unless contraindicated.	Sipping of water aids passage of NG tube into esophagus.
16. With tube just above oropharynx, instruct client to flex head forward, take a small sip of water, and swallow. Advance tube 2.5 to 5 cm (1 to 2 inches) with each swallow of water. If client is not allowed fluids, instruct to dry swallow or suck air through straw. Advance tube with each swallow.	Flexed position closes off upper airway to trachea and opens esophagus. Swallowing closes epiglottis over trachea and helps move the tube into the esophagus. Swallowing water reduces gagging or choking. Water can be removed later from stomach by suction.

STEP	RATIONALE
17. If client begins to cough, gag, or choke, withdraw slightly and stop tube advancement. Instruct client to breathe easily and take sips of water.	Tubing may accidentally enter larynx and initiate cough reflex. Gagging is eased by swallowing water. Risk for aspiration increases if vomiting occurs.

• ***Critical Decision Point***
If vomiting occurs, assist client in clearing airway; oral suctioning may be needed. Do not proceed until airway is cleared.

STEP	RATIONALE
18. If client continues to cough during insertion, pull tube back slightly.	Tube may enter larynx and obstruct airway.
19. If client continues to gag, check back of pharynx using flashlight and tongue blade.	Tube may coil around itself in back of throat and stimulate gag reflex.
20. After client relaxes, continue to advance tube desired distance.	Tip of tube should be within stomach to decompress properly.
21. Once tube is correctly advanced remove tape used to mark length of tube, place the prepared split tape with nonsplit side on nose. Anchor with one of split ends while checking tube placement.	Tube should be partially anchored before placement is checked.
22. Checking tube placement: Check institutional policy for preferred methods for checking tube placement.	
a. Ask client to talk.	Client is unable to talk if NG tube has passed through vocal cords.
b. Inspect posterior pharynx for presence of coiled tube.	Tube is pliable and can coil up in back of pharynx instead of advancing into esophagus.
c. Aspirate gently back on syringe to obtain gastric contents, observing color (see illustration).	Gastric contents are usually cloudy and green, but may be off-white, tan, bloody, or brown in color. Aspiration of contents provides means to measure fluid pH and thus determine tube tip placement in gastrointestinal tract. Other common aspirate colors include the following: duodenal placement (yellow or bile stained), esophagus (may or may not have saliva-appearing aspirate).

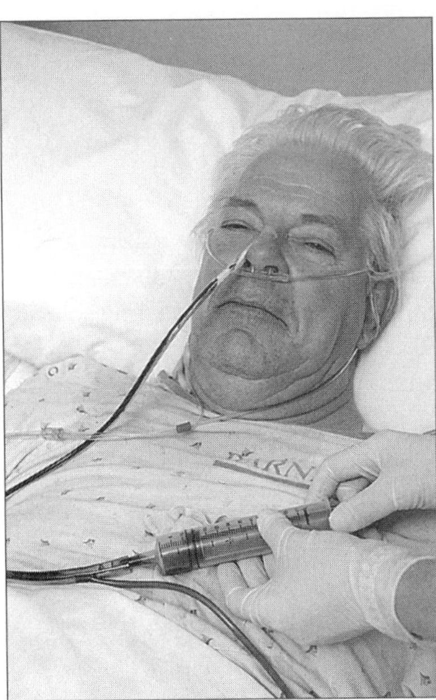

STEP **22c** Aspiration of gastric contents.

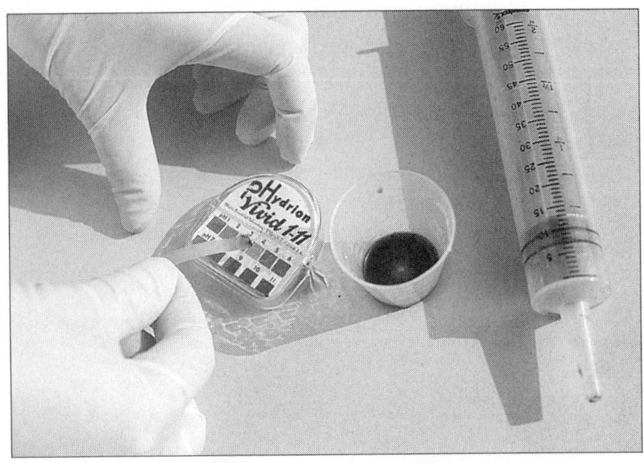

STEP **22d** Checking pH of gastric aspirate.

STEP	RATIONALE
d. Measure pH of aspirate with color-coded pH paper with range of whole numbers from 1 to 11 (see illustration).	Gastric aspirates have decidedly acidic pH values, preferably 4 or less, compared with intestinal aspirates, which are usually greater than 4, or respiratory secretions, which are usually greater than 5.5 (Metheny and others, 1993, 1994, 1998).

• ***Critical Decision Point***
Be sure to use gastric (Gastrocult) pH test and not Hemoccult test.

STEP	RATIONALE
e. If tube is not in stomach, advance another 2.5 to 5 cm (1 to 2 inches) and repeat Steps 22a-d to check tube position.	Tube must be in stomach to provide decompression.
23. Anchoring tube:	
a. After tube is properly inserted and positioned, either clamp end or connect it to drainage bag or suction machine.	Drainage bag is used for gravity drainage. Intermittent suction is most effective for decompression. Client going to the operating room often has tube clamped.
b. Tape tube to nose; avoid putting pressure on nares.	Prevents tissue necrosis. Tape anchors tube securely.
(1) Before taping tube to nose, apply small amount of tincture of benzoin to lower end of nose and allow to dry (optional). Be sure top end of tape over nose is secure.	Benzoin prevents loosening of tape if client perspires.
(2) Carefully wrap two split ends of tape around tube (see illustration).	
(3) Alternative: Apply tube fixation device using shaped adhesive patch (see illustration).	
c. Fasten end of NG tube to client's gown by looping rubber band around tube in slip knot. Pin rubber band to gown (provides slack for movement).	Reduces pressure on nares if tube moves.
d. Unless physician orders otherwise, head of bed should be elevated 30 degrees.	Helps prevent esophageal reflux and minimizes irritation of tube against posterior pharynx.
e. Explain to client that sensation of tube should decrease somewhat with time.	Adaptation to continued sensory stimulus.
f. Remove gloves and wash hands.	Reduces transmission of microorganisms.
24. Safety:	
a. Once placement is confirmed, place a mark, either a red mark or tape, on the tube to indicate where the tube exists in the nose.	The mark or tube length is to be used as a guide to indicate whether displacement may have occurred.
b. Measurement of the tube length from nares to connector is an alternate method.	
c. If tube length is the method used, document the tube length in the client record.	
25. Tube irrigation:	
a. Wash hands and apply gloves.	Reduces transmission of microorganisms.
b. Check for tube placement in stomach (see Step 22). Reconnect NG tube to connecting tube.	Prevents accidental entrance of irrigating solution into lungs.
c. Draw up 30 ml of normal saline into Asepto or catheter-tip syringe.	Use of saline minimizes loss of electrolytes from stomach fluids.
d. Pinch or clamp NG tube. Disconnect from connecting tubing, and lay end of connection tubing on towel.	Reduces soiling of client's gown and bed linen.

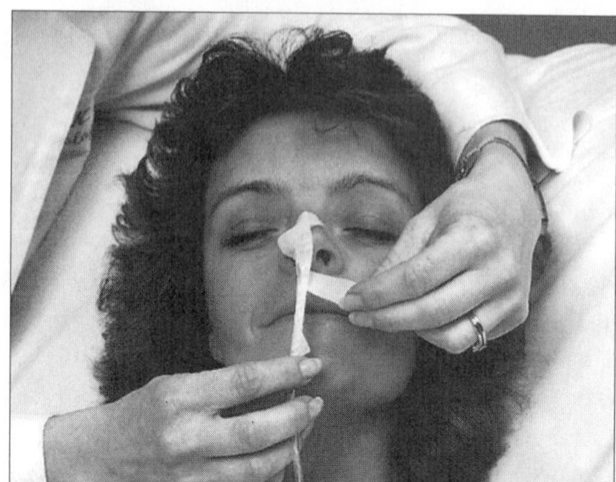

STEP **23b(2)** Tape is crossed over and around NG tube.

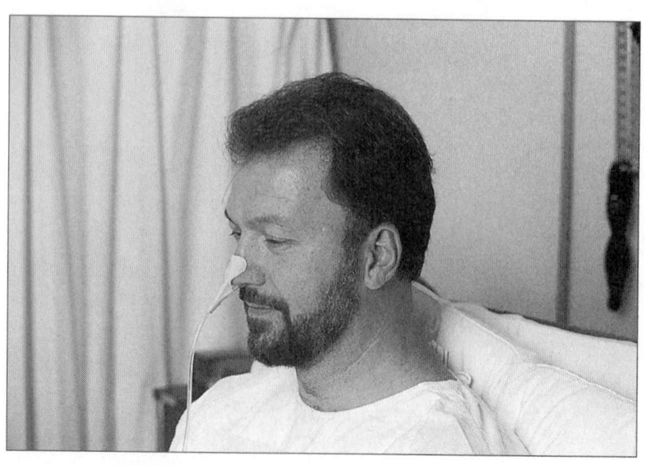

STEP **23b(3)** Client with tube fixation device.

STEP	RATIONALE
e. Insert tip of irrigating syringe into end of NG tube. Leave tube or remove clamp. Hold syringe with top pointed at floor, and inject saline slowly and evenly. Do not force solution.	Position of syringe prevents introduction of air into vent tubing, which could cause gastric distention. Solution introduced under pressure can cause gastric trauma.

- ***Critical Decision Point***

Do not introduce saline through blue colored "pigtail" air vent of Salem sump tube.

STEP	RATIONALE
f. If resistance occurs, check for kinks in tubing. Turn client onto left side. Repeated resistance should be reported to surgeon.	Tip of tube may lie against stomach lining. Repositioning on left side may dislodge tube away from the stomach lining. Buildup of secretions will cause distention.
g. After instilling saline, immediately aspirate or pull back slowly on syringe to withdraw fluid. If amount aspirated is greater than amount instilled, record the difference as output. If amount aspirated is less than amount instilled, record the difference as intake.	Irrigation clears tubing, so stomach should remain empty. Fluid remaining in stomach is measured as intake.
h. Reconnect NG tube to drainage or suction. (If solution does not return, repeat irrigation.)	Reestablishes drainage collection; may repeat irrigation or repositioning of tube until NG tube drains properly.
i. Remove gloves and wash hands.	Reduces transmission of microorganisms.
26. Discontinuation of NG tube:	
a. Verify order to discontinue NG tube.	Physician's order required for procedure.
b. Explain procedure to client, and reassure that removal is less distressing than insertion.	Minimizes anxiety and increases cooperation. Tube passes out smoothly.
c. Wash hands and apply disposable gloves.	Reduces transmission of microorganisms.
d. Turn off suction and disconnect NG tube from drainage bag or suction. Remove tape from bridge of nose and unpin tube from gown.	Have tube free of connections before removal.
e. Stand on client's right side if right-handed, left side if left-handed.	Allows easiest manipulation of tube.
f. Hand the client facial tissue; place clean towel across chest. Instruct client to take and hold a deep breath.	Client may wish to blow nose after tube is removed. Towel may keep gown from getting soiled. Airway will be temporarily obstructed during tube removal.
g. Clamp or kink tubing securely and then pull tube out steadily and smoothly into towel held in other hand while client holds breath.	Clamping prevents tube contents from draining into oropharynx. Reduces trauma to mucosa and minimizes client's discomfort. Towel covers tube, which can be an unpleasant sight. Holding breath helps to prevent aspiration.
h. Measure amount of drainage, and note character of content. Dispose of tube and drainage equipment.	Provides accurate measure of fluid output. Reduces transfer of microorganisms.
i. Clean nares and provide mouth care.	Promotes comfort.
j. Position client comfortably and explain procedure for drinking fluids, if not contraindicated.	Depends on physician's order. Sometimes clients are allowed nothing by mouth (NPO) for up to 24 hours. When fluids are allowed, the order usually begins with a small amount of ice chips each hour and increases as client is able to tolerate more.
27. Clean equipment and return to proper place. Place soiled linen in utility room or proper receptacle.	Proper disposal of equipment prevents spread of microorganisms and ensures proper exchange procedures.
28. Remove gloves and wash hands.	Reduces transmission of microorganisms.

EVALUATION

STEP	RATIONALE
1. Observe amount and character of contents draining from NG tube. Ask if client feels nauseated.	Determines if tube is decompressing stomach of contents.
2. Palpate client's abdomen periodically, noting any distention, pain, and rigidity and auscultate for the presence of bowel sounds. Turn off suction while auscultating.	Determines success of abdominal decompression and the return of peristalsis. The sound of the suction apparatus may be transmitted to abdomen and be misinterpreted as bowel sounds.

STEP	RATIONALE
3. Inspect condition of nares and nose.	Evaluates onset of skin and tissue irritation.
4. Observe position of tubing.	Determines if tension is being applied to nasal structures.
5. Ask if client feels sore throat or irritation in pharynx.	Evaluates level of client's discomfort.

UNEXPECTED OUTCOMES AND RELATED INTERVENTIONS

- Client develops abdominal distention, vomiting, or absence of drainage from tube.
  - Assess patency of tube and irrigate tube as needed.
- Client complains of sore throat from dry, irritated mucous membranes.
  - Perform oral hygiene more frequently.
  - Ask physician whether client can suck on ice chips or throat lozenges or chew gum.
- Client develops chronic inflammation and erosion of nasal mucosa.
  - Consider removal of tube and reinsertion into opposite naris (physician's order necessary).
- Client develops signs of fluid volume deficit.
  - Report decreased urine output, poor skin turgor, or excessive loss of secretions to physician.
- Client develops signs and symptoms of pulmonary aspiration, indicating tube displacement into airway. Client exhibits fever, shortness of breath, pulmonary congestion.
  - Contact physician, and prepare for chest x-ray examination to be obtained. NG tube will be removed.

RECORDING AND REPORTING

- Record length, size, and type of gastric tube inserted and through which nostril it was inserted.
- Record client's response to tube insertion, any symptoms that could indicate malposition, client's status after tube taped into position, and whether tube is clamped or connected to drainage device.
- Record pH readings that were obtained to indicate correct placement and color of secretions withdrawn from tube.
- Record difference between amount of normal saline instilled and amount of gastric aspirate removed on intake and output (I&O) sheet.
- Record in nurses' notes or flow sheet amount and character of contents draining from NG tube every shift.

GERONTOLOGICAL CONSIDERATIONS

- Check for ill-fitting dentures, and remove them for the client's safety and comfort during the insertion.
- Oral and nasal mucosal drying may be present. Be sure that the tube is adequately lubricated for insertion.

HOME CARE CONSIDERATIONS

- Clients are seldom sent home with NG suction. If client is discharged receiving tube feedings, clients and family caregivers should be taught how to manage tube and administer feedings correctly (see Chapter 22).

Critical Thinking Exercises

1. You are beginning to remove a fecal impaction on a 78-year-old client. The client's heart rate before the start of the procedure was 90 beats per minute and regular. You begin to break up the hardened fecal mass and remove a small amount of stool. The client expresses discomfort, and you reassess the pulse rate. The pulse is now 70 beats per minute. What should you do?
2. A client has been admitted to your hospital unit after a multivehicle accident. The emergency department report states that he has had a pelvic fracture. He is ordered on bed rest and is only allowed to move by turning. What type of bedpan might this client be able to use?
3. You walk into the room to find a nurse's aide administering a soap suds enema to a client who is scheduled for abdominal surgery. The client complains of cramping, and the aide explains, "Cramping is just normal; try to hold the fluid." Is this an appropriate response? If not, what should you do?
4. Mr. Benz has had an NG tube in place for 2 days following major abdominal surgery. When you go in to check the tube, you palpate Mr. Benz's abdomen, noting that it is distended and tight. Mr. Benz states that he feels "very full." When you irrigate the NG tube, you are not able to withdraw the normal saline you instilled. What should you further assess? What is occurring?

References

Doughty DB, Jackson DB: *Gastrointestinal disorders: Mosby's clinical nursing series,* St. Louis, 1993, Mosby.

Ebersole P, Hess P: *Toward healthy aging: human needs and nursing response,* ed 4, St. Louis, 1998, Mosby.

Lueckenotte AG: *Gerontological nursing,* ed 2, St. Louis, 2000, Mosby.

Metheny N and others: Effectiveness of pH measurements in predicting feeding tube placement: an update, *Nurs Res* 42(6):324, 1993.

Metheny N and others: Visual characteristics of aspirates from feeding tubes as a method for predicting tube location, *Nurs Res* 43:282, 1994.

Metheny N and others: pH, color, and feeding tubes, *RN* 61(1):277, 1998.

Moppett S: Administration of an enema, *Nurs Times* 95:insert 2p, 1999.

Mosimann F, Cornu P: Are enemas given before abdominal operations useful? A prospective randomized trial, *Eur J Surg* 164(7):527, 1998.

Prather CM, Ortiz-Camacho CP: Evaluation and treatment of constipation and fecal impaction in adults, *Mayo Clin Proc* 73(9):881, 1998.

Saltzstein R, Quebbeman L, Melvin JL: Anorectal injuries incident to enema administration: a recurring avoidable problem, *Am J Phys Med Rehabil* 67:186, 1988.

Sorrentino SA: *Mosby's textbook for nursing assistants,* ed 5, St. Louis, 2000, Mosby.

Thompson WG and others: Functional bowel disease and functional abdominal pain, *Gastroenterol Int* 5:75, 1992.

26

Ostomy Care

Skills

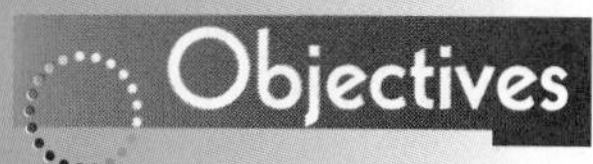

Objectives

Mastery of content in this chapter will enable the nurse to:

- Define the key terms listed.
- Identify types of bowel and bladder diversions.
- Explain differences in color and consistency of drainage based on the location of an ostomy.
- Discuss factors influencing enterostomy drainage.
- Describe methods used to maintain skin integrity during pouching of ostomies.
- Pouch an incontinent urinary diversion.
- Irrigate a colostomy.
- Catheterize a urinary diversion.

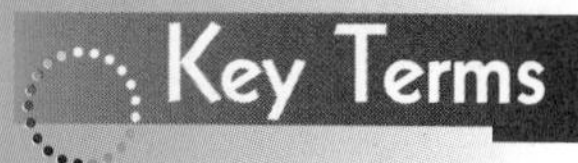

Key Terms

Anastomotic	Noncontinent (incontinent) diversion
Colon conduit	Nosocomial infection
Colostomy	Ostomy
Continent ostomy or diversion	Peristalsis
Cystectomy	Peristomal
Effluent	Skin barrier
Enterostomy	Stent
Ileal conduit	Stoma
Ileostomy	Ureterostomy
Intubation	Urinary diversion
Maceration	Urostomy
Maculopapular	

Certain diseases or conditions require surgical intervention to create an opening into the abdominal wall for fecal or urinary elimination. A portion of intestinal mucosa or segment of ureter is brought out to the abdominal wall, and a stoma, or opening, is formed to allow feces or urine to drain. An **ostomy** is an opening made to allow passage of urine or feces. The piece of intestine that is brought out onto the client's abdomen is called a **stoma.** An **enterostomy** is any surgical procedure that produces an artificial stoma in a portion of intestine through the abdominal wall. The drainage from the stoma is often called **effluent.** The forms of enterostomy are ileostomy, which involves the ileum of the small intestine, and colostomy, which can involve various segments of the colon (Figure 26-1). Ostomies can be temporary or permanent and continent or noncontinent. The surgical procedures (see Figure 26-2) involved in creating a stoma for urinary drainage are called **urinary diversions,** for which two categories of urinary diversions exist, continent and noncontinent (incontinent). Clients who have a **noncontinent (incontinent) diversion** cannot control when the urine exits from their stoma and therefore must wear an external urinary ostomy pouch at all times. Examples of noncontinent urinary diversions are an **ileal conduit** and other forms of ureterostomies (Figure 26-2). Continent urinary diversion surgery creates an internal pouch where urine is stored. Clients who have **continent diversions,** such as the Kock or Indiana pouch, do not need to wear an external ostomy pouch over their urinary stoma. Instead, these clients are taught to insert a catheter into their stoma to drain out the urine periodically throughout the day (see Skill 26-5).

For diseases or conditions of the bowel, the location of the ostomy determines the consistency of stool passed. An **ileostomy** bypasses the entire large intestine; thus stools are liquid and frequent, and contain digestive enzymes. The same fecal characteristics hold true for a colostomy of the ascending colon. A **colostomy** of the transverse colon generally results in a thicker, formed stool. The sigmoid colostomy emits stool almost identical to that normally passed through the rectum. A person with any of the above incontinent ostomies must cover the stoma with a disposable or reusable pouch to collect the effluent.

Ostomies that emit frequent liquid stools must be pouched at all times. The pouch must be emptied throughout the day. Skin care is vital to prevent irritation from fecal irritants.

A colostomy in the transverse colon has to be pouched at all times. The regularity of bowel movements is unpredictable. The transverse colostomy cannot be managed by daily irrigation. Because of its anatomical location, a sigmoid colostomy can be managed (no fecal output between irrigations) by irrigation. Scheduled irrigations of the descending or sigmoid colostomy allow the person to empty the bowel and may eliminate the need for a pouch (see Skill 26-2). Some clients continue to wear pouches for a feeling of security and in case of fecal spillage between irrigations. Irrigation is optional since many clients prefer natural bowel evacuation.

Over the past years, many developments have occurred in the field of pediatric gastrointestinal surgery that have improved survival rates for neonates having gastrointestinal ostomy surgery. Because pediatric clients have unique needs, refer to the articles that give a more in-depth explanation of these surgical procedures and the associated care (Boarini, 1989; Brown and Ricketts, 1994; Bastawrous and others, 1995; Foster, 1995; Hull and Erwin-Toth, 1996).

Figure 26-2 illustrates the two types of urinary diversions: noncontinent and continent. Some examples of noncontinent urinary diversions are ileal or colonic conduit and ureterostomy. The ileal loop may be called an ileal conduit. The surgical procedure may or may not involve **cystectomy** (removal of the bladder). For an ileal conduit, usually 6 to 8 inches of ileum are separated from the bowel. One end is used to create an external stoma, usually in the lower right quadrant, and the other end is suture closed. The ureters are internally im-

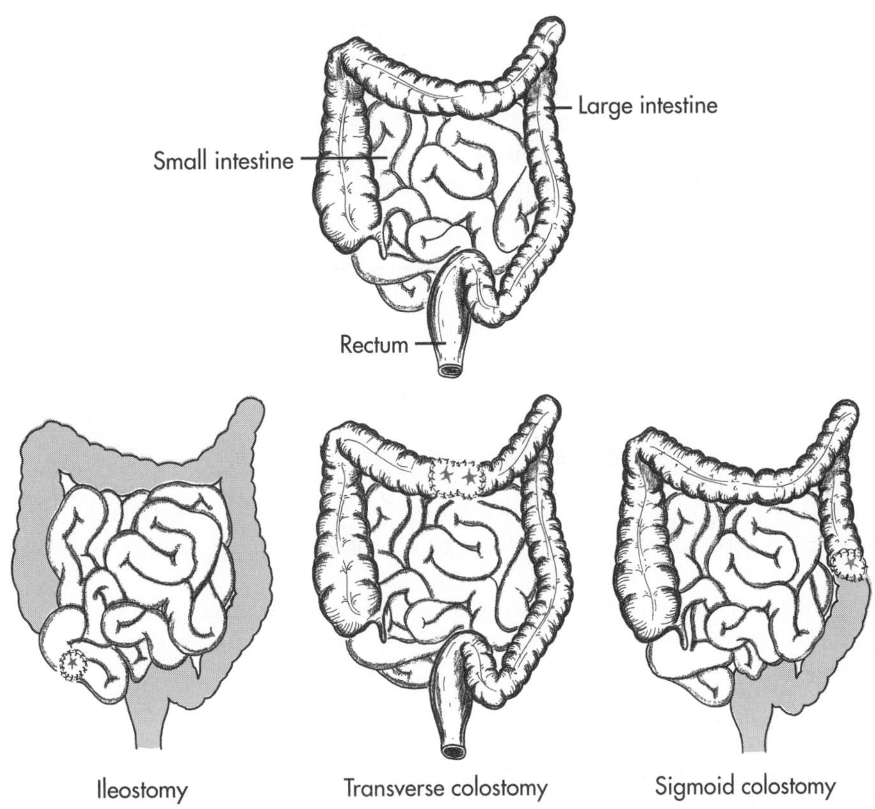

FIGURE **26-1** Types of enterostomies: ileostomy, transverse colostomy, and sigmoid colostomy.

planted into this piece of bowel. The client must wear an external ostomy pouch or appliance at all times to collect the urine. The rest of the bowel is sutured together so the client has normal bowel movements as before surgery.

An **ureterostomy** involves bringing the end of one or both ureters directly to the abdominal surface. An ureterostomy is difficult to pouch, may become occluded in certain body positions, or may become obstructed, with no urine flow. Irritation of the skin from leakage of urine is a common problem. The ureterostomy is the type of urinary diversion usually done in neonates (Boarini, 1989). **Continent ostomy or urinary diversions** include the Kock urinary reservoir/pouch, Indiana pouch (see Figure 26-2), and the Neobladder procedures, such as the Camay procedure.

Regardless of the type of ostomy, a threat to body image may be perceived (Quayle, 1994; Walsh and others, 1995; Kluka and Kristijanson, 1996; Piper and Mikols, 1996; Piper, Mikols, and Grant, 1996). Researchers have shown that clients with ostomies have concerns about stool leakage and odor, body image changes, social support, self-care, health and life expectations, and surgical complication management. Some other concerns the client may have are fears of mutilation, rejection by friends or family, and even a loss of normal sexual function (Golis, 1996). Foul-smelling odors, spillage or leakage of liquid stools or urine, and the inability to regulate

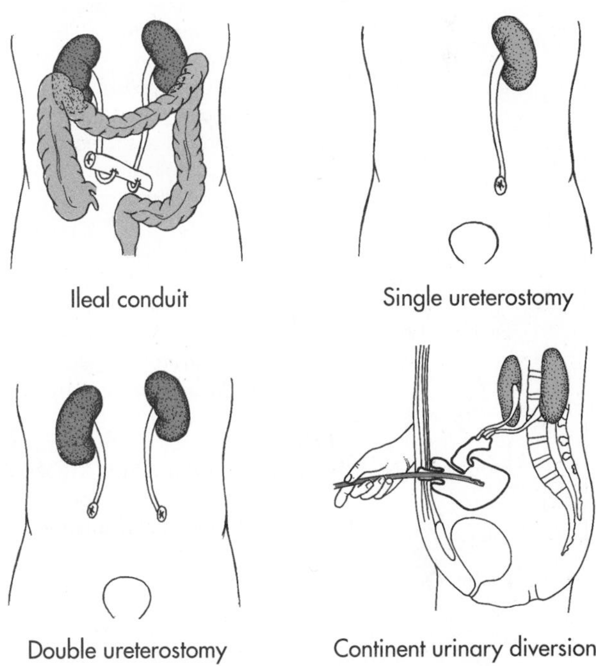

FIGURE **26-2** Types of ureterostomies: ileal loop, single ureterostomy, double ureterostomy, continent urinary diversion (Indiana pouch).

bowel movements give the client a sense of powerlessness and loss of self-esteem.

Education and counseling of clients with ostomies is a major intervention for the nurse (Piper and Mikols, 1996; Mowdy, 1998). To assist clients in caring for their own ostomies, instruction for clients should begin on admission during the preoperative period and resume early postoperatively as the client's physical condition permits. A clinical pathway for a client with an ostomy in the home care setting allows assistance in returning the client to independence (Figure 26-3). The nurse must help the client to understand that a normal lifestyle is possible with an ostomy.

OSTOMY CLINICAL PATH

PATIENT ______________ **ID #** ______________ **DATE** ______________
Medical diagnosis ______________ **ICD-9 code** ______________
SOC: ______________ **Discharge date:** ______________ **Care Coordinator:** ______________

GOALS:
PHYSIOLOGIC – Patient will achieve optimal bowel function without complications. Patient's wound will heal with no sign of infection.
PSYCHOLOGIC – Patient will demonstrate a level of acceptance of modified lifestyle.
COGNITIVE – Patient/Primary care person will demonstrate independence with ostomy care.
Outcome Achieved

	Y/N DATE VC
Problem: **ALTERATION IN BOWEL FUNCTIONS**	
1. optimal bowel function without complications	1. ______
Problem: **POTENTIAL/ACTUAL SKIN IMPAIRMENT R/T SURGICAL INCISION/OSTOMY EFFLUENT**	
1. verbalizes/demonstrates wound care	1. ______
2. verbalizes s/s of infection	2. ______
3. verbalizes/demonstrates stoma/peristomal skin care	3. ______
4. achieves/maintains intact skin	4. ______
Problem: **KNOWLEDGE DEFICIT R/T OSTOMY**	
1. verbalizes A & P of bowel	1. ______
2. verbalizes/demonstrates appliance removal	2. ______
3. verbalizes/demonstrates wafer preparation	3. ______
4. verbalizes/demonstrates wafer application	4. ______
5. verbalizes pouch application	5. ______
6. verbalizes/demonstrates clip use	6. ______
7. verbalizes/demonstrates pouch care	7. ______
8. verbalizes odor control/flatus release	8. ______
9. verbalizes potential complications	9. ______
10. verbalizes frequency of change	10. ______
11. verbalizes balanced diet	11. ______
12. verbalizes supply sources	12. ______
13. verbalizes activity levels	13. ______
14. achieves independence with ostomy care	14. ______
Problem: **ALTERATION IN BODY IMAGE**	
1. verbalizes fears/demonstrates appropriate coping mechanisms	1. ______
2. demonstrates adjustment to ostomy by active participation in care as able	2. ______
3. discusses activities resumed	3. ______
4. demonstrates ability to cope with illness	4. ______
Problem: **KNOWLEDGE DEFICIT R/T MEDICATIONS/SAFETY**	
1. verbalizes/demonstrates knowledge and compliance with medications	1. ______
2. verbalizes/demonstrates safety measures	2. ______

Code: Outcome Achieved
Y = yes
N = no
VC = variance code 1, 2, or 3

1. patient 2. environment 3. agency

____
Patient signature

____
Case manager signature

FIGURE **26-3** Ostomy care clinical pathway. (From Mitchel JV: A clinical pathway for ostomy care in the home: process and development, *J Wound Ostomy Continence Nurs* 25(4):203, 1998.)

Skill Performance Guidelines

1. Know how to assess your client's stoma (Box 26-1).
2. Know what type of effluent is expected from the ostomy. Some ostomies, such as an ileostomy, normally have liquid drainage. Due to normal enzymes in the small bowel an ileostomy drainage is most damaging to skin. Copious output may result in dehydration and electrolyte imbalance. An ileal conduit, though draining urine, normally has mucus because the bowel still produces mucus.
3. Know if the ostomy is continent or noncontinent (incontinent). This information indicates to the nurse whether the lack of spontaneous drainage signals a problem (i.e., noncontinent ostomy) or whether it requires insertion of a catheter to drain the effluent (i.e., continent ostomy). Just because a client has a stoma does not mean that the drainage will spontaneously flow from it. Clients who have

Box 26-1 ABCD's of Stoma Assessment and Pouching

A IS FOR ASSESSMENT

Number of stoma(s)
- How many stomas does your client have?

Stoma location
- Where on the abdomen is your client's stoma?
- What part of the bowel is the stoma?
- Is the stoma near structures that will impact on care?

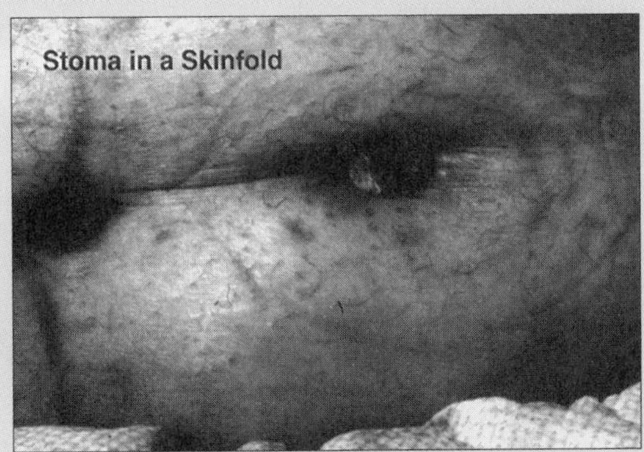

Stoma in or near a skinfold. (Courtesy ConvaTec, Princeton, NJ.)

Stoma type
- Is this a matured stoma?
- What is the length or protrusion of the stoma?
  - Bud, flush, or spout

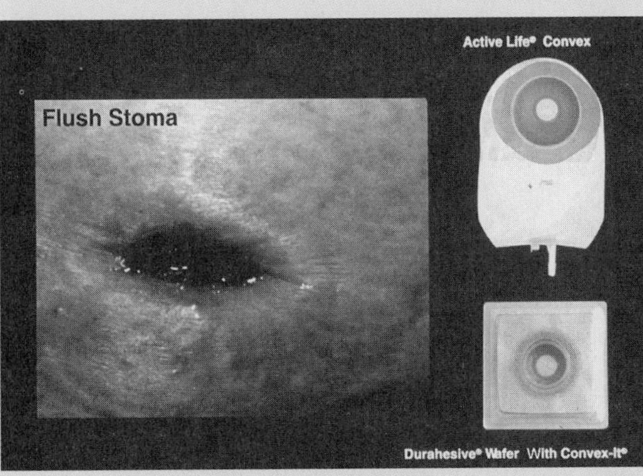

Normal flush stoma. (Courtesy ConvaTec, Princeton, NJ.)

Stoma shape
- What shape is the client's stoma?
  - Round, oval, regular/irregular

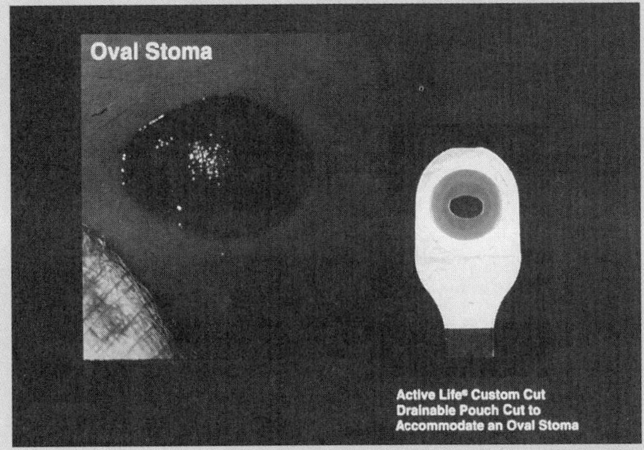

Stoma of oval shape. (Courtesy ConvaTec, Princeton, NJ.)

Stoma viability
- How do you monitor stoma viability?
  - Color, tissue turgor, bleeding

Stoma construction
- How is stoma made?
  - End, loop, double barrel
- What is the direction of the stoma lumen?

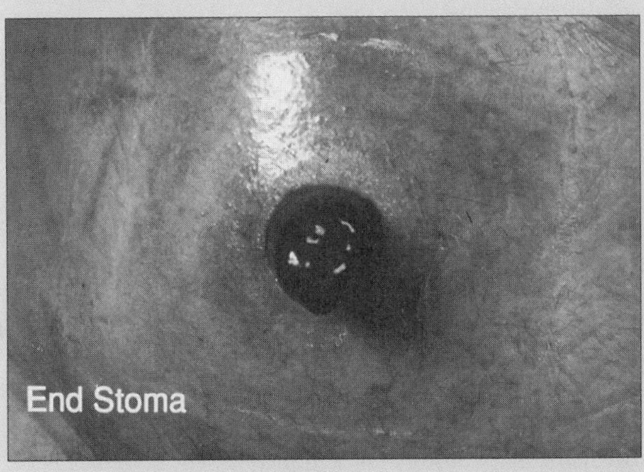

End stoma (bud type). (Courtesy ConvaTec, Princeton, NJ.)

From Ayello: The ABCD's of stoma assessment and pouching (Personal correspondence, 2000)

Continued

Box 26-1 ABCD's of Stoma Assessment and Pouching—cont'd

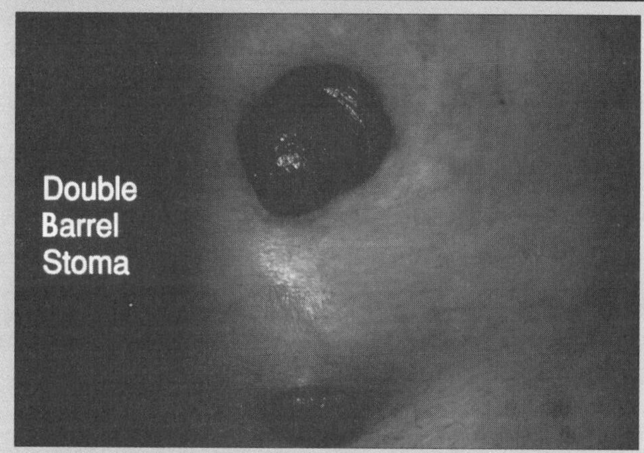

Double barrel stoma. (Courtesy ConvaTec, Princeton, NJ.)

A IS FOR ASSESSMENT—cont'd

Stoma drainage
- Is this a continent or incontinent stoma?
- What is the normal amount and consistency of stoma output?

Stoma size
- What size is the stoma?
- How do I measure it?

B IS FOR BOARDS

Wound, Ostomy, Continence Nurses (WOCN)
1550 S Coast Highway, Suite 201
Laguna Beach, CA 92651
(888) 224-9626
Fax (714) 376-3456
www.wocn.org

C IS FOR COMPLICATIONS

Bleeding
Necrosis
Prolapse
Hernia
Laceration
Irritation
Retraction
Stenosis

D IS FOR DIFFERENT AND DETERMINING POUCHING SYSTEMS

Differences in pouching systems
- Fecal versus urinary
- Adhesive versus non-adhesive
- One piece versus two piece
- Precut versus cut to fit
- Disposable versus reusable
- Drainable (open ended) versus closed end (non-drainable)

Determining pouching systems
- Is the correct skin barrier and pouch being used?
- Does the skin barrier and pouch fit correctly?
- How do you measure the stoma and determine the correct pouching system sizing for each product?
- Is the skin barrier intact?
- Are there any peristomal skin problems or abdominal contours that will alter the pouching system needed?
- How often does this pouching system need to routinely be changed?
- When should the pouch be emptied?

From Ayello: The ABCD's of stoma assessment and pouching (Personal correspondence, 2000).

continent ostomies (Kock or Indiana pouches) need to have the stoma intubated with a catheter periodically during the day to drain the fecal or urine contents (Hull and Erwin-Toth, 1996) (see Skill 26-5).

4. Know the client's usual elimination pattern so the client can return to or maintain a usual schedule while receiving nursing care.
5. Know the client's routine for self-care of the ostomy. A client who has independently cared for an ostomy should be encouraged to resume self-care as soon as possible.
6. Know the equipment options available. Various types of equipment are used for different types of stomas, ostomy drainage, and skin irritations.

Skill 26-1 Pouching an Enterostomy

Immediately after surgical diversion or removal of a portion of bowel, it is necessary to place a pouch over the newly created stoma because in some noncontinent ostomies effluent may begin immediately. The pouch collects all effluent and protects the skin from irritating drainage. A pouch with its **skin barrier** should fit comfortably, cover the skin surface around the stoma, and create a good seal. The postoperative pouch should allow visibility of the stoma.

The technique of pouching a newly formed stoma differs from techniques used to pouch a stoma several days or weeks

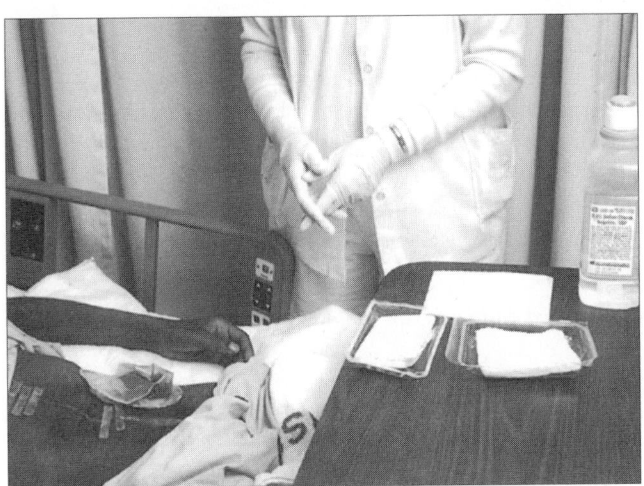

FIGURE **26-4** Ostomy pouch near suture line.

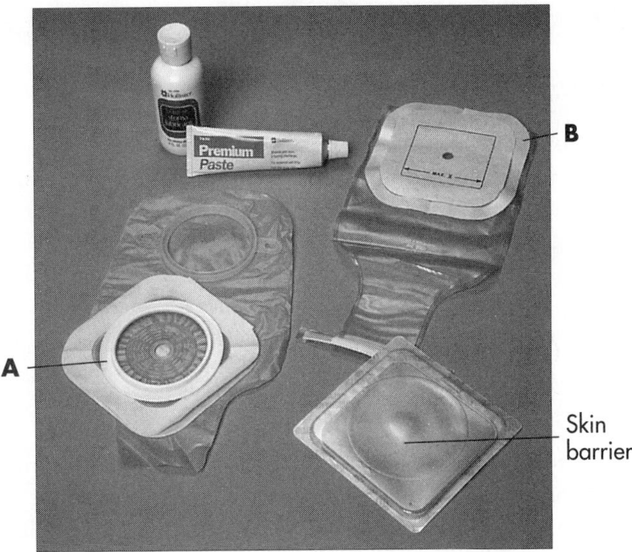

FIGURE **26-5** Examples of some pouching systems. **A,** Two-piece detachable system. (NOTE: The skin barrier would need to be custom cut by the client according to self-stoma size obtained by measurement.) The pouch opening is already precut by the manufacturer to fit the size of the flange on the skin barrier. **B,** One-piece pouch with skin barrier attached.

old. The new stoma is edematous during the postoperative healing process. An incision line from the bowel resection may lie close to or around the stoma (Figure 26-4). The stoma itself often has a series of small stitches around its perimeter. A pouch and its skin barrier must be applied so that they do not constrict the stoma or traumatize healing tissues. Initially the pouch over a postoperative colostomy may not need to be emptied frequently because drainage is diminished or lacking. Several days may pass before a client's normal elimination pattern returns. In the case of an ileostomy, the client will have frequent stools when **peristalsis** returns.

Many types of pouches and skin barriers are available (Bradley and Pupiales, 1997). Some pouches have skin barriers directly preattached and are called one-piece pouching systems. Some of these one-piece pouches already are precut to size by the manufacturer, whereas others must be custom cut to size for the client's stoma measurement. Other systems are two separate pieces. The pouch can be applied to the skin barrier by attaching it to the flange (a plastic ring) on the barrier. Often the skin barrier needs to be custom cut to the client's specific stoma size. For two-piece systems the skin barrier with flange must be used with the corresponding size pouch that fits that flange *from the same manufacturer* to use the system correctly without leakage. Nurses should understand how to use each of these different pouching systems (Figure 26-5). Modifications or usual pouching techniques for stenosed stomas and retracted stomas have been described (Wagner and Osgood, 1998; Bonham and Schaffner, 1999).

Delegation Considerations

This skill should not be delegated to assistive personnel. The one exception in some agencies is that care of established enterostomies may be delegated to assistive personnel. The care provider should be instructed in the expected amount, color, and consistency of drainage from the enterostomy. In addition, the care provider should report changes in the client's stoma and surrounding skin integrity.

Equipment

- Pouch, clear drainable colostomy/ileostomy in correct size for two-piece system (see Figure 26-5, *A*) or custom cut-to-fit one-piece type with attached skin barrier (see Figure 26-5, *B*)
- Pouch closure device, such as a clamp
- Adhesive remover (optional)
- Clean disposable gloves
- Ostomy deodorant
- Gauze pads or washcloth
- Towel or disposable waterproof barrier
- Basin with warm tap water
- Scissors
- Skin barrier such as sealant wipes or wafer
- Tape or ostomy belt

Step	Rationale

Assessment

1. Auscultate for bowel sounds. — Documents presence of peristalsis.
2. Observe existing skin barrier and pouch for leakage and length of time in place. Depending upon type of pouching system used (such as opaque pouch), nurse may have to remove pouch to fully observe stoma. Clear pouches permit viewing of stoma without their removal. — Determines likelihood of pouch loosening from stoma and failing to collect effluent.

- ***Critical Decision Point***
  Intact skin barriers with no evidence of leakage do not need to be changed daily and can remain in place for 3 to 5 days (Ayello, 2000).

3. Observe stoma for color, swelling, trauma, and healing; stoma should be moist and reddish pink. Assess type of stoma. Stomas can be flush with the skin or be a budlike protrusion on the abdomen. (An example of a normal bud stoma can be found in Box 26-1.) — Stoma characteristics should be one of the factors to consider when selecting an appropriate pouching system.

- ***Critical Decision Point***
  Stoma should be measured with each pouching system change to determine correct size of equipment needed. Follow each ostomy pouch manufacturer's directions and measuring guide as to which size ostomy pouch to use based on client's actual stoma measurement size.

4. Observe abdominal contour and abdominal incision (if present). — Relationship of abdominal contour to stoma determines proper placement of pouch (see illustration).
5. Observe effluent from stoma and record of intake and output. Ask client about skin tenderness. — Plan on changing skin barrier pouch at times of less effluent output. Generally avoid changing after meals, when gastrocolic reflux increases chance of fecal effluent output.
6. When assessing skin for irritation, check that pouching system is not leaking. — Leaking may indicate need for different type of pouch or sealant.

- ***Critical Decision Point***
  Because of stomal and abdominal characteristics, some clients may need convexity in their ostomy pouching system to avoid leakage (see illustrations for Step 8) (Rolstad and Boarini, 1996).

7. To minimize skin irritation, avoid unnecessary changing of entire pouching system. A one-piece pouch with attached skin barriers or the skin barrier of a two-piece pouching system should be changed every 3 to 7 days, *not* daily. — Pouches should be emptied when one-third to one-half full because weight of contents may dislodge skin seal, and ostomy drainage is irritating to the skin. Also, pouches collect flatus (gas), which needs to be expelled because it can disrupt skin seal.

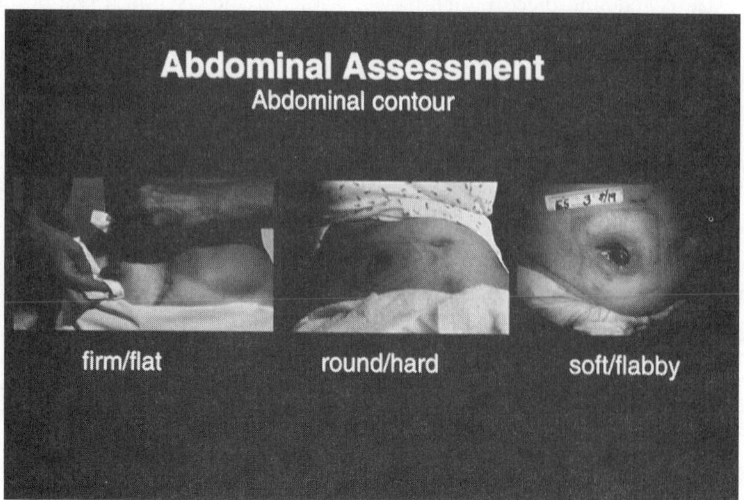

STEP **4** Relationship of abdominal contour to stoma. (Courtesy ConvaTec, Princeton, NJ.)

STEP	RATIONALE

- ***Critical Decision Point***
  Do not put holes in pouch for flatus to escape. Instead encourage client to empty pouch of flatus.

8. Assess abdomen for best type of pouching system to use. Consider:
   a. Contour and **peristomal** plane

Determines pouching system selection and need for other equipment.

A firm/flat and round/hard abdomen usually needs a flexible or soft pouching system, whereas a flabby or soft abdomen usually needs a firmer system (see illustration in Step 4). Convexity may be needed for stomas that are retracted or in skinfolds, and different pouching systems are needed (see illustration).

   b. Presence of scars, incisions
   c. Location and type of stoma

- ***Critical Decision Point***
  Pouching system options include the following:
  - *Adhesive and nonadhesive systems, which are also available for both urinary and fecal drainage.*
  - *One-piece pouch with skin barrier already attached; precut pouch and skin barrier; or two-piece pouch system, which consists of pouch that can detach from skin barrier, which remains around client's stoma for several days. Bottom of ostomy pouch is either open ended, which is closed only with a clip or has a rubber band or some other type of closure device between emptying, or closed ended, in which end of pouch is sealed closed. One-piece pouches should be open-ended pouches that can be opened periodically to empty effluent without removing pouch from around stoma.*
  - *Two-piece pouches give client choice of using either an open-ended or closed-ended pouch. This is because client can remove pouch from skin barrier to empty effluent.*

9. Assess the client's condition as to the best type of pouching system to use. Assess vision, dexterity or mobility, and cognitive function.

Clients with poor vision may benefit by using yellow-tinted sunglasses to reduce glare and improve contrast and by using magnification mirrors (Jeffries and MacKay, 1997). Clients who also have mobility problems or spinal cord injuries may benefit by using equipment that has a longer pouch, which is easier to independently empty when sitting (Edgar, 1999). Clients who have difficulty using their hands or who have limited vision may find a one-piece system or a precut pouch and skin barrier more desirable to use; others prefer being able to keep the skin barrier in place for several days, changing just the pouch, and therefore prefer the two-piece system. Even clients who are blind can be taught to change their own ostomy equipment (Ramos and Glosson, 1996).

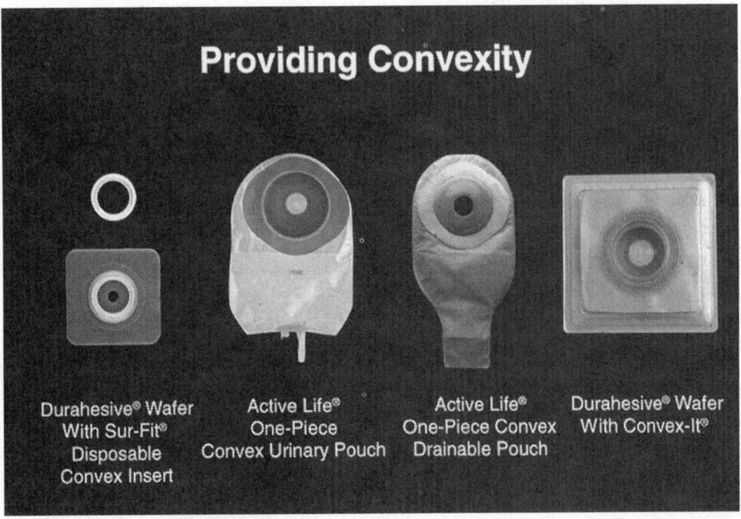

STEP **8a** Devices used to provide abdominal convexity. (Courtesy ConvaTec, Princeton, NJ.)

STEP	RATIONALE
10. After skin barrier and pouch removal, assess skin around stoma, noting scars, folds, skin breakdown, and peristomal suture line if present.	Determines need for barrier paste to increase adherence of pouch to skin or to fill in irregularities.
11. Determine client's and family's emotional response and knowledge and understanding of an ostomy and its care (Northouse and others, 1999).	Assists in determining extent to which client is able to participate in care and need for teaching and information clarification.

NURSING DIAGNOSIS

Defining characteristics from the assessment data may reveal the following nursing diagnoses for clients requiring this skill:

- Constipation
- Diarrhea
- Risk for impaired skin integrity
- Ineffective individual coping
- Deficient knowledge regarding ostomy self-care
- Acute pain

Related factors are individualized based on client's condition or needs.

PLANNING

STEP	RATIONALE
1. **Expected outcomes** following completion of procedure:	
▪ Client denies discomfort.	Stomach and surrounding skin intact.
▪ Stoma is moist and reddish pink. Skin is intact and free of irritation; sutures are intact.	Normal findings in client with postoperative enterostomy that is healing. Stoma initially is edematous and shrinks over next 6 to 8 weeks.
▪ Stoma is functioning with moderate amount of liquid or soft stool and flatus in pouch. (Flatus is noted by bulging of pouch in absence of drainage; flatus initially indicates return of peristalsis after surgery.)	Snug seal around stoma has been attained. Skin is free of irritation.
▪ Client observes stoma and steps of procedure carefully.	Reveals acknowledgment of body alteration and interest in self-care.
▪ Client asks questions about procedure and may attempt to assist with pouch change.	Asking to assist indicates readiness to learn and to begin self-care.
2. Explain procedure to client; encourage client's interaction and questions.	Lessens client's anxiety and promotes client's participation.
3. Assemble equipment, and close room curtains or door.	Optimizes use of time; conserves client's and nurse's energy. Provides privacy.

IMPLEMENTATION

STEP	RATIONALE
1. Position client either standing or supine and drape. If seated, position client either on or in front of toilet.	When client is supine, there are fewer skin wrinkles, which allows for ease of application of pouching system; maintains client's dignity.
2. Wash hands and apply disposable gloves.	Reduces transmission of microorganisms.
3. Place towel or disposable waterproof barrier under client.	Protects bed linen.
4. Remove used pouch and skin barrier gently by pushing skin away from barrier. An adhesive remover may be used to facilitate removal of skin barrier.	Reduces skin trauma. Improper removal of pouch and barrier can irritate client's skin and can cause skin tears.
5. Cleanse peristomal skin gently with warm tap water using gauze pads or clean washcloth; do not scrub skin; dry completely by patting skin with gauze or towel.	Avoid use of soap because it leaves a residue on skin that interferes with pouch adhesion to skin. Skin must be dry as skin barrier; pouch does not adhere to wet skin. If blood appears on gauze pad, do not be alarmed. If rubbed, stoma may ooze some blood as a result of cleaning process. Bleeding into pouch is abnormal. Stoma's surface is highly vascular mucous membrane.

STEP	RATIONALE
6. Measure stoma for correct size of pouching system needed using the manufacturer's measuring guide (see illustration).	Ensures accuracy in determining correct pouch size needed. Stoma shrinks and does not reach usual size for 6 to 8 weeks.
7. Select appropriate pouch for client based on client assessment. With a custom cut-to-fit pouch, use an ostomy guide to cut opening on the pouch $\frac{1}{16}$ to $\frac{1}{8}$ inch larger than stoma before removing backing. Prepare pouch by removing backing from barrier and adhesive. With ileostomy, apply thin circle of barrier paste around opening in pouch; allow to dry (see illustrations *A* to *C*).	Paste facilitates seal and protects skin. Size of pouch opening keeps drainage off skin and lessens risk of damage to stoma during peristalsis or activity. Pouch and skin barrier are changed whenever leaking. Change when client is comfortable; before a meal is better because this avoids increased peristalsis and chance of evacuation during pouch change. Can also be changed before or after tub bath or shower. Stool is alkaline, and this irritates skin; fecal bacteria can colonize on skin and increase risk of infection.

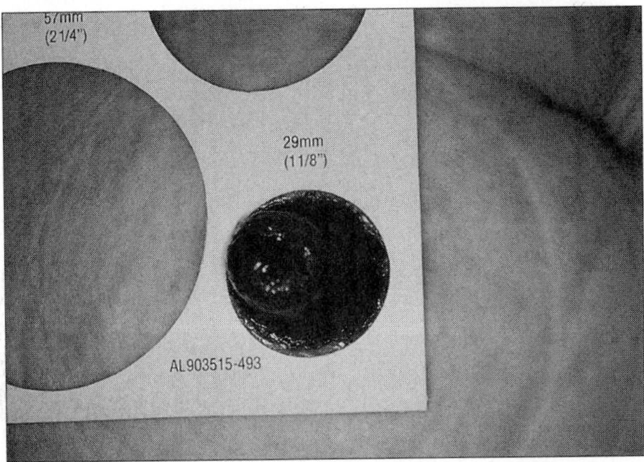

STEP **6** Measuring an ostomy.

A

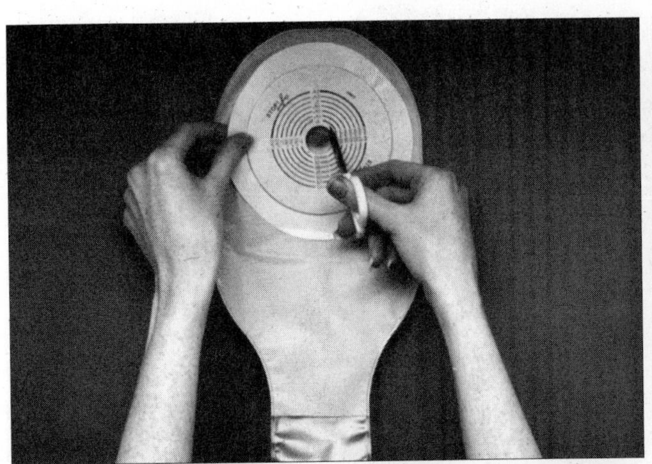

B

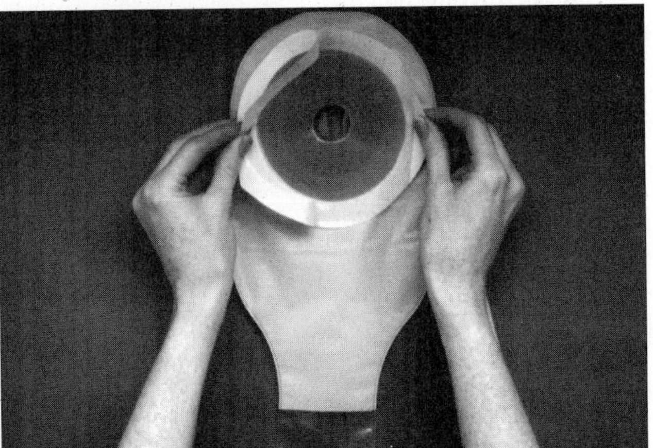

C

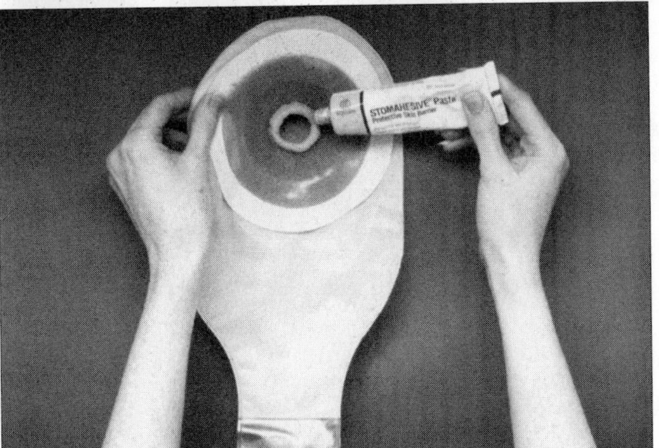

STEP **7** **A,** Cut-to-fit, one-piece drainable ostomy pouch. **B,** Removing the backing paper for the barrier of a one-piece pouch. **C,** Applying barrier paste to a one-piece ostomy pouch. (Courtesy ConvaTec, Princeton, NJ.)

STEP	RATIONALE

- ***Critical Decision Point***
  If client has large amount of liquid stool from an ileostomy, consider using a "high-output" pouch that will contain this effluent and reduce frequency of pouch emptying.

8. Apply skin barrier and pouch. If creases next to stoma occur, use barrier paste to fill in; let dry 1 to 2 minutes.

- ***Critical Decision Point***
  When applying skin barrier to stoma that is close to client's abdominal incision, skin barrier may have to be trimmed to fit.

a. For one-piece pouching system:
   (1) Use skin sealant wipes on skin directly under adhesive skin barrier or pouch; allow to dry. Press adhesive backing of pouch and/or skin barrier smoothly against skin, starting from the bottom and working up and around sides. — Ensure smooth, wrinkle free seal.
   (2) Hold pouch by barrier, center over stoma, and press down gently on barrier; bottom of pouch should point toward client's knees (see illustration).
   (3) Maintain gentle finger pressure around barrier for 1 to 2 minutes.
b. If using two-piece pouching system:
   (1) Apply barrier-paste flange (barrier with adhesive) as in steps above for one-piece system. Then snap on pouch and maintain finger pressure (see illustration). — Creates wrinkle-free, secure seal; decreases irritation from adhesive on skin. Some two-piece pouching systems may have a snapping or clicking sound that occurs when attaching pouch to skin barrier.
c. For both pouching systems gently tug on pouch in a downward direction. — Determines that pouch is securely attached.

9. Apply nonallergenic paper tape around pectin skin barrier in a "picture frame" method. Half of the tape should be on skin barrier and half on client's skin. Some clients may prefer a belt attached to the pouch for extra security rather than tape. — "Picture framing" pectin skin barrier adds to security of keeping pouch system attached securely.

- ***Critical Decision Point***
  Make sure client who chooses to wear an ostomy belt does not have the belt too tight. To check for appropriate tightness, two fingers should fit comfortably placed between belt and client's skin.

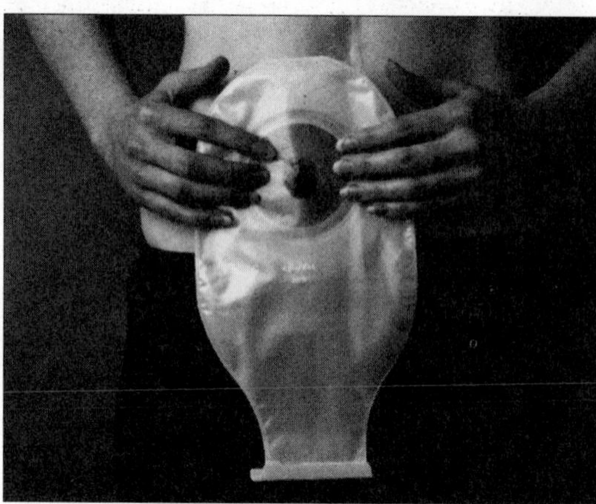

STEP **8a(2)** Applying a one-piece pouch. (Courtesy ConvaTec, Princeton, NJ.)

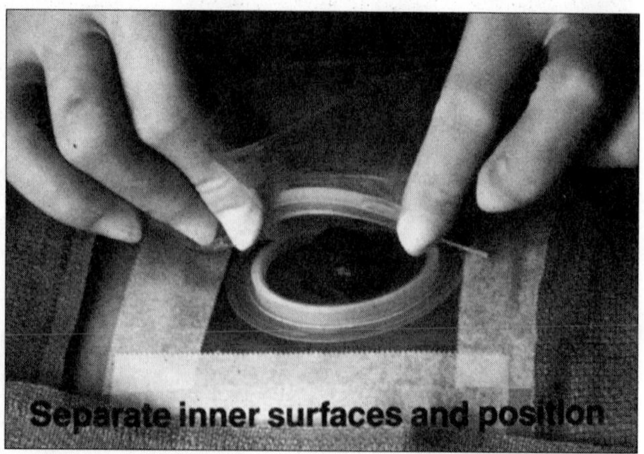

STEP **8b(1)** Application of barrier-paste flange. (Courtesy ConvaTec, Princeton, NJ.)

Step	Rationale
10. Although many ostomy pouches are odor-proof, some nurses and clients like to add a small amount of ostomy deodorant into pouch. Do not use "home remedies," which can harm stoma, to control ostomy odor. Do not make hole in pouch to release flatus.	Causes damage to pouch and defeats purpose of odor-proof pouch.

- ***Critical Decision Point***
  Aspirin should never be added to ostomy pouch. It can cause stomal bleeding.

Step	Rationale
11. Fold bottom of drainable open-ended pouches up once and close using a closure device such as a clamp (or follow manufacturers' instructions for closure).	Maintains secure seal to prevent leaking.
12. Properly dispose of old pouch and soiled equipment. Client may also request spraying of room air freshener in room if needed.	Lessens odors in room.
13. Remove gloves and wash hands.	Reduces transmission of microorganisms.
14. Change one- or two-piece pouch every 3 to 7 days unless leaking; pouch can remain in place for tub bath or shower; after bath, pat adhesive dry.	Avoids unnecessary trauma to skin from too-frequent changes. Drying ensures adhesion of pouch.

- ***Critical Decision Point***
  Sometimes nonallergic paper tape needs to be reapplied after showering or bathing.

Evaluation

Step	Rationale
1. Ask if client feels discomfort around stoma.	Determines presence of skin irritation.
2. Note appearance of stoma around skin and existing incision (if present) while pouch is removed and skin is cleansed. Reinspect condition of skin barrier and adhesive.	Determines condition of tissues and progress of healing. Determines presence of leaks.
3. Auscultate bowel sounds, and observe characteristics of stool.	Determines return of peristalsis and bowel elimination.
4. Observe client's nonverbal behaviors as pouch is applied. Ask if client has any questions about pouching.	May indicate emotional response to stoma and readiness for teaching. Determines level of understanding of procedure.

Unexpected Outcomes and Related Interventions

- Skin around stoma is irritated, has burning sensation.
  - Assess stoma as mucosal layer of stoma separates from skin.
  - May be caused by undermining of pouch seal by fecal contents.
  - May indicate an allergic reaction, which can be manifested by erythema and blistering, usually confined to one area immediately under allergen.
  - Remove pouch more slowly.
  - Obtain referral for enterostomal therapy (ET/WOCN) nurse.
- Necrotic stoma is manifested by purple or black color, dry instead of moist texture, failure to bleed when washed gently, or presence of tissue sloughing.
  - Assess circulation to stoma.
  - Determine presence of excessive edema or excessive tension on bowel suture line.
- Client complains of irritation and burning around stoma.
  - Assess skin for breaks in integrity, skin inflammation, **maceration,** or infection.
- Client refuses to view stoma or participate in care.
  - Obtain information about ostomy support groups in community.
  - Refer client and family to other volunteer clients with an ostomy in community for individual support.
  - Knowledge and acceptance by staff facilitate understanding and adjustment.

Recording and Reporting

- Chart type of pouch and skin barrier applied.
- Record amount and appearance of stool or drainage in pouch, size of stoma, color of stool, texture, condition of peristomal skin, and sutures.
- Document abdominal distention and excessive tenderness, nature of bowel sounds.
- Record client's level of participation and need for teaching.
- Report any of the following to nurse in charge and/or physician:
  - Abnormal appearance of stoma, suture line, peristomal skin, character of output, absence of bowel sounds
  - No flatus in 24 to 36 hours and no stool by third day.

Teaching Considerations

- Include family members or significant other in teaching because this may facilitate client's readiness to learn (Northouse and others, 1999).
- Client's readiness to learn may be judged, for example, by willingness to look at stoma and asking questions. If client is apprehensive about touching or looking at stoma, have client hold gauze pad over stoma and clean around stoma (Aron and others, 1999).
- Some clients acknowledge stoma with minimal emotional difficulty; some may never completely adjust to it. Individualize care according to client's situation and circumstances (Cohen, 1991).
- Teach client to avoid constipation by eating a balanced diet and having adequate fluids (Ayello and others, 1999).
- Client should be given a teaching manual with steps clearly stated, or audiotaped instructions. With client who has learning disability, a "picture book" of the steps may be more appropriate.
- Adult clients may wear usual clothes because abdominal peristalsis pushes stool out of stoma, and snug clothes do not interfere with effluent emptying into external pouch. Tight girdles and undergarments, however, should not be worn without consent of surgeon. For babies, one-piece garments are preferred because they can deter baby from pulling off ostomy pouch.

Pediatric Considerations

- Because most ostomy surgery done on neonates is for emergency situations, often no time is available for preoperative selection of stoma site. Most stomas, however, are temporary with stoma being "taken down" (removed or closed) when baby is about 1 year old. Colostomies are the most frequent type of stomas in neonates. They are usually done because baby has necrotizing enterocolitis (NEC), Hirschsprung's disease, or imperforate anus (Boarini, 1989; Brown and Ricketts, 1994).
- Although normal stoma color is red, a temporary change in stoma color to white or purple may occur when baby is crying (Boarini, 1989).
- Neonates often have multiple stomas on their tiny abdomens that may be the result of corrective bowel surgeries. Select a cut-to-fit pouch that allows multiple stoma openings in skin barrier, yet still fits on neonate's tiny abdomen (Brown and Ricketts, 1994).
- Because babies swallow large amounts of air while sucking, it is normal to expect considerable amounts of flatus. Make sure pouch can accommodate increased amount of flatus or be prepared to release flatus frequently (Brown and Ricketts, 1994).
- Use equipment that is designed by manufacturers for use with pediatric clients (Brown and Ricketts, 1994). The preterm baby's skin is immature and thus has a weaker cohesion between dermis and epidermis layers of skin. Therefore it is more permeable, leading to a greater risk of toxicity from absorption of products and an increased risk for damage from stripping of skin (Boarini, 1989).
- Usually a baby triples its birth weight in the first year. Stoma does not delay baby's growth. As baby grows in size, so too does stoma. Therefore stoma should be measured frequently and appropriate adjustments in pouching and skin barrier size be made accordingly (Boarini, 1989).
- Whenever possible, adolescents requiring an ostomy benefit from presurgical contact with other adolescents who have an ostomy (Erwin-Toth, 1999).
- Brown and Ricketts (1994) have described characteristics of pouch skin barriers for pediatric clients:
  - Flexible to cover infant's rounded abdominal contour.
  - Thin enough to avoid undermining of stool beneath skin barrier.
  - Large enough to accommodate multiple stomas in one skin barrier.
  - Stoma prolapse occurs more frequently in pediatric clients because of the increase in intraabdominal pressure that occurs with crying (Brown and Ricketts, 1994).

Gerontological Considerations

- Evaluate older adult's cognitive status for understanding ostomy self-care instructions.
- Evaluate older adult's motor and visual ability to prepare ostomy equipment. For clients who are unable to custom cut the size of their skin barriers, consider having barriers precut by ostomy equipment supplier or using a precut two-piece system (Jeffres and MacKay, 1997).
- Avoid hot water and harsh soaps when washing the peristomal skin.
- Older clients need teaching about change in number of eliminations (from an incontinent ostomy) that would be normal on a daily status.
- Financial concerns about cost of ostomy supplies and reimbursement may be an important issue for clients on Medicare (Halvorson and Kertz, 1996).

Home Care Considerations

- Client should understand that although nurse may have used sterile gauze to clean stoma, it is *not* necessary to use sterile gauze. In fact, gauze is not needed at all; a washcloth or any soft material can be used.
- If client is returned to the home setting, a clinical pathway can assist in developing individualized client interventions designed to increase client's and family's ability to care for the ostomy (Mitchel, 1998).
- Evaluate client's home toileting facilities. This includes:
  - Presence of adequate toileting facilities in client's home
  - Privacy
  - Flushing toilet facilities
  - Number and location of toileting facilities
  - Number of other people living with client who must share toileting facilities

Skill 26-2 Irrigating a Colostomy

The purpose of colostomy irrigation is to cleanse the bowel of feces before tests or surgical procedures, to relieve constipation, or to establish a pattern of regular bowel elimination after ostomy surgery. Irrigation of a colostomy is a simple procedure that clients can learn. The muscular quality of the colon allows it to be safely irrigated with a relatively large amount of fluid. Clients who perform irrigations at home learn to establish an irrigation routine so that regular evacuation of the bowel occurs without stomal discharge between irrigations. Irrigations for achieving regular bowel evacuation can be achieved only with descending and sigmoid end colostomies. A study by Leong and Yunos (1999) found that clients who irrigated their colostomy had improved continence, less cost for equipment, and fewer problems with sleeping, sex, and skin complications.

Irrigating an ileostomy is rarely necessary, except in cases of food blockage near the stomal outlet. Then, a gentle lavage may be performed, but only by a qualified person such as an enterostomal therapy (ET) nurse. An ileostomy produces a liquid drainage containing a high concentration of electrolytes such as sodium, chloride, potassium, magnesium, and bicarbonate. Because excessive lavage could lead to a serious fluid and electrolyte imbalance, normal saline is used.

Delegation Considerations

This skill should not be delegated to assistive personnel.

Equipment

- Ostomy irrigation set that consists of an irrigation solution bag and tubing with a fluid control clamp and cone tip
- Irrigation sleeve (with belt tabs or stick-on ring and end-closure device)
- Water-soluble lubricant
- Ostomy pouch and skin barrier or stoma cap cover
- Ostomy deodorant
- Clean disposable gloves
- Toilet facilities that include a flushable toilet, a hook or some device to hold the irrigation container, toilet tissue, and running water (that is suitable for use)

For Clients Who Are Bedridden

- Bedpan
- Towels
- Waterproof pad

Step	Rationale
Assessment	
1. Assess frequency of defecation, character of stool, placement of stoma, abdominal distention, and nutritional pattern.	May indicate need to irrigate to stimulate elimination function; consistency of stool varies along length of gastrointestinal (GI) tract.
2. Assess time when client normally irrigates colostomy. In the case of a new ostomy, confer with physician about when irrigations can begin. Obtain written order. Confer with client for best time to irrigate.	Maintains established routine for bowel emptying. Irrigation initiates attempt to establish regular bowel emptying. Bowel must be totally healed so irrigation fluid will not cause perforation. This usually occurs 3 to 7 days after surgery.
3. Review orders for diagnostic or surgical procedures involving the bowel.	Procedures may indicate need to cleanse bowel of fecal contents or delay starting irrigation procedure.
4. Assess client's understanding of procedure and ability to perform techniques.	Determines level of participation to expect from client and level of explanations nurse should provide and if irrigation is appropriate for client.

Nursing Diagnosis

Defining characteristics from the assessment data may reveal the following nursing diagnoses for clients requiring this skill:

Anxiety
Constipation
Deficient knowledge regarding irrigation management

Related factors are individualized based on client's condition or needs.

STEP	RATIONALE

PLANNING

1. **Expected outcomes** following completion of procedure:
   - Large amount of flatus, formed stool, and fluid returns. Client denies abdominal pain or cramping. Spillage of stool does not occur between irrigations. — Absence of abdominal discomfort indicates that irrigant was instilled at proper rate.
   - Client performs irrigation procedure with minimal emotional distress. — Ability to perform irrigation strengthens client's sense of control.
   - Client understands and can perform procedure with minimal assistance. — Client is ready to perform self-care.
2. Explain procedure and anticipated responses (e.g., some abdominal cramping) to client; encourage client's participation and questions. — Lessens anxiety and promotes client's participation.
3. Assemble equipment, and close room curtains or door. — Optimizes use of time; conserves client's and nurse's energy. Provides privacy.

IMPLEMENTATION

1. Position client: — Allows for placement of irrigation sleeve into toilet or bedpan.
   a. On toilet or in chair in front of toilet, if ambulatory.
   b. On side, with head slightly elevated, if unable to be out of bed.

   • ***Critical Decision Point***
   Assess if client is capable of sitting on toilet. Make sure end of irrigation sleeve is sufficiently into toilet to prevent stool from getting on floor or client.

2. Apply disposable gloves. — Reduces transmission of microorganisms.
3. For adult clients, fill irrigation bag with 500 to 1000 ml warm irrigation solution (either tap water or normal saline); clear tubing of air (see illustration); 500 to 1000 ml is sufficient to distend the colon and effect evacuation. Start with 500 ml. — Allows solution to slowly enter colon and avoids cramping. Cold irrigation solution could trigger syncope and bowel cramping; hot water could damage stoma and intestinal mucosa. Air entering the colon may trigger cramping.

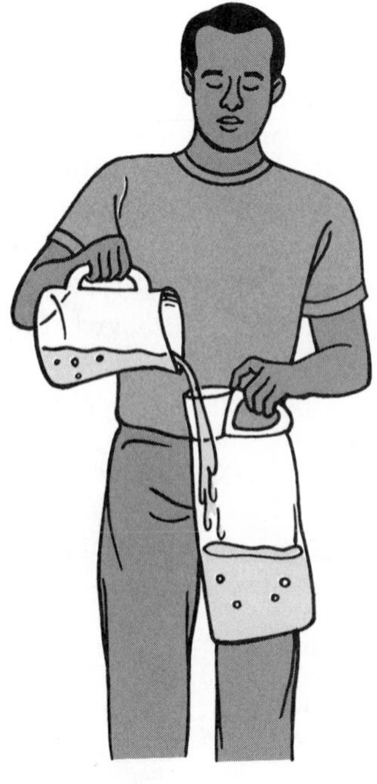

STEP 3 Filling irrigation bag.

STEP	RATIONALE

- ***Critical Decision Point***
  Do not use tap water for irrigations if tap water in region is not suitable for drinking. Replace with bottled water.

STEP	RATIONALE
4. Hang irrigation solution container on a hook so that end of bag is no higher than client's shoulder height when sitting or 18 to 20 inches (45 to 50 cm) above stoma (see illustration).	This position prevents too high a pressure and reduces possibility of bowel damage.
5. Remove used pouch by gently pushing skin from adhesive and barrier; properly dispose of used pouch (save clamp, if attached to pouch) and remove gloves and wash hands.	Prevents skin irritation; controls odor in room.
6. Apply irrigation sleeve over stoma; tip of sleeve should rest in water in toilet or in bedpan (see illustration).	Directs flow of stool into toilet or bedpan; if in toilet, also controls odor and splashing.
7. Apply gloves, lubricate cone tip, reach through top of irrigation sleeve, and hold cone tip snugly against stomal opening (see illustration *A*). *Do not* force cone into stoma or try to put entire cone into stoma. Start inflow of solution. Adjust direction of cone to facilitate inflow of solution. Illustration *B* shows client performing self-irrigation; gloves are not required for client.	Prevents trauma to stoma; cone tip avoids perforation of bowel. Cone aids in retaining solution during inflow. Aiming flow of solution toward direction of bowel aids inflow.

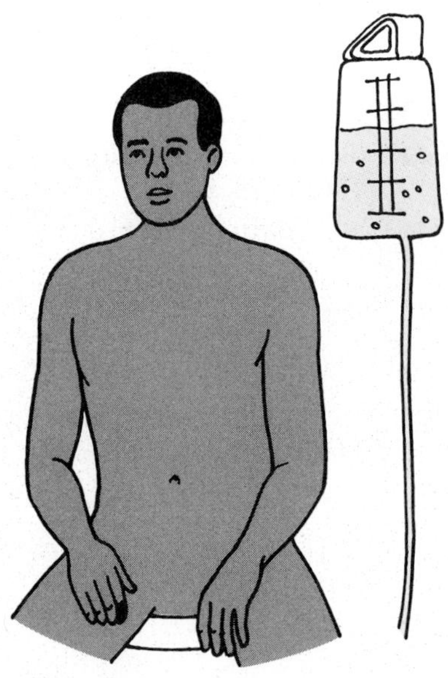

STEP **4** Position of irrigation bag.

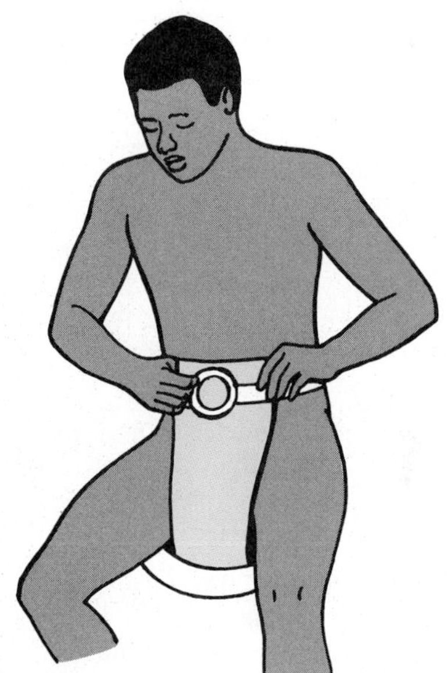

STEP **6** Irrigation sleeve applied over stoma.

A

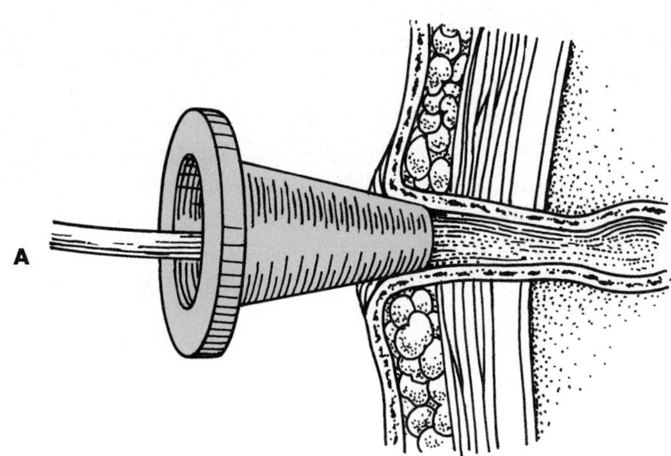

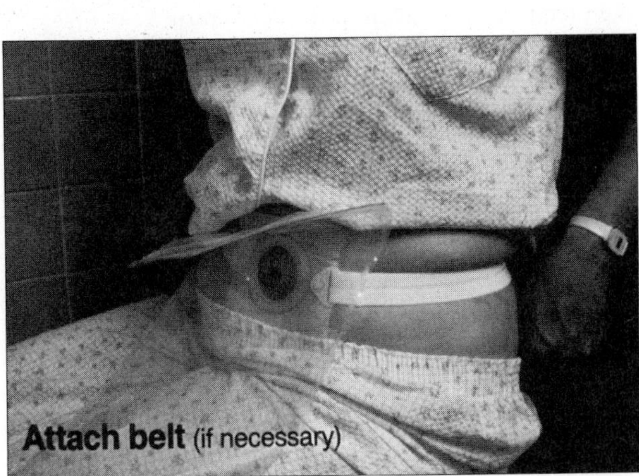

B

STEP **7** **A,** Irrigation cone against stoma opening. **B,** Ostomy irrigation. (**B** courtesy ConvaTec, Princeton, NJ.)

STEP	RATIONALE

- ***Critical Decision Point***

  Only use a cone tip to do irrigations. Do not *use a tube without a cone tip. It carries a higher risk for perforation of colon.*

Step	Rationale
8. Allow solution to flow in over 5- to 10-minute period.	Avoids rapid distention of bowel; if cramping or nausea occurs, stop the inflow of solution until either subsides; have client take a few slow, deep breaths.
9. After desired amount of solution has entered colon, clamp tubing, and remove cone. Discard gloves. Close top of irrigation sleeve.	Avoids sudden backflow of solution from stoma.
10. Allow 15 to 20 minutes for initial evacuation; apply gloves. Dry tip of irrigation sleeve, and close bottom (use ostomy pouch clamp or rubber band). Fold sleeve up and over top as per manufacturer's specific directions for each brand of irrigation sleeve; leave in place for 30 to 45 minutes. Discard gloves. Client may walk around.	Prevents leakage; optimizes evacuation of stool. Entire procedure should take approximately 1 hour. Assists in evacuation of stool.
11. Apply gloves; unclamp sleeve, empty any fecal contents; remove sleeve. Rinse with liquid cleanser and cool water. Hang sleeve to dry.	Maintains sleeve in clean condition for future use.

- ***Critical Decision Point***

  Most irrigation sleeves are meant to be reused. Do not throw out reusable irrigation sleeves after each use. This is very costly.

Step	Rationale
12. Apply new colostomy pouch or stoma cap covering per procedure (see Skill 26-1).	Avoids soiling of clothes or skin irritation from accidental leakage.
13. Remove gloves and wash hands.	Reduces transmission of microorganisms.

EVALUATION

Step	Rationale
1. Inspect volume and character of fecal material and fluid that return after irrigation.	Determines if solution is retained. If client is dehydrated, bowel may absorb irrigation solution and fecal output will be limited or nil. Character and amount of stool reveal success in evacuation.
2. Note client's response during irrigation. Assess client's radial pulse. Ask if cramping or abdominal pain is felt.	Reveals tolerance of irrigation.
3. Ask client to describe steps of procedure.	Evaluates client's learning.

UNEXPECTED OUTCOMES AND RELATED INTERVENTIONS

- Client retained all of solution with no return.
  - Decrease rate of fluid instillation.
  - Determine that solution is not too cold.
  - Determine that client is not dehydrated.
- Client experiences pain during insertion and during or after administration.
  - Assess abdomen for hardness, tenderness, and bowel sounds.
  - Assess any output through ostomy for small amount of blood. Pulse may be weak, and rate may change from baseline.
- Client experiences diarrhea or spillage between irrigation.
  - Assess for medication interaction.
  - Modify client's diet to include roughage.
  - Consult with ET/WOCN nurse.
- Client is unable to explain or perform procedure.
  - Provide additional client education.

RECORDING AND REPORTING

- Record procedure, time of irrigation, volume, and type of solution, amount and type of return, and client's tolerance.
- Record reapplication of skin barrier and pouch and condition of stoma and skin.
- Report symptoms of extreme discomfort, onset of severe diarrhea, poor results, or excessive bleeding to nurse in charge or physician.

TEACHING CONSIDERATIONS

- Client should be instructed in community resources such as ostomy groups, home health agencies, and suppliers.
- Clients should be given a teaching manual with steps clearly stated, or audiotaped instructions.
- Tell clients if they travel in a foreign country that if they cannot drink the water, they should not irrigate with it.

PEDIATRIC CONSIDERATIONS

- Irrigations to regulate bowel movements are not usually done for pediatric clients.
- Sometimes irrigations of the distal ostomy limb are done for clean-out purposes for pediatric clients with Hirschsprung's disease.
- Amount of irrigation solution used differs from amount used for adults. Physician orders the amounts of irrigation solution to use, usually based on pediatric client's weight and size.
- See also Pediatric Considerations for Skill 26-1.

GERONTOLOGICAL CONSIDERATIONS

- Assess client's willingness to do ostomy self-irrigations. This takes a time commitment to be able to perform the skill correctly.
- Assess client's physical ability to do ostomy self-irrigations. Motor and/or visual limitations may make it difficult but not impossible for client to do procedure. Some adaptations in irrigation technique may need to be made to enable older clients with motor and/or visual limitations to successfully do self-irrigation.
- Some older adults become upset if they do not have a daily bowel movement. With some irrigation routines, irrigation is not done daily; therefore the client will not have a daily bowel movement. Client needs to understand and accept this.
- See also Gerontological Considerations for Skill 26-1.

HOME CARE CONSIDERATIONS

- Assess home environment for bathroom privacy for ostomy care.
- Establish scheduled time (approximately 1 hour) for uninterrupted ostomy care.
- Irrigation sleeve may be attached by a belt, stick on, or by snapping directly onto the flange of the skin barrier. For home care, two-piece system is easier to use and more cost-effective; it allows client to remove pouch from flange and then attach irrigation sleeve, then snap on a clean pouch or stoma cap when evacuation is completed.
- See also Home Care Considerations for Skill 26-1.

Skill 26-3 Pouching a Noncontinent Urinary Diversion

Because urine flows continuously from a noncontinent urinary diversion, a urinary pouch is usually placed over the opening immediately after surgery. Placement of the pouch may be more challenging than the enterostomy because urine flow keeps the skin moist and in the immediate postoperative period urinary **stents** may be in place in the stoma.

The stoma of a urinary diversion is normally red or pink. It is made from a portion of the gastrointestinal tract, either the ileum or the colon, and has the same mucosal surface. Ideally the stoma should protrude ½ to ¾ inch above the skin. An ileal conduit is usually located in the right lower quadrant; a **colon conduit** is usually located in the left lower quadrant. Ureterostomies are usually performed in infants, and a conduit is performed when the child approaches school age (see Figure 26-2).

DELEGATION CONSIDERATIONS

The skill of pouching a noncontinent urinary diversion should not be delegated to assistive personnel. Care of an established noncontinent urinary diversion can be delegated. The care provider must be informed about the baseline assessment findings of the client's ostomy and when to report changes. In addition, the care provider must also be informed about expected output.

EQUIPMENT

- Pouch, urinary (with antireflex flap) and skin barrier (Figure 26-6)

  NOTE: Use two-piece system (pouch and flange) if stents are present (Figure 26-7); use measuring guide to measure the stoma to determine the correct size of pouch and skin barrier.
- Bedside urinary drainage bag
- Clean nonsterile disposable gloves (sterile gloves optional)
- Hand-held hair dryer
- Sterile gauze pads
- Towel or disposable waterproof barrier
- Basin with warm tap water
- Scissors
- Skin-sealant wipes
- Sterile forceps (if stents present)
- Vinegar

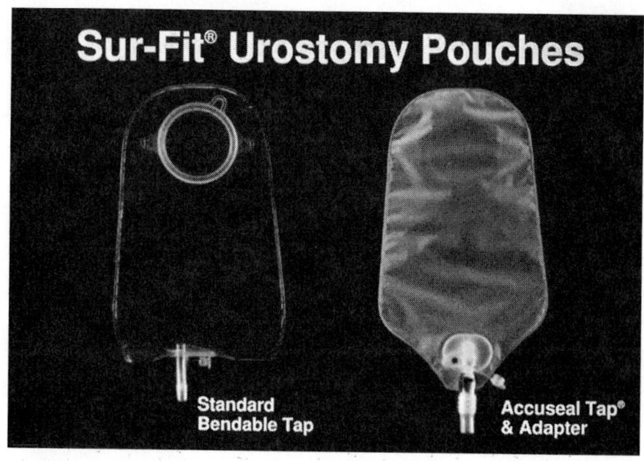

FIGURE **26-6** Types of pouches. (Courtesy ConvaTec, Princeton, NJ.)

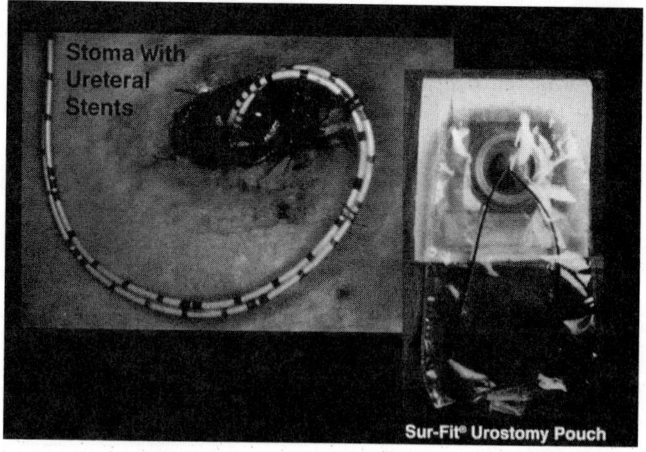

FIGURE **26-7** Stoma with stents present viable, matured transverse loop colostomy and normal peristomal skin and pouch. (Courtesy Hollister, Inc, Libertyville, Ill.)

STEP	RATIONALE
ASSESSMENT	
1. Check pouch for leakage; length of time in place; ask client about skin tenderness or discomfort. Check stoma for color, healing. Check abdominal incision (if present) for relationship to stoma for proper placement of pouch. To prevent skin irritation, one-piece pouch or skin barrier from two-piece system should be changed, if not leaking, every 3 to 7 days, or when checking for skin irritation. Stoma should be moist and reddish pink; immediately after surgery it is edematous and usually has urinary stents in place (see illustration).	Pouches should be emptied when one-third to one-half full because weight of urine in pouch may weaken or dislodge skin seal.

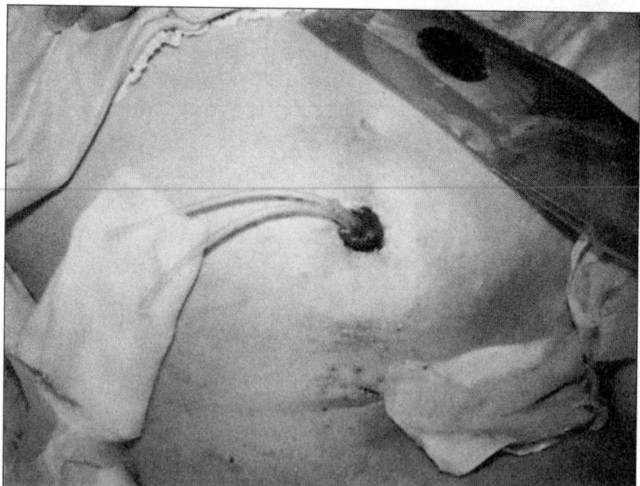

STEP **1** Urinary stoma with stents. (From Broadwell DC, Jackson BL: *Principles of ostomy care,* St. Louis, 1982, Mosby.)

STEP	RATIONALE
2. Observe output from stoma. Immediately after surgery, ureteral stents are in place and remain for up to 10 to 14 days. The physician then removes the stents.	Urinary output must be monitored on all postoperative clients with urinary diversions to monitor renal status and patency of stents; output should never be less than 30 ml/hr. Stents are used to maintain patency of ureters at **anastomotic** sites. These stents are sutured in place with dissolvable sutures.
3. Assess abdomen for best type of pouch to use. After pouch is off, assess skin around stoma, observing scars, folds, skin breakdown; also check peristomal suture line if present.	Maximizes secure fit and minimizes chance of leakage. Pouch and skin barrier are changed with any leakage. Determines need for barrier paste and additional intervention.

STEP	RATIONALE
4. Determine client's emotional response, knowledge, and understanding of ostomy. Determine client's family and other significant support.	Helps determine extent client is able to participate in care, and need for teaching. Helps anticipate discharge needs.

NURSING DIAGNOSIS

Defining characteristics from the assessment data may reveal the following nursing diagnoses for clients requiring this skill:

Disturbed body image
Risk for impaired skin integrity
Deficient knowledge regarding ostomy self-care

Related factors are individualized based on client's condition or needs.

PLANNING

STEP	RATIONALE
1. **Expected outcomes** following completion of procedure:	
▪ Stoma is moist, reddish pink, oozes blood only slightly if rubbed. Peristomal skin is free of irritation and is intact. Sutures are intact, and incision is well approximated.	Normal findings for postoperative urinary diversion.
▪ Urine drains freely from stents or stoma. Urine is yellowish with mucous shreds and is without foul odor. Volume of output is within acceptable limits (30 ml/hr).	These are normal findings in postoperative phase. The mucosal surface of the stoma is easily traumatized. Mucous shreds are normal when bowel is used as urinary diversion. Urine should flow freely if unobstructed.
▪ Client denies discomfort.	Reflects ongoing healing without complications.
▪ Client, family member, or significant other is willing to view stoma and asks questions about procedural steps.	Shows adjustment to body image change and willingness to learn self-care.
2. Assemble equipment.	Optimizes use of time; conserves client's and nurse's energy.
3. Close room curtains or door.	Provides privacy.
4. Explain procedure to client; encourage client's participation and questions.	Lessens anxiety and promotes client's participation.

IMPLEMENTATION

STEP	RATIONALE
1. Position client standing or supine and drape. Some clients may prefer to do pouch change while sitting because this may make it easier for them to see stoma. However, when skin barrier and pouch are applied in sitting position, skin may have folds and and wrinkles. Because of this, skin barriers and pouches applied with client in sitting position may leak.	When client is supine, fewer wrinkles occur, allowing for ease of pouch application; maintains client's dignity.
2. Prepare pouch by removing backing from barrier and adhesive; if using cut-to-fit, cut opening $\frac{1}{16}$ to $\frac{1}{8}$ inch larger than stoma before removing backing. Some urinary pouches have special skin barrier that melts and forms secure seal around base of stoma. This is referred as a "turtle neck" effect and will not harm stoma.	Barrier facilitates seal and protects skin; size of opening keeps urine off skin and lessens risk of maceration with skin irritation; avoids risk of damage to stoma. Stoma shrinks and does not reach optimal size for 6 to 8 weeks. Pouch and skin barrier is changed whenever leaking. Change when client is comfortable; better time is in morning on arising because urinary output is reduced.
3. Wash hands and apply gloves.	Reduces transmission of microorganisms.

Step	Rationale
4. Place towel or disposable waterproof barrier under client. Tightly roll several gauze pads separately (should resemble tampon). (*Option:* If gauze pads [called "wicks"] come in contact with stents, roll with sterile gloves on. Place wicks on sterile barrier [can use inside of gauze wrapper].)	Protects bed linen. Rolled gauze pads used to absorb urine during pouch change.
5. Remove used pouch carefully and gently by pushing skin away from barrier. If stents are present, *do not pull on them.* Immediately place a wick or sterile gauze pad over stomal opening. If stents are present, place sterile gauze pad underneath tips.	Reduces risk of trauma to skin and risk of injury to ureters if stents are present; jerking irritates skin and can cause skin tears. Keeps urine from leaking onto skin. Immediately after surgery copious mucus exists over stoma since bowel has not adjusted to presence of urine.
6. Cleanse peristomal skin gently with warm tap water using gauze pads; do not scrub skin.	Avoid soap. It leaves residue on skin, which interferes with pouch adhesion. Pouch does not adhere to wet skin. Stents are sutured in place to decrease risk of damage. If blood appears on gauze pad used to cleanse skin, do not be alarmed because stomal surface may ooze blood if rubbed. Bleeding into pouch is abnormal. Doing a vinegar soak removes uric acid crystals that may be deposited on peristomal skin.

• ***Critical Decision Point***

If uric acid crystals are present on skin, apply washcloth with a vinegar soak (one-third vinegar and two-thirds warm water) to peristomal skin. Rinse with warm tap water, and dry completely by patting skin with dry gauze or towel. Can use hand-held dryer set on cool. If copious mucus is on surface of stoma, carefully remove while stabilizing stents with sterile forceps.

Step	Rationale
7. Wick stoma continuously during pouch measurement and change. Place tip of gauze at stomal opening. Measure stoma.	Using a wick at stoma tip prevents peristomal skin from becoming wet with urine during pouching-change procedure.
a. If creases form next to stoma, use barrier paste or seal to fill in; let dry 1 to 2 minutes.	Flattening of creases with paste or seal creates smooth surface for pouch placement.

• ***Critical Decision Point***

For some clients, a pouch system with convexity may be needed.

Step	Rationale
b. Apply skin sealant in circular area around base of stoma to any skin not protected by barrier; let dry. Hold pouch by barrier, center over stoma and stents, and press down gently on barrier. Bottom of pouch should be angled slightly to attach to bedside urinary drainage bag. Use another skin sealant on skin coming in contact with adhesive; allow to dry. Press adhesive backing smoothly against skin starting from the bottom and working up and around sides. Never use a karaya skin barrier with a urinary diversion.	Urine renders karaya in skin barrier ineffective and results in leakage.

STEP	RATIONALE
c. Maintain gentle finger pressure around barrier for 1 to 2 minutes.	Helps to ensure molding and adherence of skin barrier.
d. If using two-piece pouch, apply flange (barrier with adhesive) as above, then snap on pouch. If the client is mostly out of bed and ambulatory, apply pouch vertically.	Urine drains almost continuously. Flange waterproofs any skin that may contact urine. Creates wrinkle-free secure seal. Angling pouch avoids uneven twisting, which can disrupt seal. Prevents trauma to skin.
8. During the night, open drain spout, attach specific manufacturer adapter piece to end of pouch, and then attach this to bedside urinary bag. Place bag at a point close to foot of bed.	Constant flow of urine results in frequent emptying; overfilling of pouch may break skin seal. Placing bag at foot of bed maximizes straight drainage that avoids urine accumulation in pouch.

- ***Critical Decision Point***
  Know the specific urinary equipment that is being used. Many urinary pouches need an adapter piece that is specific to their brand to attach urinary pouch to bedside urinary drainage bag. Even within some manufacturers, adapter piece varies with different types of urinary pouches available.

STEP	RATIONALE
9. Properly dispose of used pouch and soiled equipment.	Avoids odor in room.

- ***Critical Decision Point***
  Do not throw used pouch and skin barrier into toilet. Most pouching equipment clogs toilet.

STEP	RATIONALE
10. Remove gloves; wash hands.	Reduces transmission of microorganisms.
11. Change skin barrier and pouch every 3 to 7 days unless leaking; pouch can remain in place for tub bath or shower; after bath pat adhesive dry or use hand-held dryer on cool.	Avoids unnecessary trauma to skin from too-frequent changes. Drying ensures adhesion of pouch.

EVALUATION

STEP	RATIONALE
1. Observe appearance of stoma, peristomal skin, and suture line during pouch change.	Determines condition of stoma and peristomal skin and progress of wound healing.
2. Evaluate character and volume of urinary drainage.	Determines if stoma or stents are patent. Character of urine can reveal degree of concentration and alterations in renal function.

- ***Critical Decision Point***
  Mucus is a normal finding in urine from an ileal conduit or colon conduit. Other sediment in urine needs to be evaluated.

STEP	RATIONALE
3. Ask if client notes discomfort around stoma.	Evaluates presence of skin irritation.
4. Observe client's, family member's, or significant other's willingness to view stoma and ask questions about procedure.	Determines level of adjustment and understanding of stoma care and pouch application.

Unexpected Outcomes and Related Interventions

- Peristomal skin is irritated, reddened, tender, or has overgrowth.
  - Keep peristomal skin dry.
  - Determine if client has an allergy to barrier and adhesive or infection.
  - Remeasure stoma and opening of pouch.
  - Culture any drainage.
- No urinary output for several hours or output is less than 30 ml/hr. Urine has foul odor.
  - Determine patency of stents or stoma.
  - Obtain urine specimen for culture and sensitivity to test for possible infection (Chapter 41).
  - Notify physician.
- Client reports burning sensation around base of stoma.
  - Assess for presence of yeast infection around stoma which causes itching, burning; appears as reddened area with **maculopapular** rash.
  - Notify physician.
  - Apply medicated cream if ordered.
- Client, family member, or significant other is unable to observe stoma, ask questions, or participate in care.
  - Adjustment takes time, and process of grieving is individualized.
  - Further client education may be needed.

Recording and Reporting

- Record type of pouch, time of change, condition and appearance of stoma and peristomal skin, and character of urine.
- Record urinary output.
- Document client's, family's, or significant other's reaction to stoma, and level of participation. Some clients may have sexual dysfunction as a result of surgical exploration in perineal area.
- Report abnormalities in stoma or peristomal structures and absence of urinary output to nurse in charge or physician.

Teaching Considerations

- Use opportunity to teach whenever doing pouch change even if client does not appear interested. *Do not* force client to look at stoma; allow time for adjustment.
- Teach clients significance and importance of drinking at least 2 qt of water daily and of keeping urine acidic through intake of acid ash foods such as cranberry juice, cereals, and poultry. Clients need to check this with physician (Walsh, 1992).
- Teach clients that some mucus in urine is expected, but they should report any blood in their urine, excessively cloudy urine, chills, fever, and back pain to their physician.
- Client should be given a teaching manual with steps clearly stated, or audiotaped instruction.
- Clients should be given a list of equipment and name, address, and phone number of a supplier in their community.

Pediatric Considerations

- In neonates, urinary diversions are less common than fecal ostomies (Boarini, 1989).
- The type of **urostomy** done in neonates is usually an ureterostomy. Because these stomas are very tiny, are flush to the skin, and are often in skin creases in the flank area, they are *very* difficult to pouch and maintain a good intact seal with skin barrier and pouch. Sometimes parents may decide not to use an ostomy pouching system. Because urine is less erosive to the skin than fecal effluent, some parents can opt to use diapers with good skin care to manage their baby's urostomy (Boarini, 1989).

Gerontological Considerations

- Some older clients feel that they can cope with continuous flow of urine from stoma by decreasing amount of fluid they drink so they will have less output. This can be very dangerous to client's health. Client needs appropriate teaching to change this misconception.
- Limitations in physical and visual ability may require adjustments in self-ostomy routine.

Home Care Considerations

- At home, pouch spout should be opened and connected to straight drainage at night. Make sure client understands that using wrong adapter piece causes leakage.
- Many different types of pouching systems are available. Some are one-piece and others two-piece. All disposable pouches are odor-proof, and most have an antireflux valve. Clients should be encouraged to find a pouch that they can apply easily and that satisfies them.
- Clients should avoid placing pouches in extremely hot or cold locations since temperature may affect barrier and adhesive materials.
- Advise clients when they travel to always keep spare ostomy supplies with them in case luggage gets lost.
- While swimming, clients may find that applying waterproof tape to skin barrier and/or wearing an ostomy belt prevents pouch and skin barrier from becoming dislodged.
- See also Home Care Considerations given for Skill 26-2.

Skill 26-4 Catheterizing a Noncontinent Urinary Diversion

Catheterization is performed to screen for infection and is the only way to obtain an accurate culture and sensitivity specimen (Chapter 41). When necessary to obtain a specimen from a urinary diversion, the best method is to insert a sterile double-tip catheter into the stoma. Obtaining a specimen from the pouch does not provide an accurate finding.

With the use of strict aseptic technique, catheterization is relatively safe and easy. To prevent trauma of tissues, the nurse should understand how the stoma and ureteral tract are constructed.

Reflux of urine can cause infection. Incorrect pouch placement, the use of a urinary pouch without an antireflux valve, stagnant urine, or large volumes of urine promote reflux. The risk for reflux of urine into the ureter can be reduced by attaching straight drainage to the urinary pouch during sleep or when high urinary output is expected. A client must understand the importance of draining the pouch frequently and using clean technique during stomal and skin care.

Delegation Considerations

This skill should not be delegated to assistive personnel.

Equipment

Urinary catheterization supplies (may be contained in prepackaged sterile catheter kit or may need to be gathered separately). All items must be sterile.

- 14 to 16 Fr red rubber catheter (most use a double-tip catheter)
- Water-soluble lubricant
- Povidone-iodine swabs
- Sterile disposable gloves
- Sterile specimen container
- Gauze pads
- Bed protection barrier
- Towels
- Urinary diversion pouch (if client is using one-piece system; if using two-piece system, pouch can be snapped off for procedure)
- Nonsterile disposable gloves

Step	Rationale
Assessment	
1. Determine need to perform catheterization to obtain a sterile specimen from urinary diversion; note signs and symptoms of urinary tract infection (UTI) such as elevated temperature, chills, foul-smelling urine, elevated white blood cell (WBC) count.	Urinary diversion may pose risk for reflux of urine back to kidneys, resulting in infection.
2. Obtain physician's order for catheterization.	Invasive procedure requires physician's order.
3. Assess client's understanding of need for procedure and how procedure is done.	Determines willingness to cooperate and indicates extent of explanation nurse should provide.

Nursing Diagnosis

Defining characteristics from the assessment data may reveal the following nursing diagnoses for clients requiring this skill:

Risk for infection

Deficient knowledge regarding urinary diversion catheterization

Related factors are individualized based on client's condition or needs.

Planning

Step	Rationale
1. **Expected outcomes** following completion of procedure:	
▪ No bacteria are present in urine.	No infection is present.
▪ Skin and stoma are intact, without signs of irritation.	Urinary pouch is intact.
▪ Client describes risks of infection and techniques to prevent infection.	Demonstrates client's learning.

Step	Rationale
2. Assemble equipment.	Optimizes use of time; conserves client's and nurse's energy.
3. Close room curtains or door.	Provides privacy.
4. Explain procedure to client; if possible, attempt to obtain specimen when client is due to change pouch if using one-piece system.	Lessens anxiety and promotes client's cooperation. Changing pouch too frequently can result in skin breakdown.

Implementation

Step	Rationale
1. Position client sitting, if possible, and drape towel across pelvic area.	Gravity facilitates flow of urine. Maintains client's dignity. Towel absorbs urine.
2. Wash hands and open barrier. Prepare several gauze wicks and place on edge of barrier. Apply nonsterile gloves.	Reduces transmission of microorganisms; wicks absorb urine from stomal opening.
3. Remove used pouch according to Skill 26-3, Implementation, Steps 5 through 9.	Protects skin from trauma.
4. Remove and discard gloves. Open sterile catheterization set according to instructions, or open needed equipment and place on sterile barrier. If not using catheterization kit, place gauze pad on sterile field and squeeze small amount of lubricant onto gauze. If possible, have client wick stoma while waiting by placing a sterile gauze over stoma.	Avoids contamination.
5. Apply sterile gloves. Cleanse "face" of stoma with povidone-iodine swabs using circular motion from center outward. Using new swab each time, repeat twice.	Removes surface bacteria.
6. Allow some urine to flow out of stoma.	Flushes povidone-iodine off face of stoma. Iodine in specimen alters results.
7. Lubricate catheter with water-soluble lubricant.	Lubricant facilitates passage of catheter through stoma.
8. Remove lid from specimen container. Place distal end of catheter into specimen container. Hold catheter in container with nondominant hand.	Only a few drops of urine are obtained; care should be used to direct all into container.
9. With dominant hand, gently insert catheter 2 to 2½ inches (5 to 6.5 cm) into stoma. If using a double-tip catheter, insert the catheter into the stoma first, then gently advance the inner catheter. Do not force catheter, redirect course as needed. Use gentle but firm pressure similar to regular catheterization of urethra. Have client cough or turn slightly to facilitate passage of catheter.	Care must be taken to avoid perforation. Some resistance is common at muscle level in conduit. Allow catheter to enter slowly. May relax abdominal muscles.
10. Maintain container below level of stoma. Have client cough as needed. Urine may flow around and through catheter. This is acceptable, but only urine from catheter is desired. Normally, wait 5 minutes; if no urine is in container, pinch catheter and remove; direct urine "trapped" in catheter into cup.	Facilitates drainage of urine. Only 3 to 5 ml of urine is needed for culture and sensitivity studies.
11. After withdrawing catheter, place gauze pad over stoma.	Keeps skin dry.
12. Apply lid to specimen container. Remove gloves, and label specimen with required information.	Prevents accidental spillage. Labeling ensures acceptance of specimen by laboratory and processing.
13. Reapply new pouch.	Pouch is necessary to contain urine; proper technique is important to avoid skin and stoma irritation.
14. Remove used pouch and equipment and dispose of properly.	Avoids unpleasant odor in room and eliminates source of bacterial colonization.
15. Wash hands, and send specimen to laboratory at once.	Avoids transmission of infection. Allowing urine to sit for long periods at room temperature affects laboratory results.

STEP	RATIONALE
EVALUATION	
1. Refer to laboratory report, and compare results of culture and sensitivity with normal expected findings. Remember that mucus is a normal finding in the urine of a client with an ileal or colon conduit.	Determines presence of infection. If contamination appears likely, second specimen will need to be sent.
2. Observe stoma and peristomal area for skin breakdown.	Exposure of skin to urine increases the risk of skin breakdown.
3. Check that urinary pouch and skin barrier are intact with no leakage.	A properly applied pouch and skin barrier that are the correct size minimize chance of leakage.
4. Ask client about signs and symptoms of UTI.	

UNEXPECTED OUTCOMES AND RELATED INTERVENTIONS

- Culture reveals evidence of bacteria in urine.
  - Notify physician.
  - Initiate prescribed medications.
  - Encourage fluids.
- Skin or stoma reveals complications.
  - Provide additional skin care.
  - Culture any drainage.
- Client is unable to describe risks of infection.
  - Provide increased client education.

RECORDING AND REPORTING

- Record time specimen collected, client's tolerance of procedure, and appearance of urine, skin, and stoma.
- Report results of laboratory test to nurse in charge or physician.

TEACHING CONSIDERATIONS

- Explain common symptoms of UTI: flank pain, dark or bloody urine, foul-smelling urine, fever, nausea.
- Encourage client to maintain fluid intake, and notify physician if symptoms of infection develop.
- Instruct client or primary caregiver about clean technique during pouch application.
- Reinforce importance of fluid intake (2 L/day).

Skill 26-5 Maintaining a Continent Diversion

Continent diversions can be done to contain either urine or stool. These newer surgical procedures provide clients with the option of having an ostomy that does not spontaneously drain effluent, but rather must be drained from the internal pouch by the client. Figure 26-8 shows an example of an internal pouch created for a continent stool diversion. A more detailed description of the surgical procedure done to create an internal pouch for stool diversions can be found in the article by Hull and Erwin-Toth (1996). The pouch is emptied when the client inserts a catheter or tube into the external stoma to drain the stool. Because the ostomy is continent, the client does not have to wear an external ostomy pouch over the external stoma.

A continent urinary diversion is a reservoir or pouch that collects urine. Urine is evacuated only when a catheter is inserted into the stoma to empty the urine. This is unlike a conventional urinary diversion such as an ileal conduit, which serves only as a passageway for urine to flow to the outside of the abdomen. Many techniques are available for construction of a continent urinary diversion using various portions of the small and/or large bowel (see Figure 26-2). Depending on the surgical technique used, the continent urinary diversion may be a Kock pouch, an Indiana continent urinary diversion, or some other type (Atta, 1991).

Because this reservoir is continent, the client does not have to wear an external pouch. The reservoir is intubated (or catheterized) at scheduled times to drain urine, and it must be irrigated. The opening (called a stoma) into the reservoir generally is placed in the right lower quadrant of the abdomen below where an ileal conduit would be. The stoma is flush with the skin or slightly budded and is reddish pink. Skinfolds and creases do not present the same type of problem as they would with an ileal conduit (Cavas and Makay, 1991).

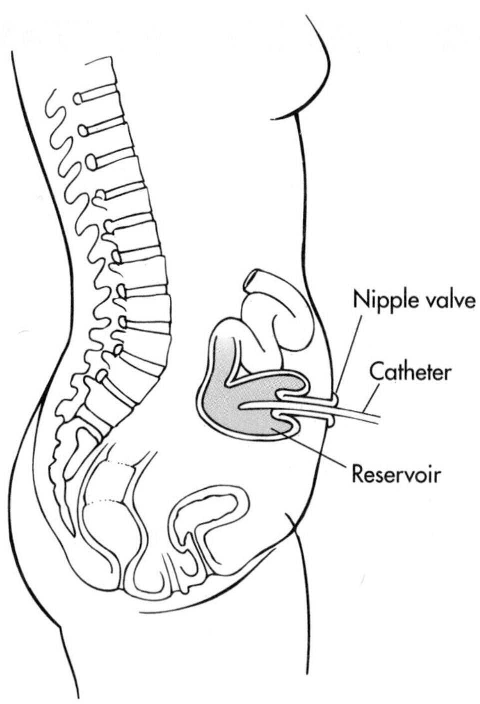

FIGURE **26-8** A catheter is inserted and secured in the pouch before conclusion of the operation. (Modified from Hull TL, Erwin-Toth P: The pelvic pouch procedure and continent ostomies: overview and controversies, *J Wound Ostomy Continence Nurs* 23(3):156, 1996.)

DELEGATION CONSIDERATIONS

The skill of maintaining a continent diversion should not be delegated to assistive personnel.

EQUIPMENT

Varies with recovery phase.

Postoperative Care to 3 Weeks

- Sterile normal saline (NS)
- Sterile catheter tip irrigating syringe
- Sterile gauze pads
- Sterile gloves
- Povidone-iodine swabs
- Sterile specimen cup
- Sterile water
- Towels

Postoperative Care 4 to 6 Weeks

- Sterile NS
- Sterile catheter tip irrigating syringe
- Sterile gauze pads
- Sterile gloves
- Povidone-iodine swabs
- Sterile basin
- Sterile 14 to 16 Fr red rubber catheter
- Water-soluble lubricant
- Stoma cover (commercial or adhesive strip or nonstick dressing)
- Liquid antimicrobial soap
- Towels

STEP	RATIONALE
ASSESSMENT	
1. Observe all tubes for intactness and patency, nature of drainage, and connection to appropriate collection system. Label all collecting bags with origin of urine or drainage contained in them. Keep intake and output record.	Clients return immediately after surgery with a catheter in stoma. Avoids errors in input and output record. Minimal acceptable urine output is 30 ml/hr from all sources.

- ***Critical Decision Point***
  If client had a continent urinary diversion, then ureteral stents that exit through stoma or another site on abdomen will also be present; stents are connected to a separate drainage system. Usually another large tube (e.g., a cecostomy) is placed into pouch for extra drainage.

STEP	RATIONALE
2. Observe stoma for color, peristomal skin for maceration, and condition of all external suture lines.	Determines potential circulatory problems and reflects healing progress.
3. Assess bowel sounds and lung sounds. Assess serum values of chloride and creatinine.	Manipulation of large portions of bowel may lead to an ileus. Underventilation by client after surgery may lead to respiratory complications. Immediately after surgery, intestinal segment used for reservoir may absorb chloride and hydrogen ions. Creatinine measures effectiveness of kidney function (Golomb, Klutke, and Raz, 1989).
4. Palpate lightly around stoma, noting any localized tenderness or guarding.	May be sign of infection along internal suture lines.
5. Determine client's emotional response, knowledge, and understanding of continent reservoir or pouch; determine family and other significant support.	Helps determine extent client is able to participate in care, and need for teaching. Assists in anticipating discharge needs.

NURSING DIAGNOSIS

Defining characteristics from the assessment data may reveal the following nursing diagnoses for clients requiring this skill:

- Impaired elimination (either urinary or bowel)
- Disturbed body image
- Risk for impaired skin integrity
- Deficient knowledge regarding ostomy self-care

Related factors are individualized based on client's condition or needs.

PLANNING

STEP	RATIONALE
1. **Expected outcomes** following completion of procedure:	
▪ Stoma is moist, reddish pink, and oozes blood only slightly if rubbed. Peristomal skin is free of irritation and intact. Sutures are intact, and incision is well approximated. Client denies discomfort.	These are normal findings in postoperative phase. Reflects ongoing healing without complications.
▪ Effluent is normal depending on type of continent diversion:	
• Urine drains freely from stents, stomal catheter, or **intubation** catheter. Urine is yellowish with mucous shreds and is without foul odor. Volume of output is within acceptable limits.	Mucous shreds are normal when bowel is used as reservoir. Urine should flow freely if unobstructed.
• Stool is brown, may be semiformed.	
▪ Client has no pain at stoma or peristomal skin.	Pain might be an indicator of infection.
▪ Client, family member, or significant other is willing to view stoma and asks questions about procedural steps.	Shows adjustment to body image change and willingness to learn self-care.
▪ Client is able to intubate and irrigate pouch before discharge.	Reflects comprehensive teaching. Continent diversion requires a knowledgeable client to maintain optimal functioning. If unable to care for self, client is at risk for complications.
2. Assemble equipment.	Optimizes use of time; conserves client's and nurse's energy.
3. Close room curtains or door.	Provides privacy.
4. Explain procedure to client; encourage client's interaction and questions.	Lessens anxiety and promotes client's participation.

IMPLEMENTATION

Postoperative Care to 3 Weeks

STEP	RATIONALE
1. Position client supine or sitting, and drape with towels.	Facilitates instilling NS into reservoir; sitting is a better position for drainage. Maintains client's dignity.

Step	Rationale
2. Wash hands and open sterile equipment. Remove lid from sterile specimen cup, and place lid with open side up. Pour 20 to 30 ml sterile NS into sterile specimen cup. Open sterile syringe and povidone-iodine swabs and position them for use.	Reduces transmission of microorganisms.
3. Put on sterile gloves, and draw 20 to 30 ml sterile NS into syringe. Cleanse connection point of indwelling stomal catheter and drainage tubing with povidone-iodine swabs using a circular motion; use each swab once; wait 30 seconds.	Reduces risk of **nosocomial infection.**
4. Disconnect catheter and tubing and gently irrigate stomal catheter by infusing saline; do not contaminate tip of drainage tubing.	Large numbers of internal anastomotic sites require strict asepsis during postoperative phase.

- ***Critical Decision Point***

  Do not aspirate because this increases risk of damage to internal suture lines. Irrigation maintains patency of stomal catheter because large amount of mucus is secreted initially by reservoir (Davidson and others, 1990).

Step	Rationale
5. Reconnect drainage system. Record volume used for irrigation. For urinary diversions, subtract this from total urine output at end of each shift. Follow agency protocol for changing bedside urinary drainage bags.	Keeps accurate urinary output record. Reduces risk of colonization of microorganisms.
6. Using remaining povidone-iodine swabs, cleanse "face" of stoma around catheter. Use another swab, and cleanse skin around base of stoma; allow to dry 30 seconds and gently remove iodine with a gauze pad moistened with sterile water.	Mucus accumulates on face of stoma and seeps onto skin. Maintains skin integrity and reduces risk of infection. Some clients are allergic to iodine.
7. Discard soiled equipment; remove gloves. Maintain sterile specimen cup and sterile NS and water containers for next irrigation. Label these with date, time, and nurse's initials. NOTE: Hospital protocols vary; generally, immediately after surgery continent diversions are irrigated every 2 to 4 hours to maintain patency of stomal catheter, allowing urine to drain freely.	Reduces transmission of microorganisms. Maintains sterility of cup so it can be used for 8 hours; helps reduce costs. Some supplies can stay at bedside for 8 hours if strict aseptic technique is followed; this helps contain costs.

Postoperative Care 4 to 6 Weeks

Step	Rationale
1. Follow steps 1 and 2 in preceding section. Omit setting up sterile specimen cup.	Generally stomal catheter is removed the third postoperative week.
2. Open sterile basin, and maintain inside of wrapper as sterile field. Pour 30 to 60 ml of sterile NS into basin. Open gauze pads onto sterile wrapper; squeeze small amount of water-soluble lubricant onto gauze pad. Open wrapper of sterile red catheter for use, or place catheter onto sterile basin wrapper.	Maintains strict aseptic technique to reduce risk of nosocomial infection during recovery phase.
3. Apply sterile gloves, and draw 30 to 60 ml of sterile NS into syringe. Cleanse "face" of stoma with povidone-iodine swab starting from center and using circular movements to outer edge; wait 30 seconds.	Reduces risk of nosocomial infection; removes any accumulation of mucus.
4. Lubricate tip of catheter well. Insert into stoma by gently rotating during insertion; insert until urine starts to drain.	Reduces trauma to continence mechanism (valve) during insertion; some resistance to insertion is normal as catheter passes through layer of abdominal fascia. Client may need to change position to facilitate insertion. Taking slow, deep breaths also helps (Davidson and others, 1990).

STEP	RATIONALE
5. If no effluent starts to drain, problem solving is needed. The illustration can be used to help solve problem of inadequate effluent from pouch. For example, try moving catheter in and out slightly. If this is unsuccessful, irrigate pouch as in Skill 26-2, Implementation, Step 7. If this is a scheduled time for irrigation, proceed after effluent has drained and irrigate with 30 to 60 ml of sterile NS; allow to drain.	Mucus may plug the catheter. Continent diversions must be irrigated at regular intervals.
6. Before withdrawing catheter, have client cough three or four times, then slowly remove.	Positive pressure inside abdomen clears residual urine from pouch and continence valve; clears mucus from catheter.
7. Gently cleanse peristomal skin with gauze pads and liquid antimicrobial soap; rinse; pat dry.	Reduces bacterial colonization and removes any dried mucus to maintain skin integrity.
8. Cover stoma with stomal covering.	Some leakage of effluent occurs until full recovery from surgery; mucus will always be produced.
9. Discard soiled equipment; remove gloves. Maintain sterile NS; label with date, time, and nurse's initials.	Reduces transmission of microorganisms. Some equipment can stay at bedside for 8 hours if strict aseptic technique is followed; this helps reduce costs.
10. Record output and amount used for irrigation.	Keeps accurate output record.
NOTE: Postoperative week 3: Stoma is intubated every 2 to 3 hours and once at night to drain urine; it is irrigated every 4 hours. Schedule should be known to client and to all caregivers. A time card at bedside facilitates this. Weeks 4 through 6: Intubate every 4 hours and as needed (PRN) at night; irrigate twice a day (bid) and PRN. Fully recovered client with continent urinary diversion must intubate (or be intubated if unable to do) every 4 hours and PRN at night; irrigate bid and PRN. Physician's protocols may vary somewhat.	The scheduled intubation times allow for gradual expansion of the pouch. Pouches or reservoirs vary as to maximum amount of urine they can hold after complete recovery; may range from 150 to 600 ml. Reservoirs constructed from bowel always secrete mucus and must be routinely irrigated.

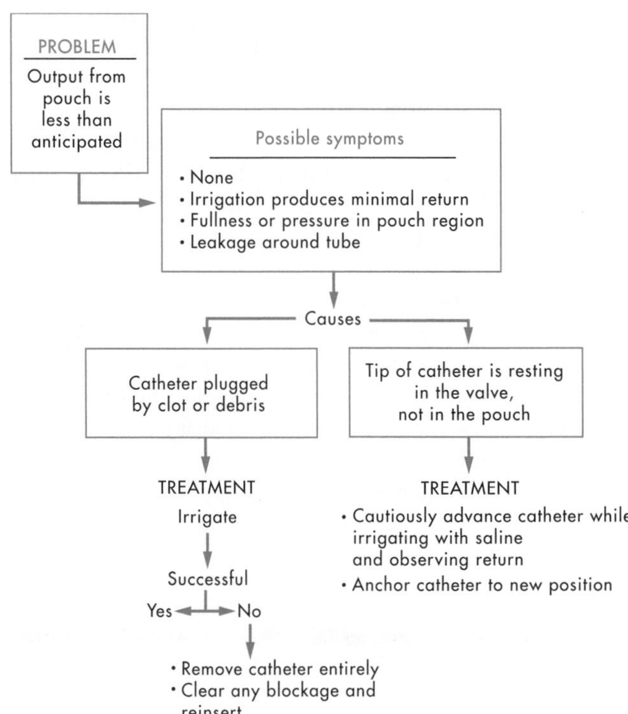

STEP 5 Problem solving when output from the pouch is lower than anticipated. (Modified from Hull TL, Erwin-Toth P: The pelvic pouch procedure and continent ostomies: overview and controversies, *J Wound Ostomy Continence Nurs* 23(3):156, 1996.)

STEP	RATIONALE
EVALUATION	
1. Note appearance of stoma, peristomal skin, and abdominal suture lines.	Determines condition of stoma and peristomal skin and progress of wound healing.
2. Evaluate character and volume of output.	Determines if stomal catheter, stents, and residual catheter (e.g., cecostomy tube) are patent. Alerts nurse for need to irrigate stomal catheter. Minimal urinary output is 30 ml/hr.
3. Palpate for discomfort over pouch site and over peristomal skin.	May indicate large amount of residual urine or infection. Determines if any skin irritation is present.
4. Observe client's, family member's, or significant other's willingness to participate in care.	Determines level of adjustment, need for teaching, and risk for complications.

UNEXPECTED OUTCOMES AND RELATED INTERVENTIONS

- Continence valve leaks excessively and continuously after stomal catheter is removed.
  - Replace valve.
  - Empty reservoir more often to avoid overdistention.
- Catheter cannot be inserted.
  - Remove catheter and start again.
  - Pouch may be overdistended; empty pouch more frequently.
- Stool is especially thick.
  - Encourage client not to take a laxative but rather to increase daily fluid intake, including intake of prune juice (Hull and Erwin-Toth, 1996).
- See also Unexpected Outcomes and Related Interventions for Skill 26-1.

RECORDING AND REPORTING

- Record time of irrigation and/or intubation, size of catheter used, ease of intubation, amount of NS used, amount and character of output, and client's tolerance.
- Document client's and family's responses and their level of participation in care.
- Report abnormalities of stoma and peristomal skin.

TEACHING CONSIDERATIONS

- Give instruction according to client's level of understanding and ability and readiness.
- Use the opportunity to teach whenever doing pouch irrigation or intubation even if client does not appear interested. Do not force client to look at stoma; allow time for adjustment.
- Include family member or significant other in teaching if possible.
- Client should be given a teaching manual with steps clearly stated, or audiotaped instructions. For someone with a learning disability, a "picture book" of steps may be more appropriate.
- Client should be given a list of equipment and name, address, and phone number of a supplier in the community.
- Teach clients that some mucus in urine is expected; they should report any blood in urine, excessively cloudy urine, chills, fever, and back pain to physician immediately.
- Teach clients to *not* use petroleum-based products for lubricating the catheter because this increases risk of infection; client may use plain warm tap water or water-soluble lubricant (preferred). May use plain warm tap water to irrigate after week 6 (this may vary with physician's protocol).

GERONTOLOGICAL CONSIDERATIONS

- Clients should be carefully assessed preoperatively for their suitability for having a continent diversion. Clients must have physical, visual, and mental ability to intubate stoma and drain internal pouch on prescribed schedule.

HOME CARE CONSIDERATIONS

- Teach clients proper care of intubation catheters: After use, rinse inside to clear any mucus and wash with warm, soapy water; rinse well inside and out; suspend catheter so that it hangs to dry. Dry completely, and keep in a clean plastic bag or toothbrush holder container.
- Clients must always carry their catheter with them.

Critical Thinking Exercises

1. Your client has had a colostomy for 6 years; today you are making a home visit, and he complains that lately he is having cramping during irrigations. How would you assess this problem?
2. Your client is experiencing leaking around the ileostomy skin barrier. What actions should you take?
3. Describe the importance of using a wick when changing a pouch of a client with a noncontinent urinary diversion.

References

Aron S, and others: Self perceptions about having an ostomy: a postoperative analysis, *Ostomy Wound Manage* 45(4):46, 1999.

Atta MA: A new technique for continent urinary reservoir reconstruction, *J Urol* 145:960, 1991.

Ayello: The ABCD's of stoma assessment and pouching, Personal correspondence, 2000.

Bastawrous AAL and others: Trends in pediatric ostomy surgery: intestinal diversion for necrotizing enterocolitis and biliary diversion for biliary hypoplasia syndromes, *J Wound Ostomy Continence Nurs* 22(6):280, 1995.

Boarini JH: Principles of stoma care for infants, *J Enterostom Ther* 16(1):21, 1989.

Bonham P, Schaffner A: Management of extensive peristomal ulcers around a retracted stenotic ileal conduit stoma site, *J Wound Ostomy Continence Nurs* 26(5):276, 1999.

Bradley M, Pupiales M: Essential elements of ostomy care, *Am J Nurs* 97(7):38, 1997.

Broadwell DC, Jackson BL: *Principles of ostomy care,* St. Louis, 1982, Mosby.

Brown KC, Ricketts RR: Current management of the neonatal patient with an ostomy, *Progressions* 6(3):3, 1994.

Cavas M, Makay S: The Indiana pouch, *AORN J* 54:494, 1991.

Cohen A: Body image in the person with a stoma, *J Enterostom Ther* 18:68, 1991.

Davidson MW and others: Continent Indiana reservoir: nursing management, *Ostomy Wound Manage* 31:50, 1990.

Edgar LVL: Elective colostomy in the patient with a spinal cord injury: an ET nurse's perspective, *Journal of WOCN* 26(1):18, 1999.

Erwin-Toth P: The effect of ostomy surgery between the ages of 6 and 12 years on psychosocial development during childhood, adolescence, and young adulthood, *J Wound Ostomy Continence Nurs* 26(2):77, 1999.

Foster ME: Surgical options for managing chronic fecal incontinence in children, *Progressions* 7(1):13, 1995.

Golis AM: Sexual issues for the person with an ostomy, *J Wound Ostomy Continence Nurs* 23:1, 1996.

Golomb J, Klutke CG, Raz S: Complications of bladder substitution and continent urinary diversion, *Urology* 34:329, 1989.

Halvorson ML, Kertz JM: Changes in Medicare reimbursement for ostomy supplies: an overview, *J Wound Ostomy Continence Nurs* 23:26, 1996.

Hull TL, Erwin-Toth P: The pelvic pouch procedure and continent ostomies: overview and controversies, *J Wound Ostomy Continence Nurs* 23(3):156, 1996.

Jeffres C, MacKay AT: Improving stoma management in the low-vision patient, *J Wound Ostomy Continence Nurs* 24(6):302, 1997.

Kluka S, Kristijanson LJ: Development and testing of the ostomy concerns scale: measuring ostomy-related concerns of cancer patients and their partners, *J Wound Ostomy Continence Nurs* 23(3):166, 1996.

Leong AFPK, Yunos ABM: Stoma management in a tropical country: colostomy irrigation versus natural evacuation, *Ostomy Wound Manage* 45(11):52, 1999.

Mitchel JV: A clinical pathway for ostomy care in the home: process and development, *J Wound Ostomy Continence Nurs* 25(4):200, 1998.

Mowdy S: The role of the WOC nurse in an ostomy support group, *J Wound Ostomy Continence Nurs* 25(1):51, 1998.

Northouse LL and others: The concerns of patients and spouses after the diagnosis of colon cancer: a qualitative analysis, *J Wound Ostomy Continence Nurs* 26(1):8, 1999.

Piper B, Mikols C: Predischarge and postdischarge concerns of persons with an ostomy, *J Wound Ostomy Continence Nurs* 23(2):105, 1996.

Piper B, Mikols C, Grant TRD: Comparing adjustment to an ostomy for three groups, *J Wound Ostomy Continence Nurs* 23(4):197, 1996.

Quayle BK: Making positive choices: body image and the new ostomy patient, *Ostomy Wound Manage* 40:4, 1994.

Ramos L, Glosson A: Teaching ostomy care to a patient who is blind, *J Wound Ostomy Continence Nurs* 23(4):235, 1996.

Rolstad BS, Boarini J: Principles and techniques in the use of convexity, *Ostomy Wound Manage* 42:1, 1996.

Wagner VP, Osgood SB: Patient with a recessed, stenosed stoma located in an irregular, pendulous abdomen and the presence of pseudo-verrucous lesions, *J Wound Ostomy Continence Nurs* 25(5):261, 1998.

Walsh BA and others: Multidisciplinary management of altered body image in the patient with an ostomy, *J Wound Ostomy Continence Nurs* 22(5):227, 1995.

Walsh BA: Urostomy and urinary pH, *J Enterostom Ther* 19:110, 1992.

27

Body Mechanics, Transfer, and Positioning

Skills

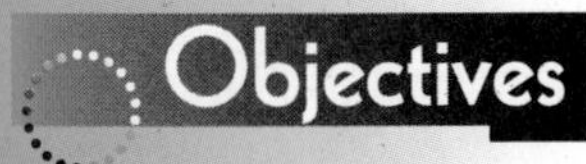

Objectives

Mastery of content in this chapter will enable the nurse to:

- Define the key terms listed.
- Describe body mechanics and its importance in caring for clients.
- Describe normal body alignment for standing, sitting, and lying down.
- Assess for alterations in body alignment.
- Describe procedures for lifting.
- Describe positioning techniques for the supported Fowler's, supine, prone, side-lying, and Sims' positions.
- Describe the procedures for helping a client to move up in bed, helping a client to a sitting position, logrolling a client, and transferring a client from a bed to a chair.
- Describe the procedure for a three-person carry.

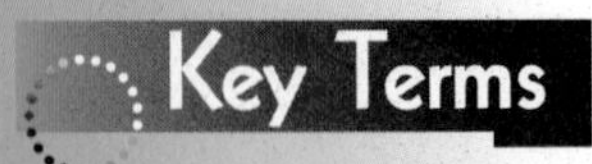

Key Terms

Balance	Hemiplegia
Base of support	Hoyer lift (mechanical/ hydraulic lift)
Body alignment	Leverage
Body mechanics	Line of gravity
Center of gravity	Logrolling
Drawsheet	Orthostatic hypotension
Footboard	Paralysis
Footdrop	Paresis
Friction	Posture
Gravity	Proprioceptive function
Hand rolls	Weight
Hemiparesis	

The rate of injuries in occupational settings has increased during recent years. More than half of these injuries are back injuries and the direct result of unsafe lifting and bending techniques (Gassett, Hearne, and Keelan, 1996). The most common back injury is strain of the lumbar muscle group, which includes the muscles surrounding the lumbar vertebrae. Muscle injury to this area affects the person's ability to bend forward, backward, and side to side. In addition, the ability to rotate the hips and lower back from left to right and right to left is decreased. By becoming knowledgeable about safe, efficient lifting techniques, nurses can promote safe transferring of clients without causing injury to the client's or the nurse's musculoskeletal systems.

Health care providers are required to provide employees with safety information and training to use when transferring, positioning, and lifting clients. The Occupational Safety and Health Administration (OSHA) has identified standards on back safety and guidelines on the prevention of musculoskeletal injuries (OSHA, 2000).

Before lifting, the nurse should assess the **weight** to be lifted and what assistance, if any, is needed. If help is needed, the nurse should assess if a second person is adequate or if mechanical assistance is needed. Once the amount of needed assistance is determined, these steps are followed:

- Tighten stomach muscles and tuck pelvis; this provides **balance** and protects the back.
- Bend at the knees; this helps to maintain the nurse's **center of gravity** and lets the strong muscles of the legs do the lifting.
- Keep the weight to be lifted as close to the body as possible; this action places the weight in the same plane as the lifter and close to the center of gravity for balance.
- Maintain the trunk erect and knees bent so that multiple muscle groups work together in a synchronized manner (Gassett, Hearne, and Keelan, 1996).
- Avoid twisting. Twisting can overload your spine and lead to serious injury.
- The best height for lifting vertically is approximately 2 feet off the ground and close to the lifter's center of gravity (Gassett, Hearne, and Keelan, 1996).

The muscles associated primarily with movement are located near the skeletal region, where leverage results in movement. **Leverage** is an inducing or compelling force. Leverage occurs when specific bones, such as the humerus, ulna, and radius, and the associated joints, such as the elbow joint, act together as a lever. Thus force is applied to one end of the bone to lift a weight while another point tends to rotate the bone in the direction opposite that of the applied force. The skeletal muscles that attach to the bones of leverage provide the necessary strength to move the object.

Muscles associated primarily with maintaining **posture** are short and shaped like a feather because they converge obliquely at a common tendon. Muscles of the lower extremities, trunk, neck, and back are associated primarily with posture. These muscle groups work together to stabilize and support body weight when a person is standing or sitting.

Body mechanics is the coordinated effort of the musculoskeletal and nervous systems to maintain balance, posture, and **body alignment** during lifting, bending, moving, and performing activities of daily living. Body mechanics also facilitates body movement so that a person can carry out a physical activity without using excessive muscle energy. The application of body mechanics and transfer and positioning are basic nursing skills.

Positioning to maintain correct body alignment is essential to prevent complications. These complications include pressure ulcers (see Chapter 7), which can develop in 24 hours and require months of time and thousands of dollars to correct (Lueckenotte, 2000); and contractures and **footdrop,** which can occur within a few days when muscles, tendons, and joints become less flexible because of lack of mobility and incorrect alignment.

The force of **gravity** pulls an unsupported, weakened foot into a footdrop position, and calf muscles and heel cords shorten, complicating future attempts at walking. Pillows placed under the knees or an elevated knee gatch can produce knee and hip contractures. A sagging mattress increases the risk of hip contractures. These knee and hip contractures can cause future gait and posture problems, making mobility more difficult.

Some clients are at especially high risk for complications of improper positioning and have increased risk of injury during transfer. A number of pathological factors and congenital or acquired postural abnormalities alter alignment, mobility, or both. Pathophysiological mechanisms altering bone formation or joint mobility present special risks, as does impaired muscle development, which results in muscle wasting and weakness. Central nervous system (CNS) damage may result in motor impairment, proprioceptive loss, or cognitive dysfunction, all of which affect mobility. Direct trauma also affects body mechanics.

The application of proper body mechanics, alignment, and the use of transfer and positioning techniques assist the client in achieving an optimal level of independence without resultant injury to the health care provider. Too often the client develops complications independent of illness because the principles of alignment, body mechanics, transfer, and positioning are not followed. Improper alignment of the dependent client can result in pressure ulcers, joint contractures, or injuries that may take months to correct or that may even result in permanent disability. The loss of independence can result in the client needing assistance in the home or even being required to live in a nursing home. The ability to maintain independence is also important in preventing social isolation and maintaining body alignment essential to well-being.

Skill Performance Guidelines

1. Know the physiological influences on body alignment and mobility that affect clients throughout the life span. The greatest impact of the physiological changes on the musculoskeletal system is observed in the early and later years of life. In the child the major consequences of decreased muscle activity are loss of muscle strength, endurance, muscle mass, and joint mobility; bone demineralization; and contracture. Inactive older adults are at risk for muscle atrophy, loss of bony mass, contractures of joints, and pressure ulcers.
2. Know the pathological conditions that affect a client's body alignment and mobility. Postural abnormalities can affect body mechanics. For example, a client with severe kyphosis may not be able to lift an object safely because the center of gravity is not aligned. Diseases affecting bone formation (e.g., osteoporosis) alter body alignment and mobility. Degenerative joint diseases (e.g., osteoarthritis), impaired muscle development (e.g., muscular dystrophy), and central nervous system damage (e.g., **paralysis**) can interfere with normal body alignment and mobility. Therefore the client's risk of musculoskeletal injury is increased.
3. Know history of underlying conditions such as chronic disease (e.g., diabetes, chronic obstructive pulmonary disease) or malnutrition. Clients with underlying chronic conditions are at risk for skin breakdown and other hazards of immobility and as a result require more frequent position changes.
4. Control factors that can indirectly affect body mechanics by altering the safety of the environment. Cluttered hallways and bedside areas increase the client's risk of falling (see Chapters 4 and 39).
5. Use an organized, systematic approach to assess and improve body mechanics. Continued nursing assessment promptly identifies risks to normal body alignment and promotes immediate nursing interventions.
6. Know the client's fluid balance status. Dehydration or edema may require more frequent position changes because clients with alterations in fluid balance are prone to skin breakdown. In addition, identify the client with incontinence or profuse sweating. Moisture from incontinence or sweating can decrease tensile strength and alter skin resiliency to external forces.
7. Know the client's range of joint motion (ROJM). Contractures or spasticity limit joint and muscle mobility; the nurse must take care not to position the limb in an unnatural way. This could result in injury to or dysfunction of the affected limb (see Chapter 28).
8. Determine the client's level of sensory perception. Loss of sensation increases vulnerability to the hazards of immobility. Clients with decreased sensation must have their positions evaluated and changed frequently to avoid damage to the integumentary and musculoskeletal systems.
9. Know the client's baseline vital signs. The client with low blood pressure may not be able to tolerate sudden position changes and is at risk of fainting while transferring from bed to chair. Along with vital signs it is necessary to assess the client's cognitive status and stage of psychological adaptation to illness. Both factors affect the ability to learn and participate in transfer and positioning.

Skill 27-1 Maintaining Body Alignment

The term *body alignment* refers to the conditions of the joints, tendons, ligaments, and muscles in various body positions. When the body is aligned, whether standing, sitting, or lying, no excessive strain is placed on these structures. Body alignment means the body is in line with the pull of gravity and contributes to body balance. Without this balance, the center of gravity is displaced, which increases the force of gravity and predisposes the person to falls and injuries.

Body balance is achieved when a wide **base of support** exists, the center of gravity falls within the base of support, and a vertical line can be drawn from the center of gravity through the base of support. Body balance also is enhanced by posture. The better aligned the posture, the greater the balance. Clinical nursing activities require the nurse to maintain body alignment. It is essential for the nurse to provide an opportunity for the client to observe correct posture and to identify the client's learning needs for maintaining body alignment. In addition, the nurse needs to identify trauma, muscle damage, or nerve dysfunction in the client.

Delegation Considerations

The skills of maintaining body alignment and mechanics can be delegated to assistive personnel. Clients who have spinal cord trauma usually require transfer and moving by professional nurses. Be sure to caution caregiver to maintain proper body mechanics. Provide caregiver with information regarding client's individual needs for body alignment and proper body mechanics.

Step	Rationale
Assessment	
1. Observe alignment of client in standing, sitting, or lying position.	Determines if client assumes normal body alignment.
2. Standing (see illustration): a. Head is erect and at midline. b. Shoulders and hips are straight and parallel. c. Vertebral column appears straight when viewed posteriorly.	Maintains body alignment in relation to body's normal center of gravity.
d. Lateral observation indicates head is erect and spinal curves are aligned in reverse-S pattern.	In reverse-S pattern, cervical vertebrae are anteriorly convex, thoracic vertebrae are posteriorly convex, and lumbar vertebrae are anteriorly convex.

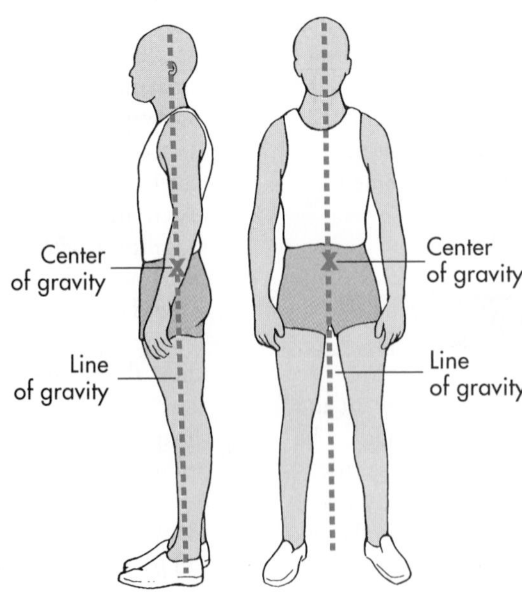

STEP 2 Body alignment when standing.

STEP	RATIONALE
e. Lateral observation indicates that abdomen is comfortably tucked in and knees and ankles are slightly flexed.	Maintains abdomen and trunk directly over body's center of gravity.
f. Arms are comfortably positioned at each side.	
g. Feet are placed slightly apart, with toes pointed forward.	Produces broad base of support and improves balance.
h. Center of gravity is located midline and forms vertical line from middle of forehead to midpoint between feet.	Laterally, **line of gravity** runs vertically from middle of skull to posterior one third of foot.

• ***Critical Decision Point***
A pregnant woman's center of gravity is more anterior to adapt to normal weight gain and growing fetus. Thus she leans slightly backward, and spinal column is slightly swaybacked (see illustration).

STEP	RATIONALE
3. Sitting (see illustration):	
a. Head is erect, and vertebrae are in straight alignment.	Prevents stress on intravertebral joints.
b. Body weight is evenly distributed on buttocks and thighs.	Prevents increased pressure over bony prominences and reduces damage to underlying musculoskeletal system.
c. Thighs are parallel and in horizontal plane.	Maintains flexion of hips and provides broad base of support.
d. Both feet are supported on floor, and ankles are comfortably flexed.	Maintains plantar flexion and reduces risk of footdrop.

• ***Critical Decision Point***
If client is unable to flex one or both knees, nurse should make sure that elevated legs are supported and ankles are flexed.

STEP	RATIONALE
e. A 2.5- to 5-cm (1- to 2-inch) space is maintained between edge of seat and popliteal space on posterior surface of knee.	Ensures that no excessive pressure is placed on popliteal artery or nerve, which could decrease circulation or impair nerve function.

• ***Critical Decision Point***
Clients at risk for thrombophlebitis (see Chapter 28), such as postoperative or postpartum clients or clients taking anticoagulants or medication that can increase platelet production, should be taught to maintain space between edge of chair and popliteal space and not to cross their legs (Phipps, Sands, and Marek, 1999).

STEP	RATIONALE
f. Client's forearms should be supported on armrest, in lap, or on table in front of chair.	Reduces force of gravity on shoulder joint and chance of accidental shoulder dislocation.

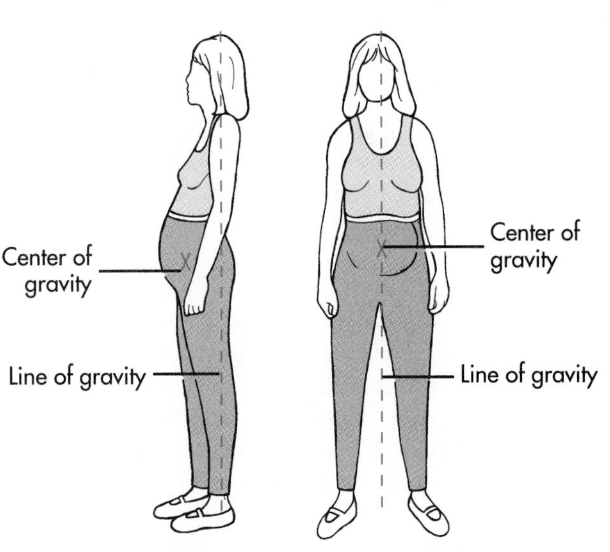

STEP **2h** Center of gravity in pregnant woman.

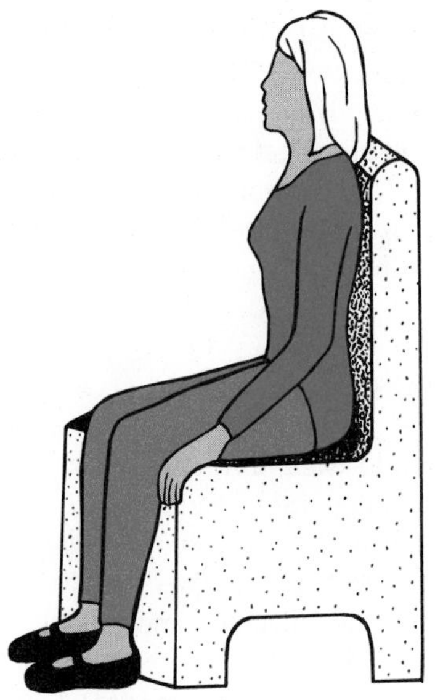
STEP **3** Center of gravity when sitting.

Step	Rationale
4. Lying (see illustration):	
a. Client is in lateral position, with positioning supports removed.	Allows nurse to observe spinal alignment and any pressure points.
b. Client's body should be supported by adequate mattress.	Reduces strain on joints and ligaments.
c. Vertebral column should be in alignment without observable curves.	Allows for even distribution of body weight.

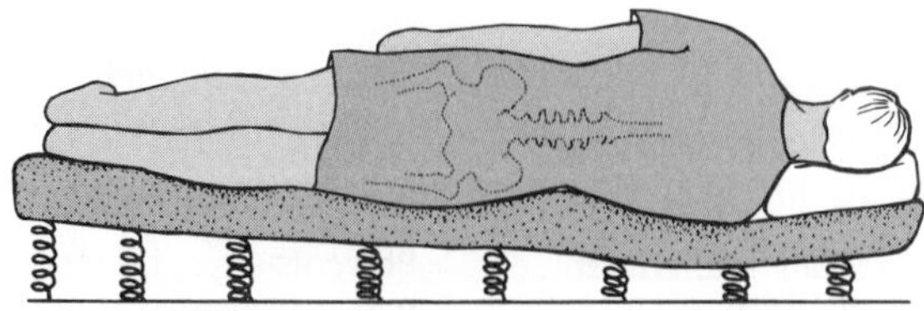

STEP **4** Body alignment in lateral position.

- ***Critical Decision Point***
  Clients with lower or upper extremity weakness, decreased sensation, paralysis, or immobilization are at risk for musculoskeletal trauma because of uneven or prolonged distribution of body weight and must have their positions changed frequently.

Nursing Diagnosis

Defining characteristics from the assessment data may reveal the following nursing diagnoses for clients requiring this skill:

- Impaired physical mobility
- Deficient knowledge concerning body mechanics
- Deficient knowledge concerning proper positioning
- Risk for activity intolerance
- Risk for disuse syndrome
- Risk for impaired skin integrity
- Risk for injury

Related factors are individualized based on client's condition or needs.

Planning

Step	Rationale
1. **Expected outcomes** following completion of procedure:	
▪ Body is positioned without skin surfaces being exposed to undue pressure.	Extremities are not crossed or aligned to cause pressure.
▪ While sitting, lying, or standing, client aligns body straight and in correct position.	Avoids strain on musculoskeletal structures.
▪ Client is able to explain benefits of body alignment.	Increases likelihood of good postural habits being followed.
2. Instruct client or caregiver in proper body alignment for standing, sitting, or lying.	Provides client or caregiver with necessary knowledge to identify potential altered body alignment.

Implementation

Step	Rationale
1. Demonstrate to client and caregiver correct body alignment for standing, sitting, and lying.	Demonstration is reliable technique for teaching psychomotor skills and enables client and caregiver to ask questions.
2. Provide opportunity for return demonstration.	Allows evaluation of client or family learning.
3. Discuss with client and caregiver the hazards of prolonged immobility on body alignment and mobility (see Chapter 7).	Alerts client and caregiver to early assessment factors associated with incorrect body alignment and impaired mobility.
4. Provide client and caregiver with resources (e.g., community health agency, physician) to contact when mobility or body alignment is impaired.	Alerts resource persons to assist with minor problems of body alignment before severe, irreversible problems occur.

STEP	RATIONALE
EVALUATION	
1. Inspect skin surfaces.	Reveals pressure sites.
2. Have client demonstrate body alignment for standing, sitting, and lying.	Return demonstration reveals if learning occurred.
3. Ask client to describe benefits of body alignment.	Evaluates cognitive learning.

Unexpected Outcomes and Related Interventions

- Incorrect body alignment is indicated by poor posture or decreased joint mobility.
  - Indicates need for follow-up learning activities.
  - Instruct caregivers to step back and view the client's body alignment and look for signs of discomfort.
- Damage to skin and musculoskeletal system (e.g., pressure sore, contracture) occurs.
  - Review plan of care with client and caregiver and modify as needed.
  - Post turning schedule above client's bed as a reminder.
  - Initiate steps to treat developing pressure sore (see Chapter 7).

Recording and Reporting

- Record information presented to client and client's progress toward learning selected knowledge.
- Report information taught to client at change of shift.
- Record time and position change of client throughout shift.

Teaching Considerations

- Shorter clients should be taught to use a footstool when sitting.
- Teach family members or friends of clients who are permanently disabled proper body mechanics, alignment, transfer, and positioning techniques. Provide family members and caregivers a turning schedule for the client.
- Clients at risk for thrombophlebitis should be taught not to cross their legs and the signs and symptoms of this complication (see Chapter 28).
- If client has cognitive or sensory impairment, is a young child, is severely debilitated, or is immobilized or confined to bed, family is primary focus of instruction (see Skills 27-2 and 27-3).

Pediatric Considerations

- Teach parents that the use of play activities such as painting or drawing on a large sheet of paper placed on the bed or wall can encourage movement. Play activities to encourage ambulation include push/pull toy (toddler) and wagon (school age) (Wong and others, 1999).

Gerontological Considerations

- Older adult clients may take smaller steps with feet closer together and may be at risk for falling.
- During aging process, cervical vertebrae may become more flexed, and kyphotic posture may result (McCance and Huether, 1998).

Home Care Considerations

- Teach family members or friends of clients who are permanently disabled proper body mechanics and proper body alignment.
- Bed must be at caregiver's waist level.
- Teach family members or friends to place clients in positions that maintain musculoskeletal alignment and reduce pressure on bony prominences.
- Provide family members and caregivers a turning schedule for the client.

Long-Term Care Considerations

- Long-term care clients may have special devices or appliances such as eggcrate cushions or air mattresses to increase comfort. Make sure these appliances or devices are smooth and wrinkle-free when assessing proper body alignment of the client.
- Clearly label all reusable padding or special mattresses with client's name.

Skill 27-2 Using Safe and Effective Transfer Techniques

Transferring is a nursing skill that helps the dependent client or the client with restricted mobility attain positions to regain optimal independence as quickly as possible. Physical activity maintains and improves joint motion, increases strength, promotes circulation, relieves pressure on skin, and improves urinary and respiratory functions. It also benefits the client psychologically by increasing social activity and mental stimulation and providing a change in environment. Thus mobilization plays a crucial role in the client's rehabilitation.

One of the major concerns during transfer is the safety of the client and the nurse. The nurse prevents self-injury by using correct posture, minimal muscle strength, and effective body mechanics and lifting techniques.

The nurse must be aware of the client's motor deficits, ability to aid in transfer, and body weight. As a rule of thumb, nurses should always get assistance if in doubt about their ability to transfer a client.

Many special problems must be considered in transfer. A client who has been immobile for several days or longer may be weak or dizzy or may develop **orthostatic hypotension** (a drop in blood pressure) when transferred. A client with neurological deficits may have **paresis** (muscle weakness) or paralysis unilaterally or bilaterally, which complicates safe transfer. A flaccid arm may sustain injury during transfer if unsupported. As a general rule, a nurse should use a transfer belt and obtain assistance for mobilization of such clients.

Delegation Considerations

The skills of effective transfer techniques can be delegated to assistive personnel. Clients who are transferred for the first time after prolonged bed rest, extensive surgery, critical illness, or spinal cord trauma usually require a nurse's supervision. The care provider must be instructed to seek assistance when moving or lifting heavy objects and must be informed about individual client's mobility restrictions, changes in blood pressure, or sensory alterations that may affect safe transfer.

Equipment

- Transfer belt, sling or lap board (as needed), nonskid shoes, bath blankets, pillows
- Wheelchair: Position chair at 45-degree angle to bed, lock brakes, remove footrests, lock bed brakes
- Stretcher: Position at right angle (90 degrees) to bed, lock brakes on stretcher, lock brakes on bed
- Mechanical/hydraulic lift: Use frame, canvas strips or chains, and hammock or canvas strips

Step	Rationale
Assessment	
1. Assess physiological capacity to transfer and cognitive ability to understand.	Determines neuromuscular integrity for transfer and special adaptive techniques that are necessary. Clients with impaired cognition may require more assistance to transfer.
a. Muscle strength (legs and upper arms)	Immobile clients have decreased muscle strength, tone, and mass. Affects ability to bear weight or raise body.
b. Joint mobility and contracture formation	Immobility or inflammatory processes (i.e., arthritis) may lead to contracture formation and impaired joint mobility.
c. Paralysis or paresis (spastic or flaccid)	Client with central nervous system (CNS) damage may have bilateral paralysis (requiring transfer by swivel bar, sliding bar, **Hoyer lift**) or unilateral paralysis, which requires belt transfer to "best" side. Weakness (paresis) requires stabilization of knee while transferring. Flaccid arm must be supported with sling during transfer.
d. Bone continuity (trauma, amputation)	Clients with trauma to one leg or hip may be non–weight-bearing when transferred. Amputees may use sliding board to transfer.
2. Assess presence of weakness, dizziness, or postural hypotension.	Determines risk of fainting or falling during transfer. Immobile clients may have decreased ability for autonomic nervous system to equalize blood supply, resulting in orthostatic hypotension, which is a drop of 15 mm Hg or more in blood pressure when rising from sitting position.
3. Assess level of endurance:	
a. Assess ability to use arms and legs for moving up and down in bed and repositioning.	Estimates ability to participate in transfer.

STEP	RATIONALE
b. Assess level of fatigue during activity.	Ability to transfer may be limited by fatigue. Strength may be evaluated by participation in activities of daily living (ADLs). Planned rest periods before transfer may enhance function.
c. Assess vital signs.	Vital sign changes such as increased pulse and respiration may indicate activity intolerance (see Chapter 9).
4. Assess client's **proprioceptive function** (awareness of posture and changes in equilibrium):	Determines stability of client's balance for transfer.
a. Ability to maintain balance while sitting in bed or on side of bed	Determines risk of fainting or falling during transfer.
b. Tendency to sway to or position self to one side	Clients with brain dysfunction may have proprioceptive losses. This may cause them to lean to one side or lose balance during transfer.
5. Assess client's sensory status:	Determines influence of sensory loss on ability to make transfer. Visual field loss decreases client's ability to see in direction of transfer. Peripheral sensation loss decreases proprioception. Clients with visual and hearing losses need transfer techniques adapted to deficits. Clients with cerebrovascular accident (CVA) may lose area of visual field, which profoundly affects vision and perception.

• ***Critical Decision Point***
Clients with ***hemiplegia*** *also may "neglect" one side of the body (inattention to or unawareness of one side of body or environment), which distorts perception of the visual field.*

STEP	RATIONALE
a. Adequacy of central and peripheral vision	
b. Adequacy of hearing	
c. Loss of peripheral sensation	
6. Assess client's level of comfort:	Pain may reduce client's motivation and ability to be mobile. Pain relief before transfer enhances client participation.
a. Pain	
b. Muscle spasm	
7. Assess client's cognitive status.	Determines client's ability to follow directions and learn transfer techniques.

• ***Critical Decision Point***
Clients with head trauma or CVA may have perceptual cognitive deficits that create safety risks. If client has difficulty in comprehension, simplify instructions and maintain consistency.

STEP	RATIONALE
a. Ability to follow verbal instructions	May indicate clients at risk for injury.
b. Short-term memory	Clients with short-term memory deficits may have difficulty with transfer, initial learning, or consistent performance.
c. Appropriateness of response	
d. Recognition of physical deficits and limitations to movement	
8. Assess client's level of motivation:	Altered psychological states reduce client's desire to engage in activity.
a. Client's eagerness versus unwillingness to be mobile	
b. Whether client avoids activity and offers excuses	
9. Assess previous mode of transfer (if applicable).	Determines mode of transfer and assistance required to provide continuity. Transfer belts should be used with hemiplegic clients being transferred for the first time and all other high-risk clients.
10. Assess client's specific risk of falling when transferred.	Certain conditions increase client's risk of falling or potential for injury. Neuromuscular deficits, motor weakness, calcium loss from long bones, cognitive and visual dysfunction, and altered balance increase risk of injury.

STEP	RATIONALE
11. Assess special transfer equipment needed for home setting. Assess home environment for hazards.	Transfer ability at home is greatly enhanced by prior teaching of family and support persons, assessment of home for safety risks and functionality, and provision of applicable aids.

NURSING DIAGNOSIS

Defining characteristics from the assessment data may reveal the following nursing diagnoses for clients requiring this skill:

- Activity intolerance
- Impaired physical mobility
- Impaired skin integrity
- Risk for injury
- Acute or chronic pain

Related factors are individualized based on client's condition or needs.

PLANNING

STEP	RATIONALE
1. **Expected outcomes** following completion of procedure:	
▪ Client dangles legs or sits without dizziness, weakness, or orthostatic hypotension.	Precautions during transferring prevent vascular compromise.
▪ Client tolerates increased activity.	Gradual increase in number of transfers and period of time out of bed increases tolerance and endurance.
▪ Client can bear more weight.	Repeated transfers usually result in improved endurance and greater independence of client.
▪ Client transfers without injury.	Proper techniques avoid injury.
▪ Client is more motivated to be mobile.	
▪ Client transfers with minimal or no assistance.	Tolerance to activity improves.
▪ Client's skin remains intact, without redness.	Absence of pressure ulcer formation.
2. Explain procedure to client. Repeat instructions simply and with continuity to client with cognitive dysfunction.	Promotes understanding and cooperation, reducing anxiety.

IMPLEMENTATION

STEP	RATIONALE
1. Wash hands.	Reduces transfer of microorganisms.
2. Assist client to sitting position (bed at waist level):	
a. Place client in supine position.	Enables nurse to assess client's body alignment continually and to administer additional care, such as suctioning or hygiene needs.
b. Face head of bed at a 45-degree angle and remove pillows.	Proper positioning reduces twisting of the nurse's body when moving the client. Pillows may cause interference when the client is sitting up in bed.
c. Place feet apart with foot nearer bed behind other foot continuing at a 45-degree angle to the head of the bed.	Improves nurse's balance and allows transfer of body weight as client is moved to sitting position.
d. Place hand farther from client under shoulders, supporting client's head and cervical vertebrae.	Maintains alignment of head and cervical vertebrae and allows for even lifting of client's upper trunk.
e. Place other hand on bed surface.	Provides support and balance.
f. Raise client to sitting position by shifting weight from front to back leg.	Improves nurse's balance, overcomes inertia, and transfers weight in direction in which client is moved.
g. Push against bed using arm that is placed on bed surface.	Divides activity between nurse's arms and legs and protects back from strain. By bracing one hand against mattress and pushing against it as client is lifted, part of weight that would be lifted by nurse's back muscles is transferred through nurse's arms onto mattress.

STEP	RATIONALE
3. Assist client to sitting position on side of bed with bed in low position:	
a. With client in supine position, raise head of bed 30 degrees.	Decreases amount of work needed by client and nurse to raise client to sitting position.
b. Turn client onto side, facing nurse on side of bed on which client will be sitting (see illustration).	Prepares client to move to side of bed and protects from falling.
c. Stand opposite client's hips. Turn diagonally so nurse faces client and far corner of foot of bed.	Places nurse's center of gravity nearer client. Reduces twisting of nurse's body because nurse is facing direction of movement.
d. Place feet apart in a wide base of support with foot closer to head of bed in front of other foot.	Increases balance and allows nurse to transfer weight as client is brought to sitting position on side of bed.
e. Place arm nearer head of bed under client's shoulders, supporting head and neck.	Maintains alignment of head and neck as nurse brings client to sitting position.
f. Place other arm over client's thighs (see illustration).	Supports hip and prevents client from falling backward during procedure.
g. Move client's lower legs and feet over side of bed. Pivot toward rear leg, allowing client's upper legs to swing downward.	Decreases **friction** and resistance. Weight of client's legs when off bed allows gravity to lower legs, and weight of legs assists in pulling upper body into sitting position.
h. At same time, shift weight to rear leg and elevate client (see illustration).	Allows nurse to transfer weight in direction of motion.

- ***Critical Decision Point***
  Remain in front until client regains balance and continue to provide physical support to weak or cognitively impaired client.

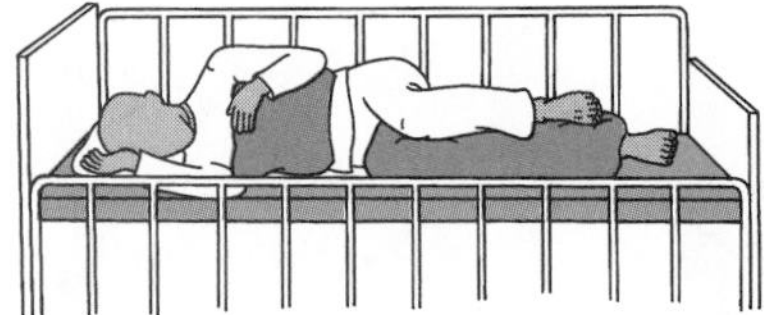

STEP **3b** Side-lying position.

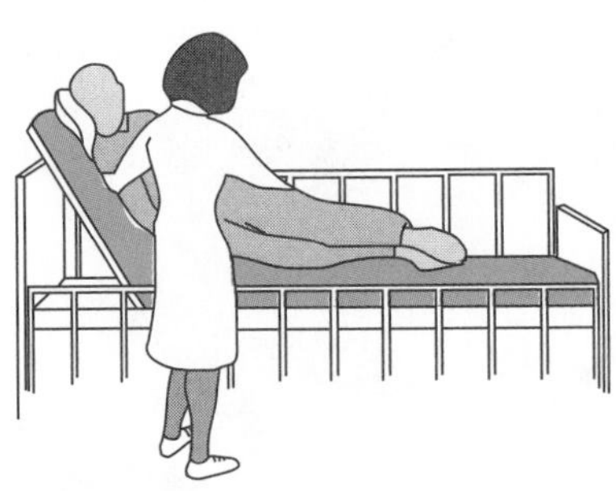

STEP **3f** Nurse places arm over client's thigh.

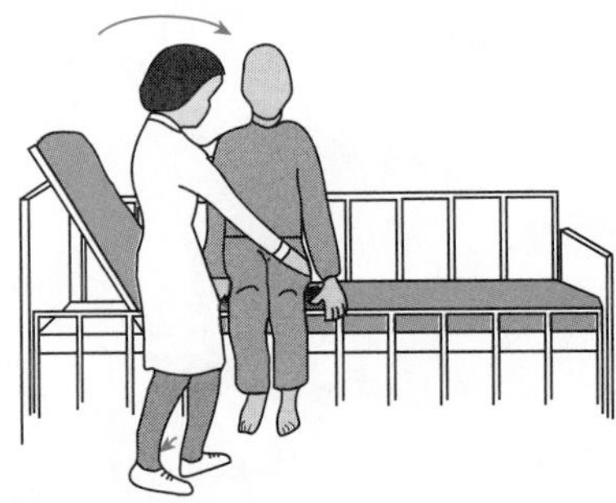

STEP **3h** Nurse shifts weight to rear leg and elevates client.

STEP	RATIONALE
4. Transferring client from bed to chair with bed in low position:	
a. Assist client to sitting position on side of bed. Have chair in position at 45-degree angle to bed.	Positions chair within easy access for transfer.
b. Apply transfer belt or other transfer aids.	Transfer belt allows nurse to maintain stability of client during transfer and reduces risk of falling (Owens, Welden, and Kane, 1999). Client's arm should be in sling if flaccid paralysis is present.

- ***Critical Decision Point***
  A battery-operated mechanical lift can assist the client to a standing position comfortably without undue physical stress on the nurse.

Step	Rationale
c. Assist client to apply stable nonskid shoes. Weight-bearing or strong leg is placed forward, with weak foot back.	Nonskid soles decrease risk of slipping during transfer. Always have client wear shoes during transfer; bare feet increase risk of falls. Client will stand on stronger, or weight-bearing, leg.
d. Spread feet apart.	Ensures balance with wide base of support.
e. Flex hips and knees, aligning knees with client's knees (see illustration).	Flexion of knees and hips lowers nurse's center of gravity to object to be raised; aligning knees with client's allows for stabilization of knees when client stands.
f. Grasp transfer belt from underneath.	Transfer belt is grasped at client's side to provide movement of client at center of gravity. Clients with upper extremity paralysis or paresis should never be lifted by or under arms.

- ***Critical Decision Point***
  A transfer belt or walking belt with handles should be used in place of the under-axilla technique. The under-axilla technique has been found to be physically stressful for nurses and uncomfortable for clients (Owens, Welden, and Kane, 1999).

Step	Rationale
g. Rock client up to standing position on count of three while straightening hips and legs and keeping knees slightly flexed (see illustration). Unless contraindicated, client may be instructed to use hands to push up if applicable.	Rocking motion gives client's body momentum and requires less muscular effort to lift client.

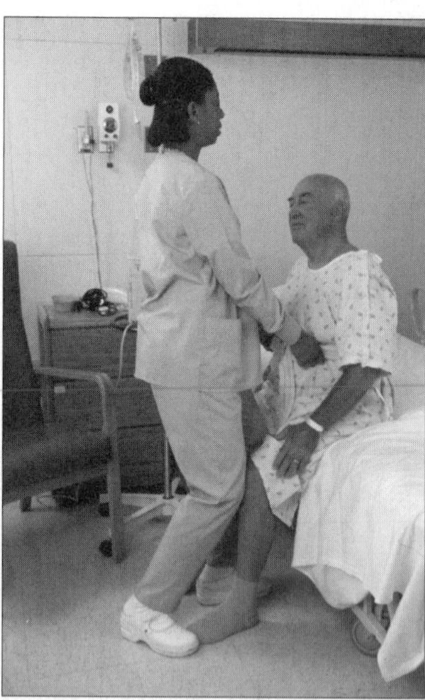

STEP **4e** Nurse flexes client's hips and knees, aligning knees with client's knee.

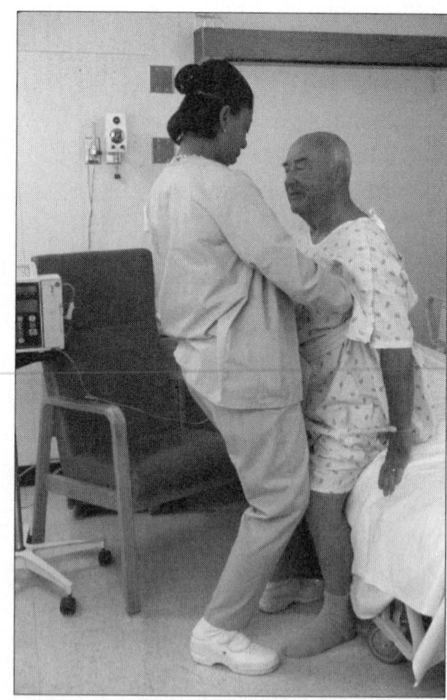

STEP **4g** Nurse rocks client to standing position.

Step	Rationale
h. Maintain stability of client's weak or paralyzed leg with your knee.	Ability to stand can often be maintained in paralyzed or weak limb with support of knee to stabilize.
i. Pivot on foot farther from chair.	Maintains support of client while allowing adequate space for client to move.
j. Instruct client to use armrests on chair for support and ease into chair (see illustration).	Increases client stability.
k. Flex hips and knees while lowering client into chair (see illustration).	Prevents injury to nurse from poor body mechanics.

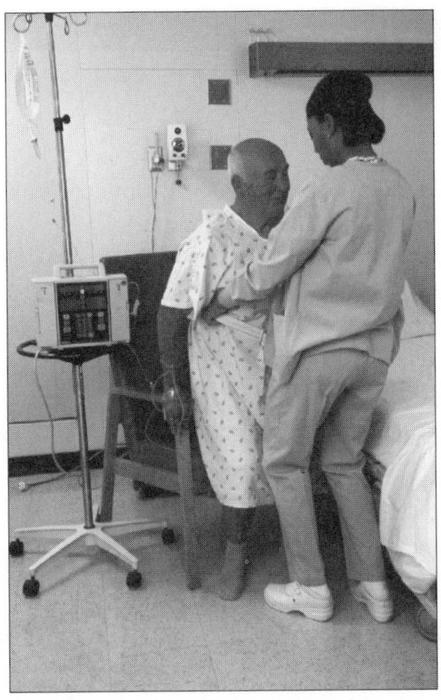

STEP **4j** Client uses armrests for support.

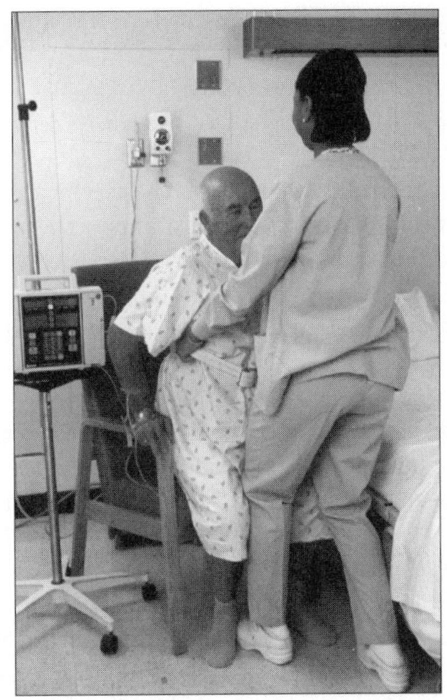

STEP **4k** Nurse eases client into chair.

STEP	RATIONALE
l. Assess client for proper alignment for sitting position. Provide support for paralyzed extremities. Lap board or sling will support flaccid arm. Stabilize leg with bath blanket or pillow.	Prevents injury to client from poor body alignment.
m. Praise client's progress, effort, and performance.	Continued support and encouragement provide incentive for client perseverance.
5. Perform three-person carry from bed to stretcher (bed at stretcher level):	
a. Three nurses stand side by side facing side of client's bed, with client lying supine.	Prevents twisting of nurses' bodies. Client's alignment is maintained.
b. Each person assumes responsibility for one of three areas: head and shoulders, hips and thighs and ankles.	Distributes client's body weight evenly.
c. Each person assumes wide base of support with foot closer to stretcher in front and knees slightly flexed.	Increases balance and lowers center of gravity of person lifting.
d. Arms of lifters are placed under client's head and shoulders, hips and thighs, and ankles, with fingers securely around other side of client's body (see illustration).	Distributes client's weight over forearms of lifters.

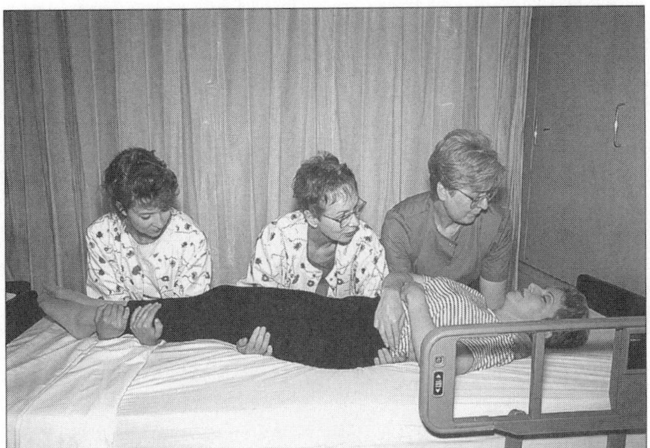

STEP **5d** Proper positioning of lifters during three-person transfer.

Step	Rationale
• ***Critical Decision Point*** *Spinal cord injuries must be stabilized before transfer.*	
e. Lifters roll client toward their chests. On count of three, client is lifted and held against nurses' chests.	Moves workload over lifters' base of support. Enables lifters to work together and safely lift client.
f. On second count of three, nurses step back and pivot toward stretcher, moving forward if needed.	Transfers weight toward stretcher.
g. Nurses gently lower client onto center of stretcher by flexing knees and hips until elbows are level with edge of stretcher.	Maintains nurses' alignment during transfer.
h. Nurses assess client's body alignment, place safety straps across body as necessary, and raise side rails.	Reduces risk of injury from poor alignment or falling.
6. Use mechanical/hydraulic lift to transfer client from bed to chair:	
a. Bring lift to bedside.	Ensures safe elevation of client off bed. (Before using lift, be thoroughly familiar with its operation.)
b. Position chair near bed, and allow adequate space to maneuver lift.	Prepares environment for safe use of lift and subsequent transfer.
c. Raise bed to high position with mattress flat. Lower side rail.	Allows nurse to use proper body mechanics.
d. Keep bed side rail up on side opposite nurse.	Maintains client safety.
e. Roll client away from nurse.	Positions client for use of lift sling.
f. Place hammock or canvas strips under client to form sling (see illustration). With two canvas pieces, lower edge fits under client's knees (wide piece), and upper edge fits under client's shoulders (narrow piece).	Two types of seat are supplied with mechanical/hydraulic lift: hammock style is better for clients who are flaccid, weak, and need support; canvas strips can be used for clients with normal muscle tone. Hooks should face away from client's skin. Place sling under client's center of gravity and greatest portion of body weight.
g. Raise bed rail.	Maintains client safety.
h. Go to opposite side of bed and lower side rail.	

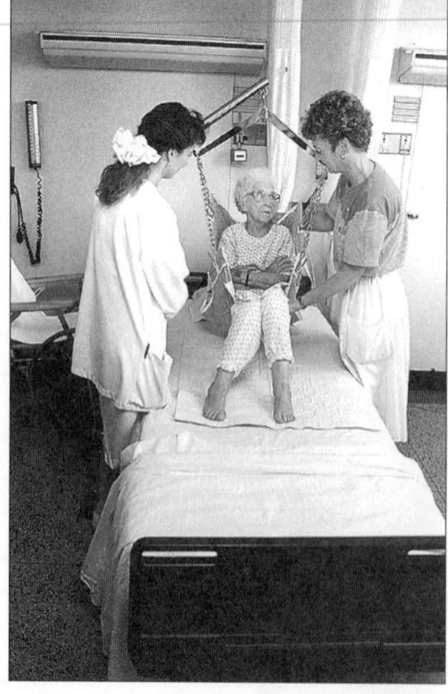

STEP **6f** Proper placement of sling under client.

Step	Rationale
i. Roll client to opposite side and pull hammock (strips) through.	Completes positioning of client on mechanical/hydraulic sling.
j. Roll client supine onto canvas seat.	Sling should extend from shoulders to knees (hammock) to support client's body weight equally.
k. Remove client's glasses, if appropriate.	Swivel bar is close to client's head and could break eyeglasses.
l. Place lift's horseshoe bar under side of bed (on side with chair).	Positions lift efficiently and promotes smooth transfer.
m. Lower horizontal bar to sling level by releasing hydraulic valve. Lock valve.	Positions hydraulic lift close to client. Locking valve prevents injury to client.
n. Attach hooks on strap (chain) to holes in sling. Short chains or straps hook to top holes of sling; longer chains hook to bottom of sling.	Secures hydraulic lift to sling.
o. Elevate head of bed.	Positions client in sitting position.
p. Fold client's arms over chest.	Prevents injury to client's arms.
q. Pump hydraulic handle using long, slow, even strokes until client is raised off bed.	Ensures safe support of client during elevation.
r. Use steering handle to pull lift from bed and maneuver to chair.	Moves client from bed to chair.
s. Roll base around chair.	Positions lift in front of the chair in which client is to be transferred.
t. Release check valve slowly (turn to left) and lower client into chair (see illustration).	Safely guides client into back of chair as seat descends.
u. Close check valve as soon as client is down and straps can be released.	If valve is left open, boom may continue to lower and injure client.
v. Remove straps and mechanical/hydraulic lift (see illustration).	Prevents damage to skin and underlying tissues from canvas or hooks.
w. Check client's sitting alignment and correct if necessary.	Prevents injury from poor posture.
7. Wash hands.	Reduces transmission of microorganisms.

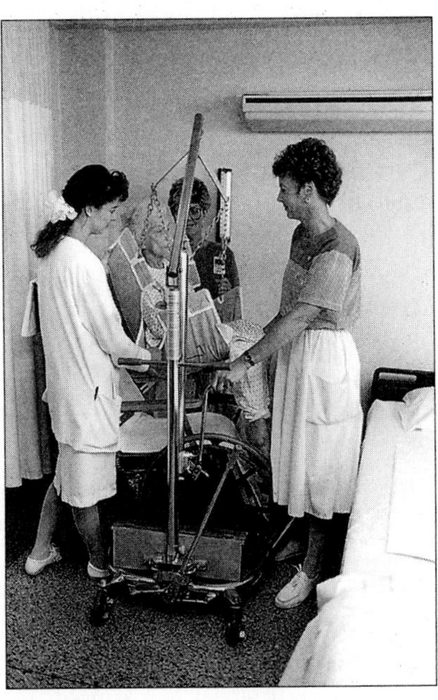

STEP **6t** Use of hydraulic lift to lower client into chair.

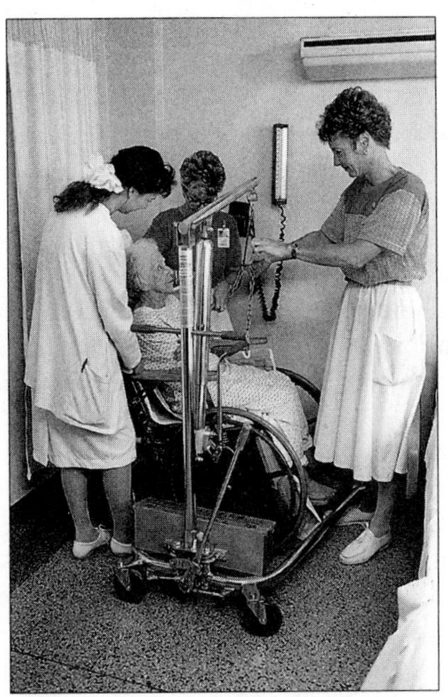

STEP **6v** Removal of hydraulic lift.

Step	Rationale
Evaluation	
1. Monitor vital signs. Ask if client feels fatigued.	Evaluates client's response to postural changes and activity.
2. Observe for correct body alignment and presence of pressure points on skin.	Minimizes risk of immobility complications.
3. Note client's behavioral response to transfer.	Reveals level of motivation and self-care potential.
4. Ask if client experienced pain during transfer.	Determines need for additional pain control or alteration in technique of transferring.

Unexpected Outcomes and Related Interventions

- Client is unable to comprehend and follow directions for transfer.
  - Cognitive impairment affects learning and retention.
  - Reassess continuity and simplicity of instruction.
  - Transfers may be difficult when client is fatigued or in pain; assess prior to transfer (allow for a rest period before transferring, or medicate for pain if indicated).
- Client sustains injury on transfer.
  - Indicates improper transfer technique was used.
  - Evaluate incident that caused injury (e.g., assessment inadequate, change in client status, or improper use of equipment).
  - Complete incident report according to institution policy.
- Client's level of weakness does not permit active transfer.
  - Physical impairments require increased assistance from nursing personnel.
  - Increase bed activity and exercise to heighten tolerance.
- Client continues to bear weight on non–weight-bearing limb.
  - Certain conditions (e.g., hip fractures) need to be non–weight bearing through healing process.
  - Reassess client's understanding of weight-bearing status.
- Client is unable to stand for time required in transfer.
  - Results from increased fatigue, orthostatic hypotension, or pain.
  - Provide for adequate assistance during transfer.
- Localized areas of erythema develop that do not disappear quickly.
  - Implement pressure ulcer prevention strategies (see Chapter 7).
  - Provide frequent skin care.

Recording and Reporting

- Record procedure, including pertinent observations: weakness, ability to follow directions, weight-bearing ability, balance, ability to pivot, number of personnel needed to assist, amount of assistance (muscle strength) required.
- Report any unusual occurrence to nurse in charge. Report transfer ability and assistance needed to next shift or other caregivers. Report progress or remission to rehabilitation staff (physical therapist, occupational therapist).

Teaching Considerations

- For many clients the return to home is coupled with enhanced psychological well-being and increased levels of motivation and ability for self-care function. Appropriate teaching of self-care skills and use of aids to maximize ability enhance outcome.
- Teach family and client transfer skills. Information should include principles of body mechanics and hazards of immobility. Incorporate return demonstration in discharge planning.

Pediatric Considerations

- Whenever possible, transporting child by stretcher, stroller, or wheelchair outside confines of room will increase environmental stimuli and provide social contact with others. The child will benefit from frequent visitors, clocks and calendars, and a program of diversional therapy.

Gerontological Considerations

- Immobilized older adult clients are at risk of developing complications that affect all body systems. These complications include muscle atrophy, contractures, pressure ulcers, cardiovascular and respiratory problems, constipation, urinary stasis, and mental confusion.
- Use a turning sheet to avoid shearing force on the older adult client who has fragile skin.

Home Care Considerations

- Transfer ability at home is greatly enhanced by prior teaching of family and support persons, assessment of home for safety risks and functionality, and provision of applicable aids.
- Family or support person should practice transfer in hospital to achieve success before taking client home. Alternatively, client (if living alone) should practice transfer skills in bed that will be used at home. Client should be taught to transfer to chair with arms for ease of rising and sitting.
- Home should be free of hazards (e.g., throw rugs, electric cords, slippery floors). If wheelchair is used, access must be possible through all doors, and space for transfer must be available in bedroom and bathroom (see Chapter 39).

- Aids that enhance transfer ability are shower stools, commode elevators, handrails on tub, and nonskid shower surface. Many self-care devices are available for wheelchair-bound clients or clients with weak or poor muscle function. These are best prescribed by occupational or physical therapist; however, many medical supply stores can provide excellent information and catalogs of such supplies.

LONG-TERM CARE CONSIDERATIONS

- Long-term care clients may have contractures and need special attention to transfer safely and devices (e.g., extra pillows, padding) to ensure comfort while sitting in a chair.

Skill 27-3 Moving and Positioning Clients in Bed

Correct positioning of clients is crucial for maintaining body alignment and comfort, preventing injury to the musculoskeletal system, and providing sensory, motor, and cognitive stimulation. A client with impaired mobility, decreased sensation, impaired circulation, or lack of voluntary muscle control can develop damage to the musculoskeletal system while lying down. The nurse must minimize this risk by maintaining unrestricted circulation and correct body alignment while moving, turning, or positioning the client.

DELEGATION CONSIDERATIONS

The skills of moving and positioning clients in bed can be delegated to assistive personnel. The caregiver should be instructed about any moving and positioning restrictions (e.g., avoid prone position or client has one-sided weakness).

EQUIPMENT

- Pillows
- Footboard (optional)
- High-top sneakers
- Trochanter roll
- Sandbag
- Hand rolls
- Side rails

STEP	RATIONALE
ASSESSMENT	
1. Assess client's body alignment and comfort level while client is lying down.	Provides baseline data for later comparisons. Determines ways to improve position and alignment.
2. Assess for risk factors that may contribute to complications of immobility:	Increased risk factors require client to be repositioned more frequently.
a. Paralysis: **hemiparesis** resulting from cerebrovascular accident (CVA); decreased sensation	Paralysis impairs movement; muscle tone changes; sensation is affected. Because of difficulty in moving and poor awareness of involved body part, client is unable to protect and position body part for self.
b. Impaired mobility: traction or arthritis or other contributing disease processes	Traction or arthritic changes of affected extremity result in decreased range of joint motion (ROJM).
c. Impaired circulation: arterial insufficiency	Decreased circulation predisposes client to pressure sores.
d. Age: very young, older adult	Premature and young infants require frequent turning because their skin is fragile. Normal physiological changes associated with aging predispose older adults to greater risks for developing complications of immobility.
3. Assess client's level of consciousness.	Determines need for special aids or devices. Clients with altered levels of consciousness may not understand instructions and may be unable to help.
4. Assess client's physical ability to help with moving and positioning: age, level of consciousness, disease process, strength, ROJM, and coordination.	Enables nurse to use client's mobility, strength and coordination. Determines need for additional help. Ensures client and nurse safety.

Step	Rationale
5. Assess for presence of tubes, incisions, and equipment (e.g., traction).	Will alter positioning procedure and type of positions to use.
6. Assess ability and motivation of client, family members, and primary caregiver to participate in moving and positioning client in bed in anticipation of discharge to home.	Determines approach needed for instruction.

Nursing Diagnosis

Defining characteristics from the assessment data may reveal the following nursing diagnoses for clients requiring this skill:

- Activity intolerance
- Impaired physical mobility
- Impaired skin integrity
- Risk for impaired skin integrity

Related factors are individualized based on client's condition or needs.

Planning

Step	Rationale
1. **Expected outcomes** following completion of procedure:	
▪ Client retains ROJM.	Correct positioning allows client to achieve optimal joint mobility and alignment.
▪ Client's skin shows no evidence of breakdown.	Frequent position changes decrease risk of skin breakdown.
▪ Client's comfort is increased.	Proper positioning reduces stress on joints.
▪ Client's level of independence in completing activities of daily living (ADLs) is increased.	Maintaining good body alignment and joint mobility increases client's level of independence and overall mobility. Client with inadequate joint mobility may need assistance to carry out ADLs.
2. Raise level of bed to comfortable working height.	Raises level of work toward nurse's center of gravity.
3. Remove all pillows and devices used in previous position.	Reduces interference from bedding during positioning procedure.
4. Get extra help as needed.	Provides for client and nurse safety.
5. Explain procedure to client.	Helps to decrease anxiety and increase cooperation.

Implementation

Step	Rationale
1. Wash hands.	Reduces transmission of infection.
2. Close door to room or close bedside curtains.	Provides for client privacy.
3. Put bed in flat position.	Provides easy access to client and allows nurses to reposition client without working against gravity.

- ***Critical Decision Point***
  Before flattening bed, account for all tubing, drains, and equipment to prevent dislodgment or spillage if caught in mattress or bed frame as bed is lowered.

Step	Rationale
4. Move immobile client up in bed (one nurse):	
a. Place client on back with head of bed flat. Stand on one side of bed.	Enables nurse to assess body alignment. Reduces gravity's pull on client's upper body.

- ***Critical Decision Point***
  Check physician's orders before positioning client. Some positions may be contraindicated in certain situations (e.g., spinal cord injury, respiratory difficulties, certain neurological conditions, and presence of incisions, drains, or tubing).

Step	Rationale
b. Remove pillow from under head and shoulders and place pillow at head of bed.	Prevents striking client's head against head of bed.

Step	Rationale
c. Begin at client's feet. Face foot of bed at 45-degree angle. Place feet apart with foot nearest head of bed behind other foot (forward-backward stance). Flex knees and hips as needed to bring arms level with client's legs. Shift weight from front to back leg, and slide client's legs diagonally toward head of bed.	Positioning is begun at client's legs because they are lighter and easier to move. Facing direction of movement ensures proper balance. Shifting nurse's weight reduces force needed to move load. Diagonal motion permits pull in direction of force. Flexing knees lowers nurse's center of gravity and uses thigh muscles rather than back muscles.
d. Move parallel to client's hips. Flex knees and hips as needed to bring arms level with client's hips.	Maintains nurse's correct body alignment. Brings nurse closest to object to be moved and lowers center of gravity. Uses thigh muscles rather than back muscles.
e. Slide client's hips diagonally toward head of bed.	Aligns client's hips and feet.
f. Move parallel to client's head and shoulders. Flex knees and hips as needed to bring arms level with client's body.	Maintains nurse's proper body alignment. Brings nurse closer to object to be moved. Lowers nurse's center of gravity. Uses thigh muscles rather than back muscles.
g. Slide arm closest to head of bed under client's neck, with hand reaching under and supporting client's opposite shoulder.	Supports client's head and neck, maintaining alignment and preventing injury during movement.
h. Place other arm under client's upper back.	Supports client's body weight and reduces friction during movement.
i. Slide client's trunk, shoulders, head, and neck diagonally toward head of bed.	Realigns client's body on one side of bed.
j. Elevate top side rail as appropriate. Move to other side of bed and lower side rail.	Upper rails protect client from falling out of bed. Use of all four side rails can increase risk of injury.
k. Repeat procedure, switching sides until client reaches desired position in bed.	
l. Center client in middle of bed, moving body in same three sections.	Maintains proper body alignment. Provides ample room for turning, positioning, and other nursing activities.
5. Assist client in moving up in bed (one or two nurses):	
a. Place client on back with head of bed flat.	Enables nurse to assess body alignment. Reduces gravity's pull on client's upper body.
b. Remove pillow from under head and shoulders and place pillow at head of bed.	Prevents striking client's head against head of bed.
c. Face head of bed.	Facing direction of movement prevents twisting of nurse's body while moving client.
(1) Each nurse should have one arm under client's head and shoulders and one arm under client's thighs.	Provides support across length of client's body.
(2) Alternative position: position one nurse at client's upper body. Nurse's arm nearest head of bed should be under client's head and opposite shoulder; other arm should be under client's closest arm and shoulder. Position other nurse at client's lower torso. The nurse's arms should be under client's lower back and torso.	Prevents trauma to client's musculoskeletal system by supporting shoulder and hip joints and evenly distributing weight.
d. Place feet apart, with foot nearest head of bed behind other foot (forward-backward stance).	Wide base of support increases nurse's balance. Stance enables nurse to shift body weight as client is moved up in bed, thereby reducing force needed to move load.
e. When possible, ask client to flex knees with feet flat on bed.	Decreases friction and enables client to use leg muscles during movement.
f. Instruct client to flex neck, tilting chin toward chest.	Prevents hyperextension of neck when moving client up in bed.
g. Instruct client to assist moving by pushing down with feet on bed surface.	Reduces friction. Increases client mobility. Decreases nurse's workload.
h. Flex knees and hips, bringing forearms closer to level of bed.	Increases balance and strength by bringing nurse's center of gravity closer to client. Uses thighs instead of back muscles.
i. Warn client to push with heels and elevate trunk while breathing out, thus moving toward head of bed on count of three.	Prepares client for move. Reinforces assistance in moving up in bed. Increases client cooperation. Breathing out avoids Valsalva maneuver.

STEP	RATIONALE
j. On count of three, rock and shift weight from front to back leg. At the same time client pushes with heels and elevates trunk.	Rocking enables nurse to improve balance and overcome inertia. Shifting nurse's weight counteracts client's weight and reduces force needed to move load. Client's assistance reduces friction and nurse's workload.
6. Move immobile client up in bed with **drawsheet** or pullsheet (two nurses):	
a. Place drawsheet or pullsheet under client, extending from shoulders to thighs.	Supports client's body weight and reduces friction during movement.
b. Place client on back with head of bed flat.	Even distribution of weight makes lift easier.
c. Position one nurse at each side of client.	Distributes weight equally between nurses.
d. Grasp drawsheet or pullsheet firmly near client.	
e. Place feet apart with forward-backward stance. Flex knees and hips. Shift weight from front to back leg, and move client and drawsheet or pullsheet to desired position in bed.	Facing direction of movement ensures proper balance. Shifting weight reduces force needed to move load. Flexing knees lowers nurses' center of gravity and uses thighs instead of back muscles.
7. Realign client in correct body alignment.	Prevents injury to musculoskeletal system. Nurses may assist client to one of the positions listed here.
a. Position client in supported Fowler's position (see illustration):	

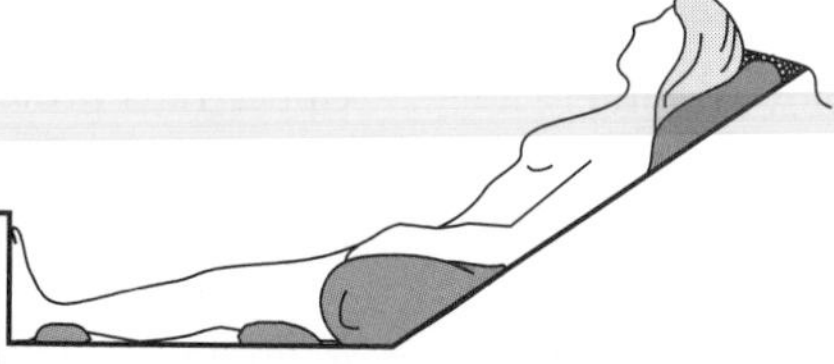

STEP **7a** Footboard in place (Fowler's position).

STEP	RATIONALE
(1) Elevate head of bed 45 to 60 degrees.	Increases comfort, improves ventilation, and increases client's opportunity to socialize or relax.
(2) Rest head against mattress or on small pillow.	Prevents flexion contractures of cervical vertebrae.
(3) Use pillows to support arms and hand if client does not have voluntary control or use of hands and arms.	Prevents shoulder dislocation from effect of downward pull of unsupported arms, promotes circulation by preventing venous pooling, and prevents flexion contractures of arms and wrists.
(4) Position pillow at lower back.	Supports lumbar vertebrae and decreases flexion of vertebrae.
(5) Place small pillow or roll under thigh.	Prevents hyperextension of knee and occlusion of popliteal artery from pressure from body weight.
(6) Place small pillow or roll under ankles.	Prevents prolonged pressure of mattress on heels.

- ***Critical Decision Point***

  *To keep feet in proper alignment, place **footboard** at bottom of client's feet, apply high-top sneakers on client's feet, or use other devices to maintain dorsiflexion.*

STEP	RATIONALE
b. Position hemiplegic client in supported Fowler's position:	
(1) Elevate head of bed 45 to 60 degrees.	Increases comfort, improves ventilation, and increases client's opportunity to relax.
(2) Position client in sitting position as straight as possible.	Counteracts tendency to slump toward affected side. Improves ventilation and cardiac output; decreases intracranial pressure. Improves client's ability to swallow and helps to prevent aspiration of food, liquids, and gastric secretions.

STEP	RATIONALE
(3) Position head on small pillow with chin slightly forward. If client is totally unable to control head movement, hyperextension of the neck must be avoided.	Prevents hyperextension of neck. Too many pillows under head may cause or worsen neck flexion contracture.
(4) Provide support for involved arm and hand on overbed table in front of client. Place arm away from client's side and support elbow with pillow.	Paralyzed muscles do not automatically resist pull of gravity as they do normally. As a result, shoulder subluxation, pain, and edema may occur.

- ***Critical Decision Point***
  Position flaccid *hand in normal resting position with wrist slightly extended, arches of hand maintained, and fingers partially flexed; may use section of rubber ball cut in half; clasp client's hands together.*

- ***Critical Decision Point***
  Position spastic *hand with wrist in neutral position or slightly extended; fingers should be extended with palm down or may be left in relaxed position with palm up.*

STEP	RATIONALE
(5) Flex knees and hips by using pillow or folded blanket under knees.	Ensures proper alignment. Flexion prevents prolonged hyperextension, which could impair joint mobility.
(6) Support feet in dorsiflexion with firm pillow, footboard, or high-top sneakers.	Prevents footdrop. Stimulation of ball of foot by hard surface has tendency to increase muscle tone in client with extensor spasticity of lower extremity.
c. Position client in supine position:	
(1) Place client on back with head of bed flat.	Necessary for placing client in supine position.
(2) Place small rolled towel under lumbar area of back.	Provides support for lumbar spine.
(3) Place pillow under upper shoulders, neck, or head.	Maintains correct alignment and prevents flexion contractures of cervical vertebrae.
(4) Place trochanter rolls or sandbags parallel to lateral surface of client's thighs.	Reduces external rotation of hip.
(5) Place small pillow or roll under ankle to elevate heels (see illustration in Step 7a).	Reduces pressure on heels, helping to prevent pressure sores.
(6) Place footboard or firm pillows against bottom of client's feet, or place high-top sneakers on client's feet.	Maintains feet in dorsiflexion. Prevents footdrop.
(7) Place pillows under pronated forearms, keeping upper arms parallel to client's body (see illustrations).	Reduces internal rotation of shoulder and prevents extension of elbows. Maintains correct body alignment.

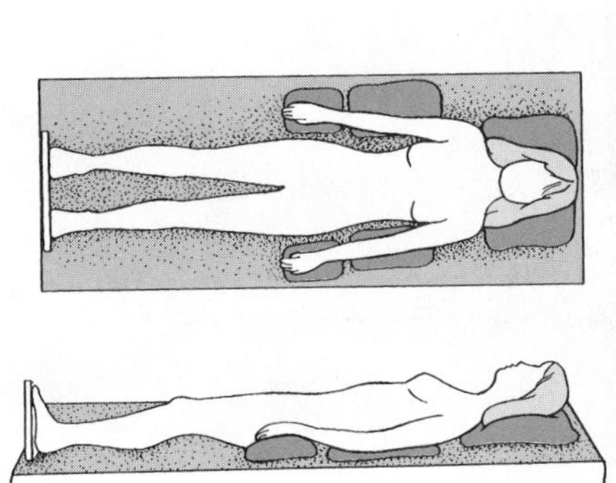
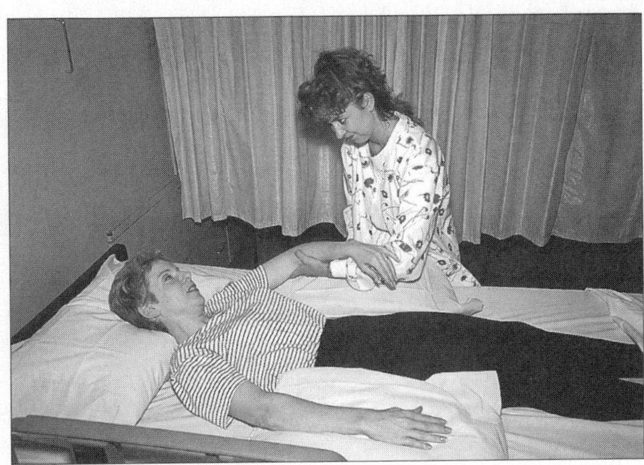

STEP **7c(7)** Supine position with pillows in place.

STEP	RATIONALE
(8) Place **hand rolls** in client's hands. Consider physical therapy referral for use of hand splints.	Reduces extension of fingers and abduction of thumb. Maintains thumb slightly adducted and in opposition to fingers.
d. Position hemiplegic client in supine position:	
(1) Place head of bed flat.	Necessary for positioning in supine position.
(2) Place folded towel or small pillow under shoulder or affected side.	Decreases possibility of pain, joint contracture, and subluxation. Maintains mobility in muscles around shoulder to permit normal movement patterns.
(3) Keep affected arm away from body with elbow extended and palm up. (Alternative is to place arm out to side, with elbow bent and hand toward head of bed.)	Maintains mobility in arm, joints, and shoulder to permit normal movement patterns. (Alternative position counteracts limitation of ability of arm to rotate outward at shoulder [external rotation]. External rotation must be present to raise arm over head without pain.)

- ***Critical Decision Point***

  Position affected hand in one of recommended positions for flaccid or spastic hand.

STEP	RATIONALE
(4) Place folded towel under hip of involved side.	Diminishes effect of spasticity in entire leg by controlling hip position.
(5) Flex affected knee 30 degrees by supporting it on pillow or folded blanket.	Slight flexion breaks up abnormal extension pattern of leg. Extensor spasticity is most severe when client is supine.
(6) Support feet with soft pillows at right angle to leg.	Maintains foot in dorsiflexion and prevents footdrop. Pillows prevent stimulation to ball of foot by hard surface, which has tendency to increase muscle tone in client with extensor spasticity of lower extremity.
e. Position client in prone position:	
(1) Roll client to one side.	Prepares client for positioning.
(2) Roll client over arm positioned close to body, with elbow straight and hand under hip. Position on abdomen in center of bed.	Positions client correctly so alignment can be maintained.
(3) Turn client's head to one side, and support head with small pillow (see illustration).	Reduces flexion or hyperextension of cervical vertebrae.
(4) Place small pillow under client's abdomen below level of diaphragm (see illustration).	Reduces pressure on breasts of some female clients and decreases hyperextension of lumbar vertebrae and strain on lower back. Improves breathing by reducing mattress pressure on diaphragm.
(5) Support arms in flexed position level at shoulders.	Maintains proper body alignment. Support reduces risk of joint dislocation.
(6) Support lower legs with pillow to elevate toes (see illustration).	Prevents footdrop. Reduces external rotation of legs. Reduces mattress pressure on toes.

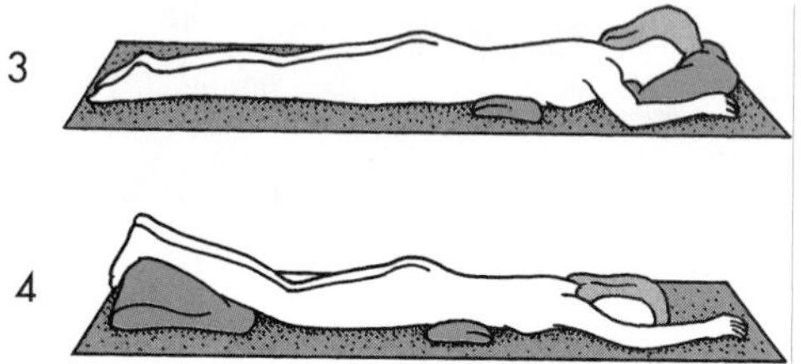

STEP **7e(3-4)** Prone position with pillows in place.

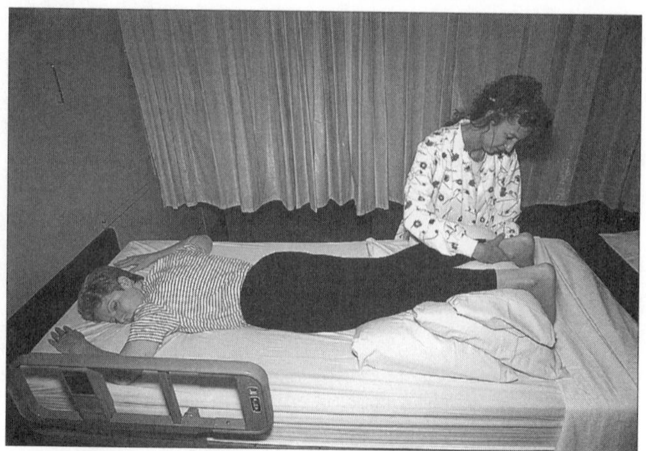

STEP **7e(6)** Prone position with pillows supporting lower legs.

STEP	RATIONALE
f. Position hemiplegic client in prone position:	

• ***Critical Decision Point***
Increase frequency of positioning if pressure areas begin to appear, joint mobility becomes impaired or worsened, or client complains of discomfort. Consult with physical and occupational therapists as needed.

STEP	RATIONALE
(1) Move client toward unaffected side.	Ensures proper alignment in center of bed when client is rolled onto abdomen.
(2) Roll client onto side.	
(3) Place pillow on client's abdomen.	Prevents sagging of abdomen when client is rolled over; decreases hyperextension of lumbar vertebrae and strain on lower back.
(4) Roll client onto abdomen by positioning involved arm close to client's body, with elbow straight and hand under hip. Roll client carefully over arm.	Prevents injury to affected side.
(5) Turn head toward involved side.	Promotes development of neck and trunk extension, which is necessary for standing and walking.
(6) Position involved arm out to side, with elbow bent, hand toward head of bed, and fingers extended (if possible).	Counteracts limitation of arm's ability to rotate outward at shoulder (external rotation). External rotation must be present to raise arm over head without pain.
(7) Flex knees slightly by placing pillow under legs from knees to ankles.	Flexion prevents prolonged hyperextension, which could impair joint mobility.
(8) Keep feet at right angle to legs by using pillow high enough to keep toes off mattress and by applying high-top sneakers.	Maintains feet in dorsiflexion.
g. Position client in 30 degree lateral (side-lying) position:	
(1) Lower head of bed completely or as low as client can tolerate.	Provides position of comfort for client and removes pressure from bony prominences on back.
(2) Position client to side of bed opposite direction client is to be turned.	Provides room for client to turn to side.
(3) Turn client onto side. To turn helpless client onto side, flex client's knee that will not be next to mattress. Place one hand on client's hip and one hand on client's shoulder.	Use of leverage makes turning to side easy.

• ***Critical Decision Point***
Clients at risk for pressure ulcer development require the 30-degree lateral position (see Chapter 7).

STEP	RATIONALE
(4) Roll client onto side toward nurse.	Rolling decreases trauma to tissues. In addition, client is positioned so leverage on hip makes turning easy.
(5) Place pillow under client's head and neck.	Maintains alignment. Reduces lateral neck flexion. Decreases strain on sternocleidomastoid muscle.
(6) Bring dependent shoulder blade forward.	Prevents client's weight from resting directly on shoulder joint.
(7) Position both arms in slightly flexed position. Upper arm is supported by pillow level with shoulder; other arm, by mattress.	Decreases internal rotation and adduction of shoulder. Supporting both arms in slightly flexed position protects joint. Ventilation is improved because chest is able to expand more easily.
(8) Bring dependent hip slightly forward.	30 degree lateral position reduces pressure on trochanter.
(9) Place small tuck-back pillow behind client's back. (Make by folding pillow lengthwise. Smooth area is slightly tucked under client's back.)	Provides support to maintain client on side.

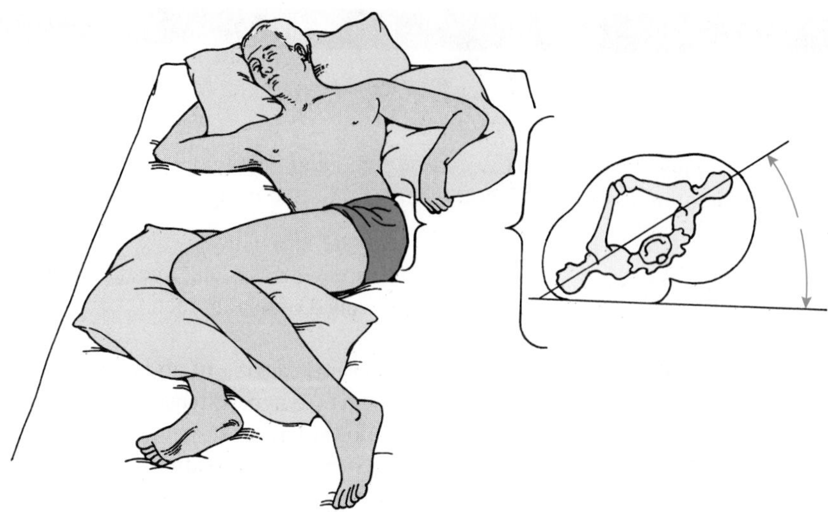

STEP **7g(10)** Lateral position with pillows in place.

STEP	RATIONALE
(10) Place pillow under semiflexed upper leg level at hip from groin to foot (see illustration).	Flexion prevents hyperextension of leg. Maintains leg in correct alignment. Prevents pressure on bony prominence.
(11) Place sandbag parallel to plantar surface of dependent foot. Place high-top sneakers on client's feet.	Maintains dorsiflexion of foot. Prevents footdrop.
h. Position client in Sims' (semiprone) position:	
(1) Lower head of bed completely.	Provides for proper body alignment while client is lying down.
(2) Place client in supine position.	Prepares client for position.
(3) Roll client on side and position in lateral position, lying partially on abdomen, with dependent shoulder lifted out and arm placed at client's side.	Client is rolled only partially on abdomen.
(4) Place small pillow under client's head.	Maintains proper alignment and prevents lateral neck flexion.
(5) Place pillow under flexed upper arm, supporting arm level with shoulder.	Prevents internal rotation of shoulder. Maintains alignment.
(6) Place pillow under flexed upper legs, supporting leg level with hip.	Prevents internal rotation of hip and adduction of leg. Flexion prevents hyperextension of leg. Reduces mattress pressure on knees and ankles.
(7) Place sandbags parallel to plantar surface of foot (see illustration) or apply high-top sneakers.	Maintains foot in dorsiflexion. Prevents footdrop.

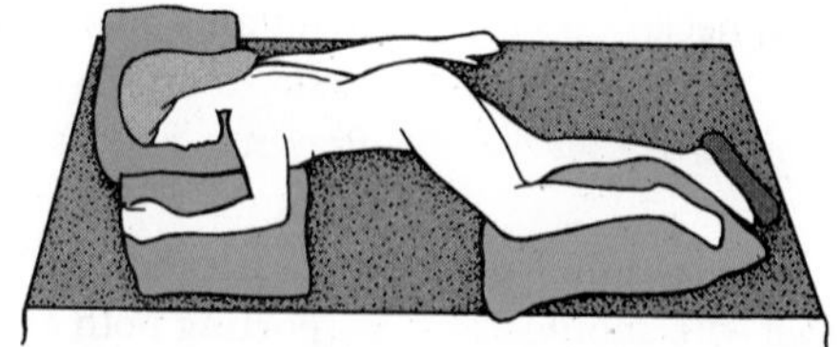

STEP **7h(7)** Sandbag supporting foot in dorsiflexion.

i. **Logrolling** the client: (two nurses)

- ***Critical Decision Point***

  A nurse should supervise and aid assistive personnel when there is a physician's order to logroll a client. Clients who have suffered from a spinal cord injury or are recovering from neck, back, or spinal surgery often need to keep the spinal column in straight alignment to prevent further injury.

STEP	RATIONALE
(1) Place small pillow between client's knees.	Prevents tension on the spinal column and adduction of the hip.
(2) Cross client's arms on chest.	Prevents injury to arms.
(3) Position a nurse on each side of bed.	Distributes weight equally between nurses during turning.
(4) Fanfold or roll the drawsheet or pullsheet, along side of client that will be turning.	Provides strong handles to grip the drawsheet or pullsheet without slipping.
(5) With one nurse grasping pull sheet at shoulders and lower hips, roll the client as one unit in a smooth, continuous motion on the count of three. The second nurse assists in supporting client's back.	This maintains proper alignment by moving all body parts at the same time, preventing tension or twisting of the spinal column.
(6) Nurse on the opposite side of the bed places pillows along the length of the client for support (see illustration).	Maintains client in side-lying position.
(7) Gently lean the client as a unit back towards the pillows for support (see illustration).	Ensures continued straight alignment of spinal column, preventing injury.
8. Wash hands.	Reduces transmission of infection.

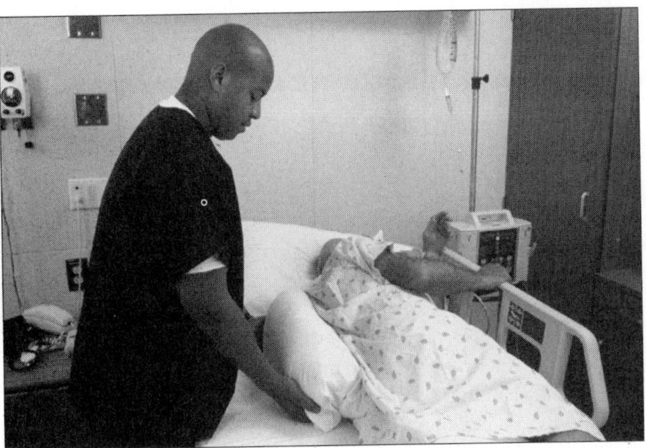

STEP **7i(6)** Place pillows along client's back for support.

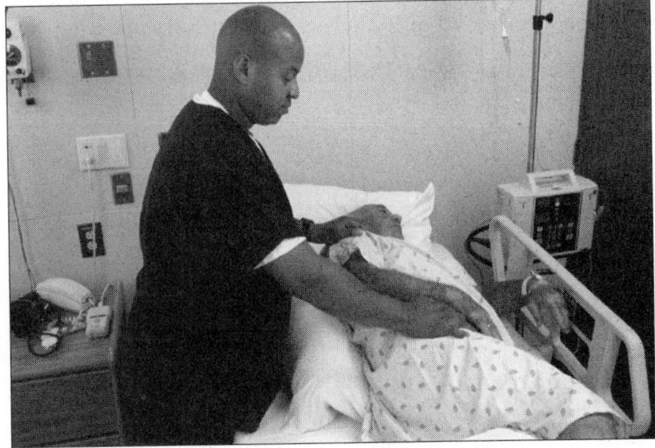

STEP **7i(7)** Gently lean client as a unit against pillows.

EVALUATION

1. Assess client's body alignment, position, and level of comfort.	Determines effectiveness of positioning. Additional supports (e.g., pillows, bath blankets) may be added or removed to promote comfort and correct body alignment.
2. Measure ROJM (see Chapter 28).	Determines if joint contracture is developing.
3. Assess for areas of erythema or breakdown involving skin.	Provides ongoing observation regarding client's skin and musculoskeletal systems. Indicates complications of immobility or improper positioning of body part.

UNEXPECTED OUTCOMES AND RELATED INTERVENTIONS

- Joint contractures develop or worsen.
  - Improper positioning results in shortening of muscles.
  - Increase range of motion to affected and immobilized areas.
- Skin shows areas of erythema and breakdown.
  - Increase frequency of repositioning.
  - Place turning schedule above client's bed.
- Client avoids moving.
  - Medicate with analgesia as ordered by physician to ensure client's comfort before moving.
  - Allow pain medication to take effect before proceeding.

RECORDING AND REPORTING

- Record procedure and observations (e.g., condition of skin, joint movement, client's ability to assist with positioning).
- Report observations at change of shift and document in nurses' notes.

Teaching Considerations

- Include family in explanations, especially when caring for infant, young child, or confused or unconscious client.
- Teach client ways to assist with positioning.
- Provide opportunity for return demonstration.
- Teach client and family signs and symptoms of pressure sores and contractures.

Pediatric Considerations

- Children should be encouraged to be as active as their condition and restrictive devices allow. Opportunity, materials, or objects to stimulate activity and encouragement and participation of others must be available.
- Children who are unable to move will need passive exercise and movement (see Chapter 28).

Gerontological Considerations

- Position older adult client to avoid strain on joints, tendons, ligaments, and muscles.
- Older adult clients must be repositioned every 2 hours, and a regular program of ROJM exercises must be maintained.

Home Care Considerations

- Assess ability and motivation of client, family members, and primary caregiver to participate in moving and positioning client in bed.
- Assess home to determine compatibility of environment with assistive devices (e.g., overbed trapeze, Hoyer lift, hospital bed).
- Assess skin for pressure areas and friction burns.

Long-Term Care Considerations

- Clients who have maintained bed rest for a long period of time may revert back to a favorite position. Frequently assess these clients, and turn more often as needed.
- Use lift (draw) sheets as often as possible to prevent shearing force on fragile skin.
- Allow client to assist with moving and positioning whenever possible to promote independence.

Critical Thinking Exercises

1. Mr. Clark is a 37-year-old man who suffered a spinal cord injury in a motor vehicle accident. He was admitted on your shift. Before looking at the physician's orders, what do you think would be the safest technique to move Mr. Clark from side to side? What important information concerning body alignment, positioning, and transfer should be included in the report to the oncoming nurse?
2. Your client assignment for the day is a 5-year-old girl with decreased mobility related to the application of a full spica (body) cast. Describe several nursing interventions to increase her mobility, keeping in mind the special needs relative to her age group.
3. Mrs. Swain has just undergone extensive abdominal surgery. What assessment parameters need to be considered before moving and positioning her in bed? What precautions should the nurse take before transferring Mrs. Swain to the chair?
4. A 73-year-old woman has been admitted to your unit with bilateral pneumonia. Past medical history reveals an old cerebrovascular accident (CVA) with right hemiplegia with flaccid paralysis. What assessment parameters need to be considered before moving and positioning her in bed? Describe proper body alignment and transfer techniques for this client.

References

Elkin M, Perry A, Potter P: *Nursing interventions and clinical skills,* St. Louis, 1999, Mosby.

Gassett R, Hearne B, Keelan B: Ergonomics and body mechanics in the work place, *Orthop Clin North Am* 27(4):861, 1996.

Lueckenotte A: *Gerontologic nursing,* ed 2, St. Louis, 2000, Mosby.

McCance K, Huether S: *Pathophysiology: the biologic basis for disease in adults and children,* ed 3, St. Louis, 1998, Mosby.

Occupational Health and Safety Administration (OSHA): Ergonomics standard proposal, *Federal Register* 29 CFR Part 1910, January 24, 2000, (www.osha-slc.gov/SLTC/ergonomics/index.html).

Owens B, Welden N, Kane J: What are we teaching about lifting and transferring patients? *Res Nurs Health* 22:3, 1999.

Phipps W, Sands J, Marek J: *Medical-surgical nursing: concepts and clinical practice,* ed 6, St. Louis, 1999, Mosby.

Wong DL and others: *Whaley and Wong's nursing care of infants and children,* ed 6, St. Louis, 1999, Mosby.

28

Exercise and Ambulation

Skills

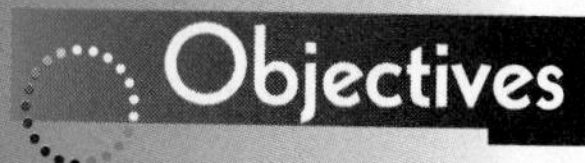

Objectives

Mastery of content in this chapter will enable the nurse to:

- Define the key terms listed.
- Discuss indications for assisting with ambulation or using devices to assist with ambulation.
- Discuss indications for performing range-of-motion and isometric exercises.
- Describe measures to minimize orthostatic hypotension.
- Identify significant assessment data to be noted before assisting with ambulation and range-of-motion and isometric exercises.
- Demonstrate the following skills on selected clients: assisting with ambulation, assisting with ambulation with the use of an ambulation aid, assisting with range-of-motion exercises, assisting with isometric exercises, applying elastic stockings, and instituting measures to minimize orthostatic hypotension.
- Develop teaching plans for selected clients for safety precautions to use at home while using an ambulation aid, applying and monitoring effects of elastic stockings and pneumatic compression devices, and performing range-of-motion and isometric exercises.

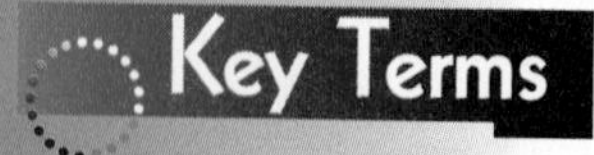

Key Terms

Abduction
Active range-of-motion exercises
Active-assisted range-of-motion exercises
Activity tolerance
Adduction
Atrophy
Bed rest
Circumduction
Contractures
Crutch gait
Crutch palsy
Dangling
Deep vein thrombosis
Dorsal
Dorsiflexion
Eversion
Exercises
Extension
External rotation
Flexion
Footboard
Gait
Gait belt
Hyperextension
Immobility
Internal rotation
Inversion
Isometric contractions
Isometric exercise
Isotonic exercises
Joint
Lateral flexion
Mobility
Opposition
Orthostatic hypotension
Osteoblastic
Osteoclastic
Passive range-of-motion exercises
Plantar flexion
Pronation
Radial flexion
Resistive isometric exercises
Rotation
Supination
Thrombus
Ulnar flexion

Mobility refers to a person's *ability* to move about freely, and **immobility** refers to a person's *inability* to move about freely. Mobility and immobility are best understood as the end points of a continuum, with many degrees of partial mobility in between. Some clients move back and forth on the mobility-immobility continuum, but for other clients, immobility is absolute and continues for an indefinite period.

The ability to move body parts independently is a function most people take for granted. The level of mobility has a significant impact on an individual's physiological, psychosocial, and developmental well-being (Hamilton and Lyon, 1995). When there is an alteration in mobility, many body systems are at risk for impairment. Impaired mobility can result in altered cardiovascular functioning such as **orthostatic hypotension,** disrupt normal metabolic functioning, produce disuse atrophy, increase risk for pulmonary complications such as pneumonia, promote the development of pressure ulcers, and affect urinary elimination, giving rise to the development of renal calculi and urinary tract infections (McCance and Huether, 1998; Potter and Perry, 2001).

The severity of the impairment related to immobility depends on the client's age, overall health status, nutritional status, and the degree of immobility experienced. For example, pronounced effects of immobility develop more quickly in older adult clients with chronic illnesses than they do in younger clients. Older adults are at greater risk for developing orthostatic hypotension, syncope, confusion, increased risk of fractures, and functional incontinence as a result of decreased mobility from **bed rest** (Hamilton and Lyon, 1995). Alterations in mobility can have profound psychosocial and developmental effects. Immobilization may lead to emotional, intellectual, sensory, and sociocultural responses. For adults, immobility may alter employment, family role functions, and social interactions. Such changes can lead to altered self-concept and lowered self-esteem. Children also are affected by immobility. Activity for them is a way of releasing energy and expressing themselves. When deprived of physical activity, children become restless and may even show signs of anger and aggression (Wong and others, 1999).

Changes in a client's mobility can result from various health problems. Examples of medical conditions that can alter mobility are musculoskeletal conditions such as fractured extremities or muscle sprains, neurological conditions such as spinal cord trauma, degenerative neurological conditions such as myasthenia gravis, and head injuries. Some clients may actually be immobilized for therapeutic reasons (e.g., prescribed bed rest, reduced activity). Nursing measures attempt to maintain and/or restore optimal mobility as well as to decrease the hazards associated with immobility. Frequent repositioning, deep breathing and coughing exercises, muscle and joint exercises, increased fluid intake, and dietary intake of foods containing fiber are measures that help to reduce the hazards of immobility.

The authors acknowledge the contribution of Mary Mercer to this chapter in previous editions of this text.

Skill Performance Guidelines

1. Check the physician's orders to determine the client's activity level and type of **exercises** or assistive device to be used. This action must be done to protect the physician and nurse legally and to determine the frequency of intervention and type of ambulation or exercise to be used.
2. Know the client's past medical history. The nurse should know why the client needs assistance with ambulation and any contraindication or limits to exercise.
3. Know the client's normal range for vital signs. Vital signs vary. Exercise and mobility can be fatiguing and stressful, so a set of baseline vital signs is necessary.
4. Assess baseline muscle strength. The client may need muscle-strengthening exercises before ambulation.
5. Assess baseline **joint** function. This knowledge helps the nurse to determine whether range-of-motion exercises are needed and provides a baseline for comparison of joint function after range-of-motion exercises are performed.
6. Obtain and become familiar with the type of assistive device to be used. Nurses need to know proper preparation and use of devices to be able to teach clients to use them safely and correctly.
7. Prepare the client. The client may be afraid of falling during ambulation so schedule other activities so that the client is not fatigued. Obtain extra personnel, safety devices, and flat, nonskid shoes for the client.
8. Determine the type and frequency of intervention. Activity that is appropriate for one day or one shift can change, resulting in an increased or decreased need for assistance with ambulation or a change in the type of intervention.
9. Know the client's home care plan. The client may need to continue the exercise regimen or use an assistive device at home.

Skill 28-1 Performing Range-of-Motion Exercises

Regardless of whether the cause of immobility is permanent or temporary, the immobilized client must receive some type of exercise to prevent excessive muscle **atrophy** and joint **contractures.** The total amount of activity required to prevent disuse syndrome is about 2 hours for every 24-hour period, but this activity must be scheduled throughout the day to prevent the client from remaining inactive for long periods.

Exercise prevents some of the complications of immobility and helps to prepare a client for ambulation. The nurse may use range-of-motion (ROM) exercise, **isometric exercise** (see Skill 28-2), and **resistive isometric exercises** to help the client maintain muscle and joint function.

ROM exercises put each joint through as full a range of motion as possible without causing discomfort. ROM exercises may be *active, passive,* or *active-assisted.* **Active range-of-motion exercises** are defined as exercises the client is able to perform independently, and **passive range-of-motion exercises** are performed for the client by someone else. **Active-assisted range-of-motion exercises** are performed by a client with some assistance. A client who is weak or partially paralyzed may be able to move a limb partially through its range of motion. In this case the nurse can help the client perform active-assisted ROM exercises by helping the client finish the full ROM. Another form of active-assisted ROM exercise is when a client uses the strong arm to exercise the weaker or paralyzed arm.

ROM exercises are the same regardless of whether the client can do the exercises independently or some degree of assistance is required by the client. Active ROM exercises should be encouraged if the client's health status allows because they involve the client in self-care and increase independence, self-control, and self-esteem. Active and active-assisted ROM exercises help to prevent muscular atrophy and joint contracture. Passive ROM exercises help to maintain joint function but do not result in sufficient muscle tension to maintain muscle tone. Active ROM exercises can be incorporated into activities of daily living (ADLs) (Table 28-1) as well as into children's play activities (Wong and others, 1999). Examples of exercise through play include having the child act like a butterfly or throw a bean bag or wadded piece of paper into a trash can or at a target.

Delegation Considerations

The skill of performing range-of-motion exercises can be delegated to assistive personnel. Clients with spinal cord or orthopedic trauma usually require exercise by professional nurses or physical therapists. Caregivers must be instructed to perform exercises slowly and to provide adequate support to each joint being exercised. In addition, caregivers need to be reminded not to exercise joints beyond the point of resistance or to the point of fatigue or pain.

Table 28-1 Incorporating Active Range-of Motion Exercises Into Activities of Daily Living

Joint Exercised	Activity of Daily Living	Movement
Neck	Nodding head yes	Flexion
	Shaking head no	Rotation
	Moving right ear to right shoulder	Lateral flexion
	Moving left ear to left shoulder	Lateral flexion
Shoulder	Reaching to turn on overhead light	Flexion
	Reaching to bedside stand for book	Extension
	Scratching back	Hyperextension
	Rotating shoulders toward chest	Abduction
	Rotating shoulders toward back	Adduction
Elbow	Eating, bathing, shaving, grooming	Flexion, extension
Wrist	Eating, bathing, shaving, grooming	Flexion, extension, hyperextension, abduction, adduction
Fingers and thumb	All activities requiring fine motor coordination (e.g., writing, eating, hobbies)	Flexion, extension, abduction, adduction, opposition
Hip	Walking	Flexion, extension, hyperextension
	Moving to side-lying position	Flexion, extension, abduction
	Moving from side-lying position	Extension, adduction
	Rolling feet inward	Internal rotation
	Rolling feet outward	External rotation
Knee	Walking	Flexion, extension
	Moving to and from side-lying position	Flexion, extension
Ankle	Walking	Dorsiflexion, plantar flexion
	Moving toe toward head of bed	Dorsiflexion
	Moving toe toward foot of bed	Plantar flexion
Toes	Walking	Extension, hyperextension
	Wiggling toes	Abduction, adduction

Step	Rationale
Assessment	
1. Review client's chart to determine client's medical history and obtain physician's order if needed.	Any type of joint problem, cardiac problem, or other condition that may be aggravated by energy expenditure or joint movement indicates the need to discuss ROM exercises with client's physician. Therefore the nurse must use some judgment in deciding whether to institute exercises independently or to consult the physician before beginning exercises.
2. Assess baseline joint function.	Assessment of baseline joint formation is important for evaluating later ROM capabilities.
a. Observe client's ability to perform ROM exercises during normal ADLs.	Allows nurse to observe client's functional abilities in using extremities.
b. During initial ROM exercises assess for the following:	
(1) Any limitation in normal ROM or any unusual increase in mobility of joint	Decreased ROM may indicate arthritis, inflammatory process, or contracture (Potter and Perry, 2001).
(2) Any signs of redness or increased heat in skin overlying joint	May indicate joint problem that contraindicates ROM exercises or may indicate inflammatory joint disease more commonly known as arthritis (McCance and Huether, 1998).
(3) Tenderness in or around joint	May indicate inflammatory process.

STEP	RATIONALE
(4) Crepitus produced by motion of joint	Crepitus, a crunching or grating sensation that is audible or palpable when the joint is moved, is an indicator of a pathological condition within the joint (Phipps, Sands, and Marek, 1999).
(5) Deformities	Deformities suggest bony enlargement (e.g., degenerative joint disease) or contracture.
3. Assess client's or caregiver's understanding of ROM exercises to be used.	Allows client to verbalize concerns and identifies educational needs of client or caregiver.

NURSING DIAGNOSIS

Defining characteristics from the assessment data may reveal the following nursing diagnoses for clients requiring this skill:

- Activity intolerance
- Fatigue
- Impaired physical mobility
- Deficient knowledge regarding ROM exercise techniques
- Pain (acute, chronic)
- Risk for impaired skin integrity

Related factors are individualized based on client's condition or needs.

PLANNING

STEP	RATIONALE
1. **Expected outcomes** following completion of procedure:	
▪ Range of joint motion is within normal limits or client's baseline range for each joint.	Indicates full joint mobility and decreases risk of contracture formation.
▪ Client denies discomfort during exercises.	Joints are exercised safely.
▪ Client demonstrates ROM during ADLs.	Incorporation of teaching into routine care makes skill relevant to client's needs.
2. Explain procedure and reason for performing ROM exercises.	Relieves client's anxiety and encourages cooperation and participation.
3. Assist client to comfortable position.	Positioning allows easy access to joints for complete ROM.

IMPLEMENTATION

STEP	RATIONALE
1. Wash hands.	Reduces transmission of microorganisms.
2. Fully expose only limb to be exercised.	Provides privacy and avoids embarrassing client. Joint unencumbered can move in full ROM.
3. Raise bed to comfortable position and stand on side of bed of joints to be exercised.	Maintains proper body mechanics to prevent back strain as exercises are carried out.
4. Be sure ROM exercises are performed slowly and gently.	Prevents joint strain.

- ***Critical Decision Point***
  Older adults may need ROM exercises in two or more sessions to control fatigue.

STEP	RATIONALE
5. When performing ROM exercises, support joint by holding distal and proximal areas adjacent to joint (see illustration), by cradling distal portion of extremity (see illustration), or by using cupped hand to support joint (see illustration).	Support is provided to joint while ROM exercises are performed.
6. Begin following exercises in sequence outlined. Each movement should be repeated five times during exercise period. NOTE: Discontinue exercise if client complains of discomfort or if there is resistance or muscle spasm.	It is easiest to perform exercises in head-to-toe format.

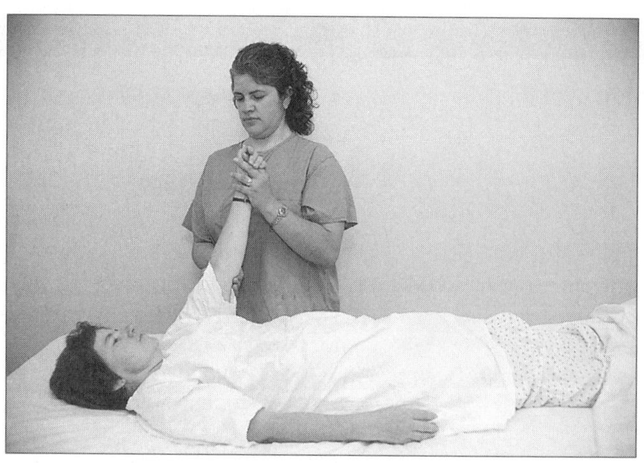

STEP **5(1)** Support joint by holding distal and proximal areas adjacent to joint.

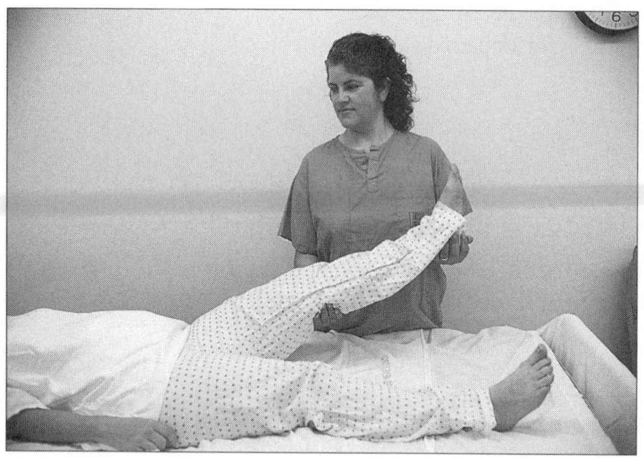

STEP **5(2)** Support joint by cradling distal portion of extremity.

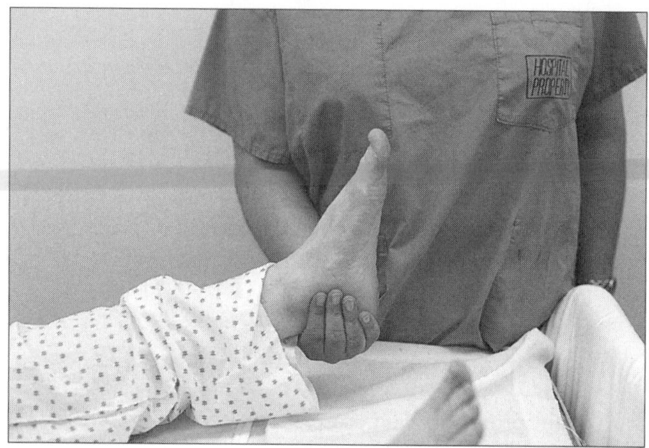

STEP **5(3)** Support joint by using cupped hand to support joint.

STEP	RATIONALE
a. Neck	
(1) **Flexion:** Bring chin to rest on chest (ROM: 45 degrees) (see illustration).	If flexion contracture of neck occurs, client's neck is permanently flexed with chin to or actually touching chest. Ultimately, client's total body alignment is altered and visual field is changed. Contractures can significantly limit the functioning of the client (Phipps, Sands, and Marek, 1999).
(2) **Extension:** Return head to erect position (ROM: 45 degrees) (see illustration).	
(3) **Hyperextension:** Bend head as far back as possible (ROM: 10 degrees) (see illustration).	
(4) **Lateral flexion:** Tilt head as far as possible toward each shoulder (ROM: 40 to 45 degrees) (see illustration).	

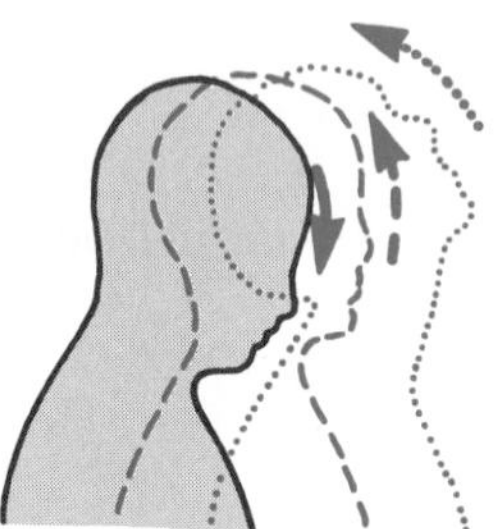

STEP **6a(1-3)** Flexion, extension, and hyperextension of neck.

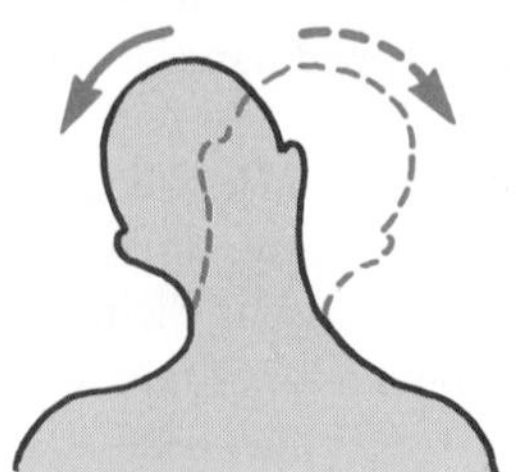

STEP **6a(4)** Lateral flexion of neck.

STEP	RATIONALE
(5) **Rotation:** Rotate head in circular motion (ROM: 360 degrees) (see illustrations).	

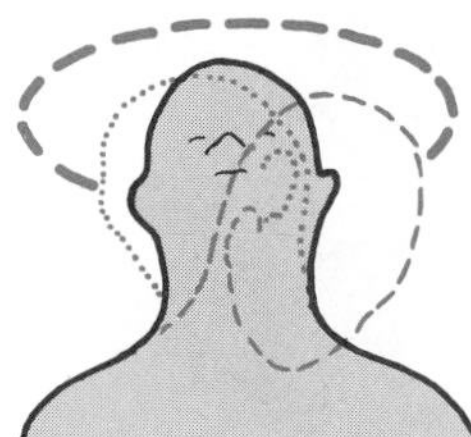

STEP **6a(5a)** Rotate head in circular motion.

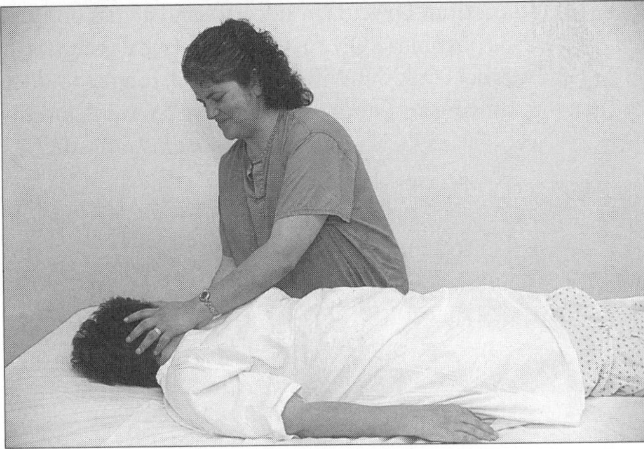

STEP **6a(5b)** Rotate head in circular motion with client in supine position.

b. Shoulder

(1) **Flexion:** Raise arm from side position forward to above head (ROM: 180 degrees) (see illustration).

Exercising shoulder effectively increases power of deltoid muscle. This strength will help if client needs to use an ambulation device, such as crutches, later.

(2) **Extension:** Return arm to position at side of body (ROM: 180 degrees).

(3) **Hyperextension:** Move arm behind body, keeping elbow straight (ROM: 45 to 60 degrees) (see illustration).

(4) **Abduction:** Raise arm to side to position above head with palm away from head (ROM: 180 degrees) (see illustration).

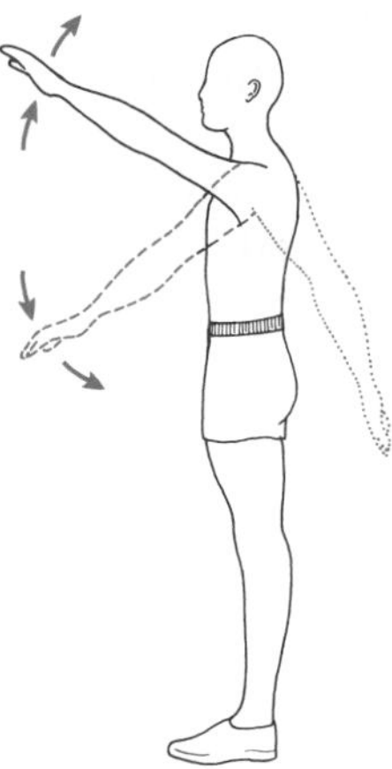

STEP **6b(3)** Hyperextension of shoulder.

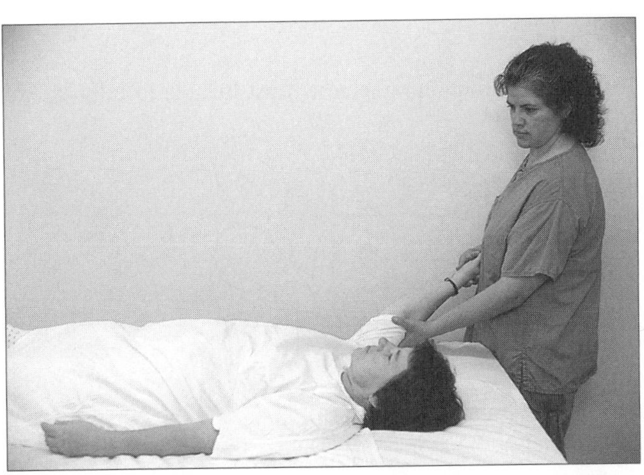

STEP **6b(1)** Flexion of shoulder.

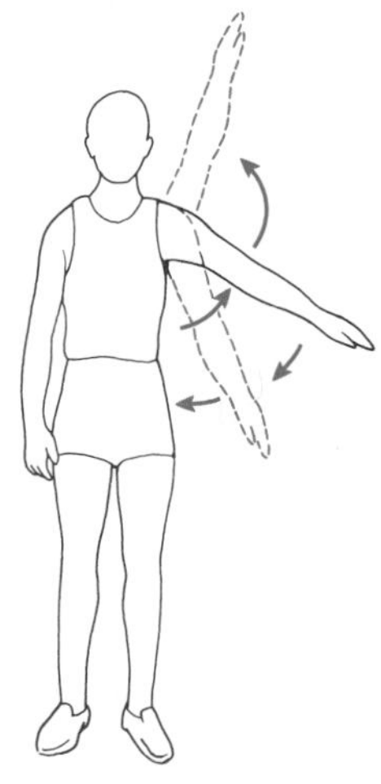

STEP **6b(4)** Abduction and adduction of shoulder.

STEP	RATIONALE

(5) **Adduction:** Lower arm sideways and across body as far as possible (ROM: 320 degrees) (see illustration).
(6) **Internal rotation:** With elbow flexed, rotate shoulder by moving arm until thumb is turned inward and toward back (ROM: 90 degrees) (see illustration).

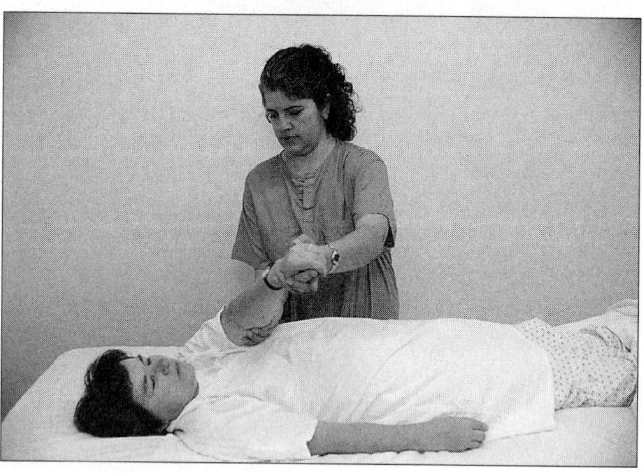

STEP **6b(5)** Adduction of shoulder.

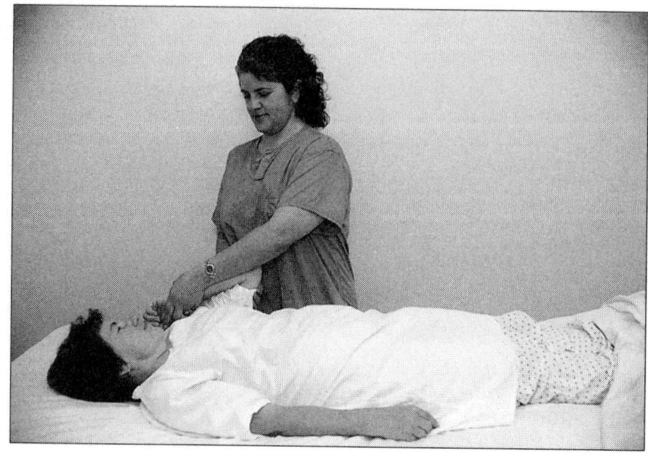

STEP **6b(6)** Internal rotation of shoulder.

(7) **External rotation:** With elbow flexed, move arm until thumb is upward and lateral to head (ROM: 90 degrees) (see illustration).
(8) **Circumduction:** Move arm in full circle. Circumduction is a combination of all movements of ball-and-socket joint (ROM: 360 degrees) (see illustration).

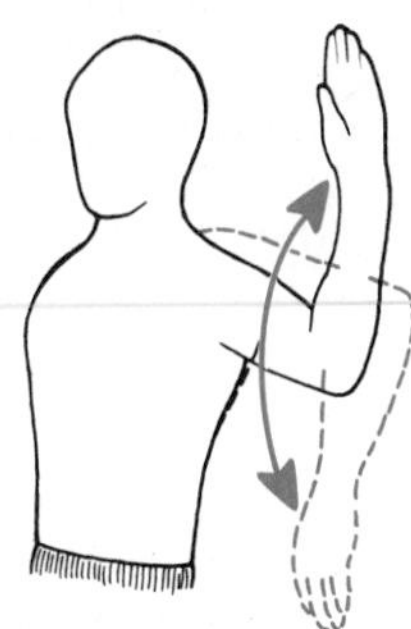

STEP **6b(7)** Rotation of shoulder.

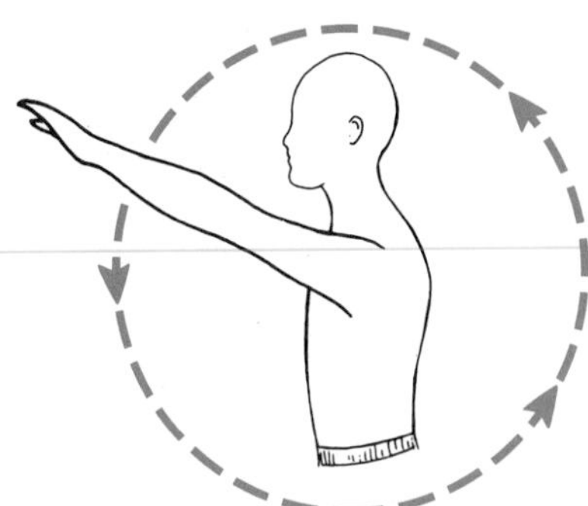

STEP **6b(8)** Circumduction of shoulder.

c. Elbow
(1) **Flexion:** Bend elbow so that lower arm moves toward its shoulder joint and hand is level with shoulder (ROM: 150 degrees) (see illustration).
(2) **Extension:** Straighten elbow by lowering hand (ROM: 150 degrees) (see illustration).
(3) **Hyperextension:** Bend lower arm back as far as possible (ROM: 10 to 20 degrees).

For optimal functioning, elbow must be able to fully extend and flex.

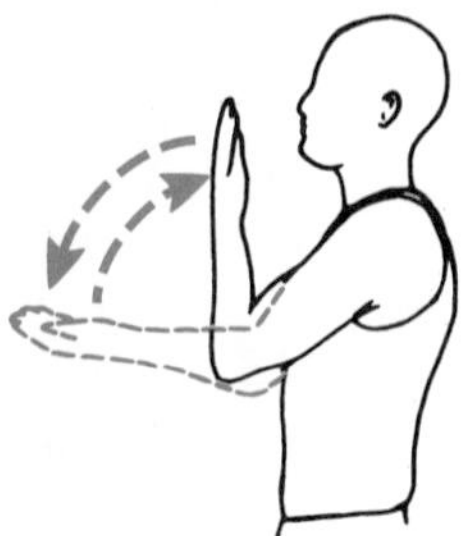

STEP **6c(1-2)** Flexion and extension of elbow.

STEP	RATIONALE

d. Forearm

(1) **Supination:** Turn lower arm and hand so that palm is up (ROM: 70 to 90 degrees) (see illustration).

(2) **Pronation:** Turn lower arm so that palm is down (ROM 70 to 90 degrees) (see illustration).

For optimal functioning, forearm must be able to rotate from supination to pronation.

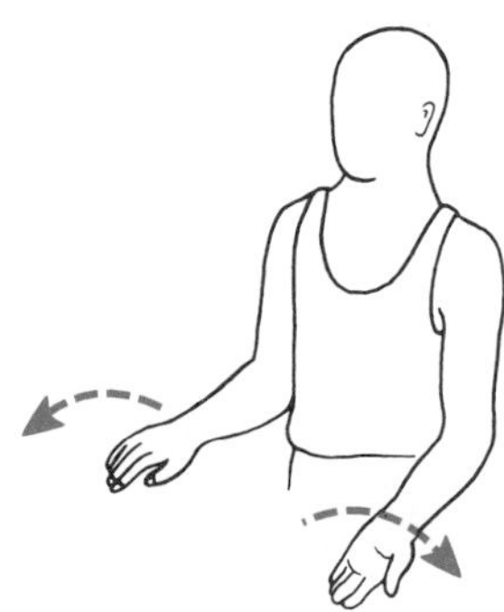

STEP **6d(1-2)** Supination and pronation of forearm.

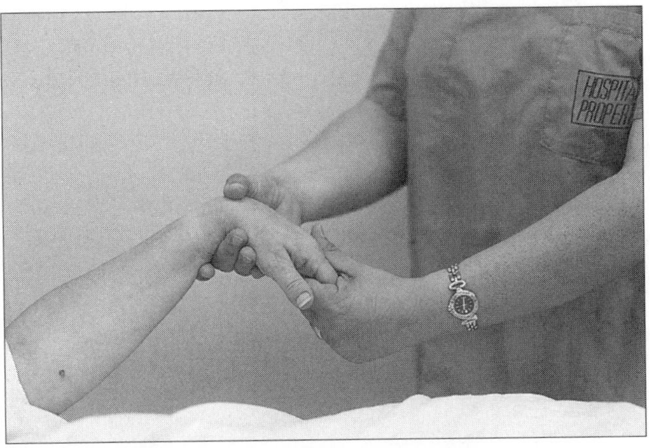

STEP **6e(1)** Flexion of wrist.

e. Wrist

(1) **Flexion:** Move palm toward inner aspect of forearm (ROM: 80 to 90 degrees) (see illustration).

(2) **Extension:** Move fingers so fingers, hands, and forearm are in same plane (ROM: 80 to 90 degrees).

(3) **Hyperextension:** Bring **dorsal** surface of hand back as far as possible (ROM: 80 to 90 degrees) (see illustration).

(4) **Abduction (radial flexion):** Bend wrist medially toward thumb (ROM: up to 30 degrees) (see illustration).

(5) **Adduction (ulnar flexion):** Bend wrist laterally toward fifth finger (ROM: 30 to 50 degrees) (see illustration).

Wrist strength is necessary to be able to use crutches.

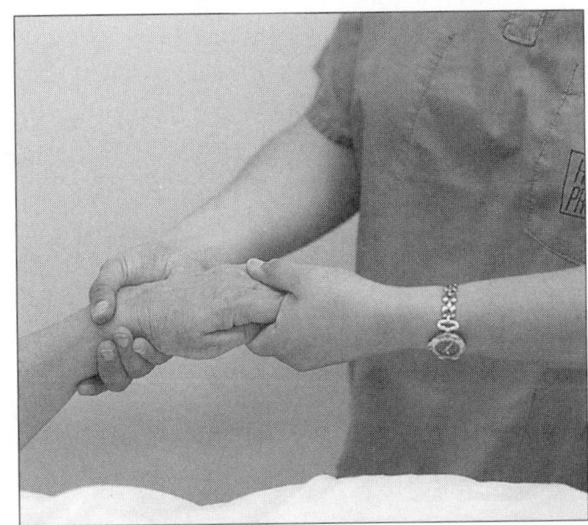

STEP **6e(4)** Abduction (radial flexion) of wrist.

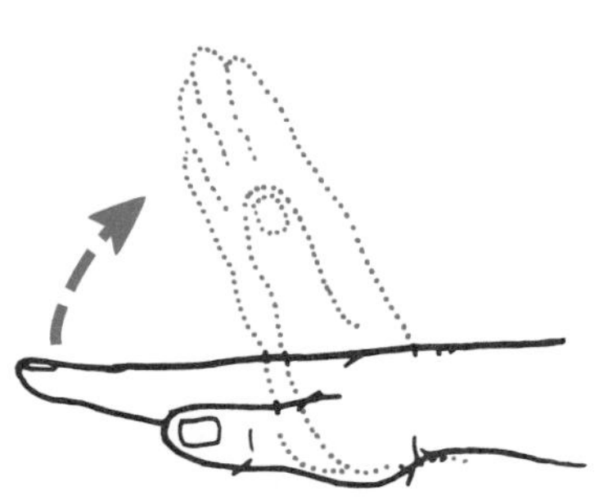

STEP **6e(3)** Hyperextension of wrist.

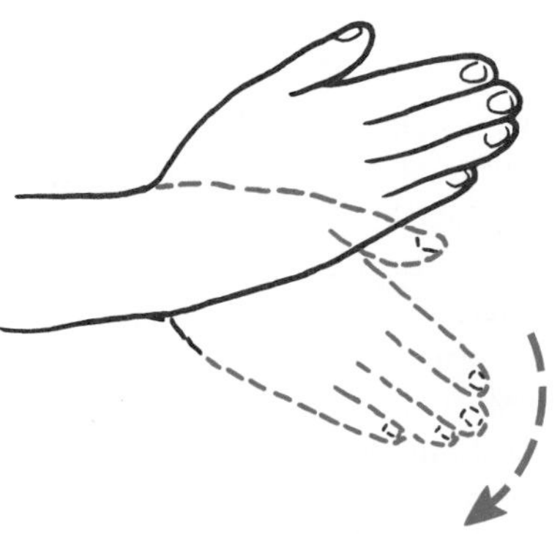

STEP **6e(5)** Adduction (ulnar flexion) of wrist.

STEP	RATIONALE
f. Fingers (1) **Flexion:** Make fist (ROM: 90 degrees) (see illustration). (2) **Extension:** Straighten fingers (ROM: 90 degrees). (3) **Hyperextension:** Bend fingers back as far as possible (ROM: 30 to 60 degrees) (see illustration). (4) **Abduction:** Spread fingers apart (ROM: 30 degrees) (see illustration). (5) **Adduction:** Bring fingers together (ROM: 30 degrees) (see illustration).	Flexibility of fingers and thumb is necessary to grasp items (e.g., holding onto crutch).

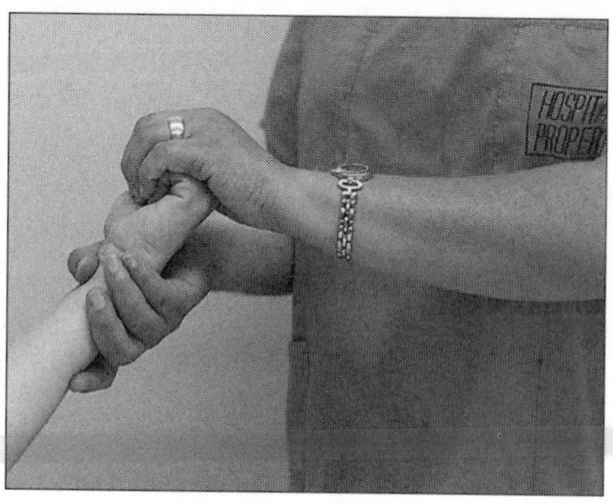

STEP **6f(1)** Flexion of fingers.

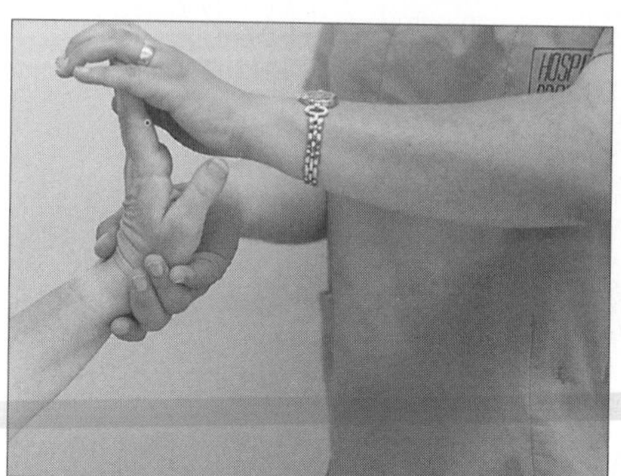

STEP **6f(3)** Hyperextension of fingers.

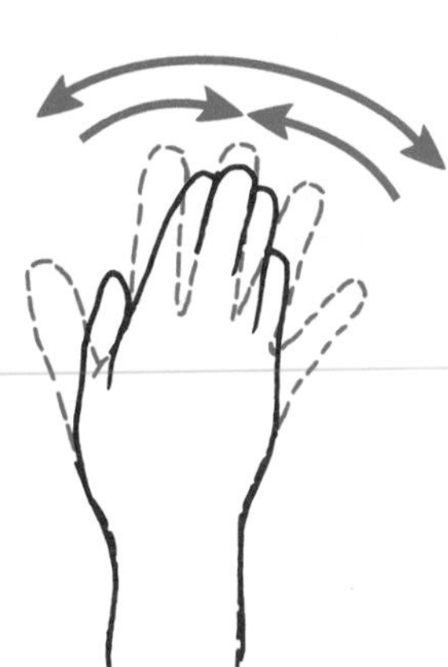

STEP **6f(4-5)** Abduction and adduction of fingers.

STEP	RATIONALE
g. Thumb (1) **Flexion:** Move thumb across palmar surface of hand (ROM: 90 degrees) (see illustration). (2) **Extension:** Move thumb straight away from hand (ROM: 90 degrees). (3) **Abduction:** Extend thumb laterally (usually done when placing fingers in abduction and adduction) (ROM: 30 degrees). (4) **Adduction:** Move thumb back toward hand (ROM: 30 degrees). (5) **Opposition:** Touch thumb to each finger of same hand (see illustration).	Flexibility of thumb maintains coordination for fine motor activities.

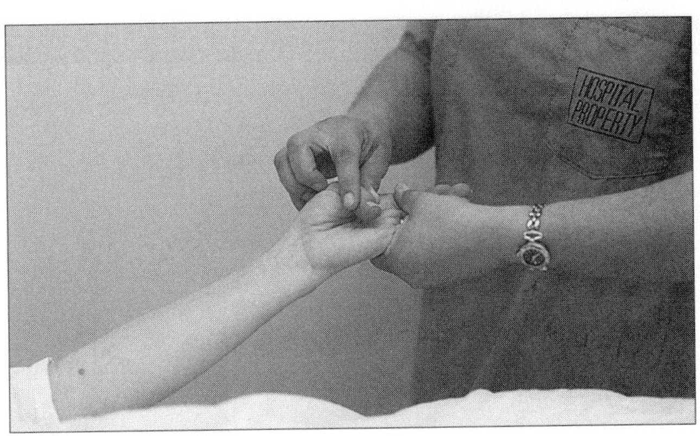

STEP **6g(1)** Flexion of thumb.

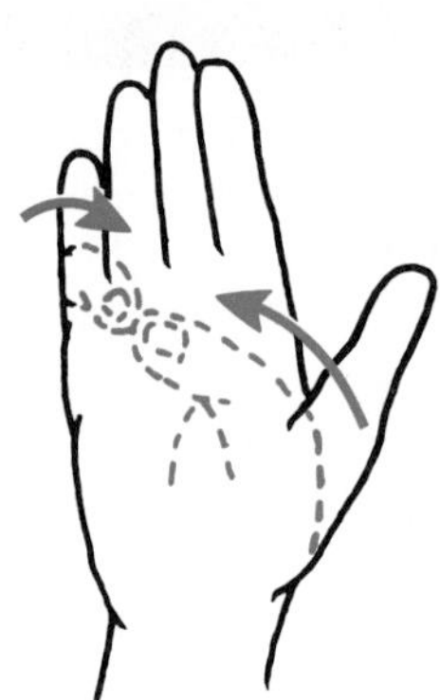

STEP **6g(5)** Opposition of thumb.

STEP	RATIONALE
h. Hip (1) **Flexion:** Move leg forward and up (ROM: 90 to 120 degrees) (see illustration). (2) **Extension:** Move leg back beside other leg (ROM: 90 to 120 degrees) (see illustration). (3) **Hyperextension:** Move leg back (ROM: 30 to 50 degrees) (see illustration). (4) **Abduction:** Move leg laterally away from body (ROM: 30 to 50 degrees) (see illustration). (5) **Adduction:** Move leg back toward medial position and beyond if possible (ROM: 30 to 50 degrees) (see illustration).	Contracture of hip can cause unsteady gait or difficulty ambulating.

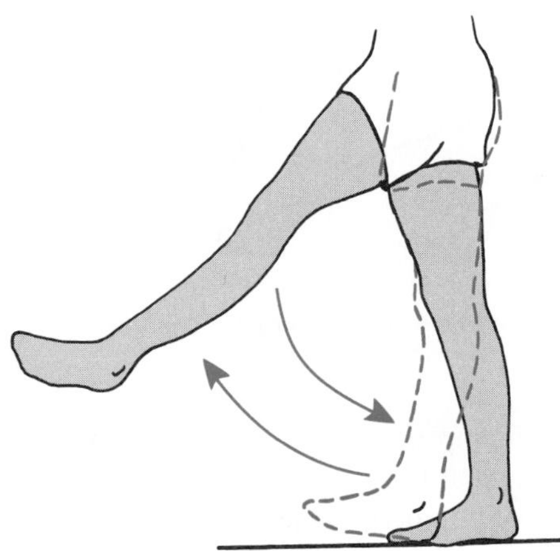

STEP **6h(1-2)** Flexion and extension of hip.

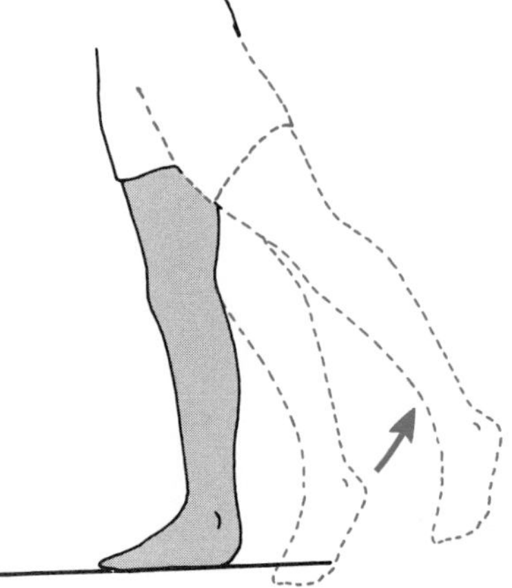

STEP **6h(3)** Hyperextension of hip.

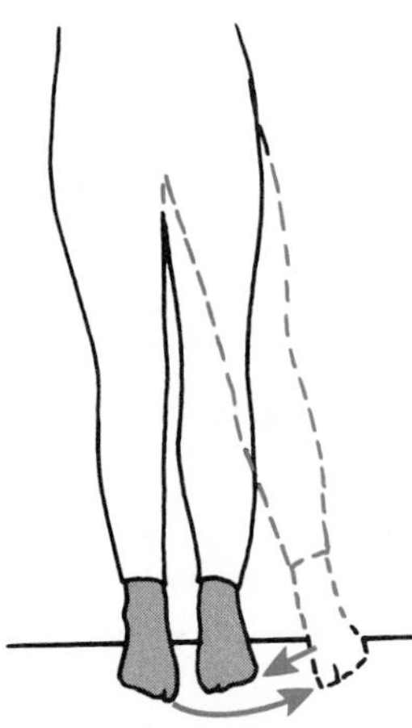

STEP **6h(4-5)** Abduction and adduction of hip.

STEP	RATIONALE
(6) **Internal rotation:** Turn foot and leg toward other leg (ROM: 90 degrees) (see illustration).	
(7) **External rotation:** Turn foot and leg away from other leg (ROM: 90 degrees) (see illustration).	
(8) **Circumduction:** Move leg in circle (ROM: 360 degrees) (see illustration).	

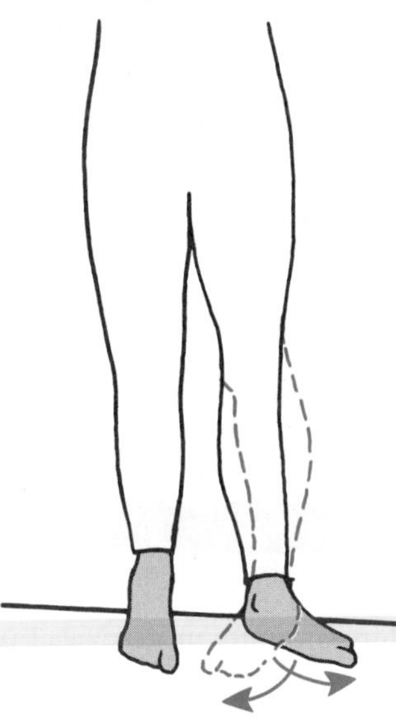

STEP **6h(6-7)** Internal and external rotation of hip.

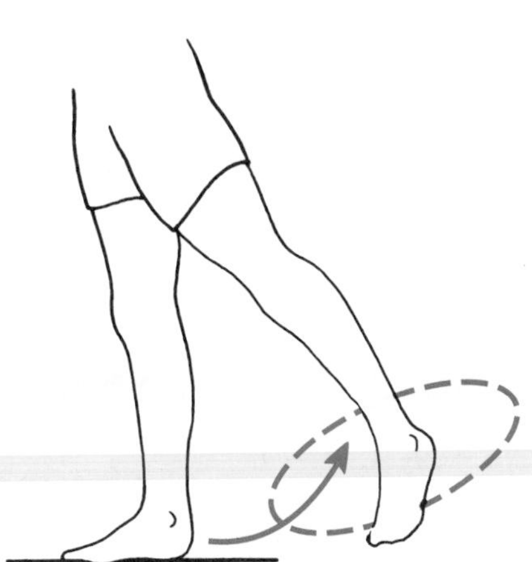

STEP **6h(8)** Circumduction of hip.

STEP	RATIONALE
i. Knee	
(1) **Flexion:** Bring heel toward back of thigh (ROM: 120 to 130 degrees) (see illustration).	Flexibility of knee is necessary to lift objects and to ambulate.
(2) **Extension:** Return leg to floor (ROM: 120 to 130 degrees) (see illustration).	

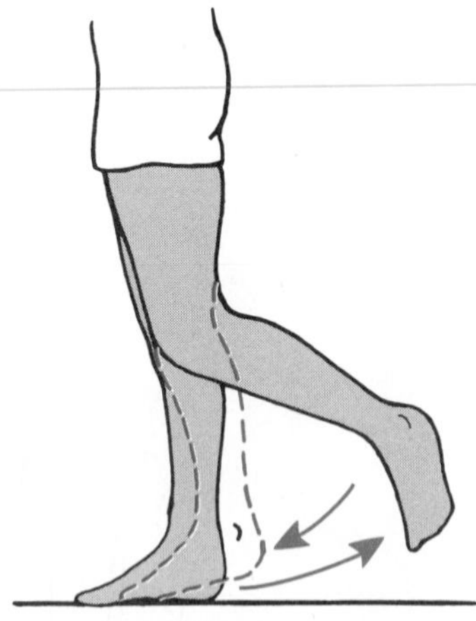

STEP **6i(1-2)** Flexion and extension of knee.

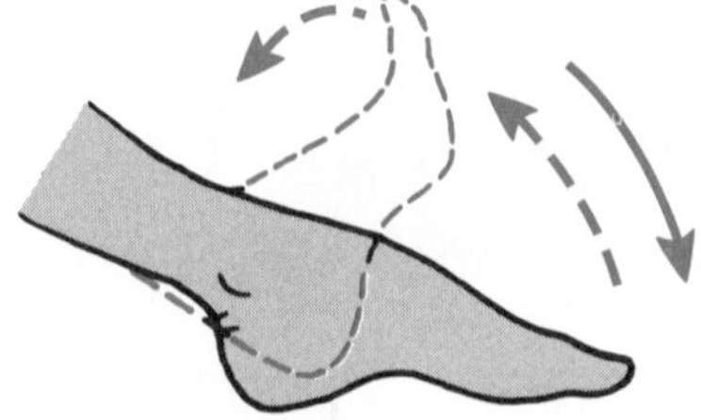

STEP **6j(1-2)** Dorsiflexion and plantar flexion of ankle.

STEP	RATIONALE
j. Ankle	
(1) **Dorsiflexion:** Move foot so toes are pointed upward (ROM: 20 to 30 degrees) (see illustration).	Deformity of ankle can impair client's ability to walk. A common, debilitating, and at times preventable contracture is footdrop. When footdrop occurs, the foot is permanently fixed in plantar flexion (Potter and Perry, 2001).
(2) **Plantar flexion:** Move foot so toes are pointed downward (ROM: 45 to 50 degrees) (see illustration).	

STEP	RATIONALE
k. Foot (1) **Inversion:** Turn sole of foot medially (ROM: 10 degrees or less) (see illustration). (2) **Eversion:** Turn sole of foot laterally (ROM: 10 degrees or less) (see illustration). (3) **Flexion:** Curl toes downward (ROM: 30 to 60 degrees) (see illustration). (4) **Extension:** Straighten toes (ROM: 30 to 60 degrees) (see illustration). (5) **Abduction:** Spread toes apart (ROM: 15 degrees or less) (see illustration). (6) **Adduction:** Bring toes together (ROM: 15 degrees or less) (see illustration).	Adequate ROM in feet allows client to walk.

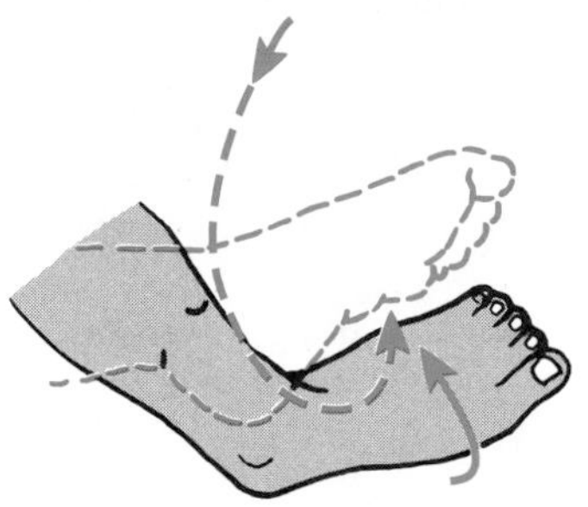

STEP **6k(2)** Eversion of foot.

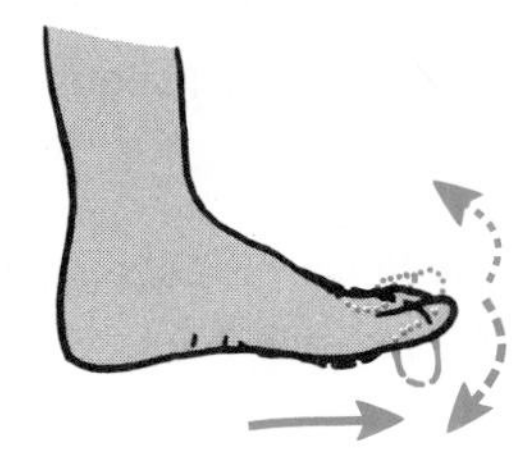

STEP **6k(3-4)** Flexion and extension of toes.

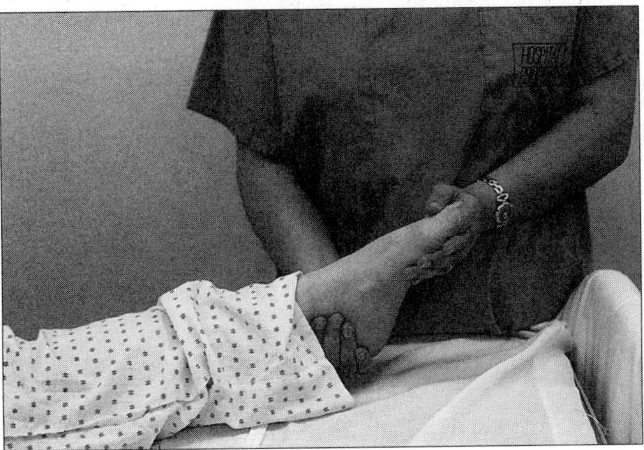

STEP **6k(1)** Inversion of foot.

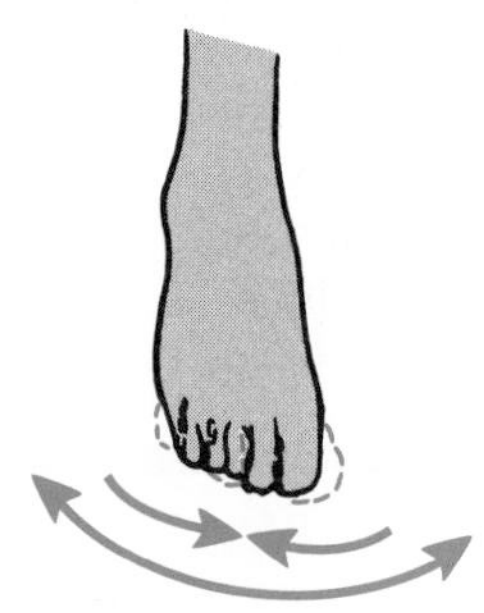

STEP **6k(5-6)** Abduction and adduction of toes.

7. Reposition client to position of comfort and wash hands.

EVALUATION

STEP	RATIONALE
1. Observe range of motion of various joints as compared to baseline range of those joints.	Determines whether exercises have had desired effect of increasing or maintaining joint mobility.
2. Ask for client's subjective statements regarding experience (e.g., complaints of discomfort, level of fatigue).	Evaluates client's tolerance of exercise. Develop schedule for implementing the performance of ROM exercises based on client's tolerance and fatigue level.
3. Determine degree of assistance required to perform exercises.	Establishes guidelines to maximize self-care ability.
4. Ask client to independently perform exercises.	Determines that client performs exercises correctly.

Unexpected Outcomes and Related Interventions

- Client experiences discomfort on ROM exercise.
  - Stop ROM exercises.
  - Notify physician if you suspect inflammation or infection.
- Resistance is encountered when performing ROM exercise.
  - Do not force movement of joint.
- Spastic muscle contraction develops during ROM exercises.
  - Stop movement of affected part.
  - Place continuous gentle pressure on muscle group until it relaxes.
  - Then restart exercises, using slower steady movement.

Recording and Reporting

Report and record:

- Joints exercised.
- Type of exercise.
- Extent to which joints can be moved.
- Any joint abnormalities.
- Client's subjective statements regarding tolerance of activity.
- Nurse's objective observation of tolerance.
- Report immediately to nurse in charge or physician if there is resistance on performance of ROM exercises, if client complains of pain on movement of joint, or if there are signs of swelling, redness, or heat in joint.

Teaching Considerations

- Instruct client to exercise only to point of resistance and to stop if pain is experienced.
- Provide opportunity for return demonstration.

Pediatric Considerations

- Children should have ROM exercises incorporated into play activities to encourage participation (Wong and others, 1999).

Gerontological Considerations

- Inform client that studies have demonstrated that nonstrenuous exercise (such as active ROM) may improve memory or the ability to recall for up to 30 minutes or more (Dawe and Moore-Orr, 1995).
- Encourage active ROM as soon as client's condition warrants independent activity.
- Be aware of chronic conditions (i.e., congestive heart failure, chronic obstructive pulmonary disease, hypertension) that may limit client's ability to participate in ROM exercises. Monitor fatigue, pain, and respiratory functioning frequently.

Home Care Considerations

- Assess family or primary caregiver's ability, availability, and motivation to assist client with exercises that client is unable to perform independently.
- Assist family or primary caregiver to arrange home environment to promote exercise program (e.g., space allocation, lighting, temperature, safety precautions).

Long-Term Care Considerations

- Develop a schedule for implementing the performance of ROM, preferably the same time each day.
- Consult with physical therapist for additional assistance or exercises and client's response to ROM exercises.

Skill 28-2 Performing Isometric Exercises

In addition to ROM exercises, some immobilized clients may be able to perform muscle-strengthening exercises. These include isotonic (dynamic), isometric (static), and resistive exercises. **Isotonic exercises** cause muscle contraction and change in muscle length. Examples of isotonic exercises are walking, performing aerobics, and moving arms and legs against light resistance. These types of exercises can have a positive effect on heart and lung function, improve muscle tone, and have beneficial effects on the entire body if performed properly (Thibodeau and Patton, 1997). Some individuals, however, are unable to tolerate such increases in activity. For these individuals, isometric exercises are more appropriate. Isometric exercises involve tightening or tensing of muscles without moving body parts **(isometric contractions).** They increase muscle tension but do not change the length of muscle fibers. Isometric exercises are easily accomplished by an immobilized client in bed. Both isotonic and isometric exercises help to prevent muscular atrophy and combat osteoporosis.

Isometric exercises may also be resistive. **Resistive isometric exercises** are those in which the individual contracts the muscle while pushing against a stationary object or resisting the movement of an object (Borgman-Gainer, 1996). Examples of resistive isometric exercises are performing push-ups, pushing against a **footboard** to move up in bed, and hip lifting. In hip lifting, the individual, who is in a sitting position, pushes with the hands against a sitting surface such as a chair to raise the hips. Resistive isometric exercises help to promote muscular strength and provide the necessary stress for bone maintenance and growth. Without sufficient stress against bone, **osteoclastic** activity (activity by cells responsible for bone tissue absorption) increases over **osteoblastic** activity (activity by bone-forming cells). The result is demineralization of the bone and eventual osteoporosis.

DELEGATION CONSIDERATIONS

The skill of performing isometric exercises can be delegated to assistive personnel. Clients with cardiovascular disease require evaluation by a nurse when initially performing these exercises. Instruct caregiver that the amount of time and frequency of isometric exercises should be gradually increased over a period of 4 to 5 days.

STEP	RATIONALE
ASSESSMENT	
1. Review client's chart for contraindications to isometric exercises.	Isometric exercises raise blood pressure and pulse. The presence of a preexisting medical condition, especially if a history of cardiac problems is present, may be a contraindication (Borgman-Gainer, 1996).
2. Assess client's baseline vital signs.	Isometric exercises may raise blood pressure. Documentation of baseline vital signs is necessary to determine whether exercises cause a deterioration in vital signs (McCance and Huether, 1998)
3. Assess client's baseline muscle strength: a. Ask client to perform task against resistance (e.g., push one foot against palm of hand). b. Assess grasp strength by having client grasp nurse's hands. Note whether hand grasps are equal. c. Have client grasp two fingers of nurse's right hand with client's left hand and two fingers of nurse's left hand with client's right hand. d. Observe client's ability to do daily activities (e.g., whether client has adequate strength to bathe self, pull self up in bed, move from bed to chair). e. Obtain client's subjective statements related to muscle strength. Does client feel weaker?	Enables nurse to compare muscle strength before and after exercise.
4. Assess client's nutritional status.	Proper nutrition is essential if client is to be able to perform exercises. Promotion of protein anabolism involves conservation and replenishment of energy stores (Lueckenotte, 2000).
5. Assess client's or caregiver's understanding of isometric exercises to be used.	Allows client to verbalize concerns and identifies educational needs of client or caregiver.

NURSING DIAGNOSIS

Defining characteristics from the assessment data may reveal the following nursing diagnoses for clients requiring this skill:

- Activity intolerance
- Fatigue
- Impaired physical mobility
- Deficient knowledge regarding exercises
- Pain (acute, chronic)

Related factors are individualized based on client's condition or needs.

PLANNING

STEP	RATIONALE
1. **Expected outcomes** following completion of procedure:	
▪ Client will gradually increase number of exercise repetitions.	Client will gradually become stronger and be able to increase number of repetitions. Isometric exercises increase muscle tone, (Borgman-Gainer, 1996).
▪ Vital signs will remain stable.	Documents client's **activity tolerance.**
2. Explain procedure and demonstrate exercises.	Relieves anxiety and encourages client cooperation.
3. Assist client to comfortable position.	Reduces stress and promotes client participation.

STEP	RATIONALE

IMPLEMENTATION

1. Provide privacy.

Prevents client embarrassment.

2. Instruct client to perform the following isometric exercises as prescribed and to gradually increase repetitions. Muscle groups used for walking should be exercised isometrically four times per day until client is ambulatory. Muscle group is tightened (contracted) for 8 seconds, then completely relaxed for several seconds (Borgman-Gainer, 1996). Repeat 8 to 10 times for each muscle group during each exercise session several times a day. Exercises are as follows:

Gradual build-up of exercise repetitions improves both muscle strength and endurance (Borgman-Gainer, 1996).

- ***Critical Decision Point***

  Clients doing isometric exercises should be taught to exhale while exerting effort. Many persons hold their breath (Valsalva maneuver), which increases intrathoracic pressure, causing a decrease in venous return to heart. However, when the breath is released, intrathoracic pressure decreases, causing a large surge of blood to return to the heart and increase the cardiac workload (Borgman-Gainer, 1996).

a. Quadriceps isometric exercises:

For person to ambulate and get out of chair, large muscles of thigh (quadriceps) must be strong enough for client to extend knees and stabilize them.

(1) Assist client to supine recumbent position.

(2) Instruct client to press back of the knee against mattress while trying to lift heel from bed (see illustration).

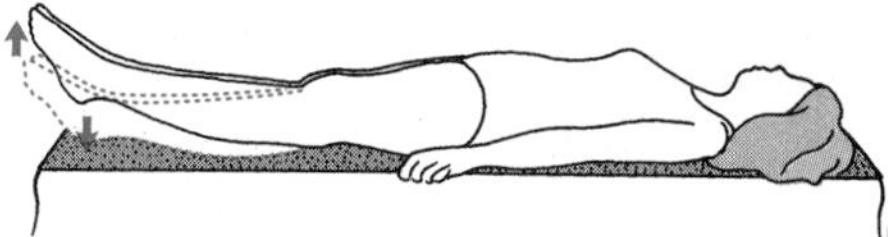

STEP **2a(2)** Lift heels while pressing back of knees against mattress.

(3) Hold muscles tightly contracted for 8 seconds and then relax completely for several seconds.

Nurse can assist client in learning this exercise by placing hand between the back of client's knee and mattress and asking client to press hand against mattress with the back of the knee.

(4) Repeat.

b. Gluteal muscle isometric exercises:

Improves client's balance when sitting.

(1) Assist client to supine position.

(2) Instruct client to pinch buttocks muscles together and hold for 8 seconds and then relax completely for several seconds (see illustration).

(3) Repeat.

c. Abdominal muscle isometric exercises:

Improves trunk stability.

(1) Have client pull abdominal muscles in as tightly as possible (see illustration).

(2) Hold for 8 seconds. Release muscles gradually.

(3) Repeat.

STEP **2b(2)** Pinch gluteal muscles together.

STEP **2c(1)** Pull abdominal muscles in tightly.

STEP	RATIONALE
d. Foot muscle isometric exercises: (1) Instruct client to move foot in a circle in all directions and flex foot toward and away from knee.	Increases muscle activity in leg and thereby promotes venous return to heart.
e. Hand muscle isometric exercises: (1) Obtain sponge rubber ball. (Size of ball depends on size of client's hand.) (2) Have client grip ball with entire hand five to ten times. (3) Dig each fingertip, one at a time, into ball five to ten times each. (4) Gradually increase frequency of exercise until client can grip ball and exercise once or twice a day.	Strengthens grip to hold onto crutch or walker more effectively.
f. Biceps isometric exercises: (1) Have client raise arms to shoulder height and interlock fingertips of both hands. (2) Try to pull hands apart using arm muscles. (3) Hold for 8 seconds. (4) Relax muscles. (5) Repeat.	Strengthens biceps and thereby helps with ambulation if ambulatory assistive device is used.
g. Triceps muscle isometric exercises (see illustration): (1) Have client raise arms to shoulder height. (2) Make fist with one hand and place against palm of other hand. (3) Push hands together as hard as possible for 8 seconds. (4) Relax and repeat after 2 minutes.	Strengthens triceps to assist with transfer techniques and use of crutches or walker. 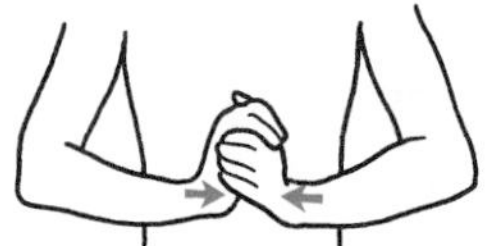 STEP 2g Triceps muscle isometric exercises.
3. Instruct client to perform the following resistive isometric exercises: a. Triceps muscle resistive isometric exercises (see illustration); (1) Assist client to sitting position on edge of bed or in chair. If mattress is soft, blocks or books are placed on bed under client's hands. (2) Instruct client to try to lift buttocks off bed or seat of chair by pressing down on mattress or chair seat with hands. (3) Hold muscles tight for 8 seconds, then relax. (4) Repeat.	To use crutches or walker effectively, client must have enough strength in the triceps to extend and stabilize the elbows while lifting or shifting body weight. 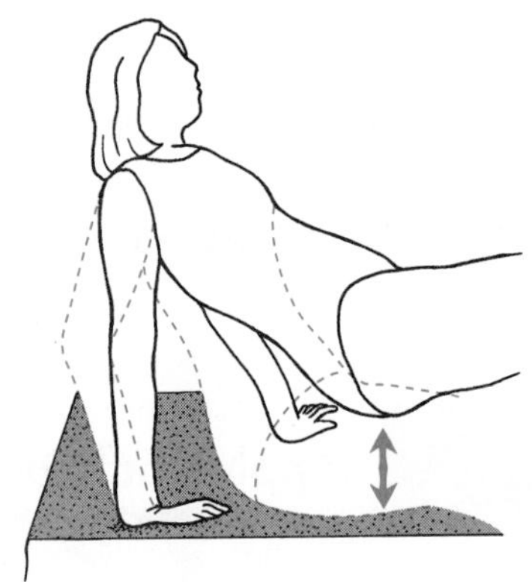 STEP 3a Triceps muscle resistive isometric exercises.
b. Quadriceps muscle resistive isometric exercises: (1) Have client push feet against footboard. (2) Hold muscles tight for 8 seconds, then relax. (3) Repeat.	Builds strength, size, and shape of leg muscles and provides stress against bone that is needed to maintain a balance between osteoblasts and osteoclasts. Without sufficient stress, the osteoclastic activity increases over the osteoblastic activity and bone demineralization occurs.

Step	Rationale

Evaluation

Step	Rationale
1. Observe client's ability to perform exercises.	Demonstrates client's learning.
2. Evaluate client's level of energy, muscular strength, and comfort following exercises.	Determines whether client is performing exercises accurately and whether the exercises are increasing muscle strength.
3. Obtain vital signs.	Determines client's tolerance to activity.

Unexpected Outcomes and Related Interventions

- Client is unable to perform exercises. Client may be too weak.
  - Continue ROM exercises and reposition client to try to increase strength.
  - Make sure nutrition and rest are adequate.
- Client is unwilling to perform exercises.
  - Lack of understanding of significance of exercises may be the problem.
  - Stress importance of the exercises.
- Muscular strength is not increasing.
  - Client may not be performing exercises as described or as often as instructed.
  - Stress importance of following routine.
- Client's blood pressure and heart rate increase significantly during exercises.
  - Client may not be able to tolerate procedure.
  - Discontinue exercises and consult physician.

Recording and Reporting

Report and record:
- Type of isometric exercises used.
- Length of time contractions held.
- Number of repetitions of each exercise.
- Assessment of client's muscular strength and comfort after exercises.
- Client's subjective statements regarding muscular strength.
- Client's ability to perform exercises.

Teaching Considerations

- Instruct client to perform exercises before regular activities, such as breakfast or work. Building exercises into routine activities increases likelihood of adherence to exercise program.
- Instruct client to gradually increase exercise activity each day.

Pediatric Considerations

- Exercises can be incorporated into a child's activity plan.
- Children are more likely to exercise as part of a game or in groups as opposed to exercising alone (Wong and others, 1999).

Gerontological Considerations

- Physical exercise is important for older adults to maintain health, preserve functional status, and improve general quality of life (Lueckenotte, 2000).
- For the older adult who has not previously participated in exercise, it is important to start with only 5 minutes of exercise and gradually work up to a 20 to 30 minute daily routine (Lueckenotte, 2000).
- Encourage older adults to drink water before and after exercising.
- Senior centers have exercise programs geared toward older adults some of whom may have varying degrees of independence and chronic illnesses.

Skill 28-3 Applying Elastic Stockings

Thrombophlebitis is one of the most common venous disorders. Thrombophlebitis is the development of a **thrombus** or clot along with inflammation of a vein; it may be classified as superficial or deep. Superficial thrombophlebitis may be caused by varicose veins or intravenous (IV) medications. However, after injury or surgery, clients are at risk for **deep vein thrombosis** (DVT). Complications of DVT are pulmonary embolism, occurring approximately 50% of the time, and increased susceptibility to recurrent DVT (Phipps and others, 1999). Because DVT usually occurs during a client's recovery phase, nurses need to employ various interventions to try to prevent this potentially fatal complication (Blondin and Titler, 1996).

Three elements (commonly referred to as Virchow's triad) contribute to the development of DVT: hypercoagulability of the blood, venous wall damage, and stasis of blood flow (Phipps and others, 1999). Elastic stockings help reduce two of the elements: blood stasis and venous wall injury. First, they promote venous return by maintaining pressure on superficial veins to prevent venous pooling, thereby reducing the risk of clot formation in the lower extremities. Second, it has been suggested that elastic stockings prevent passive dilation of the veins, thereby decreasing the risk of endothelial tears. An increased incidence of DVT has been found in clients in whom the venous diameter had increased. In such cases, the endothelial layer can tear.

Delegation Considerations

The skill of applying elastic stockings may be delegated to assistive personnel. The nurse initially assesses the client's lower extremities to determine size of elastic stockings and observes for any signs and symptoms of impaired circulation. The nurse should also instruct clients to avoid activities that promote poor circulation, such as allowing the client to cross the legs, wear garters, or roll the elastic stocking part way down the leg. Caregivers also need to be instructed on signs and symptoms of allergic reactions to elastic (e.g., redness, itching, irritation). Finally, assistive personnel must be instructed to inform the nurse if one calf appears larger than the other, a calf is red and/or warm to the touch, or the calf is painful.

Equipment

- Tape measure
- Talcum powder
- Elastic support stockings
- Bath basin, washcloth, towel, and soap (optional)

Step	Rationale
Assessment	
1. Assess client for risk factors in Virchow's triad:	Potential candidates for elastic stockings are clients who have an alteration in one of the elements of Virchow's triad (Blondin and Titler, 1996; Collier, 1999; Phipps and others, 1999).
a. *Hypercoagulability:* All clients with clotting disorders, fever, dehydration, pregnancy and/or first 6 weeks postpartum if the woman was confined to bed, or oral contraceptive use (especially if client smokes).	Hypercoagulability increases tendency for blood to clot.
b. *Venous wall abnormalities:* Local trauma, orthopedic surgeries, major abdominal surgery, varicose veins, atherosclerosis.	Venous wall abnormalities can impair circulation or traumatize blood cells, both of which increase client's risk of clotting.
c. *Blood stasis:* Immobility, obesity, pregnancy.	Stasis facilitates clotting.

- ***Critical Decision Point***
  Discourage clients from activities that promote venous stasis (e.g., crossing legs, wearing garters, elevating legs on pillows). When possible, have clients elevate legs to improve venous return.

Step	Rationale
2. Observe for signs, symptoms, and conditions that might contraindicate use of elastic stockings:	
a. Dermatitis or open skin lesion	Elastic stockings may aggravate a skin condition or cause it to spread. Also the physician may want medication and dressing applied to the lesion.
b. Recent skin graft	Recent skin grafts are delicate and should not be dislodged (Phipps and others, 1999).
c. Disproportionately large thighs	Elastic stockings may not fit correctly, causing excessive pressure and constriction around thighs, and act as a tourniquet, thereby reducing venous return as well as decreasing circulation (Blondin and Titler, 1996; Collier, 1999).
d. Decreased circulation in lower extremities as evidenced by cyanotic, cool extremities and/or gangrenous conditions affecting the lower limb(s)	Elastic stockings may further impede circulation (Phipps and others, 1999).
3. Obtain physician's order.	May be needed for reimbursement reasons.
4. Assess client's or caregiver's understanding of application of elastic stockings.	Identifies potential educational needs of client or caregiver.

STEP	RATIONALE
5. Assess the condition of client's skin and circulation to the legs (i.e., presence of pedal pulses, edema, discoloration of the skin, temperature, lesions, or cuts).	Identifies a baseline for skin integrity and the quality of peripheral pulses in lower extremities. Prevention is the best medicine to avoid the development of thrombophlebitis. Early application of elastic stockings and pneumatic compression stockings (Skill 25-4) can be instrumental in preventing this complication.

- ***Critical Decision Point***

  Thrombophlebitis can develop in the lower extremities. Clinical manifestations of thrombophlebitis vary according to the size and location of the thrombus. Signs and symptoms of superficial thrombosis include palpable veins and the surrounding area being tender to touch, reddened, and warm. There may be a slight temperature elevation. Edema of the extremity may or may not occur. Signs and symptoms of DVT include a swollen extremity; pain, warm, cyanotic skin, and temperature elevation. However, 50% of all clients are asymptomatic (Phipps and others, 1999). Although Homan's sign (pain in calf on dorsiflexion of foot) has been an assessment parameter in the past, it is not a reliable sign. Fewer than 20% of clients exhibit a positive Homan's sign (Phipps and others, 1999).

6. Assess client's or caregiver's understanding of proper care of elastic stockings.	Identifies potential educational needs of client or caregiver.

NURSING DIAGNOSIS

Defining characteristics from the assessment data may reveal the following nursing diagnoses for clients requiring this skill:

- Activity intolerance
- Ineffective peripheral tissue perfusion
- Decreased cardiac output
- Impaired physical mobility
- Deficient knowledge regarding application of elastic stockings
- Risk for impaired skin integrity

Related factors are individualized based on client's condition or needs.

PLANNING

1. **Expected outcomes** following completion of procedure:	
▪ Client shows no evidence of skin irritation or thrombophlebitis.	Ensures that there are no side effects that would impair the client's circulatory system or skin.
▪ Client is able to demonstrate application of elastic stockings.	Verifies correct psychomotor learning.
▪ Client has reduction of edema in lower extremities.	Decreases venous pooling in lower extremities.
2. Explain procedure and reasons for applying stockings.	Reduces anxiety and encourages client cooperation.
3. Use tape measure to measure client's legs to determine proper stocking size.	Stockings must be measured according to manufacturer's directions. Elastic stockings come in two lengths: knee length and thigh length. The choice of length depends on the physician's order. If too large, stockings will not adequately support extremities. If too small, stockings may impede circulation.

- ***Critical Decision Point***

  Compare client's measurements with the manufacturer's sizing chart. The optimum stocking pressure is 20 to 30 mm Hg at the ankle, decreasing to 8 mm Hg at the middle to upper thigh. This change in pressure produces the greatest increase in venous flow velocity that is both safe and practical (Collier, 1999; Phipps and others, 1999).

IMPLEMENTATION

1. Wash hands.	Reduces transmission of microorganisms.
2. Position client in supine position. Elevate head of bed to comfortable level.	Promotes good body mechanics for nurse. Client position eases application. Also the stockings should be applied before the client stands to prevent stagnation of blood in the lower extremities.

STEP	RATIONALE
3. If necessary, bathe legs and dry thoroughly. Apply small amount of talcum powder to legs and feet, provided client does not have sensitivity to talcum powder.	Talcum powder reduces friction and allows for easier application of stockings.
4. Apply stockings:	
a. Turn elastic stocking inside out by placing one hand into sock, holding toe of sock with other hand, and pulling (see illustration).	Allows easier application of stocking.
b. Place client's toes into foot of elastic stocking, making sure that sock is smooth (see illustration).	Wrinkles in sock can cause constrictions and impede circulation to lower region of extremity (Collier, 1999).
c. Slide remaining portion of sock over client's foot, being sure that the toes are covered. Make sure the foot fits into the toe and heel position of the sock. Sock will now be right side out (see illustration).	If toes remain uncovered, they will become constricted by elastic and their circulation can be reduced.
d. Slide sock up over client's calf until sock is completely extended. Be sure sock is smooth and no ridges or wrinkles are present (see illustration).	
e. Instruct client not to roll socks partially down.	Rolling sock partially down has a constricting effect and can impede venous return.
5. Reposition client to position of comfort and wash hands.	Maintains proper body alignment and promotes comfort. Reduces transmission of microorganisms.
6. Remove stockings at least once per shift.	Believed to prevent venous valve incompetency.

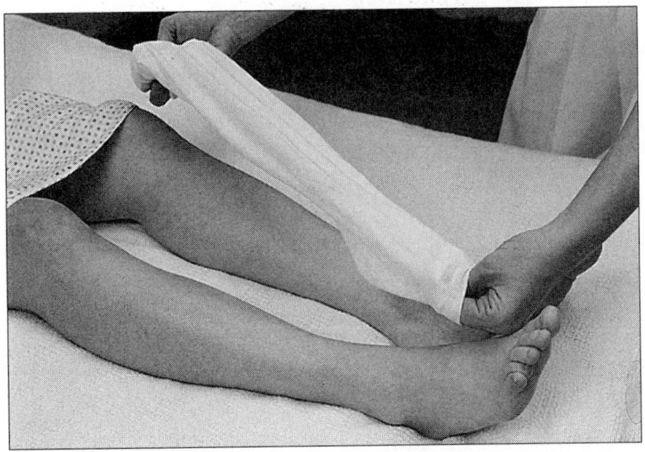

STEP **4a** Turn stocking inside out; hold toe and pull through.

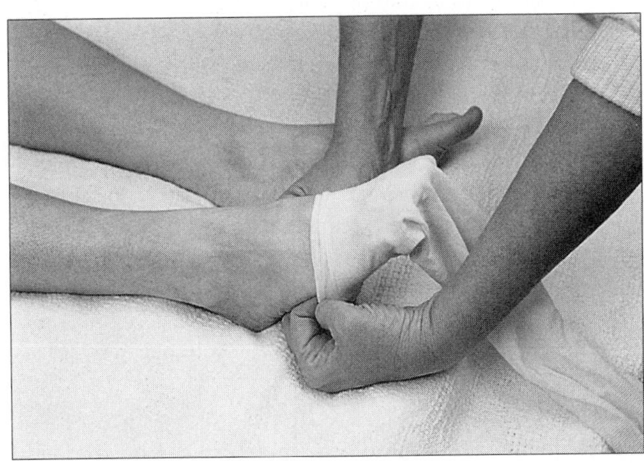

STEP **4b** Place toes into foot of stocking.

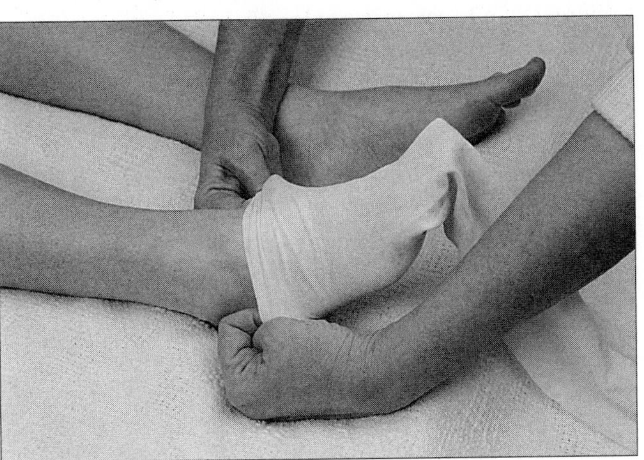

STEP **4c** Slide remaining portion of sock over foot.

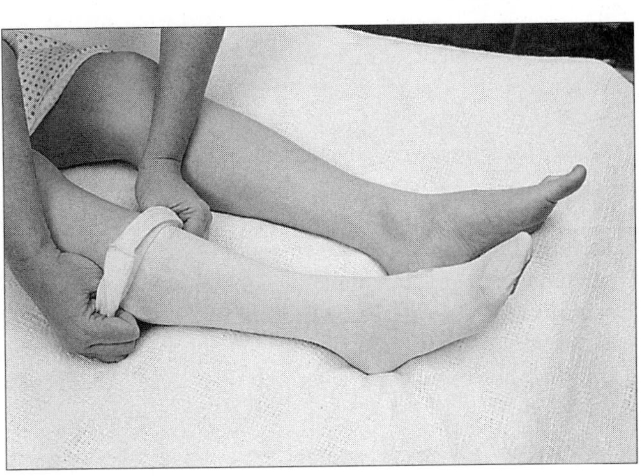

STEP **4d** Slide sock up leg until completely extended.

STEP	RATIONALE
EVALUATION	
1. Inspect stockings to make sure there are no wrinkles or binding at top of stocking.	Wrinkles lead to increased pressure and alter circulation.
2. Observe circulatory status of lower extremities. Observe color, temperature, and condition of skin.	Ensures circulatory status in lower extremities has not been compromised.
3. Observe client's reaction to stockings.	Ensures client is adapting to stockings and is not experiencing any discomfort.
4. Observe client or caregiver apply stockings.	Determines ability to perform skill accurately.

UNEXPECTED OUTCOMES AND RELATED INTERVENTIONS

- Skin reaction to elastic stockings develops.
  - Observe for evidence of redness, skin lesions, and client's subjective complaint of itching or burning.
  - Some clients may have skin reaction to material used in elastic stockings and may indicate an allergic reaction.
- Decrease in circulation in lower extremities develops.
  - Assess for coolness in lower extremities, cyanosis decrease in pedal pulses, decrease in blanching, and numbness or tingling sensation.
  - Check that elastic stockings are not too small or have wrinkles or folds that impede circulation.
  - Notify physician immediately, signs and symptoms may indicate obstruction of arterial blood flow.
- Deep vein thrombosis is suspected.
  - Because clinical signs may be vague, an order for more sensitive radiology tests should be obtained from a physician. Doppler ultrasound, a non-invasive test, may be carried out to rule out the presence of thrombosis (Brough, 1998).
  - Lower extremities should not be massaged because of potential for dislodging thrombus.
- Pulmonary embolism develops.
  - Signs and symptoms include tachypnea, shortness of breath, anxiety, pleuritic chest pain, cough, hemoptysis, tachycardia, and signs of right ventricular failure (i.e., distended neck veins) (Phipps and others, 1999).
  - Notify physician immediately.
  - Monitor vital signs.
  - Administer supplemental oxygen as ordered.

RECORDING AND REPORTING

Report and record:

- Stocking length and size.
- Time of stocking application and condition of skin before application.
- Circulatory status and condition of skin of lower extremities before stocking application.
- Time stockings are removed during shift.
- Condition of skin and circulatory status after removal.
- Calf or thigh circumferences (daily if client is at risk for thrombophlebitis).
- Immediately report signs of thrombophlebitis or impeded circulation in lower extremities to charge nurse or physician.

TEACHING CONSIDERATIONS

- Provide time for client to perform return demonstration of application of elastic stockings.
- Instruct client to launder stockings every 2 days with mild detergent and lay flat to dry.
- Recommend client to have two pair of stockings so that a clean set is available at all times.

PEDIATRIC CONSIDERATIONS

- Elastic stockings are not generally used with younger children.

GERONTOLOGICAL CONSIDERATIONS

- Perform comprehensive assessment of older adults. Normal physiological aging can mask the signs and symptoms of venous insufficiency (Galindo-Ciocon, 1995).
- Older adults may need assistance in applying elastic stockings because of decreased strength or arthritic changes in the hands.

HOME CARE CONSIDERATIONS

- Assess if client is adhering to prescribed use of stockings. Potential reasons for discontinuing use are expense, cosmetic concerns, discomfort, and difficulty with application.
- Stockings must be laundered every other day; therefore, more than one pair is needed.
- Stockings should be removed at least twice a day and circulation and inspection of the skin should be carried out by the client.

LONG-TERM CARE CONSIDERATIONS

- Stockings will lose elasticity over time and should be replaced at least every 6 months depending on proper care and use.
- Client should be measured periodically for proper fit of stockings.

Skill 28-4 Applying Pneumatic Compression Device

Prevention is the best method to reduce the risk of deep vein thrombosis secondary to immobility. Early ambulation remains the most effective preventive measure (Phipps and others, 1999). However, there are times when early ambulation is not an option, particularly in the critically ill client. Early application of elastic stockings (Skill 28-3) and sequential pneumatic compression stockings (SPC), along with low-dose heparin therapy have been reported as successful means to prevent the development of deep vein thrombosis (Blondin and Titler, 1996; Phipps and others, 1999).

Sequential pneumatic compression stockings can be used alone or, more often, in conjunction with elastic stockings. These devices consist of an air pump, connecting tubing, and extremity sleeves that sequentially inflate and deflate chambers within the stocking (Figure 28-1). The intermittent pumping action drives superficial blood into deep veins, where it is evacuated proximally by the venous valves, thus removing pooled blood and preventing both venous stasis and the accumulation of clotting factors.

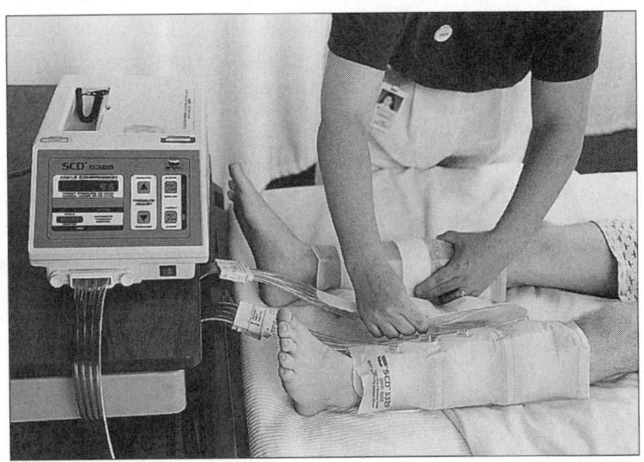

FIGURE **28-1** Sequential pneumatic compression stockings.

Delegation Considerations

The skill of applying pneumatic compression stockings may be delegated to assistive personnel. The nurse initially assesses the client's lower extremities to determine accurate application of pneumatic compression stockings and observes for any signs and symptoms of impaired circulation. The nurse instructs clients to avoid activities that promote poor circulation, such as allowing the client to cross the legs, wear garters, or roll the elastic stocking part way down the leg. Caregivers also need to be instructed on signs and symptoms of allergic reactions to elastic (e.g., redness, itching, irritation). Finally, assistive personnel must be instructed to inform the nurse if one calf appears larger than the other, a calf is red and/or warm to the touch, or the calf is painful.

Equipment

- Tape measure
- Disposable leg sleeve(s)
- Tubing assembly
- Pneumatic compression device (motor)

Step	Rationale
Assessment	
1. Assess client for risk factors in Virchow's triad to determine the need for compression stockings: a. *Hypercoagulability:* All clients with clotting disorders, fever, dehydration, pregnancy and/or first 6 weeks postpartum if the woman was confined to bed, or oral contraceptive use (especially if client smokes) b. *Venous wall abnormalities:* Local trauma, orthopedic surgeries, major abdominal surgery, varicose veins, atherosclerosis. c. *Blood stasis:* Immobility, obesity, pregnancy.	Potential candidates for elastic stockings are clients who have an alteration in one of the elements of Virchow's triad (Blondin and Titler, 1996; Collier, 1999; Phipps and others, 1999).
2. Observe for signs, symptoms, and conditions that might contraindicate use of sequential pneumatic compression stockings:	
a. Dermatitis or open skin lesion	SPC stockings may aggravate a skin condition or cause it to spread. Also, the physician may want medication and dressing applied to the lesion.

STEP	RATIONALE
b. Recent skin graft	Recent skin grafts are delicate and should not be dislodged (Phipps and others, 1999).
c. Decreased circulation in lower extremities as evidenced by cyanotic, cool extremities, and/or gangrenous conditions affecting the lower limb(s)	Application of SPCs may further impede circulation (Phipps and others, 1999).
3. Obtain physician's order.	May be needed for reimbursement reasons.
4. Assess client's or caregiver's understanding of purpose of SPC stockings.	Identifies potential educational needs of client or caregiver.
5. Assess the condition of client's skin and circulation to the legs (i.e., presence of pedal and popliteal pulses, edema, discoloration of the skin, temperature, lesions, or cuts).	Identifies a baseline for skin integrity and the quality of peripheral pulses in lower extremities.

NURSING DIAGNOSIS

Defining characteristics from the assessment data may reveal the following nursing diagnoses for clients requiring this skill:

- Activity intolerance
- Ineffective peripheral tissue perfusion
- Decreased cardiac output
- Impaired physical mobility
- Deficient knowledge regarding purpose of SPC stockings
- Risk for impaired skin integrity

Related factors are individualized based on client's condition or needs.

PLANNING

STEP	RATIONALE
1. **Expected outcomes** following completion of procedure:	
▪ Client shows no evidence of skin irritation or thrombophlebitis.	Ensures that there are no side effects indicating impairment of the client's circulatory system or skin.
▪ Client has reduction of edema in lower extremities.	Stockings decrease venous pooling in lower extremities.
2. Explain procedure and reasons for applying stockings.	Reduces anxiety and encourages client cooperation.
3. Use tape measure to measure client's legs to determine proper stocking size.	SPC stockings must be measured according to manufacturer's directions. SPC stockings come in two lengths: knee length and thigh length. The choice of length depends on the physician's order.

IMPLEMENTATION

STEP	RATIONALE
1. Wash hands.	Reduces transmission of microorganisms.
2. Position client in supine position. Elevate head of bed to comfortable level.	Promotes good body mechanics for nurse. Client position eases application. Also the stockings should be applied before the client stands to prevent stagnation of blood in the lower extremities.
3. Remove SPC stockings from plastic, unfold, and flatten.	
4. Arrange the SPC stocking under the client's leg according to the leg position indicated on the inner lining of the stocking (see illustration).	Ensures straight and even application.
5. Apply SPC stockings:	
a. Place client's leg on SPC stocking.	
b. Back of ankle should line up with the ankle marking on inner lining of stocking.	Correct application of SPC stockings is important for proper functioning.
c. Position back of knee with the popliteal opening (see illustration).	Prevents pressure on popliteal artery.

- ***Critical Decision Point***
  If client is wearing elastic stockings, eliminate any wrinkles and folds before applying SPC stockings.

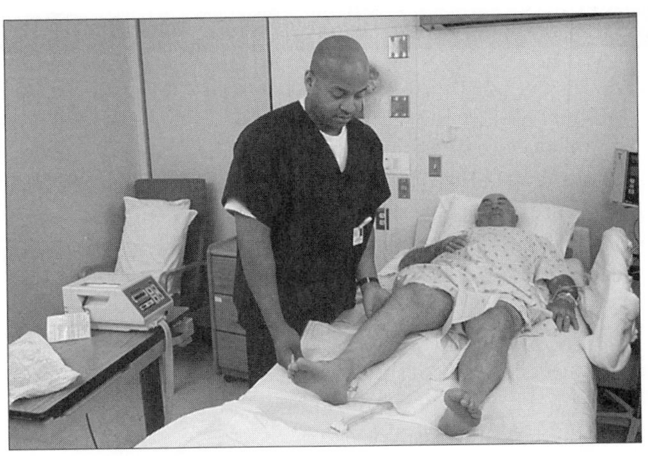

STEP 4 Correct leg position on inner lining.

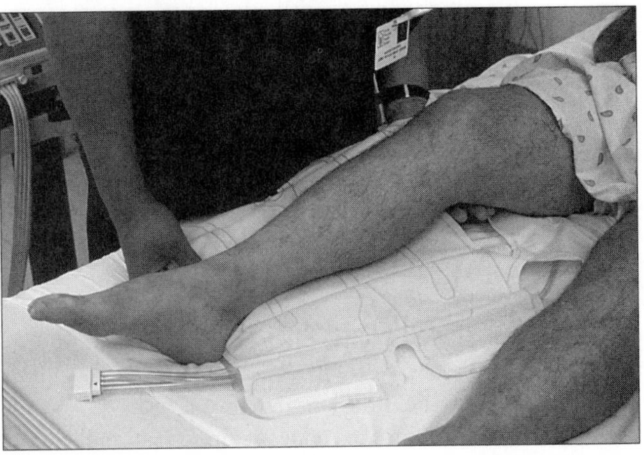

STEP 5c Position back of client's knee with the popliteal opening.

STEP	RATIONALE
d. Wrap SPC stockings securely around client's leg.	Secure fit needed for adequate compression.
e. Check fit of SPC stockings by placing two fingers between client's leg and stocking (see illustration).	Ensures proper fit and prevents constriction, which could impede circulation.
6. Attach SPC stockings' connector to plug on mechanical unit. Arrows on connector line up with arrows on plug from mechanical unit (see illustration).	

- ***Critical Decision Point***
  Make sure tubing and connection site are visible. Check for kinks or twisting of tubing to avoid a potential pressure ulcer.

STEP	RATIONALE
7. Turn mechanical unit ON. Green light indicates unit is functioning properly.	Power source initiates sequential compression cycle.
8. Monitor functioning of SPC stockings through one full cycle of inflation and deflation.	Ensures proper functioning of unit and determines if SPC stockings are too loose or constricting.
9. Reposition client to position of comfort.	Maintains proper body alignment and promotes comfort.

- ***Critical Decision Point***
  To reduce risk of injury disconnect client from SPC stockings when transferring in and out of bed.

STEP	RATIONALE
10. Wash hands.	Reduces transmission of microorganisms.

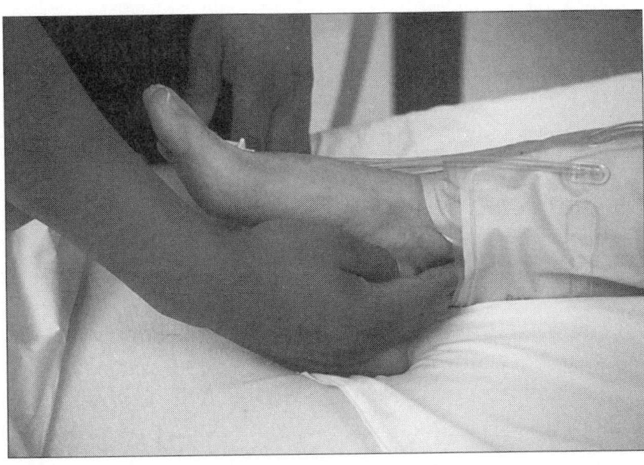

STEP 5e Check fit of SPC stocking.

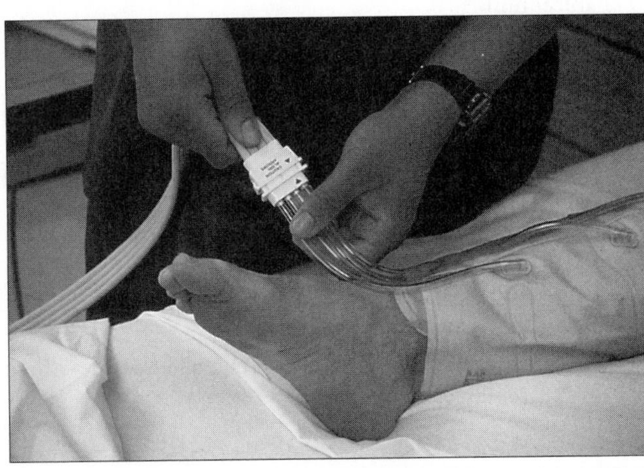

STEP 6 Align arrows when connecting to mechanical unit.

STEP	RATIONALE
EVALUATION	
1. Inspect SPC stockings for kinks or twisting in tubing.	Ensures proper functioning of unit.
2. Observe circulatory status of lower extremities. Observe color, temperature, and condition of skin.	Ensures circulatory status in lower extremities has not been compromised.
3. Observe client's reaction to SPC stockings.	Ensures client is adapting to stockings and is not experiencing any discomfort.

UNEXPECTED OUTCOMES AND RELATED INTERVENTIONS

- Skin reaction to SPC stockings develops.
  - Observe for evidence of redness, skin lesions, and client's subjective complaint of itching or burning.
  - Remove SPC stockings and notify physician.
- Decrease in circulation in lower extremities develops.
  - Assess for coolness in lower extremities, cyanosis, decrease in pedal pulses, decrease in blanching, and numbness or tingling sensation.
  - SPC stockings may be too small or secured too tightly around client's leg and impede circulation. Loosen SPC stockings and assess frequently.
  - Notify physician and anticipate radiological study to rule out obstruction. Signs and symptoms may indicate obstruction of arterial blood flow.
- Alarm on mechanical unit is activated.
  - Troubleshoot: check for kinks in tubing, air leaks, and that all connections are secure.
  - Get a new mechanical unit if there is failure to find reason for alarm.
- Deep vein thrombosis develops.
  - Because clinical signs may be vague, an order for more sensitive radiology tests should be obtained from a physician. Doppler ultrasound, a non-invasive test, may be carried out to rule out the presence of thrombosis (Brough, 1998).
  - Lower extremities should not be massaged because of potential for dislodging thrombus.
- Pulmonary embolism develops.
  - Signs and symptoms include tachypnea, shortness of breath, anxiety, pleuritic chest pain, cough, hemoptysis, tachycardia, and signs of right ventricular failure (i.e., distended neck veins) (Phipps and others, 1999).
  - Notify physician immediately.
  - Monitor vital signs.
  - Administer supplemental oxygen as ordered.

RECORDING AND REPORTING

Report and record:

- Date and time of SPC stocking application and condition of skin before application.
- Circulatory status and condition of skin of lower extremities before stocking application.
- SPC stocking length and size.
- Time SPC stockings are removed (at least once per shift).
- Condition of skin and circulatory status after removal.
- Calf or thigh circumferences (daily if client is at risk for thrombophlebitis).
- Immediately report signs of thrombophlebitis or impeded circulation in lower extremities to charge nurse or physician.

TEACHING CONSIDERATIONS

- Provide family caregiver time for client to provide return demonstration of SPC stockings.
- Instruct on troubleshooting if alarm is activated on mechanical unit.

PEDIATRIC CONSIDERATIONS

- SPC may be used occasionally in this client population.
- Observe younger children frequently because of the potential for an electrical hazard. Keep mechanical unit out of reach of child (Wong and others, 1999).
- Keep cords and tubing away from child's reach.

GERONTOLOGICAL CONSIDERATIONS

- Older adults may experience wasting of muscles because of the aging process; therefore, it is essential to measure these clients carefully to ensure proper fit.
- Reinforce need for the older client to call for help before transferring from bed to prevent entanglement with cord or tubing from mechanical unit.

HOME CARE CONSIDERATIONS

- Instruct caregiver or client on troubleshooting when mechanical unit alarms.
- Instruct caregiver or client to have mechanical unit serviced and checked for proper functioning by the manufacturer at least every 6 months.
- SPC sleeves should be checked periodically for air leaks and wear and tear.

LONG-TERM CARE CONSIDERATIONS

- SPC sleeves may lose their elasticity from long-term use. Check frequently for wear and tear.
- Check for proper fit. Sleeves may become too tight or loose if client's weight fluctuates.

Skill 28-5 Changing Client's Position to Minimize Occurrence of Orthostatic Hypotension

Orthostatic or postural hypotension is a drop in blood pressure that occurs when the client changes from a horizontal to a vertical position (e.g., when the client rises from a lying to a sitting position or from a sitting to a standing position). A drop in blood pressure of approximately 15 mm Hg in systolic pressure and 10 mm Hg in diastolic pressure with symptoms of dizziness, pallor, or fainting indicates orthostatic hypotension (Winslow and others, 1995). Immobilized clients and those undergoing prolonged bed rest are at risk for orthostatic hypotension. In the immobilized client, there is decreased circulating fluid volume, pooling of blood in the lower extremities, and decreased autonomic response. As a result the client experiences decreased venous return and decreased central venous pressure and stroke volume with a subsequent drop in blood pressure (McCance and Huether, 1998).

Although orthostatic hypotension cannot be prevented, its effects can be minimized. Interventions are directed toward maintaining muscle tone to increase venous return to the heart and to decrease stasis of blood in the lower extremities. Two interventions to help clients maintain muscle tone are the previously mentioned ROM and isometric exercises (see Skills 28-1 and 28-2) and the application of elastic and sequential pneumatic compression stockings (see Skills 28-3 and 28-4) (Borgman-Gainer, 1996). Another intervention to reduce the effects of orthostatic hypotension is to help the client become progressively mobile as soon as possible (i.e., sitting in an upright [90-degree] position in bed, sitting on the side of the bed with legs in a dependent position and wiggling the feet [**dangling**], transferring from bed to chair, or walking) (Phipps and others, 1999; Winslow and others, 1995). However, before a client is helped out of bed, certain client assessments must be made and necessary safety precautions taken.

Delegation Considerations

The skill of position changing to minimize orthostatic hypotension may be delegated to assistive personnel. Before delegating this skill, the nurse must first determine that assistive personnel know how to safely ease a dizzy or fainting client into a sitting position in a chair or on the floor. The nurse also instructs personnel about the client's baseline blood pressure. Be sure that assistive personnel know that if the client complains of nausea; dizziness, or increased pallor or diaphoresis that the client should be immediately returned to the bed or chair. Caregivers must also be instructed to be sure the client is wearing safe, nonskid-soled shoes, that the environment is free of clutter, and that there is no moisture on the floor.

Equipment

- Elastic stockings (if ordered)
- Sequential pneumatic compression stockings (if ordered)
- Robe
- Safety belt
- Nonskid shoes or slippers

Step	Rationale
Assessment	
1. Review client's chart to assess previous activity level, vital signs, and current activity order.	Determines how long client has been assigned to bed rest and the current activity order. The longer a client has been immobile, the greater the risk for orthostatic hypotension.
2. Obtain client's vital signs in supine position.	Provides baseline for comparison when client changes from supine to upright position. Dizziness and/or a decrease of 15 mm Hg in systolic blood pressure and 10 mm Hg in diastolic blood pressure when upright is indicative of postural hypotension (Winslow and others, 1995).
3. Assess client's environment for potential safety hazards before ambulation or transfer (e.g., wet floor, clutter).	Protects client from falls and other injuries.

Nursing Diagnosis

Defining characteristics from the assessment data may reveal the following nursing diagnoses for clients requiring this skill:

- Activity intolerance
- Decreased cardiac output
- Fatigue
- Impaired physical mobility
- Risk for injury

Related factors are individualized based on client's condition or needs.

STEP	RATIONALE

PLANNING

Step	Rationale
1. **Expected outcomes** following completion of procedure: ▪ Client will have no symptoms of orthostatic hypotension: dizziness, decrease in blood pressure greater than 15 mm Hg (systolic) to 10 mg Hg (diastolic) when assuming upright position.	Client is able to maintain a stable blood pressure during transfer.
2. Explain procedure and reasons for getting client out of bed.	Reduces anxiety and encourages client cooperation.
3. Assess whether another staff member is needed before transferring or ambulating client.	Prevents accidental lifting injuries to client and nurse.

• ***Critical Decision Point***

Use caution (seek assistance) when attempting to transfer or ambulate a client who has recently been given an antihypertensive, narcotic medication, or who has an epidural pain catheter in place.

Step	Rationale
4. Explain to client the importance of reporting any symptoms of dizziness, lightheadedness, or seeing spots.	Allows caregivers to quickly place client in a safe position.
5. Explain to client or caregiver the importance of maintaining adequate hydration by drinking 1500 to 2000 ml of liquid every 24 hours unless contraindicated (Radwanski and Hoeman, 1996).	Hydration improves circulating blood volume and reduces risk of orthostatic blood pressure change (Radwanski and Hoeman, 1996).

IMPLEMENTATION

Step	Rationale
1. Wash hands.	Reduces transfer of microorganisms.
2. Place bed in low position.	Have bed as close to floor as possible in case client becomes dizzy and falls.
3. Slowly raise head of bed to high Fowler's position and obtain client's blood pressure.	Raising head of bed slowly allows body to adjust to change in position. Note whether blood pressure decreases or client complains of dizziness when changing from supine to upright position.
4. Observe client for signs of orthostatic hypotension: nausea, pallor, dizziness, seeing spots, or lightheadedness.	Indicates orthostatic hypotension. Procedure may need to be postponed until client is able to tolerate high Fowler's position without signs and symptoms of orthostatic hypotension (Winslow and others, 1995).
5. Assist client to sit with legs dangling over side of bed for 1 to 3 minutes. Have client wiggle feet and move legs intermittently while dangling the legs. Avoid pressure on the backs of the knees (Winslow and others, 1995).	Allows autonomic nervous system to adapt to postural change. Decreases pooling of blood in the legs while dangling. Prevents decrease of venous return (Winslow and others, 1995).
6. Continue to talk with client and assess for orthostatic hypotension.	Decrease in blood pressure and increase in heart rate may occur for as long as 2 minutes after position changes (Winslow and others, 1995).
7. If there are no signs of dizziness or lightheadedness, assist client to stand, transfer to a chair, or ambulate.	Absence of dizziness or lightheadedness indicates that it is safe to attempt to transfer client to chair or to ambulate.
8. Wash hands.	Reduces transfer of microorganisms.

EVALUATION

Step	Rationale
1. Observe client for signs of orthostatic hypotension.	Dizziness can indicate reduced blood pressure, and the nurse must safely guide client into chair or back to bed.
2. Recheck client's blood pressure while client is sitting the first few times client is mobile.	Indicates how well the client is tolerating the activity.

UNEXPECTED OUTCOMES AND RELATED INTERVENTIONS

- Client becomes lightheaded and begins to fall.
  - Gently ease client to floor to prevent injury to nurse and client.

RECORDING AND REPORTING

Report and record:

- Supine and upright blood pressures.
- Any changes in respiratory rate, skin color, or temperature noted when client is placed in upright position.
- Client's subjective statements regarding tolerating upright position.
- If client sat in chair, note length of time client was able to sit and how well activity was tolerated. Recheck and document blood pressure while client is sitting up.
- If client ambulates, note distance walked, stability of gait, any assistance needed, and how procedure was tolerated.
- Report immediately if client sustains injury or is unable to tolerate activity.

TEACHING CONSIDERATIONS

- Instruct client or caregiver on the importance of having the client wear shoes with a nonslip surface during transfer or ambulation.
- Instruct client or caregiver on the importance of slow, gradual position change (Radwanski and Hoeman, 1996).
- Instruct client to report any symptoms of dizziness, lightheadedness, or seeing spots.

PEDIATRIC CONSIDERATIONS

- Children who have volume losses resulting in dehydration have an increased potential for orthostatic hypotension (Wong and others, 1999).
- Maintain hydration and provide safety precautions to prevent falls.
- When assisting a child, be sure to assess weight correctly-looks can be deceiving.

GERONTOLOGICAL CONSIDERATIONS

- Older adults who have volume losses or have undergone prolonged bed rest have greater risk for hypotension with postural change.
- Provide 1500 to 2000 ml of fluid every 24 hours unless contraindicated to ensure hydration (Radwanski and Hoeman, 1996).
- Clients using medications to reduce blood pressure are at greater risk for orthostatic hypotension.

HOME CARE CONSIDERATIONS

- Instruct client about symptoms of orthostatic hypotention.
- Instruct client to make postural changes slowly.
- Instruct caregiver on use of a gait belt for transfer of client.
- Instruct caregiver on proper body mechanics.

Skill 28-6 Assisting With Ambulation

Clients who have been immobile for even a short time may require assistance with ambulation. Assistance may mean walking alongside the client while providing support (Figure 28-2) or the client may require the use of an assistive device to aid in ambulation. An assistive device may be ordered to increase stability, to support a weak extremity, or to reduce the load on weight-bearing structures such as hips, knees, or ankles. These devices range from standard canes, which provide minimal support, to crutches and walkers, which can be used by clients who are unable to bear complete weight on the lower extremities or who bear weight on only one lower extremity. Selection of the appropriate device depends on the client's age, diagnosis, muscular coordination, and ease of maneuverability (Borgman-Gainer, 1996). Use of assistive devices may be temporary, such as during recuperation from a fractured extremity or orthopedic surgery, or permanent, such as in the case of a client with paralysis or permanent weakness of the lower extremities.

Canes are lightweight, easily movable devices that extend about waist high and are made of wood or metal. Canes help to maintain balance by widening the base of support. They are indicated for clients with hemiparesis and are used to ease the strain on weight-bearing joints. Canes are not recommended for clients with bilateral leg weakness; for such clients, crutches or a walker are more appropriate (Borgman-Gainer, 1996). There are three types of commonly used canes. The

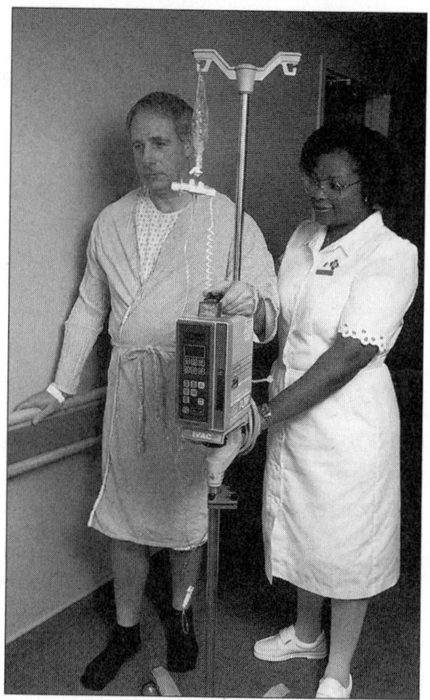

FIGURE **28-2** Assisting a client with ambulation.

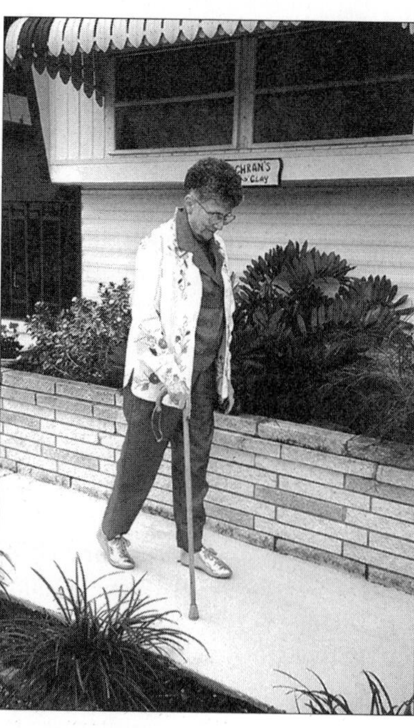

FIGURE **28-3** Standard crook cane.

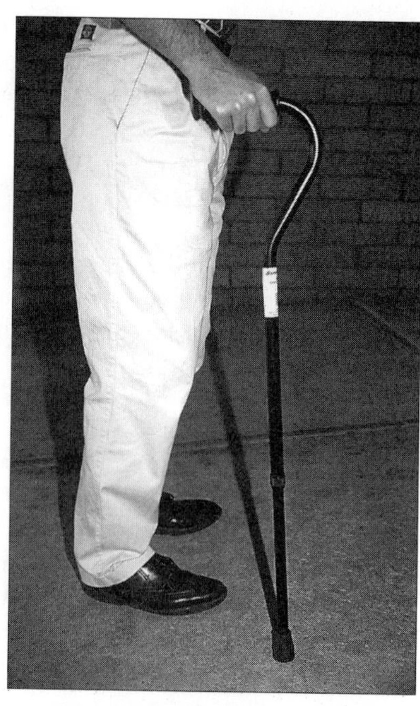

FIGURE **28-4** T-handle cane.

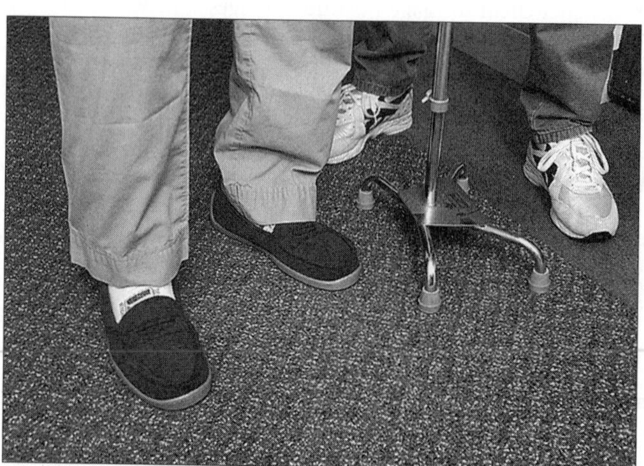

FIGURE **28-5** Quad cane.

standard crook cane provides the least support and is used by clients requiring only minimal assistance to walk. It has a half-circle handle, which allows it to be hooked over chairs (Figure 28-3). The *T-handle cane* has a bent shaft and a straight-shaped handle with grips, which makes it easier to hold. It provides greater stability than the standard cane and is especially useful for clients with hand weakness (Figure 28-4). The *tripod cane* (pyramid cane) has three legs and the *quad cane* has four legs; the additional legs provide a wide base of support. These types of cane are useful for clients with unilateral, partial, or complete leg paralysis. They also have the advantage of standing alone, freeing the arms to help the client rise from a chair (Borgman-Gainer, 1996) (Figure 28-5).

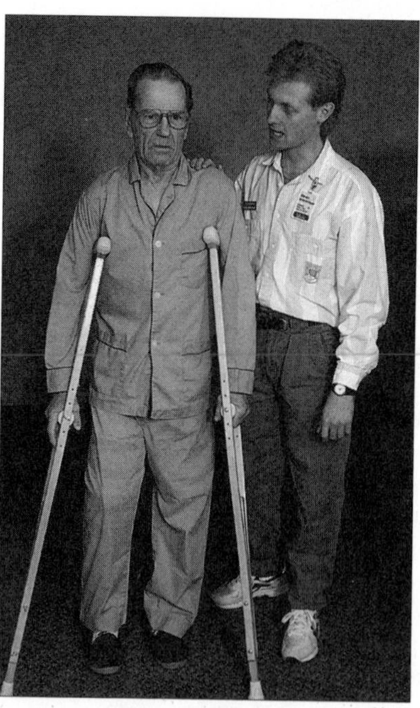

FIGURE **28-6** Axillary crutch.

A crutch is a wooden or metal staff that reaches from the ground almost to the axilla. Crutches are used to remove weight from one or both legs. They are used by clients who must transfer more weight to their arms than is possible with canes. There are three types of crutches: *axillary, Lofstrand* or *Canadian,* and *platform.* The axillary crutch is frequently used by clients of all ages on a short-term basis (Figure 28-6).

The Lofstrand crutch has a hand grip and a metal band that fits around the client's forearm. Both the metal band and the hand grip are adjusted to fit the client's height. This type of crutch is useful for clients with a permanent disability, such as paraplegia. The metal arm band stabilizes and assists in guiding the crutch. The band offers other advantages as well. First, the encircling arm band allows clients to use their hands for other activities, such as opening doors, without dropping the crutches. Second, the anterior opening of the band allows clients to free themselves of the crutches if a fall occurs.

The Canadian crutch is like the Lofstrand only it has an additional cuff for the upper arm to give added support. The platform crutch is used by clients who are unable to bear weight on their wrists. It has a horizontal trough on which clients can rest their forearms and wrists and a vertical handle for the client to grip.

A walker is an extremely light, movable device, about waist high, consisting of a metal frame with handgrips, four widely placed, sturdy legs, and one open side. Because it has a wide base of support, the walker provides great stability and security. A walker can be used by a client who is weak or who has problems with balance (Borgman-Gainer, 1996) (Figure 28-7). In addition to the standard walker, there are several other models available: a foldable version that is easy to transport, one with a fold-down seat, and one with wheels on the front legs. Walkers with wheels are useful for clients who have difficulty lifting the walker as they walk because of limited balance or endurance. The disadvantage, however, is that the walker can roll forward when weight is applied (Borgman-Gainer, 1996).

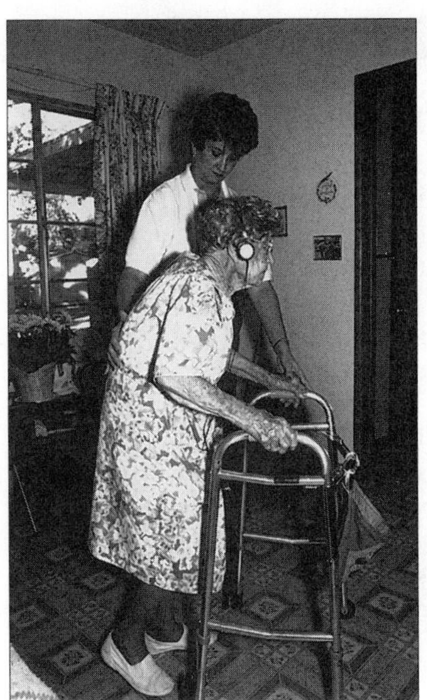

FIGURE **28-7** Walker.

Delegation Considerations

The skill of assisting clients with ambulation may be delegated to assistive personnel. Before delegating this skill, the nurse determines that assistive personnel know how to safely ease a dizzy or fainting client into a sitting position in a chair or on the floor. Be sure that assistive personnel know that if the client complains of nausea, dizziness, or has increased pallor or diaphoresis that the client should be immediately returned to the bed or chair. Caregivers must also be instructed to be sure the client is wearing safe, nonskid-soled shoes, that the environment is free of clutter, and that there is no moisture on the floor.

Equipment

- Ambulation device (crutch, walker, cane)
- Safety device **(gait belt)** (Figure 28-8)
- Well-fitting, flat, nonskid shoes for client
- Robe or sweatpants

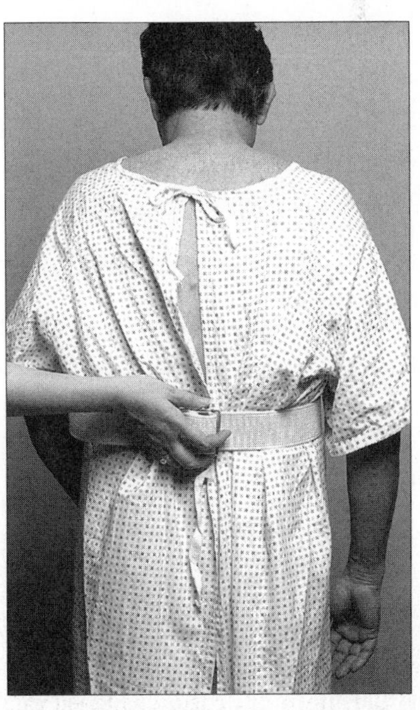

FIGURE **28-8** Walking belt.

Step	Rationale
Assessment	
1. Review client's chart including:	
a. Client's medical history	Certain medications, chronic illness, and history of falling may influence the client's ability to ambulate independently.
b. Client's previous activity level	Identifies client's previous activity level. Client may tire easily or be prone to orthostatic hypotension if bed rest has been prolonged.
c. Current activity order	Verifies if an ambulation aid is needed and specifies amount of activity permitted.
2. Assess client's physical readiness:	
a. Assess client's vital signs and orientation to time, place, and person.	Ambulation following immobility can be fatiguing and stressful. Baseline vital signs offer a means for comparison after exercise. The oriented client is able to understand instructions.
b. Assess ROM, muscle strength, and whether there is the presence of foot deformities.	Determines if client has enough flexibility and muscle strength to ambulate safely and if client needs muscle-strengthening exercises. Determines if any foot deformities are present to affect ambulation.
c. Assess client for any visual, perceptual, or sensory deficits.	Determines if client can use assistive device safely. Ambulation after immobility can be fatiguing and stressful.
d. Assess environment for potential threats to client safety.	Protects client from potential injury.
e. Assess client for discomfort.	Client may be in pain or may fear pain resulting from exercise. If necessary, administer analgesic before exercise.
3. Assess client's or caregiver's understanding of technique of ambulation to be used.	Allows client to verbalize concerns. Clients who have been immobile for a long time may be hesitant to ambulate. Caregiver may be hesitant to learn how to assist with ambulation.
4. Determine optimal time for ambulation.	Client's personal habits must be considered when planning activities.
5. Assess degree of assistance client needs.	For safety, another person may be needed initially to assist with client ambulation. Allow the client as much independence as possible.

Nursing Diagnosis

Defining characteristics from the assessment data may reveal the following nursing diagnoses for clients requiring this skill:

- Activity intolerance
- Ineffective peripheral tissue perfusion
- Decreased cardiac output
- Fatigue
- Impaired physical mobility
- Risk for impaired skin integrity
- Risk for injury

Related factors are individualized based on client's condition or needs.

Planning

Step	Rationale
1. **Expected outcomes** following completion of procedure:	
▪ Client will ambulate without episode of injury.	Appropriate level of assistance on device ensures client's safety.
▪ Client is able to ambulate without excessive fatigue or dizziness.	Assistive device chosen requires minimal exertion.
▪ Client will demonstrate correct assigned **gait.**	Demonstrates learning.
▪ Client will resume social and self-care activities.	Progressive ambulating activities increase client's endurance and independence.

STEP	RATIONALE
2. Prepare client for procedure:	
a. Explain reasons for exercise and demonstrate specific gait technique to client or care giver.	Teaching and demonstration enhance learning, reduce anxiety, and encourage cooperation.
b. Decide with client how far to ambulate.	Determines mutual goal.
c. Schedule ambulation around client's other activities.	Schedule rest periods between activities so client does not become too fatigued.
d. Place bed in low position and slowly assist client to upright position. Let client sit or stand for a few minutes until balance is gained.	Prevents orthostatic hypotension and potential injuries. If client becomes dizzy when position is changed from supine to upright, refer to Skill 28-4 for measures to minimize orthostatic hypotension.
e. Care must be taken if the client has IV tubings or a Foley catheter. Obtain an IV pole with wheels that can be pushed as the client walks. Urinary catheter drainage bags must stay at or below the level of the bladder, so a second person may be needed to assist.	Allows client to ambulate unencumbered. Urine in tubing must not reenter bladder, which would increase infection risk.

• ***Critical Decision Point***

Remove obstacles from pathways, including throw rugs, and wipe up any spills immediately. Avoid crowds. Crowds increase the risk of the crutch, cane, or walker being kicked or jarred and the client losing balance.

STEP	RATIONALE
3. If ambulation device is used, make sure it is appropriate height:	Promotes optimal support and stability.
a. *Crutch measurement:* Includes three areas: client's height, distance between crutch pad and axilla, and angle of elbow flexion. Use one of two methods:	
(1) *Standing:* Position crutches with crutch tips at point 4 to 6 inches (10 to 15 cm) to side and 4 to 6 inches in front of client's feet and crutch pads $1\frac{1}{2}$ to 2 inches (4 to 5 cm) below axilla.	Radial nerve passes under axillary area superficially. If crutch is too long, it can cause pressure on axilla and radial nerve. Injury to radial nerve causes paralysis of elbow and wrist extensors, commonly called **crutch palsy.** Also, if crutch is too long, shoulders are forced upward and client cannot push body off the ground. If ambulation device is too short, client will be bent over and uncomfortable (Borgman-Gainer, 1996).
(2) *Supine:* Crutch pad should be 3 to 4 finger widths under axilla with crutch tips positioned 6 inches (15 cm) lateral to client's heel (Borgman-Gainer, 1996) (see illustration).	
(3) Instruct client to report any tingling or numbness in the upper torso.	May mean crutches are being used incorrectly or that they are wrong size.

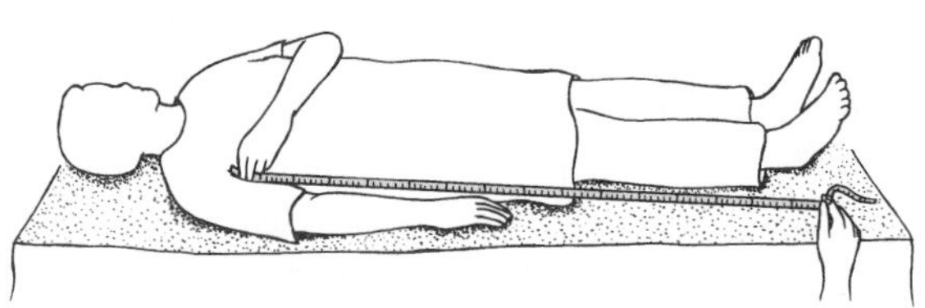

STEP **3a(2)** Supine method.

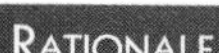

STEP	RATIONALE

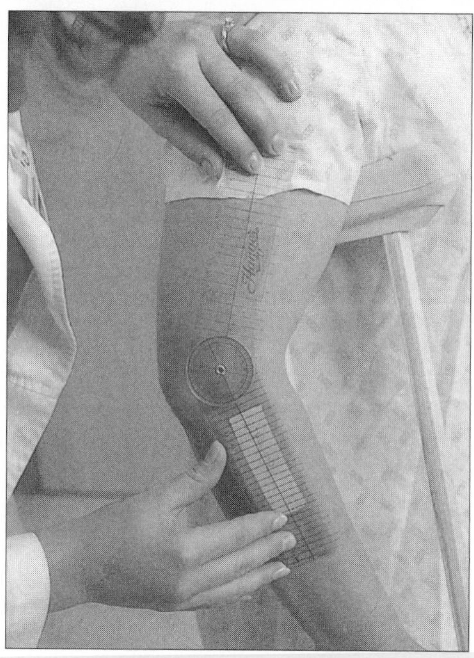

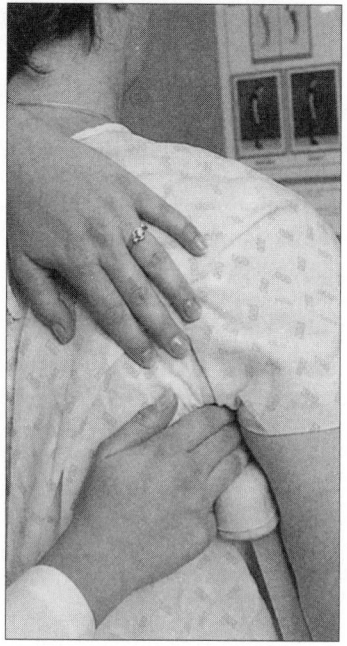

STEP **3a(4)** Top of crutch.

STEP **3a(5)** Elbows flexed.

STEP	RATIONALE
(4) Following correct crutch adjustment, two or three fingers should fit between top of crutch and axilla (see illustration).	Adequate space prevents crutch palsy.
(5) With either measurement method, elbows should be flexed 15 to 30 degrees. Elbow flexion is verified with goniometer (see illustration).	Angle ensures arms can push body off ground.
(6) In addition to overall *length* of axillary crutch, *height* of handgrip is important. Both dimensions are adjustable on well-made crutch, and the ability to adjust these dimensions is an important feature for a growing child. Handgrip should be adjusted so that the client's elbow is slightly flexed.	If handgrip is too low, radial nerve can be damaged even if overall crutch length is correct because extra length between handgrip and axillary bar can force bar up into axilla as client stretches down to reach handgrip. If handgrip is too high, client's elbow is sharply flexed, and strength and stability of arms are decreased.
b. *Cane measurement:* Client should hold cane on uninvolved side 4 to 6 (10 to 15 cm) inches to side of foot. Cane should extend from greater trochanter to floor. Allow approximately 15 to 30 degrees of elbow flexion.	Offers most support when on stronger side of body. Cane and weaker leg work together with each step. If cane is too short, client will have difficulty supporting weight and be bent over and uncomfortable. As weight is taken on by hand and affected leg is lifted off floor, complete extension of elbow is necessary (Borgman-Gainer, 1996).
c. *Walker measurement:* Upper bar of walker should be slightly below client's waist. Elbows should be flexed at approximately 15 to 30 degrees when client is standing within walker with hands on handgrips.	
4. Make sure the ambulation device has rubber tips.	Rubber tips prevent the device from slipping.
5. Make sure surface client will walk on is clean, dry, and well-lighted. Remove any objects that might obstruct the pathway.	Prevents injuries.

STEP	RATIONALE

IMPLEMENTATION

Assisted Ambulation With One Nurse

Step	Rationale
1. Follow Skill 28-5 to minimize effects of orthostatic hypotension.	Helps client gain balance before attempting ambulation and ensures that client will not become faint while walking.
2. Apply gait belt if unsure of client's stability and assist client to standing position; observe balance.	Prevents injury. Gait belt encircles client's waist and has space for nurse to hold while client walks. If client appears weak or unsteady, return client to bed.
3. Have client take a few steps while nurse is positioned on client's stronger side. If an assistive device (e.g., cane, walker) is used, then nurse stands on client's weak side.	If client has hemiplegia (one-sided paralysis) or hemiparesis (one-sided weakness), stand next to client's unaffected side and support client by placing arm closest to client on the walking belt.
4. Grasp walking belt in middle of client's back.	Provides support at waist so client's center of gravity remains midline.
5. Take a few steps forward with client. Then assess for strength and balance.	Ensures client has satisfactory strength and balance to continue.
6. If client becomes weak or dizzy, return client to bed or chair, whichever is closer.	Allows client to rest.
7. If client begins to fall, gently ease client to floor by holding firmly onto gait belt, stand with feet apart to provide broad base of support, extend leg, and let client slide against it to the floor. As client slides, nurse bends knees to lower body.	Nurse can cause more damage to self and client by trying to catch client.

Assisted Ambulation With Two Nurses

Step	Rationale
1. Follow Steps 1 and 2, *Assisted Ambulation With One Nurse.*	
2. Stand on either side of client.	
3. Both nurses grasp walking belt in middle of client's back.	Provides secure grip for each nurse.
4. Step forward in unison with client, keeping speed and step size same as client's.	Ensures stability of client.
5. Gradually increase distance walked.	Strengthens muscles, increases endurance, and prevents client from becoming too fatigued.
6. Follow Steps 6 and 7, *Assisted Ambulation With One Nurse.*	

Ambulation With Assistive Devices

Step	Rationale
1. Assist client in crutch-walking by choosing appropriate **crutch gait:**	To use crutches, client supports self with hands and arms; therefore strength in arm and shoulder muscles, ability to balance body in upright position, and stamina are necessary. Exercises such as squeezing a rubber ball, raising and lowering both arms in a slow and rhythmic manner while holding weights, push-ups, and pull-ups will assist in strengthening the upper extremities. The type of gait the client uses in crutch-walking depends on amount of weight client is able to support with one or both legs.
a. Four-point gait:	This is the most stable of crutch gaits because it provides at least three points of support at all times. Requires bearing weight on both legs. Often used when client has some form of paralysis, such as for spastic children with cerebral palsy (Wong and others, 1999). May also be used for arthritic clients.

STEP	RATIONALE
(1) Begin in tripod position. Crutches are placed 6 inches (15 cm) in front and 6 inches to side of each foot. The client's weight should be placed on the handgrips, not under the arms (see illustration).	Improves client's balance by providing wide base of support. Client should have a posture of erect head and neck, straight vertebrae, and extended hips and knees.
(2) Move right crutch forward 4 to 6 inches (10 to 15 cm) (see illustration *A*). (3) Move left foot forward to level of left crutch (see illustration *B*). (4) Move left crutch forward 4 to 6 inches (10 to 15 cm) (see illustration *C*). (5) Move right foot forward to level of right crutch (see illustration *D*). (6) Repeat above sequence.	Crutch and foot position is similar to arm and foot position during normal walking.

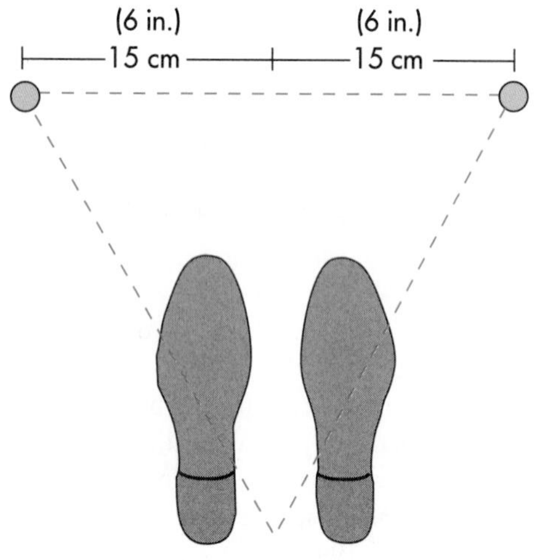

STEP **1a(1)** Tripod position.

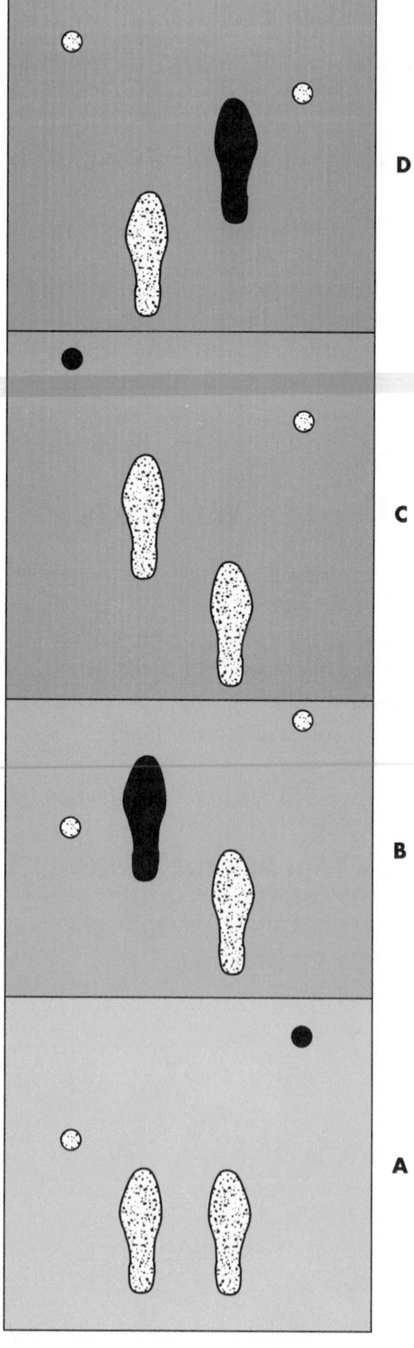

STEP **1a(2-5)** Four-point gait.

STEP	RATIONALE
b. Three-point gait:	Requires client to bear all weight on one foot. Weight is borne on uninvolved leg and then on both crutches. Affected leg does not touch ground during early phase of three-point gait. May be useful for client with broken leg or sprained ankle.
(1) Begin in tripod position (see illustration *A*).	Improves client's balance by providing wide base of support.
(2) Advance both crutches and affected leg (see illustration *B*).	
(3) Move stronger leg forward (see illustration *C*).	
(4) Repeat sequence.	
c. Two-point gait:	Requires at least partial weight-bearing on each foot. Is faster than the four-point gait. Requires more balance because only two points support body at one time (Borgman-Gainer, 1996).
(1) Begin in tripod position (see illustration *A*).	Improves client's balance by providing wide base of support.
(2) Move left crutch and right foot forward (see illustration *B*).	Crutch movements are similar to arm movement during normal walking.
(3) Move right crutch and left foot forward (see illustration *C*).	
(4) Repeat sequence.	

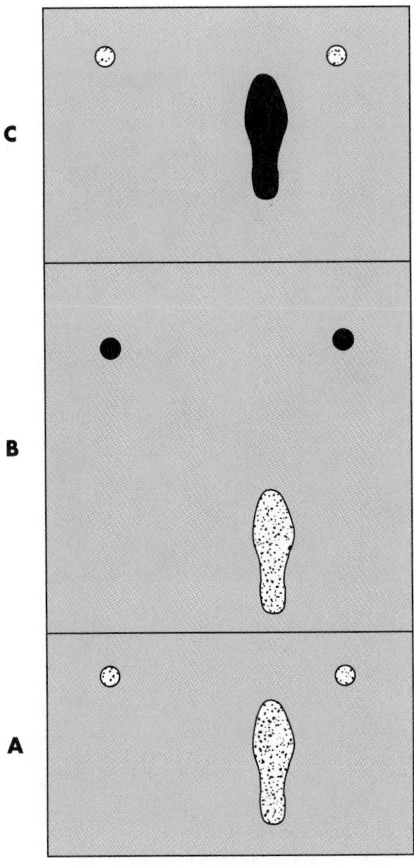

STEP **1b** Three-point gait.

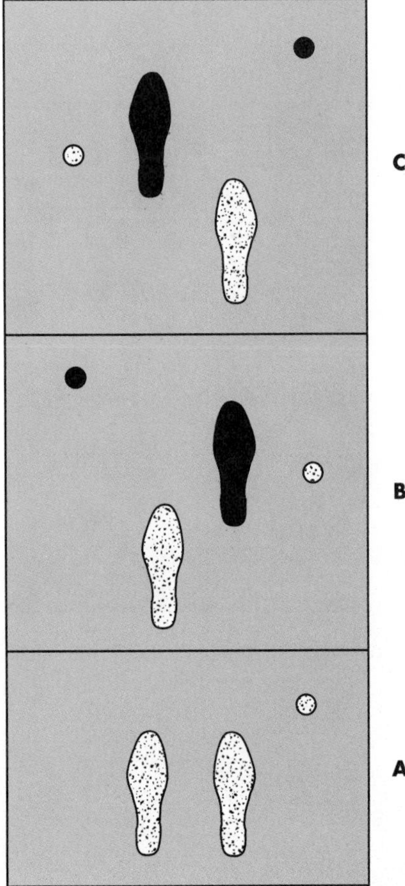

STEP **1c** Two-point gait.

Step	Rationale
d. Swing-to gait:	
(1) Begin in tripod position.	Frequently used by clients whose lower extremities are paralyzed or who wear weight-supporting braces on their legs.
(2) Move both crutches forward.	This is the easier of the two swinging gaits. It requires the ability to partially bear body weight on both legs (Borgman-Gainer, 1996).
(3) Lift and swing legs to crutches, letting crutches support body weight.	
(4) Repeat two previous steps.	
e. Swing-through gait:	
(1) Begin in tripod position.	Requires that client have the ability to bear partial weight on both feet (Borgman-Gainer, 1996).
(2) Move both crutches forward.	Initial placement of crutches is to increase the client's base of support so that when the body swings forward, the client is moving the center of gravity toward the additional support provided by the crutches.
(3) Lift and swing legs through and beyond crutches.	
2. Assist client in climbing stairs with crutches:	
a. Begin in tripod position.	Improves client's balance by providing wide base of support.
b. Client transfers body weight to crutches (see illustration).	Prepares client to transfer weight to unaffected leg when ascending first stair.
c. Client advances unaffected leg to stair (see illustration).	Crutch adds support to affected leg. Client then shifts weight from crutches to unaffected leg.

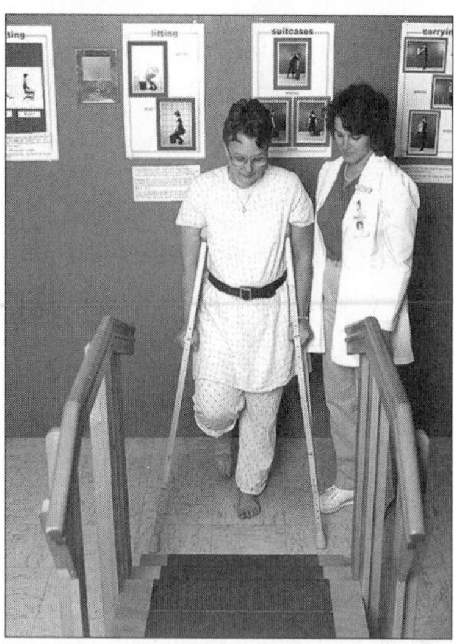

STEP **2b** Transfer body weight to crutches.

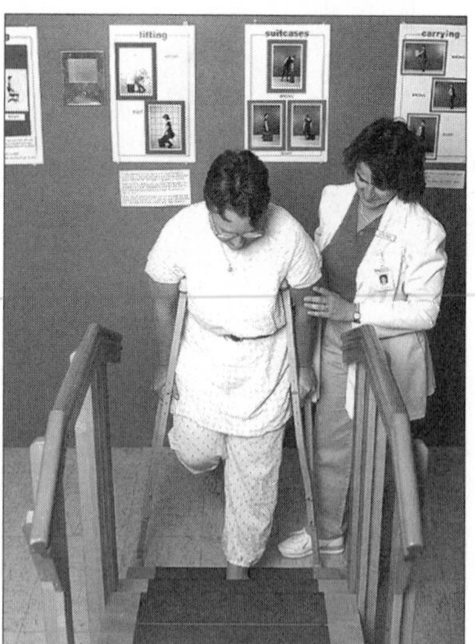

STEP **2c** Advance unaffected leg to stair.

STEP	RATIONALE
d. Both crutches are aligned with unaffected leg on stairs (see illustration).	Maintains balance and provides wide base of support.
e. Repeat sequence until client reaches top of stairs.	
3. Assist client in descending stairs with crutches:	
a. Begin in tripod position.	Improves client's balance by providing wide base of support.
b. Client transfers body weight to unaffected leg (see illustration).	Prepares client to release support of body weight maintained by crutches.
c. Move crutches to stair and instruct client to begin to transfer body weight to crutches (see illustration) and move affected leg forward.	Maintains client's balance and base of support.
d. Client moves unaffected leg to stair and aligns with crutches (see illustration).	Maintains balance and provides base of support.
e. Repeat sequence until stairs are descended.	

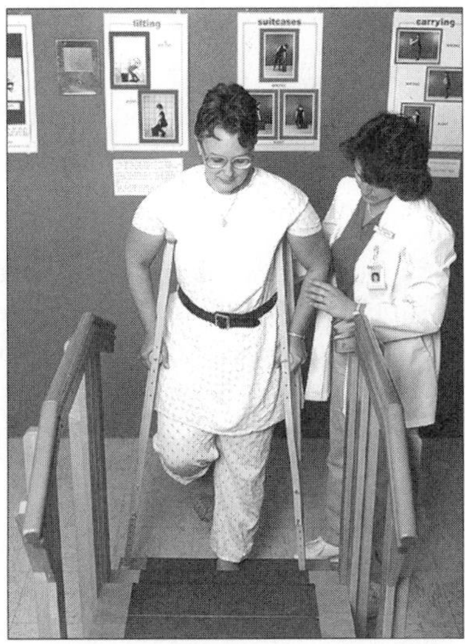

STEP **2d** Align crutches with unaffected leg.

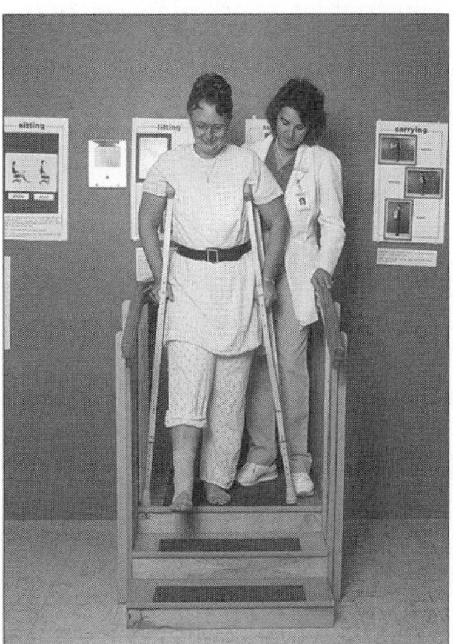

STEP **3b** Body weight is transferred to unaffected leg.

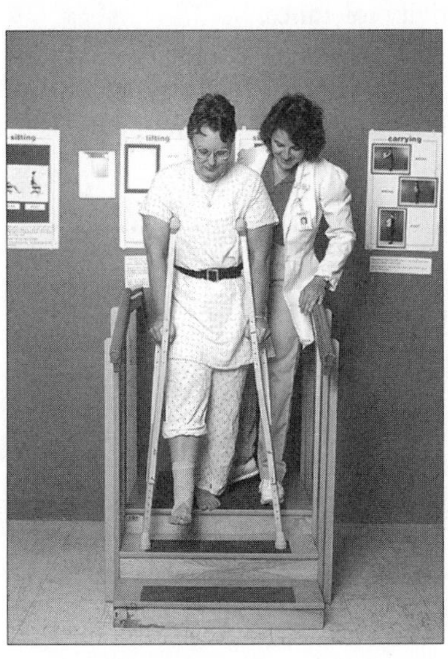

STEP **3c** Transfer weight to crutches.

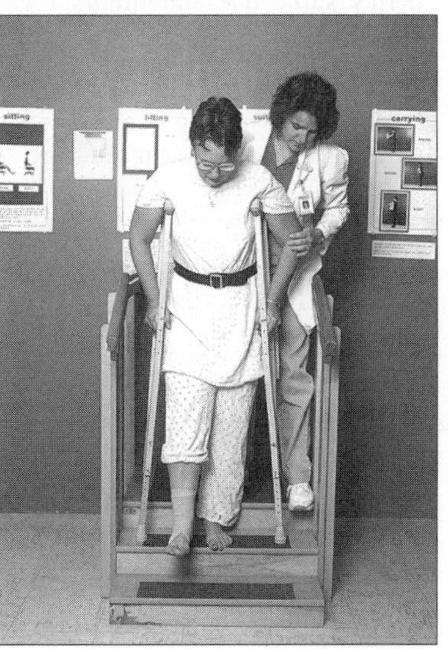

STEP **3d** Move unaffected leg and align crutches.

Step	Rationale
4. Assist client in ambulating with walker:	Walker is used by clients who are able to bear partial weight. Walkers do need to be picked up, so client does need sufficient strength to be able to pick up walker. Four-wheeled model, which does not need to be picked up, is not as stable.
a. Have client stand in center of walker and grasp handgrips on upper bars.	Client balances self before attempting to walk.
b. Lift walker, move it 6 to 8 inches (15 to 20 cm) forward, and then set it down, making sure all four feet of the walker stay on the floor. Take a step forward with either foot. Then follow through with the other leg.	Provides broad base of support between walker and client. Client then moves center of gravity toward the walker. Keeping all four feet of the walker on the floor is necessary to prevent tipping of the walker.
c. If there is unilateral weakness, after the walker is advanced, instruct the client to step forward with the weaker leg, support self with the arms, and follow through with the uninvolved leg. If client is unable to bear weight on one leg, after advancing walker have the client swing onto it, supporting weight on hands.	
5. Assist client in ambulating with cane (same steps are taught whether standard or quad canes are used):	
a. Begin by placing cane on the side opposite the involved leg.	Provides added support for the weak or impaired side.
b. Place cane forward 6 to 10 inches (15 to 25 cm), keeping body weight on both legs.	Distributes body weight equally.
c. Move involved leg forward, even with the cane.	Body weight is supported by cane and uninvolved leg.
d. Advance uninvolved leg past cane.	Body weight is supported by cane and involved leg.
e. Move involved leg forward, even with uninvolved leg.	Aligns client's center of gravity. Returns client's body weight to equal distribution.
f. Repeat these steps.	

Evaluation

1. After ambulation, obtain client's vital signs, heart rate, respiratory rate, and temperature; observe skin color, and ask about the client's energy level.	Evaluates how client tolerated procedure and evaluates whether there was progress in ambulation. Assesses stage of client's illness and degree of convalescence when evaluating the process.
2. Evaluate client's subjective statements regarding experience.	Evaluates activity tolerance.
3. Evaluate gait of client, observing body alignment in standing position and balance.	Determines if client is correctly using supportive aids for ambulation. Keep in mind the client's previous manner of ambulating when assessing gait.
4. Observe client's ability to perform self-care activities.	

Unexpected Outcomes and Related Interventions

- Client will be unable to ambulate.
  - Possible reasons include fear of falling, physical discomfort, upper body muscles that are too weak to use ambulation device, and lower extremities that are too weak to support body.
  - Initiate isometric exercise program to strengthen upper body muscles.
- Client sustains injury.
  - Obstacles in client's path, incorrect technique used, or proper safety precautions not taken.
  - Notify physician. Return client to bed if injury stable.

Recording and Reporting

Record and report:

- Type of gait the client used.
- Amount of assistance required.
- Distance walked.
- Client's tolerance of activity.
- Immediately report any injury sustained during attempts to ambulate, alteration in vital signs, or inability to ambulate to nurse in charge or physician.

Teaching Considerations

- If a walker is used, the client is taught to examine the frame daily. When inspecting a walker, the client should observe for signs of bending or deformation of the frame, protruding screws that can scratch, and loose or missing screws that weaken the joints of the frame. Handgrips should be assessed for any cracks or signs of being loose.
- Clients should be instructed to use the arms of a chair rather than the walker to give them leverage when getting up from a chair; the walker is likely to tip if used for this purpose.
- Blistering or soreness of the hands can result from continual pressure between the hand and the handle of a crutch. Advise client to release pressure intermittently and wear gloves or pad the handle to reduce friction.

Pediatric Considerations

- For rehabilitation of a small child who has not yet learned to walk or who is unsteady, special crutches with three or four legs provide needed stability to allow the child to maintain an upright posture and learn to walk (Wong and others, 1999).

Gerontological Considerations

- The older adult may require additional time in the morning before resuming activities.

Home Care Considerations

- Client should be instructed on how to use the ambulation aid on various terrains (e.g., carpet, stairs, rough ground, inclines). Client should also be instructed on how to maneuver around obstacles such as doors and how to use the aid when transferring to and from a chair, toilet, tub, and chair (Borgman-Gainer, 1996).

Long-Term Care Considerations

- Safety and maintenance checks of ambulation devices should be done on a routine basis.
- Periodic assessments should be performed to ensure that the client is using the ambulation device properly.

Critical Thinking Exercises

1. An elderly client is admitted to the hospital for a fractured left hip resulting from a fall at home. The client has just undergone total hip replacement. What potential risk factors in the Virchow's triad could this client potentially experience? What should be assessed before applying elastic and/or SPC stockings?
2. A 66-year-old male has suffered from bilateral fractured femurs and is expected to remain in traction on bed rest for several weeks. Describe two nursing interventions to help minimize orthostatic hypotension in this client.
3. After removing a client's elastic support stockings, the nurse notes an area on the right leg that is reddened and warm to the touch. What could these signs signify, and what steps should the nurse take?
4. An elderly woman underwent extensive abdominal surgery four days ago. She seems rather anxious, and her heart rate has increased considerably over baseline. She complains of shortness of breath and pleuritic chest pain. What do these signs and symptoms indicate? What is the appropriate nursing intervention at this time?

References

Blondin M, Titler M. Deep vein thrombosis and pulmonary embolism. Prevention: what role do nurses play? *Medsurg Nurs* 5(3):205, 1996.

Borgman-Gainer M. Independent function: movement and mobility. In Hoeman S, editor: *Rehabilitation nursing: process and application,* ed 2, St Louis, 1996, Mosby.

Brough E: Deep vein thrombosis, *Prof Nurs* 13(10):687, 1998.

Collier M: Brevet tx: anti-embolism stockings for prevention and treatment of DVT, *Brit J Nurs* 8(1):44, 1999.

Dawe D, Moore-Orr R: Low-intensity, range of motion exercise: invaluable nursing care for elderly patients, *J Adv Nurs* 21(4):675, 1995.

Galindo-Ciocon D: Nursing care of elders with leg edema, *J Gerontol Nurs* 21(2):7, 1995.

Hamilton L, Lyon P: A nursing-driven program to preserve and restore functional ability in hospitalized elderly patients, *J Orthop Nurs Assoc* 25(4):30, 1995.

Lueckonette AG: *Gerontologic nursing,* ed 2, St Louis, 2000, Mosby.

McCance K, Huether S: *Pathophysiology: the biologic basis for disease in adults and children,* ed 3, St Louis, 1998, Mosby.

Phipps W, Sands JK, Marek JF: *Medical-surgical nursing: concepts and clinical practice,* ed 6, St Louis, 1999, Mosby.

Potter P, Perry A: *Fundamentals of nursing: concepts, process, and practice,* ed 5, St Louis, 2001, Mosby.

Radwanski M, Hoeman S: Geriatric rehabilitation nursing. In Hoeman S, editor: *Rehabilitation nursing: process and application,* ed 2, St Louis, 1996, Mosby.

Thibodeau G, Patton K: *Structure and function of the body,* ed 4, St Louis, 1997, Mosby.

Winslow E, Lane L, Woods R: Dangling: a review of relevant physiology, research, and practice, *Heart Lung* 24(4):263, 1995.

Wong D and others: *Whaley and Wong's nursing care of infants and children,* ed 6, St Louis, 1999, Mosby.

29

Orthopedic Measures

Skills

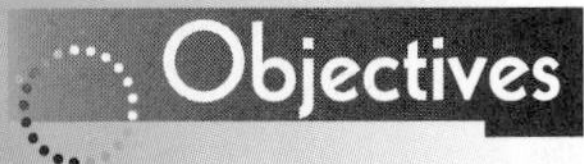

Mastery of content in this chapter will enable the nurse to:

- Define the key terms listed.
- Explain benefits of the use of casts for clients with musculoskeletal injuries.
- Describe how to assist in application of casts.
- Describe neurovascular assessments of a client in specific casts.
- Describe techniques for drying casts.
- Describe toileting techniques for clients in casts and traction.
- Describe turning and positioning techniques for clients in casts.
- Describe elements of client education for the client with a cast and after removal of a cast.
- Explain the purposes of placing clients in skin or skeletal traction.
- Describe client conditions requiring the use of each form of skin or skeletal traction.
- Describe steps for applying each form of skin or skeletal traction.

Key Terms

Cast
Cast brace
Cast saw
Cast shoe
Cast stabilization
Cast syndrome
Casting tape
Cervical halter
Compartment syndrome
Countertraction
Crepitation
External fixation
Four-poster cast
Harris splint
Minerva jacket
Neurovascular assessment
Pearson attachment
Pelvic belt
Pelvic sling
Petaling
Pulleys
Reduction
Sheet wadding
Spica cast
Spreader bar
Stockinette
Thomas splint
Traction
Traction boot
Walking heel
Webril
Weight holder

Clients in a cast or traction are susceptible to problems that can affect all body systems. Depending on the extent of a client's injury or illness, an orthopedic device may affect a single body part or the entire body. Alterations in the client's level of mobility require extensive nursing care.

The adequacy of central and peripheral circulation to the injured area must be carefully assessed, because delivery of oxygen and removal of wastes are vital for bone healing, muscle growth and strength, and regaining mobility. Color, temperature, and capillary refill assessments provide data about the adequacy of circulation to the injured extremity. Inflammation, cellulitis, or edema may indicate venous stasis or infection.

Integumentary tissues inside and outside the cast must remain healthy and well nourished. Assessment of the tissues detects pressure, inflammation, or lesions that could lead to infection or pressure sores. Gentle and thorough cleansing of skin, careful drying, and lubrication with lotions provide moisture and stimulation to the integumentary tissues to maintain a healthy state.

Turning, positioning, and range-of-joint-motion (ROJM) exercise help to maintain the health of integumentary and musculoskeletal tissues of individuals in casts. After application of a cast, especially a **spica cast** or body cast (Figure 29-1) or **Minerva jacket,** the client must be turned from side to side and prone to facilitate thorough drying of the cast. Turning the client every 2 to 3 hours while keeping the damp cast uncovered facilitates drying. Turning also aids circulation throughout the body, decreases the development of renal calculi, and prevents the development of decubitus ulcers. Placement of pillows, rolls, or blankets helps the client to maintain the side-lying or prone position. In addition, musculoskeletal tissues maintain strength through regularly performed active ROJM exercises with or without resistance or weight. Quadriceps-, gluteus-, triceps-, biceps-, and hamstring-setting exercises, performed routinely and steadily, help to maintain muscle mass and tone (see Chapter 28).

A major challenge for nurses caring for clients in body, spica, or Minerva jacket casts is to maintain respiratory function. While turning facilitates moving air and fluids in the airways, it is also vital that clients be encouraged to breathe deeply and cough. Bed rest over time affects respiration, resulting in decreased ventilation and alveolar collapse. Clients with altered mobility who develop respiratory complications may require respiratory therapy and at times administration of antibiotics. Preventive nursing care measures should be sufficient to avoid such necessities.

Additional challenges center around intake and maintenance of functions of the gastrointestinal and genitourinary systems. Clients in casts or traction who are confined to bed frequently develop anorexia, constipation, and at times fecal impaction. Maintaining a high (3000 ml or more) fluid intake plus a high-bulk or high-residue diet fosters proper bowel elimination. Fluid intake also facilitates renal circulation and urinary output to lessen the possibility of a urinary tract infection or renal calculi.

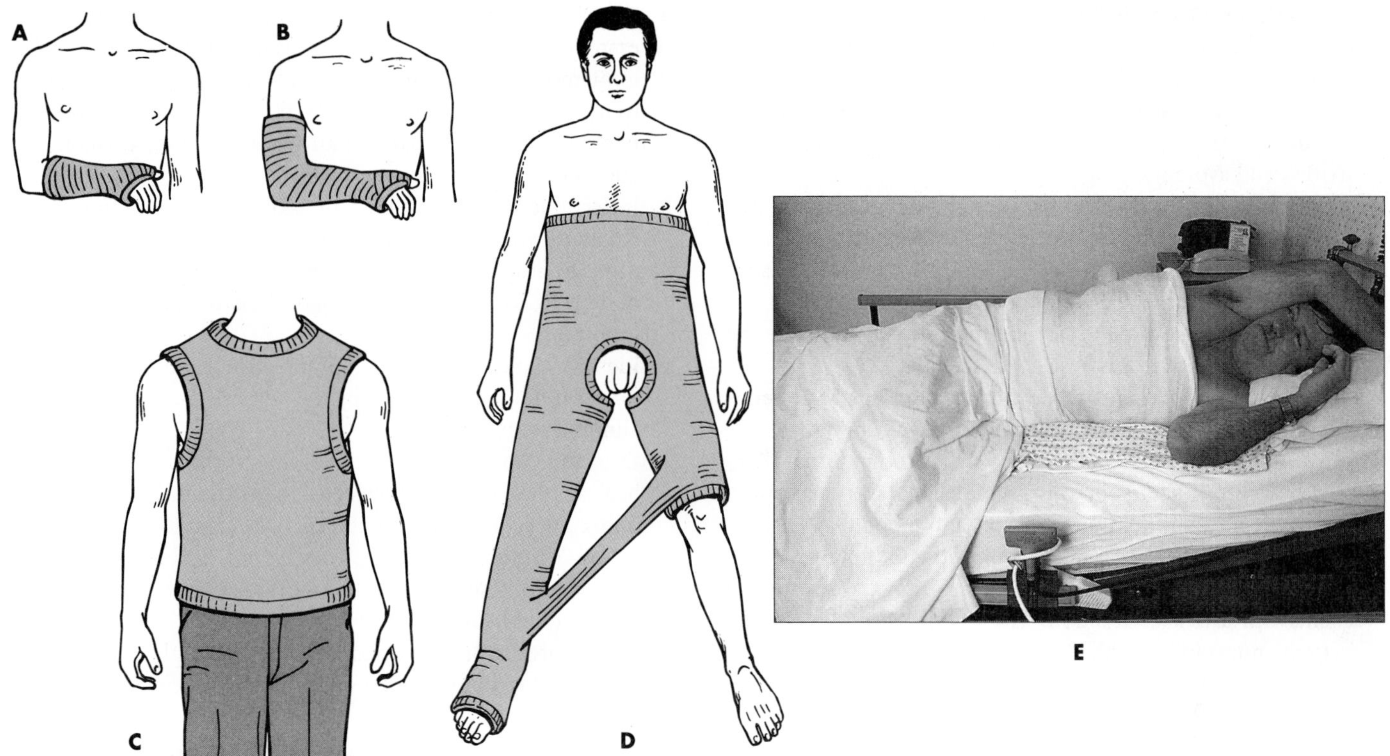

FIGURE **29-1** Types of casts. **A,** Short arm cast. **B,** Long arm cast. **C,** Plaster body jacket cast. **D,** One-and-a-half hip spica cast. **E,** Body cast.

Clients immobilized in casts or traction may lose weight. Diets should be high in protein, carbohydrates, vitamins, bulk, and fluids and should contain a moderate amount of fat, unless contraindicated. Because of individual metabolic and endocrine stress responses, the client will experience catabolism with muscle mass loss for a period of 10 to 20 or more days. Remodeling of bone, a process by which bone resorption and bone deposit occurs, is governed by hormones and stress placed on the bone. When serum calcium levels decrease, parathyroid hormone (PTH) is released. This stimulates osteoclast activity (bone resorption), calcium is released from the bone, and the serum calcium level rises. This can lead to poor bone replacement and the development of osteoporosis and renal calculi. With an elevated serum calcium level, calcitonin from the thyroid gland is released, bone resorption is suppressed, and calcium salts are deposited in the bone matrix.

Motor and sensory functions are greatly affected when a client is placed in a cast. Motor changes may lead to muscle and joint weakness from disuse or pressure. Sensory changes, also from pressure or trauma, may lead to complaints of pain, numbness, and tingling. When such sensory signs are present, they may be relieved by changing the client's position. It is essential to monitor for the five P's (pain, pallor, pulselessness, paresthesia, and paralysis) of neurovascular status, because permanent damage may result if the circulation is not restored or pressure is not removed (Kunkler, 1999). Bivalving, or cutting the cast, removes the pressure or tightness and increases circulation. Motor weakness may be restored to normal ranges through ROJM exercises and physical therapy. Full muscle function returns slowly, and consistent performance of exercises is required.

Traction is a force or pull applied to the bones directly or indirectly to overcome deformity and to help restore alignment. When bones are fractured, muscle spasms pull the distal fragments out of their normal positions, often resulting in misalignment and overriding of the bones. Sufficient pull must be applied to the injured tissues to overcome muscle spasms and thus permit the bones to realign themselves in the usual anatomical positions. In situations of severe muscle spasms, marked deformity, or displacement, traction must be applied directly to the distal fragments by means of a strong nail or pin to which traction is applied through a bar, ropes, pulleys, and weights. Such skeletal traction may be applied to one or more bones, including the bones of the skull, upper and lower extremities, and pelvic bones.

Traction to the skin, also known as "skin traction," is applied indirectly to the bones through skin around the structure. Skin traction is typically between 5 and 7 pounds and is commonly used for minor trauma or immediate immobilization before surgery. Because of the lower tolerance of skin tissues, this traction is applied for shorter periods, with less weight, and at times can be interrupted. **Neurovascular assessment** is essential to ensure that circumferential dressings (dressings that encircle an extremity) do not impede circulation or place pressure on neurological tissue. Skeletal traction, when used for severe trauma, is applied for longer periods, requires much heavier weights, and is never interrupted.

Clients in traction or those with casts who are confined to bed may become easily tired during the day and may take short, frequent naps. Thus they may be less sleepy at night and may lie awake past their usual bedtime. To offset this syndrome, clients should remain active, engage in stimulating activities, and avoid napping during the day.

Immobilized clients often experience complications of immobility such as skin breakdown and pulmonary emboli. Clients with fractures may develop complications such as fat embolism syndrome (FES), **compartment syndrome,** or osteomyelitis. Expert nursing care can minimize or eliminate the threat to the client from these complications.

Psychologically, clients in casts or traction may experience alterations in self-concept and body image. They may lose some independence, mobility, and work income during therapy; however, if clients perceive these changes as temporary, they usually regain full independence and mobility.

Knowledge of normal mobility and the findings from the nursing assessment enable the nurse to provide care to the client with a cast or traction. The following guidelines can help the nurse individualize the client's care plan.

Skill Performance Guidelines

1. Identify the client's dietary preferences. Wound healing and repair of bone and tissues require additional nutritional intake. Providing foods the client can enjoy meets these additional nutritional needs.
2. Determine the limits of ROJM to the casted extremity or extremity in traction. Although it is important to maintain joint mobility, the nurse must not move the affected extremity beyond the limits imposed by the cast or traction. Excessive movement can impair wound healing, extremity alignment, and new bone growth.
3. Determine the client's level of independent functioning. Knowing what the client is capable of doing enables the nurse to properly plan for assisting the client with activities of daily living (ADLs) such as bathing, eating, dressing, and grooming.
4. Identify the client's normal elimination patterns. Restrictions on mobility imposed by the cast or traction can alter elimination patterns.
5. Determine the client's understanding of the normal bone-healing process. This knowledge assists the nurse in developing a teaching plan for the client to care for the casted extremity at home.
6. Identify the results of recent laboratory tests. Serum calcium and phosphorus are two minerals that compose callus, the precursor to bone ossification. Hemoglobin, hematocrit, and red blood cell levels will decrease in blood loss anemia.
7. Determine the frequency and type of analgesics ordered for the client by the physician. The client may experience acute, continuous pain and/or muscle spasms during the first 4 to 7 days (the acute inflammatory stage) and thus require 24-hour administration of analgesics and/or muscle relaxants during this time.

Skill 29-1 Assisting With Cast Application

A **cast** is an externally applied structure used to hold musculoskeletal tissues in a specific position to permit healing of injuries or fractures or to align malpositioned tissues, such as in clubfoot or congenital hip dislocation. The rigidity of the cast overcomes the tension, tone, or rotational forces of the muscles or bones for the time required to heal or align the diseased or injured tissues. Because a cast holds tissue in the position in which it is applied, it must be applied carefully and properly to achieve the goals for its use.

Casts are made from plaster of Paris or synthetic materials (Figure 29-2). A plaster of Paris cast has multiple roles of open-weave cotton saturated with calcium sulfate crystals. These casts are heavier than synthetic casts and can take 24 to 72 hours with no weight bearing or application of pressure to dry. Plaster of Paris is easy to mold and shape around unstable fractures. Synthetic casts are composed of polyester and cotton material, which is impregnated with a water-activated polyurethane resin. Synthetic casts are also made of fiberglass or plastic. Although the newer synthetic casts are more expen-

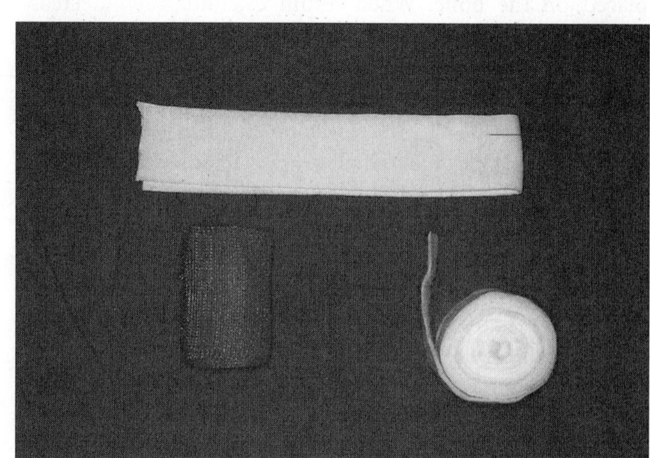

FIGURE **29-2** Plaster roll and padding material.

sive than plaster, they can withstand contact with water without crumbling. These casts are lightweight, set in 15 minutes, and can sustain weight bearing or pressure in 15 to 30 minutes.

Client safety is important as the nurse helps apply the cast. The nurse provides optimal skin care to the client before, during, and after cast application. The nurse cleans the extremity, removing dirt, glass, or debris beneath the cast that would irritate the skin. After application of the cast, the nurse ensures that plaster crumbs are removed and rough edges are "petaled" to prevent skin breakdown.

Delegation Considerations

Assessment of the client's condition should not be delegated to assistive personnel. However, the skill of assisting with cast application may be delegated to assistive personnel. Inform assistive personnel to avoid positioning that increases client discomfort, and inform and assist care provider, as needed, in the proper method of assisting with cast application.

Equipment

NOTE: Equipment may be preassembled on "cast cart."

- Plaster rolls (sizes include 2-, 3-, 4-, and 6-in rolls) or cast materials such as fiberglass, casting tape, or plastic, depending on purpose of cast or specific client condition
- Padding material (felt, **stockinette, sheet wadding, Webril,** or other material; available in various thicknesses and lengths)
- Plastic-lined bucket or basin filled three-fourths full with warm water
- Disposable gloves and aprons
- Scissors
- Paper or plastic sheets
- **Cast saw** (if old cast is to be removed)
- Cart, chair, fracture table

Step	Rationale
Assessment	
1. Assess client's previous health status, including conditions affecting wound healing (e.g., diabetes, peripheral vascular disease, malnutrition, age).	Health status influences healing of tissues enclosed by cast.
2. Assess client's understanding of upcoming cast application.	Relieves client's anxiety and helps nurse determine whether additional information is needed.
3. Assess condition of tissues to be in the cast, including circulation (pulse, color, temperature) to extremities, range of motion, and sensation. Note presence of skin breakdown, bruising, rash, and irritation. Skin of babies, children, and older adults may contain less subcutaneous fat.	Determines need for additional skin care before cast application. Provides baseline for close observation after cast is applied.
• ***Critical Decision Point*** *Clients with skin breakdown or skin lesions may not be candidates for casting.*	
4. Determine client's pain status. a. Administer analgesic per physician order. b. Administer muscle relaxant per physician order.	Fractures are painful; client responses vary, as does need for an analgesic. Administration of medications 30 minutes prior to procedure can lessen discomfort.
5. Determine extent to which client will be able to use casted extremity.	Predicts degree of assistance needed for self-care and/or ambulation.

Nursing Diagnosis

Defining characteristics from the assessment data may reveal the following nursing diagnoses for clients requiring this skill:

- Bathing/hygiene, dressing/grooming, and toileting self-care deficit
- Risk for impaired skin integrity
- Risk for peripheral neurovascular dysfunction
- Ineffective peripheral tissue perfusion
- Impaired home maintenance
- Impaired physical mobility
- Deficient knowledge regarding casting procedure
- Acute pain
- Risk for injury

Related factors are individualized based on client's condition or needs.

STEP	RATIONALE
PLANNING	
1. **Expected outcomes** following completion of procedure:	
▪ Client initially experiences only slight edema, soreness, mild pain, and some limitation of active range of joint motion (ROJM) from being in cast.	Cast limits normal function of affected tissues.
▪ Skin of tissues below cast is warm and of normal color with capillary refill of 3 seconds or less. Client verbalizes no abnormal or unusual sensations and is able to move fingers or toes below casted part.	Neurovascular function to body part is maintained (Kunkler, 1999).
▪ Skin around proximal and distal cast edges remains intact without irritation.	Skin is free of pressure and friction from cast edges (Beare and Myers, 1998).
▪ Client is able to perform limited ROJM actively.	Other joints should move without impairment.
▪ Client has some impaired function in mobility initially.	Cast may be heavy, or it may impair mobility because of size or area of body in cast.
▪ Client uses assistance with usual activities of daily living (ADLs) if head, neck, or upper extremity is in cast.	Cast can interfere with ability to dress, feed, or bathe oneself.
▪ Client verbalizes increase in comfort after cast in place.	Injured tissues and bone are stabilized.
▪ Client demonstrates cast-care techniques.	Demonstrates learning.
2. Instruct client, parent, and other assistants how they can facilitate application of cast by maintaining affected part in desired position.	Cast will hold tissues in the position in which they are held during cast application. Client teaching reduces anxiety and increases cooperation.
IMPLEMENTATION	
1. Administer analgesic before cast application: by mouth (PO), 30 to 40 minutes before; intramuscularly (IM), 20 to 30 minutes before; intravenously (IV), 2 to 5 minutes before. Administer muscle relaxant 30 minutes before cast application if spasms are present.	Reduces pain during cast application. Provides optimal analgesic effect. Muscle spasms may be more effectively treated with skeletal muscle relaxants than with narcotics.
2. Wash hands and apply gloves. Use latex-free gloves if there is risk of an allergic reaction.	Reduces transmission of microorganisms. Synthetic cast can leave gluelike resin on hands. Prevents exposure to latex allergen (Baumann, 1999).
3. Position client as needed; client may be lying, sitting, or standing, depending on type of cast and tissues to be casted.	Parts to be put in cast must be supported and in optimal position for cast application.
4. Prepare skin for cast if necessary; may involve cleansing with soap and water, changing dressing, and trimming long hair. Use gentle strokes to maintain skin integrity.	Reduces complications to underlying tissues after casting. Gentle manipulation prevents pain or additional injury.
5. Explain that client may experience warmth during the cast application process.	Plaster gives off heat from a chemical reaction when drying.
6. Depending on type of cast material being applied, do *one* of the following:	
a. Submerge plaster roll under water in a casting bucket or plastic basin until bubbles stop, then squeeze slightly and give roll to person applying cast.	Dampened plaster rolls are unrolled and molded to fit part being casted. Some have resin for easy moldability.
b. Submerge synthetic cast roll in lukewarm water for 10 to 15 seconds. Squeeze to remove excess water.	Initiates chemical reaction that produces heat and hardens tape.
7. Hold body part or parts to be put in cast in position requested by person applying cast (see illustrations).	Support of body part may involve applying slight manual traction, if desired, to maintain optimal position.
8. Hold body part while **casting tape** is applied and molded. Synthetic tape is applied with slight tension. When wrapping is completed, gently compress with hands.	Casting tape is impregnated with synthetic adhesive or glass fiber materials, which dry quickly and are lightweight. Compression promotes bonding of cast layers.

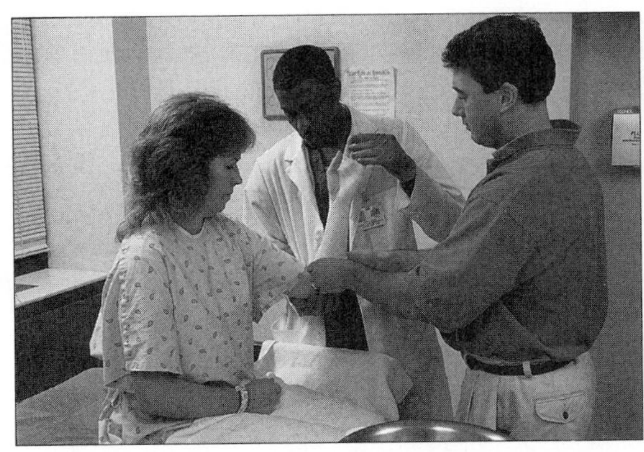
A

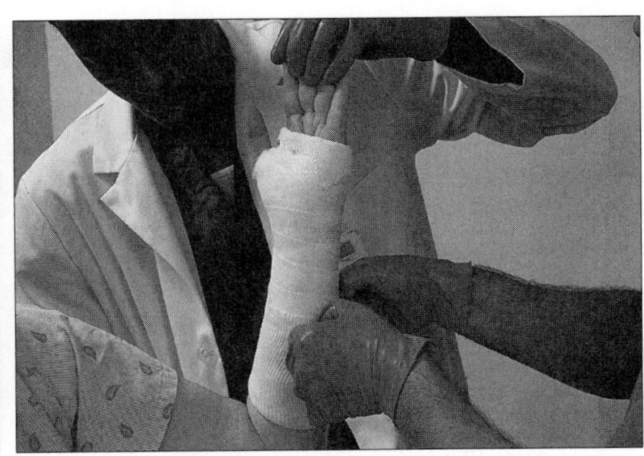
B

STEP **7** Assistant supports client's extremity as cast is applied.

STEP	RATIONALE
9. Continue to supply dampened rolls of plaster, synthetic cast roll, or cast tape or to hold parts as necessary until cast is finished. Should be able to insert two fingers between cast and limb.	Plaster must be of sufficient thickness to give strength to cast. More than two fingers' space in cast indicates cast is too loose and will not support limb, and less than two fingers' space indicates cast may be too tight and inhibit circulation.
10. Supply **walking heal** cast, **cast brace,** bar, or other **cast stabilization** material as requested by physician or practitioner.	Ambulation (after cast dries) may be permitted with partial weight bearing (see Chapter 28), which is facilitated by walking **cast shoe,** heel or sole. Bars stabilize spica cast, or "posts" (metal poles) stabilize **"four-poster" cast.** Brace can be incorporated into cast to aid in maintaining joint motion and mobility.
11. Ensure that the stockinette, Webril, or other casting material is applied evenly and smoothly to prevent wadding and lumping. Damp plaster is then unrolled over padding to hold it securely outside cast. Assist with "finishing" by folding stockinette or other padding down over outer edge of cast to provide smooth edge.	Smooth edges lessen possible skin irritation. By finishing cast with stockinette, later **"petaling"** with tape is not required when cast is dry.
12. Supply scissors to trim plaster rolls around thumb, fingers, and toes as necessary.	Cast should be snug but should not constrict joint movement or circulation.
13. Depending on tissues casted:	
a. Place damp cast on cloth-covered pillows (two to three) to prevent deformation or pressure points as it sets. Maintain elevation above heart level as long as neurovascular assessments are normal (see Evaluation section). If ice is applied, place to the side rather than the top of the cast to prevent indentations.	Pillows prevent cast from hardening in undesirable position. Elevation enhances venous return and decreases edema. If there is evidence of neurovascular deficit, then lower to the heart level to negate the effects of gravity (Beare and Myers, 1998).

• ***Critical Decision Point***

Handle casted extremity with palms only until the cast is dry. Fingers can cause indentations that can lead to pressures areas.

STEP	RATIONALE
b. Place casted tissues in sling, making sure sling just holds, and does not encase, cast.	Covering (encasing) impedes air movements and delays drying.
14. Remove and dispose of gloves.	Reduces transmission of microorganisms.
15. Cover client or reclothe as needed, leaving damp, casted areas uncovered.	Covering blocks air movement, delays drying, and retains heat, which can lead to skin damage with plaster (Beare and Myers, 1998).
16. Assist with transfer of client to stretcher or wheelchair for return to nursing unit, to prepare client for discharge. May accompany client to room and assist with transfer to bed if necessary. Client may have cast applied in room.	Safety in transfer requires use of pillows to support cast, side rails, restraints, and sufficient personnel to support client and cast. Safety in transfer requires more than one person to accompany client in body, spica, long arm, long leg, and Minerva jacket cast to prevent falls.

STEP	RATIONALE
17. Clean equipment (bucket, scissors, cast saw), and return to storage area; discard used materials. Wash hands.	Facilitates use of equipment and treatment area for next client. Reduces transmission of infection.
18. Explain purposes of exposure for faster drying, use of fans or lights to facilitate drying, use of elevation if pertinent, or application of ice bags if ordered.	Casts must dry from inside out for thorough drying. Fans should not be used in open areas or under cast; organisms may be blown in to cause infection. Hot blow dryers or heat lamps can burn tissues. Elevation and use of ice decreases edema formation.

- ***Critical Decision Point***
  Synthetic casts are dry or set by time of transfer, because they set in 7 to 15 minutes. Soft tissues around affected area may swell from processes of "reducing" or manipulating before cast was applied.

19. Reposition client every 2 to 3 hours. Do not rest cast heel on pillow.	Prevents any one area of the cast from receiving continuous pressure. Avoids indentation of cast.
20. Inform client to notify personnel of any alteration in sensation, abnormal sensation, or inability to move fingers or toes in affected extremity.	Pressure within a casted extremity may increase with edema and lead to compartment syndrome. Compartment syndrome occurs when pressure within the muscle compartment increases as a result of edema, bleeding, or decreased venous return. The fascia covering the muscle group acts as a tourniquet directing the pressure to structures within the compartment: nerves, blood vessels, and muscle tissue. Neurovascular assessments are used to determine development of compartment syndrome (Beare and Myers, 1998).
21. Cover cast with watertight plastic when bathing client. May use blow dryer on *cool* setting to dry damp areas of synthetic cast.	Plaster of Paris cast will crumble if wet. If a blow dryer is used on hot setting, it may cause the outer portion to dry while the inner section of the cast remains wet, leading to mildew development.

EVALUATION

1. Observe client for signs of pain or anxiety: severe edema, uncontrollable pain, inability to move body parts distal to cast, pain on passive motion of distal body parts, hyperventilation, swallowing air (aerophagia), tachycardia, and blood pressure elevation.	These are signs of development of compartment syndrome, **"cast syndrome,"** or severe claustrophobia from snugness of cast (common for clients in spica or body cast).
2. Perform neurovascular assessment every 1 to 2 hours for the first 24 hours: pain, pallor, pulselessness, paresthesia, paraplegia (Table 29-1). Compare neurovascular status with preapplication neurovascular assessment.	Neurovascular status determines circulation and oxygenation of tissues, functioning, and viability of neurological tissues (Kunkler, 1999).

- ***Critical Decision Point***
  Deterioration in neurovascular status requires immediate action, because irreversible tissue death occurs within 4 to 12 hours of inadequate oxygenation.

3. Observe for edema distal to cast. Older adults may have concurrent dependent edema because of health state.	Edema results from trauma or venous stasis. Rarely, heat of plaster drying contributes to development of edema.
4. Assess temperature of tissues above and below cast. Older adult clients frequently have cooler-than-usual extremities because of decreased peripheral circulation.	Warmth of tissues distal to cast usually indicates adequate perfusion.

- ***Critical Decision Point***
  Older adult clients may have slow or even poor capillary refill because of peripheral vascular conditions; use more than one neurovascular assessment to determine circulatory adequacy.

5. Compare tissues in cast with contralateral tissues to determine current condition.	Comparison with normal tissues assists in forming judgment of neurovascular status.

Table 29-1 5 P's of Neurovascular Assessment

Criteria	Assessment	Rationale
Pain	Determine amount and severity of pain if present. Ask client for descriptions; avoid coaching client with words to describe pain.	Manipulation and reduction may produce dull, aching pain as a result of pressure on nerve endings. Clients vary in perception and tolerance of pain. Pain on passive motion, unrelenting pain, or pain out of proportion is investigated further because it may signify compartment syndrome. Sudden increase in pain may signify thrombus formation.
Pallor	Observe color of tissues distal to cast. Older adult clients may have bluish color normally; however, no other signs of circulatory compromise should be present.	Pink indicates arterial pressure is normal, whitish color signifies decreased arterial supply, and bluish color signifies venous stasis.
Pulselessness	When possible, palpate distal pulse of casted extremity; note presence and strength of pulse. Assess capillary refill by pressing on toenail or fingernail (if cast is on extremity), releasing, and noting "pinking" of nail; nail should "pink up" in 3 seconds or less (Figure 29-3).	Weak or absent pulse may indicate decreased circulation to casted area. Blanching on pressure with subsequent capillary refill is indicative of arterial perfusion. Capillary refill is too sluggish if refill takes more than 3 seconds. It takes 2 seconds to say "capillary refill" slowly and 4 seconds to repeat it once (Beare and Myers, 1998).
Paresthesia	Assess for numbness, tingling, or abnormal sensations.	May indicate nerve damage and/or development of compartment syndrome.
Paraplegia	Assess for motion.	May indicate nerve damage and/or development of compartment syndrome.

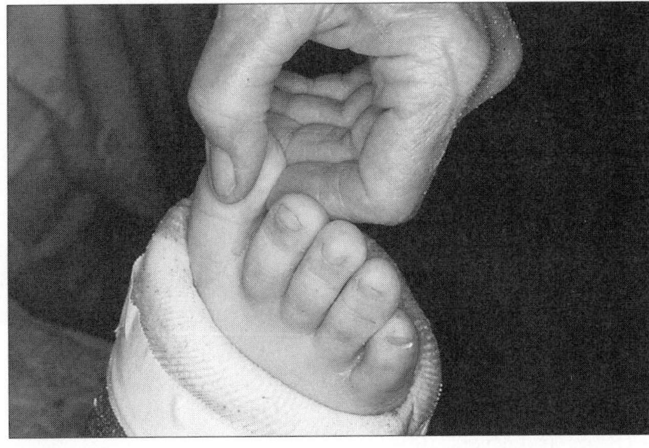

FIGURE **29-3** Assessing capillary refill. The nail bed is compressed. When released it should "pink up" in 3 seconds or less.

Step	Rationale
6. Inspect condition of skin around edges of cast. If skin irritation is evident, "petal" the edge of the cast by overlapping strips of tape or moleskin over the edge.	This area is susceptible to pressure and friction.
7. Ask client to move parts in ROJM if possible; note if client is unable to do active ROJM of uncasted areas. Older adult clients may have stiffness of joints or edema from other health conditions.	Range of motion should be performed within limitations imposed by cast. Only tissues out of cast can, or should, be moved.
8. If client cannot do *active* ROJM to contiguous tissues, perform *passive* ROJM on these joints, noting responses or complaints of increased pain.	Passive movements decrease edema and demonstrate ability of part to be moved. However, inability to perform active ROJM and increased pain during passive movement may signify development of compartment syndrome and should be reported.

STEP	RATIONALE
9. Ask client to describe sensations or feelings of tissues in cast. Listen for descriptions such as pins and needles, asleep, numb, burning, tingling, or throbbing; do not prompt client by using those words.	May signify pressure or hypoxia to neurological tissues, affecting normal transmission of nerve impulses.
10. Smell the cast edges; a sour smell is normal.	Detects early sign of infection (foul odor).
11. After cast is dry and set, observe client performing cast care.	Return demonstration objectively measures client's learning.

Unexpected Outcomes and Related Interventions

- Client experiences malunion or malposition of affected parts because of insufficient **reduction** (placement) in cast.
  - Ensure that cast is snug and not loose.
  - Report loose cast to physician; reapplication will likely be needed.
- Client experiences nonunion as a result of local or systemic factors, such as infection, foreign objects in area, diabetes, or malnutrition.
  - Treat infection, maintain normal blood sugar level, and provide adequate nutrition.
- Client develops osteomyelitis if open wound was present at time of casting.
  - A window may be cut in cast to inspect and dress wound. *Do not* discard window cutout. Tape in place.
- Client develops pressure ulcer over bony prominence.
  - Cast may be split, windowed, bivalved, or removed by physician.
- Client experiences muscle weakness.
  - Exercise limb within limits of cast. Physician may order physical therapy.
- Client experiences cold extremity, decreased capillary refill, swelling, pallor, diminished pulse, numbness, tingling, or altered motion of distal parts as a result of decreased circulation or neurological functioning distal to cast.
  - If symptoms remain, notify physician. Bivalving and splitting underlying soft dressing or removal may be necessary to prevent permanent damage (Beare and Myers, 1998).
- Client experiences skin irritation at cast edges, or cast begins to fray.
  - Apply "petals" to further protect cast. Small pieces of adhesive tape 2.5 to 5.0 cm (1 to 2 inches) are cut and taped smoothly over edge of cast.
- Client in body or hip spica cast develops nausea, vomiting, feeling of abdominal fullness or pain, indicating cast syndrome where the duodenum is compressed between the superior mesenteric artery and the spine.
  - Change the client from the supine to the prone position.
  - Notify physician and prepare to either cut abdominal window or bivalve cast (Sprague, 1998).
- Client is unable to demonstrate cast care.
  - Reinstruction is necessary. Adapt teaching interventions to fit client situation.

Recording and Reporting

- Record application of cast and condition of skin and circulation. Report abnormal or untoward findings from neurovascular assessments; report the following *immediately:* bluish color to distal parts, marked increase in edema or pain, delayed capillary refill (longer than 3 seconds), inability to palpate distal peripheral pulses if originally palpable, increased numbness or tingling, cold tissues, and inability to move tissues actively.
- Record odor and drainage from cast: Report to physician. Draw circle on cast around drainage site. Record time and date on circle.

Teaching Considerations

- Clients in casts may be more comfortable than when not in cast if deformity or **crepitation** (the sound heard when fractured ends rub against each other) is present.
- Teach client to realign pillows to promote cast drying when client is repositioned.
- Teach client about effects of pressure from cast on underlying skin and tissue.
- Prepare client for itching sensations under cast. Client should avoid sticking objects down or in cast to scratch, because these objects can cause breaks in underlying skin and subsequent infections. May require medication to control the itching.
- If client must use crutches, instruct in crutch-walking techniques (see Skill 28-5).
- Teach client proper ROJM and isometric exercises for affected extremity.
- Caution client against drying wet cast with hair dryer; this can cause plaster to crack or skin underneath to be damaged.

Pediatric Considerations

- Synthetic casts come in a variety of colors. Allow child to choose color.
- Teach parents or other caregivers to protect cast from moisture or unnecessary wear. Plastic wrap placed around perineal area during urination or defecation prevents soiling.
- If child has clubfoot, parents and child should be taught that frequent cast changes are necessary. Cast changes accommodate normal bone and tissue growth and correction of abnormality.

- Babies in casts for treatment of clubfoot have limited maneuverability.
- Children are particularly prone to placing objects into cast to scratch. They must be monitored closely. Assess edges of cast to ensure small objects have not been inserted. Antihistamines and a hair dryer set to cool can be used to control itching (Hart and Kester, 1999).
- Babies or children may signify pain through crying or restlessness. Gastric distention may occur in child who repeatedly screams and cries with fracture and cast application (Wong and others, 1999).
- Providing child with a doll that has same type of cast as child is helpful in reducing anxiety, as well as being a teaching tool.
- Child in body cast or spica cast may find it easier to self-feed from prone position with tray adjacent to child or on floor (Wong and others, 1999).
- Casts are removed earlier in babies and children because of speedy healing and to facilitate muscle and joint function.
- Encourage child to sleep on opposite side of fracture.

Gerontological Considerations

- Older nonverbal clients may signify pain through crying, agitation, or restlessness.
- Lightweight, synthetic casts are better for older adult clients. Cast is less restrictive, and light weight helps clients maintain better balance.
- Plaster of Paris casts on older adults may have less plaster, to aid in moving or lifting.
- Age-related decreased muscle strength in older adults is a result of loss of skeletal muscle and may cause difficulty in ambulating with a cast.
- Older adult clients may have reduced sensation and be less able to detect compression (Ebersole and Hess, 1998).
- Bone healing (remodeling cycle) takes longer to complete and rate of mineralization slows down in older adult clients (McCance and Huether, 1998).
- There is loss of bone density with aging, which predisposes client to fractures.
- Older adults' skin heals about 50% more slowly than that of younger adults, tears more easily because of decreased collagen, and loses its elasticity, and the dermal layer becomes thinner as a result of decreased subcutaneous fat (Ebersole and Hess, 1998).

Home Care Considerations

- Client is instructed that rest, ice, and elevation of affected extremity will help reduce swelling.
- Client must inspect cast and petal rough edges to reduce risk of trauma to underlying skin and need for cast changes.
- Client must inspect cast daily for foul odor, which indicates skin excoriation or infection under cast.
- Client must inspect skin daily for pressure or friction areas.
- Client must inspect cast daily for cracks or changes in alignment.
- Client must keep plaster of Paris cast dry. When bathing, casted extremity must not be submerged because cast absorbs water, loses structural integrity, and crumbles, If cast becomes wet, dry immediately.
- Synthetic casts may be cleaned with warm water and mild soap.
- Client must notify physician of any clinical manifestation of complications: fever, unrelieved pain, foul odor, or complaints that cast is too tight or rubbing skin.

Skill 29-2 Assisting With Cast Removal

Cast removal consists of removing the cast and padding with a mechanical device such as a cast saw (Figure 29-4). The nurse must prepare for this procedure so the client remains still and cooperates during cast removal. The removal of a cast is painless but can be noisy. A child or confused client may need to be gently restrained during the procedure to prevent injury by the equipment. After the cast is removed, the nurse provides appropriate skin care.

Delegation Considerations

Assessment of the client's condition should not be delegated to assistive personnel. However, the skill of cast removal may be delegated to assistive personnel. Inform personnel to treat skin tissues carefully following cast removal.

Equipment

- Cast saw
- Plastic sheets or papers
- Cold water enzyme wash
- Skin lotion
- Basin, water, washcloths, and towels
- Scissors
- Clean gloves

A
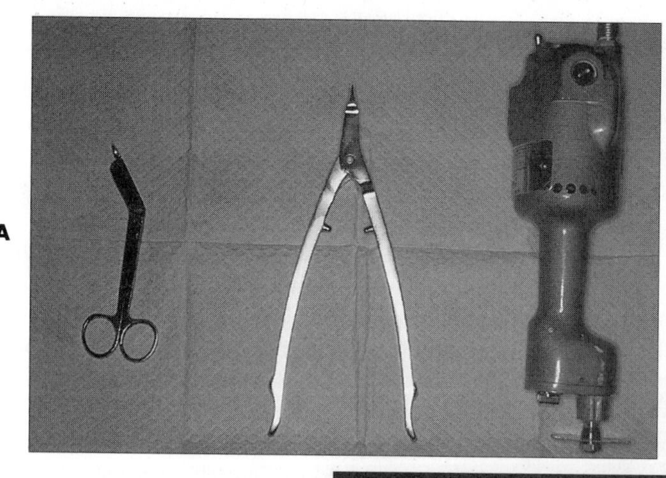

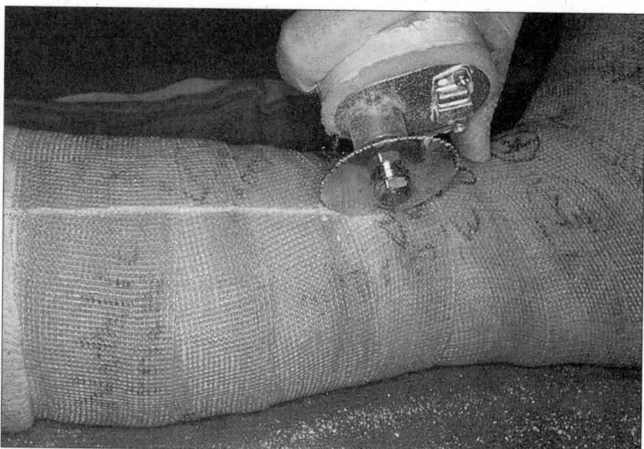
B

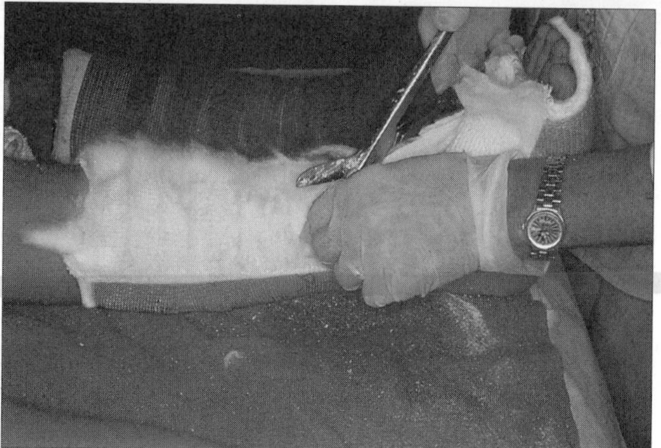
C

FIGURE **29-4** **A,** Equipment for removing a cast. *Left to right:* scissors, cast spreader, cast saw. **B,** Cast saw is used to remove cast. To bivalve a cast, it is cut longitudinally on either side and the wadding is cut with scissors. The two halves may be secured together with an elastic wrap, or the top is removed and the bottom shell of the cast becomes a posterior splint. **C,** Cutting through wadding under cast with scissors.

STEP	RATIONALE
ASSESSMENT	
1. Assess client's understanding of and response to upcoming cast removal.	Helps develop a teaching plan that aids in reducing anxiety.
2. Assess client's physical readiness for cast removal (client's physical findings, physician's orders, x-ray examination results).	Determines level of healing, readiness to remove cast, and need for supportive care after removal.
3. Ask client if any itching or irritation under cast is felt.	Indicates healing and accumulation of dried skin layers.

NURSING DIAGNOSIS

Defining characteristics from the assessment data may reveal the following nursing diagnoses for clients requiring this skill:

- Risk for impaired skin integrity
- Deficient knowledge regarding cast removal
- Anxiety
- Risk for injury

Related factors are individualized based on client's condition or needs.

Step	Rationale
Planning	
1. **Expected outcomes** following completion of procedure:	
▪ Client incurs no underlying tissue or skin injury; there is buildup of dry, dead skin. Client skin remains intact.	Cast is removed safely. Layers of dead skin cells that accumulate are removed over time without scrubbing.
▪ Client verbalizes understanding of normal physical sensations and procedural steps of cast removal.	Understanding lessens anticipatory anxiety.
▪ Client is able to describe and demonstrate level of activity and weight bearing allowed following cast removal.	Allows client to safely assume activity at home.
▪ Client is able to explain skin care measures.	Allows client to assume self-care.
2. Explain physical sensations to expect during cast removal. Cast saw vibrates cast loose; client will feel heat and vibration.	Explanation minimizes fear of possible injury.
3. Describe procedural steps for cast removal: appearance of saw, vibration sensations, removal of outer cast, appearance of padding, cleansing of skin.	Client is prepared to witness and participate in procedure.
Implementation	
1. Apply gloves if drainage is anticipated, and assist person removing cast by positioning, turning, and holding cast and tissues in cast.	Prevents injury from saw. Use latex-free gloves if there is risk of an allergic reaction (Baumann, 1999).
• ***Critical Decision Point*** *Instruct client to remain still during cast removal.*	
2. After removal of cast and padding, inspect tissues for general condition, redness, warmth, and drainage.	May signify inflammation or infection of tissues.
3. If skin is intact, gently apply cold water enzyme wash to skin; let stay on skin 15 to 20 minutes.	Helps dissolve or emulsify dead cells and fatty deposits on tissues. Prevents injury to delicate tissue.
• ***Critical Decision Point*** *Do not scrub skin, because this may traumatize delicate tissue and lead to skin breakdown. It may take several days before all residue is removed from skin.*	
4. After elapsed time, gently wash off enzyme wash; if possible, immerse tissues in basin or tub to aid in removal of tissue debris without undue rubbing or pressure.	Removes as much debris as possible.
5. After patting tissues dry (avoid rubbing), apply generous coating of skin lotion, gently massaging into skin.	Rubbing could traumatize tender tissues. Lotion lubricates skin.
6. Obtain physician's order to gently put joints through active and passive range of joint motion (ROJM). Clarify level of activity allowed.	Joints and muscles will be stiff and weak. Activity is resumed slowly to avoid reinjury.
7. Assist in transfer of client for return to room or for discharge if anticipated.	
8. All equipment and casts should be cleaned or discarded according to standard precautions. Remove gloves. If cast is soiled with blood, discard as biohazard waste.	Reduces transmission of microorganisms.
Evaluation	
1. Observe underlying skin.	Reveals condition of skin.
2. Assess client's verbal and nonverbal responses.	Expressions, tone of voice, and movement reveal level of anxiety or fear.
3. Ask client to explain ordered exercise plan and demonstrate exercises.	Demonstrates learning.
4. Have client explain and perform skin care.	Demonstrates learning of self-care.

Unexpected Outcomes and Related Interventions

- Underlying skin may be scratched from friction of saw.
  - Remind client to remain still during cast removal.
- Client becomes tense and restless and withdraws from cast saw.
  - Provide further explanation and support.
- Client experiences extensive edema, pain, or limited use of affected tissues.
  - Client may have transient symptoms after cast removal. Instruct client to:
    - Elevate body part if edema returns.
    - Use nonnarcotic analgesics every 4 hours for up to 24 hours if needed.
    - Slowly perform ROJM exercises every 4 hours. (If marked weakness exists, physician may order client to receive physical therapy or to use sling or immobilizer for 1 to 2 days for continued rest.)
- Client is unable to perform activities of daily living (ADLs) and exercises due to nonunion or pain.
  - Physician will assess the fracture site by x-ray film.
- Client is unable to explain self-care measures.
  - Reinstruct or clarify as needed.

Recording and Reporting

- Record cast removal, condition of tissues formerly in cast, and person removing cast in nurses' notes.
- Report changes in movement, severe swelling, and increased pain to physician.

Teaching Considerations

- Inform client that amount of cellular debris under cast depends on length of time tissues are in cast and overall skin integrity.
- Instruct client to use caution with tender skin areas or joints.
- Instruct client to call physician if unable to perform ADLs, if excessive edema occurs, if client experiences limited use of joints or muscles, or if mobility is affected. If client is treated for congenital deformity with repeated cast changes, instruct when next cast change is due; give client written appointment.
- Provide client with scheduled exercises to increase mobility and muscle strength.

Pediatric Considerations

- Babies and children may be frightened of cast saw. Demonstration of saw before removal of cast may alleviate anxiety.

Gerontological Considerations

- Older adult clients may experience marked stiffness or weakened muscles, depending on length of time in cast.
- Older adult client's skin is drier, thinner, and more fragile than that of a baby, child, or younger adult.

Home Care Considerations

- Client should have chair or bed with pillows to elevate extremity for intermittent edema.
- Suggest regular use of moisturizers for dry, scaly skin of casted extremity.
- Assess client's environment for potential safety risks.
- After cast is removed, teach client to dangle prior to ambulation, to proceed slowly with ambulation, and to gradually increase the time and distance ambulated.
- Client is provided instructions regarding muscle relaxants and analgesics if prescribed.

Skill 29-3 Assisting With Application of Skin Traction

Skin traction is one of the two basic types of traction used for the treatment of fractured bones and correction of orthopedic abnormalities. Skin traction applies pull to an affected body structure by straps attached to the skin around the structure. For traction to be effective, five general principles of care must be implemented (Box 29-1). Recovery is facilitated through immobilization and alignment of body parts. The nurse provides safe care through skillful application of traction. The following are the major forms of skin traction, with some variation within some of the types.

1. Bryant's traction—vertically held type of bilateral traction to the legs (Figure 29-5, *A*). This type of traction can be used for children weighing less than 40 lb. Adhesive strips are applied to the lateral surfaces of each leg and wrapped with elastic bandages to secure them in place. A **spreader bar** is attached to the strips and then to ropes, **pulleys,** and weights. Bryant's traction, known as Gallow's traction in England, is used for children with fractures of the femur. After the muscle spasms are overcome and the fragments are aligned with some evidence of union, the child is removed from traction and placed in a spica cast to continue recovery and for callus formation to progress. Children may remain in Bryant's traction for only 7 to 10 days.
2. Buck's extension—horizontally applied unilateral or bilateral traction (Figure 29-5, *B*). Buck's traction is applied

Box 29-1 Five General Principles of Traction Care

1. Maintain the Established Line of Pull

This line is along the axis of the bone. Weights will hang freely, not hitting the bed or resting on the floor. The position of the weights is rechecked if the level of the bed is altered. The nurse avoids (1) bumping against the weights when walking near the bed and (2) allowing the weights to sway; both movements can cause pain for the client in traction. It is preferred that the weights not hang over the client; if this is necessary, the nurse tapes the ropes so the weights will not fall on the client.

2. Prevent Friction to the Skin

Traction rope rests in the groove of the pulley and moves easily. The rope is monitored for fraying. The nurse securely ties the knots in the traction rope and tapes the rope ends well. The rope knots are not lodged against the pulley because this will interfere with the line of pull. For the same reason the nurse ensures that the pulley, spreader bar, and foot plate do not rest against the foot of the bed.

3. Maintain Countertraction

To provide traction the nurse ensures that countertraction is maintained. If the weight of the client's body is to provide the countertraction, the body will not interfere with the direction of pull. For instance, the feet of a client in Buck's traction will not touch the foot of the bed; or if the client is in cervical traction, the head will not touch the head of the bed.

4. Maintain Continuous Traction Unless Ordered Otherwise

The nurse will not remove traction without physician approval. To change the client's position in bed, the nurse will not lift or adjust the weights if traction is continuous. For intermittent traction the nurse gently places and slowly removes the weights, avoiding jerking or suddenly moving the weights that could jar the patient.

5. Maintain Correct Body Alignment

The client will have correct body alignment while lying centered in the bed. The nurse must ensure that the patient does not angle the body or lean off the side of the bed because the line of traction pull would then be changed or interrupted.

Modified from Beare PG, Myers JL: *Principles and practice of adult health nursing,* ed 3, St. Louis, 1998, Mosby.

in one of two ways: adhesive strips are applied to the lateral surfaces of the limb or limbs (usually one leg or forearm) and wrapped with elastic bandages, or a commercially prepared foam boot with Velcro straps is applied. A spreader bar is attached to the adhesive strips as in Bryant's traction or to the foam boot and then to ropes, pulleys, and weights. Buck's extension provides temporary immobilization of hip fracture until open reduction and internal fixation (ORIF) can be performed. It is also used to reduce muscle spasms, contractures, and dislocations and occasionally as an interim treatment for lumbosacral muscle spasms causing low back pain.

3. Cotrel's traction—skin traction consisting of two separate forms: head halter and pelvic belt (Figure 29-5, *C*). Cotrel's traction is used occasionally as a preoperative treatment to help straighten spinal curvatures before insertion of skeletal rods for correction of scoliosis. The pull in opposite directions on the head and pelvis helps to overcome the deforming muscle pull causing the curvature. **Cervical halter** traction and **pelvic belt** traction are explained later in this section.
4. Dunlop's traction—simultaneous horizontal form of Buck's extension to the humerus with an accompanying vertical Buck's extension to the forearm (Figure 29-5, *D*). The horizontal Buck's extension is the "treating" traction for fractures of the humerus, whereas the vertical Buck's extension is primarily used to maintain the forearm in the desired position relative to the humerus.
5. Cervical (head halter)—traction involving a specially shaped halter with cutout areas for the ears, face, and top of the head (Figure 29-6, *A*). The halter cups the chin and has straps leading from the occipital skull area that attach to the chin portion and then connect to one or two spreader bars on either side of the head; the bar or bars are then attached to ropes, pulleys, and weights. Cervical traction should be used only for degenerative or arthritic conditions of the cervical vertebrae, not for fractures of the vertebrae. Because cervical traction must be removed occasionally for client safety and care and because this traction does not result in total spinal immobilization, it is unsafe and potentially dangerous for a client with a fracture of cervical vertebrae. Release of the weights in such a situation could lead to trauma to the spinal cord and paralysis.
6. Pelvic belt—traction consisting of a girdlelike belt that fits around the lumbosacral and abdominal areas, fastening in the middle of the abdomen with pressure-sensitive straps or buckles (Figure 29-6, *B*). The belt has long straps that attach to a wide spreader bar beyond the feet; the bar is then connected to ropes, pulleys, and weights. The client is placed in Williams' position (supine with the head of the bed slightly elevated and the knees bent) to decrease the stress on the lumbosacral spine. This pelvic belt, or lumbosacral traction, is used for clients with low back pain, muscle spasms, and a ruptured nucleus pulposus (herniated or ruptured disk). This traction basically serves to keep the client in bed, thus relieving inflammation and irritation of the injured nerves or muscles. It does not overcome the herniation of the nucleus pulposus. Newer management principles rely on maintaining mobility rather than on promoting bed rest. Additional treatments, including diathermy, use of muscle relaxant drugs, and physical therapy, are used in conjunction with this traction.
7. **Pelvic sling** (Weil sling)—traction consisting of a hammocklike belt wherein the sling cradles the pelvis in its boundaries for treatment of one or more fractures of the pelvic bones. The sling is attached on each side to a pin threaded through a sewn tunnel; each pin is then placed in a grooved spreader bar attached to ropes, pulleys, and weights. The sling applies gentle inward pressure to the injured tissues, thereby providing comfort and security to the client (Figure 29-6, *C*).

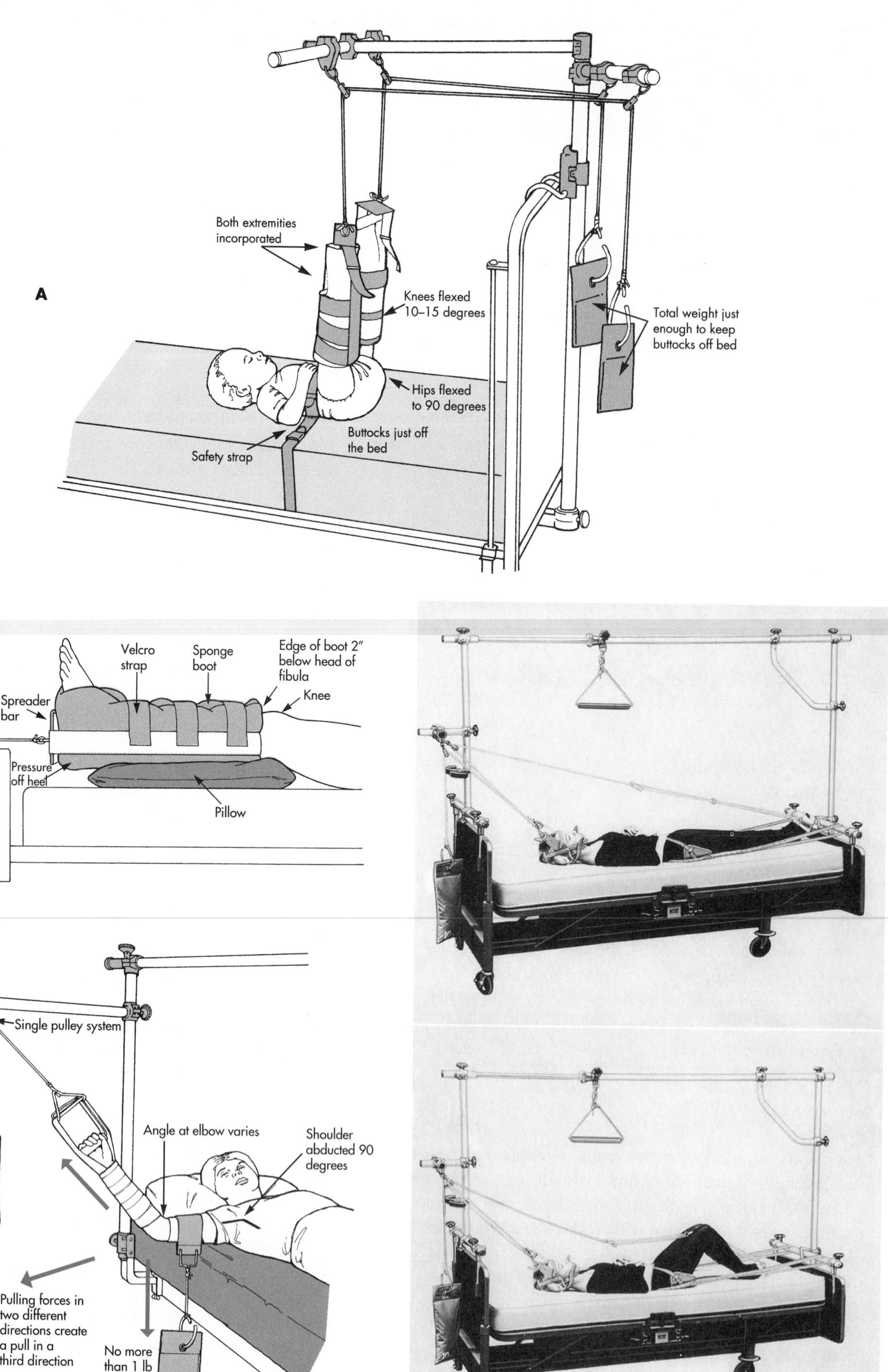

FIGURE **29-5** **A,** Bryant's traction. **B,** Buck's extension. **C,** Cotrel's traction. **D,** Dunlop's traction. (**A, B,** and **D** from Folcik M, Carini-Garcia G, Birmingham J: *Traction: assessment and management,* St. Louis, 1994, Mosby.)

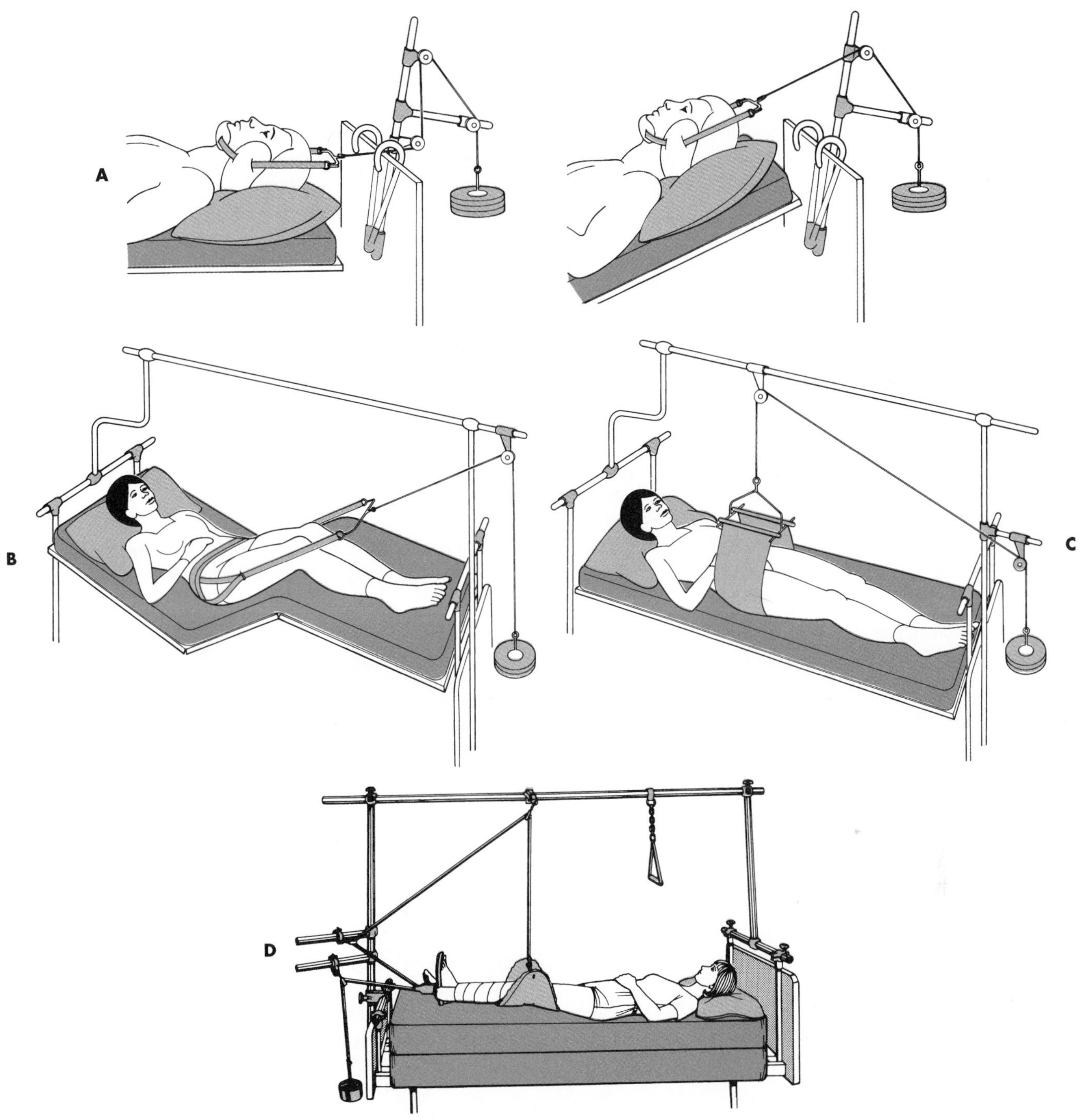

FIGURE **29-6** **A,** Cervical halter skin traction. **B,** Pelvic belt traction (skin). **C,** Pelvic sling (skin). **D,** Russell's traction. (**A, B,** and **C** from Beare PG, Myers JL: *Principles and practice of adult health nursing,* ed 3, St. Louis, 1998, Mosby. **D** from Phipps W and others: *Medical-surgical nursing: concepts and clinical practice,* ed 6, St. Louis, 1999, Mosby.)

8. Russell's traction—modification of Buck's extension using Newton's second law of thermodynamics (for each force in one direction there is an equal force in the opposite direction) to double the amount of pull through the arrangement of ropes, pulleys, and weights (Figure 29-6, *D*). Russell's traction may also be used in skeletal traction.

Because skin tissues and subcutaneous attachments cannot tolerate great amounts of weight without losing strength and continuity, skin traction uses weights varying from 1 to 2 lb for children in Bryant's traction to 7 to 10 lb for cervical skin traction. Average weights are 5 to 7 lb for Buck's extension, 7 to 10 lb for Dunlop's traction, 10 to 15 lb for pelvic belt traction (weight is distributed over the entire pelvis and lower back), and 10 to 20 lb for a pelvic sling (the sling is really a form of hammock suspension rather than traction).

Each form of skin traction mentioned above has a usual or "classic" position used for the majority of clients in that traction. Variations may be needed to treat a specific injury or condition. If pertinent, these variations are noted in the discussion of each type of traction.

Delegation Considerations

Assessment of the client and the status of traction should not be delegated to assistive personnel. However, the skill of assisting with application of skin traction may be delegated to assistive personnel. Inform assistive personnel of the necessary restrictions in positioning client and in application/removal of weights.

Equipment

- Ropes, pulleys, weights, **weight holder** (ropes are nylon for strength; weights vary from 1 to 5 lb—have several of each weight) (Babies, children, and older adults require less weight than do young adults)
- Bed frame for attachment of traction or portable frames that attach to bed
- One or more spreader bars
- Adhesive-backed moleskin
- Elastic bandages
- Heel or elbow protectors (optional)
- Knee sling for Russell's traction, traction boot for Buck's extension, cervical halter, or pelvic belt or sling
- Wastebasket with plastic bag liner

Step	Rationale
Assessment	
1. Assess condition of client's overall health, including degree of mobility and current medical conditions such as diabetes, peripheral vascular disease, or peripheral neuropathy.	Determines client's health state and ability to tolerate traction.
2. Assess condition of specific tissues to be placed in traction; note skin condition, excessive hair, bruises, rash, varicose veins, ulcers, dermatitis, or other lesions.	Determines ability of local tissues to tolerate traction.
• ***Critical Decision Point*** *Irritated or broken skin should not have skin traction placed over the damaged tissues.*	
a. Cervical halter: Assess occipital area of head, ears, chin, and neck.	Each type of traction predisposes client to area at risk for skin breakdown.
b. Bryant's traction: Assess one or both legs.	
c. Buck's extension: Assess one or both legs.	
d. Dunlop's traction: Assess arm and forearm.	
e. Pelvic belt: Assess lower back and abdomen.	
f. Pelvic sling: Assess back and abdomen.	
g. Russell's traction: Assess lower limbs.	
h. Cotrel's traction includes head halter and pelvic belt and is not considered separately.	
3. Assess client's understanding of reason for traction.	Determines concerns, acceptance, and need for instruction.
4. Assess client's level of pain.	Serves as baseline for later comparison and evaluation. Pain and spasms should be relieved by traction.
5. Assess client's neurovascular status.	Serves as baseline for later comparison and evaluation.

Nursing Diagnosis

Defining characteristics from the assessment data may reveal the following nursing diagnoses for clients requiring this skill:

- Bathing/hygiene, dressing/grooming, and toileting self-care deficit
- Risk for impaired skin integrity
- Risk for peripheral neurovascular dysfunction
- Ineffective peripheral tissue perfusion
- Impaired home maintenance
- Impaired physical mobility
- Deficient knowledge regarding the type and use of traction
- Acute pain

Related factors are individualized based on client's condition or needs.

Planning

Step	Rationale
1. **Expected outcomes** following completion of procedure:	
▪ Client participates in bathing and feeding.	Activities are performed safely and without injury.

STEP	RATIONALE
▪ Skin around straps and moleskin, halter, boot, or sling remains intact, without irritation.	Skin is free of pressure and/or pulling.
▪ X-ray studies confirm satisfactory alignment of fracture fragments with or without evidence of beginning callus formation (evidence of callus may not become apparent for 7 to 10 days or longer) if client is in traction for fracture.	Objective evidence is required for comparison with subjective relief of symptoms.
▪ Client describes purpose of traction and follows activity restrictions.	Client learns and accepts need for restrictions.
▪ Client verbalizes increase in comfort after traction application.	Injured tissues and bone are stabilized.
▪ As a result of being in one specific type of skin traction, one of the following occurs.	
a. Cervical halter: Client notes relief of spasms and pain in neck and back of neck and head (may require administration of muscle relaxant and narcotic medications while in traction).	Each type of traction is designed to relieve muscle spasms; restore alignment or lessen shortening, overriding, or rotation; relieve pain; and increase comfort.
b. Bryant's traction: Child is able to maintain positioning with distraction by parents or caregivers.	
c. Buck's extension: Client is able to maintain leg in alignment. Older adult clients with severe hip pain noticeably relax.	Immobilization decreases pain. Pull of traction may decrease muscle spasms.
d. Dunlop's traction: Same result occurs as for Buck's extension (used for upper extremity).	
e. Pelvic belt: Client notes lessening of spasms of lumbosacral muscles, possibly slight lessening of sensory signs of pressure on sciatic nerve (numbness, tingling, or pins and needles radiating down back of leg to toes), and possibly less pressure in vertebral area at site of injury.	Pull may lessen pressure on spinal or peripheral nerves, thereby alleviating symptoms.
f. Pelvic sling: Client experiences almost immediate comfort and relief from pelvic and abdominal discomfort, pain, and feeling of "coming apart."	Sling compresses tissues together. Clients are very comfortable in sling and develop sense of security while in it.
g. Russell's traction: Client notes lessening of pain in hip area (if traction is for hip trauma), relief of muscle spasms, and ease in ability to maintain more normal anatomical position of leg and thigh.	Russell's traction exerts double pull with less weight than Buck's extension because of pulley arrangement.
h. Cotrel's traction: Client experiences some straightening of curvature of spine.	
▪ Sufficient time in traction (varying from 1 to 10 or more days) elicits symptom relief. Continuous skin traction is limited to 7 to 10 days.	Time is required for inflammation to abate and tissues to regain more normal functions. Prolonged continuous skin traction leads to skin breakdown.
▪ Neurovascular status remains stable. Distal skin tissue remains warm and of a normal color with capillary refill of 3 seconds or less. Client verbalizes no abnormal sensations and is able to move fingers or toes distal to fracture site.	There is no evidence of increased pressure within the muscle compartment and no neurovascular deficit (Kunkler, 1999).
▪ Client verbalizes understanding of procedure, including traction setup and mobility restrictions.	Promotes cooperation and reduces anxiety.

IMPLEMENTATION

STEP	RATIONALE
1. Administer narcotic for acute pain and muscle relaxant for spasms in advance of traction application.	Allowing drugs to reach peak effect at time of traction application will reduce pain and resultant muscle spasm.
2. Prepare client and area of body to be in traction:	

STEP	RATIONALE
a. Cervical halter: Cleanse face and neck; shave man unless he has beard.	Lessens irritation under cervical halter.
b. Bryant's traction: Cleanse both legs gently if necessary (change diaper if necessary for baby).	Prevents irritation under traction strips and bandages.
c. Buck's extension: Wash affected leg (or legs) very gently and dry carefully. Do not shave legs.	Shaving may create micronicks that could become inflamed under traction strips.
d. Dunlop's traction: Cleanse arm and forearm gently as needed.	Prevents irritation under straps and bandages.
e. Pelvic belt: Check back and iliac crests for lesions.	Prevents skin breakdown or irritation in areas where belt is positioned.
f. Pelvic sling: Ask female client to void before being placed in sling if no catheter is in place.	Sling must be removed for placement of fracture bedpan. Male client can use urinal with no change in position of sling.
g. Russell's traction: Cleanse lower extremity to knee as needed.	Prevents irritation under bandages.
3. Position client as requested by physician: a. Cervical halter: client flat on back. b. Bryant's traction: child flat on back. c. Buck's extension: client on back; head of bed flat or elevated no more than 30 degrees. d. Dunlop's traction: client flat on back. e. Pelvic belt: client flat on back. f. Pelvic sling: client flat on side or back. g. Russell's traction: client on back; head of bed slightly elevated.	Position varies with part of body to be placed in traction, plus effects of weight and gravity. Body parts are kept anatomically aligned.
4. Assist with application of specific cervical halter, adhesive strips and elastic bandages, Buck's traction, and pelvic belt or sling as needed. Nurse may be asked to hold client in desired position or apply halter, strips, or elastic bandages while physician and other assistants hold client's tissues in desired positions.	For lower extremity, adhesive strips are applied beginning below head of fibula on lateral surface of leg to avoid pressure over peroneal nerve. Ensures proper alignment of body parts under traction. Elastic bandages are applied from distal to proximal to prevent trapping of blood and to promote venous return (Byrne, 1999) (see Chapter 37).

• ***Critical Decision Point***
Pressure on peroneal nerve as a result of bandages or traction boot can cause footdrop.

STEP	RATIONALE
a. Ensure that boot size is correct. Traction boot should fit snugly (not too tight or too loose).	Too tight leads to pressure to skin, peroneal nerve, and vascular structures. Too loose leads to slipping and lack of traction force.
b. Heel must be properly seated in traction boot. Do not pad at heel. Cut out heel section of foam boot if necessary.	Prevents pressure over heel.
c. Do not apply traction boot over pneumatic compression devices. Foot pumps may be used.	Causes undue pressure on tissues and negates effects of compression device (Byrne, 1999).
5. Assist with attachment of spreader bars, ropes, and pulleys. Ropes are tied securely in knots, passed in grooves of pulleys to weights, and are not frayed (see Box 29-1).	Provides proper weighted traction for extremity alignment.
6. When all traction materials and spreader bars are in place, weights are placed on weight holder and attached to loop in rope. The weights are then *lowered slowly and gently* until rope is taut. Physician determines exact amount of weight to be applied and position to be maintained for majority of time by client (clients should have written orders for specific traction weights, bed position, and turning regimen when pertinent).	Traction is slowly established to avoid involuntary muscle spasms or pain for client. Weight should be sufficient to create enough pull to overcome muscle spasms but not to cause distraction or marked increase in pain.

Step	Rationale
7. Before physician leaves, assess client's position and ask about additional permissible positions for client and bed.	Ensures safety of care and position for effective traction.
a. Cervical halter: Client stays flat on back, or head of bed may be elevated 15 to 20 degrees if ordered.	Angle of pull may allow head to be up to use body weight as **countertraction.**
b. Bryant's traction: Baby or child must stay on back at all times; buttocks are held slightly off bed if traction weight is correct amount.	Child cannot turn to side or abdomen, because traction would be ineffective and reinjury could occur.
c. Buck's extension: Client is primarily on back; may be allowed to turn to unaffected side for brief periods (10 to 15 minutes).	Positioning on side permits back care and rest to tissues.
d. Dunlop's traction: Client must lie on back. Bed may be tilted on low shock blocks toward side opposite traction. Head of bed is kept flat.	Tilting uses body for some countertraction.
e. Pelvic belt: Client lies on back; knee portion of bed (Gatch) and head of bed may be raised to hips and knees are flexed at 45-degree angles (Williams' position).	Flexion of hips and knees relaxes lumbosacral muscles to lessen spasms.
f. Pelvic sling: Client lies on back when in sling; sling should have enough weight attached to raise buttocks slightly off bed. If sling is off, it can be used carefully as turning sheet if client's fractures permit side lying.	Hammock effect of sling is most effective with client on back. Sling must be removed for placement of bedpan.
g. Russell's traction: Client lies on back; head of bed may be elevated 30 to 45 degrees, depending on injury.	Low-Fowler's position creates most effective traction pull.
h. Cotrel's traction: Client must lie flat on back.	
8. For safety, raise upper side rails as appropriate. Client's in Bryant's traction should always have someone in attendance.	Promotes client safety.
9. Gather unused materials, and return to storage areas. Wash hands.	Promotes safety and cleanliness. Reduces transmission of microorganisms.

Evaluation

Step	Rationale
1. Observe client's participation in self-care.	Client may refrain from activity unnecessarily or may try to do too much.
2. Assess condition of skin around traction straps or bandages.	Ensures early identification of irritation or breakdown.
3. Inspect entire traction setup and functioning: observe all knots, ropes in pulleys, correct weights on weight holder; whether apparatus is hanging freely and not resting on floor; position of halter, sling, belt, and other material for specific traction; bedclothes not interfering with traction apparatus; and proper body alignment.	Reassessment is necessary to determine if traction is functioning as designed or desired or to make needed adjustments. Malfunctioning traction interferes with healing.
4. Ask if client understands mobility restrictions.	Feedback demonstrates learning.
5. Ask if client is experiencing pain, spasms, or muscle burning (or ask parents of young child). Young children may cry when weights are initially applied but soon cease crying.	Indicates misalignment of bones or presence of muscle spasms. Initial reaction may be slight increase in soreness or pain until client is able to relax and allow traction to perform as designed.
6. Assess neurovascular status 15 minutes after application of skin traction and every 1 to 2 hours for 24 hours, then extend to every 4 hours if client is stabilizing (see Skill 29-1, Evaluation, Step 2).	Provides objective data concerning peripheral perfusion to tissues. If skin traction is applied too tightly, then pressure is applied to nerves and vascular structures, resulting in a potentially irreversible deficit.
7. Skin traction is released every 4 to 8 hours with skin condition assessed and care given. Wash, pat dry, lubricate skin, and apply a light dusting of powder before reapplication of traction.	Prevents pressure sores and gives early feedback regarding skin condition. Skin traction may *not* be removed if it is immobilizing a fracture.

Unexpected Outcomes and Related Interventions

- Child in Bryant's traction continues to turn to abdomen and disrupts traction.
  - Encourage family to stay with child and distract. Provide toys to distract child.
- Client experiences increased pain, soreness, or stiffness from pull applied to injured tissues.
  - Medicate with analgesics.
- Client suffers frequent or severe muscle spasms from muscle irritation.
  - Administer skeletal muscle relaxants.
- Client experiences displaced alignment (evident on x-ray film) if fracture is present.
  - Maintain proper weights, alignment, and positioning.
- Client experiences sense of claustrophobia or being "held down" in one or another type of traction.
  - Explain intervention to client, and monitor client frequently.
  - Administer antianxiety medication.
- Cervical halter: Client has pain in temporomandibular joint and chin or may develop headaches.
  - Consult with MD to shorten straps between chin and occipital part of halter to direct pull from occipital area and away from chin and jawline.
  - Client should describe the pull as from the back of neck, not the chin.
- Bryant's traction: Baby or child develops edema of feet. Peripheral pulses are not palpable.
  - Remove bandages and reapply.
- Buck's extension: Client develops pressure area on heel, or client is unable to dorsiflex or evert foot in traction if **traction boot,** adhesive straps, or elastic bandages exert pressure over head of fibula.
  - Reapply traction and reassess neurovascular status within 15 minutes.
- Dunlop's traction: Client experiences pressure on elbow, or client is unable to approximate thumb to rest of fingers and may complain of numbness of thumb or tingling along sides of thumb and index finger, or demonstrates capillary refill over 3 seconds in nail beds.
  - Elastic bandage is too tight over radial nerve at wrist.
  - Elastic bandage should be removed from forearm *only* and rewrapped more loosely; symptoms should then be reevaluated for alleviation or continuance.
- Pelvic belt: Client experiences marked increase in pain or numbness or other sensory pressure signs when in belt.
  - Remove traction to ease complaints.
- Pelvic sling: Client becomes very dependent on sling and refuses to allow its discontinuance or becomes anxious when out of sling.
  - Weaning may be required and involves releasing sling for short to longer periods of time to permit adjustment to being out of sling.
- Russell's traction: Client has pain behind knee or nonpalpable popliteal pulse.
  - Readjust to prevent pressure to popliteal area.
- Client experiences burning, weeping, or drainage under adhesive strips or moleskin because of possible allergy or hypersensitivity.
  - Remove traction.

Recording and Reporting

- Record assessment of skin underneath traction apparatus and nursing interventions to maintain skin integrity.
- Record neurovascular assessment of bilateral body parts (see Skill 29-1, Evaluation, Step 2).
- Record length of time client is in or out of specific traction. NOTE: Clients in cervical halter and pelvic belt traction are usually in 1 to 2 hours, out 1 to 2 hours, and out to sleep.

Teaching Considerations

- Explain that traction may increase muscle weakness, spasms, and pain in older adult clients.
- When traction time is decreased or discontinued, client is taught to ambulate slowly within medical guidelines, gradually increasing length of time out of bed and distance walked.
- Client should be taught to notify physician of undesirable signs, such as marked increase in pain, muscle spasms, and increased numbness. Symptoms may signify reinjury or insufficient healing.

Pediatric Considerations

- Babies and children have immature musculoskeletal tissues and are almost constant "movers."
- Babies and children in Bryant's traction must sleep in traction; it is rarely removed once established, except to loosen elastic bandages for marked edema of feet.
- Bryant's traction is used infrequently because of the alteration in perfusion as a result of gravitational forces and the circumferential bandages. Vasospasm and avascular necrosis may occur (Wong and others, 1999).
- Assess under child for small misplaced objects such as toys.

Gerontological Considerations

- Older adults may have keratoses, rashes, or other lesions that could become irritated in skin traction.
- Older adults may have long-standing conditions of musculoskeletal tissues such as arthritis or gout that could lead to inflamed tissues and skin breakdown.
- Older and chronically ill clients may have increased need for position changes resulting from limitations due to osteoporosis, osteomalacia, weakened muscles, or increased risk of skin breakdown.
- Older adults' skin heals more slowly, tears more easily, loses its elasticity, and becomes thinner than that of a younger

adult (Ebersole and Hess, 1998). An alternating air pressure mattress or foam overlay on the bed may be used to decrease the risk of skin breakdown.

HOME CARE CONSIDERATIONS

- If client is to be discharged to home, relatives or caregivers should be instructed on care needs (including home traction) and mode of ambulation.
- After traction is discontinued, client is taught to dangle before ambulation; to proceed slowly with ambulation; and to gradually increase the time and distance ambulated.
- Home environment must be assessed and adapted to accommodate hospital bed and traction.
- Integrity of traction should be inspected daily—weights hang freely, traction ropes rest in groove of pulley, and client's body is not allowed to interfere with countertraction. In many cases the client's body is the countertraction.
- Client is provided instructions regarding use of muscle relaxants and analgesics if prescribed.

Skill 29-4 Assisting With Insertion of Pins, Wires, or Nails for Skeletal Traction

Skeletal traction is the second kind of traction used for the treatment of fractures or correction of orthopedic abnormalities. As with skin traction, skeletal traction may be applied to one or several bones. Skeletal traction begins externally but continues internally directly through the bones. Weights are then attached to the skeletal pin, wire, or nail via ropes and pulleys. Amounts of weights for skeletal traction vary from 10 lb for Dunlop's skeletal traction, to 20 to 25 lb for cervical traction, to 30 to 40 lb for balanced suspension to the femur. Amounts of weights used are also dictated by age, overall condition of the client in traction, and the purpose of the traction.

The procedure can also involve **external fixation,** which consists of a metal frame that secures pins inserted through the bone above and below a fracture site. The external fixation stabilizes a fracture with hardware visible outside the body. It fosters the healing of complex fractured bones, usually in the lower extremities.

Skeletal traction is often used when continuous traction is desired to properly immobilize, position, and align a fractured bone during the healing process. The nurse provides safe care after skillful application of traction. Common forms of skeletal traction include the following:

1. Balanced-suspension skeletal traction (BSST) to the femur—traction used for displaced or overriding fractures of the femur. Balanced suspension brings about relief of muscle spasms, realignment of the fracture fragments, and callus formation (Figure 29-7). This form of traction is used less frequently because of the length of time required for hospitalization when it is used as the major form of treatment. It is now used primarily before surgical implantation of an internal fixation pin, plate, or nail until the client's condition or other injuries stabilize to permit surgery. Balanced suspension involves the use of splints under the thigh and leg to suspend them off the bed, with a Steinmann pin or Kirschner wire supplying the traction (Figure 29-8, *A* and *B*). The pin or wire is drilled through the upper tibia and attached to a spreader, which is then attached to ropes, pulleys, and weights (Figure 29-8, *C*). Sufficient weights are hung to overcome the quadriceps and hamstring muscle spasms; sometimes weights of 30 to 40 lb or more may be required initially. Suspension weights may be 7 to 8 lb, and they are balanced by 7 to 8 lb of countertraction.

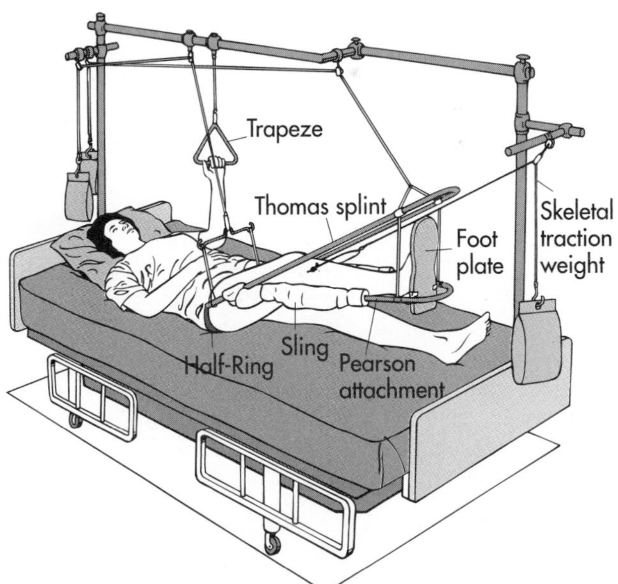

FIGURE 29-7 Balanced-suspension skeletal traction. Traction in long axis of right thigh is applied by means of Kirschner wire through proximal portion of tibia. Limb is supported by Thomas splint beneath thigh and Pearson attachment beneath leg. Foot plate attachment prevents footdrop. Weights apply countertraction to upper end of Thomas splint and suspend its lower end. By using the left arm and leg as shown, client can shift position of the hips without change in amount of traction.

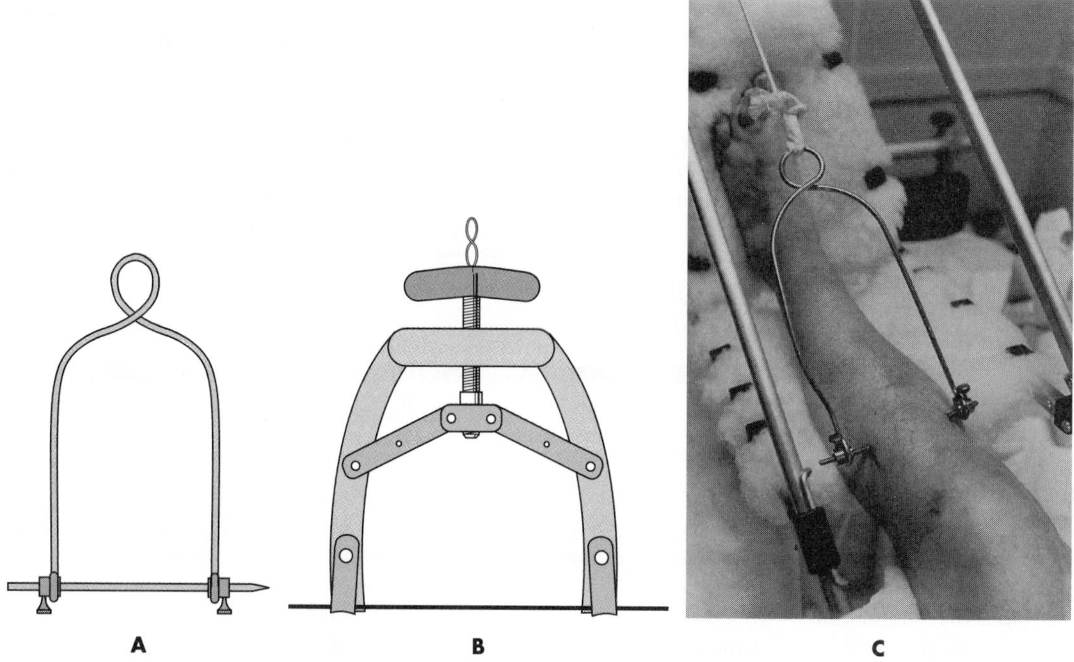

FIGURE 29-8 A, Kirschner wire and tractor. B, Steinmann pin and holder. C, Steinmann pin placed in tibial plateau for treatment of distal femoral fracture. (C from Phipps W and others: *Medical-surgical nursing: concepts and clinical practice,* ed 6, St. Louis, 1995, Mosby.)

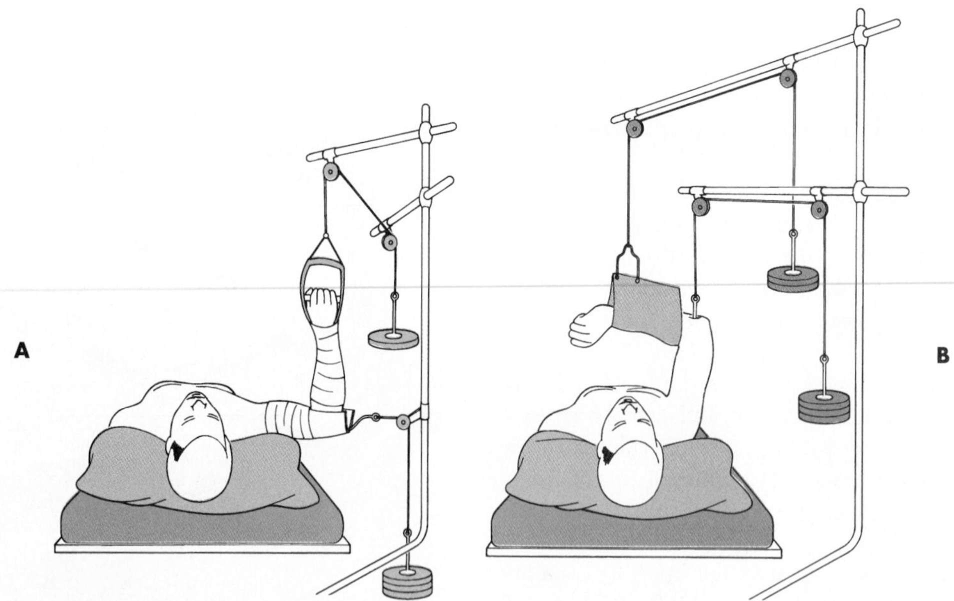

FIGURE 29-9 A, Side-arm traction (skin/skeletal). B, Overhead 90-90 traction (skeletal). (From Beare PG, Myers JL: *Principles and practice of adult health nursing,* ed 3, St. Louis, 1998, Mosby.)

2. Upper extremity traction:

   Side-arm traction—skeletal form of Dunlop's traction (Figure 29-9, *A*). The difference consists mainly of a pin drilled through the lower humerus (instead of the horizontal Buck's extension mentioned previously) and attached to a spreader, ropes, pulleys, and weights. The forearm is held in vertical Buck's extension, as it would be in Dunlop's skin traction. Side-arm skeletal traction is used for severe fractures, in which the greater pull permitted with the skeletal pin is required to overcome muscle spasms, resulting in effective alignment and union.

   Overhead 90-90 traction—humerus is placed at 90 degrees to the trunk, and elbow is flexed at 90 degrees. A sling supports the forearm. A Kirschner wire is placed through the olecranon process of the ulna (Figure 29-9, *B*).
3. External fixation—commonly used form of skeletal traction involving the use of one of a variety of frames to

hold pins drilled into or through bones (Figures 29-10 and 29-11). External fixation is frequently used with comminuted fractures having soft-tissue injury. External fixation frames are used for skull and facial fractures, ribs, all bones of the upper and lower extremities, and pelvic bones. Frames may fit on one side of a bone or bones or may be attached to pins on either side of an injured limb.

4. Skull tong traction—traction involving the use of one of a variety of tongs (Crutchfield, Vinke, Gardner-Wells, or Barton) drilled into the skull or placed below the scalp and attached to ropes, pulleys, and weights (Figure 29-12). This type of traction is used for fractures of cervical vertebrae and involves the use of special beds or turning frames to facilitate nursing care. Halo traction is used for neurologically intact clients to prevent further spinal cord damage (Figure 29-13).

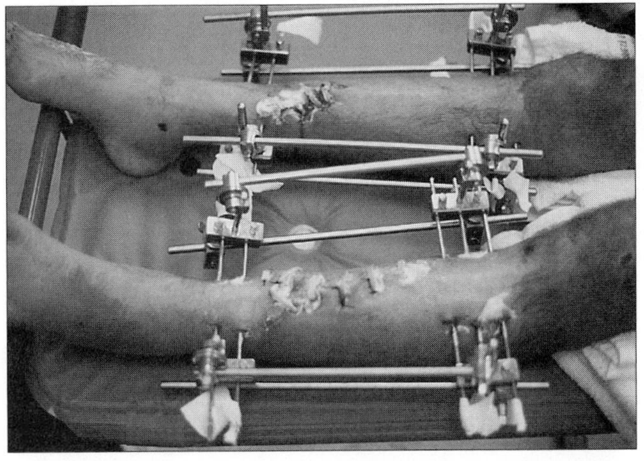

FIGURE 29-11 Bilateral Hoffman devices for treatment of comminuted fractures of tibia/fibula.

A

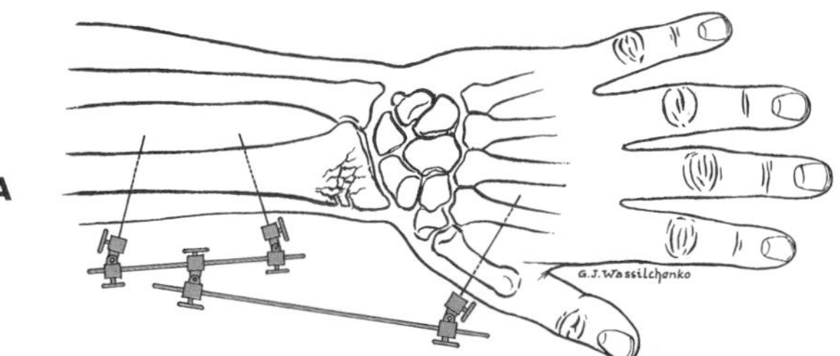

B

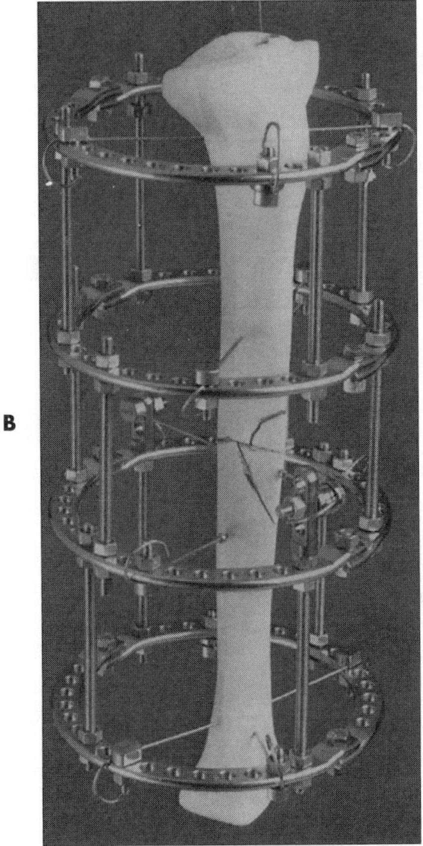

FIGURE 29-10 External fixators. **A,** Roger Anderson fixator. **B,** Ilizarhov fixator for treatment of comminuted fractures. (**B** from Phipps W and others: *Medical-surgical nursing: concepts and clinical practice,* ed 6, St. Louis, 1999, Mosby.)

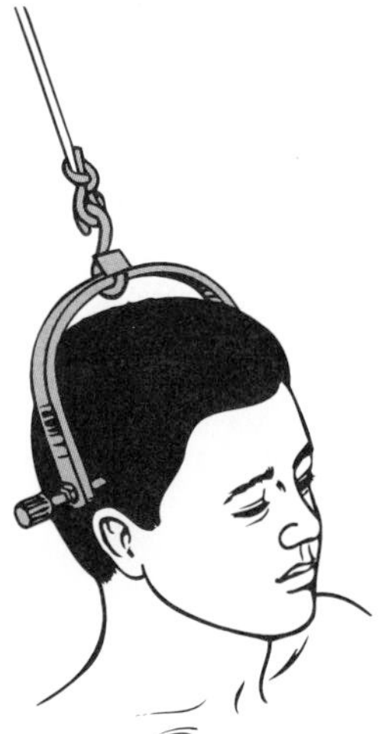

FIGURE 29-12 Gardner-Wells tongs for stabilization of cervical vertebral fractures.

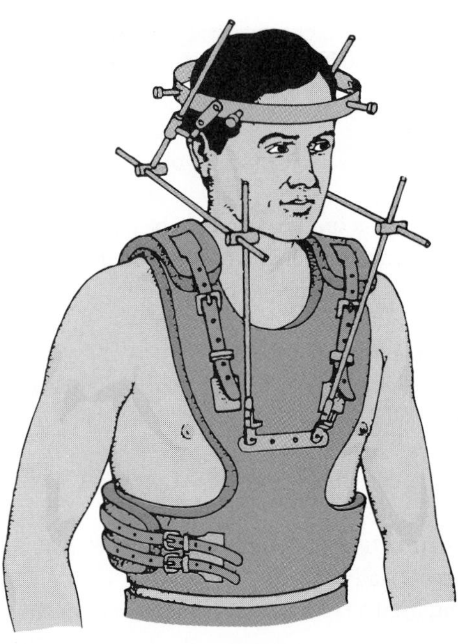

FIGURE 29-13 Halo vest. (From Beare PG, Myers JL: *Principles and practice of adult health nursing,* ed 3, St. Louis, 1998, Mosby.)

Delegation Considerations

Assessment of the client's condition and status of traction should not be delegated to assistive personnel. However, the skills of assisting with insertion of skeletal pins and pin site care may be delegated to assistive personnel who are adequately trained in principles of surgical asepsis. Instruct personnel in signs and symptoms associated with infection or inflammation at pin insertion site.

Equipment

- Sterile gloves for physician (use latex-free gloves if there is a risk of allergic reaction)
- Wastebasket with plastic liner
- Antiseptic ointment
- Skin preparation solutions as desired

Balanced-Suspension Skeletal Traction

- Sterile tray for insertion of Kirschner wire or Steinmann pin (secure from operating suite)
- Local anesthetic of physician's choice, usually 1% to 2% lidocaine
- **Thomas splint** or **Harris splint**
- **Pearson attachment**
- Foot support
- Trapeze bar
- Ropes, pulleys, weights, weight holders
- Towels, felt, stockinette
- Drill and extension cord if needed
- Adhesive tape

Upper Extremity Skeletal Traction

- Sterile tray with Kirschner wire or Steinmann pin (secure from operating suite)
- Adhesive strips or moleskin
- Elastic bandages
- Handgrip bar
- Ropes, pulley, weights, and weight holders
- Low shock blocks (optional)
- Local anesthetic of physician's choice, usually 1% to 2% lidocaine

External Fixation

- External fixator, usually Hoffman or Roger Anderson apparatus, Vital fixator, AO fixator, Ilizarhov, or other fixator (see Figures 29-10 and 29-11)
- Sterile tray with pins for insertion (secure from operating room)

Skull Tong Traction

- Tongs: Crutchfield, Vinke, Gardner-Wells, Barton, or Halo traction frame (see Figures 29-12 and 29-13)
- Sterile tray: Usually traction is applied in operating room
- Drill and extension cord if needed

Pin Care

- Sterile applicators
- Normal saline solution or hydrogen peroxide/normal saline solution in 1:1 solution or plain hydrogen peroxide
- Sterile containers
- Sterile gauze barrier (optional)
- Topical antibiotic ointment (optional)
- Clean gloves

Step	Rationale
Assessment	
1. Assess overall health condition of client, including mobility status.	Determines client's health state and ability to tolerate bed rest and skeletal traction.
2. Carefully assess specific tissues to be placed in skeletal traction. Note marked edema, rash, or other open lesions.	Determines ability of tissues to tolerate traction. Skeletal pin goes through skin to bone and out through skin.
3. Assess client's knowledge of upcoming traction, application, and purposes.	Determines willingness and ability to participate in care.
4. Assess client's level of pain.	Used as baseline for later comparisons.
5. Observe client's nonverbal behaviors and questions.	May reveal anxiety about impending procedure.

Nursing Diagnosis

Defining characteristics from the assessment data may reveal the following nursing diagnoses for clients requiring this skill:

- Bathing/hygiene, dressing/grooming, and toileting self-care deficit
- Risk for impaired skin integrity
- Risk for peripheral neurovascular dysfunction
- Risk for infection
- Impaired physical mobility
- Deficient knowledge regarding traction
- Acute pain
- Anxiety
- Risk for injury

Related factors are individualized based on client's condition or needs.

Step	Rationale
Planning	
1. **Expected outcomes** following completion of procedure:	
▪ Client participates in bathing and feeding.	Activities are performed safely, without injury. Client reduces risk of complications of immobility.
▪ Client maintains bowel and bladder function.	A fracture bedpan and/or urinal are used to facilitate elimination functions.
▪ Client's skin remains intact without redness, inflammation, or purulent drainage, especially over pressure points, proximal end of Thomas splint, and pin sites.	Indicates no development of pressure sores or infection. A small amount of clear drainage is expected from pin sites (McKenzie, 1999).
▪ Client demonstrates adequate neurovascular functioning in extremity. Distal skin tissues remain warm and of a normal skin color with capillary refill of 3 seconds or less. Client verbalizes no abnormal sensations and is able to move fingers or toes below fracture site.	Adequate neurovascular functioning is essential to the health and well-being of the extremity (Kunkler, 1999).
▪ Client retains range of joint motion (ROJM) in unaffected extremities and verbalizes understanding of activity restrictions. Demonstrates use of trapeze.	Routine exercise prevents contractures and muscle wasting.
▪ Client describes purpose of skeletal traction and follows activity restrictions.	Demonstrates learning and acceptance of restrictions.
▪ Client experiences reduced pain and muscle spasm.	Alignment of fracture reduces stress on bone fragments and adjoining muscle groups.
▪ Client does not become tense or withdrawn.	Demonstrates absence of anxiety.
▪ Client complies with restrictions imposed by traction apparatus. A fracture bedpan, as opposed to a regular-sized bedpan, is provided.	No injury is sustained.
Implementation	
1. Initial traction setup	
a. Position client according to physician's request. Nurse or other assistant may be asked to support tissues to be placed in traction. Client will most often be on back with head of bed slightly elevated. Client will be flat in bed for Dunlop's skeletal traction.	Ensures proper alignment during and after traction application.
b. Physician performs skin preparation and discards materials in wastebasket.	Reduces possibility of wound and bone infection.
c. Physician injects local anesthetic into sites as desired. Nurse and other assistants support client, limb, or other tissues to be placed in traction. Burr holes may be drilled in the outer layer of the skull for placement of tongs.	Anesthetic acts quickly to create painless area. Client will feel pressure of pin being drilled through or into bones and will hear drill but should feel no pain.
d. Provide encouragement and praise during drilling of pin tracts.	Reduces client anxiety.
e. Assist (usually by holding spreader bar, splint, or Pearson attachment) while physician continues to use drill to insert number of pins or nails desired for traction. Support area of joints not at injury site. Do not move distal portion unnecessarily.	Movement can cause severe pain or additional trauma.
2. Prepare specific traction setups (see Skill 29-3):	
a. Balanced-suspension skeletal traction (BSST)	
(1) For lower extremity traction: Assist with placement of Thomas or Harris splint, Pearson attachment, foot support, ropes, pulleys, and weights. Gently lower weights to establish traction. Apply antiseptic ointment to pin exit sites, and cover with sterile split dressing.	Splint and attachment are usually previously prepared for quick use. Foot plate prevents footdrop. Ointment and dressings are applied to cover open wounds to prevent infection.

Step	Rationale
(2) For side-arm traction: Assist with application of Buck's extension to forearm, place handgrip, and establish skin traction by *slowly* lowering weights until rope is taut (see Figure 29-9, *A*).	Skin traction allows forearm to remain in vertical position without undue effort from client.
(3) For 90-90 traction: Assist with preparing sling for forearm (see Figure 29-9, *B*).	
(4) Assist with application of spreader to hold skeletal pin; tie rope to spreader and thread through pulleys to weight holder and weights. Slowly lower weights until rope is taut. Place shock blocks if requested. Apply antiseptic ointment to pin exit sites and cover with sterile split dressing.	Amount of weight depends on severity of client's injury. Amounts vary from 5 to 10 or more pounds. Shock blocks allow one side of bed to be raised to help client maintain desired position. Ointment and sterile split dressings are applied to prevent infection.
(5) Attach trapeze bar, and instruct on use.	Allows the client to assist in movement and to maintain upper body muscle tone.
b. External fixation	
(1) Hold affected tissues or limb while physician attaches and tightens fixator screws or clamps. Apply antiseptic ointment to pin exit sites and cover with sterile split dressing.	Proper tension or tightness to pins is vital to prevent twist or torque, which would delay healing. Ointment and sterile split dressings are applied to prevent infection.
c. Skull tong traction	
(1) Client's cervical vertebrae are maintained in proper alignment with a Thomas cervical collar. Collar remains in place until skull tong traction is surgically placed. Traction is applied by weights ordered by physician.	Maintains proper cervical vertebrae alignment, thus reducing further injury and/or paralysis to the cervical segment of the spinal cord.
3. Assess client's initial reaction or response to traction before physician leaves.	Adjustments may be required immediately.
4. Raise side rails if appropriate.	Provides for client's safety.
5. Gather equipment and supplies, and return to proper storage places. Wash hands.	Provides for safety and cleanliness and prevents transmission of infection.
6. Pin care (After traction procedure, nurse needs to discuss with physician whether pin care will be performed. Type and frequency of pin site care varies according to physician preference and institutional policy.)	Although there are commonalities in care, there are currently no accepted clinical standards for pin site care. Some institutions have policies outlining pin site care, and others permit pin site care only with a physician's orders. There is no research to support the effectiveness of pin site care in preventing infections (McKenzie, 1999).
a. Wash hands and apply clean gloves.	Reduces transmission of infection. Use latex-free gloves if there is risk of an allergic reaction.
b. Remove old split gauze dressing around pins, and discard in receptacle. Note condition of tissues around pin site.	Evaluates ongoing condition of tissues. Can ensure early identification of infection.
c. Prepare supplies and apply new gloves.	Aseptic technique reduces infection transmission.
d. Begin by cleaning pins on one side of extremity, then do same on other side. Never touch one pin site with material used on another.	Prevents cross contamination.
e. Dip sterile cotton-tipped applicator into sterile container of one half hydrogen peroxide and one half saline, maintaining sterile environment. Place applicator by the pin and roll it along the skin, away from insertion site. Clean outward in a circular fashion from the pin. Dispose of applicator.	Remove crusts from pin site. Crusts can obstruct drainage, which leads to bacterial buildup. (Some institutions use only hydrogen peroxide or only saline.) Povidone-iodine may traumatize tissues and has a caustic effect on stainless steel pins (McKenzie, 1999).
f. Dip a new sterile applicator in normal saline; roll applicator across skin away from pin.	Removes peroxide solution to reduce skin irritation.

STEP	RATIONALE
g. Using a sterile applicator, apply a small amount of topical antibiotic ointment to pin site and cover with a sterile 2 × 2 split gauze dressing. (NOTE: some physicians leave site uncovered.)	Antiinfective reduces bacterial growth.
h. Repeat procedure for other pin site.	
7. Discard supplies. Remove and dispose of gloves. Wash hands.	Reduces transmission of infection.

EVALUATION

1. Evaluate entire traction setup and functioning: observe that knots are not caught in pulleys and that ropes are running straight through pulleys; observe ropes for fraying; evaluate that correct weight is hanging (do not add or remove weight without physician order) and dangling freely; determine that linens are not interfering with traction apparatus; and observe client's body alignment.	Determines if traction is functioning as desired. Anything that inhibits the smooth movement of the traction rope in the pulley will disrupt the traction and may lead to nonunion. Poor body alignment may lead to discomfort and affect proper bone healing.
2. Determine client's response to traction; client should begin to note relief of pain, sense of comfort, and lessening of muscle spasms.	Skeletal traction takes longer for client to note relief of symptoms because of increased tissue trauma.
3. Evaluate for presence of pain and muscle spasms.	Determines need for analgesics, muscle relaxants, and success of traction in stabilizing fracture.
4. Inspect pin sites for drainage or inflammation.	Recognizes early signs of infection.
5. Assess for other indicators of infection, such as fever; elevated white blood count; continuous, dull, aching pain; redness; or warmth in extremity.	Recognizes early signs of osteomyelitis.
6. Perform neurovascular assessment (see Skill 29-1, Evaluation, Step 2).	Determines peripheral perfusion to tissues, as well as client's sensation and voluntary motor activity.
7. Assess for indicators of hypoxemia, such as restlessness or agitation.	Recognizes early signs of fat embolism syndrome (FES).
8. Assess skin, especially around ankle, elbow, foot, or distal tibia, for fracture blisters. Do not rupture blister. Apply hydrocolloid dressing to ruptured blister.	Fracture blisters are associated with severe or twisting type fractures. Intact skin provides a barrier to prevent infection. Hydrocolloid dressing maintains a moist, clean environment (McCann and Gruen, 1997).

UNEXPECTED OUTCOMES AND RELATED INTERVENTIONS

- Skeletal pin moves or slides in pin tract, leading to increased risk of infection or nonunion.
  - Notify physician.
- Client experiences delayed union, malunion, or nonunion.
  - Ensure that proper amount of weight is continuously maintained.
  - Provide proper nutrition.
  - Notify physician of infection.
- Client has severe edema, marked increase in pain, inability to actively move joints, or increased pain on passive movement, indicating compartment syndrome.
  - Notify physician immediately.
- Client develops infection at pin site or at fracture site with development of osteomyelitis.
  - Maintain aseptic technique; notify physician; and administer ordered antibiotics.
- Client experiences prolonged bleeding or frank hemorrhage.
  - Chronically ill or older clients may have preexistent iron-deficiency anemia made worse by bleeding or hemorrhage. Replacement of blood loss may be required. Autologous transfusion (see Chapter 20) is frequently the treatment of choice.
- Client experiences nerve damage:
  - Peroneal nerve: footdrop with inability to evert and dorsiflex foot.
    - Notify physician.

- Radial or median nerve at wrist with inability to approximate thumb and fingers (radial) and numbness and tingling of thumb, index, middle fingers (median) with wristdrop.
    - Loosen elastic bandage at wrist for side-arm traction.
    - Reposition sling at wrist for overhead 90-90 traction.
    - Notify physician.
- Client experiences FES (more common in fractures of long bones) with symptoms of hypoxemia: restlessness, decreased level of orientation, disorientation, tachycardia, tachypnea, dyspnea, hypotension, and petechial rash over upper chest and neck.
    - Maintain stability and immobilization of fracture to prevent FES.
    - Notify physician and treat with oxygen.
- Client experiences deep vein thrombosis with possible pulmonary embolus.
    - Teach client calf-pump exercises, maintain sequential compression devices or foot pumps, and give ordered anticoagulant as preventive measures.
    - Do not massage lower extremity.
    - Notify physician. If symptoms of pulmonary embolus evident, elevate head of bed if conscious, administer oxygen, and notify physician *immediately*.
- Client experiences declining voluntary motor responses.
    - Notify physician.

Recording and Reporting

- Record in nurses' notes type of traction applied, persons applying traction, site to which traction was applied, time of application, amount of weights, and client's initial response.
- Record all findings of neurovascular assessment (see Skill 29-1, Evaluation, Step 2) every 1 to 2 hours or as ordered.

Teaching Considerations

- Before discharge, client is taught use of ambulatory aid (cane, walker, or crutches); written instructions are given to client and significant others.
- Client is provided written instructions for home care maintenance, especially if being discharged with external fixation (pin site care, elevate extremity when sitting or lying to prevent edema formation).
- Client is provided dietary instructions if necessary.
- Client is taught to notify physician of undesirable signs, including increase in pain, muscle spasms, increased numbness or tingling, appearance of drainage, redness, or soreness at operative or traction pin sites.

Pediatric Considerations

- Blood loss from a fracture can become critical more quickly in the child than the adult because blood volume in the adult is 60% of total body weight and 70% to 85% in the child (Wong and others, 1999).
- Bone remodeling is at its maximum rate at approximately 2½ years of age (McCance and Huether, 1998).
- Parents are taught that babies may cry when traction is established.
- Children may experience boredom, regression, and interference with school work. Parents and other caregivers must look for ways to divert the child's attention and support the child. Schoolwork should be obtained from school and the child assisted when able to perform tasks. Parents are counseled regarding regression to decrease their anxiety.
- Physical activity is essential for growth and development in the child. Immobility may result in increased anxiety. Behaviors that may be demonstrated are restlessness, depression, regression, lack of concentration, dependence, acting out, and outbursts of crying or temper tantrums (Wong and others, 1999).
- Children should be assured that someone will always be available to assist them while they are in traction.

Gerontological Considerations

- Older adult clients may suffer from diabetes or peripheral vascular disease, adding risks to use of traction.
- An overhead trapeze may assist the older client in maintaining upper body strength and in facilitating hygiene and repositioning.

Home Care Considerations

- After traction is discontinued, client is taught to dangle prior to ambulation, to proceed slowly with ambulation, and to gradually increase the time and distance ambulated.
- Client is provided instructions regarding use of muscle relaxants and analgesics if prescribed.

Critical Thinking Exercises

1. Mr. Byrd had a hip spica cast applied 4 hours ago. He asks you to use a hair dryer on hot and high to hasten the drying of his plaster of Paris cast. What do you do?
2. Mr. Byrd is complaining of itching beneath the cast and asks you to get him a coat hanger so that he can scratch. How do you respond?
3. Mrs. Casey fell at home and broke her hip. She is placed in Buck's extension skin traction overnight until a surgical repair can be done. During the night, she complains that the traction boot is too tight. What do you do?
4. Mr. Russell just returned from surgery for placement of balanced-suspension skeletal traction (BSST). He looks at the apparatus in dismay and asks how you will ever change his bed linens. How would you respond?

References

Baumann NH: Latex allergy: an orthopaedic case presentation and considerations in patient care, *Orthop Nurs* 18(3):15, 1999.

Beare PG, Myers JL: *Principles and practice of adult health nursing,* ed 3, St. Louis, 1998, Mosby.

Byrne T: The setup and care of a patient in Buck's traction, *Orthop Nurs* 18(2):79, 1999.

Ebersole P, Hess P: *Toward healthy aging: human needs and nursing response,* ed 5, St. Louis, 1998, Mosby.

Folcik M, Carini-Garcia G, Birmingham J: *Traction: assessment and management,* St. Louis, 1994, Mosby.

Hart KM, Kester K: Supracondylar fractures in children, *Orthop Nurs* 18(3):23, 1999.

Kunkler CE: Neurovascular assessment, Orthop Nurs 18(3):63, 1999.

McCance KL, Huether SE: *Pathophysiology: the biologic basis for disease in adults and children,* ed 3, St. Louis, 1998, Mosby.

McCann S, Gruen G: Fracture blisters: a review of the literature, *Orthop Nurs* 16(2):17, 1997.

McKenzie LL: In search of a standard for pin site care, *Orthop Nurs* 18(2):73, 1999.

Phipps W and others: *Medical-surgical nursing: concepts and clinical practice,* ed 6, St. Louis, 1999, Mosby.

Sprague J: Cast syndrome: the superior mesenteric artery syndrome, *Orthop Nurs* 17(4):12, 1998.

Wong DL and others: *Whaley and Wong's nursing care of infants and children,* ed 6, St. Louis, 1999, Mosby.

30

SUPPORT SURFACES AND SPECIAL BEDS

Skills

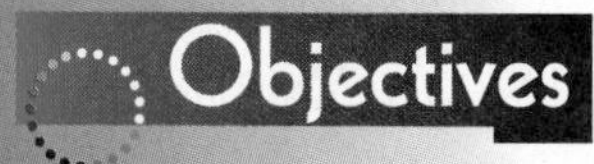

Objectives

Mastery of content in this chapter will enable the nurse to:

- Define the key terms listed.
- Identify the different types of support surfaces used to prevent pressure ulcer formation.
- Explain why preventive nursing care is still essential when using special mattresses and beds.
- Describe guidelines to follow when placing clients on special mattresses and beds.
- Compare and contrast differences between mattress overlays and mattress replacements.
- Describe mechanisms by which skin breakdown can occur on either an air-suspension or an air-fluidized bed, a bariatric bed, a Rotokinetic bed, or a support surface mattress.
- Describe correct placement of a client on an air-fluidized bed, an air-suspension bed, a bariatric bed, a Rotokinetic bed, or a support surface mattress.

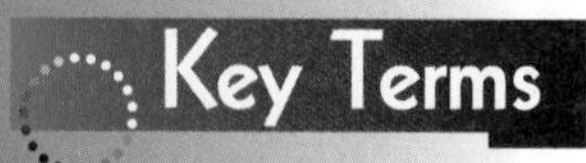

Key Terms

Air-fluidized bed	Kinesthetic
Air-suspension bed	Morbidly obese
Bariatric bed	Orthopedic
Flotation pads	Pressure ulcers
Friction	Rotokinetic bed
Immobility	Shearing

Despite the increasing technological advances in the world of medicine, pressure sores remain a major health care problem causing suffering to clients and increasing health care costs. Although a multidisciplinary team approach is key, all agree that nurses are at the forefront of prevention and treatment of pressure ulcers in health care settings (Phillips, 1997). **Pressure ulcers** are defined by the National Pressure Ulcer Advisory Panel (NPUAP) as lesions caused by unrelieved pressure against soft tissue, usually over some bony prominence. Pressure ulcers can occur among those in any age group or ethnic population, regardless of socioeconomic status (Phipps, Sands, and Marek, 1999). The occurrence of pressure ulcers is a serious and expensive health care problem in the United States, where an estimated 1 million persons are affected. The cost to treat an ulcer is approximately $2000 to $3000, and more than $6.4 million is spent annually on the treatment of ulcers (Tourtual and others, 1997). With the challenges of health care reform to improve quality while reducing costs, it is essential for the nurse to identify clients at risk for breakdown. Factors that contribute to pressure ulcer formation are both extrinsic (e.g., moisture, friction, and shear) and intrinsic (e.g., malnutrition, loss of sensation, impaired mobility, aging skin, impaired mental status, infection, incontinence, and low arteriolar pressure) (Bulechek and McCloskey, 1999).

Nurses have always been responsible for caring for persons with pressure ulcers. Historically, frail debilitated older adults were presumed to inevitably acquire pressure ulcers. New knowledge and technology, including special beds and mattresses, and vigorous systematic assessment provide ways to prevent ulcers (Fulmer and Abraham, 1998).

The major cause of pressure ulcers is unrelieved pressure. The greater the pressure and the longer the pressure is applied, the greater the likelihood that a pressure ulcer will develop. To stay healthy, body tissues require an adequate supply of oxygen and nutrients and removal of carbon dioxide and other waste products of metabolism. This requires maintenance of adequate blood flow through the capillaries. When external pressure on the tissues exceeds 32 mm Hg (the capillary closing pressure), the network of capillaries collapses, and the supply of oxygen and nutrients to the cells, as well as removal of metabolic waste products, is interrupted. As a result, there is tissue ischemia and, if unrelieved, tissue death or necrosis (Monahan and Neighbors, 1998).

When a client is confined to a bed, the tissues between the skeleton and supporting bed surface become compressed and the blood vessels within the tissues become occluded. A client lying supine on a hospital bed may exert as much as 150 mm Hg pressure (2.9 psi) on skin and soft tissue. Once pressure reaches more than 78 mm Hg for a period of time, a person usually feels discomfort and changes position. However, the client with altered sensation or one who cannot move independently is at risk for pressure ulcers of superficial and deep tissues unless pressure is significantly reduced. Pressures in excess of 20 to 40 mm Hg for prolonged periods can cause tissue injury (Koziak, 1961). The principle behind pressure-relief strategy is dispersing the load to relieve pressure at regular intervals. At-risk clients left sitting in chairs can develop deeper and more serious pressure sores than those left in a bed because a greater pressure is being exerted on a smaller surface area, the buttocks. A client lying in bed has the pressure distributed over a greater surface area but is also at risk for developing pressure ulcers over bony prominences because they receive greater pressure than other parts of the body (Phillips, 1997).

Special beds and mattresses have been designed to reduce the hazards of immobility to the skin and musculoskeletal system. These support surfaces have differing purposes, including pressure reduction, pressure relief, repositioning, and support of the morbidly obese client. These support surfaces are used in acute, rehabilitative, long-term, and home care settings. It is important to understand the difference between a pressure-reducing and a pressure-relieving support surface. The former reduces the interface pressure between the body and support surface below 32 mm Hg. Pressure-reducing devices reduce the interface pressure, but not necessarily below capillary closing pressure (Agency for Health Care Policy and Research, 1994). Pressure-reducing surfaces (e.g., fiber-filled and foam overlays, gel or water support systems, air-filled mattresses, low air loss and air-fluidized supports) increase the area of the body in contact with the surface thereby spreading the load and reducing the effects of pressure. Pressure-relieving systems move under the client and reduce the amount of pressure being applied to any one area at regular intervals. An example of this system is an alternating system where air is pumped by a motor into an overlay or mattress (Phillips, 1997).

Frequent repositioning, which temporarily relieves pressure, is the backbone of preventative protocols. No bed or mattress totally eliminates the need for competent nursing care. Although useful, turning devices can still injure soft tissues, requiring a nurse to be especially observant for signs of pressure formation (Bulechek and McCloskey, 1999).

With the use of high technology, the incidence of pressure ulcer formation should be reduced. However, these devices need to be implemented along with frequent repositioning, meticulous skin care, and nutrition adequate in vitamin C, protein, and hydration. These concepts, along with good nursing judgment, will bring nursing closer to the goal of eliminating pressure ulcers from all health care settings.

Skill Performance Guidelines

1. Know the reason for the client's reduced mobility. A totally immobilized client benefits from support devices other than those used for a partially immobile client.
2. Perform client assessment to determine selection of appropriate special mattresses and beds.
3. Continue to provide basic preventive care measures against the hazards of **immobility,** for example, turning, correct positioning, skin assessment and care, or range-of-motion exercises (when allowed).
4. Use proper body mechanics when positioning or working with clients.
5. Follow all safety measures to prevent injury to the client from accidental falls or improper positioning when placing them on special beds or mattresses.
6. Encourage clients to remain as mobile as possible within the limits of their physical conditions and prescribed activity levels.
7. Educate care provider about the advantages/disadvantages and methods of operation of all support devices to ensure their proper use in all settings.
8. Perform baseline nutritional and fluid balance assessment.
9. Collaborate with health care professionals who have expertise in this area.
10. Anticipate need to consult with social service or home health department regarding third-party reimbursement, as well as arrangements for delivery to and care of special beds in the home.

Skill 30-1 Placing a Client on a Support Surface Mattress

Numerous support surfaces that are designed to reduce pressure on tissues overlying bony prominences are available. The wide acceptance of these devices has led many nurses to recommend their use as common preventive measures for clients with reduced mobility and risk for developing pressure ulcers. Most of the devices are easy to apply and keep clean. The extent to which the devices actually relieve pressure and prevent skin breakdown is highly variable. Few systematic studies exist that consistently find one surface is better than others. Although good and frequent repositioning can do much to prevent pressure ulcers, it may still be necessary to provide a support surface that reduces pressure over bony prominences (Bulechek and McCloskey, 1999).

The types of support surfaces can be categorized as mattress (or wheelchair) overlays, mattress replacements, or specialty beds. Mattress overlays and mattress replacements are considered to be either static (e.g., foam, gels) or dynamic (e.g., alternating pressure surfaces). Specialty beds are described as either low air loss or air fluidized (Bulechek and McCloskey, 1999).

A **flotation pad** is constructed of a silicone or polyvinyl chloride gel encased in a vinyl-covered square. The pad serves as an artificial layer of fat to protect bony surfaces such as the sacrum and greater trochanters. One type of flotation pad can be used for wheelchair clients.

One type of air mattress is fully integrated into the hospital bed. This bed surface may be adjusted to the client's comfort level by adding or removing air through buttons within the client's reach, or it can automatically adjust pressures to the client's position and movement when in the automatic mode. A bedsheet is always used to cover an air mattress to prevent skin from touching the plastic surface.

There are two types of foam mattresses. One is the foam mattress overlay, which may have either a flat smooth surface, foam rubber peaks (egg-crate variety, shown in Figure 30-1), or a cut surface. It is placed on top of the bed mattress, and usually the nurse places a sheet over the foam mattress pad overlay to prevent soiling and provide ease of cleaning. The second type is the foam specialty mattress, which completely replaces the hospital mattress and is covered by a loose-fitting cover intended to protect the mattress and minimize friction and shear. The foam mattresses are designed more for comfort rather than pressure relief.

Several types of air mattresses can be used to reduce pressure on skin surfaces. The static type is made of vinyl plastic and contains a series of undulating tubes running the entire length of the device (Figure 30-2). More complex air mattresses contain several layers of tubes or support cells. A static mattress is inflated with a simple air blower after placing the mattress on a bed. An alternating air mattress connects with a pressure cycling device that intermittently inflates and deflates sections of the mattress, creating a cycling effect that minimizes pressure on bony prominences (Phillips, 1997). Use a static mattress if a client can assume a variety of positions without bearing weight on a pressure ulcer. Use a dynamic support if the client cannot assume a variety of positions and if the client fully compresses a static mattress (Agency for Health Care Policy and Research [AHCPR], 1994).

Another available option is an air mattress that replaces the conventional mattress. These mattresses may also be fully integrated into the bed (Figure 30-3).

Another intervention is a dry static flotation mattress system that may be overlaid on either the bed (Figure 30-4) or wheelchair (Figure 30-5). Through a system of controlled dynamics, low pressures are maintained by distributing pressure across the client's body surface. Thus friction and shear are minimized.

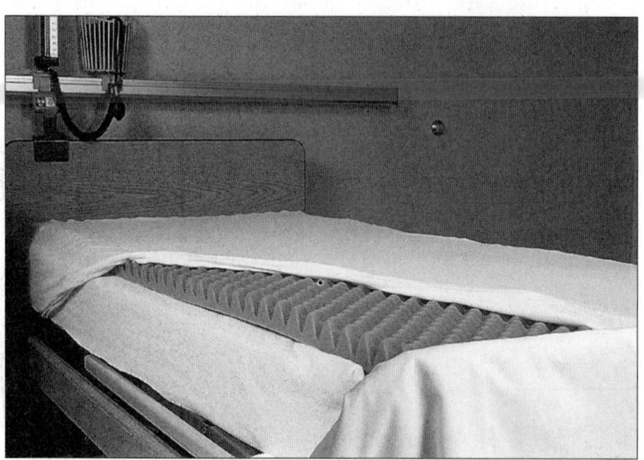

FIGURE **30-1** "Egg-crate" foam overlay is primarily for comfort.

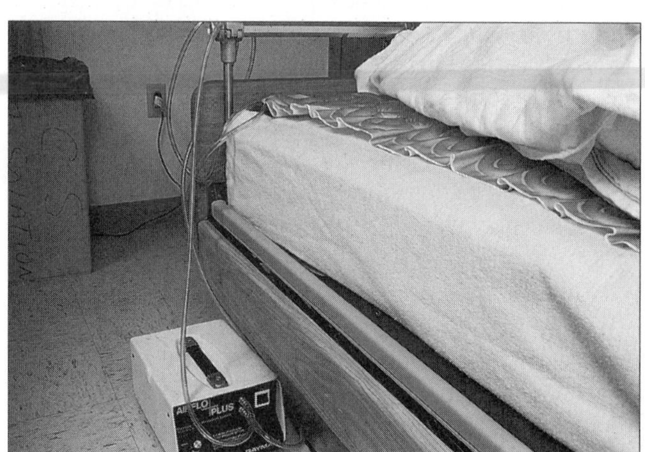

FIGURE **30-2** Air mattress.

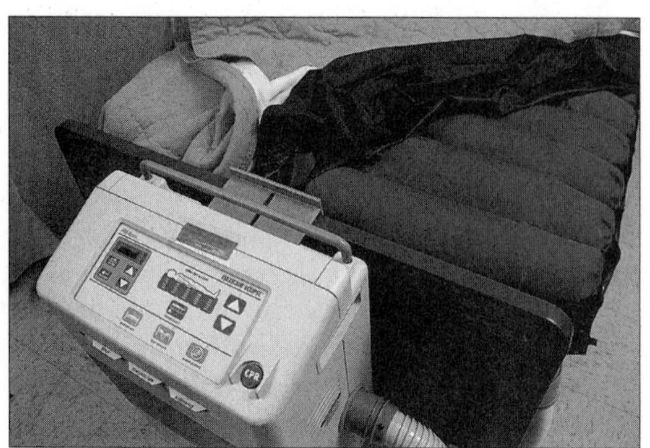

FIGURE **30-3** Integrated air mattress.

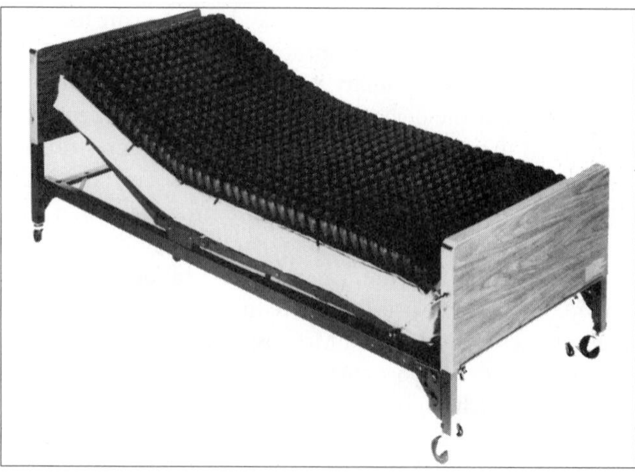

FIGURE **30-4** ROHO dry flotation mattress system. (Courtesy Crown Therapeutics, Inc, Belleville, Ill.)

Water mattresses, similar to those available for home use, are available in a variety of configurations with or without a heating unit, or the mattress may rest on top of a regular bed mattress. When a water mattress is used, the filling may be completed by the nurse, delegated to assistive personnel, or by the service company representative when supplied by a rental agency. As with the air mattress, a sheet is always placed over the water mattress.

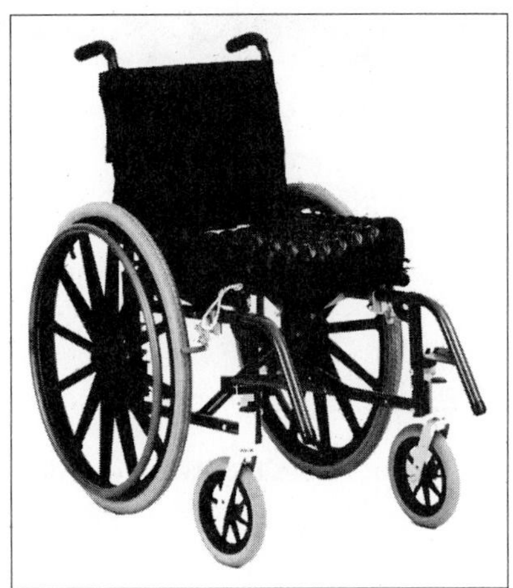

FIGURE **30-5** ROHO dry flotation mattress system for clients in wheelchairs. (Courtesy Crown Therapeutics, Inc, Belleville, Ill.)

DELEGATION CONSIDERATIONS

The skill of applying a support mattress can be delegated to assistive personnel. The caregiver must routinely inspect the client's skin over bony prominences and heels for signs of pressure and report when changes in the client's skin are observed. Instruct the caregiver to continue regular turning and repositioning of the client and to seek assistance for client position changes as necessary. Also instruct on proper method for applying each device.

EQUIPMENT

- Risk assessment tool (see Chapter 7)
- Mattress support surface of choice: bed with integrated surface, replacement mattress, or overlay
- Sheet(s)
- Disposable gloves (if soiled linen is being handled)

STEP	RATIONALE
ASSESSMENT	
1. Wash hands.	Reduces transmission of microorganisms.
2. Determine client's risk for pressure ulcer formation using a validated assessment tool (Lewis, Heitkemper, and Dirksen, 2000). Risk factors for pressure ulcers include nutritional deficits, shear stress, friction, alterations in mobility and perception, moisture, and abnormal serum albumin and hemoglobin levels (Phipps, Sands, and Marek, 1999).	Nurse can institute use of support surfaces as preventive measure against pressure ulcers. (NOTE: A medical order is required for reimbursement in the United States but not in Canada.)

• ***Critical Decision Point***
Clients with unstable conditions may not tolerate turning or positioning required for the application of a support surface mattress.

STEP	RATIONALE
3. Perform skin assessment to determine baseline. Inspect condition of skin, especially over dependent sites and bony prominences.	Data provide baseline to determine change in skin integrity or change in existing pressure ulcer.
4. Assess client's understanding of purpose of support surface.	Misconceptions can affect client's cooperation in use of mattress.
5. Assess client's level of comfort.	Provides baseline to determine client's comfort level. Nerve endings related to touch, temperature, and limb positioning are found in the skin (Phillips, 1997).

• ***Critical Decision Point***
Clients experiencing pain may require administration of pain medication before application of support surface of choice or transfer to another bed.

STEP	RATIONALE
6. Verify physician's order for type of support surface.	In the United States, mattress may be placed before physician's order is received, unless there is a question that it will be ordered. Physician's order is required to ensure third-party payment of support surface. (NOTE: Physician's order is not required in Canada.)

NURSING DIAGNOSIS

Defining characteristics from the assessment data may reveal the following nursing diagnoses for clients requiring this skill:

- Anxiety
- Risk for infection
- Deficient knowledge regarding use of support surface mattress
- Impaired physical mobility
- Pain (acute, chronic)
- Risk for impaired skin integrity
- Impaired skin integrity
- Ineffective peripheral tissue perfusion

Related factors are individualized based on client's condition or needs.

PLANNING

STEP	RATIONALE
1. **Expected outcomes** following completion of procedure:	
▪ Skin is without erythema or mottling.	Mottling represents hypoxia, which is an abnormal physiological response in tissues under pressure (Potter and Perry, 1999).
▪ Existing pressure ulcer shows signs of healing.	Skin remains free of new pressure ulcers. Support surface does not interfere with circulation to dependent areas.
▪ Client expresses sense of comfort.	Localized areas of discomfort have been eliminated by equalized pressures.
▪ Client is removed from therapeutic surface when risk for pressure ulcers decreases.	Provides for efficient, cost-effective care while maintaining high-quality outcomes.
2. Explain purpose of mattress and method of application to client.	Relieves anxiety and promotes cooperation.
3. Apply gloves (should be worn if linens are soiled or wet). Obtain assistance as needed.	Gloves prevent contact with body fluids. Assistance reduces risk of friction and shear in transfer to new surface.

IMPLEMENTATION

• ***Critical Decision Point***

Perform application of support surface mattress or transfer to bed in an organized, efficient manner. Clients whose medical conditions are unstable may not tolerate prolonged periods of position change (i.e., lying flat or turning from side to side). Turning an acutely ill client to the lateral side may cause complications such as increased oxygen demand and hypotension (Bulechek and McCloskey, 1999).

STEP	RATIONALE
1. Close room door or bedside curtain.	Provides client privacy and considerate care during application of mattress to bed or transfer to alternate bed.
2. Apply support surface to bed or prepare alternate bed (bed may be occupied or unoccupied).	
a. Mattress replacement:	
(1) Apply mattress to bed frame after removing standard hospital mattress.	Hospital mattress needs to be stored. In some instances, mattress replacements may be standard procedure.
(2) Apply sheet over mattress. Keep linens between surfaces to a minimum.	Sheet reduces soiling. Multiple layers decrease surface effectiveness.

Step	Rationale
b. Air mattress/overlay:	
(1) Apply deflated mattress flat over surface of bed mattress. (There may be directions on pad indicating which side to place up.)	Provides smooth, even surface.
(2) Bring any plastic strips or flaps around corners of bed mattress.	Secures air mattress in place.
(3) Attach connector on air mattress to inflation device. Inflate mattress to proper air pressure determined by air pump or blower.	Mattresses vary as to requiring one-time or continuous inflation cycle. Manufacturer's directions indicate desired air pressure designed to distribute client's body weight evenly. Directions are included with each mattress.
(4) Place sheet over air mattress, being sure to eliminate all wrinkles.	Prevents soiling of mattress and reduces direct contact of skin with plastic surface.
(5) Check air pumps to be sure pressure cycle alternates.	Alternating airflow mattress produces intermittent cycling, inflating only parts of mattress at any one time. Intermittent cycle continually alternates pressure against skin and soft tissue.
(6) Keep sharp objects away from air mattress.	Tears can cause loss of air, making mattress ineffective.
(7) Assist client with transferring in and out of bed.	Mattress surface may be slippery.
c. Integrated air-surface bed:	
(1) Obtain and make bed.	In some instances bed may be available in all client rooms; if not, an ordering system exists to obtain one as needed (see agency policy).
(2) Place switch in the "prevention" mode.	In the "prevention" mode, surface pressures change automatically with client position to equalize pressure and eliminate points of pressure.

- ***Critical Decision Point***
  Beds are equipped with a cardiopulmonary resuscitation (CPR) switch to instantly lower head section from an elevated position and to deflate the mattress to provide a firm surface for chest compressions (see illustration).

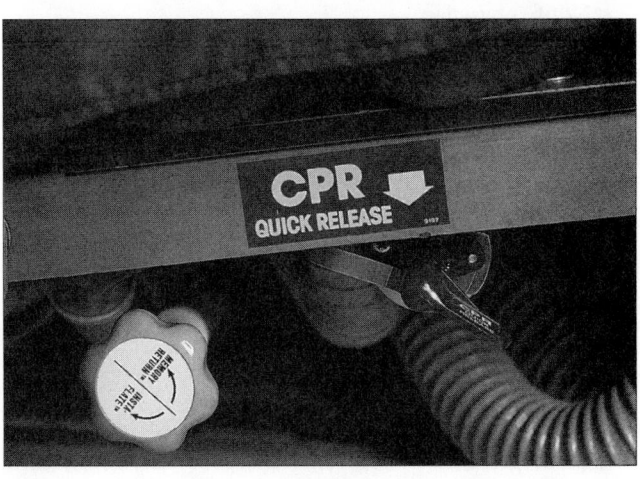

CPR quick-release switch.

Step	Rationale
d. Water mattress (supplemental and self-contained):	
(1) Apply unfilled supplemental mattress flat over the surface of standard bed mattress. (Self-contained water mattress would replace bed mattress.)	Provides a smooth, even surface.
(2) Bring any plastic strips or flaps around corners of bed mattress.	Secures water mattress in place.

STEP	RATIONALE
(3) Attach connector on water mattress to water source and fill mattress to level recommended by manufacturer. Follow manufacturer's directions regarding temperature of water. Mattress should be filled in close proximity to water source. Manufacturer's directions (enclosed with mattress) indicate desired water level designed to distribute client's body weight evenly (usually determined by client weight or height and weight).	Proper water temperature prevents loss of body heat as client lies on mattress.
(4) Place sheet over water mattress, being sure to eliminate all wrinkles.	Reduces soiling of mattress and prevents direct contact of skin with plastic surface.
(5) Keep sharp objects away from mattress.	Tears and punctures result in loss of water, making mattress ineffective.
e. Position client comfortably as desired over support surface. Reposition routinely.	Location of existing pressure ulcer might influence type of positioning.
f. Remove gloves and wash hands.	Reduces transmission of microorganisms.

EVALUATION

1. Reinspect condition of client's skin at routine intervals.	Determines if pressure sores develop or if the condition of existing sores changes.
2. Reassess client's risk for pressure ulcer formation at routine intervals.	Documents change in status, which is critical for evaluating continued need for therapeutic surface.
3. Evaluate client's level of comfort.	If pressure-relief mattress is effective, client generally experiences less discomfort.
4. Evaluate inflation of mattress periodically.	Regular inspection of mechanical components of mattress ensures proper functioning.

UNEXPECTED OUTCOMES AND RELATED INTERVENTIONS

- Skin develops areas of erythema, mottling, swelling, and tenderness.
  - Modify skin care regimen.
  - Increase frequency of skin assessment.
  - Increases types of pressure-relief interventions.
  - Consult with skin care expert.
  - Notify physician.
- Existing pressure areas fail to heal or increase in size or depth.
  - Modify skin care regimen.
  - Consult with skin care expert.
  - Notify physician.
- Client expresses discomfort while on support surface.
  - Evaluate need for analgesia or mild sedation.
  - Modify support surface selected.
  - Notify physician.
- Bed or mattress develops leak (air, water, gel).
  - Identify source of leak.
  - Review equipment instructions.
  - Follow manufacturer's guidelines.

RECORDING AND REPORTING

- Record type of support surface applied, extent to which client tolerated procedure, and condition of client's skin in nurses' notes or skin assessment flow sheet.
- Report evidence of pressure ulcer formation to nurse in charge or to physician.

TEACHING CONSIDERATIONS

- Explain risks of immobility to client and family members (see Chapter 28).
- Instruct in positioning and pressure relief.
- Explain risks for pressure ulcers.
- Explain purpose and function of the pressure-relief surface. Include reminder that the surface augments care and does not replace the need for turning and pressure-relief maneuvers.
- Explain precautions regarding sharp objects, fire hazard, and other concerns.
- Reeducate client about need for support surface and discuss alternatives, including client's right to refuse a recommended surface.

GERONTOLOGICAL CONSIDERATIONS

- Implement preventive measures because aging skin is drier, thinner, and less pressure sensitive, increasing the risk of skin breakdown (Lueckenotte, 2000).

HOME CARE CONSIDERATIONS

- Most of the devices covered in this section may be adapted for home use on a standard twin bed or hospital bed.
- Selection should be based on client needs and environmental audit. For example, the client on total bed rest who smokes would not be an ideal candidate for a foam mattress because of the potential for fire; the client with pets that sleep in the bed may not be suited for a water- or air-filled mattress because of the risk of puncture.
- Reimbursement varies by surface type and payer source.
- There needs to be more information related to prevalence of pressure ulcers in homebound clients (AHCPR, 1992).

PEDIATRIC CONSIDERATIONS

- There are various pain assessment tools developed specifically for use in children. Parents can also be helpful in assisting the child in expressing pain and treatment preferences (Bulechek and McCloskey, 1999).

LONG-TERM CARE CONSIDERATIONS

- Pressure ulcers are a major concern for older adults in health care facilities and at home. Many residents acquire pressure ulcers in the hospital or at home before nursing home admission (Ignatavicius, 1998).
- Nurse needs to make an accurate, time-efficient assessment of resident's pain in a long-term setting (Ignatavicius, 1998).

Skill 30-2 Placing a Client on an Air-Suspension Bed

Air-suspension beds are indicated for clients who are immobile or otherwise confined to the bed. The **air-suspension bed** supports a client's weight on air-filled cushions. The bed minimizes pressure and reduces shear in a low–air-loss system (Figure 30-6). If a client has large stage III or stage IV pressure ulcers on multiple turning surfaces, a low–air-loss bed or air-fluidized bed may be indicated (Agency for Health Care Policy and Research, 1994).

For clients requiring high air loss under a given body part, for example, under the buttocks, high–air-loss cushions may be substituted. High air loss provides for selective drying while not having the effect of substantially increasing insensible fluid losses.

It is also possible to adapt the air-suspension beds to individual client needs with specialty cushions for positioning, foot support, and lateral arm supports. Clients usually require less analgesia while on the bed. Another adaptation of the air-suspension bed is the kinetic low–air-loss bed. This bed is marketed widely to intensive care areas and has the ability to provide a pressure-relief surface while rotating continuously approximately 30 to 35 degrees. This surface should not be used with a client who has an unstable spine or who is in traction.

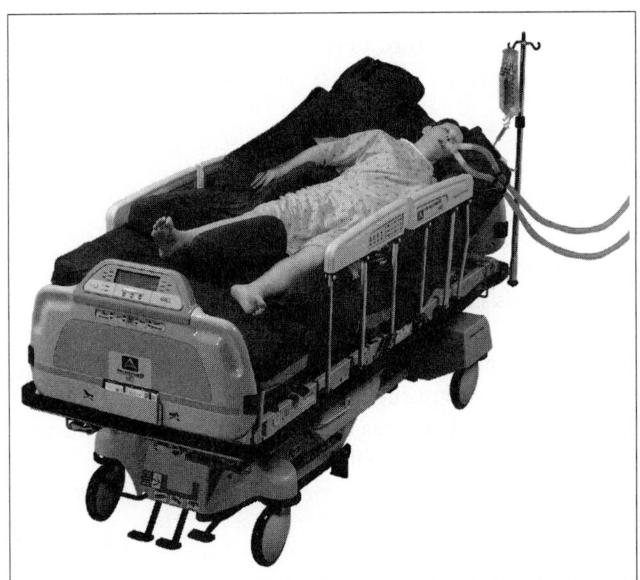

FIGURE 30-6 Air-suspension bed. (TriaDyne II Critical Care Healing System courtesy Kinetic Concepts, Inc., San Antonio, Tex.)

DELEGATION CONSIDERATIONS

The skill of placing a client on an air-suspension bed can be delegated to assistive personnel. The caregiver must routinely inspect the client's skin over bony prominences and heels for signs of pressure and report when changes in the client's skin are observed. The caregiver should be instructed in when to seek assistance for client position changes; in specifics regarding applying, cleaning, and maintaining support surface; and to report if client becomes disoriented, becomes restless, or complains of nausea.

EQUIPMENT

- Air-suspension bed (KinAir, Therapulse, Flexicare, Mediscus, Biodyne, RestCue)
- Gore-Tex sheet (supplied by rental company)
- Disposable bed pads, if indicated
- Disposable gloves (optional)

STEP	RATIONALE

ASSESSMENT

Step	Rationale
1. Identify clients who would benefit from air-suspension therapy, such as immobilized or burn clients.	Beds effectively minimize pressure on fragile tissues and dependent body parts. Selected for clients who require pressure relief for treatment of or prevention of pressure ulcers.

- ***Critical Decision Point***
  This surface should not be used with a client who has an unstable spine or who is in traction.

Step	Rationale
2. Assess client for pain.	Helps to anticipate client's need for analgesic prior to transfer. Serves as baseline for change in condition. Premedicate client before repositioning to decrease energy expenditure during turning (Bulechek and McCloskey, 1999).
3. Review client's medical orders.	In the United States a physician's order is needed to receive third-party reimbursement for cost of bed.
4. Wash hands and apply gloves. Assess condition of client's skin, paying particular attention to potential pressure sites and any existing skin lesions.	Prevents spread of microorganisms. Data provide baseline to determine any change in client's condition while on bed.
5. Assess client's level of consciousness.	Baseline used to detect change while client is on bed. Clients who are unconscious are at increased risk for pressure ulcers (Bulechek and McCloskey, 1999).
6. Assess client's and caregiver's understanding of purpose of bed.	Bed inflation is maintained by one or two blowers, which make a sound that may create anxiety for the client.
7. Review client's serum electrolyte levels in medical record, if available.	Baseline data used to compare with subsequent laboratory results to determine electrolyte imbalances.
8. Check medical record to see if client needs to be weighed frequently.	Scales are available in some air-suspension beds and available as underbed units for clients who need to be weighed frequently or for those who cannot be moved for weighing.

NURSING DIAGNOSIS

Defining characteristics from the assessment data may reveal the following nursing diagnoses for clients requiring this skill:

Anxiety
Deficient fluid volume
Impaired home maintenance management
Deficient knowledge regarding use of support surface mattress
Impaired physical mobility
Pain (acute, chronic)
Impaired skin integrity
Risk for impaired skin integrity
Kinesthetic sensory/perceptual alterations
Ineffective peripheral tissue perfusion

Related factors are individualized based on client's condition or needs.

PLANNING

Step	Rationale
1. **Expected outcomes** following completion of procedure:	
▪ Skin remains warm, clean, and intact, or existing lesions show evidence of healing.	Skin is free from pressure effects of immobility.
▪ Client rates comfort level as acceptable.	Bed's surface is soft, minimizing pain stimulation.
▪ Client remains alert and oriented or shows no change in level of orientation.	Client does not experience sensory perceptual changes from flotation.
2. Explain procedure and purpose of bed to client and caregiver.	Reduces anxiety and promotes client's cooperation.
3. Wash hands, and prepare necessary equipment and supplies.	Reduces transmission of microorganisms.
4. Review instructions supplied by bed manufacturer.	Promotes safe and correct use of bed.

STEP	RATIONALE
5. For clients with severe to moderate pain, premedicate approximately 30 minutes before transfer.	Promotes client's comfort and ability to cooperate during transfer to bed. Decreases client's energy expenditure.
6. Obtain any additional personnel needed to transfer client to bed.	Ensures client's safety by having sufficient personnel to assist in transferring.

IMPLEMENTATION

STEP	RATIONALE
1. Close client's room door or bedside curtain.	Maintains client's privacy during transfer.
2. Explain steps of transfer.	Reduces anxiety and helps client be a part of decision making during maneuvering.
3. Transfer client to bed using appropriate transfer techniques (see Chapter 27). Bed surface may be slippery, and transfers should not be attempted without assistance.	Appropriate transfer techniques maintain alignment and reduce risk of injury during procedure. Company representative will adjust bed to client's height and weight.
Check lateral client surfaces for reddening (e.g., lateral ankles, thighs, shoulder).	Gore-Tex sheet may cause pressure from hammocking if applied too tightly to bed.
4. Turn bed on by depressing switch; regulate temperature.	Suspension minimizes pressure against skin's surface and reduces friction and shear force.
5. Position client and perform range-of-motion (ROM) exercises as appropriate.	Promotes comfort and reduces contracture formation. The bed reduces pressure on skin, but clients must still be turned and exercised to avoid joint deformity or contractures.
6. To turn clients, position bedpans, or perform other therapies, turn on instaflate setting. Once procedure is completed, release instaflate.	Instaflate firms the bed surface to facilitate turning and handling client. Client will not receive pressure relief while bed is in this mode.
7. In emergencies when resuscitation is required, press cardiopulmonary resuscitation (CPR) switch to deflate bed immediately (see Skill 30-1). Be aware that transport units are available to maintain inflation during interruption of primary power source.	Creates firm surface against which cardiopulmonary resuscitation can be performed.
8. Remove gloves. Wash hands.	

EVALUATION

STEP	RATIONALE
1. Inspect condition of client's skin periodically while client is on bed.	Evaluates healing progress of any existing pressure sores. Determines if any new pressure areas are forming.
2. Ask client to rate level of comfort on a scale of 0 to 10.	Flotation effects of bed minimize pain stimuli.
3. Assess client's orientation.	Determines onset of perceptual changes.

UNEXPECTED OUTCOMES AND RELATED INTERVENTIONS

- Existing areas of skin breakdown or pressure areas fail to heal or increase in size or depth.
  - Modify skin care regimen.
  - Consult with skin care expert.
  - Notify physician.
- Client is restless or agitated.
  - Evaluate the need for analgesia or mild sedation.
  - Modify support surface selected.
  - Notify physician.
- Client becomes disoriented or complains of nausea.
  - Administer sedation or antiemetic.
  - Modify support surface selected.
  - Notify physician.
- Bed or mattress develops air leak.
  - Maintain client safety.
  - Identify source of leak.
  - Review equipment instructions.
  - Follow manufacturer's guidelines.
  - Change equipment.

RECORDING AND REPORTING

- Record transfer of client to bed, tolerance of procedure, and condition of skin in nurses' notes or skin assessment flow sheet.
- Report changes in condition of skin and electrolyte levels to physician.
- Record teaching provided and client and/or caregiver response.
- Report restlessness or change in orientation.

TEACHING CONSIDERATIONS

- Explain function and purpose of air-suspension therapy.
- Explain the need to continue to change position at intervals to diminish the effects of immobility.
- Explain the need for adequate fluid intake, because bed surface may be drying and may cause dehydration.

GERONTOLOGICAL CONSIDERATIONS

- When hospitalized, some older adult clients may experience misperceptions of their environment that may be intensified by the constant flotation of the air-suspension bed. Proprioception abnormalities affecting older adults are the result of nervous system and muscle changes (Lueckenotte, 2000).

HOME CARE CONSIDERATIONS

- A version of the bed is available for home use for rent or purchase; bed rental company is responsible for proper cleaning.
- Instruct family on importance of maintaining client hydration.
- Instruct family regarding the need to provide client's skin care.

Skill 30-3 Placing a Client on an Air-Fluidized Bed

An **air-fluidized bed** (Figure 30-7) is designed to distribute a client's weight evenly over its support surface. The bed minimizes pressure and reduces **shearing** force and **friction** through the principle of fluidization. Fluidization is created by forcing a gentle flow of temperature-controlled air upward through a mass of fine ceramic microspheres. The microspheres fluidize and take on the appearance of boiling milk and all the properties of a fluid. The client lies directly on a polyester filter sheet that allows air to pass through but does not allow the microspheres to escape. Clients feel as though they are floating on a surface like a warm waterbed. The contact pressure of the client's body against the filter sheet stays at 11 to 16 mm Hg.

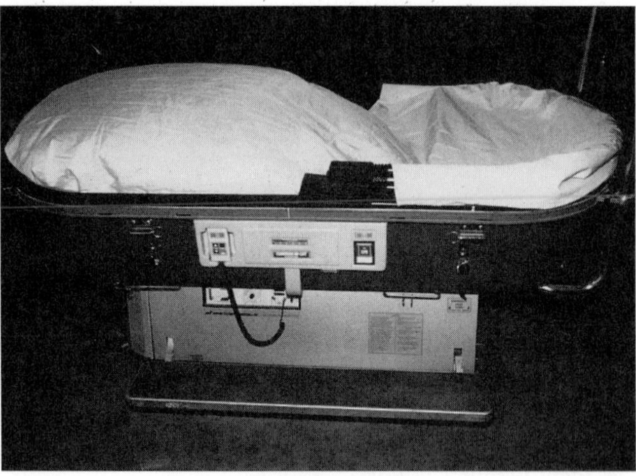

FIGURE 30-7 Clinitron bed.

Air-fluidized beds are useful in the care of clients who require minimal movement to prevent skin damage by shearing force and for clients who experience significant pain when being turned or positioned. Clients who can benefit from the bed include burn clients, those who have undergone extensive skin grafts or who have existing pressure ulcers, and victims of multiple trauma. Clients tend to perspire and lose body fluids while on the bed (Bryant and others, 2000). The surface of the filter sheet warms; as clients perspire, moisture is quickly absorbed into the circulating microspheres. Diaphoresis can go undetected, and thus insensible fluid loss may not be noticed until a client develops fluid and electrolyte imbalances. This individual is often already compromised in relation to hydration, fluids, and electrolytes; therefore the client's fluid balance status should be carefully monitored.

Conventional fluidized beds do not allow for head-of-bed position changes. Foam wedges are used to elevate the head. There are also combinations of fluidized and air suspension to lift the upper body while the lower body stays in a fluidized bed surface. The weight of the bed structure makes transport extremely difficult. A pediatric version of this bed is available.

DELEGATION CONSIDERATIONS

The skill of placing a client on an air-fluidized bed can be delegated to assistive personnel. The caregiver must routinely inspect the client's skin over bony prominences and heels for signs of pressure and report when changes in the client's skin are observed. The caregiver should be instructed in when to seek assistance for client position changes; in specifics regarding applying, cleaning, and maintaining support surface; and to report if client becomes disoriented, becomes restless, or complains of nausea.

EQUIPMENT

- Air fluidized bed (Clinitron, Fluidair, Skytron)
- Foam positioning wedges
- Filter sheet (supplied by rental company)
- Disposable gloves (optional)

STEP	RATIONALE

ASSESSMENT

1. Wash hands. — Reduces transmission of organisms.
2. Perform pressure ulcer risk assessment to identify clients who would benefit from air-fluidized therapy. — Selected for clients who must not move because of risk of increased pain or trauma (see Chapter 7).

    - ***Critical Decision Point***
      The bed may not provide a stable surface for clients requiring skeletal traction.

3. Assess condition of client's skin; pay particular attention to potential pressure sites and any existing pressure ulcers. — Data provide baseline to determine any change in client's condition while on bed.
4. Review client's medical orders. — Physician's order needed to receive third-party reimbursement for cost of bed (not required in Canada).
5. Assess client's level of comfort. — Helps to anticipate client's need for analgesic before transfer. Serves as baseline for change in condition.
6. Assess client's level of orientation. — Baseline used to detect change while client is on bed. Flotation effect may cause altered sensory perceptions.
7. Assess client's and family members' understanding of purpose of bed. — Bed is large and makes sound when air blower is operating, which may create anxiety for client.
8. Review client's serum electrolyte levels in medical record (if available). — There is a tendency for clients to lose body fluids through diaphoresis. Baseline data are used to compare with subsequent laboratory results to determine electrolyte imbalances.
9. Identify clients at risk for complications of air-fluidized therapy: — Allows nurse to anticipate need for frequent monitoring once client is placed on support surface.
    a. Older adult clients may become dehydrated from the airflow, which may increase insensible fluid losses.
    b. Clients receiving enteric tube feedings are at risk for aspiration due to the inability to elevate head of bed, which is limited to placing foam wedges under client's head and shoulders.
    c. Clients who have limited ability to change positions and who are susceptible to dehydration may have tenacious pulmonary secretions that are difficult to remove.
    d. Clients with specific positioning requirements such as elevating head of bed are limited to use of foam wedges.

    - ***Critical Decision Point***
      The prone position should never be attempted.

NURSING DIAGNOSIS

Defining characteristics from the assessment data may reveal the following nursing diagnoses for clients requiring this skill:

- Anxiety
- Risk for imbalanced body temperature
- Risk for deficient fluid volume
- Ineffective health maintenance
- Impaired home maintenance management
- Risk for infection
- Deficient knowledge regarding use of support surface mattress
- Impaired physical mobility
- Pain (acute, chronic)
- Kinesthetic sensory/perceptual alterations
- Risk for impaired skin integrity
- Impaired skin integrity
- Ineffective peripheral tissue perfusion

Related factors are individualized based on client's condition or needs.

STEP	RATIONALE

PLANNING

Step	Rationale
1. **Expected outcomes** following completion of procedure:	
▪ Skin remains warm, clean, and intact, or there is evidence of healing of pressure ulcers.	Skin is free from pressure effects of immobility.
▪ Client rates comfort level as acceptable.	Bed's surface effective in promoting comfort.
▪ Skin remains well hydrated, with good turgor; mucous membranes are moist; and electrolyte levels are in normal range.	Client's fluid and nutrient intake balance any insensible fluid loss from being on bed.
▪ Client remains alert and oriented or shows no change in level of consciousness.	Client does not experience sensory perceptual changes from flotation.
2. Explain procedure and purpose of bed to client and family.	Reduces anxiety and promotes client's cooperation.
3. Review instructions supplied by bed manufacturer.	Promotes safe and correct use of bed.
4. For clients with severe to moderate pain, premedicate approximately 30 minutes before transfer.	Promotes client's comfort and ability to cooperate during transfer to bed. Decreases client's energy expenditure (Bulechek and McCloskey, 1999).
5. Obtain any additional personnel needed to transfer client to bed.	Ensures client's safety by having sufficient personnel to assist in transferring.

IMPLEMENTATION

Step	Rationale
1. Close client's room door or bedside curtain.	Maintains client's privacy during transfer.
2. Explain steps of transfer.	Reduces anxiety and helps client be a part of decision making during maneuvering.
3. Wash hands and apply gloves (if bed linens or surface is soiled).	Reduces transmission of microorganisms.
4. Transfer client to bed using appropriate transfer techniques (see Chapter 27).	Appropriate transfer techniques maintain alignment and reduce risk of injury during procedure.

• ***Critical Decision Point***

Never attempt to place a client in a face-down position on an air-fluidized bed. Suffocation may occur.

Step	Rationale
5. Turn fluidization cycle on by depressing switch; regulate temperature.	Fluidization minimizes pressure against skin's surface and reduces friction and shear force when client moves.
6. Position client for comfort, and perform range-of-motion (ROM) exercises as appropriate.	Promotes comfort and reduces contracture formation. The bed reduces pressure on skin, but clients must still be turned and exercised to avoid joint deformity or contractures.
7. To turn clients, position bedpans, or perform other therapies, stop fluidization. Once procedure is completed, set to continuous fluidization.	Stopping fluidization provides firm, molded support that facilitates turning and handling client. Continuous fluidization provides permanent fluid support.
8. In emergencies when resuscitation is required, press cardiopulmonary resuscitation (CPR) switch and unplug unit to defluidize bed immediately (see Skill 30-1).	Creates firm surface against which cardiopulmonary resuscitation can be performed. Unplugging bed prevents automatic start of fluidization, which occurs 30 minutes after cycle is stopped.
9. Remove gloves and wash hands.	Reduces transmission of infection.

EVALUATION

Step	Rationale
1. Inspect condition of client's skin periodically while on bed, and monitor risk assessment.	Evaluates healing progress of any existing pressure ulcers. Determines if any new pressure areas are forming.
2. Ask client to rate ability to rest.	Bed surface is soft and conforming, minimizing pain stimulation.
3. Review client's serum electrolyte levels, monitor body temperature, and note hydration status of skin and mucous membranes.	Factors may reveal fluid and electrolyte losses.
4. Measure client's level of orientation.	Determines onset of perceptual changes.

Unexpected Outcomes and Related Interventions

- Existing areas of skin breakdown or pressure areas fail to heal or increase in size or depth.
  - Modify skin care regimen.
  - Consult with skin care expert.
  - Notify physician.
- Client's skin and mucous membranes are dehydrated.
  - Provide oral fluids unless contraindicated.
  - If electrolyte levels are also abnormal, notify physician.
  - Monitor client's intake and output.
  - Provide intravenous fluids as ordered.
- Client is restless or agitated.
  - Evaluate the need for analgesia or mild sedation.
  - Modify support surface selected.
  - Notify physician.
- Client becomes disoriented or complains of nausea.
  - Administer sedation or antiemetic.
  - Modify support surface selected.
  - Notify physician.
- The filter sheet develops a tear.
  - Inspect sheets for source of tear.
  - Mend tears with adhesive tape as per manufacturer's guidelines until a new bed can be provided.
  - Avoid use of additional sheets because they interfere with optimal bed performance.
  - Maintain client safety.

Recording and Reporting

- Record transfer of client to bed, tolerance to procedure, and condition of skin in nurses' notes or skin assessment flow sheet.
- Report changes in condition of skin and electrolyte levels to nurse in charge or to physician.
- Report teaching provided and client and/or caregiver response.
- Report change in orientation.

Teaching Considerations

- Explain function and purpose of air-fluidized therapy.
- Explain that client will require assistance to change positions.
- Explain the need to maintain adequate hydration of client.

Gerontological Considerations

- Older adult clients are at increased risk for dehydration.
- When hospitalized, older adult client may experience significant misperceptions of their environment that may be intensified by the flotation of the air-fluidized bed.

Home Care Considerations

- Beds weigh between 1700 and 2100 pounds; therefore the company leasing the bed needs to inspect the home for accessibility and structural support.
- Consult with social worker or case manager to determine third-party reimbursement.

Skill 30-4 Placing a Client on a Bariatric Bed

A nursing adjunct in the care of the **morbidly obese** client (a person who weighs more than 100 lb above ideal weight) is the bariatric bed (Figure 30-8), a safe, adaptable surface. The **bariatric bed** is capable of allowing upright or sitting positioning, client transport, and in-bed scales. The bed is equipped with hand controls that allow self-positioning and facilitate independence for the obese client. Since the bariatric bed is capable of supporting weights up to 850 pounds, it provides a stable balanced surface that limits hospital liability should the standard bed frame collapse or the electric motor burn out.

The full-function hand controls allow the nurse caring for the obese client to change the bed position and thus facilitate care while reducing risk of staff injury while moving the client. The in-bed scale provides the nurse with a means of obtaining accurate weights and thus improves health care and client dignity. The bed is slightly wider than a standard hospital bed, yet it is within the guidelines for standard door width, which allows movement into and out of a room without difficulty.

A limitation of this bed is the lack of pressure reduction or relief in the mattress. The at-risk obese client should have some type of pressure-relief mattress placed on the bariatric bed. Usual choices for pressure relief are the 4-inch foam, static air, or alternating air mattress overlays.

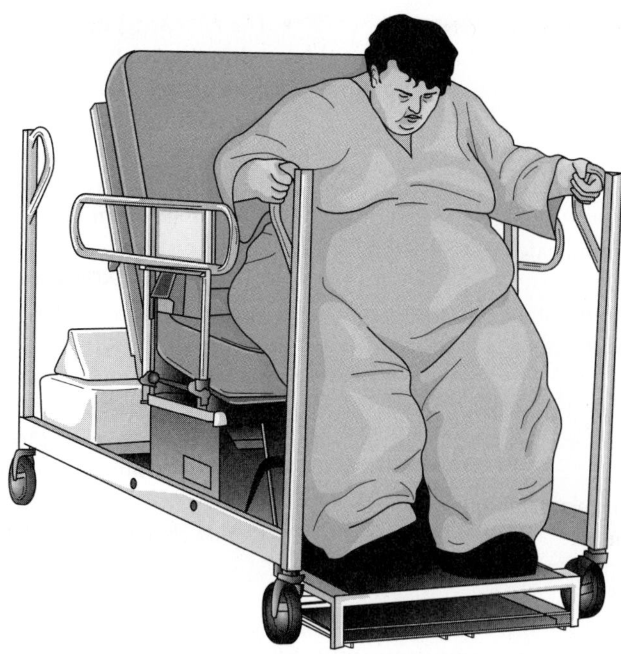

FIGURE 30-8 The bariatric bed eliminates unnecessary client transfers. (Courtesy Burke, Inc, Mission, Kan.)

Delegation Considerations

The skill of placing a client on a bariatric bed can be delegated to assistive personnel. The number of people needed to assist in safe client transfer from traditional to bariatric bed must be determined. The caregiver must routinely inspect the client's skin over bony prominences and heels for signs of pressure and report when changes in the client's skin are observed. The caregiver should be instructed in when to seek assistance for client position changes and in specifics regarding applying, cleaning, and maintaining support surface.

Equipment

- Bariatric bed
- Pressure-relief mattress overlay
- Sheets
- Overhead frame (optional)

Step	Rationale
Assessment	
1. Identify clients who would benefit from the bariatric bed system; assess their mobility status.	Selected for clients who are morbidly obese and who have the potential of being independent in positioning with assistance of a stable surface.
2. Assess condition of client's skin, paying particular attention to potential pressure sites and skinfolds. Determine the need for client to have pressure-relief mattress placed on the bariatric bed.	Data provide baseline to determine any change in client's condition while on the bed.
3. Assess client's and family members' understanding of purpose of bed.	Improves client and family compliance.
4. Review client's medical orders.	In the United States, a physician's order is needed to receive third-party reimbursement for cost of bed.
5. Assess need for client to be weighed.	Scales are available in many bariatric beds or as underbed scales for beds without in-bed scales.

STEP	RATIONALE

NURSING DIAGNOSIS

Defining characteristics from the assessment data may reveal the following nursing diagnoses for clients requiring this skill:

- Risk for caregiver role strain
- Ineffective health maintenance
- Impaired home maintenance management
- Deficient knowledge regarding use of support surface mattress
- Impaired physical mobility
- Impaired skin integrity
- Ineffective peripheral tissue perfusion
- Risk for impaired skin integrity

Related factors are individualized based on client's condition or needs.

PLANNING

Step	Rationale
1. **Expected outcomes** following completion of procedure:	
▪ Client is independent for position changes.	Bed surface is adaptable by hand-operated controls.
▪ Skin remains intact, or existing lesions show evidence of healing.	Skin is free from pressure effects of immobility.
▪ Client remains free of injury.	Bed is stable to allow for positioning without tipping or bending.
2. Explain procedure and purpose of bed to client and family.	Reduces anxiety and promotes client's cooperation.
3. Review instructions supplied by bed manufacturer.	Promotes safe and correct use of bed.

• ***Critical Decision Point***
Do not exceed weight limits indicated by the manufacturer.

Step	Rationale
4. For clients with severe to moderate pain, medicate approximately 30 minutes before transfer.	Promotes client's comfort and ability to cooperate during transfer to bed. Decreases client's energy expenditure (Bulechek and McCloskey, 1999).
5. Obtain any additional personnel needed to transfer client to bed.	Ensures safety of client and staff by having sufficient personnel to assist in transferring.

IMPLEMENTATION

• ***Critical Decision Point***
Use of this bed is contraindicated in clients with spinal cord injuries.

Step	Rationale
1. Close client's room door or bedside curtain.	Maintains client's privacy during transfer.
2. Explain steps of transfer.	Reduces anxiety and helps client be part of decision making during maneuvering.
3. Wash hands and put on gloves (if needed) before assisting client to bed using appropriate transfer techniques (see Chapter 27). Depending on client's mobility status, it may be necessary to call for assistance.	Appropriate transfer techniques maintain alignment and reduce risk of injury to client and health care workers during procedure.
4. Cover and position client, and place hand controls within reach. Be certain that the out-of-bed alarm is on, if needed. Attach overhead frame if needed.	Allows for maximal client independence. Alerts caregiver that client has left the bed surface.
5. Remove gloves and wash hands.	Reduces transmission of microorganisms.

EVALUATION

Step	Rationale
1. Inspect condition of client's skin periodically while client is on bed.	Evaluates healing of any existing pressure ulcers. Determines if any new pressure areas are forming.
2. Ask client to rate sense of comfort and safety. Encourage range of motion (ROM) by client.	Bed frame is stable for movement and position changes.
3. Evaluate client's risk for injury.	Surface is balanced and allows maximal client independence.
4. Evaluate client's ability to move in bed.	Evaluates effectiveness of bed and education to promote independence.

UNEXPECTED OUTCOMES AND RELATED INTERVENTIONS

- Existing areas of skin breakdown or pressure areas fail to heal or increase in size or depth.
  - Modify skin care regimen.
  - Consult with skin care expert.
  - Notify physician.
- Client is unable to operate bed for position changes independently.
  - Reassess client's level of independence and ability to understand instructions.
  - Reinstruct client and family in how to operate the bed.
  - Provide for return demonstration regarding bed operation.

RECORDING AND REPORTING

- Record transfer of client to bed, tolerance of procedure, and condition of skin in nurses' notes or skin assessment flow sheet.
- Report changes in condition of skin to nurse in charge or physician.

TEACHING CONSIDERATIONS

- Explain function and purpose of bariatric bed.
- Explain function and purpose of pressure-relief mattress overlay used.
- Explain the need to continue to change position at intervals to diminish effects of immobility.

Skill 30-5 Placing a Client on a Rotokinetic Bed

The **Rotokinetic bed** is used to maintain skeletal alignment while providing constant rotation. It is used in the care of spinal cord–injured and multitrauma clients. The support structure of the bed outlines the body parts and maintains proper alignment when secured properly. The bed rotates from side to side at a 60- to 90-degree angle every 7 minutes. Turning angles may be adjusted to meet the client's needs. Constant rotation reduces pressure ulcer development and stimulates body systems. It is recommended that the bed stay in the rotation mode for at least 20 hours a day. There is an emergency gatch that can quickly interrupt rotation when needed.

The constant motion may lead to sensory distress for the client, especially older adults. This may be associated with the constant kinetic stimulation, the limited visual field, and inner ear disequilibrium. The nurse must be mindful of these complications and provide necessary emotional support. A physician's order is required for third-party payment.

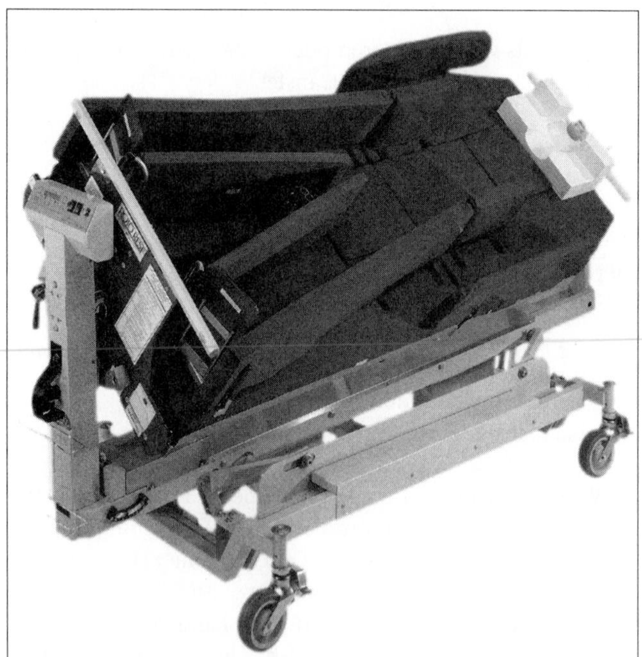

FIGURE 30-9 Rotokinetic bed. (KCI RotoRest Delta bed courtesy Kinetic Concepts, Inc, San Antonio, Tex.)

DELEGATION CONSIDERATIONS

The skill of placing a client on a Rotokinetic bed should not be delegated to assistive personnel. Because this type of bed is frequently used for clients with spinal cord injuries, other aspects of the client's care may be delegated to assistive personnel. When providing care to clients on the Rotokinetic bed, the caregiver must routinely inspect the client's skin over bony prominences and heels for signs of pressure and report when changes in the client's skin are observed. The caregiver should be instructed in when to seek assistance for client position changes and to report immediately if the client becomes disoriented or anxious or complains of nausea.

EQUIPMENT

- Rotokinetic bed with support packs, bolsters, and safety straps (Figure 30-9)
- Top sheet
- Pillow cases for bolsters

STEP	RATIONALE

ASSESSMENT

Step	Rationale
1. Wash hands.	Reduces transmission of microorganisms.
2. Assess condition of client's skin; pay particular attention to potential pressure sites and any existing pressure ulcers.	Data provide baseline to determine any change in client's condition while on bed.
3. Review client's medical orders.	Physician's order is needed to receive third-party reimbursement for cost of bed (not required in Canada).
4. Assess client's level of comfort.	Helps to anticipate client's need for analgesic before transfer. Serves as a baseline for change in condition.
5. Assess client's level of orientation.	Baseline used to detect change while client is on bed. Constant motion may lead to sensory distress.
6. Assess client's and family members' understanding of purpose of bed.	Appearance and movement of bed may create anxiety for client and family members.

NURSING DIAGNOSIS

Defining characteristics from the assessment data may reveal the following nursing diagnoses for clients requiring this skill:

- Anxiety
- Ineffective health maintenance
- Impaired home maintenance management
- Risk for infection
- Deficient knowledge regarding the use of Rotokinetic bed
- Impaired physical mobility
- Impaired skin integrity
- Risk for impaired skin integrity
- Kinesthetic sensory/perceptual alterations
- Ineffective peripheral tissue perfusion

Related factors are individualized based on client's condition or needs.

PLANNING

Step	Rationale
1. **Expected outcomes** following completion of procedure:	
▪ Skin remains intact without evidence of abnormal reactive hyperemia or mottling.	Skin is free from pressure effects of immobility.
▪ Existing pressure ulcers show evidence of healing.	Client is experiencing benefits of bed.
▪ Client's musculoskeletal system is properly aligned and free of contractures.	Device provides support and alignment to trunk and extremities.
▪ Client's breath sounds improve from baseline assessment or remain clear to auscultation.	Client's pulmonary congestion is improving or absent.
▪ Client remains alert, oriented, and cooperative.	Client does not experience sensory perceptual changes from bed positions.
▪ Client denies nausea or dizziness.	Motion of bed is not negatively affecting client.
▪ Client's blood pressure remains consistent with baseline vital signs.	Client not experiencing cardiovascular disturbances.
2. Explain procedure and purpose of bed to client and family.	Reduces anxiety and promotes cooperation.
3. Review instructions supplied by bed manufacturer.	Promotes safe and correct use of bed.
4. For clients with severe to moderate pain, medicate approximately 30 minutes before transfer.	Promotes client's comfort and ability to cooperate during transfer to bed. Decreases client's energy expenditure (Bulechek and McCloskey, 1999).
5. Obtain any additional personnel needed to transfer client to bed.	Ensures client's safety.

IMPLEMENTATION

Step	Rationale
1. Close client's room door or bedside curtain.	Maintains client's privacy during transfer.
2. Place Rotokinetic bed in horizontal position and remove all bolsters, straps, and supports. Close posterior hatches.	

STEP	RATIONALE
3. Unplug electrical cord. Lock gatch.	Prevents accidental rotation during transfer.
4. Maintaining proper alignment, transfer client to Rotokinetic bed.	Reduces risk of further tissue injury during transfer. May need physician available to assist in transfer.
5. Secure thoracic panels, bolsters, head and knee packs, and safety straps.	Maintains proper alignment and prevents sliding during rotation.
6. Cover client with top sheet.	Maintains client dignity.
7. Plug bed in.	
8. Have company representative set optional angle as ordered by physician. May gradually increase rotation.	Rotational angle is determined by physician based on the client's overall condition and tolerance to constant motion.
9. Increase degree of rotation gradually according to client's tolerance.	Gradually increasing rotation may prevent nausea and dizziness.
10. It is difficult to maintain eye contact when talking with clients during rotation. Provide adequate space for caregivers and family to move around the bed to facilitate communication.	Allows opportunity to meet client's psychosocial needs.
11. The bed may be stopped for assessment and procedures. To stop the bed, permit bed to rotate to the desired position, turn the motor off, and push knob into a lock position. If necessary, the bed can be manually repositioned.	Allows nurse to assess client.
12. Inform client that there may be a sensation of light-headedness or falling. However, reassure client that he or she will not fall because the pads are positioned to prevent this and are checked by two people to ensure proper placement.	Informing client of what to expect will decrease his or her anxiety.

- ***Critical Decision Point***
  Manual rotation may cause nausea or dizziness if done too rapidly. Keep bed stopped for no longer than 30 minutes.

EVALUATION

1. Inspect condition of skin (occiput, ears, axillae, elbows, sacrum, groin, and heels) and musculoskeletal alignment every 2 hours.	Evaluates healing process of any existing pressure ulcers and determines effectiveness of Rotokinetic therapy.
2. Inspect client's pressure ulcers for evidence of healing.	Evaluates healing process.
3. Observe alignment and range of motion of all joints.	Determines if complications (e.g., atelectasis) have developed.
4. Auscultate lung sounds every shift, and compare with baseline.	
5. Determine client's level of orientation once per shift while on bed.	Evaluates if sensory overload has developed from excess kinetic stimulation.
6. Ask whether client is experiencing nausea or dizziness.	Determines if client experiences orthostatic hypotension from position rotation.
7. Monitor blood pressure.	

UNEXPECTED OUTCOMES AND RELATED INTERVENTIONS

- Existing areas of skin breakdown or pressure areas fail to heal or increase in size or depth.
  - Modify skin care regimen.
  - Consult with skin care expert.
  - Notify physician.
- Client experiences orthostatic hypotension.
  - Notify physician.
  - Stop motion of the bed.
  - Monitor client's vital signs.
- Client becomes disoriented, confused, and anxious.
  - Reorient client to person, time, and place.
  - Provide audio stimulation via radio or compact disc player.
  - Provide television adapted for Rotokinetic bed (available from manufacturer).
  - Provide prescribed medication for motion sickness.
- Client develops abnormal lung sounds.
  - Increase frequency for pulmonary hygiene measures.
  - Notify physician.
  - Possible use of incentive spirometry.

- Bed fails to rotate.
  - Provide for client safety.
  - Position bed in flat position.
  - Transfer client to another surface until a new bed is provided.
  - Notify manufacturer.

Recording and Reporting

- Describe condition of skin before placement on the Rotokinetic bed. A photograph may be taken to document skin condition and provide a baseline for later assessments for progress in healing.
- Indicate time of transfer to Rotokinetic bed and degree of rotation.
- Document subjective data indicating response to the constant rotation and presence/absence of dizziness, nausea, or blood pressure changes.
- A flow sheet may be used to document routine assessment and care, including the length of time the bed rotation stopped. The bed needs to be rotating at least 20 hours out of every 24 hours and stopped for no more than 30 minutes at a time.

Teaching Considerations

- Explain function and purpose of Rotokinetic bed.
- Explain that client may feel sensation of light-headedness or falling. However, client will not fall because pads are positioned to prevent this.

Gerontological Considerations

- Older adults are at increased risk for sensation of light-headedness or dizziness.

Critical Thinking Exercises

1. Ms. L., an alert 40-year-old client, is admitted to your unit after sustaining multiple trauma from an auto accident and right lower lobe pneumonia. The physician has ordered a Rotokinetic bed. Ms. L. becomes quite anxious at the appearance of the bed. The assistive personnel overheard Ms. L. talking to family members about recent experiences with inner ear disturbances. What assessments and nursing actions should take place?
2. Mr. T., 62-year-old retired schoolteacher, has been in a skilled nursing facility receiving rehabilitation for several months following his recent cerebrovascular accident (CVA). The doctor has ordered an air-suspension bed because he is developing pressure ulcers over bony prominences. Mr. T. begins experiencing a small amount of nausea and restlessness when initially placed on the air-suspension bed. Mr. T. tells the assistive personnel, "Nurse, I am afraid that I will fall out of this bed when it tilts. Will I?" What actions should the nurse implement for Mr. T.'s nausea and anxiety?
3. A 72-year-old Asian American who resides in a nursing home, Mrs. W., is transferred to acute care. She is independent and requires minimal assistance with her activities of daily living (ADLs). She has a history of severe, painful osteoarthritis and is maintained on tube feedings for a chronic esophageal problem. After 2 days in the hospital, she is placed on an air-fluidized bed for ease of turning after developing a pressure ulcer on her coccyx.
   a. What impact does her culture have on expression of pain, and what is the nurse's response?
   b. What special considerations are necessary because of Mrs. W.'s tube feeding requirement?
   c. What would be the nurse's response if the client suddenly became agitated, confused, and complained of a "sinking feeling"?
   d. What nursing assessments and laboratory values are significant while the client is on this bed?

References

Agency for Health Care Policy and Research: *Pressure ulcers in adults: prediction and prevention,* Clinical practice guideline No. 3, Rockville, Md, 1992, U.S. Department of Health and Human Services.

Agency for Health Care Policy and Research, Panel for the Treatment of Pressure Ulcers: *Treatment of pressure ulcers,* Clinical practice guideline No. 15, AHCPR Pub No. 95-0652, Rockville, Md, 1994, U.S. Department of Health and Human Services.

Bryant RA and others: Pressure ulcers. In Bryant RA, editor: *Acute and chronic wounds: nursing management,* ed 2, St. Louis, 2000, Mosby.

Bulechek G, McCloskey J: *Nursing interventions: effective nursing treatments,* ed 3, St. Louis, 1999, Mosby.

Elkin M, Perry A, Potter, P: *Nursing interventions and clinical skills,* St. Louis, 2000, Mosby.

Fulmer T, Abraham, I: Rethinking geriatric nursing, *Nurs Clin North Am* 33(3):387, 1998.

Ignatavicius D: *Introduction to long term care nursing: principles and practice,* Philadelphia, 1998, FA Davis.

Koziak M: Etiology of decubitus ulcers, *Arch Phys Med Rehabil* 42:19, 1961.

Lewis S, Heitkemper M, Dirksen S: *Medical-surgical nursing: assessment and management of clinical problems,* ed 5, St. Louis, 2000, Mosby.

Lueckenotte A: *Gerontologic nursing,* ed 2, St. Louis, 2000, Mosby.
Monahan FD, Neighbors M: *Medical-surgical nursing: foundations for clinical practice,* ed 2, Philadelphia, 1998, WB Saunders.
Phillips J: *Pressure sores,* New York, 1997, Churchill Livingstone.
Phipps WJ, Sands JK, Marek JF, editors: *Medical-surgical nursing: concepts and clinical practice,* ed 6, St. Louis, 1999, Mosby.
Potter P, Perry A: *Basic nursing: a critical thinking approach,* ed 4, St. Louis, 1999, Mosby.
Tourtual DM and others: Predictors of hospital-acquired heel pressure ulcers, *Ostomy Wound Manage* 43(9):24, 1997.

31

MEDICAL ASEPSIS

Skills

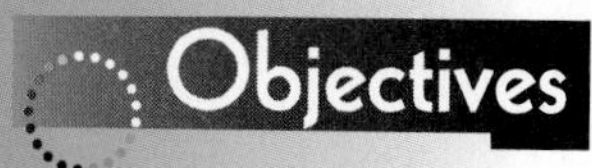

Mastery of content in this chapter will enable the nurse to:

- Define the key terms listed.
- Discuss how critical thinking applies in the prevention of the transmission of infection.
- Explain the difference between medical and surgical asepsis.
- Identify nursing care measures intended to break the chain of infection.
- Explain how each element of the infection chain contributes to infection.
- Describe factors that can influence nursing staff compliance with hand washing.
- Perform proper procedures for hand washing.
- Perform correct isolation techniques.

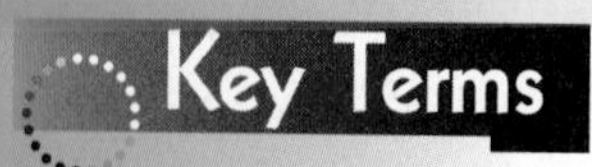

Asepsis
Aseptic technique
Colonized
Contamination
Immunocompromised
Infection
Invasive procedure
Isolation
Medical asepsis
Microorganism
Nosocomial infection
Pathogen
Standard precautions
Surgical asepsis
Transmission-based precautions

Infection control practices that reduce and/or eliminate sources and transmission of infection help to protect clients and health care providers from disease. Clients in all health care settings are at risk for acquiring infections because of lower resistance to infectious microorganisms, exposure to an increased number of and more types of disease-causing organisms, and the performance of invasive procedures. Clients in acute care or ambulatory care facilities have an increased risk of acquiring infections. **Nosocomial infections** are those that develop as a result of a stay or visit in a health care facility and the infection was not present or incubating at the time of admission (Bobo, 1994). A hospital is one of the most likely settings for acquiring a nosocomial infection because of staff, clients, and environmental factors that support a high population of virulent strains of microorganisms, that are resistant to antibiotics. Most nosocomial infections are transmitted by health care workers and clients as a result of direct contact during the delivery of care activities. Nurses must pay close attention to washing their hands after contact with clients or equipment.

In all settings, clients and their families must be able to recognize sources of infection and be able to institute protective measures. Nurses are in a position to influence positively others' behavior and to change their own behavior through health education (Goldrick and Turner, 1994). Client and family teaching should include information concerning signs and symptoms of infections, modes of transmission, and methods of prevention.

Although protection of the client is an obvious priority, nurses are at risk for contact with infectious materials or exposure to a communicable disease. Knowledge of the infectious process and disease transmission and critical thinking skills associated with aseptic techniques and barrier protection cannot be overemphasized. The nurse must be able to use judgment when caring for any client who has the risk of acquiring or transmitting an infection. The nurse must know the infectious organism and how it is transmitted, the actions needed to protect the client, and the steps to take to ensure protection from exposure to the microorganism. Today's nurse plays a vital role in the prevention and control of infections.

The mere presence of a pathogen does not mean that an infection will begin. Development of an infection occurs in a cyclical process that depends on the following six elements:

1. An infectious agent or **pathogen**
2. A reservoir or source for pathogen growth
3. A portal of exit from the reservoir
4. A mode of transmission
5. A portal of entry to the host
6. A susceptible host

An infection develops if this chain remains intact (Figure 31-1). Nurses use infection control practices to break an element of the chain so that infection will not be transmitted (Table 31-1). The nurse's efforts to minimize the onset and spread of infection are based upon asepsis and the principles of aseptic technique. **Asepsis** is defined as the absence of disease-producing (pathogenic) organisms (Crow, Planchock, and Hendrick, 1994; DeCastro, Fauerback, and Masters, 1996). The two types of **aseptic technique** the nurse practices are medical and surgical asepsis.

Medical asepsis, or clean technique, includes procedures used to reduce the number of and prevent the spread of microorganisms. Hand washing, barrier techniques, and routine environmental cleaning are examples of medical asepsis. Principles of medical asepsis are commonly followed in the home, as in the case of washing hands before preparing food.

Surgical asepsis, or sterile technique, includes procedures used to eliminate all microorganisms from an area. Sterilization destroys all microorganisms and their spores (Rutala, 1996). Sterile technique is practiced by nurses in the operating room (OR), labor and delivery, and procedural areas, where sterile instruments and supplies are used. The techniques used in maintaining surgical asepsis are more rigid than those performed under medical asepsis (see Chapter 32).

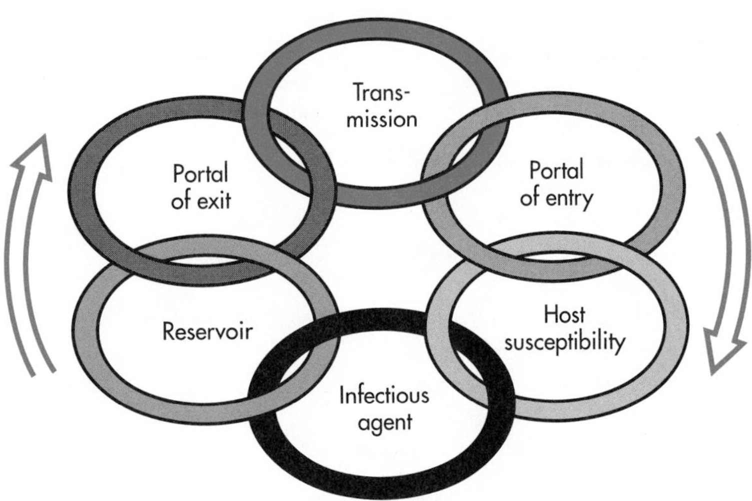

FIGURE **31-1** Chain of infection.

Table 31-1 Breaking the Chain of Infection

ELEMENT OF INFECTION CHAIN	MEDICAL ASEPTIC PRACTICES
Infectious agent (pathogenic organism capable of causing disease)	Cleanse contaminated objects. Perform cleaning, disinfection and sterilization.
Reservoir (site or source of microorganism growth)	Control sources of body fluids and drainage. Wash hands. Bathe client with soap and water. Change soiled dressings. Dispose of soiled tissues, dressings, or linen in moisture-resistant bags. Place syringes, uncapped hypodermic needles, and intravenous needles in designated puncture-proof containers. Keep table surfaces clean and dry. Do not leave bottled solutions open for prolonged periods. Keep solutions tightly capped. Keep surgical wound drainage tubes and collecting bags patent. Empty and dispose of drainage suction bottles according to agency policy.
Portal of exit (means by which microorganisms leave a site)	Respiratory Avoid talking, sneezing, or coughing directly over wound or sterile dressing field. Cover nose and mouth when sneezing or coughing. Wear mask if suffering respiratory tract infection. Urine, feces, emesis, and blood Wear disposable gloves when handling blood and body fluids. Wear gowns and eyewear if there is a chance of splashing fluids. Handle all laboratory specimens as if infectious.
Transmission (means of spread)	Reduce microorganism spread Wash hands. Use personal set of care items for each client. Avoid shaking bed linen or clothes; dust with damp cloth. Avoid contact of soiled item with uniform. Discard any item that touches the floor. Follow standard precautions or select transmission-based isolation precautions.

Continued

Table 31-1 Breaking the Chain of Infection—cont'd

Element of Infection Chain	Medical Aseptic Practices
Portal of entry (site through which microorganism enters a host)	Skin and mucosa Maintain skin and mucous membrane integrity, lubricate skin, offer frequent hygiene, turn and position. Cover wounds as needed. Clean wound sites thoroughly. Dispose of used needles in puncture-proof container. Urinary Keep all drainage systems closed and intact, maintaining downward flow.
Host (client)	Reduce susceptibility to infection. Provide adequate nutrition. Ensure adequate rest. Promote body defenses against infection. Provide immunization.

Skill Performance Guidelines

1. Remember that hand washing with an appropriate soap or antiseptic is an essential part of client care and infection prevention. (Antiseptics are recommended for use in intensive care units, the OR, and special procedure areas, or when performing or assisting with invasive procedures).
2. Always know a client's susceptibility to infection. Age, nutritional status, stress, disease processes, and forms of medical therapy can place clients at risk.
3. Recognize the elements of the chain of infection and initiate measures to prevent the onset and spread of infection.
4. Incorporate consistently the basic principles of asepsis into client care.
5. Protect fellow health care workers from exposure to infectious agents through proper use and disposal of equipment.
6. Be aware of body sites where nosocomial infections are most likely to develop (e.g., urinary or respiratory tract). This enables the nurse to direct preventive measures.

Skill 31-1 Hand Washing

The most important and most basic technique in preventing and controlling transmission of **infection** is hand washing. Hand washing is a vigorous, brief rubbing together of all surfaces of hands lathered in soap, followed by rinsing under a stream of water. The purpose is to remove soil and transient organisms from the hands and to reduce total microbial counts over time (Larson, 1995).

Contaminated hands are a prime cause of transmission of infection. For example, a nurse caring for a client who has excessive pulmonary secretions assists the client in expectorating mucus and disposes of the tissues in a bedside container. The client's roommate asks the nurse to open containers of food on the meal tray. The nurse then leaves the client's room to pour a dose of medication due in 5 minutes. If the nurse fails to wash hands before each of these actions, organisms from the first client's mucus could easily be transmitted to the roommate's food and to the medication container. Unfortunately, health care workers function in a busy environment. Client care activities are fast paced. With an increased workload, frequent interruptions in care activity, and sometimes limited access to sinks, hand-washing compliance can be a problem. Nishimura and others (1999) have found that hand-washing compliance among intensive care unit (ICU) personnel is low. After videotaping staff as they entered the ICU, the researchers found only 71% of ICU personnel washed their hands before beginning client care. *Handwashing is not optional.* It is a critical responsibility for all health care workers.

The decision regarding when hand washing should occur depends on the following: the intensity of contact with clients or contaminated objects; the degree or amount or **contamination** that could occur with that contact; the susceptibility of the client or the health care worker to infection; and the procedure or activity to be performed (Larson, 2000). For example, if a nurse touches an object that is not visibly soiled, hand washing may not be required. In contrast, prolonged and intense contact with a client's wound drainage would require thorough hand washing (Table 31-2). Larson (1995) recommends that nurses wash hands in the following situations:

1. When visibly soiled
2. Before and after client contact

Table 31-2 Guidelines for Hand Care Based on Degree of Antisepsis

TYPE OF HAND CARE	PURPOSE	METHOD
Handwash	Remove soil and transient microorganisms.	Soap or detergent for at least 10-15 seconds.
Hand antisepsis	Remove or destroy transient microorganisms.	Antimicrobial soap or detergent or alcohol-based hand rub for at least 10-15 seconds.
Surgical hand scrub	Reduce, remove or destroy transient microorganisms and reduce resident flora.	Antimicrobial soap or detergent preparation and brushing to create friction for at least 120 seconds, or alcohol-based preparation for at least 120 seconds.

Modified from Larson EL: APIC guideline for hand washing and hand antisepsis in health care settings, *Am J Infect Control* 23(4):251, 1995.

3. After contact with a source of **microorganisms** (blood or body fluids, mucous membrane, nonintact skin, or inanimate objects that might be contaminated)
4. Before the performance of **invasive procedures** such as placement of intravascular catheters or indwelling catheters (antimicrobial soap recommended)
5. After removing gloves (wearing gloves does not remove the need to wash hands)

The Centers for Disease Control and Prevention (CDC) and the U.S. Public Health Service note that washing times of at least 10 to 15 seconds (Garner, 1995) will remove most transient microorganisms from the skin. If hands are visibly soiled, more time may be needed. The frequency of washing also affects the type and number of bacteria on the hands. Larson (1995) stated that nurses who wash their hands eight times a day are less likely to carry gram-negative bacteria on their hands. Routine hand washing may be performed with soap in any convenient form (bar, leaflets, liquid, or powder). However, bar soap that remains wet or in pooled water may harbor microorganisms. The use of antimicrobial soap (antiseptic) is encouraged when nurses need to reduce total microbial counts on their hands, such as situations where nurses are in contact with children or older adult clients who are **immunocompromised** or clients who have damage to their integumentary system (wounds or bruises). In addition, an antimicrobial soap should be used before performing an invasive procedure such as care or insertion of an intravascular catheter. There are a number of effective antimicrobial soaps that contain chlorhexidine gluconate (CHG), alcohols, and iodophors. Certain antimicrobial soaps can irritate the skin, and the need for antimicrobial soap must be weighed against potential skin irritation.

An alternative to hand washing is the use of alcoholic solutions. The solutions contain alcohol in addition to products that prevent skin dryness. When hands are vigorously cleansed with the alcohol solution, a significantly greater reduction in the number of microbial counts on the hands results, when compared with traditional hand washing (Zaragoza and others, 1999). The researchers recommend that if alcohol solutions are a viable option, hand washing should precede cleansing if the hands are visibly soiled.

Delegation Considerations

Hand washing is a basic procedure that should be performed correctly by all caregivers. If you observe assistive personnel, physicians or therapists, and family caregivers incorrectly perform hand washing, reinforce the importance of the technique and the correct procedural steps.

Equipment

- Easy-to-reach sink with warm running water
- Antimicrobial or regular soap
- Paper towels or air dryer
- Clean orangewood stick (optional)

Step	Rationale
Assessment	
1. Inspect surface of hands for breaks or cuts in skin or cuticles. Note condition of nails. Artificial nails and long or unkept nails should be avoided. Report and cover any skin lesions before providing client care.	Open cuts or wounds can harbor high concentrations of microorganisms. Long nails and chipped or old polish increase number of bacteria residing on nails, requiring more vigorous hand washing. Artificial nails may increase the microbial load on hands (Larsen, 1995). Agency policy may prevent nurse from caring for high-risk clients if open lesions are present on hands.
2. Inspect hands for heavy soiling.	Requires lengthier hand washing.
3. Assess client's risk for or extent of infection, for example, white blood cell count, extent of open wounds, or known medical diagnosis.	Use of antimicrobial soaps is encouraged for clients who are immunosuppressed (Larson, 1995).

STEP | RATIONALE

NURSING DIAGNOSIS

Defining characteristics from the assessment data may reveal the following nursing diagnoses for clients requiring this skill:

This skill is required for clients having a variety of nursing diagnoses

Related factors are individualized based on client's condition or needs.

PLANNING

1. **Expected outcomes** following completion of procedure:
   - Hands and areas under fingernails are clean and free of debris. — Transient bacteria have been removed.

IMPLEMENTATION

1. Push wristwatch and long uniform sleeves above wrists. Avoid wearing rings. If worn, remove during washing. — Provides complete access to fingers, hands, wrists. Wearing of rings increases number of microorganisms on hands (Garner, 1995).
2. Be sure fingernails are short, filed, and smooth. — Many microorganisms on hands come from the subungual region (beneath the fingernails).
3. Stand in front of sink, keeping hands and uniform away from sink surface. (If hands touch sink during hand washing, repeat.) — Inside of sink is a contaminated area. Reaching over sink increases risk of touching edge, which is contaminated.
4. Turn on water. Turn faucet on (see illustration) or push knee pedals laterally or press pedals with foot to regulate flow and temperature.
5. Avoid splashing water against uniform. — Microorganisms travel and grow in moisture.
6. Regulate flow of water so that temperature is warm. — Warm water removes less of the protective oils than hot water.
7. Wet hands and wrists thoroughly under running water. Keep hands and forearms lower then elbows during washing. — Hands are the most contaminated parts to be washed. Water flows from least to most contaminated area, rinsing microorganisms into sink.
8. Apply a small amount of soap or antiseptic, lathering thoroughly (see illustration). Soap granules and leaflet preparations may be used. — The use of antiseptic exclusively can be drying to the hands and cause skin irritations.

   - ***Critical Decision Point***
     The decision whether to use an antiseptic or not should be dependent on the procedure to be performed and the client's immune status.

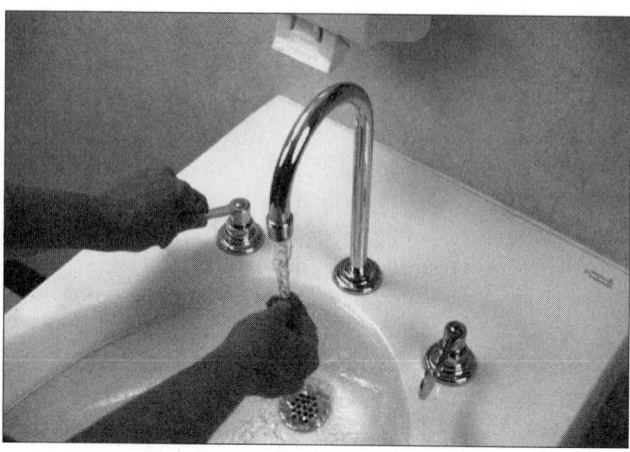

STEP 4 Turning on water.

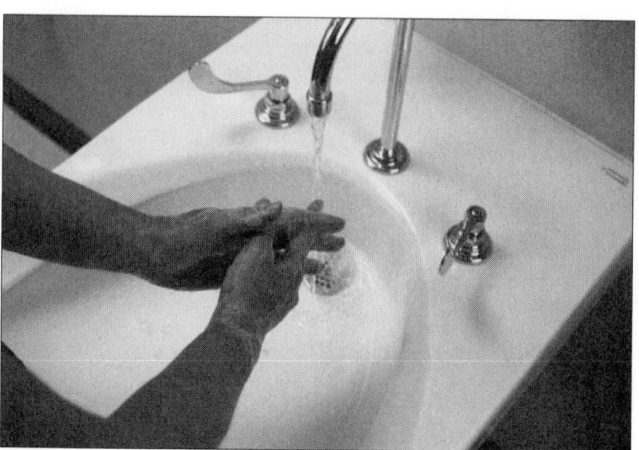

STEP 8 Lathering hands thoroughly.

Step	Rationale
9. Wash hands using plenty of lather and friction for at least 10 to 15 seconds. Interlace fingers and rub palms and back of hands with circular motion at least 5 times each. Keep fingertips down to facilitate removal of microorganisms.	Soap cleanses by emulsifying fat and oil and lowering surface tension. Friction and rubbing mechanically loosen and remove dirt and transient bacteria. Interlacing fingers and thumbs ensures that all surfaces are cleansed.
10. Areas underlying fingernails are often soiled. Clean them with fingernails of other hand and additional soap or clean orangewood stick.	Area under nails can be highly contaminated, which will increase the risk for infections for the nurse or the client.
• ***Critical Decision Point*** *Do not tear or cut skin under or around nail.*	
11. Rinse hands and wrists thoroughly, keeping hands down and elbows up (see illustration).	Rinsing mechanically washes away dirt and microorganisms.
12. Dry hands thoroughly from fingers to wrists and forearms with paper towel, single-use cloth, or warm air dryer.	Drying from cleanest (fingertips) to least clean (forearms) area avoids contamination. Drying hands prevents chapping and roughened skin.
13. If used, discard paper towel in proper receptacle.	Prevents transfer of microorganisms.
14. To turn off hand faucet, use clean, dry paper towel, avoiding touching handles with hands (see illustration). Turn off water with foot or knee pedals (if applicable).	Wet towel and hands allow transfer of pathogens by capillary action.

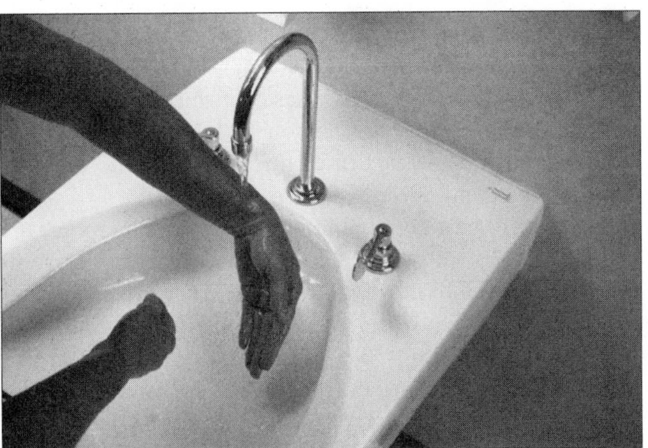

STEP **11** Rinsing hands.

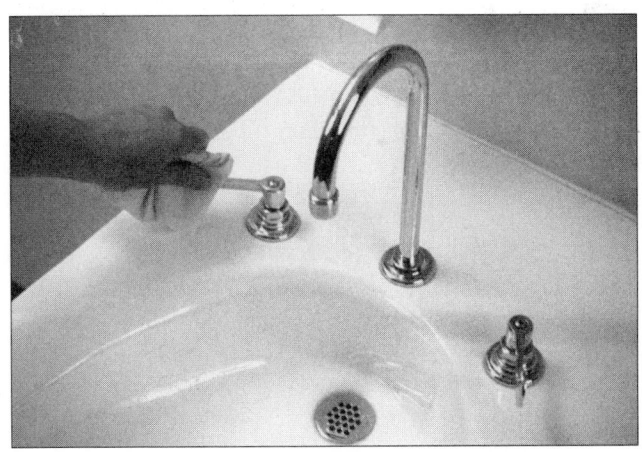

STEP **14** Turning off faucet.

Evaluation

1. Inspect surface of hands for obvious signs of dirt or other contaminants.	Determines if hand washing is adequate.

Unexpected Outcomes and Related Interventions

- Hands or areas under fingernails remain soiled.
  - Nurse must repeat handwashing.
- Repeated use of soaps or antiseptic may cause dermatitis or cracked skin.
  - Requires methods to alleviate complications of hand washing: Rinse and dry hands thoroughly, avoid excessive amounts of soap or antiseptic, try various products, use hand lotions or barrier creams (small individual-use containers are preferred because large containers have been associated with nosocomial infections).
  - Wear gloves. (This should be on a temporary basis because glove wearing can increase bacterial growth and may increase latex allergies among clients and health care workers.)

Recording and Reporting

- It is not necessary to record or report this procedure.
- Report any dermatitis to employee health and/or infection control per your agency's policy.

TEACHING CONSIDERATIONS

- Instruct the client and primary caregiver in proper techniques and situations for hand washing.
- Clients are aware of the importance of hand washing (McGuckin and others, 1999). It has been shown that when clients are educated about the risks of infection in hospitals, they can play an important role in improving hand-washing compliance by reminding health care workers to wash their hands.

GERONTOLOGICAL CONSIDERATIONS

- The impact of infections is much greater in older adults. This is especially true in elderly day-care centers where incidence of acute respiratory infection is high. Hand washing by staff attending the elderly is of utmost importance and should be an ongoing continuing education requirement (Falsey, 1999).

HOME CARE CONSIDERATIONS

- Evaluate client and primary caregiver to determine their understanding of the transmission of microorganisms and their ability and motivation to perform hand washing according to medical asepsis.
- Evaluate the hand-washing facilities in the home to determine the possibility of contamination, proximity of the facilities to the client, and the ability to maintain supplies and equipment.

Skill 31-2 Caring for Clients Under Isolation Precautions

There is a risk of transmitting nosocomial infection or infectious disease among clients or health care workers. When a client has a known source of infection, health care workers follow specific infection control practices and preventions.

Box 31-1 Standard Precautions (Tier One)* for Use With All Clients

- Standard precautions apply to blood, all body fluids, secretions, excretions, nonintact skin, and mucous membranes.
- Hands are washed if contaminated with blood or body fluid, immediately after gloves are removed, between client contact, and when indicated to prevent transfer of microorganisms between clients or between clients and environment.
- Gloves are worn when touching blood, body fluid, secretions, excretions, nonintact skin, mucous membranes, or contaminated items. Gloves should be removed and hands washed between client care.
- Masks, eye protection, or face shields are worn if client care activities may generate splashes or sprays of blood or body fluid.
- Gowns are worn if soiling of clothing is likely from blood or body fluid. Wash hands after removing gown.
- Client care equipment is properly cleaned and reprocessed, and single-use items are discarded.
- Contaminated linen is placed in leakproof bag and is handled to prevent skin and mucous membrane exposure.
- All sharp instruments and needles are discarded in a puncture-resistant container. CDC recommends that needles be disposed of uncapped or a mechanical device be used for recapping.
- A private room is unnecessary unless the client's hygiene is unacceptable. Check with infection control professional.

Modified from Centers for Disease Control and Prevention, Hospital Infection Control Practice Advisory Committee: Guidelines for isolation precautions in hospitals, *Am J Infect Control* 24:24, 1996.

*Formerly universal precautions and body substance isolation.

The majority of organisms causing nosocomial infections are found in the colonized body substances of clients, regardless of whether or not a culture has confirmed infection and a diagnosis has been made (Jackson and Lynch, 1992). Body substances such as feces, urine, mucus, and wound drainage can contain potentially infectious organisms.

Isolation or barrier precautions include the appropriate use of gowns, masks, eyewear, and other protective devices or clothing. Nurses should assess the need for barrier precautions for each task they plan and for all clients regardless of their diagnoses (Lynch, 1995). Because of increased attention to the prevention of blood-borne pathogens and tuberculosis (TB), the Centers for Disease Control and Prevention (CDC) (1988, 1994) and the Occupational Safety and Health Administration (OSHA) (1991, 1994) have stressed the importance of barrier protection.

In 1996 the Hospital Infection Control Practice Advisory Committee (HICPAC) of the CDC published revised guidelines for isolation precautions. These recommendations were based on current epidemiological information regarding disease transmission in hospitals. Although primarily intended for care of clients in acute care, the recommendations can be applied to clients in subacute care or long-term care facilities. HICPAC recommended that hospitals modify the recommendations according to their needs and as dictated by federal, state, or local regulations (Centers for Disease Control and Prevention, 1996; Garner, 1995).

The new guidelines contained two tiers of precautions. The first and most important tier (Box 31-1) is called standard precautions and is designed for care of all clients regardless of risk or presumed infection status. **Standard precautions** are the primary strategies for prevention of infection transmission. Standard precautions apply to contact with (1) blood, (2) body fluids, (3) nonintact skin, and (4) mucous membranes.

The second tier (Table 31-3) is precautions designed for care of clients who are known or suspected to be infected, or **colo-**

nized, with microorganisms transmitted by droplets, by airborne route, or by contact with contaminated surfaces or dry skin. The three types of **transmission-based precautions**—airborne, droplet, and contact—may be combined for diseases that have multiple routes of transmission, for example, chickenpox. When used either singularly or in combination, they are to be used in addition to standard precautions when required by the specific infection or colonization with a specific organism. Box 31-2 summarizes the tiers of precautions and the types of clients requiring their use.

Table 31-3 Transmission Categories (Tier Two) (for Use With Clients Infected or Colonized With Specific Organisms)

Category	Disease	Barrier Protection
Airborne precautions	For diseases transmitted by small droplet nuclei (smaller than 5 μm), such as measles, chickenpox, disseminated varicella zoster, pulmonary or laryngeal TB.*	Private room, negative airflow of at least six air exchanges per hour; respirator or mask.*
Droplet precautions	For diseases transmitted by large droplets (larger than 5 μm), such as streptococcal pharyngitis, pneumonia, and scarlet fever in infants or small children, pertussis, mumps, meningococcal pneumonia or sepsis, pneumonic plague.	Private room or cohort client; mask when closer than 3 ft from client.
Contact precautions	For diseases transmitted by direct client or environmental contact, such as colonization or infection with multidrug-resistant organisms, respiratory syncytial virus, major wound infections, herpes simplex, scabies.	Private room or cohort client; gloves, gowns.

Modified from Centers for Disease Control and Prevention, Hospital Infection Control Practice Advisory Committee: Guidelines for isolation precautions in hospitals, *Am J Infect Control* 24:24, 1996.
*See CDC TB guidelines.

Box 31-2 Synopsis of Types of Precautions of Clients Requiring the Precautions*

Standard Precautions

Use Standard Precautions for the care of all patients

Airborne Precautions

In addition to Standard Precautions, use Airborne Precautions for patients known or suspected to have serious illnesses transmitted by airborne droplet nuclei. Examples of such illnesses include:

(1) Measles
(2) Varicella (including disseminated zoster)*
(3) Tuberculosis†

Droplet Precautions

In addition to Standard Precautions, use Droplet Precautions for patients known or suspected to have serious illnesses transmitted by large particle droplets. Examples of such illnesses include:

(1) Invasive *Haemophilus influenzae* type b disease, including meningitis, pneumonia, epiglottitis, and sepsis
(2) Invasive *Neisseria meningitidis* disease, including meningitis, pneumonia, and sepsis
(3) Other serious bacterial respiratory infections spread by droplet transmission, including:
    (a) Diphtheria (pharyngeal)
    (b) Mycoplasma pneumonia
    (c) Pertussis
    (d) Pneumonic plague
    (e) Streptococcal pharyngitis, pneumonia, or scarlet fever in infants and young children
(4) Serious viral infections spread by droplet transmission, including:
    (a) Adenovirus*
    (b) Influenza
    (c) Mumps
    (d) Parvovirus B 19
    (e) Rubella

From Centers for Disease Control and Prevention, Hospital Infection Control Practice Advisory Committee: Guidelines for isolation precautions in hospitals, *Am J Infect Control* 24:24, 1996.
*Certain infections require more than one type of precaution.
†See CDC *Guidelines for Preventing the Transmission of Tuberculosis in Health-Care Facilities.*

Continued

Box 31-2 Synopsis of Types of Precautions of Clients Requiring the Precautions—cont'd

CONTACT PRECAUTIONS

In addition to Standard Precautions, use Contact Precautions for patients known or suspected to have serious illnesses easily transmitted by direct patient contact or by contact with items in the patient's environment. Examples of such illnesses include:

(1) Gastrointestinal, respiratory, skin, or wound infections or colonization with multidrug-resistant bacteria judged by the infection control program, based on current state, regional, or national recommendations, to be of special clinical and epidemiologic significance
(2) Enteric infections with a low infectious dose or prolonged environmental survival, including:
   (a) *Clostridium difficile*
   (b) For diapered or incontinent patients: enterohemorrhagic *Escherichia coli* 0157:H7, *Shigella*, hepatitis A, or rotavirus
(3) Respiratory syncytial virus, parainfluenza virus, or enteroviral infections in infants and young children
(4) Skin infections that are highly contagious or that may occur on dry skin, including:
   (a) Diphtheria (cutaneous)
   (b) Herpes simplex virus (neonatal or mucocutaneous)
   (c) Impetigo
   (d) Major (noncontained) abscesses, cellulitis, or decubiti
   (e) Pediculosis
   (f) Scabies
   (g) Staphylococcal furunculosis in infants and young children
   (h) Zoster (disseminated or in the immunocompromised host)*
(5) Viral/hemorrhagic conjunctivitis
(6) Viral hemorrhagic infections (Ebola, Lassa, or Marburg)

From Centers for Disease Control and Prevention, Hospital Infection Control Practice Advisory Committee: Guidelines for isolation precautions in hospitals, *Am J Infect Control* 24:24, 1996.
*Certain infections require more than one type of precaution.

When a client requires isolation in a private room, the nurse must remember that loneliness can easily develop. Isolation disrupts normal social relationships with visitors and caregivers. A client who suffers from an infectious disease may also experience self-concept or body image changes. Unless the nurse acts to minimize feelings of psychological and physical isolation, the client's emotional state can interfere with recovery.

DELEGATION CONSIDERATIONS

The skill of caring for clients under isolation precautions can be delegated to assistive personnel. Review with care provider the nature and type of infection a client has. Warn care provider of high risk factors for infection transmission.

EQUIPMENT

- Disposable gloves, mask, eyewear or goggles, and gown
- Other client care equipment (as appropriate)
- Soiled linen and trash receptacle

STEP	RATIONALE
ASSESSMENT	
1. Assess client and review medical history for possible indications for isolation, for example, risk factors for TB, major draining wound, or purulent productive cough. Review the precautions necessary for the specific isolation system.	Mode of transmission for infectious microorganism determines type and degree of precautions followed.
2. Review laboratory test results.	Informs nurse of type of microorganism for which client is being isolated, body fluid in which it was identified, and whether client is immunosuppressed.
3. Consider types of care measures to be performed while in client's room (e.g., medication administration or dressing change).	Enables nurse to organize care items for procedures and time spent in client's room.

STEP	RATIONALE
4. Review nursing care plan notes or confer with colleagues regarding client's emotional state and reaction/adjustment to isolation.	Determines need for things such as emotional support, and teaching.
5. Prepare all equipment needed to be taken into client's room.	Prevents nurse from making more than one trip into room.
6. Determine from nursing care plan, medical record, or significant other if client and family understand the purpose of isolation or procedures to anticipate.	Determines client's level of knowledge and need for instruction/reinforcement.
7. Before applying latex gloves, assess if the client has a known latex allergy.	Client with latex allergy can have a serious allergic or sensitivity reaction even after brief exposure to gloves.

NURSING DIAGNOSIS

Defining characteristics from the assessment data may reveal the following nursing diagnoses for clients requiring this skill:

- Ineffective protection
- Impaired social interaction
- Deficient knowledge regarding purpose of isolation
- Risk for infection

Related factors are individualized based on client's condition or needs.

PLANNING

STEP	RATIONALE
1. **Expected outcomes** following completion of procedure:	
▪ Client spontaneously engages in discussions with nurse and family. ▪ Client asks for information about disease transmission.	Active interaction reveals client's willingness and/or ability to communicate and to be taught and to understand information.

IMPLEMENTATION

STEP	RATIONALE
1. Wash hands.	Reduces transmission of microorganisms.

- ***Critical Decision Point***
  Determine appropriate barriers to apply based upon isolation category and activities to be performed for client.

STEP	RATIONALE
2. Prepare for entrance into isolation room. Choice of barrier protection depends on type of isolation and facility policy (see Table 31-3). For example, if client is on airborne precautions, apply only a special mask and keep room door closed.	Proper preparation ensures nurse is protected from microorganism exposure.
a. Apply either surgical mask or respirator around mouth and nose (type will depend on type of isolation and facility policy) (see illustrations).	Prevents exposure to airborne microorganisms or exposure to microorganisms from splashing of fluids.
b. Apply eyewear or goggles snugly around face and eyes (when needed) (see illustration).	Protects nurse from exposure to microorganisms that may occur during splashing of fluids.
c. Apply gown, being sure it covers all outer garments. Pull sleeves down to wrist. Tie securely at neck and waist (see illustration).	Prevents transmission of infection when client has excessive drainage, discharges.
d. Apply disposable gloves. (NOTE: Unpowdered latex-free gloves should be worn if the client or the health care worker has a latex allergy.) If gloves are worn with gown, bring glove cuffs over edge of gown sleeves.	Reduces transmission of microorganisms.

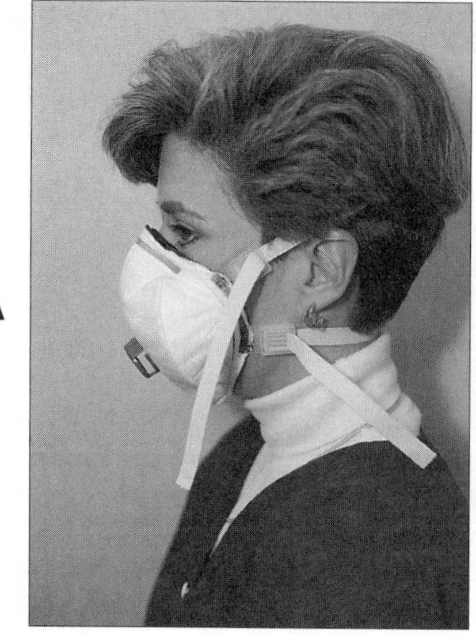

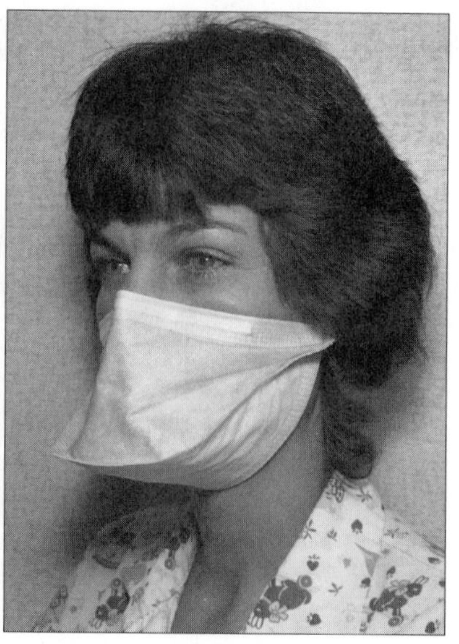

STEP **2a** **A,** Nurse wearing HEPA respirator. **B,** Nurse wearing N-95 respirator.

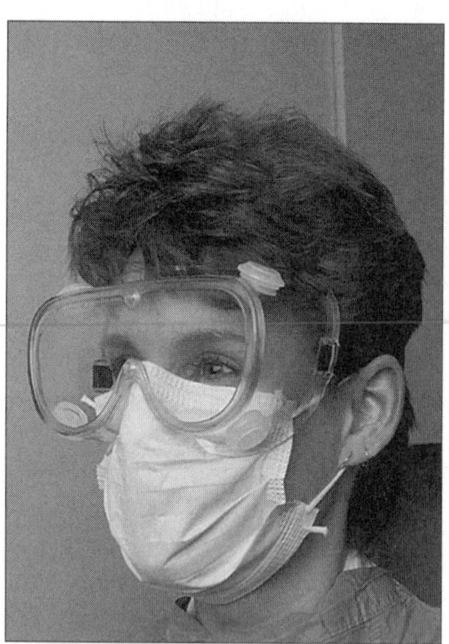

STEP **2b** Nurse wearing goggles.

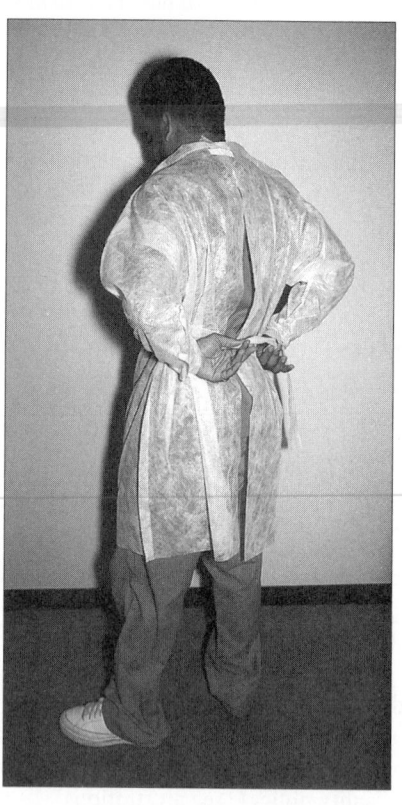

STEP **2c** Nurse tying gown.

STEP	RATIONALE
3. Enter client's room. Arrange supplies and equipment.	Prevents extra trips entering and leaving room.
4. Explain purpose of isolation and precautions necessary to client and family. Offer opportunity to ask questions. Assess for emotions that may be related to the isolation, such as loneliness or boredom, and for signs/symptoms of depression, for example, lack of appetite or difficulty sleeping.	Improves client's and family's ability to participate in care and minimizes anxiety.

Step	Rationale
5. Assess vital signs.	
a. Avoid contact of stethoscope or blood pressure cuff with infective material. Wipe off with disinfectant as needed.	If used later on other clients, increases risk of infection being transmitted.
• ***Critical Decision Point*** *If a resistant organism, for example, vancomycin-resistant* Enterococcus *(VRE) is present, equipment remains in room.*	
b. If stethoscope is to be reused, clean diaphragm or bell with 70% alcohol or liquid soap. Set aside on clean surface.	Systematic disinfection of stethoscopes with 70% alcohol or liquid soap will minimize chance of spreading infectious agents between clients (Bernard and others, 1999).
c. Individual or disposable thermometers should be used.	Prevents cross contamination.
6. Administer medications (see Chapters 17 and 18):	
a. Give oral medication in wrapper or cup.	Supplies are handled and discarded to minimize transfer of microorganisms.
b. Dispose of wrapper or cup in plastic-lined receptacle.	
c. Administer injection, being sure gloves are worn.	
d. Discard disposable syringe and uncapped needle into designated sharps container (see illustration).	Reduces risk of needle stick injury.
e. Place reusable plastic syringe (e.g., carpuject) on clean towel for eventual removal and disinfection.	Prevents added contamination of syringe.

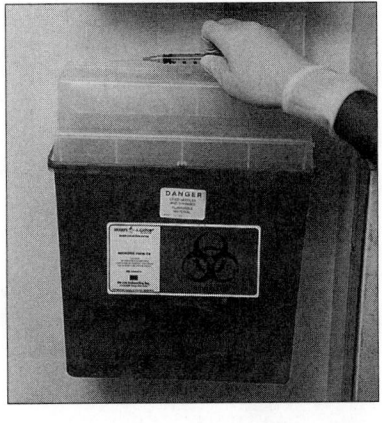

STEP **6d** Disposal of syringes and uncapped needle.

Step	Rationale
7. Administer hygiene, encouraging the client to verbalize any questions or concerns regarding isolation.	Hygiene practices further minimize transfer of microorganisms.
• ***Critical Decision Point*** *During this time, informal teaching can be provided.*	
a. Avoid allowing isolation gown to become wet; carry washbasin outward away from gown; avoid leaning against wet tabletop.	Moisture allows organisms to travel through gown to uniform.
b. Assist client in removing own gown; discard in impervious linen bag.	Reduces transfer of microorganisms.
c. Remove linen from bed; avoid contact with isolation gown. Place in impervious linen bag.	Linen soiled by client's body fluids is handled so as to prevent contact with clean items.
• ***Critical Decision Point*** *In case of excess soiling, a gown impervious to moisture should be worn.*	
d. Provide clean bed linen and set of towels.	
e. Change gloves and wash hands if they become excessively soiled and further care is necessary.	

STEP	RATIONALE
8. Collect specimens (see Chapter 41):	
a. Place specimen containers on clean paper towel in client's bathroom.	Container will be taken out of client's room, prevents contamination of outer surface.
b. Follow procedure for collecting specimen of body fluids.	
c. Transfer specimen to container without soiling outside of container. Place container in a plastic bag.	Specimens of blood and body fluids are placed in well-constructed containers with secure lids to prevent leaks during transport.
d. Check label on specimen for accuracy. Send to laboratory (warning labels may be used, depending on hospital policy).	
9. Dispose of linen, trash, and disposable items:	
a. Use single bags that are impervious to moisture and sturdy to contain soiled articles. Use double bag if necessary for heavily soiled linen or heavy wet trash.	Linen or refuse should be totally contained to prevent exposure of personnel to infective material.
b. Tie bags securely at top in knot (see illustration).	

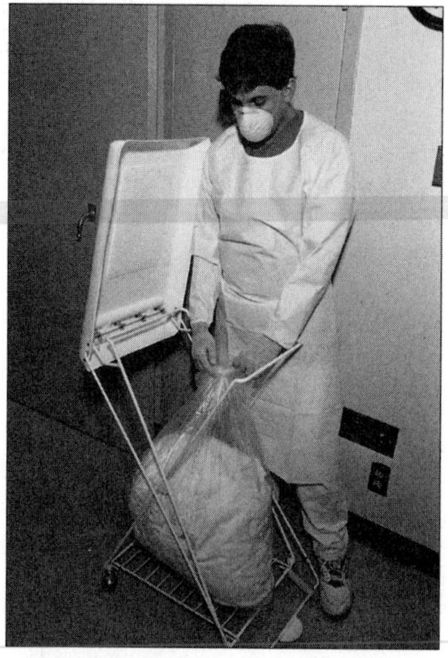

STEP **9b** Tie bags.

STEP	RATIONALE
10. Remove all reusable pieces of equipment. Clean any contaminated surfaces with hospital approved disinfectant (Bonilla and others, 1996) (see agency policy).	All items must be properly cleaned, disinfected, or sterilized for reuse.
11. Resupply room as needed. Have staff colleague hand new supplies to you.	Limiting trips of personnel into and out of room reduces nurse's and client's exposure to microorganisms. Quality time should be spent with the client when in the room.
12. Leave isolation room. Remember, order of removal of protective barriers depends on what is worn in room. This sequence describes steps to take if all barriers were required to be worn.	
a. Remove gloves. Remove one glove by grasping cuff and pulling glove inside out over hand (see illustration). Discard glove. With ungloved hand, tuck finger inside cuff of remaining glove and pull it off, inside out (see illustration).	Technique prevents nurse from contacting contaminated glove's outer surface.
b. Untie *top* mask string and then bottom strings, pull mask away from face and drop into trash receptacle (Do not touch outer surface of mask).	Ungloved hands will not be contaminated by touching only mask strings.

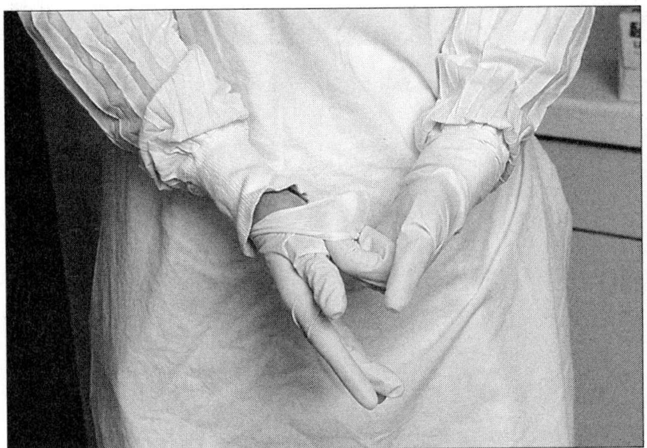

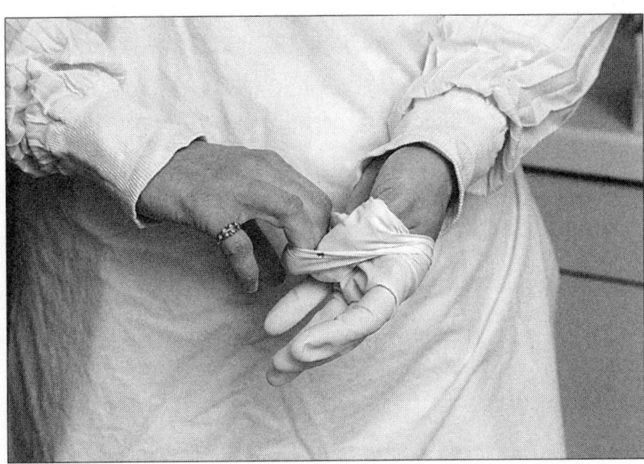

STEP **12a** Removal of gloves.

STEP	RATIONALE
c. Untie neck strings, then back strings of gown. Allow gown to fall from shoulders. Remove hands from sleeves without touching outside of gown. Hold gown inside at shoulder seams and fold inside out (see illustration); discard in laundry bag.	Hands do not come in contact with soiled front of gown.

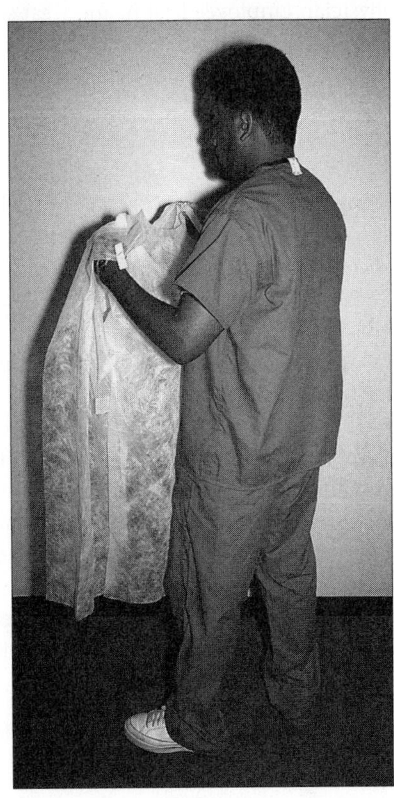

STEP **12c** Removal of gown.

STEP	RATIONALE
d. Remove eyewear or goggles.	Hands have not been soiled.
e. Wash hands for a minimum of 10 seconds.	
f. Retrieve wristwatch and stethoscope (unless it must remain in room) and record vital sign values on notepaper.	Clean hands can contact clean items.
g. Explain to client when you plan to return to room. Ask whether client requires any personal care items. Offer books, magazines, audiotapes.	Diversions help to minimize boredom and feeling of social isolation.

STEP	RATIONALE
h. Leave room and close door, if necessary. Door should be closed if client is in negative airflow room.	

EVALUATION

1. While in room, ask if client has had sufficient opportunity to discuss health problems, course of treatment, or other topics important to client.	Measures client's perception of adequacy of discussions with caregivers.

UNEXPECTED OUTCOMES AND RELATED INTERVENTIONS

- Client avoids social and therapeutic discussions.
  - Confer with family and/or significant other and determine best approach to reduce client's sense of loneliness and depression.
- Client or health care worker may have an allergy to latex gloves.
  - Notify physician/employee health, and treat sensitivity or allergic reaction appropriately.
  - Use latex-free gloves for future care activities.

RECORDING AND REPORTING

- Document procedures performed and client's response to social isolation in nurses' progress notes. Also document any client education performed and reinforced.

TEACHING CONSIDERATIONS

- Visitors and family members are taught by the nurse to follow the recommended isolation precautions when visiting client. They are also taught appropriate use of barrier techniques for home caregiving.

PEDIATRIC CONSIDERATIONS

- Isolation creates sense of separation from family and loss of control. Strange environment adds to confusion child feels during isolation. Preschoolers are unable to understand cause-effect relationship for isolation. Older children may be able to understand cause but still fantasize. Children require simple explanations, for example, "You need to be in this room to help you get better." All barriers to be used must be shown to child. Parents must be actively involved in any explanations. Nurses let child see their faces before applying masks so that child does not become frightened.

GERONTOLOGICAL CONSIDERATIONS

- Isolation also can be a particular concern for older adults, especially those who have signs and symptoms of confusion or depression. Many times clients become more confused when they are confronted with a nurse using barrier precautions or when they are left in a room with the door closed. Nurse must assess need for closing door (negative airflow room) along with safety of client and additional safety measures that may need to be taken. Older adults should be assessed for signs of depression such as loss of appetite or decrease in verbal communications. If necessary, this should be brought to attention of health care team for appropriate interventions.

HOME CARE CONSIDERATIONS

- Although isolation precautions followed in the hospital are not directly applicable to home care, caregivers should be aware of potential sources of contamination in home.

Critical Thinking Exercises

1. When Joe enters Mr. Nesbitt's room he begins to conduct a physical assessment. As he turns Mr. Nesbitt to check the condition of his skin, he notices moisture on his hand. Joe looks more closely and realizes the moisture is from an open, oozing lesion on Mr. Nesbitt's sacral area. After assessing the wound, Joe quickly checks the position and function of Mr. Nesbitt's indwelling urinary catheter and then washes his hands before leaving Mr. Nesbitt's room. What elements of the infection chain were intact or broken as a result of Joe's care?
2. Tamara is caring for two clients in the same room, Mrs. Lee and Mrs. Myer. Tamara enters the room and begins to help Mrs. Lee position more comfortably. She administers an intramuscular (IM) injection to Mrs. Lee and straightens out her bed linen. Mrs. Myer calls for assistance, and Tamara inspects the condition of Mrs. Myer's intravenous catheter. At what point should Tamara have washed her hands?
3. Which of the following measures help to control or prevent a reservoir of growth for microorganisms: avoidance of shaking bed linen, disposing of used needles, keeping a surgical drainage tube patent?
4. When a client is placed on droplet precautions, what protective barriers are necessary?

References

Bernard L and others: Bacterial contamination of hospital physicians' stethoscopes, *Infect Control Hosp Epidemiol* 20(9):626, 1999.

Bobo L: The microbiologic environment. In Soule B, Larson E, Preson G, editors: *Infection and nursing practice: prevention and control,* St. Louis, 1994, Mosby.

Bonilla HF and others: Long-term survival of vancomycin-resistant *Enterococcus faecium* on a contaminated surface, *Infect Control Hosp Epidemiol* 17(12)770, 1996.

Centers for Disease Control: Update: universal precautions for prevention of transmission of human immunodeficiency virus, hepatitis B virus, and other bloodborne pathogens in health care setting, *MMWR Morbid Mortal Wkly Rep* 37(24):377, 1988.

Centers for Disease Control and Prevention: Guidelines for preventing the transmission of mycobacterium tuberculosis in health-care facilities, *Fed Regis* 59(208):54242, 1994.

Centers for Disease Control and Prevention, Hospital Infection Control Practice Advisory Committee: Guidelines for isolation precautions in hospitals, *Am J Infect Control* 24:24, 1996.

Crow S, Planchock N, Hedrick E: Antisepsis: disinfection and sterilization. In Soule B, Larson E, Preston G, editors: *Infection and nursing practice: prevention and control,* St. Louis, 1994, Mosby.

DeCastro M, Fauerback L, Masters L: Aseptic technique. In Olmsted R, editor: *APIC infection control and applied epidemiology,* St. Louis, 1996, Mosby.

Falsey A and others: Evaluation of a handwashing intervention to reduce respiratory illness rates in senior day-care centers, *Infect Control Hosp Epidemiol* 20(3):200, 1999.

Garner B: Infection control. In Meeker MH, Rothrock JC, editors: *Alexander's care of the patient in surgery,* St. Louis, 1995, Mosby.

Garner J: Isolation systems. In Olmsted R, editor: *APIC infection control and applied epidemiology,* St. Louis, 2000, Mosby.

Goldrick B, Turner J: Education and behavior change in prevention and control of infection. In Soule B, Larson E, Preston G, editors: *Infection and nursing practice: prevention and control,* St. Louis, 1994, Mosby.

Jackson M, Lynch P: Body substance isolation, *Infect Control Hosp Epidemiol* 13(14):191, 1992.

Larson EL: APIC guideline for handwashing and hand antisepsis in health care settings, *Am J Infect Control* 23(4):251, 1995.

Larson E: Antiseptic. In Olmsted R, editor: *APIC infection control and applied epidemiology,* St. Louis, 2000, Mosby.

Lynch P: Barrier precautions and personal protection. In Soule B, Larson E, Preston G, editors: *Infections and nursing practices,* St. Louis, 1995, Mosby.

McGuckin M and others: Patient education model for increasing handwashing compliance, *Am J Infect Control* 27(4):309, 1999.

Nishimura S and others: Handwashing before entering the intensive care unit: what we learned from continuous video-camera surveillance, *Am J Infect Control* 27(4):367, 1999.

Occupational Safety and Health Administration: Occupational exposure to bloodborne pathogens: final rule, 29 CFR 1919:1030, *Fed Regis* 56:64003, 1991.

Occupational Safety and Health Administration: Respiratory protection, *Fed Regis* 59(219):58884, 1994.

Rutala W: Disinfection and sterilization of patient-care items, *Infect Control Hosp Epidemiol* 17(6):377, 1996.

Zaragoza M and others: Handwashing with soap or alcoholic solutions? A randomized clinical trial of its effectiveness, *Am J Infect Control* 27(3):258, 1999.

32

Sterile Technique

Skills

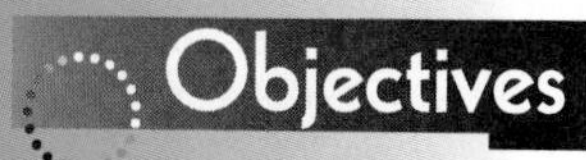

Objectives

Mastery of content in this chapter will enable the nurse to:

- Define the key terms listed.
- Discuss settings where surgical aseptic techniques may be used.
- Describe conditions when surgical asepsis should be used.
- Identify principles of surgical asepsis.
- Explain the importance of organization and caution when using surgical aseptic techniques.
- Apply and remove a cap and mask correctly.
- Identify individuals at risk for latex allergy.
- Apply sterile gloves using open glove method.
- Prepare a sterile field.
- Apply a sterile drape correctly.

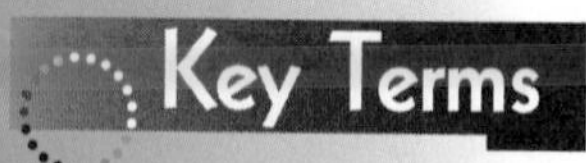

Key Terms

Asepsis
Latex allergy reaction
Microorganisms
Pathogenic microorganisms
Standard precautions
Sterile
Sterile field
Strike through
Surgical asepsis
Transmission-based precautions

Surgical asepsis or aseptic techniques and practices are designed to render and maintain objects and areas free from **pathogenic microorganisms** (Crow, Planchock, and Hendrick, 1995). As in medical **asepsis,** hand washing with an appropriate cleanser or antiseptic is essential before the initiation of an aseptic procedure. Surgical asepsis does require more precautions than medical aseptic technique (see Chapter 31). Any break in technique could result in contamination, increasing the client's risk for an infection. Although surgical asepsis is commonly practiced in operating rooms (ORs), labor and delivery areas, and major diagnostic or special procedure areas, the nurse may use surgical aseptic techniques at the client's bedside (Box 32-1) in three primary situations:

- During procedures that require intentional perforation of a client's skin (e.g., insertion of intravenous [IV] catheters and administration of injections [see Chapter 19 and 18])
- When the skin's integrity is broken due to a surgical incision or burns
- During procedures that involve insertion of devices or surgical instruments into normally sterile body cavities (e.g., insertion of a urinary catheter [see Chapter 24])

Box 32-1 Principles of Surgical Asepsis

1. All items used within a sterile field must be sterile.
2. A sterile barrier that has been permeated by punctures, tears, or moisture must be considered contaminated.
3. Once a sterile package is opened, a 2.5-cm (1-inch) border around the edges is considered unsterile.
4. Tables draped as part of sterile field are considered sterile only at table level.
5. If there is any question or doubt of an item's sterility, the item is considered to be unsterile.
6. Sterile persons or items contact only sterile areas; unsterile persons or items contact only unsterile areas.
7. Movement around and in the sterile field must not compromise or contaminate the sterile field.
8. A sterile object or field out of the range of vision or an object held below a person's waist is contaminated.
9. A sterile object or field becomes contaminated by prolonged exposure to air; stay organized, and complete any procedure as soon as possible.

The skills in this chapter can be used at the client's bedside; portions of Skills 32-1 and 32-2 also can be practiced in the OR, labor and delivery, and procedure areas. Chapter 34 describes additional skills specific to the OR and labor and delivery areas. A nurse in an OR follows a series of steps toward **sterile** technique, such as applying a mask, protective eyewear, and a cap; performing a surgical hand scrub; applying a sterile gown; and applying sterile gloves using the closed method. In contrast, a nurse performing a sterile dressing change at a client's bedside or in the home setting may only wash the hands and apply sterile gloves using the open method. Regardless of the procedures followed in different settings, the use of surgical asepsis depends on the nurse developing a surgical aseptic awareness. The nurse must always recognize the importance of strict adherence to aseptic principles (Roth, 1996). All individuals involved in surgical asepsis have a responsibility to provide and maintain a safe environment by following aseptic principles (AORN, 1996). The nurse can be an excellent role model and client advocate, reinforcing proper practice when another caregiver breaks technique.

In treatment areas and at the bedside, it is important to have a client's full cooperation to minimize contamination of a work area. The nurse must prepare a client before any procedure. Certain clients may fear moving or touching objects during a sterile procedure, whereas others may even try to assist. The nurse explains how a procedure is to be performed and what a client can do to avoid contaminating sterile items, including avoiding sudden body movement, refraining from touching sterile supplies, and avoiding coughing or talking over a sterile area.

The Centers for Disease Control and Prevention (CDC) (1996) has established standard precautions as the minimum standard for infection control (see Chapter 31). **Standard precautions** should be used for potential contact with blood and certain body fluids (peritoneal, pericardial, pleural, cerebrospinal fluid [CSF], vaginal, seminal, and amniotic). These are considered infectious for human immunodeficiency virus (HIV), hepatitis B virus (HBV), hepatitis C virus (HCV), and other blood-borne pathogens. Standard precautions also apply to body fluids containing visible blood. The use of standard precautions calls for the wearing of masks in combination with eye protection devices such as goggles or glasses with solid side shields whenever splashes, spray, splatter, or droplets of blood or other potentially infectious fluids may be generated. These barriers keep the eyes, nose, and mouth free from exposure. Similarly, gowns are to be worn when there is risk of being splattered with blood or other infectious materials. All health care institutions should ensure that personal protective equipment and instructions for their use are provided to all employees (Soule, Larson, and Preston, 1995; Meeker and Rothrock, 1999).

In addition to standard precautions, **transmission-based precautions** are a second tier of precautions used, either singularly or in combination, when required by a specific infection or colonization of an organism (see Chapter 31). For example, when a client requires airborne or droplet precautions, the nurse will wear a mask.

Skill Performance Guidelines

1. Always follow standard precautions with all clients.
2. Always review your agency's policies and procedures before conducting a sterile procedure.
3. Always assess the client's potential for infection before choosing the barrier to be used, such as masks or caps.
4. Use barrier techniques to decrease the transmission of **microorganisms** from health care personnel and the environment to the client.
5. Remember that hand washing is essential before initiating any sterile procedure.
6. Incorporate the principles of surgical asepsis when conducting any sterile procedure.

Skill 32-1 Applying and Removing Cap, Mask, and Protective Eyewear

Although masks and caps are usually worn in surgical procedure areas (e.g., the operating room), there are certain surgical aseptic procedures performed at a client's bedside that might require these barriers. For example, it may be an agency's policy for a nurse to wear a mask during the changing of a central line dressing or insertion of a peripherally inserted central catheter (PICC). Other policies might require that a nurse wear a mask and a cap to secure hair during dressing changes on a client with extensive burns. When there is a risk for the nurse to be exposed to splattering of blood or body fluid, there is also the need to apply protective eyewear.

The nurse should assess the client's potential for acquiring an infection before applying a mask (e.g., does the client have a large open wound, does the nurse have a respiratory infection, is the client immunosuppressed). If a mask is worn, it should be changed if it becomes moist or soiled (e.g., splattered with blood). Nurses may choose to wear a surgical cap to secure loose hair that might contaminate a sterile area (Meeker and Rothrock, 1999). As in all situations that require protection from splatters from blood or body fluid, the nurse should follow standard precautions (see Chapter 31).

Delegation Considerations

The skill of applying and removing cap, mask, and protective eyewear can be delegated to assistive personnel. However, the procedures performed at a client's bedside that require cap and mask generally cannot be delegated (refer to specific skill for recommendations). Assistive personnel should learn how to be available to hand off additional sterile equipment or assist with client positioning. The RN determines if protective barriers are necessary for the other staff.

Equipment

- Mask (different types are available for people with different skin sensitivities)
- Paper surgical cap (NOTE: Use only if hospital policy requires, or use to secure hair if there is a possibility of contamination of a sterile field)
- Hairpins, rubber bands, or both
- Protective eyewear (e.g., goggles or glasses with appropriate side shields)

STEP	RATIONALE

ASSESSMENT

1. Consider type of sterile procedure to be performed, and consult agency's policy for use of mask/caps/eyewear.	Not all sterile procedures require mask, cap, or eyewear.
2. If you have symptoms of a cold or respiratory infection, either avoid participating in procedure or apply a mask.	A greater number of pathogenic microorganisms reside within the respiratory tract when infection is present.
3. Assess the client's actual or potential risk for infection when choosing barriers for surgical asepsis (e.g., older adult, neonatal client or immunocompromised client).	Some clients are at a greater risk for acquiring an infection, so nurse uses additional barriers.

NURSING DIAGNOSIS

Defining characteristics from the assessment data may reveal the following nursing diagnoses for clients requiring this skill:

Risk for infection

Ineffective protection

Related factors are individualized based on client's condition or needs.

PLANNING

1. **Expected outcomes** following completion of procedure:	
▪ Client will not develop signs of localized infection.	Indicates lack of microorganism transfer to client and sterile field.
2. Prepare equipment and inspect packaging for integrity and exposure to sterilization.	Ensures availability of equipment and sterility of supplies before procedure begins.

IMPLEMENTATION

1. Applying cap	
a. If hair is long, comb back behind shoulders and arrange on crown of head.	Cap must cover all hair entirely.
b. Secure hair in place with pins.	Long hair should not fall down or cause cap to slip and expose hair.
c. Apply cap over head as you would apply hairnet. Be sure all hair fits under cap's edges (see illustration).	Loose hair hanging over sterile field or falling dander may result in contamination of objects on sterile field.

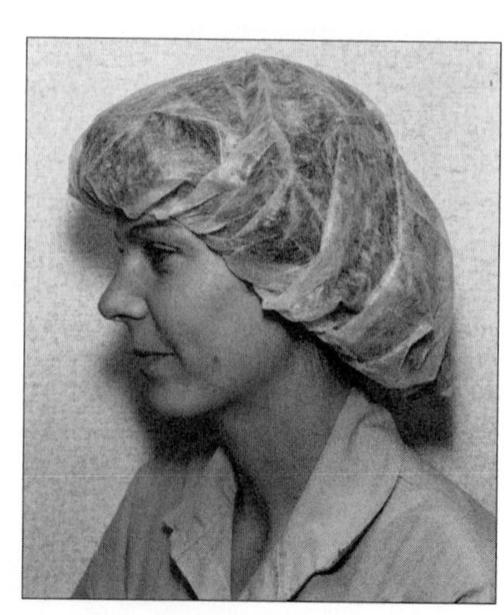

STEP 1c Apply cap over head, covering all hair.

STEP	RATIONALE
2. Applying mask	
a. Find top edge of mask, which usually has a thin metal strip along edge.	Pliable metal fits snugly against bridge of nose.
b. Hold mask by top two strings or loops, keeping top edge above bridge of nose.	Prevents contact of hands with clean facial portion of mask. Mask will cover all of nose.
c. Tie two top strings at top of back of head, over cap (if worn), with strings above ears (see illustration).	Position of ties at top of head provides tight fit. Ties over ears may cause irritation.
d. Tie two lower ties snugly around neck with mask well under chin (see illustration).	Prevents escape of microorganisms through sides of mask as nurse talks and breathes.
e. Gently pinch upper metal band around bridge of nose.	Prevents microorganisms from escaping around nose.

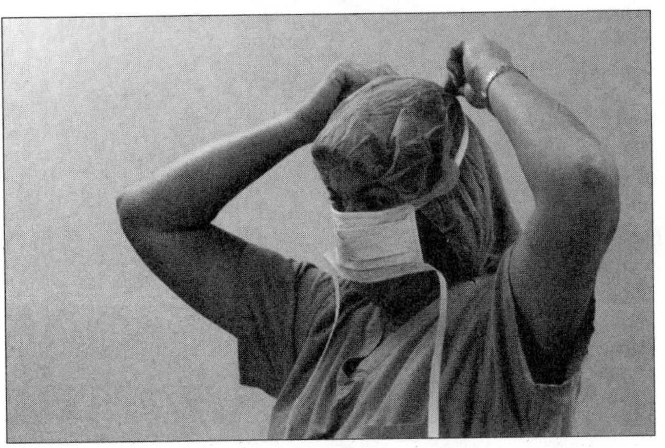

STEP **2c** Tie top strings of mask.

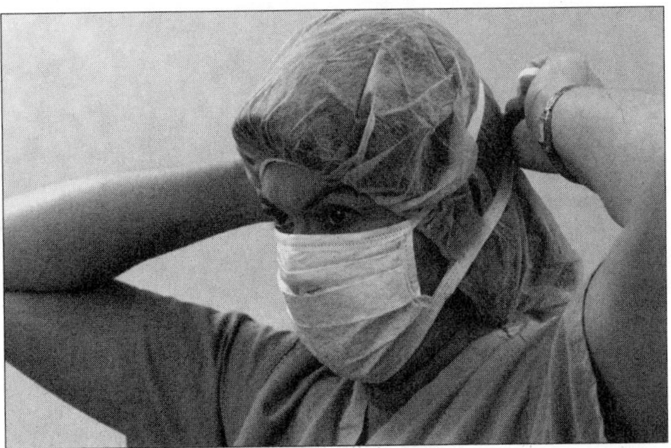

STEP **2d** Tie bottom strings of mask.

STEP	RATIONALE
3. Applying protective eyewear	
a. Apply protective glasses, goggles, or shield comfortably over eyes, and check that vision is clear (see illustration).	Positioning can affect clarity of vision.
b. Be sure eyewear fits snugly around forehead and face.	Ensures eyes are fully protected.

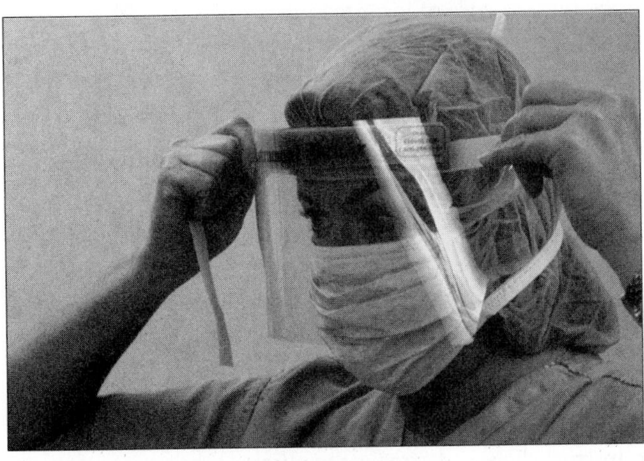

STEP **3a** Apply shield over cap.

STEP	RATIONALE
4. Disposing of cap and mask and removing eyewear	
a. Remove gloves first, if worn (see Skill 32-3).	Prevents contamination of hair, neck, and facial area.
b. Untie bottom strings of mask first.	Prevents top part of mask from falling down over nurse's uniform. Contaminated surface of mask could then contaminate uniform.

Step	Rationale
c. Untie top strings of mask and remove mask from face, holding ties securely. Discard mask in proper receptacle (see illustrations).	Avoids contact of nurse's hands with contaminated mask.

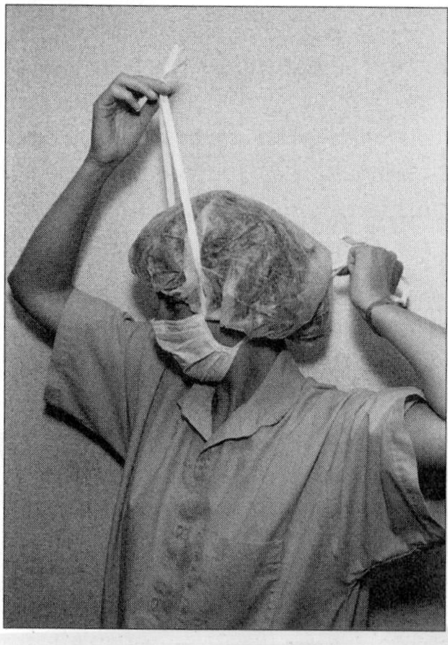

A

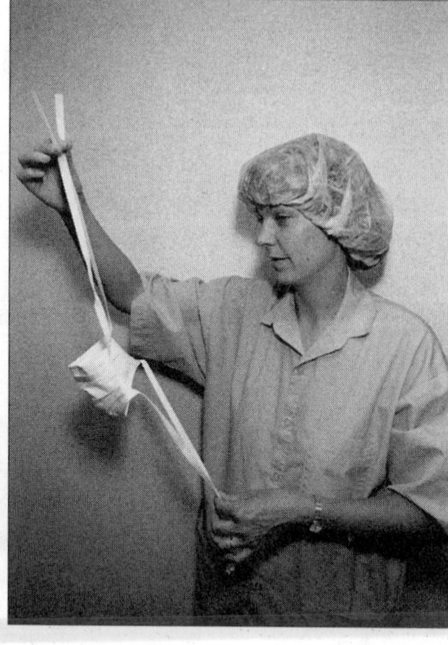

B

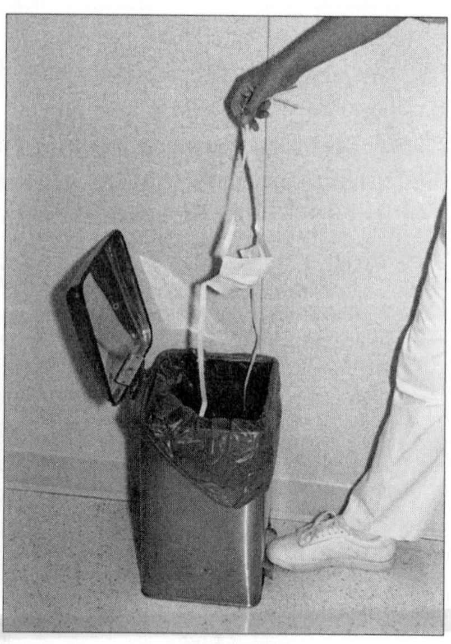

C

STEP **4c** **A**, Untying top mask strings. **B**, Removing mask from face. **C**, Discarding mask.

Step	Rationale
d. Remove eyewear, avoiding placing hands over soiled lens.	Prevents transmission of microorganisms.
e. Grasp outer surface of cap and lift from hair.	Minimizes contact of hands with hair.
f. Discard cap in proper receptacle, and wash hands.	Reduces transmission of infection.

Evaluation

Step	Rationale
1. Following procedure, assess area of body treated for drainage, tenderness, edema, or change in temperature or color of skin (infection usually develops 2 to 3 days after exposure to organism).	Rules out presence of localized infection.

Unexpected Outcomes and Related Interventions

- Redness, heat, edema, pain, or purulent drainage develops at wound or treatment site, indicating possible infection.
  - Notify physician of change in condition of affected area, and initiate appropriate treatments as ordered.
  - If there is a pattern or trend in clients developing similar infection, infection control team will investigate.

Recording and Reporting

- No recording or reporting is required for this set of skills. Record specific procedure performed in nurses' progress notes, and describe client's status, for example, condition of surgical site, appearance of intravenous central catheter site.

Home Care Considerations

- Instruct caregiver as to specifics of when to apply cap, mask, and protective eyewear.
- Determine ability of caregiver to safely implement sterile procedure.
- Instruct client and caregiver to observe for signs of infection.

Skill 32-2 Preparing a Sterile Field

When performing sterile aseptic procedures, the nurse must have a work area in which objects can be handled with minimal risk of contamination. A **sterile field** serves such a purpose. It is an area considered free of microorganisms and may consist of a sterile kit or tray, a work surface draped with a sterile towel or wrapper, or a table covered with a large sterile drape (Crow, Planchock, and Hendrick, 1995). Sterile drapes establish a sterile field around a treatment site, such as a surgical incision, venipuncture site, or site for introduction of an indwelling urinary catheter. Drapes also provide a work surface for placing sterile supplies and for manipulating items with sterile gloves. Drapes are available in cloth, paper, and plastic. They may be wrapped in individual sterile packages or included within sterile kits or trays. Most are fluid resistant. Many styles, shapes, and sizes are available to accommodate different areas or body parts to be covered. For example, a fenestrated drape has a slitlike opening in it to expose only the perineal area during urinary catheter insertion.

Many sterile items come prepackaged within containers that serve as both sterile fields and work areas for the nurse. For example, bladder catheterization kits and tracheal suction kits contain sterile items that can be moved within the tray and containers into which sterile solutions can be poured. Once a sterile field is created, it is the responsibility of the nurse to perform the procedure and to be sure the field is not contaminated.

The skill of preparing a sterile field incorporates skills of opening sterile packages, preparing a sterile drape, adding sterile supplies to a field, and pouring sterile solutions.

Delegation Considerations

The procedures performed at clients' bedsides that require use of a sterile field generally should not be delegated (refer to specific skill for recommendations). However, assistive personnel may assist in positioning clients and obtaining extra supplies.

Equipment

- Sterile gloves
- Sterile drape or kit that is to be used as a sterile field
- Sterile gown (see agency's policy)
- Disposable cap and mask (see agency's policy)
- Sterile supplies and solutions specific to the procedure
- Waist-high table/countertop surface
- Protective eyewear

Step	Rationale
Assessment	
1. Verify that procedure requires surgical aseptic technique.	Some procedures require medical rather than surgical aseptic technique.
2. Assess client's comfort, oxygen requirements, and elimination needs before preparing for procedure.	Certain procedures for which sterile field is prepared may last a long time. Nurse anticipates client's needs so that client can relax and avoid any unnecessary movement that might disrupt procedure.

- ***Critical Decision Point***

  Position client for maximum comfort and ease of breathing. Additional staff may be needed to assist with positioning so client does not contaminate sterile field.

Step	Rationale
3. Check sterile package integrity for punctures, tears, discoloration, moisture, or any other signs of contamination. If using commercially packaged supplies or those prepared by agency, check for sterilization indicator.	The inspection of packaging ensures that only sterile items are presented to sterile field (AORN, 1996).
4. Anticipate number and variety of supplies needed for procedure.	Not all sterile kits contain sufficient amounts or types of supplies. Failure to have necessary supplies causes nurse to leave sterile field, increasing risk of contamination.

STEP	RATIONALE

NURSING DIAGNOSIS

Defining characteristics from the assessment data may reveal the following nursing diagnoses for clients requiring this skill:

Risk for infection

Ineffective protection

Related factors are individualized based on client's condition or needs.

PLANNING

STEP	RATIONALE
1. **Expected outcomes** following completion of procedure:	
▪ The field is not contaminated. Client not exposed to microorganisms.	Nurse uses correct surgical aseptic practice.
2. Complete all other priority tasks before beginning procedure.	Sterile fields should be prepared as close as possible to time of use to reduce potential for contamination (AORN, 1996).
3. Prepare equipment at bedside.	Ensures availability before the procedure and prevents break in sterile technique. (NOTE: that povidone-iodine and chlorhexidine are not considered sterile solutions and require separate work surfaces for prepping.)
4. Ask visitors to step out briefly during procedure. Discourage movement by staff who will assist with procedure.	Traffic or movement can increase potential for contamination through spread of microorganisms by air currents.
5. Position client comfortably for specific procedure to be performed. If a body part is to be examined or treated, position client so part is accessible. Have assistive personnel assist with positioning as needed.	Client should be able to lie still in one position comfortably during procedure. Movement can cause contamination of sterile items.
6. Explain to client purpose of procedure and importance of sterile technique.	Ensures client's ability to cooperate. Teaching before procedure eliminates need to talk during procedure, which can cause air-droplet contamination of sterile area.

IMPLEMENTATION

STEP	RATIONALE
1. Apply cap, mask, protective eyewear, and/or gown as needed (consult agency's policy).	Controls spread of airborne microorganisms.
2. Select a clean, flat, dry work surface above waist level.	A sterile object below a person's waist is considered contaminated.
3. Wash hands thoroughly (decision whether to use soap or antiseptic depends on procedure).	Reduces transmission of infection.
4. Preparing sterile work surface	
a. Sterile commercial kit or tray containing sterile items	
(1) Place sterile kit or package containing sterile items on clean, dry, flat work surface above waist level.	Items placed below waist level are considered contaminated.
(2) Open outside cover, and remove kit from dust cover. Place on work surface.	Inner kit remains sterile.
(3) Grasp outer surface of tip of outermost flap.	Outer surface of package is considered unsterile. There is a 2.5-cm (1-inch) border around any sterile drape or wrap that is considered contaminated.
(4) Open outermost flap away from body, keeping arm outstretched and away from sterile field (see illustration).	Reaching over sterile field contaminates it.
(5) Grasp outside surface of edge of first side flap.	Outer border is considered unsterile.
(6) Open side flap, pulling to side, allowing it to lie flat on table surface. Keep your arm to side and not over sterile surface (see illustration).	Drape or wrapper should lie flat so it will not accidentally rise up and contaminate inner surface or sterile contents.

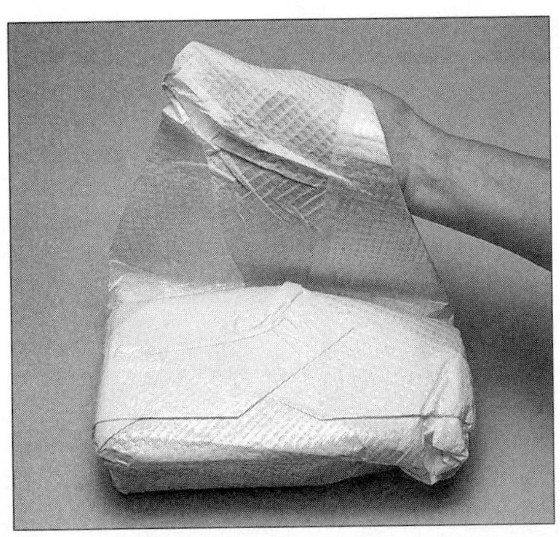

STEP **4a(4)** Open outermost flap of sterile kit away from body.

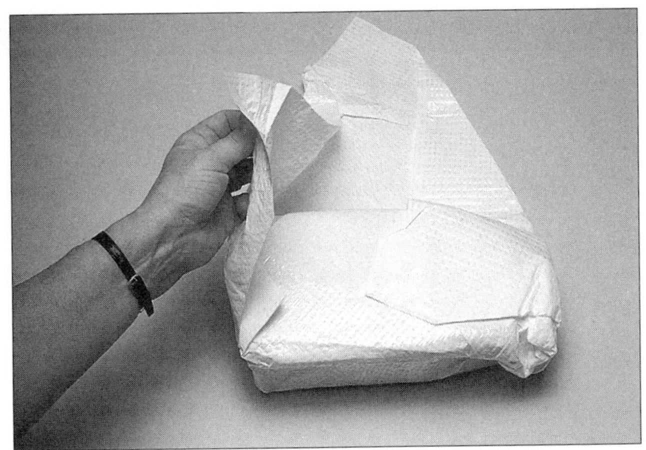

STEP **4a(6)** Open first side flap, pulling to side.

STEP	RATIONALE
(7) Repeat steps for second side flap (see illustration).	
(8) Grasp outside border of last and innermost flap (see illustration).	Outer border is considered unsterile.
(9) Stand away from sterile package and pull flap back, allowing it to fall flat on table (see illustration).	Never reach over a sterile field.

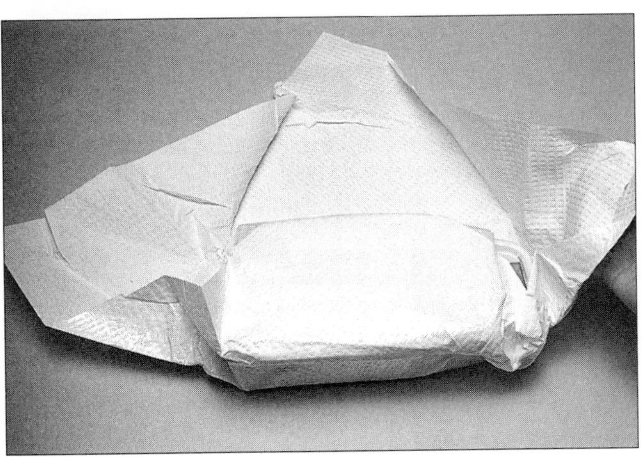

STEP **4a(7)** Open second side flap, pulling to side.

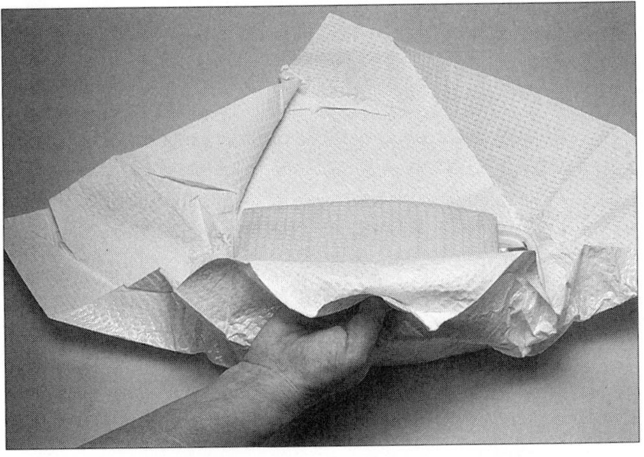

STEP **4a(8)** Open last and innermost flap.

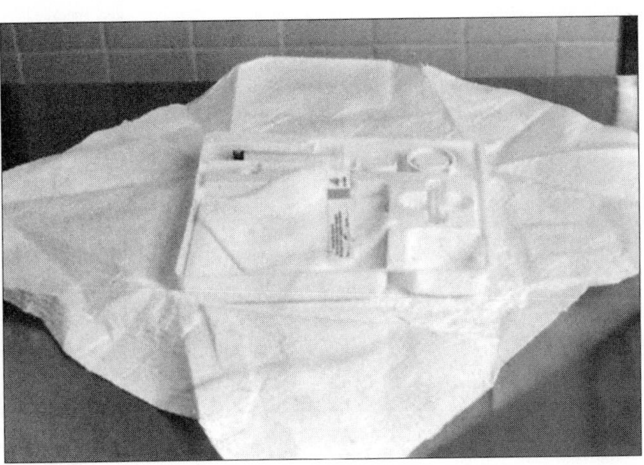

STEP **4a(9)** Sterile kit fully open.

STEP	RATIONALE
b. Sterile linen-wrapped package	
(1) Place package on clean, dry, flat work surface above waist level.	Items placed below waist level are considered contaminated.
(2) Remove tape seal and unwrap both layers as with sterile kit above (see illustration).	Linen-wrapped items have two layers. The first is a dust cover. The second layer must be opened to view chemical indicator. If item is dropped on floor, it is considered contaminated.

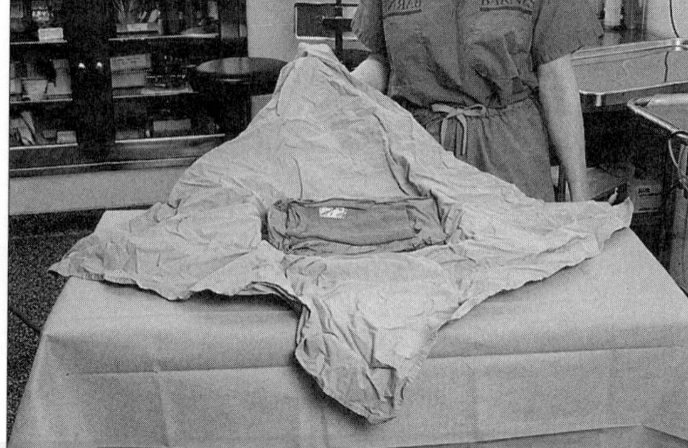

STEP **4b(2)** Open linen-wrapped sterile package.

STEP	RATIONALE
(3) Use opened package wrapper as sterile field.	Inner surface of wrapper is considered sterile.
c. Sterile drape	
(1) Place pack containing sterile drape on flat, dry surface and open as described (see Steps 4a(2) through 4a(9)) for sterile package.	Ensures sterility of packaged drape.
(2) Apply sterile gloves (optional, see agency policy).	A sterile object remains sterile only when touched by another sterile object.
(3) Grasp folded top edge of drape with fingertips of one hand. Gently lift drape up from its wrapper without touching any object.	If a sterile object touches any nonsterile object, it becomes contaminated.
(4) Allow drape to unfold, keeping it above waist and work surface and away from body. (Discard wrapper with other hand.)	Object held below person's waist is contaminated.
(5) With other hand, grasp adjacent corner of drape. Hold drape straight over work surface (see illustration).	Drape can now be properly placed with two hands.

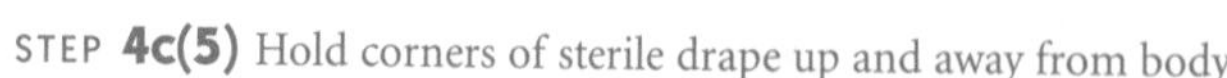

STEP **4c(5)** Hold corners of sterile drape up and away from body.

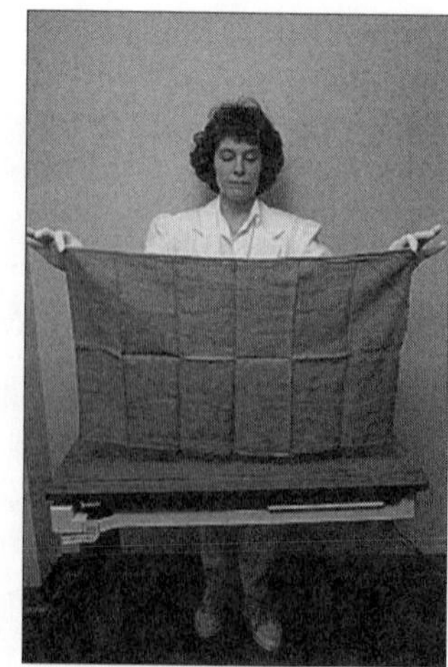

STEP	RATIONALE
(6) Holding drape, first position the bottom half over top half of intended work surface (see illustration).	Prevents nurse from reaching over sterile field.
(7) Then allow top half of drape to be placed over bottom half of work surface (see illustration). A flat draped area is now available for placement of sterile supplies.	Creates flat sterile work surface.

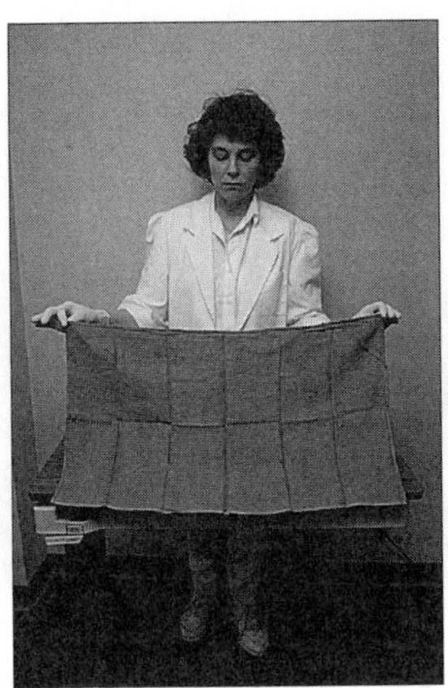

STEP **4c(6)** Position bottom half of sterile drape over top half of work surface.

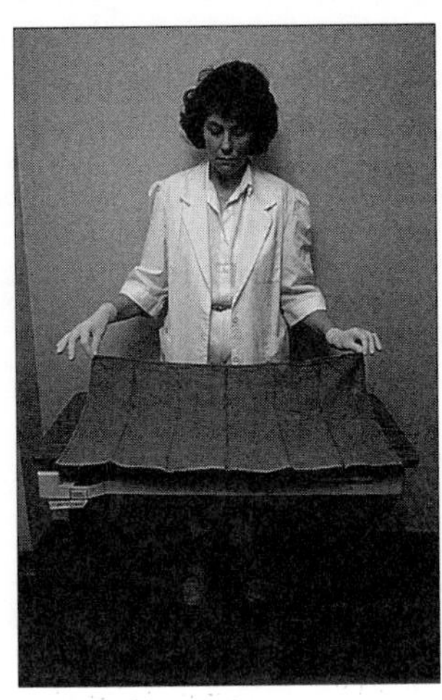

STEP **4c(7)** Allow top half of drape to be placed over bottom half of work surface.

STEP	RATIONALE
5. Adding sterile items	
a. Open sterile item (following package directions) while holding outside wrapper in nondominant hand.	Frees dominant hand for unwrapping outer wrapper.
b. Carefully peel wrapper over nondominant hand.	Item remains sterile. Inner surface of wrapper covers hand, making it sterile.
c. Being sure wrapper does not fall down on sterile field, place item onto field at an angle (see illustration). Do not hold arm over sterile field.	Secured wrapper edges prevent flipping wrapper and contaminating contents of sterile field (AORN, 1996).
• ***Critical Decision Point*** *Do not flip or throw objects onto sterile field.*	
d. Dispose of outer wrapper.	Prevents accidental contamination of sterile field.

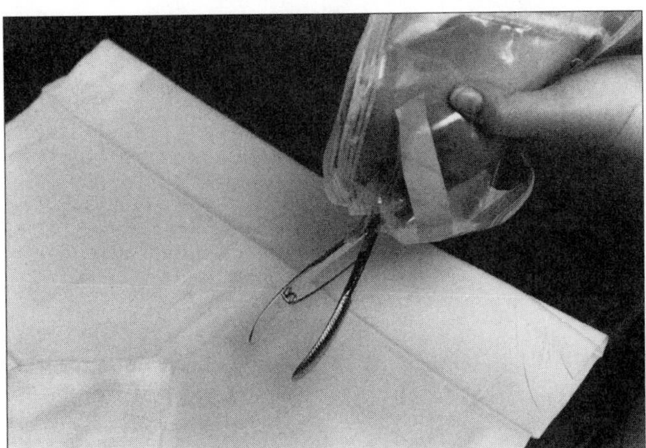

STEP **5c** Adding item to sterile field.

STEP	RATIONALE
6. Pouring sterile solutions	
a. Verify contents and expiration date of solution.	Ensures proper solution and sterility of contents.
b. Be sure receptacle for solution is located near table/work surface edge. Sterile kits have cups or plastic molded sections into which fluids can be poured.	Prevents reaching over sterile field during pouring of solution.
c. Remove seal and cap from bottle in an upward motion.	Prevents contamination of the bottle lip.
d. With solution bottle held away from field and bottle lip above inside of sterile receiving container, slowly pour entire contents of solution container (see illustration).	Edge and outside of bottle are considered contaminated. Slow pouring prevents splashing. Sterility of contents cannot be ensured if cap is replaced.

• ***Critical Decision Point***

*When liquids permeate sterile field or barrier, it is called **strike through,** resulting in contamination.*

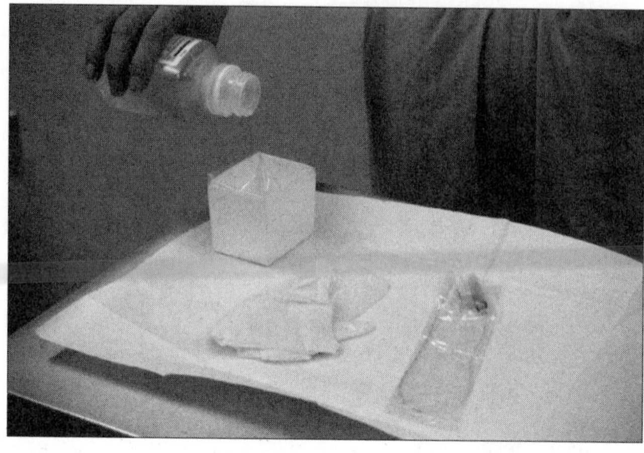

STEP **6d** Pouring solution into receiving container on sterile field.

EVALUATION

1. Observe for break in sterile technique.	Break in sterile field requires the nurse to set up new sterile field.

UNEXPECTED OUTCOMES AND RELATED INTERVENTIONS

- Sterile field comes in contact with contaminated object or liquid splatters onto drape causing strike through.
  - Discontinue field preparation and start over with new equipment.
- Sterile item falls off sterile field.
  - Open package containing new sterile item and add to field, unless field becomes contaminated.

RECORDING AND REPORTING

- No recording or reporting is required for this set of skills. Record sterile procedure performed in nurses' progress notes, and describe client's status, for example, condition of surgical site, appearance of intravenous central catheter site.

HOME CARE CONSIDERATIONS

- In the home setting most care will be performed in a clean environment. In the event that a sterile environment is ordered, client and family need to be aware of the principles that apply to the sterile environment. For example, family can be taught how to correctly use package wrapper as a sterile drape/barrier when applying a sterile dressing, or family can be taught correct procedure for removing sterile item from package without contaminating item.
- Assess client's and family's understanding and ability to provide a sterile environment when needed to perform a specific procedure.

Skill 32-3 Open Gloving

Gloves help prevent the transmission of pathogens by direct and indirect contact. Nurses apply sterile gloves before performing sterile procedures such as inserting urinary catheters, changing dressings on central intravenous (IV) catheters, or applying sterile dressings. It is important to select the proper-size glove. The gloves should not stretch so tightly over the fingers that they can easily tear, yet they should be tight enough that objects can be picked up easily. Sterile gloves are available in sizes, such as sizes 6, 6 ½, and 7. However, in most clinical areas sterile gloves in "one size fits all" are available.

It is important to choose not only the right size of glove but also the correct material. Many clients and health care workers have known allergies to latex, the natural rubber used in most gloves and other medical products (Association for Professionals in Infection Control and Epidemiology, Inc., 1996). Box 32-2 lists individuals who are at risk for latex allergy. Latex proteins enter the body in various ways—through skin or mucous membranes, intravascularly, or via inhalation. The cornstarch powder used to make latex gloves slip on easily over the hands is a carrier of the latex proteins (Burt, 1998). When gloves are applied or removed, the cornstarch particles become airborne and can remain so for hours. The latex can then be inhaled or settle on clothing, skin, or mucous membranes. Reactions to latex can be mild to severe (Box 32-3). For individuals at high risk or with suspected sensitivity to latex, it is important to choose latex-free or synthetic gloves. More health care institutions are implementing latex-safe environments for workers (Kim and others, 1998).

Once gloves are applied, the nurse should always be conscious of the position of the hands during procedures. If a sterile glove touches a clean, a contaminated, or a questionably contaminated object, it becomes unsterile. It is helpful to interlock the fingers and hold the hands together in front of the body and above waist level while waiting to handle sterile items. If a tear develops in a sterile glove, the nurse applies a new glove immediately.

Box 32-2 Individuals at Risk for Latex Allergy

Spina bifida.
Congenital or urogenital defects.
History of indwelling catheters or repeated catheterizations.
History of using condom catheters.
High latex exposure (e.g., health care workers, housekeepers, food handlers, tire manufacturers, workers in industries that use gloves routinely).
History of multiple childhood surgeries.
History of food allergies.

Modified from Gritter M: The latex threat, *Am J Nurs* 98(9):26, 1998; and Kim KT and others: Implementation recommendations for making health care facilities latex safe, *AORN J* 67(3):615, 1998.

Box 32-3 Levels of Latex Reactions

Contact dermatitis—a nonallergic response characterized by skin redness and itching.
Type IV hypersensitivity—cell-mediated allergic reaction to chemicals used in latex processing. Reaction can be delayed up to 48 hours, including redness, itching, and hives. Localized swelling, red and itchy or runny eyes and nose, and coughing may develop.
Type I hypersensitivity—a true latex allergy that can be life-threatening. Reactions vary based on type of latex protein and degree of individual sensitivity, including local and systemic. Symptoms include hives, generalized edema, itching, rash, wheezing, bronchospasm, difficulty breathing, laryngeal edema, diarrhea, nausea, hypotension, tachycardia, and respiratory or cardiac arrest.

Modified from Gritter M: The latex threat, *Am J Nurs* 98(9):26, 1998.

Delegation Considerations

The skill of applying and removing sterile gloves can be delegated to assistive personnel. However, many procedures that require the use of sterile gloves cannot be delegated to assistive personnel. (Refer to specific skill for recommendations.)

Equipment

- Package of proper-size sterile gloves; latex or synthetic nonlatex (NOTE: Hypoallergenic, low-powder, and low-protein latex gloves may still contain enough protein to cause an allergic reaction [Burt, 1998])

Step	Rationale
ASSESSMENT	
1. Consider the type of procedure to be performed, and consult institutional policy on use of sterile gloves.	Ensures proper use of sterile gloves when needed.
2. Consider client's risk for infection. For example, preexisting condition and size or extent of area being treated.	Directs nurse to follow added precautions (e.g., use of additional protective barriers) if necessary.
3. Examine glove package to determine if it is dry and intact.	Torn or wet package is considered contaminated.
4. Inspect condition of hands for cuts, open lesions, or abrasions. Lesions harbor microorganisms and should be covered with an impervious dressing.	When strict surgical asepsis is used, presence of such lesions may prevent nurse from participating in procedure.
5. Assess client for the following risk factors before applying latex gloves: a. Previous reaction to the following items within hours of exposure: adhesive tape, dental or face mask, golf club grip, ostomy bag, rubber band, balloon, bandage, elastic underwear, IV tubing, rubber gloves, condom. b. Personal history of asthma, contact dermatitis, eczema, urticaria, rhinitis. c. History of food allergies, especially avocado, banana, peach, chestnut, raw potato, kiwi, tomato, papaya. d. Previous history of adverse reactions during surgery, dental procedure. e. Previous reaction to latex product.	Determines level of client's risk for latex allergy.

NURSING DIAGNOSIS

Defining characteristics from the assessment data may reveal the following nursing diagnoses for clients requiring this skill:

- Risk for infection
- Risk for injury
- Ineffective protection

Related factors are individualized based on client's condition or needs.

Step	Rationale
PLANNING	
1. **Expected outcomes** following completion of procedure:	
▪ Client will not develop signs or symptoms of infection after procedure.	Indicates microorganisms not introduced into sterile body cavities or sites (such as skin or urinary tract).
▪ Client will not develop latex sensitivity or **latex allergy reaction.**	Client at risk for latex allergy is not exposed to latex proteins.
2. Select correct fit and type of gloves.	There is less chance of contamination if correct size of gloves is worn.

• ***Critical Decision Point***

Synthetic nonlatex gloves are necessary for clients at risk or if nurse has sensitivity or allergy to latex.

Step	Rationale
3. Place glove package near work area.	Ensures availability before procedure.

STEP	RATIONALE

IMPLEMENTATION

1. Glove application
   a. Perform thorough hand washing. — Reduces number of bacteria on skin surfaces and reduces transmission of infection.
   b. Remove outer glove package wrapper by carefully separating and peeling apart sides (see illustration). — Prevents inner glove package from accidentally opening and touching contaminated objects.

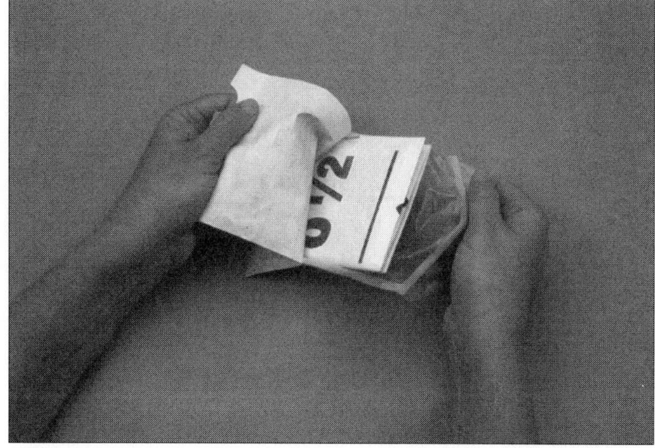

STEP **1b** Open outer glove package wrapper.

   c. Grasp inner package and lay it on clean, dry, flat surface at waist level. Open package, keeping gloves on wrapper's inside surface (see illustration). — Sterile object held below waist is contaminated. Inner surface of glove package is sterile.
   d. Identify right and left glove. Each glove has a cuff approximately 5 cm (2 inches) wide. Glove dominant hand first. — Proper identification of gloves prevents contamination by improper fit. Gloving of dominant hand first improves dexterity.
   e. With thumb and first two fingers of nondominant hand, grasp edge of cuff of glove for dominant hand. Touch only glove's inside surface (see illustration). — Inner edge of cuff will lie against skin and thus is not sterile.

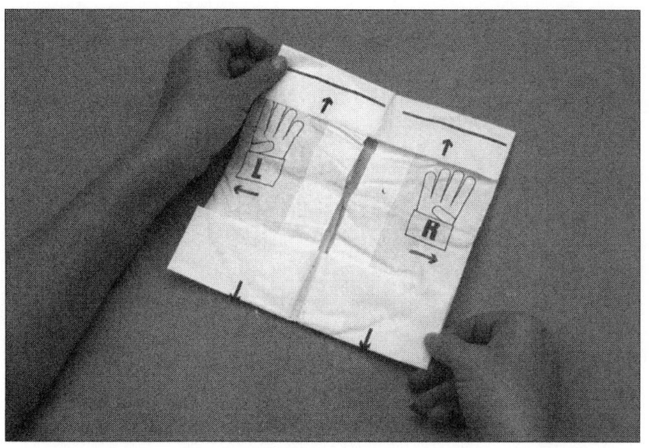

STEP **1c** Open inner glove package on work surface.

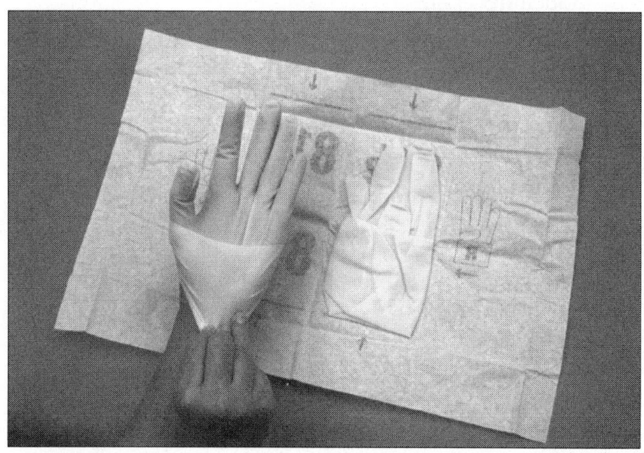

STEP **1e** Pick up glove for dominant hand and insert fingers, pull glove completely over dominant hand.

STEP	RATIONALE

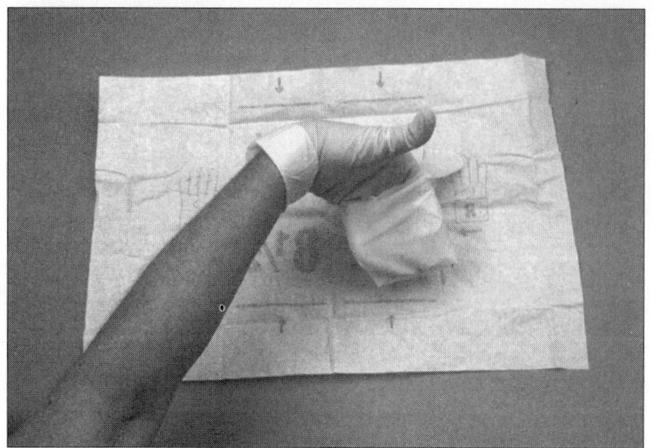

STEP **1g** Pick up glove for nondominant hand.

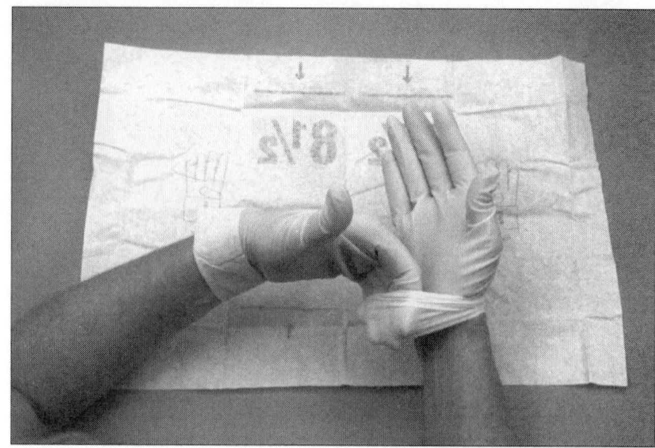

STEP **1h** Pull second glove over nondominant hand.

STEP	RATIONALE
f. Carefully pull glove over dominant hand, leaving cuff and being sure cuff does not roll up wrist. Be sure thumb and fingers are in proper spaces (see illustration for Step 1e).	If glove's outer surface touches hand or wrist, it is contaminated.
g. With gloved dominant hand, slip fingers underneath second glove's cuff (see illustration).	Cuff protects gloved fingers. Sterile touching sterile prevents glove contamination.
h. Carefully pull second glove over nondominant hand (see illustration).	Contact of gloved hand with exposed hand results in contamination.

• ***Critical Decision Point***

Do not allow fingers and thumb of gloved dominant hand to touch any part of exposed nondominant hand. Keep thumb of dominant hand abducted back.

STEP	RATIONALE
i. After second glove is on, interlock hands together, above waist level. The cuffs usually fall down after application. Be sure to touch only sterile sides (see illustration).	Ensures smooth fit over fingers.
2. Glove disposal	
a. Grasp outside of one cuff with other gloved hand; avoid touching wrist.	Minimizes contamination of underlying skin.
b. Pull glove off, turning it inside out. Discard in receptacle (see illustration).	Outside of glove does not touch skin surface.
c. Take fingers of bare hand and tuck inside remaining glove cuff. Peel glove off inside out. Discard in receptacle.	Fingers do not touch contaminated glove surface.
d. Wash hands thoroughly.	This protects health care worker from contamination resulting from any unseen tears or pinholes in gloves, also removing powder from hands helps to prevent skin irritations.

STEP	RATIONALE

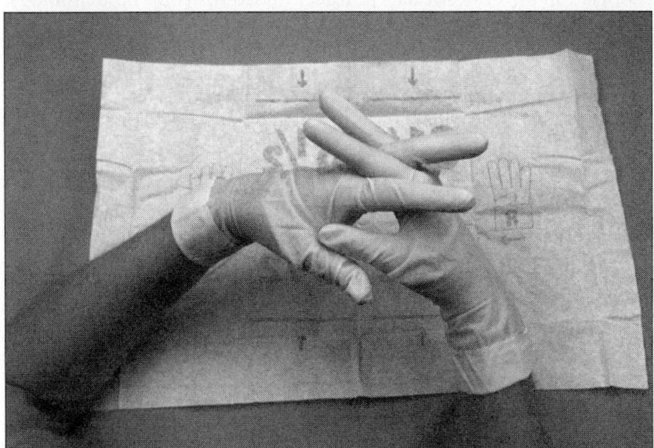

STEP **1i** Interlock gloved hands.

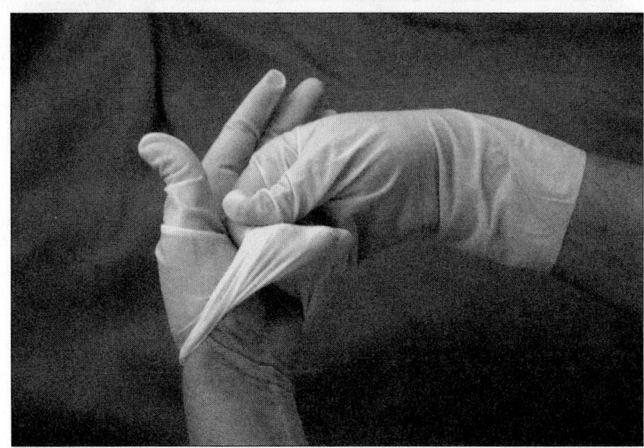

STEP **2b** Carefully remove first glove by turning it inside out.

EVALUATION

1. Assess client for signs of infection, focusing on area treated. — Improper technique may contribute to development of an infection.

UNEXPECTED OUTCOMES AND RELATED INTERVENTIONS

- Client develops localized signs of infection—for example, urine becomes cloudy or odorous; wound becomes painful, edematous, reddened with purulent drainage.
  - Contact physician and implement appropriate treatments as ordered.
- Client develops systemic signs of infection—for example, fever, malaise, increased white blood cell count.
  - Contact physician and implement appropriate treatments as ordered.
- Client develops allergic reaction to latex (see Box 32-3).
  - Immediately remove source of latex.
  - Bring emergency equipment to bedside. Have epinephrine injection ready for administration, and be prepared to initiate IV fluids and oxygen.

RECORDING AND REPORTING

- It is not necessary to record application of gloves. Record specific procedure performed and client's response and status.
- In the event of a latex allergy reaction, record client's response in nurses' notes and vital sign flow sheet. Note type of response and client's reaction to emergency treatment.

TEACHING CONSIDERATIONS

- Nurse or client with a known latex allergy should wear a medical alert bracelet or tag and carry a wallet card stating "latex allergy."
- Individuals with known latex allergies should carry a quick-acting oral antihistamine and an epinephrine autoinjector at all times.

Critical Thinking Exercises

1. Jean is a student nurse preparing to change a client's surgical wound dressing. She has opened her sterile dressings and prepared the appropriate topical solutions for cleansing the wound. Just before she begins to apply sterile gloves a student colleague comes to the door and asks Jean to help her move a client. What should Jean do?
2. You observe a nurse colleague preparing a sterile field for an indwelling catheter insertion. The nurse begins to pour a solution into the plastic container inside the catheter kit. You notice that the container is positioned in the center of the sterile field. Is there a potential problem? If so, what might you do?
3. Why do you remove gloves before removing your mask following completion of a sterile procedure?
4. The nurse enters the client's room to begin a series of procedures: measurement of urine for intake and output, irrigation of a nasogastric tube, insertion of a peripheral intravenous catheter, and measurement of the client's blood pressure. Which procedure requires use of sterile gloves?

References

Association for Professionals in Infection Control and Epidemiology, Inc: *APIC infection control and applied epidemiology,* St. Louis, 1996, Mosby.

Association of Operating Room Nurses. Recommended practices for maintaining a sterile field, *AORN Journal* 64(5):811, 1996.

Burt S: What you need to know about latex allergy, *Nursing* 28(10): 33, 1998.

Centers for Disease Control and Prevention, Hospital Infection Control Practice Advisory Committee: Guidelines for isolation precautions in hospitals, *Am J Infect Control* 24:24, 1996.

Crow S, Planchock N, Hendrick E: Antisepsis: disinfection and sterilization. In Soule B, Larson E, Preston G, editors: *Infection and nursing practice: prevention and control,* St. Louis, 1995, Mosby.

Gritter M: The latex threat, *Am J Nurs* 98(9):26, 1998.

Kim KT and others: Implementation recommendations for making health care facilities latex safe, *AORN J* 67(3):615, 1998.

Meeker MH, Rothrock JC: *Alexander's care of the patient in surgery,* ed 11, St. Louis, 1999, Mosby.

Roth A: Infection prevention in the operating room, *Asepsis* 18(1):12, 1996.

Soule B, Larson E, Preston G, editors: *Infection and nursing practice: prevention and control,* St. Louis, 1995, Mosby.

33

Preoperative and Postoperative Care

Skills

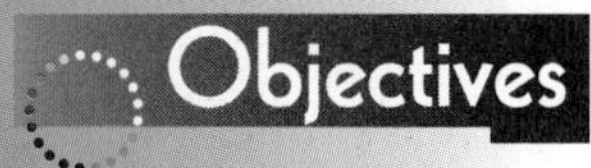

Objectives

Mastery of content in this chapter will enable the nurse to:

- Define the key terms listed.
- Describe the activities needed to prepare a client for surgery.
- Explain the rationale for preoperative procedures.
- Discuss cultural differences that might affect the implementation of preoperative and postoperative procedures.
- Adequately prepare a client for surgery.
- Describe the benefits of structured preoperative teaching.
- Explain the rationale for each of the four postoperative exercises.
- Successfully instruct a client in performing postoperative exercises.
- Identify the benefits and risks associated with shaving a surgical site.
- Correctly prepare a surgical site.
- Discuss the differences in nursing assessment during the immediate postoperative period and the convalescent phase of recovery.
- Conduct an assessment of a postoperative client.

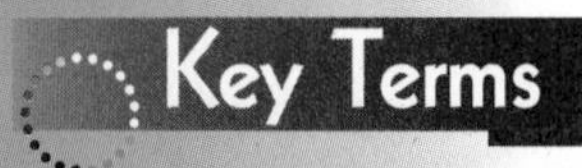

Key Terms

Analgesia
Anesthesia
Aspiration
Atelectasis
Coagulopathies
Conscious sedation
Decompression
Dehiscence
Ecchymosis
Evisceration
Hemostasis
Hemovac drain
Homans' sign
Hypovolemic shock
Incentive spirometer
Informed consent
Jackson-Pratt drain
Malignant hyperthermia
Paralytic ileus
Penrose drain
Phlebothrombosis
Postanesthesia care unit (PACU)
Postoperative
Postural hypotension
Preoperative
Preoperative checklist
Pulmonary edema
Renal insufficiency
Thrombophlebitis
Urinary retention
Venous thrombosis

Any form of surgery is a stressful event, whether it is a major surgical procedure occurring in a large medical center or a minor procedure taking place in an outpatient center. The client must frequently make the decision to undergo a procedure that is associated with pain, possible disfigurement, dependence, or even the threat of death. Physiologically, the more complex the surgery, the more likely a client will undergo changes in most major body systems. The nurse uses a variety of skills to help the surgical client adequately prepare for the physiological and psychological stressors of surgery.

During the **preoperative** phase the nurse performs a thorough assessment of the client's physical and emotional status. Coordination of a variety of diagnostic tests ensures that the surgeon and the anesthesia care provider have the information needed to determine the client's risks during surgery and the postoperative period. In preparation for surgery, the nurse instructs the client and family concerning **postoperative** care in compliance with the Joint Commission on Accreditation of Health Organizations (JCAHO) client and family education standards (Box 33-1). This enables the client and family to actively participate in the recovery process. Certain procedures, such as surgical skin preparation (see Skill 33-3), the insertion of an indwelling catheter (see Chapter 24) or nasogastric (NG) tube (see Chapter 25), may be performed to protect the client from risks associated with surgery.

It is imperative that the nurse inquire about cultural practices and religious beliefs that may alter the client's

Box 33-1 JCAHO Client and Family Education Standards

The client's learning needs, abilities, preferences, and readiness to learn are assessed.

The assessment considers cultural and religious practices, emotional barriers, desire and motivation to learn, physical and cognitive limitations, language barriers, and the financial implications of care choices.

When called for by the age of the client and the length of stay, the hospital assesses and provides for client's academic education needs.

Clients are educated about the safe and effective use of medication, according to law and their needs.

Clients are educated about the safe and effective use of medical equipment.

Clients are educated about potential drug-food interactions, and are provided counseling on nutrition and modified diets.

Clients are educated about rehabilitation techniques to help them adapt or function more independently in their environment.

Clients are informed about access to additional resources in the community.

Clients are informed about when and how to obtain any further treatment they may need.

Modified from Joint Commission on Accreditation of Healthcare Organizations: *Accreditation manual for hospitals,* Chicago, 1997, The Commission.

and/or family's acceptance of perioperative teaching and procedures. The nurse remains nonjudgmental and adapts the client's care to encompass these practices and beliefs whenever possible. Each client's plan of care is individualized to provide an improved state of wellness and to maximize the ultimate level of independence. The nurse also communicates pertinent information to all members of the health care team so that the client receives comprehensive and holistic care.

During the postoperative phase, when the client returns from the operating room (OR), the nurse is initially responsible for assessing the client's physical status to monitor any changes during the recovery process. Once the client's condition stabilizes, the nurse focuses efforts on returning the client to a functional level of wellness as soon as possible within the limitations created by surgery. The speed of a client's recovery depends on how effectively the nurse can anticipate potential complications, initiate necessary supportive and preventive therapies, and actively involve the client and family in the recovery process.

If the client is to be admitted for same-day surgery, the preoperative assessment and teaching of postoperative exercises may be done several days prior to surgery. This may be done by the surgeon's office nurse or, more typically, by the preoperative nurse in the outpatient department. The nurse obtains the client's signature on the operative permits and sees that blood work, electrocardiogram (ECG), and any other ordered procedures are done.

Skill Performance Guidelines

1. Know the type and nature of any previous surgery. Anatomical and physiological alterations may affect the client's health care needs.
2. Identify the factors and conditions that may increase a client's risks during surgery. Preoperative preparation and postoperative care depend upon the knowledge of these risk factors.
3. Know the rationale for and extent of impending surgery. Each type of surgical procedure requires a different type of nursing care.
4. Administer pain relief therapies according to the client's needs perioperatively. Pain can slow the surgical client's recovery.
5. Encourage the client's independence as soon as possible during the postoperative period. This minimizes the occurrence of postoperative complications.
6. Anticipate how surgery will affect the client's ability to return home to a functional lifestyle. Early discharge planning, client education, referral to community resources, and rehabilitation measures are needed to prepare the client to return home.
7. Identify cultural and religious beliefs and practices that may affect clients' and/or family members' reactions to the surgical experience, such as who can give consent, blood transfusions, and disposal of body parts, including hair.

Skill 33-1 Preparing the Client for Surgery

Preparing the client for surgery involves activities and procedures that help to decrease anxiety, to ensure client safety, and to decrease the risks of complications. A thorough nursing assessment is needed to document baseline data for future comparisons, to determine teaching needs, and to identify clients at risk for complications during the perioperative experience.

Anxiety can interfere with the effectiveness of **anesthesia** and the ability of clients to actively participate in their care. The nurse provides information to clients about what will occur during the perioperative experience, as well as what sensations the client can expect to feel. Knowing that medication for nausea and **analgesia** will be prescribed as needed will help to decrease the client's anxiety. Demonstration of a caring attitude toward the client, family members, and significant others can increase feelings of trust and reduce anxiety (Figure 33-1). Sedatives are frequently prescribed to inpatients to aid in sleep the night before surgery, and preoperative medications are administered the day of surgery to promote relaxation.

Client safety is ensured through a number of interventions and activities. **Informed consent** is required by law to help protect clients' rights, their autonomy, and their privacy. Failure to obtain informed consent may result in charges of "assault and battery or negligence" (Brick, 1996) being brought against the health care providers. The client should be given information by the surgeon about the extent and type of

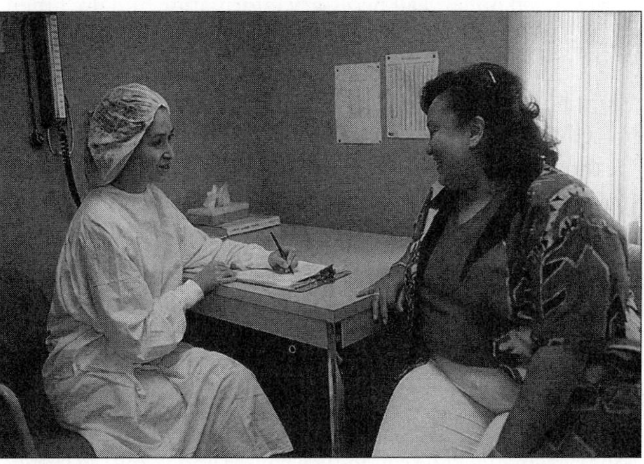

FIGURE 33-1 Nurse establishes a trusting relationship with client.

Table 33-1 Information Needed for Informed Consent

PARAMETERS	EXAMPLES
Name of procedure/surgery	Abdominal hysterectomy under general anesthesia.
Description of procedure/surgery	Removal of uterus only through an incision in the abdominal wall at the top of the pubic hairline done while unconscious.
Person performing the procedure/surgery	Doctor Richard Jones assisted by Doctor William Smith.
Benefits of procedure/surgery	To remove uterus with fibroids and stop excessive bleeding. Abdominal route is necessary due to anticipated adhesions from prior abdominal surgery.
Potential risks and adverse effects of procedure/surgery	Risks of hemorrhage and infection from surgery, risks of excessive sedation and allergic reaction to drugs used with general anesthesia, accidental damage to bladder, intestines, and/or nerves controlling these organs.
Approximate length of time for procedure/surgery	About 1 hour; 1 to 2 hours in recovery room.
Approximate length of time needed for recovery	3 to 4 days on surgical unit; 4 to 6 weeks before resuming physically stressful work.
Alternative treatments	Removal of uterus vaginally, radiation to shrink fibroids.
Consequences of refusing treatment	Continuation of pain and vaginal bleeding, risk of developing anemia. After menopause, fibroids should regress.

surgery, alternative therapies, usual risks and benefits and consequences of not having surgery in a nonthreatening manner as outlined in *A Patient's Bill of Rights* developed by the American Hospital Association (Dunn, 1999) (Table 33-1). The client or the client's legal guardian must sign a surgical consent form that includes this information. If the client's cultural practices include male dominance, as in most Asian and Middle Eastern cultures (Geissler, 1998), the female client and her husband, father, or oldest brother may also need to sign the consent. The consent must also be signed by a witness to verify that the person who signed the consent is the client so named or his legal guardian. It is the nurse's ethical (not legal) responsibility, acting as the client's advocate, to ensure that the client understands the information and that the form has been signed and witnessed before the client receives preoperative medication.

Client safety is also promoted by restricting activity after administration of sedatives and by completion of a **preoperative checklist** (Figure 33-2) to ensure that all procedures have been carried out and all necessary information and documentation for safe delivery of care is in the client's chart.

The risks for postoperative complications are decreased in a number of ways, some of which are specific to the type of procedure. For example, any client with a surgical incision of the thorax or abdomen will be encouraged to use an **incentive spirometer** postoperatively to reduce the incidence of **atelectasis.** Skin preparation and deep breathing and coughing exercises are examples of other procedures used to reduce complications. Food and fluids are usually withheld for 4 to 8 hours before surgery requiring general anesthesia to minimize the risk of **aspiration.** The client may need to be allowed nothing by mouth (NPO) even when spinal or epidural anesthesia is administered. Hypotension due to autonomic nervous system blockade can induce nausea and vomiting (Lewis, Heitkemper, and Dirkson, 2000). Clients who are dehydrated or are at risk for hypovolemia will have intravenous fluids ordered. Medications may be given to decrease respiratory and gastrointestinal (GI) secretions, as an adjunct to anesthesia, and to decrease the risk of infection and development of stress ulcers. Low-residue and clear liquid diets, enemas, and cathartics are ordered for clients before undergoing bowel surgery. Povidone-iodine douches may be used before many gynecological procedures. Eye drops may need to be instilled before ophthalmic surgery. Clients who smoke should be encouraged to stop the use of all tobacco products for at least 30 days before surgery. Nicotine delays wound healing and increases the risk of wound infection by constricting blood flow (Centers for Disease Control and Prevention [CDC], 1999). Clients whose blood work indicates a low hemoglobin level and/or abnormal electrolyte levels or **coagulopathies** may require inpatient therapy before surgery.

Because many clients are admitted on the day of surgery, much of the preoperative preparation is often the responsibility of the client or the primary caregiver. It is important therefore that the hospital preadmission nurse or a nurse in the surgeon's practice be designated to provide adequate instructions. This client teaching should include any food and fluid restrictions, which medications, if any, are permitted on the morning of surgery and the need for surgical site preparation, such as enemas, laxatives, or skin cleansing the evening before surgery. It is also important to include action to be taken if any of these instructions are mistakenly omitted. Written instructions are a useful adjunct to teaching because the client and/or family can refer to them for any points that are unclear or forgotten. Videos and pamphlets are also useful adjuncts in preparing clients and their families. The admitting nurse in the surgical unit must assess the client's adherence to instructions.

A-1c PREOPERATIVE/PREPROCEDURAL CHECKLIST

• File with other A-1c's of same date. •

PROCEDURE: ______

DATE OF PROCEDURE: ______

1. Place initials in appropriate box: YES, NO, N/A (not applicable, or was not ordered). Each item must have an entry.
2. Explain any "No." This can be done in the space after the item or in the "Comments" section. Use back of form, if needed.
3. To give more information on any item, use the space after the item. If more space is needed, use the "Comments" section or back of form.

DATE

HOSP. NO.

NAME

BIRTHDATE

ADDRESS

IF NOT IMPRINTED, PLEASE PRINT DATE, HOSP. NO., NAME AND LOCATION.

YES	NO	N/A	
			Special information (e.g., blind, O_2, combative)
			Preoperative orders written.
			(If "NO", Dr. ______ notivied at ______ date/time.)
			Consent complete and in medical record.
			Allergies (or NKA) labelled on cover of medical record.
			Specify Allergies:
			Isolation label on cover of medical record. Specify type.
			Ordered lab results in medical record.
			Urinalysis results in medical record.
			Chest x-ray completed. (Report in medical record: Yes____ No____)
			EKG in medical record.
			Type and cross/screen (circle) done. Date drawn:
			History and physical in medical record.
			Forms complete and in medical record:
			1. Nursing documentation with assessment, VS, and wt./ht.
			2. IV Solution Administration Cardex.
			3. Medication Administration Cardex.
			Addressograph plate on cover of medical record. All volumes to procedure, if required.
COMMENTS:			
			Blood band on patient and legible. Specify location ______ and blood band #______
			Identification band on patient and legible. Specify location:
			Bathed and in proper attire.
			Nail polish, makeup, and hairpins removed.
			Jewelry removed. Specify item(s) removed and disposition:
			Prosthesis removed: hearing aid, dentures, eye glasses, contact lenses (circle).
			Other: Disposition:
			Anti-embolism stockings on.
			Sequential compression device sleeves on and controller to OR.
			NPO since:
			Teaching completed and documented.
			Preps/tests completed as ordered. Specify:
			Voided/catheterized (circle). Time:
			Medication(s) given.
			Medication(s)/article(s) sent with patient. Specify:
COMMENTS:			

Date	Initials	Signature and Title of Individuals Filling Out Form
Date	**Initials**	**Signature of RN Sending Patient to Procedure**

41006/4-93/H7528 THE UNIVERSITY OF IOWA HOSPITALS AND CLINICS

A 1c | B CLIN. NOTES | C LABORATORY | D XRAY EXAM | E CONSULTATION | F SPEC. EXAM | G THERAPY | H PATHOLOGY | I DIAGNOSIS

FIGURE **33-2** Preoperative/preprocedural checklist. (Courtesy University of Iowa Hospitals and Clinics.)

Delegation Considerations

The skills of assessment and teaching that are part of preparing the client for surgery should not be delegated to assistive personnel. Assistive personnel may administer an enema or a douche, obtain vital signs, apply antiembolism stockings, and assist clients in removing clothing, jewelry, and prostheses. Personnel should be instructed in any precautions needed for assigned client.

Equipment

- Stethoscope
- Informed consent form
- Preoperative checklist
- Enema set and prescribed solution (if ordered—see Chapter 25)
- Douche set and prescribed solution (if ordered)
- Intravenous (IV) solutions and equipment (if ordered—see Chapter 19)
- Indwelling catheter set (if ordered—see Chapter 24)
- Antiembolism stockings (if ordered—see Skill 28-3)
- Medications (if ordered—see Chapter 18)

Step	Rationale
Assessment	
1. Determine ability of client to answer questions regarding health history and pending surgery.	Identifies reliability of client and need to supplement with information from family members or significant others. May indicate need for further information for informed consent.
2. Obtain nursing history (Table 33-2).	Provides information regarding risk factors and past patterns of behavior.
3. Perform physical examination (see Table 33-2 and Chapter 10).	Provides baseline data for future assessments and interventions. Also confirms or disputes information from history and may uncover new information.

- ***Critical Decision Point***

  If client is having emergency surgery, nurse focuses on assessment of primary body systems affected.

Step	Rationale
4. Identify risk factors (see Table 33-2).	Allows for anticipation of possible complications and planning for interventions to reduce risks. Allergies, particularly to latex, can be life threatening.
5. Ask about client's and family members' expectations of surgery and care to be provided. Include questions concerning fears, cultural practices, and religious beliefs, if applicable.	Allows nurse to anticipate client's/family's priorities and to adapt plan so that appropriate instruction and support can be given.
6. Assess client's preoperative orders.	Identifies specific procedures and diagnostic tests to be done and medications to be given.

Nursing Diagnosis

Defining characteristics from the assessment data may reveal the following nursing diagnoses for clients requiring this skill:

Anxiety
Fear
Disturbed body image
Risk for infection
Ineffective airway clearance
Ineffective breathing pattern
Impaired gas exchange
Acute pain
Ineffective tissue perfusion
Risk for aspiration
Impaired physical mobility
Deficient knowledge regarding the surgical experience
Risk for impaired skin integrity
Impaired oral mucous membrane
Risk for perioperative-positioning injury

Related factors are individualized based on client's condition or needs.

Table 33-2 Assessment of the Surgical Client

Assessment Category	Key Criteria
Nursing history	Previous personal/family experience with surgery and anesthesia (malignant hyperthermia)
Physical examination	Client's and family's perceptions and understanding of surgery
Risk factors	Medication history (prescription, over-the-counter [OTC], and herbal remedies)
	Physical or mental impairments
	Mobility limitations
	Prostheses (including hearing aids)
	Allergies (including drugs, food, latex, and environmental)
	Smoking habits
	Alcohol ingestion
	Family support and coping mechanisms
	Occupation
	Emotional health
	Temperature, blood pressure, pulse and respiratory rates
	Height and weight
	Oxygen saturation
	Electrocardiogram
	Laboratory values (e.g., Hgb, K+, glucose, coagulation studies)
	Radiology and diagnostic test findings
	General system review:
	Head and neck
	Integument
	Thorax and lungs
	Heart and vascular
	Abdomen
	Neurological status
	Age
	Nutrition
	Radiotherapy, chemotherapy, medications that depress immune system
	Fluid and electrolyte balance
	Preexisting infection
	Chronic respiratory disease (emphysema, bronchitis, asthma)
	Immunological disorders (leukemia, acquired immunodeficiency syndrome)
	Allergies (drugs, food, latex, or other environmental factors)

Step	Rationale
Planning	
1. **Expected outcomes** following completion of procedure:	
▪ Client can state what surgical procedure is being performed and risks and benefits of surgery.	Identifies readiness to sign informed consent.
▪ Client participates in preoperative and postoperative care.	Preoperative preparations were effective.
▪ Client states anxiety is decreased.	Anxiety may interfere with effectiveness of teaching and of anesthesia.
2. Prepare client's chart using preoperative checklist, and assemble equipment as needed.	Ensures that all preoperative procedures will be completed.
3. Explain procedures, and allow client, family members, and significant others to ask questions and express concerns.	Decreases anxiety and increases cooperation.

STEP	RATIONALE

IMPLEMENTATION

Step	Rationale
1. Orient client to room or presurgical (holding) area.	Decreases anxiety and promotes feelings of control.
2. Assist with informed consent. Act as client advocate as needed, including any culturally sensitive issues. Witness form if allowed by agency.	Surgery cannot be legally performed without client receiving information about need and extent of the surgery, alternatives, risks, and benefits. Client and/or family may be afraid to ask questions or express concerns regarding diverse practices.
3. Check medical record, and review or complete preoperative checklist (see Figure 33-2).	Ensures that pertinent laboratory and diagnostic test results are available and that all preoperative preparations are completed.

- ***Critical Decision Point***
  Clients who are illiterate can sign with a mark if properly witnessed. Minors, unless married or declared emancipated, or individuals considered incompetent cannot legally sign a consent form. Parent or legal guardian must provide consent. Some cultures do not allow female members to give consent (Geissler, 1998).

Step	Rationale
4. Provide preoperative teaching, including explanation of postoperative exercises (see Skill 33-2), skin preparation (see Skill 33-3), pain control measures (see Chapter 5), and postoperative care in recovery room and nursing division (see Skill 33-4).	Decreases anxiety and promotes cooperation in care.
5. Instruct client on need and rationale for ingesting nothing by mouth (NPO) for 4 to 8 hours before surgery.	GI tract should be empty to decrease risk of vomiting and aspiration.

- ***Critical Decision Point***
  Client may brush teeth but should not swallow water. Client may take oral medications with sips of water (30 ml) if they are specifically ordered to be taken preoperatively (i.e., antiarrhythmic or seizure medications). All other oral medications are withheld. The nurse must check postoperative orders to ensure that scheduled medications unrelated to surgery are not forgotten.

Step	Rationale
6. Assess that any preoperative orders for enemas, douches, and skin preparations have been followed. Insert IV and/or indwelling catheter if ordered.	May delay or postpone surgery if not completed. IV and/or indwelling catheter may be inserted in holding or preanesthesia area.
7. Provide for hygiene measures, ensuring client privacy. Instruct client to remove all clothing, including undergarments, and to apply disposable cap and hospital gown with opening in back.	Prevents client's hair from contaminating sterile surfaces and provides easy access to client's body in operating room (OR).
8. Instruct client to remove hairpins, clips, wigs, hairpieces, jewelry, including rings used in body piercing, and makeup (including nail polish and acrylic nails). Religious medals may be pinned to gown if agency policy permits. In some institutions, acrylic nails or nail polish may be removed from only one finger if a pulse oximeter is used. Check institution's policy.	Hair appliances and jewelry anywhere on the body may become dislodged and cause injury during positioning and intubation (Armstrong, 1998). Rings may decrease circulation in fingers. Makeup, nail polish and false nails impede assessment of skin and oxygenation. In addition, acrylic nails may harbor pathogenic organisms (Association of Operating Room Nurses [AORN], 1999).

- ***Critical Decision Point***
  Wedding rings that cannot be removed may be taped in place. Be careful not to create tourniquet effect with tape around finger.

Step	Rationale
9. Assist client in removing prostheses, including dentures and oral appliances, glasses and contact lenses, artificial limbs and eyes, artificial eyelashes, and hearing aids. Inventory items and give to family members or have security lock them up. Document list of items and their location in preoperative checklist and/or nurses' notes per agency policy.	Prostheses can be lost or damaged during surgery and could cause injury. Oral appliances may occlude airway.

STEP	RATIONALE

- ***Critical Decision Point***
  If client will be required to follow instructions in the OR, hearing aid may be left in place. Decision may be made to leave wig or dentures in place until entering OR suite if removal will cause embarrassment. Check agency policy.

STEP	RATIONALE
10. Secure all valuables or give to family member or significant other. Have release form signed if required by agency.	Valuables may be lost or stolen.
11. Apply antiembolism stockings as ordered (see Skill 28-3)	Promotes venous return and reduces risk of thrombus formation.
12. Assess vital signs immediately before going to OR.	Abnormal vital signs may indicate conditions that increase risk for surgery.

- ***Critical Decision Point***
  Vital signs not within normal range or client's baseline must be reported to physician and may require surgery to be postponed. Document abnormal vital signs and any action taken in nurses' notes and/or preoperative checklist according to agency policy.

STEP	RATIONALE
13. If client does not have an indwelling catheter, assist him or her in voiding before receiving preoperative medication.	Prevents incontinence and bladder distention during surgery and **urinary retention** with overflow postoperatively. Preoperative medication may cause drowsiness and decreased voiding sensation.
14. Administer preoperative medications as ordered. (These medications may be given in preoperative or holding area. Check preoperative orders.)	Reduces pain, anxiety, respiratory secretions, and amount of anesthesia required. Promotes relaxation. Antibiotics may be ordered prophylactically.

- ***Critical Decision Point***
  Check that informed consent is signed before giving medications. Times on consent form and on medication administration record (MAR) must attest to this. Preoperative medications may alter level of consciousness and make the consent invalid.

STEP	RATIONALE
15. Client is placed on bed rest with side rails up and call light within reach and is told not to get out of bed without assistance.	There is an increased chance of injury in attempting to ambulate to void when client is sedated and unattended.

EVALUATION

STEP	RATIONALE
1. Have client describe surgical procedure and its benefits and risks.	Confirms level of knowledge needed to sign informed consent.
2. Compare all assessment data with client's baseline and expected normals.	Evaluates client's risk for complications and possible need to postpone surgery.
3. Have client repeat preoperative instructions and demonstrate postoperative exercises.	Provides evidence that client understands preoperative instructions and can perform exercises.
4. Monitor client for signs and symptoms of anxiety and ask how client and family are feeling.	Increased heart rate and blood pressure, dilated pupils, dry mouth, increased sweating, and muscle rigidity or shaking are responses to stress and anxiety. Asking client about feeling gives permission to express concerns, which can be further explored.

UNEXPECTED OUTCOMES AND RELATED INTERVENTIONS

- Client is unable to give consent, and family member is unavailable.
  - In emergency situations, telephone consent from next of kin may be obtained. Two persons must witness oral consent.
  - Documentation must include explanation of situation and fact that oral consent was obtained and so witnessed.
  - At the earliest opportunity, person giving oral consent must sign a written consent. Signed telegram or signed fax may also be considered oral consent. Follow agency policy.

- Vital signs are above or below client's baseline or expected range.
  - This may indicate infection, anxiety, pain, or cardiovascular dysfunction, which increases surgical risk.
  - Clients who are dehydrated or malnourished may require hydration with IV solutions (see Chapter 19), parenteral nutrition (see Chapter 23), or antibiotic therapy before surgery.
- Informed consent not signed and witnessed. Physician did not provide information and/or ensure that consent form was signed.
  - Client is not ready for surgery. Client must sign consent before administration of preoperative medications or any medication that alters central nervous system.
- Client did not remain NPO, which may indicate that the client did not understand instructions or forgot.
  - Notify surgeon and anesthesiologist. Surgery may be postponed or cancelled.
- Client unable to state instructions or demonstrate postoperative exercises.
  - Assessment of client's level of understanding or method of instruction was insufficient. Revision of instruction and reteaching is necessary.
- Client did not void prior to receiving preoperative medication.
  - Perhaps client did not need to void or was unable to void. Assess for bladder distention. If distended, client can use urinal or bedpan or may need order to be catheterized (see Chapter 24).

Recording and Reporting

- Document all preoperative preparations in nurses' notes and/or checklist.
- Document client's condition on transfer to OR in nurses' notes and/or on flow sheet.
- Report and record any abnormal assessment findings, lack of signed and witnessed consent form, or failure of client to maintain NPO status and action taken.
- Report and record client's cultural practices and/or religious beliefs that affect perioperative care and any modification of care planned.

Teaching Considerations

- JCAHO client and family education standards are guidelines that should ensure that client, family member, and/or primary caregiver be taught about surgical procedure, healing process, sutures, dressing, drains, feeding tubes, pain control, and diet with rationale for each. Adults learn best when they understand the purpose or meaning of what is being taught (JCAHO, 1997).

Box 33-2 Teaching Methods Based on Client's Developmental Capacity

Infant

Keep routines (feeding, bathing) consistent.

Hold infant firmly while smiling and speaking softly to convey sense of trust.

Have infant touch different textures (soft fabric, hard plastic).

Toddler

Use play to teach procedure or activity (handling examination equipment, applying bandage to doll).

Offer picture books that describe story of children in hospital or clinic.

Use simple words such as *cut* instead of *laceration* to promote understanding.

Preschooler

Use role playing, imitation, and play to make it fun for preschoolers to learn.

Encourage questions and offer explanations. Use simple explanations and demonstrations.

Encourage children to learn together through pictures and short stories of how to perform hygiene.

School-Age Child

Teach psychomotor skills needed to maintain health. (Complicated skills, such as learning to use a syringe, may take considerable practice.)

Offer opportunities to discuss health problems and answer questions.

Adolescent

Help adolescent learn about feelings and need for self-expression.

Use teaching as collaborative activity.

Allow adolescents to make decisions about health and health promotion (safety, sex education, substance abuse).

Use problem solving to help adolescents make choices.

Young or Middle Adult

Encourage participation in teaching plan by setting mutual goals.

Encourage independent learning.

Offer information so that adult can understand effects of health problem.

Older Adult

Teach when client is alert and rested.

Involve adult in discussion or activity.

Focus on wellness and the person's strength.

Use approaches that enhance sensorially impaired client's reception of stimuli.

Keep teaching sessions short.

PEDIATRIC CONSIDERATIONS

- Parents should be involved in preoperative preparation to decrease children's anxiety. Preadmission programs to prepare parents and children for same-day surgery have been shown to decrease anxiety in both parents and children.
- Hospital programs that involve well-prepared parents during anesthesia induction in OR "virtually eliminated the need for heavy preoperative sedation—and shortened the child's postop recovery period" (Fennell, 1999).
- Preoperative preparation should take into consideration developmental level of child; for example, toys and games may be used to demonstrate preoperative procedures (Box 33-2).

GERONTOLOGICAL CONSIDERATIONS

- Physiological changes that occur with aging may require admission to hospital before surgery for additional diagnostic tests and stabilization of condition (Table 33-3).

Table 33-3 Physiological Factors That Place Older Adult Clients at Risk for Surgery

ALTERATIONS	RISKS	NURSING IMPLICATIONS
CARDIOVASCULAR		
Degenerative change in myocardium and valves	Reduces cardiac reserve.	Assess baseline vital signs.
Rigidity of arterial walls and reduction in sympathetic and parasympathetic innervation to heart	Predisposes client to postoperative hemorrhage and rise in systolic and diastolic blood pressure.	Instruct client on techniques for performing leg exercises and proper turning.
Increase in calcium and cholesterol deposits within small arteries; arterial walls thickened	Predisposes client to clot formation in lower extremities.	
PULMONARY		
Rib cage stiffens and enlarges	Reduces vital capacity.	Instruct client on proper technique for coughing and deep-breathing exercises.
Reduced diaphragm excursion	Greater residual capacity or volume of air left in lung after normal breath increases, reducing amount of new air brought into lungs with each inspiration.	
Lung tissue less distensible; alveoli enlarged	Reduces blood oxygenation.	
RENAL		
Reduced blood flow to kidneys	Increases danger of shock when blood loss occurs.	Determine baseline urinary output for 24 hours.
Reduced glomerular filtration rate and excretory times	Limits ability to remove drugs or toxic substances.	
Reduced bladder capacity	Voiding frequency increases, and larger amount of urine stays in the bladder after voiding. Sensation of need to void may not occur until bladder is filled.	Instruct client to notify nurse immediately when sensation of bladder fullness develops. Keep call light or bedpan within easy reach.
NEUROLOGICAL		
Sensory losses, including reduced tactile sense, increased pain tolerance	Client less able to respond to early warning signs of surgical complications.	Orient client to surrounding environment. Observe for nonverbal signs of pain.
Decreased reaction time	Client becomes confused easily after anesthesia.	
METABOLIC		
Lower basal metabolic rate	Reduces total oxygen consumption.	
Reduced number of red blood cells and hemoglobin levels	Reduces ability to carry adequate oxygen to tissues.	Administer necessary blood products.
Change in total amounts of body potassium and water volume	Greater risk for fluid or electrolyte imbalance.	Monitor electrolyte levels.

Box 33-3 Postanesthesia and Ambulatory Surgery Discharge Criteria

Postanesthesia Discharge Criteria

Patient awake (or baseline)
Vital signs stable
No excess bleeding or drainage
No respiratory depression
Oxygen saturation >90%
Report given

Ambulatory Surgery Discharge Criteria

All postanesthesia care unit (PACU) discharge criteria met
No intravenous (IV) narcotics for last 30 minutes
Minimal nausea and vomiting
Voided (if appropriate to surgical procedure/orders)
Able to ambulate if age-appropriate and not contraindicated
Responsible adult present to accompany patient
Discharge instructions given and understood

- Age-related changes such as decreased vision, hearing, and short-term memory may require presence of family members or primary caregiver during preoperative preparation.

Home Care Considerations

- Clients admitted on day of surgery must be instructed about NPO status, skin preparation, and procedures such as enemas and douches before admission. Often enemas or douches are done at home.
- Clients having surgery performed in ambulatory surgery centers must be accompanied by family member or friend to allow for discharge after procedure (Box 33-3).

Skill 33-2 Demonstrating Postoperative Exercises

Structured preoperative teaching has a positive influence on a surgical client's recovery (Shuldham, 1999). The nurse provides information and teaches skills that help clients understand the surgical experience and participate actively in the recovery process. Ideally a client should have adequate time to learn about the surgical experience (Lancaster, 1997). In the past, teaching occurred the evening before surgery when clients were most anxious. But due to cost reduction efforts, many clients are admitted to the hospital or ambulatory surgery center on the day of surgery. Preoperative teaching done at this time may not be highly effective because of the client's high anxiety level. Health care institutions are realizing the value of preparing clients well in advance so that clients gain the knowledge and skills needed to participate in their own care (Dunn, 1998). Clients now frequently receive instruction before admission to a hospital or an outpatient surgical clinic. Teaching booklets and videotapes are available to supplement any instruction a nurse provides.

Postoperative exercises include diaphragmatic breathing and effective coughing, turning, and leg exercises. The use of incentive spirometry to encourage voluntary deep breathing through an apparatus that provides visual feedback may also be included. The physician may order incentive spirometry for clients especially at risk for atelectasis or pneumonia (chronic smokers or clients on prolonged bed rest). During the discussion of these exercises, the nurse explains the relationship between the exercises and the physiological principles that make them important. Through specific explanations and guided practice the nurse helps develop client commitment to the recovery process. The nurse demonstrates the exercises and then continues to coach the client through several return practice sessions. Commitment to the exercise regimen is evidenced by the client's independent practice.

Whenever possible the nurse includes family members or other significant persons in the practice sessions. Frequently these individuals are with the client during the postoperative period and can thus serve as coaches. The nurse also provides clients with information about the sensations typically experienced after surgery, such as incisional pain, nausea, tightness of dressings, and what can be done to alleviate them. The information helps clients interpret realistically the events that occur in the postoperative period. As a result, clients are able to decrease anxiety, conserve their energies, and attend to performing the exercises that assist in their recovery.

Delegation Considerations

The skill of teaching postoperative exercises should not be delegated to assistive personnel. Assistive personnel can reinforce and assist clients in performing postoperative exercises. Assistive personnel should know any precautions unique to a particular client and when to report if the client is unable or unwilling to perform the exercises correctly.

Equipment

- Pillow (optional; used to splint the incision when coughing to reduce discomfort)
- Incentive spirometer
- Elastic stockings or pneumatic compression cuffs (see Chapter 28)

STEP	RATIONALE

ASSESSMENT

1. Assess client's risk for postoperative respiratory complications: identify presence of chronic pulmonary condition (e.g., emphysema, chronic bronchitis, or asthma); any condition that affects chest wall movement, such as obesity, advanced pregnancy, thoracic or abdominal surgery; history of smoking; and presence of reduced hemoglobin level.

General anesthesia predisposes client to respiratory problems because lungs are not fully inflated during surgery; cough reflex is suppressed, and mucus collects within airway passages. Postoperatively, inadequate lung expansion can lead to atelectasis and pneumonia. Chronic lung conditions create greater risk for developing respiratory complications. Smoking damages ciliary clearance and increases mucus secretion. A reduced hemoglobin level can lead to reduced oxygen delivery.

- ***Critical Decision Point***

  Assess and report to physician and/or anesthesiologist if client has had a cold or upper respiratory infection within past week.

2. Assess client's ability to deep breathe and cough by placing hand on client's abdomen, having client take a deep breath, and observing movement of shoulders, chest wall, and abdomen. Observe chest excursion during a deep breath. Ask client to cough into tissue after taking a deep breath.

Reveals maximum potential for chest expansion and ability to cough forcefully; serves as baseline to measure client's ability to perform exercises postoperatively. Diaphragmatic breathing allows for complete lung expansion and improved ventilation and increases blood oxygenation. Deep breathing also allows air to pass by partially obstructing mucus plugs, thus increasing force with which to expel mucus plug (Potter and Perry, 1998). Coughing loosens secretions and helps to remove them from pulmonary alveoli and bronchi.

3. Assess client's risk for postoperative thrombus formation (older adults, immobilized clients, clients with personal or family history of clots, and women over 35 who smoke and are taking birth control pills are most at risk). Observe for positive **Homans' sign** (which may or may not be present) by monitoring calf pain when dorsiflexing client's foot with knee flexed (see Skill 10-11). Observe for calf pain, redness, swelling, or vein distention, usually unilaterally. Compare legs for bilateral equality.

For a thrombus to form, venous stasis, involving hypercoagulability and vein trauma must exist simultaneously (Lewis, Heitkemper, and Dirkson, 2000). Following general anesthesia, circulation is slowed, causing a greater tendency for clot formation. Immobilization results in decreased muscular contraction in lower extremities, which promotes venous stasis. The physical stress of surgery creates a hypercoagulable state in most individuals. Manipulation and positioning during surgery may inadvertently cause trauma to leg veins.

- ***Critical Decision Point***

  If a thrombus is suspected, notify physician and refrain from manipulating extremity any further. Surgery will usually be postponed. Antiembolism stockings or pneumatic compression cuffs may be ordered for clients at risk for thrombus formation (Chapter 28).

4. Assess client's ability to move independently while in bed.

Clients confined to bed rest, even for limited periods, will need to turn regularly. Determines existence of any mobility restrictions.

5. Assess client's willingness and capability to learn exercises; note factors such as attention span, anxiety level, level of consciousness, language skills, and level of pain, if any.

Capacity to learn depends on readiness, ability, and learning environment.

- ***Critical Decision Point***

  Highly anxious clients or those in severe pain have difficulty learning and performing postoperative exercises.

6. Assess family members' or significant others' willingness to learn and to support client postoperatively.

Family's or significant other's presence postoperatively can be potential motivating factor for client's recovery; family member or significant other can coach clients on exercise performance.

7. Assess client's medical orders preoperatively and postoperatively.

May require adaptations in way exercises are performed.

STEP	RATIONALE

NURSING DIAGNOSIS

Defining characteristics from the assessment data may reveal the following nursing diagnoses for clients requiring this skill:

Risk for infection
Ineffective airway clearance
Ineffective breathing pattern
Impaired gas exchange
Acute pain
Ineffective tissue perfusion
Impaired physical mobility
Nausea
Risk for impaired skin integrity
Impaired memory

Related factors are individualized based on client's condition or needs.

PLANNING

1. **Expected outcomes** following completion of procedure:
   - Client is able to correctly deep breathe, use incentive spirometer, cough, turn, and perform leg exercises throughout postoperative period.

     Client's ability to perform exercises should reduce risk of postoperative complications.
   - Postoperatively, chest excursion meets or exceeds preoperative level.

     Turning, deep breathing, and coughing exercises help client maintain full lung expansion and clear airways postoperatively.
   - Lungs are clear to auscultation preoperatively and postoperatively.

     Absence of secretions reduces risk for postoperative pneumonia.
   - Negative Homans' sign, no redness in lower extremities, and client denies pain or tenderness in lower extremities.

     Leg exercises prevent circulatory and mobility problems postoperatively.
   - Client initiates exercises spontaneously.

     Client values importance of exercises to recovery.
2. Prepare equipment as needed.
3. Prepare room for teaching.

   Quiet, private area free from distractions enhances client's ability to learn.

IMPLEMENTATION

Teach Diaphragmatic Breathing

1. Assist client to comfortable semi-Fowler's or high-Fowler's position with knees flexed. If client chooses to sit, assist to side of bed or to upright position in chair. If client is sitting in a chair, knees should be at or higher than hips. Use stool if necessary.

   Upright position facilitates diaphragmatic excursion by using gravity to keep abdominal contents away from diaphragm. Prevents tension on abdominal muscles, which allows for greater diaphragmatic excursion.

   - ***Critical Decision Point***
     Postoperatively, client can usually be positioned upright with head of bed elevated. If client must remain flat in bed, stress that exercises can still be performed.
2. Stand or sit facing client.

   Client will be able to observe breathing exercises performed by nurse.
3. Instruct client to place palms of hands across from each other along lower borders of anterior rib cage; place tips of third finger lightly together. Demonstrate for client (see illustration).

   Position of hands allows client to feel movement of chest and abdomen as diaphragm descends and lungs inside chest wall expand.
4. Have client take slow, deep breaths, inhaling through nose, and pushing abdomen against hands. Tell client to feel middle fingers separate as client inhales. Explain that client will feel normal downward movement of diaphragm during inspiration. Explain that abdominal organs descend as chest wall expands. Demonstrate for client.

   Slow, deep breath allows for more complete lung expansion than is ordinarily done and prevents panting or hyperventilation. Inhaling through nose warms, humidifies, and filters air. Explanation and demonstration focus on normal ventilatory movement of chest and abdominal wall. Client learns to understand how diaphragmatic breathing feels.

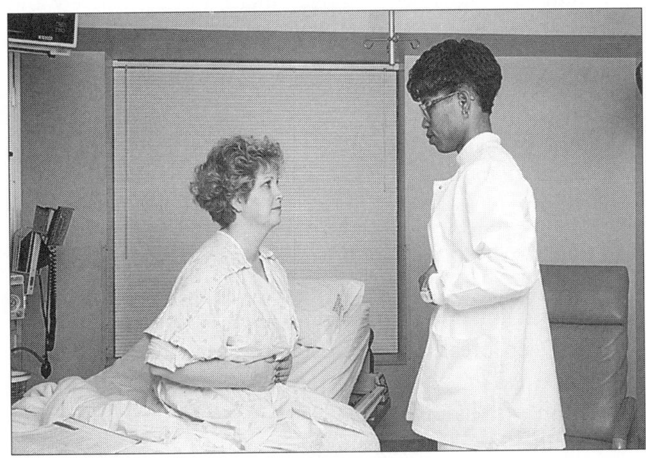

STEP **3** Client and nurse practicing deep breathing.

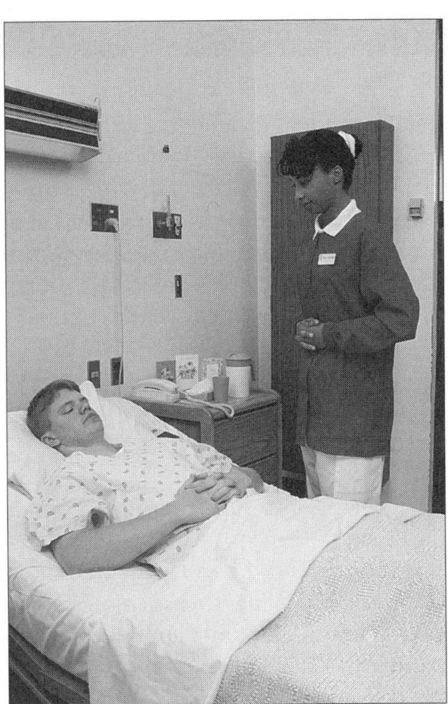

STEP **6** Deep breathing exercise—placement of hands on upper abdomen during inhalation. (From *Mosby's medical, nursing, and allied health dictionary,* ed 5, St. Louis, 1998, Mosby.)

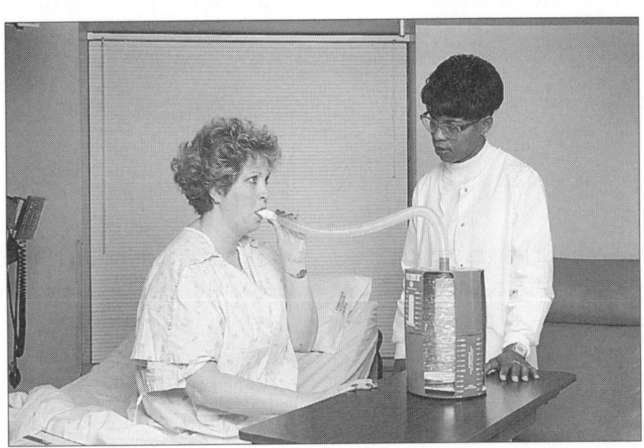

STEP **8** Client demonstrates incentive spirometry.

STEP	RATIONALE
5. Avoid using chest and shoulder muscles while inhaling, and instruct client in same manner.	Using auxiliary chest and shoulder muscles during breathing increases useless energy expenditures and does not promote full lung expansion.
6. Take a slow, deep breath and hold for count of 3, and then slowly exhale through mouth as if blowing out a candle (pursed lips). Explain that client will feel middle fingertips touch as chest wall contracts (see illustration).	Allows for gradual, controlled expulsion of air.
7. Repeat breathing exercise three to five times.	Allows client to observe slow, rhythmic breathing pattern.
8. Have client practice exercise. Client is instructed to take 10 slow, deep breaths every 2 hours while awake during postoperative period until mobile. Another option is to have client use incentive spirometry (see illustration).	Repetition of exercise reinforces learning. Regular deep breathing will prevent or minimize postoperative respiratory complications. Incentive spirometer gives a visual incentive to breathe as deeply as possible.

STEP	RATIONALE

Teach Controlled Coughing

1. Explain importance of maintaining an upright position.
   Position facilitates diaphragm excursion and enhances thorax and abdominal expansion.
2. Demonstrate coughing. Take two slow, deep breaths, inhaling through nose and exhaling through pursed lips.
   Deep breaths expand lungs fully so that air moves behind mucus and facilitates effective coughing.
3. Inhale deeply a third time and hold breath to count of 3. Cough fully for two to three consecutive coughs without inhaling between coughs. (Tell client to push all air out of lungs.)
   Consecutive coughs help remove mucus more effectively and completely than one forceful cough.

- ***Critical Decision Point***
  Coughing may be contraindicated after brain, spinal, or eye surgery due to an increase in intracranial pressure.

4. Caution client against just clearing throat instead of coughing deeply.
   Clearing throat does not remove mucus from deeper airways.
5. If surgical incision is to be either thoracic or abdominal, teach client to place pillow over incisional area and place hands over pillow to splint incision (see illustration). During breathing and coughing exercises, press gently against incisional area for splinting and support (see illustration).
   Surgical incision cuts through muscles, tissues, and nerve endings. Deep breathing and coughing exercises place additional stress on suture line and cause discomfort. Splinting incision with hands or pillow provides firm support and reduces incisional pulling and pain.
6. Client continues to practice coughing exercises, splinting imaginary incision. The client is instructed to cough two to three times every 2 hours while awake.
   Value of deep coughing with splinting is stressed to effectively expectorate mucus with minimal discomfort.
7. Instruct client to examine sputum for consistency, odor, amount, and color changes and to notify nurse if any changes are noted.
   Sputum consistency, odor, amount, and color changes may indicate the presence of a pulmonary complication such as pneumonia.

- ***Critical Decision Point***
  For clients with preexisting pulmonary disease, know usual character of mucus to determine if change has occurred.

Teach Turning

1. Instruct client to assume supine position and move toward left side of bed. This is easily accomplished by bending knees and pressing heels against mattress to raise buttocks (see illustration).
   Positioning begins on left side of bed so that turning to right side will not cause client to roll off bed's edge. Buttocks lift prevents shearing force from body moving against sheets.

- ***Critical Decision Point***
  If client has decreased strength of mobility on the left side, have client assume position on right side of bed. Pull sheet can also be used by the nurse to turn client.

2. Have client place the right hand over incisional area to splint it.
   Splinting incision supports and minimizes pulling on suture line during turning.

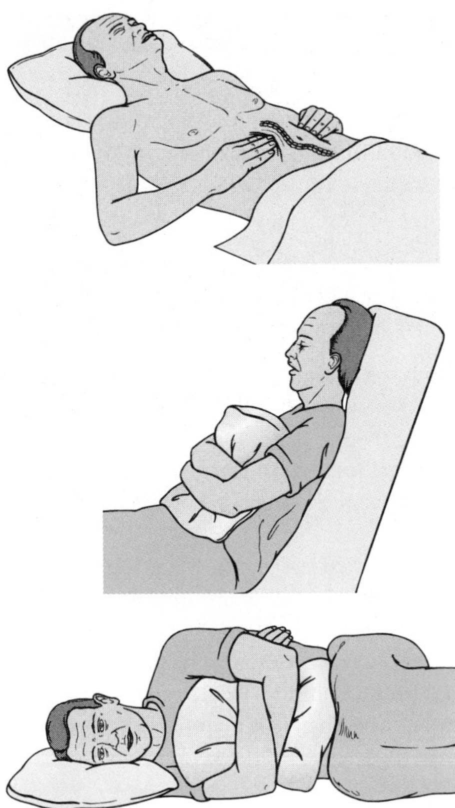

STEP **5(a)** Techniques for splinting incision when coughing or moving. (From Lewis S, Heitkemper M, Dirkson S: *Medical-surgical nursing: assessment and management of clinical problems,* ed 5, St. Louis, 2000, Mosby.)

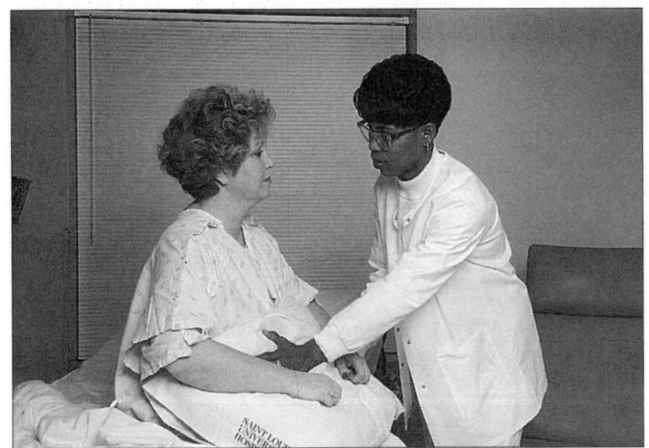

STEP **5(b)** Client splinting abdomen with pillow.

STEP	RATIONALE
3. Instruct client to keep right leg straight and flex left knee up (see illustration).	Straight leg stabilizes the client's position. Flexed left leg shifts weight for easier turning.

- ***Critical Decision Point***
  Some clients, such as those who have had back surgery or vascular repair, may be restricted from flexing their legs postoperatively. Client may be restricted from turning or may need assistance for positioning (see Chapter 27).

STEP	RATIONALE
4. Have client grab right side rail with left hand, pull toward right, and roll onto right side.	Pulling toward side rail reduces effort needed for turning.
5. Instruct client to turn every 2 hours while awake. If client is unable to perform above maneuver, note in chart that staff or primary caregiver must turn client every 2 hours. May need to place pillows behind client to help maintain side-lying position.	Reduces risk of vascular complications by contraction of leg muscles around veins to improve venous return. Also reduces pulmonary complications by shifting mucus to prevent consolidation.

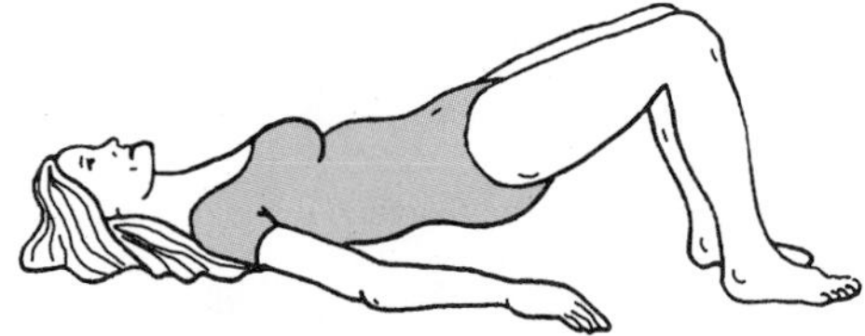

STEP **1** Buttocks lift. (From Lowdermilk D, Perry S, Bobak I: *Maternity nursing,* ed 5, St. Louis, 1999, Mosby).

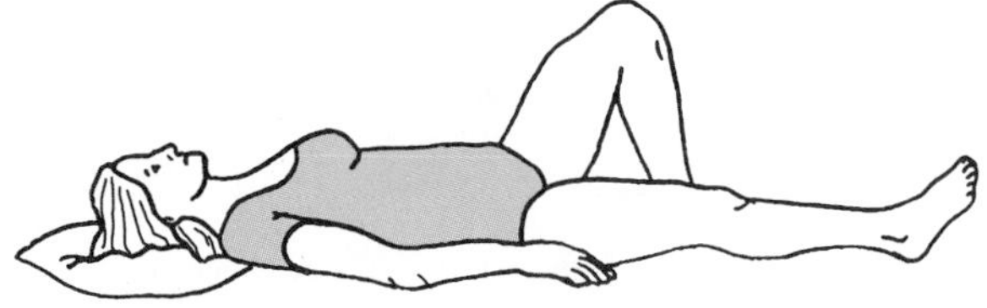

STEP **3** Leg position when turning. (From Lowdermilk D, Perry S, Bobak I: *Maternity nursing,* ed 5, St. Louis, 1999, Mosby).

STEP	RATIONALE

Teach Leg Exercises

1. Have client assume supine position in bed. Demonstrate leg exercises by performing passive range-of-motion exercises and simultaneously explaining exercise.

Provides for normal anatomical position of lower extremities and normal joint motion of each joint of lower extremities.

- ***Critical Decision Point***

  *If client's surgery involves one or both lower extremities, surgeon must order leg exercises in postoperative period. Leg unaffected by surgery can be safely exercised unless client has preexisting **phlebothrombosis** (blood clot formation) or **thrombophlebitis** (inflammation of vein wall).*

2. Rotate each ankle in complete circle. Instruct client to draw imaginary circles with big toe (see illustration). Repeat five times.

Ankle circle exercises maintain joint mobility and promote venous return.

3. Alternate dorsiflexion and plantar flexion by moving both feet up and down. Direct client to feel calf muscles contract and relax alternately (see illustration). Repeat five times.

Calf pumping stretches and contracts gastrocnemius muscles, which enhances venous return.

4. Client continues leg exercises by alternately flexing and extending knees (see illustration). Repeat five times.

Quadriceps setting exercises contract muscles of upper legs and maintains knee mobility and improves venous return to the heart.

5. Client alternately raises each leg from bed surface, client begins by keeping leg straight and then bends hip and knee joint (see illustration). Repeat five times.

Leg raises promote contraction and relaxation of quadriceps muscles and promote hip and knee movements by keeping leg straight and then bends hip and knee joints.

- ***Critical Decision Point***

  If client is unable to perform exercises, note on Kardex that staff or primary caregiver must do passive range of motion to lower extremities every 2 hours while awake. Alternatively, notify surgeon and request an order for pneumatic compression cuffs (see Chapter 28).

6. Have client continue to practice exercises at least every 2 hours while awake. Client is instructed to coordinate turning and leg exercises with diaphragmatic breathing, incentive spirometry, and coughing exercises.

Repetition of exercise sequence reinforces learning. Establishes routine for exercises that develops habit for performance. Sequence of exercises should be leg exercises, turning, deep breathing, and coughing. Exercises prior to coughing should enhance ability to move secretions so that they may be expectorated.

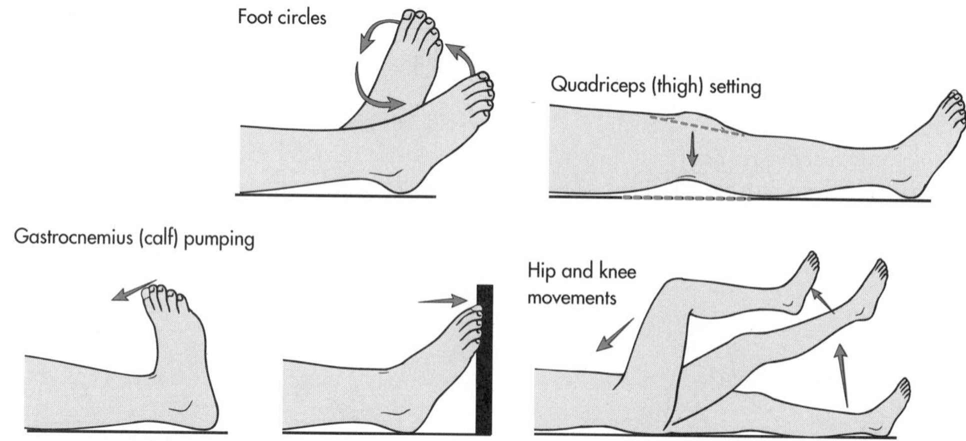

STEPS **2-5** Leg exercises. (From Lewis S, Heitkemper M, Dirkson S: *Medical-surgical nursing: assessment and management of clinical problems,* ed 5, St. Louis, 2000, Mosby.)

Step	Rationale
Evaluation	
1. Observe client performing all four exercises independently.	Provides opportunity for practice and return demonstration of exercises. Ensures client has learned correct technique.
2. Observe family members' or significant other's ability to coach client.	Family member or significant other can assist positively or interfere with correct technique.
3. Evaluate client's chest excursion.	Determines extent of lung expansion.
4. Auscultate client's lungs.	Breath sounds reveal if airways are clear.
5. Assess for Homans' sign.	Negative sign usually indicates that no venous thrombosis is present.

Unexpected Outcomes and Related Interventions

- Client is unable to perform exercises correctly.
  - Additional instruction is needed.
  - Anxiety, pain, and fatigue alter client's performance.
  - Client may benefit from stress reduction techniques and pain management strategies.
- Client is unwilling to perform exercises due to incisional pain of thorax or abdomen (deep breathing and coughing, turning) or due to surgery in lower abdomen, groin, buttocks, or legs (leg exercises).
  - Instruct client to ask for pain medication 30 minutes before performing postoperative exercises or use patient-controlled analgesia (PCA) immediately before exercising.
- Client develops pulmonary complications such as atelectasis postoperatively. Breaths shallow, cough ineffective.
  - Notify physician, start oxygen as ordered, and increase frequency of coughing exercises.
- Client develops circulatory complications such as venous stasis or thrombophlebitis postoperatively. Leg exercises inadequate.
  - Notify physician and place client on bed rest with affected leg elevated as ordered.
  - Continue to have client do exercises with unaffected leg.

Recording and Reporting

- Record physical assessment findings in nurses' notes or flow sheet.
- Report and record any assessed complications and action taken.
- Record which exercises have been demonstrated to client and whether or not client can perform exercises independently.
- Report and record any problem client has in practicing exercises to nurse assigned to client on next shift.

Teaching Considerations

- Clients do better with combination of procedural explanations, skills teaching, and psychosocial support (Shuldham, 1999).
- Explain postoperative exercises to client and primary caregiver, including their importance to recovery and physiological benefits. Adults learn best when they understand how they will benefit from activity.

Pediatric Considerations

- Parents should encourage and allow children to move within limits posed by surgery.
- Adolescents should receive same preoperative instructions and teaching as adults to support their developmental stage. Adolescents are searching for identity, and treating them with respect will enhance their self-esteem and independence and should increase compliance.
- Children's normal responses of crying and moving extremities will maintain lung expansion and peripheral circulation. Therefore teaching coughing, deep breathing, and leg exercises is not usually necessary for young children.
- Children need family members and/or nursing staff to assume coach's role of reminding and encouraging.

Gerontological Considerations

- Changes related to aging such as decreased vision, hearing, and short-term memory may affect teaching effectiveness. Shorter sessions with frequent reinforcement and use of teaching aids with large print may be necessary. Including family members or primary caregiver in teaching sessions is strongly encouraged. Take time to instruct client properly.
- Aging process decreases ventilatory capacity and increases risk for respiratory complications.
- Aging process decreases muscle mass, thus decreasing energy level and increasing risk of venous stasis.

Home Care Considerations

- Review coughing, deep breathing, abdominal splinting, relaxation, and leg exercises before admission to hospital or surgical clinic and after discharge.

Skill 33-3 Preparing the Surgical Site

The body's first line of defense against infection is intact skin. A break in the integrity of the skin as a result of a surgical incision can become a potential source of infection. Before surgery, the skin overlying the proposed surgical site is thoroughly cleansed to minimize skin contamination and the risk of postoperative wound infection. Preparation of the incisional area sometimes begins the evening before surgery and involves washing the skin (Centers for Disease Control and Prevention [CDC], 1999). For same day surgery, clients may be asked to do this at home.

The skin is cleansed by scrubbing with an antimicrobial soap (e.g., chlorhexidine) two or more times. The client can perform the scrubbing during either a bath or shower. If an enema is given in preparation for surgery, the final shower or bath should be given after the enema. The client also may be required to shampoo hair if surgery involves the head, neck, or even the upper chest.

Hair removal should be performed only as necessary. Hair can be removed by use of a depilatory, clipping, or wet shaving. The Centers for Disease Control and Prevention (CDC) recommends use of a depilatory or clippers for hair removal to minimize skin abrasions and cuts (CDC, 1999). Shaving the surgical site removes hair that serves as a reservoir for bacterial growth. However, evidence shows that infection can form in small cuts made by a razor. Wound infection occurs more often in clients who are shaved preoperatively than clients who are not shaved. Shaving, if necessary, is usually done immediately before the operation in the OR or holding area to reduce the time for potential bacterial growth. The procedure may be done by a nurse or surgical technician.

Delegation Considerations

The skill of preparing the surgical site can be delegated to assistive personnel after assessment of client's risk for bleeding tendencies, condition of client's skin prior to site preparation, and client's level of cooperation. Personnel should know information to report to RN after completion of procedure.

Equipment

- Portable lamp or extra light source
- Bath blanket
- Towel or waterproof pad
- Disposable gloves

Depilation

- Depilatory cream
- Basin with liquid antiseptic soap mixed with water

Clipping

- Electric clippers (used to remove short hair)
- Scissors (used to remove long hair)
- Cotton balls, applicators, and antiseptic solution as needed

Wet Shave

- Disposable razor
- Clean basin with warm water
- Gauze sponges (4 × 4 inches)
- Basin with liquid antiseptic soap mixed with water (avoid using povidone-iodine for clients with allergies to iodine or shellfish)
- Washcloth
- Cotton balls, cotton applicators, and antiseptic solution as needed

Step	Rationale
Assessment	
1. Inspect general condition of skin.	Preexisting lesions, irritations, or infection increase chance for postoperative wound infection.
• ***Critical Decision Point*** *If lesions, irritations, or signs of skin infection are present, shaving should not be done.*	
2. Assess for allergy to iodine or shellfish.	Povidone-iodine solutions should not be used if client is allergic to iodine. Shellfish contain iodine.
3. Assess for bleeding tendency by reviewing client's medication history and coagulation laboratory values (prothrombin time [PT], partial thromboplastin time [PTT]).	Presence of bleeding tendency would contraindicate use of a razor. Medications such as aspirin and warfarin (Coumadin) increase clotting time. Prednisone causes skin to be thin and friable.

STEP	RATIONALE
4. Review physician's order or agency's procedure book for specific area to be shaved.	Extent of area for hair removal depends on site of incision, nature of surgery, and physician's preference. Area is always larger than actual incision to ensure wide perimeter with minimal bacteria.
5. Assess client's understanding and acceptance of purpose for hair removal.	Client may be anxious regarding removal of hair and implications regarding change in appearance.

- ***Critical Decision Point***
  Certain cultures and religious groups have restrictions on removal and disposal of body hair. The nurse should ask client and/or family.

NURSING DIAGNOSIS

Defining characteristics from the assessment data may reveal the following nursing diagnoses for clients requiring this skill:

- Acute pain
- Risk for infection
- Risk for impaired skin integrity
- Disturbed body image

Related factors are individualized based on client's condition or needs.

PLANNING

STEP	RATIONALE
1. **Expected outcomes** following completion of procedure:	
▪ Client's skin is free of all hair over surgical area.	Skin prepared for surgical incision.
▪ Skin is free of visible cuts, nicks, and areas of inflammation.	Less likelihood of skin infections developing.
▪ Client denies burning, discomfort, or itching.	Skin intact without abrasions, cuts, or allergy to disinfectant used.
2. Prepare equipment at client's bedside.	
3. Explain procedure, extent of hair removal, and rationale for removal of hair over large surface area.	Promotes cooperation and minimizes anxiety because client may think incision will be as large as shaved site.

- ***Critical Decision Point***
  Scissors may be used to trim especially long hair. Never dispose of client's scalp hair without permission, since this is considered personal property. Some clients use their hair for a wig. In some facilities a separate consent form must be signed for shaving hair on head.

IMPLEMENTATION

STEP	RATIONALE
1. Wash hands.	Reduces transmission of microorganisms.
2. Close room doors or bedside curtains, raise bed to high position, and position lamp or extra light source.	Provides client privacy. Bed position prevents nurse from having to bend over for long periods. Promotes correct body mechanics and decreases back injury. Direct and tangential lighting enhances visual inspection of skin surface.
3. Position client comfortably with surgical site accessible. Rearrange drapes as necessary.	Hair removal and skin preparation can take several minutes. Nurse should have easy access to hard-to-reach areas. Prevents unnecessary exposure of body parts.
4. Apply disposable gloves.	Use of disposable gloves safeguards client and nurse, minimizing nurse's exposure to blood-borne pathogens.
5. Depilatory hair removal:	
a. Apply depilatory cream to area; be sure entire area is adequately covered.	Hair removal by depilation leaves skin intact and free from cuts. If the client is not sensitive to the depilatory, it is a safer method of hair removal than shaving.

Step	Rationale
b. Wait required number of minutes, and then wipe off cream.	Hair is removed simultaneously when wiping off depilatory.
c. Wash skin with antiseptic soap, and rinse thoroughly.	Removes microorganisms from the skin.
6. Hair clipping:	
a. Using a towel, lightly dry area to be clipped.	Removes moisture, which interferes with clean cut of clippers.
b. Hold clippers in dominant hand, about 1 cm (1/2 inch) above skin, and cut hair in direction it grows. Clip small area at a time.	Prevents pulling on hair and abrasion of skin.
c. Lightly brush off cut hair with towel.	Removes contaminated hair and promotes comfort. Improves visibility of area being clipped.
d. When clipped area is over body crevices, for example, umbilicus or groin, clean crevices with cotton-tipped applicators or cotton ball dipped in antiseptic solution, then dry.	Removes secretions, dirt, and hair clippings, which harbor microorganisms.
7. Wet shave:	
a. Place towel or waterproof pads under body part to be shaved.	Prevents soiling of bed linen.
b. Drape client with bath blanket, leaving only area to be shaved at one time (10 to 20 cm [4 to 8 inches]) exposed.	Prevents unnecessary exposure of body parts and reduces client's anxiety.
c. Adjust lamp.	Provides maximum skin illumination.
d. Lather skin with gauze sponges dipped in antiseptic soap.	Softens hair and reduces friction from razor.
e. Shave small area at a time. With nondominant hand hold gauze sponge to stabilize skin. Hold razor at 45-degree angle in dominant hand, and shave hair in direction it grows. Use short, gentle strokes (see illustration).	Shaving small areas minimizes cutting skin; shaving in direction hair grows prevents pulling.

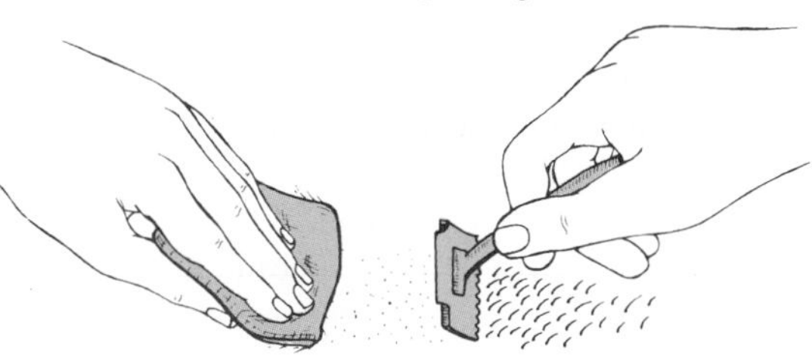

STEP **7e** Shaving.

Step	Rationale
f. Rinse razor in basin of water as soap and hair accumulate on blade. Change and discard blades as they become dull.	Maintains clean, sharp razor edge to promote client's comfort and reduces risk of cuts and abrasions.
g. Rearrange bath blanket as each portion of shave is completed.	Maintains client's comfort and privacy.
h. Use washcloth and warm water to rinse away remaining cut hair and soap solution. Change water as needed.	Reduces skin irritation and potential contamination; allows good visualization of skin.
i. If shaved area is over body crevices, for example, umbilicus or groin, cleanse with cotton-tipped applicators or cotton balls dipped in antiseptic solution.	Removes secretions, dirt, and remaining hair clippings, which harbor microorganisms.
j. Dry shaved areas with towel, and dry crevices with dry cotton-tipped applicators or cotton balls.	Reduces maceration of skin from retained moisture.
k. Discard waterproof towel or pad.	Reduces spread of microorganisms.
l. Observe skin closely for any nicks or cuts.	Any break in skin integrity increases risk of wound infection.
8. Tell client when procedure is completed.	Relieves client's anxiety.
9. Clean and dispose of equipment according to policy. Do not recover razor blade. Razor handle with blade is discarded into contaminated sharps holder. Dispose of gloves.	Reduces spread of infection and reduces risk of injury from contaminated razor blades. Occupational Safety and Health Administration (OSHA) guidelines require gloves to be worn, razor blades to be disposed of safely, and reusable items to be sterilized.
10. Wash hands.	Reduces spread of microorganisms.

STEP	RATIONALE
EVALUATION	
1. Inspect condition of skin after completion of hair removal.	Determines if there is remaining hair or if skin was cut.
2. Question if client feels burning, discomfort, or itching.	Indicates presence of skin cut, irritation, or allergic response.

UNEXPECTED OUTCOMES AND RELATED INTERVENTIONS

- Client's skin is not totally clear of all hair.
  - Exceptionally thick hair is difficult to remove the first time. Additional depilatory or another shave is necessary.
- Client's skin becomes cut, nicked, or inflamed.
  - Blade may be dulled, angle of blade was not correct, or too much pressure was applied. Even minor skin wounds can become infected. Notify surgeon.
- Client experiences burning or itching over shaved site.
  - If allergic response noted, call physician for antihistamine order.

RECORDING AND REPORTING

- Record procedure, area clipped or shaved, and condition of skin before and after in nurses' notes.
- Report any skin alterations, nicks, or cuts in skin to surgeon. Skin problems may require cancellation of surgery.

PEDIATRIC CONSIDERATIONS

- The face and neck of children are not usually shaved.
- Parents may want to save hair if child's head is shaved.

GERONTOLOGICAL CONSIDERATIONS

- Skin changes that occur with aging make skin more susceptible to irritation and injury, which increases risk for infection.

HOME CARE CONSIDERATIONS

- Some surgeons may encourage clients to use a chlorhexidine skin cleanser or soap product containing hexachlorophene at home before an elective procedure.

Skill 33-4 Performing Postoperative Care of the Surgical Client

Nursing care of the postoperative surgical client is divided into two phases. During both phases the nurse must make comprehensive and detailed assessments of the client's condition. The effects of anesthesia and the physiological stressors imposed by surgery can place the client at risk for a variety of physiological alterations. It is also important for the nurse to facilitate communication among all members of the health care team, the client, and the client's family or significant other.

The first phase of postoperative care takes place during the immediate recovery period. For hospitalized clients this extends from the time the client leaves the operating room (OR) to the time the client has stabilized in the recovery room (RR), postanesthesia room (PAR), or **postanesthesia care unit (PACU)** and has been transferred to the nursing division. For an ambulatory surgical client, the first phase of recovery normally lasts 1 to 2 hours before discharge home. The first phase is the most critical postoperative phase for assessing aftereffects of anesthesia, airway clearance, cardiovascular complications, temperature control, and neurological function. The client's condition can change rapidly. The nurse in the recovery area must make timely, intelligent, and accurate assessments to select the most appropriate measures of care for the client.

Each hospital has its own policies directing the process for recovering clients during the immediate postoperative period. Frequently, for example, clients undergoing cardiac or central vascular repair transfer from the OR to an intensive care unit. In this situation the client is not sent to the RR/PACU area. The conditions of these clients are potentially so unstable as to require the monitoring available only in an intensive care unit.

The second phase of recovery is the postoperative convalescent period. This period extends from the time the client is discharged from the RR or PACU to the time the client is discharged from the hospital for inpatient clients. Outpatient surgical clients undergo convalescence at home. All clients who have undergone surgical procedures have similar postoperative needs. However, nursing care becomes very individualized and depends on the nature of the client's surgery, preexisting medical conditions, the onset of complications, and the speed of recovery. Not all surgical clients recover at the same rate. During the convalescent period the nurse begins preparation for discharge and actively includes client, family, and significant others in the process. The nurse promotes the client's independence, educates the client and/or family about any limitations imposed by surgery, and provides resources needed for the client to assume an improved state of wellness.

Delegation Considerations

The skill of initiating and managing postoperative care of the client should not be delegated to assistive personnel. Assistive personnel may obtain vital signs, apply nasal cannula or oxygen mask, and provide comfort and hygiene measures. Personnel should be instructed to report specific changes in client's vital signs, behavior, or level of consciousness. In addition, personnel should be instructed in liters of oxygen per minute ordered for each client and to report if flow meter differs from order.

Equipment

Phase 1: Immediate Recovery Period

- Stethoscope, sphygmomanometer, or Dinamapp automatic blood pressure machine
- Thermometer
- Pulse oximeter and monitor
- Intravenous (IV) fluid poles and IV fluids ordered
- Emesis basin
- Oxygen equipment such as mask, nasal cannula, tubing, and oxygen regulator
- Continuous suction equipment (to suction airway)
- Intermittent suction (for nasogastric [NG] tube suction if ordered)
- Dressing supplies
- Warmed blankets
- Graduated container for measuring output
- Additional equipment for physical assessment as ordered

Phase 2: Postoperative Convalescent Period

- Stethoscope, sphygmomanometer, thermometer
- IV fluid poles and IV fluids ordered
- Intermittent external pneumatic compression equipment (if ordered)
- Emesis basin
- Washcloth and towel
- Waterproof pads
- Equipment for oral hygiene
- Pillows
- Facial tissue
- Oxygen equipment (if ordered)
- Continuous suction equipment (for airway suction and wound drainage systems if ordered)
- Intermittent suction (for NG suction if ordered)
- Dressing supplies
- Orthopedic appliances (if skeletal traction ordered)
- Graduated containers for measuring output

Step	Rationale
Assessment	
Phase 1: Immediate Recovery Period	
1. Receive report from circulating nurse, including procedure performed, range of vital signs, any complications, estimated blood loss (EBL), other fluid loss, fluid replacement, type of anesthesia, medications given, type of airway and size, extent of surgical wound, and any preoperative medical and/or nursing diagnoses.	Determines client's general status and allows nurse to anticipate need for special equipment, nursing care, and activities in RR/PACU.
• ***Critical Decision Point*** *Clients' usual first complaint is of pain. Know how much sedative and/or analgesic has already been given and how long ago.*	
2. Upon client's arrival in RR/PACU, obtain report from surgeon and anesthesia provider.	Review provides detailed analysis of client's physiological status, allowing nurse to make appropriate observations and interventions. Provides baseline data to determine any change in condition.
3. Consider type of surgery client underwent, restrictions to movement, and type of anesthesia used.	Influences type of assessments nurse initiates, type of complications to observe for, and specific nursing interventions needed.
4. After receiving report, perform a thorough client assessment, including respiratory, cardiac, neurological, gastrointestinal (GI), genitourinary (GU), and fluid status. Monitor client's temperature, surgical site and drains, skin integrity, comfort, safety, and anxiety level.	Provides baseline for further postoperative evaluations. Identifies priority-nursing interventions.

STEP	RATIONALE

- ***Critical Decision Point***
  Be sure to turn client on side (when possible) to observe underlying skin and accumulation of blood or serous drainage not visible otherwise.

Phase 2: Convalescent Period

1. Obtain phone report from nurse in RR/PACU.

   Preliminary report allows nurse to prepare hospital room with necessary supplies and equipment for client's special needs.

2. Upon client's arrival at division, collect more detailed report from nurse accompanying client.

   Detailed report helps nurse plan appropriate assessment and nursing care measures. Data provide baseline to detect any change in client's condition.

3. Review client's chart for information pertaining to type of surgery, complications, medications administered, preoperative medical risks, baseline vital signs and client's usual medications given/not given preoperatively.

   Nature of surgery, intraoperative complications, and presence of medical risks dictate complications for which to observe. Vital signs provide means to measure postoperative changes. List of client's usual medications may necessitate a call to physician for orders concerning timing and dose of drugs not given preoperatively.

4. Review postoperative orders.

   Offers additional guidelines for type of care to provide.

NURSING DIAGNOSIS

Defining characteristics from the assessment data may reveal the following nursing diagnoses for clients requiring this skill:

Ineffective airway clearance
Ineffective breathing pattern
Impaired gas exchange
Deficient knowledge regarding postoperative care
Acute pain
Ineffective peripheral tissue perfusion
Risk for aspiration
Impaired physical mobility
Disturbed body image
Impaired verbal communication
Acute confusion
Impaired skin integrity
Deficient fluid volume
Excess fluid volume
Ineffective thermoregulation
Impaired spontaneous ventilation
Ineffective protection
Disturbed sensory/perception: visual, auditory
Impaired swallowing
Urinary retention

Related factors are individualized based on client's condition or needs.

PLANNING

1. **Expected outcomes** following completion of procedure:
   - Client's vital signs, including oxygen saturation, remain within previous baseline or normal expected range.

     No occurrence of cardiovascular, pulmonary, or thermoregulatory changes except those expected from effects of anesthetic or analgesic.
   - Client reports relief of discomfort after analgesic or other pain relief measures.

     Pain relief measures effectively alter client's reception or perception of pain.
   - Surgical wound remains intact without redness, edema, **ecchymosis,** or discharge. If opaque dressing covers incision, dressing remains dry and intact.

     Indicates wound healing without signs of bleeding or infection.
   - Breath sounds remain clear to auscultation; cough is clear.

     Postoperative exercises and activity promote lung expansion and alveolar stability.
   - Normal bowel sounds present within 48 to 72 hours after bowel or abdominal surgery and/or general anesthetic. Normal bowel sounds are heard within 24 hours in cases of minor surgery.

     Indicates return of intestinal peristalsis.

STEP	RATIONALE
▪ Intake and output remain relatively in balance.	Adequate urinary elimination maintained. Fluid intake (IV and/or by mouth [PO]) adequately maintained.
▪ Legs remain without signs and symptoms of thrombophlebitis.	Postoperative leg exercises and early ambulation minimize venous stasis and clot formation.
▪ Client is able to discuss recovery and discharge plans. Verbalizes no specific physical complaints.	Client coping with physical and psychological stress of surgery.
2. Prepare the equipment as necessary at bedside, and test equipment for function.	Prepared for use if needed.
3. Explain to client all procedures you are to perform and rationale for each. On nursing division include family members and/or significant other in explanations. In ambulatory surgery centers, families are allowed at the bedside during recovery period.	Involves client in plan of care and minimizes anxiety. As recovery progresses, client is able to make more choices regarding how procedures should be performed. Family can serve as coach and can help client remember explanations given.

IMPLEMENTATION

Phase 1: Immediate Recovery Period

STEP	RATIONALE
1. Wash hands.	Reduces transmission of microorganisms.
2. Check equipment setup in cubicle of RR/PACU.	All equipment must be operational and ready to use on client's arrival.
3. As client enters RR/PACU on stretcher, immediately attach oxygen tubing to regulator, hang IV fluids, check IV flow rates, and attach pulse oximeter (see Skill 9-6). Connect any drainage tubes to gravity drainage, continuous or intermittent suction as ordered. Attach cardiac monitor. Ensure indwelling catheter and bag are in drainage position and patent.	Maintaining oxygenation and circulation are two priorities. Inhaled oxygen improves percentage delivered to alveoli. Pulse oximeter provides information on arterial oxygen saturation. IV fluids maintain circulatory volume and provide route for emergency drugs. Drainage tubes must remain patent and in proper position to allow fluid to drain.
4. Conduct complete assessment of all vital signs. Compare findings with client's normal baseline. Continue assessing vital signs at least every 15 minutes until client stabilizes. Provide warm blankets as needed for client comfort.	Vital signs can reveal onset of postoperative complications, for example, respiratory depression, hypothermia or hyperthermia, pulse irregularity, or hypotension. Respiratory depression can result from anesthetics. Hypotension can result from anesthetics or acute blood loss. Acute blood loss may lead to **hypovolemic shock** with signs of reduced blood pressure, elevated heart and respiratory rates, pale skin, and restlessness. General anesthetic may affect temperature-regulating center, and lower metabolic rate causes hypothermia. **Malignant hyperthermia** is a rare inherited condition that develops after receiving an anesthetic and is a medical emergency.

• ***Critical Decision Point***

*If client underwent a short procedure under IV sedation/analgesia (**conscious sedation**), check agency policy for sedation recovery guidelines. The RN monitoring a client who receives conscious sedation/analgesia should have no other responsibilities that require the nurse to leave the client unattended or compromise continuous client monitoring (AORN, 1997). Vital signs, oxygen saturation, auscultation of breath sounds and heart rhythm, and level of consciousness should be documented every 15 minutes during the immediate recovery period (American Society of Anesthesiologists, 1996).*

STEP	RATIONALE
5. Maintain patent airway:	
a. Position client on side with head facing down and neck slightly extended (see illustration). Never position client with hands over chest (reduces chest expansion).	Extension prevents occlusion of airway at pharynx. Downward position of head moves tongue forward, and mucus or vomitus can drain out of mouth, preventing aspiration.

STEP	RATIONALE
b. Place small folded towel under client's head. If client is restricted to supine position, elevate head of bed approximately 10 to 15 degrees, extend neck, and turn head to side. Have emesis basin available if client becomes nauseated.	Supports head in extended position. Prevents aspiration if client should vomit.
c. Clients with spinal anesthetic should be positioned supine, without elevation of head, for up to 24 hours. Fluids should be encouraged.	To prevent spinal headache from loss of cerebrospinal fluid. Increased IV or PO fluids aids body in replacing cerebrospinal fluid.

- ***Critical Decision Point***
  If client is not able to hyperextend neck, turn head to side if possible, suction oropharynx (Chapter 13) frequently.

STEP	RATIONALE
d. Encourage client to deep breathe and cough on awakening.	Promotes lung expansion and expectoration of mucus secretions.
e. Suction artificial airway and oral cavity as secretions accumulate.	Clears airways of secretions.
f. Once gag reflex returns, client spits out oral airway (see illustration). Do not tape oral airway.	Indicates client can clear airway independently. If airway is taped, client will gag and may obstruct airway.

- ***Critical Decision Point***
  Due to shorter half-life of drugs used today, many clients have oral airway removed before leaving OR. PACU nurse must assess that respiratory effort is adequate; otherwise airway may need to be replaced, and client may need a ventilator.

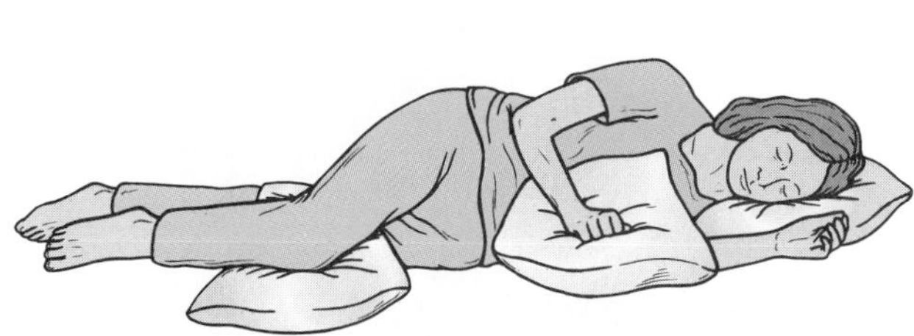

STEP **5a** Position of client during recovery from general anesthesia. (From Lewis S, Heitkemper M, Dirkson S: *Medical-surgical nursing: assessment and management of clinical problems,* ed 5, St. Louis, 2000, Mosby.)

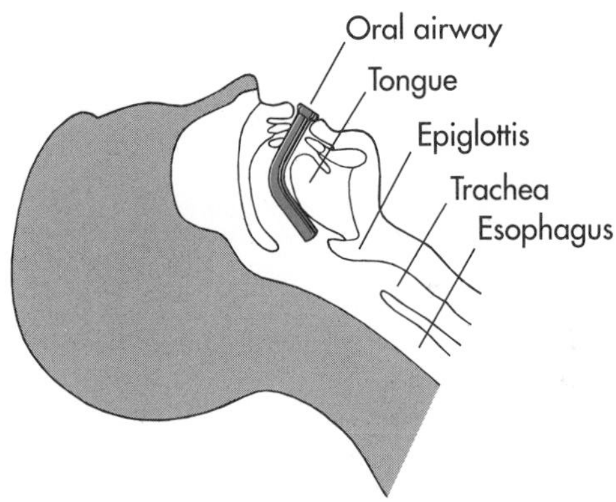

STEP **5f** Oral airway position before removal.

STEP	RATIONALE
6. Call client by name in moderate tone of voice. If there is no response, attempt to arouse client by touching or gently moving a body part. Explain that client is in RR/PACU.	Determines client's level of consciousness and ability to follow commands.
7. Assess circulatory perfusion by inspecting color of nail beds, mucous membranes, and skin. Palpate for skin temperature. Test for capillary refill.	Pink or normal color of skin, nail beds, and mucous membranes and brisk (less than or equal to 3 seconds) capillary refill indicate adequate perfusion. Warm extremities reveal adequate circulation.
8. Observe condition of dressing and drains for any evidence of bright red blood. Also look underneath client for any pooling of bloody drainage.	Hemorrhage from surgical wound usually occurs within first few hours, indicating that a blood vessel was incompletely tied or cauterized during surgery. When dressing becomes saturated, blood oozes down client's side and collects underneath client.

STEP	RATIONALE
9. Inspect surgical area for swelling or discoloration. Note condition of surgical dressing, including amount, color, odor, and consistency of drainage. Mark dressing with circle around drainage using a black pen. Place time of marking and check area every 10 to 15 minutes, marking any changes and noting vital signs.	A spread of an inch or more per three checks warrants call to surgeon because it could indicate hemorrhage. Determines extent of fluid loss and condition of underlying wound. Size, location, and depth of wound influence amount of drainage (see Chapter 35).
10. Reinforce pressure dressing or change simple dressing as ordered and needed. Make observations of condition of incision, surrounding tissue, and amount and color of any drainage if incision is exposed or covered with transparent dressing.	Pressure dressing helps to maintain **hemostasis** (termination of bleeding) and to absorb drainage. Changing dressings immediately postoperatively can disrupt wound edges and aggravate drainage. First dressing changes most often occur 24 hours postoperatively and are usually done by physician. Minor surgical wounds may not have dressings but simply skin closure or may be covered with transparent dressing, which allows for observation of incision and surrounding tissue.
11. Inspect condition and contents of any drainage tubes and collecting devices. Note character and volume of drainage (see illustration). See Chapter 35 for other types of drains and collection devices.	Determines drainage tube patency and extent and character of wound drainage.

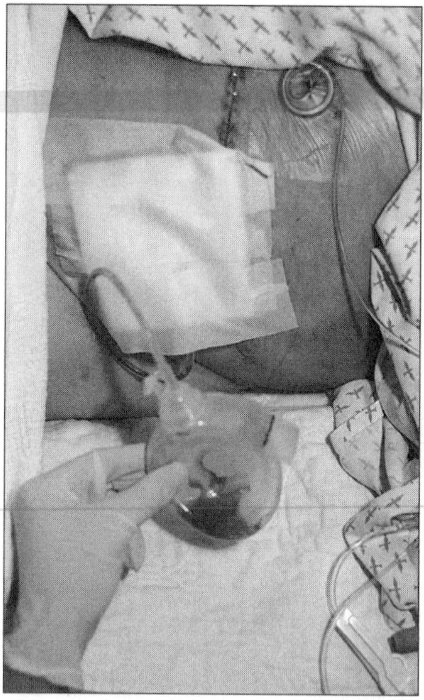

STEP **11** Jackson-Pratt drain charged (collapsed) and client's wound.

STEP	RATIONALE
12. Observe patency and intactness of urinary catheter system (if present). Note volume and character of urine.	Patent drainage system prevents bladder distention. Urine volume monitors renal function and perfusion. Decreased output (less than 30 ml/hr in an adult) is an early sign of hypovolemic shock.
13. If NG tube is present, irrigate periodically (see Chapter 25) with normal saline, if ordered.	Maintains patency of tube to ensure gastric **decompression** (removal of pressure caused by gas or liquid). Normal saline is isotonic and will not increase loss of fluid and electrolytes from stomach.
14. Continue monitoring of IV fluid rates. Observe IV site for signs of infiltration, such as swelling, edema, redness, warmth, discomfort, and leakage of IV fluid.	Continuous regular infusion of IV fluids maintains client's fluid intake to maintain adequate hydration and circulatory function.
15. As client awakens, provide mouth care by placing moistened washcloth to lips, swabbing oral mucosa with dampened swab, or applying petrolatum to lips. Sips of tap water and ice chips may also be ordered.	Client remains at risk for aspiration and should not be given fluids to rinse mouth. Moist cloth, swab, or sips of water and/or ice chips can be soothing to dry mucosa.

Step	Rationale
16. Assess level of pain as client awakens. Provide pain medication as ordered and when vital signs have stabilized (Joint Commission on Accreditation of Healthcare Organizations [JCAHO], 1999).	Pain can increase the stress response and interfere with postoperative exercises. Pain medication can further depress vital signs if effect of anesthetic is still present. Client with spinal anesthesia is unable to feel sensation below level of spinal cord. Client will need pain medication as regional anesthetic wears off.
17. Encourage client to practice ankle circles and calf-pumping exercises.	These leg exercises encourage venous return. If spinal or epidural anesthetic was used, leg exercises help effects of regional anesthetic to wear off once drug has been substantially metabolized by liver.
18. Explain to client how he or she is progressing and that plans for transfer to a nursing division are being made.	Helps client remain oriented to surroundings and recovery activities.
19. Once all physiological signs have stabilized, contact physician for order to release client to nursing division. Measure all intake and output (I&O) prior to transferring client to nursing division.	Physician is responsible for dictating level of observation and care required by client. Intake and output while in PACU is important baseline information to include in report to nurse in nursing division.

- ***Critical Decision Point***

If client is to be discharged to home, ensure that client has someone to drive him or her home and to observe client for signs and symptoms of complications. Review with client and driver reportable signs and symptoms and emergency care needed (Box 33-4).

Phase 2: Convalescent Period

Step	Rationale
1. Make final check of equipment setup in client's room, including emesis basin and waterproof pads. Be sure bed is placed in high horizontal position and to side so that stretcher can easily be moved beside bed.	During transfer, client's status may change, necessitating quick interventions upon arrival. Availability of equipment ensures smooth transfer process.
2. Upon arrival at client's room assist RR/PACU staff, and use three-person carry or slide board to transfer client to bed (see Chapter 27).	Technique avoids strain on nurses' back muscles and maintains client's safety.
3. Once client is transferred to bed, immediately attach any existing oxygen tubing, hang IV fluids, check IV flow rate, attach NG tube to suction, and place indwelling catheter in drainage position.	Maintains client's oxygenation, circulation, and elimination functions. Allows for frequent monitoring of I&O. Provides for client's comfort. Prevents potentially contaminated urine backflow into sterile bladder, thus decreasing incidence of bladder infections.
4. Conduct complete assessment of all vital signs. Compare findings with vital signs in recovery area and client's baseline values. Continue monitoring as ordered.	Client should be stabilized once transferred to nursing division. Change in vital signs can reveal early onset of postoperative complications.

- ***Critical Decision Point***

Report to the anesthesiologist and/or physician any findings deviating from previous assessment.

Step	Rationale
5. Maintain client's airway:	
a. Position client on side (if allowed); if client remains sleepy or lethargic, keep head extended.	Positioning minimizes chances of aspiration.

Box 33-4 Client Teaching for Ambulatory Surgical Clients

- Physician's office telephone number (24-hour answer)
- Surgery center's telephone number
- Follow-up appointment, date, time
- Review of prescribed medications
- Guidelines related to specific surgery
  Dressing and wound care
  Activity restrictions
- Guidelines related to anesthesia
  Dietary
  Activity restrictions
- Warning signs of complications

STEP	RATIONALE
b. Encourage deep breathing and coughing using pillow as an incisional splint every 1 to 2 hours.	Promotes lung expansion and expectoration of mucus.
6. Be sure any drainage tubes are connected to proper suction or drainage device. If NG tube is present, irrigate as ordered and connect to proper drainage device (see Chapter 25).	Maintains drainage tube patency so that wound beds remain dry for healing. Occlusion of NG tube can lead to abdominal distention, vomiting, and aspiration.
7. Assess client's surgical dressing for intactness and presence and character of drainage. Reinforce as ordered. If no dressing present, inspect condition of wound (see Chapter 35).	Wound can hemorrhage quickly during early postoperative period. Observations of wound and dressings provide data to measure progress of wound healing.

- ***Critical Decision Point***
  If unable to change dressing, mark area of drainage and label with time, date and initials. Record frequency of reinforcement. Never use felt tip marker to mark dressing since ink can bleed into gauze, contaminating incision site.

STEP	RATIONALE
8. Assess for bladder distention if client does not have indwelling catheter. Offer bedpan if client senses urge to void (see Chapter 24).	Anesthetics and analgesics depress sensation of bladder fullness. Client may still have no sensations below level of spinal or epidural anesthetic.

- ***Critical Decision Point***
  Initiate measures to stimulate voiding within 4 hours of surgery or removal of indwelling catheter to prevent urinary retention with overflow.

STEP	RATIONALE
9. Measure and record all sources of fluid intake and output (IV, irrigation fluids, ice chips, PO fluids; Foley/voided urine, NG drainage, wound drainage, and excessive perspiration).	Assists in monitoring fluid and electrolyte balance.
10. Position client for comfort, maintaining airway and correct body alignment. Avoid positioning on surgical wound site or with pressure on popliteal space.	Good positioning reduces stress on suture line and decreases risks of aspiration and impaired circulation. Comfortable position helps client relax.
11. Encourage client to continue with leg exercises every 1 to 2 hours. If client is unable or unwilling to do them, nurse should do passive range of motion.	Leg exercises increase venous return, which decreases risk of thrombophlebitis. Range-of-motion exercises maintain joint mobility.
12. If ordered, apply elastic stockings or pneumatic compression cuffs to lower extremities and attach to compressor (see Skill 28-3). Explain to client that compression cuffs will inflate and deflate intermittently.	Increases venous return. Explanation decreases anxiety and fosters cooperation.
13. Explain to client that you have completed all observations and that you will ask family members or significant other to enter room. Place bed in lowest position, and call light within reach, and raise side rails.	Promotes client's orientation and sense of well-being. Lowest position minimizes injury should client become confused and try to get out of bed. Call light and side rail positioning ensure client's safety as effects of anesthetic continue to diminish.
14. Explain client's general status to family and/or significant other, describe purpose of any equipment in room, and explain reason for frequent observations and procedures.	Family and significant others are normally anxious to learn about client's status. Unfamiliar sights (equipment and client's appearance) can be anxiety provoking. Family's and significant other's understanding can promote their participation in client's care.

- ***Critical Decision Point***
  It can be helpful to give family simple tasks to perform, such as wiping client's face with washcloth and coaching postoperative exercises.

STEP	RATIONALE
15. Refer to recovery record to determine if pain medication was administered. Administer analgesic if vital signs remain stable or initiate patient-controlled analgesia (PCA), if ordered (see Skill 5-3). Always ask client to rate the severity of pain on an analog scale and to indicate the amount of analgesic he or she wants (JCAHO, 1999).	Pain relief is essential for client to be able to begin postoperative exercises. Pain may sometimes lower blood pressure, thus giving analgesics may restore vital signs to normal levels. Client is best judge of his or her pain. Pain scale helps to make this experience more objective for nurse to understand.

STEP	RATIONALE
16. Provide oral hygiene, and repeat as needed.	Maintenance of moist mucous membranes facilitates expectoration of secretions and promotes comfort.
17. As client stabilizes over the next hours or days, perform the following measures:	
a. Have client participate in postoperative exercises.	Promotes pulmonary and circulatory function to minimize onset of postoperative complications.
b. Encourage use of incentive spirometer if ordered. Watch client use spirometer first few times to judge efficacy of breathing pattern. Chart level to which client can achieve.	Promotes lung expansion. Can monitor progress and encourage client to inhale more deeply.
c. Begin activity orders. Assess vital signs first time client sits or stands to judge tolerance.	Early ambulation promotes circulation, lung expansion, and peristalsis. Sudden positional changes can cause **postural hypotension.**
d. Monitor bowel sounds every 4 to 8 hours. Must wait to have at least hypoactive bowel sounds before advancing diet beyond ice chips. Begin dietary orders slowly according to client's tolerance. Medicate with antiemetic if client is nauseated. Give analgesic with antiemetic until client is eating well.	Promotes normal fluid and electrolyte balance, restores nutritional intake, and promotes normal GI function and wound healing. Analgesics often cause nausea on an empty stomach.
e. Assist client in assuming normal urinary voiding pattern (see Chapter 24). Male clients may need assistance to stand to void. Female clients may need to sit on bedpan in bed or chair so legs can be bent and dangling or helped to bathroom.	Promotes normal urinary elimination and prevents bladder distention and urinary retention with overflow. A more natural position may help client to void.

- ***Critical Decision Point***

  If client does not void within 8 hours after surgery or bladder becomes distended, notify physician. Urinary catheter may have to be inserted.

STEP	RATIONALE
f. Closely monitor progress of wound healing, and change dressings as ordered.	Wound infection occurs most often within 3 to 6 days postoperatively. Wound **dehiscence** occurs most often 3 to 11 days postoperatively.

- ***Critical Decision Point***

  Delayed wound healing may result in wound dehiscence or ***evisceration.*** *This occurs most frequently after coughing, sneezing, vomiting, or getting up from a sitting position. Caution should be observed when client performs these activities. Remind client to use pillow to splint incision during these activities. Evisceration is a medical emergency (see Chapter 35).*

STEP	RATIONALE
g. Monitor and maintain wound drainage devices, such as **Jackson-Pratt, Hemovac,** or **Penrose drains.** Jackson-Pratt and Hemovac drainage systems must be emptied whenever they are half full of drainage or air and be recharged (compressed to discharge air) (see illustration).	Wound drainage devices promote healing from inside to outside and relieve pressure on suture line. Compressing a flexible closed container and then plugging drainage hole creates negative suction pressure.
h. Monitor drainage for color, consistency, and amount every 4 to 8 hours. Compare to previous assessment.	Drainage should progress from sanguineous to serosanguineous to serous in color, become more watery, and decrease in amount as wound heals.
18. Gradually increase client's involvement in decision making and in any explanations about surgery and related implications.	Promotes client's sense of control and independence. Encourages feeling of self-esteem.
19. Teach client and family signs and symptoms of complications such as infection, dehiscence, excessive bleeding, and nutrition for wound healing and wound care if needed.	Early discharge necessitates client and family involvement because complications often occur after client goes home.
20. Discuss with client and family or significant other plans for discharge.	Discharge planning is continuous process, beginning with client's admission.

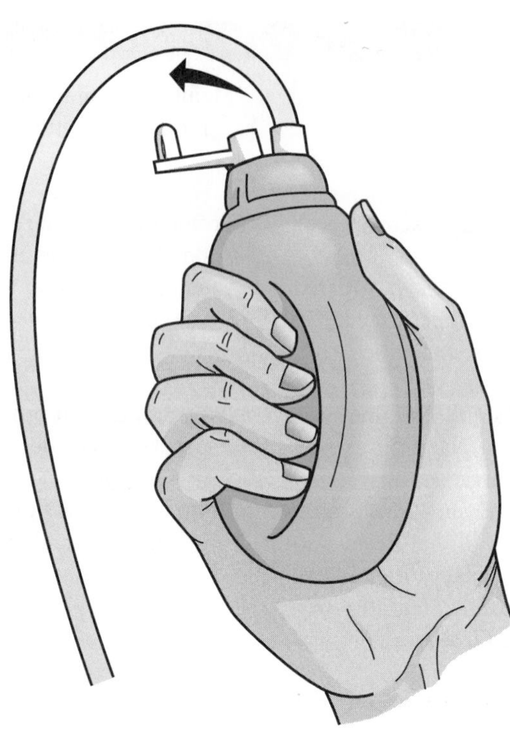

STEP 17g Charging a Jackson-Pratt drainage system.

Step	Rationale
21. Prepare to make referral for home health or convalescent care as client's condition dictates. Get order from physician.	If client continues to need nursing care or rehabilitation after discharge, physician's order is necessary. Referral provides continuity of care.

Evaluation

Step	Rationale
1. Compare all vital sign assessment measurements with client's baseline and expected normals.	Allows nurse to evaluate client's respiratory, cardiovascular, and thermoregulatory status throughout recovery.
2. Evaluate effects of pain-relief measures, such as positioning, and use of analgesics.	Determines level of comfort achieved and effectiveness of pain-relief measures.
3. Monitor changes in surgical wound at least every shift.	Provides data for nurse to measure progress of wound healing.
4. Monitor lung sounds following postoperative exercises.	Determines status of airways.
5. Auscultate bowel sounds at least each shift.	Allows nurse to evaluate return of peristalsis and diet tolerance.
6. Monitor intake and output balance for each shift.	Can indicate onset of fluid imbalances.
7. Discuss with client general level of comfort and progress toward recovery.	Gives client sense of participation in care. Client's perceptions can also be helpful in noting onset of complications. Reveals readiness to learn about discharge.
8. Conduct physical assessments appropriate for client's unique type of surgery.	Allows nurse to monitor course of recovery.

Unexpected Outcomes and Related Interventions

- Vital signs are above or below client's baseline or expected range.
  - Alterations may result from anesthetic effects, pain, or surgical complications such as hypovolemic shock, airway obstruction, fluid and electrolyte imbalances, or malignant hyperthermia. Malignant hyperthermia (MH) is caused by use of certain anesthetic agents and usually occurs during or immediately after surgery. Often involves personal or family history of MH (Stolworthy and Haas, 1998).

- Client continues to experience incisional pain.
  - Factors such as anxiety, isolation, and fatigue may heighten client's pain perception. Analgesic ordered may be of insufficient dosage.
  - Call physician for additional analgesic orders.
- Abnormal or absent breath sounds are auscultated. This may be due to bronchial constriction or mucus secretions in large airways immediately postoperatively or result of atelectasis a day or more later.
  - Notify physician and request order for incentive spirometer, if not already ordered.
  - Encourage client to turn, deep breathe, and cough more often.
  - Investigate history of asthma or allergic response to medication when wheezing or stridor is auscultated.
- Client complains of calf tenderness; exhibits positive Homans' sign, redness and edema in lower extremity.
  - These are signs and symptoms of **venous thrombosis** or thrombophlebitis. Notify physician, and anticipate orders for bed rest, leg elevation, and heparin drip.
  - Do not massage affected leg.
  - Continue to have client do leg exercises with unaffected leg.
- Bowel sounds are absent or decreased.
  - **Paralytic ileus** can develop as common complication after bowel or abdominal surgery. Intestinal motility may return slowly depending on anesthetic effects.
  - Keep IV in place.
  - Encourage turning and ambulation.
  - Assess for bowel sounds and flatus every 4 hours.
  - Report findings to physician.
- Client develops fever, tenderness, and pain at wound site; increased white blood cell count or purulent drainage is present.
  - These are signs and symptoms of wound infection. Notify physician, and anticipate orders for culture of wound drainage and IV antibiotics.
- Client reports feeling something in wound "give way." Increased serosanguineous drainage is noted.
  - May indicate wound dehiscence or evisceration. Report wound dehiscence and/or evisceration to surgeon immediately because it could be life threatening.
  - If evisceration has occurred, cover abdominal contents with sterile gauze saturated with sterile normal saline and prepare client for emergency surgery.
- Intake and output measurements reflect imbalance.
  - Indicates possible fluid volume excess or deficit. Client is at risk for electrolyte imbalance, **pulmonary edema,** and **renal insufficiency**.
  - Continue to monitor strict I&O, and contact physician if 24-hour totals continue to reflect imbalance.
- Client is unable to discuss discharge plans or has negative view of recovery.
  - May indicate client is coping poorly with stress of surgery. Discuss discharge plans and instructions with significant family member or friend.
  - Encourage client to express fears and concerns.
  - Refer client to support group if appropriate.
  - Notify physician, and request referral for counseling if necessary.

Recording and Reporting

- Document client's arrival in RR/PACU or nursing division; record vital signs, assessment findings, and all nursing measures initiated in nurses' notes. Continue documentation every 15 minutes until stable, then every 30 minutes times 2, every hour times 4, then every 4 to 8 hours as condition warrants.
- Record vital signs and I&O on appropriate flow sheets.
- Report any abnormal assessment findings and signs of complications to nurse in charge and/or physician.

Teaching Considerations

- If client had spinal or epidural anesthetic, remind family or significant other that loss of extremity movement is normal for several hours.
- Reinforce preoperative teaching regarding coughing, deep breathing, and leg exercises and information concerning ambulation and pain control.
- Instruct client and primary caregiver to identify signs and symptoms and appropriate actions for infection, respiratory, circulatory, or GI difficulties, and wound disruptions.
- Provide important phone numbers to client and primary caregiver for use in event of emergency and for follow-up care on discharge.
- Teach client about appropriate wound care and diet recommendations.
- Inform client of any activity restrictions.

Pediatric Considerations

- Parent-child separation should be kept to minimum time possible. When a parent cannot be present, it is important to leave a favorite possession with child.
- Nurse must be alert for allergic responses and signs and symptoms of malignant hyperthermia in children who have not been exposed to drugs or anesthetic agents. Family history of allergies makes child at high risk for experiencing similar reactions.
- Vomiting is a major concern in young children due to increased risk of fluid and electrolyte imbalances and risk of aspiration. Vomiting is also more likely because surgery in children is often necessitated by accidental injuries without benefit of status of ingesting nothing by mouth (NPO).
- Mandatory fluid intake guidelines are not usually necessary because of aggressive fluid replacement in children.

- Voiding before discharge from ambulatory surgery is not usually required for young children.
- Undermedicating young children may be based on myth that narcotics are more dangerous for infants. The fact is that "by 3-6 months of age, healthy infants can metabolize opioids similarly to older children" (Wong, 1997). Observing the normalizing of vital signs and behavior after administration of analgesics is a valuable clue that pain really existed before treatment (Wong, 1997).

Gerontological Considerations

- The ability of older adults to tolerate surgery depends on extent of physiological changes that have occurred with aging, presence of any chronic diseases, and duration of surgical procedure.
- Risk-versus-benefit ratio for older adults looks at quality-of-life issues concerning increased operative risk and risk of complications versus potential benefit to client from surgery (Nusbaum, 1996).
- Undermedicating older adults is common. Asking clients to rate their pain before and after administration of analgesics and asking what numerical rating is acceptable to them are better methods of individualizing care.

Home Care Considerations

- Teach primary caregiver about any postoperative exercises, home modifications, or activity limitations.
- If client is discharged with dressing changes, bedroom or bathroom is usually an ideal location for procedure. Have primary caregiver perform return demonstration of dressing change.

Critical Thinking Exercises

1. A 66-year-old client is receiving intravenous (IV) fluid and electrolyte replacements in preparation for tomorrow's surgery. He is requesting opioid analgesics every 4 hours for pain and has not signed the operative consent form. How could the nurse obtain a valid consent for surgery?
2. An obese, 40-year-old female client smokes two packs of cigarettes per day and has been taking birth control pills "for years." She is scheduled for an abdominal hysterectomy. Which postoperative exercises should the nurse emphasize the most? Give rationale.
3. A client has signed the operating room (OR) permit and has given evidence that he is informed about the surgery. After he has received his preoperative medications, he confides to the nurse that he really does not want this surgery. What should the nurse do?
4. A postoperative client with an IV of 5% dextrose in 0.45% sodium chloride has an order to discontinue the IV. What client parameters must the nurse consider before following this order?

References

American Society of Anesthesiologists: Practice guidelines for sedation and analgesia by nonanesthesiologists, *Anesthesiology* 84:459, 1996.

Armstrong M: A clinical look at body piercing, *RN* 61(9):26, 1998.

Association of Operating Room Nurses: *Standards and recommended practices for perioperative nursing,* Denver, 1997, The Association.

Association of Operating Room Nurses: *Standards and recommended practices for perioperative nursing,* Denver, 1999, The Association.

Brick J: Informed consent and perioperative nursing, *AORN J* 63(1):258, 1996.

Centers for Disease Control and Prevention: *Guidelines for prevention of surgical site infections,* Atlanta, 1999, Hospital Infection Control Programs, US Department of Health and Human Services.

Dunn D: Preoperative assessment criteria and patient teaching for ambulatory surgery patients, *J Perianesth Nurs* 13(5):274, 1998.

Dunn D: Exploring the gray areas of informed consent, *Nursing* 29(7):41, 1999.

Fennell MD: Parents in, you bet! *RN* 62(12):38, 1999.

Geissler E: *Pocket guide to cultural assessment,* St. Louis, 1998, Mosby.

Joint Commission on Accreditation of Healthcare Organizations: *Accreditation manual for hospitals,* Chicago, 1997, The Commission.

Joint Commission on Accreditation of Healthcare Organizations: *Accreditation manual for hospitals,* Chicago, 1999, The Commission.

Lancaster KA: Patient teaching in ambulatory surgery, *Nurs Clin North Am* 32(2):417, 1997.

Lewis S, Heitkemper M, Dirkson S: *Medical-surgical nursing, assessment and management of clinical problems,* ed 5, St. Louis, 2000, Mosby.

Lowdermilk D, Perry S, Bobak I: *Maternity nursing,* ed 5, St. Louis, 1999, Mosby.

Mosby's medical, nursing, and allied health dictionary, ed 5, St. Louis, 1998, Mosby.

Nusbaum N: How do geriatric patients recover from surgery? *South Med J* Vol 89(10):950-957, 1996.

Potter P, Perry A: *Basic nursing: a critical thinking approach,* ed 4, St. Louis, 1998, Mosby.

Shuldham C: A review of the impact of pre-operative education on recovery from surgery, *Int J Nurs Stud* 36:171, 1999.

Stolworthy C, Haas RE: Malignant hyperthermia: a potentially fatal complication of anesthesia, *Semin Perioper Nurs* 7(1):58, 1998.

Wong D: *Whaley and Wong's essentials of pediatric nursing,* ed 5, St. Louis, 1997, Mosby.

34

Intraoperative Care

Skills

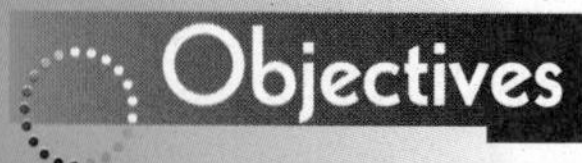

Objectives

Mastery of content in this chapter will enable the nurse to:

- Define the key terms listed.
- Describe the meaning of a sterile conscience.
- Describe the roles of a registered nurse in the operating room.
- Identify guidelines for use of sterile technique in the operating room.
- Correctly perform surgical hand washing.
- Correctly don a sterile surgical gown.
- Correctly apply sterile gloves using the closed technique.

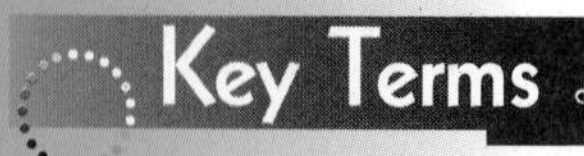

Key Terms

Asepsis
Aseptic technique
Circulating nurse
Contamination
Perioperative
Registered Nurse First Assistant (RNFA)
Scrub nurse
Sponge
Sterile
Sterile conscience
Sterile field
Strike through
Surgical scrub

The **perioperative** role of the nurse working in the operating room (OR) suite encompasses the client's surgical experience from the preoperative throughout the intraoperative period and into the postoperative phase (see Chapter 33). The standards of clinical practice that registered nurses follow within the OR are designed to provide an optimal level of care that ensures the client's safety and comfort (AORN, 1999a). In addition, the nurse exercises judgment, critical thinking, and interpersonal communication skills in applying the nursing process to ensure clients receive appropriate nursing care during the perioperative experience.

Members of the surgical team may include the surgeon, **registered nurse first assistant (RNFA),** certified registered nurse anesthetist (CRNA) and/or physician anesthesiologist, circulating nurse and scrub nurse, and surgical technologist. The intraoperative phase begins when the client enters the OR suite and ends with admission to the postanesthesia care unit (PACU). During the intraoperative phase, the registered professional nurse assumes the role of either first assistant to the surgeon, scrub nurse, or circulating nurse. The RNFA is a nurse with advanced education (including a clinical practicum or internship) who assists the surgeon with the surgical procedure, performing a combination of nursing and medical functions (Box 34-1). The **scrub nurse** (Box 34-2) provides the surgeon with instruments and supplies, disposes of soiled sponges, and accounts for sponges, needles, and instruments on the surgical field. Registered nurses, licensed practical nurses, or surgical technologists may assume the scrub nurse role. The **circulating nurse** (Box 34-3) is always a registered nurse and is considered to be the charge nurse in the room (AORN, 1995). The circulating nurse assumes responsibility and accountability for maintaining client safety and continuity of quality care. This includes supervising the conduct of the nonprofessional staff. The circulating nurse is also an assistant to the first assistant, scrub nurse, and surgeon.

It is essential that perioperative nurses fully understand and follow the principles of **aseptic technique.** The over-all goal of **asepsis** is to minimize contamination of the surgical wound. Before the client reaches the OR, supplies, instruments, and equipment must be thoroughly sterilized to remove all microorganisms. Members of the surgical team follow specific guidelines for performing a **surgical scrub** and

Box 34-1 Role and Responsibilities of a Registered Nurse First Assistant

The RNFA role is an expansion of the traditional perioperative nursing role and areas of responsibility will overlap. Responsibilities specific to the practice of first assisting include:

- Providing surgical exposure (assists in retraction of tissues and suctioning of surgical field)
- Providing hemostasis (control of bleeding)
- Handling tissue safely
- Using surgical instruments and suturing
- Performing wound closure
- Applying human anatomical and physiological considerations in practice; recognizes structure, function and location of tissues and organs; manipulates tissues accordingly to avoid injury

Adapted from Johnson CR and others: RN first assistant certification; clinical internship; job descriptions; insurance coverage; specialty assembly, *AORN J* 64(1):115-118, 1996.

Box 34-2 Role of the Scrub Nurse

- Assists circulating nurse in preparing OR, opening supplies
- Performs surgical hand scrub and dons sterile gown and gloves
- Sets up sterile field with procedure-appropriate supplies and instruments, verifying all are in working order
- Performs **sponge,** sharp, and instrument counts with circulating nurse before incision is made
- Gowns and gloves surgeons and assistants as they enter the OR
- Assists surgeons with sterile draping of client
- Keeps sterile field orderly and monitors progress of procedure and any breaks in aseptic technique
- Passes instruments and supplies to surgeons and assistants
- Handles surgical specimens per institutional policy
- Constantly monitors location of all sponges and sharps in the field and performs closing sponge, sharp, and instrument counts with circulating nurse.

donning surgical attire before handling **sterile** items. The special preparation of the client's skin before application of sterile drapes helps reduce the numbers of microorganisms around the surgical incision. The **scrub nurse** and surgeons create a **sterile field** around the surgical wound and maintain it throughout the procedure in accordance with strict aseptic principles. The surgical procedure itself finally ends with sterile application of dressings.

All OR personnel must develop a **sterile conscience,** or personal commitment to safe, quality client care. A sterile conscience means a nurse must know what is sterile, what is unsterile, and how to keep sterile and unsterile items apart. The practice of strict aseptic technique requires discipline, integrity, honesty, and assertiveness concerning any shortcomings in aseptic practice. The scrub nurse, who accidentally touches the faucet with one hand, while rinsing rescrubs the hands; the circulating nurse, who accidentally touches a sterile item, has it removed from the field; the surgeon who contaminates a sterile glove, has the affected glove changed. These are all examples of following one's sterile conscience.

During the postoperative phase, the registered nurse assists in transferring the client to the recovery room or postanesthesia room. The OR nurse is an important resource in planning the client's postoperative care.

Box 34-3 Role of the Circulating Nurse

- Organizes and prepares OR before start of case; checks to see equipment works properly
- Gathers supplies for case and opens sterile supplies for scrub nurse
- Counts sponges, sharps, and instruments with scrub nurse before incision is made
- Sends for client at appropriate time
- Conducts preoperative client assessment, including the following:
  - Explains role and identifies client
  - Reviews medical record and verifies procedure and consents
  - Confirms dentures and prostheses removed
  - Confirms client's allergies, nothing by mouth (NPO) status, laboratory values, electrocardiogram (ECG), x-ray films, skin condition, circulatory and pulmonary status
- Safely transfers client to operating table and positions client according to surgeon preference and procedure type
- Applies return electrode pad to client if electrocautery used; may prepare client's skin; may apply ECG electrodes for local case
- Explains briefly to client what the circulating nurse and the scrub nurse are doing
- Assists surgical team by tying gowns and arranging tables
- Assists anesthesiologist during induction and extubation
- Continuously monitors procedure for any breaks in aseptic technique or to anticipate needs of the team; opens additional sterile supplies for scrub nurse; ensures standard precautions maintained
- Handles surgical specimens per institutional policy
- Documents care on perioperative nurse's notes
- Performs sponge, sharp, and instrument counts with scrub nurse at beginning of wound closure

Skill Performance Guidelines

1. All items used within a sterile field must be sterile.
2. Gowns used by scrub persons must be sterile before donning. Once in place, gowns are considered sterile from the front chest and shoulders to table level and on the sleeves to 2 inches (5 cm) above the elbow.
3. Sterile persons must keep hands in sight, above waist level and below neckline to avoid **contamination.**
4. When wearing a sterile gown, arms should *not* be folded with hands tucked in the axillary region. This area is not considered sterile once the gown is donned. Perspiration can lead to **strike through,** or contamination that occurs when moisture permeates a sterile barrier.
5. Draped tables should be considered sterile only at table level. Sides of the drape extending below table level are unsterile.
6. All personnel moving around or within a sterile field must do so in a manner consistent with maintaining the sterility of that field. Scrubbed persons move from sterile areas to other sterile areas, contacting a sterile field only with sterile gowns and gloves. Unscrubbed persons should always stay at least 1 foot away from the sterile field while keeping it in constant view and should contact only unsterile areas.
7. All sterile supplies and equipment should be grouped around the sterile-draped client.
8. Unsterile persons must avoid reaching over the sterile field.
9. Scrubbed persons should remain close to the sterile field. When changing position, they should turn face to face or back to back.

Skill 34-1 Surgical Hand Washing

The skin is a major potential source of microbial contamination. Although scrubbed members of the surgical team wear sterile gloves, the skin of their hands and forearms should be cleaned preoperatively to reduce the number of microorganisms in the event of glove tears (AORN, 1999b). The skin can never be rendered sterile; however, it can be made surgically clean through scrubbing. Surgical hand washing is necessary for nurses working in OR suites, delivery rooms, and in special diagnostic and procedure areas. The purposes of a surgical hand scrub are:

- To remove debris and transient microorganisms from the nails, hands, and forearms
- To reduce the resident microbial count to a minimum
- To inhibit rapid rebound growth of microorganisms (AORN, 1999b)

The Association of Operating Room Nurses (AORN) recommends a 2- to 3-minute surgical scrub to effectively reduce microbial counts on the hands before each surgical procedure (AORN, 1999b). Exceptions to the rule include procedures such as bronchoscopies, laryngoscopies, esophagoscopies, and certain laser procedures. These procedures require only a thorough hand washing of 3 to 5 minutes.

For maximum elimination of bacteria, the nurse removes all rings, watches, and bracelets and keeps fingernails short, clean, healthy, and free of artificial nails (Salisbury, and others, 1997). Brushes are used during scrubbing. Some experts caution that too much brushing removes outer layers of the epidermis, thereby exposing bacterial flora in the deeper skin layers.

If harsh soaps are used, the nurse's skin can become irritated, providing an environment for additional microorganism growth. Antiseptic solutions such as chlorhexidine gluconate, iodophors, and triclosan improve removal of bacteria from the hands and arms.

Delegation Considerations

Surgical hand washing is performed by a scrub nurse or RNFA. The role of the scrub nurse can be delegated to a surgical technologist or licensed practice nurse. Nonlicensed personnel can assist the RN in the circulating role by setting up gown and glove supplies, opening sterile supplies, setting up sterile fields, and running errands under the direction of the RN.

Equipment

- Deep sink with foot or knee controls for dispensing water and soap (faucets should be high enough for hands and forearms to fit comfortably)
- Antiseptic detergent (nonirritating, broad-spectrum, fast-acting, effective in reducing skin microorganisms, and having a residual effect) (AORN, 1999b)
- Surgical scrub brush with plastic nail pick
- Paper mask and cap or hood
- Sterile towel
- Scrub suit attire
- Protective eyewear (glasses or goggles)

Step	Rationale
Assessment	
1. Consult institutional policy regarding required length of time for hand wash.	Guidelines vary regarding ideal time needed for surgical scrub.
2. Be sure fingernails are short, clean, and healthy. Artificial nails should be removed.	Long nails and chipped or old polish increase number of bacteria residing on nails. Long fingernails can puncture gloves, causing contamination. Artificial nails may harbor gram-negative microorganisms and fungus.

- ***Critical Decision Point***
  Nail polish should be removed if chipped or worn longer than 4 days because there is a tendency after that time for the nails to harbor greater numbers of bacteria (AORN, 1999b).

Step	Rationale
3. Inspect condition of cuticles, hands, and forearms for presence of abrasions, cuts, or open lesions.	Cuts, abrasions, exudative lesions, and hangnails tend to ooze serum, which may contain pathogens. Broken skin permits microorganisms to enter various layers of the skin, providing deeper microbial breeding grounds (AORN, 1999b).
4. Be sure if wearing a two-piece pants and top scrub suit, that the top is secured at the waist and tucked into the pants.	Prevents brushing against sterile areas.

Nursing Diagnosis

Defining characteristics from the assessment data may reveal the following nursing diagnoses for clients requiring this skill:

Risk for infection
Risk for injury

Related factors are individualized based on client's condition or needs.

Step	Rationale
Planning	
1. **Expected outcomes** following completion of procedure: ▪ Client will not develop signs of surgical wound infection.	Indicates microorganisms are not transferred to the client and sterile field.
2. Prepare equipment.	Ensures availability before the procedure.
3. Remove watch, rings, and bracelets.	Jewelry harbors microorganisms and interferes with access to all surfaces of skin to be cleaned.
4. Be sure sleeves are above elbows and uniform is fitted or tucked at waist.	Scrubbed hands and arms can become contaminated by brushing against loose garments.
Implementation	
1. Apply surgical attire: shoe covers, cap or hood, face mask, and protective eyewear (Chapter 32).	Mask prevents escape into air of microorganisms that can contaminate hands. Other protective wear prevents exposure to blood and body fluid splashes during the procedure.
2. Turn on water using knee or foot controls and adjust to comfortable temperature.	Knee or foot controls prevent contamination of hands after scrub.
3. Wet hands and arms under running lukewarm water and lather with detergent up to 2 inches above elbows (see illustration). (Hands need to be held above elbows at all times.)	Water runs by gravity from fingertips to elbows. Hands become cleanest part of upper extremity. Keeping hands elevated allows water to flow from least to most contaminated areas. Washing a wide area reduces risk of contaminating overlying gown that the nurse later applies.
4. Rinse hands and arms thoroughly under running water. **Remember to keep hands above elbows.**	Rinsing removes transient bacteria from fingers, hands, and forearms.
5. Under running water, clean under nails of both hands with file. Discard after use (see illustration).	Removes dirt and organic material that harbor large numbers of microorganisms.
6. Wet brush and apply antimicrobial detergent. Scrub the nails of one hand with 15 strokes. Holding brush perpendicular, scrub the palm, each side of the thumb, and fingers, and the posterior side of the hand with 10 strokes each. The arm is mentally divided into thirds and each third is scrubbed 10 times (see illustration). Entire scrub should last at least 2 to 3 minutes (AORN, 1999b). Rinse brush and repeat the sequence for the other arm. A two-brush method may be substituted. Check institution's policy.	Scrubbing loosens resident bacteria that adhere to skin surfaces. Ensures coverage of all surfaces. Scrubbing is performed from cleanest area (hands) to marginal area (upper arms).

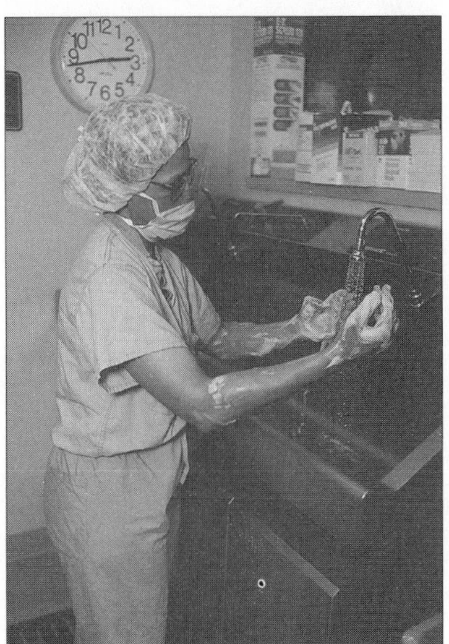

STEP **3** Prescrub wash/rinse.

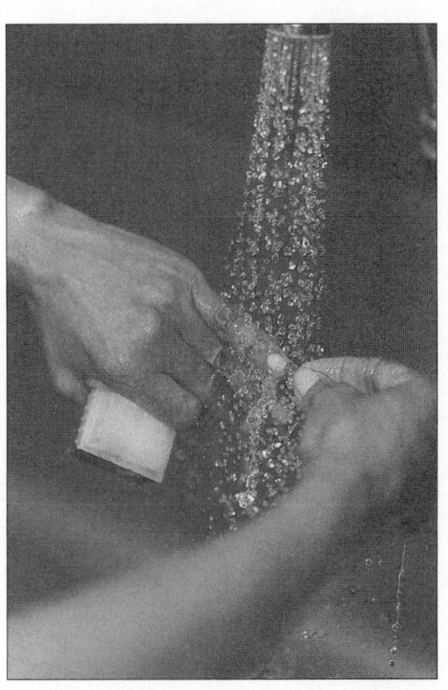

STEP **5** Cleaning under fingernails.

Step	Rationale
7. Discard brush and rinse hands and arms thoroughly (see illustration). Turn off water with foot or knee control and back into room entrance with hands elevated in front of and away from the body.	After touching skin, brush is considered contaminated. Rinsing removes resident bacteria. Prevents accidental contamination.
8. Bending slightly forward at the waist, use a sterile towel to dry one hand thoroughly moving from fingers to elbow. Dry in a rotating motion (see illustration). Dry from cleanest to least clean area.	Drying prevents chapping and facilitates donning of gloves. Leaning forward prevents accidental contact of arms with scrub attire.
9. Repeat drying method for other hand, using a different area of the towel or a new sterile towel (see illustration).	Prevents accidental contamination.

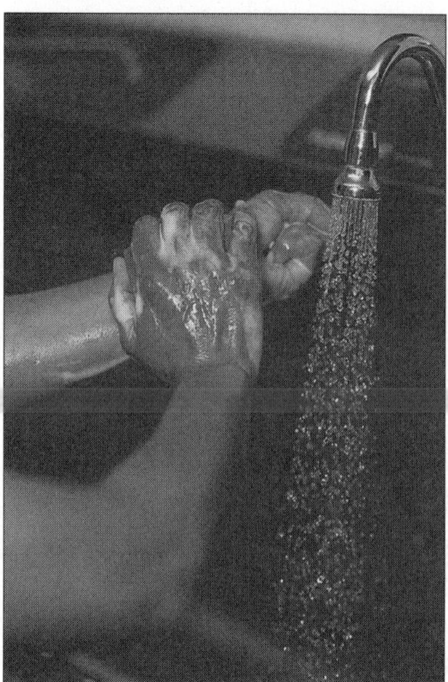

STEP **6** Scrubbing forearms.

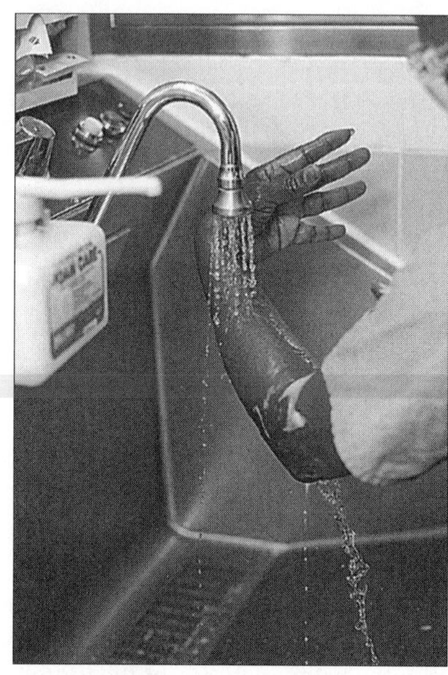

STEP **7** Rinsing arm.

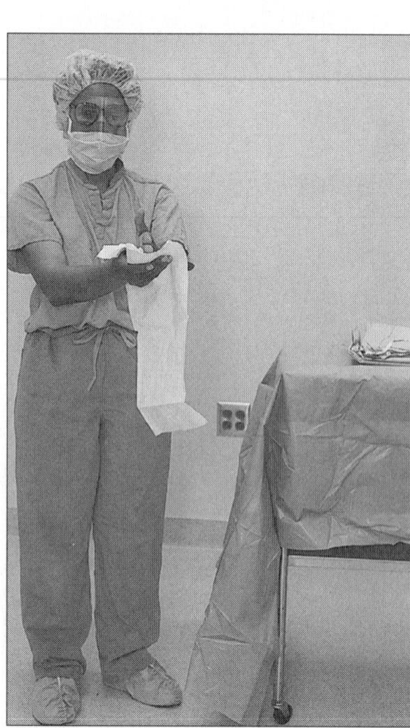

STEP **8** Drying sequence.

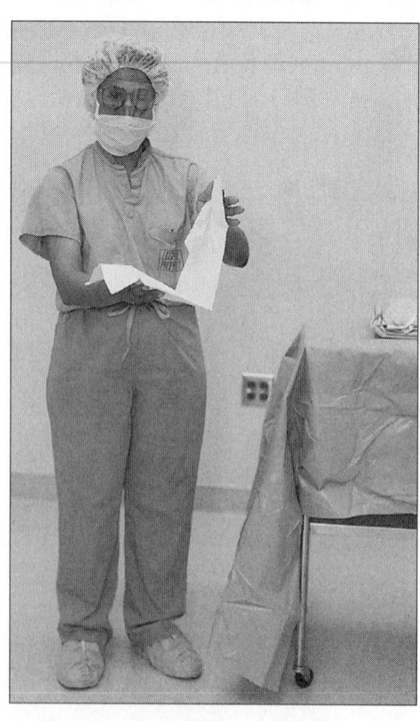

STEP **9** Repeating drying method for other hand.

STEP	RATIONALE
EVALUATION	
1. Observe the client for signs of localized wound infection (usually occurs 2 to 3 days post-op).	Signs of infection include redness, heat, swelling, pain, and drainage.

UNEXPECTED OUTCOMES AND RELATED INTERVENTIONS

- Redness, heat, swelling, pain, or drainage may develop at surgical site as a result of infection. Institute appropriate wound care (see Chapter 35).
- In the event a pattern of surgical wound infections occurs, the hospital infection control team will monitor trends from the operating rooms in an effort to trace origin. This may include cultures of nails and hands of staff, soap dispensers, etc.

RECORDING AND REPORTING

- No recording is required for hand washing. Record area and description of surgical site postoperatively to provide baseline for monitoring wound.

Skill 34-2 Donning a Sterile Gown and Gloves (Closed Gloving)

There are semirestricted and restricted areas within traditional OR suites, ambulatory surgical units, and special procedure areas where personnel must wear special surgical attire. The human body is a major source of microbial contamination. Wearing surgical attire helps to prevent the transmission of microorganisms from personnel to clients. Scrub gowns, hair coverings, masks, and protective eyewear offer barriers to contamination. **Surgical attire should be worn only within the surgical suite.** If it is worn outside the OR, it should be covered or changed before the person reenters the area. Street clothes are not worn in the restricted areas of the surgical suite.

The scrub suit offers a high-level of cleanliness and hygiene within the surgical environment (AORN, 1999c). A clean scrub suit (dress or pants and top) (Figure 34-1) is worn to contain bacterial shedding from the thoracic and abdominal skin. If a two-piece pants and top is worn, the top must be secured at the waist, tucked into the pants, or fit close to the body to prevent brushing against sterile areas. Scrub suits should be changed daily or whenever they become visibly soiled or wet by blood, body fluid, sweat, or food. Sleeves should be short enough to allow for surgical hand washing (scrubbing) to 2 inches above the elbow. A warm-up jacket may be worn after scrubbing by a circulating nurse if desired.

All possible head and facial hair (including sideburns and necklines) should be covered when one is in the semirestricted and restricted areas of the surgical suite (AORN, 1999c). A clean, low-lint surgical hat or hood should be the first piece of OR attire that is donned to prevent hair from collecting on the scrub clothes. A clean hat should be worn each day.

Shoe covers may be worn inside the OR for sanitation purposes. Knee-high shoe covers may be worn as personal protective equipment for cases in which large amounts of fluid or blood may be lost. All shoe covers should be removed on leaving the restricted areas of the suite, and new shoe covers may be put on when returning to the OR. Clean shoe covers should be worn each day and should be changed if they become

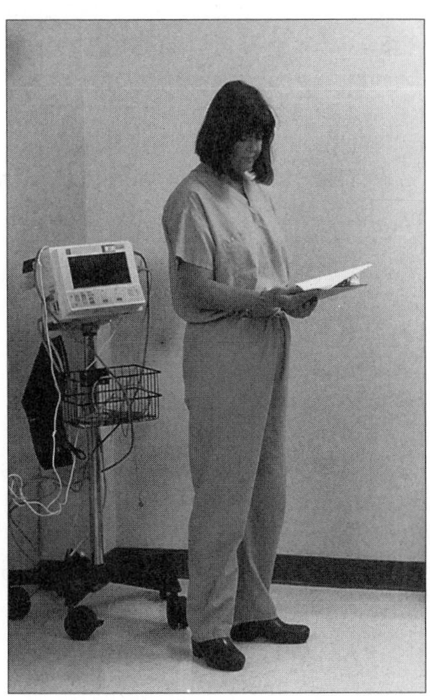

FIGURE 34-1 Nurse in scrub suit.

soiled. Sandals are not recommended in the OR because they are not considered safe.

Masks must be worn in specified restricted areas of the surgical suite. Examples of restricted areas include rooms with open sterile supplies and areas designed to sterilize instruments. The purpose of the mask is to filter organisms from exhaled air. The mask should be secured over the nose, along the sides of the face, and under the chin to prevent venting or the escape of air (see Chapter 32). As a mask becomes moist, its effectiveness decreases because bacteria can pass through it. Surgical masks should be changed between procedures and should not be allowed to hang around the neck, harboring bacteria from the nasopharyngeal airway. Use of a double mask provides a barrier rather than a filter and is unacceptable (Garner, 1995). Only mask strings should be touched when removing a mask to reduce contamination of hands by bacteria from the airway.

Protective eyewear is worn to reduce the incidence of contamination of mucous membranes of the eyes, nose, and mouth whenever contamination can be anticipated as a result of splashes, sprays, or splatters of blood droplets or other infectious material. If the nurse is the scrub nurse or first assistant, the risk of splashing is very high. Protective eyewear includes goggles or glasses with solid side shields or chin-length face shields.

Jewelry should not be worn in the surgical suite. Rings, watches, and necklaces serve as reservoirs for bacteria. Dangling earrings that hang outside the cap can fall onto the sterile field.

When a scrub nurse or RNFA enters the operating room, it becomes necessary to apply a sterile gown and gloves, using the closed method. Gloves should fit properly to ensure ease of handling of the OR instruments and supplies. It is also important for the nurse to know his or her own risk of latex sensitivity (see Chapter 32). The selection of latex-free gloves eliminates risk of an allergic response. Before donning the gown and gloves, a complete surgical scrub (Skill 34-1) must be performed.

Delegation Considerations

Application of a sterile gown and gloves is usually performed by a scrub nurse or RNFA. The role of a scrub nurse can be delegated to a surgical technologist or licensed practical or licensed vocational nurse. See agency policy for level of staff working in sterile procedure areas. Technologists can assist in setting up sterile gown and glove packages.

Equipment

- Package of proper-sized sterile gloves (latex-free if nurse or client has sensitivity or allergy)
- Sterile pack containing sterile gown (prepared by circulating nurse)
- Surgical hat or hood, mask, and footwear
- Equipment needed for surgical hand washing (Skill 34-1)
- Protective eyewear/face shield

Step	Rationale
Assessment	
1. Inspect condition of cuticles and hands for cuts, open lesions, or abrasions.	Lesions harbor microorganisms and may prevent nurse from performing procedure.
2. Check fingernails per procedure in Skill 34-1.	Fingernails harbor microorganisms.
3. Choose proper size and type of glove. Latex-free glove is preferred.	Ill-fitting gloves impede the ability to grasp objects and provide an opportunity for needle punctures. Skin sensitivities may occur with latex gloves. Powder in latex gloves can be inhaled and cause an allergic response.
4. Choose proper size and type of gown.	Ill-fitting gown may impede movement of nurse's extremities.

Nursing Diagnosis

Defining characteristics from the assessment data may reveal the following nursing diagnoses for clients requiring this skill:

Risk for infection

Related factors are individualized based on client's condition or needs.

Planning

Step	Rationale
1. **Expected outcomes** following completion of procedure:	
▪ No break in surgical technique will occur. Client is not exposed to microorganisms.	Nurse maintains aseptic practice and does not contaminate gown or gloves.

STEP	RATIONALE
2. Prepare for surgical hand washing. Alert personnel in OR suite or treatment area that scrubbing is to begin. (Personnel will prepare gown and glove packs.)	Circulating nurse or technician must be available to assist nurse with gowning once scrub is completed.

IMPLEMENTATION

STEP	RATIONALE
1. Perform surgical hand scrub (Skill 34-1).	
2. Enter operating suite, keeping elbows bent away from scrub suit and hands above waist. Dry hands with sterile towel provided by circulating nurse.	Prevents hands from touching contaminated object. Prevents wetting scrubs with water.
3. Ask circulating nurse to assist by opening sterile gown pack (packed inside out) and glove package on a clean, dry, flat surface (see illustration).	Gown's outer surface remains sterile. Gloves remain sterile in package.
4. Reach down to sterile gown package; pick up the gown, grasping the inside surface of gown at the collar.	The hands are not completely sterile. The inside surface of the gown will contact the skin's surface and is thus considered contaminated.
5. Lift folded gown directly upward and step back away from table.	Provides wide margin of safety, avoiding contamination of gown.
6. Holding folded gown, locate neckband. With both hands, grasp inside front of gown just below neckband.	Clean hands may touch inside of gown without contaminating outer surface.
7. Hold gown at arm's length away from your body. Allow gown to unfold, keeping inside of gown toward body. Do not touch outside of gown with bare hands.	Outside of gown remains sterile.
8. With hands at shoulder level, slip both arms into armholes simultaneously (see illustration). Ask circulating nurse to bring gown over shoulders by reaching inside to arm seams. Gown is pulled on, leaving sleeves covering hands.	Careful application prevents contamination. Gown covers hands to prepare for closed gloving.

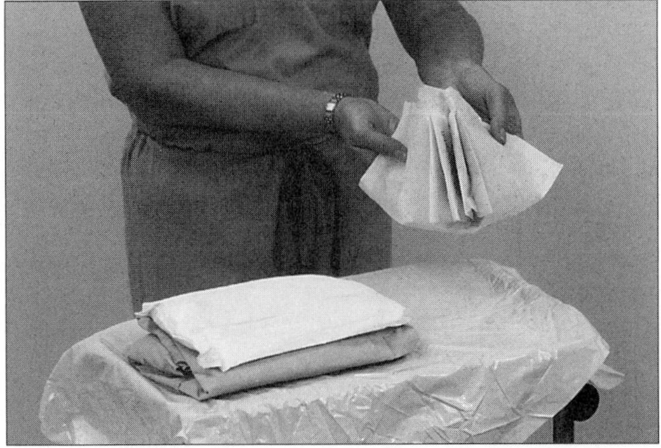

STEP 3 Circulating nurse opening sterile gown package.

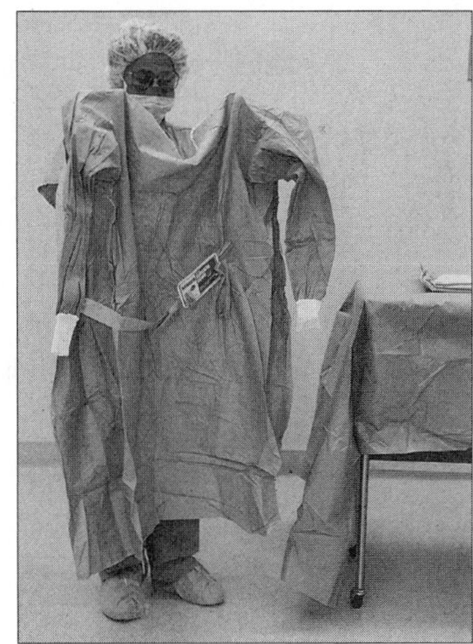

STEP 8 Placing arms in sleeves.

STEP	RATIONALE
9. Have circulating nurse securely tie back of gown at collar and waist (see illustration). (If gown is a wrap-around style, sterile flap to cover gown is not touched until the nurse has gloved.)	Gown must completely enclose underlying garments.
10. Apply gloves using the closed-glove method:	
a. With hands covered by gown sleeves, open inner sterile glove package (see illustration).	Hands remain clean. Sterile gown cuff will touch sterile glove surface.

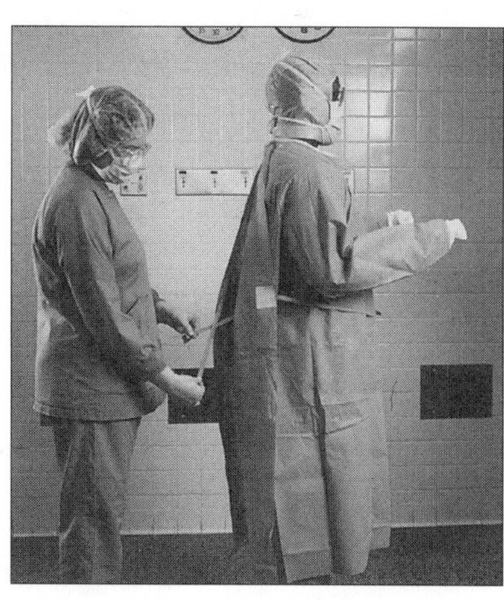

STEP **9** Circulating nurse ties scrub gown.

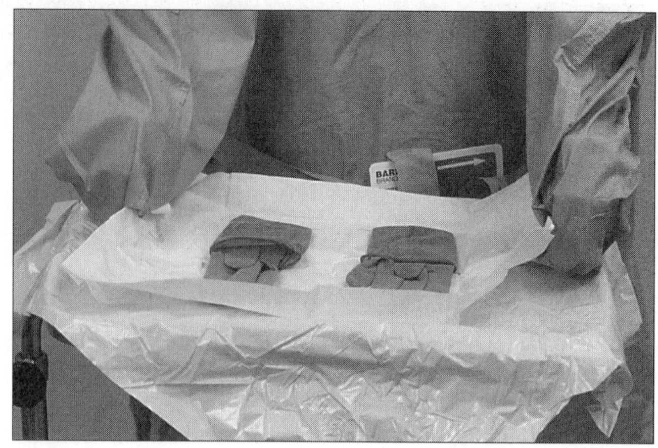

STEP **10a** Nurse opens glove package.

STEP	RATIONALE
b. With nondominant hand inside gown cuff, pick up glove for the dominant hand by grasping folded cuff.	Sterile gown touches sterile glove.
c. Extend dominant forearm with palm up and place palm of glove against palm of dominant hand. Glove fingers will point toward elbow.	Positions glove for application over cuffed hand, keeping glove sterile.
d. While holding glove cuff through gown with dominant hand on which it is placed, grasp back of glove cuff with nondominant hand and turn glove cuff over end of dominant hand and gown cuff (see illustration).	
e. Grasp top of glove and underlying gown sleeve with covered nondominant hand. Carefully extend fingers into glove, being sure glove's cuff covers gown's cuff.	Seal created by glove cuff over gown prevents exit of microorganisms over operative sterile field.
f. Glove nondominant hand in same manner, reversing hands (see illustration). Use gloved dominant hand to pull on glove.	Sterile touches sterile.
• ***Critical Decision Point*** *Keep hand inside sleeve.*	
g. Be sure fingers are fully extended into both gloves.	Ensures that nurse has full dexterity while using gloved hand.

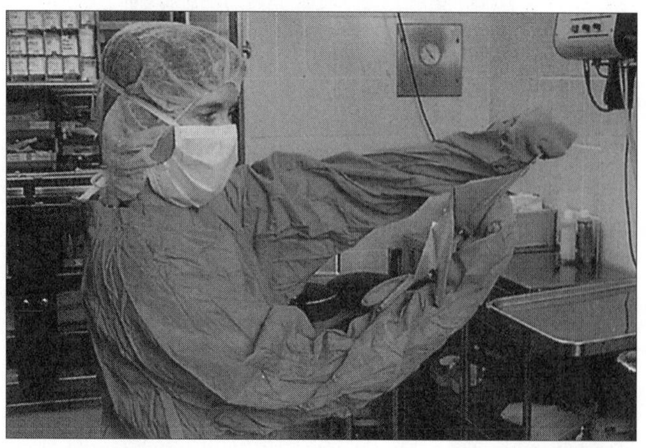

STEP **10d** Glove applied as hands remain inside cuff.

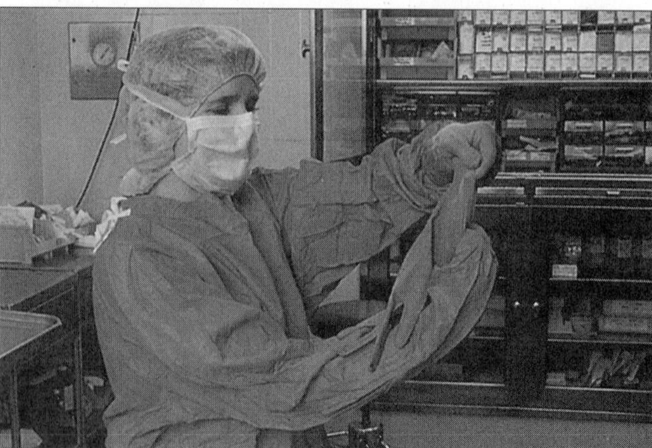

STEP **10f** Second glove applied.

STEP	RATIONALE
11. For wraparound sterile gowns: take gloved hand and release fastener or ties in front of gown.	Front of gown is sterile.
12. Enclose ties or snaps in a sterile towel and hand the towel to sterile team member to stands still (see illustration). Allowing margin of safety, turn around one-half turn to the left, covering back with extended gown flap. Take back tie from team member and secure tie to gown.	Contact with team member could contaminate gown and gloves. Sterile gown must enclose all non-sterile garments.

- ***Critical Decision Point***

  On disposable sterile gowns, there is often a disposable tab attached to the tie that can be passed to a nonsterile team member for turning.

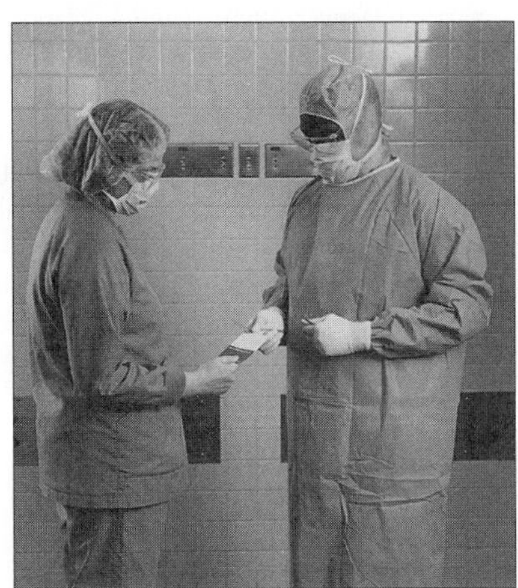

STEP **12** Turning wrap-around gown.

EVALUATION

1. Observe for break in sterile technique.	There is no break in sterile technique. Nurse is not required to reglove or apply a second gown.

UNEXPECTED OUTCOMES AND RELATED INTERVENTIONS

- Both gloves become contaminated during a procedure. Regown and reglove or have a sterile member of the team do the regloving.
- One glove becomes contaminated during a procedure. Use open gloving method to reglove (see Chapter 32).
- Client develops signs of infection—redness, heat, swelling, pain, and drainage at surgical site, as a result of contamination of glove. Implement appropriate wound care (see Chapter 35).

RECORDING AND REPORTING

- Record the area and description of surgical site postoperatively to provide baseline for monitoring wound.
- Special forms are available for operative procedures to record name and role of each health care professional in OR. Document that either no breach in sterile technique was observed or reported or that technique was broken.

TEACHING CONSIDERATIONS

- Instruct client and family or significant other to observe surgical site for signs of infection.

Critical Thinking Exercises

1. You notice a colleague who is working in an endoscopy procedure area. He enters the sterile room and applies a sterile gown. He holds his hands down straight at his sides and is careful not to come in contact with other staff members. Has he done anything wrong? If so, what must he do?
2. A colleague tells you that your scrubbed arm hit the faucet, but you did not feel it. What would you do in this situation?
3. Why is it important before performing a surgical hand wash and before applying sterile gloves that the nurse inspect the condition of the hands and fingernails?

References

Association of Operating Room Nurses: Position statement: resolution on the necessity for the registered nurse in the operating room. In *AORN standards and recommended practices for perioperative nursing,* Denver, 1995, The Association.

Association of Operating Room Nurses: Position statement: statement on mandate for the registered professional nurse in the perioperative practice setting. In *AORN standards, recommended practices, and guidelines,* Denver, 1999a, The Association.

Association of Operating Room Nurses: Recommended practices for surgical hand scrubs. In *AORN standards and recommended practices for perioperative nursing,* Denver, 1999b, The Association.

Association of Operating Room Nurses: Recommended practices for surgical attire. In *AORN standards and recommended practices for perioperative nursing,* Denver, 1999c, The Association.

Garner BD: Infection control. In Meeker MH, Rothrock J, editors: *Alexander's care of the patient in surgery,* ed 10, St. Louis, 1995, Mosby.

Johnson CR and others: RN first assistant certification; clinical internship; job descriptions; insurance coverage; specialty assembly, *AORN J* 64(1):115-118, 1996.

Salisbury DM and others: The effect of rings on microbial load of health care workers' hands, *Am J Infect Control* 25(2):24-27, 1997.

35

Wound Care and Irrigations

Skills

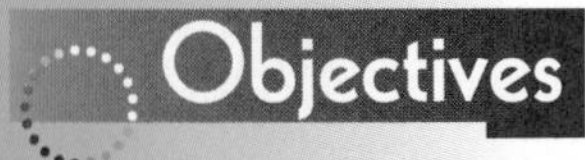

Mastery of content in this chapter will enable the nurse to:

- Define the key terms listed.
- Discuss the body's response during each stage of the wound-healing process.
- Differentiate between primary and secondary intention.
- Explain factors that impair or promote normal wound healing.
- Administer a wound irrigation.
- Remove sutures or staples.
- Demonstrate care of a wound-drainage system.

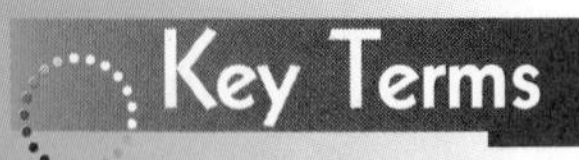

Dehiscence
Eschar
Evisceration
Granulation tissue
Healing ridge
Hemostasis
Hemovac drain
Irrigation
Jackson-Pratt (JP) drain
Keloid
Penrose drain
Primary intention
Secondary intention
Staples
Tertiary intention

Proper wound care is necessary to promote an intact skin layer during healing. The integumentary system is the body's first line of defense against invasion by infectious microorganisms. The skin defends the body in other ways by serving as a sensory organ for pain, touch, and temperature. It has an acid pH, which is often called the "acid mantle."

The skin or integument, the largest external organ, has two layers: the epidermis and the dermis (Figure 35-1). The outer layer, the epidermis, has five layers. The outermost layer, the stratum corneum, consists of flattened dead keratinized cells. The thin layer of the stratum corneum prevents dehydration of underlying cells and is a physical barrier to the entry of certain chemicals. The barrier is selective; it does allow absorption of topical medications in paste form. The next layers in the epidermis are the stratum lucidum, stratum granulosum, and stratum spinosum. The innermost layer of the epidermis, the stratum germinativum, is sometimes called the basal layer. It is from this single layer of keratinocytes that cells migrate up toward the stratum corneum. An important feature of the stratum germinativum are the epidermal protrusions, or "peaks and valleys," that point downward into the dermis. They provide resiliency and integrity to the skin structure. Also found in this layer are the melanocytes, which are the cells that give the skin its color. The area that separates the epidermis from the

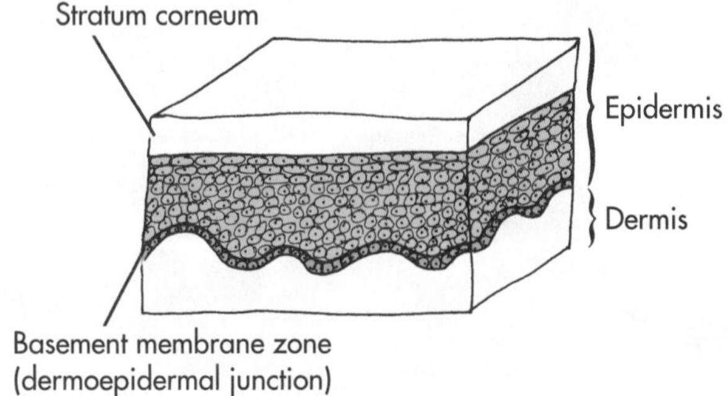

FIGURE **35-1** Layers of the integument.

Box 35-1 Stages of Wound Healing (Full-Thickness Wounds)

INFLAMMATORY STAGE

Starts when skin integrity is impaired and continues from 4 to 6 days.

- **Hemostasis**—Blood vessels constrict, gathering of platelets stops bleeding. Clots form a fibrin matrix. Scab forms, preventing entry of infectious organisms.
- Inflammatory response—Increases blood flow to wound and vascular permeability to plasma, resulting in localized redness and edema.
- White blood cells arrive at wound.
    - *Neutrophils* ingest bacteria and small debris, then die in a few days and leave enzyme exudate, which either attacks bacteria *or* interferes with tissue repair.
    - *Monocytes* become macrophages.
    - *Macrophages* clean cell of debris by phagocytosis; aid in wound repair by recycling normal amino acids and sugars.
- Epithelial cells move from wound margins to base of clot or scab (for period of approximately 48 hours).

PROLIFERATIVE STAGE

Closure begins on day 3 or 4 of defensive stage and continues for 2 to 3 weeks.

- Fibroblasts—Function with help of vitamins B and C; oxygen and amino acids synthesize collagen.
- Collagen—Provides strength and structural integrity to the wound.
- Contraction—Occurs only in open wounds and greatly reduces healing time because it reduces the amount of matrix that must be produced to fill the wound.
- Epithelial cells—Differentiate to duplicate damaged cells (e.g., intestinal mucosal cells acquire their columnar appearance).

REMODELING PHASE

This is the final phase in full-thickness wound healing and may continue for 1 year or more.

Data from Waldrop J, Doughty DB: Wound healing physiology. In Bryant RA: *Acute and chronic wounds: nursing management,* ed 2, St. Louis, 2000, Mosby.

dermis is called the dermoepidermal junction or the basement membrane zone.

Beneath the epidermis is the dermis. The dermis contains no skin cells. Collagen (a tough fibrous protein layer), blood vessels, and nerves compose the dermal layer. Collagen composes about 70% of the dermis and is therefore extremely important in wound healing. The dermis restores the physical properties of the skin and its structural integrity. Restoration of both the epidermal and dermal layers is necessary to promote healing. Risk of local or systemic infection, impaired circulation, and breakdown of tissue directly influence the ability of the dermal layer to heal (Bonier, 1985).

Physiologically, wound healing occurs in the same way for all clients, with skin cells and some tissues (including the vascular tissues) regenerating quickly and others regenerating slowly or not at all. The latter group includes cells of the liver, renal tubules, and central nervous system neurons.

Wound healing in the adult skin is complex and involves a series of physiological processes among cells and tissues (Box 35-1). The role of each cell type during phases of healing contributes to tissue restoration (Martin, 1997). These processes can be affected by the location, severity, and extent of the injury. In addition, there are underlying factors that inhibit the ability of cells and tissues to regenerate, return to normal structure, or resume normal functioning (Box 35-2).

The color of an open wound represents the balance between necrotic and new scar tissue (Cuzzell, 1997). A wound that is healing well is red or pink in color (Table 35-1). Necrotic wounds are without proper circulation and provide an excellent medium for bacterial growth, resulting in wound infections.

Collagen deposition begins in the inflammatory phase and peaks during the proliferative phase. It is important for nurses to assess for the accumulation of this new tissue (Cooper, 2000). This **"healing ridge"** is an "induration beneath the skin extending to about 1 cm ($\frac{1}{2}$ inch) on each side of the wound" (Hunt, 1979) (Figure 35-2). It is usually present directly under the suture line between days 5 and 9 (Cooper, 2000). Absence of the healing ridge may indicate a wound at risk for dehiscence or infection (Hunt, 1979) (Figure 35-3).

Types of healing are **primary intention, secondary intention,** and **tertiary intention.** Healing by primary intention is expected when the edges of a clean surgical incision remain close together. The wound heals quickly, and tissue loss is minimal or absent (Waldrop and Doughty, 2000). The skin cells quickly regenerate, and capillary walls stretch across under the suture line to form a smooth surface as they join.

Box 35-2 Underlying Factors That Inhibit Wound Healing

EXTERNAL

Trauma
Scalds and burns, both physical and chemical
Animal bites or insect stings

INTERNAL

Pressure
Vascular compromise; arterial, venous or mixed
Immunodeficiency
Malignancy
Connective tissue disorders
Metabolic disease, including diabetes
Nutritional deficiencies

QUALITY OF LIFE

Pain
Psychosocial issues

IATROGENIC

Adverse effects of medications or treatments

From Keast DH, Orsted H: The basic principles of wound care, *Ostomy Wound Manage* 44(8):24, 1998.

Table 35-1 Wound Color

Black wounds	Black eschar represents full-thickness tissue destruction. It is also common with stage III and IV pressure ulcers and the gangrenous lesions secondary to peripheral vascular disease. Moisture-retentive dressings or synthetic dressings are contraindicated. These wounds are usually treated conservatively. As long as the wound is noninfected and eschar is dry and intact, the wound may be left alone. If the client is ambulatory, chemical enzymes may be used as an alternative for debridement. However, this treatment may not be as effective as debridement in some clients.
Yellow wounds	Devitalized tissue in the presence of moisture results in yellow, cream-colored, or gray necrotic slough, which is usually accompanied by purulent drainage. For clients with a low infection risk, the use of moisture-retentive dressings enhances debridement. These moisture-retentive dressings may include wet-to-dry dressings, as well as hydrocolloids or alginates.
Red wounds	Red wounds occur when the yellow slough is removed. The red color is the result of an increasing amount of red or pink granulation tissue. The goal in red wound management is to select a dressing that maintains a clean and slightly moist wound environment and minimizes damage to healing tissue.

Data from Cuzzell J: Choosing a wound dressing, *Geriatr Nurs* 18(6):260, 1997.

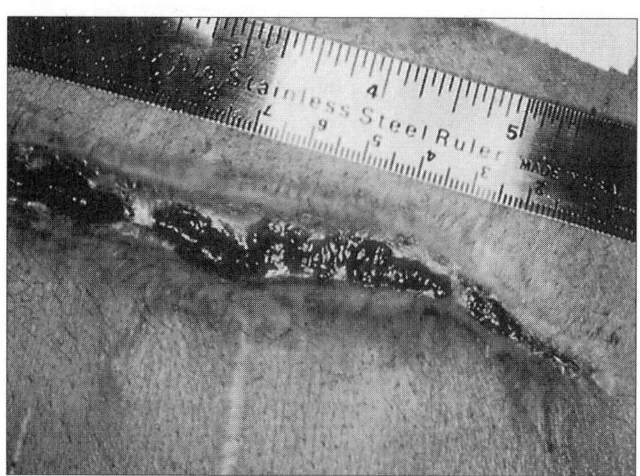

FIGURE **35-2** Surgical wound with epithelialization occurring: epithelial healing ridge apparent. (From Bryant RA, editor: *Acute and chronic wounds,* ed 2, St. Louis, 2000, Mosby.)

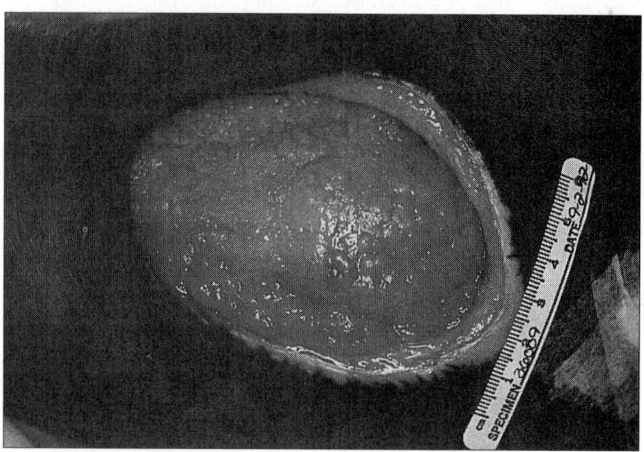

FIGURE **35-4** Open wound with granulating base.

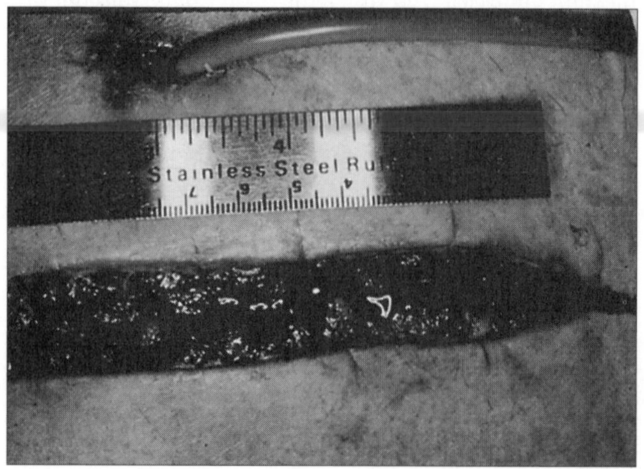

FIGURE **35-3** Surgical wound lacking evidence of healing epithelial ridge. (From Bryant RA, editor: *Acute and chronic wounds,* St. Louis, 1992, Mosby.)

Wounds that are left open and allowed to heal by scar formation are classified as healing by secondary intention (Waldrop and Doughty, 2000). There is tissue loss and open, jagged wound edges. **Granulation tissue** gradually fills in the area of the defect with scar tissue (Figure 35-4). This process is typical of severe laceration or massive surgical intervention with skin loss. The risk of infection is directly related to the length of time it takes for the body surface to be covered with an intact skin layer. In secondary intention there is some gap between the edges. A thin fibrinous exudate covers the edges of the wound, prevents bacterial invasion, and coagulates surface bleeding. New capillaries are supported by connective tissue. This form of healing results in a thicker surface closure. The slowness of this process places the client at greater risk for infection and collection of body fluids that must be drained to permit healing. Some clients who heal by secondary intention may develop an excessive amount of connective tissue in the scar surface. This tissue is known as **keloid.** Other developments may include the formation of a fistula in response to the presence of bacteria in the wound.

Healing by tertiary intention is sometimes called delayed primary intention or closure. It occurs when surgical wounds are not closed immediately but left open for 3 to 5 days to allow edema or infection to diminish. Then the wound edges are sutured or stapled closed. Scarring is usually minimal (Maklebust and Palleschi, 1996). During the healing process a wound may have some type of dressing covering it.

The initial dressing is not removed for direct wound inspection until a physician writes a medical order to remove it. Certain situations and some institutional policies govern who changes the dressing the first time. Special attention is paid to maintaining the position of drains during dressing changes (Waldrop and Doughty, 2000). An analgesic, as ordered, should be administered 30 to 45 minutes before changing the dressing. However, the nurse's assessment determines the best time for analgesic administration before wound care. Skin cleansing in the area of the suture line or drain site is indicated when an excessive amount of drainage occurs. The presence of wound exudate is an expected stage of epithelial cell growth.

Recently a new method, vacuum-assisted closure (VAC), for wound healing is being investigated. VAC uses controlled negative pressure on wounds. Negative pressure stretches and distorts the cells within the wound, pulling them close together. It is believed that this distortion causes the epithelial cells to multiply rapidly and form granulation tissue (Mendez-Eastman, 1998). In addition, biochemical mediators stimulate the growth of new blood vessels to improve circulation to the region. There have been good results with VAC on chronic wounds; such as stasis ulcers and stage III and IV pressure ulcers. This technique appears to decrease the time it takes to heal stubborn, chronic wounds (Mendez-Eastman, 1998).

Meticulous hand washing and proper infection control procedures before and after removing soiled dressings, coupled with proper wound-cleansing procedures, limit the risk of nosocomial infection. Using clean gloves prevents exposure

Table 35-2 Wound Cleansing Protocol

MECHANICAL FORCE	HIGH PRESSURE	LOW PRESSURE
Phase of healing	Inflammatory	Proliferative
Wound base characteristics	• Presence of necrotic tissue (eschar, fibrin slough), debris, or other particulate matter • Significant bacterial burden • Moderate/large amount of exudate • Residue from wound care products	• Presence of granulation tissue or new epithelial cells • Non/minimum serous or sero-sanguinous exudate • Residue from wound care products
Clinical outcome(s)	• Loosen, soften, and remove devitalized tissue from wound • Separate eschar from fibrotic tissue/fibrotic tissue from granulating base • Remove wound care product residue	• Prevent trauma to viable wound tissue • Remove wound care product residue
Solutions	• Normal saline • Wound cleansers • Amount depends on size of wound	• Normal saline • Amount depends on size of wound
Delivery systems*	• 35 cc syringe/19 gauge angiocath • Irrijet® DS • Pleurovac	• Pouring saline directly from bottle • Bulb syringe • Piston syringe

From Barr JE: Principles of wound cleansing, *Ostomy Wound Manage* 7A(suppl 41):15S, 1995.
*This is not an all-inclusive list of delivery systems available. Inclusion does not imply endorsement.

from body fluids, exudate, or bloody drainage from a wound. Wound cleansing "delivers a fluid or cleansing solution to the wound surface by means of a specific mechanical force and assists with the separation and removal of necrotic debris, particulate matter, bacteria, and residue of wound care products" (Barr, 1995b). Effective wound cleansing can be accomplished by using an appropriate cleansing solution that does not harm the tissue and is delivered by adequate mechanical cleansing force action of either soaking, scrubbing, or irrigation (Barr, 1995b). Irrigation is the method of wound cleansing most used by nurses.

Irrigation uses the mechanical force (either high or low) of a stream of solution to loosen particulate matter on the wound surface. The phase of wound healing and goal of wound cleansing determine whether high pressures (which are measured in psi, or pounds per square inch) (4 to 15 psi) or low irrigation (less than 4 psi) is used (Barr, 1995b) (Table 35-2). A commonly used high-pressure irrigation system is a 35-ml syringe with a 19-gauge needle or angiocath, which delivers a psi of 8 (Agency for Health Care Policy and Research [AHCPR], 1994). This nursing intervention is used for wounds on any part of the torso or extremities. In addition to cleansing an area, prescribed medications may be introduced in solution form. Principles of basic wound irrigation include the following:

1. Cleanse in a direction from the least contaminated area to the most contaminated.
2. When irrigating, all the solution flows from the least contaminated to the most contaminated area.

When administering an irrigation, be sure that the flow of irrigation moves from the area being cleansed to an area that is both distal to and lower than that area. In wound care the

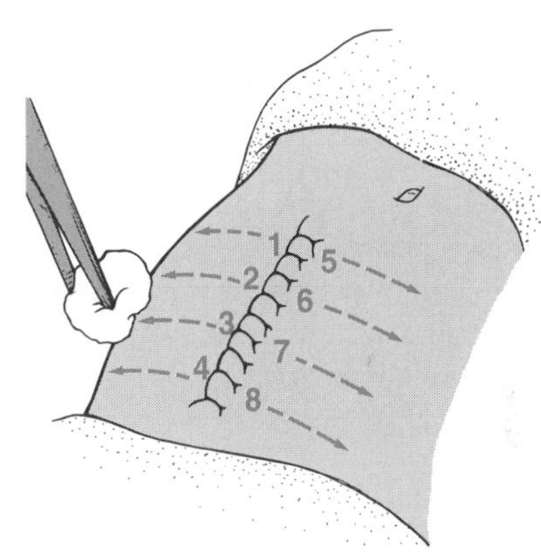

FIGURE **35-5** Method of cleansing the suture line area.

area being cleansed is considered "clean" and the surrounding skin surfaces are considered "contaminated" without respect to whether the wound is infected. Within the wound the flow is directed from healthy tissue toward infected tissue. Irrigating solutions are sterile. In the event that the irrigant has caustic or irritating properties, protect the skin with a skin protectant product and place the collection basin close to the area of the exiting fluid.

The suture line is the "least contaminated" area and is always cleansed first (Figure 35-5). The center is the most important part of the suture line; therefore clean the suture line itself by starting at the center of the suture line and working toward one end. With another sterile swab or gauze, start at the center of the incision and work toward the other end. All other cleansing involves moving from one end to the other on each side of the incision on the skin surrounding the incision. Work in straight lines, moving away from the suture line with

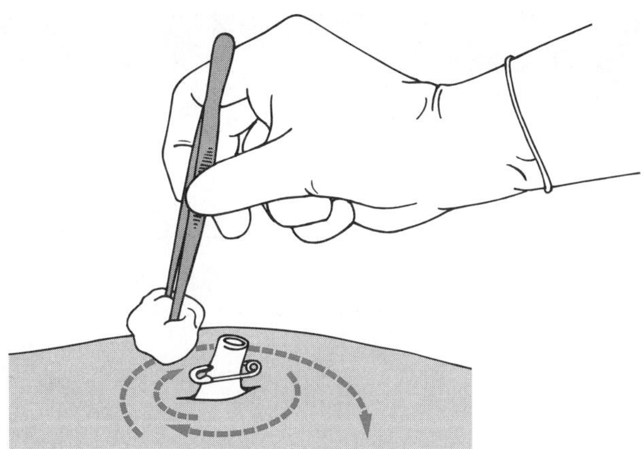

FIGURE **35-6** Cleansing a drain site.

each successive stroke. Use a sterile 2 × 2 gauze containing antiseptic or an antiseptic swab for each stroke.

The drain site is cleansed using a circular stroke starting with the area immediately next to the drain (Figure 35-6). With each new swab start immediately next to drain and attempt to cleanse a little further out from the drain.

Skill Performance Guidelines

1. Know the client's age. With age, vascular changes occur, collagen tissue is less pliable, and scar tissue is tighter. Because the epidermodermal junction becomes flatter in older adults, their skin tears more easily from mechanical trauma such as tape removal.
2. Know the client's nutritional status. Tissue repair and infection resistance are directly related to adequate nutrition, including proteins, carbohydrates, lipids, vitamins, and minerals (Pontieri-Lewis, 1997; Brylinsky, 1995). Clients who are malnourished are at increased risk of wound infections and wound infection–related sepsis (Pontieri-Lewis, 1997).
3. Beware of risks of obesity. Inadequate vascularization decreases delivery of nutrients and cellular elements required for healing. The client is at greater risk for wound infection and dehiscence or evisceration.
4. Identify factors that decrease oxygenation, such as decreased hemoglobin level and smoking. Adequate oxygenation at the tissue level is essential for white blood cell (WBC) activity and phagocytosis, for fibroblast proliferation and collagen synthesis, and for reepitheliaziation (Barr, 1995a). Small wounds heal more quickly when exposed to air. Tissue repair is negatively influenced by a hematocrit value below 33% and a hemoglobin value below 10 g/100 ml. Hemoglobin level is reduced and oxygen release to tissues is reduced in smokers.
5. Know the types of medications prescribed. Steroids reduce inflammatory response and slow collagen synthesis. Cortisone depresses fibroblast activity and capillary growth. Chemotherapy depresses bone marrow.
6. Identify the presence of chronic diseases or chronic trauma, such as diabetes or radiation. Decreased tissue perfusion and failure to release oxygen to tissues result from diabetes. In radiation therapy, wound healing is most effective when surgery is performed within 4 to 6 weeks of irradiation before the anticipated vascular scarring and fibrosis.
7. Unwounded skin is always stronger than healed skin that has been wounded.

Skill 35-1 Performing Wound Irrigation

Wound cleansing and irrigation is accomplished using sterile technique (surgical wounds) or clean technique (some chronic wounds). The cleansing solution is introduced directly into the wound with either a syringe, syringe and catheter, shower, or whirlpool. When a syringe is used, the tip should remain 2.5 cm (1 inch) above the wound. If the client has a deep wound with a narrow opening, a soft catheter is attached to the syringe to permit the fluid to enter the wound. Irrigation should not cause tissue injury or discomfort. Fluid retention is avoided by positioning the client on the side to encourage the flow of the irrigant away from the wound. With small wounds, it is often helpful to use a 35-ml syringe with a 19-gauge needle attached to facilitate optimal pressure for cleansing with minimal risk of tissue injury (Rodeheaver, 1990). Ambulatory clients may benefit from the use of a hand-held shower for wound cleansing, holding the shower spray approximately 12 inches (30 cm) from the wound. If the force applies too much pressure for the client's comfort, a clean washcloth may be tied around the showerhead to disperse the force. An alternative is the shower table (Figure 35-7), frequently used in burn and trauma wound care, which allows cleansing in the acute care area. For clients who require mechanical debridement and cleansing but cannot tolerate the above methods, the whirlpool is a useful method. The whirlpool procedure is frequently performed by or with the assistance of physical therapists, who then help apply dressings.

There are two types of wound irrigation: high-pressure and pulsatile high-pressure lavage. High-pressure irrigation is the cleansing of a necrotic wound with irrigating fluid delivered at 8 to 12 pounds per square inch (psi), such as with a 35-ml syringe and a 19-gauge angiocatheter. This procedure provides force to remove wound debris without damaging healthy tissue. Pulsatile high-pressure lavage is an alternative to high-pressure irrigation. It is the use of a machine to deliver intermittent high-pressure irrigation, combined with suction to remove the irrigant and wound debris (Ramundo and Wells, 2000). A whirlpool is also commonly used to remove bacteria and debris from the surface of large wounds. In addition, a whirlpool will soften and loosen adherent necrotic tissue and cleanse and remove wound exudate.

Wound irrigations promote wound healing through removing debris from a wound surface, decreasing bacterial counts, and loosening and removing eschar. **Eschar** is "thick, leathery, necrotic, devitalized tissue" (Agency for Health Care Policy and Research [AHCPR], 1994). Solutions used for irrigations include normal saline, warm water, or mild wound cleansers such as Cara Klenz, Saf Clens, and Biolex. Skin cleansers are not the same as wound cleansers and should not be indiscriminately substituted for them.

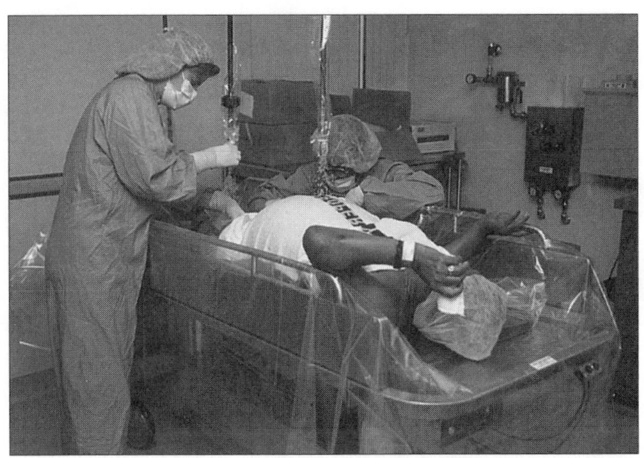

FIGURE **35-7** Shower table.

Delegation Considerations

Check institutional policy and the state's Nurse Practice Act regarding which wound care interventions can be delegated to assistive personnel. The skill of wound irrigation should not be delegated to assistive personnel. However, cleansing of chronic wounds using clean technique can be delegated. Assistive personnel must always be instructed specifically what to report when a wound is cleansed (e.g., wound color, presence of bleeding, drainage, pain).

Equipment

- Irrigant/cleansing solution (volume 1.2 to 2 times the estimated wound volume)
- Irrigation delivery system, depending on amount of pressure desired: sterile irrigation 35-ml syringe with sterile soft angiocath or 19-gauge needle (AHCPR, 1994) or hand-held shower or whirlpool
- Irrigation syringes: 35-ml syringe with 19-gauge angiocatheter
- Clean gloves
- Sterile gloves
- Waterproof underpad, if needed
- Dressing supplies (Table 35-3)
- Disposable waterproof bag
- Gown
- Goggles
- Extra towels and padding (to use to protect bed)

Table 35-3 Common Wound Dressing Categories

Category	Description	Indications	Side Effects	Examples
Absorptive fillers	Variety of product types including absorptive powders, pastes, and beads; highly absorptive; oxygen permeable Requires secondary cover dressing	• Absorption in full-thickness wounds with moderate to heavy exudate • Autolytic debridement of yellow slough in deep wounds with uneven wound beds • Odor control • Hydrophilic cleansing action and reduction of surface bacteria	• Will desiccate wound and cause further damage if exudate is minimal • Some products may be difficult to remove if wound is deep with tunneling	Bard Absorption Dressing Chronicure Comfeel Powder Duoderm Paste and Granules HydraGran

From Cuzzell J: Choosing a wound dressing, *Geriatr Nurs* 18(6):260, 1997.

Continued

Table 35-3 Common Wound Dressing Categories—cont'd

Category	Description	Indications	Side Effects	Examples
Alginates	Nonwoven mass of calcium-sodium alginate fibers that form moisture-retentive gel on contact with wound fluid; moisture-retentive; nonocclusive; varying levels of absorbency; nonadhesive; available in pads and ropes for packing Requires secondary cover dressing to secure	• Absorption of heavy to moderate wound exudate in superficial and deep wounds • Autolytic debridement of yellow slough • Infected wounds (after appropriate intervention and with close monitoring of wound progress) • "Filler" for deep or tunnelling wounds (rope form) • Hemostasis	• May contribute to wound desiccation if wound exudate is minimal and gel dries (saturate with saline to soften) • Contraindicated for use on third-degree burns • Limited hemostatic properties	CURASORB Kaltostat Sorbsan
Foams	Semipermeable polyurethane foam dressings that have varying barrier properties; moisture-retentive; conformable; available in pads and pillows for filling wound cavities; available in adhesive and nonadhesive forms Some products require tape or secondary cover dressing to secure	• Absorption of moderate to heavy exudate in superficial and deep wounds • Protection of friable peri-wound skin (non-adhesive pads) • Infected wounds (after appropriate intervention and with close monitoring of wound progress) • Autolytic debridement of yellow slough • Padding of tracheostomy sites • Padding and protection of high trauma areas (pretibial area, forearms, etc.)	• May promote wound dehydration and desiccation if exudate is minimal • Contraindicated for sinus tracts	Allevyn CURAFOAM Flexzan LyoFoam MitraFlex
Gauze (Woven)	Absorbent, 100% meshed cotton fabric woven into squares, rolls, and packing strips; available in sterile and nonsterile packing	• Protection of surgical wounds • Mechanical debridement of yellow slough (wet-to-dry gauze) • Autolytic debridement (saline-moistened gauze) • Absorption of minimal to heavy exudate in superficial and deep wounds • "Filler" for packing dead space in large, deep wound cavities • Infected wounds (moistened or impregnated with topical antimicrobials)	• May adhere to healthy tissue and cause injury on removal • Some products may shed, leaving lint in wound	Curity Gauze Sponges KERLIX Super Sponge KLING gauze rolls NUGAUZE packing strips
Hydrocolloids	Conformable material made of gelatin, pectin and carboxymethylcellulose particles suspended in adhesive base; moisture-retentive; highly occlusive; wafers are available in regular and extra-thin forms and in variety of shapes	• Autolytic debridement of minimal to moderate amount of yellow slough • Protection of high-friction areas • Protection from exogenous contamination [excellent barrier function] • Absorption of minimal to moderate exudate in superficial and shallow full-thickness wounds • Fibrinolytic activity (venous leg ulcers)	• Occlusive properties can promote infection in high-risk patients (especially anaerobic infection) • Contraindicated for third-degree burns • May promote hypertrophic granulation tissue • Some products leave residue in wound on removal • Some products have an unpleasant odor on dressing removal	Comfeel Cutinova DuoDERM Restore Tegasorb

Table 35-3 Common Wound Dressing Categories—cont'd

CATEGORY	DESCRIPTION	INDICATIONS	SIDE EFFECTS	EXAMPLES
Hydrogels	Semipermeable hydrophilic polymers composed primarily of water or glycerin; available in both sheet and gel forms; moisture-retentive Require secondary cover dressing to secure	• Absorption of minimal to moderate exudate in superficial and deep wounds • Autolytic debridement of yellow slough and softening of black eschar • Pain relief in radiation-damaged tissue and superficial burns • Ultrasound treatments • Gel forms can be used as filler for deep wounds	• Not indicated for heavily exuding wounds • May contribute to peri-wound maceration • May promote growth of yeast	Carrington Gel Geliperm IntraSite Gel Nu-Gel Vigilon
Transparent films	Transparent polyurethane and polyethylene films coated with adhesive; semipermeable; moisture vapor transmission rates vary with product type; moisture-retentive; nonabsorptive	• Protection of high-friction areas (heels, beneath restraints, Stage 1, etc.) • Autolytic debridement of yellow slough in shallow wounds • IV sites • Covering dressing for fillers and other, more absorptive dressing materials	• Not recommended for wounds with moderate or heavy exudate • May cause skin tears or adhesive stripping of peri-wound skin • Contributes to peri-wound maceration and yeast colonization if exudate collects • Contraindicated in infected wound	Bioclusive OpSite Tegaderm

STEP	RATIONALE
ASSESSMENT	
1. Review physician's order for irrigation of open wound and type of solution to be used.	Open wound irrigation requires medical order including type of solution(s) to use (Waldrop and Doughty, 2000).
2. Assess recent recording of signs and symptoms related to client's open wound:	
a. Extent of impairment of skin integrity, including size of wound (measure length, width, and depth). Wounds should be measured in cm and in the following order: length, width, and depth (Cooper, 2000).	This assesses volume of irrigation solution needed. Data also used as baseline to indicate change in condition of wound.
b. Elevation of body temperature.	May indicate response to infection (Keast and Orsted, 1998).
c. Drainage from wound (amount and color). Amount can be measured by part of dressing saturated or in terms of quantity (e.g., scant, moderate, copious).	Expect amount to decrease as healing takes place. Serous drainage is clear; sanguineous or bright red drainage indicates fresh bleeding; serosanguineous drainage is pink; purulent drainage is thick and yellow, pale green, or white (Cuzzell, 1997).
d. Odor. Must state that there is no odor if none is present. More frequent cleansing is needed if wound has a foul odor (AHCPR, 1994).	Strong odor indicates infectious process.
e. Wound color (see Table 35-1).	Color represents a balance between necrotic tissue and new scar tissue. Proper selection of wound products, based on the color of the wound, facilitates removal of necrotic tissue and promotes new tissue growth (Cuzzell, 1997).
f. Consistency of drainage.	Leukocytes produce thick drainage (Barr, 1995a).
g. Culture reports.	Remember that chronic wounds healing by secondary intention are often colonized.

STEP	RATIONALE
h. Stage of healing of the client's wound.	Client's wound characteristics determine type and amount of pressure to use during irrigation.
i. Dressing: dry and clean; evidence of bleeding, profuse drainage.	Provides an initial assessment of present wound drainage.
3. Assess comfort level or pain, and identify symptoms of anxiety.	Discomfort may be related directly to wound or indirectly to muscle tension or immobility. Anxiety results from multiple factors (e.g., surgery, diagnosis, awaiting pathology reports) and anticipation of unknown nursing interventions (e.g., first wound irrigation).
4. Assess client for history of allergies to antiseptics, tapes, or dressing material.	Known allergies suggest application of a sample of prescribed antiseptic as skin test before flushing wound with large volume of solution.

NURSING DIAGNOSIS

Defining characteristics from the assessment data may reveal the following nursing diagnoses for clients requiring this skill:

- Impaired skin integrity
- Impaired tissue integrity
- Pain (acute, chronic)
- Risk for injury

Related factors are individualized based on client's condition or needs.

PLANNING

STEP	RATIONALE
1. **Expected outcomes** following completion of procedure:	
▪ Client is comfortable after wound irrigation.	Premedication, gently administered irrigation, application of clean dressing, and repositioning client ensure comfort.
▪ Wound begins to heal; dressing is clean and dry; wound is free of drainage and inflammation, or drainage is decreased in amount or type (e.g., less bloody or serous as opposed to serosanguineous).	Healing progresses in absence of debris and presence of protective covering.
▪ Skin integrity is maintained; no redness, edema, or inflammation noted in surrounding tissue.	No further skin and tissue damage has resulted from wound irrigation.
2. Explain procedure of wound irrigation and cleansing.	Information will reduce client's anxiety.
3. Administer prescribed analgesic 30 to 45 minutes before starting wound irrigation procedure.	Increased comfort level permits client to move more easily and be positioned to facilitate wound irrigation.
4. Position client.	
▪ Position comfortably to permit gravitational flow of irrigating solution through wound and into collection receptacle (see illustration).	Directing solution from top to bottom of wound and from clean to contaminated area prevents further infection. Positioning client during planning stage provides bed surfaces for later preparation of equipment.
▪ Position client so that wound is vertical to collection basin. Place container in basin of hot water.	
▪ Place padding or extra towels.	Protects bedding.
▪ Expose wound only.	Prevents chilling of client.

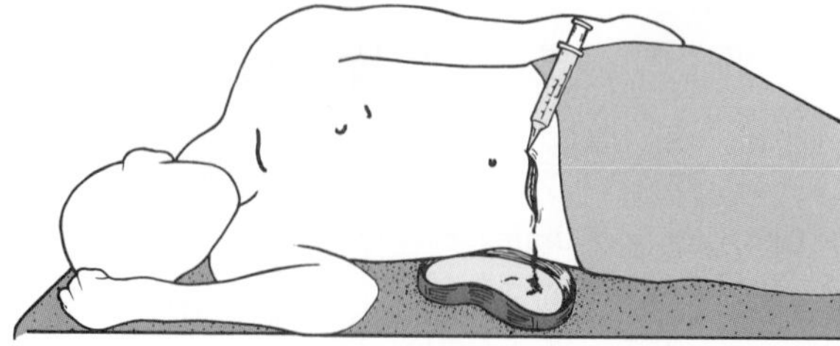

STEP 4 Client position for wound irrigation.

Step	Rationale
Implementation	
1. Warm irrigation solution to approximate body temperature.	Warmed solution increases comfort and reduces vascular constriction response in tissues.
2. Wash hands.	Reduces transmission of microorganisms.
3. Form cuff on waterproof bag, and place it near bed.	Cuffing helps to maintain large opening, thereby permitting placement of contaminated dressing without touching refuse bag itself.
4. Close room door or bed curtains.	Maintains privacy.
5. Apply gown and goggles.	Protects nurse from splashes or sprays of blood and body fluids (Centers for Disease Control and Prevention [CDC], 1996).
6. Apply clean gloves, and remove soiled dressing and discard in waterproof bag. Discard gloves.	Reduces transmission of microorganisms.
7. Prepare equipment; open sterile supplies.	
8. Apply sterile gloves.	Prevents transfer of microorganisms to wound surface.
9. To irrigate wound with wide opening:	
a. Fill 35-ml syringe with irrigation solution.	Flushing wound helps remove debris and facilitates healing by secondary intention.
b. Attach 19-gauge angiocatheter	Provides ideal pressure for cleansing and removal of debris (Ramundo and Wells, 2000).
c. Hold syringe tip 2.5 cm (1 inch) above upper end of wound and over area being cleansed.	Prevents syringe contamination. Careful placement of the syringe prevents unsafe pressure of the flowing solution.
d. Using continuous pressure, flush wound; repeat Steps 9a, b, and c until solution draining into basin is clear.	Clear solution indicates all debris has been removed.
10. To irrigate deep wound with very small opening:	
a. Attach soft angiocatheter to filled irrigating syringe.	Catheter permits direct flow of irrigant into wound. Expect wound to take longer to empty when opening is small.
b. Lubricate tip of catheter with irrigating solution; then gently insert tip of catheter and pull out about 1 cm (½ inch).	Removes tip from fragile inner wall of wound.

- ***Critical Decision Point***
  Do not force catheter into the wound because this could cause tissue damage.

Step	Rationale
c. Using slow, continuous pressure, flush wound.	Use of slow mechanical force of a stream of solution loosens particulate matter on the wound surface and promotes healing (Barr, 1995b).

- ***Critical Decision Point***
  CAUTION: Splashing may occur during this step.

Step	Rationale
d. Pinch off catheter just below syringe while keeping catheter in place.	Avoids contamination of sterile solution.
e. Remove and refill syringe. Reconnect to catheter and repeat until solution draining into basin is clear.	

- ***Critical Decision Point***
  Pulsatile high-pressure lavage may be the irrigation of choice for necrotic wounds. The amount of irrigant is wound-size dependent. Pressure settings on the device should remain between 8 and 15 psi. The nurse should use pulsatile high-pressure lavage on exposed blood vessels, muscle, tendon, and bone. This type of irrigation should not be used with graft sites and should be used with caution in clients receiving anticoagulant therapy (Ramundo and Wells, 2000).

Step	Rationale
11. To cleanse wound with hand-held shower:	Useful for clients able to shower with assistance or independently. May be accomplished at home. A shower table (see Figure 35-7, p. 1009) is helpful for bed-bound or acutely ill clients.
a. With client seated comfortably in shower chair, adjust spray to gentle flow; water temperature should be warm.	

Step	Rationale
b. Cover showerhead with clean washcloth if needed.	Reduces pressure released at shower head.
c. Shower for 5 to 10 minutes with shower head 12 inches (30 cm) from wound.	Ensures wound is thoroughly cleansed.
12. To cleanse wound with whirlpool:	
a. Adjust water level and temperature; add prescribed cleansing agent.	Wound is hypersensitive to hot temperature.

- ***Critical Decision Point***
  To avoid tissue damage, position client so that water jets are not directly over clean granulating wound tissue.

Step	Rationale
b. Assist client into whirlpool, or place extremity into whirlpool.	
c. Allow client to remain in whirlpool for prescribed interval.	Ensures thorough wound cleansing.

- ***Critical Decision Point***
  Clients who are confused, have poor activity tolerance, or have impaired mobility should never be left alone in the whirlpool.

Step	Rationale
13. When indicated, obtain cultures (see Chapter 41) after cleansing with nonbacteriostatic saline.	Routine culturing of open wounds is not recommended by AHCPR (1994). AHCPR (1994) recommends using quantitative bacterial cultures (tissue biopsy or wound fluid by needle aspiration) rather than swab cultures, which often detect only surface bacterial contaminants.

- ***Critical Decision Point***
  Consider culturing a wound if it has a foul, purulent odor; inflammation surrounds the wound; a nondraining wound begins to drain; or client is febrile.

Step	Rationale
14. Dry wound edges with gauze; dry client if shower or whirlpool is used.	Prevents maceration of surrounding tissue from excess moisture.
15. Apply appropriate dressing (see Chapter 36).	Maintains protective barrier and healing environment for wound.
16. Remove gloves, mask, goggles, and gown.	Prevents transfer of microorganisms.
17. Assist client to comfortable position.	
18. Dispose of equipment and soiled supplies, and wash hands.	Reduces transmission of microorganisms.

Evaluation

Step	Rationale
1. Assess type of tissue in wound bed.	Identifies wound healing progress and determines type of wound cleansing needed.
2. Inspect dressing periodically.	Determines client's response to wound irrigation and need to modify plan of care.
3. Evaluate skin integrity.	Determines if extension of wound has occurred.
4. Observe client for signs of discomfort.	Client's pain should not increase as a result of wound irrigation.
5. Observe for presence of retained irrigant.	Retained irrigant is a medium for bacterial growth and subsequent infection.

Unexpected Outcomes and Related Interventions

- Bleeding or serosanguineous drainage appears.
  - Flush wound during next irrigation using less pressure.
  - Notify physician of bleeding.
- Retained fluid and debris appear.
  - Increase amount of fluid used during irrigation.
  - Increase amount of pressure when flushing wound.
  - Make sure wound is clear of retained fluid and debris before applying dressing.

- Increased pain or discomfort occurs.
  - Decrease force of pressure during wound irrigation.
  - Assess client for need for additional analgesia before wound care.
  - Assess client for need for additional analgesia if discomfort increases.
- Suture line opening extends.
  - Notify physician.
  - Reevaluate amount of pressure to use for next wound irrigation.

Recording and Reporting

- Record wound irrigation and client response on progress notes.
- Immediately report any evidence of fresh bleeding, sharp increase in pain, retention of irrigant, or signs of shock to attending physician.
- At change of shift, report expected and unexpected outcomes that have actually occurred.

Teaching Considerations

- Instruct and provide written handouts to client and primary caregiver to observe wound care, and provide time for return demonstrations.
- Explain the need for specialized supplies such as irrigating solutions and dressings and the need to maintain asepsis when performing care.
- Instruct client and caregiver where and how additional supplies are obtained.
- Instruct client and primary caregiver about signs of improper wound healing and wound infection.
- Stress aseptic technique.
- Assess client's and primary caregiver's understanding of need for and methods of wound care.
- Teach client and caregiver how to make normal saline, especially if cost is an issue. Normal saline can be made by using 2 teaspoons of salt in 1 L (1 q) of boiling water (Barr, 1995b).
- Provide written instruction on dressing change.
- Client may need to receive wound care management in a free-standing wound care clinic. Be sure client has directions to clinic and knows where to park and where to obtain dressing supplies.

Pediatric Considerations

- Pediatric clients may be very frightened. They might verbally and physically try to prevent nurse from cleaning wound. Having child active in parts of procedure or working out child's feelings about wound irrigation using play therapy on a doll with a wound may help child to be more cooperative with procedure.
- Skin on neonates is immature and can easily be damaged from pressure and wound care products. Check that products are approved for use with this population. Remember that in neonates the skin readily absorbs products.
- Topical anesthetic solutions (e.g., lidocaine, adrenaline, and tetracycline [LAT] and tetracycline-phenylephrine [tetraphen]) applied to wounds supply short-term (10 to 15 minutes) anesthesia (Wong and others, 1999).
- Assess need for pain management. Provide pain management before performing wound irrigation (Wong and others, 1999).

Gerontological Considerations

- Wound irrigations can be traumatic, frightening, and painful to some older clients. Nurse should assess client's cooperation before doing a wound irrigation. Nurse should be mindful of client's cognitive level of understanding when performing a wound irrigation.
- Older adult's skin has increased potential for irritation from products used and increased risk for infection (Cuzzell, 1997).
- Older skin loses many of its normal characteristics; therefore it is more easily damaged from trauma due to the cleaning process (Ebersole and Hess, 1998; Lueckenotte, 2000).

Long-Term Care Considerations

- Centers with subacute care units often provide specialized wound care. Client may need subacute care because of poor or delayed wound healing (Sorrentino and Gorek, 1999).

Home Care Considerations

- Assess client's home environment to determine adequacy of facilities for performing wound care; check especially for adequate lighting, running water, and storage of supplies.
- Tell client and caregiver that because normal saline has no preservatives, the bottle should be labeled with day and time, and it should be thrown out 24 to 48 hours after it is first opened or made (Barr, 1995b).
- Wound care is planned in conjunction with client's total rehabilitation goals. The objective of wound care management in a subacute care setting is to return client to the home environment (Beshara, Jameson, and Barr, 2000).

Skill 35-2 Performing Suture and Staple Removal

Institutional policy determines whether *only* the physician or the physician *and* nurse may remove sutures and staples. The physician's written order is always obtained before implementing either skill. The time of removal is based on the stage of incisional healing and the extent of surgery.

Sutures and staples are generally removed within 7 to 10 days after surgery if healing is adequate. Retention sutures usually remain in place 14 to 21 days. Timing the removal of sutures and staples is important. They are left in long enough to ensure initial wound closure with enough strength to support internal tissues and organs. Leaving them in too long increases the risk of infection at the puncture sites. The physician determines and orders removal of all sutures or staples at one time or removal of every other suture or staple as the first phase, with the remainder removed in the second phase.

Sutures are threads of wire or other materials used to sew body tissues together. Sutures are placed within tissue layers in deep wounds and superficially as the final means for wound closure. The deeper sutures are usually an absorbable material that disappears in several days.

Staples are made of stainless steel wire. Their use is restricted by the location of the incision, because there must be adequate distance between the skin and structure that lie below the skin, including bone and vascular structures. The cosmetic result may not be as desirable as that obtained with finer suture material. Staples do provide ample strength. Removal requires a sterile staple extractor and maintenance of aseptic technique.

The client's history of wound healing, site of wound, tissues involved, and the purpose of the sutures determine the suture material selected. For example, a client with repeated abdominal surgeries might require wire sutures for greater strength to promote wound closure.

The physician and/or nurse judge whether to remove all sutures if any sign of suture line separation is evident during the process of suture or staple removal. It is not uncommon to remove every other suture initially, removing the balance several days to a week later.

Delegation Considerations

This skill should not be delegated to assistive personnel. Instruct care provider on signs and symptoms to report following suture removal.

Equipment

- Disposable waterproof bag
- Sterile suture removal set (forceps and scissors) or sterile staple extractor
- Sterile applicators or antiseptic swabs
- Steri-Strips or butterfly adhesive strips
- Clean gloves
- Sterile disposable gloves

Step	Rationale
Assessment	
1. Identify client with need for suture or staple removal: check physician's order.	Removal of sutures or staples is a dependent intervention. Adequate healing should have taken place within this time frame.
a. Review specific directions related to suture or staple removal.	Indicates specifically which sutures are to be removed (e.g., every other suture).
b. Determine history of conditions that may interfere with healing.	
(1) Conditions that place client at risk for impaired healing include advanced age, cardiovascular disease, diabetes, immunosuppression, radiation, obesity, smoking, poor cellular nutrition, very deep wounds, and infection.	Preexisting health disorders affect speed of healing and may result in dehiscence.
2. Assess client for history of allergies.	Determines if client is sensitive to antiseptic.
3. Inspect skin integrity of suture line for uniform closure of wound edges, normal color, and absence of drainage and inflammation.	Indicates adequate wound healing for support of internal structures without continued need for sutures or staples.

STEP	RATIONALE

- ***Critical Decision Point***
  If wound edges are separated or signs of infection are present, wound has not healed properly. Notify physician because sutures or staples may need to remain in place and/or other wound care initiated.

NURSING DIAGNOSIS

Defining characteristics from the assessment data may reveal the following nursing diagnoses for clients requiring this skill:

Impaired skin integrity
Risk for impaired skin integrity
Risk for infection

Related factors are individualized based on client's condition or needs.

PLANNING

1. **Expected outcomes** following completion of procedure:
   - All suture material or staples are removed. — Removes source of infection or irritation from retained sutures.
   - Suture line is intact. — Wound is healing and does not require protective dressings.
2. Explain to client that suture removal is usually not a painful procedure but that client may feel pulling or tugging of the skin. — Gains client cooperation and reduces anxiety.

IMPLEMENTATION

1. Close curtains or room door. — Provides privacy.
2. Position client comfortably, while exposing suture line. — Prepares area for staple or suture removal.
   - ***Critical Decision Point***
     For client who is highly anxious or who has an extensive wound, consider need to administer analgesic 30 minutes before suture removal.
3. Ensure direct lighting is on suture line. — Aids visibility and correct placement of forceps or extractor during removal process, ultimately reducing soft tissue injury.
4. Wash hands. — Reduces risk of infection.
5. Place cuffed refuse disposable bag within easy reach. — Provides for easy disposal of contaminated dressings and prevents passing items over sterile work area.
6. Prepare sterile field with dressing change supplies: — Allows nurse to freely handle sterile supplies.
   a. Open sterile suture removal tray or staple extract tray and slide contents onto prepared field, maintaining sterility of inside surface of wrapper or tray (see Chapter 32).
   b. Open sterile antiseptic swabs and place on inside surface of tray.
   c. Open sterile glove package, exposing cuffed ends.
7. Apply clean gloves. Carefully remove dressing, and discard dressing and clean gloves in prepared refuse disposal bag. — Reduces transmission of infection.
8. Inspect wound (see illustration). — Determines adequacy of wound healing.
9. Apply sterile gloves, if required by policy. — Allows nurse to handle sterile supplies.
10. Cleanse sutures or staples and healed incision with antiseptic swabs. — Removes surface bacteria from incision and sutures or staples.

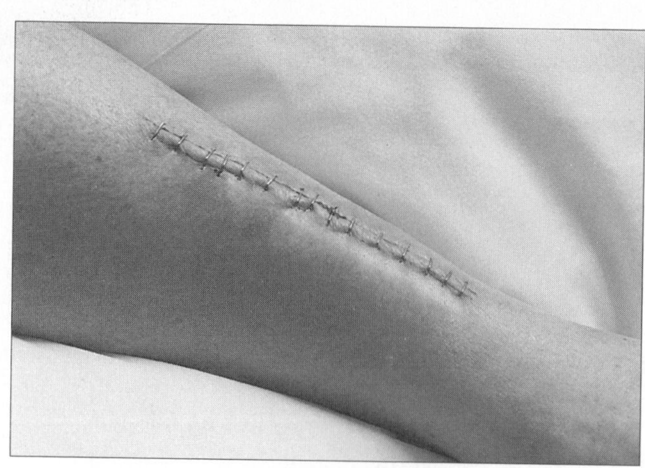

STEP **8** Suture line secured with staples.

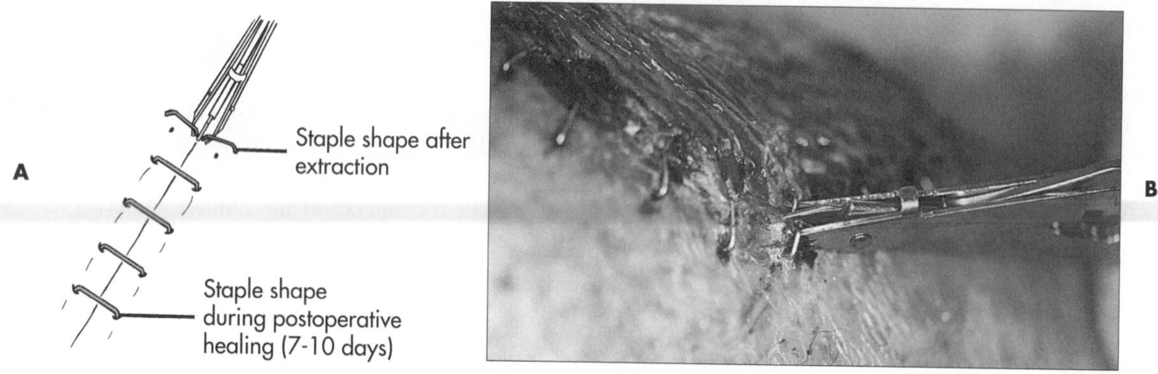

STEP **11a** Staple extractor placed under staple.

STEP	RATIONALE
11. Remove staples:	
a. Place lower tips of staple extractor under first staple. As you close handles, upper tip of extractor depresses center of staple, causing both ends of staple to be bent upward and simultaneously exit their insertion sites in the dermal layer (see illustrations).	Avoids excess pressure to suture line and secures smooth removal of each staple.
b. Carefully control staple extractor.	Avoids suture-line pressure and pain.
c. As soon as both ends of staple are visible, move it away from skin surface and continue on until staple is over refuse bag (see illustration).	Prevents scratching tender skin surface with sharp pointed ends of staple for comfort and infection control.
d. Release handles of staple extractor, allowing staple to drop into refuse bag.	Avoids contaminating sterile field with used staples.
e. Repeat Steps a through c until all staples are removed.	

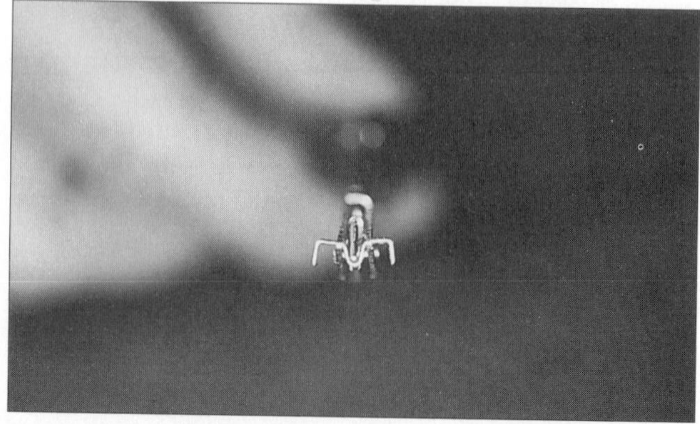

STEP **11c** Metal staple removed by extractor.

STEP	RATIONALE
12. Remove intermittent sutures* (see illustration):	
a. Place gauze a few inches from suture line. Grasp scissors in dominant hand and forceps in nondominant hand.	Gauze serves as receptacle for removed sutures. Placement of scissors and forceps allows for efficient suture removal.

- ***Critical Decision Point***
  Placement of scissors and forceps is very important. Avoid pinching the skin around the wound when lifting up the suture. Likewise, avoid cutting the skin around the wound by accident when snipping the suture.

b. Snip suture,* close to skin surface, at end distal to knot (see illustration). Be sure ends are completely severed by gently lifting exposed end away from skin.	Releases suture.

- ***Critical Decision Point***
  Never snip both ends of suture; there will be no way to remove half of suture situated below the surface.

c. Grasp knotted end with forceps and in one continuous smooth action remove entire suture (see illustration). Place removed suture on gauze.	Smoothly removes suture without additional tension to suture line.

- ***Critical Decision Point***
  Never pull exposed surface of any suture into tissue below epidermis. The exposed surface of any suture is considered contaminated.

*Each suture has a knot. Each interrupted suture is secured with its own knot. Knots are lined up on same side of incision.

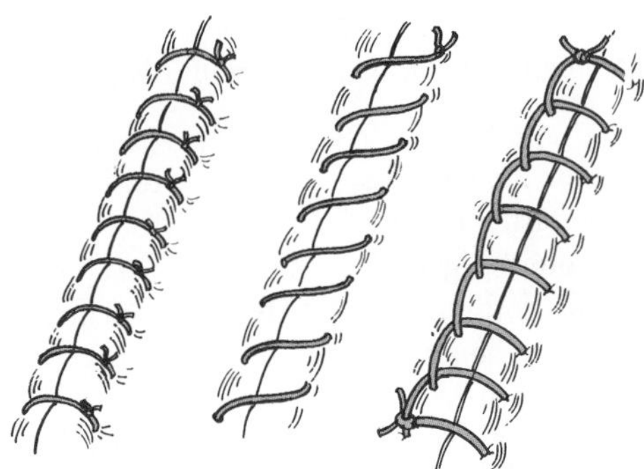

STEP **12** *Left,* Intermittent; *middle,* continuous; *right,* blanket.

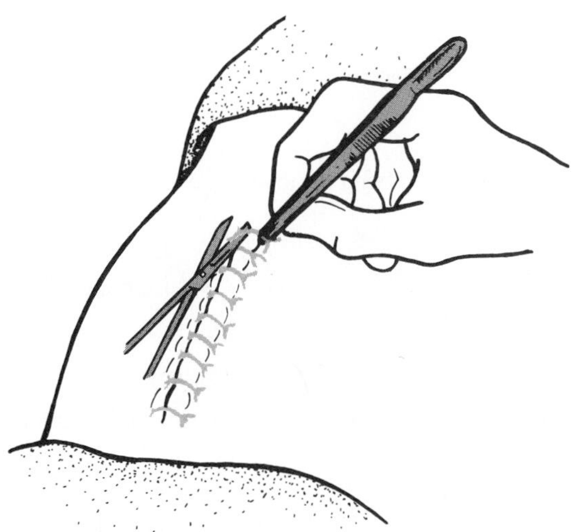

STEP **12b** Removal of intermittent suture. Nurse cuts suture as close to skin as possible, away from the knot.

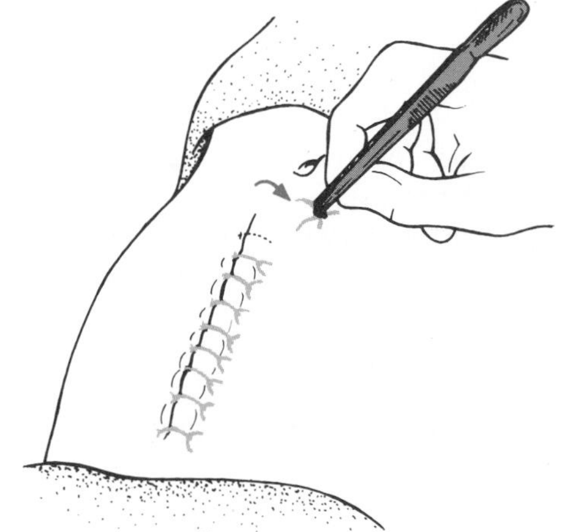

STEP **12c** Nurse removes suture and never pulls the contaminated stitch through tissues.

Step	Rationale
d. Repeat Steps a through c until every other suture has been removed.	
e. Observe healing level. Based on observations of wound response to suture removal and physician's original order, determine whether remaining sutures will be removed at this time. If so, repeat Steps a through c until all sutures have been removed.	Determines status of wound healing and if suture line will remain closed after all sutures are removed.
f. If any doubt, stop and notify physician.	
13. Remove continuous sutures, including blanket stitch sutures (see illustration for Step 12):	
a. Place sterile gauze a few inches from suture line. Grasp scissors in dominant hand and forceps in nondominant hand.	Gauze serves as receptacle for removed sutures. Placement of scissors and forceps allows for efficient suture removal.
b. Snip first suture close to skin surface at end distal to knot.	Releases suture.
c. Snip second suture on same side.	Releases interrupted sutures from knot.
d. Grasp knotted end and remove first line of spiral in continuous smooth action, pulling away from severed end. Place suture on gauze compress.	Smoothly removes sutures without additional tension to suture line.
e. Repeat Steps a through d in consecutive order until the entire line has been removed.	
14. Inspect incision site and identify any trouble areas. Gently wipe suture line with antiseptic swab to remove debris and cleanse wound.	Reduces risk of further incision line separation.

- ***Critical Decision Point***

  Make sure that all of the suture has been removed and that no part of it has been retained in the client's wound.

Step	Rationale
15. If *any* separation greater than 2 stitches or 2 staples in width is apparent, place supportive butterfly closure across area to maintain contact between wound edges.	Prevents further wound separation.
16. Apply light dressing or expose to air if no clothing will come in contact with suture line. Instruct client about applying own dressing if it will be needed at home.	Healing by primary intention eliminates need for dressing.
17. Discard all contaminated materials, and remove and dispose of gloves.	Reduces transmission of infection.
18. Route reusable items such as staple extractor for resterilization, and wash hands.	Reduces transmission of infection.

Evaluation

Step	Rationale
1. Assess site where sutures or staples were removed; inspect condition of soft tissues, including skin. Look for any pieces of removed suture that were left behind.	Sources of infection have been removed.
2. Determine if client has pain along incision.	Determines comfort level. Can indicate if suture material remains in skin.

Unexpected Outcomes and Related Interventions

- Retained suture
  - Assess suture line closely to determine if any suture material remains.
  - Notify physician.
  - Instruct client to notify physician if signs of suture line infection develop following discharge from agency.
- Wound separation or drainage secondary to healing problems
  - Leave remaining sutures or staples in place.
  - Place supportive butterfly closures across suture line.
  - Notify physician.

Recording and Reporting

- Record on client's progress note *number* of sutures or staples removed and appearance of wound. Indicate that entire suture was removed.
- Report time sutures were removed, level of healing of wound, and client's response to suture removal.
- Notify physician immediately of any of the following findings: suture line separation, **dehiscence, evisceration,** bleeding, or purulent drainage.

Teaching Considerations

- Crusting from around sutures can be removed with half-strength hydrogen peroxide as long as skin is intact.
- Teach client to observe for any sign of separation of wound edges before removing remaining sutures.
- Have client apply own dressing and inspect suture line for continued healing. Continue instruction on resumption of bathing and showering activities, prevention of abdominal strain during defecation, and provision of adequate nutrition and ambulation.
- Explain gradual suture line skin color changes (e.g., in light-tone clients from red to natural color).
- Teach client not to put additional stress on suture line from such activities as lifting or bending (Maklebust and Palleschi, 1996). Client with abdominal surgery or injury must avoid lifting heavy packages or equipment for several weeks.
- Instruct primary caregiver and client to maintain clean technique when treating suture line and changing dressings.
- Instruct client that sometimes there may be a small amount of drainage from wound immediately after suture removal.

Pediatric Considerations

- Assistance may be needed to keep babies from moving during the suture removal procedure.
- Topical anesthetic solutions (e.g., lidocaine, adrenaline, and tetracycline [LAT] and tetracycline-phenylephrine [tetraphen]) applied to wounds supply short-term (10 to 15 minutes) anesthesia (Wong and others, 1999).

Gerontological Considerations

- Older adults may need reassurance about suture removal procedure. Depending on their mental status, they may not understand procedure.
- Older skin may be at higher risk for dehiscence after sutures are removed.

Skill 35-3 Performing Drainage Evacuation

A wound heals only if drainage does not accumulate in the wound bed. Removal of even small amounts of drainage is accomplished by either a closed or open drain system. The drain may be inserted directly through the suture line into the wound or through a small stab wound near the suture line into the wound.

An open drain system (e.g., a **Penrose drain** [Figure 35-8]) removes drainage from the wound and deposits it onto the skin surface. A safety pin is inserted through this drain, outside the skin, to prevent the tubing from moving into the wound.

To remove the Penrose drain the physician advances the tubing in stages as the wound heals from the bottom up. Nursing interventions include caution to prevent accidental removal of the drain during dressing changes and to protect skin surfaces in direct contact with the irritating drainage. Because of the danger of accidental dislodgement and the need to assess the drain placement accurately, Penrose drains that are covered with gauze pads are usually managed by the nurse and are not delegated to assistive personnel. Some Penrose drains are contained within wound pouches.

A closed drain system (e.g., the **Jackson-Pratt [JP] drain** [Figure 35-9]), **Hemovac drain** (Figure 35-10), VacuDrain, or Constavac relies on the presence of a vacuum (Box 35-3) to withdraw accumulated drainage through multiple perforations in clear plastic tubing into the closed reservoir, suction bladder, or bag (Box 35-3). The closed system ensures dry skin but operates only if the tubing is patent and a vacuum exists. Drainage is emptied periodically from the reservoir, and the vacuum is reestablished.

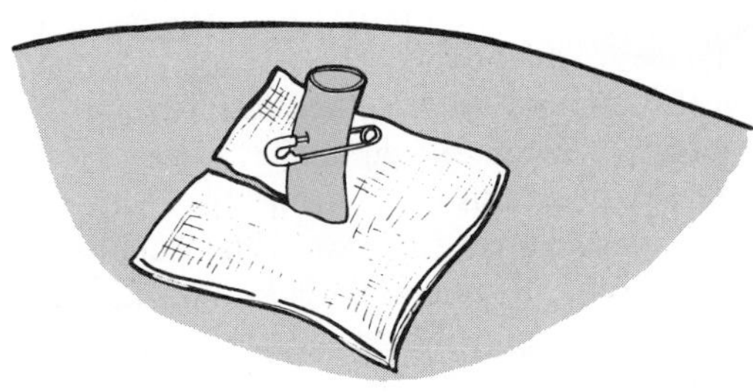

FIGURE 35-8 Penrose drain with a drain-split gauze.

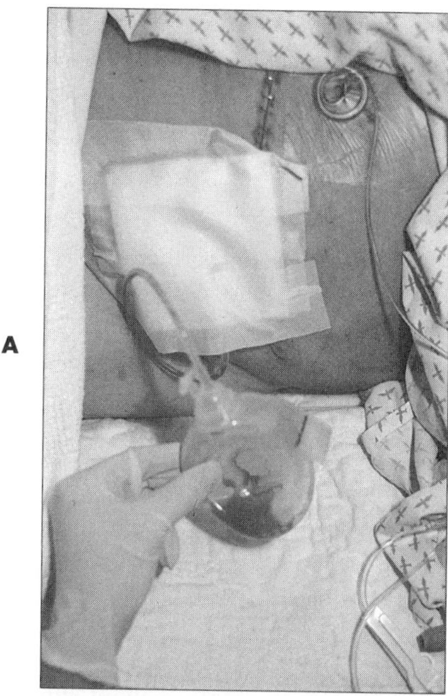

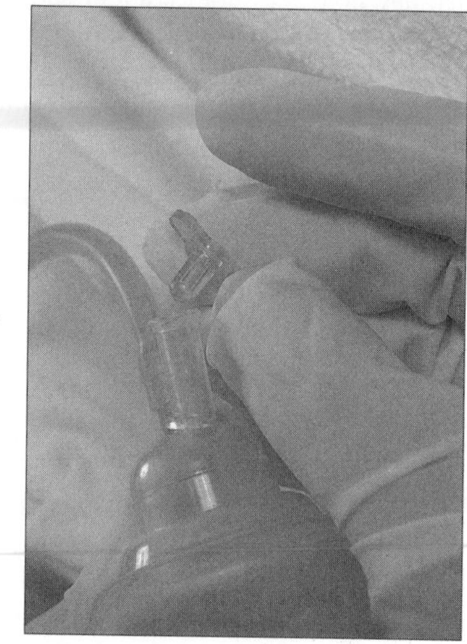

FIGURE **35-9** **A**, Jackson-Pratt wound drainage system. **B**, Emptying Jackson-Pratt device.

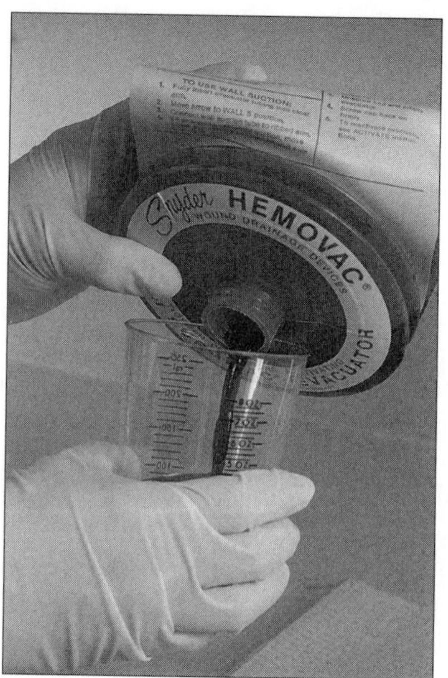

FIGURE **35-10** To come.

Box 35-3 Attaching Wound Suction Devices to Wall Suction

HEMOVAC

- Connect graduated adapter to emptying port and then to wall suction tubing.
- Set suction level as prescribed or on *low* if suction level not specified.

JACKSON-PRATT

- Attach connecting adapter to suction tubing.
- Set suction level as prescribed on *low* setting if not specified.
- Attach tubing with graduated connector to open port, and secure with tape.

DELEGATION CONSIDERATIONS

Assessment of wound drainage and maintenance of drains and the drainage system should not be delegated to assistive personnel. However, assistive personnel may empty a closed drainage container or pouch, measure the amount of drainage, and report the amount on the client's intake and output (I&O) record. The nurse should assist the staff in reviewing I&O procedure.

EQUIPMENT

- Graduated measuring cylinder
- Alcohol sponge
- Gauze sponges
- Goggles
- Sterile specimen container, if culture is needed
- Sterile dressings or pouch, if drain is needed
- Clean disposable gloves
- Safety pin(s)

STEP	RATIONALE

ASSESSMENT

1. Identify presence, location, and purpose of closed wound drain and drainage system as client returns from surgery. Assess drainage present on client's dressing.
   Drainage tubing may be placed within wound or through small surgical incision near major wound.
2. Identify *number* of wound drain tubes and what drainage each one ought to be draining. Label each drain tube with a number or label.
   Assigning a labeling system to each drain helps with consistent documentation when client has multiple drainage tubes.
3. Assess if drain tube needs self-suction, wall suction, or no suction by checking physician's orders.
   Some drain tubes such as Hemovacs can be used with self-suction or wall suction.
4. Inspect system to determine presence of one straight tube or Y-tube arrangement with two tube insertion sites.
   To plan skin care and identify quantity of sterile dressing supplies.
5. Inspect system to ensure proper functioning. A complete systematic inspection should include the insertion site, drainage moving through tubing in direction of reservoir (tubing patent), airtight connection sites, and presence of any leaks or kinks in the system.
   Properly functioning system maintains suction until reservoir is filled; drainage is no longer being produced or accumulated. Tension on drainage tubing increases injury to skin and underlying muscle.

   • ***Critical Decision Point***
   Attach drainage tubing with tape and a safety pin to client's gown so that it does not pull on insertion site.

6. Be sure Penrose drain has a sterile safety pin in place. Penrose drains may be covered with a gauze dressing or a closed wound container.
   Pin prevents drain from being pulled below the skin's surface.
7. Identify type of drainage container client has.
   Determines frequency for emptying drainage.

NURSING DIAGNOSIS

Clustering of defining characteristics from the assessment data may reveal the following nursing diagnoses for clients requiring this skill:

- Impaired skin integrity
- Risk for infection
- Risk for injury

Related factors are individualized based on client's condition or needs.

PLANNING

1. **Expected outcomes** following completion of procedure:
   - Wound healing continues.
     Client will be comfortable, and epithelialization will continue in the absence of infectious pathogens or accumulated debris.
   - Vacuum is reestablished.
     Suction system is intact.
   - Tubing is patent.
     Fluid is draining away from wound.
2. Explain procedure to client.
   Promotes client's cooperation.

IMPLEMENTATION

1. Close room door or bedside curtains.
   Provides privacy.
2. Wash hands and apply gloves.
   Reduces transmission of microorganisms.
3. Place open specimen container or measuring graduate on bed between you and client.
   Permits measuring and discarding of wound drainage.

Step	Rationale
4. When emptying evacuator, maintain asepsis while opening port:	Avoids entry of pathogens.
a. Hemovac (see Figure 35-10):	
(1) Open plug on port indicated for emptying drainage reservoir.	Vacuum will be broken, and reservoir will pull air in until chamber is fully expanded.
(2) Tilt evacuator in direction of plug.	Drains fluid toward plug.
(3) Slowly squeeze two flat surfaces together while draining into sterile laboratory specimen container if culture is ordered and remainder into graduated cylinder. Cover specimen container.	Prevents splashing of contaminated drainage.
(4) Hold uncovered alcohol sponge in dominant hand; place evacuator on flat surface with open outlet facing upward; continue pressing downward until bottom and top are in contact; hold surfaces together with one hand, quickly cleanse opening and plug with other hand, and immediately replace plug; secure evacuator on client's bed.	Compression of surface of Hemovac creates vacuum. Cleansing of plug reduces transmission of microorganisms into drainage evacuation.
(5) Check evacuator for reestablishment of vacuum, patency of drainage tubing, and absence of stress on tubing.	Facilitates wound drainage and prevents tension on drainage tubing.
b. Jackson-Pratt evacuator (see Figure 35-9, *A*):	
(1) Open emptying port on opposite side of bulb-shaped reservoir (see Figure 35-9, *B*).	
(2) Compress bulb over drainage container.	Empties drainage and reestablishes vacuum.
(a) Cleanse ends of emptying port with alcohol sponge while continuing to compress container. Replace cap immediately. Secure evacuator below wound site with safety pin through indicated perforation to client's gown.	Reduces transmission of microorganisms into drainage evacuator and prevents tension on drainage tubing.
5. Place and secure drainage reservoirs to prevent any pull on tubing insertion sites.	Pinning drainage tubing to client's gown will prevent tension or pulling on tubing and insertion site.

• ***Critical Decision Point***
Be sure there is slack in tubing from reservoir to wound.

Step	Rationale
6. Route labeled specimen to laboratory if ordered by physician *or* if purulence is noted.	Allows for culture testing to reveal infection.
7. Discard soiled supplies, remove gloves, and wash hands.	Reduces transmission of microorganisms.
8. Apply new sterile gloves, and proceed with dressing change (see Chapter 36) around drain site and inspection of skin if indicated or ordered. Split-drain sponge dressings are often used around drain tubes (see illustrations) and then covered with gauze. Penrose drains are either covered with gauze dressings or a wound pouch.	Prevents entrance of bacteria into surgical wound.
9. Discard contaminated materials and wash hands.	Reduces transmission of microorganisms.

Evaluation

Step	Rationale
1. Observe for drainage in drainage evacuator.	Indicates presence of vacuum, patency of tubing, and functioning of drainage evacuator.

• ***Critical Decision Point***
Clots or large collections of debris may prohibit drainage flow. An area especially prone to clogging from drainage is the Y site in the drainage tubing.

A 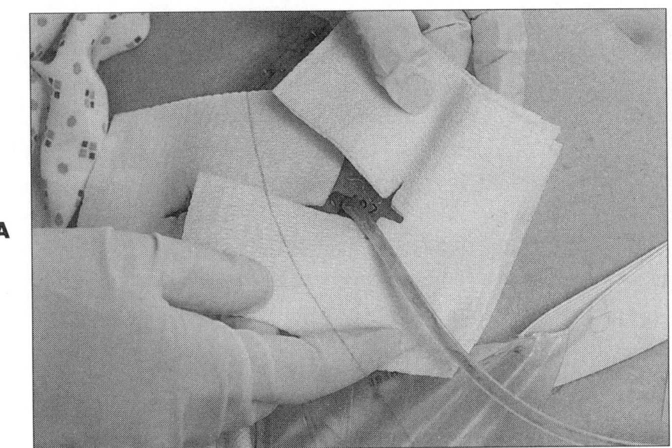

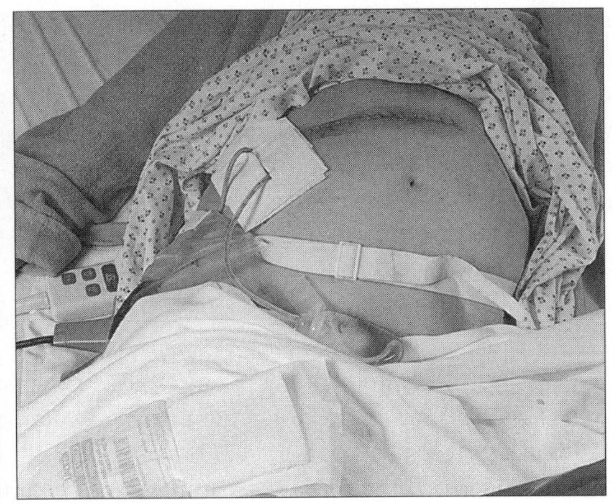 B

STEP **8** **A,** Jackson-Pratt (JP) drain-split gauze dressing. Applying split-drain dressing around a JP drain tube. **B,** Split-drain dressing in place around a JP drain tube.

STEP	RATIONALE
2. Inspect wound for drainage or collection of drainage fluid under the skin, causing a seroma.	Drainage should not be significant under suture line. Indicates inadequate functioning of drainage evacuator. New wound drainage appears very red at first and later changes to lighter color.
3. Empty drainage system and measure drainage.	Drainage collection reservoir is emptied every 8 to 12 hours and as needed for large drainage volume. The nurse collects diagnostic specimen in the presence of unexpected purulence or pungent odor, reports findings to physician, and records in progress note.
4. Assess client's level of comfort.	Procedure should not increase client's pain.

Unexpected Outcomes and Related Interventions

- Wound becomes infected.
  - Notify physician about the presence of signs of infection: purulent drainage, increased white blood cell (WBC) count, and temperature elevation.
  - Use aseptic technique when changing dressings.
- Bleeding appears.
  - Determine amount of bleeding, and notify physician if excessive.
  - Assess for tension on client's drainage tubing.
  - Secure tubing to prevent pulling and pain.
- Client experiences pain.
  - Assess client's level of pain.
  - Medicate client.
  - Stabilize drainage tubing to reduce tension and pulling against incision.
  - Notify physician if signs of wound infection are present.
- Drainage evacuator system is not accumulating drainage.
  - Assess drainage tubing for clots.
  - Assess drainage system for air leaks or kinks.
  - Notify physician.

Recording and Reporting

- Record results of emptying wound drainage evacuator and dressing change (when performed) on progress notes and I&O record. Note characteristics of drainage; measure volume and discard.
- Quickly report to the physician:
  - Sudden change in amount of drainage, either output or absence of drainage flow
  - Pungent odor of drainage or new evidence of purulence
  - Severe pain
  - Dislodgement of the drainage tube
- Report presence of functioning drainage evacuator and emptying frequency at a change-of-shift report to nurse.

Teaching Considerations

- Instruct client about anticipated postoperative drainage, expected progress of wound healing and drainage volume, and estimated date of removal of drain as volume diminishes.
- Instruct client in how to empty and record amount of drainage.
- Unexplained dark red drainage is major concern to any client. Being aware of what to expect reduces anxiety.
- Instruct primary caregiver and client in how to change dressings located around drain site.
- Instruct client to wear loose-fitting clothes.
- Instruct client to keep drain lower than waist level when ambulating, sitting, or lying down.
- Instruct client not to pull or tug on tubing; secure drain with safety pin.

Pediatric Considerations

- Have parents help to prevent pediatric clients from dislodging drainage tubes.

Gerontological Considerations

- Be aware that older adult clients with large amounts of drainage will need additional fluid intake because they are more apt to become dehydrated.
- Measures may need to be taken to prevent a confused client from pulling out drain collector.

Home Care Considerations

- Dispose of drainage in commode.
- Wear clean gloves, and wash hands after procedure.
- Provide written instructions on drain care.
- Arrange for home health nurse if needed.

Critical Thinking Exercises

1. You plan to irrigate a client's sacral pressure ulcer with a 35-ml syringe and a 19-gauge needle. How do you protect yourself from exposure to microorganisms?
2. It is your client's sixth postoperative day. When assessing the wound you note that several sutures remain. What actions do you take?
3. A client has two Jackson-Pratt drainage collectors on the left side of the abdomen. What nursing assessments should be made to ensure proper functioning of this system? Can any aspects of care for this type of drain collector be delegated? Explain the rationale for your answer.

References

Agency for Health Care Policy and Research (AHCPR): *Treatment of pressure ulcers,* Clinical practice guideline No. 15, AHCPR Pub No. 95-0653, Rockville, Md, 1994. U.S. Department of Health and Human Services, Public Health Service.

Barr JE: Physiology of healing: the basis for the principles of wound management, *Medsurg Nurs* 5(4):387, 1995a.

Barr JE: Principles of wound cleansing, *Ostomy Wound Manage* 7A(suppl 41):15S, 1995b.

Beshara M, Jameson G, Barr B: Practice development in acute and long-term care settings. In Bryant RA: *Acute and chronic wounds: nursing management,* ed 2, St. Louis, 2000, Mosby.

Bonier P: Wound care forum: an unusual alternative, *Am J Nurs* 85:418, 1985.

Bryant RA, editor: *Acute and chronic wounds,* St. Louis, 1992, Mosby.

Bryant RA, editor: *Acute and chronic wounds,* ed 2, St. Louis, 2000, Mosby.

Brylinsky CM: Nutrition and wound healing: an overview, *Ostomy Wound Manage* 41(10):14, 1995.

Centers for Disease Control and Prevention: Guideline for isolation precautions in hospitals, *Am J Infect Control* 24:24, 1996.

Cooper DM: Assessment, measurement, and evaluation: their pivotal roles in wound healing. In Bryant R, editor: *Acute and chronic wounds,* ed 2, St. Louis, 2000, Mosby.

Cuzzell J: Choosing a wound dressing, *Geriatr Nurs* 18(6):260, 1997.

Doughty DB: Principles of wound healing and wound management. In Bryant R, editor: *Acute and chronic wounds,* St. Louis, 1992, Mosby.

Ebersole P, Hess P: *Toward healthy aging: human needs and nursing response,* St. Louis, 1998, Mosby.

Hunt TK: Disorders of repair and their management. In Hunt TK, Dunphy JE, editors: *Fundamentals of wound management,* New York, 1979, Appleton-Century Crofts.

Keast DH, Orsted H: The basic principles of wound care, *Ostomy Wound Manage* 44(8):24, 1998.

Lueckenotte AG: *Gerontologic nursing,* ed 2, St. Louis, 2000, Mosby.

Maklebust J, Palleschi M: Promoting surgical wound healing, *Nursing* 26(6):24C, 1996.

Martin P: Wound healing: aiming for perfect skin regeneration, *Science* 276(5309):75, 1997.

Mendez-Eastman S: When wounds won't heal, *RN* 61(1):20, 1998.

Pontieri-Lewis V: The role of nutrition in wound healing, *Medsurg Nurs* 6(4):187, 1997.

Potter P, Perry A: *Fundamentals of nursing: concepts, process, and practice,* ed 4, St. Louis, 1997, Mosby.

Ramundo J, Wells J: Wound debridement. In Bryant RA: *Acute and chronic wounds: nursing management,* ed 2, St. Louis, 2000, Mosby.

Rodeheaver GT: Controversies in topical wound management: wound cleansing and wound disinfection. In Krasner D, editor: *Chronic wound care,* King of Prussia, Pa, 1990, Health Management Publications.

Sorrentino SA, Gorek B: *Long-term care assistants,* ed 3, St. Louis, 1999, Mosby.

Waldrop J, Doughty DB: Wound healing physiology. In Bryant RA: *Acute and chronic wounds: nursing management,* ed 2, St. Louis, 2000, Mosby.

Wong DL and others: *Whaley and Wong's nursing care of infants and children,* St. Louis, 1999, Mosby.

36

Dressings

Skills

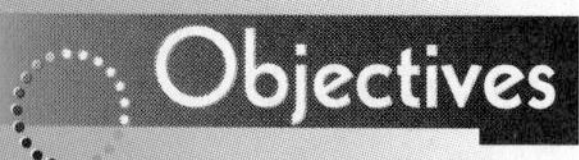

Objectives

Mastery of content in this chapter will enable the nurse to:

- Define the key terms listed.
- Properly assess a wound.
- Choose the correct dressing for a wound.
- Understand the technique of a dressing application.
- State advantages and disadvantages of the types of dressings used.
- Correctly apply dry, wet-to-dry, pressure, and synthetic dressings.

Key Terms

Dead space
Debridement
Dehiscence
Epithelialization
Erythema
Evisceration
Excoriated
Exudate
Granulation
Hydrocolloid
Hydrogel
Macerated
Neovascularization
Primary dressing
Pseudomonas aeruginosa
Secondary dressing

Wound characteristics identified during assessment along with treatment goals determine the type of dressing needed (Agency for Health Care Policy and Research [AHCPR], 1994) (Box 36-1). Wounds heal best in a moist environment. The concept of moist wound healing revolutionized wound management and served as a catalyst for the development of many moisture-retentive dressings (see Skills 36-4 through 36-7).

In addition, another major change in wound care is the treatment of postsurgical dressings. Although the initial dressing is a sterile dressing, subsequent dressing changes may be clean rather than sterile. This change in practice is due to the fact that research has demonstrated no difference in wound infection rate and the practice results in lower costs for dressing supplies (Stotts and others, 1997). Dressings that come in direct contact with the wound bed are called **primary dressings. Secondary dressings** are used to cover or hold primary dressings in place.

Dressings serve several functions, including maintenance of a moist environment (Field and Kerstein, 1994), protection from outside contaminants, protection from further injury, prevention of the spread of microorganisms, increased client comfort, and control of bleeding. Therefore the ideal dressing will be based on the purpose of the dressing. For example, to control bleeding, a dressing must be applied with pressure. When a wound has drainage, the dressing must be highly absorbent. Another factor to consider when choosing a dressing is ease of application. The dressing should conform to body contours and should be durable but flexible, cost-effective, able to absorb or contain exudate, easily removed without damage to the healing surface, and acceptable in appearance (Bolton and Rijswijk, 1991).

When changing a dressing the nurse must be knowledgeable about wound healing to differentiate a normal or expected appearance from abnormal changes. Assessment of the exudates absorbed by the dressing provides valuable diagnostic information.

Primary healing takes place when tissue is cleanly cut and the margins are reapproximated. Repair should occur without complication. New capillary circulation bridges the wound quickly in 3 to 4 days, and once normal tissue oxygenation is achieved, the wound is considered to be healed. A wound closed for primary healing is most susceptible to infection during the first 4 days.

Healing by secondary intention occurs when a wound is left open. Healing results in the formation of **granulation** tissue from the bottom of the wound and eventual **epithelialization** from the sides of the wound to close the defect made by the wound. Burns, infected wounds, and deep pressure ulcers heal in this manner (Wysocki, 1995; Keast and Orsted, 1998).

The type of dressing used depends on the wound characteristics and the goal of wound management, which can be wound **debridement** or wound healing. Various types of dressings can be applied to wounds (Krasner, 1992a, 1992b,

Box 36-1 AHCPR 1994 Dressing Recommendations

- Use a dressing that keeps the ulcer bed continuously moist. Wet-to-dry dressings should be used only for debridement and are not considered continuously moist saline dressings.
- Use clinical judgment to select a type of moist wound dressing suitable for the ulcer. Studies of different types of moist wound dressings showed no differences in pressure ulcer healing outcomes.
- Choose a dressing that keeps the surrounding (periulcer) intact skin dry while keeping the ulcer bed moist.
- Choose a dressing that controls exudate but does not desiccate the ulcer bed.
- Consider caregiver time when selecting a dressing.
- Eliminate wound dead space by loosely filling all cavities with dressing material. Avoid overpacking the wound.
- Monitor dressings applied near the anus, because they are difficult to keep intact.

1995; Erwin-Toth and Hocevar, 1995; Motta, 1995). Given the many types of dressings that are now available, the nurse may find it difficult to decide which dressing is best to use on a particular wound. Some nurses may find the decision tree in Figure 36-1 helpful in selecting the appropriate dressing to care for a particular wound (Maklebust and Palleschi, 1996).

Woven gauze dressings, the oldest and most common type, do not interact with wound tissues and thus cause little wound irritation (Aronovitch, 1995). Gauze comes in a variety of sizes and shapes. The nurse applies gauze either wet or dry, depending on whether the wound needs debridement, a moist healing environment, or a covering to prevent trauma.

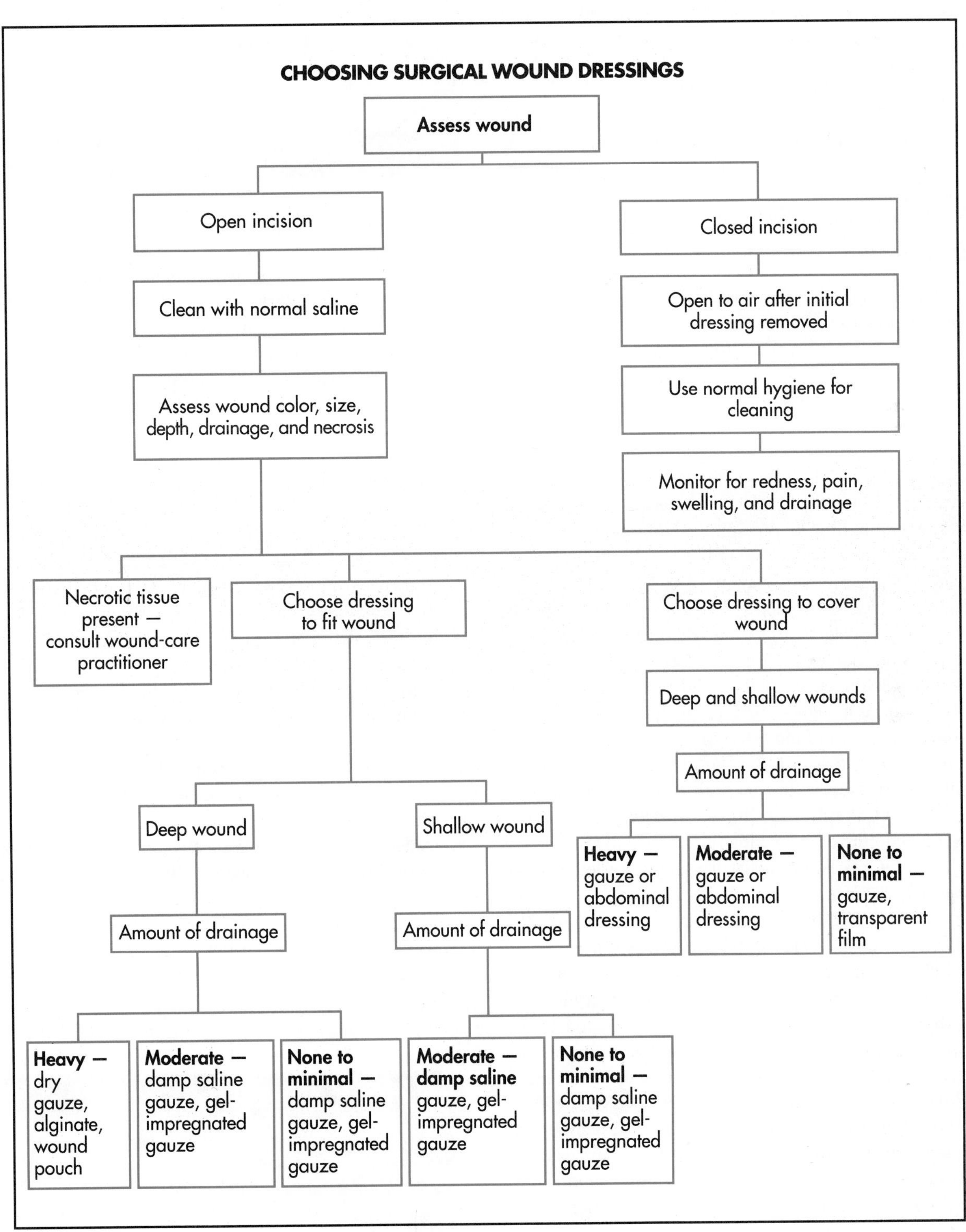

FIGURE 36-1 Flow chart for dressing selection.

Wet-to-dry dressings are used for wounds requiring debridement (see Skill 36-2). The nurse moistens the gauze layer that touches the wound surface (primary dressing). This dressing should not be so moist that it will never dry out. The moistened gauze increases the absorptive ability of the dressing to collect exudate and wound debris. This then is covered with a secondary dressing layer that is dry. When the inner moistened gauze dressing is dried, it is then removed from the wound. As the gauze is pulled from the wound, the wound tissue that has adhered to the gauze is removed, thus effectively debriding the wound. Wet-to-dry dressings are an example of mechanical nonselective debridement and are effective in cleansing infected and necrotic wounds (Johnson, 1992). To maintain the moist environment needed for wound healing, wet-to-wet (damp-to-damp or moist-to-moist) dressings rather than dry dressings should be used in a clean granulating wound.

Telfa gauze dressings contain a shiny, nonadherent surface on one side. When used as a contact layer the Telfa gauze usually does not stick to incisions or wound openings. Drainage passes through the nonadherent surface to the softened gauze above.

The **hydrocolloid** dressings (DuoDERM, Comfeel, Restore, RepliCare, and others) represent a category of hydroactive dressings (see Skill 36-5). These dressings provide a moist environment for wound healing while facilitating the softening and subsequent removal of wound debris. The dressing promotes wound healing by providing an occlusive protective barrier that absorbs drainage from the wound into the dressing. In addition, the dressing stays in place through an adhesive backing, reduces local pain, and may be used with wound **exudate** absorbers (e.g., DuoDerm granules) to increase time between dressing changes (Krasner, 1992a).

Hydrogel dressings (e.g., Vigilon, Biolex, Nu-Gel, IntraSite Gel, Saf-Gel) have a high moisture content (95%) causing them to swell and retain fluid (see Skill 36-5). They are useful over clean, moist, or **macerated** tissues. The dressing provides a nonadherent, protective barrier with the ability to absorb wound drainage (Krasner, 1992b). These dressings are very soothing and cooling, thus making them especially useful for painful burn wounds. A secondary dressing is needed to hold these dressings in place.

Foam dressings (e.g., Allevyn, LYOfoam, Reston, Epi-Lock, BIOPATCH, CURAFORM) absorb light-to-heavy amounts of exudate, are conformable, and can easily be made to fit a wound. These properties make them especially useful for treating leg ulcers.

Dressings are also available as thin, self-adhesive elastic films (e.g., Op-Site, Bioclusive, Blisterfilm, Acu-derm, Tegaderm, PRO-CLUDE, Polyskin) (see Skill 36-4). The dressing is a synthetic permeable membrane that acts as a temporary second skin. This type of dressing has several advantages: (1) it adheres to undamaged skin to contain exudate and minimize wound contamination, (2) it serves as a barrier to external fluids and bacteria but allows the wound surface to "breathe," (3) it promotes a moist environment that speeds epithelial cell growth, and (4) it can be removed without damaging underlying tissues (Krasner, 1992a). Other advantages are that it allows the client to shower, and it permits direct observation of the wound. A disadvantage of such a dressing is that it cannot debride an infected wound. The film is ideal for small, superficial wounds. This type of dressing can be used to autolytically debride a necrotic wound. It is also useful as a dressing over an intravenous catheter site. The transparent film allows the nurse to assess the wound without removing the dressing.

Skill Performance Guidelines

1. Know the goal of management for the wound. For example, certain dressings can be used to debride wounds, whereas others can be used to maintain a moist wound environment necessary for granulation tissue to fill in the wound defect in a clean wound.
2. Know the cause or type of wound. Wounds caused by vascular insufficiency, diabetes, pressure, trauma, and surgery are all very different and must have an individualized treatment plan (Baranoski, 1995). Not knowing the cause of the wound can have serious negative effects if the nurse uses treatments that are contraindicated for certain types of wounds.
3. Know the expected amount and type (Box 36-2) of wound exudate or drainage. Wounds that have large amounts of drainage require more frequent dressing changes or need dressings that are capable of absorbing large amounts of drainage. Such wounds include fresh postoperative sites, open wounds, and fistulae.
4. Know the type of dressing ordered. Wet-to-dry dressings require more equipment than do dry dressings. Pressure dressings require elastic bandages to maintain the pressure.
5. Determine if wound drainage tubes are present. This prevents their accidental dislocation when the old dressing is removed (see Skill 35-3).
6. Determine the presence of any further break in skin integrity adjacent to the wound. Breaks in skin integrity further increase the client's risk for infection.
7. The location of the wound, the care setting that the client is in, and the client's level of activity influence the decision of what dressing to use.

Box 36-2 Types of Wound Exudate

- *Serous,* which is a clear, watery plasma
- *Sanguineous,* which indicates fresh bleeding
- *Serosanguineous,* which is a pale, more watery drainage than sanguineous drainage
- *Purulent,* which is a thick, yellow, green, or brown drainage

Skill 36-1 Applying a Dry Dressing

A dry dressing may be chosen for management of a wound healing by primary intention with little drainage. The dressing protects the wound from injury, prevents introduction of bacteria, reduces discomfort, and speeds healing.

Dry dressings are most commonly used for abrasions and nondraining postoperative (primary intention healing) incisions. The dry dressing does not debride the wound and should not be selected for wounds requiring debridement. It is not appropriate for an open wound that is healing by secondary intention. If a dry dressing adheres to a wound, the nurse should moisten the dressing with sterile normal saline or water before removing the woven gauze. Moistening the dressing in this manner decreases the adherence of the dressing to the wound and reduces the risk of further trauma to the wound.

Delegation Considerations

The skill of applying a dry dressing may be delegated to assistive personnel. The caregiver must be informed about the signs of infection and poor wound healing and immediately report the findings for further assessment. The care of acute new wounds and those that require sterile technique for dressing change generally remain within the domain of nursing practice. The *assessment* of the wound should not be delegated to assistive personnel even if the dressing change is delegated to assistive personnel.

Equipment

- Gloves, clean or sterile (check institution policy)
- Dressing set (sterile), scissors, forceps (may be optional, check institution policy)
- Sterile drape (optional)
- Gauze dressings, sterile
- Sterile basin (optional)
- Antiseptic ointment (if ordered)
- Cleansing solution such as sterile saline or water
- Tape, ties, or bandage as needed (include nonallergic tape if necessary)
- Waterproof bag
- Extra gauze dressings
- Abdominal (ABD) pads
- Adhesive remover (optional)
- Measurement device (optional): tape measure, camera
- Protective gown, mask, goggles

Step	Rationale
Assessment	
1. Assess size of wound to be dressed.	Assists nurse in planning for proper type and amount of supplies needed.
2. Assess location of wound.	Wound location alerts nurse to dressing type needed and if assistance is needed to hold dressings in place.
3. Assess client's level of comfort.	Removal of dry dressing can be painful; client may require pain medication before dressing change to allow drug's peak effect during procedure.
4. Assess client's knowledge of purpose of dressing change.	Determines level of support and explanation required by client.
5. Assess need and readiness for client or family member to participate in dressing wound.	Prepares client or family member if dressing must be changed at home.
6. Review medical orders for dressing change procedure.	Indicates type of dressing or applications to use.
7. Identify clients with risk factors for wound-healing problems, including:	Physiological changes due to aging, chronic illness, poor nutrition, medications, and cancer treatments have the potential to affect wound healing (Barr, 1995).
a. Aging	Physiological changes of aging alter the immune system, resulting in decreased resistance to pathogens.
b. Prematurity	The skin of premature babies is not mature and does not have the immune functions of normal skin.
c. Obesity	Subcutaneous tissue has diminished vascularity.

Step	Rationale
d. Diabetes	Vascular changes associated with diabetes reduce blood flow to peripheral tissues; also leukocyte malfunction occurs secondary to hyperglycemia.
e. Compromised circulation	Results in inadequate supply of nutrients, blood cells, and oxygen to wound.
f. Poor nutritional state	Impairs stages of inflammation and collagen formation states.
g. Immunosuppressive drugs	Decreases inflammatory response and decreases collagen synthesis.
h. Irradiation in area of wound	Decreases blood supply to tissues.
i. High levels of stress	Increased cortisol levels reduce number of lymphocytes and decrease inflammatory response.
j. Steroids	Slows rate of epithelialization and **neovascularization** and inhibits contraction.

Nursing Diagnosis

Defining characteristics from the assessment data may reveal the following nursing diagnoses for clients requiring this skill:

- Risk for infection
- Impaired skin integrity
- Deficient knowledge regarding dressing application
- Acute pain

Related factors are individualized based on client's condition or needs.

Planning

Step	Rationale
1. **Expected outcomes** following completion of procedure:	
▪ Client's wound is free of infection; drainage begins to diminish in amount, and wound closure is progressing.	Indicates wound is healing appropriately.
▪ Client reports minimal discomfort.	Indicates dressing procedure and choice are appropriate.
▪ Client explains method of dressing application.	Indicates learning has occurred.
2. Explain procedure to client.	Decreases client's anxiety.
3. Assess need for pain medication.	Dressing change is better tolerated by client if pain medication has been administered before dressing change.

Implementation

Step	Rationale
1. Close room or cubicle curtains. Wash hands. Apply gown, goggles, and mask if risk of spray exists.	Provides for privacy and reduces transmission of microorganisms.
2. Position client comfortably and drape to expose only wound site. Instruct client not to touch wound or sterile supplies.	Draping provides access to the wound yet minimizes unnecessary exposure.
3. Place disposable bag within reach of work area. Fold top of bag to make cuff. Put on clean disposable gloves.	Ensures easy disposal of soiled dressings. Prevents contamination of bag's outer surface. Prevents transmission of infectious organisms.
4. Remove tape: pull parallel to skin, toward dressing. Remove remaining adhesive from skin.	Pulling tape toward dressing reduces stress on suture line or wound edges. Tape located over hair areas should be removed in direction of hair growth to reduce irritation and discomfort.
5. With gloved hand remove dressings. Keep soiled undersurface from client's sight.	Appearance of drainage may be upsetting to client.
6. Observe appearance of drainage on dressing. If drains are present, slowly and carefully remove dressings one layer at a time. Assess for odor. Assess the wound.	Provides qualitative assessment of drainage and assessment of wound's condition. Avoids accidental removal of drain.

STEP	RATIONALE

- ***Critical Decision Point***
  Dressings that are heavily saturated with exudate indicate a need to add more absorbent gauze dressing to the wound.

STEP	RATIONALE
7. Describe the appearance of the wound and any indicators of wound healing to the client.	Wounds may appear unsettling and frightening to clients, it is helpful for the client to know that the wound appearance is as expected and what healing is taking place.
8. Dispose of soiled dressings in disposable bag. Remove gloves by pulling them inside out. Dispose of in bag and wash hands.	Reduces transmission of microorganisms to other persons.
9. Open sterile dressing tray or individually wrapped sterile supplies. Place on bedside table (see illustration).	Sterile dressings remain sterile while on or within sterile surface. Preparation of all supplies prevents break in technique during dressing change.
10. Open cleansing solution and pour over sterile gauze.	Keeps supplies sterile. Solution may be packaged to spray/pour directly on wound. Microorganisms move from nonsterile environment through dressing package to dressing itself by capillary action (see Chapter 32).

- ***Critical Decision Point***
  If sterile drape or gauze packages become wet from solution, repeat preparation of supplies.

STEP	RATIONALE
11. Put on gloves, clean or sterile depending on institution policy.	Sterile gloves allow handling of sterile supplies without contamination. Some researchers have demonstrated no difference in wound healing and less cost when clean techniques were used for open gastrointestinal surgical wounds instead of sterile technique (Stotts and others, 1997).
12. Inspect wound for appearance, drains, exudate, and integrity (see illustration). Gently palpate wound edges for drainage, bogginess, or client report of increased pain. Measure wound size (length, width, and depth [if indicated]) (see Chapter 35). Avoid contact with contaminated material.	Indicates status of healing.

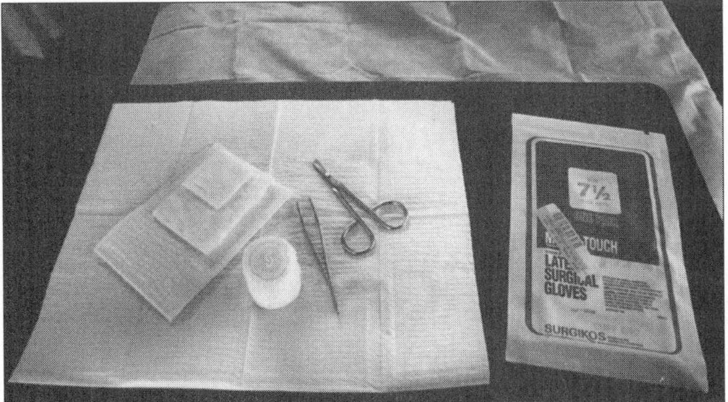

STEP **9** Sterile dressing supplies.

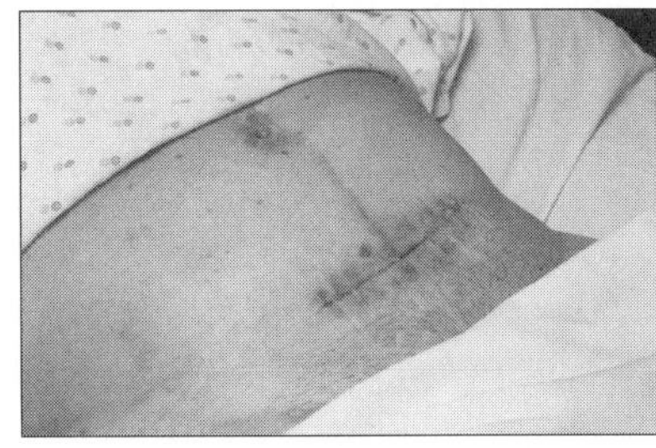

STEP **12** Abdominal wound.

STEP	RATIONALE
13. Cleanse wound (see Chapter 35):	
a. Use separate swab for each cleansing stroke, or spray wound surface.	Prevents contaminating previously cleaned area.
b. Clean from least contaminated area to most contaminated.	Cleansing in this direction prevents introduction of organisms into wound.
14. Use dry gauze to blot in same manner as in Step 13 to dry wound.	Drying reduces excess moisture, which could eventually harbor microorganisms.
15. Apply antiseptic ointment if ordered, using same technique as for cleansing.	Helps reduce growth of microorganisms.

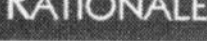

STEP	RATIONALE
16. Apply dry sterile dressings to incision or wound site:	
a. Apply loose woven gauze as contact layer.	Promotes proper absorption of drainage.
b. Cut 4 × 4 gauze flat to fit around drain if present or use precut split drain flat.	Secures drain and promotes drainage absorption at site (see Skill 35-3).
c. Apply additional layers of gauze as needed.	Layering ensures proper coverage and optimal absorption.
d. Apply thicker woven pad (e.g., surgi-pad, abdominal dressing).	This type of dressing is often used for postoperative wounds. It is more effective in wound healing for postoperative cardiac and abdominal wounds (Wikblad and Anderson, 1995; Cannavo and others, 1998).
17. Secure dressing with tape, Montgomery ties or straps (which are applied perpendicular to the wound) (see illustration), or binder.	Supports wound and ensures placement and stability of dressing.

- ***Critical Decision Point***

If areas of redness appear from tape, paper tape or alternatives, such as elastic bandage, Kerlix, or a binder may be used to secure dressing. Sometimes strips of a hydrocolloid dressing are placed on the skin under the Montgomery ties to further protect the skin.

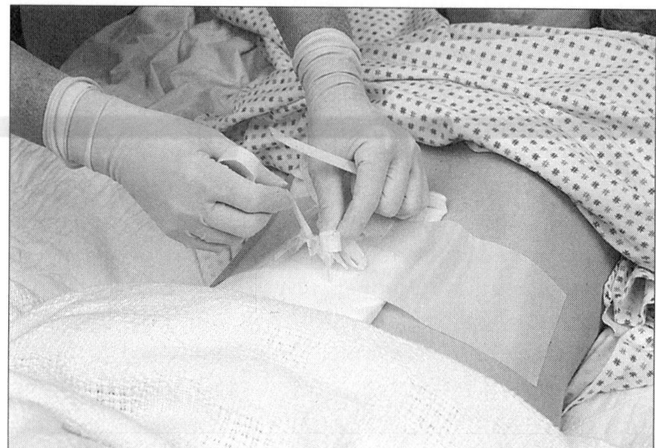

STEP **17** Securing Montgomery ties.

STEP	RATIONALE
18. Remove gloves, gown if worn, and dispose of them in bag. Dispose of all supplies. Remove goggles if worn.	Reduces transmission of microorganisms. Clean environment enhances client comfort.
19. Assist client to comfortable position.	Promotes client's sense of well-being.
20. Wash hands.	Reduces transmission of microorganisms.

EVALUATION

STEP	RATIONALE
1. Inspect condition of wound and presence of any drainage.	Determines rate of healing.
2. Ask if client notes discomfort during procedure.	Pain may be early indication of wound complication or result of dressing pulling tissue.
3. Inspect condition of dressing at least every shift.	Determines status of wound drainage.
4. Ask client to describe steps and techniques of dressing change.	Evaluates client's learning.

UNEXPECTED OUTCOMES AND RELATED INTERVENTIONS

- Wound drainage increases.
  - Increase frequency of dressing changes.
  - Notify physician, who may consider drain placement or alternate dressing method.
- Wound bleeds during dressing change.
  - Observe color and amount of drainage.
  - If excessive, may need to apply pressure.
  - Notify physician.

- Client reports sensation that "something has given way under the dressing."
  - Remove dressing and inspect wound for **dehiscence** or **evisceration.**
  - Protect wound. Cover with sterile moist dressing.
  - Instruct client to lie still.
  - Notify physician.
- Client is unable to describe proper application of dressing.
  - Provide additional teaching or support.
  - Obtain services of home health care agency if needed.

Recording and Reporting

- Report and record:
  - Appearance of wound and drainage
  - Change in wound characteristics, especially drainage amount, to physician
  - Unexpected appearance of wound drainage or accidental removal of drain within an hour to physician
  - Type of dressing applied in client's medical record
  - Tolerance of client to dressing change during shift change
- Record frequency of dressing change and supplies needed on care plan.
- Write nurse's initials, date, and time of dressing change on the new dressing or tape in ink (not marker).

Teaching Considerations

- Wounds out of client's reach and vision require assistance from another caregiver.
- Explain expected wound appearance, what should be reported, and risks of improper wound care.
- After demonstrating wound care, allow client or caregiver to perform dressing change with and without supervision.

Pediatric Considerations

- Check that dressings products are safe to use on pediatric clients, especially on premature infants.
- Pediatric clients may be fearful of dressing changes. Obtaining client's cooperation and/or having another person available to keep child from moving during dressing change procedure may be needed (Wong and others, 1999).
- Older child may need something to do during dressing changes. Listening to music or watching video helps to relieve some of the boredom or stress during procedure (Wong and others, 1999).

Gerontological Considerations

- Dressing change procedure may be a source of pain and misunderstanding for a confused or disoriented client.
- Normal aging results in loss of thickness, elasticity, vascularity, and strength of skin tissue. As a result, there is an increased risk for skin tear when removing adhesive from older adult's skin (Lueckenotte, 2000).
- Normal aging changes of skin tissue may also delay wound-healing process (Lueckenotte, 2000).

Home Care Considerations

- Assess extent of wound or incision in relation to client's level of activity to determine type of dressing that will achieve desired purpose.
- Assess area where procedure will be performed for adequate lighting. Determine if a table or cabinet is available on which sterile supplies may be placed with reasonable security.

Long-Term Care Considerations

- Centers with subacute care units often provide specialized wound care. Clients are admitted to center for continued wound care management (Sorrentino and Gorek, 1999).
- Be sure dressing is secure so that client can actively participate in physical therapy and other activities that increase independence (Sorrentino and Gorek, 1999).

Skill 36-2 Applying a Wet-to-Dry Dressing

Wet-to-dry dressings are gauze moistened with an appropriate solution. For this reason, wet-to-dry dressings are sometimes called moist- or damp-to-dry dressings because this terminology more accurately describes what the dressing should be. In clinical practice, these terms (wet-to-dry, moist-to-dry, damp-to-dry) are considered synonymous.

The primary purpose of wet-to-dry dressings is to mechanically debride a wound. The moistened contact layer of the dressing (primary dressing) increases the absorptive ability of the dressing to collect exudate and wound debris (Provan and Phillips, 1991). As the dressing dries, it adheres to the wound and debrides the wound of the tissue when the dressing is removed. One must *take care not to apply a dressing so wet that it remains wet continuously* (Table 36-1). A dressing that is too wet may cause tissue maceration and bacterial growth. It also does not dry out and therefore does not remove the necrotic tissue when being removed from the wound. The moistened gauze must be covered with a secondary dressing layer that is dry.

Woven gauze should be used to pack wounds (Aronovitch, 1995). Principles for correctly packing a wound can be found in Box 36-3. Commonly used wetting agents include normal saline and lactated Ringer's solution, which are isotonic solu-

Table 36-1 Problems Associated With Wounds Requiring Debridement

PROBLEM	NURSING ACTIVITIES
Solutions used may be irritating to healthy skin around wound.	Protect healthy skin with protective barrier, such as stomahesive, or apply topical ointments, such as zinc oxide. If zinc oxide is used, it should be removed with mineral oil.
Wound becomes excessively dry.	Continually moist dressing (with a physician's order) might be tried. Eliminate fine mesh gauze and lightly pack wound with fluffy gauze dampened with prescribed solution.
Wound is deep, and retention of dressing in cavity is suspected.	Irrigate wound copiously with prescribed solution to loosen dressing for removal. Use continuous "ribbon" or strip of gauze to dress deep wounds.
Wound drainage is damaging healthy tissue.	Protect healthy tissue with skin barrier, such as a hydrocolloid. Wounds with large amounts of drainage may benefit from occlusive drainage collection device.
Client's skin is irritated by tape.	Use hydrocolloid under tape, use Montgomery ties as needed, use fabric tape that has multidirection stretch, secure dressing with binder, or wrap with roll gauze if on extremity.

Box 36-3 Principles for Packing a Wound

- Use the wound characteristics to decide what type of packing is appropriate.
- Make sure the packing material can be safely used to pack a wound.
- Moisten the packing material with a noncytotoxic solution such as normal saline. Never use cytotoxic solutions to pack a wound.
- If using woven gauze, fluff it before packing it into the wound.
- Loosely pack the wound.
- Do not let the packing material drag or touch the surrounding wound tissue before you put it into the wound.
- Fill all the wound dead space with the packing material.
- Pack the wound until you reach the wound surface; never pack the wound higher than the wound surface.

tions that aid in mechanical debridement. Acetic acid is effective against ***Pseudomonas aeruginosa*** but is toxic to fibroblasts in standard dilutions.

Povidone-iodine, usually one-quarter to one-half strength, is a rapid-acting antimicrobial agent for cleansing *intact* skin. It should never be used on a healthy granulating wound bed. This agent should be used only in select situations for short term use. In open wounds, this solution is toxic to fibroblasts and has questionable efficacy in infected wounds (Andrews, 1994). Other antibiotic solutions may be ordered, although their use is controversial. See Chapter 35 for a more detailed discussion of appropriate solutions to use to clean wounds. Because they can harbor microorganism growth, solutions should be discarded 24 to 48 hours after opening and replaced with fresh solutions. All solution bottles must be clearly labeled with date and time of opening.

Delegation Considerations

The skill of applying a wet-to-dry dressing should not be delegated to assistive personnel. Some aspects of wound care such as changing the top dressing may be delegated to assistive personnel. The *assessment* of the wound should not be delegated to assistive personnel even if a portion of the dressing change is delegated to others.

Equipment

- Sterile gloves
- Dressing set (scissors and forceps)
- Sterile drape (optional)
- Thin, fine-mesh gauze or packing strip (Figure 36-2)
- Gauze dressings and pads
- Sterile solution (as prescribed) to moisten dressing
- Waterproof pad
- Sterile solution such as saline
- Clean disposable gloves
- Tape, ties, or bandage as needed
- Waterproof bag
- Adhesive remover
- Protective gown, mask, goggles (used when spray from wound is a risk)

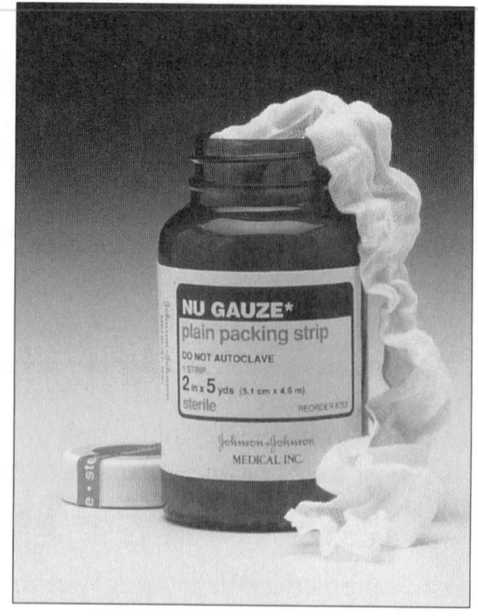

FIGURE **36-2** Packing strip gauze.

STEP	RATIONALE

ASSESSMENT

Step	Rationale
1. Assess location and size of wound to be dressed (see Skill 36-1, Assessment, and Chapter 35).	Allows nurse to determine supplies needed and if assistance is required.

NURSING DIAGNOSIS

Defining characteristics from the assessment data may reveal the following nursing diagnoses for clients requiring this skill:

- Risk for infection
- Impaired skin integrity
- Deficient knowledge regarding wet-to-dry dressings
- Acute pain

Related factors are individualized based on client's condition or needs.

PLANNING

Step	Rationale
1. **Expected outcomes** following completion of procedure:	
▪ Exudate and necrotic debris are decreased; wound becomes clean with granulation tissue present.	Indicates progress in wound healing.
▪ Client describes minimal discomfort.	Pain medication and positioning are effective.
▪ Client explains procedure correctly.	Indicates learning has occurred.
2. Explain procedure to client. Instruct client not to touch sterile supplies.	Relieves anxiety and promotes understanding of dressing change. Prevents contamination of supplies.
3. Position client to allow access to area to be dressed.	Facilitates application of dressing.
4. Plan dressing change to occur 30 minutes following administration of analgesic.	Analgesia alleviates the discomfort associated with proper wet-to-dry dressing technique. Pain medications given at least 30 minutes prior to dressing change can reduce discomfort and increase client cooperation (Cuzzell, 1997).

IMPLEMENTATION

Step	Rationale
1. Close room curtain or door, and keep sheet or gown draped over body parts not requiring exposure.	Provides privacy.
2. Make cuff at top of disposable waterproof bag, and place within reach of work area.	Cuff prevents accidental contamination of top of outer bag.
3. Place waterproof pad under client where dressing is to be changed.	Prevents soiling of bed linens.
4. Wash hands thoroughly. Put on mask, goggles, and moistureproof gown if spray potential. Put on clean disposable gloves and remove tape or bandage or untie Montgomery ties. Remove tape by loosening end and pulling gently parallel to skin and toward dressing.	Prevents transmission of infectious organisms. Reduces tension against wound edges.
5. With gloved hand or forceps, lift old outer secondary cover dressings off first, then remove the inner dressing (called the primary dressing) that is in direct contact with the wound bed. Keep soiled undersurface away from client's sight. Gently remove this inner dressing, and inform client about possible discomfort. Because of this, premedication before this procedure may be necessary.	Purpose of dressing is to remove necrotic tissue and exudate. Appearance of drainage may be upsetting to client.

- ***Critical Decision Point***

  Inner primary dressing if applied properly will have dried and will adhere to underlying tissues; do not moisten it. This is a very critical point! It is incorrect technique and a common error by some clinicians to moisten the dried gauze prior to removing it so it does not stick to the wound. This defeats the purpose of using this type of dressing (Cuzzell, 1997).

STEP	RATIONALE
6. Observe character of drainage on dressings and condition of the wound bed. Check for bleeding or unexpected odor.	Provides assessment of wound's condition. Presence of bleeding during this type of dressing change is an indication that healthy tissue is being injured (Cuzzell, 1997). An odor indicates the presence of an infection.
7. Dispose of soiled dressings in prepared waterproof bag.	Reduces transmission of microorganisms.
8. Remove disposable gloves by pulling them inside out, and dispose of them properly.	Reduces transmission of microorganisms.
9. Prepare sterile dressing supplies.	Reduces risk of break in sterile technique resulting in contamination.

- ***Critical Decision Point***

  Open or "fluff" the woven gauze that will be placed directly against the wound bed. Sometimes "packing strip" may be used to pack the wound (see Figure 36-2). When using packing strip, with a sterile scissor cut the amount of dressing that is anticipated to be used to pack the wound. Do not let the packing strip touch the side of the bottle. Pour prescribed solution over the packing gauze or strip to moisten it. Contact layer must be totally moistened to increase dressing's absorptive abilities (Cuzzell, 1997).

STEP	RATIONALE
10. Put on sterile gloves.	Allows handling of sterile supplies without contamination.
11. Inspect wound for type of tissue, color, characteristics of drainage, presence and type of sutures, and presence of any drains.	Provides assessment of wound healing.
12. Cleanse wound with prescribed solution. Clean from least to most contaminated area.	Assists in debridement and cleanses wound of debris.
13. Wring out excess fluid and apply moist fluffed woven-mesh gauze or packing strip directly onto wound surface without having the gauze touch the surrounding skin (see illustration *A*).	Moist gauze absorbs drainage and adheres to debris (Barr, 1995). The inner gauze should be moist but not dripping wet. The moist gauze must be able to dry in the wound. Having the inner gauze too wet so it does not dry is a common error in technique for this type of dressing.

- ***Critical Decision Point***

  If wound is deep, gently lay gauze over wound surface with forceps until all surfaces are in contact with moist gauze and the wound is loosely filled with the moistened woven gauze. Fill the wound but avoid packing the wound too tightly or having the gauze extend beyond the top of the wound (see illustration B).

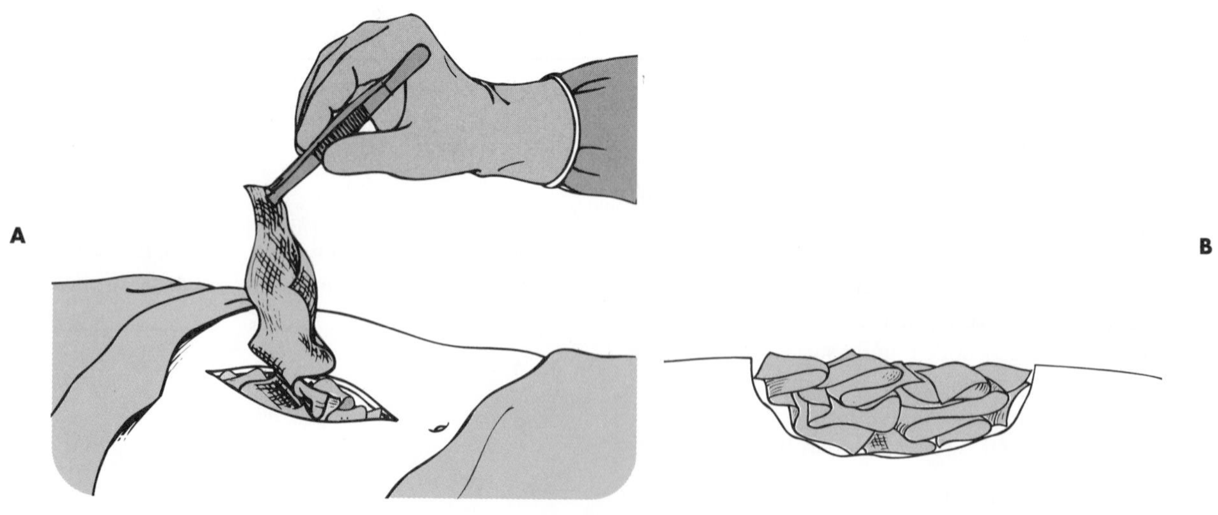

STEP **13** **A,** Packing wound. **B,** Wound packed loosely.

STEP	RATIONALE
14. Make sure any **dead space** from sinus tracts, undermining, or tunneling is loosely packed with gauze.	Do not overpack the wound too tightly; it can cause wound trauma when the dressing is removed (Cuzzell, 1997).
15. Apply dry sterile gauze over wet gauze.	Dry layer pulls moisture from wound.
16. Cover the packed wound with a secondary dressing such as an ABD pad, surgi-pad, or gauze (see illustration).	Protects wound from entrance of microorganisms.

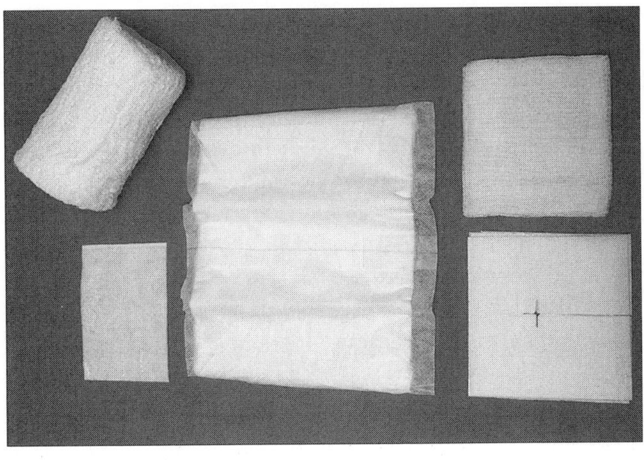

STEP **16** Secondary wound dressings.

STEP	RATIONALE
17. Apply roll gauze (for circumferential dressings) (see illustrations) or Montgomery ties. For application of Montgomery ties or straps (see Skill 36-1):	Secures dressing in place. Montgomery tie allows for frequent dressing changes without removal of adhesive tape.
a. Expose adhesive surface of tape end.	
b. Place ties on opposite sides of dressing.	
c. Adhesive may be placed directly on client's skin or skin barrier may be used.	Skin barrier (strips of a hydrocolloid dressing) protects intact skin from stretch and tension of adhesive tape.
d. Lace ties across dressing.	Secures dressing.

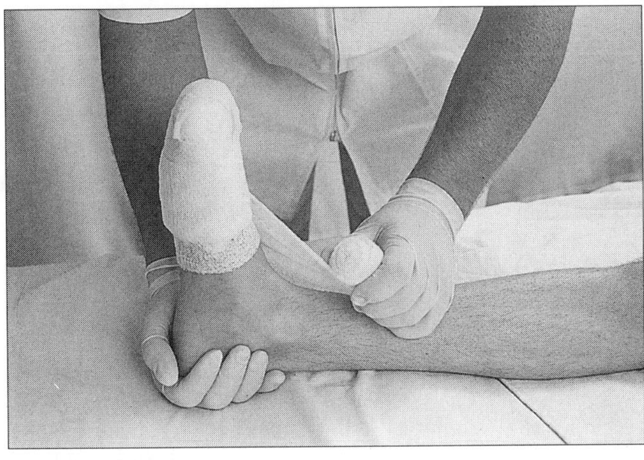

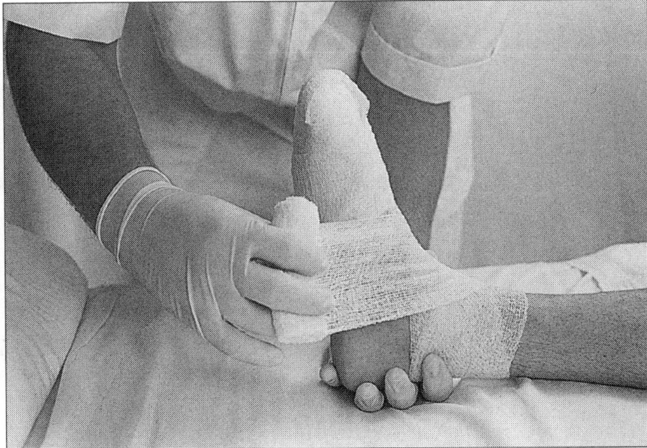

STEP **17** Application of roll gauze.

STEP	RATIONALE
18. Remove and dispose gloves and cover gown (optional). Remove goggles.	
19. Assist client to comfortable position.	Restores client's sense of well-being.
20. Wash hands thoroughly.	Reduces transfer of microorganisms.

Step	Rationale
Evaluation	
1. Observe wound for healing.	Monitoring wound characteristics provides evidence of wound healing.
2. Ask if client has pain during procedure.	Determines client's comfort level and need for pain management.
3. Inspect status of dressing at least every shift.	Evaluates extent of drainage and integrity of dressing.
4. Ask client to describe wound care method.	Evaluates level of client's understanding of procedure.

Unexpected Outcomes and Related Interventions

- Wound eschar toughens.
  - Eschar may require surgical debridement before resumption of wet-to-dry dressing changes.
- Character of wound drainage changes (increases, purulent).
  - Monitor client for signs of infection.
  - Notify physician.
  - Obtain wound culture if ordered.
- Skin around wound margins becomes red, macerated, or **excoriated.**
  - The outer layer of the wet-to-dry dressing is too moist.
- Client is unable to describe proper application of dressing.
  - Provide additional teaching or support.
  - Obtain services of home care agency if needed.

Recording and Reporting

- Report brisk, bright red bleeding or evidence of wound dehiscence or evisceration to physician immediately.
- Report wound appearance and characteristics of drainage at shift change.
- Record wound appearance, color, presence and characteristics of exudate, type and amount of dressings used, and tolerance of client to procedure.
- Write date and time dressing applied on tape in ink (not marker).

Teaching Considerations

- Explain risks of improper wound care.
- Explain expected appearance of wound and what should be reported.
- Wounds out of client's reach and vision require assistance for learning self-care.
- After demonstrating wound care, allow client or family member to perform dressing change with supervision.

Gerontological Considerations

- See Gerontological Considerations for Skill 36-1.

Pediatric Considerations

- See Pediatric Considerations for Skill 36-1.

Home Care Considerations

- Ability of caregiver and amount of time needed to change a particular dressing should be considered when selecting a dressing procedure in the home care setting. "In the home care setting, caregivers may choose more expensive dressing materials to reduce the frequency of dressing changes" (Agency for Health Care Policy and Research [AHCPR], 1994).

Skill 36-3 Applying a Pressure Bandage

A pressure bandage is a temporary treatment for the control of excessive bleeding. The bleeding is usually sudden and not anticipated. It may follow surgical intervention, or it may be a life-threatening occurrence related to accidental trauma, stabbing, suicide attempt, or other injury. Following application of the pressure dressing itself, sandbags are placed adjacent to the dressing to augment pressure.

An adult weighing 154 lb (70 kg) has a total volume of 5 L of circulating blood. All nursing actions must be rapidly and effectively executed when excessive blood loss occurs. Once pressure has been applied, it must continue until definitive actions can be executed by the health care team. Surgical repair is most often the option of choice.

Delegation Considerations

The skill of applying a pressure dressing should not be delegated to assistive personnel. However, aspects of care for clients who have a pressure dressing in place may be delegated. The caregiver must be informed as to the need to observe the pressure dressing to make sure that it remains in place and that there is no visible bleeding from the site. Assistive personnel should be instructed to observe under the patient for bleeding as well. The *assessment* of the wound, condition of the pressure dressing, and the circulation status distal to the pressure dressing should not be delegated to assistive personnel even if the dressing change is delegated to others.

Equipment

- Sterile gauze
- Gauze roll bandage
- Adhesive tape
- Gloves
- Sandbags
- Protective gown, mask, goggles (used when spray from wound is a risk)

Step	Rationale
Assessment	
1. Identify clients at risk for unexpected bleeding: a. Traumatic injury b. Donor graft site c. Arterial puncture sites d. Postoperative wounds e. Wounds after surgical debridement	Nurse should be familiar with conditions associated with unexpected bleeding to rapidly respond to bleeding.
Phase I: Immediate Action—First Nurse	
1. Identify client with sudden hemorrhage: a. Locate external bleeding site.	Maintaining asepsis and privacy are considered only if time and severity of blood loss permit inclusion of these activities. NOTE: Wounds to the groin area can result in large amounts of blood loss, which is not always visible.
b. Apply direct pressure immediately.	Hemostasis maintained as supplies are prepared.
2. Seek assistance.	Bandage must be quickly secured.
Phase II: Applying Pressure Bandage—Second Nurse	
1. Quickly observe location of bleeding.	Bleeding source determines method and supplies needed for applying pressure bandage. *Arterial bleeding* is bright red and gushes forth in waves, related to heart rhythm; if vessel is very deep, flow will be steady. *Venous bleeding* is dark red and flows smoothly. *Capillary bleeding* is oozing of dark red blood; self-sealing controls this bleeding. *Hemorrhage* is loss of a large amount of blood either externally or internally in short period of time.
2. Quickly observe area underneath client for blood.	Blood will flow with gravity to the lowest point. Frequently a large volume of blood may be underneath client and not initially visible.
3. Quickly assess client's pulse, blood pressure, skin color, anxiety/restlessness, and changes in level of consciousness. Reassess every 5 to 15 minutes until client is stabilized.	Findings of tachycardia, hypotension, diaphoresis, restlessness, and diminished urinary output indicate impending hypovolemic shock.

Nursing Diagnosis

Defining characteristics from the assessment data may reveal the following nursing diagnoses for clients requiring this skill:

- Ineffective peripheral tissue perfusion
- Decreased cardiac output
- Impaired skin integrity
- Deficient fluid volume

Related factors are individualized based on client's condition or needs.

Step	Rationale

Planning

1. **Expected outcomes** following completion of procedure:
   - Bleeding is temporarily controlled. — Source of bleeding is controlled with pressure.
   - Circulation to distal parts is adequate. — Blood flow to periphery is maintained.
   - Fluid loss is minimal.
   - Client's blood pressure and pulse remain within normal range. — Loss of blood is controlled.

Implementation

Step	Rationale
1. Apply clean gloves. *If client's condition permits,* wash hands, apply clean gloves, and provide privacy.	Maintaining asepsis and privacy are considered only if time and severity of blood loss permit inclusion of these activities.
2. First person presses on site of bleeding. Second person unwraps roller bandage and places within easy access.	Hemostasis maintained as supplies are prepared. Pressure dressing provides interim control of bleeding.
3. Second person quickly cuts 3 to 5 lengths of adhesive tape and places them within easy reach.	Bandage must be quickly secured.
4. In *simultaneous coordinated actions:*	
a. Rapidly cover bleeding area with many thicknesses of gauze compresses. First person slips fingers out as other nurse exerts adequate pressure to continue controlling bleeding.	Gauze is absorbent. Layers provide bulk against which local pressure can be applied to bleeding site.

- ***Critical Decision Point***
  As soon as possible elevate extremity or area of bleeding. Elevation assists in decreasing the rate of blood loss.

Step	Rationale
b. Adhesive strips are placed 7 to 10 cm (3 to 4 inches) beyond width of dressing with even pressure on both sides of nurse's fingers as close as possible to central bleeding source. Secure tape on distal end, pull tape across dressing, and maintain firm pressure as proximate end of tape is secured.	Tape exerts downward pressure, promoting hemostasis. To ensure blood flow to distal tissues and prevent tourniquet effect, adhesive tape must not be continued around entire extremity.

- ***Critical Decision Point***
  Do not tape around circumference.

Step	Rationale
c. Remove fingers and quickly cover center of area with third strip of tape.	Provides pressure to source of bleeding.
d. Continue reinforcing area with tape as each successive strip is overlapped on alternating sides of center strip.	Prevents tape from loosening.
e. When pressure bandage is on extremity, apply roller gauze: apply two circular turns tautly on both sides of fingers that are pressing gauze. Compress over bleeding site. Simultaneously remove finger pressure and apply roller gauze pressure over center. Continue with figure-eight turns. Secure end with two circular turns and strip of adhesive.	Roller gauze acts as pressure bandage, exerting more even pressure over extremity.

- ***Critical Decision Point***
  Start pressure bandage from distal to proximal.

Step	Rationale
5. Remove gloves and wash hands.	Reduces the spread of microorganisms.

STEP	RATIONALE

EVALUATION

1. Immediately evaluate client to determine response to pressure dressing. Observe for:
   a. Control of bleeding — Effective pressure bandage controls bleeding without blocking distal circulation.
   b. Adequacy of circulation (distal pulse, skin characteristics) — Determines level of perfusion to distal body parts.
   c. Estimated volume of blood loss (e.g., count number of dressings used, weigh saturated dressing) — Determines blood and fluid replacement needs.
   d. Vital signs — Identifies client's adaptation to blood loss and early stages of hypovolemic shock.

UNEXPECTED OUTCOMES AND RELATED INTERVENTIONS

- Excessive pressure is exerted that results in pain, weak or absent pulses, edema of distal body part, or tissue necrosis.
  - Release pressure slightly, and monitor distal circulation every 5 to 10 minutes.
- Uncontrolled hemorrhaging progresses to fluid and electrolyte imbalance, tissue hypoxia, confusion, hypovolemic shock, cardiac arrest, and death.
  - Initiate intravenous (IV) therapy (physician's order is required) for fluid replacement.
  - Initiate nothing-by-mouth (NPO) order because surgical intervention may be needed.
  - Apply pressure to pressure point as needed; place client in Trendelenburg position; provide warmth.
  - Monitor vital signs every 5 to 15 minutes (apical, distal rate, blood pressure).
  - Monitor dressing for signs of bleeding.
  - Reinforce dressing with tape as needed to prevent seepage. If dressing is saturated, replace only top layers so as not to disturb any clot formation at the wound site.

RECORDING AND REPORTING

- Report immediately to physician present status of client's bleeding control, time bleeding was discovered, estimated blood loss, nursing interventions (including effectiveness of applied pressure bandage), apical and distal pulses, blood pressure, sensorium level, signs of restlessness, and need for physician to administer to client without delay.
- Record and implement physician's verbal orders in response to above reporting. (NOTE: Institutional policy on telephone/verbal orders varies.)
- Shift-change report includes emergency situation, intervention and evaluation as reported to physician, and need for continuous bedside monitoring of bleeding control, distal pulse, vital signs, IV, consciousness level, oxygenation or hypoxia, and anxiety level.
- Record on progress note exact findings and care administered in relation to application of pressure bandage.

TEACHING CONSIDERATIONS

- Explain purpose of pressure bandage.
- Explain need to monitor vital signs.
- Explain need for client to remain quiet and stay in position to reduce bleeding.

PEDIATRIC CONSIDERATIONS

- Child will calm down if care providers and family remain calm.

GERONTOLOGICAL CONSIDERATIONS

- Due to the normal changes of aging, the older adult has an increased risk for vascular and tissue changes distal to the pressure dressing. Therefore assess skin and pulse distal to the pressure bandage frequently.

HOME CARE CONSIDERATIONS

- At home client may apply pressure with clean towels or linen.
- Emergency system (911) should be activated.
- Client should be positioned to promote elevation of affected body part (if extremity) and promote relaxation.
- If a puncture wound occurs from a penetrating object (e.g., knife, toy, building materials), do not remove the object. Removal of object will cause more rapid blood loss and may damage underlying structures.

Skill 36-4 Applying a Transparent Dressing

A film dressing is a "clear, adherent, nonabsorptive, polymer-based dressing that is permeable to oxygen and water vapor but not to water" (Agency for Health Care Policy and Research [AHCPR], 1994) (Figure 36-3). Polyurethane moisture and vapor-permeable film dressing were developed to manage superficial wounds. They are often used following laparoscopic surgery.

Transparent dressings can also be used for autolytic debridement of small wounds. Pain and discomfort are diminished with the use of a transparent dressing, and the film conforms well to different body contours. Therefore bodily movement is less restricted. Transparent dressings may be with or without adhesives.

With the use of a transparent dressing, a moist exudate forms over the wound surface, which prevents tissue dehydration and allows for rapid, effective healing by speeding epithelial cell growth. Because these dressings are clear, the wound can be visualized without removing the dressing. For best results these dressings should be used on clean, debrided wounds that are not actively bleeding. The film should be applied wrinkle free but not stretched over the skin. Should the fluid accumulation take on a white, opaque appearance with **erythema** of the surrounding tissue, one must assume an infectious process is under way, and the dressing should be removed and a wound culture obtained.

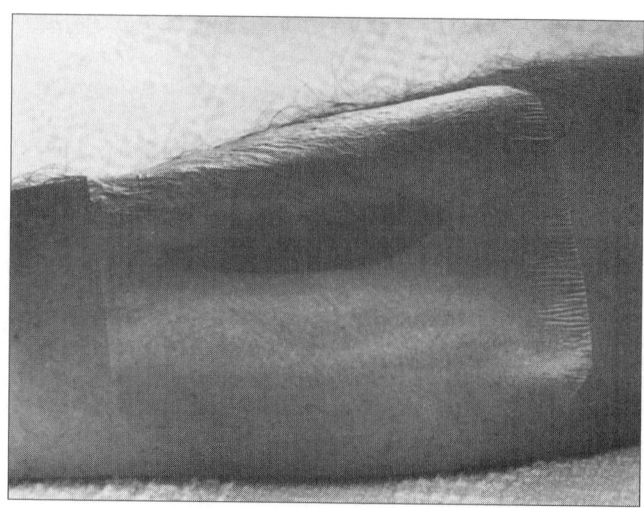

FIGURE **36-3** Transparent dressing.

Delegation Considerations

The skill of applying a transparent dressing may be delegated to assistive personnel. However, the care of acute new wounds and those that require sterile technique for dressing change generally remain within the domain of nursing practice. The *assessment* of the wound should not be delegated to assistive personnel even if the dressing change is delegated to others.

Equipment

- Sterile gloves (optional)
- Dressing set (optional)
- Sterile saline or other agent (as ordered)
- Clean disposable gloves
- Cotton swabs
- Waterproof bag for disposal
- Mineral oil (optional)
- Transparent dressing (size as needed)
- Sterile gauze pads (4 × 4 inches)
- Skin preparation materials (optional)
- Protective gown, mask, goggles (used when spray from wound is a risk)

Step	Rationale
Assessment	
1. Assess location and size of wound to be dressed (see Chapter 35).	Allows nurse to determine supplies and assistance needed.
2. Review physician's orders for frequency and type of dressing change.	Physician orders frequency of dressing changes and special instructions.
3. Assess client's level of comfort.	Client who is comfortable during procedure is less likely to move suddenly, causing wound or supply contamination. Dressing change procedure can be painful, and client may need pain management.

STEP	RATIONALE
4. Assess client's knowledge of purpose of dressing.	Identifies client's learning needs.
5. Assess risk for impaired wound healing (see Chapter 35).	

NURSING DIAGNOSIS

Defining characteristics from the assessment data may reveal the following nursing diagnoses for clients requiring this skill:

Impaired skin integrity
Acute pain
Risk for infection

Related factors are individualized based on client's condition or needs.

PLANNING

STEP	RATIONALE
1. **Expected outcome** following completion of procedure:	
▪ Wound heals rapidly with little pain and mobility restriction for client.	Dressing effective in preventing infection and promoting healing.
2. Explain procedure to client.	Relieves anxiety and promotes understanding of healing process.
3. Position client to allow access to dressing site.	Facilitates application of dressing.

IMPLEMENTATION

STEP	RATIONALE
1. Close door or cubicle curtains; keep sheet or gown draped over body parts not requiring exposure.	Provides privacy and decreases transfer of microorganisms.
2. Cuff top of disposable waterproof bag, and place within reach of work area.	Cuff prevents accidental contamination of tip of outer bag.
3. Wash hands and put on clean disposable gloves. Moistureproof gown, mask, and eye goggles are worn when risk of spray exists.	Reduces transmission of infectious organisms from soiled dressings to nurse's hands.
4. Remove old dressing. For easier removal, ease off using cotton swab soaked in mineral oil, or secure piece of tape to corner of dressing and pull back slowly across dressing in direction of hair growth.	Reduces excoriation or irritation of skin following dressing removal.
5. Dispose of soiled dressings in waterproof bag, remove disposable gloves by pulling them inside out, dispose of them in waterproof bag, and wash hands.	Reduces transmission of microorganisms.
6. Prepare sterile dressing supplies.	Reduces risk of break in sterile technique.
7. Pour saline or prescribed solution over 4 × 4 sterile gauze pads.	Maintains sterility of dressing.
8. Apply gloves (sterile if institution policy).	Allows nurse to handle dressings.
9. Cleanse area gently with moist 4 × 4 sterile gauze pads, or spray with wound cleanser.	Reduces introduction of organisms into wound.
10. Pat dry skin around wound thoroughly with dry 4 × 4 sterile gauze pads. Transparent dressing with adhesive backing does not adhere to damp surface.	Nonadhesive transparent dressing clings to moist wound surface.
11. Inspect wound for tissue type, color, odor, and drainage; measure if indicated.	Appearance indicates state of wound healing.

- ***Critical Decision Point***

  If wound has a large amount of drainage, choose another dressing that can absorb this amount of wound drainage rather than transparent film dressing, which can absorb only light-to-moderate amounts of drainage.

STEP	RATIONALE
12. Apply transparent dressing according to manufacturer's directions (see Figure 36-3). *Film should not be stretched during applications.* Avoid wrinkles in film.	Wrinkles would provide tunnel for exudate drainage.

- ***Critical Decision Point***
  Know specific characteristics of the brand of film dressing you are applying. Some film dressings can be removed during application process and reapplied to correct application errors such as being applied too tight or too loose with wrinkles.

STEP	RATIONALE
13. Remove gown and goggles. Remove gloves by pulling inside out, and discard in prepared bag.	Reduces risk of microorganism transfer.
14. Assist client to comfortable position.	Enhances client comfort and relaxation.
15. Discard soiled dressing change materials properly and wash hands.	Reduces transmission of microorganisms.

EVALUATION

1. Inspect condition of wound on ongoing basis.	Determines status of wound healing. Wound can be easily viewed.
2. Evaluate client's level of comfort.	Determines if pain resulted from procedure.

UNEXPECTED OUTCOMES AND RELATED INTERVENTIONS

- Wound becomes infected.
  - Dressing changes may need to be done more frequently.
  - Different type of dressing may be required.
  - Obtain wound culture per agency policy.
- Dressing does not stay in place.
  - Evaluate size of dressing used for adequate wound margin (1 to 1½ inches [2.5 to 3.75 cm]).
  - Client's skin may be too dry or too moist.
- Skin tears can occur with this type of dressing.
  - Adhesive backing may be too strong for fragile skin.
  - Consider other dressing type.

RECORDING AND REPORTING

- Report unusual observations immediately, then chart what was reported and when.
- Record characteristics of wound; color, odor, viscosity, and amount of drainage; and application of dressing in nurses' notes.
- Write date and time on a sticker, and place on peripheral aspect of dressing.

TEACHING CONSIDERATIONS

- Explain wound-healing process with film dressing.
- Explain need to change dressing should edges loosen.
- Explain to client and family that collection of wound fluid under dressing is not "pus," but normal interaction of body fluids with dressing.
- Allow client or caregiver to demonstrate dressing change should self-care need be identified.

PEDIATRIC CONSIDERATIONS

- Adhesive backing may cause skin tears on premature babies' immature skin (Wong and others, 1999).
- To remove: raise one edge of dressing and pull parallel to skin to loosen adhesive.
- Children may find this procedure more tolerable if they know that the longer the dressing is left on, the easier it is to remove (Wong and others, 1999).

GERONTOLOGICAL CONSIDERATIONS

- Adhesive backing may be too strong for the skin of older adults. Do not use a film dressing that has an adhesive backing that has a stronger bond to the epidermis than the epidermis has to the dermis (Lueckenotte, 2000).

HOME CARE CONSIDERATIONS

- Wound may be cleansed in shower, if approved by physician.
- Client may shower or bathe with dressing in place.
- Many types of transparent dressings exist. Explore types with client, and recommend type client finds easy to work with and has access to.
- Make sure client has a source of dressing supplies for purchase after discharge.

Skill 36-5 Applying a Hydrocolloid or Hydrogel Dressing

Hydrocolloid dressings can be used for a variety of reasons. These include (1) maintaining a moist wound environment for healing of clean, shallow to moderately deep wounds, (2) autolytic debriding of necrotic wounds, (3) protecting high-friction areas on intact skin, (4) protecting from contamination, and (5) providing absorption of minimal amount of exudates in superficial and shallow wounds (Cuzzell, 1997). For example, the dressing may be applied beneath Montgomery ties or on bony prominences to prevent shearing or friction injuries, including pressure ulcers (see Chapter 7). Pain and discomfort are diminished with the use of a hydrocolloid dressing. Their "cushioning" effect provides protection to the wound and skin beneath bony prominences. These adhesive-backed dressings conform well to different body contours. Hydrocolloids come in the form of granules, paste, or wafer dressings.

With the use of a hydrocolloid dressing, wound exudate is absorbed into the dressing, forming a jellylike substance next to the wound surface. The dressing maintains a moist, insulated environment that promotes rapid, effective healing.

A hydrogel dressing is a semipermeable "water-based nonadherent, polymer based dressing that has some absorptive properties" (Agency for Health Care Policy and Research [AHCPR], 1994). These dressings are available in several forms including a "sheet" (Figure 36-4, *A* and *B*), amorphous gels (see illustration for Implementation, Step 14b, on p. 1049), and impregnated gauze that can be placed in the wound. They can serve the same functions as a hydrocolloid dressing (Cuzzell, 1997).

Hydrogel dressings facilitate wound debridement by rehydration; they absorb exudate and encourage healing by maintaining a moist wound-healing environment. The gel dressings are nonadherent and must be covered with a secondary dressing to hold them in place. The hydrogels may be used over leg ulcers, pressure ulcers, and burns. They can also be used to protect skin from radiation.

The hydrocolloid or hydrogel dressings are used frequently over venous stasis ulcers, arterial ulcers, and pressure ulcers. Hydrocolloid dressings are one of the most frequently used dressings for pressure ulcers in home and long-term care settings (Meehan, O'Hara, and Morrison, 1999). When used in combination with wound exudate absorbers, these dressings are useful over stage III pressure ulcers (see Chapter 7). Hydrogels do not stick to the wound and can be easily removed. Their "cooling" and soothing properties make them especially useful on painful wounds such as burns.

Delegation Considerations

The skill of applying a hydrocolloid or hydrogel dressing should not be delegated to assistive personnel.

Equipment

- Sterile gloves (optional)
- Dressing set (optional)
- Sterile saline or other cleansing solution (as ordered)
- Clean disposable gloves
- Waterproof bag for disposal
- Hydrocolloid dressing (size as needed) or hydrogel dressing
- Sterile gauze pads (4 × 4 inches)
- Protective gown, mask, goggles (used when spray from wound is a risk)

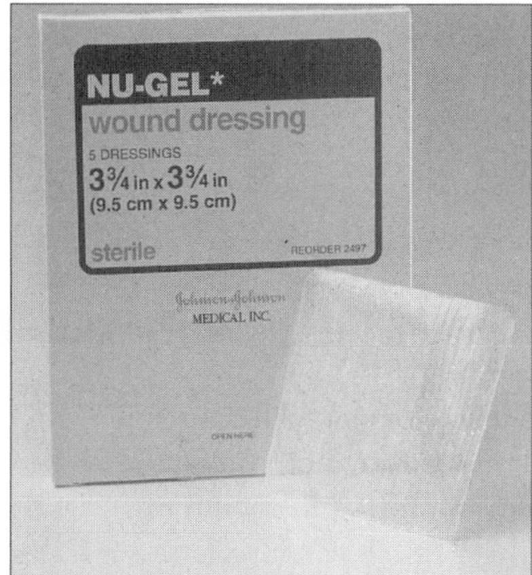

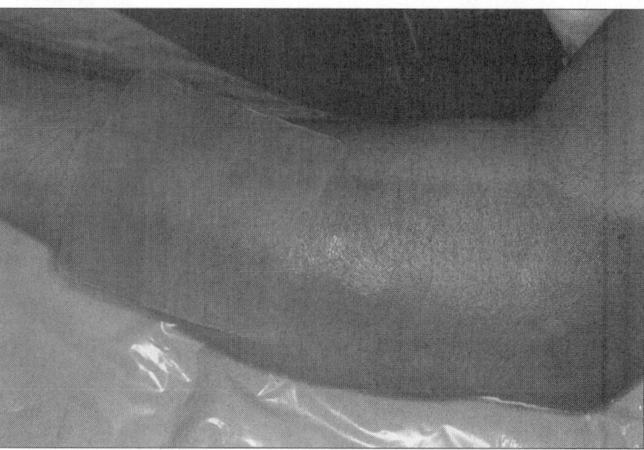

FIGURE **36-4** Types of hydrocolloid or hydrogel dressings.

STEP	RATIONALE

ASSESSMENT

1. Assess wound location and size of wound to be dressed (see Skill 36-1, Assessment and Chapter 35). — Allows nurse to determine supplies and assistance needed.
2. Determine the type of hydrocolloid dressing.

   - ***Critical Decision Point***
     Some brands of hydrocolloid dressings are available in custom shapes and sizes to better fit certain difficult body parts such as the sacrum, heels, or elbows. The variety of shapes aids in flexibility of dressing selection and better dressing adherence.

3. Review physician's orders for frequency and type of dressing change. — Physician orders mode of therapy.
4. Assess client's level of comfort. — Client who is comfortable during procedure is less likely to move suddenly, causing wound or supply contamination. Some dressing change procedures can cause client discomfort, and pain management may be necessary.
5. Assess client's knowledge of purpose of dressing. — Identifies client's learning needs.

NURSING DIAGNOSIS

Defining characteristics from the assessment data may reveal the following nursing diagnoses for clients requiring this skill:

Impaired skin integrity
Deficient knowledge regarding hydrocolloid dressing application
Acute pain
Risk for infection

Related factors are individualized based on client's condition or needs.

PLANNING

1. **Expected outcomes** following completion of procedure:
   - Wound heals rapidly with little pain and mobility restriction for client. — Dressing effective in preventing infection and promoting healing.
   - Wound exudate is adequately absorbed. — Dressing is effective in exudate management for draining wounds.
   - Client explains procedure correctly. — Indicates learning has occurred.
2. Explain procedure to client. — Relieves anxiety and promotes understanding of healing process.
3. Position client to allow access to dressing site. — Facilitates application of dressing.

IMPLEMENTATION

1. Close room door or cubicle curtains. — Provides for client privacy.
2. Expose wound site, and cover client with bath blanket. — Draping provides access to wound while minimizing exposure.
3. Cuff top of disposable waterproof bag, and place within reach of work area. — Cuff prevents accidental contamination of top of outer bag. Nurse should not reach across sterile field.
4. Wash hands and put on clean disposable gloves. Moistureproof gown, mask, and goggles are worn when risk of spray exists. — Reduces transmission of infectious organisms.
5. Remove old dressing. For easier removal, ease off dressing with adhesive remover, and pull back slowly across dressing in direction of hair growth. Use caution to avoid contact of adhesive remover with the wound. — Reduces irritation and possible injury to skin.

Step	Rationale
6. The hydrocolloid dressing interacts with wound fluids and forms a soft whitish-yellowish gel, which is hard to remove and may have a faint odor.	This is a normal occurrence with hydrocolloid dressings and should not be confused with pus or purulent exudate or malodorous infected wounds (Cuzzell, 1997).
7. Dispose of soiled dressings in waterproof bag. Remove disposable gloves by pulling them inside out, and dispose of them in waterproof bag. Avoid having client see old dressing because the site of wound drainage may be upsetting to the client.	Reduces transmission of microorganisms.
8. Prepare sterile dressing supplies.	Reduces risk of break in sterile technique.
9. Pour saline or prescribed solution over 4 × 4 sterile gauze pads.	Maintains sterility of dressing.
10. Put on gloves, sterile if required by policy.	Allows nurse to handle dressings.
11. Cleanse area gently with moist 4 × 4 sterile gauze pads, swabbing exudate away from wound, or spray with wound cleanser (see also Chapter 35).	Reduces introduction of organisms into wound.
12. Thoroughly pat area dry with dry 4 × 4 sterile gauze pads.	Dressing will not adhere to damp surface. Hydrocolloid dressing has adhesive backing.
13. Inspect wound for tissue type, color, odor, and drainage. Measure wound size and depth (see also Chapter 35).	Appearance indicates state of wound healing.

- ***Critical Decision Point***
  For some brands of hydrocolloid wafers, size of dressing used should be larger than wound size by a 1- to 1 ½-inch margin beyond wound end.

Step	Rationale
14. Apply dressing.	
a. Apply hydrocolloid dressing according to manufacturer's directions. Apply hydrocolloid granules or paste before wafer dressing in deeper wounds.	*Dressing should not be stretched during application.* Avoid wrinkles that would provide tunnel for exudate drainage. Hydrocolloid granules assist in absorbing drainage to increase wearing time of dressing.

- ***Critical Decision Point***
  Edges may be notched to help mold around wound. Consider using custom shapes to better conform to certain parts of the body such as heels, elbows, and sacrum. If necessary, apply tape around the edges of the hydrocolloid dressing to assist in keeping the dressing in place.

Step	Rationale
b. Apply amphorous gels approximately ¼- to ½-inch thick across wound surface (see illustration), or put hydrogel sheet over wound bed (see Figure 36-4, *B*). Cover with secondary dressing such as gauze, hydrocolloid, or foam.	Fluid gels take form of cavity type of wounds. A secondary dressing must be used with a hydrogel to hold it in place; it has no adhesive.

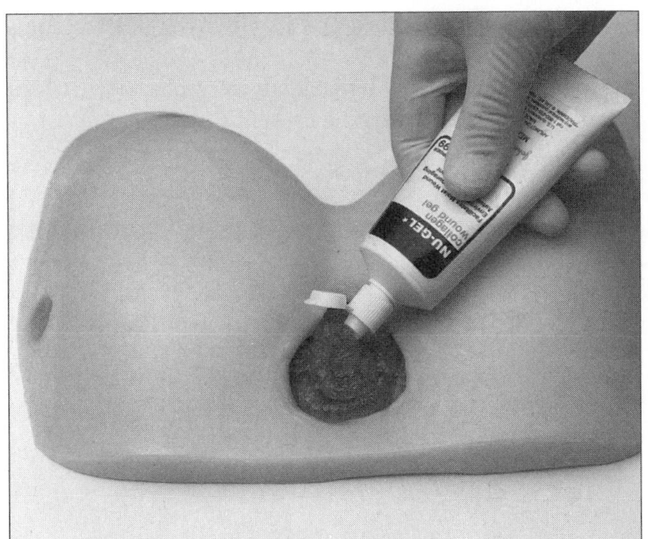

STEP **14b** Hydrogel amorphous gel.

STEP	RATIONALE
15. Remove sterile gloves by pulling them inside out, and discard in prepared bag.	Reduces transfer of microorganisms.
16. Assist client to comfortable position.	Enhances client comfort and relaxation.
17. Discard soiled dressing change materials properly. Wash hands.	Reduces transmission of microorganisms.

EVALUATION

1. Inspect condition of wound on ongoing basis.	Determines status of wound healing.
2. Evaluate client's level of comfort.	Determines if pain resulted from procedure.
3. Ask client to describe wound care method.	Evaluates client's level of learning.

UNEXPECTED OUTCOMES AND RELATED INTERVENTIONS

- Wound becomes infected.
  - Dressing changes may need to be done more frequently.
  - Different type of dressing may be required.
  - Discontinue use of dressing.
- Dressing does not stay in place.
  - Evaluate size of dressing used for adequate margin (1- to 1½-inch [2.5 to 3.75 cm]), or dry skin more thoroughly before reapplication.
  - Consider custom shapes for difficult body parts. "Picture frame" the edges of the hydrocolloid dressing using tape.
- Wound develops more necrotic tissue and increases in size.
  - In rare instances, wounds do not tolerate hypoxia induced by hydrocolloid dressings. In these clients use should be discontinued.
- Wound drainage is more than dressing can absorb.
  - Change type of dressing to one that can absorb amount of wound drainage.
- Client is unable to describe proper application of dressing.
  - Provide additional teaching or support.
  - Obtain services of home care agency if needed.

RECORDING AND REPORTING

- Report unusual observations immediately, then chart what was reported and when.
- Record characteristics of wound tissue type, color, odor, viscosity and amount of drainage and application of dressing in client's medical record.
- Write date, time, and nurse's initials in ink (not marker) on the dressing.

TEACHING CONSIDERATIONS

- Instruct client and family regarding proper handling of hydrocolloid dressing to avoid contamination of sterile adhesive surface.
- Advise client and family that fluid that may collect under dressing will have an odor and may appear purulent but is *not* an infection with purulent drainage but a normal occurrence as a result of the interaction of the hydrocolloid with wound fluid.
- Hydrogel dressings will feel cool when first applied.

PEDIATRIC CONSIDERATIONS

- See Pediatric Considerations for Skills 36-1, 36-2, and 36-4.

GERONTOLOGICAL CONSIDERATIONS

- See also Gerontological Considerations for Skills 36-1, 36-2, and 36-4.
- Avoid early and frequent removal of a hydrocolloid dressing to reduce injury to surrounding intact skin.

HOME CARE CONSIDERATIONS

- Dressing is easily applied and readily adaptable for home use.
- Dressing may not be available at every pharmacy. Client may need assistance locating dressing.

Skill 36-6 Applying a Foam Dressing

A foam dressing is "a sponge like polymer dressing that may or may not be adherent; it may be impregnated or coated with other materials and has some absorptive properties" (Agency for Health Care Policy and Research [AHCPR], 1994). These hydrophilic dressings are used in full-thickness wounds with minimal to moderate amounts of drainage. Foam dressings absorb moderate to heavy exudates in superficial or deep wounds, protect friable periwound skin, provide autolytic debridement, pad and protect high-trauma areas (e.g., pretibial area, forearms), and can be used with infected wounds following appropriate intervention and close monitoring of wound healing (Cuzzell, 1997). More heavily draining wounds may be covered with foam dressings when absorptive wound fillers are also used. These dressings require a secondary dressing to secure the foam in place, or they may be secured with tape or a sheet of flexible tape.

The foam dressings protect the wound surface while maintaining a moist, insulated environment. The result is a well-hydrated wound bed that can heal rapidly with little discomfort to the client. Application directions for the different brands of foam dressings vary. The nurse should read and follow the specific directions for the particular brand of foam dressings that is being used.

Delegation Considerations

The skill of applying a foam dressing should not be delegated to assistive personnel.

Equipment

- Sterile gloves (optional)
- Dressing set (optional)
- Cleansing solution (as ordered) or sterile saline
- Waterproof bag
- Foam dressing
- Sterile gauze pads (4 × 4 inches)
- Wound measurement devices (tape measure, tracing paper, camera)
- Protective gown, mask, goggles (used when spray from wound is a risk)

Step	Rationale
Assessment	
1. Assess wound location, drainage, and size of wound to be dressed (see Skill 36-1, Assessment and Chapter 35).	Allows nurse to determine supplies and assistance needed. Do not use foam dressings on nonexuding wounds. Most foam dressings are designed to absorb moderate amounts of wound drainage.
2. Assess client's level of comfort.	Client who is comfortable during procedure is less likely to move suddenly, causing wound or supply contamination. Dressing change procedure can be painful. Client may need pain management during this procedure.
3. Review physician's orders for frequency and type of dressing change.	Physician orders mode of therapy; nurse frequently suggests dressings for local management of wound.
4. Assess client's knowledge of purpose of dressing.	Identifies client's learning needs.
5. Identify client's risk for poor wound healing (see Skill 36-1, Assessment, Step 7).	

Nursing Diagnosis

Defining characteristics from the assessment data may reveal the following nursing diagnoses for clients requiring this skill:

- Impaired skin integrity
- Deficient knowledge regarding wound care
- Acute pain

Related factors are individualized based on client's condition or needs.

STEP	RATIONALE
PLANNING	
1. **Expected outcomes** following completion of procedure:	
▪ Wound heals rapidly with little pain or mobility restriction for client.	Dressing effective in preventing infection and promoting healing.
▪ Wound exudate is adequately absorbed.	Dressing is effective in exudate management for draining wounds.
▪ Client explains procedure correctly.	Indicates learning has occurred.
2. Explain procedure to client.	Relieves anxiety and promotes understanding of healing process.
3. Position client to allow access to dressing site.	Facilitates application of dressing.
IMPLEMENTATION	
1. Close room door or cubicle curtains.	Provides for client privacy and decreases transfer of microorganisms.
2. Expose wound site and drape client.	Draping provides access to wound while minimizing exposure.
3. Cuff top of disposable waterproof bag and place within reach of work area.	Cuff prevents accidental contamination of top of outer bag.
4. Wash hands and put on clean disposable gloves. If a risk of spray exists, apply protective gown, goggles, and mask.	Reduces transmission of infectious organisms.
5. Remove old dressing. For easier removal, ease off, pulling back slowly.	Reduces irritation and possible injury to intact skin. Foam dressing may fall off on its own as wound heals underneath.

• ***Critical Decision Point***

Check removal directions for specific brand of foam dressing that is being used. Some brands need to have old dressing soaked or moistened for removal.

STEP	RATIONALE
6. Dispose of soiled dressings in waterproof bag. Remove disposable gloves by pulling them inside out, and dispose of them in waterproof bag.	Reduces transmission of microorganisms.

• ***Critical Decision Point***

Do not confuse normal discoloration that occurs with some brands of foam dressings as a sign of infection or deterioration of wound.

STEP	RATIONALE
7. Prepare sterile dressing supplies.	Reduces risk of break in sterile technique.
8. Pour saline or prescribed solution over 4 × 4s, or open spray wound cleanser.	Maintains sterility of dressing. With some brands of foam dressings, wound must be thoroughly irrigated to remove all of old dressing.
9. Apply gloves (sterile if required by policy).	Allows nurse to handle dressings.
10. Cleanse area gently with moist 4 × 4s, swabbing exudate away from wound, or spray wound directly (see Chapter 35).	Reduces introduction of organisms into wound.
11. Blot excess moisture from wound surface; dry intact skin around wound.	Periwound skin should be kept dry.
12. Inspect wound for tissue type, color, odor, and drainage; obtain wound measurements (see Chapter 35).	Appearance indicates state of wound healing. Measurements provide a basis for monitoring wound closure.
13. *Apply foam dressing according to manufacturer's directions.* Application techniques differ for different brands of foam dressings.	Most foam dressings should be applied smoothly; avoid wrinkles. May be used with absorptive dressings to accommodate more highly draining wounds.
a. Make sure you know which side of foam dressing should be placed towards wound bed and which side should be facing away from wound bed.	Check with manufacturer as to which types of secondary dressings to avoid when covering foam dressing that could reduce effectiveness of foam dressing.

STEP	RATIONALE
b. With some brands, dressings can be trimmed to fit wound size, whereas other brands of dressings cannot be cut.	Some brands of foam dressings need slight tension on the dressing while being applied. Some brands of foam dressings need to be covered with a secondary dressing.
c. Know removal and application characteristics of specific brand of foam dressing you are using.	
14. Remove gloves by pulling inside out, and discard in prepared bag.	Reduces risk of microorganism transfer.
15. Assist client to comfortable position.	Enhances client comfort and relaxation.
16. Discard soiled dressing change materials properly.	Reduces transmission of microorganisms.
17. Wash hands.	Reduces risk of microorganism transmission.

EVALUATION

1. Inspect condition of wound, especially amount of exudate, on ongoing basis.	Determines status of wound healing.
2. Evaluate client's level of comfort.	Determines if pain resulted from procedure.
3. Ask client to explain wound care method.	Evaluates client's level of learning.

UNEXPECTED OUTCOMES AND RELATED INTERVENTIONS

- Wound becomes infected.
  - Dressing changes may need to be done more frequently.
  - Different type of dressing regimen may be required.
- Dressing does not stay in place.
  - Evaluate size of dressing used for adequate margin.
  - Dressing may be secured with roll gauze, tape, transparent dressing, or dressing sheet.
- Wound increases in size.
  - Evaluate appropriateness of wound care protocol, and look for other impediments to wound healing.
- Wound exudate is not adequately absorbed.
  - Consider using a different type of dressing for more heavily draining wounds.
  - Foam dressings may be used over wound exudate absorbers.
- Client is unable to describe proper application of dressing.
  - Provide additional teaching or support.
  - Obtain services of home health care agency if needed.

RECORDING AND REPORTING

- Report unusual observations immediately; then chart what was reported and when.
- Record characteristics of wound; color, odor, viscosity, and amount of drainage; and application of dressing in nurses' notes.
- Graph wound surface area or volume if wound is a chronic wound.
- Write nurse's initials, date, and time of dressing change on the new dressing or tape in ink (not marker).

TEACHING CONSIDERATIONS

- Explain expected wound appearance with use of foam dressing.
- Explain frequency of dressing changes required.
- Instruct client and caregiver to observe wound for signs and symptoms of infection.
- Because application technique can vary with different brands, tell client and caregiver not to purchase a brand different from the one for which nurse gave them. If a different brand must be used, client and caregiver should check with nurse for any additional instructions or modification in foam dressing removal and application technique needed.

PEDIATRIC CONSIDERATIONS

- See Pediatric Considerations given for Skill 36-1.

GERONTOLOGICAL CONSIDERATIONS

- See Gerontological Considerations given for Skill 36-1.

HOME CARE CONSIDERATIONS

- See Home Care Considerations given for Skills 36-1 and 36-5.

Skill 36-7 Applying Absorption and Alginate Dressings

Absorption dressings can contain large amounts of wound exudate. They may take the form of pastes, granules, sheeting, or rope. This group of dressings include calcium alginate materials (see Figure 36-5, *A*), which are manufactured from natural material (seaweed) and are known for their absorptive properties, forming a gel over the wound surface as exudate is contained. The exudate absorbers are nonadhesive, nonocclusive dressings that can be used in combination with other dressings. These dressings are appropriate for full-thickness wounds with moderate to high amounts of drainage. Deep tracking wounds can safely be packed with calcium-sodium alginate preparation, which allows easy removal with little risk of retained dressing deep in the wound cavity. Calcium-sodium alginate dressings may be further useful in control of wound odor, achieving hemostasis, and control of pain (Cuzzell, 1997).

Generally absorption and alginate dressings require a secondary dressing, and that dressing can be changed as needed (Cuzzell, 1997). The typical frequency of dressing changes is daily to once or twice a week.

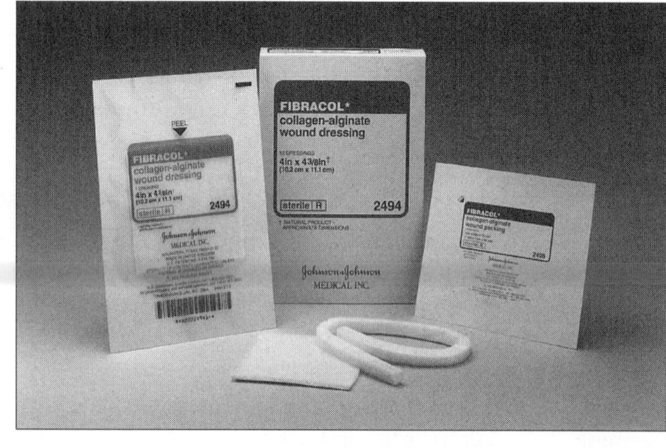

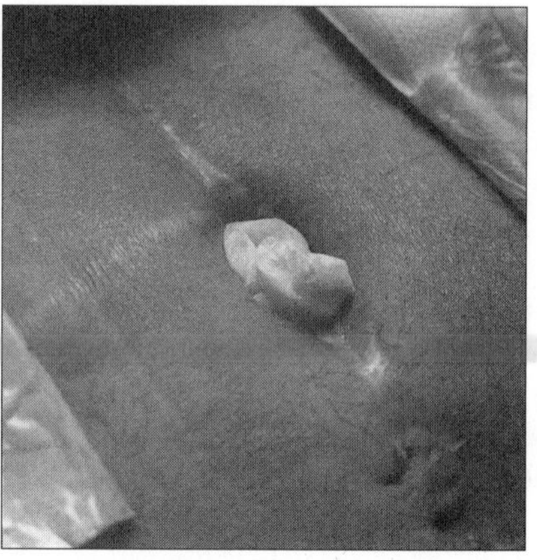

FIGURE **36-5** **A,** Example of alginate dressing package. Alginate sheet *(left)* and alginate rope *(right)*. **B,** Alginate dressing placed in an abdominal wound.

Delegation Considerations

The skill of applying absorption and alginate dressings should not be delegated to assistive personnel.

Equipment

- Sterile gloves (optional)
- Dressing set (optional)
- Sterile saline or other wound cleanser (as ordered)
- Clean disposable gloves
- Waterproof bag for disposal
- Absorption dressing
- Sterile gauze pads (4 × 4 inches)
- Irrigation tray
- Secondary dressing of choice
- Protection gown, mask, goggles (used when spray from wound is a risk)

Step	Rationale
Assessment	
1. Assess wound location, drainage, and size of wound to be dressed (see Chapter 35).	Allows nurse to determine supplies and assistance needed. Do not use alginate or absorption dressings on nonexuding wounds. Most of these dressings are designed to absorb moderate to large amounts of wound drainage and therefore should not be used in wounds with minimal or no drainage. For some brands the dressing technique may need to be further modified if the wound is infected (Cuzzell, 1997).

STEP	RATIONALE
2. Review physician's orders for frequency and type of dressing change.	Physician orders frequency of dressing changes and special instructions.
3. Assess client's level of comfort.	Client who is comfortable during procedure is less likely to move suddenly, causing wound or supply contamination.
4. Assess client's knowledge of purpose of dressing.	Identifies client's learning needs.

Nursing Diagnosis

Defining characteristics from the assessment data may reveal the following nursing diagnoses for clients requiring this skill:

Impaired skin integrity

Acute pain

Related factors are individualized based on client's condition or needs.

Planning

STEP	RATIONALE
1. **Expected outcomes** following completion of procedure:	
▪ Wound heals rapidly with little pain or mobility restriction to client.	Dressing effective in preventing infection and promoting healing.
▪ Wound drainage is contained, and skin surrounding wound remains intact.	Dressing effective in controlling wound exudate.
2. Explain procedure to client.	Relieves anxiety and promotes understanding of healing process.
3. Position client to allow access to dressing site.	Facilitates application of dressing.

Implementation

STEP	RATIONALE
1. Close room door or cubicle curtains.	Provides for client privacy and reduces transmission of organisms.
2. Expose wound site and cover client.	Draping provides access to wound while minimizing exposure.
3. Cuff top of disposable waterproof bag, and place within reach of work area.	Cuff prevents accidental contamination of top of outer bag.
4. Wash hands and put on clean disposable gloves. If risk of spray exists, apply protective gown, goggles, and mask.	Reduces transmission of infectious organisms from soiled dressings to nurse's hands.
5. Remove old dressing and dispose of in waterproof bag. Remove gloves.	Reduces transmission of microorganisms.

• ***Critical Decision Point***

Do not confuse residual gel substance in wound bed that occurs with some brands of alginate dressings with pus. Gel in wound bed is not a sign of infection or deterioration of wound.

STEP	RATIONALE
6. Prepare sterile dressing supplies.	Reduces risk of break in sterile technique.
7. Pour saline or cleansing solution over 4 × 4s.	Maintains sterility of dressing. With most brands of alginate dressings, wound must be thoroughly irrigated to remove all of old dressing.
8. Put on gloves, sterile if required by policy, and cleanse area gently with 4 × 4s (see Chapter 35).	Aseptically irrigating the wound *gently* effectively removes any residual dressing gel without injuring newly formed delicate granulation tissue that is forming in healing wound bed without introducing organisms into wound.

STEP	RATIONALE
9. Inspect wound for tissue type, color, odor, and drainage; measure wound (see Chapter 35).	Appearance and measurements indicate state of wound healing.
10. Apply absorption or alginate dressing according to the manufacturer's directions (see Figure 36-5, *B*).	Application techniques differ for different brands of dressings. For most brands of alginate dressings, dressing can be cut or folded to fit wound. For others, it is important not to completely fill wound bed with dressing, but rather to allow space for alginate dressing to expand to fill wound bed.
a. Fill wound cavity, but fill one-half to two-thirds full to allow for expansion with absorption.	For some brands the alginate dressing should be applied moist, and for others it should be dry. Some brands need a secondary dressing that extends at least 1¼-inches from wound edges.
b. Apply secondary dressing, if needed (check manufacturer's directions).	Some secondary dressings may reduce effectiveness of alginate or absorption dressing (Cuzzell, 1997).
11. Remove gloves by pulling inside out, and discard in prepared bag.	Reduces risk of microorganism transfer.
12. Assist client to comfortable position.	Enhances client comfort and relaxation.
13. Discard soiled dressing change materials properly. Wash hands.	Reduces transmission of microorganisms.

EVALUATION

1. Inspect condition of wound on ongoing basis; note drainage and odor.	Change in wound condition may require new therapy.
2. Note length of time before dressing needed to be changed.	Dressing is intended for moderately to highly draining wounds. If wound is dry, an alternative dressing should be chosen, for example, a hydrogel.

UNEXPECTED OUTCOMES AND RELATED INTERVENTIONS

- Wound dressing is dry and adherent when removed.
  - Wound drainage has diminished, and an alternative dressing should be considered.
- Client is unable to describe proper application of dressing.
  - Provide additional teaching or support.
  - Obtain services of home health care agency if needed.

RECORDING AND REPORTING

- Report unusual characteristics immediately.
- Record wound characteristics and measurements in client's medical record.
- Graph wound surface area or volume if wound is a chronic wound.
- Write nurse's initials, date, and time of dressing change on the new dressing or tape in ink (not marker).

TEACHING CONSIDERATIONS

- Instruct client and caregiver to observe wound for signs and symptoms of infection.
- Explain expected wound appearance with use of dressing. Instruct client and caregiver in appearance of alginate dressings because dressing becomes a gelatinous mass when maximal absorption has occurred.
- Dressing may have a "low tide" or fishy odor when removed.
- Explain frequency of dressing changes required. Often the dressing is not changed daily.
- Because application technique can vary with different brands, tell client and caregiver not to purchase a brand different from the one for which nurse gave them instructions. If a different brand must be used, client and caregiver should check with nurse for any additional instructions or modifications in alginate or absorption dressing removal and application technique needed.

PEDIATRIC CONSIDERATIONS

- See Pediatric Considerations given for Skill 36-1.

GERONTOLOGICAL CONSIDERATIONS

- See Gerontological Considerations given for Skill 36-1.

HOME CARE CONSIDERATIONS

- See Home Care Considerations given for Skills 36-1 and 36-5.

Critical Thinking Exercises

1. Your client has ordered wet-to-dry dressings for debridement of a wound healing by secondary intention. In the change-of-shift report, the nurse tells you that during dressing changes the wound bled. What do you think about the nurse's statement? How do you plan to do this dressing change during your shift?
2. A client has a large, draining wound that is being cared for with an alginate dressing. When removing the old dressing, the nurse notices a "fishy" smell from the jellylike substance in the wound. Based on this assessment, what clinical decision should the nurse make?
3. Your home care client keeps removing the dressing because the dressing is moist and she thinks a dry environment is better to heal the wound. How should the nurse answer?

References

Agency for Health Care Policy and Research (AHCPR): *Treatment of pressure ulcers,* Rockville, Md, 1994, Clinical practice guideline No. 15, U.S. Department of Health and Human Services, Public Health Service.

Andrews LW: The perils of povidone-iodine use, *Ostomy Wound Manage* 23(1):68, 1994.

Aronovitch S: Selecting the best dressing sponge, *Nursing* 25(7):52, 1995.

Baranoski S: Wound assessment and dressing selection, *Ostomy Wound Manage* 41(7A Suppl):7S, 1995.

Barr JE: Physiology of healing: the basis for the principles of wound management, *Medsurg Nurs* 4(5):387, 1995.

Bolton L, Rijswijk L: Wound dressings: meeting clinical and biological needs, *Dermatol Nurs* 3(3):146, 1991.

Cannavo M and others: A comparison of dressings in the management of surgical abdominal wounds, *J Wound Care* 7(2):57, 1998.

Cuzzell J: Choosing a wound dressing, *Geriatr Nurs* 18(6):260, 1997.

Erwin-Toth P, Hocevar BJ: Wound care: selecting the right dressing, *Am J Nurs* 95:46, 1995.

Field CK, Kerstein MD: Overview of wound healing in a moist environment, *Am J Surg* 167(1A suppl):2S, 1994.

Johnson A: A short history of wound dressings, *Ostomy Wound Manage* 38(2):36, 1992.

Keast DH, Orsted H: The basic principles of wound care, *Ostomy Wound Manage* 44(8):24, 1998.

Krasner D: Resolving the dressing dilemma: selecting wound dressings by category, *Plast Surg Nurs* 12(1):22, 1992a.

Krasner D: Using a hydrogel, foam and dressing retention sheet, *Ostomy Wound Manage* 38(3):28, 1992b.

Krasner D: Wound care: how to use the red-yellow-black system, *Am J Nurs* 5:44, 1995.

Lueckenotte AG: *Gerontologic nursing,* ed 2, St. Louis, 2000, Mosby.

Maklebust J, Palleschi M: Promoting surgical wound healing, *Nursing* 26(6):24c, 1996.

Meehan M, O'Hara L, Morrison YM: Report on the prevalence of skin ulcers in a home health agency population, *Adv Wound Care* 12(9):459, 1999.

Motta GJ: Moistening up for good healing, *Nursing* 25:32H, 1995.

Provan A, Phillips TJ: An overview of moist wound dressings: the under cover story, *Dermatol Nurs* 3(6):393, 1991.

Sorrentino SA, Gorek B: *Long-term care assistants,* ed 3, St. Louis, 1999, Mosby.

Stotts NA and others: Sterile versus clean technique in postoperative wound care of patients with open surgical wounds, *J Wound Ostomy Continence Nurs* 24(1):10, 1997.

Wikblad K, Anderson B: A comparison of three wound dressings in patients undergoing heart surgery, *Nurs Res* 44(5):312, 1995.

Wysocki AB, Bryant, RA: Skin. In Bryant RA: *Acute and chronic wounds: nursing management,* St. Louis, 2000, Mosby.

Wysocki AB: A review of the skin and its appendages, *Adv Wound Care* 8:53, 1995.

37

Binders and Bandages

Skills

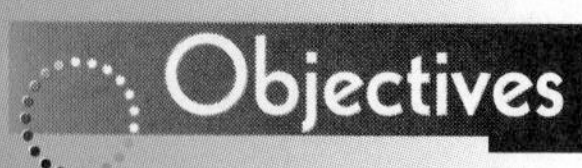

Objectives

Mastery of content in this chapter will enable the nurse to:

- Define the key terms listed.
- Discuss the purposes of binders and bandages.
- Describe the precautions for use of binders and bandages.
- Demonstrate correct technique for applying turned bandages.
- Demonstrate correct application of binders.
- Describe the elements to document when applying binders and bandages.

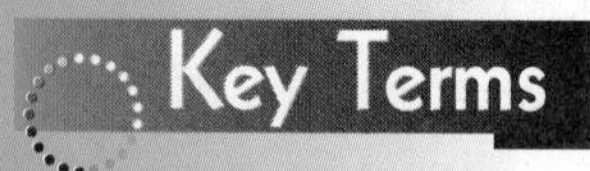

Key Terms

Binder
Chronic venous insufficiency
Elastic bandage
Excoriation
Maceration

Binders and elastic bandages applied over dressings can provide extra protection and therapeutic benefits by:

1. Creating pressure over a body part (e.g., a compression bandage applied over venous leg ulcers)
2. Immobilizing a body part (e.g., an elastic bandage applied around a sprained ankle)
3. Supporting a wound (e.g., an abdominal binder applied over a large abdominal incision and dressing)
4. Reducing or preventing edema (e.g., a breast binder used to minimize swelling between skin and tissue layers after a mastectomy)
5. Securing a splint (e.g., a bandage applied around hand splints for correction of deformities)
6. Securing dressings (e.g., elastic webbing applied around leg dressings after a vein stripping)
7. Maintaining the position of special equipment for applying traction (e.g., Buck's extension) (see Chapter 29)
8. Enabling the client to participate in effective respiratory functions of deep breathing, coughing, and clearing of airway sections (e.g., an abdominal binder used to support local incisions, reducing the pain from respiratory maneuvers)

Elasticized bandages are available in rolls of various widths and materials, including gauze, elasticized knit, elastic webbing, flannel, and muslin. Gauze bandages are lightweight and inexpensive, mold easily around contours of the body, and permit air circulation to prevent skin **maceration.** Flannel and muslin bandages are thicker than gauze and thus stronger for supporting or applying pressure. A flannel bandage also insulates to provide warmth. **Elastic bandages** conform well to body parts but can also be used to exert pressure over a body part. Elastic compression bandages are categorized as either long-stretch or short-stretch (Reichardt, 1999). Long-stretch bandages provide sustained compression regardless of a client's activities. Short-stretch bandages provide compression only when a client activates his or her calf muscle pump, as in walking. Gauze and elastic bandages are used to secure dressings on extremities, amputation stumps, and the hand (Table 37-1). In addition, elastic bandages are used for compression therapy on lower extremities to promote the return of blood from the peripheral veins to the central circulation.

Binders are bandages made of large pieces of material specially designed to fit a specific body part. Most binders are made of elastic, cotton, muslin, or flannel. The most common type of binder is the abdominal binder. Breast binders continue to be used in limited circumstances.

An abdominal binder supports large abdominal incisions that are vulnerable to tension or stress as the client moves or coughs (Figure 37-1). A breast binder looks like a tight-fitting sleeveless vest. Although used less often because of changes in surgical techniques, the breast binder helps to reduce swelling of tissues following major breast surgery. The binder conforms to the shape of the chest wall and is available in different sizes. Breast binders can provide support after breast surgery or exert pressure to reduce lactation in a woman after childbirth. The nurse secures a binder with Velcro strips, metal fasteners, or safety pins.

Skill Performance Guidelines

1. The nurse who applies a bandage or binder can loosen or readjust it as necessary. The nurse should have a physician's order before loosening or removing a bandage or binder applied by a physician.
2. Assess the status of circulation frequently below a site where a bandage has been applied.
3. Assess the status of ventilation frequently when an abdominal binder or breast binder has been applied.
4. Correctly applied binders or bandages should not cause injury to underlying and nearby body parts and should not create discomfort or reduce ventilatory expansion.

Table 37-1 Types of Bandage Turns

TYPE	DESCRIPTION	PURPOSE OR USE
Circular	Bandage turn overlapping previous turn completely 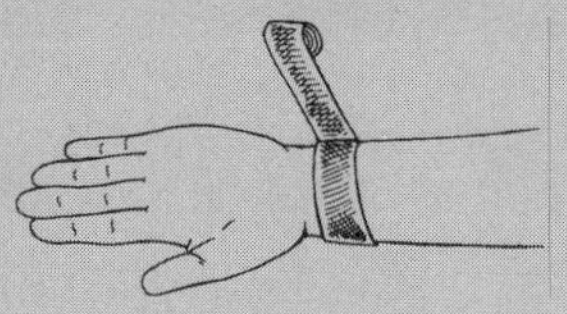 Circular turns.	Anchors bandage at the first and final turn; covers small part (finger, toe)
Spiral	Bandage ascending body part with each turn overlapping previous one by one-half or two-thirds width of bandage 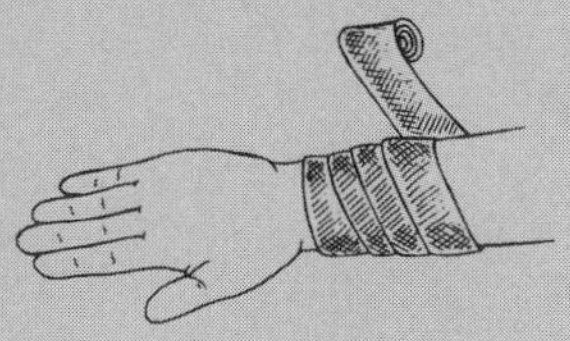 Spiral turns.	Covers cylindrical body parts such as wrist or upper arm
Spiral-reverse	Turn requiring twist (reversal) of bandage halfway through each turn 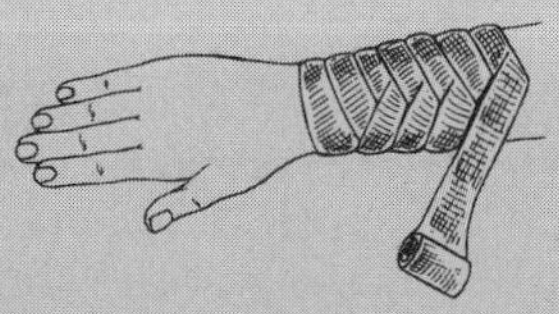 Spiral-reverse turns.	Covers cone-shaped body parts such as the forearm, thigh, or calf; useful with nonstretching bandages such as gauze or flannel
Figure eight	Oblique overlapping turns alternately ascending and descending over bandaged part; each turn crossing previous one to form figure eight 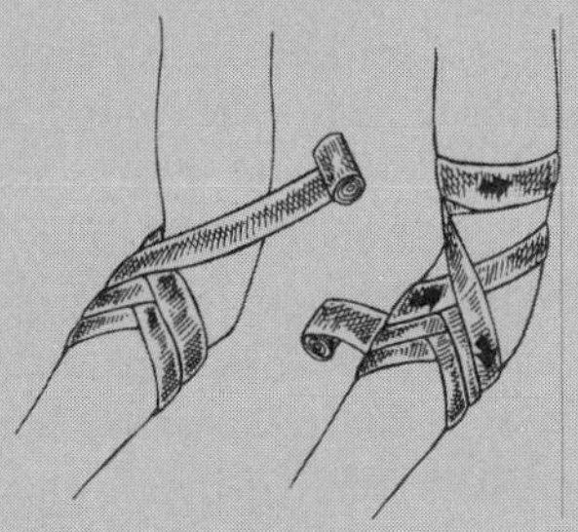 Figure-eight turns.	Covers joints, applies low-grade pressure for venous return; snug fit provides excellent immobilization
Recurrent	Bandage first secured with two circular turns around proximal end of body part; half turn made perpendicular up from bandage edge; body of bandage brought over distal end of body part to be covered with each turn folded back over on itself 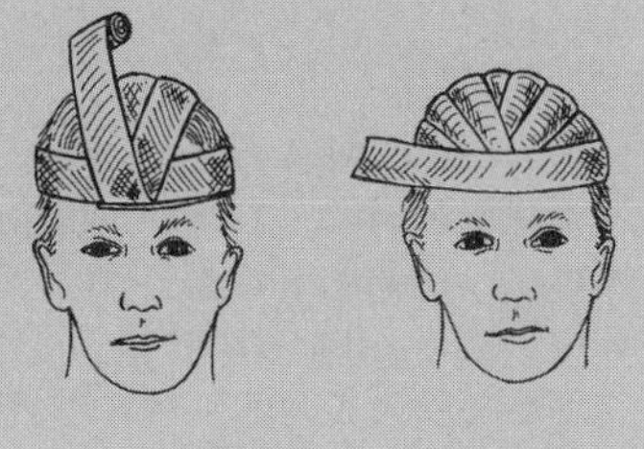 Recurrent turns.	Covers uneven body parts such as head or stump

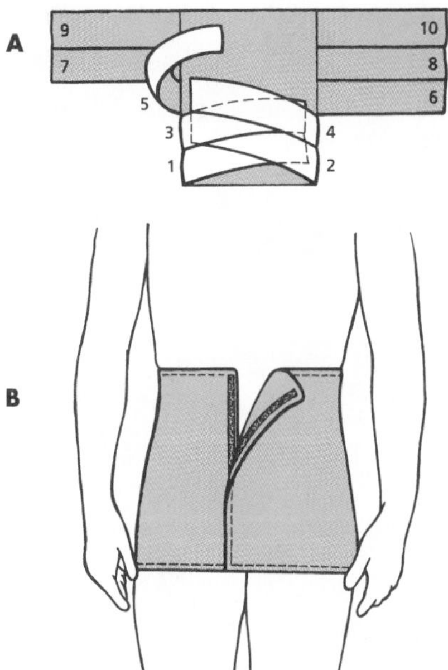

FIGURE **37-1** Abdominal binders. **A,** Scultetus binder with crossover strap closures. **B,** Straight binder with Velcro closure.

Skill 37-1 Applying Gauze and Elastic Bandages

Both gauze and elastic bandages can be used to hold dressings securely in hard-to-cover areas. For example, a dressing covering the length of a client's lower leg will be held in place more firmly when the dressing is surrounded by a well-secured gauze bandage. An elastic bandage is also used to apply compression to an area. Elastic compression is used most often on the lower extremities to prevent edema and to support varicosities. Many clients use elastic bandages to reduce dependent edema in the extremities. Continuous compression therapy, the treatment of choice for **chronic venous insufficiency,** has multiple therapeutic benefits (Box 37-1). The principle of compression therapy is consistent with Laplace's law of physics. Following the natural shape of the lower leg, gradient compression therapy delivers higher pressures at the ankle (smaller radius) with a decline in pressure at the knee (larger radius). This provides for normal venous flow (Reichardt, 1999). Continuous compression therapy typically involves the application of four layers of bandages, designed to apply 40 mm Hg of pressure at the ankle and to remain in place without slipping (Moffatt and O'Hare, 1995). Nurses require advanced training to apply continuous compression bandages, which is beyond the scope of this text.

Box 37-1 Therapeutic Benefits of Continuous Compression Therapy

- Alleviation of venous hypertension
- Increased return of venous blood to the central circulation and heart
- Stimulation of fibrinolysis
- Removal of sodium from subcutaneous tissue
- Reduction of local edema
- Increased local oxygenation
- Promotion of an environment favorable for wound healing

Modified from Reichardt LE: Venous ulceration: compression as the mainstay of therapy, *J Wound Ostomy Continence Nurs* 26(1):39, 1999.

Other uses of elastic bandages include support of the knee, ankle, elbow, and wrist in conditions such as strains and sprains (Phipps, 1995; Moffatt and O'Hare, 1995; Reichardt, 1999). When fully stretched, an elastic bandage extends to 3 yards (270 cm). Shorter lengths of $1\frac{1}{2}$ yards (135 cm) are available for bandaging the wrist or a child's foot or knee. Gauze bandages likewise come in a variety of lengths. Gauze and elastic bandages are available in widths ranging from 2 inches (5 cm) to 8 inches (20 cm).

When selecting gauze or elastic bandages to secure a dressing, the type of bandage turn and selected width are determined by the size and shape of the body part to be bandaged. For example, 3- and 4-inch bandages are most commonly used for the adult leg. A smaller 2-inch bandage would be used for the wrist.

Gauze and elastic bandages come supplied in a roll with an inner and outer surface. In preparation for bandaging, the outer surface is placed next to the skin and then rolled around the surface to be covered. Even tension is applied during application. When an elastic bandage is applied to an extremity, the bandage is started at the site farthest from the heart (distal) and proceeds toward the heart (proximal).

Delegation Considerations

The skill of applying an elastic bandage for compression should not be delegated to assistive personnel. The skill of applying bandages to secure nonsterile dressings can be delegated following assessment. Caution care providers to report when a client complains of pain, numbness, or tingling after a bandage has been applied.

Equipment

- Correct width and number of gauze or highly elastic bandages
- Clips or adhesive tape
- Disposable gloves, if wound drainage is present

Step	Rationale
Assessment	
1. Review client's medical record and nursing prescriptions for specific orders related to application of elastic bandage. Note area to be covered, type of bandage required, frequency of change, and previous response to treatment.	Specific prescription may direct procedure, including such factors as extent of application (e.g., toe to knee, toe to groin) or duration of treatment.
2. Inspect skin of area to be bandaged for alterations in integrity as indicated by presence of abrasion, discoloration, or chafing. Pay close attention to areas over bony prominences.	Altered skin integrity may contraindicate use of elastic bandage to be applied directly to the skin because of applied pressure. May require gauze cover dressing before bandage is applied.
3. Inspect any surgical dressing.	Surgical dressing replacement or reinforcement precedes application of any bandage.

- ***Critical Decision Point***

  If incision/wound is to be covered by a bandage, it should be covered entirely to avoid soiling of bandage and irritation of wound.

Step	Rationale
4. Observe adequacy of circulation by noting surface temperature, skin color, pulses (distal to area to be bandaged), presence of edema, and sensation and movement of body parts to be wrapped.	Comparison of area before and after application of bandage is necessary to ensure continued adequate circulation. Impairment of circulation may result in pain, coolness to touch when compared with opposite side of body, cyanosis or pallor of skin, diminished or absent pulses, edema or localized pooling, and numbness and/or tingling of body part.
5. Assess client's comfort level using visual analog scale of 0 to 10 (see Chapter 5), and note any other objective signs of discomfort.	Provides baseline to determine effects of therapy and client's response.
6. Assess for size of bandage.	
a. Gauze or basic elastic bandage to secure a dressing: Assess size of area to be covered. Each successive role of gauze/elastic should overlap previous layer. Smaller widths used for upper extremities, larger widths for lower extremities.	Proper size bandage avoids bulkiness and ensures adequate coverage.
b. Elastic bandage to provide simple compression: Assess circumference of lower extremity before or shortly after client gets out of bed in the morning or after client has been in bed for at least 15 minutes. Select width that will cover and overlap without bulkiness.	Assures clinician that dependent edema is at a minimum, so true leg circumference can be estimated (Reichardt, 1999). Compression bandages not applied correctly may produce pressures that are either too low or too high to promote venous return.
7. Identify client's and primary caregiver's present knowledge level of skill if bandaging will be continued at home.	Ensures that planning and teaching are individualized.

Nursing Diagnosis

Defining characteristics from the assessment data may reveal the following nursing diagnoses for clients requiring this skill:

- Impaired physical mobility
- Impaired tissue integrity
- Deficient knowledge regarding bandage application
- Pain (acute, chronic)

Related factors are individualized based on client's condition or needs.

Step	Rationale

Planning

1. **Expected outcomes** following completion of procedure:
   - Client states pain or discomfort is decreased or absent. — Indicates proper application of elastic bandage without excess pressure or compression that could impair local blood flow.
   - No tingling or numbness is noted by client. — Bandage is not causing pressure on peripheral nerves or arterial circulation.
   - Distal parts (toes, fingers) feel warm (symmetrically) to touch, pulse is present, no cyanosis or blanching is present, and motion is not unnecessarily impaired. — Indicates adequate circulation to distal regions.
   - Localized edema is reduced. — Elastic bandage promotes venous return.
   - Client applies bandage correctly. — Demonstrates learning and ensures continuity of care after discharge.
2. Explain procedure to client. Reinforce during teaching that smooth, even pressure will be applied to improve venous circulation, prevent clot formation, reduce or prevent swelling, immobilize body part, secure surgical dressings, and provide pressure. — Increased knowledge needed to promote cooperation, reduce anxiety, and ensure correct technique for self-application.
3. Teach skill to client or significant other when bandage will be applied in the home. — Reduces anxiety and ensures continuity of care.

Implementation

1. Close room door or curtains. — Maintains client's comfort and dignity.
2. Assist client to assume comfortable, anatomically correct position, lying in bed. — Maintains alignment. Facilitates application of bandage in anatomical position.
3. Wash hands and apply gloves if drainage is present. — Reduces transmission of microorganisms.

   • ***Critical Decision Point***
   With client in bed, elevation of dependent extremities for 20 minutes before elastic bandage application will enhance venous return.

4. Apply bandage
   a. Gauze or elastic bandage to secure dressing:
      (1) Hold roll of bandage in dominant hand and use other hand to lightly hold beginning layer of bandage at distal body part. While rolling bandage around body part, continue transferring roll to dominant hand as bandage is wrapped (see illustration). — Maintains appropriate and consistent bandage tension.

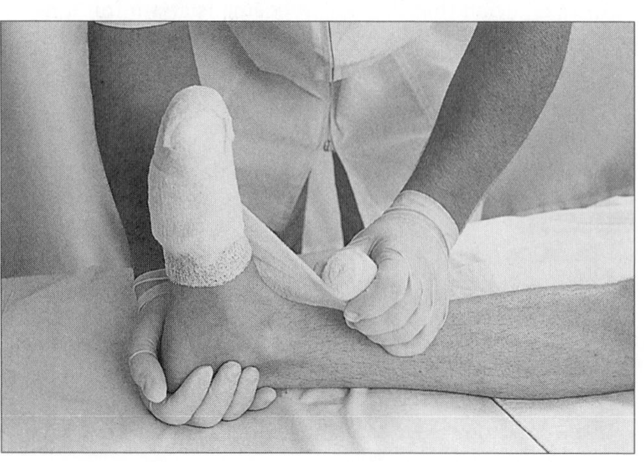

STEP **4a(1)** Nurse applies roller gauze to foot.

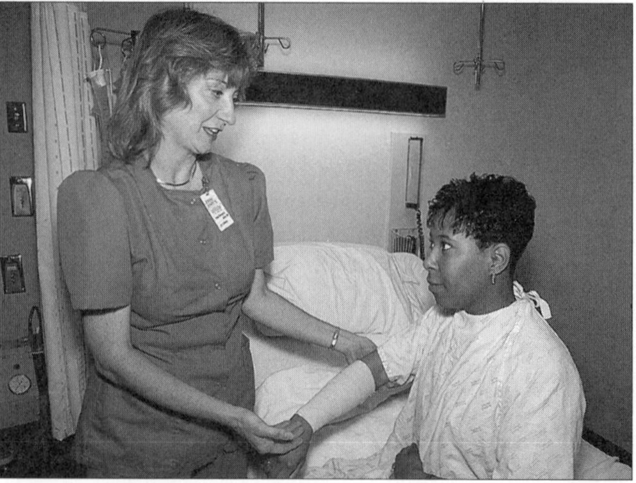

STEP **4a(1a)** Nurse checks temperature of skin below site of bandage application.

STEP	RATIONALE
• ***Critical Decision Point*** *Except in cases where toes or fingers are treated because of wounds, toes or fingertips should remain uncovered and visible for follow-up circulatory assessment (see illustration).*	
(2) Apply bandage from distal point toward proximal boundary using variety of turns to cover various shapes of body parts (see Table 37-1). (For bandaging of amputation stump, see illustration.)	Bandage is applied in manner that conforms evenly to body part and promotes venous return.
(3) While unrolling elastic bandage, stretch bandage slightly.	Maintains uniform bandage tension.
• ***Critical Decision Point*** *Avoid wrapping bandage too tightly because this may cause numbness and tingling from impaired circulation and/or pressure on peripheral nerves.*	
(4) Overlap turns by one-half to two-thirds width of bandage roll.	Prevents uneven bandage tension and circulatory impairment.
(5) Secure first bandage with clip or tape before applying additional rolls.	Maintains a smooth bandage surface.
(6) Apply additional rolls without leaving any uncovered skin surface. Secure last bandage applied.	Prevents wrinkling or loose ends.

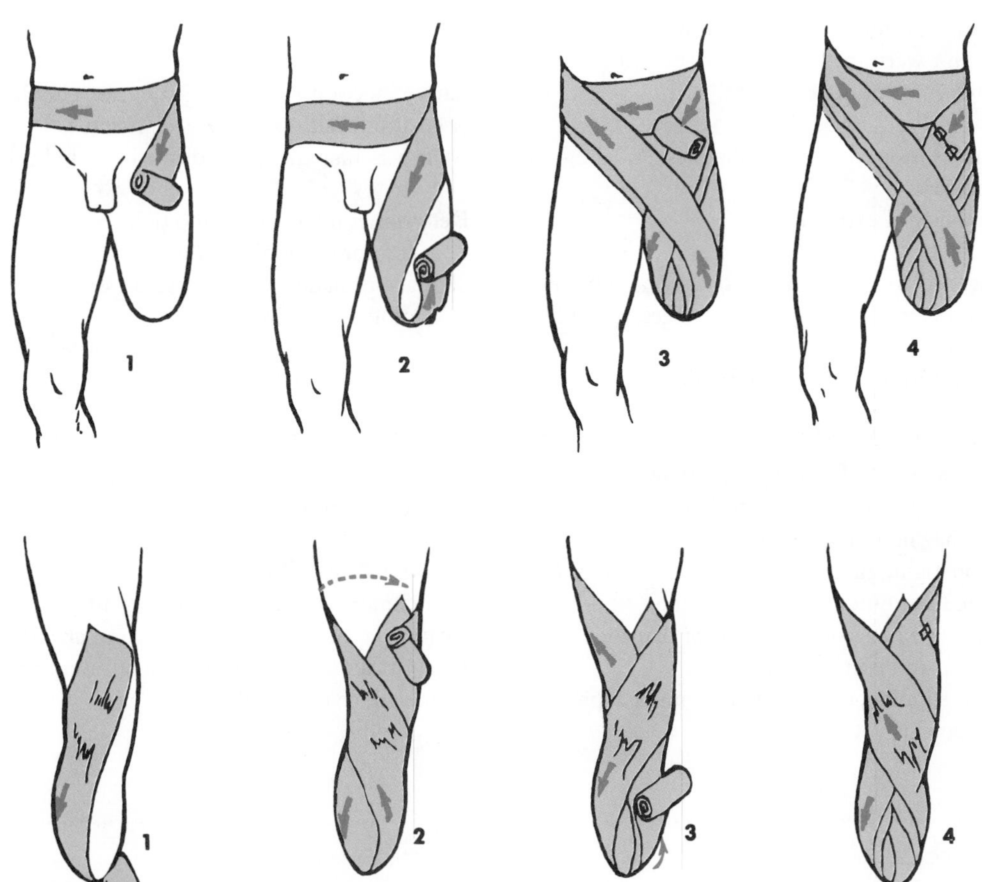

STEP **4a(2)** *Top,* Correct method for bandaging midthigh amputation stump. Note that bandage must be anchored around patient's waist. *Bottom,* Correct method for bandaging midcalf amputation stump. Note that bandage need not be anchored around the waist. (From Williamson V: Amputation of the lower extremity: an overview, *Orthop Nurs* 11(2):55, 1992.)

STEP	RATIONALE
b. Elastic bandage for simple intermittent compression:	
(1) Have client lie in bed with leg slightly elevated.	Promotes venous return during application.
(2) Hold roll of bandage in dominant hand and use other hand to lightly hold beginning layer of bandage at distal body part. While rolling bandage around body part, continue transferring roll to dominant hand as bandage is wrapped.	Maintains appropriate and consistent bandage tension.
(3) Apply the highly elastic conformable bandage using a figure-eight turn. Apply from distal (just above toes) to most proximal boundary.	Applies up to 17 mm Hg pressure at the ankle to promote venous return (Reichardt, 1999).
(4) Stretch bandage slightly while applying.	Maintains uniform tension.
(5) After applying only one layer of bandage, secure with tape or clips.	Prevents excess pressure over limb. Continuous pressure bandage using multiple layers requires trained clinician to apply.
5. Remove gloves if worn, and wash hands.	Reduces transmission of microorganisms.
6. Remove and reapply elastic bandage once every 8 hours unless otherwise directed by physician.	Single layer bandage can slip easily, causing excess pressure where bandage rests.

EVALUATION

1. Evaluate distal circulation when bandage application is complete and at least twice during 8-hour period.	Measurements determine if bandage is applied too tightly, compromising circulation or movement.
a. Observe skin color for pallor or cyanosis.	
b. Palpate skin for warmth.	
c. Palpate pulses and compare bilaterally.	Early detection and management of circulatory impairment ensures healthy neurovascular status.
d. Ask if client is aware of pain, numbness, tingling, or other discomfort.	Neurovascular changes indicate impaired venous return.
e. Observe mobility of extremity.	Determines if bandage is too tight, which restricts movement, or if joint immobility is attained.
2. Evaluate as needed for wrinkles, looseness, or tightness; client discomfort or itchiness; and changes, including drainage.	Slippage of bandage can cause pressure on underlying tissue, leading to impaired circulation or pressure on nerves.
3. Have client demonstrate bandage application.	Return demonstration validates client's learning.

UNEXPECTED OUTCOMES AND RELATED INTERVENTIONS

- Circumferential ridging develops with deep indentations into skin; client may note tingling, numbness, or pain.
  - Bandage is too tight, causing impaired circulation. Remove and wait 30 minutes before reapplying.
- Extremity distal to wrap is cool, cyanotic, or blanched.
  - Notify physician, and remove bandage.
- Dressing is loose, slipping, or improperly wrapped, providing improper support.
  - Reapply.
- Extremity has decreased range of joint motion.
  - Notify physician.

RECORDING AND REPORTING

- Document condition of wound, integrity of dressing, application of bandage, circulation, and client's comfort level.
- Report any changes in neurological or circulatory status to nurse in charge or physician.

TEACHING CONSIDERATIONS

- Applying elastic bandage to oneself is difficult. Teach significant other if treatment will continue after hospitalization.
- Unless total immobilization is prescribed for client, instruct on proper range-of-motion exercises. Encourage client to practice regularly.

PEDIATRIC CONSIDERATIONS

- Use adhesive tape rather than loose clips or safety pins to fasten bandage on small child or infant.

Gerontological Considerations

- As clients age, skin becomes more fragile, which increases their susceptibility to skin breakdown. Once skin/tissue injury occurs, wound healing is delayed. Assess these clients more frequently for evidence of skin breakdown or decrease in circulation over the areas covered by and distal to the bandage.

Home Care Considerations

- Advise client on best resources for obtaining bandage supplies. Consult with home health care nurse as needed.
- Assess client and primary caregiver's ability, motivation, and availability to participate in bandaging procedure.
- Assess client's understanding of bandaging and willingness to leave bandage in place.
- Assess client's environment to determine potential for permitting bandaged area to remain free from contaminants.
- The elastic bandage is washable and is placed in large folds over a line to dry. Do not use an electric dryer because bandage can shrink.

Skill 37-2 Applying an Abdominal Binder and a Breast Binder

Binders are indicated for the support of underlying muscles and large incisions. The muscles and viscera surrounding an operative site may require support during the postoperative period to reduce trauma and edema. This promotes healing and permits a client to move more freely without additional discomfort. The basic shape of an abdominal binder is a rectangle that is wide enough to extend from the groin to the waistline and long enough to encircle the abdomen with an overlap for closure. Breast binders are made in the form of tight-fitting vests.

Delegation Considerations

The skill of applying a binder can be delegated to assistive personnel. The assessment of the client should be conducted before binder application.

Equipment

- Gloves, if wound drainage present

Abdominal Binder

- Correct size cloth/elastic straight binder
- Safety pins (6 to 8) unless Velcro closure or metal fasteners are attached

Breast Binder

- Correct size binder
- Safety pins (approximately 12) unless Velcro closure is attached

Step	Rationale
Assessment	
1. For client who needs support of abdomen, observe ability to breathe deeply, cough effectively, and turn or move independently.	Baseline assessment determines client's ability to breathe and cough. Impaired ventilation of lung can lead to alveolar atelectasis and inadequate arterial oxygenation.
2. Determine if client has allergy to adhesive tape.	Contraindicates use of tape to secure binder.
3. Inspect skin for actual or potential alterations in integrity. Observe for irritation, abrasion, skin surfaces that rub against each other, and allergic response to adhesive tape used to secure dressing.	Actual impairments in skin integrity can be worsened with application of a binder. Binder can cause pressure and **excoriation.**
4. Inspect any surgical dressing for intactness, presence of drainage, and coverage of incision. Change any soiled dressing before applying binder.	Dressing replacement or reinforcement precedes application of any binder. If left uncovered, a wound can be damaged from rubbing of binder.
5. Assess client's comfort level, using visual analog scale of 0 to 10 (see Chapter 5) and noting any other objective signs and symptoms.	Data will provide baseline to later determine effectiveness of binder placement.

STEP	RATIONALE
6. Gather necessary data regarding size of client and appropriate binder to use (see manufacturer's guidelines).	Ensures proper fit of binder.

NURSING DIAGNOSIS

Defining characteristics from the assessment data may reveal the following nursing diagnoses for clients requiring this skill:

- Impaired physical mobility
- Impaired skin integrity
- Ineffective breathing pattern
- Impaired tissue integrity
- Deficient knowledge regarding binder application
- Acute pain

Related factors are individualized based on client's condition or needs.

PLANNING

STEP	RATIONALE
1. **Expected outcomes** following completion of procedure:	
▪ Client's respirations are unrestricted. Coughing is effective, and secretions are expectorated.	Ability to fully expand lungs and cough must continue after application of binder to enhance oxygenation and avoid pulmonary complications.
▪ Client is able to move within prescribed limits and states pain is absent or reduced.	Support to incision from binder promotes comfort during turning, ambulation, or deep breathing.
▪ Client's suture line is intact, with no drainage or separation.	Binder decreases tension on suture line to promote healing. Snug support helps maintain intact suture line.
2. Explain procedure to client.	Promotes client's understanding and cooperation.
3. Teach skill to client or significant other.	Reduces anxiety and ensures continuity of care after discharge.

IMPLEMENTATION

STEP	RATIONALE
1. Close curtains or room door.	Maintains client's comfort and dignity.
2. Wash hands and apply gloves (if likely to contact wound drainage).	Reduces transmission of microorganisms.
3. Apply abdominal binder:	
a. Position client in supine position with head slightly elevated and knees slightly flexed.	Minimizes muscular tension on abdominal organs.
b. Assist client in rolling on side away from nurse toward raised side rail while firmly supporting abdominal incision and dressing with hands.	Reduces pain and discomfort.
c. Place binder flat on bed, right side up. Fanfold far side of binder toward midline of binder. (For a scultetus binder, be sure tails are smoothly placed against client's side as far side is fanfolded.	Gathers binder together so client can roll over with minimal effort.
d. Place fanfolded ends of binder under client.	Permits placement and centering of binder with minimal discomfort.
e. Instruct or assist client in rolling over folded binder.	Positions client over binder.
f. Unfold and stretch ends out smoothly on far side of bed. Then stretch out ends on near side of bed.	Smooth, even binder maintains skin integrity and comfort.
g. Instruct client to roll back into supine position.	Facilitates an even application of binder over abdomen.
h. Adjust binder so that supine client is centered over binder, using symphysis pubis and costal margins as lower and upper landmarks.	Centers support from binder over abdominal structures, which reduces incidence of decreased lung expansion while ensuring adequate wound support.
i. If client is very thin, pad iliac prominences with gauze bandage.	Reduces pressure on prominences.

STEP	RATIONALE
j. Close binder. Pull one end of binder over center of client's abdomen. While maintaining tension on that end of binder, pull opposite end of binder over center and secure with Velcro closure tabs, metal fasteners, or horizontally placed safety pins.	Provides continuous wound support and comfort.

- ***Critical Decision Point***
  Recheck client's ability to breathe deeply and cough effectively. Shallow respirations, continuing after a tight binder has been loosened, may indicate beginning of serious respiratory problems, including alveolar atelectasis and pulmonary embolus, among others.

STEP	RATIONALE
k. Assess client's comfort level.	Helps determine effectiveness of binder placement.
l. Adjust binder as necessary.	Promotes comfort and chest expansion.
4. Apply breast binder:	
a. Have client lie supine with head elevated 45 degrees.	Facilitates normal anatomical position of breasts and eases application of binder.
b. Thoroughly wash and dry under pendulous breasts before applying a breast binder.	Reduces risk of growth of microorganisms.
c. Assist client in placing arms through binder's armholes.	Eases binder placement process.
d. Lightly pad area under breasts with 4 × 4 gauze dressing if necessary.	Prevents skin contact with undersurface.
e. Using Velcro closure tabs or horizontally placed safety pins, secure binder at nipple level first. Continue closure process above and then below nipple line until entire binder is closed (see illustration).	Horizontal placement of pins may reduce risk of uneven pressure or localized irritation. Applying support at nipple line ensures even alignment of breasts.

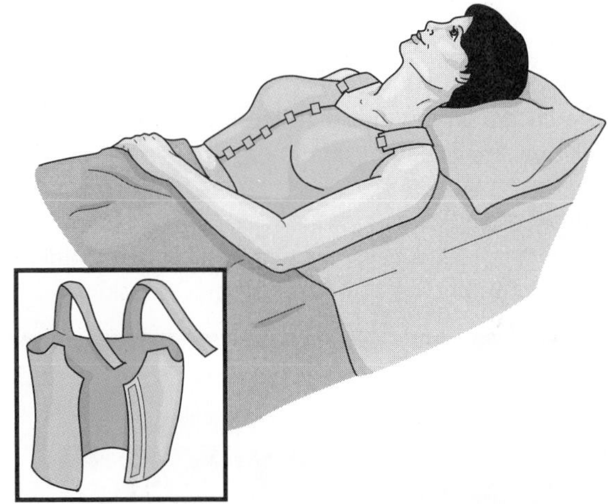

STEP **4e** Client with breast binder applied. (From Sorrentino SA: *Mosby's textbook for nursing assistants,* ed 5, St. Louis, 2000, Mosby.)

STEP	RATIONALE
f. Make appropriate adjustments, including individualizing fit of shoulder straps and pinning waistline darts to reduce binder size.	Maintains support to client's breasts.
g. Instruct and observe skill development in self-care related to reapplying breast binder.	Self-care is integral aspect of discharge planning. Skin-integrity and comfort-level goals are ensured.
5. Remove gloves and wash hands.	Prevents cross infections.

EVALUATION

STEP	RATIONALE
1. Observe site for skin integrity, circulation, and characteristics of the wound. Remove binder and surgical dressing to assess wound characteristics at least every 8 hours.	Determines that binder has not resulted in complications (e.g., rubbing or abrasion of skin, disruption of wound).
2. Evaluate comfort level of client, using visual analog scale of 0 to 10, and note any other objective signs and symptoms.	Binders should not increase discomfort.
3. Evaluate client's ability to ventilate properly, including deep breathing and coughing, every 4 hours.	Identifies any impaired ventilation and potential pulmonary complications.

STEP	RATIONALE
4. Identify client's need for assistance with activities such as hair combing, dressing, and ambulating.	Mobility of upper extremities may be limited, depending on severity and location of incision.

Unexpected Outcomes and Related Interventions

- Impaired breathing as evidenced by shallow, rapid respirations leads to ineffective oxygenation.
  - Remove and then reapply binder.
- Tight binder impairs circulation to tissues.
  - Remove and then reapply binder.
- Skin integrity is impaired, resulting from uneven pressure and irritation.
  - Remove binder.
  - Administer skin care as appropriate.
  - Consult with physician, and reapply if appropriate.
- Pain and discomfort are increased.
  - Binder or dressing support may be applied incorrectly. Remove and reapply.

Recording and Reporting

- Record type and application of binder, condition of skin, circulation, integrity of underlying dressing, and client's comfort level.
- Report any complications (e.g., pain, skin irritation, impaired ventilation) to nurse in charge.
- Report reduced lung expansion to physician immediately.

Teaching Considerations

- Instruct client that a properly fitting brassiere that extends to lower rib cage and has front closure may be substituted for breast binder.
- Consider client's dexterity in reapplying binder to self, opportunities to practice skill, and need to teach significant other.

Pediatric Considerations

- Use adhesive tape rather than loose clips or pins to fasten binder on small child or infant.

Gerontological Considerations

- As clients age, skin becomes more fragile, which increases their susceptibility to skin breakdown. Once skin/tissue injury occurs, healing is delayed. Assess these clients more frequently for evidence of skin breakdown over area covered by binder.

Home Care Considerations

- Assess primary caregiver's understanding, ability, and motivation to participate in application of binder.
- Assess client's understanding of purpose of binder and willingness to permit binder to remain in place.
- Abdominal and breast binders are washable and are placed over a line to dry.

Critical Thinking Exercises

1. After applying an elastic bandage to a client's right lower leg, you check the client's dorsal pedal pulse, temperature of skin, and capillary refill. The client states the bandage feels "a bit too tight." Your assessment reveals a pulse equal in strength to the left leg, warm skin, and capillary refill in less than 2 seconds. What should your actions be?
2. Mr. Niles has had major surgery involving the abdominal cavity. He requires dressing changes every 4 to 6 hours as a result of copious drainage. Mr. Niles is obese, and the physician decides to provide an abdominal binder to prevent the risk of trauma to the suture line when Mr. Niles coughs. What consideration must be made in applying a binder for Mr. Niles?
3. About 2 hours after applying Mr. Niles's binder you return and note that respirations are shallow and at a rate of 28 breaths per minute, compared with 18 breaths per minute when the binder was first applied. What should you do?

References

Lewis S, Collier I, Heitkemper M: *Medical-surgical nursing: assessment and management of clinical problems,* ed 4, St. Louis, 2000, Mosby.

Moffatt CJ, O'Hare L: Venous leg ulceration: treatment by high compression bandaging, *Ostomy Wound Manage* 41(4):16, 1995.

Phipps J and others: *Medical-surgical nursing: concepts and clinical practice,* ed 5, St. Louis, 1995, Mosby.

Reichardt LE: Venous ulceration: compression as the mainstay of therapy, *J Wound Ostomy Continence Nurs* 26(1):39, 1999.

Sorrentino SA: *Mosby's textbook for nursing assistants,* ed 5, St. Louis, 2000, Mosby.

Williamson V: Amputation of the lower extremity: an overview, *Orthop Nurs* 11(2):55, 1992.

38

HOT AND COLD THERAPY

Skills

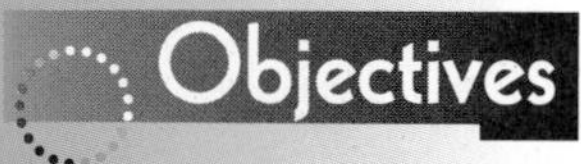

Objectives

Mastery of content in this chapter will enable the nurse to:

- Define the key terms listed.
- Identify the effects of heat and cold on the client.
- Differentiate the types of injuries or conditions that benefit from hot and cold applications.
- Identify the risks to clients related to hot and cold applications.
- Explain common guidelines used to protect clients who receive hot and cold applications.
- Correctly apply hot and cold applications.

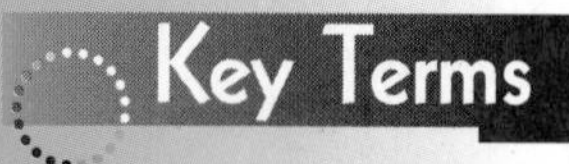

Key Terms

Compress
Conduction
Cryotherapy
Evaporation
Insulator
Neuropathy
Piloerection
Sitz bath
Vasoconstriction
Vasodilation

The local application of heat and cold to body parts can have a beneficial effect. To use heat and cold therapies safely, the nurse must understand how the body normally responds to temperature variations and the risks connected with these applications.

Exposure to heat or cold causes both systemic and local responses. The hypothalamus acts as the thermostat of the body to maintain body temperature at approximately 37° C, or 98.6° F. Systemically, when the skin is exposed to warm or hot temperatures, **vasodilation** and perspiration occur to promote heat loss. As perspiration evaporates from the skin, cooling occurs. In **cryotherapy,** when the skin is exposed to cool or cold temperatures, the systemic response includes **vasoconstriction** and **piloerection** to conserve heat. Shivering occurs in response to cooler temperatures, producing heat through muscular contraction.

The local response to heat and cold results from changes in blood vessel size, which affect blood flow to the exposed area. This physiological response explains the effectiveness of hot and cold therapies (Table 38-1).

When receptors for heat or cold are stimulated, sensory impulses travel via somatic afferent fibers to the hypothalamus and cerebral cortex. The cerebral cortex makes a person aware of temperature sensations. The person can then adapt as necessary to maintain normal body temperature; if cold, the person can put on additional clothing, or if warm, the person can cool down by bathing the face with a tepid damp cloth. The hypothalamus simultaneously controls physiological reflexes needed to regulate normal body temperature. The body also has a protective reflex response for exposure to temperature extremes. Exposure to an extremely hot or cold stimulus sends impulses traveling to the spinal cord, synapsing at the spinal cord, and returning by way of motor nerves to cause withdrawal from the stimulus. The person becomes aware of the discomfort as withdrawal occurs.

Sensory adaptation to local temperature extremes can occur quickly within the body. Although a person may initially feel a temperature extreme, once the sensory receptors adapt, the person may become unaware of any temperature variation. Eventually excessive heat causes a burning sensation; excessive cold causes a numbing sensation before pain is sensed. Because of this physiological phenomenon, the risk of tissue injury from hot and cold applications is great. Certain clients are more at risk than others for injury from hot and cold applications (Table 38-2). The nurse plays an important role in maintaining the client's safety in the application of heat and cold. The nurse must always have an order for a hot or cold application, and the order should include the desired temperature to be used when settings can be controlled (Table 38-3). In health care agencies, central supply departments typically set temperatures on hot and cold devices. Because many of these therapies can be used at home, the nurse must instruct clients and their families in the proper use of these therapies.

When using hot or cold therapies, the nurse can use either dry or moist applications. The selection of dry or moist application is determined by the nature of temperature **conduction** and the result desired from therapy. Temperature travels from an external source such as a **compress** or water pad to the skin's surface. A substance that conducts temperatures poorly is a good **insulator** and thus a protector for skin and tissues. For example, cloth placed over a heating pad insulates the skin from hot temperature extremes. Plastic, which is the external covering for most commercial heating pads, and the fluid in moist compresses both conduct heat well, thus placing the client at risk for injury during heat applications. However, there are distinct advantages to using both dry and moist applications (Table 38-4). The nurse should be familiar with the effects of each application type.

Skill Performance Guidelines

1. Protect damaged skin. Exposed layers of skin are more sensitive to temperature variations than intact skin.
2. Time all applications carefully. A person tolerates temperature extremes better when the duration of exposure is

Table 38-1 Therapeutic Effects of Heat and Cold Applications

Therapy	Physiological Responses	Therapeutic Benefit	Examples of Conditions Treated
Heat	Vasodilation	Improves blood flow to injured body part, promotes delivery of nutrients and removal of wastes, decreases venous congestion in injured tissues	Inflamed or edematous body part; new surgical wound; infected wound; arthritis, degenerative joint disease; localized joint pain, muscle strains; low pack pain, menstrual cramping; hemorrhoidal, perianal, and vaginal inflammation; local abscesses
	Reduced blood viscosity	Improves delivery of leukocytes and antibodies to wound site	
	Reduced muscle tension	Promotes muscle relaxation and reduces pain from spasm or stiffness	
	Increased tissue metabolism	Increases blood flow; provides local warmth	
	Increased capillary permeability	Promotes movement of waste products and nutrients	
Cold	Vasoconstriction	Reduces blood flow to injured body part, prevents edema formation, reduces inflammation	Immediately after direct trauma such as sprains, strains, fractures, muscle spasms, after superficial lacerations or puncture wound; after minor burns; when malignancy is suspected in area of injury or pain; after injections; for arthritis, joint trauma
	Local anesthesia	Reduces localized pain by slowing or blocking peripheral nerve conduction	
	Reduced cell metabolism	Reduces enzyme function and oxygen needs of tissues	
	Increased blood viscosity	Promotes blood coagulation at injury site	
	Decreased muscle tension	Prevents muscles spasm by decreasing spasticity/tone and relieves pain	

Data from Stitik T, Nadler S: I. When—and how—to use cold most effectively, *Consultant* 38(12):2881, 1998; and Stitik T, Nadler S: II. When—and how—to apply the heat, *Consultant* 39(1):144, 1999.

Table 38-2 Conditions That Increase Risk of Injury From Heat and Cold Application

Condition	Risk Factors
Areas with little body fat	Thinner layers in children increase risk of burns; older adults have reduced sensitivity to painful stimuli.
Open wounds, broken skin, stomas	Subcutaneous and visceral tissue more sensitive to temperature variations; also contain no temperature receptors and fewer pain receptors than normal skin.
Areas of edema or immature scar tissue	Reduced sensation to temperature stimuli because of thickening of skin layers from fluid buildup or scar formation.
Peripheral vascular disease (e.g., diabetes, arteriosclerosis)	Body's extremities are less sensitive to temperature and pain stimuli because of circulatory impairment and local tissue injury; cold applications would further compromise blood flow.
Confusion or unconsciousness	Reduced perception of sensory or painful stimuli.
Spinal cord injury	Alteration in nerve pathway preventing reception of sensory or painful stimuli.
Abscessed tooth or appendix	Infection highly localized; application of heat may cause rupture with systemic spread of microorganisms.

Data from Stitik T, Nadler S: I. When—and how—to use cold most effectively, *Consultant* 38(12):2881, 1998; and Stitik T, Nadler S: II. When—and how—to apply the heat, *Consultant* 39(1):144, 1999.

short (10 to 20 minutes). Prolonged exposure can injure tissues and eliminate the benefits of therapy (Stitik and Nadler, 1998). Keep a timer or clock close by so that the client can help the nurse time applications.

3. Know the temperature of the application being used. Many devices, such as heating pads or water flow pads, have thermostats to regulate temperature. Always check the temperature of moist compresses applied directly to the skin.
4. Certain body parts, such as the extremities or perineum, are more sensitive than others to temperature extremes. The nurse can modify the intensity of heat and cold when sensitive skin areas are being treated.

Table 38-3 Temperature Ranges for Hot and Cold Applications

Temperature	Centigrade Range (degrees)	Fahrenheit Range (degrees)
Hot	37-41	98-106
Warm	34-37	93-98
Tepid	26-34	80-93
Cool	18-26	65-80
Cold	10-18	50-65

Table 38-4 Choice of Dry or Moist Warm Application

TYPE	ADVANTAGES	DISADVANTAGES
Moist application	Reduces drying of skin and softens wound exudate Conforms well to body area being treated Penetrates deeply into tissue layers Lessens sweating and insensible fluid loss	Can cause maceration of the skin with prolonged exposure Cools rapidly because of moisture evaporation Creates greater risk for burns to skin because moisture conducts heat
Dry application	Less likely to burn skin Does not cause skin maceration Retains temperature longer because not influenced by evaporation	Increases body fluid loss through sweating Does not penetrate deep into tissue Causes increased drying of skin

5. Check the client frequently during a hot or cold application. The condition of the skin indicates whether tissue injury is occurring. Be observant for signs of excessive redness, maceration, or blistering.
6. Know the client's risk for injury from heat or cold. Certain clients are more predisposed to injury than others (see Table 38-2).
7. Do not allow the client to adjust temperature settings. It is common for the client to adapt to a temperature extreme and then think that the temperature should be adjusted.
8. Never position the client so that the client cannot move away from the temperature source. This avoids the risk of injuries from temperature exposure. The hospitalized client should always have a call light within reach.
9. Do not leave the client unattended if the person is unable to sense temperature changes or move away from the temperature source. The nurse is responsible for the client's safety.
10. Discourage the client from moving an application. This may cause injury to an unprotected area of the body and decrease the effectiveness of therapy.

Skill 38-1 Applying a Moist Hot Compress to an Open Wound

A hot compress is a section of sterile or clean gauze moistened with a prescribed heated solution (i.e., normal saline, sterile water) and applied directly to an open wound or the skin's surface. A sterile compress is necessary only when there is a break in skin integrity. Commercially packaged sterile, premoistened compresses are available in some agencies. They require the use of a special infrared lamp to heat. Plain sterile or clean gauze can be heated by adding the gauze to a container of warmed solution. Often the nurse applies an aquathermia heating pad over a compress to deliver a continuous, controlled source of heat to improve the application's therapeutic effects (see Skill 38-3). Moist hot compresses are used to improve circulation, relieve edema, promote consolidation of exudate in a wound, and promote comfort.

DELEGATION CONSIDERATIONS

The client should be assessed, and the purpose of the treatment explained. If there are no risks or complications, this skill can be delegated to assistive personnel. The caregiver should be cautioned to maintain proper temperature of the application throughout the treatment and to keep the application in place for only the length of time specified in the physician's order. The caregiver should report when treatment is complete so that an evaluation of the client's response can be made.

EQUIPMENT

- Prescribed solution warmed to appropriate temperature
- Sterile gauze dressings or commercially prepared compresses
- Sterile container for solution
- Dry bath towel
- Disposable gloves
- Sterile gloves
- Waterproof pad
- Ties or tape
- Aquathermia or electric heating pad (optional)
- Bath blanket

STEP	RATIONALE

ASSESSMENT

1. Refer to physician's order for type of compress, location and duration of application, desired temperature, and institutional policies regarding temperature of compress. — Ensures safe and correct application.
2. Inspect condition of exposed skin and wound on which compress is to be applied. — Provides baseline to determine changes in skin during heat application.

 • ***Critical Decision Point***
 Very thin or damaged skin is more susceptible to injury from heat. Nonintact skin and drainage from wounds are indications to wear gloves.

3. Assess client's extremities for sensitivity to temperature and pain by measuring light touch, pinprick and temperature sensation (see Chapter 10). — Clients insensitive to heat or cold sensations must be monitored closely during treatment.

 • ***Critical Decision Point***
 Diabetic clients, victims of stroke, spinal cord injury, and clients with peripheral ***neuropathy*** *are particularly at risk for thermal injury (Stitik and Nadler, 1999).*

4. Refer to medical record to identify any systemic contraindications to heat application. — Heat causes vasodilation, which aggravates active bleeding. Heat applied to localized area of acute inflammation or tumor may cause rupture or activate cell growth (Stitik and Nadler, 1999).

 • ***Critical Decision Point***
 Use caution when there is an area of active bleeding or inflammation.

5. Assess client's understanding of application and its purpose. — Determines need for health teaching.

NURSING DIAGNOSIS

Defining characteristics from the assessment data may reveal the following nursing diagnoses for clients requiring this skill:

- Ineffective peripheral tissue perfusion
- Impaired physical mobility
- Impaired skin integrity
- Deficient knowledge regarding moist heat applications
- Pain (acute, chronic)
- Risk for injury
- Sensory perceptual alterations (tactile)

Related factors are individualized based on client's condition or needs.

PLANNING

1. **Expected outcomes** following completion of procedure:
   - Affected site is pink and warm to touch immediately after application. — Vasodilation increases blood flow to site.
   - After multiple applications, wound shows signs of healing (e.g., granulation; reduced edema, inflammation, drainage). — Moist heat increases blood flow, enhances white blood cell infiltration, and removes waste products from cells (Stitik and Nadler, 1999).
   - Client denies burning sensation. — Indicates appropriate temperature applied.
   - Client able to safely apply therapy. — Measures level of learning.
2. Assemble equipment and supplies. — Organization of supplies prevents unnecessary delays in procedure.
3. Explain steps of procedure and purpose to client. Describe sensations to be felt, such as decreasing warmth and wetness. Explain precautions to prevent burning. — Minimizes client's anxiety and promotes cooperation during procedure.

STEP	RATIONALE
IMPLEMENTATION	
1. Close door if in private room, and/or close bedside curtains.	Decreases drafts, thus decreasing the transmission of microorganisms. Provides for client privacy.
2. Assist client in assuming comfortable position in proper body alignment, and place waterproof pad under area to be treated.	Compress remains in place for several minutes. Limited mobility in uncomfortable position causes muscular stress. Pad prevents soiling of bed linen.
3. Expose body part to be covered with compress, and drape client with bath blanket.	Prevents unnecessary cooling and exposure of body part.
4. Wash hands.	Reduces transmission of microorganisms.
5. Prepare compress:	Ensures orderly procedure.
a. Pour solution into sterile container.	
b. If using portable heating source, warm solution. Commercially prepared compresses may remain under infrared lamp until just before use. Open sterile packages, and drop gauze into container to become immersed in solution.	Compresses must retain warmth for therapeutic benefit.

- ***Critical Decision Point***
  Temperature must be tested by applying sterile solution to nurse's forearm (without contaminating solution).

STEP	RATIONALE
6. Prepare aquathermia pad (if needed) (see Skill 38-3).	Temperature usually pre-set by central supply department, ensures safe application.
7. Apply disposable gloves. Remove any existing dressing covering wound. Dispose of gloves and dressings in proper receptacle.	Reduces transmission of microorganisms.
8. Assess condition of wound and surrounding skin. Inflamed wound appears reddened, but surrounding skin is less red in color.	Provides baseline to determine skin changes following compress application.

- ***Critical Decision Point***
  If skin surrounding wound is reddened, application may be contraindicated.

STEP	RATIONALE
9. Apply sterile gloves.	Allows nurse to manipulate sterile dressing and touch open wound.
10. Pick up one layer of immersed gauze, wring out any excess solution, and apply it lightly to open wound and avoid surrounding skin.	Excess moisture macerates skin and increases risk of burns and infection. Skin is sensitive to sudden change in temperature.
11. In few seconds, lift edge of gauze to assess for redness.	Increased redness indicates burn.
12. If client tolerates compress, pack gauze snugly against wound. Be sure all wound surfaces are covered by hot compress.	Packing of compress prevents rapid cooling from underlying air currents.
13. Cover moist compress with dry sterile dressing and bath towel. If necessary, pin or tie in place. Remove sterile gloves.	Dry sterile dressing will prevent transfer of microorganisms to wound via capillary action caused by moist compress. Towel insulates compress to prevent heat loss.
14. Apply aquathermia or waterproof heating pad over a towel (optional) (see Skill 38-3). Keep it in place for desired duration of application.	Provides constant temperature to compress.

- ***Critical Decision Point***
  Removing hot compress after 20 minutes and then reapplying in 15 minutes if desired maintains vasodilation and positive therapeutic effects. Local application of heat for more then 20 minutes may result in reflex vasoconstriction (Stitik and Nadler, 1999).

STEP	RATIONALE
15. If an aquathermia pad is *not* used to maintain temperature of application, change hot compress using sterile technique every 5 minutes or as ordered during duration of therapy.	Prevents cooling and maintains therapeutic benefit of compress.

STEP	RATIONALE
16. After prescribed time, apply disposable gloves and remove pad, towel, and compress. Reassess wound and condition of skin, and replace dry sterile dressing as ordered.	Continued exposure to moisture will macerate skin. Prevents entrance of microorganisms into wound site.
17. Assist client to preferred comfortable position.	Maintains client's comfort.
18. Dispose of equipment and soiled compress. Wash hands.	Reduces transmission of microorganisms.

EVALUATION

1. Inspect affected area covered by compress and heating pad every 5 to 10 minutes.	Assists in determining effects of application.
2. Ask every 5 to 10 minutes if client notices any unusual burning sensation not felt before application.	It may be difficult to assess burn merely by color changes if wound is inflamed or drainage is present.
3. Have client explain and demonstrate application.	Evaluates client's understanding of and ability to perform procedure.

UNEXPECTED OUTCOMES AND RELATED INTERVENTIONS

- Presence of redness or tenderness at affected site. Increased redness and tenderness are signs of first-degree burns.
  - Reduce temperature.
  - Assess for skin breakdown.
- Client complains of burning and discomfort. Individuals vary in their tolerance to heat and pain.
  - Extreme temperature for client to tolerate—reduce temperature.
- Client unable to explain or apply compress correctly.
  - Reinstruction or clarification needed.

RECORDING AND REPORTING

- Record procedure, noting type, location, and duration of application, as well as solution and temperature.
- Record condition of wound and skin before and after treatment and client's response to therapy.
- Record any instructions given and client's ability to explain and perform procedure.
- Report unusual findings to nurse in charge or physician.

TEACHING CONSIDERATIONS

- If heat applications are to be continued after discharge, have client or family member give a return demonstration before discharge.
- Teach client to gently pack wound to avoid discomfort.
- Caregivers and clients need to be taught that careful assessment is needed for clients with reduced sensation to determine if temperature of compress is too hot.

PEDIATRIC CONSIDERATIONS

- The skin of infants and children is thin and fragile and therefore easily damaged. Use special caution in this population (Wong and others, 1999).

GERONTOLOGICAL CONSIDERATIONS

- The older adult client who is receiving long-term steroid therapy or is malnourished can develop thin, fragile skin, which is more easily damaged.
- The older adult may have impaired circulation to a given skin region or impaired sensation for pain/or temperature (Lueckenotte, 2000).

HOME CARE CONSIDERATIONS

- When necessary, assess availability of primary caregiver to assist client in application of compress, caregiver's understanding of purpose of procedure, and willingness of caregiver to comply with procedure and not leave client with compress in place beyond prescribed time limit.
- Assess physical environment to determine existence of adequate facilities to prepare hot compress and provide for sterile technique.

Skill 38-2 Assisting With Warm Soaks and Sitz Baths

Moist heat application also includes the use of warm baths, soaks, and sitz baths. A warm bath or soak usually involves immersion of a body part into a warmed solution. Warm soaks and sitz baths are used to promote circulation, reduce edema and inflammation, promote muscle relaxation, debride wounds, and apply medicated solutions. If a body part is too large to immerse, a soak can be accomplished by wrapping the affected body part in a dressing saturated with the prepared, warmed solution.

A **sitz bath** is given by use of a special tub or chair basin that allows a client to sit in water without immersing the legs, feet, and upper trunk (Figure 38-1). Sitz basins are disposable and especially easy to use in the home. Clients who have undergone perineal or rectal surgery, who have had an episiotomy during childbirth, or who have painful hemorrhoids or perineal inflammation may benefit from a sitz bath.

When preparing a soak or bath, the nurse should remember that the heated solution is in direct contact with the client's skin. It is very important to check water temperature carefully to prevent burns. It is also desirable to keep the solution temperature constant to enhance the moist heat's therapeutic effects. Whenever heated solution is added to a soak basin or bath, the client's body part should be removed and then reimmersed once the solution has mixed.

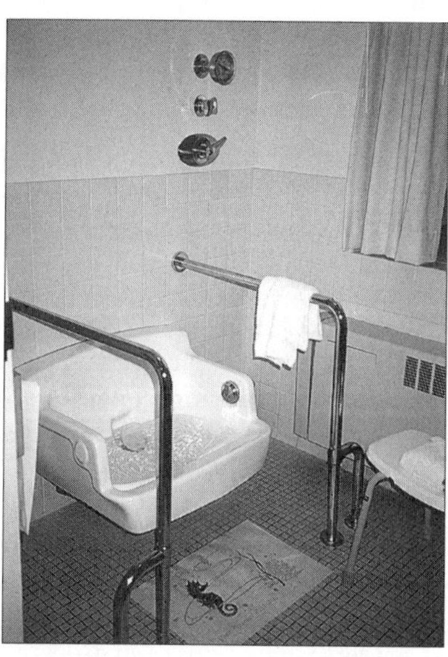

FIGURE **38-1** Sitz bath.

Delegation Considerations

The client should be assessed, and the purpose of the treatment explained. If there are no risks or complications, this skill can be delegated to assistive personnel. The caregiver should be cautioned to maintain proper temperature of the application throughout the treatment and to keep the application in place for only the length of time specified in the physician's order. The caregiver should report when treatment is complete so that an evaluation of the client's response can be made.

Equipment

- Clean basin, tub, or sitz bath (basin may need to be sterile if body part to be soaked has open wound)
- Prescribed solution warmed to proper temperature (tap water is commonly used for sitz baths)
- Bath towel
- Bath blanket
- Absorbent gauze or cloth rolls (optional)
- Prescribed medication (if ordered)
- Waterproof pad for soak
- Gloves

Step	Rationale
Assessment	
1. Check physician's order for desired solution, body part to be soaked, and desired temperature as per institutional policy.	Ensures safe use of moist heat.
2. Refer to medical record to determine client's risk for reduced temperature sensation.	Certain conditions alter conduction of sensory impulses that transmit temperature and pain stimuli.
3. Refer to medical record to identify any systemic contraindications to immersion in warm baths.	Certain cardiovascular conditions and side effects of certain medications place clients at risk for sudden changes in blood pressure and blood flow caused by vasodilation.

- ***Critical Decision Point***

  Clients with history of myocardial infarction, angina pectoris, or hypotension and those using nitroglycerin transdermal patch or ointment are at risk for sudden changes in blood pressure caused by vasodilation.

STEP	RATIONALE
4. Assess and document client's blood pressure and pulse.	Establishes a baseline for comparison.
5. Assess and document condition of skin of body part to be immersed.	Identifies thin or sensitive skin that is prone to injury from temperature extremes. Provides baseline to determine changes in skin during therapy. Identifies open wound, which necessitates use of sterile technique.

- ***Critical Decision Point***
  Sitz baths are frequently used for episiotomy wounds in female clients. Inspect condition of suture line.

STEP	RATIONALE
6. Assess and document client's ability to position self in bath/soak.	Determines level of assistance needed to place client into sitz bath and to remove at end of treatment.
7. Assess and document client's level of comfort using a visual analog scale.	Provides baseline for client's comfort level. Soak or bath may soothe inflamed or injured body parts (Stitik and Nadler, 1999).
8. Assess and document client's understanding of therapy and its purpose.	Determines need for health teaching.

Nursing Diagnosis

Defining characteristics from the assessment data may reveal the following nursing diagnoses for clients requiring this skill:

Ineffective peripheral tissue perfusion
Impaired physical mobility
Impaired skin integrity
Deficient knowledge regarding sitz bath/warm soaks
Pain (acute, chronic)
Risk for injury
Disturbed sensory perception (tactile)

Related factors are individualized based on client's condition or needs.

Planning

STEP	RATIONALE
1. **Expected outcomes** following completion of procedure:	
▪ Client's skin is pink and warm to touch immediately after soak.	Vasodilation increases blood flow to area.
▪ Client will relate a measurable decrease in pain.	Moist heat reduces edema/inflammation and relaxes stiff and strained muscles. Heat applications cause pain signals to be overridden as they enter dorsal horn of spinal column and decreases pain perception in cerebral cortex (Stitik and Nadler, 1999).
▪ Blood pressure and pulse are within client's normal range.	No systemic vascular changes occurred. The goal of therapy is to achieve a localized vascular response.
▪ Client correctly uses heat application.	Demonstrates learning.
2. Prepare equipment and supplies.	Organization of supplies prevents unnecessary delays in procedure.
3. Explain steps of procedure and purpose to client.	Minimizes client's anxiety and promotes cooperation during procedure.

Implementation

STEP	RATIONALE
1. Close door in private room, and/or close bedside curtains.	Maintains privacy.
2. Wash hands.	Reduces transmission of microorganisms.
3. Fill basin or tub with warmed solution. Check temperature.	Checking for correct temperature reduces risk of burns.

- ***Critical Decision Point***
  Test temperature of solution by applying small amount to forearm.

STEP	RATIONALE
4. For soaks, position client comfortably and place waterproof pad under area to be treated.	Prevents soiling of bed linen or clothing.
5. Assist client to immerse body part in tub or basin.	Prevents falls.
6. Cover client with bath blanket or towel as desired.	Prevents chilling and enhances client's ability to relax.
7. Maintain constant temperature throughout 15- to 20-minute soak:	Ensures proper therapeutic effect.
a. Keep large sheet or blanket over container or basin.	Prevents heat loss through **evaporation.** Therapeutic effects of soak can be obtained only from constant temperature.
b. After 10 minutes, remove body part from soak, check to see that skin is not burned, empty cooled solution, add newly heated solution, and reimmerse body part.	Maintains constant therapeutic temperature. Presence of burn contraindicates completing the soak. Adding warmed solution to basin with body part immersed can cause burn.
8. After 15 to 20 minutes, remove client from soak or bath; dry body parts thoroughly. (Clean gloves are required if drainage is present.)	Avoids chilling. Enhances client's comfort.
9. Assist client into comfortable position.	Maintains comfortable environment for client.
10. Drain solution from basin or tub. Clean tub and place in proper storage area. Dispose of soiled linen and gloves (if used); wash hands.	Reduces transmission of microorganisms.

EVALUATION

1. Inspect condition of body part or wound immersed for redness, burns, and pain.	Evaluates effectiveness of treatments and risk for potential injury.
2. Question client regarding presence of burning sensation, severity of pain, and general response to therapy.	Determines if client was exposed to temperature extreme, resulting in burn. Evaluates client's subjective response to therapy.
3. Assess vital signs if client complains of dizziness or light-headedness.	Determines if vascular response to vasodilation has occurred.
4. Ask client to demonstrate procedure and explain purpose of soak or sitz bath.	Measures level of learning.

UNEXPECTED OUTCOMES AND RELATED INTERVENTIONS

- Client's skin is reddened and sensitive to touch. Extreme warmth caused burning of skin layer.
  - Discontinue warm soak immediately.
  - Notify physician.
- Client experiences hypotension and complains of dizziness, nausea, and light-headedness. This is a result of systemic vasodilation.
  - Lower client to floor to avoid a fall.
  - Discontinue treatment immediately.
  - Notify physician.
  - Monitor and document vital signs and mental status.
- Client is unable to explain purpose of procedure or uses soak/bath incorrectly.
  - Reinstruction or clarification is required.

RECORDING AND REPORTING

- Record procedure, including temperature and duration of soak, in nurses' notes.
- Record condition of body part before and after therapy and client's response.
- Record preprocedure and postprocedure vital signs.
- Record any instruction given and client's success in demonstrating procedure.
- Report all client complaints and any unusual observations (e.g., change in vital signs) to nurse in charge or physician.

TEACHING CONSIDERATIONS

- Client may resume therapy at home and should understand risks of burns. Explain risks of using warm baths and methods to ensure safety.
- If heat applications are to be continued after discharge, have client or family member give a return demonstration before discharge.

PEDIATRIC CONSIDERATIONS

- The skin of infants and children is thin and fragile and therefore easily damaged. Use special caution in this population. Remain with children during procedure for safety and effectiveness (Wong and others, 1999).

GERONTOLOGICAL CONSIDERATIONS

- Older adult clients, whose aging process has resulted in loss of subcutaneous tissue and fat and consequently the insulating effect of these substances, may experience alterations in thermoregulation (Lueckenotte, 2000).
- In some clients, such as frail, older clients with cardiac conditions, it may be necessary to monitor vital signs throughout procedure.

HOME CARE CONSIDERATIONS

- When necessary, assess availability of primary caregiver to assist client. If caregiver is not available, evaluate client as to ability, willingness, and understanding of preparing soaks or baths.
- Assess home environment to determine adequacy of facilities for use by client. Medical equipment companies may be contacted for assistance in determining best product for client.

Skill 38-3 Applying Aquathermia and Heating Pads

Aquathermia and heating pads are common forms of dry heat therapy used in health care settings and in the home (Figure 38-2). Both are covered and applied directly to the skin's surface, and for this reason extra precautions are needed to prevent burns. The aquathermia pad (water flow pad) consists of a waterproof rubber or plastic pad connected by two hoses to an electrical control unit that has a heating element and motor. Distilled water circulates through hollowed channels in the pad to the control unit where water is heated (or cooled). The nurse can adjust the temperature setting by inserting a plastic key into the control unit. In most health care institutions, the central supply department sets the temperature regulators to the recommended temperature, approximately 40.5° to 43° C (105° to 109.4° F). Because of the constant temperature control, aquathermia pads tend to be safer than heating pads. If distilled water in the unit runs low, the nurse simply adds more distilled water to the reservoir at the top of the control unit. Rubber and plastic conduct heat, so the pad should be encased in a towel or pillowcase to avoid direct exposure to the skin.

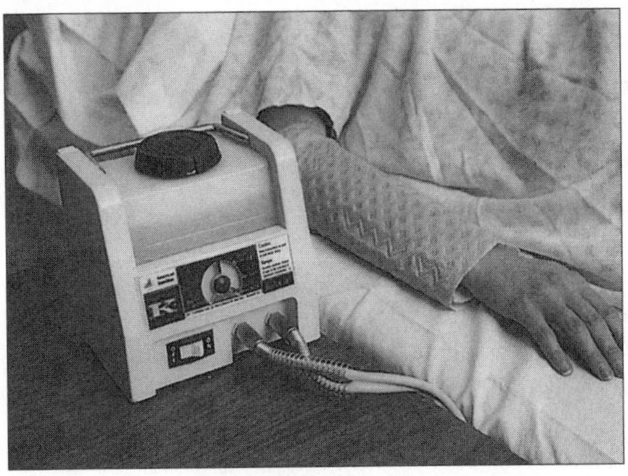

FIGURE 38-2 Aquathermia pad.

The conventional heating pad consists of an electric coil enclosed in a waterproof cover. A cotton or flannel cloth covers the outer pad. The pad connects to an electrical cord that has a temperature-regulating unit for high, medium, or low settings. Because it is so easy to readjust temperature settings on heating pads, clients should be instructed not to turn the setting higher once they have adapted to the temperature. It is wise to avoid ever using the highest setting.

DELEGATION CONSIDERATIONS

The client should be assessed, and the purpose of the treatment explained. If there are no risks or complications, this skill can be delegated to assistive personnel. The caregiver should be cautioned to maintain proper temperature of the application throughout the treatment and to keep the application in place for only the length of time specified in the physician's order. The caregiver should report when treatment is complete so that an evaluation of the client's response can be made.

EQUIPMENT

- Aquathermia or heating pad
- Electrical control unit
- Distilled water (for aquathermia pad)
- Bath towel or pillowcase
- Tape, ties, or gauze roll

Step	Rationale
Assessment	
1. Refer to physician's order for location of application and duration of therapy. Institutional policy usually sets recommended temperature.	Order required to help ensure client's safety.
2. Assess condition of skin over which pad is to be applied.	Provides baseline to determine change in skin condition after heat application.
3. Assess level of discomfort and range of motion if client is being treated for muscle sprain.	Provides baseline to determine if pain relief is achieved.
4. Assess area to be treated for sensitivity to temperature, light touch, and pain (see Chapter 10).	Determines if client is insensitive to heat extremes.
5. Check electrical plugs and cords for obvious fraying or cracking.	Prevents injury from accidental electrical shock.
6. Determine client's or family members' knowledge of procedure, including steps for application and safety precautions.	Heating pads are frequently used in home. Assessment determines extent of health teaching required.

Nursing Diagnosis

Defining characteristics from the assessment data may reveal the following nursing diagnoses for clients requiring this skill:

- Ineffective peripheral tissue perfusion
- Impaired physical mobility
- Impaired skin integrity
- Deficient knowledge regarding moist heat applications
- Pain (acute, chronic)
- Risk for injury
- Disturbed sensory perception (tactile)

Related factors are individualized based on client's condition or needs.

Step	Rationale
Planning	
1. **Expected outcomes** following completion of procedure:	
▪ Skin is pink and warm to touch after application.	Vasodilation from heat exposure increases blood flow to affected part.
▪ Client reports less discomfort of inflamed tissues or strained muscles.	Heat applications lower pain perception by stimulating large-diameter sensory nerve fibers and blocking pain impulses of smaller nerve fibers (Stitik and Nadler, 1999).
▪ Client may be able to move strained muscles more freely.	Heat reduces stiffness and improves range of motion (Stitik and Nadler, 1999).
▪ Client correctly applies pad.	Documents learning.
2. Prepare equipment and supplies.	Organization of supplies prevents unnecessary delays in procedure.
3. Explain procedure and precautions.	Improves likelihood of client's compliance with therapy.
Implementation	
1. Close door if in private room and/or close bedside curtains.	Provides for client's privacy.
2. Wash hands, and position client comfortably so area to be treated may be exposed.	Reduces transfer of microorganisms. Client must be able to assume position for several minutes during application.
3. For aquathermia or uncovered heating pad, cover or wrap affected area with bath towel or enclose pad with pillowcase.	Prevents heated surface from touching client's skin and increasing risk for injury to client's skin.

- ***Critical Decision Point***
  Do not pin the wrap to pad because this may cause a leak in device.

STEP	RATIONALE
4. Place pad over affected area (see Figure 39-2), and secure with tape, tie, or gauze as needed.	Pad delivers dry warm heat to injured tissues. Pad should not slip onto different body part.

- ***Critical Decision Point***
  Never position client so that client is lying directly on pad. This position prevents dissipation of heat and increases risk of burns.

STEP	RATIONALE
5. Turn heating pad on to low or medium setting, and check temperature of aquathermia pad.	Prevents exposure of client to temperature extremes.
6. Monitor condition of skin every 5 minutes during application, and question client regarding sensation of burning.	Determines if heat exposure is resulting in burn.
7. After 20 to 30 minutes (or time ordered by physician), remove pad and store.	Continued exposure will result in burns. Some clients should not have access to pad without supervision.
8. Assist client in returning to preferred comfortable position, dispose of soiled linen, and wash hands.	Promotes relaxing environment. Reduces spread of microorganisms.

EVALUATION

STEP	RATIONALE
1. Inspect condition of skin exposed to heat.	Evaluates response of skin to heat exposure.
2. Ask client if strained muscle or inflamed area continues to be painful.	Heat reduces edema and relieves pain from muscle stiffness and spasm (Stitik and Nadler, 1999).
3. Note if client is able to move strained muscle with less comfort.	Heat relaxes strained muscle.

- ***Critical Decision Point***
  Do not have client actively exercise muscle to evaluate results of therapy. Active exercise can aggravate muscle strain.

STEP	RATIONALE
4. Observe client apply pad.	Measures level of learning.

UNEXPECTED OUTCOMES AND RELATED INTERVENTIONS

- Skin is reddened and sensitive to touch. Symptoms indicate first-degree burn.
  - Remove the pad, and reassess in 5 to 10 minutes.
  - If symptoms continue, notify nurse in charge or contact physician.
- Edema and inflammation are increased. Applying heat too soon after an injury can increase edema through vasodilation.
  - Notify nurse in charge or contact physician.
- Body part is painful to move. Movement stretches burn-sensitive nerve fibers in skin.
  - Discontinue aquathermia or heating pad use. Wait for swelling to resolve before attempting to reapply.
  - Notify nurse in charge or contact physician.
- Client applies heat incorrectly or is unable to relate precautions.
  - Reinstruct client as necessary.

RECORDING AND REPORTING

- Record site of application, duration of therapy, and client's response.
- Describe any instruction given and client's success in demonstrating procedure.
- Report changes in skin integrity such as burns.

TEACHING CONSIDERATIONS

- Highlight safety precautions as they are followed during application.

PEDIATRIC CONSIDERATIONS

- The skin of infants and children is thin and fragile and therefore easily damaged. Use special caution in this population (Wong and others, 1999).

GERONTOLOGICAL CONSIDERATIONS

- Older adults are more at risk for burns because of loss of heat sensation. Check site frequently during all treatments.

HOME CARE CONSIDERATIONS

- Assess client and primary caregiver as to understanding, ability, and motivation to comply with procedure.
- Assess home environment for facilities to comply with implementation of procedure.

Skill 38-4 Applying Cold Applications

Application of cold, or cryotherapy, can be accomplished through many therapeutic modalities, such as moist cold compresses, chemical or cold packs, electromechanical or compression devices, or immersion of a body part into a cold soak. This form of therapy is used to treat localized inflammatory responses that lead to edema, hemorrhage, muscle spasm, or pain (see Table 38-1). Cold can exert a profound physiological effect on the body, reducing inflammation caused by injuries to the musculoskeletal system (Stitik and Nadler, 1998). Because reduction of inflammation is the primary goal, cryotherapy is the treatment of choice for the first 24 to 48 hours after an injury.

Vasoconstriction resulting from cold application reduces blood flow to the injured part and thus reduces fluid accumulation and slows bleeding and hematoma formation associated with trauma. The lower temperature also suppresses muscle spasm and produces a local anesthetic response. When used appropriately, cold applications can significantly lessen pain and immobility by reducing swelling of injured tissues (Murphy and Tkach, 1996; Stitik and Nadler, 1998). This is an important point for nurses to know when deciding on the choice of heat or cold for the treatment of acute injuries. Cold is also indicated as an adjunct analgesic for chronic pain and spasticity control. It can also be used as an analgesic after arthroscopic surgical procedures (Cohn, Draeger, and Jackson, 1989).

A cold compress usually consists of a commercial cold pack, a gauze dressing, or a washcloth that has been immersed in iced or chilled solution to achieve the desired temperature. The compress may be sterile or clean; however, a clean compress is most commonly used. Any open wounds require sterile applications. A variety of sizes or thicknesses of gauze can be used, depending on the site of injury. For example, a cold compress to the eye requires thicker gauze that fits a small area to maintain a cold temperature. Thin gauze works more effectively for larger areas such as the face.

Ice bags and cold packs come in a variety of sizes to fit different body parts (Figure 38-3). When a commercial ice bag or cold pack is unavailable, the client can use a plastic bag or glove filled halfway with crushed ice (Murphy and Tkach, 1996). The bag or glove should be squeezed to expel air, which hampers cold conduction (McConnell, 1998).

There are electrically controlled cooling devices that work much like an aquathermia pad (see Skill 38-3). The cooling pad has the advantage of delivering a constant cool temperature. This type of machine can be recommended as an alternative aid to postoperative pain management in clients undergoing certain orthopedic surgeries (Cohn, Draeger, and Jackson, 1989). Cold modalities that simultaneously provide compression are extremely effective in treating acute musculoskeletal injuries that are associated with soft-tissue swelling. Elevating the extremity during treatment further augments venous return. A person who undergoes treatment with one of these devices is simultaneously receiving all four components of the rest, ice, compression, and elevation (RICE) method for managing this type of injury.

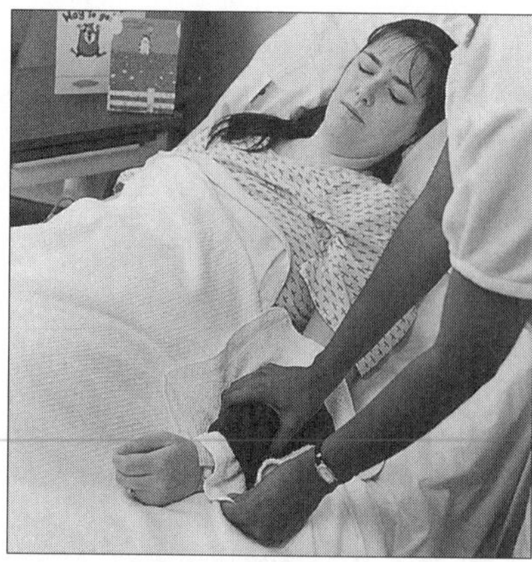

FIGURE 38-3 Placement of ice pack (or bag) on extremity.

Delegation Considerations

The client should be assessed, and the purpose of the treatment explained. If there are no risks or complications, this skill can be delegated to assistive personnel. The caregiver should be cautioned to maintain proper temperature of the application throughout the treatment and to keep the application in place for only the length of time specified in the physician's order. The caregiver should report when treatment is complete so that an evaluation of the client's response can be made.

Equipment

- Cold compress
- Absorbent gauze (clean or sterile) folded to desired size
- Clean or sterile basin with ice and water at desired temperature
- Bath towel or absorbent pad
- Two pairs of disposable or sterile gloves (according to agency policy)
- Cool water flow pad
- Cooling pad and electrical pump
- Compression device with appropriate extremity attachments
- Tapes, ties, gauze roll, or elastic wrap bandage
- Ice bag or collar with water
- Ice pack
- Towel or pillowcase
- Cloth ties or tape
- Gloves (if blood or body fluids are present)

STEP	RATIONALE

ASSESSMENT

1. Refer to physician's order for location and duration of application. — Physician's order is required for all cold applications.
2. Inspect and document condition of injured or affected part. Gently palpate area. — Provides baseline for determining change in condition of injured tissues.

   - ***Critical Decision Point***
     Keep injured part immobilized and in alignment. Movement can cause further injury to strains, sprains, or fractures.

3. Consider time in which injury occurred. — Cold should be applied quickly after an injury to prevent edema. Application of cold is most effective if started within 24 hours of injury.
4. Ask client to describe severity and character of pain using a visual analog scale. — Provides baseline for determining pain relief with therapy.
5. Assess area to be treated for sensitivity to temperature, light touch, and pain and for adequate circulation (see Chapter 10). — Determines if client is insensitive to cold extremes.
6. Assess client's understanding of procedure. — Determines need for health teaching.

NURSING DIAGNOSIS

Defining characteristics from the assessment data may reveal the following nursing diagnoses for clients requiring this skill:

Impaired physical mobility
Impaired skin integrity
Deficient knowledge regarding moist cold applications
Pain (acute, chronic)
Risk for injury
Ineffective peripheral tissue perfusion

Related factors are individualized based on client's condition or needs.

PLANNING

1. **Expected outcomes** following completion of procedure:
   - Affected area is slightly pale and cool to touch. — Result of vasoconstriction.
   - Extent of edema is decreased. — Cold reduces blood flow to affected part, reducing edema formation (Stitik and Nadler, 1998).
   - Client relates measurable decrease in pain. — Cold creates local anesthetic effect (Cohn, Draeger, and Jackson, 1989).
   - Client correctly states how to apply cold compress and provides demonstration. — Documents learning.
2. Prepare equipment and supplies. — Organization prevents unnecessary delays.
3. Explain procedure and precautions. — Improves likelihood of client's compliance with therapy.

IMPLEMENTATION

1. Close room door and bedside curtain. — Provides privacy for client.
2. Wash hands. — Reduces spread of microorganisms.
3. Position client carefully, keeping body part in proper alignment and exposing only area to be treated. — Prevents further injury to body part. Avoids unnecessary exposure of body parts, maintaining client's comfort and privacy.

   - ***Critical Decision Point***
     In cases of strains, sprains, or fractures, extremity or body part should remain aligned to prevent further injury.

STEP	RATIONALE
4. Place towel or absorbent pad under area to be treated.	Prevents soiling of bed linen.
5. Apply disposable gloves.	Reduces spread of infection.
6. Cold compress:	
a. Check temperature of solution, and submerge gauze into filled basin at bedside; wring out excess moisture.	Extreme temperature can cause tissue damage. Dripping gauze is uncomfortable to client.
b. Apply compress to affected area, molding it gently over site.	Ensures that cold is directed over site of injury.
7. Electrically controlled cooling device:	
a. Wrap cool water flow pad around body part (see illustration).	Ensures even application of cold temperature.
b. Be sure correct temperature is set.	Ensures effective therapy.
c. Secure with elastic wrap bandage, gauze roll, or ties.	

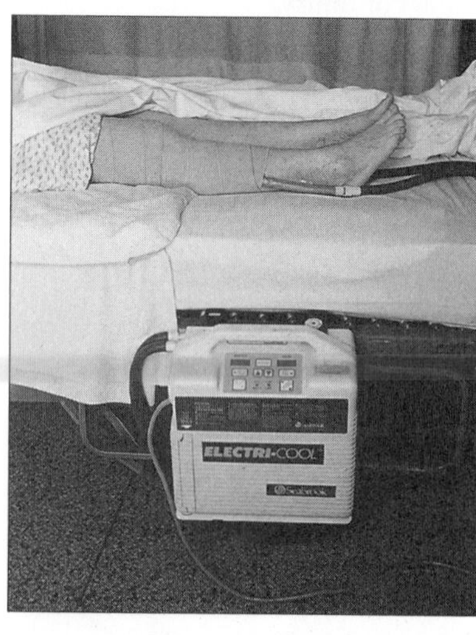

STEP **7a** Cooling device.

STEP	RATIONALE
8. Prepare ice bag or collar:	
a. Fill bag with water, secure cap, and invert.	Checks for leaks.
b. Empty water, and then fill bag two-thirds full with small ice chips.	Bag can be more easily molded over body part.
c. Release excess air from bag by squeezing its sides before securing cap.	Excess air interferes with cold conduction (McConnell, 1998).
d. Wipe bag dry.	Prevents skin maceration.
e. Apply snugly over area. Secure with tape as needed.	Cold should be directly over injury.
9. Prepare ice pack:	
a. Commercial packs are squeezed or kneaded.	Releases alcohol-based solution to create cold temperature.

• ***Critical Decision Point***
Moisture may form on outside of bag if room temperature is warm. This does not indicate a leak.

STEP	RATIONALE
b. Apply pack directly over area. Cover prepared bag or pack with towel or pillowcase.	Cold should be applied directly over injury. Protects client's tissue and absorbs condensation (McConnell, 1998). Prevents direct exposure of cold against client's skin.

• ***Critical Decision Point***
Do not reapply ice pack to red or bluish areas; continual use of ice pack makes ischemia worse.

STEP	RATIONALE
10. Remove gloves and dispose of in proper container.	Reduces transfer of microorganisms.
11. Check condition of skin every 5 minutes for duration of application:	Determines if there are adverse reactions to cold. These include mottling, redness, burning, blistering, and numbness (Stitik and Nadler, 1998).
a. If area is edematous, sensation may be reduced, and extra caution must be used during cold therapy.	

STEP	RATIONALE
b. Numbness and tingling are common sensations with cold applications and indicate adverse reactions only when severe and coupled with other symptoms. Stop when client complains of burning sensation or skin begins to feel numb.	When applying cold, skin will initially feel cold, followed by relief of pain. As cryotherapy continues, client will feel a burning sensation, then pain in the skin, and finally numbness (Stamford, 1996; Stitik and Nadler, 1998).
12. After 15 to 20 minutes (or as ordered by the physician), apply clean gloves, remove compress or pad, and gently dry off any moisture.	Drying prevents maceration of skin. Prolonged application of cold can result in diminished blood flow and tissue ischemia or compensatory vasodilation to provide warmth to area being treated (Stitik and Nadler, 1998).

• ***Critical Decision Point***
Areas with little body fat (such as knee, ankle, and elbow) do not tolerate cold as well as fatty areas (such as thigh and buttocks). For bony areas, decrease time of cold application to lower range.

STEP	RATIONALE
13. Assist client to comfortable position.	Maintains relaxing environment.
14. Empty basin, dry, and store. Dispose of soiled linen and gloves; wash hands.	Reduces transfer of microorganisms.

EVALUATION

STEP	RATIONALE
1. Inspect affected area for changes in condition of skin.	Determines reaction to cold compress application.
2. Palpate affected area gently.	Determines level of edema.
3. Question client about level of comfort.	Determines if pain has been relieved.
4. Ask client to apply cold application and explain risks of treatment.	Measures level of learning.

UNEXPECTED OUTCOMES AND RELATED INTERVENTIONS

- Skin takes on mottled, reddened, or bluish purple appearance as a result of prolonged exposure.
  - Stop the treatment.
  - Notify nurse in charge or physician.
  - Injury from prolonged exposure requires different therapy.
- Client complains of burning type of pain and numbness.
  - Stop the treatment because these are signs of ischemia.
  - Notify nurse in charge or physician.
- Client is unable to describe application or use compress correctly.
  - Reinstruction and clarification are necessary.

RECORDING AND REPORTING

- Record procedure, including type, location, duration of application, and client's response, in nurses' notes. Documents therapy provided and client's response.
- Describe any instruction given and client's success in demonstrating procedure. Documents client's response to teaching efforts.
- Report undesirable changes in condition of skin to nurse in charge or physician. Injury from prolonged exposure requires different therapy.

TEACHING CONSIDERATIONS

- Injuries requiring this type of therapy usually occur away from health care settings. Clients active in sports should know steps to take to minimize extent of injury.

PEDIATRIC CONSIDERATIONS

- A greater metabolic rate and larger trunk in relation to rest of body make children more prone to hypothermia (Thomas, 1996). Exercise caution with young clients.
- Infants have an unstable temperature control mechanism, so mottling of extremities is common and may not indicate an adverse reaction if this symptom is seen alone (Thomas, 1996).

GERONTOLOGICAL CONSIDERATIONS

- Older adults are more at risk for tissue damage due to loss of cold sensation. Check site frequently during all treatments.

HOME CARE CONSIDERATIONS

- Clean cloth can be used in home setting as long as there is no open wound.
- Assess client and primary caregiver as to understanding, ability, and motivation to comply with procedure.
- Assess client's home environment for adequacy of facilities with which to implement procedure.
- An ice pack can be improvised by placing ice cubes in a zippered plastic bag or by using a bag of frozen peas or corn. Place a thin towel between bag and skin.

Skill 38-5 Caring for Clients Requiring Hypothermia or Hyperthermia Blankets

The hypothermia-hyperthermia blanket raises, lowers, or maintains body temperature through conductive heat or cold transfer between the blanket and the client. When operated manually, the unit maintains a set temperature regardless of the client's temperature. Because the client's temperature is assessed using conventional thermometers, the unit's temperature is manually adjusted to reach a different temperature setting.

When operating in the automatic setting, the unit continually monitors the client's temperature using a thermistor probe (rectal, skin, or esophageal). Temperature heating and cooling cycles alternate to achieve and maintain the desired temperature.

Clients can have high, prolonged fevers from infectious and neurological diseases and as side effects from anesthesia. When there is difficulty controlling a fever in a client, one measure is the use of a hypothermia (cooling) blanket. Hypothermia blankets are fluid-filled rubberized blankets that circulate cooled solution (usually distilled water) through the blanket. When the client lies on the device, the cooling blanket helps to reduce the client's body temperature (Figure 38-4).

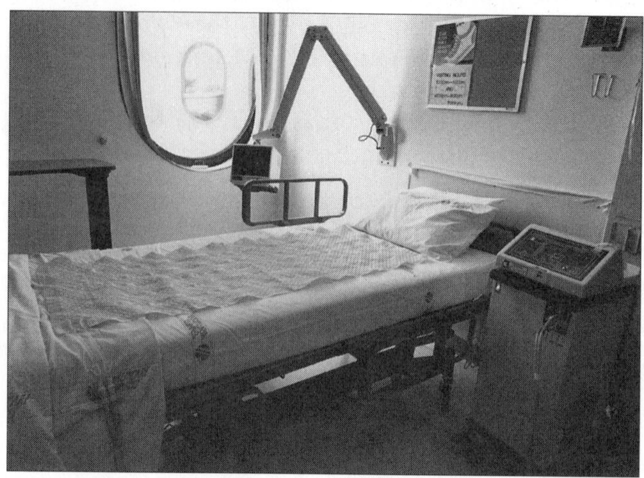

FIGURE **38-4** Hypothermia cooling blanket before sheet applied to bed.

Conversely, clients whose body temperature is abnormally low due to extreme exposure to cold or due to hypothermia induced for neurological or cardiac surgery require a hyperthermia (warming) blanket to assist the body in returning to near-normal temperature. In the case of hyperthermia or rewarming therapy, a warmed solution is circulated through the blanket to help return the client's body temperature to normal.

Delegation Considerations

The client should be assessed, and the purpose of the treatment explained. If there are no risks or complications, this skill can be delegated to assistive personnel. The caregiver should be cautioned to maintain proper temperature of the application throughout the treatment and to discontinue the application as specified in the physician's order. The caregiver should report when treatment is complete so that an evaluation of the client's response can be made.

Equipment

- Hypothermia or hyperthermia blanket with control panel and rectal probe
- Sheet or thin bath blanket
- Distilled water to fill the units if necessary
- Disposable gloves
- Rectal thermometer

Step	Rationale
Assessment	
1. Refer to physician's order and double-check that client's current body temperature requires use of hypothermia or hyperthermia blanket.	Institution of therapy requires physician's order.
2. Assess vital signs, neurological status, mental status, and peripheral circulation.	Establishes baseline data to use for comparison during therapy.
3. Verify that other, less intensive measures cannot return client's body temperature to normal.	Use of hypothermia and hyperthermia blanket is not without risk and should be instituted only when other measures are not effective (Henker, 1999).

- ***Critical Decision Point***
  Antipyretic therapy should be attempted for fever. Physiological manifestations of fever include increased oxygen consumption, increased heart rate, increased cardiac output, and elevated levels of catecholamines, which can be detrimental to seriously or critically ill clients (McKenzie, 1998, Henker, 1999).

STEP	RATIONALE
4. Assess client's skin on ears, hands, fingers, heels, sacrum, and other bony prominences before therapy. Inspect scrotal surface of male client.	These areas are more exposed to blanket and consequently are at greater risk for injury. Baseline data enable nurse to quickly determine if injury to skin is result of therapy.

NURSING DIAGNOSIS

Defining characteristics from the assessment data may reveal the following nursing diagnoses for clients requiring this skill:

- Ineffective peripheral tissue perfusion
- Impaired physical mobility
- Impaired skin integrity
- Deficient knowledge regarding implications of hypothermia or hyperthermia blanket
- Pain (acute, chronic)
- Risk for injury
- Fever
- Disturbed sensory perception (tactile)

Related factors are individualized based on client's condition or needs.

PLANNING

STEP	RATIONALE
1. **Expected outcomes** following completion of procedure:	
▪ Temperature is within normal range.	Indicates that therapy is effective.
▪ Absence of shivering with hypothermia blanket.	Shivering increases metabolic rate and heat production but also increases oxygen consumption. This mechanism contributes to body temperature elevation and can cause client's body temperature to rise (Henker, 1999). In addition, shivering causes vasoconstriction, which can injure skin of distal body regions (McKenzie, 1998).
▪ Skin clear without signs of injury or burns.	Distal regions of client's skin are at greatest risk for injury from blanket. Indicates that treatment is causing no adverse effects.
2. Explain procedure to client.	Increases cooperation and reduces anxiety.
3. Position client comfortably.	
4. Prepare blanket according to agency policy and manufacturer's instructions.	Agencies have specific policies as to who should maintain equipment in functional order. Each type of blanket varies from one manufacturer to another. Manufacturer's instructions are located on machine. Read before using.

IMPLEMENTATION

STEP	RATIONALE
1. Wash hands and apply gloves.	Reduces transmission of microorganisms.
2. Take baseline temperature, pulse, respirations, and blood pressure.	Provides baseline for determining response to therapy.
3. Apply lanolin or mixture of lanolin and cold cream to client's skin where it will touch blanket.	Helps protect skin from heat and cold sensations.
4. Turn on blanket, and observe that cool or warm light is on. Precool or prewarm blanket, setting pad temperature to desired level.	Verifies that blanket is correctly set to assist in reducing (cool) or increasing (warm) client's body temperature. Prepares blanket for prescribed therapy.
5. Verify that pad temperature limits are set at desired safety ranges.	Safety ranges prevent excessive cooling or warming. The blanket automatically shuts off when preset body temperature is achieved.
6. Cover the hypothermia or hyperthermia blanket with a thin sheet or bath blanket.	Protects client's skin from direct contact with blanket, thus reducing risk of injury to skin. Sheet or blanket covers plastic and provides insulation between client and appliance.

Step	Rationale
7. Position hypothermia or hyperthermia blanket under client.	Provides wide distribution of blanket against client's skin.

- ***Critical Decision Point***
  When using blanket for hypothermia, placement of blanket under client provides potential for formation of pressure ulcers because of the combination of pressure and decreased blood flow in the skin.

Step	Rationale
a. Wrap client's hands and feet in gauze.	This reduces risk of thermal injury to body's distal areas.
b. Elevate scrotum off blanket surface with towels.	Protects sensitive tissue from direct contact with cold.
8. Lubricate rectal probe and insert into client's rectum.	When using hypothermia or hyperthermia blanket, it is imperative that nurse continuously monitor client's core internal (rectal) temperature.
9. Turn and position client regularly to protect from pressure ulcer development and impaired body alignment (see Chapter 27). Keep linens free of perspiration and condensation.	Client has an increased risk of pressure ulcer development because of skin moisture created by blanket and client's body temperature (Henker, 1999).
10. Double-check fluid thermometer on control panel of blanket before leaving room.	Verifies that pad temperature is maintained at desired level.
11. Remove gloves and wash hands.	Reduces transmission of microorganisms.

Evaluation

Step	Rationale
1. Monitor client's temperature and vital signs every 15 minutes during first hour, every 30 minutes during second hour, and every hour of therapy thereafter.	Provides continuous evaluation of response of client's body temperature to therapy during initial and continual therapy.
2. Evaluate automatic temperature control every 30 minutes visually and every 4 hours by taking client's rectal temperature with glass thermometer.	Ensures removal of hypothermia or hyperthermia blanket when client's temperature returns to desired level. Decreases risk of subnormal body temperature. Verifies accuracy of rectal probe and automatic temperature control device.

- ***Critical Decision Point***
  It is generally accepted to discontinue hypothermia treatment when the client's core temperature is 1° F above desired temperature.

Step	Rationale
3. Observe skin for indications of burns, change in color, and other signs of injury.	Hypothermia and hyperthermia blankets have the potential to cause skin injuries.
4. Observe client for signs of shivering.	Early signs of shivering, which may harm client, include electrocardiographic changes, facial muscle twitching, or hyperventilation.
5. Determine client's level of comfort.	Therapy has the potential to cause discomfort. Prompt assessment reduces risk for severe injuries.

Unexpected Outcomes and Related Interventions

- Client's core body temperature decreases or rises rapidly. This indicates that temperature is too extreme and might produce injury to client.
  - Adjust blanket temperature no more than 1° F every 15 minutes to avoid complications.
- Client's core temperature remains unchanged.
  - Client may need hypothermic or hyperthermic treatment of additional sites, such as axilla, groin, and neck, in addition to those covered by blanket.
  - Discuss use of an antipyretic with physician.
- Client begins to shiver. Shivering increases metabolic rate and heat production, causing client's core body temperature to rise, and increases oxygen consumption.
  - Increase the temperature to a more comfortable range, and assess if shivering decreases.
  - If shivering continues, stop treatment and notify physician.
- Skin breaks down, indicating that client's skin may have received thermal injury (frostbite or burn) from blanket.
  - Stop treatment.
  - Notify physician.

RECORDING AND REPORTING

- Record baseline data: vital signs, neurological and mental status, status of peripheral circulation and skin integrity when therapy was initiated. This will document client's status before instituting therapy.
- Note type of hyperthermia-hypothermia unit used; control settings (manual or automatic, and temperature settings); date, time, duration, and client's tolerance of treatment.
- Chart on temperature graphic repeated measurements of vital signs to document response to therapy.
- Report any unexpected outcome to physician. Further treatment may be needed.

TEACHING CONSIDERATIONS

- Clients and their families need to be instructed not to move client off blanket.

PEDIATRIC CONSIDERATIONS

- A greater metabolic rate and larger trunk in relation to rest of body make children more prone to hypothermia (Thomas, 1996). Exercise caution with young clients.
- Infants have an unstable temperature control mechanism, so mottling of extremities is common and may not indicate an adverse reaction.

GERONTOLOGICAL CONSIDERATIONS

- Older adults are more at risk for tissue damage because of loss of cold sensation. Check client frequently during all treatments.

Critical Thinking Exercises

1. Your teenage client requires a cold application to the left ankle for 48 hours because of a sprain suffered during a soccer game. What instructions would you provide for applying a cold pack at home?
2. Your client has been diagnosed with severe muscle strain of the lower back, and the physician has ordered heat applications to the back for 48 hours. What discharge instructions will you provide?
3. What criteria do you use to decide whether to use hot or cold therapy?

References

Cohn B, Draeger R, Jackson DW: The effects of cold therapy in the postoperative management of pain in patients undergoing anterior cruciate ligament reconstruction, *Am J Sports Med* 17(3):344, 1989.

Henker R: Evidence-based practice: fever-related interventions, *Am J Crit Care* 8(1):481, 1999.

Lueckenotte AG: *Gerontologic nursing,* ed 2, St. Louis, 2000, Mosby.

McConnell E: Clinical do's & don'ts: applying cold treatment, *Nursing* 28(6):26, 1998.

McKenzie NE: Fever: upping the body's thermostat, *Nursing* 28(10):41, 1998.

Murphy P, Tkach T: The heat is on: treating heat related emergencies, *J Emerg Med Serv* 21(6):54, 1996.

Stamford B: Giving injuries the cold treatment, *Physician Sports Med* 24(3):99, 1996.

Stitik T, Nadler S: I. When—and how—to use cold most effectively, *Consultant* 38(12):2881, 1998.

Stitik T, Nadler S: II. When—and how—to apply the heat, *Consultant* 39(1):144, 1999.

Thomas D: Assessing children: it's different, *RN* 59(4):38, 1996.

Wong DL and others: *Whaley and Wong's nursing care of infants and children,* ed 6, St. Louis, 1999, Mosby.

39

Home Care Safety

Skills

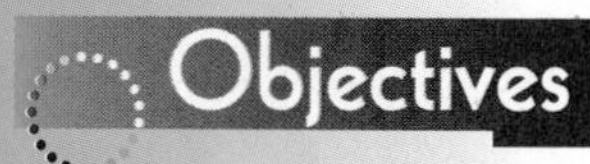

Objectives

Mastery of content in this chapter will enable the nurse to:

- Define the key terms listed.
- Identify clients at risk for accidents.
- Promote self-care of clients in the home.
- Describe factors within a home environment that create risks for injury for clients.
- Perform a home safety risk assessment.
- Identify interventions that will modify the home environment for physical safety.
- Identify interventions to reduce safety risks for clients with sensory, cognitive, and mental status alterations.
- Recommend strategies to ensure safe drug administration within the home.

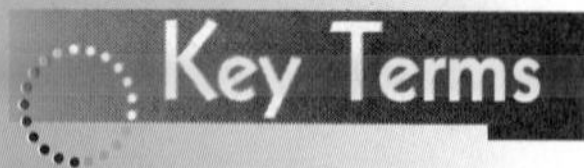

Key Terms

Alzheimer's disease
Dementia
Polypharmacy
Reminiscing
Respite care

Safety implies that people feel secure in their surroundings. In Maslow's hierarchy of needs, safety includes security, stability, protection, and freedom from fear and anxiety (Maslow, 1954). Thus safety has both a physical and an emotional component. For example, if a wheelchair-bound client has removed door frames to allow for better bathroom access, the physical improvements will enhance the client's confidence to maneuver within the home. When a person's environment is safe, the potential to provide self-care is maximized. In addition, the client will emotionally feel less anxious about interacting within the environment.

Accidents are a common health problem in the United States, Canada, and other nations. Billions of dollars are spent annually as a result of accidents in the home. These accidents occur as a result of environmental threats and limitations and disabilities experienced by individuals. Accident prevention often begins with making timely and adequate home repairs. However, many clients do not have the resources needed to ensure a safe home environment by keeping the home in good repair. The nurse plays an important role in improving a client's safety conscience, whatever resources the client may bring to a situation. The nurse collaborates with clients, family members, and other health care providers in the community in finding the best approaches for meeting a client's safety needs. The ultimate goal is to create an environment in which the client and family can provide self-care safely and effectively.

A nurse faces many situations when assisting clients in making their homes safe environments to live in. Nurses care for clients who develop serious physical and emotional limitations and who are unable to fully recover before having to return home. In many cases it may take clients weeks, months, or years to recover from traumatic injuries. For example, the nurse must face basic questions such as can clients reach the things they need if they are bed or chair bound? Is the immediate environment safe for other family members? What care requirements does the client have that cannot be easily accomplished in the home environment? Anticipation of the client's needs is essential so that clients and families can adapt their home environment as necessary. Home care nurses must continually be alert for safety factors that place clients at risk for injury. Family caregiving is on the rise as more people are providing ongoing support to family members and friends in the home. The home care nurse becomes very adept at partnering closely with clients and family members so that the client's nursing care needs can be met within the home without disrupting normal lifestyles unnecessarily. Finally, nurses in any setting must assess for patterns of health care problems (e.g., falls, burns, or medication errors) that may point to safety problems in the home.

Home care clients include the chronically ill, disabled children with physical and mental impairment, victims of acute medical illness and traumatic accidents, and the terminally ill. One group of clients that has significant risk for experiencing threats to safety within the home are older adults because of the physiological changes that accompanying aging, including a slower reaction time; muscular weakness; reduced pain perception; reduced visual acuity, depth perception, and color discrimination; and reduced hearing acuity. Because of older adults' vulnerability, it becomes the nurse's responsibility to restore pattern, order, and environmental predictability to a client's personal life space as possible (Ebersole and Hess, 1998). Despite older adults' risks, they learn how to negotiate their environments relatively well and are usually more aware of potential dangers. Thus older adults may often be more cautious than younger persons and are amenable to changes that bring a sense of security and safety. However, the onset of an acute illness can change this and may require special effort to restore the older adult's sense of security.

There is a percentage of the older adult population affected by cognitive and mental status alterations such as **dementia,** delirium, or **Alzheimer's disease.** The nature and implications of behavioral manifestations for each of these syndromes is beyond the scope of this textbook. However, it is important to recognize that if an older adult suffers memory loss, confusion, poor orientation, or reduced attention span, accidents can easily occur. Care providers are challenged with the choice of maintaining a person's autonomy versus taking steps to prevent accidents or injuries that ensure the person's physical safety and protection (Lueckenotte, 2000).

Clients of all ages have safety risks when they experience alterations that impair their mobility, sensory function, or cognitive thought processes. If a loss or reduction in a persons' ability to function within the environment occurs suddenly, the person may resist environmental changes, attempting to deny any limitations. In this case, the client may try to initiate self-care actions without needed guidance or modification to the environment. For the client whose functional loss has been gradual, the accommodation may require only minimal revision. However, for the client whose alteration has been gradual and unnoticed by the client, such as with Alzheimer's disease, more aggressive revisions may be needed from the client, family, and/or nurse.

Lueckenotte (2000) defines preventive safety as the interruption of a sequence of events that could result in an accident. To successfully prevent or reduce the number of accidents in the home, it is necessary to consider what predisposes a person to an accident and how the environment can be modified to minimize the risk. The skills within this chapter are focused on helping clients retain their independence while implementing preventive safety measures within the home.

Skill Performance Guidelines

1. Any changes in a client's home environment should be made to retain as much of the client's independence and ability to provide self-care as possible.
2. Before recommending any revisions to clients' home environment, it is necessary to know their preferences, values, and financial resources.
3. Whenever possible, let the client be the final decision maker in the types of alterations to be made.
4. Reinforce with family or friends who assume the role of caregiver the importance of preserving client autonomy as much as possible.
5. Any modifications to the home environment should be made after considering clients' physical strengths and remaining functional abilities instead of their disabilities.
6. Promoting self-care is the goal of maintaining or establishing a safe environment.

Skill 39-1 Modifying Safety Risks in the Home Environment

The home environment should be a place that is healthy, comfortable, and safe. People want to be able to move about freely within their homes, regardless of the home's size, and to have a sense of control over daily living routines. This requires maintenance of personal space and a sense of privacy. Ebersole and Hess (1998) point out that older adults in particular maintain a sense of personal space by clutter and placement of personal items. However, all persons create a personal space in their homes with which they can identify and maneuver about without having to think about every action or movement.

Clients requiring home care have often experienced physical alterations that create deficits requiring changes to be made in their home environment. In the case of older adults, the progressive physical changes of aging can create the same type of need. The changes should complement the client's remaining strengths. For example, if a client has poor balance but good upper arm strength, modifications could be made so that the client can safely walk or move throughout the house, ascend and descend stairs, and enter and exit a bathtub or shower. Side rails along hallways and stairwells and grab bars in the bathroom are good solutions. A nurse who cares for a client who requires changes in the home environment must respect the concept of personal space. Making changes too rapidly without the client's consent may cause more problems than benefits. The nurse must appreciate the arrangement of the client's space within the home and not move things or suggest modifications without permission. Knowing the rooms the client most frequently uses can help in making the adjustments that will most likely create a safe environment.

An important part of making changes in the home environment is conducting a safety assessment. The home safety assessment covers all major living areas and helps to identify which changes are of greater priority than others. Frequently the nurse consults with physical and occupational therapists on the type of adjustments necessary. Well-planned environmental changes can reinforce the capabilities rather than the disabilities of a client. Independence can be enhanced to secure a better quality of life for clients and family members.

Delegation Considerations

Some of the principles that are involved in changing the home environment are both practical and commonsense in approach. Assistive personnel such as home health aides often interact with clients and make suggestions for ways to make the home safer. However, an RN is best qualified to conduct a thorough home safety assessment and to determine what alterations or revisions are preferred on the basis of the client's physical and/or cognitive limitations. The RN briefs assistive personnel on cognitive enhancing techniques (e.g., keeping calendars up to date) and on approaches to ensure client safety.

Equipment

- Home safety checklist

STEP	RATIONALE
ASSESSMENT	
1. Review previous physical findings, or conduct an assessment of the client's vision, hearing, musculoskeletal, and neurological function (see Chapter 10).	May reveal sensory alterations or problems with strength, coordination, or balance that predispose client to injury.
2. Determine if client has had a history of falls or other injuries within home. Be specific in your assessment. Follow this acronym, SPLATT: *S*ymptoms at time of fall *P*revious fall *L*ocation of fall *A*ctivity at time of fall *T*ime of fall *T*rauma postfall (Lueckenotte, 2000)	Key symptoms can be helpful in identifying cause for fall. Onset, location, and activity associated with fall provide further details on causative factors and how future falls might be prevented.
3. Have client who has had near fall or actual fall maintain a fall diary (Box 39-1).	Information in fall diary is very helpful in determining antecedents and consequences of falling (Lueckenotte, 2000).
4. Review any risk factors client may have for being predisposed to accidents within home:	
a. Known visual impairment	Reduced visual function may alter client's balance, prevent clear perception of objects along client's normal walkways, or interfere with adaptation to the dark or glaring light.
b. Hearing impairment	Prevents client from hearing normal environmental sounds clearly as a source of orientation. Also prevents clear perception of any home-installed alarms (e.g., smoke alarm).
c. Neuromuscular dysfunction (e.g., lower-extremity weakness, unsteady gait, impaired balance, poor ankle dorsiflexion)	Factors predispose clients to fall. Recurrent falls are associated with difficulty standing up from a chair (Corbett and Pennypacker, 1992). Poor ankle dorsiflexion impairs reflex to right oneself during phases of a fall (Tideiksaar, 1998).
d. Reduced energy or fatigue	Predisposes to falls.
e. Incontinence	Frequent trips to bathroom often cause client with other deficits to accidentally trip or fall over barriers.
f. History of stroke, diabetes, or spinal cord injury	Conditions cause changes in peripheral sensation of extremities, preventing client from perceiving hot or cold extremes.
g. Postural hypotension, palpitations, difficulty breathing, or shortness of breath.	Dizziness of light-headedness predisposes to falls.
5. Determine if client has a fear of falling. Possible indicators include apprehension during ambulation (observed in facial expressions), sweating or trembling while ambulating, clutching persons or objects while ambulating, reluctance to change position or ambulate, and new onset of wobbly, reduced mobility after a fall (Gray-Micelli, 1997).	Fear of falling occurs variably in older adult population (Arfken and others, 1994; Gray-Micelli, 1997). Clinicians believe that fear of falling causes individual to take unnatural precautions that may predispose client to fall.

- ***Critical Decision Point***
  Use family as a resource in assessment. Family may witness accident trends or patterns.

Box 39-1 Fall/Near Fall Diary

- Obtain a spiral notebook, or keep several pieces of 8½ × 11 inch paper together. Across the longest edge of the paper, write the headings: "Date," "Time of Fall," "Activity at Time of Fall," "Symptoms," and "Injury."
- As soon as possible after a fall has occurred, complete information under each heading.
- If a family member witnesses the fall, have him or her record on a separate page what was observed.
- Have listed in the fall diary an emergency contact number for clients to call in case a fall results in a serious injury.
- Have client who has experienced a fall bring diary to the health care provider's office at the next scheduled visit.

Modified from Lueckenotte A: *Gerontologic nursing,* ed 2, St. Louis, 2000, Mosby.

Step	Rationale
6. With client and family as active participants, conduct home safety assessment:	Provides comprehensive review of all areas within home that may pose barriers and hazardous situations.
a. Front and back entrances	
(1) Are walkways to the front/back door even and free from holes or cracks?	Entrances may pose barriers in surfaces over which client must walk.
(2) Are home entrances well lighted, including walkways?	Poorly lit areas prevent individuals from seeing variations in walking surface.
(3) Does client have nonskid strips/safety treads or bright-colored paint on outdoor steps? What colors are most easily seen by client?	Nonskid surfaces cause fewer slips on stairs. Color on steps permits individual to see edges, accommodating for any reduced depth perception.
(4) Are doormats in good repair with nonskid backing and tapered edge?	
(5) Can client open and close all doors easily?	Act of opening and closing door can cause a fall.
(6) Is there a sturdy handrail on both sides of stairs leading to entrance?	Handrails provide greater support while ascending and descending stairs.
(7) Are steps in good condition with even, flat surfaces?	
(8) Does client have a shelf or bench by front/back door to place grocery bags or other packages to make entry easy?	
b. Kitchen	
(1) Does client wear clothing with short or close-fitting sleeves when cooking?	Kitchen is one of the most hazard-oriented rooms in house and poses serious hazards for fire. Client learns importance of staying attentive when cooking and minimizing risks.
(2) Does client always stay in kitchen when cooking?	
(3) Does client have a loud timer to signal when food is cooked?	
(4) Does client keep stove top and oven clean and grease free?	
(5) Are stove control dials easy to see and use?	
(6) Is easy-to-use fire extinguisher close at hand?	

- ***Critical Decision Point***
  Have client walk through steps of how to use extinguisher.

Step	Rationale
(7) Are there emergency numbers for police, fire, and poison control posted on or near telephone?	Emergency phone numbers and extinguisher ensure quick response should fire break out.
(8) Can items in kitchen cabinets and shelves be reached without climbing on a stool or chair? Is step stool sturdy and in good repair?	Climbing on step stools or chairs poses risks for falls.
(9) Is there adequate lighting over sink, stove, and work areas?	Poor lighting may make it difficult to see control knobs or dials or provides inadequate illumination when using sharp knives or utensils.
(10) Does client wipe up spills on floor immediately?	
(11) Are kitchen throw rugs and mats slip resistant?	
c. Bathrooms	
(1) Can bathroom door lock be unlocked from both sides of door?	Bathroom is also a hazard-oriented room. Wet floors and tub or shower bottoms can be very slippery, creating risk of falls.
(2) Is tub or shower equipped with nonskid mats, abrasive strips, or surfaces that are not slippery?	
(3) Does bathroom floor have nonslip surface or rug with nonskid backing?	
(4) Does client avoid using slippery bath oils when bathing?	Use of bath oils can make tub surface slippery and increase risk of falls.

- ***Critical Decision Point***
  If client uses oils, recommend draining tub and placing towel in bottom of tub before attempting to get out.

Step	Rationale
(5) Do bathtub and shower have at least one grab bar that is different color than that of the wall?	Grab bars provide extra support while maneuvering into and out of tubs or showers.
(6) Is client careful not to place towels on grab bars?	
(7) Does shower have stable stool or chair and hand-held sprayer?	Shower stool allows client to sit while showering.
(8) Are cold and hot water faucets clearly marked, and is temperature on water heater 120° F or lower?	Accidental burns can occur from exposure to hot water.
d. Bedroom	
(1) Is a night-light placed in bedroom and/or bath?	Older adults have poor night vision.
(2) Is a working smoke detector just outside bedroom door?	Alarm situated just outside bedroom can awaken person early enough to escape fire.
(3) Can client turn on light without having to get out of bed in the dark?	Getting out of bed, without proper lighting or ability to adjust to light changes, and reaching for necessary objects can predispose client to fall.
(4) Is flashlight kept near bedside in case of power outage?	
(5) Is furniture arranged to provide clear path from bed to bathroom?	Obstructed path creates barrier that can cause tripping and falls.
(6) Does client who smokes ever smoke in bed?	Person who smokes in bed can fall asleep and accidentally drop cigarette, causing fire in bed linen.
(7) Is phone with emergency numbers within easy reach of bed?	Clients may develop physical symptoms while in bed, requiring easy access to phone.
(8) Are other alarm systems available? Push buttons that call for help? Nursery listening devices for invalid clients?	Alarm systems placed in readily accessible location can alert family/caregivers when person requires immediate assistance.
e. Living room/family room	
(1) Are electrical cords removed from under furniture and carpeting?	Clients can easily trip or fall over electrical cords, clutter, loose rugs, and furniture. The common walkway through the house should be clutter and barrier free.
(2) Can client turn on light without having to walk into dark room?	
(3) Are lamp, extension, or phone cords kept out of the way of traffic?	
(4) Are hallways and walkways free from objects and clutter?	
(5) Are loose area rugs securely attached to floor and not placed over carpeting? (For best safety, consider removal of throw rugs.)	
(6) Is furniture arranged in each room so that client can walk around easily?	
(7) Is all furniture steady and without sharp edges?	
(8) Can client sit and stand up easily from couches or chairs?	Some physical conditions make it difficult to bend at knees and hips, making it hard to sit in low chairs or couches.
f. Around the house	
(1) Are all living areas and stairways well lighted?	Good lighting helps persons to see any barriers or uneven walking surfaces.
(2) Is flooring or carpeting throughout house in good repair?	Frayed carpet or irregular surfaces can cause tripping and result in a fall.
(3) Are all thresholds level with floor or no more than ½ inch in height?	
(4) Is there a light switch at both top and bottom of stairs?	Prevents individual from having to walk a portion of stairs in dark.
(5) Does lighting produce glare or shadows on stairs?	Older adults are sensitive to glare.
(6) Do handrails run continuously from top to bottom of flights of stairs?	

STEP	RATIONALE
(7) Are step coverings in good condition?	
(8) Are all stairs kept free of clutter?	
g. General fire safety	
(1) Does client have properly working smoke detectors? (2) Does client or caregiver routinely check detector alarms to be sure batteries are good?	Smoke alarms properly located, well functioning, and with batteries replaced twice a year, can provide timely alert for fire.
• ***Critical Decision Point*** *Check to see when battery was last changed.*	
(3) Does client have several emergency exit plans in case of fire?	Exit plan helps persons to anticipate route of escape when fire does occur. Exit should be route that is not barred by difficult-to-open locks or any physical barriers.
(4) Has family determined a meeting place in event of emergency, such as at mailbox in front of home or parking area in front of house?	Use of a common emergency meeting location provides an efficient method for determining that all family members are safely out of the house.
(5) Does client use portable space heaters? Are they kept 3 feet away from flammable items?	Heaters, furnaces, and chimneys pose risks for fire.
(6) Is furnace area free of things that can catch on fire?	
(7) Does a qualified professional check furnace and chimney annually?	
h. General electrical safety	
(1) Are electrical cords in good condition, not frayed, spliced, or cracked?	Damaged cords can short-circuit and lead to fire.
(2) Are electrical cords kept away from water?	Use of any appliance or device that is exposed to water creates risk for electrical shock.
(3) Does client use extension cord/outlet extenders with built-in circuit breaker or fuse?	Prevents overloading of circuit that can lead to fire.
(4) Do all wall outlets and switches have cover plates?	
(5) Does client use light bulbs of correct wattage for each fixture?	Use of excessive wattage can lead to fire.
(6) Is fuse box (main electrical box for all electrical lines in home) easily accessible and clearly labeled?	In event of emergency, fuse box should be easy to access so that proper circuit can be cut off.
(7) Are lamp switches easy to turn to avoid burns from hot lightbulbs?	
i. Carbon monoxide prevention	
(1) Are furnace flues checked regularly for patency?	Common cause of carbon monoxide toxicity (Droscher and others, 1999).
(2) Is there a carbon monoxide detector in home?	
7. Assess client's financial resources; determine monthly income used for ongoing expenses.	Determines potential for making repairs to home. May reveal need for low-cost community service support.
8. Assess client's and family member's willingness to make changes. Has client accepted limitations that pose risk for injury? Determine how important functional independence is for client.	Nurse's attempt to improve safety within home can be perceived as intrusive. If it can be shown that necessary revisions to home environment will preserve independence, client may participate more willingly.

NURSING DIAGNOSIS

Defining characteristics from the assessment data may reveal the following nursing diagnoses for clients requiring this skill:

- Ineffective health maintenance
- Health-seeking behaviors regarding home safety
- Impaired home maintenance
- Impaired memory
- Impaired physical mobility
- Deficient knowledge regarding home safety risks
- Risk for injury
- Disturbed sensory perception (visual, auditory, and/or tactile)

Related factors are individualized based on client's condition or needs.

Step	Rationale

Planning

1. **Expected outcomes** following completion of procedure:
   - Client and/or family will describe potential environmental risks within home that may predispose to accidents. — During home safety assessment nurse instructs client on those risks that are of greatest concern.
   - Client and/or family will initiate actions to correct environmental risks, making home safer. — Client sees value in altering living environment.
   - Client will remain free of injury. — Environmental barriers are reduced or removed to minimize injuries.
2. Prioritize with client and family environmental barriers that pose greatest risk. — Client's own physical and/or cognitive deficits will make certain environmental risks more hazardous. Prioritization helps client make best choices.
3. Recommend calling in reliable contractor if major home repairs are necessary. — Ensures repairs are made safely and correctly.

Implementation

1. Take steps to reduce physical hazards that can predispose to falls:
   a. Paint edges of concrete stairs bright yellow, orange, or white. — This highlights visual target for client to see edge of stairs more clearly.
   b. Rearrange furniture to open up space through hallway, living room, family room, and bedroom. — Creates unobstructed pathway for ambulation.
   c. Reduce clutter within living areas, including footstools, flower pots, extension cords, and children's toys.
   d. Remove all doormats and area rugs and replace with mat or carpet that has nonskid backing. — Reduces chance of client slipping when stepping on rug surface.
   e. Pad floor and use specialized tile that absorbs impact of falls. — Cushions person's fall.
   f. Use low-rise beds, or use futon beds or a mattress on the floor. — Lowers distance to floor surface.
   g. Have enough electrical outlets installed to be able to plug light or electronic device (e.g., TV, video) into nearby outlet. — Prevents need to run extension cords across walkways.
   h. Have any rough edges on flooring or carpeting repaired. — Reduces risk of tripping over rough surface.
   i. Install nonskid strips on surface of bathtub and/or shower stall. — Reduces chances of slipping on tub/shower stall surface.
   j. Have grab bar installed in studs at tub, toilet, and/or shower (see illustration). Have client select vertical or horizontal placement if choice available. — Bar provides stability for maneuvering in bathroom.

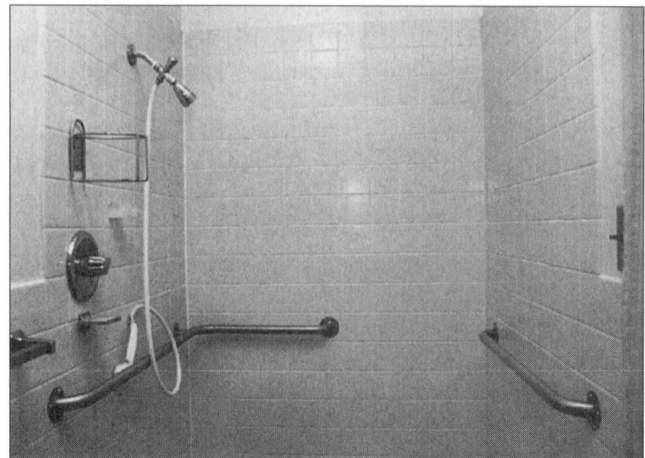

STEP **1j** Grab bars installed in a shower. (From Lueckenotte A: *Gerontologic nursing,* St. Louis, 1996, Mosby.)

STEP	RATIONALE
• ***Critical Decision Point*** *Be sure bar is a different color than that of wall for easy visibility*	
k. Have handrails installed along the side of any stairway (see illustration). Be sure stairways are well lighted, with switches at top and bottom of steps.	Older adults have difficulty seeing edges of stairs.

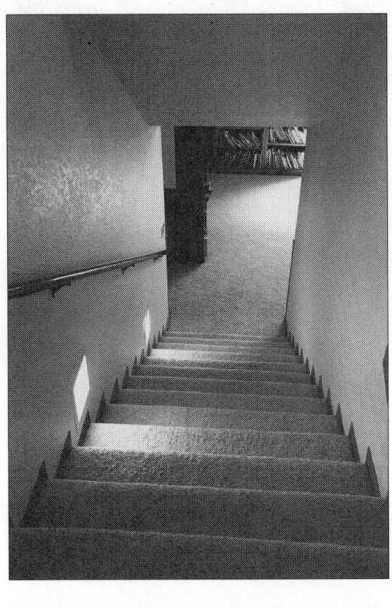

STEP **1k** Handrails installed along stairways provide security for clients with visual, balance, and coordination problems.

STEP	RATIONALE
l. Install appropriate broad-beam lighting for outside walkways.	
m. Keep a lighted phone easily accessible, next to the client's bed.	Prevents client from having to get up out of bed, often in the dark.
2. Have client use padding or types of clothing that will cushion bony prominences, especially high-risk bony prominences (e.g., hips).	Helps to absorb impact of falling body.
3. Make modifications to promote safe practice of activities of daily living:	
a. Provide direct light source in areas where client reads, cooks, uses tools, or conducts hobby work. High-intensity light on object or surface that is involved works best.	Older adults require three times as much light to see objects as they did when they were in their twenties (Ebersole and Hess, 1998).
• ***Critical Decision Point*** *Avoid fluorescent lighting because it can create excessive glare.*	
b. Consider satin and nongloss finishes for walls, cabinets, and countertops in kitchen. Have sheer curtains or adjustable shades in other living areas.	Reduces glare, to which older adults are very sensitive.
c. Apply colored tape or paint to color code controls of stove, oven, dryer, toaster, and other appliances.	Clients with reduced visual acuity may adjust appliance to wrong setting, creating potential risk of fire or burning.
d. Consider installing lazy Susans and pull-out drawers with glide mechanisms in kitchen cabinets. Also install C-ring handles in lower cabinets.	Makes access to food and kitchen supplies easier.
4. Take steps to eliminate fire hazards:	
a. Have smoke detectors installed near each bedroom, kitchen, and in basement of home. Be sure detector is on each floor of home.	Fires most frequently start in basement near furnace, dryer, or electrical wiring; kitchen; or in living areas where extensive wiring can be found. Alarm should be close by to alert client and family when sleeping.

STEP	RATIONALE
b. Have client select fire extinguisher that is easy to handle and manipulate (see illustration). Ask client to read instructions and discuss its proper use.	Older adult or client with disability may have difficulty gripping mechanisms on certain extinguishers.

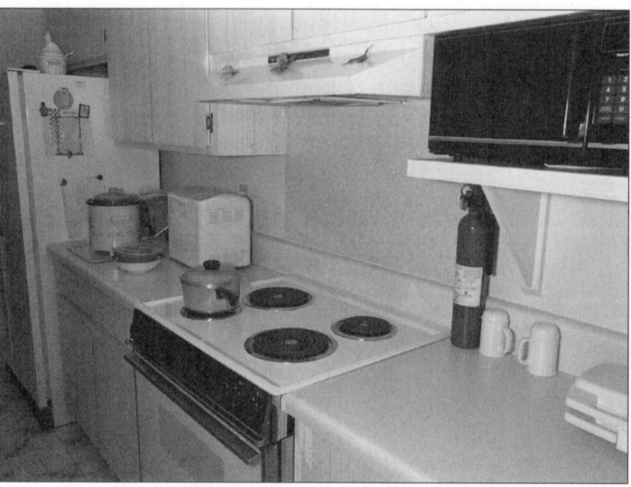

STEP 4b Fire extinguisher accessible in kitchen.

STEP	RATIONALE
c. Have area around furnace cleared of any flammable items.	Reduces risk for fire.
d. Instruct client to never place portable space heater within 3 feet of flammable items. Have client buy model that turns off automatically as soon as change in position occurs (Lueckenotte, 2000).	Intense heat can ignite flammable items easily. Safety device can shut off heater and prevent ignition of fire.
e. Have client make appointments for maintenance of furnace and chimney cleaning in appropriate season.	Furnace maintenance prevents short circuits and fires. Accumulation of creosote on chimney walls can lead to fire.
f. Have client check lightbulb wattage in all fixtures.	Ensures proper wattage being used.
g. Have client establish routine during cooking that keeps client in kitchen. Be sure cooking range is kept clean and items such as potholders and towels are kept away from burners.	Food cooking on stove can easily boil over or begin to burn when unattended.
h. If client is a smoker, review need to keep ashtrays clean and emptied as much as possible. Placing a small amount of water or sand in bottom of ashtray is useful if client is visually impaired.	Client with reduced vision may be unable to tell if cigarette, cigar, or match has extinguished.
i. Caution client against smoking in bed, smoking in a chair when there is a possibility of falling asleep, and smoking after taking a mind-altering medication.	Risks factors for burns as well as fire.
5. Take steps to reduce chances of injury from burns:	
a. Have setting on hot water heater adjusted to 120° F or lower. To check water temperature, let water run until steam is noted, fill container, and check temperature with a meat thermometer.	Scalds are typically caused from bathing and showering when hot water tank temperatures are in excess of 140° F or 60° C (Harper and Dickson, 1995).
b. Instruct client to always turn cold water on first.	Prevents direct exposure to hot water.
c. Install touch pads on lamps.	Light can be easily turned on without risk of touching hot light bulb.
d. Use color codes of red for hot and blue for cold on water faucets. (If client cannot distinguish colors, choose two that are easily distinguished.)	Prevents accidental burning from turning on wrong faucet.
6. Take steps to prevent carbon monoxide exposure in the home:	
a. Have condition of furnace venting checked annually just before time of season when furnace is turned on.	Improper venting prevents escape of carbon monoxide, a poisonous gas. Carbon monoxide combines irreversibly with hemoglobin, preventing formation of oxyhemoglobin and reducing oxygen supply to tissues.

Step	Rationale
b. Caution clients against using a gas stove or barbecue grill for heating inside of home.	Both are sources of carbon monoxide.
c. Have carbon monoxide detector installed in home.	Detector alarms when carbon monoxide reaches unsafe levels.

Evaluation

Step	Rationale
1. Have client and family member(s) identify safety risks that were revealed in home safety assessment.	This will demonstrate what client recognizes as a risk and its relative importance for changing.
2. During follow-up visits to home ask client to discuss plans for making any modifications and observe what changes have been implemented.	Evaluates extent to which client sees risks as potentially harmful and complies with suggested changes.
3. During follow-up visit or call, ask if client has experienced any falls or other injuries within home.	May reveal if risks have been eliminated, depending on client's previous history of injury.

Unexpected Outcomes and Related Interventions

- Client and family do not acknowledge all of risks revealed on home safety assessment.
  - Determine if there is reluctance to make changes due to limited resources, disbelief concerning need to make changes, or fear of loss of autonomy.
  - Review implications of risks on client's safety and welfare.
- Client fails to make changes agreed on in previous plan.
  - Determine reason for failure to make changes.
  - Help prioritize greatest risks.
- Client suffers fall within home and is found unconscious or displaying signs of serious injury.
  - Call 911, immobilize any suspected fractured extremity with a splint or board and elastic wrap bandage, and apply ice to injured area. Following a fall, monitor client's pulse and blood pressure and perform a neurological assessment.
- Client is found having suffered a serious burn within home.
  - Assess extent of burn, keep covered with a clean cloth or sheet, and arrange to take to emergency department or call 911.

Recording and Reporting

- Retain copy of home safety assessment in client's home health record.
- Record any instruction provided, client's response, and changes made within environment in progress notes.

Teaching Considerations

- Family caregivers may benefit from learning how to safely assist client in ambulating or transferring from bed to chair or wheelchair to chair, depending on client's mobility limitations.
- Instruct client and caregiver in what to do in case client falls, including access to emergency assistance and how to prevent further injury. Many communities have a service available that is designed for persons who live alone. The service company provides a small device worn around client's neck and a special monitor connected to client's telephone. Client can summon help by pressing button on device if phone is inaccessible. When alarm is received by company, call is initiated to client to assess possibility of false alarm. If there is no answer, the company will contact family members, friends, or a rescue squad to check on client. This service is a valuable option to frail older adults who are competent to live alone or be left at home while family members are away.

Pediatric Considerations

- Children with muscular dystrophies and spinal cord injuries will require use of a wheelchair. Child's wheelchair is smaller than an adult's, so movement along one level of home should not be too difficult. Creative thinking may be needed when homes have more than one level. Ultimately you want child to be part of family life.

Gerontological Considerations

- If client is wheelchair bound, there may be a need to lower light switches and other control devices within easy reach. Similarly, kitchen cabinets and other storage closets can be redesigned for access. A high-rise toilet with vertically hinged arm support allows client to transfer sideways from wheelchair to toilet seat (Shamberg and Shamberg, 1995). Another option is placing a bedside commode (with bedpan removed) over a conventional toilet seat. Commode level is usually higher than toilet. Then commode can also be moved near the bed for nighttime use.

Skill 39-2 Adapting the Home Setting for Clients With Cognitive Deficits

An important aspect of safety is a person's ability to perform routine activities of daily living (ADLs) and to make the correct decisions necessary to conduct home management activities. Home management includes use of the telephone, cleaning, shopping, money management, meal preparation, and taking medication. A person who is unable to perform these activities or who requires assistance from another may have physical disabilities and/or cognitive limitations. When the limitations are cognitive, a person's autonomy is clearly threatened. Family members often misunderstand certain behaviors associated with cognitive and mental changes and become concerned as to whether the individual can function safely within the home. The nurse may enter into situations where decisions must be made as to whether a client is competent to perform self-care.

It is a myth that all older adults experience cognitive dysfunction. However, it is the older adult that the nurse most commonly cares for with cognitive dysfunction and who needs support within the home to remain functional. Making the right decisions about safety within the home and the care that will be required depends on an accurate assessment of mental health, physical health, social and economic status, functional status, and environmental characteristics (Solomon, 1988; Ebersole and Hess, 1994). The difficulty lies in distinguishing between normal and diverse characteristics of aging and pathological conditions (Ebersole and Hess, 1998).

Making accurate assessments of older adults' mental status and cognitive function takes considerable practice. Mental status is an overlap between affective and cognitive function. A person may have certain mental processes intact (e.g., orientation to name, time, and place), while at the same time other processes are diminished or compromised (e.g., short-term memory of life events). Assessment of a client's level of orientation alone is not an accurate indicator of cognitive functioning (Palmateer and McCartney, 1985; Ebersole and Hess, 1998).

To complicate the issue of differentiating mental status and cognitive changes, it must be remembered that older adults commonly suffer from depression. Depression is an emotional disorder that can result in cognitive impairment (Lueckenotte, 2000). It can occur alone or in combination with cognitive disorders such as dementia. Depression can also occur secondarily to isolation when the older adult is home bound and has few social visitors.

This skill does not cover the complexity of assessing the full range of cognitive dysfunction in older adults. Instead it attempts to give the nurse guidelines for how to help clients who have varying degrees of cognitive dysfunction make adaptations to preserve their ability to function safely within the home. Similarly the skill addresses techniques for the family to use in assisting older adults.

Delegation Considerations

This skill should not be delegated to assistive personnel.

Equipment

- Mini-Mental State examination
- Calendar
- Paper for making lists
- Bulletin board or poster board (optional)

Step	Rationale
Assessment	
1. Conduct client's assessment over short period of time, and be sensitive to client's sensory needs or disabilities.	Improves likelihood of gathering relevant data (Ebersole and Hess, 1998).
2. Be sure the room in which you meet with client and family is well lit with minimal outside noises or interruptions. Speak clearly and in normal tone of voice.	An optimal environment for the assessment of the client's cognitive and mental status will provide a more valid assessment.
3. Ask client to describe own level of health and how it affects the ability to maintain self-care skills (e.g., bathing, dressing, eating, toileting).	Question will require client to attend to one topic. Allows nurse to assess attention and concentration. Also determines if client is fully perceptive of physical capabilities.

- ***Critical Decision Point***

  Family members may be used to confirm description. Do not create situation in which client feels you are not listening to his or her views.

STEP	RATIONALE
4. Ask how the client is doing with home management responsibilities. Questions that may be asked include, "To give me an idea of how you manage at home, tell me what bills you pay each month. Can you tell what each one is for? Can you tell me about your normal day—when do you get up, eat meals? Do you have problems getting dressed or bathing?	Provides good comparison of client and family perceptions. Interaction will help to measure short-term memory, judgment, and problem solving.
5. Assess medications client takes. Review number and type of medications, purpose as prescribed, time of day taken, and dosages. Give special attention to pain medications, anticonvulsants, antihypertensives (especially beta-adrenergic blockers), Lasic, digoxin, aspirin, and anticoagulants.	Older adults frequently suffer drug interactions from **polypharmacy,** concurrent prescribing of multiple medications. Select drugs and/or combinations of drugs can place client at risk for side effects that may increase chances of injury as a result of physical or cognitive changes.
6. Determine if client has family member or friend who assists with self-care or home management responsibilities. Does client perceive satisfaction in caregiver's support? What level of satisfaction does caregiver perceive?	Role of family caregiver can be stressful. Determines availability of resource to client and quality of that support.
7. During discussion, observe client's dress, nonverbal expressions, appearance, and cleanliness.	Conditions such as depression and dementia can result in client's inability to attend to personal appearance.

- ***Critical Decision Point***
  Do not confuse behavioral changes with lack of available resources to maintain hygiene. Also be aware of signs and symptoms of abuse (Box 39-2). Report to appropriate social service agency.

STEP	RATIONALE
8. Observe immediate home environment, is it well kept and orderly?	Behavioral changes associated with cognitive dysfunction may be first detected in disorderly home and inappropriate placement of objects (e.g., carton of orange juice placed inside kitchen cabinet instead of refrigerator).
9. If you suspect a cognitive or mental status change, complete a Mini-Mental State examination (e.g., Folstein's mini-mental).	Screening examination will measure orientation, attention and calculation, recall, language, and intelligence.

NURSING DIAGNOSIS

Defining characteristics from the assessment data may reveal the following nursing diagnoses for clients requiring this skill:

- Acute confusion
- Ineffective health maintenance
- Ineffective role performance
- Disturbed thought processes
- Caregiver role strain
- Impaired home maintenance
- Impaired memory
- Risk for injury
- Self-care deficit (feeding, toileting, bathing/hygiene, dressing/grooming)

Related factors are individualized based on client's condition or needs.

Box 39-2 Warning Signs of Abuse

DOMESTIC ABUSE

Injuries or trauma inconsistent with reported cause
Multiple injuries involving head, face, neck, breasts, abdomen and genitalia
Burns
Human bites
Client reports eating or sleeping disorders, anxiety, panic attacks, low self-esteem, depression, sense of helplessness

ELDER ABUSE

Injuries or trauma inconsistent with reported cause, e.g.
Hematomas, bruises, burns, fractures
Prolonged interval between injury and medical treatment
Dependence on caregiver
Physically and/or cognitively impaired
Combative
Wandering
Verbally belligerent

Data from All A: A literature review: assessment and intervention in elder abuse, *J Gerontol Nurs* 20(7):25, 1994; Campbell J, Humphreys J: *Nursing care of survivors of family violence,* ed 2, St. Louis, 1993, Mosby; Pace H, Hoag-Apel C: Stemming the tide of domestic violence. *Point of View Magazine* 33(3):12, 1996.

STEP	RATIONALE

PLANNING

1. **Expected outcomes** following completion of procedure:
   - Client is able to complete home management responsibilities within existing limitations.
     Modifications are made that help client apply remaining cognitive functions.
   - Client receives appropriate combination of medications for diagnosed conditions.
     Environmental aids enable client to follow prescribed medication regimen.
   - Caregiver describes techniques to use in helping client perform self-care and home management activities.
     Instruction will prepare caregiver with variety of caregiving techniques.
   - Caregiver uses techniques that help client complete self-care and home management activities.
     Caregiver preserves client's autonomy and maximizes client's functionality.
2. If client has difficulty with self-care skills, refer family to homemaker services and **respite care** as appropriate.
   Provides additional resource to either deliver direct personal care to client or to provide caregiver temporary rest away from continuous responsibilities.
3. If client has physical disability affecting fine motor skills, consult with physical and/or occupational therapist.
   Can offer assistive devices to make bathing, dressing, writing, and feeding easier (see illustration).

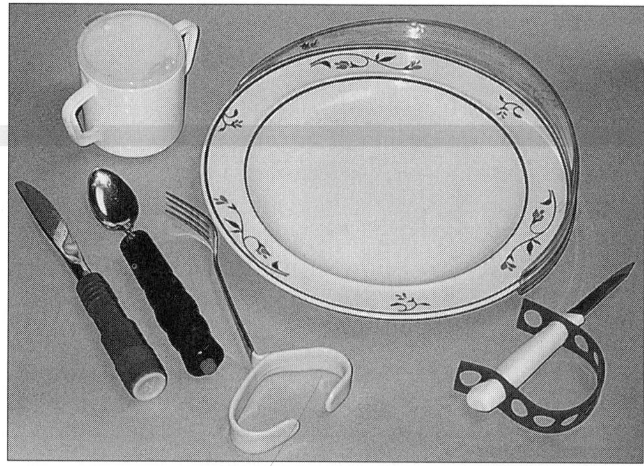

STEP **3** Assistive feeding devices.

4. Consider client's level of cognitive impairment before implementing strategies that will require changes in living environment. Some clients may require only minor adaptations, and others will depend more on assistance of caregivers.
   Retention of client's independence and autonomy is ultimate goal.
5. Determine best time of day for approaches that result in desired response.
   Client may be more alert and responsive in morning versus afternoon or vice versa.

IMPLEMENTATION

1. If client has difficulty remembering when to perform tasks (e.g., paying bills, taking medicines) help to create a list or post reminder notes in a conspicuous location (e.g., bulletin board, front of refrigerator), provide a medication container organized by days of week, recommend a wristwatch with alarm to signal during medication times.
   Memory function in older adults tends to be preserved for relevant, well-learned material (Lueckenotte, 2000). Lists will help client overcome memory loss.
2. When client has difficulty completing tasks such as writing checks for bills or bringing groceries into home to store, reduce steps it takes to complete task. Find ways to consolidate steps or simplify task.
   Prevents frustration in completing task and/or forgetting step that leads to task being unfinished.

STEP	RATIONALE
3. Help client and caregiver determine routine schedule for daily activities such as eating, bathing, daily exercise, home management activities, and napping. Have large calendar posted in conspicuous area to write in appointments or special planned events.	Consistency creates sense of security and keeps client more easily oriented to daily activities. Routines are important in providing security, but client must also have option of making changes as necessary.
4. Instruct caregiver to focus on client's abilities rather than disabilities.	Helps to retain dominant skills (Burgener, Shimer, and Murrell, 1993).
5. Have caregiver assist with setting-up activities so that client can complete task (e.g., chopping up vegetables before actual cooking, placing wash basin on table in bedroom for sponge bath, placing clothes to wear for the day on bed, unpacking groceries on countertop for eventual storage, arranging food on plate with items in clockwise orientation—vegetables at 9, salad at 3, meat at 6).	Helps client master task even though unable either physically or cognitively to perform all steps.
6. Discuss with client, caregiver, and physician or primary care provider options for scheduling multiple medications:	Drugs may cause physiological changes that create risk for injury.
a. Administer drugs likely to cause confusion at nighttime.	

• ***Critical Decision Point***
Do not recommend this if client has nocturia.

STEP	RATIONALE
b. Space antihypertensives and antiarrhythmics at different times to minimize side effects.	These drugs may cause blood pressure changes and dizziness, thus increasing risk of falls.
c. Reduce number of different pain medications used.	
d. Give Lasix (diuretic) early in day and not at night.	Diuretic effect occurs during the day while client is awake.
7. Instruct caregiver in how to use simple and direct communication:	Relays care and support through therapeutic communications techniques.
a. Use a calm and relaxed approach.	
b. Use eye contact and touch.	
c. Speak in simple words and short sentences.	
d. Use nonverbal gestures that complement verbal messages.	

• ***Critical Decision Point***
Be sure client can contribute to discussion. Caregiver should not dominate discussion.

STEP	RATIONALE
8. Keep clocks, calendars, and personal mementos (e.g., pictures, scrapbooks, special personal gifts from loved ones) situated throughout rooms within the home.	Reinforces reality orientation when client's memory is failing.
9. Have caregiver routinely orient client to who caregiver is and what activities they are going to complete.	This strategy is useful in clients with progressive dementia. This improves their productivity and responses (Lueckenotte, 2000).
10. Be sure client has regular naps or rest periods during the day.	Fatigue can add to any mental status changes. Gives client energy to perform planned activities.
11. Have caregiver encourage and support frequent visits by family and friends. Instruct caregiver in how to use humor and **reminiscing** of favorite stories to promote social interaction.	Participation in social activities prevents boredom and restlessness.

EVALUATION

STEP	RATIONALE
1. During a follow-up visit, ask client to review the home management activities completed the morning of that day, as well as the previous day.	Determines client's ability to recall events and evaluates if planned activities were completed.

Step	Rationale
2. Review with client and caregiver revised schedule for medication administration.	Evaluates understanding of regimen.
3. Have caregiver keep track of doses client takes over a 1-week period.	Tracking doses will confirm if client is adherent to regimen.
4. Ask caregiver to describe ways that will increase client's success in completing home management and self-care activities.	Measures learning.
5. Have caregiver show schedules of daily routines and review specific approaches used. Observe environment for presence of reality orientation cues.	Determines caregiver's success in applying information and making environmental changes.

Unexpected Outcomes and Related Interventions

- Client fails to complete daily activities as planned.
  - Further modifications may be needed to help client be successful. Reassess what occurred when a task was not completed. Caregiver and client conflict could have played a role rather than client being unable cognitively to complete task.
- Client experiences drug interaction from multiple medications.
  - Have physician evaluate client's medication regimen. Recommend feasibility of pharmacy consult.
- Caregiver is unable to describe/implement techniques that will improve client's orientation and ability to complete activities.
  - Reinstruction and discussion are necessary.
  - Support for caregiver may be necessary before caregiver can learn how to support someone else.
  - Consider that caregiver may not be able to provide necessary support; other options may need to be analyzed.

Recording and Reporting

- Record assessment of client's cognitive and mental status, recommended interventions, and client's and caregiver's response in progress notes.
- Report to physician any change in client's behavior that might reflect a decline in cognitive or mental status.

Teaching Considerations

- Instruct caregiver in signs and symptoms to expect for clients suffering from dementia and Alzheimer's disease. If client's functionality continues to decline, caregiver may choose to learn more ADL support skills (e.g., how to assist with hygiene, dressing, transfer and turning, toileting).

Pediatric Considerations

- Children with cognitive impairment are often not aware of inherent dangers during play and other activities. Parental supervision is critical.

Gerontological Considerations

- Many clients experience progressive loss of function, requiring constant adaptations and adjustments.
- Stress created for caregiver by older adult demonstrating problematic behaviors may be eliminated if awareness of meaning of behaviors and methods of managing these is encouraged (Lueckenotte, 2000).

Skill 39-3 Medication and Medical Device Safety

Clients frequently must manage the administration of medications and the use of medical devices such as syringes, blood glucose monitoring equipment, dressing supplies, and even intravenous devices. This includes administration, storage, and disposal. Safety is critical in ensuring that medications are administered correctly, devices are used properly, and equipment is cleaned and/or removed as waste. Infection control is just one principle the client and/or caregiver must learn to ensure a safe environment within the home.

One of the nurse's responsibilities within the home environment is to assist the client with sensory, mobility, or cognitive deficits. Clients who require special consideration include those with acute sensory or neurological impairment, clients with chronic illness such as diabetes or arthritis, and older adults who frequently have physical limitations that make manipulation of medical devices and dispensing of medications difficult. For example, clients with arthritic hands are sometimes unable to open medication containers because of the lack of strength in the hands and the pain created by pressure on the joints. This skill reviews steps to take to ensure safe use of medications and medical devices. Chapter 40 addresses how to instruct clients in medication use.

Delegation Considerations

Assessment of the client's risks in using medical devices and in administering medication should not be delegated to assistive personnel. The RN is best equipped to identify the adaptations needed within the home based on the client's limitations. However, assistive personnel, such as home health aides, will frequently be in a situation to be able to see how clients use these adaptations. Assistive personnel can learn how to make suggestions that further ensure client safety regarding the use of basic infection control practices, and how to dispose of sharps, needles, and contaminated supplies.

Equipment

- Colored marking pens
- Labels
- Puncture-resistant sharps container or 2-L soda bottle with cap
- Duct or adhesive tape
- Assistive devices (e.g., syringe magnifier)

Step	Rationale
Assessment	
1. Assess client's sensory, musculoskeletal, and neurological function (see Chapter 10).	Helps to reveal any deficits that may affect preparation and use of medications or medical devices.
2. If family caregiver provides routine assistance, assess his or her function as above.	
3. Assess client's medication regimen and length of time client has been receiving each drug.	Determines complexity of medication regimen and extent to which client should be familiar with regimen.
4. Ask client to show you where medications are stored in home. Look at each container.	Allows nurse to assess conditions and labeling of containers.

- ***Critical Decision Point***
  Note temperature of storage area. Medications should not be stored in extreme heat. Insulin should be kept in a cool place.

Step	Rationale
5. Have client describe daily schedule for drug administration and whether there are any problems in following that schedule.	Helps to reveal client's adherence to or misunderstanding of instructions (see Chapter 40).
6. If client self-administers injections, ask to see where those supplies are stored and what is used to dispose of used syringes and needles.	Determines sterility of equipment and whether method of disposal creates risk to client or family for needle-stick injuries.
7. If client uses a glucose-monitoring device, ask to see where monitor, lancets, and glucose strips are stored. Also ask about how client disposes of lancets.	Allows nurse to examine cleanliness of equipment, sterility of lancets, and condition of glucose strips. Sharps should be disposed of in puncture-proof container.

Step	Rationale
8. If client applies dressings to a wound, ask to see where dressings are stored and determine how client disposes of soiled dressings.	Determines if dressings supplies are kept clean and are properly discarded.

Nursing Diagnosis

Defining characteristics from the assessment data may reveal the following nursing diagnoses for clients requiring this skill:

- Ineffective health maintenance
- Health-seeking behaviors regarding medication safety
- Noncompliance (sharps disposal)
- Risk for infection
- Risk for injury
- Deficient knowledge regarding medication and medical device safety

Related factors are individualized based on client's condition or needs.

Planning

1. **Expected outcomes** following completion of procedure:
   - Client and caregiver will discuss principles of medication safety. — Nurse provides knowledge base for safe medication administration.
   - Client and caregiver will be able to prepare medications independently. — Adaptations are made to accommodate client's and/or caregiver's deficits in handling and manipulating equipment.
   - Client and caregiver will identify correct conditions for storing medications, medical devices, and supplies. — Instruction focuses on infection control measures.
   - Client and caregiver will dispose of used medical equipment and supplies correctly. — Appropriate receptacles and methods for disposal are made available.

Implementation

Step	Rationale
1. Instruct client and caregiver in principles to ensure medications are safe to use:	Medications must be of full strength and used for the appropriate pharmacological reason to have therapeutic benefit.
a. Never take a medicine prescribed for another member of household.	
b. Do not take any medicine more than a year old or past expiration date on container.	Expired medication may be toxic or no longer effective.
c. Do not place different medicines in same container.	Prevents accidental "mix-up" of medications and medication error.
d. Always finish a prescribed medication; do not save for a future illness.	
2. Recommend approaches to facilitate preparation of medications:	
a. For clients with weakened grasp or pain of hands and fingers, have local pharmacist place medications in a screw-top container.	Tops of child-proof containers are difficult to remove, especially if hand and finger grasp are weakened.

• ***Critical Decision Point***

If client has children or grandchildren who have easy access to medication storage area or client's purse, be sure medications are stored in secure place.

Step	Rationale
b. For clients with visual alterations, have pharmacy type larger labels on all medication containers.	Ensures client is able to read drug name and dosage schedule clearly.
c. For clients who are legally blind, have braille labels placed on medication containers.	Labels embossed with drug name, strength, and prescription numbers can be easily read by client trained in use of braille.

STEP	RATIONALE
d. For clients taking multiple medications, a color-coding system may be useful. For example, colors could be used for drugs that are to be taken at the same time. Tops of bottle caps can be marked with a colored marking pen.	Technique may help to ensure correct drugs and doses are taken at correct times of day.
e. Provide specially designed syringes with large numerals or syringe magnifier for clients with visual alterations (see illustration).	Ensures accurate dose of drug is prepared in syringe.
f. For clients who have difficulty manipulating syringes, offer a spring-loaded needle insertion aid.	Delivers injection safely without manipulation of plunger.

- ***Critical Decision Point***
  If client or caregiver suffers a needle-stick injury, wash the affected area thoroughly with soap and water, then dry. Record incident.

g. Instruct caregivers on how to properly draw up prescribed volume of medication into syringe. When necessary, have caregiver prepare extra prefilled syringes for client's use when caregiver is absent.	Ensures caregiver knows proper preparation techniques. Ensures client has access of injections.

- ***Critical Decision Point***
  Refer to medication insert or pharmacist as to whether doses can be stored in syringe over several hours or days. Keep all prefilled insulin syringes refrigerated and use within 21 days (Rice, 2000).

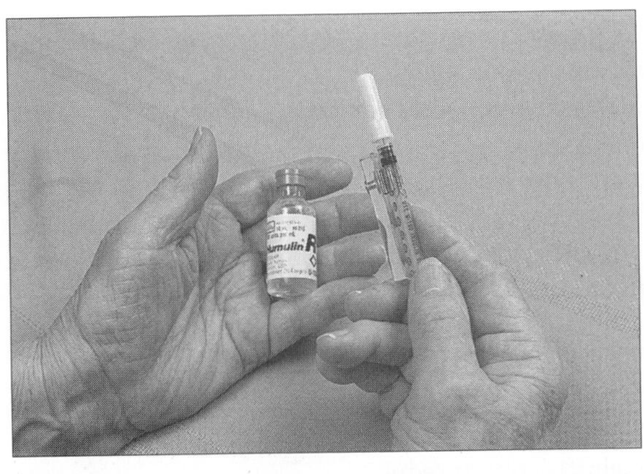

STEP **2e** Syringe with magnifier.

3. Recommend approaches to ensure medications and supplies are properly stored:	
a. Store medications in a safe place, preferably in the kitchen.	Moisture in bathroom may cause medications to decompose.
b. Keep liquid medications and parenteral drugs, especially insulin, in a cool place.	Prevents decomposition of drug.

- ***Critical Decision Point***
  Insulin may be stored in refrigerator, but it is not necessary. The vial in use can be stored at room temperature for up to 30 days without losing potency (Rice, 2000). If it is stored in refrigerator, be sure drug is kept in a bin or container, away from food. An unused supply of insulin vials should be stored in refrigerator to maintain potency.

c. Keep medical supplies such as syringes, dressing supplies, and glucose meter in airtight container (e.g., plastic storage bin) and stored in cool place, such as bedroom closet.	Ensures supplies are not exposed to moisture or other contaminants.
4. Review for client and caregiver the proper techniques for disposal of medications, "sharps," and disposable medical supplies:	
a. Discard unused portions of drugs or outdated drugs in sink or toilet.	Ensures that no one in household uses drug not prescribed for their use or drugs that will be ineffective pharmacologically.

Step	Rationale
b. Obtain sharps container from medical supply store or intravenous (IV) equipment supplier. (If finances are limited, have client use a small-neck plastic bottle, such as a soda bottle.) Dispose of all needles and lancets in container.	Puncture-proof container prevents exposure to contaminated needle stick. Small-neck container makes it difficult for anyone to easily retrieve a used needle or sharp.
c. Caution against filling container to a point where needles protrude out opening. Discard when three-fourths full, securing top with duct tape or adhesive tape.	Prevents needle sticks.
d. Store sharps container in an area inaccessible to children.	Prevents injury to child.
e. Dispose of soiled dressings, used glucose testing reagent strips, and IV tubing in a separate, sealed, plastic garbage bag. Then place in second plastic bag (double bagged) and discard appropriately as trash.	Prevents contamination with other items in home. Minimizes chances of caregiver being exposed to infectious waste.
f. Consult local public health department or community authorities regarding proper way to dispose of waste.	Most communities have strict guidelines for waste disposal.

Evaluation

Step	Rationale
1. Have client and/or caregiver describe steps to take to ensure medications are safe to use.	Demonstrates learning.
2. Observe client and/or caregiver prepare and administer a medication dose.	Evaluates ability to physically manipulate medications and necessary equipment.
3. Observe home setting for location of medications and supplies.	Evaluates client's and/or caregiver's adherence to recommendations.
4. Have client describe how sharps or medical equipment is discarded.	Demonstrates learning.
5. Do pill counts (pills remaining in containers) at successive intervals, such as twice a week for 2 weeks.	Verifies client takes correct number of medications over a period of time.

Unexpected Outcomes and Related Interventions

- Client and/or caregiver is unable to recall principles for safe use of drugs.
  - Reinstruction may be necessary, or client and caregiver may need chance to ask more questions regarding benefit of precautions.
  - Offer written, simple, and clear instructions.
- Client and/or caregiver has difficulty or is unable to prepare and self-administer a medication.
  - Further assistance may be necessary in setting up equipment, offering assistive aids, or explaining steps to prepare medication.
- Medications and medical devices are not stored in a secure or appropriate location.
  - Client may choose to store items conveniently rather than safely or may have limited resources. Reinstruction and discussion are necessary.
- Sharps and disposable medical equipment are not disposed of properly.
  - Reinstruction is required.
  - Arrange to provide appropriate containers.
- An excess or insufficient number of pills are found in pill container during pill count.
  - Incorrect dosage is being taken. Review with client daily drug prescribed. Reevaluate use of dosage reminders.

Recording and Reporting

- Record instructions and recommendations to client and caregiver and results of return demonstrations in progress notes.

Teaching Considerations

- Instruct clients in care of linen. Use of lancets or application of dressings may cause soiling of client's linen supply. Infected or soiled linen should be kept in a separate, leakproof plastic bag. Contaminated items should be washed separately from household laundry in hot water with 1 cup of bleach and detergent for *two* regular wash cycles.

Critical Thinking Exercises

1. Mr. Pinetta has experienced a stroke, causing partial paralysis of his right side. Following rehabilitation, he is unable to walk without dragging his right foot. He is able to move his right arm but has limited use of his right hand. What is important for you, the nurse, to assess in regard to Mr. Pinetta's ability to use his bathroom safely?
2. Mr. O'Connor has a progressive memory loss and lives alone. How might you better ensure his ability to self-administer his antihypertensive and diuretic medications safely?
3. If a client tells you that he disposes of insulin syringes and needles in a used milk carton, what advice would you give, and why?

References

All A: A literature review: assessment and intervention in elder abuse, *J Gerontol Nurs* 20(7):25, 1994.

Arfken C and others: The prevalence and correlates of fear of falling in elderly persons living in the community, *Am J Pub Health* 84(4):565, 1994.

Burgener SC, Shimer R, Murrell L: Nursing care of cognitively impaired, institutionalized elderly, *J Gerontol Nurs* 17:37, 1993.

Campbell J, Humphreys J: *Nursing care of survivors of family violence,* ed 2, St. Louis, 1993, Mosby.

Corbett C, Pennypacker B: Using a quality improvement team to reduce patient falls, *J Health Qual* 15(5):38, 1992.

Droscher MJ et al: Heating oil company responses to inquiries concerning carbon monoxide toxicity, *Annals of Emergency Medicine* 33(4):406, 1999.

Ebersole P, Hess P: *Toward healthy aging,* ed 4, St. Louis, 1994, Mosby.

Ebersole P, Hess P: *Toward healthy aging,* ed 5, St. Louis, 1998, Mosby.

Gray-Micelli D: Falling among older individuals: exploring psychological issues, *Advances for Nurse Practitioners* 5:7, 1997.

Harper RD, Dickson WA: Reducing the burn risk to elderly persons living in residential care, *Burns* 21(3):205, 1995.

Lueckenotte A: *Gerontologic nursing,* St. Louis, 1996, Mosby.

Lueckenotte A: *Gerontologic nursing,* ed 2, St. Louis, 2000, Mosby.

Maslow A: *Motivation and personality,* ed 2, New York, 1954, Harper and Row.

McDougall GJ: A review of screening instruments for assessing cognition and mental status in older adults, *Nurs Pract* 15:11, 1990.

Pace H, Hoag-Apel C: Stemming the tide of domestic violence. *Point of View Magazine* 33(3):12, 1996.

Palmateer LM, McCartney JR: Do nurses know when patients have cognitive deficits? *J Gerontol Nurs* 11(2):6, 1985.

Rice R: *Home health nursing practice,* ed 3, St. Louis, 2000, Mosby.

Shamberg S, Shamberg A: Reentry begins at home, *Rehab Management* 8(5):24, 1995.

Solomon D: National Institutes of Health consensus development conference statement: geriatric assessment methods for clinical decision-making, *J Am Geriatr Soc* 36(4):342, 1988.

Tideiksaar R: *Falls in order persons: prevention and management,* ed 2, Baltimore, 1998, Health Professions Press.

40

HOME CARE TEACHING

Skills

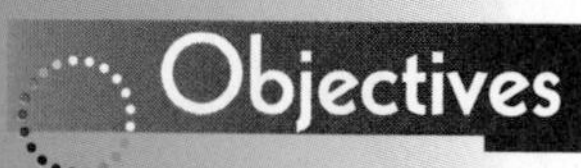

Objectives

Mastery of content in this chapter will enable the nurse to:

- Define the key terms listed.
- Identify factors that alter clients' learning abilities.
- Discuss the collaborative nature of home health care teaching.
- Assess safety factors that may impair or prohibit the client's skill performance in the home setting.
- Discuss situations and conditions that require client and/or family skills performance to support and achieve health maintenance.
- Understand variances in teaching strategies in the home setting.
- Identify factors that influence clients' learning and skill performance of home care.
- Implement and evaluate appropriate learning strategies that support positive client outcomes.

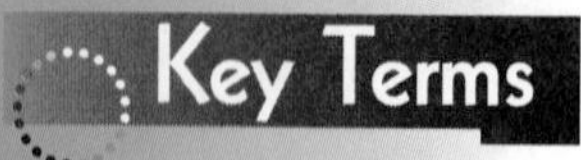

Key Terms

Antipyretic
Clean technique
Dementia
Enteral nutrition
Febrile
Gastrostomy feeding tube
High Fowler's position
Hypothermia
Hypoxia
Infusion pump
Intake and output (I&O) record
Medical asepsis
Nasal cannula
Nasogastric feeding tube
Over-the-counter drug
Oxygen therapy
prn
Transtracheal oxygen therapy (TTOT)

Changes in the health care delivery system in recent times have shifted the site of care delivery from the acute inpatient setting to the home health care arena. Although acute and long-term care settings continue to provide services along the spectrum of the health care continuum, more frequently than in past decades, clients recover from or are treated for illnesses in the home environment. The psychosocial, emotional, and financial issues surrounding the ongoing needs of individuals and families dealing with chronic or episodic illnesses are often best managed in the home setting as well.

The home care nurse is faced with a diverse client population with varying levels of acuity of illness. Techniques and treatments that a few years ago were strictly provided in a general hospital are now commonplace in home health care.

The development and maintenance of successful treatment plans for home care teaching skills must be done in collaboration with the prescribing physician, the client, family or designated caregivers, pharmacists, and organizations that provide and maintain equipment. Very often a variety of other social services and/or health-related organizations are also involved in making the client's home care plan successful. The home care nurse not only teaches and assesses the client's health status but also identifies, coordinates, and intervenes with the various services and resources that are required to support the client's successful health maintenance. Teaching will not achieve positive outcomes if the client has an unidentified barrier to following through, such as lack of transportation or inadequate funds for medication and equipment. The client's cultural beliefs or values may also conflict with teaching approaches. In addition to the understanding and ability of the nurse to perform a skill and teach it, the home care nurse must assess all intrinsic and extrinsic factors that could affect the client's ability to comply with self-care.

Client education is a major component of home health care. When the home care nurse successfully teaches aspects of self-care maintenance, clients and families may attain an improved quality of life, fewer physician visits, reduction in overall costs of health care, and may gain more control over an illness.

Skill Performance Guidelines

1. Consider the client's and caregiver's physical, cognitive, emotional, cultural, environmental, and social resources in regard to successful learning and skill performance.
2. Present information in an understandable and orderly manner directed toward the client's and caregiver's learning style and abilities.
3. Individualize the teaching care plan based on the physical, psychosocial, and cognitive abilities of the client and caregiver.
4. Assess if a skill can be safely performed in the home setting. A care partner may be required for some skills to be safely in the home setting.
5. Assess home environment for hygiene facilities to support successful self-care management.
6. Consider other persons in the household who positively or negatively influence the client's self-care modalities.

Skill 40-1 Teaching Clients to Measure Body Temperature, Blood Pressure, and Pulse

Teaching Clients to Measure Body Temperature

To practice health maintenance for themselves and their family members, clients need to know how to measure body temperature. An elevation in body temperature can be an early warning sign of serious health problems. Clients susceptible to temperature alterations should know how to measure their temperatures correctly so that they can seek medical attention early when alterations occur. Parents must know how to measure their children's temperature because children can develop seriously high fevers very quickly. Because older adults have impaired temperature-control mechanisms, the caregiver should know the techniques for temperature measurement. Nurses can teach clients the skills of measuring body temperature and lowering temperature when a **febrile** episode occurs at home and medical care is not immediately accessible.

There are a variety of body temperature measurement tools available for use. The mercury in-glass thermometer is becoming less available because of environmental health and safety regulations. However, the glass thermometer is still very common in the home setting. The disposable, single-use thermometer and the tympanic membrane thermometer are newer devices with varying prevalence in the home setting. The small electronic digital thermometers are less expensive and more readily available than some of the newer types mentioned and perhaps allow for safer use than the glass thermometer. This section will deal with the instruction of the client or family in the use of glass thermometers, which most families have available in the home. The need for the use of an oral, rectal, or stubby (axillary) thermometer will be determined before use depending on the client's age and health status. Having all three types of these inexpensive items at home allows for a variety of client possibilities and needs. (See Chapter 9 for a review of vital signs assessment.)

Delegation Considerations

The skill of teaching clients to measure body temperature, blood pressure, and pulse can be delegated to assistive personnel. After the client or caregiver has demonstrated competency with the skill, a nurse must clarify: the appropriate route and device for the client to measure body temperature; any special considerations for positioning a client for vital sign measurement; client history of or risk of abnormal vital signs; preferable pulse site; appropriate limb for blood pressure (BP) measurement; appropriate size BP cuff for designated extremity; frequency of specific vital sign measurements; and the need to report abnormalities to the client's physician or health care provider.

Equipment

Instruct client on purchase and selection of glass thermometer. If available in market, assist with selection of alternative device (refer to Chapter 9 for measurement technique). Determine need for oral, rectal, or stubby thermometer before purchase if finances are limited.

- Soft tissue
- Lubricant (for rectal measurement)
- Paper and pencil if frequent measurements are to be taken
- Disposable gloves (for rectal temperature taken by a caregiver)

Step	Rationale
Assessment	
1. Assess client's ability to manipulate and read thermometer by having client read temperature values and shake thermometer down. Client who wears eyeglasses should wear them while reading thermometer.	Physical restrictions in handling or reading thermometer may require nurse to instruct family member or significant other instead of client. Visual acuity impairment may prevent client from being able to read thermometer.
2. Assess client's knowledge of normal temperature range and symptoms and common causes of fever and **hypothermia.**	Identifies client's ability to initiate preventive health measures and recognize alterations in body temperature.
3. Assess client's knowledge of criteria to determine appropriate type of thermometer to be used in varying situations (see Chapter 9).	Determines knowledge of age-related or medical conditions that would make oral or rectal temperature measurement detrimental to client.
4. If client has had experience in measuring temperature, ask for demonstration of technique.	Allows nurse to assess client's knowledge and use of safety precautions, aseptic technique, and time period for insertion.

STEP	RATIONALE

NURSING DIAGNOSIS

Defining characteristics from the assessment data may reveal the following nursing diagnoses for clients requiring this skill:

- Impaired home maintenance
- Health-seeking behaviors (temperature measurement)
- Hyperthermia
- Hypothermia
- Deficient knowledge regarding specific temperature measurement
- Risk for imbalanced body temperature
- Risk for infection
- Ineffective thermoregulation

Related factors are individualized based on client's condition or needs.

PLANNING

Step	Rationale
1. **Expected outcomes** following completion of procedure:	
▪ Client is able to correctly measure own or family member's temperature.	Indicates skills are effectively learned.
▪ Client demonstrates proper cleaning and storage of equipment.	
▪ Client states factors affecting temperature, signs and symptoms of fever and hypothermia, and measures to take.	Cognitive learning is achieved.
2. Select setting in home where client is most likely to measure temperature.	Practicing in same environment where skill is routinely performed facilitates comprehension and learning.
3. Discuss and demonstrate with client or family member proper way to position client before thermometer insertion; instruct family member to remain with client if age or physical status requires.	Promotes client's understanding of comfort and safety principles, as well as technique to ensure accurate measurement.

IMPLEMENTATION

Step	Rationale
1. Demonstrate steps and provide rationale for steps to client or caregiver.	Demonstration is best technique for teaching psychomotor skill. Adults learn best when they understand purpose of procedure.
2. Have client perform each step with guidance from nurse. Do not rush client.	Nurse is able to correct errors in technique as they occur and discuss implications.

• ***Critical Decision Point***
Discuss normal temperature range for adult or child.

Step	Rationale
3. Discuss effects of smoking and hot and cold liquids or foods on oral temperature readings.	Client must understand factors that can alter temperature readings.
4. Discuss common symptoms of fever: warm, dry, flushed skin; feeling warm; chills; piloerection; malaise; and restlessness.	Client must be able to recognize onset of fever in self or family member.
5. Discuss common signs and symptoms of hypothermia: cool skin, uncontrolled shivering, loss of memory, and signs of poor judgment.	Persons with inadequate home heating, older adults, or those unaware of potential dangers of cold conditions are at risk.

• ***Critical Decision Point***
Teach client to take temperature after chills/shivering subsides to obtain a true temperature.

Step	Rationale
6. Discuss importance of notifying physician when temperature elevations occur, and review common therapies for temperature reduction that are safe to perform at home.	Clients must understand danger of high temperature elevations. Use of antipyretics, sponging with tepid water, and drinking fluids are unlikely to cause complications.

STEP	RATIONALE
7. Provide set of written guidelines for client's reference to promote client confidence in ability to implement the skill independently, and offer guidance regarding when additional action (such as notifying physician) should be taken.	Some clients need instructions written out in clear, concise statements or pictures to minimize anxiety and support appropriate actions for health maintenance.

EVALUATION

STEP	RATIONALE
1. Have client independently demonstrate technique for temperature measurement, including ability to read thermometer three separate times.	Feedback through independent demonstration of psychomotor skill is best means of evaluating mastery of skill.
2. Observe client clean and store equipment.	
3. Ask client to identify normal temperature range and influence of smoking and hot and cold liquids or foods on oral readings; discuss safety implications for temperature measurement.	Measures cognitive learning.
4. Have client describe common signs and symptoms of fever and hypothermia and methods for control.	Measures cognitive learning.

UNEXPECTED OUTCOMES AND RELATED INTERVENTIONS

- Client is unable to measure temperature or clean thermometer correctly.
  - Plan for client to demonstrate next temperature measurement under observation.
  - If home health nurse is visiting client, plan for a repeat demonstration during a scheduled visit.
  - Ask client to describe any difficulties experienced while performing temperature measurement and review and/or redesign learning component with demonstration of that part of the skill.
- Client is unable to explain factors affecting temperature, common signs and symptoms of fever and hypothermia, or measures to lower fever.
  - Use a different teaching strategy.
  - Repeat instruction pertaining to signs and symptoms of fever, measures to lower fever, and factors affecting body temperature.

RECORDING AND REPORTING

- Record information taught and client's response in home care record.

TEACHING CONSIDERATIONS

- Nurse may demonstrate on self or family member. Using client for demonstration prevents client from being able to observe entire procedure.
- Instruct client to maintain a written record of temperature readings along with time of day measured if routine temperature taking is part of plan of care.
- Instruct client or family to never use rectal thermometer after rectal surgery, with client who has a rectal disorder such as tumor or severe hemorrhoids, or with client who cannot be positioned for proper thermometer placement.
- Instruct client or family never to force thermometer into rectum and if client complains of rectal pain after insertion to notify physician and observe for rectal bleeding.
- Use caution in recommending aspirin or any other **over-the-counter drug** or **antipyretic** medicine in clients whose conditions contraindicate their use (e.g., gastric ulcer, bleeding tendencies, risk of Reye's syndrome in children, allergic reactions, drug interactions, liver or kidney dysfunction). Physician contact before use of antipyretics, even over-the-counter types, is recommended.
- Instruct to never use alcohol to lower fever. Inhaled fumes can be noxious, especially to young children and older adults.
- Instruct caregiver in safety measures for children and very debilitated clients, including remaining with client and assisting with maintaining safe and proper placement of thermometer.

PEDIATRIC CONSIDERATIONS

- Stage of growth and development of child will determine site of measurement and type of equipment used (see Chapter 9).
- When using glass thermometers in particular, but as a general rule for any equipment type, younger child should never be left unattended during procedure.

GERONTOLOGICAL CONSIDERATIONS

- Median oral temperature of older adults is 36° C (96.8° F); therefore temperature considered within normal range may reflect a fever in the older adult (Ebersole and Hess, 1999).
- Older adults are more sensitive to temperature changes and have a tendency to demonstrate symptoms of delirium or dementia with variations of body temperature, more frequently than younger adults.
- Altered internal temperature regulation or dehydration may be seen in frail, debilitated clients. Temperature measurement becomes very important to prevent severe states of hypothermia or hyperthermia.

- Teaching sessions should involve client actively with discussion of activity. Learning will be best accomplished when client is rested and alert. Sessions may be shorter in duration depending on factors such as fatigue.
- Consider common age-related sensory changes in the older adult, and direct teaching strategies to compensate for any alterations, such as a magnifying glass to read thermometer.

HOME CARE CONSIDERATIONS

- Assess temperature and ventilation of environment to determine existence of any condition that may influence client's temperature.
- Assess for safe storage of mercury-in-glass thermometer to protect from breakage.
- A digital thermometer may work best, because decreased visual acuity or poor lighting in environment may impair client's ability to properly read thermometer.

TEACHING CLIENTS TO MEASURE BLOOD PRESSURE

Clients learn to measure blood pressure to assist in the monitoring of health, to assess medication regimen effectiveness, or as part of a rehabilitation or exercise program. Clients with underlying physical ailments such as cardiac, kidney, or vascular disease may be susceptible to wide variations in their blood pressure. They should know how to correctly measure this indicator of their health status so they can seek medical attention early when alterations outside their acceptable ranges occur. Nurses can teach clients the skills of measuring arterial blood pressure and the important issues surrounding unusual readings of this measurement. Specific actions to be taken to reduce the chance of negative outcomes that are possible with poorly controlled blood pressure are equally important to the teaching plan (see Chapter 9).

Various types of electronic blood pressure reading devices are commercially available for home care use. These devices produce a blood pressure measurement without needing to use a stethoscope. A cuff around the arm or even a fingertip device is used, and a reading is displayed electronically for the client. When teaching blood pressure measurement using conventional equipment is not possible, these types of equipment may be used. Issues surrounding calibration and accuracy of electronic equipment need to be investigated before the client makes a purchase.

EQUIPMENT

- Mercury or aneroid sphygmomanometer
- Bladder and cuff: bladder should completely encircle arm without overlapping; cuff should be secure and fit snugly
  Average measurements:
  a. Width of bladder
     Adult: 12 to 13 cm (4¾ to 5¼ inches)
     Obese arm: 15 to 16 cm (6 to 6½ inches)
     Infant: 6 to 8 cm (2½ to 3¼ inches)
  b. Length of bladder:
     Adult: 22 to 23 cm (8¾ to 9¼ inches)
     Obese arm: 30 cm (12 inches)
     Infant: 12 to 13 cm (4¾ to 5¼ inches)
- Stethoscope (two-headed teaching stethoscope is ideal)
- Pen and paper for recording

STEP	RATIONALE
ASSESSMENT	
1. Assess client's abilities to manipulate and properly place cuff, to handle and read measurement gauge, and to properly place and hear through stethoscope.	Physical restrictions in handling, seeing, or hearing when using equipment may require nurse to instruct family member instead of client.
2. Assess client's knowledge of normal blood pressure range and symptoms and common causes of hypotension and hypertension.	Identifies client's ability to know when to initiate preventive health measures and recognize alterations in BP.
3. Assess client's knowledge of what BP measures, any specific medical issues that affect it, and why an awareness of variations are important to client's well-being.	Identifies client's understanding of potential cause-and-effect relationships of poorly controlled BP variations for health status.
4. If client has had experience in measuring BP, ask for demonstration of technique.	Allows nurse to assess client's knowledge and skill performance.
5. Determine best site for BP assessment. Avoid applying cuff to arm with intravenous (IV) fluids infusing or with an infusion catheter in place, in the presence of arteriovenous shunt, when breast or axillary surgery has been performed on that side, if arm or hand has been traumatized or diseased, or in presence of lower arm cast or bulky bandage.	Application of pressure from inflated bladder can temporarily impair blood flow and compromise circulation in extremity that already has impaired circulation.

STEP	RATIONALE
6. Assess home environment for quiet place to measure BP.	Ensures more accurate detection of BP.

- ***Critical Decision Point***
  Eliminate extraneous noise, such as television and conversation.

NURSING DIAGNOSIS

Defining characteristics from the assessment data may reveal the following nursing diagnoses for clients requiring this skill:

- Decreased cardiac output
- Deficient fluid volume
- Excess fluid volume
- Ineffective health maintenance
- Health-seeking behaviors (BP measurement)
- Deficient knowledge regarding blood pressure monitoring

Related factors are individualized based on client's condition or needs.

PLANNING

STEP	RATIONALE
1. **Expected outcomes** following completion of procedure:	
▪ BP is accurately monitored by client.	Learning has occurred.
▪ BP is within range expected for client for client's age and condition.	Cardiovascular status is stable at level that is acceptable for client.
▪ Client explains purpose and implications of therapies and describes which alterations in BP require communication with physician to evaluate changes in treatment regimen.	Measures cognitive learning.
2. Encourage client to perform measurements on routine schedule for a long-term monitoring plan.	Daily activities and many extrinsic and intrinsic factors affect BP fluctuations.
3. Encourage client to avoid exercise, caffeine, and smoking for 30 minutes before assessment.	These factors can cause false elevations in BP.
4. Have client perform measurement in a comfortable position, with feet flat on floor, and in warm and quiet environment.	Maintains client's comfort during measurement. Systolic and diastolic BP increase significantly with crossed-leg position (Foster-Fitzpatrick and others, 1999).
5. In teaching phase, explain procedure to client and have client rest at least 5 minutes before measurement.	Reduces anxiety that can falsely elevate readings. BP readings taken at different times can be objectively compared when all are assessed with client at rest.
6. Have client describe symptoms that would benefit from performing a BP measurement to evaluate possible causes of symptoms.	Measures learning of health status alterations that may need medical intervention.

IMPLEMENTATION

STEP	RATIONALE
1. Discuss with client the best sites for assessing BP: brachial and popliteal artery. For self-measurement, brachial artery is almost always used.	Most accessible sites are easiest to measure for accuracy of assessment. Appropriate site selection will promote accuracy in reading and minimize potential for trauma.

- ***Critical Decision Point***
  If client is recovering from trauma to upper or lower arm tell client not to use this extremity for BP measurement as there may be poor amplification of sounds or compromised circulation.

STEP	RATIONALE
2. Demonstrate steps for skill performance (see Chapter 9): palpation of artery, positioning of cuff, wrapping of cuff, placement of stethoscope, inflation and release of cuff, listening.	Demonstration is best technique for teaching psychomotor skill.
3. Describe sounds of measurement and relationship to observation of gauge as BP reading. Caution client about level and length of time appropriate for cuff inflation.	Learning is supported with appropriate information being received. Prolonged inflation of cuff may damage circulation of limb.

Step	Rationale
4. Have client manipulate all equipment away from limb.	Proper equipment utilization is required for accurate skill performance.
5. Have client attempt each step of skill on nurse or family member.	Nurse can correct any errors in technique as they occur.
6. Have client demonstrate techniques on self. Do not allow multiple repetitive attempts on any one limb.	Repeated attempts may affect measurement because of anxiety and repeated circulatory restriction.
7. Identify that skill performance teaching may need to be accomplished slowly, attempting each step of skill at different times until comfort is gained.	Psychomotor, cognitive, and affective learning may be impaired if teaching is attempted too quickly rather than in incremental steps.
8. Have client perform skill under observation and record readings. Use a double-headed stethoscope to verify accuracy of reading, or nurse should perform BP reading after client's attempt.	Verification of accuracy promotes confidence in client's abilities to successfully measure BP.
9. Utilize instructions with written or pictorial guide.	References for client will promote confidence for independent performance.

Evaluation

Step	Rationale
1. Observe client demonstrate technique for BP measurement on at least three different occasions.	Feedback through independent demonstration of psychomotor learning is best means to evaluate.
2. Ask client if blood pressure is within desired range.	Determines client's ability to know when blood pressure obtained is within proper range.
3. Ask client to describe reason for blood pressure monitoring and any related medications (e.g., antihypertensives) or treatment (e.g., diet and exercise).	Determines client's understanding of blood pressure monitoring and related therapies.

Unexpected Outcomes and Related Interventions

- Client or family member is unable to utilize this measurement method due to inability to manipulate equipment or accurately hear or palpate BP.
  - Indicates need for alteration in teaching plan.
  - Review skill performance and recording of BP measurements client has performed in between home care nursing visits.
- Client has difficulty in explaining purposes or implications of therapy.
  - Reinstruction is required.
- Blood pressure is inaudible or difficult to obtain.
  - Have client wait 1 or 2 minutes and repeat attempt.
  - If pressure is still inaudible or difficult to obtain, try alternative methods: use other arm, consider changing equipment for measurement.

Recording and Reporting

- Record teaching and client responses in home care record.
- Record BP in home care record and home documentation system developed.
- Instruct client and/or family to report abnormal readings to physician.

Teaching Considerations

- Nurse should demonstrate on self or family member. Using client for total demonstration prevents client from being able to observe entire procedure. Nurse explains rationale for each step during demonstration.
- Client needs to be educated about risks for hypertension (see Chapter 9).
- Client needs to understand specifics of treatment regimen, including potential side effects and interactions of any drug therapies.
- Appropriate cuff size must be used (adult, large adult, thigh, or pediatric) to provide accuracy.
- As long as cuff is inflated, client will feel numbness or tingling in arm because of reduced blood flow.
- Improper care and storage of equipment can affect accuracy of measurement.
- Instruct client that if it is difficult to hear the pressure, cuff may be too loose or not the correct size; stethoscope may not be over arterial pulse, or tubing may be too long; cuff may have been deflated too quickly or too slowly; or cuff may not have been pumped high enough for systolic readings.

PEDIATRIC CONSIDERATIONS

- Understand that accurate BP readings may be difficult if infant or young child is not cooperative in procedure. Assistance from others in the form of cajoling or providing diversionary tactics may be needed.
- Young children will be more apt to cooperate if allowed to manipulate and/or play with equipment before procedure. Another suggested technique is to perform procedure first on parent or other person significant to child to allow observation of role modeling that procedure is safe for child to undergo.

GERONTOLOGICAL CONSIDERATIONS

- Musculoskeletal changes such as arthritis or other joint conditions may impair abilities to position limb comfortably and/or perform fine motor skills required for client to measure blood pressure (Lueckenotte, 2000).
- Older adults, especially those who are frail, have lost upper arm mass, requiring attention to selection of a smaller BP cuff.
- Older adults have an increased systolic pressure related to decreased vessel elasticity.
- Possible alterations in hearing or visual acuity associated with changes of aging or disease processes may negatively affect client's performance of this skill.

HOME CARE CONSIDERATIONS

- Assess home noise level to select a room that will provide a quiet environment for assessing BP.
- Consider electronic BP cuff for home use if client or caregiver has hearing difficulties (Rice, 1996).

TEACHING CLIENTS TO ASSESS THEIR OWN PULSE

Certain clients can benefit from knowing how to assess their own pulse. Persons taking medications that specifically affect heart function already have symptoms of heart disease and are susceptible to side effects of the medications. By being able to assess their own pulse rate and rhythm correctly, these clients can detect complications of their disease and any undesirable effects of their medications. Clients can thus seek prompt medical attention before serious problems occur.

Another group of clients who should learn how to assess their own pulse are those undergoing cardiovascular rehabilitation. For example, clients who have had myocardial infarction undergo exercise training to improve the strength of their heart muscle. Pulse rate and rhythm are the criteria used to determine how well these clients tolerate exercise.

There are also many healthy persons who actively exercise and who can learn about their health from measuring their own pulse. Exercise tolerance can vary depending on environmental conditions, intake of certain foods, and the overall physical condition of a person. By measuring pulse rate and rhythm, a person can learn how the body responds to strenuous exercise and when to cease further physical activity.

EQUIPMENT

- Wristwatch or clock with second hand
- Paper and pencil

STEP	RATIONALE
ASSESSMENT	
1. Identify client's knowledge of purpose for assessing pulse and level of interest in performing skill.	Aids in identifying client's motivation to regularly assess pulse after learning skill. Also allows nurse to assess client's understanding of physical conditions and knowledge of medications prescribed.
2. Assess client's ability to feel arterial pulse by having client palpate own or nurse's artery. (Nurse palpates pulse of client or self simultaneously to see if client can successfully feel pulse wave.)	Physical impairment in sensation may necessitate nurse instructing family member or significant other instead of client.
3. If client reports having measured own pulse before, ask client to demonstrate technique for assessing pulse.	Reveals client's level of skill in assessing pulse.

NURSING DIAGNOSIS

Defining characteristics from the assessment data may reveal the following nursing diagnoses for clients requiring this skill:

Anxiety
Decreased cardiac output
Deficient fluid volume
Excess fluid volume
Impaired home maintenance management
Health-seeking behaviors (pulse measurement)
Deficient knowledge regarding obtaining pulse

Related factors are individualized based on client's condition or needs.

Step	Rationale
Planning	
1. **Expected outcomes** following completion of procedure:	
▪ Client is able to measure own pulse rate and rhythm correctly.	Indicates skill was effectively learned.
▪ Client identifies normal range of pulse rate.	Cognitive learning was achieved.
▪ Client discusses importance of assessing pulse and best time for measurement.	
▪ Client discusses abnormalities and steps to take.	Client learns preventive health actions.
2. Select setting in home that client is most likely to use when assessing pulse.	Practicing in same environment in which skill is routinely performed facilitates comprehension and learning.
Implementation	
1. Discuss with client the best sites for assessing pulse: radial and carotid.	Most accessible sites are easiest to palpate for accuracy of assessment.

• ***Critical Decision Point***

If carotid is chosen, caution client against vigorously massaging neck while attempting to locate pulse or attempting to locate both arteries at the same time. Stimulation of carotid sinus could lead to reflex slowing of heart rate from vagal stimulation. In addition, simultaneous occlusion of both carotid arteries further decreases blood to brain, resulting in fainting.

Step	Rationale
2. Demonstrate steps for palpating pulse (see Chapter 9): position on wrist or neck, locate artery, use fingertips for palpation, compress artery, palpate pulse before counting, count pulse, and calculate pulse rate.	Demonstration is best technique for teaching psychomotor skill.
a. Instruct use of gentle pressure; reinforce not to press hard over pulse sites.	Pressing too hard may occlude the artery.
b. Instruct in use of watch or clock with a second hand to count pulses.	Ensures correct timing of pulse.
c. Instruct to count for a full 60 seconds, starting with second hand at 12:00 position.	To reduce confusion, forgetfulness about time period, or starting point used for pulse measurement. A full 60-second count increases accuracy of measure.
3. Have client perform each step with nurse's guidance (see illustration).	Nurse can correct any errors in technique as they occur.
4. Discuss normal desired pulse range, purpose for monitoring pulse, and when pulse should be measured.	Client must be able to identify pulse alterations.

• ***Critical Decision Point***

Discuss importance of notifying physician and withholding medication dose when pulse alterations occur. Client must understand preventive measures to take and physician's directions to be followed if alterations in pulse develop.

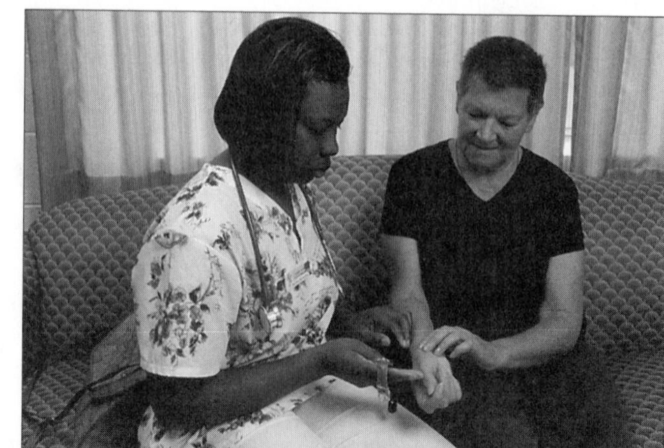

STEP **3** Nurse observing client checking pulse.

Step	Rationale
Evaluation	
1. Observe client independently demonstrate technique for pulse assessment and calculate pulse rate and rhythm three times.	Feedback through independent demonstration of psychomotor skill is best means of evaluating learning of skill.
2. Have learner take radial pulse rate of nurse or other person at same time nurse is taking pulse of the individual.	Concomitant pulse taking will verify learner is able to accurately accomplish this skill.
3. Ask client to identify reasons for assessing pulse, normal pulse rate range, and steps to take when abnormalities are found.	Measures client's cognitive learning.
4. Ask client to reiterate instructions regarding withholding of medication in response to critical changes in pulse rate.	Confirms understanding of specific medical instructions received regarding withholding of certain prescribed medications with specific pulse rates.
5. Ask client to state time of day and activity level before pulse taking if purpose of measuring is for possible medication dosage adjustment.	Demonstrates understanding of relationships of time of day and activity levels with pulse rate variation.

Unexpected Outcomes and Related Interventions

- Client is unable to palpate pulse or count rate correctly.
  - May result from sensory alteration or inability to locate artery or palpate it correctly. Clients with preexisting dysrhythmias often have difficulty learning to count pulse correctly.
  - Plan a repeat demonstration and return demonstration to evaluate client ability to perform skill.
  - Teach skill to a friend or family member.
- Client is unable to discuss information related to pulse assessment.
  - Anxiety, lack of interest, language barriers, or method of instruction may interfere with learning.
  - Review client's pulse assessment recording sheet to assess for significant issues or medication noncompliance.

Recording and Reporting

- Record information taught and client's response in home care record.
- Have client develop and use a written record of pulse rate, rhythm, time of taking, and whether medications are to be withheld with certain variations.

Teaching Considerations

- Physicians will recommend whether drug dose should be withheld in event of pulse alteration. Clients taking thyroid medications are often instructed to withhold medications when pulse is above 100 beats per minute; propranolol (Inderal) or digitalis often is withheld if pulse is below 60 beats per minute. Specific drug dosage instructions are to be confirmed with physician, and documented in home care record, and written for client.
- Pulse rate is usually assessed before medications are taken and before and during exercise.
- Nurse may demonstrate on self or family member. Using client for entire demonstration prevents client from being able to observe entire procedure. Nurse explains rationale for each step during demonstration.

Pediatric Considerations

- Femoral pulse is best site for palpation of pulse for infant or toddler. Although carotid pulse reading is more easily obtained than radial, which is usually used for adults, when teaching nonmedical caregivers, the potential for occluding carotid artery and creating hypoxia should be avoided.
- In infants, pulse can be observed (do not palpate) and counted on anterior fontanel.

Gerontological Considerations

- Musculoskeletal changes such as arthritis or other joint conditions may impair abilities to palpate pulse for 60 seconds because of discomfort caused by positioning. Provide client with options for comfortable resting position of limbs when measuring pulse.
- Be aware of possible changes in visual acuity and ensure environment and equipment used (clock or watch) support clear visualization.

Skill 40-2 Using Home Oxygen Equipment

Home **oxygen therapy** is usually administered via a **nasal cannula** and, more recently, through a reservoir nasal cannula, which stores oxygen in a chamber during the expiratory phase of respirations (Rice, 1996), and a Venturi mask. When a client has a permanent tracheostomy, however, a T tube, tracheostomy collar, or **transtracheal oxygen therapy (TTOT)** is used. TTOT is a newer method of oxygen administration that delivers oxygen directly into the trachea using a scoop catheter. In the home the main consideration is the oxygen delivery source; the three types used are (1) compressed oxygen, (2) oxygen concentrators (Figure 40-1, Table 40-1), and (3) liquid oxygen (Figure 40-2 *A*, *B*).

Compressed oxygen requires the delivery of several large oxygen tanks to the home. Each tank lasts approximately 50 hours at 2 L/min. Liquid systems use a small portable tank that is filled from a reservoir in the home. The oxygen concentrator method extracts oxygen from the room air and supplies oxygen to the client at prescribed flow rates. Table 40-2 shows how long a liquid oxygen system will last depending on the prescribed flow rate. Home oxygen therapy is often paid for by governmental or private insurance if there are written orders prescribed by the physician. Specific guidelines must be met before Medicare coverage can begin (Box 40-1).

Clients requiring home oxygen need extensive teaching so that they can continue their oxygen therapy efficiently and safely. In preparation the home care nurse must coordinate efforts with the client, physician, caregivers, oxygen supply vendor, and payer. The nurse must set aside sufficient time for client and family teaching so proper oxygen therapy can be performed safely and accurately in the home. Ultimately, the home care nurse is responsible and accountable for determining the validity of safe and effective home oxygen administration.

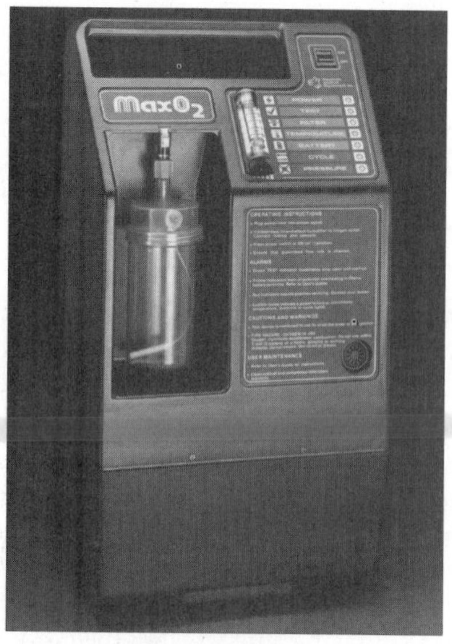

FIGURE 40-1 Oxygen concentrator. (Courtesy Mountain Medical Equipment Inc, Littleton, Colo.)

Table 40-1 Home Oxygen Systems

Primary Use	Advantages	Disadvantages
Compressed Gas Cylinders		
Intermittent therapy, such as for exercise or sleep only	100% oxygen, relatively inexpensive, no loss of gas during storage, relatively portable, delivery of up to 15 L/min	Bulky, possibly unsightly, frequent refilling necessary with continuous use
Liquid Oxygen Systems		
High-liter flows and active clients	100% oxygen, conveniently portable, portable units refilled at home, delivery of up to 6 L/min	Usually weekly delivery necessary for refill, evaporates if not used, potential for frostbite at connections and if liquid is spilled
Concentrators		
Moderate-liter flows and clients with limited mobility inside or outside home	Fixed monthly cost, minimal interruption of household by supplier, no refills of "main tank," most units with delivery of up to 4 or 5 L/min	Oxygen concentration decreases as liter flow increases (usually 85% to 90%), power supply necessary, increasing electrical costs, second system for portability necessary (usually gas cylinders)

From Dettenmeier PA: *Pulmonary nursing care,* St. Louis, 1992, Mosby.

A

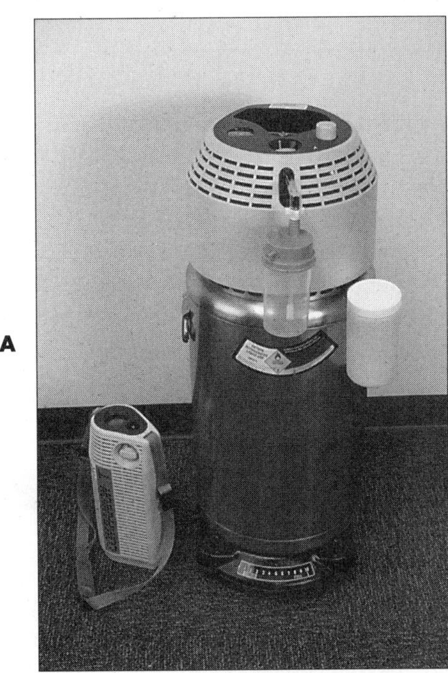

B

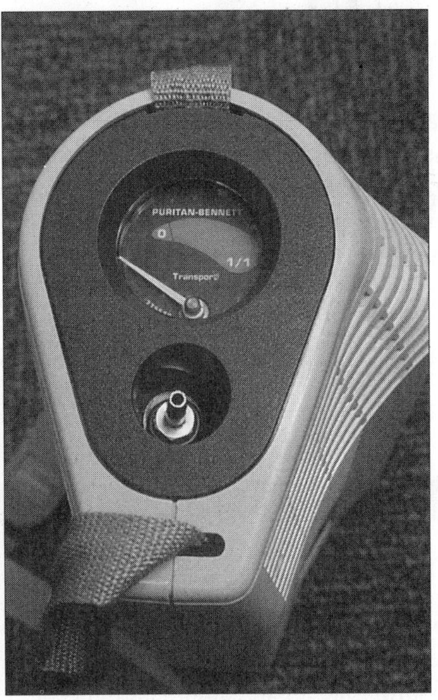

FIGURE **40-2** **A,** Liquid oxygen container. **B,** Control panel.

Table 40-2 Liquid Oxygen Timetable

L/MIN	STATIONARY RESERVOIRS 17,000 L	STATIONARY RESERVOIRS 25,000 L	PORTABLE UNITS 500 L	PORTABLE UNITS 1000 L
1	248 hr	396 hr	7 hr	14 hr
2	124 hr	198 hr	3 hr	7 hr
3	83 hr	134 hr	2 hr	4½ hr
4	61 hr	99 hr	1½ hr	3½ hr
5	40 hr	80 hr	—	—
6	—	—	1 hr	2 hr

When oxygen cylinders are used, the following formulas are used to determine the length of time a tank will last.

FOR E CYLINDERS

Pressure on cylinder gauge (PSI) − 500 psi (safety factor) × 0.3 (E cylinder factor) ÷ L/min = minutes

FOR H CYLINDERS

Pressure on cylinder gauge (PSI) − 500 psi (safety factor) × 3.1 (H cylinder factor) ÷ L/min = minutes

EXAMPLE: E cylinder reads 1500 psi
Liter flow rate is 4 L/min
1500 − 500 × 0.3 ÷ 4 = ?
1000 × 0.3 ÷ 4 = ?
300 ÷ 4 = ?
75 minutes, or 1 hour 15 minutes

NOTE: Do not allow oxygen cylinder pressure to fall below 500 psi, or the client may run out of oxygen.

Box 40-1 Medicare Qualifications for Home Oxygen Therapy

PaO_2 ≤55 mm Hg or SaO_2 ≤85% or PaO_2 = 56 to 59 mm Hg *and*
Dependent edema suggesting congestive heart failure *or*
Cor pulmonale as evidenced on ECG *or*
Erythrocytosis as evidenced by hematocrit >56%

NOCTURNAL OXYGEN THERAPY

PaO_2 ≤55 mm Hg during sleep *or*
PaO_2 falls more than 10 mm Hg during sleep *or*
SaO_2 ≤85% during sleep or falls more than 5% during sleep

EXERCISE OXYGEN THERAPY

PaO_2 ≤55 mm Hg during exercise *or*
SaO_2 ≤85% during exercise

PaO_2, arterial oxygen tension (partial pressure); SaO_2, oxygen saturation in blood; ECG, electrocardiogram.

Delegation Considerations

This skill should not be delegated to assistive personnel. The nurse assumes accountability for appropriate assessment and implementation of home oxygen therapy by the client or appropriate caregiver after teaching has occurred.

Equipment

- Nasal cannula (see Skill 11-1) or other prescribed delivery device
- Oxygen tubing
- Liquid oxygen
- In home: Liberator
- Portable system: Stroller
- Cylinders
- In home: H tanks
- Portable system: E cylinder
- Concentrator for home system

Step	Rationale
Assessment	
1. Determine client's or family's ability to use oxygen equipment correctly while in hospital (if appropriate and possible), and assess for appropriate use of equipment in home.	Physical or cognitive impairments may necessitate instructing family member or significant other how to operate home oxygen equipment.
2. Assess home environment for adequate electrical service.	Continuous O_2 therapy must not be interrupted.
3. Assess client's and/or family's ability to observe for signs and symptoms of **hypoxia:** apprehension, anxiety, decreased ability to concentrate, decreased levels of consciousness, increased fatigue, dizziness, behavioral changes, increased pulse, increased respiratory rate, pallor, and cyanosis.	Hypoxia can occur at home when client uses oxygen. It can be caused by worsening of client's physical problem or another underlying condition such as change in respiratory status.
4. Observe client's or family's ability to use prescribed oxygen therapy.	Enables nurse to determine specific components of skill that client or family can easily complete.
5. Determine appropriate resource in community for equipment and assistance.	Ensures repair service availability, readily available assistance, and additional equipment for clients with home oxygen systems.
6. Determine appropriate back-up systems, if compressor is used, in event of power failure (e.g., notify local emergency medical service [EMS]).	Many municipalities require that clients who have home oxygen equipment notify EMS before bringing the equipment home. When there is a power outage, EMS will call the home and in some cases the home is on priority list for having power restored.

Nursing Diagnosis

Defining characteristics from the assessment data may reveal the following nursing diagnoses for clients requiring this skill:

- Ineffective peripheral tissue perfusion
- Anxiety
- Impaired home maintenance
- Ineffective breathing pattern
- Deficient knowledge regarding home oxygen therapy

Related factors are individualized based on client's condition or needs.

Planning

Step	Rationale
1. **Expected outcomes** following completion of procedure:	
▪ Client receives oxygen at the prescribed rate.	O_2 system set up correctly.
▪ Client and family will verbalize purpose and correct use of home oxygen.	Provides measurable criteria to determine client's and family's level of understanding.
▪ Client and family will demonstrate how to set up oxygen system.	Provides return demonstration of skills needed to use home oxygen system.

Step	Rationale
▪ Client and family will be able to verbalize safety guidelines for oxygen use. ▪ Client and family will be able to verbalize emergency plan of care.	Provides measure of client's and family's understanding of oxygen use.
2. Explain procedure to client and family.	Reinforces teaching received. Enables client and family to ask questions.

Implementation

Step	Rationale
1. Wash hands.	Reduces transmission of microorganisms.
2. Demonstrates steps for preparation and completion of oxygen therapy.	Demonstration is reliable technique for teaching psychomotor skill and enables client to ask questions.
3. Prepare Liberator and Stroller for use:	
a. Place Liberator in clutter-free environment (see Figure 40-2, *A*).	30-L Liberator replaces $3\frac{1}{2}$ compressed oxygen cylinders.

• ***Critical Decision Point***
Check oxygen levels of both Liberator and Stroller by depressing button at lower right corner and reading dial (see Figure 40-2, B*).*

Step	Rationale
b. Equipment vendor and nurse should instruct client or caregiver how frequently Liberator and Stroller must be filled. Refilling occurs automatically and takes a few seconds to a minute, depending on amount of oxygen required to fill Stroller.	Ensures timely and effective use of remaining oxygen supply and allows time for refill. Small Liberator has 4-hour capacity, whereas large Stroller has 8-hour capacity.
c. When necessary, refill Stroller: turn bayonet-coupling lock on Stroller 45 degrees (see illustration 3c [A]). Insert female adapter (Liberator) into male adapter (Liberator) (see illustration 3c [B]).	Allows secure connection between Liberator and Stroller to prevent leakage of oxygen into room air.

A
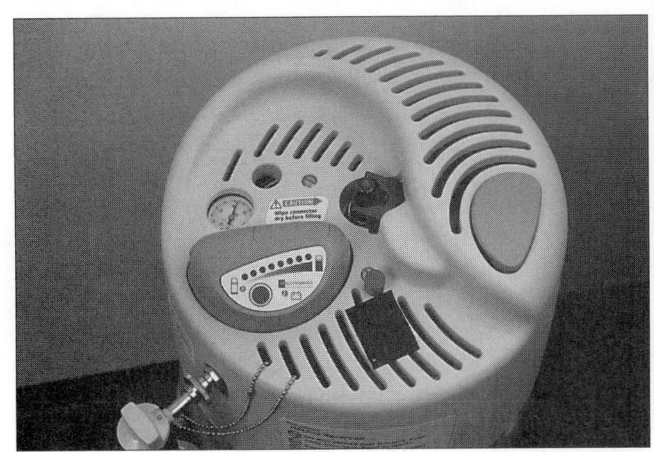

B
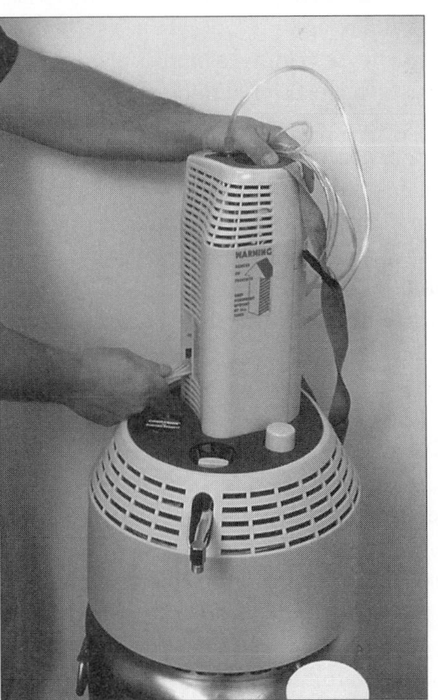

STEP **3c** **A,** Turn Bayonet coupling lock. **B,** Insertion of Liberator into liquid oxygen container.

STEP	RATIONALE
d. Select prescribed rate and lock flow meter.	Ensures delivery of prescribed amount of oxygen and prevents client from changing oxygen flow rate.
e. Connect appropriate oxygen delivery device and oxygen tubing to Stroller (see Chapter 11) (see illustration).	Connects oxygen source to delivery method.

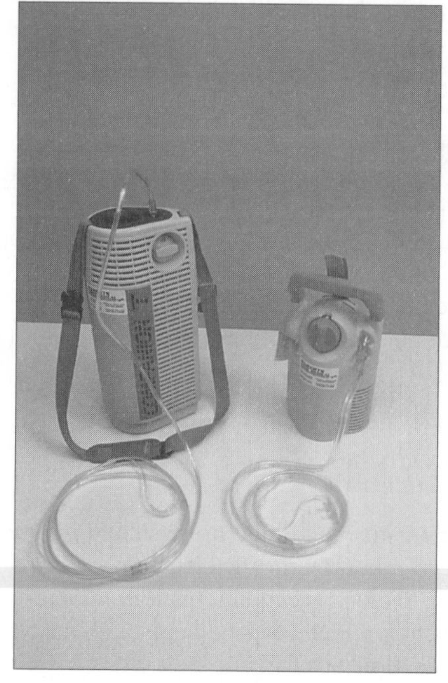

STEP 3e Oxygen delivery device and tubing connected to Stroller.

STEP	RATIONALE
f. Place Stroller on cart.	Allows client to ambulate freely without expending energy to carry Stroller.
4. Have client or family member perform each step with guidance from nurse. Provide written material for reinforcement and review.	Allows nurse to correct any errors in technique and discuss their implications.
5. Instruct client or family to notify physician if signs or symptoms of hypoxia or respiratory tract infection (e.g., fever, increased sputum, change in color of sputum, foul sputum odor) occur.	Respiratory tract infections increase oxygen demand and may affect oxygen transfer from lungs to blood. Can create severe exacerbation of client's pulmonary disease.
6. Discuss emergency plan: power loss, natural disaster, acute respiratory distress; call 911 and notify physician and agency.	Ensures appropriate response and can prevent worsening of client's condition.
7. Wash hands.	Reduces transmission of microorganisms.
8. Record teaching plan, information given to client, and validation of learning.	Provides written documentation of teaching plan for client and family. Documents client learning.

EVALUATION

STEP	RATIONALE
1. Client receives oxygen at prescribed rate.	Determines that client and family are able to correctly monitor oxygen delivery.
2. Ask client about ease or problems associated with home oxygen.	Determines ability of client or family to deal with stressors associated with home oxygen use. Also indicates client's risk for inappropriate oxygen use.
3. Ask client and family to state safety guidelines, emergency precautions, and emergency plan.	Determines client's knowledge of what to do if power fails, there is a failure in equipment, or client's status worsens.

Unexpected Outcomes and Related Interventions

- Client has signs and symptoms associated with hypoxia (see Assessment, Step 3).
  - Determine if oxygen delivery device and oxygen source are delivering oxygen properly.
  - Determine if prescribed oxygen flow rate is set properly.
  - Assess client for change in respiratory status, such as airway plugging, respiratory tract infection, or bronchospasm.
  - Instruct client and family when to notify physician of signs of hypoxia.
- Client uses unsafe practices with oxygen therapy, uses oxygen around fire or cigarette smoking, or sets incorrect flow rate.
  - Reinforce client education and perform follow-up reassessment.

Recording and Reporting

- Record in home care record teaching plan preparations for teaching client to use home oxygen.
- Record in home care record information given to client or family and any validation of learning.
- Communicate client's or family's learning progress to other health care providers involved.

Teaching Considerations

- Potential for oxygen desaturation and decreased oxygen delivery to brain impairs client's ability to remember previous learning. Thus nurse should provide more opportunity and written or pictorial instructions to reinforce previous learning of teaching plan.
- Instruct client to observe level of oxygen in canister tank and to use portable tank when client goes out.
- Instruct client and family in the dangers of oxygen use with smoking, gas stove, or fires of any kind.
- Instruct client to fill plastic humidity bottle with distilled water every 24 hours. Tap water should not be used. Effective humidification of home oxygen is essential for respiratory mucus flow and secretion removal (Fell and Boehm, 1998).
- Instruct client and caregiver to check mask and tubing by placing hands or face over mask or cannula to feel air flow and to check to be sure mask is not too tight; it can leave marks on skin. Apply cotton or gauze sponge at pressure points.
- Instruct client to keep a bell handy for notifying primary caregiver when help is needed.

Pediatric Considerations

- Equipment must be kept out of reach of the child and/or other children in home. Manipulation of dials or flow meters could have disastrous effects on oxygen delivery process.

Gerontological Considerations

- Older adults have less efficient respiratory systems and less surface area for gas exchange, so their response to decreased oxygen and infection may cause cerebral anoxia and they may experience confusion. They may be unable to recognize respiratory problems or problems with delivery system; therefore they must have frequent contact with a designated caregiver.

Home Care Considerations

- Provide two complete sets of tubing so that there is equipment available for use while the other is being cleansed or repaired.
- Assess home for availability of three-pronged outlet for compressor to prevent electric shock.
- Client, family, and visitors must understand danger of and refrain from smoking cigarettes or having any source of fire near oxygen system.
- Some clients are able to manage portable oxygen system but are unable to fill portable system and require assistance.

Skill 40-3 Teaching Home Tracheostomy Care and Suctioning

The indications for performing tracheostomy care and suctioning in the home are similar to tracheostomy care and suctioning in the hospital except for one key variable: the use of principles of **medical asepsis** or **clean technique.** In the hospital, principles of surgical asepsis are used because the client is more susceptible to infection and because more virulent or pathogenic microorganisms are usually present than in the home setting. In the home setting the majority of clients use clean technique.

However, not all home care clients should use clean technique. The nurse must use good nursing judgment in choosing clients who are candidates for using clean or aseptic technique. The immunocompromised client, who is at risk for severe infections, may need to continue to receive suctioning using principles of surgical asepsis. A client receiving care from visiting nurses or other caregivers who have contact with other clients (or institutions) should be suctioned by the nurse using sterile technique. Infected (not colonized) clients should be suctioned using sterile technique until the infection is resolved. Caregivers who are infected with viral, bacterial, or fungal microorganisms should suction using principles of surgical asepsis. All caregivers should use standard precautions when suctioning. Clients living in nonhygienic (nonclean) conditions should be suctioned using sterile technique whenever possible, in hopes of preventing infection.

Caring for a tracheostomy at home begins in the hospital with teaching and return demonstration. The client usually learns better when less invasive techniques such as stoma care precede more invasive techniques such as inner cannula care and suctioning. The nurse continually develops, implements, and evaluates the teaching plan based on client performance. Some clients and their families learn quickly, whereas others do not. Therefore teaching should begin as soon as it is feasible. It is imperative that clients and their families have the ability to suction before discharge; otherwise, arrangements to provide 24-hour care are necessary before discharge.

Delegation Considerations

This skill should not be delegated to assistive personnel. The nurse assumes accountability for appropriate assessment and implementation of home oxygen therapy by the client or appropriate caregiver after teaching has occurred.

Equipment

- Suction machine with connecting tube (Figure 40-3)
- Clean gloves
- 3 small basins
- Hydrogen peroxide, water (boiled preferred over tap)
- Normal saline
- Clean 4 × 4 gauze pads (nonshredding)
- Appropriate size of sterile or clean and disinfected catheter (diameter should be no greater than half the diameter of the trach tube)
- Tracheostomy care kit or clean 4 × 4 gauze pads (nonshredding)
- Water-soluble lubricant
- Small nylon bottle brush or pipe cleaners
- Cotton-tipped applicators
- Tracheostomy ties (twill ⅜-inch preferably)
- Mirror
- Wet washcloth or paper towel
- Dry cloth, towel, or paper towel
- Protective eyewear (optional)
- Trash bag (plastic, nonleaking preferred)
- Disposable apron (optional)

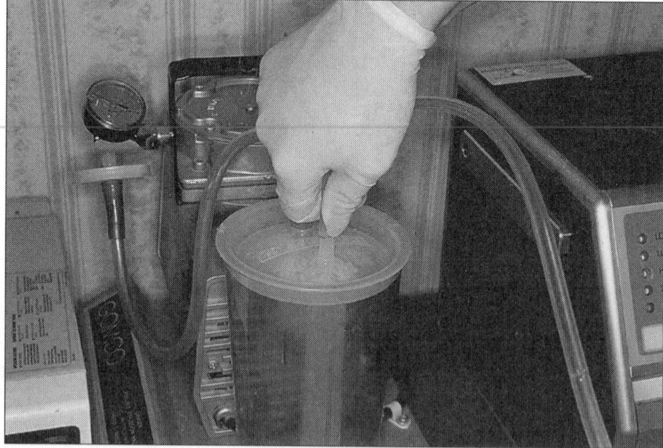

FIGURE 40-3 Suction machine.

Step	Rationale
Assessment	
1. Assess client's ability to properly perform tracheostomy care and suctioning.	Physical and cognitive impairment may necessitate instructing family member or significant other to perform tracheostomy care and suctioning. An emergency situation may also require family member or significant other to suction.

Step	Rationale
2. Assess client and family member's knowledge and ability to observe for signs and symptoms of need to perform:	
a. Tracheostomy care, including excess peristomal secretions, excess intratracheal secretions, soiled or damp tracheostomy dressing/ties, and diminished airway through tracheostomy tube.	Signs and symptoms are related to presence of secretions at stoma site or within tracheostomy tube.
b. Suctioning, including gurgling, tactile fremitus, wheezes or crackles on inspiration or expiration, restlessness, ineffective coughing, absent or diminished breath sounds, tachypnea, cyanosis, acutely decreased level of consciousness, hypertension or hypotension, tachycardia or bradycardia, acutely shallow respirations, or acute dyspnea.	Physical signs and symptoms result from lower airway obstruction and tissue hypoxia.
3. Assess client's and family's ability to observe for factors that normally influence tracheostomy airway functioning.	Allows client to accurately evaluate need to perform trach tube suctioning.
4. Assess client's understanding of and ability to perform own tracheostomy care and suctioning.	Allows nurse to identify potential need for instruction.
5. Observe client or family member performing complete trach tube care and suctioning.	Allows nurse to determine which specific components of skill client or family member can easily complete and which are more difficult and require more instruction.

Nursing Diagnosis

Defining characteristics from the assessment data may reveal the following nursing diagnoses for clients requiring this skill:

- Risk for caregiver role strain
- Impaired verbal communication
- Ineffective airway clearance
- Ineffective breathing pattern
- Deficient knowledge regarding tracheostomy care
- Risk for infection

Related factors are individualized based on client's condition or needs.

Planning

Step	Rationale
1. **Expected outcomes** following completion of procedure:	
▪ Client is able to identify signs and symptoms indicating need for trach care and suctioning.	Allows nurse to objectively measure client's learning and to modify teaching plan as necessary.
▪ Client can state factors that normally influence tracheostomy airway functioning.	Tracheostomy can impair normal airway clearance, humidification, and gas exchange.
▪ Client can correctly demonstrate complete trach tube care and suctioning in controlled setting.	Provides documentation of client's ability to perform procedure.
▪ Client is able to identify signs of stoma inflammation or respiratory tract infection, and when to notify physician.	Measures cognitive learning.
▪ Lower and upper airways are cleared of secretions, as evidenced by absent or diminished crackles, wheezes, tactile fremitus, and gurgles in large airways; return of absent or diminished breath sounds; normalization of vital signs; increased depth of respirations; absence of cyanosis; and decreased dyspnea.	Suctioning is successful.
▪ Stoma site is clean and free of infection; inner cannula is free of secretions.	Tracheostomy care is successful.
2. Select setting in home that client is most likely to use when completing trach tube care.	Practicing skill in same setting where skill will be routinely performed facilitates comprehension and learning.
3. Discuss and demonstrate with client proper position for procedure (high-Fowler's position in front of a mirror).	Promotes client's understanding of comfort and safety principles and facilitates visibility.

STEP	RATIONALE
IMPLEMENTATION	
1. Verify physician orders for suctioning.	
2. Wash hands.	Reduces transmission of microorganisms.
3. Demonstrate step-by-step preparation and completion of tracheostomy tube suctioning.	Demonstration is reliable technique for teaching psychomotor skill and enables client to ask questions throughout procedure.
4. Prepare suction equipment according to manufacturer's directions. a. Place machine on level surface. b. Plug into grounded outlet. c. Set suction pressure between 100 and 120 mm Hg.	Preparation of equipment ensures orderly procedure.
5. Place client in **high Fowler's position.**	Promotes lung expansion and allows client to view procedure.
6. Fill basin with ½ cup water or normal saline.	
7. Apply gloves.	Reduces transmission of microorganisms.
8. Connect suction catheter to suction apparatus, and check that equipment is functioning by suctioning small amount of fluid from basin.	Prepares suction. Ensures proper equipment function before catheter insertion and lubricates internal catheter.

• ***Critical Decision Point***
Encourage client to cough.

9. In an adult insert catheter without applying suction. If resistance (carina) is met, pull catheter back 1 cm.	Prevents trauma to tracheal tissues.
10. Apply intermittent suction, 5 to 10 seconds, by placing and releasing thumb over catheter vent, and slowly withdraw catheter while rotating it between thumb and forefinger (see illustration). Reapply oxygen or humidifying device.	Intermittent suction and rotation of catheter prevent injury to tracheal mucosal lining and hypoxia.

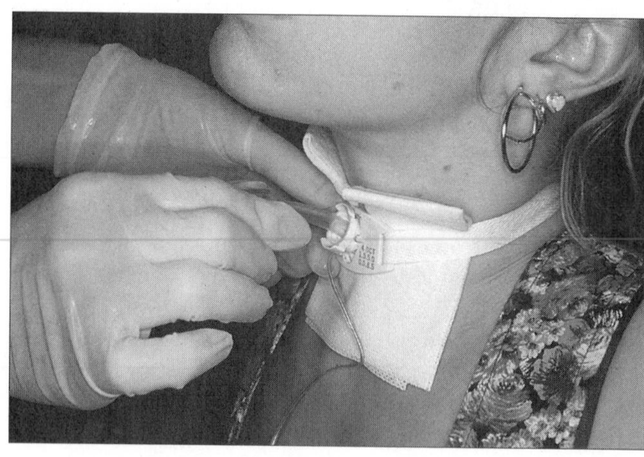

STEP **10** Applying suction to catheter in tracheostomy tube.

• ***Critical Decision Point***
Before continuing suction allow client to rest and encourage client to take two to three deep breaths to reduce oxygen loss and prevent hypoxia.

11. Using continuous suction, rinse catheter with basin fluid until clean. Repeat steps as needed to remove secretions.	Removes secretions from catheter. Promotes patent catheter.
12. Suction nasal and oral pharynx if needed (see Chapter 13). *Do not reinsert catheter into trachea after oral or nasal suction.*	Removes secretions from upper airway.
13. Rinse catheter as described.	Removes secretions from catheter. Reduces transmission of microorganisms.

Step	Rationale
14. At conclusion of procedure have client take two to three deep breaths.	Reduces oxygen loss and prevents hypoxia.
15. Disconnect suction catheter, coil, and discard. If catheter is to be cleaned and disinfected, set aside.	

Trach Care

Step	Rationale
1. To clean inner cannula, place impervious trash bag near work site and create a clean field for equipment; place the three basins on the field.	Ensures maintenance of standard precautions.
2. Pour hydrogen peroxide in one container and water or normal saline in second container. Pour hydrogen peroxide or normal saline in third container with 4 × 4 gauze pads.	Prepares work area for cleansing of trach tube.
3. Remove old tracheostomy bib or dressing and discard using standard precautions.	Reduces transmission of microorganisms.
4. Remove and discard contaminated gloves.	
5. Apply clean gloves.	Reduces transmission of microorganisms.
6. Using presoaked 4 × 4 gauze sponges and damp applicators, gently wash skin around stoma, under trach ties and flanges (see illustration).	Removes secretions that predispose client to localized infection.
7. Dry exposed outer cannula and skin with dry trach gauze or towel.	Prevents moist environment for organism growth.
8. Unlock and remove inner cannula; place in hydrogen peroxide and allow to soak.	Removes secretions and encrustations adhered to inner cannula.
9. Using nylon brush or pipe cleaners, gently scrub inner cannula.	Removes crusted secretions that adhere to tube.
10. Rinse inner cannula thoroughly with normal saline or water for at least 15 seconds; shake off excess solution.	Removes hydrogen peroxide from inner cannula. Remaining solutions could cause airway or stoma irritation.
11. Examine patency of cannula; if not clean, repeat cleansing process. Replace inner cannula in position and lock.	Ensures patent airway.
12. Change ties (see Chapter 13).	

- ***Critical Decision Point***
  Client is at risk for tube coming out as ties are changed. In home another trach tube with stylet for insertion should always be present.

Step	Rationale
13. Apply fresh trach dressing (see illustration).	Protects skin around stoma from pressure breakdown and collects secretions.

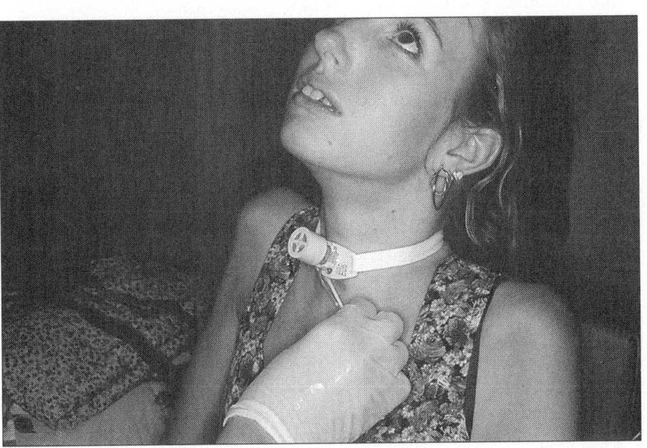
STEP **6** Cleansing area around tracheal stoma.

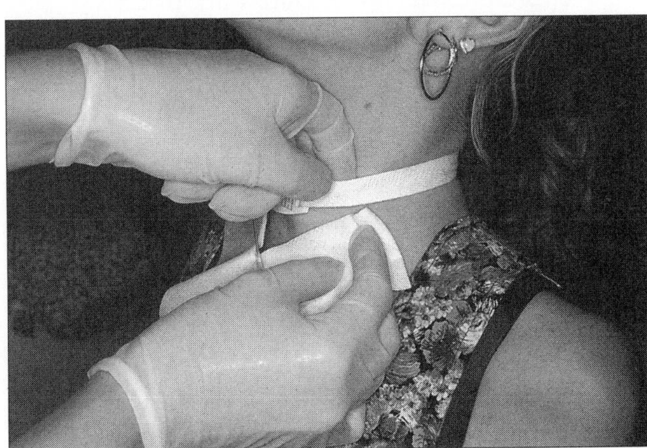
STEP **13** Applying clean tracheostomy dressing.

STEP	RATIONALE
14. Clean reusable supplies in warm soapy water. Rinse thoroughly and dry between two layers of clean paper towels. Store supplies in loosely closed clear plastic bag.	Prevents transmission of microorganisms. Air must circulate, or humidity in bag can promote microorganism growth.
15. Remove and discard gloves. Wash hands.	Reduces transmission of microorganisms.
16. Reusable supplies should be disinfected at least weekly. To disinfect supplies use one of the methods described here:	Removes organisms and reduces risk for infection.
a. Method 1: Boil reusable (boilable) supplies for 15 minutes. Allow to cool and dry.	
b. Method 2: Soak reusable supplies in equal parts of vinegar and water for 30 minutes. Remove, rinse thoroughly, and dry.	
c. Method 3: Soak reusable supplies in prepared solutions of quaternary ammonium chloride compounds according to manufacturer's instructions. Rinse and dry.	Reduces transmission of microorganisms.
17. Have client or family member perform each step with guidance from nurse.	Adult learners learn best by active participation, and nurse can correct any errors in technique as they occur and discuss their implications.
18. Discuss signs and symptoms of: a. Stomal infection (redness, tenderness, drainage). b. Respiratory tract infection (fever, increased sputum, change in color of sputum, foul sputum odor, increased cough, chills, night sweats).	Client must be able to recognize onset of inflammation or infections early so that timely ordering and administering of antibiotics can reduce risk of more serious infections.

- ***Critical Decision Point***

  Discuss importance of notifying physician when prolonged stoma inflammation or respiratory infection occurs. Client must understand implications of upper respiratory tract infection.

EVALUATION

1. Ask client to state all signs of stomal or respiratory tract infection.	Prompt identification of symptoms results in early treatment and decreases risk of complications that may lead to hospital readmission.
2. Observe client demonstrate technique for trach tube care and suctioning.	Feedback through independent demonstration of psychomotor skill is reliable method to evaluate learning.

UNEXPECTED OUTCOMES AND RELATED INTERVENTIONS

- Stoma site is reddened or hard, with or without drainage.
  - Evaluate cleaning regimen for continued use of clean technique.
  - Increase tracheostomy care frequency.
- Copious colored secretions are present around stoma or when client is suctioned.
  - Use sterile technique for suctioning and tracheostomy inner cannula care.
  - Evaluate for adequate humidity (use room humidifier or tracheostomy collar humidity, if needed) (see Chapter 11).
  - Notify physician.
- Bloody secretions are suctioned.
  - Evaluate suctioning technique, suctioning frequency, and size of catheter used.
  - Identify other signs of infection.
- No secretions are suctioned.
  - Evaluate fluid status, need for increased humidity.
  - Determine if appropriate size of suction catheter is used.
  - Reassess suction frequency.
- Trach tube comes out.
  - Replace trach tube.
  - Activate emergency medical service system if needed.
- Skin breakdown is present at stoma site.
  - Assess site for pressure areas or site infection.
  - Remove pressure source.

RECORDING AND REPORTING

- Record in client record the teaching done and accuracy of care delivered by client or family member.
- Develop a system of recording to be used by client or caregiver to provide information that compliance is achieved or maintained.

Teaching Considerations

- Families of tracheostomy clients must know how to obtain emergency assistance within their community.
- Client may need mirror to visualize stomal area.
- If at all possible, a family member or other caregiver in home should learn procedure in event emergency assistance is required or client's level of debilitation makes self-care improbable.
- Loss of upper airway functions with tracheostomy can predispose client to greater secretions.
- Ideally, home care nurse should participate in discharge teaching in hospital.

Pediatric Considerations

- Many physicians order child to receive 10% to 15% higher oxygen before tracheostomy tube changes.
- Infants and young children have smaller diameter airway. Awareness of level of parent's anxiety surrounding performance of this skill will require frequent support and assistance by home care nurse until independence and comfort level are achieved.

Gerontological Considerations

- Manual dexterity may be limited due to arthritic changes of upper extremities.
- Skin integrity may be compromised and at risk for breakdown from secretions and/or tape.
- Older adults have lost some properties of elastic recoil and may have greater difficulty in clearing airway secretions through cough. As a result they require more suctioning and airway care and have increased risk of infection.

Home Care Considerations

- Procedure must be performed at least daily in home setting. When tracheal secretions are copious, client or family member must perform procedure more frequently (such as every 4 hours).
- Clients may benefit from proper room humidification. Be sure humidifier is clean and in optimal operating condition.
- Water in humidifier may grow *Pseudomonas,* and container must be cleaned daily.

Skill 40-4 Helping Clients With Self-Medication

Clients who are prescribed drug regimens at home often fail to take medications correctly. Difficulty in taking prescribed medications regularly exists for several reasons: clients stop taking medications once symptoms subside; regimens involving multiple drugs are confusing; the consequences of not taking mediation are poorly understood; prescriptions are costly; and many clients fear addiction. A large portion of clients who do not comply are older adults, who frequently suffer sensory and mobility problems that interfere with the ability to prepare and take medications correctly.

The following skill is actually an outline to help prepare clients for following drug regimens in the home.

Delegation Considerations

This skill should not be delegated to assistive personnel. However, assistive personnel, such as home health aides, are often in a situation to be able to see how clients are self-administering medications. Assistive personnel can learn how to make suggestions that further ensure client safety regarding use of infection-control practices, disposal of sharps and needles, and disposal of contaminated supplies.

Equipment

- Medication
- Liquid to take with medication
- Medication administration record or computer printout
- Container for daily or weekly preparation
- Measuring devices as needed (e.g., medicine cup, teaspoon)
- Teaching tools (e.g., charts, written instructions, color codes)

Step	Rationale
Assessment	
1. Assess client's cognitive, sensory, and motor function; level of consciousness, sight, hearing, touch, literacy, swallowing ability, ambulatory ability, activity tolerance, and willingness to cooperate.	Cognitive, sensory, and motor deficits may influence client's ability to take or prepare prescribed medication correctly and to participate in instruction.
2. Assess resources client has to obtain medications when needed.	Lack of financial resources or transportation are two major factors that will negatively affect compliance with self-medication regimen.

Step	Rationale
3. Assess client's learning readiness and abilities.	Presence of significant illness, frailty, or suggestion of or presence of confusion will affect teaching plan. Reliance on caregiver for learning and implementation (if available) may be necessary on a short- or long-term basis.
4. Assess client's knowledge regarding medication therapy: names of drugs, how to administer, purpose or action, daily doses and times taken, side effects to expect, and what to do if problems occur.	Reveals client's level of understanding and need for instruction.
5. Assess family member's knowledge of medication therapy: why client takes medication, daily doses, side effects, and what to do if problems arise.	Family member or support person is important resource to help client comply with therapy.
6. Assess client's belief in need for drug therapy. Consider cultural values, religious beliefs, personal experiences with medications, and significant others' values about drugs.	Many factors influence client's willingness to follow drug regimen.
7. Check client's prescribed medications: Has more than one physician prescribed medications? Are medications obviously inappropriate? Are labels clearly marked? Are time schedules confusing? Do different drugs look alike? Does client store medications together or out of original containers?	Assists nurse in determining sources of confusion affecting client's compliance. Noncompliance with medication therapy (especially in older adults) may be aggravated by multiple chronic conditions, which are often treated with multiple medications sometimes prescribed by more than one physician (Lueckenotte, 2000).
8. Assess client's understanding of effects and interactions between prescribed medications, with ingestion of certain foods, and with over-the-counter drugs.	Medication interactions, including those with over-the-counter drugs and certain foods, can seriously affect effectiveness and/or create negative side effects.

Nursing Diagnosis

Defining characteristics from the assessment data may reveal the following nursing diagnoses for clients requiring this skill:

- Anxiety
- Ineffective health maintenance
- Health-seeking behaviors (self medication)
- Ineffective family therapeutic regimen management
- Deficient knowledge regarding drug administration

Related factors are individualized based on client's condition or needs.

Planning

Step	Rationale
1. **Expected outcomes** following completion of procedure:	
▪ Client is able to state purpose of each medication and why it is beneficial.	Demonstrates cognitive learning.
▪ Client identifies common side effects and relief measures.	
▪ Client is able to state when to notify physician about drug problems.	
▪ Client reads each label and explains when each drug should be taken.	
▪ Client demonstrates self-administration of medication by prescribed route (see illustrations).	Demonstrates skill achieved.
2. Prepare environment for teaching session: a. Select room that is well lit. b. Provide comfortable seating. c. Be sure client is close and can see nurse clearly. d. Control sources of noise and distractions.	Room environment should be designed to minimize existing sensory alterations. Comfortable environment free of distractions promotes client's attention.

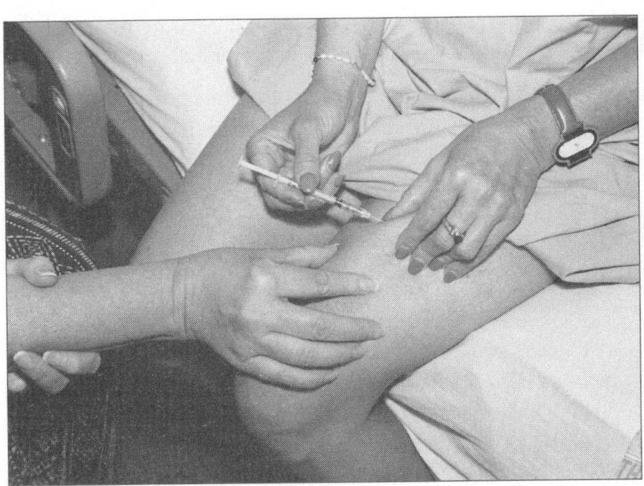
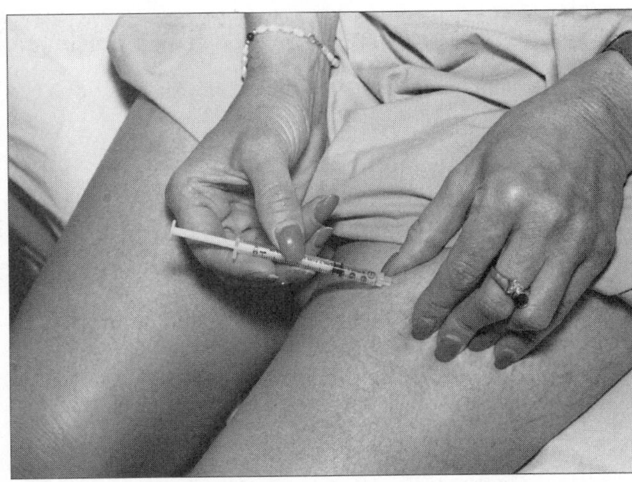

STEP 1 Client demonstrating self-injection technique.

STEP	RATIONALE
3. Prepare teaching materials: a. Materials should be printed in large bold letters. b. Illustrations of safety guidelines should be provided. c. Written schedules or individualized instruction sheets are helpful.	Teaching materials should be designed to meet client's learning needs and client's capacity to learn.
4. Be sure clients who wear glasses or hearing aids do so during teaching session.	Use of glasses or hearing aids increases client's sensory perception and increases likelihood of attending to teaching session and understanding content.
5. Consult with physician to review medications client is receiving and to simplify regimen if possible.	Review of medications can help minimize risk of drug interactions from multiple medications and ensures accuracy of medication regimen. Simplification of regimen can improve compliance, particularly related to daily frequency of prescribed doses.
6. Arrange teaching time so that family members may participate (see illustration).	Family can serve as positive resource to client.

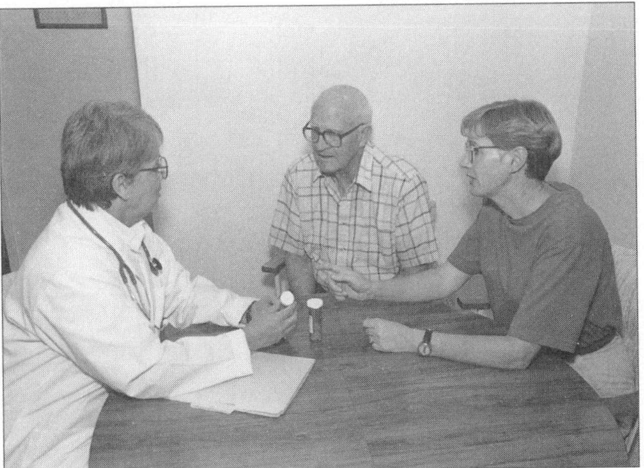

STEP 6 Family participating in self-medication teaching program.

IMPLEMENTATION

STEP	RATIONALE
1. Present information clearly and concisely:	Improves client's ability to attend and understand.
a. Face learner; be sure nurse's face is illuminated. b. Use short sentences and speak in slow, low-pitched voice.	Client with hearing loss or visual problem will be able to see nurse's expressions and hear voice more clearly.
c. Provide descriptions in understandable terms.	Prevents confusion of terminology.

STEP	RATIONALE
2. Provide frequent pauses so that client can ask questions and express understanding of content.	Increases client's participation in learning process. Ongoing feedback assures nurse that client is acquiring information.

- ***Critical Decision Point***
  Discuss the following content: purpose of drugs and their positive effects, how drug works and why it helps, dosage schedules and rationale, common side effects, what to do to relieve side effects, what to do if dose is missed, when to call with problems, who to call with problems, drug safety guidelines, and implications when medications are not taken.

STEP	RATIONALE
3. Provide frequent, short teaching sessions. Learning about multiple medication regimen will require several teaching sessions.	Client needs to learn extensive amount of information. Improves client's attention and retention of information discussed. Reference to charts, written information, and other teaching tools as a resource will assist client in learning.

- ***Critical Decision Point***
  Review previous information, and ask client to recall and relay previously taught information before proceeding to new teaching area.

STEP	RATIONALE
4. Be sure to include teaching about prescribed and over-the counter medications that are used on a **prn** basis.	Consideration of knowledge and accessibility of these medications must be given, because prn drugs are not included in routine, prepared medication delivery systems (i.e., daily or weekly pillbox systems).
5. Provide client with special charts, diagrams, or learning aids (see illustration).	Simplest mechanism for reminding clients of when to take medications improves compliance.

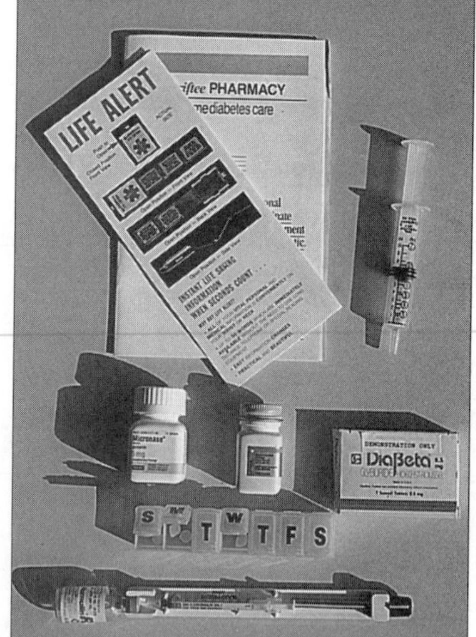

STEP **5** Examples of aids for client self-medication administration.

STEP	RATIONALE
6. Offer assistance as client practices preparing medication (e.g., "Let's prepare the medications you will take with your meals; or prepare the medicines you take first in the morning").	Nurse can observe client's ability to read labels correctly and prepare all medications for prescribed times.
7. Have pharmacy provide clear, large-print labels for medication bottles if appropriate.	Improves client's ability to read and follow directions.
8. Have pharmacy provide containers that client can open independently if manual dexterity is limited.	Most pharmacies dispense pills in "childproof" containers, which the client with limited mobility of fingers/hands may find difficult to manipulate or open.

- ***Critical Decision Point***
  If there are pets or small children in home or children who frequently visit home, help client establish a "safe place" for medication, to reduce risk of accidental ingestion by pets or children.

Step	Rationale
9. Facilitate arrangements for pharmacy to receive written prescriptions in a timely fashion if required for dispensing and to deliver medications at home if client is unable to reach facility.	Availability of drugs influences compliance.

Evaluation

Step	Rationale
1. Ask client and family member to explain information about each drug: purpose, actions, reason/maximum frequency of use of either prescribed or over-the-counter drug, side effects and interactions, and foods or over-the-counter drugs to avoid.	Feedback measures client's cognitive learning.
2. Identify client's problem-solving initiatives if unsure of action to be taken (e.g., call health care provider, refer to printed information for resources).	Developing techniques to gain information and solve problems will assist in client compliance and reduce potential problems from medication regimen.
3. Have client or family member prepare doses for all prescribed medications.	Indicates client's and family member's understanding of dosages and schedules.
4. Ask client about any questions.	Offers opportunity for clarification and minimizes any remaining confusion or misunderstanding.

Unexpected Outcomes and Related Interventions

- Client makes errors in preparing medications or is unable to recall and/or explain information discussed in teaching sessions.
  - Client requires additional instruction and/or teaching materials that client can consult when information is forgotten or unclear.
  - Written instructions need to be at reader's level of understanding. Some commercially prepared booklets may contain instructions that are too complex or contain medical jargon that is difficult to understand.
  - Pictures, color coding, diagrams, and tape recorded instructions need to be considered as creative teaching tools for the reading or sight impaired.
  - Periodically observe client demonstrate medication administration.
- Self-medication plan is not possible due to client's self-care deficits—very commonly in relation to changes in mentation.
  - Alternate plan, which may rely on others, is developed to provide administration of home medication regimen.

Recording and Reporting

- Document instruction provided and learning outcomes achieved by client in home care record.
- Develop system of recording to be used by client or family member to provide information that compliance is achieved or maintained.
- Develop a client recording mechanism of dosage schedules and self-monitoring of regimen.

Teaching Considerations

- See Chapter 39 for guidelines for drug safety.
- If it is difficult to plan a separate teaching session, instruct client while administering medications.
- Repetition, reinforcement, and positive feedback must be elements of teaching plan.
- Assessment of an appropriate amount of information taught at each session is critical so as not to overwhelm client with task at hand.
- Examples of learning aids include homemade calendars for each week that contain plastic bags containing medications to take at specific times, egg cartons divided into color-coded sections with medications for the day, clock faces for clients who cannot read or see clearly, color coding for drug types (e.g., blue for sedative, red for pain pill), and pillboxes that identify days of the week and times of day.

Pediatric Considerations

- All medications must be kept safely out of reach of children.
- Caregivers should not compare medications to treats, even artificially sweetened varieties, because this could add to risk of child overdosing by mistaking medicine for candy.
- All medications in homes with small children must be placed in safe, secure, out-of-reach location.

GERONTOLOGICAL CONSIDERATIONS

- Older adults commonly have reduced visual and hearing acuity and difficulty understanding language because high-frequency tones are less perceptible.
- C.pacity for learning new information remains as we age (in the absence of **dementia**); however, additional time needed to accomplish learning has been demonstrated in research studies. Allow adequate time and number of teaching sessions to support successful learning.
- Memory loss related to aging does not eliminate ability to learn all components of self-medication management. The confusion that may occur in some older adults, associated with a variety of environmental, emotional, physiological, social, and/or psychiatric circumstances, may be identified in isolated, homebound older adult client and will severely affect success of teaching client to comply with self-medication program.

HOME CARE CONSIDERATIONS

- Discuss proper storage of medications; some may require refrigeration.
- If client or family member can not reliably fill weekly pillbox, nurse should make arrangements with pharmacy to deliver medications weekly.

Skill 40-5 Enteral Nutrition in the Home

Enteral nutrition therapy in the home setting can be accomplished if several criteria are used to determine client eligibility (Young and White, 1992). These criteria include the client's ability to tolerate 70% of feeding intake without complications, the client's medical stability, the client's capability of performing the skills and/or having a responsible and capable caregiver, and the client or caregiver having sufficient time in a controlled environment to learn the skill. This procedure in the home setting follows the guidelines and skills described in Chapter 22. This skill focuses on the teaching of the client or caregiver in the home. The nurse may be responsible in this setting for reinsertion of **nasogastric** and **gastrostomy feeding tubes,** and the physician may be responsible for reinsertion of jejunostomy tubes. See Skills 22-1 to 22-5 for insertion and replacement procedures.

DELEGATION CONSIDERATIONS

For this skill, feeding tube insertion or medication administration should not be delegated to assistive personnel. However, administration of enteral tube feeding via syringe is a procedure that can be delegated to assistive personnel. The nurse should verify feeding tube placement before feeding and assess for residual volume. Also be sure to instruct assistive personnel to report difficulty with feeding, coughing, gagging, respiratory distress, discomfort, or vomiting.

EQUIPMENT

See Skills 22-1 and 22-2 for equipment for insertion, Skill 22-1 for placement, and Skills 22-4 to 22-5 for administration and equipment.

- Documentation records (daily weights, **intake and output [I&O]**, temperature)

STEP	RATIONALE
ASSESSMENT	
1. Assess client's health status and ability to successfully manage enteral feedings in the home.	Increases successful home management with fewer complications.
2. Assess client's or caregiver's physical, emotional, financial, and community resources.	Increases ability for self-care and home management.
3. Assess environmental conditions of home (sanitation, storage of equipment, work area, and supplies, and power source).	Ensures safe environment and decreases risks of infection and complications.
4. Assess client's and caregiver's understanding of purpose of enteral feedings and positive expected outcomes.	Understanding rationale of treatment is critical to enhancing client's and family's advice participation and cooperation.
5. Assess client's and caregiver's understanding of storage and management of equipment and supplies and where and how to obtain supplies.	Ensures safe home management and decreases risk of complications.
6. Assess client's and caregiver's ability to manipulate feeding equipment.	May require caregiver to administer all enteral feedings. Allows nurse to identify areas for teaching and support.

STEP	RATIONALE

NURSING DIAGNOSIS

Defining characteristics from the assessment data may reveal the following nursing diagnoses for clients requiring this skill:

- Imbalanced nutrition: less than body requirements
- Anxiety
- Disturbed body image
- Diarrhea
- Feeding self-care deficit
- Deficient knowledge regarding administration of enteral feedings
- Risk for aspiration

Related factors are individualized based on client's condition or needs.

PLANNING

1. **Expected outcomes** following completion of procedure:
   - Client and caregiver will verbalize the purpose of enteral feedings and enhanced nutritional health. — Provides measurable criteria to determine level of understanding.
   - Client and caregiver will demonstrate accurate administration of enteral feedings and medications. — Provides demonstration of skills needed to manage home enteral nutrition.
   - Client and caregiver will demonstrate proper use of equipment and handling of formulas. — Provides demonstration of skills needed to manage home enteral nutrition.
   - Client and caregiver will verbalize understanding of signs and symptoms and management of complications. — Provides identification of teaching needs and enables client and caregiver to ask questions.

IMPLEMENTATION

Step	Rationale
1. Wash hands.	Reduces transmission of microorganisms.
2. Discuss with client and caregiver purpose of enteral feeding and enhanced nutritional health.	Reinforces importance of regular feedings.
3. Demonstrate how to identify placement of feeding tube: aspiration of gastric fluid and checking pH of gastric fluid (see Skill 22-2).	Nasally placed tubes can be inadvertently placed in respiratory system and can migrate to esophagus or into respiratory tract. Nurse may need to check pH periodically. Aspirated secretions with low pH are strong indicator of gastric placement. However, high pH cannot differentiate between aspirated secretions obtained from respiratory and intestinal tube placements (Metheny and others, 1999).
4. Observe client and family determine placement of nasally placed tube.	Identifies areas for further teaching.

- ***Critical Decision Point***

  Discuss with client or caregiver the need to aspirate before each feeding or every 4 hours for continuous drip feedings; to delay feeding if residual exceeds the last hour's infusion or 150 ml; to return gastric contents; and to elevate the head of client's bed for 1 hour after feedings or maintain at least a 30-degree elevation for continuous feedings. Gastric distention is a major risk factor for reflux and aspiration. Preventing gastric distention reduces risk of aspiration.

Step	Rationale
5. Observe client or caregiver aspirate gastric contents.	Identifies competence and need for further teaching. Allows client and caregiver to perform skill with nurse in attendance for guidance.
6. Discuss use of medical asepsis techniques in setting up administration and changing administration sets, mixing formulas (not adding formula to hanging bag), refrigeration of unused formula, limiting amount of formula "hung" at one time to amount that can be infused in a 4- to 6-hour period (less time in warmer weather), and maintenance and care of bag.	Medical aseptic technique minimizes risk of microorganism contamination. Refrigeration and limiting "hang" time reduces microorganism proliferation. Changing administration sets every 24 hours reduces microorganism growth.

Step	Rationale
7. Observe client or caregiver mixing, administering, and storing formulas, changing administration sets, and cleaning bags.	Identifies competence and need for further teaching.

- ***Critical Decision Point***
  Discuss mixing and administration of medications via tube and flushing tube out after administration. Ensures administration of medication dose and prevents clogging of tube.

Step	Rationale
8. Observe client or caregiver administering medications and flushing tube.	Identifies competence and need for further teaching.

- ***Critical Decision Point***
  Verify that medications to be administered do not include any sublingual, enteric-coated, or sustained-release medications.

Step	Rationale
9. Discuss and observe use of **infusion pump** if client is receiving continuous feeding (see Chapter 22).	Infusion pumps provide positive pressure to ensure constant flow and prevent occlusion and gastric distention.
10. Discuss measures to stabilize feeding tube in clients with abdominal tubes and to protect skin integrity.	Prevents tube from dislodging and prevents skin breakdown.
11. Discuss measures to prevent aspiration, indicated by increased severe coughing, difficulty in breathing, or increased vomiting.	Ensures safe home management.
12. Discuss whom to contact for equipment and supplies or in case of equipment failure.	Ensures family can respond in an emergency.
13. Discuss emergency plan and actions to take for signs and symptoms of aspiration.	Ensures client's and caregiver's understanding of management of equipment, supplies, emergency plan, and collaboration.
14. Discuss whom to contact and when for signs of diarrhea, constipation, or weight loss.	
15. Wash hands.	Reduces transmission of microorganisms.

Evaluation

Step	Rationale
1. Ask client and caregiver to state purpose of home enteral nutrition therapy.	Demonstrates cognitive learning.
2. Observe client and caregiver performing medical asepsis techniques, checking tube placement, administering medications and solutions, and using equipment.	Demonstrates psychomotor learning.
3. Ask client and caregiver to state measures needed to be used to prevent complications (e.g., verification of tube position before each feeding, elevation of client during feeding, stabilization and flushing of tubing).	Ensures safe home management and identification of areas for teaching.
4. Ask client and caregiver how to remove occlusions within feeding tube and how to care for open formula cans.	Ensures safe home management and identification of areas of teaching.
5. Ask client and caregiver about management of complications (e.g., signs of intolerance: nausea, abdominal distention, diarrhea, skin problems, and fluid deficit).	Ensures safe home management and identification of areas of teaching.

Unexpected Outcomes and Related Interventions

- Displacement of feeding tube occurs.
  - Feeding tube must be repositioned and position verified before initiating any enteral feeding.
  - Have family notify home health nurse.
- Signs and symptoms of aspiration are present.
  - Stop feeding.
  - Verify tube position.
  - Notify physician.
- Client develops diarrhea.
  - Notify physician.
  - May need to change strength or type of enteral feeding.
  - May need to administer antidiarrhea agents.
- Skin surrounding stoma or tube insertion site (nares) breaks down.
  - Reposition feeding tube at nares to avoid pressure.
  - Cleanse stoma area more frequently.
  - Apply antibiotic ointment around stoma as ordered.

Recording and Reporting

- Record in home care record instructions given to client and caregivers and their response to them.
- Record specifics of enteral feeding plan, including type and size of tube in home, formula, and amounts to be administered in specific time frames.
- Client and caregivers need to document I&O, daily weights, amount of gastric fluid aspirated before each feeding (or every 4 hours if receiving continuous feeding), date and time of feedings, amount and type of formula, any additives, and date and time administration sets are changed.

Teaching Considerations

- Teaching of enteral therapy skills begins in the hospital.
- Teach primary caregiver to check placement of feeding tube before administering any feeding or medication.
- Instruct caregiver to not give feeding or medication if there is any doubt as to placement of tube.
- Instruct caregiver in method of gastrointestinal fluid pH measurement and expected range.
- Instruct caregiver to administer prescribed amount of water before and after medications to avoid clogging feeding tube.
- Carrying out performance of skills without nurse in attendance is anxiety provoking. Always leave a phone number and instructions about how to reach nurse if needed.

Pediatric Considerations

- A child's potential risk for aspiration and fluid and electrolyte imbalance is great and must be carefully monitored.

Gerontological Considerations

- Changes and limitations in sensory functioning or issues with mobility, dexterity, and fluid and caloric needs must be factored into plan of care and monitored for needs to alter prescriptions or teaching methods.

Home Care Considerations

- Assess environmental safety and sanitation of client's home to determine potential for infection or injury if tube is to be inserted for ongoing nutritional support.

Critical Thinking Exercises

1. Mr. Williams is able to demonstrate effective and accurate measurement of his wife's blood pressure when the home care nurse is observing him. When attempting this skill alone, he says he is uncomfortable with the accuracy of the results. What nursing actions would you implement to promote successful, independent skill performance?
2. During your third home care nursing visit for the purpose of teaching the client a self-medication regimen, you note that several types of pills are grouped together in one container. What actions would you take?
3. Mrs. Pickard is usually independent in caring for her husband's tracheostomy. She would like to visit grandchildren in another state, and a family friend will be caring for Mr. Pickard. You are meeting the friend; what will you tell him?

References

Dettenmeier PA: *Pulmonary nursing care,* St. Louis, 1992, Mosby.

Ebersole P, Hess P: *Toward healthy aging: human needs and nursing response,* ed 5, St. Louis, 1999, Mosby.

Fell H, Boehm M: Easing the discomfort of oxygen therapy, *Nurs Times* 94:56, Sept 1998.

Foster-Fitzpatrick and others: The effects of crossed leg on blood pressure measurement, *Nurs Res* 48:105, 1999.

Lueckenotte AG: *Gerontologic nursing,* ed 2, St. Louis, 2000, Mosby.

Metheny NA and others: pH and concentration of bilirubin in feeding tube aspirates as predictors of tube placement, *Nurs Res* 48:189, 1999.

Rice R: *Home health nursing practice: concepts and application,* ed 2, St. Louis, 1996, Mosby.

Young C, White S: Tube feeding at home, *Am J Nurs* 92(4):46, 1992.

41

Specimen Collection

Skills

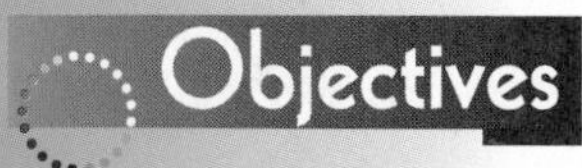

Objectives

Mastery of content in this chapter will enable the nurse to:

- Define the key terms listed.
- Explain the rationale for the collection of each specimen.
- Identify special conditions necessary for satisfactory collection of each specimen.
- Describe instructions to encourage client cooperation for successful collection of the specimen.
- Recognize the impact of sociocultural issues that may affect client's cooperation with collection of specimen.
- Identify measures to minimize anxiety and promote safety for selected techniques.
- Discuss nursing responsibilities for processing the specimen after collection.
- Chart appropriate information in the client's record after collection of the specimen.
- Discuss precautions to prevent injury to the client during specimen collection.
- Properly collect clean-voided, timed, and catheterized urine specimens.
- Correctly measure specific gravity and pH of urine.
- Correctly measure glucose, ketones, protein, and blood in urine.
- Correctly measure for the presence of occult blood in a stool specimen.
- Properly collect specimens for culture from the nose and throat, urethra and vagina, sputum, and wound.
- Correctly measure for pH and presence of occult blood in gastric drainage.
- Properly perform venipuncture.
- Properly collect specimens for blood cultures.
- Correctly measure for blood glucose from a blood specimen collected by skin puncture.
- Properly collect an arterial blood sample.
- Utilize measures recommended for preventing transmission of pathogens.

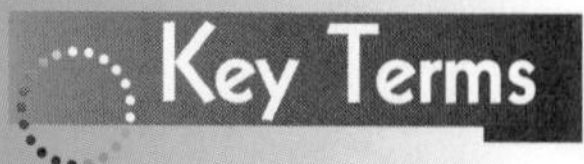

Key Terms

Acetest
Aerobic
Allen's test
Anaerobic
Aseptic technique
Aspirate
Autolet
Blood culture
Clean-voided specimen
Clinitest
Culture
Double-voided specimen
Dysuria
Ecchymosis
Expectorate
Frequency
Glucose monitoring
Guaiac test
Hematemesis
Hematoma
Hematuria
Hemoconcentration
Hemolysis
Hemostasis
Ketones
Meatus
Melena
Midstream
Occult blood
pH
Platelet
Reagent
Refractometer
Renal
Sensitivity
Specific gravity
Timed urine collection
Tourniquet
Urgency
Urinometer
Vacutainer tube
Venipuncture
Void

Proficiency in assisting with diagnostic testing and specimen analysis is important for the professional nurse. Skill and judgment in obtaining specimens affect client comfort and ensure quality of diagnostic samples and procedures. Accountability is increasing, and there is more attention to monitoring client outcomes. In addition, current health care economics insist that laboratory tests be performed accurately and in a timely manner.

Nurses often are responsible for collection of specimens. Depending on the type of specimen needed and skill required, the nurse may be able to delegate this task to the assistive personnel (AP). Laboratory examination of specimens of urine, stool, sputum, blood, and wound drainage provides important information about body functioning and contributes to the assessment of the client's health status. Laboratory test results can aid in the diagnosis of health care problems, provide information about the stage and activity of a disease process, and measure the response to therapy.

Normal values for laboratory tests can be found in reference books, but the nurse should know that each laboratory establishes its own values for each test. These values are usually readily available on the laboratory slips of the agency. Any major deviations should be discussed with the provider immediately.

Clients often experience embarrassment or discomfort when giving a sample of body excretions or secretions. Excretion is the process by which the body eliminates or sheds substances by organs or tissues, whereas secretion is the release of chemical substances manufactured by cells of glandular organs. Excretions should be handled discreetly; therefore it is important to provide the client with as much comfort and privacy as possible. Anxiety is also provoked by the invasive nature of some collection procedures or by fear of unknown test results. Clients who are given a clear explanation about the purpose of the specimen and how it is to be obtained may be more cooperative in its collection. With proper instruction many clients are able to obtain their own specimens of urine, stool, and sputum, thus avoiding embarrassment.

Laboratory tests are often expensive. The nurse can prevent unnecessary costs by using the correct procedure for obtaining and processing specimens. When there are questions about laboratory tests, the nurse should consult the institution's procedure manual or call the laboratory.

Skill Performance Guidelines

1. Consider the client's need and ability to participate in specimen collection procedures.
2. Recognize that specimen collection may cause anxiety, embarrassment, or discomfort.
3. Provide support for clients who are fearful of the results of a specimen examination.
4. Consider age-related factors that may affect client's compliance with specimen collection.
5. Recognize that children require a clear explanation of procedures and may benefit from support of parents/family members.
6. Consider sociocultural variations that may affect client's compliance with specimen collection.
7. Obtain specimens in accordance with specific prerequisite conditions (e.g., fasting, nothing by mouth [NPO]) as required.
8. Follow standard precautions (see Chapter 31) when collecting specimens of blood or other body fluids.
9. Wash hands and other skin surfaces immediately and thoroughly if they are contaminated with blood or body fluids; wash hands immediately after removing gloves.
10. Collect specimens in appropriate containers, at the correct time, in the appropriate amount.
11. Properly label all specimens with the client's identification; complete laboratory requisition as necessary.
12. Deliver specimens to the laboratory within the recommended time, or ensure that they are stored properly for later transport.
13. Use **aseptic technique** in all collections to prevent contamination, which can cause inaccurate test results.
14. Be aware of special conditions (e.g., iced specimens or special containers with preservatives) required for transport of specimens.
15. Know institutional policy regarding infection-control practices for transportation of all specimen containers of body substances.
16. Be aware that some deviations from normal values occur as a result of medications or dietary intake.
17. Follow precautions for collecting specimens from clients who are in protective isolation.

Skill 41-1 Collecting a Midstream (Clean-Voided) Urine Specimen

A common test performed on urine is a **culture** and **sensitivity** measurement. In the laboratory a few drops of urine are placed on a special medium to determine whether or not bacteria are present. Readings are made at 24- and 48-hour intervals, and the final reading is made after 72 hours. If bacteria are present, sensitivity testing reveals which antibiotics will be effective against the microorganisms.

With clients who are able to void voluntarily, the nurse collects a **midstream** urine specimen for culture and sensitivity testing. The nurse may need to assist some clients who are unable to collect specimens independently. A client begins the urinary stream and then during the middle portion of voiding collects a specimen. The initial stream flushes the urethral orifice and meatus of any resident bacteria. It is easiest for a client to obtain a **clean-voided specimen** while using toilet facilities rather than a bedpan or urinal.

Delegation Considerations

The skill of collecting a midstream (clean-voided) urine specimen may be delegated to assistive personnel. Assistive personnel must know how to cleanse urethra before obtaining specimen and how to instruct client in obtaining specimen. Assistive personnel should be instructed to report when blood, mucus, or foul odors are present in the specimen.

Equipment

- Commercial Kit (Figure 41-1) for Clean-Voided Urine Containing:
- Sterile cotton balls and/or 2 × 2 inch gauze pads, cleansing towelette, or two gauze pads
- Antiseptic solution (usually povidone-iodine solution)
- Sterile water or saline
- Sterile specimen container
- Sterile gloves
- Soap, water, washcloth, and towel
- Bedpan (for nonambulatory client), specimen hat (Figure 41-2) (if all urine needs to be measured), potty chair (for young child)
- Completed specimen identification label
- Completed laboratory requisition form

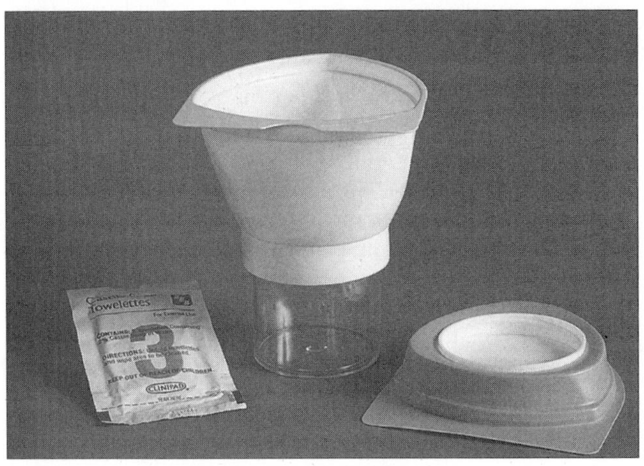

FIGURE **41-1** Clean voided specimen collection kit.

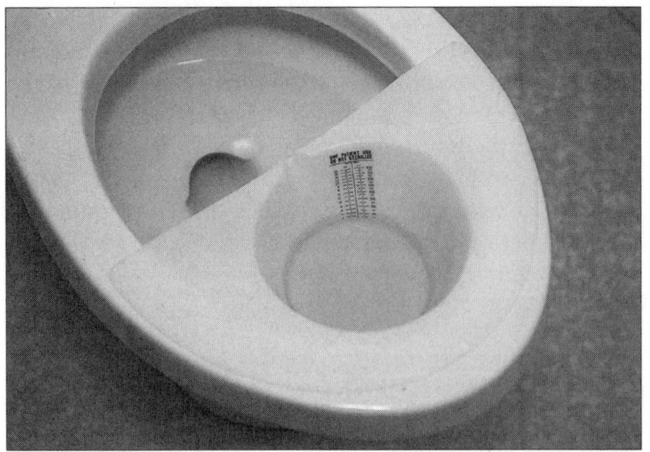

FIGURE **41-2** Specimen hat.

STEP	RATIONALE

ASSESSMENT

Step	Rationale
1. Assess client's level of understanding of purpose of test and method of collection.	Information allows nurse to clarify misunderstanding; promotes client compliance.
2. Assess client's mobility and balance in being able to use toilet facilities independently.	Determines level of assistance required by client.
3. Refer to medical record for indications of urinary infection.	Helps nurse explain purpose of specimen procedure for client.
a. Assess risks for urinary tract infection (e.g., poor perineal hygiene, improperly handled diagnostic instruments, previous urinary catheterization).	Allows nurse to anticipate need to test client's urine for bacteria.
b. Observe for signs and symptoms of urinary tract infections: frequency, urgency, dysuria, **hematuria,** flank pain, fever, and cloudy, malodorous urine.	Can suggest bacteria in urine (Meredith and Horan, 2000).
c. Refer to agency procedures for specimen collection methods.	Agency policies may vary regarding collection or handling of specimens.

NURSING DIAGNOSIS

Defining characteristics from the assessment data may reveal the following nursing diagnoses for clients requiring this skill:

- Anxiety
- Risk for infection
- Deficient knowledge regarding specimen collection
- Pain (acute)

Related factors are individualized based on client's condition or needs.

PLANNING

Step	Rationale
1. **Expected outcomes** following completion of procedure:	
▪ Client produces midstream urine specimen that is not contaminated with feces or toilet tissue.	These substances change normal characteristics of urine.
▪ Urine has normal characteristics and does not reveal bacterial growth.	Provides evidence of absence of infection.
▪ Client will discuss purpose and benefits of midstream urine collection.	Discussion can be used to evaluate client's learning.
2. Offer client fluids to drink (if permitted) before attempting to collect specimen.	Enhances client's ability to **void.**

STEP	RATIONALE
3. Explain procedure to client and/or family member. a. Reason midstream specimen is needed b. How client/family member can assist	Promotes cooperation and participation and client may be able to independently obtain specimen.
c. How to obtain specimen free of feces and tissue	Feces and tissue alter chemical composition of specimen.
d. Use visual aids (if available) to explain procedure to client.	Because this method of urine collection is somewhat complicated, clients benefit from illustrations emphasizing midstream collection technique.

IMPLEMENTATION

STEP	RATIONALE
1. Identify client. Wash hands.	Handwashing reduces transfer of microorganisms.
2. Provide privacy for client who will give specimen in bed by closing curtain around bed or closing room door.	Privacy allows client to relax and produce a specimen more easily.
3. Give client or family member cleansing towelette or towel, washcloth, and soap to cleanse perineum, or assist client to cleanse perineum (if able).	Clients prefer to wash their own perineal areas when possible. Cleansing prevents contamination of specimen after urine passes from urethra.
4. Assist bedridden client onto bedpan (see illustration).	Provides easy access to perineal areas to collect specimen.

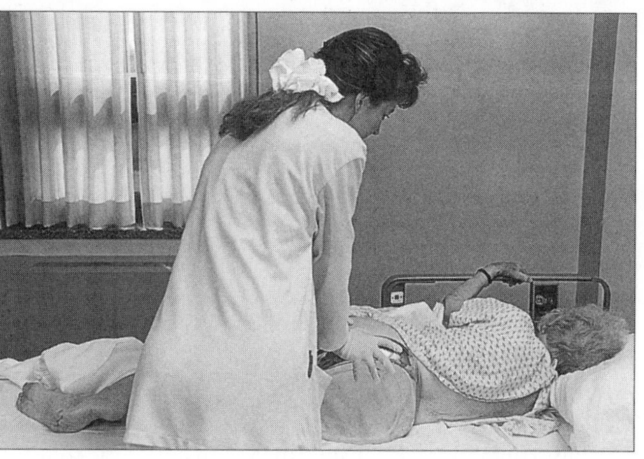

STEP 4 Nurse assisting client on a bedpan.

STEP	RATIONALE
5. Using surgical asepsis, open sterile kit or prepare sterile tray.	Maintains sterility of equipment.
6. Apply sterile gloves.	Prevents introduction of microorganisms on nurse's hands into specimen.
7. Pour antiseptic solution over cotton balls (unless kit contains prepared gauze pads in antiseptic solution).	Cotton ball or gauze is used to cleanse perineum.
8. Open specimen container and place cap with sterile inside surface up, and do not touch inside of container.	Contaminated specimen is most frequent reason for inaccurate reporting on urine cultures and sensitivities.
9. Perform urine collection by assisting or allowing client to independently cleanse perineum and collect specimen. The amount of assistance needed varies with each client. The nurse will assess client's ability to perform procedure and assist as needed.	Maintains client's dignity and comfort.
a. Male client	
(1) Either nurse or client will hold client's penis with one hand. Using circular motion and antiseptic swab, cleanse **meatus,** moving from center to outside (see illustration).	Reduces number of microorganisms at urethral meatus and moves from areas of least to most contamination (Potter and Perry, 1999).
(2) If agency procedure indicates, rinse area with sterile water and dry with cotton balls or gauze pad.	Prevents contamination of specimen with antiseptic solution.
(3) After client has initiated urine stream, pass urine specimen container into stream and collect 30 to 60 ml of urine (see illustration).	Initial urine flushes out microorganisms that normally accumulate at urinary meatus and prevents collection in specimen.

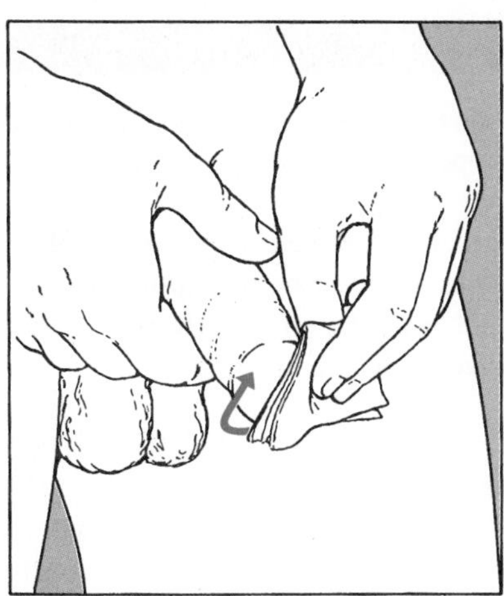

STEP **9a(1)** Cleansing urinary meatus. (Modified from Grimes D: *Infectious diseases,* Mosby's clinical nursing series, St. Louis, 1991, Mosby.)

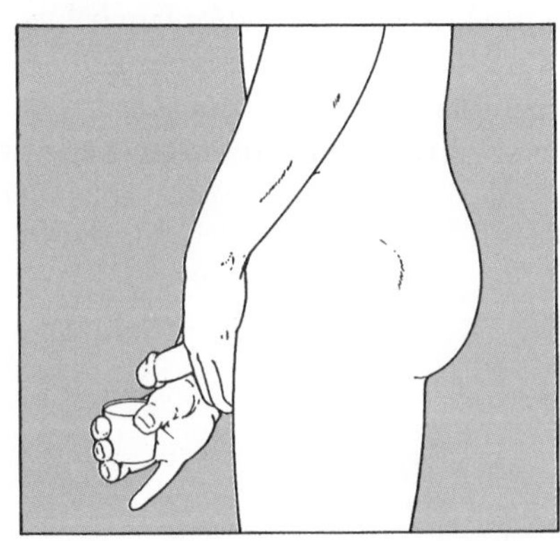

STEP **9a(3)** Collecting midstream urine specimen.

STEP	RATIONALE
b. Female client	
• ***Critical Decision Point*** *If client is menstruating place this information on laboratory slip.*	
(1) Either nurse or client will spread client's labia minora with thumb and forefinger of nondominant hand.	Provides access to urethral meatus.
(2) Use dominant hand to cleanse area with swab (cotton ball or gauze), moving from front (above urethral orifice) to back (toward anus). Using a fresh swab each time, repeat front-to-back motion three times (begin with center, then do left side, then do right side) (see illustration).	Prevents contamination of urinary meatus with fecal material.
(3) If agency procedure indicates, rinse area with sterile water and dry with cotton ball.	Prevents contamination of specimen with antiseptic solution.
(4) While continuing to hold labia apart, client should initiate urine stream into toilet or bedpan; after stream is achieved, pass specimen container into stream and collect 30 to 60 ml (see illustration).	Initial stream flushes out resident microorganisms that accumulate at urethral meatus.

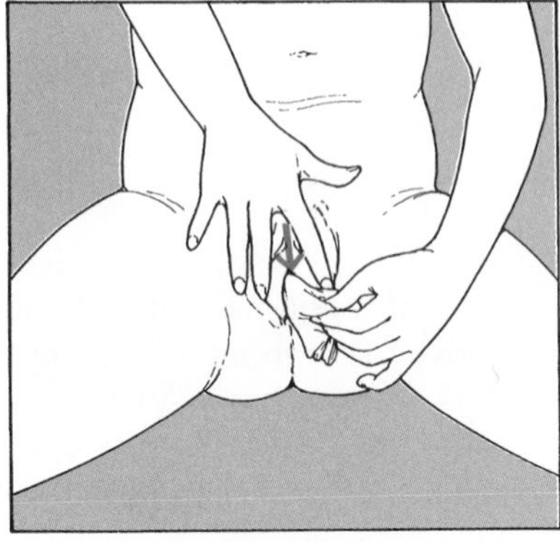

STEP **9b(2)** Cleansing urinary meatus with front-to-back motion. (Modified from Grimes D: *Infectious diseases,* Mosby's clinical nursing series, St. Louis, 1991, Mosby.)

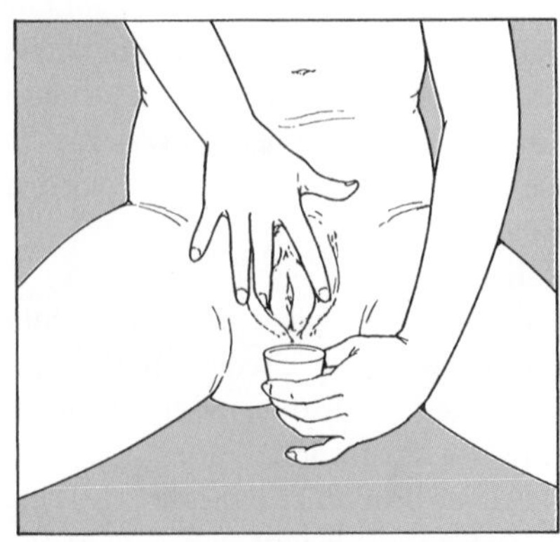

STEP **9b(4)** Collection of midstream urine specimen. (Modified from Grimes D: *Infectious diseases,* Mosby's clinical nursing series, St. Louis, 1991, Mosby.)

Step	Rationale
10. Remove specimen container before flow of urine stops and before releasing labia or penis. Client finishes voiding into bedpan or toilet.	Prevents contamination of specimen with skin flora.
11. Replace cap securely on specimen container (touch only outside).	Retains sterility of inside of container and prevents spillage of urine.
12. Cleanse urine from exterior surface of container.	Prevents transfer of microorganisms to others.
13. Dispose of bedpan (if applicable), remove and discard gloves, and wash hands.	Reduces transmission of microorganisms.
14. Label specimen and attach laboratory requisition.	Prevents inaccurate identification that could lead to errors in diagnosis or therapy.
15. Take specimen to laboratory within 15 to 20 minutes.	Because bacteria grow quickly in urine, urine not received by the laboratory within 20 minutes of collection should be refrigerated. However, refrigeration should not exceed 24 hours (Monahan and Neighbors, 1998).

Evaluation

1. Observe specimen for contaminants such as toilet paper or feces.	Contaminants prevent specimen from being used.
2. Assess client's urine culture and sensitivity report for bacterial growth.	Routine cultures identify organism(s), and sensitivity study identifies antimicrobial medications that may be effective against pathogen (Malarkey and McMorrow, 2000).
3. Ask client to describe midstream urine collection procedure.	Documents client's understanding (Potter and Perry, 1999).

Unexpected Outcomes and Related Interventions

- Urine specimen is contaminated with feces or toilet paper.
  - Repeat client instruction and collection.
  - If unable to obtain specimen through clean voiding, client may require catheterization.
- Urine specimen is accidentally discarded.
  - Repeat specimen collection.
- Client is unable to urinate on demand.
  - Offer fluids (if permitted).
  - Allow more time for urine to accumulate in bladder.
  - Try obtaining specimen after 30 minutes.
- Urine culture reveals bacterial growth (designated by colony count of more than 10,000 organisms per milliliter).
  - Report findings to provider.
  - Administer medications as ordered.
  - Monitor client for fever and **dysuria.**

Recording and Reporting

- Record appearance and odor of urine and evidence of dysuria in nurses' notes.
- Notify physician of any significant abnormalities.

Teaching Considerations

- Use visual aids to describe collection of specimen.
- Discuss signs and symptoms of urinary tract infection.
- Explain significance of cleansing genital area before collecting specimen.
- Explain to female client importance of cleansing labia from front to back.
- Discuss client's role in collecting specimen.
- Nurses should request feedback to assess client's understanding of purpose of test and directions for collecting specimen (Redman, 1997).

Pediatric Considerations

- It is not possible to obtain midstream urine collection on non–toilet-trained child; consequently, urine for culture should be obtained by use of sterile plastic urine-collecting bag that adheres to perineum (Figure 41-3). Same cleansing procedure should be followed as indicated in Step 9 of Implementation (Wong and others, 1999).

Gerontological Considerations

- Special assistance should be given to older adults. A clear and concise explanation should be given about procedure and reason for sample to be obtained. All equipment should be available at bedside to allow proceeding with obtaining specimen when client needs assistance.

Home Care Considerations

- Ideally, specimen for culture should not be collected at home because time delay before applying it to culture medium in laboratory setting would greatly enhance bacterial growth. If urine specimen is collected, it should be kept on ice until it reaches laboratory and is placed on medium.

A 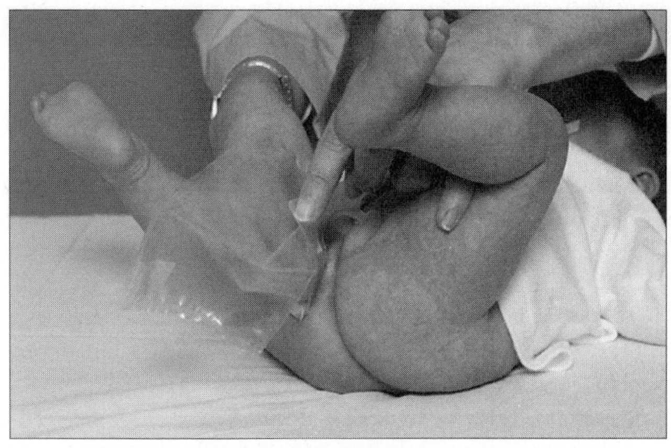

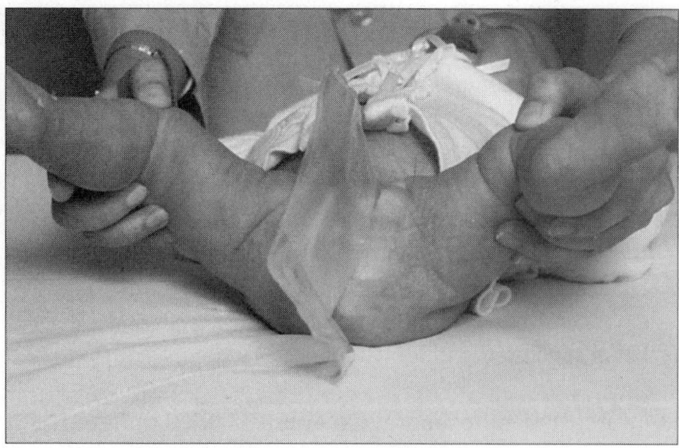 B

FIGURE **41-3** Application of urine collection bag. (From Wong DL and others: *Whaley and Wong's nursing care of infants and children*, ed 6, St. Louis, Mo, 1999, Mosby.)

Skill 41-2 Collecting a Timed Urine Specimen

Some tests of **renal** function and urine composition require urine to be collected over 2 to 72 hours. The 24-hour timed collection is most common. The tests allow for the measurement of elements such as amino acids, creatinine, hormones, glucose, and adrenocorticosteroids, whose levels change over time. A **timed urine collection** can also provide a means to measure the concentration or dilution of urine.

Timed urine collections begin after a client urinates. The nurse discards the first specimen and then collects every successive specimen until the time period has ended. Each specimen is transferred immediately to a large collection bottle kept in the client's bathroom. Any missed specimens make test results inaccurate. The client should always provide the last specimen as close as possible to the end of the collection period.

Delegation Considerations

The skill of collecting a timed urine specimen may be delegated to assistive personnel. Assistive personnel should be instructed in when timed collection is to begin and the proper way to store the specimen during the collection period. Care provider should be reminded to place signs in client's toileting area that a timed urine collection is taking place and not to discard any urine. Assistive personnel should be instructed to report when blood, mucus, or foul odors are present in the specimen.

Equipment

- Large collection bottle with cap that may contain a chemical for urine preservation (consultation with laboratory is usually necessary to obtain bottle and determine appropriate chemical additive [e.g., toluene, acetic acid])
- Bedpan, urinal, specimen hat, bedside commode, or pediatric potty chair if client does not have indwelling catheter
- Graduated measuring cup if intake and output are to be measured
- Basin large enough to hold collection bottle surrounded by ice if immediate refrigeration is required
- Completed specimen identification label
- Completed laboratory requisition with client's name, date, and time of collection
- Instructional signs that remind client and staff to save urine for timed specimen collection
- Clean disposable gloves

Step	Rationale
Assessment	
1. Determine purpose of timed urine specimen collection for client and period collection is to include.	Most collection periods are for 24 hours because this provides average excretion rate for substances such as hormones or proteins excreted in small variable amounts in urine. If these substances are to be accurately measured and yield quantities of diagnostic value, urine may need to be collected over an extended period. Challenge dose of a chemical such as insulin may be given, and then timed urine specimen collection may be begun to detect renal disorders.
2. Determine if fluid or dietary requirements or medications need to be administered in conjunction with test.	Certain substances affect excretion and levels of urinary constituents. Glucose solution may be given for glucose tolerance test. Specific amounts of fluid may be required when collecting concentration/dilution tests.
3. Determine that correct diet is being taken by client.	Client's compliance is necessary for accurate test.
4. Assess client's ability to collect specimens independently.	Because timed specimens are difficult to collect, specimen collection must be a priority in client's care (Monahan and Neighbors, 1998).
5. Assess client's or family members' understanding of purpose of test and need to collect urine over extended period.	Compliance is facilitated by degree of understanding.
6. Refer to agency policy for specimen collection procedure.	Agency policies may vary regarding collection or handling of specimens.

Nursing Diagnosis

Defining characteristics from the assessment data may reveal the following nursing diagnoses for clients requiring this skill:

Deficient knowledge regarding urine collection procedure

Related factors are individualized based on client's condition or needs.

Planning

Step	Rationale
1. **Expected outcomes** following completion of procedure:	
▪ All of client's urine voided during the time period is saved.	Necessary for satisfactory completion of test.
▪ Urine specimen is not contaminated with feces or toilet tissue.	Prevents results of urine test from being adversely affected by these substances.
▪ Urine has normal constituency.	Client is free of urinary alterations.
▪ Client explains purpose of and procedure for urine collection.	Demonstrates learning and assures compliance.
2. Have client drink two to four glasses of water about 30 minutes before timed collection is to begin (if not contraindicated).	Enables client to void old urine (collected in bladder) at time test begins.
3. Explain procedure to client and/or family member. Discuss reason for specimen collection and how client can assist. Explain that urine must be free of feces and tissue.	A client who understands procedure is more likely to cooperate and may be able to obtain specimen independently. It also prevents accidental disposal and chemical changes resulting from feces and tissue.

Implementation

Step	Rationale
1. Provide privacy for and assist the client in collecting specimen.	Clients prefer collecting specimens themselves. Timed specimens are not sterile.

STEP	RATIONALE
2. Wear gloves when handling urine.	Prevents transmission of microorganisms.
3. Discard this first specimen as test begins. Indicate time that test began on laboratory requisition.	Collection period begins with empty bladder.
4. Certain urine tests are done to measure metabolites that are unstable in urine and require special conditions be adhered to and/or that preservatives be added to the specimen container (i.e., a 24-hour urine test for catecholamines requires that hydrochloric acid be added to container by laboratory and specimen be kept refrigerated or on ice during collection). Check agency policy for specific guidelines and collection protocols (Monahan and Neighbors, 1998).	Maintains integrity of urine specimen.
5. When applicable, have client drink required amount of liquid or take ordered medication.	Required for specific types of tests to measure elimination of urine constituents.
6. Place signs on client's door and toileting area indicating that timed urine specimen collection is in progress. If client leaves unit for test or procedure, be sure that personnel in that area collect and save all urine.	Prevents uninformed persons from accidentally discarding urine specimens.
7. Measure volume of each voiding if output is to be recorded.	Measures client's fluid balance (Elkin, Perry, and Potter, 2000).
8. Place all voided urine in labeled specimen bottle with appropriate additive.	Additives preserve urine specimen and prevent deterioration.
9. Unless instructed otherwise, keep specimen bottle in specimen refrigerator or in container of ice in bathroom.	Cold temperature prevents decomposition of urine.
10. Wash hands and discard gloves after collection of each voiding.	Reduces transmission of microorganisms.
11. Encourage client to drink two glasses of water 1 hour before timed urine collection ends. If client's condition warrants fluid restrictions, be cautious in encouraging fluids.	Facilitates client's ability to void at end of period.
12. Encourage client to empty bladder during last 15 minutes of urine collection period.	Ensures urine collected for precise amount of time.
13. At end of period, send labeled specimen to laboratory with appropriate requisition.	Ensures laboratory results credited to correct client.
14. Remove signs and remind client that specimen collection period is completed.	Allows client to resume usual voiding habits.

EVALUATION

1. Intermittently during collection period, observe client's compliance with saving of all urine.	Clients often benefit from being reminded to save urine.
2. Inspect urine for contamination from feces or toilet tissue.	Ensures specimen is not contaminated.
3. Compare results of client's urinalysis with normal laboratory values.	Reveals deviations from normal and may indicate need for further testing.

UNEXPECTED OUTCOMES AND RELATED INTERVENTIONS

- A portion of urine specimen is accidentally discarded.
  - Reinforce importance of saving the total specimen.
  - Notify laboratory to determine if collection must be restarted.
- Urine specimen is contaminated by feces or toilet tissue.
  - Reinforce importance of saving total specimen.
  - Notify laboratory to determine if collection must be restarted.
  - Assist client with specimen collection as needed.
- Laboratory results reveal abnormal values for urine constituents.
  - Notify physician of findings.
  - Continue to monitor client.

RECORDING AND REPORTING

- Record starting time of urine collection in client's chart.
- Report to oncoming shift that 24-hour urine collection is in progress.
- At completion of test, record time urine collection is finished; appearance, amount, and odor of urine; and disposition of specimen to laboratory.
- Discuss abnormal test results with physician.

TEACHING CONSIDERATIONS

- Explain fluid or dietary recommendations or restrictions to client and family.
- Explain how specimen is obtained and duration of collection.
- Instruct client in how specimen is stored.

PEDIATRIC CONSIDERATIONS

- For infants and young children who are not yet potty trained, special plastic urine-collecting bags with self-adhesive are designed to attach to perineal area.
- Toilet-trained young child may not be able to void on request and may be more successful if bedpan or potty chair is placed on toilet. Use terms familiar to child such as "tinkle" or "wee wee." Enlist parent's support (Wong and others, 1999).
- Toilet-trained older child is cooperative and appreciates explanation of why specimen is needed. Provide privacy and receptacle to conceal specimen, such as a paper bag (Wong and others, 1999).

GERONTOLOGICAL CONSIDERATIONS

- A reminder should be placed in bathroom on mirror for ambulatory client.
- Verbal reminders will further enhance continuing sample collection.

HOME CARE CONSIDERATIONS

- Depending on type of specimen collected, instruct client regarding need to refrigerate specimen.

Skill 41-3 Collecting a Sterile Urine Specimen From an Indwelling Catheter

It is often necessary to collect urine specimens from a client who has an indwelling catheter. Strict aseptic technique should be used to ensure sterility and to avoid introducing infection into the urinary tract.

A urine specimen for culture tests should not be collected from a urine drainage bag unless it is the first urine to drain into a new sterile bag. Bacteria grow rapidly in drainage bags and can give a false measurement of bacteria in the urine.

DELEGATION CONSIDERATIONS

The skill of collecting a sterile urine specimen from an indwelling catheter may be delegated to assistive personnel. The client must first be assessed to determine patency and functioning of the indwelling catheter system. Assistive personnel should be instructed in the proper way to collect the specimen and when the specimen should be obtained. In addition, assistive personnel should be instructed to report when blood, mucus, or foul odors are present in the specimen.

EQUIPMENT

- 3-ml syringe with 1-inch needle (21 gauge) (for culture) or 20-ml syringe with 1-inch needle (21 gauge) (for routine urinalysis)
- Alcohol, povidone-iodine, or other disinfectant swab
- Clamp or rubber band
- Specimen container (nonsterile for routine urinalysis, sterile for culture)
- Completed specimen identification label
- Completed laboratory requisition (client's name, date, time of collection)
- Clean disposable gloves

STEP	RATIONALE
ASSESSMENT	
1. Assess client's or family members' understanding of need to collect urine from indwelling catheter.	Reveals knowledge of procedure and willingness to cooperate.
2. Assess for signs and symptoms of urinary tract infection: **frequency, urgency,** dysuria, changes in urine color or odor, hematuria, and flank pain.	Suggest bacteria in urine (Meredith and Horan, 2000).

STEP	RATIONALE
3. Assess indwelling catheter for built-in sampling port and type of material from which it is made.	Provides appropriate place for removal of urine from catheter. Port prevents leakage of urine from catheter. It is safe to insert needle directly into self-sealing rubber catheter. Silastic, silicone, or plastic catheters are not self-sealing and thus should not be punctured with needle for aspiration of urine.

Nursing Diagnosis

Defining characteristics from the assessment data may reveal the following nursing diagnoses for clients requiring this skill:

- Risk for infection
- Pain (acute)
- Toileting self-care deficit

Related factors are individualized based on client's condition or needs.

Planning

STEP	RATIONALE
1. **Expected outcomes** following completion of procedure:	
▪ Urine specimen is obtained from catheter without contamination.	Procedure is safely performed.
▪ Urinary catheter and drainage system remain intact.	There is no indication (e.g., leaking of urine) that catheter or drainage system was punctured by needle during specimen collection.
▪ Urine has normal characteristics and no bacterial growth.	Client is free of urinary abnormality. No signs of nosocomial infection.
2. Explain why catheter will need to be clamped for 30 minutes before obtaining urine specimen and why it is not obtained from drainage bag.	Prevents development of anxiety over catheter clamping and promotes understanding of need for urine to collect within bladder.
3. Explain procedure to client and/or family member. Emphasize that although syringe with needle is used to remove urine from catheter, client will not experience any discomfort.	Prevents anxiety when nurse manipulates catheter and aspirates urine with syringe and needle. Promotes client cooperation.

Implementation

STEP	RATIONALE
1. Wash hands.	Reduces transfer of microorganisms.
2. Clamp drainage tubing with clamp or rubber band for 30 minutes (see illustration).	Permits collection of fresh sterile urine in catheter tubing rather than draining into bag.

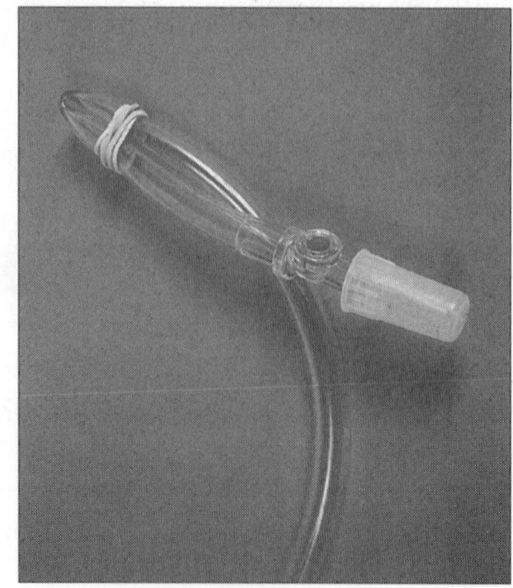

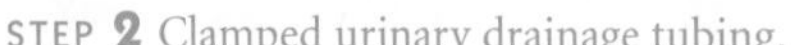

STEP 2 Clamped urinary drainage tubing.

STEP	RATIONALE
3. Return to room and inform client that procedure to collect specimen from catheter will begin.	Allows client to anticipate manipulation of urinary catheter and cope more effectively with discomfort that may occur when catheter is moved.
4. Wash hands and put on gloves.	Reduces transfer of microorganisms.
5. Position client so that catheter is easily accessible.	Allows for easy collection of specimen.
6. Cleanse entry port for needle with disinfectant swab. Wait until disinfectant is dry.	Prevents entry of microorganisms into catheter.
7. Insert needle at 45-degree angle just above where catheter is attached to drainage tube in self-sealing rubber catheter or at built-in sampling port in silastic, silicone, or plastic catheter (see illustration).	Ensures entrance of needle into catheter lumen and prevents accidental puncture of lumen leading to balloon that holds catheter in place in bladder. Aspiration of water from lumen can result in catheter slipping out of bladder.

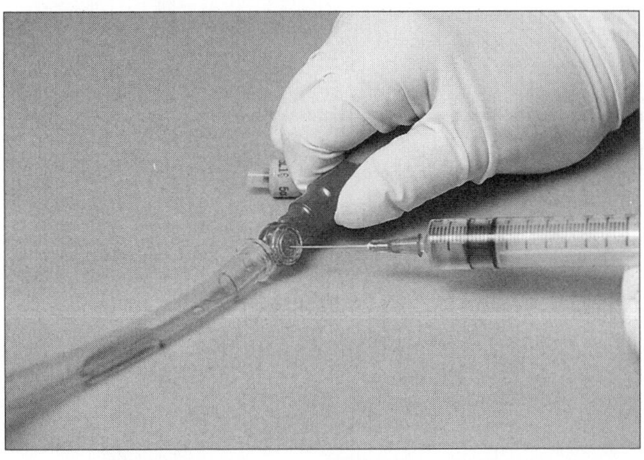

STEP 7 Insertion of needle through self-sealing port.

STEP	RATIONALE
8. Draw urine into 3-ml syringe (for culture), or draw urine into 20-ml syringe (for routine urinalysis).	Allows collection of urine without contamination. Proper volume is needed to perform test.
9. Transfer urine from syringe into sterile urine container for culture or into nonsterile urine container for routine urinalysis.	Prevents contamination of urine during transfer procedure.
10. Place lid tightly on container.	Prevents contamination of specimen by air and loss by spillage.
11. Unclamp catheter and allow urine to flow into drainage bag.	Allows urine to drain by gravity and prevents stasis of urine in bladder, which can cause much discomfort and potential damage to kidneys.
12. Dispose of soiled supplies, remove and discard gloves, and wash hands.	Reduces transmission of microorganisms.
13. Securely attach properly completed identification label and laboratory requisition to specimen.	Incorrect identification of specimen could result in diagnostic or therapeutic errors.
14. Send specimen to laboratory immediately or place in specimen refrigerator.	Transport specimen to laboratory immediately (at least within 30 minutes). If this is not possible, specimen may be refrigerated up to 2 hours (Pagana and Pagana, 1997).

EVALUATION

1. Observe characteristics of urine and any signs of client discomfort.	Symptoms need to be further explored (Meredith and Horan, 2000).
2. Observe urinary drainage system to ensure that it is intact and patent.	System must remain closed to remain sterile.
3. Compare results of client's laboratory report with normal laboratory values, and report any abnormalities to physician.	Reveals deviations from normal and indicates need for further testing and intervention.

UNEXPECTED OUTCOMES AND RELATED INTERVENTIONS

- Urine specimen is contaminated during procedure.
  - Recollect specimen.
- Lumen that leads to balloon that holds catheter in bladder is punctured.
  - Reinsert new catheter.
  - Collect specimen.
- Urine has abnormal constituents.
  - Continue to monitor client.
  - Notify physician of findings for further orders.
- Client has pain during procedure.
  - Continue to monitor client.
  - Notify physician.
  - Administer pain medication if ordered.

RECORDING AND REPORTING

- Record collection of specimen in nurses' notes or per agency policy; note time and date, appearance, odor and color of urine, and disposition to laboratory.
- Report any significant differences in urine.

Skill 41-4 Measuring Specific Gravity of Urine

Specific gravity, the concentration of dissolved substances in water, can be measured easily by the nurse in any clinical setting. At least three modes currently exist to accomplish this measurement. The most common mode is to place a **urinometer** with a mercury bulb in a cylinder containing urine. The density or concentration of urine determines the level at which the urinometer floats within the cylinder. If the urine is dilute, the urinometer tends to sink. Concentrated solutes in urine raise the level at which the urinometer floats. This test requires only a few seconds to complete and can often provide useful information about the client's state of hydration and/or kidney function and provide a parameter for the adjustment of fluid intake. Measurement of urinary specific gravity may also be evaluated with a urine dipstick (i.e., Multistix reagent test strips) or a **refractometer,** which measures the amount of light that can pass through a drop of urine (Pagana and Pagana, 1998).

DELEGATION CONSIDERATIONS

Assistive personnel may perform the measurement of specific gravity. Care provider should be instructed in how to use calibrated urinometer and report results or record on appropriate document.

EQUIPMENT

- Accurately calibrated urinometer (validate by measuring specific gravity of distilled water, which is 1.000), Multistix reagent test strips, or refractometer
- Clean, dry glass cylinder
- 20 ml urine or enough volume to fill glass cylinder two-thirds full
- Clean disposable gloves

STEP	RATIONALE
ASSESSMENT	
1. Assess client's or family member's understanding of need to test specific gravity and how test is performed.	Provides nurse with information on which to base teaching.
2. Determine client's ability to collect specimen.	Determines level of assistance required from nurse.
3. Assess client's hydration status: skin turgor, condition of mucous membranes, intake and output (I&O), integrity of fontanels (infants).	Specific gravity measures concentration of urine solutes and is affected by state of hydration (Malarkey and McMorrow, 2000).
4. Assess client's medical history for evidence of renal disease.	Renal tubular disease results in loss of capacity of kidneys to concentrate urine (Meredith and Horan, 2000).

STEP | RATIONALE

NURSING DIAGNOSIS

Defining characteristics from the assessment data may reveal the following nursing diagnoses for clients requiring this skill:
Deficient fluid volume
Excess fluid volume
Related factors are individualized based on client's condition or needs.

PLANNING

1. **Expected outcomes** following completion of procedure:
   - Specific gravity is between 1.010 and 1.025.
     Normal range of values.
   - There are no feces, blood, or toilet tissue in urine specimen.
     Feces, tissue, and menstrual blood falsely elevate specific gravity reading.
2. Explain procedure to client and/or family member. Explain that urine must be free of feces and toilet tissue.
   Understanding promotes cooperation and relieves anxiety.

IMPLEMENTATION

1. Wash hands and put on clean, disposable gloves.
   Reduces transmission of microorganisms.
2. If using urinometer, carefully pour fresh urine specimen into glass cylinder until it is two-thirds to three-quarters full.
   Cylinder must be at least two-thirds full to cause urinometer to float.
   a. Place urinometer in cylinder of urine and gently twirl top of stem.
      Prevents urinometer from adhering to sides of cylinder.
   b. Wait until urinometer stops bobbing; then with urinometer scale at eye level, read point where urine level touches calibrated scale. Read scale at lowest point of meniscus for best accuracy (see illustration). Report abnormal reading to physician.
      Concentration of dissolved solutes in urine influences depth at which urinometer floats. Point at which urine reaches scale is specific gravity.

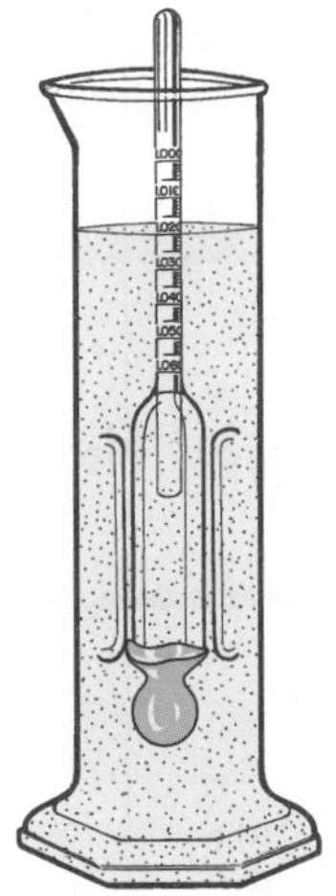

STEP **2b** Urinometer.

   c. Discard urine and wash cylinder and urinometer in cool water.
      Warm water coagulates proteins in urine and causes them to stick to glass surfaces.
3. If using Multistix reagent strips, dip end of test strip (which is impregnated with a chemical reagent) into urine sample. After specified time (indicated on label) color of strip is compared with color chart on bottle.
   Timed exposure to urine will allow reagent to measure specific gravity.

Step	Rationale
4. If using refractometer, place one drop of urine on slide and view through refractometer, which allows visualization of density of urine on calibrated scale.	
5. Remove and discard gloves, and wash hands.	Reduces transfer of microorganisms.

Evaluation

1. Observe specimen for contaminants, feces, or toilet tissue.	Ensures specimen not contaminated.
2. Compare results of client's urinalysis with normal laboratory values.	Reveals deviations from normal and indicates need for intervention.

Unexpected Outcomes and Related Interventions

- Specific gravity is less than 1.010 or greater than 1.025.
  - Continue to monitor client.
  - Report findings to physician for further orders.
- Urine contains feces or blood.
  - Repeat specimen collection.

Recording and Reporting

- Record specific gravity reading and note character of urine in nurses' notes.
- If client's I&O is being monitored, record urine volume on flow sheet.
- Special flow sheets are available for recording frequent measurements of specific gravity.
- Report abnormal values to physician.

Teaching Considerations

- Instruct client about proper method for collecting random urine specimen.
- Explain reason for measuring specific gravity.
- Discuss significance of test if client shows interest.

Pediatric Considerations

- For infants and children who are not toilet trained, the urine specific gravity may be obtained if cotton ball is left in diaper area. Cotton ball can be removed when it is well saturated to obtain specimen.

Gerontological Considerations

- When obtaining specific gravity for older adult, note any medications that may influence results of sample. Some medications may cause alteration in true values.
- When older adult is undergoing fluid restrictions, this may also have an impact on true specific gravity of urine.
- The specific gravity decreases proportionately with advancing years in normal older adult (Malarkey and McMorrow, 2000).

Skill 41-5 Measuring Chemical Properties of Urine: Glucose, Ketones, Protein, Blood, and pH

Tests for chemical properties of urine, which are a part of the routine urinalysis done by the laboratory, can be performed quickly. Normally, glucose and **ketones** are not present in the urine, and the appearance of either element generally indicates that glucose is not effectively reaching the body's cells. When this screening test for the presence of glucose in the urine is positive, other tests are used to determine the diagnosis of diabetes mellitus.

In the past, persons with diabetes mellitus routinely used urine testing of glucose to monitor the effectiveness of their medication, diet, and exercise on their blood glucose levels. Today, this practice has been largely supplanted by determination of blood glucose levels by finger sticks (Pagana and Pagana, 1998). Nevertheless, this traditional method of testing the urine for glucose is described here.

Urine testing for glucose and acetone has been used for many years to monitor glucose control by diet and insulin. The test is acceptable to clients because it is easily performed and causes no pain; however, it is being replaced by testing capillary blood, which is obtained by skin puncture of the fingertip (see Skill 41-13). This change is being made because capillary blood monitoring directly reflects current serum glucose levels and is not affected by the renal threshold for glucose or fluid volume. Hypoglycemia, which cannot be detected by urine testing, may be identified by sampling of serum glucose.

Assessing the chemical properties of urine can be done by immersing a special chemically prepared strip of paper into a clean urine specimen or by combining drops of urine with chemically prepared tablets. The change in color of the strip or tablet indicates the presence of any of these substances.

Delegation Considerations

Assistive personnel instructed in performing the skill may obtain this specimen, perform the test, and report the results of the test.

Equipment

- Specimen hat, bedside commode, bedpan, urinal, or pediatric potty chair
- Watch with second hand or digital counter
- Clean disposable gloves (if person other than client tests urine)

Reagent Tablet Testing

- 10-ml test tube
- Test tube holder
- Medicine dropper
- Clean container with 10 ml water
- Clinitest or Acetest tablets
- Tablet color chart
- Facial tissue

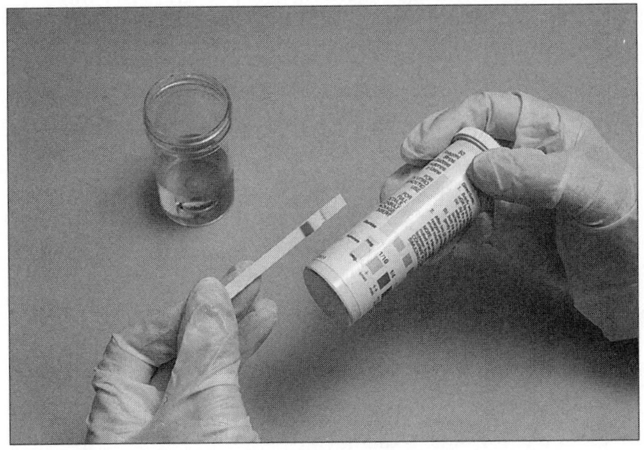

FIGURE 41-4 Testing urine using a reagent strip.

Reagent Strip Testing (Figure 41-4)

- Reagent test strip
- Test strip color chart

Step	Rationale
Assessment	
1. Determine rationale for physician request of this particular urine test.	Allows nurse to consider other significant assessments to make.
2. Assess if client or family member performs urine testing at home or if there is need for client to learn skill.	Client accustomed to testing own urine may prefer continuing to do so.
3. Determine if physician has recommended specific type of reagent test for client to use.	Variety of **reagent** strips and tablets permit fast, accurate monitoring of urine glucose and ketones.
4. Assess whether client, if diabetic, is familiar with **double-voided specimen** and uses technique regularly.	A double-voided specimen is preferable for accuracy of glucose test (Pagana and Pagana, 1998). Clients often do not perceive importance of procedure.
5. Assess type of medications client receives; check drug literature for effects on reagent strips and tablets.	Certain drug components create false-positive glucose readings. Drugs that may cause false-positive results with reagent tablets (e.g., Clinitest) but not with enzyme-impregnated strips (e.g., Clinistix, Tes-Tape) include acetylsalicylic acid, aminosalicylic acid, ascorbic acid, cephalothin, chloral hydrate, nitrofurantoin, streptomycin, and sulfonamides (Pagana and Pagana, 1998).
6. Assess client for signs and symptoms of diabetes mellitus: polydipsia, polyuria, and polyphagia.	Presence of these symptoms is often accompanied by glucosuria (Linton, Matteson, and Maebius, 2000).
7. Assess client's ability to perform urine test.	Determines level of instruction or assistance required from nurse. Diabetic clients may suffer from visual alterations or peripheral nerve damage that interfere with their ability to accurately perform test (Beare and Myers, 1998).

STEP	RATIONALE

NURSING DIAGNOSIS

Defining characteristics from the assessment data may reveal the following nursing diagnosis for clients requiring this skill:

Acute or chronic confusion
Deficient knowledge regarding urine testing procedure
Noncompliance

Related factors are individualized based on client's condition or needs.

PLANNING

STEP	RATIONALE
1. **Expected outcomes** following completion of procedure.	
▪ Client who requires daily or more frequent testing will be able to perform test independently.	Demonstrates learning and independence in own health maintenance.
▪ Test results are negative for glucose, ketones, protein, and blood; pH is between 4.5 and 8.	Urine glucose is normally negligible and is reported as none. Ketones, protein, and blood are not normally found in urine (Malarkey and McMorrow, 2000).
▪ Urine is not contaminated with feces or toilet tissue.	Demonstrates client's ability to collect urine specimen correctly.
2. Offer client fluids to drink (if permitted) about 30 minutes before collecting urine.	Enhances client's ability to void at requested times.
3. Explain procedure to client and/or family member. Discuss reason for specimen collection, how client can assist, and fact that specimen must be free of feces and tissue.	Client who understands procedure is more likely to cooperate and may be able to obtain specimen independently. Also prevents accidental disposal.

IMPLEMENTATION

STEP	RATIONALE
1. Obtain double-voided specimen when testing urine for glucose:	A fresh specimen should be used because stagnant urine that has been in bladder for several hours will not accurately reflect serum glucose level at testing (Pagana and Pagana, 1998).
a. Ask client to collect random urine specimen and discard.	Stagnant urine stored in bladder overnight or for long periods does not reveal amount of glucose and ketones excreted by kidney at time of testing.
b. Have client drink a glass of water.	Facilitates ability to void again within short time period.
c. Have client collect another specimen 30 to 45 minutes later.	Fresh specimen will provide accurate test measurements. If client is catheterized, single fresh specimen from catheter is adequate.
2. Apply gloves.	Reduces transmission of microorganisms.
3. Measure urine for glucose or ketones.	
a. Perform glucose reagent tablet test (**Clinitest** [5-drop test]):	Measures 0% to 2% glucose.
(1) Use medicine dropper to transfer 5 drops of well-mixed urine from container to clean, dry test tube. Use a 2-drop or 1-drop test with young children: 2-drop test = 2 drops urine and 10 drops water; 1-drop test = 1 drop urine and 11 drops water.	Proper volume of urine is needed to ensure proper reaction of urine to agents in tablet.
(2) Rinse dropper.	Prevents excess urine from being added to tube.
(3) Add 10 drops of water to test tube.	Reagent tablet contains sodium hydroxide, which boils in water.
(4) Add reagent tablet (Clinitest tablet) to test tube without touching to bare skin.	Combination of tablet and solution results in boiling effect. If fingers are moist, tablet will be caustic.
(5) Place tube in holder or hold tube near top.	Chemical reaction produces heat that can cause burn.

Step	Rationale
(6) Observe color change occurring as tablet boils.	Heat of reaction causes reduction of chemicals in tablet if glucose is present. Concentration of glucose determines color of urine solution.
(7) Fifteen seconds after boiling stops, shake tube gently and compare color of solution with color chart.	Comparison of color in test tube with standardized color chart indicates glucose concentration in urine. Delay in reading causes inaccuracy that can cause serious problems if treatments are initiated because of results.
(8) Rinse test tube and drain.	Tube should be dry and free of chemicals for next test.
b. Perform glucose/ketone reagent test strip test:	Strip test is often preferred over reagent tablet method.
(1) Immerse end of strip impregnated with chemical reagent into urine specimen.	Immersion exposes reagent to urine constituents. Although Diastix, Clinistix, and Tes-Tape all measure quantity of glucose in urine, measurement scales are not interchangeable.
(2) Remove strip immediately from container, and tap it gently against container's side.	Excess urine can dilute reagents.
(3) Hold strip in horizontal position.	Prevents possible mixing of chemical reagents.
(4) Time for number of seconds specified on container, and compare color of strip with color chart (see Figure 41-4, p. 1163).	Accurate interpretation of results depends on precise timing: Ketostix, 15 seconds; Clinistix, 10 seconds; Diastix, 30 seconds; Tes-Tape, 60 seconds. Compare darkest part of tape with color chart. If results exceed 0.5%, wait another 60 seconds and compare with second color chart.
(5) Dispose of reagent strip in trash.	Maintains neat environment and reduces spread of infection.
c. Perform ketone (**Acetest**) tablet test:	

- ***Critical Decision Point***
  Unnecessary if Ketostix, Multistix, or Diastix reagent test strips are used.

Step	Rationale
(1) Place Acetest tablet on white tissue.	Color of tablet changes to shades of tan or gray, which can be seen more easily on white background.
(2) Add 1 drop of urine to tablet.	Begins chemical reaction.
(3) Time for 30 seconds, and compare color of tablet with Acetest color chart.	Time required for reagent to indicate ketone bodies.
(4) Discard tablet and tissue in trash.	Reduces transmission of microorganisms.
d. Use Multistix reagent test strip to assess for chemical properties of pH, protein, glucose, ketones, and/or blood simultaneously:	Eliminates need for all previous testing discussed. Presence of these elements may indicate renal or other systemic diseases.
(1) Immerse end of chemically impregnated test strip into urine.	Exposes reagent to urine.
(2) Remove strip from container immediately, and tap it gently against side of container.	Excess urine can dilute reagents.
(3) Hold strip in horizontal position.	Prevents possible mixing of chemical reagents.
(4) Time for number of seconds specified on container, and compare color of strip with color chart (Table 41-1).	Accurate interpretation of results depends on precise timing.
4. Remove and discard gloves; wash hands.	Reduces transmission of microorganisms.

Table 41-1 Color Chart for Reagent Strip

Test	When to Read	Range of Results
pH	Anytime	5-9
Protein	Anytime	(1) to +4 (72,000 mg/dl)
Glucose	10 seconds (qualitative)	(−) to +4
	30 seconds (quantitative)	(−) to +4 (270)
Ketones	15 seconds	(−) to +3 (large)
Blood	25 seconds	(−) to +3 (large)

STEP	RATIONALE
5. Discuss test results with client.	Client should participate in care to improve understanding and compliance.

EVALUATION

1. If client is to be responsible for self-testing, have client demonstrate proficiency.	Return demonstration is best evidence of proficiency.
2. Note presence of blood, protein, glucose, or ketones in urine.	None of these substances should be in urine; pH should be slightly acidic (average, 6; normal, 4.5 to 8).
3. Observe that sample is not contaminated with feces or toilet tissue.	May affect accuracy of measurement.

UNEXPECTED OUTCOMES AND RELATED INTERVENTIONS

- Client or family member is unable to perform urine test correctly.
  - Reinforce need for specimen.
  - Repeat teaching as needed.
- Test results are positive for glucose, ketones, protein, blood, and/or alterations in pH.
  - Continue to monitor client.
  - Report findings to physician, and follow new orders.

RECORDING AND REPORTING

- Record results immediately in nurses' notes or glucose testing flow sheet
- If client is diabetic, nurse should determine if insulin should be given. If capillary glucose monitoring is impossible, urinary glucose level may be measured to determine dietary needs and insulin requirements (Malarkey and McMorrow, 2000).
- Have client in home setting record results of test on flow sheet. Encourage client to take samples at same time each day.
- Diabetic flow sheets often require charting of medications and amount of urine, as well as results of glucose and ketone tests.

TEACHING CONSIDERATIONS

- Instruct client about proper method for collecting random urine sample.
- Teach client to check expiration date on bottle of test strips.
- Teach client to store tablets in clean, dry area. Moisture can alter chemical makeup of tablets.
- Teach clients to close bottles tightly after removing reagent strips to prevent them from absorbing moisture and altering future results.
- Teach client to avoid touching test tube during boiling process.
- Explain rationale for double-voided specimen, and seek appropriate client feedback.
- Explain relationship of urinary findings of glucose with blood glucose when indicated.
- Discuss possible reasons for finding acetone, blood, and protein in urine.
- Discuss relationship of urinary pH to urinary tract infection and formation of renal calculi when appropriate.
- Have client return demonstrations on urine testing until client uses correct technique.
- Discuss client's plans for testing urine at home, if indicated.

PEDIATRIC CONSIDERATIONS

- School-age children can learn to test urine accurately, but parents should continue to provide backup.
- If reagent tablets are used, keep them away from small children. Tablets contain caustic soda, which can burn mouth and oral mucosa.
- Parents are usually very helpful in guiding young children through procedure.
- Procedures involving genitals in preschool children cause anxiety (Wong and others, 1999).

GERONTOLOGICAL CONSIDERATIONS

- Older adults may have difficulty seeing color chart.
- Older adults with musculoskeletal alterations may not have fine motor coordination necessary to obtain samples for specimen collection.
- In older adults, urine testing is considered unreliable because of age-related renal function changes (Lueckenotte, 2000).

HOME CARE CONSIDERATIONS

- Most kits sold in drug stores contain all equipment necessary for testing urine except specimen container.
- Clients at home may prefer to use large clock with second hand for timing urine tests.
- Reagent strip method is most frequently used at home (Malarkey and McMorrow, 2000).

Skill 41-6 Measuring Occult Blood in Stool

A common fecal laboratory test is the guaiac test for fecal occult blood. Fecal occult blood testing detects blood in the stool and is useful as a colorectal cancer screening test because cancers and adenomatous polyps bleed more than normal mucosa (Agency for Health Care Policy and Research [AHCPR], 1998). The test measures microscopic amounts of blood in the feces. Normally a person loses small amounts of blood daily in the feces as a result of minor abrasions of the nasopharyngeal or oral mucosa. If greater than 50 ml of blood enters the feces from the upper gastrointestinal tract, the blood can be visualized as **melena** (darkening of feces). The **guaiac test** helps to reveal blood that is visually undetectable.

The test is a useful diagnostic tool for conditions such as colon cancer, upper gastrointestinal ulcers, and localized gastric parasitic infections or intestinal irritation. The amount of bleeding increases with the size of the polyp and stage of cancer. People with small polyps (less than 1 cm in diameter) bleed scarcely more than those without polyps (AHCPR, 1998).

The test is easy to perform. Clients are often instructed in how to collect fecal specimens for the test in the home. Only a small amount of stool is needed to perform the test successfully. The most common guaiac tests are the Hemoccult slides and the Hematest tablets.

Delegation Considerations

Assistive personnel may obtain and test stool for occult blood. Care provider should be instructed to report immediately if blood is detected and not to discard stool from a positive test, so that the nurse may repeat the testing.

Equipment

- Paper towel
- Disposable gloves
- Wooden applicator

Hemoccult Test (Figure 41-5)

- Cardboard Hemoccult slide
- Hemoccult developing solution

Hematest

- Hematest tablets (tablets must be protected from moisture, heat, and light)
- Guaiac paper (reagent tablet produces blue reaction on guaiac paper if fecal smear contains blood)
- Sink with running water

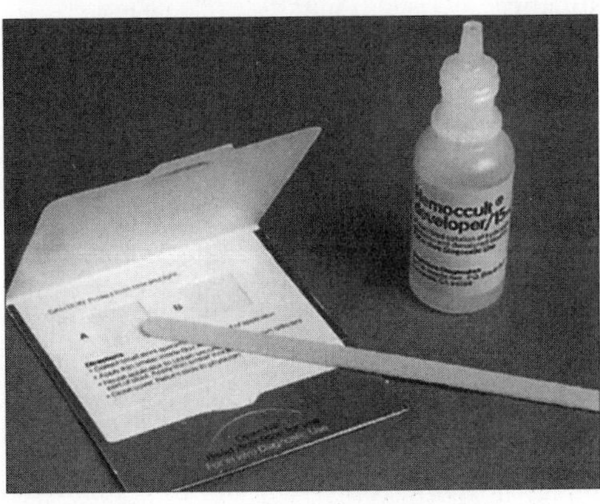

FIGURE 41-5 Hemoccult testing kit for measuring occult blood.

Step	Rationale
Assessment	
1. Assess client's or family members' understanding of need for stool test.	Provides nurse with information on which to base necessary health teaching.
2. Assess client's ability to cooperate with procedure and collect specimen.	To avoid embarrassment, clients often prefer to collect own stool specimen. Some clients require assistance.
3. Assess client's medical history for bleeding, gastrointestinal disorder, or hemorrhoids.	Routine screening can be instituted by nurse. Hemorrhoids can cause bleeding that may be misinterpreted as upper gastrointestinal bleeding.
4. Obtain client's medication history. Note drugs that can cause gastrointestinal mucosal bleeding.	Anticoagulants increase risk of bleeding in gastrointestinal tract, even from minor trauma to mucosa. Long-term use of steroids, nonsteroidal antiinflammatory drugs (NSAIDs), and acetylsalicylic acid (aspirin) can irritate mucosa.

STEP	RATIONALE
5. Refer to physician's orders for medication or dietary modifications or restrictions before test.	Specimens will be positive if contaminated by menstrual blood or hemorrhoidal blood or povidone-iodine. Diets rich in meats, green leafy vegetables, poultry, and fish may produce false-positive results. Drugs that affect results include alcohol, antiinflammatory agents, ascorbic acid (Vitamin C), and nonsteroidal agents (Chernecky and Berger, 1997).

NURSING DIAGNOSIS

Defining characteristics from the assessment data may reveal the following nursing diagnoses for clients requiring this skill:

- Anxiety
- Bowel incontinence
- Constipation
- Diarrhea
- Deficient knowledge regarding collection and testing of stool specimen

Related factors are individualized based on client's condition or needs.

PLANNING

STEP	RATIONALE
1. **Expected outcomes** following completion of procedure:	
▪ Test for **occult blood** is negative.	Client has only small amount of blood in feces because of normal nasopharyngeal and oral mucosa abrasions.
▪ Client will discuss purpose and benefits of testing stool for blood.	Documents learning.
2. Explain procedure to client and/or family member. Discuss reason for specimen collection and how client can assist. Explain that feces must be free of urine and tissue.	Client who understands procedure is more likely to cooperate and may be able to obtain specimen independently. Also prevents accidental disposal of specimen.
3. Arrange for any needed dietary or medication restrictions.	Ensures accuracy of test results.

IMPLEMENTATION

STEP	RATIONALE
1. Wash hands and apply clean disposable gloves.	Reduces transmission of microorganisms.
2. Obtain uncontaminated stool specimen.	Specimen is obtained in clean, dry container and not contaminated with urine, water, or toilet tissue.

- ***Critical Decision Point***
  Observe fecal specimen. If frank red blood is observed within stool itself, report these findings immediately.

STEP	RATIONALE
3. Use tip of wooden applicator to obtain small portion of feces.	Small specimen is sufficient for measuring blood content.
4. Measure for occult blood.	
a. Perform Hemoccult slide test:	
(1) Open flap of slide, and apply thin smear of stool on paper in first box.	Guaiac paper inside box is sensitive to fecal blood content. Occult blood from upper gastrointestinal tract is not always equally dispersed throughout stool.
(2) Obtain second fecal specimen from different portion of stool, and apply thinly to slide's second box (see illustration).	Findings of occult blood are more conclusive for gastrointestinal bleeding when entire specimen is found to contain blood.
(3) Close slide cover and turn slide over to reverse side. Open cardboard flap, and apply 2 drops of Hemoccult developing solution on each box of guaiac paper (see illustration).	Developing solution penetrates underlying fecal specimen. Blood is indicated by change in color of guaiac paper.

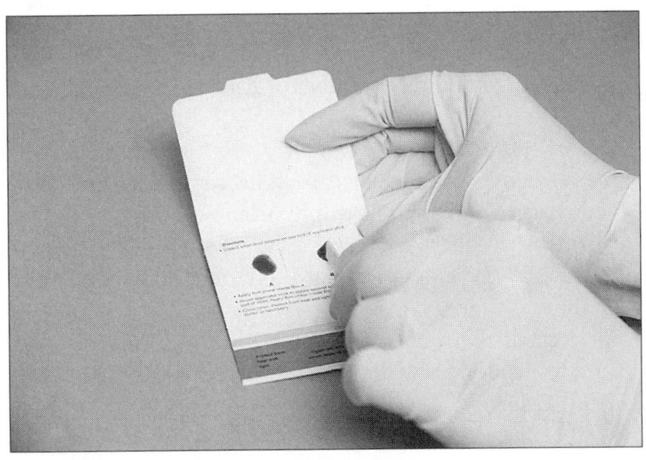

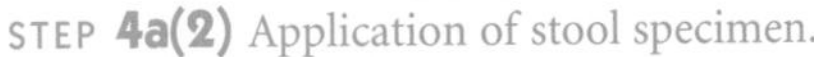
STEP 4a(2) Application of stool specimen.

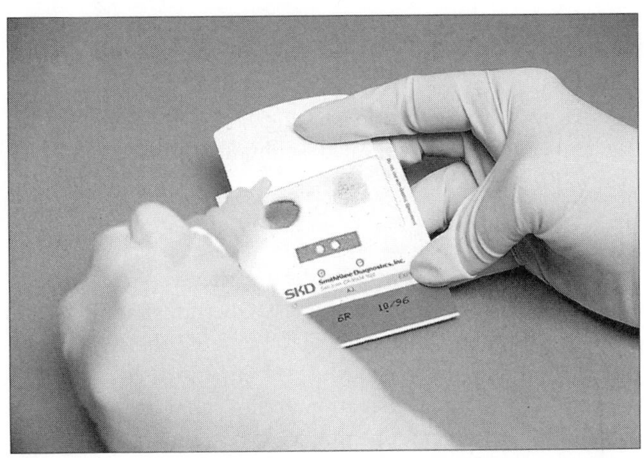

STEP 4a(3) Application of solution.

STEP	RATIONALE
(4) Read results of test after 30 to 60 seconds. Note color changes.	Bluish discoloration indicates occult blood (guaiac positive). No change in color of guaiac paper indicates negative results.
(5) Dispose of test slide in proper receptacle.	Reduces transfer of microorganisms.
b. Perform test using Hematest tablets:	
(1) Place stool on guaiac paper and Hematest tablet on top of stool specimen.	Tablet contains solid form of developing solution.
(2) Apply 2 to 3 drops of tap water to tablet, allowing water to flow onto guaiac paper.	Tap water dissolves Hematest tablet and thus dispenses developing solution over specimen and guaiac paper.
(3) Observe color of guaiac paper within 2 minutes.	Bluish discoloration is guaiac positive. Do not read color after 2 minutes. False findings may occur.
(4) Dispose of tablet and paper in proper receptacle.	Reduces transmission of microorganisms.
(5) Wrap wooden applicator in paper towel, and dispose in proper receptacle.	Reduces transmission of microorganisms.
(6) Wash hands after removing and discarding gloves.	Reduces spread of infection.

EVALUATION

1. Ask client to explain collection procedure.	Documents level of learning.
2. Note color changes in guaiac paper.	Reveals blood in feces.

• ***Critical Decision Point***
Single positive test result does not confirm bleeding or indicate colorectal cancer. For confirmed positive results, test must be repeated at least three times while client is on meat-free, high-residue diet. More in-depth diagnosis is needed with positive results.

3. Note character of stool specimen.	Certain abnormal constituents of stool may be visible.

UNEXPECTED OUTCOME AND RELATED INTERVENTIONS

- Test for occult blood is positive.
  - Continue to monitor client.
  - Notify physician.

RECORDING AND REPORTING

- Record results of test in nurses' notes.
- Record any unusual characteristics of stool in nurses' notes
- Report positive test results to physician.

TEACHING CONSIDERATIONS

- Explain rationale regarding why client should obtain specimens from two different areas of stool specimen.
- If client has been on long-term steroid or anticoagulant drug therapy, explain how these drugs may result in occult blood in stools.

- If physician orders meat-free diet before test, explain its significance to test results (red meats can cause false-positive results).
- Discuss reason for multiple testing of stool for occult blood. Clients are usually requested to obtain specimen every day for 3 days.

PEDIATRIC CONSIDERATIONS
- Children of school age and older are often very curious and may ask many questions about test. Questions should be answered honestly and at child's level of understanding. Allow child to watch, if desired, while test is performed.
- Encourage active participation in the school-age child (e.g., handling equipment, opening packages) (Wong and others, 1999).

GERONTOLOGICAL CONSIDERATIONS
- If serial fecal specimens are required, older adult may need assistance from family member or friend.

HOME CARE CONSIDERATIONS
- Many clients are instructed to collect specimens at home and return them to clinic or physician's office.
- Clients who collect specimen at home are asked to prepare slide with feces, close cardboard slide, and return it to office or clinic.
- Alert client that presence of toilet bowel cleaner, disinfectant, or deodorizer will interfere with the results (Malarkey and McMorrow, 2000).

Skill 41-7 Collecting Nose and Throat Specimens for Culture

Clients frequently have signs or symptoms of upper respiratory or sinus infections. A nose or throat culture specimen is a simple diagnostic tool for determining the nature of the client's problem. The laboratory personnel places the specimen on a culture medium to determine if pathogenic organisms will grow.

This specimen collection can cause discomfort to sensitive mucosal membranes. Likewise, collection of a throat culture may cause gagging. Clients should clearly understand how each specimen is to be collected to minimize anxiety or discomfort.

DELEGATION CONSIDERATIONS

This skill should not be delegated to assistive personnel.

EQUIPMENT
- Two sterile swabs in sterile culture tubes (flexible wire swab with cotton tip may be used for nose cultures)
- Nasal speculum (optional)
- Emesis basin or clean container (optional)
- Tongue blades
- Penlight
- Completed identification labels
- Completed laboratory requisition (date, time, name of test, source of culture)
- Facial tissues
- Clean disposable gloves

STEP	RATIONALE
ASSESSMENT	
1. Assess understanding of purpose of procedure and ability to cooperate. Nurse may need assistance to obtain throat cultures from confused, combative, or unconscious clients.	Provides basis to determine need for health teaching and need for assistance.
2. Assess condition of and drainage from nasal mucosa and sinuses.	Reveals physical signs that may indicate infection or allergic irritation. Clear drainage usually indicates allergy. Yellow, green, or brown drainage usually indicates infection.
3. Determine if client has experienced postnasal drip, sinus headache or tenderness, nasal congestion, or sore throat.	Symptoms help reveal nature of problem.
4. Assess condition of posterior pharynx.	

- ***Critical Decision Point***
  Pay particular attention to areas of inflammation or purulent drainage. Identification of inflamed or purulent areas allows nurse to swab those sites quickly.

Step	Rationale
5. Assess client for systemic signs of infection: fever, chills, and/or fatigue.	Infection originating within nasopharynx can become systemic, requiring antibiotic therapy.
6. Review physician's orders to determine if nose, throat, or both cultures are needed.	Prevents exposing client to unnecessary discomfort of repeated cultures.

Nursing Diagnosis

Defining characteristics from the assessment data may reveal the following nursing diagnoses for clients requiring this skill:

Risk for infection
Deficient knowledge regarding specimen collection
Pain (acute or chronic)

Related factors are individualized based on client's condition or needs.

Planning

Step	Rationale
1. **Expected outcomes** following completion of procedure:	
▪ There is no bacterial growth in specimens.	Absence of infection.
▪ Client does not experience bleeding of nasal mucosa.	Procedure is atraumatic.
▪ Specimen is not contaminated.	Evidenced by results of laboratory analysis.
▪ Client will discuss purpose of nose and throat cultures.	Documents learning.
2. Plan to do culture before mealtime or at least 1 hour after eating.	Because gagging may be induced by procedure, incidence of vomiting is decreased.
3. Explain procedure to client and/or family member. Discuss reason for specimen collection and how client can assist.	Understanding of procedure usually decreases anxiety and promotes cooperation.
4. Explain that client may have tickling sensation or gag during swabbing of throat. Nasal swab may create urge to sneeze. Both procedures require only a few seconds.	May help client to relax.

Implementation

Step	Rationale
1. Ask client to sit erect in bed or chair facing nurse. Acutely ill client or young child may lie back against bed with head of bed raised to 45-degree angle.	Provides easy access to nasal or oral structures.
2. Have swab in tube ready for use. Nurse may wish to loosen top so that swab can be removed easily.	Nurse should be able to grasp swab easily without danger of contaminating it. Most commercially prepared tubes have tops that fit securely over end of swab, which allows nurse to touch outer tops without contaminating swab stick.
3. Collect throat culture:	
a. Wash hands and put on gloves.	
b. Instruct client to tilt head backward. For clients in bed, place pillow behind shoulders.	Facilitates visualization of pharynx.
c. Ask client to open mouth and say "ah."	Permits exposure of pharynx, relaxes throat muscles, and minimizes gag reflex.

• ***Critical Decision Point***

If pharynx is not visualized, depress tongue with tongue blade and note inflamed areas of pharynx or tonsils. Depress anterior third of tongue only. (Illuminate with penlight as needed.) Area to be swabbed should be clearly visualized. Placement of tongue blade along back of tongue more likely initiates gag reflex. If client gags, remove tongue blade and allow client to relax before reinserting. Place pressure only on anterior third of tongue.

Step	Rationale
d. Insert swab without touching lips, teeth, tongue, cheeks, or uvula.	Poor technique will cause a false-positive result (Malarkey and McMorrow, 2000).
e. Gently but quickly swab tonsillar area side to side, making contact with inflamed or purulent sites (see illustration).	These areas contain most microorganisms.

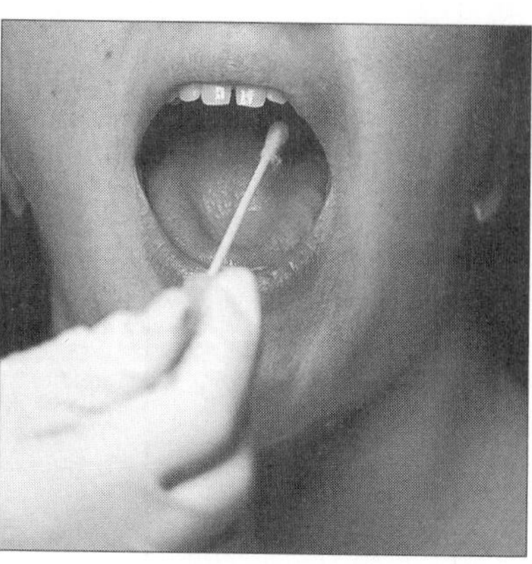

STEP **3e** Obtaining tonsillar swab.

A

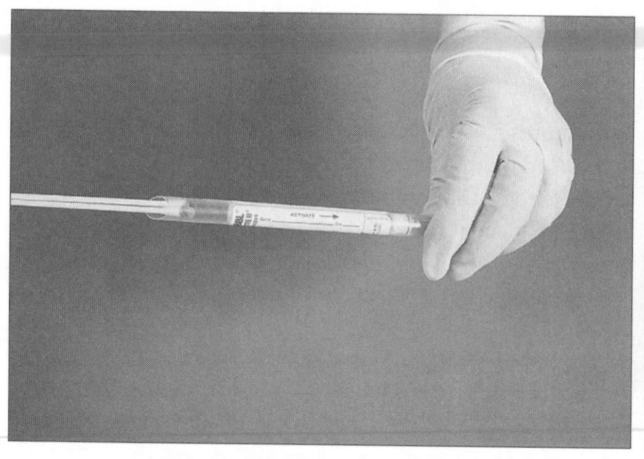

B

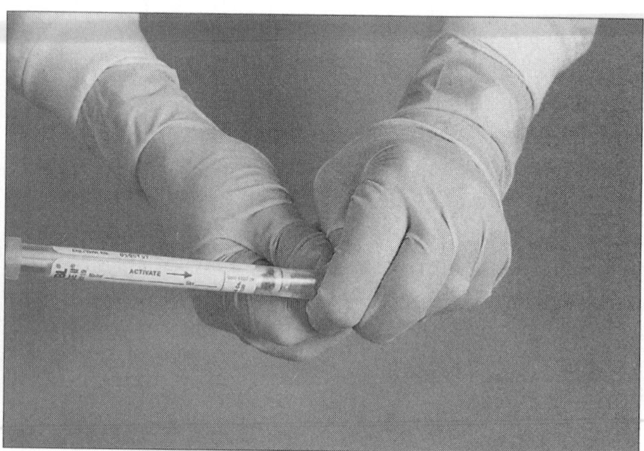

STEP **3f** **A,** Placing swab into culture tube. **B,** Crushing ampule.

Step	Rationale
f. Carefully withdraw swab without striking oral structures. Immediately place swab in culture tube. Place gauze around ampule, and crush ampule at bottom of tube. Push tip of swab into liquid medium (see illustrations).	Retains microorganisms within culture tube. Mixing swab tip with culture medium ensures life of bacteria for testing.
g. Place top on culture tube securely.	Prevents contamination from microorganisms.
h. Discard tongue depressor into trash.	Reduces transmission of microorganisms.
i. Remove gloves and discard.	
4. Collect nose culture:	
a. Wash hands and put on gloves.	
b. Encourage client to blow nose, and check nostrils for patency with penlight.	Clears nasal passages of mucus containing resident bacteria.

- ***Critical Decision Point***
  Ask client to alternatively occlude each nostril and exhale. Determines nostril with greater patency, from which specimen will be collected.

Step	Rationale
c. Ask client to tilt head back. Clients in bed should have pillow behind shoulders.	Facilitates visualization of nasal septum and sinuses (Malarkey and McMorrow, 2000).
d. Gently insert nasal speculum in one nostril (optional).	Allows retraction of mucosa for easier swab insertion.
e. Carefully pass swab through center of speculum (if used) into nostril until it reaches that portion of mucosa that is inflamed or containing exudate. Rotate swab quickly.	Swab should remain sterile until it reaches area to be cultured. Rotating swab covers all surfaces where exudate is present.
f. Remove swab without touching sides of speculum.	Prevents contamination of swab by resident bacteria.
g. Carefully remove nasal speculum (if used) and place in basin. Offer client facial tissue.	Minimizes period of time client will experience discomfort.
h. Insert swab into culture tube. Crush ampule at bottom of tube and push tip of swab into liquid medium.	Retains microorganisms within culture tube. Mixing swab tip with culture medium ensures life of bacteria for testing.
i. Place top on tube securely.	Prevents contamination from microorganisms.
j. Remove gloves, discard, and wash hands.	
5. Collection of nasopharyngeal culture:	
a. Follow Step 4, a through j, except use a special swab on a flexible wire that can be flexed downward to reach nasopharynx via nose.	Only this specially designed swab allows access to difficult-to-reach nasopharyngeal area.

• ***Critical Decision Point***

This swab must advance into nasopharynx to ensure that culture has been obtained correctly.

Step	Rationale
6. Securely attach properly completed identification label and laboratory requisition to culture tube. Agency policy may dictate type of information to place on label. Note on laboratory requisition if client is taking antibiotic or if specific organism is suspected (e.g., *Bordetella pertussis*).	Incorrect identification of specimen could result in diagnostic or therapeutic errors.
7. Send specimen to laboratory immediately or refrigerate.	Fresh specimen provides most accurate test results.

Evaluation

Step	Rationale
1. Check laboratory record for results of culture test.	Results reveal type of organisms in nose or pharynx and antibiotics most likely to be effective.

Unexpected Outcomes and Related Interventions

- Nose and throat cultures reveal bacterial growth.
  - Notify physician of findings.
  - Administer medications as ordered.
- Client experiences minor nasal bleeding.
  - Apply mild pressure and ice pack over bridge of nose.
  - Notify physician of client's condition.
- Specimen is contaminated.
  - Repeat specimen collection.

Recording and Reporting

- Record specimen collection, date, time, and disposition in nurses' notes.
- Describe appearance of nasal and oral mucosal structures in nurses' notes.
- Report unusual test results to physician.

Teaching Considerations

- Clients should be instructed that procedure is painless but the gag reflex is commonly stimulated during procedure.
- Discuss client's role in collecting specimen.
- Explain how and why specimen is being obtained.
- Discuss relationship between culture results and medication.
- Discuss reason for time delay in receiving culture results.

Pediatric Considerations

- Allowing young children to visualize and examine speculum decreases their fear of it.
- Immobilization of child's head and arms is important when obtaining nose or throat culture and should be done in firm, gentle, kind manner. Ask another nurse to assist, if necessary.
- Ask parents to act as coach with their child.

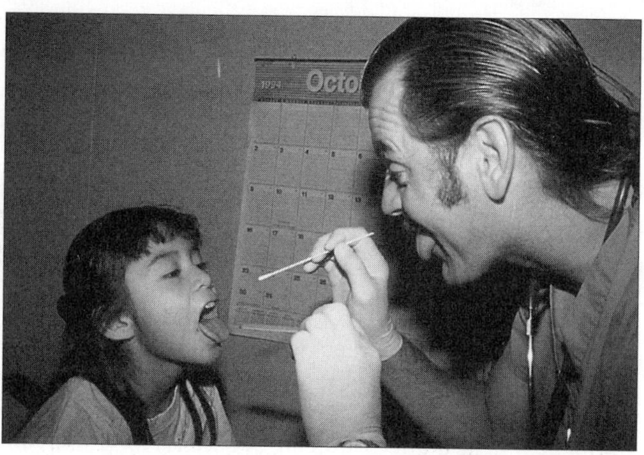

FIGURE **41-6** Preparing a child for throat culture.

- Showing tongue blade and penlight to child and demonstrating how to say "ah" helps to decrease anxiety (Figure 41-6).
- School-age child will be more cooperative if given opportunity to ask questions about procedure and results.
- Respiratory syncytial virus (RSV) is detected directly in respiratory secretions, usually obtained by nasopharyngeal aspiration (Wong and others, 1999).
- Throat cultures should not be attempted if acute epiglottitis is suspected because trauma from swab might cause increase in edema and resulting occlusion of airway (Wong and others, 1999).

Gerontological Considerations

- Older adults may need assistance in keeping mouth open to obtain specimen.
- In confused clients, assistive personnel may be necessary to hold client's hands while sample is being obtained.

Skill 41-8 Obtaining Vaginal or Urethral Discharge Specimens

Normally there is minimal discharge from the vagina or urethra. Poor hygiene practices may cause an accumulation of discharge. However, if a client develops an increased amount of discharge or if there is a change in the character of discharge from the vagina or urethra, medical follow-up is necessary.

Drainage from the vagina or urethra is normally thin, nonpurulent, whitish or clear, and small in amount. A woman will have bloody discharge during menstruation. A newborn infant may have bloody discharge from the vagina for 2 to 4 weeks after birth because of the abrupt decrease in maternal hormones at birth.

The clients most commonly requiring cultures of vaginal or urethral discharge have signs and symptoms of sexually transmitted disease or urinary tract infection. Clients suspected of having a sexually transmitted disease may be embarrassed by their condition. The nurse must show respect and understanding toward the client. If the client undergoes a complete diagnostic workup, the many questions can be exhausting and may cause anxiety. When collecting vaginal or urethral specimens, the nurse should work quickly and calmly, maintaining the client's privacy at all times.

Delegation Considerations

The skill of obtaining vaginal and urethral discharge culture samples should not be delegated to assistive personnel.

Equipment

- Sterile swab in sterile culture tube (commercially available culture tubes have swab and tube with ampule containing special transport medium)
- Sheet, blanket, or paper drape
- Clean disposable gloves
- Penlight or gooseneck lamp
- Completed identification labels
- Completed laboratory requisition (date, time, name of test, type of culture)

Step	Rationale
Assessment	
1. Assess understanding of need for culture and ability to cooperate with procedure.	Provides data on which nurse develops teaching plan.
2. Assess condition of external genitalia. Observe urethra, meatus, and vaginal orifice for redness, swelling, tenderness, and discharge that is whitish, mucoid, and purulent.	Assessment findings and specimen test results reveal nature of problem.

STEP	RATIONALE
3. Ask client if dysuria, localized pruritus of genitalia, or lower abdominal pain have been experienced.	Symptoms of urinary tract or vaginal infection.
4. If symptoms suggest sexually transmitted disease, record sexual history of client.	Determine sexual activity and if there has been sexual contact with a person known to have a sexually transmitted disease (Linton, Matteson, and Maebius, 2000). If culture results are positive, tell client to receive treatment and to have sexual partners evaluated (Pagana and Pagana, 1998).
5. Refer to physician's order to determine if culture is vaginal or urethral.	Client may require one or both types of cultures.

NURSING DIAGNOSIS

Defining characteristics from the assessment data may reveal the following nursing diagnoses for clients requiring this skill:

- Anxiety
- Deficient knowledge regarding specimen collection
- Pain (acute)
- Risk for infection

Related factors are individualized based on client's condition or needs.

PLANNING

STEP	RATIONALE
1. **Expected outcomes** following completion of procedure.	
▪ Specimen is not contaminated.	Results on laboratory test can reveal whether skin cells or mucosal cells have contaminated specimen.
▪ Vaginal or urethral cultures do not reveal growth of microorganisms.	Evidence of absence of infection.
2. Explain procedure to client and/or family member. Discuss reason for specimen collection and how client can assist. Instruct female client not to douche before culture is obtained.	Client who understands procedure is less anxious and more likely to cooperate. Douching of vaginal canal would remove discharge containing pathogens.
3. Maintain nonjudgmental attitude while obtaining data.	Demonstrates respect for client.

IMPLEMENTATION

STEP	RATIONALE
1. Wash hands.	Reduces transmission of microorganisms.
2. Draw bedside curtains or close room door. Place "Do Not Enter" sign on door (if available).	Provides privacy for client and demonstrates nurse's respect for client's well-being.
3. Assist client to proper position, raise gown, and drape body parts to be exposed:	Provides easy access to perineal area. Draping minimizes exposure of body parts, minimizing anxiety.
a. Female: Dorsal recumbent position with sheet draped over each leg and genitalia.	
b. Male: Sit on chair or bed or lie supine with sheet draped across lower trunk and genitalia.	
4. Apply clean disposable gloves.	Prevents contamination of nurse's hands from discharge.
5. Direct light source onto perineum (may not be needed for male client).	Allows better visualization of urethral or vaginal structures.
6. Open culture tube and hold swab in dominant hand.	Provides for easier manipulation of swab during culture collection.
7. Instruct client to slowly deep breathe.	Helps client to relax. Tensing of muscles around pelvic floor may cause discomfort during swabbing.
8. Obtain necessary specimens:	
a. Female	
(1) With nondominant hand, fully separate labia to expose vaginal orifice.	Exposes perineum and ensures specimen is of vaginal discharge.

Step	Rationale
(2) Touch tip of swab into discharge pool, being careful not to touch skin or mucosa along perineum or vaginal canal. If no discharge is visible, gently insert swabs 1 to 2.5 cm (½ to 1 inch) into vaginal orifice and rotate before removal.	Discharge contains the greatest concentration of microorganisms.
(3) To expose urethral meatus, use nondominant hand to pull gently on labia minora upward and back.	Allows better visualization of urethral orifice.
(4) Use clean swab, and gently apply to tip of meatus where discharge is visible. Avoid touching labia.	Discharge contains greatest concentration of microorganisms.

- ***Critical Decision Point***
  If discharge near vagina appears different from discharge along perineum, collect separate specimens from each area. If there are two organisms present, they are not cross contaminated on a single swab.

Step	Rationale
b. Male	
(1) Hold client's penis near tip with nondominant hand; if male is uncircumcised, gently retract foreskin.	Provides clear exposure of urethral meatus.
(2) Use dominant hand to hold swab. Apply gently to area of discharge at urinary meatus.	Discharge contains greatest number of microorganisms.
(3) If no discharge is apparent, physician may order swab to be introduced into urinary meatus. Hold male genitalia gently.	Excess manipulation can cause erection.
(4) Return foreskin to natural position.	Tightening of foreskin around shaft of penis can cause localized discomfort and edema and potential necrosis.
9. Return each swab to culture tube, and secure top.	Retains microorganisms within tube.
10. Remove and discard gloves.	Reduces spread of microorganisms.
11. If using commercial culture tube, wrap ampule with gauze to prevent injury to nurse's fingers while crushing. Immediately squeeze end of tube to crush ampule (see Skill 41-7, Implementation, Step 3f). Push tip of swab into fluid medium.	Medium supports life of microorganisms until culture is obtained.
12. Label each culture tube with identification label, and affix completed requisition.	Incorrect specimen identification could lead to diagnostic or therapeutic error.
13. Send specimen immediately to laboratory or refrigerate.	Bacteria multiply quickly; specimen should be analyzed quickly for accurate results.
14. Assist client to comfortable position, replace gown, and remove drape.	Reinforces client's sense of self-esteem.
15. Wash hands.	Reduces transmission of microorganisms.

Evaluation

Step	Rationale
1. Review laboratory results for evidence of pathogens.	Results will reveal type of organisms present. Certain organisms are common to vaginal tract. Urethra should be free of microorganisms.
2. Continue to monitor whether discharge is present and if so, observe color and amount.	Characteristics of discharge can indicate specific type of infection.
3. Observe specimen for presence of feces.	If feces are observed, obtain another specimen.

Unexpected Outcomes and Related Interventions

- Vaginal or urethral cultures reveal growth of pathogenic microorganisms.
  - Inform physician of findings, and follow new orders.
  - Continue to monitor client.
- Specimen is contaminated with epidermal cells.
  - Repeat specimen collection.

Recording and Reporting

- In nurses' notes record types of cultures obtained and date and time sent to laboratory.
- Describe character of discharge and appearance of vaginal orifice or urethral meatus.
- Report laboratory results to nurse in charge or physician.

Teaching Considerations

- Discuss symptoms of vaginal or urethral infection with client as appropriate.
- Explain relationship between genital discomfort and infection of vaginal or urinary tract.
- Explain time required to obtain results of culture.
- Discuss sexuality and safe sexual practices with client if appropriate.
- Clients with urethral or vaginal discharge may require instruction about perineal hygiene measures.
- If topical treatments (e.g., suppositories) are ordered, instruct client in proper administration of medication (see Chapter 17).

Pediatric Considerations

- Young child will probably desire parents' presence, whereas adolescent usually will not.
- In collection from infant or young child, another nurse can assist with specimen by gently holding child's legs apart in frog-like position. Have parent present to encourage cooperation.
- Parents should understand that obtaining specimen will not affect virginity of child.
- Be sensitive to cultural variations and beliefs pertaining to genitalia (i.e., female circumcisions).

Gerontological Considerations

- When obtaining sample from older adult, assist client to comfortable position.
- Clear explanation regarding importance of obtaining sample is extremely helpful to alleviate or diminish anxiety and to gain cooperation.

Skill 41-9 Collecting Sputum Specimens

Sputum is produced by cells lining the respiratory tract. Although production is minimal in the healthy state, disease states can increase the amount or change the character of sputum. Examination of sputum may aid in the diagnosis and treatment of several conditions ranging from simple bronchitis to lung cancer.

Suctioning may be indicated to collect sputum from the client who is unable to spontaneously produce a sample for laboratory analysis. Suctioning may provoke violent coughing, which can cause vomiting and aspiration of stomach contents, as well as induce constriction of pharyngeal, laryngeal, and bronchial muscles. In addition, suctioning may cause direct stimulation of vagal nerve fibers in the airway and may cause cardiac arrhythmias and increases in intracranial pressure (Beare and Myers, 1998).

Three major types of sputum specimens are sputum for cytology, culture and sensitivity, and acid-fast bacilli (AFB). Cytological or cellular examination of sputum may identify aberrant cells or cancer. Sputum collected for culture and sensitivity testing can be used to identify specific microorganisms and to determine antibiotics to which they are most sensitive. The AFB smear is used to support the diagnosis of tuberculosis (TB). A definitive diagnosis of TB requires a sputum culture and sensitivity.

Delegation Considerations

The skill of collecting expectorated sputum specimens may be delegated to assistive personnel. The client's respiratory status and sputum production must first be assessed. When a client's mobility is restricted, the caregiver must know how to properly position the client. If a sterile suction method is needed to obtain the sputum specimen, this skill should not be delegated to assistive personnel.

Equipment

Expectorated Specimen

- Sterile specimen container with cover
- Clean disposable gloves
- Facial tissues
- Emesis basin (optional)
- Toothbrush (optional)

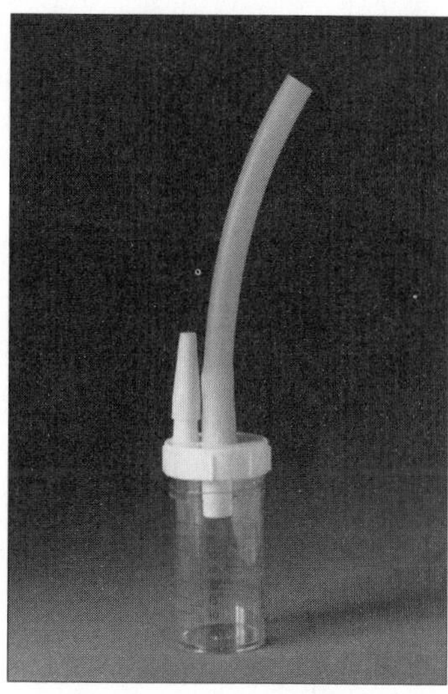

FIGURE 41-7 Sputum trap.

- Completed identification labels
- Completed laboratory requisition (date, time, name of test, source of culture)
- Small plastic bag for delivery of specimen to lab (or a container as specified by agency)

Suctioned Specimen

- Suction device (wall or portable)
- Sterile suction catheter (size 14, 16, or 18 Fr—not large enough to cause trauma to nasal mucosa)
- Sterile gloves
- Sterile saline in container
- In-line specimen container or sputum trap (Figure 41-7).
- Small plastic bag for delivery of specimen to laboratory (or a container as specified by agency)
- Oxygen therapy equipment if indicated
- Protective eye wear

STEP	RATIONALE
ASSESSMENT	
1. Check physician's orders for type of sputum analysis and specifications (e.g., amount of sputum, number of specimens, time of collection, method to obtain). Specimens for AFB require three consecutive morning samples, and cultures can take up to 8 weeks.	Specific test to be performed may dictate when or how frequently specimens are collected. Ideal time to collect sputum is early morning because bronchial secretions tend to accumulate during the night. Bacteria also accumulate as secretions pool.
2. Assess level of understanding of procedure and its purpose.	Provides baseline for nurse to establish teaching plan.
3. Assess client's ability to cough and expectorate specimens.	Adequate cough is essential in production of mucus from tracheobronchial tree. Client may have nonproductive cough associated with abdominal or chest pain. Simple clearing of throat is unacceptable.
4. Assess when client last ate a meal (or had a tube feeding). Wait 1 to 2 hours after eating.	Client may gag, vomit, and aspirate stomach contents.
5. Determine type of assistance needed by client to obtain specimen.	Positioning, postural drainage, deep breathing and coughing exercises may improve ability to cough productively. Suctioning may be indicated if client is unable to cough and expectorate.
6. Assess client's respiratory status, including respiratory rate, depth, pattern, and color of mucous membranes.	Active coughing may alter respiratory status. Respiratory status can depend on amount of sputum in tracheobronchial tree.

NURSING DIAGNOSIS

Defining characteristics from the assessment data may reveal the following nursing diagnoses for clients requiring this skill:

Ineffective airway clearance
Risk for aspiration
Ineffective breathing pattern
Risk for infection
Deficient knowledge regarding specimen collection procedures

Related factors are individualized based on client's condition or needs.

STEP	RATIONALE

PLANNING

1. **Expected outcomes** following completion of procedure:
   - Client's respirations are same rate and character as before procedure. — Specimen collection did not alter respiratory status.
   - Client is relaxed, able to answer questions (if no artificial airway present). — Suctioning tends to cause anxiety.
   - Sputum is not contaminated by saliva or oropharyngeal flora. — Sputum must originate from tracheobronchial tree for accurate results.
   - Laboratory tests fail to reveal abnormal cells or microorganisms. — Absence of infection or abnormal cells.
   - Client will discuss purpose and benefit of sputum collection. — Documents learning.
2. Explain steps of procedure and purpose. Specimen should not contain saliva. Secretions from oropharynx contain numerous bacteria that will contaminate sputum. Client who is to be suctioned should breathe normally to prevent hyperventilation. — Promotes understanding and cooperation.

   - ***Critical Decision Point***
     When client is expectorating sputum, stress importance of deep coughing and need to avoid clearing of throat. If client is to be suctioned, stress importance of relaxing and breathing at normal rate.

3. For expectorated specimen, have client rinse mouth or brush teeth with water. — Reduces number of oral contaminants that can alter test results.

   - ***Critical Decision Point***
     Client should not use mouthwash or toothpaste because they may decrease viability of microorganisms and alter culture results.

IMPLEMENTATION

1. Wash hands. — Reduces transmission of microorganisms.
2. Close curtains or room door. — Provides privacy.
3. Position client: semi-Fowler's position, sitting on side of bed or chair, standing for coughing and expectorating specimen; high or semi-Fowler's position for suctioning. — Promotes full lung expansion and facilitates ability to cough.

   - ***Critical Decision Point***
     If client has surgical incision or localized area of discomfort, have client place hands firmly over affected area or place pillow over area. Splinting of painful area minimizes muscular stretching and discomfort during coughing and thus makes cough more productive.

4. Collect specimen:
   a. Coughing and expectoration
      (1) Apply clean disposable gloves. — Reduces risk of exposure to pathogens.
      (2) Provide client with specimen container and instruct client not to touch inside. Refer to agency policy and provide type of specimen container indicated. — Prevents risk of contamination.
      (3) Instruct client to take three to four slow deep breaths. — Helps to open airways, loosen secretions, and stimulate cough reflex.
      (4) Instruct client to emphasize slow, full exhalation. — Moves secretions into large airways.
      (5) After series of deep breaths, ask client to cough after full inhalation. — Full inhalation provides force to move secretions out of airways up to pharynx.

STEP	RATIONALE
(6) Instruct client to **expectorate** sputum directly into specimen container.	Retains microorganisms in sterile container.
(7) Have client repeat coughing until an adequate amount of sputum has been collected.	Usually 2 to 10 ml ($\frac{1}{2}$ to 2 teaspoons) is required to ensure accurate analysis of specimen.
b. Suctioning	
(1) Prepare suction machine or device and determine if it functions properly.	Adequate amount of suction is necessary to **aspirate** sputum.
(2) Connect suction tube to adapter on sputum trap.	Establishes suction that passes through sputum trap to aspirate specimen.
(3) Apply sterile gloves (required only for dominant hand).	Tracheobronchial tree is sterile body cavity. Allows nurse to manipulate suction catheter without contamination.
(4) With gloved hand, connect sterile suction catheter to rubber tubing on sputum trap.	Aspirated sputum will go directly to trap instead of to suction tubing.
(5) Other hand should have glove on for application of suction. Thumb should be on trap prepared to provide suction, and trap should be covered.	
(6) Gently insert tip of suction catheter through nasopharynx, endotracheal tube, or tracheostomy tube without applying suction (see Chapter 13).	Minimizes trauma to airway as catheter is inserted.
(7) Advance catheter into trachea.	Entrance of catheter into larynx and trachea triggers cough reflex.
(8) As client coughs, apply suction for 5 to 10 seconds, collecting 2 to 10 ml sputum.	Ensures collection of sputum from deep within tracheobronchial tree. Suctioning longer than 10 seconds can cause hypoxia and mucosal damage (Beare and Myers, 1998).
(9) Remove catheter without applying suction, then turn off suction.	Suction can damage mucosa if applied during withdrawal.
(10) Detach catheter from specimen trap, and dispose of catheter in appropriate receptacle.	Decreases risk of spreading microorganisms.
5. Secure top on specimen container tightly. For sputum trap, detach suction tubing and connect rubber tubing on sputum trap to plastic adapter (see illustration).	Contains microorganisms within container, preventing exposure to personnel handling specimen.

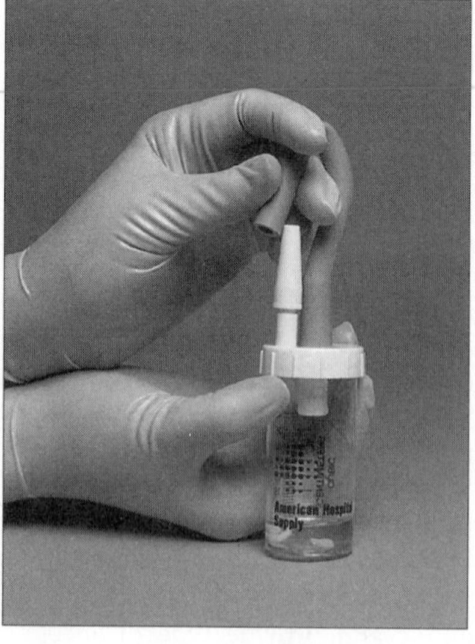

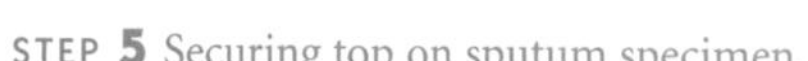

STEP 5 Securing top on sputum specimen.

STEP	RATIONALE
6. If any sputum is present on outside of container, wash it off with disinfectant.	Prevents spread of infection to persons handling specimen.
7. Offer client tissues after expectorating. Dispose of tissues in emesis basin or trash container.	Maintains cleanliness and comfort.
8. Remove and dispose of glove(s).	

Step	Rationale
9. Offer client mouth care, if desired.	Promotes comfort.
10. Wash hands.	Reduces spread of microorganisms.
11. Label specimen with identification label.	Incorrect identification could lead to diagnostic or therapeutic error.
12. Place specimen in small plastic bag (or container specified by agency) and attach requisition.	Plastic bag or container reduces risk of health care worker's exposure to sputum.
13. Send specimen immediately to laboratory or refrigerate.	Bacteria multiply quickly. Specimen should be analyzed promptly for accurate results.

Evaluation

Step	Rationale
1. Observe client's respiratory status throughout procedure, especially during suctioning.	Excessive coughing or prolonged suctioning can alter respiratory pattern and cause hypoxia.
2. Note anxiety or discomfort in client.	Procedure can be uncomfortable. If client becomes short of breath, anxiety will develop.
3. Observe character of sputum: color, consistency, odor, volume, viscosity and/or presence of blood.	Characteristics may indicate disease entities.
4. Refer to laboratory reports for test results.	Report abnormal cells or microorganisms in sputum.
5. Evaluate client's ability to describe/demonstrate sputum collection process.	

Unexpected Outcomes and Related Interventions

- Client becomes hypoxic; increased respiratory rate and effort are necessary; client feels short of breath.
  - Discontinue procedure until stable.
  - Provide oxygen therapy as needed (if ordered).
  - Notify physician of client's condition.
  - Continue to monitor client's vital signs and pulse oximetry.
- Client remains anxious or complains of discomfort from suction catheter.
  - Discontinue procedure until stable.
  - Provide oxygen therapy as needed (if ordered).
  - Notify physician of client's change in condition.
  - Continue to monitor client's vital signs and pulse oximetry.
- Specimen contains saliva.
  - Repeat specimen collection after client takes several deep breaths and coughs.
- Inadequate amount of sputum is collected.
  - Repeat specimen collection after client takes several deep breaths and coughs.
- Specimen contains blood, pathogenic organisms, or abnormal cells.
  - Report findings to physician.
- Client complains of pain when coughing to produce sputum.
  - Encourage client who is recovering from a surgical procedure to splint incision prior to coughing.
  - Obtain order for pain medication as needed (prn).
  - Inform physician of changes in client's condition.

Recording and Reporting

- Record method used to obtain specimen, date and time collected, type of test ordered, and laboratory receiving specimen in nurses' notes.
- Describe characteristics of sputum specimen.
- Describe client's tolerance of procedure.
- Report unusual sputum characteristics and client response to nurse in charge or physician.
- When laboratory reports are available, report abnormal findings. If AFB sputum culture is positive, initiate appropriate isolation techniques.
- Many agencies require nurse to note on specimen requisition if client is receiving antibiotics.

Teaching Considerations

- Nurse may demonstrate effective coughing techniques versus clearing of throat.
- Nurse can demonstrate proper splinting technique for postoperative clients.
- Explain purpose of avoiding use of mouthwashes and toothpaste before sputum expectoration (to prevent decreasing viability of microorganisms).
- Explain purpose of obtaining specimen before breakfast (specimen will be most concentrated and free of food particles).

- If aerosol treatment is indicated, teach client purpose of procedure, explaining that it will stimulate coughing and sputum expectoration.
- Nurse can teach client to avoid contaminating outside of specimen cup to reduce risk of spread of infection.

PEDIATRIC CONSIDERATIONS

- Children need very clear instructions or demonstration for deep breathing. Infants and young children will be unable to cooperate; aerosol treatment or suctioning may be indicated.
- Another nurse can assist nurse in restraining young child's head and arms during suctioning; parent may assist to give support.
- Young children often swallow secretions instead of expectorating. Use smaller catheter size for young children.

HOME CARE CONSIDERATIONS

- If client is to produce sputum specimen at home, instruct client and/or family member regarding proper technique and importance of having specimen sent to laboratory in timely manner.

Skill 41-10 Obtaining Gastric Specimens

Analysis of gastric contents can aid physicians in diagnosing and treating a number of conditions such as gastric acid irregularities, **hematemesis,** and gastrointestinal bleeding from ulcers or tumors. Gastric pH level determines the acidity of gastrointestinal secretions. Measuring gastric occult blood, which reveals bleeding in the esophagus, stomach, or duodenum, is similar to measuring stool for occult blood.

The testing of gastric specimens for occult blood and pH is relatively easy. The nurse can perform the tests on emesis or on drainage collected from an existing nasogastric tube. Inserting a nasogastric tube solely to collect gastric secretions is very unusual.

DELEGATION CONSIDERATIONS

The skill of obtaining gastric specimens may be delegated to assistive personnel. The client must first be assessed to determine patency and functioning of any gastric drainage system. The care provider must be instructed in how to empty container containing gastric secretions and how to test for pH and occult blood. The caregiver must also know when to report test results.

EQUIPMENT

- Clean disposable gloves
- Facial tissues
- Emesis basin
- Wooden applicator or 1-ml syringe
- Commercial kit with test paper for pH level and occult blood appropriate for gastric secretions
- Developing solution
- 60-ml bulb or catheter tip syringe
- Nasogastric tube and supplies for insertion (if indicated)

STEP	RATIONALE
ASSESSMENT	
1. Review physician's order to determine test and source of specimen.	Provides order when regularly testing specimen.
2. Determine presence of nasogastric tube.	Test requires aspiration of gastric secretions from nasogastric tube.
3. Assess client's level of understanding of procedure and purpose.	Provides baseline for nurse to establish teaching plan.
4. Review medications that client is receiving and foods eaten by client recently. If client has a gastric tube, review schedule for feedings and medications being administered.	Some medications and foods can cause false-positive readings for occult blood.

STEP	RATIONALE
5. Check with laboratory and physician to determine if dietary restrictions or temporary discontinuation of medications is necessary before test.	Gastric analysis for occult blood requires fasting because results depend on peroxidase activity of hemoglobin in red blood cells. Some foods contain peroxidases and cause false results.
6. Assess client for symptoms of abdominal cramping, pain, nausea, or vomiting.	Symptoms are characteristic of gastrointestinal alteration.

NURSING DIAGNOSIS

Defining characteristics from the assessment data may reveal the following nursing diagnoses for clients requiring this skill:

Anxiety
Risk for aspiration
Deficient knowledge regarding gastric specimen collection procedure

Related factors are individualized based on client's condition or needs.

PLANNING

STEP	RATIONALE
1. **Expected outcomes** following completion of procedure:	
▪ Gastric secretions are greenish to clear, with no evidence of bleeding or clots.	Greenish color results from bile secreted in duodenum.
▪ **pH** level is 1.5 to 3.0.	Gastric secretions are highly acidic. Lower gastrointestinal tract secretions are more basic.
▪ Test is negative for occult blood.	Indicates absence of bleeding in gastrointestinal tract. Positive result indicates bleeding in gastrointestinal tract.
▪ Client will discuss purpose and benefits of gastric analysis.	Documents learning.
2. Institute dietary or medication restrictions as needed.	Ensures accurate test results.
3. Explain steps of procedure to client. Emphasize that test is painless.	Reduces anxiety and promotes cooperation.

IMPLEMENTATION

STEP	RATIONALE
1. Wash hands before procedure.	Reduces transfer of microorganisms.
2. Apply disposable gloves.	Prevents risk of exposure to pathogens in bodily secretions.
3. Position client in high-Fowler's position in bed or chair.	Minimizes aspiration of gastric contents. Position relieves pressure on abdominal organs. If client is nauseated, flat position in bed or one in which client cannot sit straight may cause abdominal discomfort.
4. Close bedside curtains or door to room.	Maintains privacy.
5. Verify nasogastric tube placement (see Chapter 22).	Allows aspiration of gastric contents.
6. Obtain specimen of gastric contents by attaching bulb syringe to nasogastric tube and aspirating 5 to 10 ml; obtain sample of emesis with 1-ml syringe or wooden applicator.	Only small amount of specimen is needed for pH and occult blood testing.
7. Using applicator or syringe, apply 1 drop of gastric sample to pH test paper. Be sure that drop covers paper completely.	Paper should be completely exposed to secretions to ensure full color change.
8. Read color of pH test paper within 30 seconds, and compare with pH color guide.	Results range from 1 to 10 (depending on type of paper used). Acidic solutions are 4 or less. Basic solutions are 5 or more.
9. Apply 1 drop of gastric sample to Gastroccult blood test paper.	Sample must cover guaiac paper for test reaction to occur.

STEP	RATIONALE
10. Apply 2 drops of commercial developer solution over sample and 1 drop between positive and negative performance monitors (see illustration).	Developer initiates chemical reaction of solution with guaiac paper.

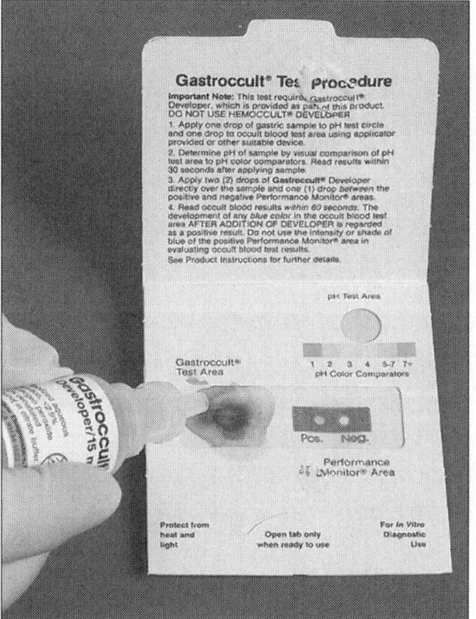

STEP **10** Applying developer solution.

STEP	RATIONALE
11. After 60 seconds, compare color of gastric sample to that of performance monitors.	Positive performance monitor turns blue in 30 seconds, and negative monitor remains white or beige. If sample turns blue, test is positive for occult blood. If sample turns green, test is negative.
12. Explain results to client.	Immediate results are obtained. Allows client to participate in care.
13. Dispose of test slide paper, wooden applicator, and 1-ml syringe in proper receptacle.	Reduces spread of infection and keeps environment clean.
14. Reconnect nasogastric tube to drainage system or clamp as ordered.	Nasogastric tube serves to decompress abdomen by promoting drainage. Clamping may be ordered to determine tolerance to stomach filling.
15. Remove and dispose of disposable gloves.	
16. Assist client to comfortable position, and offer oral hygiene.	After vomiting or removal of tube, oral hygiene promotes comfort and helps to reduce nausea.
17. Wash hands.	Reduces transmission of microorganisms.

EVALUATION

1. Observe quantity, character, and color of emesis or gastric secretions.	Characteristics can reveal abnormal status.
2. Compare test findings with normal expected results.	Determines if gastric contents are abnormally acidic or basic, or if blood is present.
3. Ask client about purpose of test.	Documents learning.

UNEXPECTED OUTCOMES AND RELATED INTERVENTIONS

- Gastric secretions may contain clots or blood. Emesis may have "coffee grounds" appearance.
  - Monitor client's vital signs.
  - Determine if client has pain.
  - Inform physician of findings.
- pH level is above or below desired range.
  - Repeat test.
  - Monitor client.
  - Inform physician of findings.
- Test is positive for occult blood.
  - Repeat test.
  - Inform physician of findings.

RECORDING AND REPORTING

- Record test performed, source of specimen, results, and disposition of specimen in nurses' notes.
- Describe characteristics of gastric contents.
- Report abnormal results to nurse in charge or physician.

TEACHING CONSIDERATIONS

- Instruct client on foods and medications that may give false test results for occult blood.
- If antacids are ordered, instruct client on proper use.

Skill 41-11 Obtaining Wound Drainage Specimens

When caring for a client with a wound, the nurse assesses the wound's condition and observes for the development of infection. Localized inflammation, tenderness, and warmth at the wound site, in addition to purulent drainage, usually signify wound infection. Infection cannot be confirmed or treated accurately unless the causative organism is identified. A specimen of wound drainage is analyzed to determine the type and number of pathogenic microorganisms.

The nurse should never collect a wound culture sample from old drainage. Resident colonies of bacteria on the skin grow in wound exudate and may not be the true causative organisms of infection. Separate techniques are used to collect specimens for measuring aerobic versus anaerobic microorganisms. Aerobic organisms grow in superficial wounds exposed to the air. Anaerobic organisms grow deep within body cavities, where oxygen is not normally present.

DELEGATION CONSIDERATIONS

Obtaining wound drainage specimens should not be delegated to assistive personnel.

EQUIPMENT

- Culture tube with swab and transport medium for aerobic culture
- Anaerobic culture tube with swab (tubes contain carbon dioxide or nitrogen gas)
- 5- to 10-ml syringe and 21-gauge needle
- Disposable gloves
- Sterile gloves
- Protective eyewear
- Antiseptic swab
- Sterile dressing materials (determined by type of dressing)
- Paper or plastic disposable bag
- Completed specimen identification label (according to institutional policy)
- Completed laboratory requisition (date, time, name of test)
- Small plastic bag for delivery of specimen to laboratory (or container specified by agency)

STEP	RATIONALE
ASSESSMENT	
1. Assess client's understanding of need for wound culture and ability to cooperate with procedure.	Nurse uses data to develop teaching plan. Wound is painful site. Collection of specimen may arouse anxiety or fear.
2. Assess client for signs of fever, chills, or excessive thirst. Note in laboratory results if white blood cell count is elevated.	Signs and symptoms indicate systemic infection.
3. Ask client about extent and type of pain at wound site. If client requires analgesic before dressing changes, ideally medication is given 30 minutes before to reach peak effect.	Pain at wound site often increases with infection.
4. Review physician's orders for **aerobic** or **anaerobic** culture.	Specimens are taken from different sites and placed in different containers, depending on type of culture.
5. Wear disposable gloves to remove any soiled dressings covering wound. Apply sterile gloves and assess condition of wound carefully. Observe for swelling, opening of wound edges, inflammation, and drainage. Palpate gently along wound edges and note tenderness or drainage. While dressing is being changed, client may prefer not to see wound or soiled dressing.	Surface of open wound is considered sterile. Sterile gloves allow nurse to palpate area without wound contamination. Signs indicate wound infection. Gloves minimize exposure to microorganisms.
6. Determine when dressing change is scheduled (see Chapter 36). This step may be performed as part of the procedure.	

STEP	RATIONALE

NURSING DIAGNOSIS

Defining characteristics from the assessment data may reveal the following nursing diagnoses for clients requiring this skill:

- Anxiety
- Risk for infection
- Risk for injury
- Deficient knowledge regarding wound drainage culture procedure
- Pain (acute or chronic)
- Impaired tissue integrity

Related factors are individualized based on client's condition or needs.

PLANNING

Step	Rationale
1. **Expected outcomes** following completion of procedure:	
▪ Wound culture does not reveal bacterial growth.	Wound remains free of pathogenic microorganisms.
▪ Culture swab is not contaminated by bacteria from skin.	Test results indicate type of cells present.
▪ Client will discuss purpose and procedure for specimen collection.	Documents learning.
2. Determine if client may receive analgesic before dressing change or specimen collection. Administer as ordered.	Minimizes discomfort during procedure.
3. Explain reason for wound culture and how it will be collected.	Promotes understanding and cooperation and eases anxiety.
4. Explain that client may feel tickling sensation when wound is swabbed.	Anticipation of expected sensations minimizes anxiety.

IMPLEMENTATION

Step	Rationale
1. Wash hands.	Reduces transfer of microorganisms.
2. Close bedside curtains or door to room.	Provides privacy.
3. Apply disposable gloves, and remove old dressing. Observe drainage. Fold soiled sides of dressing together, and then dispose of dressing in bag.	Protects hands from contact with drainage.
4. Cleanse area around wound edges with antiseptic swab. Remove old exudate.	Removes skin flora, preventing possible contamination of specimen.
5. Discard swab and dispose of soiled gloves in bag.	Reduces spread of infection.
6. Open packages containing sterile culture tube and dressing supplies.	Provides sterile field from which nurse can pick up and handle sterile supplies.
7. Apply sterile gloves.	Allows nurse to maintain sterility of items while collecting specimen.
8. Collect cultures:	
a. Aerobic culture	
(1) Take swab from culture tube, insert tip into wound in area of drainage, and rotate swab gently. Remove swab and return to culture tube. (Wrap ampule with gauze to prevent injury to nurse's fingers.) Crush ampule of medium, and push swab into fluid.	Swab should be coated with fresh secretions from within wound. Medium keeps bacteria alive until analysis is complete.
b. Anaerobic culture	
(1) Take swab from special anaerobic culture tube, swab deeply into draining body cavity, and rotate gently. Remove swab and return to culture tube. OR Insert tip of syringe (without needle) into wound, and aspirate 5 to 10 ml of exudate. Attach 21-gauge needle, expel all air, and inject drainage into special culture tube.	Specimen is taken from deep cavity where oxygen is not present. Carbon dioxide or nitrogen gas keeps organisms alive until analysis is complete. Air injected into tube would cause organisms to die.

Step	Rationale
• ***Critical Decision Point*** *Never collect exudate from skin unless it is separate culture and labeled as such.*	
9. Place each culture tube on correct specimen label.	Ensures correct results for correct client.
10. Ask another nurse to attach labels and proper requisitions to each tube. Note on specimen requisition if client is receiving antibiotics. Send specimens to laboratory immediately.	Bacteria grow rapidly. Cultures should be prepared quickly for accurate results.
11. Clean wound as ordered, and apply new sterile dressing.	Protects wound from further contamination and aids in absorbing drainage and debriding wound.
12. Remove gloves by pulling inside out, and dispose of gloves in trash. Dispose of soiled supplies according to agency policy.	Reduces spread of infection.
13. Secure dressings with tape or ties.	Keeps dressing securely in place over wound.
14. Assist client to comfortable position.	Promotes client's ability to relax.
15. Wash hands after procedure.	Reduces transmission of microorganisms.

Evaluation

1. Obtain laboratory report for results of cultures.	Report indicates if pathogenic organisms are identified.
2. Observe character of wound drainage.	Characteristics can reveal abnormal status.
3. Observe edges of wound for redness and bleeding.	Indicates trauma to healing tissue.
4. Ask client about purpose of wound culture.	Documents learning.

Unexpected Outcomes and Related Interventions

- Wound cultures reveal heavy bacterial growth.
  - Monitor client for fever, chills, or excessive thirst, which may indicate systemic infection.
  - Inform physician of findings.
- Wound culture is contaminated from superficial skin cells.
  - Monitor client for fever and pain.
  - Inform physician of findings.
  - Repeat collection of specimen as ordered.
- Client describes increased pain.
  - Provide analgesia.
  - Repeat culture.

Recording and Reporting

- Record types of specimens obtained, source, and time and date sent to laboratory in nurses' notes.
- Describe appearance of wound and characteristics of drainage in nurses' notes.
- Report any evidence of infection to nurse in charge and physician.
- Record toleration of procedure and response to analgesics.

Teaching Considerations

- Notify client before possible discomfort during procedure.
- Instruct client to inform nurse if procedure causes pain.
- Teach client to assess status of wound for changes.
- Discuss signs and symptoms of infection.

Pediatric Considerations

- If procedure is to be performed on a child and is anticipated to be painful, some agencies prefer performing procedure in area other than child's room, thus maintaining feeling that child's room is safe place (Wong and others, 1999).

Home Care Considerations

- When applicable, discuss ways to prevent infection.
- Teach client aseptic technique for self-dressing change.

Long-Term Care Considerations

- Carefully monitor wound drainage to prevent spread of infection to other residents (e.g., in a nursing home).

Skill 41-12 Collecting Blood Specimens by Venipuncture (Syringe Method, Vacutainer Method, and Blood Cultures)

Blood tests are one of the most commonly used diagnostic aids in the care and evaluation of clients. In any health care setting blood tests can yield valuable information about nutritional, hematological, metabolic, immune, and biochemical status. Tests allow physicians to screen clients carefully for early signs of physical alterations, plot the course of existing disease, and monitor responses to therapies.

The nurse is often responsible for collecting blood specimens; however, many institutions have specially trained phlebotomists who are responsible for drawing blood. Nurses must be familiar with their institution's policies and procedures and their state's Nurse Practice Act regarding guidelines for drawing blood samples.

The three primary methods of obtaining blood specimens are venipuncture, skin puncture, and arterial stick. **Venipuncture,** the most common method, involves inserting a hollow-bore needle into the lumen of a large vein to obtain a specimen. The nurse may use a needle and syringe or a special **Vacutainer tube** that allows the drawing of multiple blood samples. Because veins are major sources of blood for laboratory testing and routes for intravenous (IV) fluid or blood replacement, maintaining their integrity is essential. The nurse must be skilled in venipuncture to avoid unnecessary injury to veins.

Skin puncture, also called capillary puncture (Malarkey and McMorrow, 2000), is the least traumatic method of obtaining a blood specimen. A sterile lancet or needle is used to puncture a vascular area on a finger, toe, or heel. A drop of blood is placed on a test slide or collected within a thin glass capillary tube for laboratory analysis. Skin puncture is used to obtain blood glucose levels and blood samples in newborns.

Arterial blood gas (ABG) levels are obtained for various reasons when diagnosing a respiratory disorder. Also, ABG determinations are used in the management of clients on mechanical ventilators and during the weaning process from ventilators. Arterial blood samples are drawn from an arterial puncture (usually a radial or brachial artery) or arterial line. Complications from ABG determinations result from the trauma of arterial puncture and may include arterial occlusion from **hematoma** or thrombosis, bleeding, and infection (Malarkey and McMorrow, 2000).

Regardless of the method used to obtain a blood specimen, the nurse must anticipate the client's anxiety. The procedures can be painful, and often just the appearance of a needle is frightening, especially to children. The nurse's calm approach and skilled technique helps to limit anxiety.

Blood cultures aid in detection of bacteria in the blood. It is important that at least two culture specimens be drawn from two different sites. Because bacteremia may be accompanied by fever and chills, blood cultures should be drawn when the client is experiencing these clinical signs (Pagana and Pagana, 1998). If only one culture produces bacteria, the assumption is that the bacteria are contaminants rather than the infectious agent. Bacteremia exists when both cultures grow the infecting agent.

Because culture specimens obtained through an IV catheter are frequently contaminated, tests using them should not be performed unless catheter sepsis is suspected. Cultures should be drawn before antibiotic therapy is started, because the antibiotic may interrupt the organism's growth in the laboratory. If the client is receiving antibiotics, the laboratory needs to be notified and told what specific antibiotics the client is receiving (Pagana and Pagana, 1997).

Delegation Considerations

The skill of collecting blood specimens by venipuncture should not be delegated to assistive personnel. In many institutions phlebotomists (unlicensed or licensed) are the persons responsible for obtaining venipuncture samples. They are usually intravenous certified by the employing agency. Agency policies differ regarding personnel who may draw blood specimens.

Equipment

- Alcohol or antiseptic swab
- Disposable gloves
- Small pillow or folded towel
- Sterile gauze pads (2 × 2 inch)
- Rubber tourniquet
- Adhesive bandage or adhesive tape
- Appropriate blood tubes
- Completed identification labels according to agency policy
- Completed laboratory requisition (date, time, type of test)
- Plastic bag for delivery of specimen to laboratory (or container as specified by agency)

Syringe Method

- Sterile needles: 20- to 21-gauge for adults; 23- to 25-gauge for children; 23- to 25-gauge butterfly for older adults
- Sterile syringe of appropriate size

Vacutainer Method

- Vacutainer tube with needle holder
- Sterile double-ended needles: 20- to 21-gauge for adults; 23- to 25-gauge for children

Blood Cultures

- Povidone-iodine (Betadine) (check agency policy for specific antiseptic solution)
- 70% alcohol (check agency policy)
- Sterile needles: 20- to 21-gauge for adults; 23- to 25-gauge for children; 23- to 25-gauge butterfly for older adults
- Anaerobic and aerobic culture bottles (Figure 41-8)

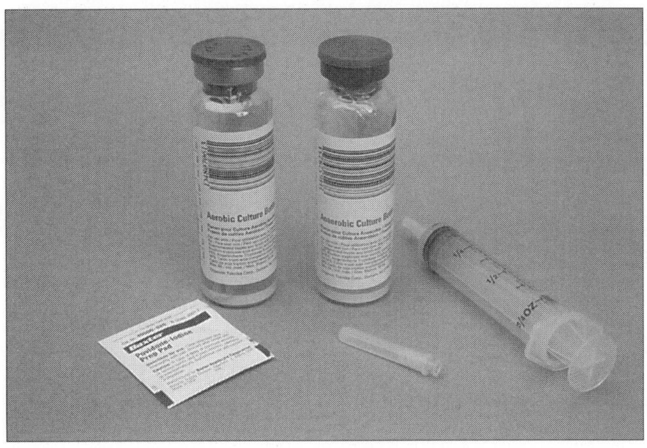

FIGURE **41-8** Blood culture.

STEP	RATIONALE
ASSESSMENT	
1. Determine understanding of purpose of procedure and method to be used.	Provides data for nurse to establish teaching plan and provide emotional support. Many clients may have past experiences that increase anxiety.
2. Determine if special conditions need to be met before specimen collection.	Some tests require meeting specific conditions to obtain accurate measurement of blood elements (e.g., fasting blood sugar, drug peak and trough level, and timed endocrine hormone levels).

- ***Critical Decision Point***
  The assurance of confidentiality is an important issue associated with testing. Disclosure of confidential information can result in discrimination in a variety of circumstances. Agencies must have clearly written and enforced policies regarding disclosure of test results and maintenance of confidentiality throughout the health care system (Ungvarski and Flaskerud, 1999).

STEP	RATIONALE
3. Assess client for possible risks associated with venipuncture: anticoagulant therapy, low **platelet** count, bleeding disorders (history of hemophilia). Review medication history.	Client history may include abnormal clotting abilities caused by low platelet count, hemophilia, or medications that increase risk for bleeding and hematoma formation.
4. Determine client's ability to cooperate with procedure.	Some clients may need assistance of another caregiver. Procedure may appear threatening to client. Reassure child that blood entering tube or syringe will not hurt (Wong and others, 1999).
5. Assess client for contraindicated sites for venipuncture: presence of IV fluids, hematoma at potential site, arm on side of mastectomy, or hemodialysis shunt.	Drawing specimens from such sites can result in false test results or may injure client. Samples taken from vein near IV infusion may be diluted or may contain concentrations of IV fluids. Postmastectomy client may have reduced lymphatic drainage in arm on operative side, increasing risk of infection from needle sticks. Arteriovenous shunt should never be used to obtain specimens because of risks of clotting and bleeding. Hematoma indicates existing injury to vessel's wall (Pagana and Pagana, 1998).
6. Review physician's orders for type of tests.	Multiple samples may be needed; physician's order is required.

STEP	RATIONALE

- ***Critical Decision Point***
  Some specimens require special collection requirements before or following specimen collection:
  - *Cryoglobulin levels: Use prewarmed test tubes.*
  - *Ammonia levels: Tube must be placed in ice for delivery to laboratory.*
  - *Lactic acid levels: Do not use tourniquet.*
  - *Vitamin levels: Avoid exposure of test tube to light.*

NURSING DIAGNOSIS

Defining characteristics from the assessment data may reveal the following nursing diagnoses for clients requiring this skill:

Anxiety
Fear
Deficient knowledge regarding blood specimen collection process
Risk for infection
Risk for injury

Related factors are individualized based on client's condition or needs.

PLANNING

Step	Rationale
1. **Expected outcomes** following completion of procedure:	
▪ Venipuncture site shows no evidence of continued bleeding or hematoma.	Indicates hemostasis achieved.
▪ Client denies anxiety or discomfort.	Removal of painful stimulus lessens anxiety. Some clients are not anxious about procedure.
▪ Laboratory tests show normal findings.	No abnormalities are found in blood elements.
▪ Client will discuss purpose, procedure, and benefits of venipuncture.	Documents learning.
2. Explain procedure to client: describe purpose of tests; explain how sensation of **tourniquet,** alcohol swab, and needle stick will feel.	Anticipatory guidance helps to reduce anxiety.

IMPLEMENTATION

Step	Rationale
1. Wash hands.	Reduces transfer of microorganisms.
2. Bring equipment to bedside.	Facilitates organized procedure.
3. Close bedside curtain or room door.	Provides for privacy.
4. Raise or lower bed to comfortable working height.	Reduces strain on nurse's back muscles and improves access to venipuncture site.
5. Assist client to supine or semi-Fowler's position with arms extended to form straight line from shoulders to wrists. Place small pillow or towel under upper arm. If in clinic or physician's office, chair with special arm extension may be used.	Helps to stabilize extremity because arms are most common sites of venipuncture. Supported position in bed reduces chance of injury to client if fainting occurs.
6. Apply disposable gloves. If glove(s) become contaminated with blood, replace with clean pair after proper disposal of contaminated gloves	Reduces risk of exposure to blood-borne bacteria.
7. Apply tourniquet 5 to 10 cm (2 to 4 inches) above venipuncture site selected (antecubital fossa site is most often used). Encircle extremity, and pull one end of tourniquet tightly over other, looping one end under other. Apply tourniquet so it can be removed by pulling end with single motion.	Tourniquet blocks venous return to heart from extremity, causing veins to dilate for easier visibility.

STEP	RATIONALE

- ***Critical Decision Point***
  Palpate distal pulse (e.g., radial) below tourniquet. If pulse is not palpable, reapply tourniquet more loosely. If tourniquet is too tight, pressure will impede arterial blood flow.

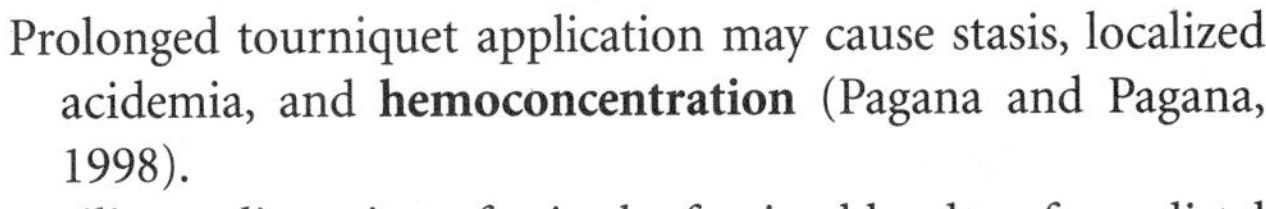

STEP	RATIONALE
8. Keep tourniquet on client no longer than 1 minute.	Prolonged tourniquet application may cause stasis, localized acidemia, and **hemoconcentration** (Pagana and Pagana, 1998).
9. Ask client to open and close fist several times, finally leaving fist clenched.	Facilitates distention of veins by forcing blood up from distal veins.
10. Instruct client to avoid vigorous opening and closing of fist.	May cause erroneous laboratory results of hemoconcentration.
11. Quickly inspect extremity for best venipuncture site, looking for straight, prominent vein without swelling or hematoma.	Straight and intact veins are easiest to puncture.
12. Palpate selected vein with fingers. Note if vein is firm and rebounds when palpated or if vein feels rigid and cordlike and rolls when palpated (see illustration).	Patent, healthy vein is elastic and rebounds on palpation. Thrombosed vein is rigid, rolls easily, and is difficult to puncture.

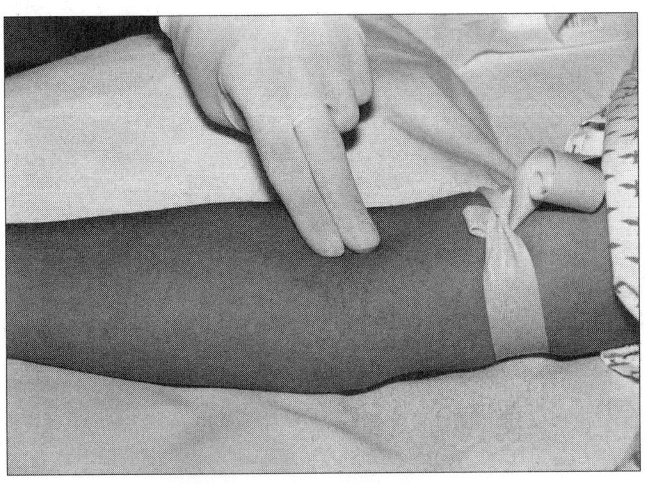

STEP **12** Palpation of vein.

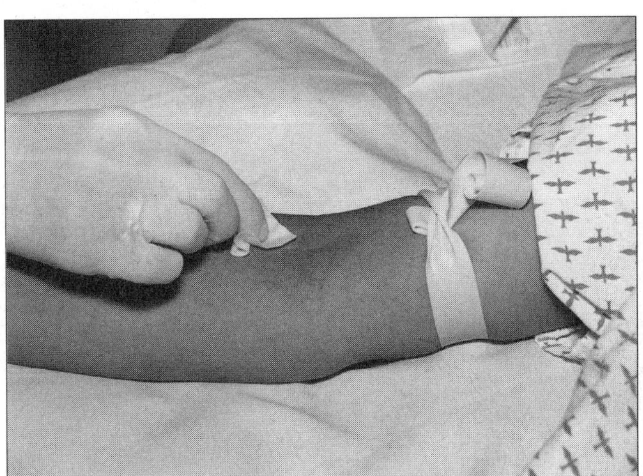

STEP **14a(2)** Cleansing site.

STEP	RATIONALE
13. Select venipuncture site. If tourniquet has been in place longer than 1 minute, remove and assess other extremity, or wait 60 seconds before reapplying. (If vein cannot be palpated or viewed easily, remove tourniquet and apply warm, wet compress over extremity for 10 minutes).	Prevents discomfort to client and inaccurate test results (Malarkey and McMorrow, 2000). Heat causes local dilation.
14. Obtain blood sample:	
a. Syringe method	
(1) Have syringe with appropriate needle securely attached.	Needle must not dislodge from syringe during venipuncture.
(2) Cleanse venipuncture site with alcohol swab (70% isopropyl alcohol is recommended), moving in circular motion from site for approximately 5 cm (2 inches) (see illustration). Allow to dry.	Antimicrobial agent cleans skin surface of resident bacteria so organisms do not enter puncture site. Allowing alcohol to dry completes its antimicrobial task and reduces "sting" of venipuncture. Alcohol left on skin can cause **hemolysis** of sample.
(a) If drawing sample for blood alcohol level or blood cultures, use only antiseptic swab rather than alcohol swab.	Ensures accurate test results.

STEP	RATIONALE
(3) Remove needle cover, and inform client that "stick" lasting only a few seconds will be felt.	Client has better control over anxiety when prepared about what to expect.

- ***Critical Decision Point***
  Observe needle for defects, such as burrs, which can cause increased discomfort and damage to the client's vein.

STEP	RATIONALE
(4) Place thumb or forefinger of nondominant hand 2.5 cm (1 inch) below site and gently pull skin taut. Stretch skin down until vein is stabilized.	Stabilizes vein and prevents rolling during needle insertion.
(5) Hold syringe and needle at 15- to 30-degree angle from client's arm with bevel up.	Reduces chance of penetrating both sides of vein during insertion. Keeping bevel up reduces vein trauma.
(6) Slowly insert needle into vein (see illustration).	Prevents puncture through vein to opposite side.
a. With experience nurse will feel "pop" as needle enters vein. If plunger is pulled back too quickly, pressure may cause vein to collapse.	
(7) Hold syringe securely, and pull back gently on plunger (see illustration).	Syringe held securely prevents needle from advancing. Pulling on plunger creates vacuum needed to draw blood into syringe.

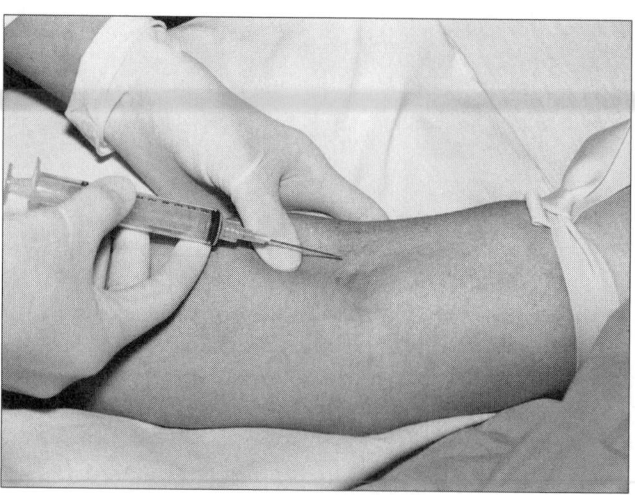

STEP **14a(6)** Inserting needle into vein.

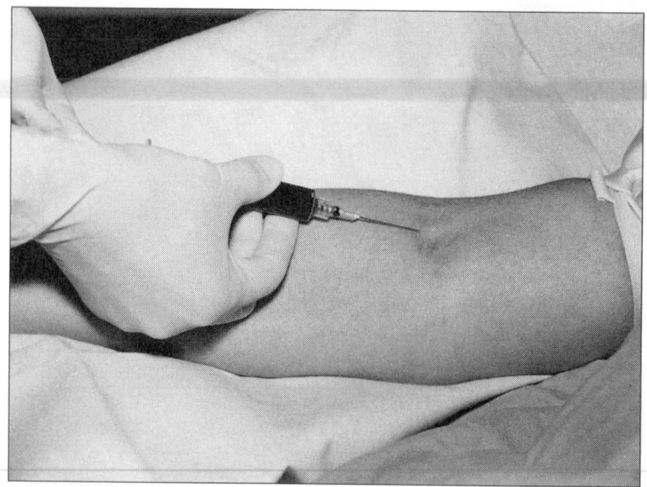

STEP **14a(7)** Pulling back on plunger.

STEP	RATIONALE
(8) Look for blood return.	If blood flow fails to appear, needle is not in vein.
(9) Obtain desired amount of blood, keeping needle stabilized.	Test results are more accurate when required amount of blood is obtained. Some tests cannot be performed without minimal blood requirement. Movement of needle increases discomfort.
(10) After specimen is obtained, release tourniquet.	Reduces bleeding at site when needle is withdrawn.
(11) Apply 2 × 2 inch gauze pad or alcohol swab over puncture site without applying pressure, quickly but carefully withdraw needle from vein, and apply pressure following removal of needle (see illustration).	Pressure over needle can cause discomfort. Careful removal of needle minimizes discomfort and vein trauma.
(12) Discard uncapped needle in proper receptacle.	Reduces risk of needle-stick injury.
b. Vacutainer method (vacuum tube system method)	
(1) Attach double-ended needle to Vacutainer tube (see illustration).	Long end of needle is used to puncture vein. Short end fits into blood tubes.
(2) Have proper blood specimen tube resting inside Vacutainer, but do not puncture rubber stopper.	Puncturing causes loss of tube's vacuum.

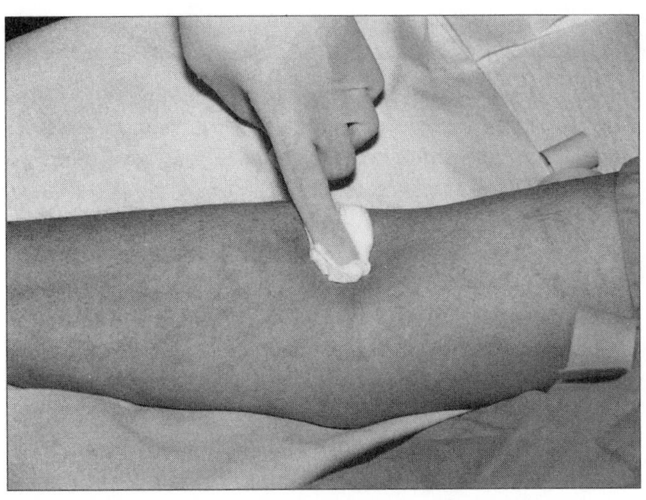

STEP **14a(11)** Application of gauze to puncture site.

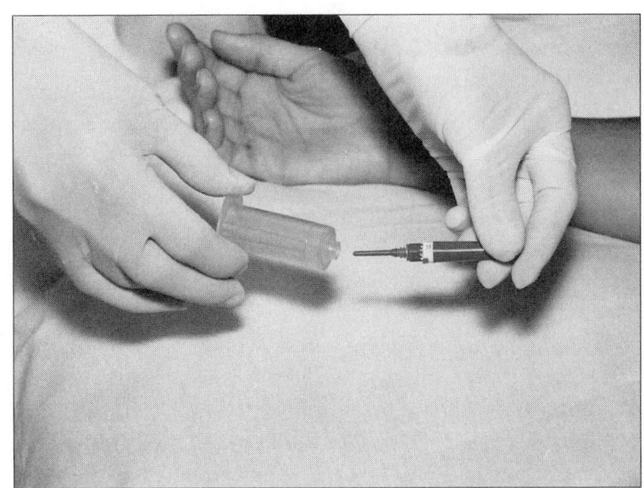

STEP **14b(1)** Attaching needle to Vacutainer tube.

STEP	RATIONALE
(3) Cleanse venipuncture site with alcohol swab, moving in circular motion out from site for approximately 5 cm (2 inches). Allow to dry.	Cleans skin surface of resident bacteria so that organisms do not enter puncture site.
(4) Remove needle cover, and inform client that "stick" lasting only a few seconds will be felt.	Client has better control over anxiety when prepared about what to expect.
(5) Place thumb or forefinger of nondominant hand 2.5 cm (1 inch) above or below site and pull skin taut. Stretch skin down until vein is stabilized.	Helps to stabilize vein and prevent rolling during needle insertion.
(6) Hold Vacutainer needle at 15- to 30-degree angle from arm with bevel up.	Reduces chance of penetrating both sides of vein during insertion. Keeping bevel up causes less trauma to vein.
(7) Slowly insert needle into vein (see illustration).	Prevents puncture on opposite side.
(8) Grasp Vacutainer securely, and advance specimen tube into needle of holder (do not advance needle in vein).	Pushing needle through stopper breaks vacuum and causes flow of blood into tube. If needle in vein advances, vein may become punctured on other side.
(9) Note flow of blood into tube (should be fairly rapid) (see illustration).	Failure of blood to appear indicates that vacuum in tube is lost or needle is not in vein.

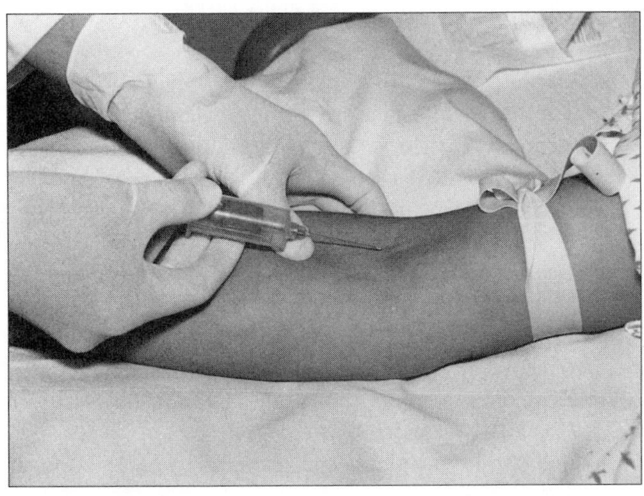

STEP **14b(7)** Inserting Vacutainer needle into vein.

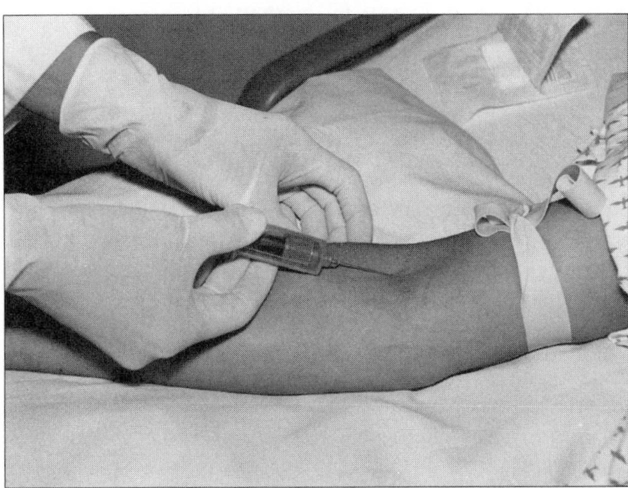

STEP **14b(9)** Blood flowing into tube.

Step	Rationale
(10) After specimen tube is filled, grasp Vacutainer firmly and remove tube. Insert additional specimen tubes as needed.	Prevents needle from advancing or dislodging. Tube should fill completely because additives in certain tubes are measured in proportion to filled tube. Tubes with additives should be inverted as soon as possible (Pagana and Pagana, 1998).
(11) After last tube is filled and removed from Vacutainer, release tourniquet.	Reduces bleeding at site when needle is withdrawn.
(12) Apply 2 × 2 inch gauze pad over puncture site without applying pressure, and quickly but carefully withdraw needle from vein.	Pressure over needle can cause discomfort. Careful removal of needle minimizes discomfort and vein trauma.
15. Immediately apply pressure over venipuncture site with gauze or antiseptic pad for 2 to 3 minutes or until bleeding stops (see Step 14a[11]). Apply pressure over site, and tape gauze dressing securely.	Direct pressure minimizes bleeding and prevents hematoma formation. Pressure dressing controls bleeding.
16. For blood obtained by syringe, transfer specimen to tubes:	
a. Using one-handed technique, insert needle through stopper of blood tube and allow vacuum to fill tube. Do not force blood into tube.	Prevents needle stick injury.
b. Alternative method is to remove needle from syringe and stopper to each test tube. Gently inject required amount of blood into each tube. Reapply stopper.	Forcing blood into tube may cause hemolysis of red blood cells.
17. Take blood tubes containing additives; gently rotate back and forth 8 to 10 times.	Additives should be mixed with blood to prevent clotting. Shaking can cause hemolysis of red blood cells, producing inaccurate test results (Pagana and Pagana, 1998).
18. Inspect puncture site for bleeding, and apply adhesive tape with gauze.	Keeps puncture site clean and controls any final oozing.
19. Check tubes for any sign of external contamination with blood. Decontaminate with 70% alcohol if necessary.	Prevents cross contamination. Reduces risk of exposure to pathogens present in blood.
20. Assist client to comfortable position.	
21. Securely attach properly completed identification label to each tube, and affix proper requisition.	Incorrect identification of specimen could result in diagnostic or therapeutic errors.
22. Dispose of needles, syringe, and soiled equipment in proper container. Do not cap needles.	Prevents cross contamination through needle sticks and contact with blood.
23. Place specimens in bag to be sent to laboratory.	
24. Remove disposable gloves after specimen is obtained and any spillage is cleaned.	Reduces risk of exposure to human immunodeficiency virus (HIV), hepatitis, and other blood-borne pathogens.
25. Wash hands after procedure.	Reduces transfer of microorganisms.
26. Send specimens immediately to laboratory.	Fresh specimen ensures accurate results.

Blood Cultures

Step	Rationale
1. Carefully prepare proposed sites with povidone-iodine (Betadine). Allow povidone-iodine to dry.	Antimicrobial agent cleans skin surface so organisms do not enter puncture site or contaminate culture.
2. Clean bottle tops of vacuum tubes or culture bottles. Check agency policy regarding cleaning with 70% alcohol after cleaning with antiseptic solution and air drying.	Ensures specimen is sterile.
3. Collect 10 to 15 ml of venous blood by venipuncture in 20-ml syringe from each venipuncture site.	Culture specimens must be obtained from two sites. If one site produces bacteria, but not the other, assumption is that bacteria in first culture may be a contaminant and not the infecting agent. When infecting agent grows in both cultures, bacteremia exists and is due to organism in culture (Pagana and Pagana, 1998).
4. Discard needle on syringe; replace with new sterile needle before injecting blood sample into culture bottle.	Maintains sterile technique and prevents contamination of specimen.

Step	Rationale
5. If both aerobic and anaerobic cultures are needed, inoculate anaerobic first (Pagana and Pagana, 1998).	Anaerobic organisms may take longer to grow (Pagana and Pagana, 1998).
6. Mix gently after inoculation.	Mixes medium and blood.
7. Immediately apply pressure over venipuncture site with gauze or antiseptic pad for 2 to 3 minutes or until bleeding stops. Apply pressure over site, and tape gauze dressing securely.	Direct pressure minimizes bleeding and prevents hematoma.
8. Label the specimen with the client's name, date, time, and tentative diagnosis. Indicate on laboratory slip any medications (e.g., antibiotics) that may affect results. Place in appropriate bag for transfer.	
9. Transport the culture bottles immediately to the laboratory (or at least within 30 minutes) (Pagana and Pagana, 1998).	

Evaluation

Step	Rationale
1. Reinspect venipuncture site.	Determines if bleeding has stopped or hematoma has formed.
2. Determine if client remains anxious or fearful.	Client may require more blood tests in future. Anxiety or concerns should be expressed and addressed.
3. Check laboratory report for test results.	Reveals constituents of blood specimen.
4. Ask client to explain purposes of tests.	Demonstrates learning.

Unexpected Outcomes and Related Interventions

- Hematoma forms at venipuncture site.
  - Apply pressure.
  - Continue to monitor client for pain and discomfort.
- Bleeding at site continues.
  - Apply pressure to site.
  - Instruct client to apply pressure.
  - Monitor client.
  - Notify physician.
- Signs and symptoms of infection at venipuncture site occur.
  - Notify physician.
  - Apply heat to site.
- Client becomes dizzy or faints during venipuncture.
  - Assist client into chair.
  - Lower client's head between knees.
  - Remain with client.
- Laboratory tests reveal abnormal blood constituents.
  - Notify physician.

Recording and Reporting

- Record date and time of venipuncture, samples obtained, and disposition of specimen.
- Describe venipuncture site.
- Report any "stat" test results to physician.
- Report any abnormal test results to physician.

Teaching Considerations

- Instruct client to apply pressure to venipuncture site briefly. Clients with bleeding disorders or those undergoing anticoagulant therapy should apply pressure for at least 5 minutes.
- Instruct client to notify nurse or physician if persistent or recurrent bleeding or expanding hematoma occurs at venipuncture site.

Pediatric Considerations

- Explain procedure to child as developmentally appropriate and provide atraumatic care (Wong and others, 1999).
- Because children often fear that loss of their blood is a threat to their lives, explain to them that their blood is continually being produced. Adhesive bandage gives them assurance that their blood will not leak out through puncture site (Wong and others, 1999).
- At times it is advantageous to draw children's blood specimens in treatment room instead of in bed or room to maintain feeling that room is safe place.
- Restrain child only as necessary to prevent injury (Wong and others, 1999).
- When performing venipuncture on children, nurse needs to explore a variety of sources for vein access: scalp, antecubital fossa, saphenous, and hand veins.
- Application of EMLA Cream may be ordered to reduce pain in infants and young children (Wong and others, 1999).

GERONTOLOGICAL CONSIDERATIONS

- Older adults have fragile veins that are easily traumatized during venipuncture. Sometimes application of warm compresses may help in obtaining samples. Using small-bore catheter also may be beneficial.

HOME CARE CONSIDERATIONS

- In home care setting a blood pressure cuff, rather than a tourniquet, can be used for venipuncture.

Skill 41-13 Measuring Blood Glucose Level After Skin Puncture (Capillary Puncture)

Obtaining capillary blood by skin puncture is an alternative when venipuncture cannot be performed or when reducing the frequency of needle sticks is desirable. The procedure is also less painful than venipuncture, and the ease of the skin puncture method to obtain blood samples makes it possible for clients to perform this procedure. Along with the development of reagent strips and home glucose monitors, the skin puncture method has revolutionized home management care of clients with diabetes. Although not all blood tests can be performed on capillary samples, it is a viable alternative to venipuncture in many situations.

Self-testing of blood glucose level can be performed by two methods. Both methods require obtaining a large drop of blood by skin puncture. A hand-held single-use lancet or one of many automatic lancet-holding devices available on the market today may be used. The blood is applied to a specially prepared chemical reagent strip.

The first method involves visually reading the reagent strip by comparing it to the color chart on the container. Examples of such strips include Chemstrip BG, Glucostix, and Trendstrips. If the color on the strip falls between two reference blocks on the chart, the results may need to be estimated. Thus accurate results of blood glucose measurement may not always be obtained.

The second type of blood glucose monitoring is done by the use of reflectance meters. A variety of meters are on the market, including the Glucometer II (Ames), Accu-check III (Boehringer Mannheim), Glucoscan 3000 (LifeScan), and One Touch (LifeScan). After a drop of blood from the skin puncture is dropped onto the reagent strip, the meter provides an accurate measurement of blood glucose level in less than 5 minutes.

The meters use a wet-wash or dry-wipe method of testing. To perform a wet wash, the user flushes the blood-coated

Table 41-2 Glucose Meters Currently Available

METER	GLUCOSE RANGE (MG/DL)	TEST STRIP USED	TEST TIME	MEMORY
Accu-Check Advantage	10-600	Advantage	40 seconds	100 readings
Accu-Check Easy	20-500	Easy Test Strips	15-60 seconds	350 readings
Accu-Check Instant	20-500	Instant Glucose	12 seconds	9 readings
Accu-Check III	20-500	Chemstrip bG	2 minutes	20 readings
CheckMate Plus	25-500	CheckMate Plus	15-70 seconds	255 readings
Diascan-S	10-600	Diascan	90 seconds	10 readings
ExacTech	40-450	ExacTech	30 seconds	Last reading recall
ExacTech RSG	40-450	ExacTech RSG	30 seconds	—
Glucometer Elite	20-500	Glucometer Elite	30 seconds	Last reading recall
Glucometer Encore	10-600	Glucometer Encore	15-60 seconds	10 readings
MediSense 2 Card	20-600	MediSense 2 or Precision Q.I.D.	20 seconds	Extended memory
MediSense 2 Pen	20-600	MediSense 2 or Precision Q.I.D.	20 seconds	Extended memory
One Touch Basic	0-600	Genuine One Touch	45 seconds	Last reading recall
One Touch Profile	0-600	Genuine One Touch	45 seconds	250 readings
Precision Q.I.D.	20-600	Precision Q.I.D.	20 seconds	Extended memory
Prestige	25-600	Prestige	20-50 seconds	—
Select GT	30-600	Select GT	50 seconds	100 readings
Supreme II	30-600	Supreme	50 seconds	100 readings
SureStep	0-500	SureStep	15-30 seconds	10 readings
Ultra +	30-600	Ultra +	45 seconds	—

Data from American Diabetes Association: 1998 Buyer's guide to diabetes products, *Diabetes Forecast* 50(10):68, 1997.

reagent strip with water before inserting the strip into the glucose meter. The dry-wipe method is somewhat simpler, requiring the user to wipe off the blood-coated reagent strip with a dry cotton ball before making a reading. Some products do not require blood to be wiped before a reading is given. The various methods allow measurement of blood glucose between 20 and 800 mg/100 ml, thus providing a sensitive measure of blood glucose level.

A variety of glucose meters are currently available (Table 41-2). The skill describes the techniques used to measure blood glucose level with a meter using the dry-wipe method. Figure 41-9 depicts an Accu-Check Easy glucose monitor. When the nurse measures blood glucose, gloves are worn according to the Centers for Disease Control and Prevention's (CDC's) standard precautions (CDC, 1996) and Occupational Safety and Health Administration's (OSHA's) recommendations (OSHA, 1991).

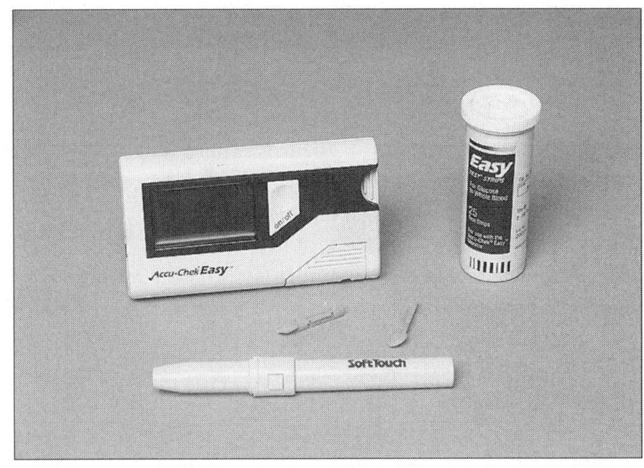

FIGURE **41-9** Accu-Check Easy glucose monitoring equipment.

Delegation Considerations

The skill of measuring blood glucose level after skin puncture (capillary puncture) may be delegated to assistive personnel who have been instructed in performing the skill. The client must first be assessed to determine that the client's need for serum glucose monitoring is appropriate for delegation. If the client's condition changes frequently, this skill should not be delegated to assistive personnel.

Equipment

- Antiseptic swab
- Cotton ball
- Sterile lancet or blood-letting device
- Heel-warming device (optional)
- Paper towel
- Glucose testing meter
- Blood glucose reagent strips (brand determined by meter used)
- Disposable gloves

Step	Rationale
Assessment	
1. Assess understanding of procedure and purpose. Determine if clients with diabetes understand how to perform test and realize importance of **glucose monitoring.**	Data set guidelines for nurse to develop teaching plan.
2. Determine if specific conditions need to be met before or after sample collection (e.g., with fasting, after meals, or after certain medications or before insulin doses).	Dietary intake of carbohydrates and ingestion of concentrated glucose preparations alter blood glucose levels.
3. Determine if risks exist for performing skin puncture (e.g., low platelet count, anticoagulant therapy, bleeding disorders).	Abnormal clotting mechanisms increase risk for local **ecchymosis** and bleeding.
4. Assess area of skin to be used as puncture site. Inspect fingers, toes, and heel. Avoid areas of bruising and open lesions.	Sides of fingers, toes, and heels are commonly selected because they have fewer nerve endings and are highly vascular. The puncture site should not be edematous, inflamed, or recently punctured because these factors cause increased interstitial fluid and blood to mix and also increase the risk of infection (Malarkey and McMorrow, 2000).
5. Review physician's order for time of frequency of measurement.	Physician determines test schedule on basis of client's physiological status and risk for glucose imbalance.
6. For diabetic client who performs test at home, assess ability to handle skin-puncturing device. If client chooses, he or she may wish to continue self-testing while in hospital.	Client's physical health may change (e.g., vision disturbance, fatigue, pain, disease process), preventing client from performing test.

STEP	RATIONALE

NURSING DIAGNOSIS

Defining characteristics from the assessment data may reveal the following nursing diagnoses for clients requiring this skill:

- Ineffective health maintenance
- Anxiety
- Deficient knowledge regarding blood glucose monitoring
- Ineffective therapeutic regimen management
- Disturbed sensory perception (tactile)

Related factors are individualized based on client's condition or needs.

PLANNING

Step	Rationale
1. **Expected outcomes** following completion of procedure:	
▪ Puncture site shows no evidence of bleeding or tissue damage.	**Hemostasis** achieved. Lancet or needle did not puncture skin too deeply.
▪ Blood glucose level is normal.	Normal fasting glucose is 70 to 120 mg/100 ml, indicating good metabolic control.
▪ Client demonstrates procedure.	Demonstrates psychomotor learning.
▪ Client explains test results.	Demonstrates knowledge.
2. Explain procedure and purpose to client and/or family. Offer client and family opportunity to practice testing procedures. Provide resources/teaching aids for client.	Promotes understanding and cooperation.

IMPLEMENTATION

Step	Rationale
1. Wash hands before procedure.	Reduces transfer of microorganisms.
2. Instruct adult to wash hands with soap and warm water, if able.	Promotes skin cleansing and vasodilation at selected puncture site. Hand washing establishes practice for client when test is performed at home.
3. Position client comfortably in chair or in semi-Fowler's position in bed.	Ensures easy accessibility to puncture site. Client will assume position when self-testing.
4. Remove reagent strip from container, and tightly seal caps.	Protects strips from accidental discoloration due to exposure to air or light.
5. Turn on glucose meter.	Activates meter.
6. Insert strip into glucose meter (see manufacturer's directions), and make necessary adjustments.	Some machines must be calibrated; others require zeroing of timer. Each meter is adjusted differently.
7. Remove unused reagent strip from meter, and place on paper towel or clean, dry surface with test pad facing up.	Moisture on strip can change its color, altering reading of final test results.
8. Apply disposable gloves.	Reduces risk of contamination by blood.
9. Choose puncture site. Puncture site should be vascular. In adult, select lateral side of finger; be sure to avoid central tip of finger, which has more dense nerve supply (Pagana and Pagana, 1998).	Ensures free flow of blood following puncture.
10. Hold finger to be punctured in dependent position while gently massaging finger toward puncture site (Malarkey and McMorrow, 2000).	Increases blood flow to area before puncture.
11. Clean site with antiseptic swab, and *allow it to dry completely.*	Alcohol can cause blood to hemolyze.
12. Remove cover of lancet or blood-letting device. Some agencies use lancet devices with an automatic blade retraction system (Microtainer Brand Safety Flow Lancet [Becton Dickinson]). This reduces the possibility of self-sticks, preventing exposure to blood-borne pathogens.	Cover keeps tip of lancet/needle sterile.

STEP	RATIONALE
13. Place blood-letting device firmly against side of finger and push release button, causing needle to pierce skin (see illustration). Hold lancet perpendicular to puncture site, and pierce finger or heel quickly in one continuous motion (do not force lancet).	Blood-letting devices are designed to pierce skin for specific depth, ensuring adequate blood flow. Perpendicular position ensures proper skin penetration.
14. Wipe away first droplet of blood with cotton ball. (See manufacturer's directions for meter used.)	First drop of blood contains tissue fluids (Malarkey and McMorrow, 2000).
15. Lightly squeeze puncture site (without touching) until large droplet of blood has formed. Some agencies use capillary tubes or pipettes to collect the blood sample, reducing risk of direct contact with blood.	Ensures proper coverage of test pad on reagent strip. Excessive squeezing of tissues during blood sample collection may contribute to pain, bruising, scarring, and hematoma formation (Malarkey and McMorrow, 2000).
16. Hold reagent strip test pad close to drop of blood, and lightly transfer droplet to test pad (see illustration). Do not smear blood. Repuncturing may be necessary if large enough droplet does not form to ensure accurate test results.	Droplet must be absorbed by test pad to ensure proper chemical reaction. Smearing causes inaccurate test results.

- ***Critical Decision Point***

  Diabetic clients frequently have peripheral vascular disease, making it difficult to produce a large droplet of blood after a finger stick. Be sure that finger is held in dependent position before stick is done to improve blood flow to area.

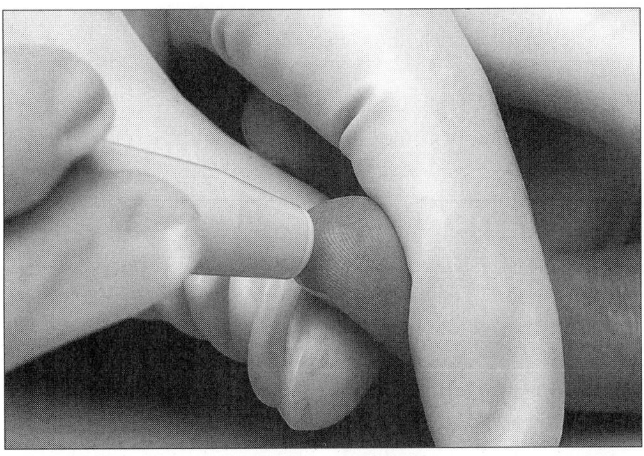

STEP **13** Piercing of fingertip.

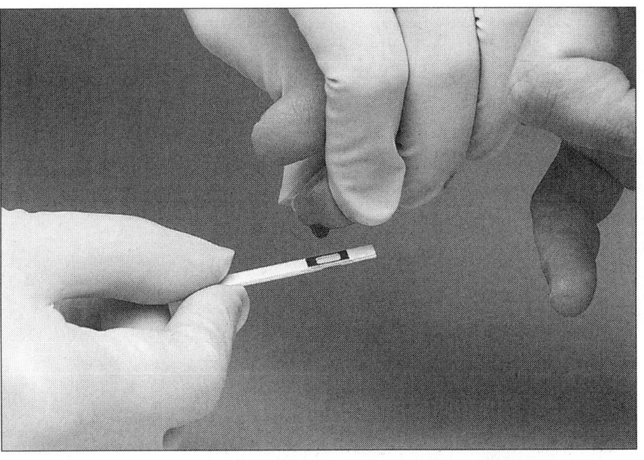

STEP **16** Transferring droplet to test pad.

STEP	RATIONALE
17. Immediately press timer on glucose meter, and place reagent strip on paper towel or on side of timer. (See manufacturer's directions for meter used.)	Blood must be exposed to test strip for prescribed time to ensure proper results. Strip should lie flat so that blood does not pool on only one part of pad.

- ***Critical Decision Point***

  Some meters, (such as One Touch [LifeScan]), require blood sample to be applied to test strip, which is already in meter.

STEP	RATIONALE
18. Apply pressure to skin puncture site.	Promotes hemostasis.
19. When timer displays 60 seconds (for Accu-Check III model), use moderate pressure to wipe blood from test pad with dry cotton ball. No blood should remain on test pad for some meters. (See manufacturer's directions for meter used.)	For meter to read glucose levels, some strips must be dry. Refer to product directions for timing used with each type of meter.

STEP	RATIONALE
20. While timer continues to count, place reagent strip into meter (see illustration).	Strip must be inserted correctly to obtain accurate reading.
21. Read meter, noting reading on display (see illustration).	Each meter has specified time for reading glucose level.

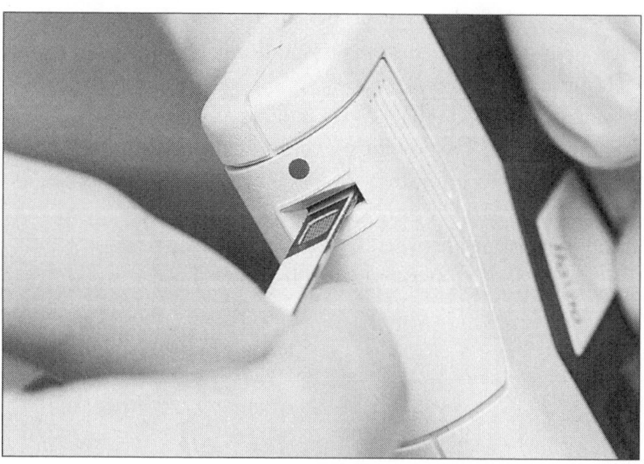

STEP 20 Placing reagent strip into meter.

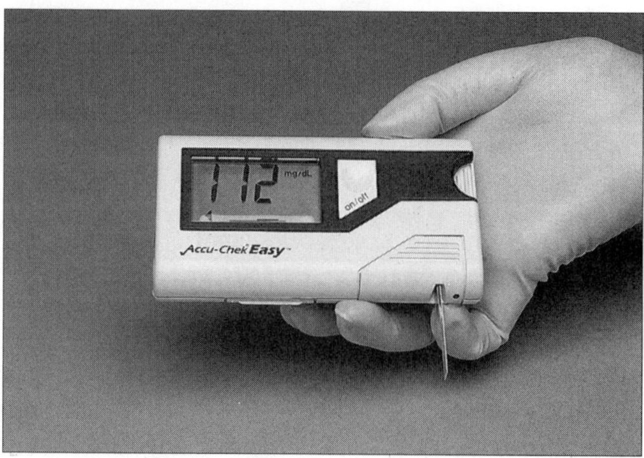

STEP 21 Reading meter.

STEP	RATIONALE
22. Turn meter off. Dispose of test strip, cotton balls, uncapped lancet or **autolet,** and platform from lancet device (if indicated) in proper receptacle.	Meter is battery powered. Proper disposal reduces spread of microorganisms. Lancets and platforms need to be disposed of after each client use.
23. Remove disposable gloves, and dispose of them properly.	
24. Wash hands.	Reduces transmission of infection.
25. Share test results with client.	Promotes participation and compliance with therapy.

EVALUATION

1. Reinspect puncture site for bleeding or tissue injury.	Can be source of discomfort.
2. Compare glucose meter reading with normal blood glucose levels.	Determines if glucose level is normal.
3. Ask client to discuss procedure.	Documents level of learning.
4. Ask client to explain test and results.	Results of test may cause anxiety. Client may misunderstand specific step of procedure.

UNEXPECTED OUTCOMES AND RELATED INTERVENTIONS

- Puncture site is bruised or continues to bleed.
  - Apply pressure.
  - Notify physician of findings.
- Blood glucose level above or below normal range.
  - Continue to monitor client.
  - Check chart to see if there are medication orders for deviations in glucose level.
  - Administer insulin or carbohydrate source as ordered, depending on glucose level.
  - Notify physician of findings.
- Glucose meter malfunctions.
  - Review instructions for glucose meter.
  - Repeat test.
- Client expresses misunderstanding of procedure and results.
  - Repeat instructions to client.
  - Have client demonstrate procedure.

RECORDING AND REPORTING

- Record procedure and glucose level in nurses' notes or special flow sheet and action taken for abnormal range.
- Describe response, including appearance of puncture site, in nurses' notes.
- Describe explanations or teaching provided in nurses' notes.
- Record and report abnormal blood glucose levels.

Teaching Considerations

- Provide information on where client with diabetes can obtain testing supplies if applicable.
- Provide client with information on where to obtain assistance if glucose meter has malfunctioned.
- Instruct client in what to do and whom to contact if glucose meter malfunctions.
- Stress importance of testing blood glucose level, particularly in diabetic clients.

Pediatric Considerations

- Young children should be allowed to choose puncture site.
- Heel and great toe are frequently used as puncture sites in infants.
- To avoid osteochondritis, puncture of heel in infant must be no deeper than 2.4 mm and should be made at outer aspect of heel (Wong and others, 1999).
- Assess for localized complications in heels of premature infants who must have blood drawn repeatedly.
- Heel warming can be used to facilitate obtaining specimen from neonate.
- Infection is the most serious complication of heel-stick puncture in infants (Malarkey and McMorrow, 2000).
- Earlobe may be used to obtain blood in older pediatric clients (Pagana and Pagana, 1998).
- Allow young child with parent to demonstrate technique; incorporate a play activity for further understanding.

Gerontological Consideration

- Warming fingertips may facilitate obtaining specimen.
- Older adults may have vision or dexterity problems that may interfere with performing self–finger stick (Lueckenotte, 2000).

Home Care Considerations

- Glucose meters may be used routinely by clients in their homes.

Long-Term Care Considerations

- Suggest client attend diabetic support group if needed.

Skill 41-14 Obtaining an Arterial Specimen for Blood Gas Measurement

Oxygenation and ventilation can be assessed by measuring arterial blood gases (ABGs). Measurement of ABGs provides valuable information in assessing and managing a client's respiratory and metabolic disturbances (Pagana and Pagana, 1998). The parameters measured include arterial blood pH, partial pressure of oxygen (PaO_2), partial pressure of carbon dioxide ($PaCO_2$), and arterial oxygen saturation (SaO_2). The ABG sample is easily obtained and can be quickly analyzed to provide the nurse with a clear picture of acid-base balance, oxygenation, and ventilation. Alterations from normal show the nurse how the client is adapting to the disease process.

Measuring ABGs aids the nurse in assessment. Nurses should check agency policy regarding who is allowed to obtain ABG samples. Many institutions allow only nurses in critical care areas to obtain ABG samples and require institutional certification of this skill. A decision to draw ABG samples frequently may be a direct result of the nurse's physical assessment (see Chapter 10).

Delegation Considerations

The skill of obtaining an arterial blood sample should not be delegated to assistive personnel.

Equipment

- 3-ml heparinized syringe
- 23- or 25-gauge needle
- Syringe cap
- Alcohol swabs (2)
- 2 × 2 inch gauze pad
- Tape
- Heparin (1:1000 solution)
- Cup or plastic bag with crushed ice
- Label with client identification
- Laboratory requisition
- Disposable gloves
- Protective eyewear
- Commercial blood gas kits are available

STEP	RATIONALE

ASSESSMENT

1. Determine need to obtain ABG sample and presence of physician's order. Signs and symptoms of alteration in respiratory status requiring sampling may include dyspnea, sudden change in respiratory rate or pattern, unequal breath sounds, unequal chest expansion, cyanosis, change in level of consciousness, self-extubation without need for immediate reintubation, and increased work of breathing.

Some situations and medical conditions place clients at risk for alteration in acid-base balance and ventilation status. Physician's order is required for ABG sample.

2. Assess for factors that influence ABG measurements:
   a. Client who has just awakened
   b. Immediately after suctioning
   c. Less than 20 to 30 minutes after oxygen therapy or ventilator setting change
   d. Client whose oxygen has not been in place continually for at least 20 to 30 minutes

Allows nurse to eliminate factors that cause inaccurate results.

3. Perform physical assessment of thorax and lungs.

Physical signs and symptoms may indicate need for ABG sample.

4. Review criteria for choosing site for ABG sample.

• ***Critical Decision Point***
Factors that contraindicate use of arterial site include amputation, contractures, localized infection, dressing or cast, mastectomy, or arteriovenous shunts.

a. Assess collateral blood flow. Perform **Allen's test:**

Allen's test is performed to assess collateral circulation before performing arterial puncture on radial artery. Positive Allen's Test ensures collateral circulation to hand in case thrombosis of radial artery occurs following puncture (Pagana and Pagana, 1998).

(1) Have client make tight fist and raise hand above heart.

Removes as much blood from hand as possible.

(2) Apply direct pressure to both radial and ulnar arteries (see illustration).

Obstructs arterial blood flow to hand.

(3) Have client lower hand and open hand (see illustration).

Fingers and hand should be pale and blanched, indicating lack of arterial blood flow.

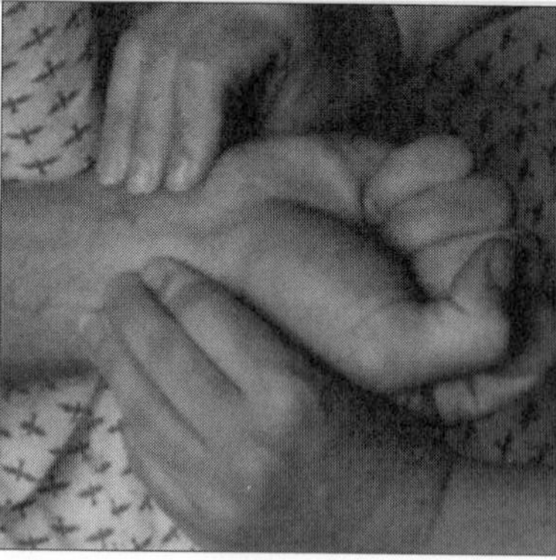

STEP **4a(2)** Applying pressure to radial and ulnar arteries.

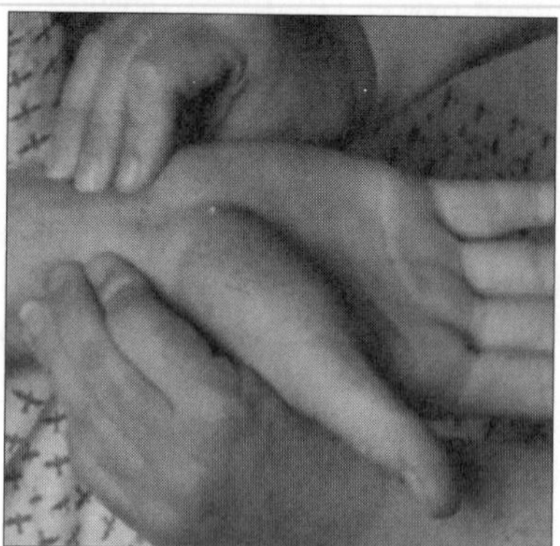

STEP **4a(3)** Client opening hand.

(4) Release pressure over ulnar artery; observe color of fingers, thumbs, and hand (see illustration).

Flushing can be seen immediately if flow through ulnar artery is good. Allen's test is positive, verifying ulnar artery alone is capable of providing blood supply to entire hand. Therefore radial artery can be used for puncture. If there is no flushing in 15 seconds, Allen's test is negative, and this test should be repeated on other arm. When both arms give a negative result, another artery (femoral) needs to be chosen for puncture (Pagana and Pagana, 1998).

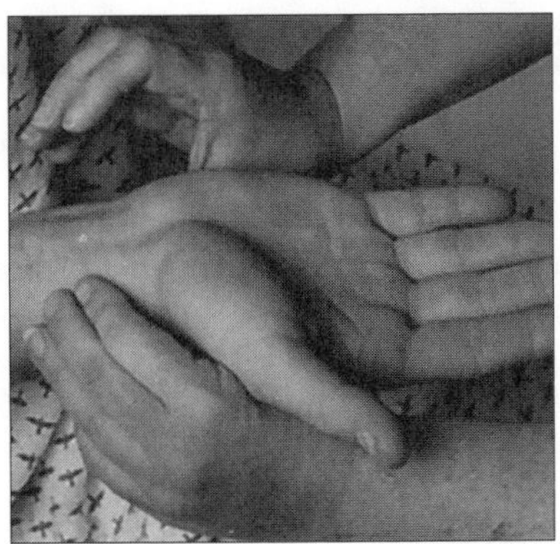

STEP **4a(4)** Releasing pressure over ulnar artery.

Step	Rationale
b. Accessibility of vessel.	Palpating, stabilizing, and performing venipuncture of superficial artery is easier. Superficial arteries are located at distal ends of extremities.
c. Tissue surrounding artery.	Muscle, tendon, and fat have decreased sensation to pain. Bony periosteum and nerves are highly sensitive to pain.
d. Arteries not directly adjacent to veins.	Help reduce chance of venous puncture and possibility of inaccurate samples.
5. Assess best arterial sites for use in obtaining specimen.	Arterial blood may be obtained from areas where strong pulses are palpable (i.e., radial, brachial, or femoral artery) (Pagana and Pagana, 1998).

• ***Critical Decision Point***
Previous puncture sites or preexisting conditions may eliminate potential sites. Artery should be easily accessible.

Step	Rationale
a. Radial artery	Safest, most accessible site for puncture; is superficial, is not adjacent to large veins, usually has adequate collateral circulation by ulnar artery, is relatively painless if periosteum is avoided, is used when Allen's test is positive.
b. Brachial artery	Has reasonable collateral blood flow, is less superficial, is more difficult to palpate and stabilize, carries increased risk of venous puncture, results in increased discomfort for client if brachial nerve is punctured, is used when radial artery is inaccessible or Allen's test is negative.
c. Femoral artery	Should not be used by nurses without specialized training. Has no adequate collateral flow if obstructed below inguinal ligament, is difficult to stabilize, is deep, and directly adjacent to femoral vein. Is best artery to use in emergency (e.g., cardiac arrest or hypovolemic shock when pulses are difficult to palpate).
6. Determine baseline ABG values for client.	Provides basis for comparison and evaluation of therapies.
7. Determine client's knowledge about ABG procedure.	Obtaining blood specimen is painful. Client who is knowledgeable will be more cooperative.

Nursing Diagnosis

Defining characteristics from the assessment data may reveal the following nursing diagnoses for clients requiring this skill:

- Anxiety
- Ineffective breathing pattern
- Impaired gas exchange
- Risk for injury
- Deficient knowledge regarding arterial blood gases
- Ineffective peripheral tissue perfusion

Related factors are individualized based on client's condition or needs.

Step	Rationale
Planning	
1. **Expected outcomes** following completion of procedure:	
▪ Client's ABG values are within normal ranges.	Determining normal values is essential for accurate interpretation.
▪ Client's extremity distal to puncture remains warm, pink, and free of pain and has adequate capillary refill.	Documents adequate arterial circulation to extremity.
▪ Client denies anxiety, and respiratory rate remains within baseline.	Anxiety can increase respiratory rate, which can alter ABG results.
▪ Client discusses ABG procedure.	Documents learning.
2. Prepare heparinized syringe (if heparinized syringes are unavailable).	Heparin mixes with specimen to prevent clotting.
3. Aspirate 0.5 ml sodium heparin (1000 units/ml) into syringe from vial or ampule.	Prevents blood sample from clotting before reaching laboratory. Excessive heparin can affect pH of arterial sample.
4. Withdraw plunger entire length of syringe and maintain asepsis.	Coats barrel of syringe with heparin.
5. Eject all heparin in barrel out of syringe.	In hub of syringe 0.15 to 0.25 ml of sodium heparin remains; 0.05 ml of sodium heparin adequately anticoagulates 1 ml of blood; 0.15 ml adequately anticoagulates 3 ml without affecting pH level.
6. Explain steps and purpose of procedure to client.	Reduces anxiety and promotes understanding and cooperation.
Implementation	
1. Wash hands and apply gloves.	Reduces transmission of infection.
2. Palpate selected radial site with fingertips.	Determines area of maximal impulse for puncture site.
3. Stabilize artery by hyperextending wrist slightly.	Reduces mobility of artery and makes insertion of needle easier.
4. Clean area of maximal impulse with alcohol swab, wiping in circular motion.	Reduces number of resident bacteria on skin's surface.
5. Hold 2 × 2 inch gauze pad with same fingers used to palpate artery.	Keeps gauze pad accessible when covering of puncture site becomes necessary.
6. Keep fingertip on artery, just above chosen puncture site.	Maintaining location of artery improves likelihood of successful puncture.
7. Hold needle bevel up and insert at 45-degree angle into artery, with bevel directed proximally. Prepare client for needle stick because radial sticks are painful. Prepared client will be less likely to withdraw arm.	Angle allows for better arterial flow into needle. Oblique hole in artery seals more easily.
8. Stop advancing needle when blood is noted returning into hub of needle or syringe.	Quick return of blood indicates that arterial flow is obtained. Prevents completely transversing needle through artery.
9. Allow arterial pulsations to pump 2 to 3 ml of blood into heparinized syringe slowly (see illustration).	Allowing pulsations to assist in filling syringe reduces presence of air bubbles in sample. Bubbles can alter ABG results.
10. When sampling is complete, hold 2 × 2 inch gauze pad over puncture site and withdraw needle.	Pad minimizes pulling of skin as needle is withdrawn.
11. Apply pressure over and just proximal to puncture site with pad (see illustration).	Insertion of needle into artery is just proximal to insertion site through skin. Gauze absorbs any blood that might ooze from site.
12. Maintain continuous pressure on and proximal to site for 3 to 5 minutes (approximately 15 minutes if client is undergoing anticoagulant therapy or has bleeding disorder) (Pagana and Pagana, 1998).	To avoid hematoma formation, hold pressure, apply pressure, or a pressure dressing to the arterial puncture site for 3 to 5 minutes (Pagana and Pagana, 1998).

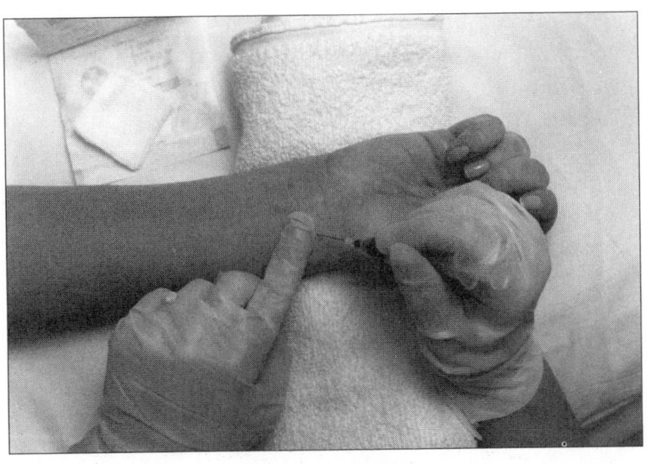

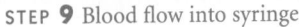

STEP **9** Blood flow into syringe.

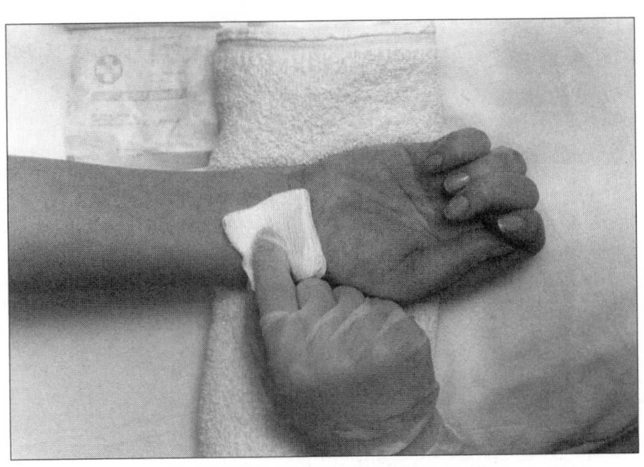

STEP **11** Application of pressure to site.

STEP	RATIONALE
13. Visually inspect site for signs of bleeding or hematoma formation.	Determines if continued need exists to exert pressure. Because an artery rather than a vein has been accessed, puncture site needs to be monitored for bleeding.
14. Palpate artery below or distal to puncture site.	Determines if pulse quality has changed, indicating alteration in arterial flow.
15. Remove gloves and wash hands.	Reduces transmission of microorganisms.
16. Expel air bubbles from syringe.	Failure to expel air from the syringe will result in falsely elevated PaO_2 and falsely decreased $PaCO_2$ (Chernecky and Berger, 1997).
17. Prepare syringe for laboratory analysis according to agency policy. Common principles include:	
a. Place client identification label on syringe.	Permits proper identification of sample for laboratory.
b. Place syringe in cup of crushed ice.	Failure to place the ABG sample in an ice bath may result in decreased pH, PaO_2, and oxygen saturation (Chernecky and Berger, 1997)
c. Attach properly labeled requisition to blood gas sample.	Prevents mislabeled specimens in laboratory. Ensures correct results received for correct client.
d. Indicate amount of any supplemental oxygen (e.g., 2 L O_2, 70% by mask, room air) on requisition.	Documents F_IO_2 (fraction of inspired oxygen) at the time specimen was collected (Linton, Matteson, and Maebius, 2000).
e. Indicate client's temperature.	Elevated body temperature decreases the oxygen saturation result (Chernecky and Berger, 1997).
18. Send sample to laboratory immediately.	A prolonged time lapse between collection and testing may result in a decreased pH (Chernecky and Berger, 1997).

EVALUATION

1. Inspect area distal to puncture site for complications.	Obstruction of artery can develop from hematoma or damage to vessel wall, reducing arterial flow (Pagana and Pagana, 1998).
2. Review results of sample as soon as possible.	Identifies any abnormality and expedites initiation of treatment.

Unexpected Outcomes and Related Interventions

- Client has abnormal ABG values.
  - Continue to monitor client.
  - Notify physician of findings and obtain further orders.
- Client has hematoma formation at puncture site.
  - Apply warm compresses to enhance absorption of blood (Pagana and Pagana, 1998).
  - Continue to monitor client.
  - Notify physician.
- Puncture site is bruised or continues to bleed.
  - Apply pressure.
  - Notify physician.

Recording and Reporting

- Record puncture site and disposition of specimen to laboratory in nurses' notes.
- Report ABG results to physician as soon as available.
- Report client's F_IO_2 and any ventilator settings (e.g., [VT], respiratory frequency [RF] mode of ventilation).
- Record results of test and condition of puncture site in nurses' notes.

Teaching Considerations

- Client is taught to report numbness, burning, and/or tingling in hand that had radial artery puncture.

Pediatric Considerations

- In neonatal and pediatric clients, capillary blood gas may also be used. Procedures are similar to those for obtaining heel sticks.
- When dealing with neonatal clients, especially premature infants, normal values for ABGs may differ from those of adults.
- Arterial blood samples from punctures are painful and cause crying and breath holding that affect the accuracy of blood gas values (decreases PO_2) (Wong and others, 1999).

Gerontological Considerations

- Special attention in interpretation of ABGs must be devoted to clients with chronic pulmonary conditions. In these clients compensatory mechanisms may allow normal pH in face of markedly elevated PCO_2.

Critical Thinking Exercises

1. A 37-year-old woman with new-onset insulin-dependent diabetes says that she is "afraid to poke myself" for blood glucose measurements and would like to know more about urine testing. What positive and negative aspects of each method would you review with her? If she opts for glucose testing by the finger-stick method, what points would you review with her to make her testing less traumatic?
2. A 62-year-old man comes in to pick up some guaiac cards for occult blood testing. As part of your assessment, you inquire about medications. He takes "something" but cannot remember the name of it. Which medication(s) and food(s) would have an impact on the occult blood test?
3. An 18-year-old woman is very anxious before an arterial blood gas test. What effect might this have on the results? How could you alleviate her anxiety?
4. What nursing strategies would you need to implement to obtain a clean-voided specimen from a very obese woman confined to bed rest?

References

American Diabetes Association: 1998 Buyer's guide to diabetes products, *Diabetes Forecast* 50(10):68, 1997.

Beare P, Myers J: *Adult health nursing,* ed 3, St. Louis, 1998, Mosby.

Centers for Disease Control and Prevention: Standard precautions, *Am J Infect Control* February 24, 1996.

Chernecky C, Berger B: *Laboratory tests and diagnostic procedures,* ed 2, Philadelphia, 1997, WB Saunders.

Elkin M, Perry A, Potter P: *Nursing interventions and clinical skills,* ed 2, St. Louis, 2000, Mosby.

Grimes D: *Infectious diseases,* Mosby's clinical nursing series, St. Louis, 1991, Mosby.

Linton A, Matteson M, Maebius N: *Introductory nursing care of adults,* ed 2, Philadelphia, 2000, WB Saunders.

Lueckenotte A: *Gerontologic nursing,* ed 2, St. Louis, 2000, Mosby.

Malarkey L, McMorrow: *Nurse's manual of laboratory tests and diagnostic procedures,* ed 2, Philadelphia, 2000, WB Saunders.

Meredith P, Horan N: *Adult primary care,* Philadelphia, 2000, WB Saunders.

Monahan F, Neighbors M: *Medical-surgical nursing: foundations for clinical practice,* ed 2, St. Louis, 1998, WB Saunders.

Occupational Safety and Health Administration: Occupational exposure to bloodborne pathogens: Final Rule 29 CFR 1919:1030, Fed Register 56:64003, 1991.

Pagana K, Pagana T: *Mosby's diagnostic and laboratory test reference,* ed 3, St. Louis, 1997, Mosby.

Pagana K, Pagana T: *Mosby's manual of diagnostic and laboratory tests,* St. Louis, 1998, Mosby.

Potter P, Perry A: *Basic nursing: a critical thinking approach,* ed 4, St. Louis, 1999, Mosby.

Redman BK: *The practice of patient education,* ed 8, St. Louis, 1997, Mosby.

Agency for Health Care Policy and Research: *Technical review 1: colorectal cancer screening,* AHCPR Pub No. 98-0033, Rockville, Md, 1998, US Department of Health and Human Services.

Ungvarski P, Flaskerud J: *HIV/AIDS: a guide to primary care management,* ed 4, St. Louis, 1999, Mosby.

Wong DL and others: *Whaley and Wong's nursing care of infants and children,* ed 6, St. Louis, 1999, Mosby.

42

Diagnostic Procedures

Skills

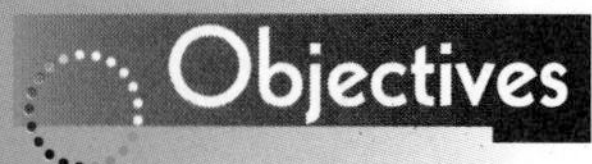

Objectives

Mastery of content in this chapter will enable the nurse to:

- Define the key terms listed.
- Identify physiological factors related to diagnostic procedures.
- Perform physical and psychological assessments related to procedures.
- Discuss the impact of high technology on multicultural clients' health care needs.
- Demonstrate organizational skills in planning procedures.
- Effectively assist the physician or other health professional with abdominal paracentesis, arteriography, bone marrow aspiration, bronchoscopy, electrocardiogram, endoscopy, lumbar puncture, magnetic resonance imaging, and thoracentesis.
- Demonstrate understanding of follow-up activities of procedures.
- Describe the responsibilities related to the procedure of the nurse, physician, and unlicensed assistive personnel.

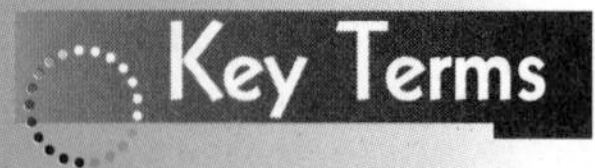

Key Terms

Abdominal girth
Ascites
Aspiration
Biopsy
Bone marrow
Cannula
Cerebrospinal fluid (CSF)
Coagulopathy
Cytologic
Fiberoptic
Foramen magnum
Herniation
Immunocompromised
Intercostal space (ICS)
Intestinal obstruction
Intraabdominal pressure
Intracranial pressure
Intravenous conscious sedation (IVCS)
Lavage
Lumens
Manometer
Medullary
Megakaryocyte
Occult blood
Peritoneal fluid
Pleural cavity
Pleural fluid
Portal hypertension
Precordial
Radiopaque
Sigmoid colon
Stopcock
Subarachnoid space
Thrombocytopenia
Tracheobronchial tree
Trocar
Varices
Viscera

Diagnostic tests are performed at the client's bedside or in specifically equipped rooms for diagnostic purposes either within the hospital or in an outpatient setting. Responsibilities of the nurse include assessing the client's knowledge of the procedure, preparing the client, providing a safe environment throughout the procedure, and providing post-procedural assessment and care. The nurse supervises care delegated to the licensed personnel. If testing was done on an outpatient basis, the nurse provides detailed printed home health care instructions. In some instances, the nurse may provide teaching regarding long-term care needs that must be performed by the patient or caregiver. Knowledge of each test and application of the nursing process ensures safe performance of the procedure.

Certain diagnostic procedures require the client to receive **intravenous conscious sedation (IVCS).** IVCS is the administration of pharmacological agents to provide a minimally depressed level of consciousness. During IVCS the client independently and continuously maintains an airway and is responsive to physical stimulation and verbal commands. The use of IVCS provides client comfort and safe effective performance during the procedure. Although a registered nurse may administer IVCS with a physician in attendance, it is the responsibility of the physician to order the appropriate drugs and dosages. Check agency policy for recommended and maximum doses of medications. Registered nurses responding to the increased number of procedures requiring conscious sedation must be knowledgeable of legal scope-of-practice issues, which are delegated and administered through state boards of nursing (Kost 1998).

When providing IVCS to the geriatric client, it is important to maintain the client's psychological well-being. Many geriatric clients are used to a daily routine and the administration of IVCS for minor procedures removes clients from their usual patterns of behavior. Physical limitations of the patient, including hearing and vision loss as well as lack of autonomy, may contribute to frustration and confusion. Geriatric patients are able to tolerate the administration of IVCS without incident as long as specific needs are identified, thorough pre-procedure assessments and explanations (Kost, 1998).

Pediatric IVCS is widely used for diagnostic and screening procedures but is not a popular technique in the operating room. It is important to consider anatomical and physiological variations, pre-procedure assessments and pharmacological techniques to safely administer IVCS to the pediatric client. During the pre-procedure assessment, the physician and nurse participating in the patient's care should answer the parent's questions in a relaxed and confident manner. Methods to aid in developing rapport with the child are based on the child's developmental stage (Kost, 1998). Children are more likely than adults to sustain a serious complication resulting from anesthesia. Such complications are often linked to either the cardiovascular or respiratory system (Zaglaniczny and Aker, 1999).

Client risks during IVCS include airway compromise, hemodynamic instability, and/or altered levels of consciousness. Emergency equipment (see Chapter 15) and staff prepared to perform emergency medical treatment must be immediately accessible in settings where IVCS is administered. After IVCS, clients need continuous monitoring of vital signs and oxygen saturation by pulse oximetry (see Chapter 11). The client's level of sedation and level of consciousness must be assessed and documented according to agency policy by an RN or delegated to a licensed practical nurse (LPN) or respiratory therapist depending on scope-of-practice guidelines as determined by state board regulatory agencies. Check agency policies regarding specific monitoring parameters and frequency both during and after the procedure.

The nurse must know legal implications related to diagnostic testing. Invasive diagnostic tests require a signed informed consent (see Chapter 33). This means the patient has received a thorough explanation and understands the risks, alternative methods of treatment, and the probability of a successful outcome of the procedure. The nurse cannot obtain the consent and can only witness the patient's signature on the form. Responsibility for obtaining the informed consent resides with the physician who is doing the procedure. In most states, children under 18 years of age are considered to be minors and require a parent or legal guardian to be informed concerning treatment needs and permission obtained before treatment (Meiner, 1999).

The nurse must record and report the client's status before, during, and after the procedure. The nurse assists the client throughout a procedure. Most of these procedures cause moderate discomfort, and the client may tolerate the procedure better if a well-informed nurse remains in attendance at the client's bedside and explains each step.

In the implementation phase of those tests performed by a physician, the physician's responsibility is outlined separately from the nurse's responsibility. There are two main reasons for this separation of duties. First, the nurse anticipates the needs of the physician to have supplies ready. Second and most important, the nurse keeps the client adequately informed of procedural details that could cause discomfort.

Skill Performance Guidelines

1. Assess client's baseline vital signs. Invasive diagnostic procedures can cause complications. Deviations from the baseline vital signs can provide early physiological data about potential complications.
2. Determine client's level of anxiety, educational level, previous experience, language barriers, and sensory deficits that may have an impact on the learning process.
3. Determine the client's knowledge and perception of actual and potential medical diagnoses.
4. Be aware of any abnormal findings that indicate or contraindicate a particular diagnostic test (e.g., prolonged clotting time or prothrombin time).
5. Be aware of a client's past history of adverse reaction to IVCS (e.g., hemodynamic instability, airway compromise, and/or altered level of consciousness).
6. Clients who have previously experienced diagnostic testing may have preconceived (positive or negative) ideas concerning the test, which may influence the amount of pre-procedure teaching and support required.
7. Be aware of clients' disabilities that might affect their ability to be positioned for certain procedures.
8. Be sensitive to cultural patterns that might influence a client's response to various procedures.
9. Certain diagnostic procedures require the client remain NPO before testing. When performing the medication history, the nurse assesses whether the client is taking medications that require an uninterrupted dosage schedule (e.g., anticonvulsants, antibiotics, or cardiac medications) and then contacts the physician.
10. If insulin or oral hypoglycemic medications have been administered to clients before diagnostic testing, arrange to have either the client's meal or other nutritional support available on completion of the test.
11. Because of age-related changes in the older adult, plan diagnostic testing schedules to provide rest periods.
12. If in doubt as to whether a laboratory specimen will be needed, collect a sterile specimen. The specimen can easily be discarded, at no cost to client, if not needed.
13. IV fluids or albumin may be given to prevent hypotension.
14. In addition to consenting for a diagnostic procedure, clients who have experienced blunt abdominal trauma should also consent for emergency abdominal surgery. Operating room personnel need to be notified of pending emergency surgery before the procedure takes place.
15. Before the procedure, determine how client will be safely transported back to the original site (i.e., home, nursing home) if the procedure is done on an outpatient basis.

Skill 42-1 Assisting With Abdominal Paracentesis

Abdominal paracentesis is a sterile, invasive procedure performed by the physician to obtain **peritoneal fluid** for diagnostic analyses or for palliative reasons, such as to reduce **intraabdominal pressure.** Two types of abdominal paracentesis include peritoneal **lavage** and abdominal **aspiration.** Common medical diagnoses requiring abdominal paracentesis include blunt trauma with possible intraabdominal bleeding and **ascites.**

Peritoneal fluid is obtained by inserting a large-bore needle or **trocar** and **cannula** into the peritoneal cavity. A three-way stopcock with polyethylene tubing or a syringe is used to draw off the fluid (Malarkey and McMorrow, 2000). The fluid aspirated is analyzed to determine the presence of bacteria, blood, fungi, glucose, and protein. Additionally, **cytologic** analyses may be done to detect tumors.

As a palliative measure, paracentesis may be performed to provide temporary relief of respiratory and abdominal discomfort caused by severe ascites. Abdominal paracentesis may be performed in the hospital at the client's bedside, the treatment room, or the physician's office in less than 30 minutes.

Delegation Considerations

The skills of assisting with abdominal paracentesis may be delegated to assistive personnel if the client is stable. Inform and assist personnel in the proper way to position the client before a diagnostic procedure. Instruct assistive personnel to take baseline, as well as post-procedure, vital signs and to report these vital signs to the nurse. Caution assistive personnel to be alert for and report signs and symptoms experienced by the client.

Equipment

- Antiseptic solution for hand washing (e.g., povidone-iodine scrub)
- Paracentesis tray, if available from central supply, which may include: antiseptic solution (e.g., povidone-iodine solution), sterile gauze sponges (4 × 4); local anesthetic solution for injection (e.g., lidocaine 1%); sterile syringes: two 3-ml, 23- to 25-gauge needles for anesthetic; four 10- to 60-ml, 19- to 21-gauge needles; small, sterile knife blade; two sterile cannula needles; sizes 10 or 12, with inner trocar, or catheter
- 2 to 3 L IV fluids as ordered
- IV tubing, usually macrodrip size with 3-way **stopcock**
- Sterile specimen containers and bag for containment
- Vacuum bottles as ordered
- Two packages of sterile gloves (check physician's preferred size)
- Masks and goggles for nurse, physician, and assistive personnel (check institution's policy)
- Sterile gauze sponges (2 × 2), tape, adhesive bandages, and antiseptic ointment
- Pain medication, if ordered (given 30 minutes before procedure)
- Laboratory requisitions and labels
- Measuring tape and marker

Step	Rationale
Assessment	
1. Determine whether client has history of being uncooperative or has severe coagulopathy, **thrombocytopenia, intestinal obstruction,** abdominal wall infection, previous multiple abdominal surgeries, or **portal hypertension** with abdominal collateral circulation.	These conditions contraindicate procedure.
2. Wash hands.	Reduces transmission of microorganisms.
3. Obtain vital signs, especially blood pressure. Check with physician regarding attainment of hematocrit, prothrombin time, partial thromboplastin time, and platelet values within 48 hours of the test.	Baseline vital signs detect changes caused by complications from drainage of large fluid volumes. Attainment of laboratory values provides a baseline to compare values because of the risk of bleeding in the post-test period (Malarkey and McMorrow, 2000).
4. Palpate client's bladder for distention or determine time of last voiding. Have client void before procedure.	Chance of bladder trauma is decreased if bladder is not distended (Malarkey and McMorrow, 2000).

STEP	RATIONALE
5. Obtain client's medication history. Determine if there are allergies to local anesthetic or antiseptic solutions that may be used or if client is receiving anticoagulants.	Common allergic reactions to anesthetic agents are central nervous system depression, respiratory difficulties, and hypotension. Allergic reactions to antiseptic solutions are usually skin irritations. Client who is receiving anticoagulants may experience hemorrhage.
6. Weigh client, assess abdomen (see Chapter 10), and measure **abdominal girth** in centimeters at largest point of abdomen. Use ink pen to mark where measuring tape lies.	Abdominal girth is measured in same place to accurately note abdominal size before and after paracentesis (Linton, and others, 2000).
7. Assess client's respiratory rate, diaphragmatic excursion, and chest wall motion.	Excess peritoneal fluid increases intraabdominal pressure, which in turn compromises respiration (Linton, and others, 2000).
8. Assess client's knowledge regarding procedure.	Client must be informed of impending procedure, its purpose, and risks.
9. Check whether client has signed written informed consent.	Most institutions require written permission for procedure.

• ***Critical Decision Point***
Do not administer an analgesic before the client gives informed consent.

10. Administer pre-procedure medication if indicated.	Clients who are anxious may benefit from pre-procedure medications.

NURSING DIAGNOSIS

Defining characteristics from the assessment data may reveal the following nursing diagnoses for clients requiring this skill:

- Anxiety
- Ineffective breathing pattern
- Risk for infection
- Risk for injury
- Deficient knowledge regarding purpose and steps of procedure
- Acute pain

Related factors are individualized based on the client's, family's, and significant others' needs.

PLANNING

1. **Expected outcomes** following completion of procedure:	
▪ Client assumes positions without problems, has few changes in vital signs, and has no complications.	Client tolerates procedure well.
▪ For peritoneal lavage and abdominal aspiration, aspirate is clear or slightly blood tinged.	Slight amount of blood-tinged drainage may be caused by irritation to tissue by needle.
▪ For therapeutic treatment of ascites by paracentesis, amount of fluid drained results in decreased abdominal girth, skin tightness, and weight.	Patients usually experience transient relief of distention (Pagana and Pagana, 1998).
▪ Client experiences increased comfort.	Distention from buildup of fluid in peritoneal space is relieved.
▪ Client has improved respiratory status.	Patients usually experience transient relief of shortness of breath (Pagana and Pagana, 1998).
2. Organize equipment on bedside table.	Ensures ease and success of procedure.
3. Prepare client for procedure:	
4. Explain purpose of and steps in the procedure.	Assists in minimizing anxiety and promoting relaxation and cooperation.
5. Have client void before procedure.	Full or distended bladder increases possibility of puncturing bladder (Chernecky and Berger, 1997).

• ***Critical Decision Point***
If client is unable to void and bladder is distended, obtain an order for catheterization.

STEP	RATIONALE
6. Client assumes position desired by physician, either semi-Fowler's in bed or sitting upright on side of bed or in chair with feet supported. Because of underlying physical condition (i.e., respiratory distress from increased fluid), client may be unable to assume required position for procedure and may require assistance of pillows or other positional devices.	These positions cause fluid to accumulate in the lower abdominal cavity and be drained more easily (SGNA, 1998) (see illustration).

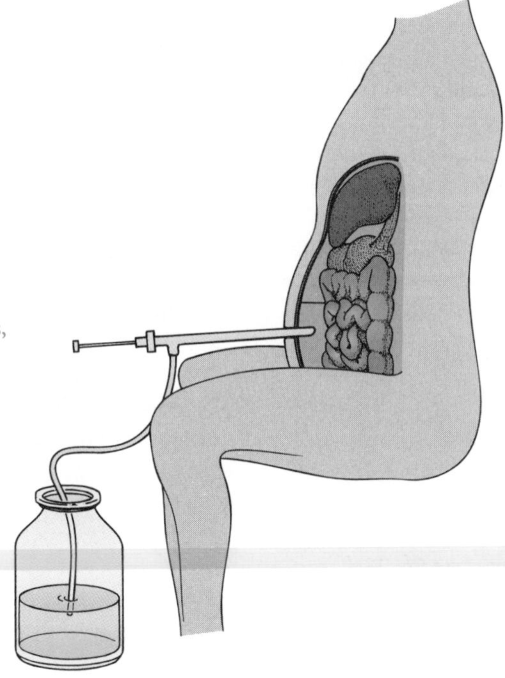

STEP 6 Paracentesis. (From Beare P, Myers J: *Adult health nursing,* ed 3, St Louis, 1998, Mosby.)

IMPLEMENTATION

NURSE'S RESPONSIBILITY

STEP	RATIONALE
1. Wash hands.	Reduces transmission of microorganisms.
2. Set up sterile tray or open sterile supplies and make accessible for physician.	Ensures maintenance of sterility throughout procedure.
3. Prepare solution to be used for lavage; attach to IV tubing.	If fluid instillation is to be performed, as with blunt abdominal trauma, fluid is ready to attach to plastic tubing after cannula is in place in abdomen.
4. Assist client through procedure:	
a. Describe steps of procedure as physician implements them.	Allows client opportunity to ask questions and helps to decrease anxiety.
b. Ensure client's comfort and assess for complications.	Assists client in tolerating procedure and identifies need to modify or discontinue procedure.
5. Assess vital signs before, every 15 minutes during and, every 15 minutes for an hour after the procedure or according to agency policy.	Identifies hemodynamic changes and possible complications of procedure. Hypotension may occur if a large volume of fluid was removed (Pagana and Pagana, 1998).
6. Implement fluid instillation for lavage:	
a. Apply clean gloves (and mask and goggles, if required).	Reduces transmission of microorganisms.
b. After IV tubing is attached to cannula, administer physician-ordered amount of fluid at prescribed rate.	Promotes infusion of prescribed fluid into peritoneum.
c. Clamp IV tubing after fluid is instilled and place drainage tubing below client's abdominal level.	Promotes gravitational drainage of fluid from peritoneal cavity.

Step	Rationale
d. Ascitic fluid is withdrawn by either gravity or vacuum drainage. Maximum amount of ascitic fluid usually allowed to drain is 1500 ml.	Permits flow of fluid or solution from abdomen. Aspiration of more than 1500 ml of fluid may cause hypovolemic shock because of the sudden shift of fluid from the circulatory system to replace the aspirated fluid (SGNA, 1998).
7. Collect any necessary laboratory specimens in sterile containers.	
8. Assess client's tolerance of procedure, including pain and mental status.	Enables nurse to evaluate client's tolerance of procedure and detects changes from pre-procedure condition.
9. Assist client in assuming comfortable position in bed.	Maintains comfort.
10. Carefully dispose of equipment, remove gloves, and wash hands. Needles and other sharp objects should be placed in special containers. Dispose of peritoneal fluid not sent to laboratory according to hospital procedure.	Controls transmission of infection. Proper disposal of sharps prevents accidental injury to personnel.

Physician's Responsibility

Step	Rationale
1. Wash hands. Prep abdomen with antiseptic solution and 4 × 4 sponges.	Reduces transmission of microorganisms.
2. Wear mask (if required), apply sterile gloves and goggles, and drape client with sterile towels.	Maintains surgical asepsis.
3. Inject local anesthetic and allow to take effect.	Provides local anesthetic to area of puncture or incision.
4. If the purpose of the paracentesis is to drain ascitic fluid or to lavage, insert the large-bore needle or trocar through a small incision between the umbilicus and the symphysis pubis.	Facilitates placement of large-bore needle or trocar into abdominal cavity for instillation and drainage of fluid. Permits the removal of blood and/or fluid specimens.
5. Attach IV tubing to the cannula and allow fluid to drain into a receptacle to a maximum of 1500 ml. (The fluid may also be aspirated, using a 60-ml syringe.) For lavage, instill prescribed amount of sterile fluid and allow it to drain.	Fluid is drained slowly, to a maximum of 1500 ml to prevent hypovolemic shock (SGNA, 1998).
6. If only specimens are needed and an incision is not made, insert 10-gauge needle attached to syringe, aspirate fluid, and place in specimen containers. Remove cannula, needle, or trocar.	Obtains sterile specimens for laboratory analysis.
7. Place manual pressure over insertion site until drainage ceases or apply pressure dressing.	Prevents excessive drainage from puncture site.
8. Place antiseptic ointment with 2 × 2 gauze sponge over insertion site.	Prevents growth of bacteria at puncture site.

Evaluation

Step	Rationale
1. Take vital signs every 15 minutes for 1 hour and then every 30 minutes for 2 hours or according to agency policy; check for stability by comparing with pre-procedure values.	Hypotension and/or shock may result because of rapid shift of fluid, potassium, and albumin from the circulation into the peritoneal cavity (Malarkey and McMorrow, 2000).
2. Monitor urinary output for 24 hours.	Verifies client's physiological status. Hematuria may indicate bladder trauma.
3. Check dressing over insertion site for bleeding or drainage.	Provides for continued observation of puncture site. May indicate accumulation of blood or fluid in abdominal cavity. A major complication of this procedure is hemorrhage (Malarkey and McMorrow, 2000).
4. Measure abdominal girth and weight.	Determines change after fluid drainage.
5. Inspect character of lavage or aspirate.	For peritoneal lavage and abdominal aspiration, aspirate is clear or slightly blood tinged.
6. Observe and question if client is having acute abdominal pain.	May indicate perforation of the bowel (Malarkey and McMorrow, 2000).

Unexpected Outcomes and Related Interventions

- Changes in client's vital signs that are not within normal limits.
  - Continue to monitor.
  - Notify physician.
- In clients with blunt abdominal trauma, injured or perforated contents may bleed into peritoneal cavity and may be observed through this procedure.
  - Monitor quantity and quality of drainage.
  - Record vital signs.
  - Notify physician of findings and obtain further orders.
- Client's aspirate or drained fluid is bright or dark red.
  - Continue to monitor aspirate drainage and vital signs.
  - Notify physician of findings.
- Client develops infection.
  - Monitor temperature and signs of chilling.
  - Assess site.
  - Notify physician of findings and obtain further orders.
- Laboratory test results, including cell counts, protein levels, and specific gravity, are not within normal limits.
  - Notify physician of findings and obtain further orders.

Recording and Reporting

Record in client's medical record:

- Time and type of procedure (aspiration or lavage).
- Name of physician.
- Color, consistency, and amount of fluid withdrawn.
- Client's tolerance of procedure (pain level, vital signs).
- Type of dressing over insertion site and whether drainage is present.
- Indicate to which laboratory specimen was sent.
- Record changes in abdominal girth, weight, and amount, color, and clarity of fluid.

Report to physician immediately any deviations from client's baseline vital signs, or if there is severe abdominal pain or excessive bloody drainage from insertion site.

Teaching Considerations

- Explain to client that procedure will be more safely performed if bladder is empty.
- Explain that although the local anesthetic will eliminate pain at the insertion site, a pressure-type discomfort may be experienced as the needle is inserted.
- Tell client with ascites that comfort will probably increase and respiration will be easier after paracentesis.
- Inform client with ascites that the procedure provides temporary decrease in abdominal distention and may need to be repeated.
- Encourage client to check with physician regarding test results.

Gerontological Considerations

- If the older adult cannot tolerate sitting at the side of the bed, he or she is placed in high Fowler's position.
- In older adults, skin is normally inelastic and thin; therefore, special care should be used when removing adhesive bandages or tape at puncture site.
- Monitor client's BP for signs of hypotension if a large volume of fluid was removed.

Home Care Considerations

- If paracentesis is done on an outpatient basis, inform client to notify physician of fever or any swelling, pain, or drainage at puncture site.
- In males, scrotal edema should be reported to the physician (SGNA, 1998).

Long-Term Care Considerations

- Be alert for signs and symptoms of hypovolemia and electrolyte imbalances, especially in the elderly.

Skill 42-2 Assisting With Angiography (Arteriography)

Angiography (arteriography) permits radiographic visualization of the vasculature of the heart and arterial system after the intravascular injection of a **radiopaque** contrast medium. Arteriography is most frequently performed to aid in the diagnosis of occlusions, stenosis, emboli or thromboses, aneurysms, tumors, congenital malformations, or trauma of the arteries of the brain, heart, lung, kidneys, or lower extremities.

A small incision or needle puncture is made in a peripheral artery (femoral, brachial, or carotid), and, under x-ray visualization, a small radiopaque catheter is threaded through the artery to the site. The iodinated contrast material is injected, and timed x-ray films are taken. A radiologist in the x-ray department usually performs the test.

Potential complications of angiography include hemorrhage or thrombosis at the catheter insertion site, infection, allergic reactions to the dye, embolism, and renal failure. Additionally, the nurse must be alert for complications related to IVCS.

Cardiac catheterization is a specialized form of angiography in which a catheter is inserted into either the left or right side of the heart to study pressures within the heart, cardiac volumes, valvular function, and patency of coronary arteries (Figure 42-1). A contrast medium is injected, and the structures and functions of the heart assessed. In right-side heart catheterizations, usually the subclavian or femoral vein is used for vascular access.

Cardiac catheterizations may be contraindicated in clients who would refuse surgery if needed, who are allergic to iodine contrast media, who are uncooperative or who cannot lie still during the entire procedure, or who are susceptible to dye-induced renal failure (Beare and Myers, 1998; Pagana and Pagana, 1998). The procedures are usually elective but may be done on an emergency basis in the event of sudden occlusion of an artery or in the case of myocardial infarction.

For both procedures, a technologist rather than the nurse usually assists the cardiologist or radiologist, and the procedures are done in the radiology department. An exception would be when IVCS is administered by an RN with a physician in attendance. Agency policies may vary.

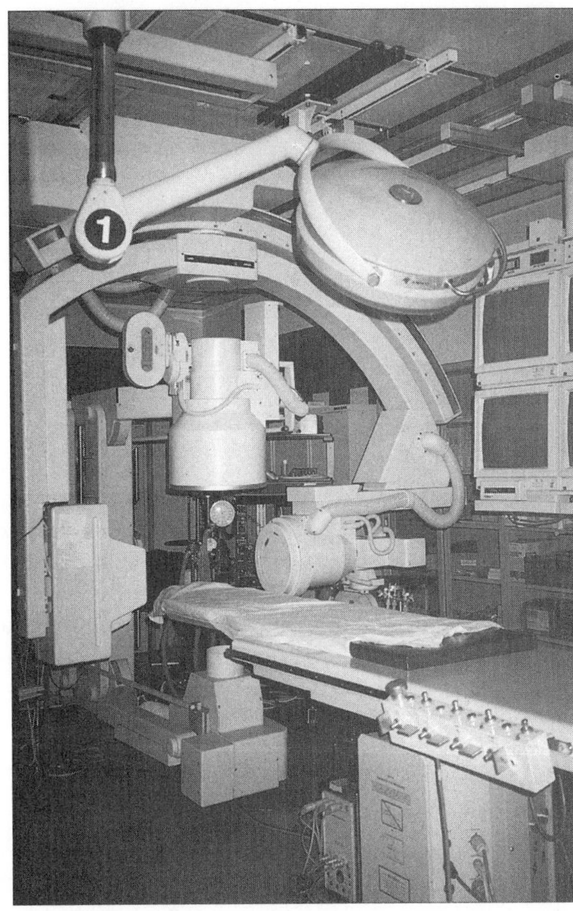

FIGURE **42-1** Cardiac catherization laboratory. (From Wong D and others: *Whaley and Wong's nursing care of infants and children,* ed 6, St Louis, 1999, Mosby.)

Delegation Considerations

The skill of assisting with angiography may be delegated to assistive personnel if the client is stable. Frequently assistive personnel may be required to accompany the client to the procedure room, and specially trained personnel assist with the specific angiography procedure. Instruct assistive personnel to take baseline, as well as post-procedure, vital signs and to report these vital signs to the nurse. Caution assistive personnel to be alert for and report signs and symptoms experienced by the client. If the client requires IVCS, delegation to assistive personnel is inappropriate.

Equipment

For either an arteriogram or a cardiac catheterization, special packs are usually available from central sterile supply. The packs contain various sizes and types of catheters for performing the procedures as well as the necessary specialized equipment.

- Sterile gown
- Sterile gloves
- Mask
- Goggles
- Intravenous equipment for IV start
- Diazepam, midazolam, or other sedative for IV sedation
- Oxygen, resuscitative equipment, pulse oximeter, cardiac monitor for IVCS

Step	Rationale
Assessment	
1. Assess client's knowledge of procedure. Encourage client to verbalize concerns.	Procedure creates physical sensations and involves visual analyses of x-ray/fluoroscope that need to be explained in detail. Patients may be anxious about the procedure and possible outcomes and may have difficulty asking questions and interpreting information. Even patients who have previously undergone this procedure, may worry about the outcome (Gulanick, and others, 1998).

• ***Critical Decision Point***
Instruct client about coughing and holding breath when asked to do so during the procedure. Coughing can sometimes eliminate potentially life-threatening dysrhythmias (VanRiper and VanRiper, 1997).

Step	Rationale
2. Obtain vital signs and peripheral pulses. Mark client's peripheral pulses before procedure. For cardiac catheterization, also auscultate heart and lungs and obtain weight.	Provides baseline data for comparison with findings during and after procedure. Marking pulses permits quicker post-procedure assessment of pulse in affected and nonaffected extremities (Pagana and Pagana, 1998).
3. Determine type of arteriogram to be performed—carotid, femoral, or brachial. If cardiac catheterization, determine whether right or left heart is being studied.	Enables nurse to anticipate client teaching needs and post-procedure interventions.

• ***Critical Decision Point***
Area of catheter insertion may need to be shaved and prepped with antiseptic just before the procedure.

Step	Rationale
4. Determine whether client has signed consent form.	The presence of a signed consent form indicates the patient has received a thorough explanation of the procedure and understands the risks and the probability of successful outcome of the procedure (Meiner, 1999).

• ***Critical Decision Point***
Consent form must be completed before administration of pre-procedural sedation or IVCS.

Step	Rationale
5. Assess that client has been NPO for 6 to 8 hours before the procedure.	Prevents possible aspiration because client is sedated. Excessive hydration causes dilution of the contrast medium, making structures more difficult to visualize.
6. Assess whether client is allergic to iodine dye. If so, notify cardiologist or radiologist. Benadryl IV may be routinely given before the procedure.	An iodine-based radiopaque contrast medium may be used during the procedure; however, a nonionic, hypoallergenic contrast medium is more frequently used (Pagana and Pagana, 1998). Clients with allergies to iodine, shellfish, or other contrast media may experience anaphylactic reactions.
7. Determine if client is taking anticoagulants.	Physician needs to be aware of and medication will need to be stopped before the procedure.
8. Obtain ordered laboratory tests, e.g., CBC, platelets, prothrombin time, electrolytes, BUN, and creatinine levels before the procedure.	Abnormal findings might contraindicate the procedure because hemorrhage and/or renal failure may be a complication. Report elevated BUN or creatinine levels because such clients are at risk for renal failure (Malarkey and McMorrow, 2000).
9. Review physician's orders for pre-procedure medications (may be given on nursing unit or in radiology department) and sedative for IVCS:	Increased sedation may be necessary in anxious or confused clients.
a. Atropine	Decreases salivary secretions and increases heart rate when bradycardia is present (Kee and Hayes, 2000).
b. Benadryl	Used prophylactically to block histamine and decrease allergic response (Kee and Hayes, 2000).
c. Pre-procedural sedative	Decreases anxiety and promotes relaxation (Pagana and Pagana, 1998).

STEP	RATIONALE
d. IVCS during procedure	Provides a minimally depressed level of consciousness yet allows client to independently and continuously maintain an airway and respond to physical stimuli and verbal commands (Kost, 1998).

NURSING DIAGNOSIS

Defining characteristics from the assessment data may reveal the following nursing diagnoses for clients requiring this skill:

- Anxiety
- Decreased cardiac output
- Fear
- Risk for infection
- Risk for injury
- Deficient knowledge regarding purpose and steps of procedure
- Acute pain

Related factors are individualized based on client's condition or needs.

PLANNING

STEP	RATIONALE
1. **Expected outcomes** following completion of procedure:	
▪ Client has no significant changes in vital signs or peripheral pulses and no allergic response.	Procedure performed without complication.
▪ Client has only minimal discomfort, which includes soreness at catheter insertion site and possible backache.	Client tolerates procedure. These are considered normal and expected.
▪ Client recovers from IVCS without respiratory complications or change in level of consciousness.	Level of sedation is appropriate.
2. Explain to client purpose of the procedure and what will happen during the procedure.	Helps to minimize client's anxiety.

IMPLEMENTATION

NURSE'S RESPONSIBILITY

STEP	RATIONALE
1. Wash hands and apply clean gloves.	Reduces transmission of microorganisms.
2. For cardiac catheterization, provide IV access using large-bore cannula.	Provides access for delivery of intravenous fluids and/or drugs.
3. Monitor vital signs, obtain weight, and palpate peripheral pulses.	Provides baseline data for comparison during and after procedure.
4. Assist client in assuming comfortable position on x-ray table.	Position may need to be maintained for 1 to 3 hours.
5. Provide support to client throughout the procedure and as x-rays are taken.	The client may be frightened by the loud noises (Pagana and Pagana, 1998).
6. Tell client that during the injection of the dye, he or she may experience some chest pain and there may be a severe hot flash that is quite uncomfortable but lasts only a few seconds (Pagana and Pagana, 1998; VanRiper and VanRiper, 1997).	Dye causes a feeling of warmth, flushing, or a metallic taste may be sensed (Malarkey and McMorrow, 2000).
7. Nurse administering IVCS monitors level of sedation and level of consciousness.	IVCS should not cause loss of consciousness.
8. Note that some clients have a tendency to cough as the catheter is placed into the pulmonary artery (Pagana and Pagana, 1998).	

STEP	RATIONALE
PHYSICIAN'S RESPONSIBILITY	
1. Wash hands and prep area of catheter insertion (femoral, carotid, or brachial) with antiseptic.	Reduces transmission of microorganisms.
2. Apply mask and goggles, sterile gown, cap, and gloves. (All technologists and assistants do the same.) Drape client with sterile drapes.	Maintains surgical asepsis.
3. Anesthetize the skin overlying the arterial puncture site.	Provides local anesthetic to area of incision or puncture.
4. Perform needle puncture of artery; insert guidewire through needle and angiographic (or cardiographic) catheter threaded over wire.	Permits access to artery and prevents coiling of catheter in artery.
5. Advance catheter to desired artery or cardiac chamber and inject contrast medium.	Permits radiographic visualization of structures, aneurysms, occlusions, or anomalies.
6. During dye injection, specialized machinery takes rapid sequence of x-rays.	Permits radiographic records of visualization of dye through artery as well as any abnormalities present.
7. For cardiac catheterization, also measure cardiac volumes and pressures; then withdraw catheter and apply pressure to puncture site for at least 5 minutes.	Provides data related to cardiac output, central venous pressure (CVP), ventricular pressures, and pulmonary artery pressure. Pressure on puncture site promotes clotting and prevents bleeding.

EVALUATION

Step	Rationale
1. Monitor vital signs and assess peripheral pulses (compare right and left) and assess affected extremity for skin color, temperature, and sensation (Gulanick, and others, 1998). Auscultate heart and lungs if cardiac catheterization done and compare findings with pre-procedure values.	Verifies client's physiological status and evaluates effect of procedure. Dressing checks and pulse checks are necessary to ensure that circulation to the affected extremity has not been impaired (VanRiper and VanRiper, 1997). Decreased peripheral pulses, coolness, mottling, pallor, pain, numbness, and tingling in affected extremity are signs of decreased tissue perfusion (Gulanick and others, 1998).
2. Apply pressure dressing or sand bag to vascular access site (Chernecky and Berger, 1997).	Promotes clotting and prevents bleeding (Chernecky and Berger, 1997).
3. Maintain client on bed rest for 4 to 8 hours.	Allows sealing of arterial puncture.
4. Keep affected extremity immobilized for 6 to 8 hours after removal of catheter (VanRiper and VanRiper, 1997). Use orthopedic bedpan for female client as needed while on bed rest.	To promote complete arterial repair (VanRiper and VanRiper, 1997).
5. Emphasize the need to lay flat for 6 to 12 hours (and possibly overnight if the catheters are left in the groin).	To decrease bleeding and promote complete arterial repair (VanRiper and VanRiper, 1997).
6. Encourage client to drink 1 to 2 liters of fluid after procedure.	To facilitate elimination of contrast material and prevent renal damage (VanRiper and VanRiper, 1997).
7. Assess client for possible delayed reaction to iodine dye (if used)—dyspnea, hives, tachycardia, and rash (Pagana and Pagana, 1998).	Reaction may occur up to 6 hours after injection of dye.
8. Assess for level of sedation, level of consciousness, and O_2 saturation.	Determines client's response to IVCS.
9. Assess post-procedure laboratory values—CBC, prothrombin time, electrolytes, BUN, and creatinine.	Changes in laboratory values may indicate the onset of complications.
10. Observe client for signs of discomfort.	May be early sign of complication.

- ***Critical Decision Point***

  If the client reports any feelings of pain, dyspnea, numbness or tingling, or other untoward symptoms, immediately report these to the physician.

Unexpected Outcomes and Related Interventions

- Client has marked changes in vital signs or peripheral pulses.
  - Continue to monitor.
  - Notify physician immediately.
  - Follow specific post-procedural orders related to findings.
- Client remains sedated with decreased respiration or blood pressure, decreased oxygen saturation, or decreased level of consciousness.
  - Continue monitoring as necessary.
  - Notify physician.
  - Follow specific post-procedural orders related to findings.
  - Administer reversal agent if ordered.
- Client has hematoma or hemorrhage present at catheter insertion site.
  - Apply pressure to site.
  - Monitor catheter site every 30 minutes for 2 to 3 hours, then as needed.
  - Notify physician.
  - Follow specific post-procedural orders related to findings.
- Client experiences flushing, itching, and uticaria.
  - Continue monitoring.
  - Assess client for anaphylaxis.
  - Monitor vital signs.
  - Notify physician.
  - Follow specific post-procedural orders related to findings.
  - Administer antihistamine if ordered.
- Client experiences cardiac dysrhythmias.
  - Follow specific post-procedural orders.
  - Monitor vital signs
  - Notify physician.
- Client develops infection/sepsis.
  - Continue to monitor temperature and vital signs.
  - Notify physician

Recording and Reporting

- Record client's status on return to nursing unit: vital signs, status of pulses for equality and symmetry, BP especially for hypotension, temperature and color of catheterized extremity, condition of IV site, and level of client responsiveness.
  - Record any drainage from puncture site, appearance of dressing, and condition of puncture site
  - If IVCS was used, record vital signs per agency policy, oxygen saturation, airway status, and level of consciousness
- Report to physician changes in vital signs, excessive bleeding or increasing hematoma at puncture site, decreased or absent peripheral pulses, altered neurological status, dysrhythmias, decreased oxygen saturation or decreased responsiveness after sedation.
  - Report to nurses on next shift all relevant physiological data, status of puncture site and dressing.

Teaching Considerations

- Before the procedure, confirm that client has made arrangements for transport home afterwards. Additionally, the client needs to be prepared to stay overnight in a hospital if complications occur or if an intervention like a percutaneous transluminal coronary angioplasty (PTCA) is necessary.
- Explain to client that, during the procedure, lying in one position for 1 to 3 hours is expected.
- If IVCS is to be used, explain to client purpose and expected effects of sedation and the post-procedural instructions regarding client's care and necessary precautions.
- Explain that the client might experience a feeling of falling when the table is rotated from side to side.
- Explain the necessity of bed rest and immobility following the procedure.
- Explain that after the procedure the client's vital signs will be taken and the puncture site will be inspected at frequent intervals.
- Some clients may experience difficulty urinating in a supine position and may require measures that stimulate voiding.
- Encourage client to check with physician regarding test results.
- Some institutions provide written discharge instructions (Figure 42-2).

Pediatric Considerations

- The pressure of catheter insertion at the selected site may cause the pediatric client to become nauseated or vomit (Zaglaniczny and Aker, 1999).
- Children who are cyanotic may have a high hematocrit. Following the administration of radiocontrast dyes (which act as osmotic diuretics), further hemoconcentration may develop (Zaglaniczny and Aker, 1999).
- Blood loss from the procedure occurs from the cutdown site and bleeding into surrounding tissues. Fluid boluses IV may be required to maintain acceptable circulating plasma volume (Zaglaniczny and Aker, 1999).
- Procedure should be performed with child under general anesthesia (Wong and others, 1999).

Gerontological Considerations

- Keep frail older adults warm to maintain core temperature at comfortable, safe levels (Worfolk, 1997).
- Inspect bony prominences of older adults frequently because such clients are more susceptible to skin breakdown from lying in one position.
- In the older adult, slight alterations in vital signs or behavior may be precursors to impending problems; therefore, skilled observations are critical (Phipps and others, 1999).
- Older adult clients may have reduced drug clearance from decreased glomerular filtration rate (GFR) and nephron activity or decreased hepatic function. Therefore the nurse must monitor the effects of narcotics and hypnotics that may interfere with breathing (Phipps and others, 1999).
- Older adults with chronic dehydration or mild renal failure are at high risk for dye-induced renal failure (Pagana and Pagana, 1998).

BARNES

POST-CARDIAC CATHETERIZATION ORDERS
FORM #234A

A-17

1. Notify intern/resident or house physician that patient has returned from the cardiac cath lab.

2. Cardiac catheterization performed by *(please check)*:
☐ RFA ☐ RFV
☐ LFA ☐ LFV

3. Record blood pressure and heart rate every 15 minutes x 4, every 30 minutes x 2, every 1 hour x 2, then every 4 hours x 24 hours if patient stable, then every shift.

4. Call house physician stat for: HR > 100 ________ or < 50 ________ bpm.
sBP > 160 ________ or < 100 ________ mmHg.

5. Mark pedal pulses distal to cardiac cath site. Monitor ☐ Rt. ☐ Lt. groin puncture site and distal pedal pulses every 15 minutes x 4, every 30 minutes x 2, every 1 hour x 2, then every 4 hours x 24 hours if patient stable.

6. Report bleeding, swelling or pain at groin puncture site or reduction or loss of distal pedal pulses to house physician and on-call cardiac cath fellow.

7. Record I & O every 8 hours for 24 hours. Notify house physician if urine output is less than 400cc in 8 hours.

8. Patients with femoral sheaths sutured in place should remain at strict bedrest with HOB < 30° and cath leg straight until sheaths removed by the cardiac cath fellow.

9. For patients with femoral sheaths removed:
   a. Patient to remain at strict bedrest for 6 hours or ________ hours after return from cath lab.
   b. The HOB may be raised to 30° one hour after return from cath lab, if there is no bleeding at puncture site and vital signs are stable.
   c. RN to remove sandbag 4 hours after return from cath lab.
   d. When period of strict bedrest is over, RN to remove groin dressing and observe puncture site for bleeding or swelling.
   e. When groin dressing removed assess puncture site and distal pedal pulse every 2 hours x 2, every 4 hours x 2, every shift for 24 hours, then daily.
   f. If bleeding or oozing noted at puncture site apply firm pressure and call the on-call cardiac cath fellow.
   g. If groin puncture site intact patient may sit at side of bed and ambulate to bathroom with assistance. Apply bandaid to site and change daily for two days.
   h. In AM patient may resume pre-cath activity level if vital signs stable and there is no bleeding or swelling at groin puncture site.

10. Orthopedic bedpan for female patients as needed while at bedrest.

11. Straight cath PRN if patient unable to urinate within 4-8 hours following cardiac cath.

12. Diet post-cardiac cath:
    a. Clear liquids for first hour if patient alert and free from nausea.
    b. Resume previous diet after one hour if patient fully awake and free from nausea, vital signs stable, and groin puncture site intact.

13. Medications post-cardiac cath:
    a. Acetaminophen 300mg and codeine 30mg (acet/codeine #3 tabs) 1 or 2 tablets po every 4 hours PRN for pain at puncture site, back pain, or headache.
    b. If allergic to codeine substitute Darvocet-N 100 1 tablet po every 4 hours PRN.
    c. Tigan suppository 200mg for nausea and/or vomiting (stat dose only).
    d. Resume previous oral medications when vital signs stable and patient free from nausea.

14. IV medications post-cardiac cath *(check and fill in blanks)*:
    a. ☐ Heparin 25,000u/250ml 1/2 NS to be resumed at (time) ______ on (date) ______ at ______ U/hr. Avoid heparin boluses for at least 12 hours following cardiac cath.
    b. ☐ Nitroglycerin 50mg/250ml D_5W at ______ mcg/min, titrate for sBP > ______ or < ______ mmHg. Wean nitroglycerin off after ______ hours.

15. Post-cardiac cath IV fluids:
    Start 1L NS or ____________ at ____________ ml/hr,
    then 1L NS or ____________ at ____________ ml/hr,
    then 1L NS or ____________ at KVO.

16. In AM: *(check one)* ☐ discontinue post-cath IVFs and resume pre-cath IVFs or
    ☐ replace with saline lock (flush each shift).

17. AM labs: ____

18. For chest discomfort/anginal equivalent, shortness of breath, nausea/vomiting, or hypotension obtain a stat ECG and contact the house physician and on-call cardiac cath fellow STAT.

19. For acute cardiac problems or puncture site bleeding contact the cardiology fellow (Dr.______________ Pager: ________) or the cardiac cath lab (2-9300). At night contact the on-call cardiology fellow in the CCU (2-5096) or the on-call cardiac cath fellow (2-2284).

20. No patient should be discharged until a note in the chart indicates that the patient's groin puncture site has been examined by the cardiac cath fellow.

21. If patient is to be discharged the morning after cardiac cath, give patient a copy of "Barnes Hospital Nursing Service Cardiac Catheterization Discharge Instructions".

22. Other orders: ____

____

____

MD: ________________________

A

FIGURE **42-2** **A,** Post-cardiac catherization (coronary angiography) orders.

Continued

BARNES HOSPITAL CARDIAC CATHETERIZATION DISCHARGE INSTRUCTIONS

C-51

The following information is intended to serve as a guide to assist with your care after discharge following cardiac catheterization.

1. Resume your normal diet immediately, unless directed otherwise by your physician.
2. It is important to limit activity of the limb site used for the catheterization for **3 days.***
   This includes, but is not limited to activities such as aerobics, swimming, jogging or running, bicycling, bowling, dancing, rowing, stair-stepping. If you are involved in activities not listed above, please ask your nurse or physician for specific instructions.
3. Avoid lifting for **2 days.***
4. Gentle walking is permissible but only on level ground.
5. No driving for **2 days.***
6. Restrict stair-climbing for **2 days**, if possible. If stair-climbing is essential, climb with your non-catheterized leg, then bring the catheterized leg up to the same step.*
7. Customary sexual activity may be resumed after **2 days**. Use postures that do not place a strain on the catheterized leg.*
8. Avoid straining for bowel movements for **7 days.** If you tend to be constipated and/or regularly strain to pass stool, please inform your nurse of this so that a stool softening medication can be ordered.
9. It is common to have some bruising or purple discoloration of the skin near the puncture site.

***(If you have received an angioplasty, atherectomy, laser, rotoblator or stent procedure extend activity restrictions to 7 days.)**

However, if any of the following occur, immediately contact your own physician, or the Barnes Hospital Emergency Department at **(314) 362-9123.**

a. Bleeding from the catheterization puncture site: apply gentle pressure with a clean gauze or cloth and call your physician or the Barnes Hospital Emergency Room immediately.
b. If a knot or lump under the skin increases in size or,
c. If bruising appears to be worsening or tracking/moving down the leg rather than disappearing.
d. If you have pain at the puncture site or in the leg used for the catheterization.
e. If the leg used for the catheterization appears pale in color and/or feels cooler to touch compared to the opposite leg.
f. If the leg used for the catheterization appears reddened, swollen and/or feels warmer to touch compared to the opposite leg.

10. You may bathe or shower the day following the catheterization. Be careful to avoid slipping as your leg may feel stiff.
11. Resume the same medications you were taking before the catheterization unless otherwise ordered by your physician.
12. If you have any questions or concerns, contact your private physician or call the Barnes Hospital Emergency Department.

My discharge instructions have been explained and a copy has been given to me.

____________________	____________________
Physician's Signature/Date and Time	*Patient/Significant Other/Signature Date and Time*
____________________	
Nurse's Signature/Date and Time	
White copy (place in chart)	***Yellow copy (patient's copy)***

1290-21 Revised 12/94

B

FIGURE **42-2 B,** Post-cardiac catherization (coronary angiography) patient discharge orders. (Courtesy Barnes-Jewish Hospital, St Louis.)

- Because of the normal aging process, an older adult is at risk for skin breakdown and joint stiffness. The client may require assistance with frequent position changes.
- Offer bedpan/urinal every 2 to 3 hours in the older adult client because of age-related changes in the urinary tract.
- Be aware that NPO status in the older adult client may result in dehydration.
- Because the older adult client may be taking multiple medications, be aware of alterations in administration schedules necessary for the diagnostic test caused by the NPO status.

Home Care Considerations

On discharge, client will be instructed to contact the physician (or affiliated emergency department) if the following occurs after cardiac catheterization:

- Bleeding from the catheterization puncture site; apply gentle pressure with a clean gauze or cloth.
- Formation of a knot or lump under the skin that increases in size.
- Worsening of a bruise or its movement down the extremity rather than disappearing.
- Pain at puncture site or in the extremity used for the catheterization.
- Pale and cool to the touch extremity where arterial puncture is made.
- Appearance of redness, swelling, or warmth of the affected extremity.
- Although bathing or showering may be allowed the day after the catheterization, the client should be cautioned to avoid slipping because the leg (if this extremity was used) may feel stiff.
- If procedure performed as outpatient, instruct client not to drive or climb stairs for 24 hours; to avoid sports, strenuous housework, and lifting for 3 days; and to avoid taking baths until wound is healed (Malarkey and McMorrow, 2000).
- After the procedure, client's urinary output needs to be monitored. Encourage fluid intake because dehydration may result from diuretic action of the dye.
- Instruct client to keep follow-up appointments.

Skill 42-3 Assisting With Bone Marrow Aspiration/Biopsy

Bone marrow aspiration is the removal of a small amount of the liquid organic material in the **medullary** canals of selected bones, in particular the sternum and the posterior superior iliac crests (Figure 42-3). In children, the proximal tibia may be used (Pagana and Pagana, 1998). A **biopsy** is the removal of a core of marrow cells for laboratory analysis. Both aspiration and biopsy are used to diagnose leukemias, certain malignancies, anemias, and **thrombocytopenia.** The marrow is examined in a laboratory to reveal the number, size, shape, and development of red blood cells (RBCs) and **megakaryocytes** (platelet precursors).

The sterile procedure is usually performed by a physician assisted by a nurse or unlicensed assistive personnel at the client's bedside and takes approximately 20 minutes. Potential complications of bone marrow aspiration or biopsy are bleeding, especially if a **coagulopathy** is present, infection, and less commonly, organ puncture. The nurse should know normal hematological laboratory values before assisting with the procedure.

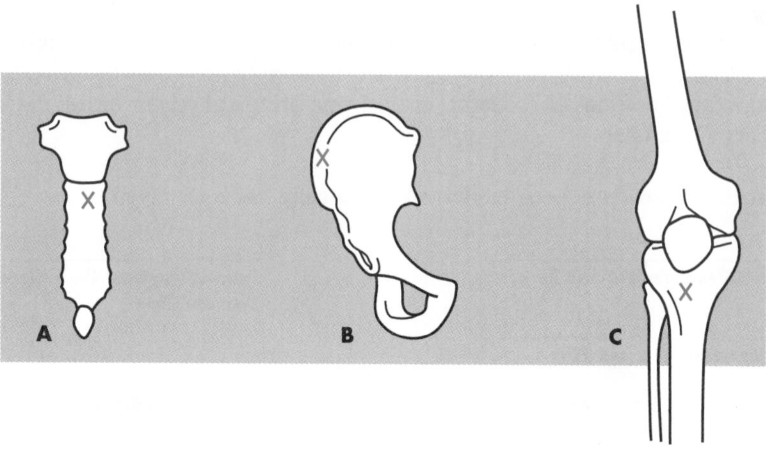

FIGURE **42-3** Anatomical sites (*X*) for bone marrow aspiration. **A,** Sternum between the second and third intercostal spaces. **B,** Iliac crest on the rim or upper posterior surface. **C,** Proximal tibia about 1 to 2 inches below the patella of the infant or small child.

Delegation Considerations

The skill of assisting with bone marrow aspiration may be delegated to assistive personnel if the client is stable. Instruct personnel on proper positioning of client during the procedure. Instruct assistive personnel to take baseline, as well as post-procedure, vital signs and to report these vital signs to the nurse. Caution assistive personnel to be alert for and report signs and symptoms experienced by the client.

Equipment

- Antiseptic solution
- Bone marrow aspiration tray, if available from central supply, which may include: antiseptic solution (e.g., povidone-iodine); gauze sponges (4 × 4); sterile towels for draping; local anesthetic solution (e.g., lidocaine 1%); sterile syringes: two 3-ml, 23- to 25-gauge needles for anesthetic; two 10- and 50-ml for marrow aspiration; two bone marrow needles with inner stylus
- Test tubes and/or glass slides
- Sterile gloves of proper size for physician
- Masks, goggles, and gowns for physician and nurse (check institution's policy) (masks are used for **immunocompromised** clients, including those receiving chemotherapy or high-dose steroid therapy)
- Gauze (2 × 2), tape, and antiseptic ointment
- Pain medication, if ordered (given 30 minutes before procedure)

Step	Rationale
Assessment	
1. Assess client's knowledge of procedure.	Client must be informed of procedure, its purposes, and risks.

- ***Critical Decision Point***
  Obtain a premedication order (i.e., sedative) if client is extremely anxious. Clients who are extremely anxious and who cannot cooperate or remain still during the procedure may require stronger sedatives (Pagana and Pagana, 1998).

Step	Rationale
2. Determines client's level of anxiety and observe verbal and nonverbal behaviors.	Highly anxious clients may be unable to cooperate with procedure.
3. Determine client's ability to assume position required for procedure and ability to remain still.	Required position depends on site used for bone marrow aspiration (e.g., for sternal or tibial biopsy use supine position; for iliac crest biopsy use prone or lateral recumbent position; for vertebral biopsy have client in a seated position). Client must maintain position without moving to avoid complications (Malarkey and McMorrow, 2000).
4. Obtain vital signs.	Provides baseline for comparison with post-procedure vital signs. A potential complication is hemorrhage, especially if client has coagulopathy (Pagana and Pagana, 1998).
5. Assess client's coagulation status: use of anticoagulants, platelet count, and prothrombin time.	Clients with coagulation disorders may not have this procedure done because of risk of excessive bleeding (Pagana and Pagana, 1998).
6. Determine purpose of procedure.	Allows nurse to determine whether aspiration or biopsy will be performed and to anticipate laboratory requisitions.
7. Check whether client has signed a consent form.	The presence of a signed consent form indicates the patient has received a thorough explanation of the procedure and understands the risks and the probability of successful outcome of the procedure (Meiner, 1999).
8. Determine whether client is allergic to antiseptic or anesthetic solutions.	Decreases chance of allergic reactions.

Nursing Diagnosis

Defining characteristics from the assessment data may reveal the following nursing diagnoses for clients requiring this skill:

Anxiety
Fear
Risk for infection
Risk for injury
Deficient knowledge regarding purpose and steps of procedure
Acute pain

Related factors are individualized based on client's condition or needs.

STEP	RATIONALE
PLANNING	
1. **Expected outcomes** following completion of procedure:	
▪ Client can assume position and has little pain.	Client tolerates procedure well.
▪ Client has no bleeding at needle insertion site.	Precautions during procedure prevent bleeding.
▪ Amount of aspirate is sufficient to perform laboratory testing.	
▪ Client explains purpose of procedure and position to be assumed.	Documents learning.
2. Explain steps of skin preparation, anesthetic injection, needle insertion, and position required.	Anticipation of expected sensations and procedural activities reduces anxiety.
IMPLEMENTATION	
NURSE'S RESPONSIBILITY	
1. Wash hands.	Reduces transmission of microorganisms.
2. Set up sterile tray or open supplies to make accessible for physician.	Maintains integrity of sterile field and promotes prompt completion of procedure.
3. Assist client in maintaining correct position (see Assessment, step 3). Reassure client while explaining procedure. Emphasize to client to remain very still and avoid sudden movement throughout the procedure.	Decreases chance of complications occurring during procedure. Explanations increase client comfort and relaxation.
4. Explain to client that pain may occur when lidocaine is injected into the tissues. Pressure may also occur when the bone marrow is aspirated.	Bone marrow aspiration is painful, but lasts for only a few moments. Pre-procedure analgesia may be given to decrease the discomfort. A deep pressure feeling may be experienced as the bone marrow is withdrawn (Chernecky and Berger, 1997).
5. Assess client's condition during procedure, including respiratory status and vital signs if indicated.	Identifies any changes that may indicate complication.
6. Note characteristics of bone marrow aspirate (e.g., amount, color).	Characteristics are used for observation, reporting, and recording.
PHYSICIAN'S RESPONSIBILITY	
1. Wash hands.	Reduces transmission of microorganisms.
2. Select site to be used for bone marrow aspiration.	Sites are chosen for direct access to area of spongy bone. These sites include anterior and posterior iliac spines, iliac crest, body of sternum, and tibia.
3. Apply sterile gloves. Disinfect skin with antiseptic solution and 4 × 4 gauze sponges. Remove gloves and discard.	Removes surface bacteria from skin at area of puncture site.
4. Apply sterile mask and goggles, then new pair of sterile gloves, and drape client with sterile towels.	Maintains surgical asepsis.
5. Inject local anesthetic and allow it to take effect.	Provides optimal effect of anesthesia at time of bone marrow aspiration.
6. Insert bone marrow needle (see illustration) with inner stylus into bone, then advance needle until it reaches area of spongy bone and remove stylus.	Stylus is stiff and has longer level to enter bone with more ease. Spongy bone is location of bone marrow.
7. Attach 10-ml syringe to needle and aspirate bone marrow. For biopsy, screw the core biopsy instrument into the bone and remove plug of tissue.	Amount aspirated is determined by purpose of procedure: small amount (approximately 0.5 to 2.0 ml) is obtained for laboratory test; larger amount, including cells, is obtained by biopsy.
8. Remove needle or biopsy instrument and apply pressure to puncture site. Apply antiseptic ointment and dressing.	Prevents bleeding from puncture site (Pagana and Pagana, 1998). Antiseptic ointment reduces bacterial growth at puncture site.

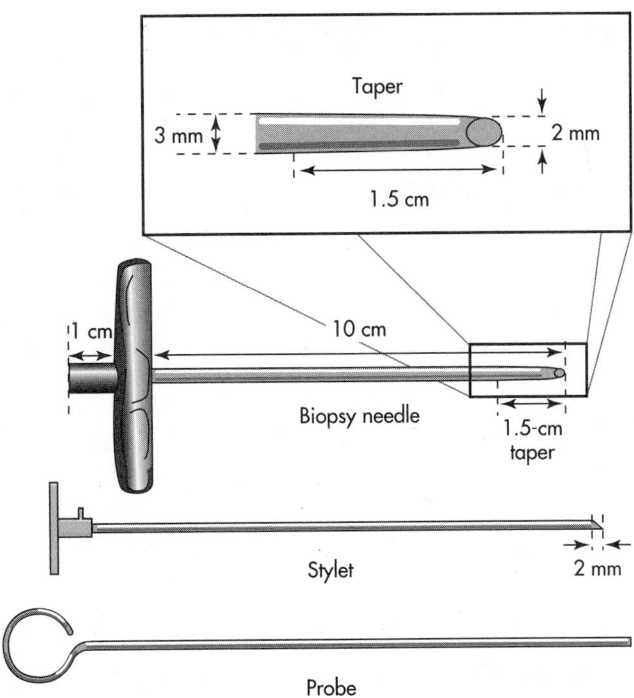

STEP 6 Bone marrow biopsy needle showing shape and size. (From Phipps W, Sands J, Marek J: *Medical-surgical nursing,* ed 6, St Louis, 1999, Mosby.)

STEP	RATIONALE
9. Place the specimen on glass slides or in test tubes.	Allows specimen to be sent for laboratory analysis.

EVALUATION

1. Monitor vital signs. Check hospital policy; may be as often as every 15 minutes for 2 hours.	Verifies client's physiological status in response to potential blood loss.
2. Inspect dressing over puncture site for bleeding, swelling, tenderness, and erythema. Inspect area under client for bleeding.	Determines further blood loss from puncture site. Infection is a potential complication, especially if the patient is leukopenic (Pagana and Pagana, 1998).

• ***Critical Decision Point***
A pressure dressing may be in place. If so, do not remove.

3. Observe client's level of comfort.	Client may require post-procedure analgesia.

UNEXPECTED OUTCOMES AND RELATED INTERVENTIONS

- Client is unable to assume correct position; moves during procedure.
  - Notify physician immediately.
  - Encourage client to remain still.
- Client experiences tenderness, erythema at bone marrow site, decreased blood pressure and increased pulse.
  - Continue to monitor vital signs and aspiration site.
  - Notify physician of findings and obtain further orders.
- Client is unable to discuss procedure.
  - Continue to provide more education or explanation as needed.

RECORDING AND REPORTING

- Record in client's chart name of procedure, location of puncture site, amount and color of marrow aspirated, duration of procedure, client's tolerance to the procedure, vital signs, pain, any complications, laboratory tests ordered, specimen sent, type of dressing over puncture site, and whether drainage is present.
- Report to physician immediately any change in vital signs beyond client's normal limits and any excessive drainage from dressing over puncture site.
- Report results of procedure to nurses on the next shift.

Teaching Considerations

- After explaining this procedure, encourage client to verbalize concerns. Many clients are anxious about procedure.
- Emphasize importance of remaining still during procedure.
- Encourage client to contact physician regarding test results.
- Teach patient to contact physician if tenderness and/or redness appear at puncture site.

Pediatric Considerations

- Test can be frightening for child because it is done behind his or her field of vision
- Conscious or unconscious sedation is usually used.
- Prepare child of preschool age before the procedure; having child recall next procedural step can serve as distraction mechanism (Wong and others, 1999).

Gerontological Considerations

- Older adults with arthritis may have difficulty sustaining the position required for the procedure.
- Assess for pain; the older adult may not ask for pain relief.
- Be aware that older adults may have specific fears and anxiety related to falling and fatigue.
- Older adults have increased infection rates because of age-related changes of decreased immunocompetence, presence of pathological conditions, and increased disability.

Home Care Considerations

- Instruct client that some persons experience tenderness at the puncture site for several days after the study and that mild analgesia may be ordered by the physician.
- Instruct client to notify physician if any redness, swelling, or signs of infection develop.
- Instruct client that mild analgesics may be needed for several days after this procedure because of tenderness at the puncture site (Pagana and Pagana, 1998).
- If client is transferred to long-term care facility, ensure thorough communication between facilities regarding results of procedure and client condition.

Skill 42-4 Assisting With Bronchoscopy

Bronchoscopy is the examination of the **tracheobronchial tree** through a lighted tube containing mirrors. The tube, or bronchoscope, most commonly used is a flexible **fiberoptic** bronchoscope. The fiberoptic bronchoscope has **lumens** for visualization and for obtaining sputum, foreign bodies, and biopsy specimens. Laser ablation of endotracheal lesions may be performed through the bronchoscope.

Bronchoscopy may be an emergency or elective procedure and is performed for diagnostic or therapeutic reasons. The main purposes of this procedure are to aspirate excessive sputum or mucous plugs that cannot be sufficiently suctioned nasotracheally, to visualize the tracheobronchial tree for assessment of abnormalities of the mucosa, and to remove foreign bodies. This procedure would be contraindicated in clients with hypercapnea and severe shortness of breath and clients with tracheal stenosis (Pagana and Pagana, 1998). Potential complications of bronchoscopy may include fever, infection, hypoxemia, laryngospasm, pneumothorax, aspiration, hemorrhage (after biopsy), and cardiac arrest. The nurse should be able to perform nasotracheal and orotracheal suctioning before assisting with the procedure.

This procedure is usually performed by a physician, usually a pulmonary specialist or surgeon, in about 30 to 45 minutes. The procedure may be performed at the bedside or in a specially equipped endoscopy room (Pagana and Pagana, 1998).

Delegation Considerations

The skill of assisting with bronchoscopy may be delegated to assistive personnel if the client is stable. Instruct personnel on proper positioning of client during the procedure. Instruct assistive personnel to take baseline, as well as post-procedure, vital signs and to report these vital signs to the nurse. Caution assistive personnel to be alert for and report signs and symptoms of respiratory distress experienced by the client and to immediately report them to the nurse. If the client requires intravenous conscious sedation (IVCS) for the bronchoscopy, delegation is inappropriate. In addition, delegation of assisting with bronchoscopy with unstable clients (i.e., those on ventilatory support or receiving blood products) is inappropriate.

Equipment

- Antiseptic solution for hand washing
- Bronchoscopy tray, if available from central supply, which may include: flexible fiberoptic bronchoscope (Figure 42-4); gauze sponges (4 × 4); local anesthetic spray (lidocaine); sterile tracheal suction catheters (see Chapter 17); diazepam, midazolam, or other sedative for IV sedation; oxygen, resuscitative equipment, pulse oximeter, cardiac monitor for IV sedation; sterile gloves; sterile water-soluble lubricating jelly. Petroleum-based lubricants should not be used because of the hazard of aspiration and subsequent pneumonia.
- Mask and goggles for physician and nurse
- Emesis basin
- Oxygen equipment

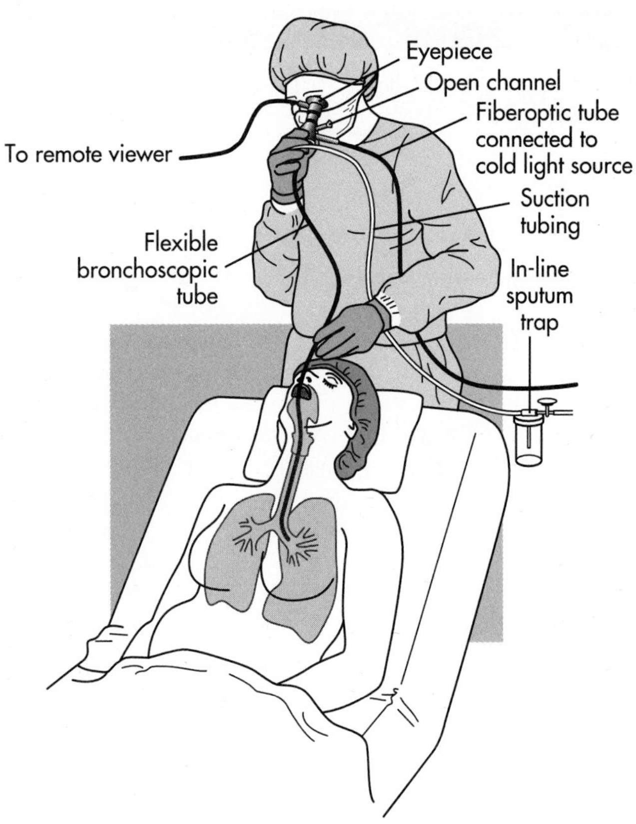

FIGURE **42-4** Flexible fiberoptic bronchoscopy.

STEP	RATIONALE
ASSESSMENT	
1. Assess client's knowledge of procedure; observe verbal and nonverbal behaviors.	Determines client's level of understanding and anxiety.
• ***Critical Decision Point*** *Because client may fear the diagnosis that may follow, allow client to verbalize feelings and concerns regarding this procedure.*	
2. Obtain vital signs and oxygen saturation.	Baseline data provides for comparison with findings during and after procedure.
3. Assess respiratory status: type of cough, sputum produced, and lung sounds.	Provides for comparison with respiratory status during and after procedure.
4. Determine purpose of procedure: for sputum aspiration, for assessment, for tissue biopsy, or for removal of foreign body.	Enables nurse to anticipate needs of client and physician.
5. Check whether client signed a consent form (check institution's policy). This must be done before administration of pre-procedural sedative or IVCS.	The presence of a signed consent form indicates the patient has received a thorough explanation of the procedure and understands the risks and the probability of successful outcome of the procedure (Meiner, 1999).
6. Determine whether client is allergic to local anesthetic used for spraying throat (lidocaine usually used).	Allergy could cause laryngeal edema or laryngospasm.
7. Assess need for pre-procedure medication (usually atropine and narcotic or sedative).	Atropine decreases secretions and inhibits vagal-stimulated bradycardia; narcotics or sedatives relieve anxiety and decrease discomfort (Pagana and Pagana, 1998).
8. If using IVCS, assess pulse and respiratory rate, blood pressure, and oxygen saturation before administration of IVCS.	Provides baseline data.

STEP	RATIONALE
9. Assess time client last ingested food. Client should have been NPO for 8 hours before procedure.	Reduces risk of aspiration.

NURSING DIAGNOSIS

Defining characteristics from the assessment data may reveal the following nursing diagnoses for clients requiring this skill:

- Anxiety
- Risk for aspiration
- Ineffective breathing pattern
- Fear
- Impaired gas exchange
- Risk for infection
- Risk for injury
- Deficient knowledge regarding purpose and steps of procedure

Related factors are individualized based on client's condition or needs.

PLANNING

STEP	RATIONALE
1. **Expected outcomes** following completion of procedure:	
▪ Client has no respiratory complications.	Client tolerates procedure well.
▪ Client has minimal pain.	Minimal trauma caused by bronchoscope.
▪ Physician is able to observe, suction, and obtain specimens from tracheobronchial tree.	Indicates that purpose of procedure was achieved.
▪ Client recovers from sedation without respiratory complications or change in level of consciousness.	Sedation adequate.
▪ Client explains procedure and position to be assumed.	Demonstrates client's understanding.
2. Explain procedure to client.	Reduces anxiety and increases cooperation.
3. Assist client in maintaining position desired by physician: semi-Fowler's or supine.	Provides maximal visualization of lower airway and adequate lung expansion.
4. Remove and safely store client's dentures.	Minimizes chance of airway obstruction.
5. Make sure client is NPO at least 8 hours before procedure.	Decreases risk of aspiration of gastric contents.

IMPLEMENTATION

NURSE'S RESPONSIBILITY

STEP	RATIONALE
1. Instruct client not to swallow local anesthetic; provide emesis basin for expectoration of local anesthetic.	
2. Assist client through procedure with explanations.	Although premedicated and drowsy, clients need to be reminded not to change position and to cooperate. Reinforce that client will be able to breathe during procedure.
3. Assess client's respiratory status during procedure: observe degree of restlessness and respiratory rate; observe capillary refill, color of nail beds, and pulse oximetery.	Bronchoscope may cause feelings of suffocation; in addition, because airway is partially occluded, client may become hypoxic during observations.
• ***Critical Decision Point*** *Oxygen is usually administered through bronchoscope.*	
4. Note characteristics of suctioned material. Small amount of bleeding in suctioned material is expected because of tissue trauma.	Information used to record and report and to make further client observations.
5. Using gloved hand, wipe client's mouth and nose to remove lubricant after bronchoscope is removed.	Promotes hygiene and comfort.
6. Do not allow client to eat or drink until the tracheobronchial anesthesia has worn off and gag reflex has returned, usually 2 hours. Use tongue depressor to touch pharynx to test for presence of gag reflex.	Prevents aspiration.

STEP	RATIONALE

PHYSICIAN'S RESPONSIBILITY

1. Wash hands. — Reduces transmission of microorganisms.
2. Spray nasopharynx and oropharynx with topical anesthetic. Lidocaine is commonly used for throat spraying. — Throat is sprayed early for anesthesia to take effect.
   - ***Critical Decision Point***
     When a client is intubated or has a tracheostomy, anesthetic spray may not be needed.
3. Attach bronchoscope to machine for light source. — Another physician, OR personnel, or nurse attaches machine cable to bronchoscope.
4. Apply goggles, mask, and sterile gloves; then introduce bronchoscope into mouth to pharynx, and pass through glottis. May use more anesthetic spray at glottis to prevent cough reflex. Pass tube into trachea and bronchi. — Bronchoscope must be passed through upper airway structures to promote visualization of lower airways. Trachea and bronchi are observed for lesions and obstructions. For intubated client, bronchoscope is passed through endotracheal tube. Adaptor accompanies bronchoscope and may be used for Ambu bag or ventilator use.
5. Obtain cytological specimens with wire brush or curette. — Cytological specimens are obtained to diagnose carcinoma.

EVALUATION

1. Monitor vital signs. — Verifies physiological response.
2. Observe character and amount of sputum. Physician may order serial sputum collection for 24 hours for cytological examination. — Sputum may be blood tinged, which indicates superficial tissue damage. Severe hemoptysis is an emergency.
3. Observe respiratory status closely. — May provide evidence of laryngeal bronchospasm (Pagana and Pagana, 1997).
4. Assess for level of sedation and level of consciousness. — Determines client's response to IVCS.
5. Assess for return of gag reflex. Gag reflex usually returns in approximately 2 hours (Pagana and Pagana, 1997). — No food or fluids are given until gag reflex returns (Chernecky and Berger, 1997).
6. Ask client to describe post-procedure normal and abnormal symptoms. — Evaluates client's understanding.

UNEXPECTED OUTCOMES AND RELATED INTERVENTIONS

- Client experiences laryngospasm and bronchospasm indicated by sudden, severe shortness of breath.
  - Call physician immediately.
  - Emergency resuscitation equipment should be readily available.
- Client experiences hypoxemia indicated by gradual shortness of breath and decreasing level of consciousness.
  - Maintain airway.
  - Monitor oxygen saturation.
  - Notify physician immediately.
- Client hemorrhages.
  - Notify physician immediately.
  - Follow specific post-procedural orders related to findings.
- Client remains sedated with decreased respiration or blood pressure, decreased oxygen saturation, or decreased level of consciousness.
  - Continued monitoring is necessary.
  - May require administration of narcotic reversal agent.

RECORDING AND REPORTING

- Record in nurse's notes name of procedure (include biopsy if performed), duration of procedure, client's tolerance of procedure and complications, and collection and disposition of specimen.
- Report excessive bleeding or respiratory difficulty after procedure or changes in vital signs beyond client's normal limits to physician immediately.
- Report results of procedure to nurses on the next shift.

TEACHING CONSIDERATIONS

- Before procedure, instruct client to perform good mouth care to decrease risk of introducing bacteria into lungs during procedure (Pagana and Pagana, 1998).
- If bronchoscopy is performed on an outpatient basis, client is kept in the department until gag reflex returns and client is able to swallow water easily (Phipps and others, 1999).

- Inform client to arrange for transportation home after an ambulatory procedure because client will not be permitted to drive for 24 hours after receiving sedation (Chernecky and Berger, 1997).
- If IVCS is to be used, explain to client purpose and expected effects of sedation and post-procedure instructions regarding client's care and necessary precautions.
- Instruct client how to perform controlled coughing techniques for obtaining sputum samples, if ordered (see Chapter 41).
- Encourage client to be involved in self-care by contacting physician regarding test results.
- Instruct client on how to obtain serial sputum specimens if ordered.

Pediatric Considerations

- In children, the procedure is most frequently performed to remove foreign bodies from larynx or trachea and is often done under general anesthesia. Client is placed in the lateral position after the procedure to prevent aspiration.
- Children are at higher risk of hypoxemia than adults because of their smaller bronchus and the bronchoscope decreasing the available breathing space (Pagana and Pagana, 1998).
- Follow-up care after the foreign body is removed includes chest physiotherapy as needed, monitoring for respiratory distress, and education of parents (Wong and others, 1999).

Gerontological Considerations

- Keep frail older adult warm to maintain core temperature at comfortable, safe levels (Worfolk, 1997).
- Be aware that NPO status in the older adult client may result in dehydration.
- Postoperative restlessness could indicate hypoxemia, not pain. Inappropriate administration of a narcotic analgesic could further deplete the body's oxygen supply (Eliopoulos, 1997).
- Elderly client may experience post-procedure pain related to positioning.
- Because of multiple medications the older adult client may be taking, be aware of alterations in administration schedules necessary as a result of the NPO status for the diagnostic test.

Home Care Considerations

- Outpatients should be instructed to notify the physician if the following symptoms develop: fever, chest pain or discomfort, dyspnea, wheezing, or hemoptysis.
- Written instructions regarding names and phone numbers of persons to contact reinforce oral instructions.
- Throat discomfort may be managed with warm saline gargles or throat lozenges (Phipps and others, 1999).

Skill 42-5 Assisting With Electrocardiogram

An electrocardiogram (ECG or EKG) is a graphic representation of the electrical impulses generated by the heart during the cardiac cycle. The electrical impulses are conducted to the body's surface, where they are detected by electrodes placed on the limbs and chest. The electrodes carry the electrical impulses to a continuously running graph that plots the ECG wave pattern. The appearance of the ECG pattern helps diagnose whether there are any abnormalities interfering with electrical conduction through the heart. The 12-lead ECG is composed of five electrodes. One electrode is placed on each of the four extremities, and one is successively placed at varying sites on the chest.

If a continuous ECG recording is needed over an extended period of time, a Holter monitor is used. A Holter monitor is a small, portable device that records electrical activity of the heart for up to 24 hours. The ECG is recorded on magnetic tape and monitors cardiac rhythm during activity, rest, and sleep.

Delegation Considerations

The skill of assisting with the electrocardiogram is routinely delegated to assistive personnel who are specifically skilled in obtaining the measurement. This procedure should only be delegated to those personnel.

Equipment

- ECG machine
- ECG leads or electrodes (self-stick adhesive)
- Electrode gel (optional)
- Alcohol wipes
- Razor

Step	Rationale

Assessment

1. Determine rationale for obtaining ECG.

ECG represents the electrical impulses during the cardiac cycle and may be done to determine baseline cardiac function (e.g., preoperative, prediagnostic testing) or when client experiences chest discomfort (Chernecky and Berger, 1997).

2. If client reports chest pain, assess character of pain thoroughly.

Pain may be related to any number of factors (e.g., positioning, trauma, GI disturbance). Characteristics will help in determining therapy.

- ***Critical Decision Point***
  Crushing substernal chest pain that radiates to jaw or arm may indicate angina or myocardial infarction. Chest pain should be brought to immediate attention of physician.

3. Assess client's knowledge of procedure; observe verbal and nonverbal behaviors. If Holter monitor is selected, client may require further explanation of how cardiac cycle is monitored.

Identifies needed education and client's anxiety level.

- ***Critical Decision Point***
  Assure the client that the flow of electric current is from the client and that nothing will be felt during the procedure (Pagana and Pagana, 1998).

4. Obtain baseline vital signs.

Provides for comparison with vital sign data at later date.

Nursing Diagnosis

Defining characteristics from the assessment data may reveal the following nursing diagnoses for clients requiring this skill:

Anxiety
Fear
Deficient knowledge regarding purpose and steps of procedure

Related factors are individualized based on client's condition or needs.

Planning

1. **Expected outcomes** following completion of procedure:
   - Client tolerates procedure without anxiety or discomfort.
     Appropriate preparation decreases anxiety.
   - Client discusses purpose and steps of procedure.
     Demonstrates client's understanding.
2. Close room door or bedside curtains.
   Provides privacy.
3. Prepare client for procedure:
   a. Remove client's clothing or lower gown to expose only the client's chest and arms. Keep the abdomen and thighs covered.
   Facilitates correct placement of cardiac leads and minimizes client's embarrassment. Improper lead placement produces artifact, which may necessitate repeating the test (Chernecky and Berger, 1997).
   b. Place client in supine position.
   Exposes client for lead placement.
   c. Instruct client to lie still without talking (12-lead ECG only) and to not cross legs.
   Body movement produces artifact, which may necessitate repeating the test (Chernecky and Berger, 1997).

Implementation

1. Wash hands.

Reduces transmission of microorganisms.

2. Cleanse and prepare skin; wipe sites with alcohol. It may be necessary to shave the chest if large amounts of hair are present. In clients who are very thin and emaciated, it may be difficult to secure electrodes because of bony structure and decreased amount of subcutaneous tissue.

Alcohol defats the skin and promotes adherence of leads (electrodes) to chest or extremity (Pagana and Pagana, 1998). Poor skin cleansing produces artifact, which may necessitate repeating the test (Chernecky and Berger, 1997).

STEP	RATIONALE
3. Apply self-sticking electrode and attach leads. (If self-sticking leads are not available, apply electrode paste to skin before attaching leads.) For 12-lead ECG: a. Chest (**precordial** leads) (see illustration): V_1—Fourth **intercostal space (ICS)** at right sternal border. V_2—Fourth ICS at left sternal border. V_3—Midway between V_2 and V_4. V_4—Fifth ICS at midclavicular line. V_5—Left anterior axillary line at level of V_4 horizontally. V_6—Left midaxillary line at level of V_4 horizontally. b. Extremities: one lead on each extremity.	Position of leads promotes proper display of ECG on paper. Electrode paste ensures electrical conduction between the skin and electrodes (Pagana and Pagana, 1998).

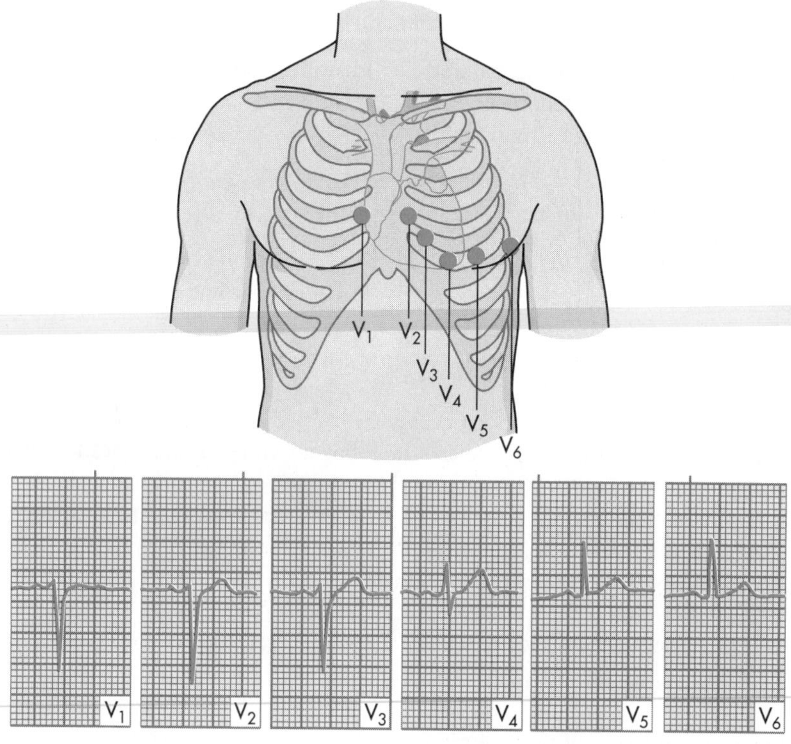

STEP **3a** Anatomical placement of precordial leads. (From Phipps W, Sands J, Marek J: *Medical-surgical nursing*, ed 6, St Louis, 1999, Mosby.)

STEP	RATIONALE
4. Obtain tracing; 12-lead ECG may be obtained without removing precordial leads. If client experiences severe chest pain, notify physician, continue to monitor cardiac activity with ECG, obtain vital signs, and remain with client.	Transfers electrocardiac conduction to ECG tracing paper for subsequent analysis by cardiologist. Chest pain experienced during the study may be correlated to an arrhythmia on the ECG (Pagana and Pagana, 1998).
5. Disconnect leads, wipe excess electrode paste from chest, and wash hands.	Promotes comfort and hygiene. Reduces transmission of microorganisms.
6. Deliver ECG tracing to appropriate laboratory or heart station.	Provides for review of ECG by cardiologist.

EVALUATION

1. Although the procedure is painless, it is important to note and document if the client is experiencing any chest discomfort during the procedure.	Determines worsening of condition.
2. Measure vital signs.	Electrocardiac changes may result in vital sign alterations.

Unexpected Outcomes and Related Interventions

- Client experiences chest pain (not result of test, but client's condition).
  - Continue to monitor.
  - Follow specific post-procedural orders related to findings.
  - Notify physician.
- Client experiences anxiety.
  - Reassess factors contributing to anxiety.

Recording and Reporting

- Record in nurse's notes when ECG was obtained (date and time) and where tracing was sent, rationale for obtaining ECG (e.g., pain, discomfort, preop, postop), and baseline vital signs.
- Report any unexpected outcomes immediately.

Teaching Considerations

- After explaining procedure, assure client that flow of electric current is from client to machine. Client will not feel anything during procedure.
- If Holter monitoring is selected, instruct client to maintain an accurate diary of activities (detailed documentation of activities and occurrence of chest pain assist in diagnoses of condition).
- Inform client that the Holter monitoring interpretation will be available in a few days.
- Encourage client to contact physician regarding test results.

Gerontological Considerations

- Be aware that medications that can affect results, including digitalis, quinidine, and barbiturates (Pagana and Pagana, 1998).

Skill 42-6 Assisting With Endoscopy

Endoscopy is any study that allows direct visualization of an internal organ or structure by means of a long, flexible fiberoptic scope with a light source attached. For visualization of the upper GI tract, esophagoscopy, gastroscopy, or duodenoscopy is performed, or more frequently, esophagogastroduodenoscopy, which permits visualization of esophagus, stomach, and duodenum in one examination. For visual examination of the lower GI tract, a proctoscopy, sigmoidoscopy, or colonoscopy may be performed. Typically, these clients receive IVCS.

Besides direct observation, endoscopy enables biopsy of suspicious tissue, polyp removal, injection of variceal blood vessels, and performance of many other procedures. Areas of stricture can be dilated and stented during endoscopy (Pagana and Pagana, 1998).

Endoscopy of the upper GI tract is indicated to diagnose lesions such as gastric or duodenal ulcers and neoplasms, to locate sources of and study upper GI bleeding and motility and identify strictures and obstructions, and to diagnose hiatal hernias and esophageal and gastric **varices.** Both upper and lower GI endoscopic examinations are performed in a specially equipped endoscopic unit.

Delegation Considerations

The skill of assisting with endoscopy may be delegated to assistive personnel if the client is stable. Instruct personnel on proper positioning of client during the procedure. Instruct assistive personnel to take baseline, as well as post-procedure, vital signs and to report these vital signs to the nurse. Caution assistive personnel to be alert for and report signs and symptoms of gastrointestinal problems or respiratory distress experienced by the client and to immediately report them to the nurse. If the client requires intravenous conscious sedation (IVCS) for the endoscopy delegation is inappropriate. In addition, delegation of assisting with endoscopy when the client has active gastrointestinal bleeding and/or is unstable is inappropriate.

Equipment

- Antiseptic solution for hand washing
- Endoscopy tray
- Fiberoptic endoscope (Figure 42-5)
- Camera
- Solutions for biopsy specimens
- Local anesthetic spray
- Tracheal suction equipment (see Chapter 13)
- Blood pressure equipment
- Sterile water-soluble jelly
- Sterile gloves for physician
- Emesis basin
- Intravenous fluid and equipment for IV start (optional)
- Diazepam, midazolam, or other sedative for IV sedation (optional)
- Oxygen, resuscitative equipment, pulse oximeter, cardiac monitor if IVCS is used
- Mask
- Gown
- Gloves
- Goggles

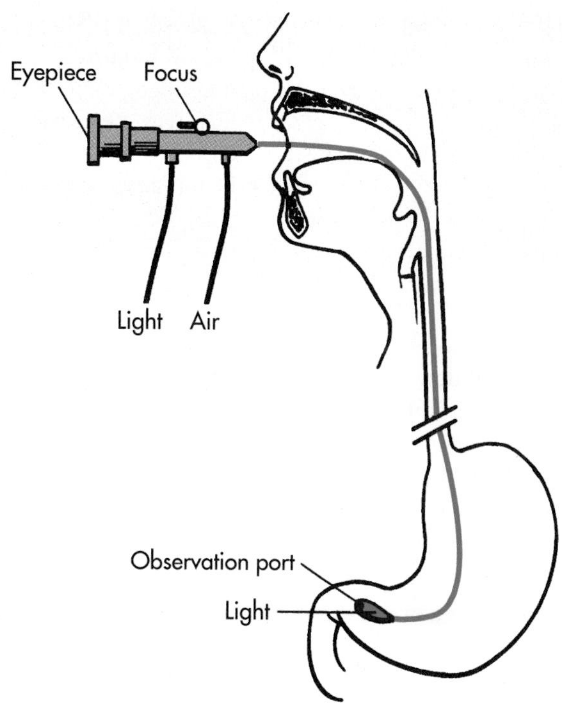

FIGURE 42-5 Stomach may be visualized by means of a fiberscope.

STEP	RATIONALE
ASSESSMENT	
1. Assess client's knowledge of procedure; observe verbal and nonverbal behaviors.	Determines client's understanding and level of anxiety.
2. Determine if GI bleeding is present. Observe character of emesis, stool, and nasogastric tube drainage.	Test is contraindicated in clients with severe upper GI bleeding because viewing lens may get covered with blood clots, preventing visualization (Pagana and Pagana, 1997).

- ***Critical Decision Point***
  If client is actively bleeding, physician may order stomach be lavaged and aspirated clear of clots before procedure is attempted.

STEP	RATIONALE
3. Determine purpose of procedure: biopsy, examination, or coagulation of bleeding sites.	Enables nurse to anticipate equipment needs.
4. Check for completion of signed consent form (check institutional policy).	The presence of a signed consent form indicates the patient has received a thorough explanation of the procedure and understands the risks and the probability of successful outcome of the procedure (Meiner, 1999).
5. Verify that client has been NPO for at least 8 hours for endoscopy of upper GI tract.	Introduction of endoscope can induce vomiting. Empty stomach reduces risk of aspiration of stomach contents (SGNA, 1998).

- ***Critical Decision Point***
  If endoscopy of the upper GI tract is an emergency procedure and client has had something to eat or drink within the last 24 hours, be sure physician is informed first.

STEP	RATIONALE
6. Obtain pulse and respiratory rate, blood pressure, and oxygen saturation before administration of IVCS.	Provides baseline data.
7. Verify that client does not have esophageal diverticulum.	Esophageal diverticulum is contraindication to endoscopy because scope can easily fall into diverticulum and perforate its wall (Pagana and Pagana, 1998).

STEP	RATIONALE
8. Review physician's orders for pre-procedure medication and IVCS:	
a. Diazepam	Decreases anxiety and promotes muscle relaxation (SGNA, 1998).
b. Meperedine	Decreases pain and induces sedation (SGNA, 1998).
c. Midazolam (given in endoscopy unit just before examination)	Produces amnesic effect; diminishes recall of events during procedure (SGNA, 1998).

NURSING DIAGNOSIS

Defining characteristics from the assessment data may reveal the following nursing diagnoses for clients requiring this skill:

- Anxiety
- Risk for aspiration
- Ineffective breathing pattern
- Fear
- Impaired gas exchange
- Risk for infection
- Risk for injury
- Deficient knowledge regarding purpose and steps of procedure
- Acute pain

Related factors are individualized based on client's condition or needs.

PLANNING

1. **Expected outcomes** following completion of procedure:	
▪ Client has little pain or discomfort, does not aspirate, and has no post-procedure bleeding.	Indicates absence of complications and tolerance of procedure.
▪ Client is without respiratory complications or change in level of consciousness.	Recovers from sedation.
▪ Client describes purposes and steps of procedure.	Documents client understanding.
2. Prepare client.	
a. Explain steps of procedure, including sensations to expect.	Nurse can relieve anxiety and answer client's questions.
b. Explain purpose and effects of IVCS.	
c. Administer pain medication or pre-procedure medication.	Promotes relaxation and reduces anxiety.

IMPLEMENTATION

NURSE'S RESPONSIBILITY

1. Wash hands and apply gloves, goggles, and mask.	Reduces transmission of organisms.
2. Remove client's dentures or other dental appliances.	Prevents dislodgment of dental structures during intubation phase.
3. Assist client in maintaining left lateral decubitus position (Pagana and Pagana, 1997).	
4. Ensure IV line is patent. RN will administer sedation for IVCS (according to institution policy).	Provides route for emergency medications.
5. Assist client through procedure:	
a. Anticipate needs and promote comfort.	Client is unable to speak after tube is passed into throat.
b. Tell client what is happening.	Reassures client about procedure and how long it will last.
c. Place tissue specimens in proper laboratory containers.	Ensures proper labeling and preparation of specimens for microscopic examination.
d. Suction if client begins to vomit or accumulate saliva.	Prevents aspiration of gastric contents or oral secretions. Ensures client safety.
e. Assist client to comfortable position, then wash hands.	Promotes rest and relaxation.

STEP	RATIONALE
PHYSICIAN'S RESPONSIBILITY	
1. Wash hands.	Reduces transmission of microorganisms.
2. Spray nasopharynx and oropharynx with local anesthetic (usually xylocaine).	Topical anesthetic decreases the gag reflex caused by passage of the endoscope (Pagana and Pagana, 1997)
3. Apply gown, mask, goggles, and gloves.	Adheres to standard precautions.
4. Attach distal end of endoscope to light source (see Figure 42-5, p. 1234).	Provides for direct visualization of upper GI tract.
5. Position client in left lateral (Sim's) position.	Provides for airway clearance if client gags and vomits gastric contents.
6. Slowly pass endoscope into mouth, esophagus, stomach, or duodenum.	Provides visualization of structures.
7. Insufflate air through endoscope into upper GI tract.	Distends GI structures for better visualization.
8. Examine or perform biopsy of structures.	Provides data from which diagnosis is made.
EVALUATION	
1. Monitor vital signs and O_2 saturation according to hospital policy. May be as often as every 15 minutes for 2 hours.	Change in vital signs can indicate new bleeding in GI tract or over-sedation.
• ***Critical Decision Point*** *Initially, after procedure, client may experience internal bleeding without visible signs of blood loss.*	
2. Assess for level of sedation and level of consciousness.	Determines client's response to IVCS.
3. Observe for pain.	Sudden abdominal pain can indicate rupture of abdominal organs.
4. Evaluate emesis or aspirate for frank or **occult blood** (see Chapter 41).	Indicates gastrointestinal bleeding.
5. Assess for return of gag reflex, usually in 2 to 4 hours (Pagana and Pagana, 1998). Provide oral hygiene when gag reflex returns.	Determines when effects of anesthetic have disappeared. Gag reflex prevents aspiration.
6. Ask client to state post-procedure dietary and activity limitations.	Evaluates understanding.

UNEXPECTED OUTCOMES AND RELATED INTERVENTIONS:

- Client has abdominal pain, fever, or bleeding.
  - Continue to monitor vital signs.
  - Notify physician of findings.
- Client develops dyspnea or aspiration pneumonia.
  - Follow specific post-procedural orders related to findings.
  - Notify physician.
- Client remains sedated with decreased respiration or blood pressure, decreased oxygen saturation, and decreased level of consciousness.
  - Continue monitoring vital signs, perform pulse oximetry.
  - Notify physician immediately.
  - Client may require administration of narcotic reversal agent.
- Client's vital signs indicate deterioration of condition.
  - Follow specific post-procedural orders related to findings.
  - Notify physician.

RECORDING AND REPORTING

- Record in nurse's notes the procedure, duration, client's tolerance, and collection and disposition of specimen.
- Report onset of bleeding, abdominal pain, dyspnea, and vital sign changes to physician
- Report to nurse in charge the duration of procedure, client's tolerance, and changes in vital signs or condition.

TEACHING CONSIDERATIONS

- Inform client of pre-procedure medication and anticipated effects.
- Explain method for endoscope insertion.
- Explain that client will be unable to speak when the endoscope is positioned in the esophagus.
- Make sure client knows not to eat or drink until gag reflex returns.
- Inform client that insertion of endoscope into mouth may cause feeling of inability to breathe. Assure client that suffocation will not occur.
- Encourage client to contact physician regarding test results.
- Some institutions may provide written discharge instructions (Figure 42-6).

DIGESTIVE DISEASE CLINICAL CENTER
ENDOSCOPY UNIT
BARNES HOSPITAL
PATIENT DISCHARGE INSTRUCTIONS

Patient Name: ____________________

OP # ____________________

You have just had a diagnostic and/or therapeutic procedure performed in the Barnes Hospital Digestive Diseases Clinical Center. Please contact your physician promptly or go to the emergency room if you develop persistent or large amounts of bleeding or persistent or increasing pain.

Private doctor's office # ____________________

Digestive Disease Clinical Center # (314) 362-5673. (8:00 a.m. - 4:30 p.m.)

After 4:30 p.m. call Barnes Hospital Operator #(314)362-5000 and ask for the G.I. Fellow "ON CALL".

Patient Instructions: Follow instructions checked

1) _______ The procedure on your GI tract required medication to assist you in relaxing. Rest at home for the remainder of the day and night. Do not drive or perform any activity that requires you to be completely alert during this recovery period. Alcohol should not be used during this period.

2) _______ Do not eat or drink until you are able to swallow without difficulty.

3) _______ Avoid roughage for 14 days (this includes nuts, popcorn, seeds, fresh fruits and raw vegetables).

4) _______ Do not take aspirin or aspirin-like products (such as Alka-Seltzer, Bufferin or Advil) for 14 days.

5) _______ Resume normal activities and diet.

6) _______ Additional instructions: ____________________

____

____

____

____

Follow-up Care:

You should call Dr. ____________________ on ____________________

Ordered by: ____________________

Issued by: ____________________

Signature indicates that you acknowledge receipt of these discharge instructions.

Patient ____________________

Responsible Party ____________________

Relationship to Patient ____________________

Date: ____________________

3160-15 New 5/88

FIGURE 42-6 Discharge orders for endoscopy. (Courtesy Barnes-Jewish Hospital, St Louis.)

PEDIATRIC CONSIDERATIONS

- Child requires sedation or general anesthesia.
- Child needs preparation for the procedure.
- Introduction of the endoscope in infants and small children who have a narrow and collapsible airway may result in respiratory distress (SGNA, 1998).

GERONTOLOGICAL CONSIDERATIONS

- Removal of dentures may cause embarrassment to client.
- Older adult clients may have reduced drug clearance from decreased glomerular filtration rate (GFR) and nephron activity or decreased hepatic function. Therefore the nurse must monitor the effects of medications given to the older adult client (Phipps, and others, 1999).
- Because of age-related changes in the older adult, the gastric mucosa is thinner, which increases the incidence of irritation and ulceration (Phipps, and others, 1999).
- Assess skin integrity of client who has been lying still on examining table. Older adult clients are at greater risk for skin breakdown.
- Keep frail older adult warm to maintain core temperature at safe, comfortable levels (Worfolk, 1997).
- When older adult client recovers from IVCS, offer bedpan/urinal every 2 to 3 hours because of age-related changes in the urinary tract.
- Be aware that NPO status in the older adult client may result in dehydration.
- Because of multiple medications the older adult client may be taking, be aware of alterations in administration schedules necessary as a result of the NPO status for the diagnostic test.
- The older adult may experience dehydration and exhaustion from test preparation. If the procedure is done on an outpatient basis, it may be helpful to have someone stay with the client.

HOME CARE CONSIDERATIONS

- Explain that client may be hoarse or have sore throat after procedure. Ice chips or anesthetic lozenges can be given after gag reflex returns.
- Instruct client to drink fluids to promote dye excretion.
- A warm tub bath may be soothing if rectal discomfort occurs after lower GI tract endoscopy.

Skill 42-7 Assisting With Lumbar Puncture

A lumbar puncture, also called a spinal puncture or spinal tap, involves the introduction of a spinal needle into the **subarachnoid space** of the spinal column. The actual procedure is performed by a physician who may be assisted by a nurse or by assistive personnel.

The purposes of a lumbar puncture are to measure **cerebrospinal fluid (CSF)** pressure in the subarachnoid space, to obtain CSF for visual and laboratory examination, and to inject anesthetic, diagnostic, or therapeutic agents. A baseline neurological assessment needs to be done to evaluate the client's strength, sensation, and leg movement.

This procedure is contraindicated if there is evidence of greatly increased **intracranial pressure** because the sudden release of pressure may cause **herniation** of the brain structures through the **foramen magnum.** This herniation compresses the brainstem, which contains the vital cardiac, respiratory, and vasomotor centers, and sudden death may result. Lumbar puncture is useful in the diagnosis of meningitis, encephalitis, brain or spinal cord tumors, and cerebral hemorrhage.

DELEGATION CONSIDERATIONS

The skill of assisting with a lumbar puncture may be delegated to assistive personnel if the client is stable. Instruct personnel on proper positioning of client during the procedure. Instruct assistive personnel to take baseline, as well as post-procedure, vital signs and to report these vital signs to the nurse. Caution assistive personnel to be alert for and report signs and symptoms experienced by the client.

EQUIPMENT

- Lumbar puncture tray, including: Antiseptic solution (e.g., povidone-iodine); ten gauze sponges (4 × 4); sterile towels; three spinal needles (various sizes) with inner obturators (5 to 12.5 cm long; infants need 5-cm needle); alcohol swabs; anesthetic agent (e.g., lidocaine 1%); syringes (3 to 5 ml); two rolled bath towels; needles ($\frac{5}{8}$ inch, 25 gauge to $\frac{1}{2}$ inch, 21 gauge)
- Sterile gloves (check physician's size)
- Masks (optional)
- Goggles (optional)
- Glass or plastic **manometer** with three-way stopcock
- Four test tubes
- Antiseptic ointment
- Band-aids or 2 × 2 gauze dressing
- Straight chair for physician

STEP	RATIONALE

ASSESSMENT

Step	Rationale
1. Assess for client's ability to understand and follow directions.	Procedure requires client to follow directions closely and assume proper position. Clients with neurological problems may have reduced level of consciousness.
2. Assess musculoskeletal flexibility of client to assume lateral decubitus (fetal) position.	Lateral decubitus position is important to place spinal needle in proper position.

- ***Critical Decision Point***
  Clients who have severe arthritic conditions or who are orthopneic may be unable to assume this position.

Step	Rationale
3. Assess client's ability to cooperate and to remain in position without excessive movement.	Movement can cause injury from spinal needle.
4. Examine medical record for contraindications of increased intracranial pressure, bleeding disorders, degenerative joint disease, or agitation.	Increased intracranial pressure may cause brain herniation. Bleeding disorders will result in prolonged bleeding into the tissues or cerebral spinal fluid. Degenerative joint disease may prevent client from attaining proper position or physician from easily entering subarachnoid space for procedure. An agitated patient may not cooperate during the procedure (Chernecky and Berger, 1997; Malarkey and McMorrow, 2000).
5. Determine whether client is allergic to medication to be used as local anesthetic agent (e.g., lidocaine).	Previous allergies to anesthetic agents should be noted so these agents may be avoided by physician.
6. Assess client's knowledge regarding procedure.	Procedure can create anxiety because of needle placement.
7. Check signed consent form (refer to institution's policy).	The presence of a signed consent form indicates the patient has received a thorough explanation of the procedure and understands the risks and the probability of successful outcome of the procedure (Meiner, 1999).
8. Obtain vital signs and neurological status of lower extremities: movement, sensation, and muscle strength (see Chapter 10).	Provides baseline data for comparison with post-procedural measurements.

NURSING DIAGNOSIS

Defining characteristics from the assessment data may reveal the following nursing diagnoses for clients requiring this skill:

- Anxiety
- Fear
- Risk for infection
- Risk for injury
- Deficient knowledge regarding purpose and steps of procedure
- Acute pain

Related factors are individualized based on client's condition or needs.

PLANNING

Step	Rationale
1. **Expected outcomes** following completion of procedure:	
▪ Small amount (1- to 2-cm circle) (½ to 1 inch) of clear or red drainage is present at puncture site.	Small amount of CSF or bloody drainage is considered normal and expected.
▪ Client does not experience post-puncture headache.	Patients who lie flat in a supine position following the lumbar puncture will be less likely to experience a post-puncture headache (Malarkey and McMorrow, 2000).
▪ Test results of CSF are normal.	Comparison of client's laboratory data with normal laboratory values shows no abnormal pressures, cells, organisms, or other constituents.
▪ Client understands procedure.	

STEP	RATIONALE
2. Explain procedure to client.	Nurse tells client in understandable terms about potential discomfort associated with procedure and length of procedure.
3. Have client empty bladder and bowel before procedure begins.	Avoids interruption of test and prevents discomfort.
4. Position client in lateral recumbent (fetal) position with head and neck flexed (see illustration).	Flexion of lumbar spine allows easy access to CSF in spinal canal (Chernecky and Berger, 1997).

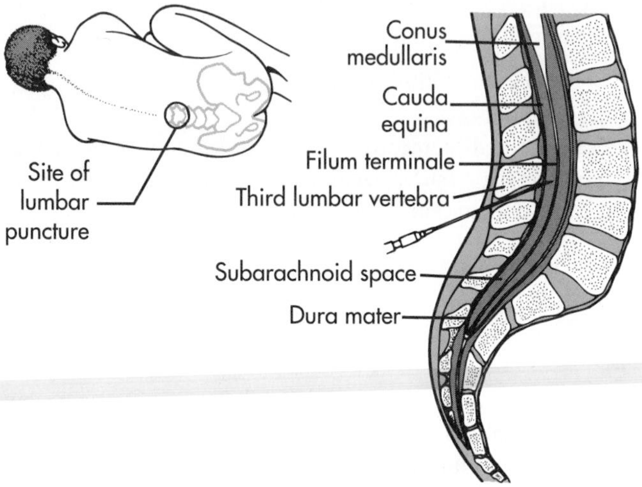

STEP 4 Client position for lumbar puncture. (Modified from Pagana K, Pagana T: *Mosby's diagnostic and laboratory test reference,* ed 5, St. Louis, 2000, Mosby.)

STEP	RATIONALE
5. Bring both arms and knees toward center of body; client may grasp knees with hands.	Gives spinal column full curvature. Spinal column should be flexed as much as possible to allow maximal space between vertebrae.
6. May place pillow between knees.	Prevents discomfort and possibility of upper leg rolling forward.
7. Be sure back is exposed.	Allows easy access to spinal column.

IMPLEMENTATION

NURSE'S RESPONSIBILITY

STEP	RATIONALE
1. Explain that client must lie in flexed position and remain still for entire procedure.	Client must remain still throughout procedure because movement may cause traumatic injury from the spinal needle within spinal column (Chernecky and Berger, 1997).
2. Position client so spine (dorsal side) is against side of bed. Hold arms and legs in flexed position.	Position allows full flexion of the spine and wider spaces between the vertebrae (Malarkey and McMorrow, 2000). Prevents sudden movement by client.
3. Caution client not to cough and to breathe slowly and deeply.	Coughing or changes in breathing may result in injury and/or inaccurate readings.
4. Explain each step that may give discomfort.	Reassure client as needles are inserted. A stinging sensation results from administration of the anesthetic. Brief pain occurs when the spinal needle penetrates the dura and enters the subarachnoid space (Malarkey and McMorrow, 2000).
5. Apply gloves in preparation for assisting with filling test tubes with CSF.	Prevents transmission of microorganisms.

STEP	RATIONALE
6. Properly label tubes with client information and name of test desired. Transport specimens to laboratory immediately.	Test tubes are numbered in sequence of collection (e.g., mark the tubes "1," "2," "3," etc). *Tube #1* is used for chemical and immunological analysis because blood or tissue fluid will not alter these test results. *Tube #2* is used for microbial analysis. *Tube #3* is used for microscopic examination of cells (Malarkey and McMorrow, 2000). Analysis must be performed promptly on freshly obtained specimens (Chernecky and Berger, 1997).
7. Assist with placement of direct pressure and gauze dressing once needle is withdrawn from puncture site.	Pressure helps minimize CSF loss and bleeding.
8. Remove gloves; wash hands thoroughly after procedure, especially if tubes with CSF have been handled.	Tubes might contain virulent organisms. Proper disposal of gloves reduces transmission of organisms.
9. Assist client in assuming comfortable position.	
10. Ask client to maintain supine or dorsal recumbent position, usually 4 to 12 hours. Check agency policy and physician's order(s). Client may turn from side to side as long is head is not raised.	Maintaining this position helps prevent headache following lumbar puncture (Malarkey and McMorrow, 2000).
11. Provide for client's comfort with medication if ordered, desirable, and not contraindicated. Use positioning, relaxation techniques if indicated.	Procedure is usually described as painful by client. Post-procedure headache may require that client be medicated.

- ***Critical Decision Point***
  If client has a CNS disorder, a sedative or analgesic may be contraindicated so as not to further cloud client's consciousness.

12. During and after procedure, observe client for:	
a. Changes in level of consciousness, pupil size and reaction, respiratory status, and vital signs.	Although an infrequent complication, increased intracranial pressure can occur (Malarkey and McMorrow, 2000). Changes in level of consciousness, pupil size and reaction, respiratory status, and vital signs indicate increasing intracranial pressure
b. Numbness, tingling, or pain radiating down legs.	May result from spinal nerve irritation.
c. Encourage client to force fluids by mouth using a straw if not contraindicated.	Needed to replace CSF lost and to resume hemodynamics. Use of straw allows client to drink while supine (Connolly, 1999; Pagana and Pagana, 1998)

PHYSICIAN'S RESPONSIBILITY

1. Wash hands.	Reduces transmission of microorganisms.
2. Set up sterile field of equipment.	Provides sterile work area.
3. Apply sterile gloves (mask and goggles optional).	
4. Prepare lumbosacral area with antiseptic solution and gauze sponges.	Prevents entry of microorganisms from skin to CSF in spinal canal.
5. Inject topical anesthetic agent.	Provides local anesthetic to skin surrounding puncture site.
6. Insert spinal needle containing an inner obturator into subarachnoid space (see illustration [p. 1240] Nurses Responsibility).	Care is taken to avoid trauma to spinal nerves.
7. After entering subarachnoid space, obturator is removed.	Allows flow of CSF from subarachnoid space.
8. Attach manometer with stopcock and read manometer for "opening pressure." Before the pressure reading is taken, ask client to relax and straighten the legs.	Manometer is calibrated in centimeters of water. Relaxing and straightening the legs reduces the intraabdominal pressure, which causes an increase in CSF pressure (Pagana and Pagana, 1998).
9. Turn stopcock to allow CSF to drip into test tubes to send for appropriate testing.	

STEP	RATIONALE
10. Remove spinal needle and place digital pressure on insertion site.	Decreases or stops CSF leakage from spinal canal. Headache follows lumbar puncture in 10% of patients and is caused by leakage of CSF at the puncture site (Monahan and Neighbors, 1998).
11. Place adhesive gauze or Band-aid over insertion site.	Ensures sterility of insertion site.

EVALUATION

1. Assess needle insertion site for drainage.	Small amount of CSF (clear) or bloody (red) drainage is considered normal.
2. Assess level of consciousness, vital signs, pupils, and respiratory status; assess numbness, tingling, and ability to move the lower extremities.	Changes may indicate complications of brain herniation or irritation of spinal nerves.
3. Ask client to describe post-procedure positioning and activity restriction.	Evaluates learning.

UNEXPECTED OUTCOMES AND RELATED INTERVENTIONS:

- Client has excessive drainage from insertion site.
  - Monitor vital signs.
  - Continue to assess insertion site.
  - Follow specific post-procedural orders related to findings.
  - Notify physician.
- Client has post-puncture headache.
  - Instruct client to lie flat in bed.
  - Encourage fluid intake of at least 1 glass per hour (unless contraindicated).
  - Administer analgesia as ordered.
- Client has pain or tingling sensation in lower extremities.
  - Compare to pre-procedure baseline assessment.
  - Continue to monitor.
  - Notify physician.
- Client develops reduced level of consciousness, dilated pupils, and increased blood pressure.
  - Maintain airway.
  - Notify physician immediately.

RECORDING AND REPORTING

- Record in nurse's notes the procedure performed including time, physician's name, client's tolerance (e.g., opening pressure, color of CSF, amount of drainage on dressing, and whether headache and leg tingling are present) and specimens sent to lab.
- Report pertinent findings to nurse in charge and to physician: changes in vital signs, nausea, vomiting, and changes in level of consciousness.

TEACHING CONSIDERATIONS

- Thoroughly explain procedure and post-procedure routine to client. Many clients have misconceptions regarding procedure. Emphasize importance of remaining flat after procedure for up to 12 hours to avoid a post-procedure spinal headache
- Teach client the importance of forcing fluids after the procedure to replace CSF removed during the lumbar puncture.
- Encourage client to contact the physician regarding test results.
- Teach client to inform physician of any unusual sensations in the legs, such as numbness and tingling.

PEDIATRIC CONSIDERATIONS

- Apply EMLA to the lumbar puncture site at least 1 hour before the procedure. Conscious or unconscious sedation is recommended for lumbar puncture (Wong and others, 1999).
- Even children who are cooperative need to be gently held to prevent trauma from involuntary, unexpected movement. Assure children that although they are trusted, holding them serves as support and as a reminder to maintain desired position (Wong and others, 1999).

GERONTOLOGICAL CONSIDERATIONS

- Older adults may have difficulty assuming the side-lying knee-to-chest position.

HOME CARE CONSIDERATIONS

- Provide written instructions to reinforce oral instructions.
- Inform client postdural puncture headache usually occurs within 48 hours of the punctured but may be delayed as long as 12 days; it is not psychological in origin (Connolly, 1999).
- Client should seek medical attention immediately if he or she suddenly complains of severe headache or has change in level of consciousness.

Skill 42-8 Assisting With Magnetic Resonance Imaging

Magnetic resonance imaging (MRI) is a noninvasive scanning technique that provides visualization of the body's organs and structures by means of magnetic forces rather than by ionizing radiation. Magnetic resonance images are picked up by computers once the client is placed inside a large electromagnet (Figure 42-7). This diagnostic study is based on the alignment of hydrogen atoms in the body and the change in alignment of those atoms by radiofrequency signals. MRI does not require exposure to ionizing radiation.

MRI may be used to assess organs, soft tissues, and anatomical structures. It allows for visualization of any present pathological condition. MRI can differentiate between benign and malignant growth as well as stage cancer or evaluate treatment response to a malignancy (Malarkey and McMorrow, 2000). The procedure is usually performed by a trained technologist in the MRI department.

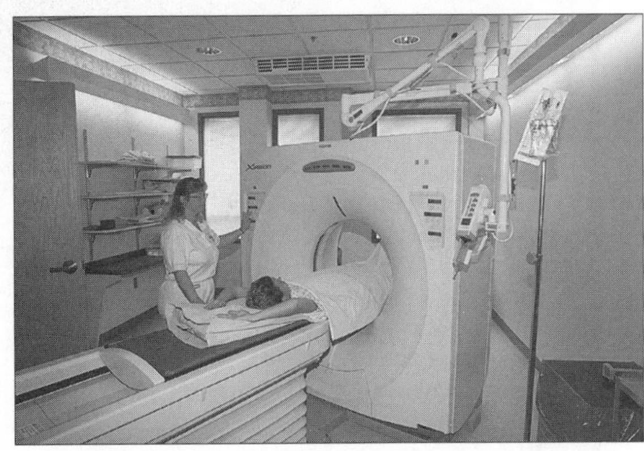

FIGURE **42-7** Magnetic resonance imaging (MRI).

Delegation Considerations

The skill of assisting with magnetic resonance imaging is routinely delegated to assistive personnel to transport the client to the diagnostic test. Transporting to MRI an unstable client or a client with invasive equipment (e.g., arterial lines, mechanical ventilation, etc.) should not be delegated to assistive personnel.

Equipment

- Contrast medium gadolinium (Magnevist) (optional); must be ordered by physician

Step	Rationale
Assessment	
1. Assess client's knowledge of purposes of and steps in the procedure.	Helps to reduce anxiety and gain cooperation.
• ***Critical Decision Point*** *MRI is contraindicated in clients who are confused or agitated.*	
2. Assess stability of client's medical condition.	Monitoring equipment and other equipment (that contains metal) cannot be used inside the scanner room.
• ***Critical Decision Point*** *Clients who are medically unstable and require continuous life-support equipment (that contains metal) are not candidates for this procedure unless specially designed monitoring equipment is available.*	
3. Obtain client's weight.	Procedure contraindicated in clients over 300 pounds. Table will not hold the weight (Pagana and Pagana, 1998).
4. Assess client for implantable metal objects such as cardiac pacemaker, aneurysm clips, inner ear implants, or history of valve replacement (before 1964) as well as those clients with medical equipment that contains metal (e.g., infusion pumps, neurostimulator or TENS unit, implanted insulin/drug pumps, or intrauterine devices) (Chernecky and Berger, 1997). Equipment is available that does not contain metal parts. Additional items that may interfere with magnetic resonance imaging are found on the informational diagram (see illustration).	Procedure is contraindicated if any of these are present because the magnet may cause movement of metal or electronic objects (Pagana and Pagana, 1998). Movement of metal objects can be detrimental to anyone within the magnetic field (Pagana and Pagana, 1997).

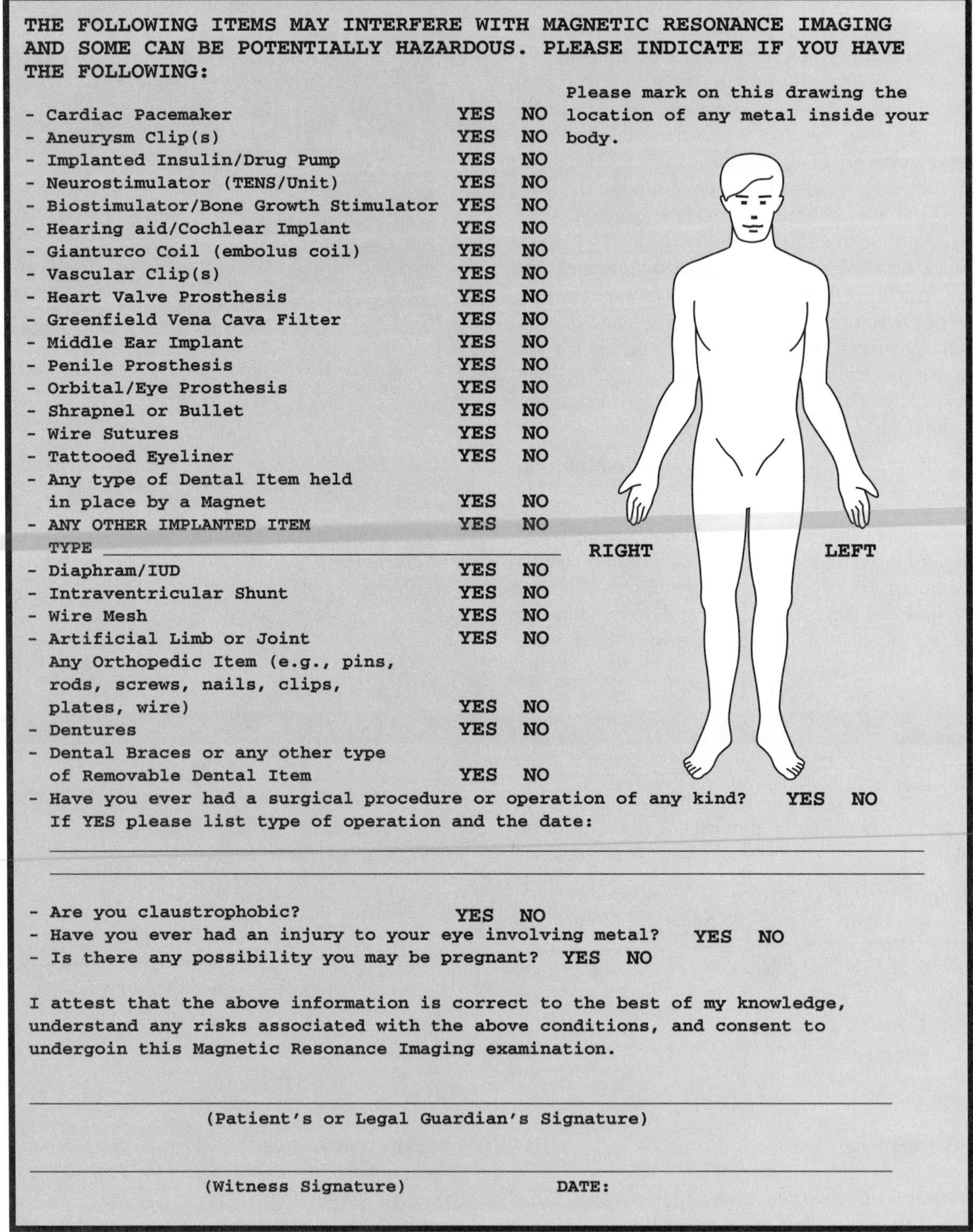

ALL INFORMATION IN SHADED BOXED AREA
MUST BE BILLED OUT PRIOR TO MRI

THE FOLLOWING ITEMS MAY INTERFERE WITH MAGNETIC RESONANCE IMAGING AND SOME CAN BE POTENTIALLY HAZARDOUS. PLEASE INDICATE IF YOU HAVE THE FOLLOWING:

- Cardiac Pacemaker YES NO
- Aneurysm Clip(s) YES NO
- Implanted Insulin/Drug Pump YES NO
- Neurostimulator (TENS/Unit) YES NO
- Biostimulator/Bone Growth Stimulator YES NO
- Hearing aid/Cochlear Implant YES NO
- Gianturco Coil (embolus coil) YES NO
- Vascular Clip(s) YES NO
- Heart Valve Prosthesis YES NO
- Greenfield Vena Cava Filter YES NO
- Middle Ear Implant YES NO
- Penile Prosthesis YES NO
- Orbital/Eye Prosthesis YES NO
- Shrapnel or Bullet YES NO
- Wire Sutures YES NO
- Tattooed Eyeliner YES NO
- Any type of Dental Item held in place by a Magnet YES NO
- ANY OTHER IMPLANTED ITEM YES NO
  TYPE ______
- Diaphram/IUD YES NO
- Intraventricular Shunt YES NO
- Wire Mesh YES NO
- Artificial Limb or Joint YES NO
  Any Orthopedic Item (e.g., pins, rods, screws, nails, clips, plates, wire) YES NO
- Dentures YES NO
- Dental Braces or any other type of Removable Dental Item YES NO

Please mark on this drawing the location of any metal inside your body.

RIGHT LEFT

- Have you ever had a surgical procedure or operation of any kind? YES NO
  If YES please list type of operation and the date:
  ______
  ______
- Are you claustrophobic? YES NO
- Have you ever had an injury to your eye involving metal? YES NO
- Is there any possibility you may be pregnant? YES NO

I attest that the above information is correct to the best of my knowledge, understand any risks associated with the above conditions, and consent to undergoin this Magnetic Resonance Imaging examination.

______
(Patient's or Legal Guardian's Signature)

______
(Witness Signature) DATE:

STEP 4 Sample check-off sheet for MRI.

STEP	RATIONALE
5. Assess client for claustrophobia.	Client may become fearful or overly anxious of becoming trapped in an enclosed or narrow place. This problem may be decreased if client uses the newer, open MR imagers (Pagana and Pagana, 1998). Procedure may be contraindicated if claustrophobia is severe and/or not relieved by sedation. Only 1% to 2% of people refuse MRI because of claustrophobia (Chernecky and Berger, 1997).
6. Assess client for pregnancy.	Long-term effects of MRI on fetus are currently unknown. MRI is contraindicated during pregnancy (Pagana and Pagana, 1998).
7. Assess client's ability to remain still throughout the procedure. Determine client's understanding of the importance of remaining in one position for the duration of the procedure. Factors that might influence client's inability to remain still include pain, alteration in mental status, claustrophobia, difficulty breathing, polyuria, and restlessness.	Any movement may produce artifacts. Client must remain still for 30 to 90 minutes. The image will be distorted by motion or movement during the procedure (Chernecky and Berger, 1997).
8. Assess for allergies to dye and contrast medium.	Prevents injury to client. If allergy is noted, ensure that client is wearing an allergy wristband and document appropriately. Intravenous injection of an allergic substance is a life-threatening condition and can result in anaphylactic shock and death.
9. Assess whether client signed a consent document (check institution's policy).	The presence of a signed consent form indicates the patient has received a thorough explanation of the procedure and understands the risks and the probability of successful outcome of the procedure (Meiner, 1999).

NURSING DIAGNOSIS

Defining characteristics from the assessment data may reveal the following nursing diagnoses for clients requiring this skill:

- Anxiety
- Fear
- Risk for injury
- Deficient knowledge regarding purpose and steps of procedure
- Pain (acute, chronic)
- Disturbed sensory perception

Related factors are individualized based on client's condition or needs.

PLANNING

1. **Expected outcomes** following completion of procedure:

▪ Client tolerates procedure with minimal discomfort.	
▪ Client can maintain position without moving.	Anxiety or sense of claustrophobia minimized.
▪ If contrast medium is used, client has no reaction to dye.	Indicates absence of complications.
▪ Satisfactory images are obtained.	Indicates that purpose of procedure was achieved.
▪ Client describes purpose and steps of procedure.	Documents understanding.

IMPLEMENTATION

NURSE'S RESPONSIBILITY

1. If possible, show client picture of MRI machine and encourage questions (see Figure 42-7).	
2. Remove all metallic objects from client, such as watch, jewelry, coins, keys, hairpins, credit cards, prostheses, and dentures. Lock away for safe keeping (Pagana and Pagana, 1998).	Metallic objects will create interference with MRI imaging (Chernecky and Berger, 1997).

STEP	RATIONALE
3. Have client put on hospital gown without snaps and void before the procedure.	Voiding promotes comfort during procedure.

TECHNOLOGIST'S RESPONSIBILITY

STEP	RATIONALE
4. If not previously performed, remove all metallic objects from client (see preceding Step 2).	Metallic objects will create artifacts on the scan, and some metal objects may move or be damaged by the magnetic field.
5. Assist client onto padded table and position comfortably.	Provides for correct positioning and for client's comfort.
6. Place special helmet around head if it is to be scanned and secure client on table with Velcro straps.	Allows for accurate imaging and helps to keep client from moving during procedure.
7. Provide client with earplugs and/or intercom or earphones.	Decreases sounds of images and allows for communication between client and technologist.
8. After examination, allow client to sit for a few moments before standing.	Decreases possibility of orthostatic hypotension (Elkin, and others, 2000).

EVALUATION

STEP	RATIONALE
1. Evaluate client's level of comfort after procedure.	Determines if complications related to positioning have occurred.

UNEXPECTED OUTCOMES AND RELATED INTERVENTIONS

- Allergic reaction to contrast medium.
  - Reaction is immediate.
  - Maintain airway.
  - Monitor client.
  - Call physician immediately and obtain further orders.
- Client is unable to maintain position during procedure.
  - Reassess and instruct client on importance of maintaining position and not moving.

RECORDING AND REPORTING

- Record in client's chart the date, time, and place MRI was performed; whether contrast medium was used; and client's tolerance of procedure.

TEACHING CONSIDERATIONS

- Inform the client that no food or fluid restrictions are necessary before or after the test.
- Instruct the client to void just before the procedure, for comfort (Pagana and Pagana, 1998).
- Explain that during the examination the client will hear the hum of the machine and a loud thumping sound when the radiowaves are turned on. Earplugs are usually available.
- Reassure client that a microphone and earphone are present in the scanner to enable communication with the staff during the scan.
- Inform client that make-up should not be worn because some products may contain metallic particles.
- Explain that client must remain motionless throughout this painless study; a slight discomfort may be experienced if contrast medium is injected.
- Inform client that a tingling sensation may be felt in teeth containing metal fillings (Pagana and Pagana, 1997).
- Tell client that no special post-procedural care is needed.

PEDIATRIC CONSIDERATIONS

- Show a picture of the machine to children unfamiliar with the equipment.
- If child is old enough to understand, explain why the test is being done, what the child will experience, and how the child can help (Wong and others, 1999).
- Explain the chin and cheek pads to a frightened child by comparing them to what astronauts need for a space flight (Wong and others, 1999).
- Emphasize to the child that the procedure is painless.
- Tell parents they may read or talk to a child in the scanning room during the procedure because no risk of radiation from the procedure exists (Pagana and Pagana, 1997).

GERONTOLOGICAL CONSIDERATIONS

- The older adult client may experience increased discomfort during and after the procedure because of lying motionless for an extended period of time.
- Keep frail older adult warm to maintain core temperature at safe, comfortable levels (Worfolk, 1997).
- Assess skin integrity of client who has been lying still on hard narrow examining table. Older adult clients are at greater risk for skin breakdown.
- Assess for joint stiffness because of decreased mobility during procedure.

- After the procedure, be aware of need to change positions slowly in older adult clients to minimize safety risks and possible postural blood pressure changes.
- Because of age-related cardiovascular changes in older adults, plan diagnostic testing schedule to provide rest periods.
- If the older adult client was required to remove sensory assistive devices (e.g., glasses, hearing aids) for diagnostic testing, provide measures to compensate for these sensory deficits and return assistive devices.

Home Care Considerations

- Inform the client that no food or fluid restrictions are necessary before or after the test.

Skill 42-9 Assisting With Thoracentesis

Thoracentesis, an invasive procedure, is performed to analyze or remove **pleural fluid** or to instill medications intrapleurally. Specimens are examined for gross appearance and consistency and for protein, glucose, amylase, lactic dehydrogenase (LDH), and cellular composition. Cytologically, specimens are examined for malignancy and cultured for pathogens. The procedure is performed by a physician and assisted by a nurse or assistive personnel using strict sterile technique. A large-bore needle is passed through the chest wall into the **pleural cavity.** Excess pleural fluid resulting from injury, infection, or disease may be removed. The primary therapeutic purpose of thoracentesis is to relive pain, dyspnea, and other signs of pleural pressure.

Diagnostically, the procedure is performed when there is evidence of pleural effusion with unknown etiology. Before the procedure, a decubitus chest x-ray is done to ensure the mobility of pleural fluid and therefore the accessibility of pleural fluid to a needle inserted into the pleural space.

The procedure is usually performed while the client is in a sitting position with one arm held upward from the chest, or more commonly, leaning over a bedside table padded with pillows. Thoracentesis can generally be performed in less than 30 minutes at the client's bedside, in a procedure room, or in the physician's office.

Delegation Considerations

The skill of assisting with a thoracentesis may be delegated to assistive personnel if the client is stable. Instruct personnel on proper positioning of client during the procedure. Instruct assistive personnel to take baseline, as well as post-procedure, vital signs and to report these vital signs to the nurse. Caution assistive personnel to be alert for and report signs and symptoms experienced by the client.

Equipment

- Antiseptic solution for hand washing
- Thoracentesis tray, if available from central supply, which may include: antiseptic solution (e.g., povidone-iodine); gauze sponges (4 × 4); sterile towels; local anesthetic solution for injection (e.g., lidocaine 1%); sterile syringes: two 3-ml, 23- to 25-gauge needles for anesthetic; two 50-ml, 14- to 17-gauge needles, 5 to 7 cm long (or 2 to 3 inches), for drainage of pleural fluid; receptacle for fluid; three-way stopcock; two-way stopcock with extension tubing; test tubes
- Sterile gloves of proper size for physician
- Masks and goggles for physician, nurse, and/or assistive personnel (check institution's policy)
- Gauze (2 × 2), tape, and antiseptic ointment
- Cough suppressant (Pagana and Pagana, 1998) or pain medication if ordered

Step	Rationale
Assessment	
1. Assess client's knowledge of procedure.	Determines level of health teaching required.
2. Assess client's ability to assume position required for procedure (see illustration).	Client must remain immobile during the procedure to prevent needle damage to the lung or pleura (Pagana and Pagana, 1998). Clients with musculoskeletal or respiratory alterations may be unable to sit on side of bed with arms draped over high bedside table.

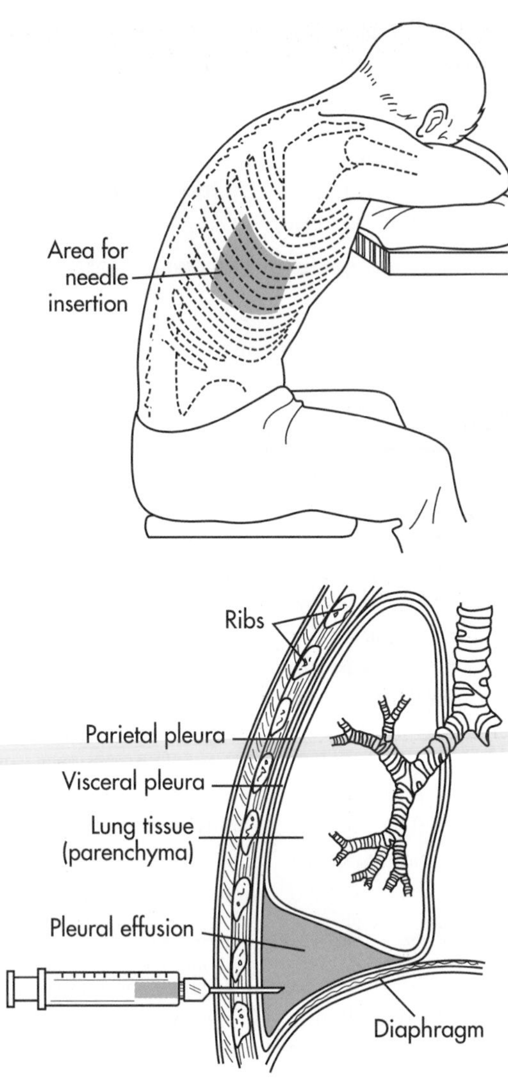

STEP 2 Thoracentesis.

Step	Rationale
3. Obtain vital signs and oxygen saturation.	Provides baseline data for comparison.
4. Be aware of client's underlying medical condition, which may indicate presence of potential bleeding problems.	May contraindicate procedure because of risk of bleeding.
5. Assess respiratory function: symmetry of chest on inspiration and expiration, respiratory difficulty, and type of cough and sputum produced.	Provides for comparison with respiratory status during and after procedure.
6. Determine purpose of procedure.	Enables nurse to anticipate needed supplies and laboratory requisitions.
7. Assess if client signed a consent form (check institution's policy).	The presence of a signed consent form indicates the patient has received a thorough explanation of the procedure and understands the risks and the probability of successful outcome of the procedure (Meiner, 1999).
8. Determine whether client is allergic to antiseptic or anesthetic solutions.	Decreases chances of complications.
9. Assess need for pre-procedure pain medication.	Procedure can be painful, and client must remain still throughout it because of potential complications.

STEP	RATIONALE

NURSING DIAGNOSIS

Defining characteristics from the assessment data may reveal the following nursing diagnoses for clients requiring this skill:

- Anxiety
- Ineffective breathing pattern
- Fear
- Impaired gas exchange
- Risk for infection
- Risk for injury
- Deficient knowledge regarding purpose and steps of procedure
- Acute pain

Related factors are individualized based on client's condition or needs.

PLANNING

Step	Rationale
1. **Expected outcomes** following completion of procedure:	
▪ Client tolerates procedure well.	Client can assume position without problems and has little discomfort.
▪ Respiratory status is improved as evidenced by nonlabored respirations, improved oxygen saturation, and improved comfort.	Optimal expansion of lungs improves gas exchange.
▪ Client describes purpose and steps of procedure as well as proper positioning.	Documents understanding.
2. Prepare client:	
a. Explain procedure.	Ensures knowledge of procedure, thus promoting cooperation and relaxation.
b. Explain that, although a local anesthetic will be given at the insertion site, the client may feel a pressure-like pain when the pleura is entered for fluid removal (Malarkey and McMorrow, 2000).	Reinforces that sensation of pressure is related to entrance of catheter into pleur and not lack of adequate anesthesia. Client should not feel pain.
c. Have client void just before procedure.	Prevents interruption of procedure and promotes client's comfort.
d. Assist client in assuming an upright position with arms and shoulders raised and supported on a padded overbed table. If unable to tolerate this position, assist client to side-lying position on the unaffected side with side to be tapped uppermost (Pagana and Pagana, 1998).	Spreads the ribs, enlarging intercostal space for needle insertion (Pagana and Pagana, 1998).

IMPLEMENTATION

NURSE'S RESPONSIBILITY

Step	Rationale
1. Wash hands.	Reduces transmission of microorganisms.
2. Set up sterile tray or open supplies to make them accessible for physician.	Prevents introduction of pathogens into the pleural space.
3. Assist client in maintaining correct position. If necessary, hold client's shoulders or sides and provide reassurance.	Prevents sudden movement on part of client.

• ***Critical Decision Point***

Emphasize the importance of remaining immobile during the procedure to prevent trauma to the visceral pleura. Client must not cough, sneeze, or breathe deeply during procedure because it could cause trauma to visceral pleura (Pagana and Pagana, 1998).

Step	Rationale
4. Assess client's pulse for reflex bradycardia, diaphoresis, and feeling of faintness (Pagana and Pagana, 1998).	Evaluates tolerance to procedure.

Step	Rationale
5. Assess client's respiratory status during procedure: rate, effort to breathe, and color of mucous membranes and nail beds.	Enables nurse to detect tolerance to procedure and possible complications.
6. After thoracentesis, assist client in assuming comfortable position in bed.	If leakage into pleural space is suspected, client is positioned recumbent with punctured chest side up.

Physician's Responsibility

Step	Rationale
1. Wash hands.	Reduces transmission of microorganisms.
2. Disinfect skin with antiseptic solution and 4 × 4s.	Removes surface bacteria on skin.
3. Apply mask, goggles, and sterile gloves and drape client with sterile towels.	Maintains surgical asepsis.
4. Inject anesthetic and allow time for it to take effect.	Provides local anesthesia at needle insertion site.
5. Palpate exact site needed for thoracentesis (most often just below angle of scapula at seventh intercostal space).	If needle is inserted too low, liver or spleen may be punctured, causing serious complications (Chernecky and Berger, 1997).
6. Attach thoracentesis needle to three-way stopcock, which is turned off to needle lumen.	Ensures that no air enters pleural space when needle is introduced.
7. Insert needle into determined site slowly until pleural space is reached and then slowly aspirate fluid. Up to 1000 ml of pleural fluid can be removed at one time.	Places needle in pleural space. Fluid is aspirated slowly to decrease complications of drawing lung tissue into needle. 1000–1200 ml of pleural fluid are usually removed at one time to prevent mediastinal shift and compromised venous return (Lewis, and others, 2000).
8. Remove needle and apply pressure and sterile dressing to puncture site.	Pressure assists in sealing puncture site. Dressing ensures sterility of site.
9. Order chest x-ray film and blood work (e.g., hematocrit and hemoglobin, serum electrolytes).	Chest x-ray may show decreased fluid level in pleural space. Blood work is performed to check cell count and electrolytes in case replacement is needed.

Evaluation

Step	Rationale
1. Note amount and color of pleural fluid. Apply small bandage over needle site. Turn client on unaffected side for 1 hour.	Characteristics are used for observation, reporting, and recording. Allows pleural puncture site to heal (Pagana and Pagana, 1998).
2. Monitor vital signs, oxygen saturation, and auscultate lung sounds. Compare with pre-thoracentesis data. Monitor for decreased lung sounds or shortness of breath (SOB) if large volume of fluid removed.	Monitors physiological status.
3. Monitor client for complications from the thoracentesis, which may include pneumothorax (e.g., acute SOB, anxiety, tachypnea), shock (e.g., hypotension, tachycardia, cool clammy skin, altered LOC), subcutaneous emphysema (e.g., swelling of soft tissues and palpation of crepitations over the affected area), and pyogenic infection (e.g., fever, tachycardia, chills). Observe for hemoptysis, anxiety, and restlessness (Pagana and Pagana, 1997).	

- ***Critical Decision Point***
  The complications of liver and spleen perforation are less common than lung perforation. Symptoms are subtle and may not be noted for several days. Symptoms include decreasing hemoglobin and hematocrit values and possibly abdominal pain.

Step	Rationale
4. Follow up on post-thoracentesis chest x-ray as indicated (Chernecky and Berger, 1997).	Determines presence of pneumothorax.
5. Note drainage on chest dressing.	Documents leakage of fluid from puncture site.
6. Ask client to describe post-procedure limitations and positioning.	Evaluates learning.

Unexpected Outcomes and Related Interventions

- Client does not assume position well.
  - Reassess and assist client in proper position.
- Client moves abruptly or coughs during procedure.
  - Reassess and instruct client on importance of maintaining position and not moving.
  - Alert physician of client's need to cough.

Recording and Reporting

- Record in nurse's notes the name of procedure, name of person performing procedure, location of puncture site, amount and color of fluid drained, duration, tolerance (e.g., vital signs, pain, respiratory status, complications), laboratory tests ordered and sent, type of dressing over puncture site, and drainage.
- Report to physician immediately.
  - Decreased respiratory function.
  - Changes in vital signs beyond normal limits.
  - Changes in post-procedure hemoglobin, hematocrit, or serum electrolyte values.
- Document completion of chest x-ray if ordered after procedure; notify physician if any complications were detected.
- Report to nurses on next shift all data that have been recorded in nurse's notes and reported to physician.

Teaching Considerations

- After explaining procedure, make certain client knows that movement or coughing could damage lung or pleura. Cough suppressant may be administered before procedure if client has cough.
- Explain to client that chest x-ray is often ordered after procedure to check for adequate lung expansion.
- Encourage client to report any dyspnea, chest pain, or cough after procedure.
- Inform the client that no food or fluid restrictions are necessary before or after the test.
- Encourage client to check with physician regarding test results.

Gerontological Considerations

- During all aspects of this procedure, be aware of ineffective breathing patterns in the older adult because of age-related changes such as reduced elastic lung recoil, declining chest expansion, reduced cough efficiency, and weaker thoracic and diaphragmatic muscles (Eliopoulos, 1997).
- During the procedure assess client pulses for reflex bradycardia; evaluate for diaphoresis and faintness (Pagana and Pagana, 1998).
- Elderly clients may demonstrate restlessness as an early indication of hypoxia.
- Age-related changes of the musculoskeletal system may restrict movement during positioning and during procedure.
- After the procedure, be aware of need to change positions slowly in older adult clients to minimize safety risks and possible postural changes.

Home Care Considerations

- Teach client symptoms of complications related to liver and spleen perforation that may not be present for several days after procedure and to notify the physician.
- Encourage client to report any dyspnea, chest pain, or cough after procedure.
- Inform the client that no food or fluid restrictions are necessary before or after the test.

Critical Thinking Exercises

1. Mr. D.L., a 52-year-old businessman has just returned from the cardiac catheterization lab. He is vomiting and his wife calls you to the bedside to tell you he is bleeding. You arrive to find Mr. L. visibly upset and sitting in a pool of blood. What do you do?
2. As you prepare to give Mr. D. his pre-procedure sedation medication for a diagnostic procedure, he quietly questions you if there are any risks or possible adverse events that might occur during the procedure. He voices uncertainty regarding having the procedure done. What is your response?
3. Your client, an elderly Old Order Amish male is scheduled for an MRI. He became ill while visiting his sister and required his first ever hospitalization. After obtaining his history, you realize he has never been exposed to high technology tests and treatments and to large electronically run environments. He is afraid of the MRI equipment. Despite your best explanations, he is threatening to leave. What do you do?

References

Beare P, Myers J: *Principles and practice of adult health nursing,* ed 2, St Louis, 1998, Mosby.

Chernecky C, Berger, B: *Laboratory tests and diagnostic procedures,* ed 4, Philadelphia, 1997, WB Saunders

Connolly, M: Postdural puncture headache, *Am J Nurs* 99(11):48, 1999.

Eliopoulos C: *Gerontological nursing,* ed 4, Philadelphia, 1997, Lippincott.

Elkin MK, Perry AG, Potter PA: *Nursing interventions & clinical skills,* ed 2, St. Louis, 2000, Mosby.

Gulanick M, Klopp A, Galanes S, Gradishar D, Puzas M: *Nursing care plans: nursing diagnosis and intervention,* ed 4, St Louis, 1998, Mosby.

Jarvis C: *Physical examination and health assessment,* ed 3, Philadelphia, 2000, WB Saunders.

Kee J, Hayes E: *Pharmacology: a nursing process approach,* ed 3, Philadelphia, 2000, WB Saunders.

Kost M: *Manual of conscious sedation,* Philadelphia, 1998, WB Saunders.

Lewis S, Heitkemper M, Dirksen S: *Medical-surgical nursing,* ed 5, St Louis, 2000, Mosby.

Linton A, Matteson M, Maebius N: *Introductory nursing care of adults,* ed 2, Philadelphia, 2000, WB Saunders.

Malarkey L, McMorrow M: *Nurse's manual of laboratory tests and diagnostic procedures,* ed 2, Philadelphia, 2000, WB Saunders.

Meiner S: *Nursing documentation,* London, 1999, SAGE Publications.

Monahan F, Neighbors M: *Medical-surgical nursing: foundations for clinical practice,* ed 2, Philadelphia, 1998, WB Saunders.

Pagana K, Pagana T: *Mosby's diagnostic and laboratory test reference,* ed 3, St Louis, 1997, Mosby.

Pagana K, Pagana T: *Mosby's manual of diagnostic and laboratory tests,* St Louis, 1998, Mosby.

Pagana K, Pagana T: *Mosby's diagnostic and laboratory test reference,* ed 5, St Louis, 2000, Mosby.

Phipps W and others, editors: *Medical-surgical nursing: concepts and clinical practice,* ed 5, St Louis, 1999, Mosby.

VanRiper S, VanRiper J: *Cardiac diagnostic tests: a guide for nurses,* Philadelphia, 1997, WB Saunders.

Wong D and others: *Whaley and Wong's nursing care of infants and children,* ed 6, St Louis, 1999, Mosby.

Worfolk J: Keep frail elders warm, *Geriatr Nurs* 97(18):7, 1997.

Zaglaniczny K, Aker J: *Clinical guide to pediatric anesthesia,* Philadelphia, 1999, WB Saunders.

43

Care After Death

Skills

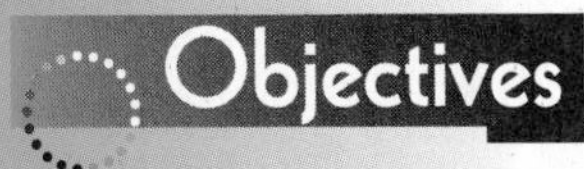

Mastery of content in this chapter will enable the nurse to:

- Define the key terms listed.
- Discuss the importance of end-of-life care for client and family comfort.
- Discuss important considerations when working with families and significant others in regard to organ and/or tissue donation.
- Describe the physiological changes after death.
- Describe postmortem care techniques.
- Correctly prepare a client's body after death.

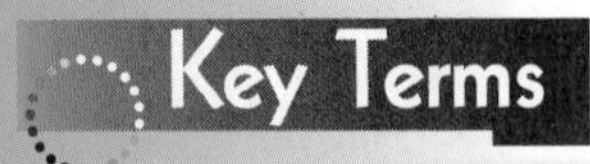

Advanced directives
Autopsy
End-of-life care
Loss
Morgue
Organ Procurement Agency (OPA)
Organ/tissue donation
Rigor mortis

Providing **end-of-life care** to a terminally ill client has a profound effect on the dying person, significant others, friends, and caregivers. The fears associated with dying are often related more to the client's sense of loneliness and isolation and family members' sense of powerlessness. Nursing care focuses on symptom management, spiritual comfort, and grief support. To be effective in providing end-of-life care, the nurse needs both a knowledge of the dying process and a degree of personal comfort in addressing death.

The nurse and other members of the health care team need to consider life support and the degree of intervention the person desires at the time of death. As part of a person's right to self-determination, every adult may accept or refuse recommended medical treatment. The Patient Self-Determination Act of 1991 requires all health care agencies serving Medicaid and Medicare clients to provide clients with information regarding advanced directives options. **Advance directives** are legal documents that allow persons to have a say in the medical treatments they will receive if unable to make decisions (Figure 43-1). The person can specify what types of treatments are acceptable or unacceptable and can also designate another person appointed as a proxy to make treatment decisions if he or she is unable to make decisions. Ideally a client has had an opportunity to discuss with family and friends his or her wishes regarding end-of-life care. For example, does the client want to be placed on a ventilator; wish to have cardiopulmonary resuscitation; wish to receive blood products? It is the nurse's responsibility to determine if the client's wishes have been assessed and if advanced directives are appropriately documented in the client record. A copy of any advanced directive document should be placed in the client's medical record.

Although it is legally mandated that health care agencies provide information related to advanced directives, studies suggest that clients and families often have a limited understanding of advanced directives and their implications. For example, once a client becomes seriously ill, what options do the family have in making decisions? If a client requires a ventilator for temporary treatment and chances of survival are good, does the advanced directive supersede and require the family to withhold treatment? Many clients have not executed advanced directives often because of confusion and misleading information (Rein and others, 1996). The nurse may well find it beneficial to discuss advanced directives with a dying person and family if the person's wishes are not clearly reflected in the record (Johns, 1996). Because agency policies and state laws differ, nurses need to be familiar with agency policies and the state laws where they are practicing (Badzek, 1992).

Another consideration as death approaches is one of **organ/tissue donation.** The 1986 Omnibus Budget Reconciliation Act (OBRA) requires a client's significant others be offered the option of organ and tissue donation (Chabalewski and Norris, 1994). Organs may be requested when the client is terminally ill but on life support. Tissues may also be requested after death. It is important for individuals to express their views about organ and tissue donation to family members. Most states now give citizens the option of signing the back of their motor vehicle license to designate their wish to be an organ or tissue donor. However, the final decision may ultimately be made by a family member. Nevertheless, a client's choice regarding organ and tissue donation can be included in an advanced directive. More people favor organ/tissue donation and express that they wish to donate their own organs/tissues when they die. Following donation, most donor families report feeling positive about the donation and report that donation has helped them in working through the grieving process. Health care providers are responsible for approaching families and significant others regarding organ and tissue donation, to let them know if their dying significant other is a potential donor, and to describe what types of organs/tissues could be donated.

There continues to be a shortage of donor organs and tissues, partly as a result of health care professionals' hesitancy to identify and approach significant others and the dying regarding organ/tissue donation (Lindsay, 1995). In health care centers in which transplants are performed, a full-time

FLORIDA LIVING WILL

INSTRUCTIONS

PRINT THE DATE

PRINT YOUR NAME

Declaration made this _____________ day of ______________________, ___________,
(day) (month) (year)

I, ________________________________, willfully and voluntarily make known my desire that my dying not be artificially prolonged under the circumstances set forth below, and I do hereby declare that:

PLEASE INITIAL EACH THAT APPLIES

If at any time I am incapacitated and

_____ I have a terminal condition, or
_____ I have an end-stage condition, or
_____ I am in a persistent vegetative state

and if my attending or treating physician and another consulting physician have determined that there is no reasonable medical probability of my recovery from such condition, I direct that life-prolonging procedures be withheld or withdrawn when the application of such procedures would serve only to prolong artificially the process of dying, and that I be permitted to die naturally with only the administration of medication or the performance of any medical procedure deemed necessary to provide me with comfort care or to alleviate pain.

It is my intention that this declaration be honored by my family and physician as the final expression of my legal right to refuse medical or surgical treatment and to accept the consequences for such refusal.

In the event that I have been determined to be unable to provide express and informed consent regarding the withholding, withdrawal, or continuation of life-prolonging procedures, I wish to designate, as my surrogate to carry out the provisions of this declaration:

PRINT THE NAME, HOME ADDRESS AND TELEPHONE NUMBER OF YOUR SURROGATE

Name: ______________________________
Address: ______________________________
______________________________ Zip Code: __________
Phone: ______________________________

PRINT THE NAME, HOME ADDRESS AND TELEPHONE NUMBER OF YOUR ALTERNATE SURROGATE

I wish to designate the following person as my alternate surrogate, to carry out the provisions of this declaration should my surrogate be unwilling or unable to act on my behalf:

Name: ______________________________
Address: ______________________________
______________________________ Zip Code: __________
Phone: ______________________________

ADD PERSONAL INSTRUCTIONS (IF ANY)

Additional instructions (optional):

SIGN THE DOCUMENT

I understand the full import of this declaration, and I am emotionally and mentally competent to make this declaration.

Signed: ______________________________

WITNESSING PROCEDURE

TWO WITNESSES MUST SIGN AND PRINT THEIR ADDRESSES

Witness 1:
Signed: ______________________________
Address: ______________________________

Witness 2:
Signed: ______________________________
Address: ______________________________

Courtesy of **Partnership for Caring, Inc.** 6/00
1035 30th Street, NW Washington, DC 20007 800-989-9455

FIGURE **43-1** Example of a living will declaration. (Courtesy of Partnership for Caring, Inc. 1035 30th Street, NW Washington, DC 20007.)

transplant coordinator is usually available to talk and meet with families. However, in other institutions, it is often the nurse who must make an organ and tissue request. Because nurses often develop close relationships with families, some organizations choose to have pastoral care workers or social workers make donation requests. However, family members often prefer to turn to the nurse for emotional support. In addition, if an unfamiliar care provider approaches a family for a donation, the experience could be more emotionally traumatic. Ideally the health care provider who knows the family best, knows when the death is expected, or has the opportunity to spend time with the family when the death is unexpected assumes the role of requestor (Wong and others, 1999). It is essential for the health care provider who makes the request to be well informed and to be able to explain all options to family members.

Basic principles to remember when making organ and tissue requests include:

- Finding the family a private place to sit while a request is being made.
- Being sure the legal decision maker in the family is involved in the request.
- Notifying the local donor registry to determine if the client qualifies. Certain disease states prohibit organ/tissue donation.
- Being sure the family is well informed of options and how the body of the deceased will be cared for.
- Not placing any pressure on the family to consent to donation.
- Being sensitive to the family's cultural and religious practices.

Symptom Management

Managing the dying client's symptoms begins with understanding that the symptoms are very real. The client's fears and anxieties often compound the effect and magnitude of symptoms, particularly that of pain and fear of suffocation (air hunger). Therefore symptom management includes not only physical care giving but psychological care giving as well. Unfortunately, clients often ask nurses for assistance in dying (Schwarz, 1999), but it is frequently an expression of the need for better pain management (Ersek and others, 1995), emotional support (Quill, 1993), or for someone to actively listen and be present (Dixon, 1997). Table 43-1 summarizes common symptoms experienced by dying clients and associated nursing interventions.

Table 43-1 Physical Signs and Symptoms Associated with the Final Stages of Dying, Rationale, and Interventions

Physical Signs and Symptoms	Rationale	Intervention (if any)
Coolness, color, and temperature change in hands, arms, feet, and legs, perspiration may be present	Peripheral circulation diminished to facilitate increased circulation to vital organs	Place socks on feet; cover with light cotton blankets; keep warm blankets on person, but *do not use electric blanket*
Increased sleeping	Conservation of energy	Spend time with the client; hold the hand; speak normally to the client even though there may be a lack of response
Disorientation, confusion of time, place, person	Metabolic changes	Identify self by name before speaking to client; speak softly, clearly, and truthfully
Incontinence of urine and/or bowel	Increased muscle relaxation and decreased consciousness	Maintain vigilance, change bedding as appropriate, use bed pads, try not to use an indwelling catheter
Congestion	Poor circulation of body fluids, immobilization, and the inability to expectorate secretions causes gurgling, rattles, bubbling	Elevate the head with pillows and/or raise the head of the bed; gently turn the head to the side to drain secretions
Restlessness	Metabolic changes and decrease in oxygen to the brain	Calm the client by speech and action; reduce light; gently rub back, stroke arms, or read aloud; play soothing music; *do not use restraints*
Decreased intake of food and fluids	Body conservation of energy for function	Do not force client to eat or drink; give ice chips, soft drinks, juice, popsicles as possible; apply petroleum jelly to dry lips, if client is a mouth breather, apply protective jelly more frequently as necessary
Decreased urine output	Decreased fluid intake and decreased circulation to kidney	None
Altered breathing pattern Fear of suffocation, air hunger	Metabolic and oxygen changes of respiratory system Decreased oxygenation	Elevate the head of bed; hold hand, speak gently to client. Administer anxiolytics, opiates as ordered to relieve pain and apprehension

Adapted from Hess PA: Loss, grief, and dying. In Beare P, Myers J: *Adult health nursing,* ed 2, St. Louis, 1994, Mosby.

Spiritual Comfort

Giving spiritual comfort means as much to most clients as meeting their physical needs. Without a purpose or sense of hope about their lives, clients' values and worth as living human beings may be doubted. The nurse seeks to help the dying client explore the meaning of his or her life, the experience of dying, and spiritual answers to life's questions as a step in comprehending the loss that death presents. The nurse develops a healing relationship with a client to mobilize hope that the experience will not lead to suffering, to find an interpretation or understanding of death, and to assist the client in using emotional and spiritual resources (Benner, 1984). For many clients, a chaplain, social worker, or member of the church can provide invaluable support.

Box 43-1 Approaches for Involving the Dying Client's Family in End-of-Life Care

- Describe and demonstrate feeding techniques and selection of foods to facilitate ease of chewing and swallowing.
- Demonstrate bathing, mouth care, straightening of linen, and other hygiene measures to family.
- Instruct family on need to enforce rest periods for client's comfort.
- Teach family to recognize signs and symptoms to expect as the client's condition worsens and information on whom to call in an emergency.
- Provide information daily with regard to the client's condition. Prepare the family for sudden changes in the client's appearance and behavior.
- Discuss ways to support the dying person and listen to needs and fears.
- Assist in planning a visitation schedule for family members to prevent client and family from becoming fatigued.
- Allow young children to visit a dying parent or grandparent if all parties consent. (Some dying clients have strong feelings about possibly traumatizing children during this transition).
- Be willing to listen to family complaints about the client's care and feelings about the client.
- Help family members learn to interact with the dying person (e.g., using attentive listening, avoiding false reassurances, conducting conversations about normal family activities or problems).
- When the family becomes fatigued with care activities, relieve them from their duties so that they can acquire needed rest and support. Refer them to resources for meals and lodging.
- As death nears, help the family stay in communication with the dying person through short visits, caring silence, touch, and telling the client of their love.
- After death, assist the family with decision making, such as selection of a mortician, transportation of family members, and collection of the client's belongings.

Grief Support

As death approaches, the family and significant others need increased support. Support for grieving families is best provided within the context of understanding the cultural, ethnic, and social factors that influence the family's feelings and beliefs about death and their relationship to the client. The nurse must remain sensitive to the limits and nature of their role as perceived by the family. During a conversation when family members are able to express their feelings and wishes is a good time for the nurse to clarify who is handling the client's affairs and what funeral arrangements are to be made. Teaching the family various coping skills will meet the family's need to be useful and involved in the loss experience (Box 43-1). Factual information about what to expect as death draws near (e.g., type of supportive care, its purpose, and expected client responses) can provide some understanding of the unknown. The nurse must be willing to give assistance and be accessible to the client and family.

Time of Death

The Uniform Determination of Death Act (UDDA) definition or a similar definition of death is now accepted in all 50 of the United States as valid and legal criteria of death. The UDDA defines death as "irreversible cessation of circulatory and respiratory functions or irreversible cessation of all function of the brain, including the brainstem" (Chabalewski and Norris, 1994). When death occurs, cellular and circulatory changes create alterations in the body's tissues (Table 43-2). These changes influence the manner in which the nurse cares for the body after death, particularly the way tissues and body parts are handled and moved. It is important for the nurse to prepare the body for viewing by family and significant others as quickly as possible. The longer a nurse waits to care for the body, the more difficult it is to make the body appear natural.

Table 43-2 Physiological Changes After Death

Change	Related Interventions
Stiffening of body (**rigor mortis**) developing 2 to 4 hours after death; involves contraction of skeletal and smooth muscle owing to lack of adenosine 5-triphosphate (ATP).	Before rigor mortis develops, position body in normal anatomical alignment, close eyelids and mouth and insert dentures in mouth.
Reduction in body temperature with loss of skin elasticity (algor mortis).	Gently remove tape and dressings to avoid tissue breakdown. Avoid pulling on skin or body parts.
Purple discoloration of skin (livor mortis) in dependent areas caused by breakdown of red blood cells.	Elevate head to prevent facial discoloration.
Body tissues soften and liquefy by bacterial fermentation.	Store body in cool place in hospital morgue or other designated area.

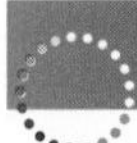

Skill Performance Guidelines

1. As it becomes obvious that a person is facing a life-threatening illness or is likely to die following an accident, determine the status of the person's advanced directives.
2. As a client's death approaches, consider if the dying person is a candidate for organ/tissue donation.
3. Following a client's death, consult agency policy regarding who is to pronounce death (e.g., attending physician or resident) and what departments (e.g., nursing supervisor, medical records) are to be notified at the time of death. Notify as directed.
4. Following a client's death, contact significant others to determine their status and to address priority needs.
5. Care for the body needs to be performed in a timely manner. If organ or tissue donation has been made, notify the **Organ Procurement Agency (OPA)** as soon as death is imminent.
6. Determine the needs and desires of the family and significant others as the body is prepared for transfer to the funeral home or **morgue.** Consult with significant others about when they want to see the deceased, if or how they want to be involved in caring for the body, and if cultural practices or spiritual beliefs of the deceased impact care of the body.
7. Consider the well-being of the roommates and others in the unit. Let the roommate know of the death and offer the opportunity to move the roommate to another location while the deceased is prepared to be removed from the room. Close door of other client rooms during body preparation and transfer.
8. Implement Standard Precautions: use protective equipment for the level of anticipated body substance exposure.
9. Ensure that the deceased's belongings are given to significant others. Follow agency policy in documenting the transfer. If there are valuables involved, having a second witness present is always a sound practice.

Skill 43-1 Care of the Body After Death

When a client's death is pronounced, the physician certifies the death in the medical record and records the time of death and a description of therapies or actions taken. The physician may request permission from the family for an autopsy. An **autopsy** or postmortem examination is performed to confirm or determine the cause of death, gather data regarding the nature and progress of a disease, study the effects of therapies on body tissues, and provide statistical data for epidemiology and research purposes. A consent form must be signed by the most immediate family member and the physician or designated requester. Autopsies are required in circumstances of unusual death (e.g., violent trauma, unexpected death in the home) as well as death occurring within a set time frame following hospitalization. Each state has guidelines for when autopsies are required. Autopsies normally do not delay burial.

Delegation Considerations

Care of the body after death can be delegated to assistive personnel. However, the nurse should recognize that often the family will expect to see the nurse more than usual to provide support. At the time of death it may be best for the nurse and assistive personnel to work together in preparing the body.

Inform care providers of any preferences the family might have because of cultural, religious, or ethnic beliefs that will influence the routine procedure of caring for the client's body.

Reinforce the importance of handling the body with respect.

Equipment

- Disposable gloves, gown, and other protective clothing
- Plastic bag for hazardous waste disposal
- Washbasin, washcloth, warm water, and bath towel
- Clean gown or disposable gown for body as indicated by agency policy
- Absorbent pads
- Syringes for removing Foley catheters
- Scissors
- Body bag or plastic shroud (consult agency procedure)
- Identification tag(s) as specified by hospital policy
- Small pillow or towel
- Paper tape, gauze dressings
- Paper bag, plastic bag, or other suitable receptacle for client's clothing, belongings, and other items to be returned to significant others
- Valuables envelope

Step	Rationale

Assessment

1. Assess for presence of family members or significant others and whether they have been informed of the client's death. Determine who is legally defined as next of kin.
   It is the physician's responsibility to notify significant others of the client's death. The nurse provides emotional support and prepares the body for viewing.
2. Approach next of kin for tissue donation or call organ/tissue request team (check agency policy). Discuss all options.
   Organ/tissue request should be performed by staff who have received appropriate training.
3. Allow time for significant others to ask questions.
   Conveys caring and concern for significant other. May provide valuable information about the response of significant others and their needs.
4. Once family has made decision, complete necessary organ/tissue donation request form.
   Federal guidelines require documentation that request has been made.
5. Assess the deceased for general condition of the body and any bandages, tubes, or equipment.
   Because of the fragility of tissues following death, tissue damage can occur easily. Most agencies have specific policies about removal of tubes, wires, and equipment.
6. Determine if an autopsy is planned.
   If an autopsy is planned, some procedures such as removal of tubes and lines may be contraindicated.

Nursing Diagnosis

Defining characteristics from the assessment data may reveal the following nursing diagnoses for clients requiring this skill:

For clients:
Risk for impaired skin integrity

For family and significant others:
Powerlessness
Dysfunctional grieving

Related factors are individualized based on the client's, family's, and significant others' needs.

Planning

1. **Expected outcomes** following completion of procedure:
   - Deceased's body will be free of skin damage.
     Care is delivered so as to prevent additional bruises, lacerations, or abrasions.
   - Significant others will express grief.
     Significant others feel support in being able to react to loss of loved one.
2. Gather or direct assistive personnel to gather needed equipment.
   Because this is often a time of emotional intensity for significant others, organization is particularly important.
3. Have body placed in a private room or have roommate moved to another area as body is being prepared.
   Provides staff with an area to make the body presentable for family to visit in private.

Implementation

1. Check with significant others about notifying other significant family members or friends.
   Following a death, significant others may have difficulty with remembering details about what to do, how to respond, and may need assistance.
2. Discuss procedure of preparing the body with significant others. Inquire if there are particular cultural or spiritual practices that should be followed.
   Having an ability to direct what is happening can increase the significant other's sense of control. Discussing personal preferences with the significant others can convey your caring and concern.

- ***Critical Decision Point***
  Significant others may want to be involved with the final preparation of the body. Being able to participate in this final aspect of care can facilitate grieving and acknowledgment of the death.

Step	Rationale
3. If tissue donation has been made, consult agency policy for specific guidelines on care of the body.	Retrieval of tissues (e.g., eyes, bone, skin) may require special preparation measures.
4. Arrange equipment at bedside.	
5. Wash hands.	Reduces transmission of microorganisms.
6. Close room door or draw bedside curtain.	Provides privacy for the deceased and significant others. Limits exposure of other clients to the person's death.
7. Apply disposable gloves and gown or protective barriers as applicable.	Body excretions may harbor infectious microorganisms. For example, withdrawal of intravenous tubing or other tubing may cause temporary bleeding.

- ***Critical Decision Point***
  If significant others are assisting in the preparation of the body, be sure they too are protected from body excretions.

Step	Rationale
8. Identify the body according to agency policy. Leave identification in place as directed in agency policy.	Ensures proper identification of the body for delivery to morgue, autopsy room, and funeral home.
9. If in keeping with agency procedures, remove all indwelling catheters, intravenous, oxygen, and other tubes. **(If an autopsy is to be performed, policy may direct to leave these devices in place.)** Dress puncture wounds with a small dressing and paper tape.	Creates a normal appearance. Paper tape minimizes skin trauma.
10. If the person wore dentures, reinsert them. If mouth fails to close, place a rolled-up towel under the chin.	It is difficult to insert dentures after rigor mortis occurs. Dentures maintain natural facial expression.
11. Position client as outlined in agency procedures. Avoid placing one hand on top of the other. Check agency policy regarding need to restrain hands and feet.	Client appears natural and comfortable. Placing one hand on top of the other can lead to discoloration of skin. Agencies often require restraining of appendages to prevent tissue damage when body is being moved.
12. Place small pillow or folded towel under the head or elevate head of bed 10 to 15 degrees.	Prevents pooling of blood in the face and subsequent discoloration.
13. Close eyes gently by grasping the eyelashes and pulling lids over corneas of eyes.	Closed eyes present a more natural appearance. Pressure on lids can lead to discoloration.
14. Wash body parts soiled by blood, urine, feces, or other drainage. (A mortician will provide a complete bath.)	Prepares body for viewing and reduces odors.
15. Place an absorbent pad under the client's buttocks.	Relaxation of sphincter muscles at time of death may cause release of urine or feces.

- ***Critical Decision Point***
  Turning a corpse sometimes leads to a breath exhaled from the body. This is a normal event.

Step	Rationale
16. Remove soiled dressings and replace with clean gauze dressings. Use paper tape.	Paper tape minimizes skin trauma. Changing dressings helps to control odors caused by microorganisms and to create a more acceptable appearance.
17. Place a clean gown on the client (agency policy may require removal before body is wrapped).	Prepares body for viewing.
18. Brush and comb client's hair. Remove any clips, hairpins, or rubber bands.	During viewing, the client should appear well-groomed. Hard objects such as pins can damage or discolor the face and scalp.
19. If significant others request viewing, place a sheet or light blanket over the body with only the head and upper shoulders exposed. Remove unneeded equipment from the room. Provide soft lighting and offer chairs.	Maintains dignity and respect for the client and significant others. Prevents exposure of body parts.

- ***Critical Decision Point***
  Determine if significant others need time alone with the deceased or would be more comfortable if a staff member remained in the room.

STEP	RATIONALE
20. After the significant others have left the room, remove all linen and the client's gown (refer to agency policy). Place body in body bag or apply the shroud as required by the agency (see illustration).	Prevents injury to skin and extremities. Avoids unnecessary exposure of body parts.

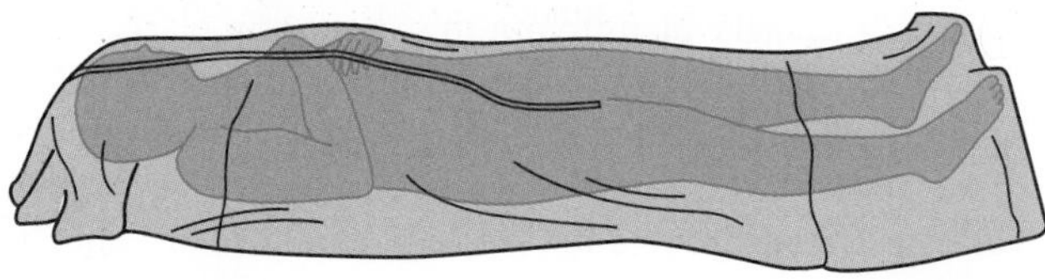

STEP **20** Body bag.

STEP	RATIONALE
21. Label the body as directed by agency policy.	Ensures proper identification of the body.
22. Arrange transportation of the body to the morgue or mortuary. If delay is anticipated before the mortician arrives, the body should be cooled in the morgue to prevent further tissue damage.	

EVALUATION

STEP	RATIONALE
1. Observe significant others' response to the loss.	Each person's response to loss is unique, and evaluation is necessary to determine the need for referral for assistance.
2. Provide significant others with the opportunity to express feelings.	Significant others often seek chance to express feelings with someone other than an immediate family member.

- ***Critical Decision Point***
  The nurse may need to find a private place for significant others so they can feel free to express their emotions.

STEP	RATIONALE
3. Note appearance and condition of client's skin during preparation of the body.	Determines if damage to tissues occurs after preparation of the body.

UNEXPECTED OUTCOMES AND RELATED INTERVENTIONS

- Family/significant others become immobilized by their grief and have difficulty functioning.
  - Consider if a member of the family is able to act as a calming presence. Enlist his or her help in explaining what to expect in after-death care.
  - Call for assistance from pastoral care workers, social work staff, or a nursing staff member who has developed a close relationship with the client/family.
- Significant others become very agitated and express their grief openly.
  - Additional support from security may be necessary.
- Lacerations, bruises, or abrasions are noted on skin surfaces of deceased. Positioning or preparation of the body results in skin injury.
  - Document according to policy.

RECORDING AND REPORTING

- Record date and time of death, time physician notified, name of physician pronouncing death, delivery of postmortem care, identification of body, consent form signed by significant other, disposition of the body, and information provided to significant others.
- Document any marks, bruises, wounds on body before death or those observed during care of the body. Reduces risk of liability for creating such marks in the care of the body after death or in transport to the morgue. Certain markings can identify the body if identification tags are lost or destroyed.
- Document how valuables and personal belongings were handled and who received them. Secure signatures as required by agency policy.

Pediatric Considerations

- Parents should be allowed to stay with the child any time of day or night. Reassure parents that everything possible was done for the child.
- Make every effort to arrange for family members, especially parents, to be with the child at the time of death, if they wish to be present (Wong and others, 1999).
- Parents frequently ask, "What will my child die from?", "What will happen when he dies?" Answer questions giving specific details of an impending death, while being sensitive to the family's cultural background and knowledge level (Martinson, 1995).
- Parents frequently ask to hold the child's body during viewing.

Gerontological Considerations

- Despite the family's grief and pain, the family must give the client permission to die, let the client know it is alright to let go and leave (Ebersole and Hess, 1998).
- Visitors should be allowed to be with the dying aged any time of day or night. Night is the most lonely and painful time.

Home Care Considerations

- As death approaches, significant others often need information about what to expect (e.g., the signs and symptoms of impending death). Encourage family to talk with client and say their last goodbyes, as the client's hearing is still often intact.
- As death approaches, the nurse needs to consider the type of support the significant others are likely to need at the time of death and make plans to put this support in place.
- Following death in the home, the nurse will need to follow agency guidelines related to body preparation and transfer of the body.
- For disposal of durable medical equipment (e.g., tubings, needles, syringes) or soiled dressings or linens, the nurse must follow the policies of the agency. The nurse may need to instruct significant others in the handling and disposal of medical waste.

Critical Thinking Exercises

1. Mr. Weiss is a client you have cared for over the last two days. His family is not able to reach the hospital at the time of his death, but they arrive shortly thereafter. You approach his daughter and ask if the family wishes to donate her father's tissues. She responds, "I didn't think you could donate anything after someone dies?" How might you respond? Is the daughter the best person to ask?
2. Mr. Weiss's daughter asks to view Mr. Weiss's body. When she enters the room she asks, "Why is that small towel placed under dad's head?" What would be your response?
3. You are preparing Mr. Weiss's body for the funeral home. As you turn him to place the body in the body bag, drainage exits from a puncture wound. What would you do?

References

Badzek L: What you need to know about the advance directives, *Nurs 92* 22(6):58, 1992.

Callanan M, Kelley P: *Final gifts: understanding the special awareness, needs, and communications of the dying,* New York, 1992, Simon & Schuster.

Chabalewski F, Norris M: The gift of life: talking to families about organ and tissue donation, *Am J Nurs* 94(6):28, 1994.

Dixon MD: The quality of mercy: reflections on provider-assisted suicide, *J Clin Ethics* 8:290-302, 1997.

Ebersole P, Hess P: *Toward healthy aging,* ed 5, St Louis, 1998, Mosby.

Ersek M and others: Priority ethical issues in oncology nursing: current approaches and future directions, *Oncol Nurs Forum* 22:803-807, 1995.

Hess PA: Loss, grief, and dying. In Beare P, Myers J: *Adult health nursing,* ed 3, St. Louis, 1998, Mosby.

Johns J: Advanced directives and opportunities for nurses, *Image* 28(2):149, 1996.

Lindsay K: Assisting professionals in approaching families for donation, *Crit Care Nurs Q* 17(4):55, 1995.

Long B, Phipps W, Cassmeyer V: *Medical-surgical nursing: a nursing process approach,* ed 3, St. Louis, 1993, Mosby.

Martinson M: Pediatric hospice nursing, *Ann Rev Nurs Res* 13:195-214, 1995.

Quill TE and others: Palliative options of last resort: a comparison of voluntarily stopping eating and drinking, terminal sedation, physician-assisted suicide, and voluntary active euthanasia, *JAMA* 278:2099-2104.

Rein A and others: Advance directive decision making among medical inpatients, *J Prof Nurs* 12(1):39, 1996.

Schwarz JK: Assisted dying and nursing practice, *Image* 31(4):367-373, 1999.

Wong D and others: *Whaley and Wong nursing care of infants and children,* ed 6, St. Louis, 1999, Mosby.

GLOSSARY

abdominal girth — The measurement of the abdomen's circumference, taken at the same place with each measurement.

abduction — Movement of an extremity away from the midline of the body.

accommodation reflex — Adjustment of the eyes for near vision, composed of pupillary constriction, convergence of the visual axes, and increased convexity of the lens.

accurate empathy — Communication technique used by nurse to show understanding of client's feelings and experiences.

Acetest — A test that measures the presence of ketone (acetone) bodies in the urine. A large quantity of acetone causes rapid change in the color of the Acetest tablet.

active listening — An interpersonal process whereby a person hears a message, decodes the meaning, and conveys an understanding about the meaning to the sender.

active range of motion — Exercises of the joints performed by an individual without assistance.

active-assisted range of motion — Exercises of the joints performed by an individual with some assistance. A nurse, for example, helps support an extremity.

activity tolerance — Kind and amount of exercise or work that a person is able to perform.

acuity charting — Documentation that quantifies the level of care required by a client in a health care setting.

acute pain — Severe pain with a rapid onset and of short duration.

A.D. — Right ear.

addiction — A compulsive physiological need for a habit-forming drug.

adduction — Movement of an extremity toward midline of the body.

adjuvant therapy — The treatment of a disease with substances that enhance the action of drugs, especially drugs that promote the production of antibodies.

adrenergic drug — A medication that mimics the effects of sympathetic nerve stimulation of the autonomic nervous system.

advance directives — A written agreement established between a client and physician to withhold heroic measures or life-sustaining treatment if the client's condition becomes irreversible.

adverse drug reactions — Nontherapeutic effects of medications.

aerobe — A microorganism that lives and grows in the presence of free oxygen.

afebrile — Without fever.

agglutinate — A process by which cells that display antigens (red blood cells, bacteria) adhere to each other, or clump together.

air embolus — A quantity of air that circulates in the bloodstream to eventually lodge in a blood vessel.

air fluidization — The process of blowing warm air through a collection of microspheres to create a fluidlike environment; used in special mattresses designed to reduce pressure against a person's skin.

air leak — Escaping air in closed chest drainage; may be client centered or within the chest tube system.

air suspension bed — A device that supports a client's weight on air-filled cushions, minimizing tissue damage from pressure and shear.

air-fluidized bed — A special bed designed to distribute weight evenly over its support surface. Fluidization is created by forcing a gentle flow of temperature-controlled air upward through a mass of fine ceramic microspheres.

airway obstruction — An abnormal condition of the respiratory system characterized by a mechanical impediment to the delivery or the absorption of oxygen in the lungs.

aldosterone — A steroid hormone produced by the adrenal cortex that causes the kidney tubules to excrete potassium and reabsorb sodium and water.

Allen's test — This test is performed to determine the collateral circulation supply in the radial and ulnar arteries.

allergen — A substance that can produce a hypersensitive reaction in the body but that is not necessarily intrinsically harmful.

allogenic — Denoting a cell type that is from the same species but genetically distinct.

alopecia — Partial or complete lack of hair.

Alzheimer's disease — Presenile dementia, characterized by progressive confusion, memory failure, disorientation, restlessness, and speech disturbances. Cause is not fully understood.

Ambu-bag — Portable resuscitation device that provides manual inflation of the lungs. An Ambu-bag is usually used with supplemental oxygen.

Ambularm™ — Battery operated, position-sensitive alarm attached to a client's leg, which alerts the staff when a client attempts to get out of bed.

American Hospital Association (AHA) — A not-for-profit association of health care provider organizations that are committed to health improvement of their communities.

The American Society of Parenteral and Enteral Nutrition (ASPEN) — An organization that provides education, support, and accreditation to individuals in the nutritional support field.

amino acid — An organic compound composed of one or more basic amino groups and one or more carboxyl groups. Amino acids are the building blocks that construct proteins and the end products of protein digestion.

amnesic syndrome — Memory impairment in the absence of other cognitive impairments.

ampule — Small sterile glass or plastic container that usually contains a single dose of solution to be administered parenterally.

anaerobic — Pertaining to absence of air or oxygen.

analgesia — A decreased or absent sensation of pain.

anaphylactic reaction — Exaggerated hypersensitivity reaction to a previously encountered antigen. It is a severe and sometimes fatal systemic reaction characterized by itching, hyperemia, angioedema, and in severe cases vascular collapse, bronchospasm, and shock.

anaphylaxis — An exaggerated hypersensitivity reaction to a previously encountered antigen. The reaction may be localized or generalized.

anastomosis — A surgical joining of two ducts or blood vessels to allow flow from one to the other.

anemia — A disorder characterized by a decrease in hemoglobin in the blood to levels below the normal range, decreased red cell production, or increased red cell destruction or blood loss.

anesthesia — The absence of normal sensation, especially sensitivity to pain.

anesthetics — Drugs or agents capable of producing a complete or partial loss of feeling.

anions — Negatively charged ions.
anthropometry — The science of measuring the human body as to height, weight, and size of component parts, including measurement of skin folds.
antianginal drug — A medication that dilates coronary arteries, improving blood flow to the myocardium to prevent angina.
anticipatory guidance — A cognitive strategy that involves use of descriptive sensory words and phrases the client is familiar with to provide an understanding of what to expect during a procedure.
antidysrhythmic — A class of medications that possesses properties for controlling abnormal cardiac rhythms, (e.g., quinidine and propranolol [Inderal]).
antiemetic — Of or pertaining to a substance or procedure that prevents or alleviates nausea and vomiting.
antipyretic — Pertaining to a substance, such as a medication, that reduces fever.
apical pulse — Measurement of the heartbeat as taken with the stethoscope placed over the apex of the heart.
apnea — An absence of spontaneous respirations.
approximate — To come together, as in the edges of a wound.
aqueous — Watery or waterlike; referring to a medication prepared with water.
areola — Referring to the areola mammae, the pigmented, circular area surrounding the nipple of each breast.
artificial airway — Plastic or rubber device inserted into the upper or lower respiratory tract to facilitate ventilation or secretion removal.
A.S. — Left ear.
ascites — Effusion and accumulation of serous fluid in the abdominal cavity.
asepsis — The absence of disease-producing (pathogenic) organisms.
aseptic technique — The methods used during client care to prevent microbial contamination. They can be either clean (medical asepsis) techniques or sterile (surgical asepsis) techniques.
aspirant — Fluid or particulate that is aspirated.
aspirate — Withdrawal of fluid or air into the barrel of a syringe or suction device.
aspiration — The entry of gastric contents into the tracheobronchial passages. This increases a client's risk for aspiratory pneumonia.
astigmatism — Abnormal condition of the eye in which the light rays cannot be focused clearly in a point on the retina because the spherical curve of the cornea is not equal in all meridians. Vision is blurred, and use of the eyes causes discomfort.
astringent — A topical substance that causes constriction of tissues upon application; commonly used for cleansing the skin.
atelectasis — An abnormal condition characterized by the collapse of lung tissue, preventing the respiratory exchange of carbon dioxide and oxygen.
atmospheric pressure — Pressure exerted by the atmosphere. (Atmospheric pressure at sea level is 760 mm Hg.)
atrophy — Wasting or diminution of size or physiological activity of a part of the body caused by disease or other influences.
A.U. — Both ears.
auscultation — The act of listening for sounds within the body to evaluate the condition of the heart, lungs, pleura, intestines, or other organs or to detect fetal heart sounds. Performed directly or most commonly through use of a stethoscope.
auscultatory gap — The temporary disappearance of Korotkoff sounds when blood pressure is being auscultated. Occurs in hypertensive clients and may cause an underestimation of blood pressure.
autoclave — An appliance used to sterilize medical instruments or other objects with steam under pressure.
autolet — A small instrument with a lancet used to obtain a capillary blood specimen.
autologous blood transfusion — Transfusion of a client's own blood through either predeposit, blood salvaged intraoperatively by a cell saver, or blood shed postoperatively.
autopsy — Examination of the deceased's body performed after a person's death to confirm or determine the cause of death.
autotransfusion — The collection, anticoagulation, filtration, and reinfusion of blood from an active bleeding site. Used in cases of trauma and major surgery.
axillary — Pertaining to the pyramid-shaped space that forms the underside of the shoulder between the upper part of the arm and the side of the chest.
backrub — The application of gentle methodical pressure to the back.
bacteremia — Presence of bacteria in the blood.
bacteriostatic — Tending to inhibit development or reproduction of bacteria.
balance — Position in which the person's center of gravity is correct so that the risk of falling is reduced.
bariatric bed — A specialized surface equipped with hand controls to allow for self-positioning, providing a stable, adaptable surface for managing the morbidly obese client.
basal energy expenditure (BEE) — The amount of energy required at rest for basic life processes such as breathing, maintaining body temperature, and cardiac function. Basal energy expenditure can be estimated or measured.
basal metabolism — Energy needed to maintain the body's basic processes such as respiration, circulation, and temperature.
base of support — Surface area on which an object rests.
bed rest — Placement of the client in bed for a prescribed period for therapeutic reasons.
BEE — Abbreviation for basal energy expenditure.
belt restraint — Type of restraint used to secure a client on a stretcher.
bile — A digestive juice secreted by the liver, stored in the gallbladder, and secreted in the small intestine to digest fat. Bile causes brown color of feces.
binder — Bandage made of a large piece of material to fit and support a specific body part.
biopsy — The removal and microscopic examination of tissue, performed to establish precise diagnosis.
blood culture — A laboratory test on serum to determine presence of infection in the blood.
blood group — Classification of blood based on the presence or absence of genetically determined antigens on the surface of the red cell.
blood plasma — The liquid portion of the blood, free of its formed elements and particles.
blood transfusion — Administration of whole blood or a blood component as cells to replace blood lost through trauma, surgery, or disease.
blood type — Blood groups identified by genetically determined antigens on the surface of red blood cells.
blood typing — Identification of genetically determined antigens on the surface of the red blood cell, used to determine a person's blood group.
blood warming coil — Device constructed of coiled plastic tubing used to warm reserve blood before massive transfusion.
body alignment — Refers to the condition of joints, tendons, ligaments, and muscles in various body positions.
body mechanics — Coordinated efforts of the musculoskeletal and nervous systems to maintain proper balance, posture, and body alignment.

bolus — 1. A round mass, specifically a masticated lump of food ready to be swallowed. 2. A large, round preparation of medicinal material for oral ingestion. 3. A dose of a medication or a contrast material injected all at once intravenously.

bone marrow — Specialized, soft tissue filling the spaces in cancellous bone of the epiphyses; responsible for red blood cell production.

borborygmus — Audible abdominal sound produced by hyperactive intestinal peristalsis.

bradycardia — An abnormality in heart rate in which the heart contracts steadily at a rate less than 60 contractions per minute.

bradypnea — Breathing that is normal in rate but abnormally slow (less than 12 breaths per minute).

broad-spectrum antibiotic — An antibiotic that is effective against a wide range of infectious microorganisms.

bronchophony — An increase in intensity and clarity of vocal resonance that may result from an increase in lung tissue density, such as in the consolidation of pneumonia.

bronchospasm — Abnormal contraction of the smooth muscles of the bronchi.

bronchus — One of several large air passages in the lungs through which pass inspired air and exhaled gases.

bruit — Abnormal sound or murmur created by turbulent blood flow heard while auscultating an organ, gland, or artery.

buccal — Of or pertaining to the inside of the cheek; surface of a tooth or gum next to the cheek.

cadence — Pace or rate of verbal communication.

calorie (Kcal) — A calorie is the amount of heat required to raise the temperature of 1 g of water 1° C at atmospheric pressure.

cancer pain — Pain that may be due to tumor progression and its related pathology and/or treatment modalities, may have a rapid or prolonged onset, varies in intensity, and can last less than or greater than 6 months.

cannula — A flexible tube containing a stiff, pointed trocar; the tube may be inserted into the body, guided by the trocar. As the trocar is removed, a body fluid may pass through the cannula.

capillary closing pressure — The amount of external pressure required to close off the blood flow to the capillaries.

carcinoma — Malignant epithelial neoplasm that tends to invade surrounding tissue and spread to distant regions of the body.

cardiac — 1. Of or pertaining to the heart. 2. Pertaining to a person with heart disease.

cardiac output — Volume of blood ejected by the ventricles of the heart in 1 minute; equal to stroke volume times heart rate.

cardiomegaly — Enlargement of the heart; typical sign of heart failure.

cardiopulmonary arrest — Sudden cessation of respirations, pulse, and circulation.

cardiopulmonary resuscitation (CPR) — Basic emergency procedure for life support, consisting of artificial respiration and manual external cardiac massage.

caries — Decay of a tooth; progressive decalcification of enamel and dentin of a tooth.

carminative — A solution to provide relief from gaseous distention.

case management — The assignment of a health care provider to assist a client by assessing need for health care and social service systems and to ensure that required services are obtained.

cast — Rigid plaster or fiberglass application molded over skin tissues to hold musculoskeletal tissues to permit healing of injuries.

cast brace — Combination of a brace within a cast at a joint.

cast saw — Saw used to cut through plaster to remove cast.

cast shoe — Shoe worn over the foot encased in plaster.

cast stabilization — Use of rods, pins, broom handles, or sticks to lend stability to a particular cast.

cast syndrome — A series of client signs indicative of an untoward (claustrophobic) reaction to being in a cast.

casting tape — Rolls of adhesive or resin-impregnated tape for use as lightweight casts.

cathartic — Drug that acts to promote bowel evacuation.

catheter hub — Plastic threaded connection at end of an intravenous catheter.

catheterization — Introduction of a rubber or plastic tube through the urethra and into the bladder.

cations — Positively charged ions.

cell cycle — The sequence of events that occurs during the growth and division of tissue cells.

center of gravity — Midpoint or center of body weight. In the adult it is the midpelvic cavity between the symphysis pubis and the umbilicus.

centigrade — Temperature scale in which 0 degrees is the freezing point of water and 100 degrees is the boiling point of water at sea level; also called Celsius.

central venous catheter (CVC) — A catheter that is threaded through the internal jugular, antecubital, or subclavian vein, usually with tip resting in the superior vena cava or right atrium.

central venous pressure (CVP) — Pressure in the great veins (superior and inferior vena cava) as blood returns to the heart.

cephalic vein — One of the four superficial veins of the upper limb.

cerebrospinal fluid — Substance contained within the four ventricles of the brain, the subarachnoid space, and the central canal of the spinal cord.

cerumen — Earwax; a waxy secretion produced by apocrine sweat glands in the external ear canal.

cervical halter — Support for the head, made of cotton material, used for traction.

chart — A client's medical record; or the act of recording data in a client's record, usually at prescribed intervals.

charting by exception — A charting methodology in which data are entered only when there is an exception from what is normal or expected. Reduces time spent documenting.

cheilosis — Disorder of the lips and mouth characterized by scales and fissures.

chemotherapeutic agent — A medication used to treat cancer, which alters the growth of a cancer cell.

chemotherapy — Use of drugs to prevent cancer cells from multiplying, invading adjacent tissue, and metastasizing.

chest physiotherapy — Physical maneuvers, including postural drainage, chest percussion, vibration, rib shaking, and cough, to improve airway mucus clearance in clients with retained tracheobronchial secretions.

chest tube — Catheter inserted through the chest wall into the intrapleural space by the physician.

chronic nonmalignant pain — Pain occurring over a prolonged period that is not caused by a malignancy.

chronic pain — Continuous or recurrent pain lasting longer than 3 months.

chronic venous insufficiency — Abnormal circulatory condition characterized by decreased return of the venous blood from the legs to the trunk of the body.

Circulating Nurse — An RN considered to be the charge nurse in the operating room during a surgical procedure.

circumduction — The circular movement of a limb; the motion of the head of a bone within an articulating cavity such as the hip joint.

clarification — An attempt to put into words vague ideas or unclear thoughts of the client to enhance the nurse's understanding or asking the client to explain what he or she means.

class II biological safety cabinet — A vertical containment or biological safety cabinet that recirculates air through a high-efficiency particulate air (HEPA) filter.

clean technique (medical asepsis) — The purposeful prevention of the transmission of microorganisms by using procedures such as hand washing and disinfection of equipment to reduce the number of microorganisms.

cleansing enema — An enema, usually soap suds, administered repeatedly until the colon is free of all formed fecal material.

clean-voided specimen — A technique used to collect a urine specimen as free from bacterial contamination as possible without catheterizing the client.

client-centered air leak — The entry of air, that originates from the client into a closed chest drainage system, as opposed to the entry of air originating from the chest drainage system itself.

Clinitest — A test that measures the amount of glucose and acetone in a urine specimen.

Clinitron bed — A special bed containing an air-fluidization mattress that conforms to the shape of a person's body to reduce pressure exerted against skin and soft tissues.

closed system suction catheter — A suction catheter that is attached to the mechanical ventilator circuit encased within a sterile sheath. The catheter system permits sterile airway suctioning without interrupting mechanical ventilation or requiring the nurse to apply sterile gloves.

coagulopathy — A pathological condition affecting the ability of the blood to coagulate.

colon — Portion of large intestine from the cecum to the rectum.

colon conduit — A surgical noncontinent (sometimes called incontinent) urinary diversion where the ureters are implanted into a 4 to 6 cm piece of large intestine that has been removed from the rest of the bowel and will now serve as a passageway for the urine. The distal end of this piece of colon is sutured closed, and the other end of the colon is brought out onto the client's abdomen as a stoma.

colonization — The reproduction of microorganisms at a specific site without the signs/symptoms of a disease or tissue invasion.

colonized — The presence of bacteria on the surface or in the tissue of a wound without indications of infection such as purulent exudate, foul odor, or surrounding inflammation. All stage II, III, and IV pressure ulcers are colonized.

colostomy — Surgical formation of an opening of the colon onto the surface of the abdomen through which fecal matter is emptied.

comforting — Any nursing action taken to promote comfort of the client, such as a back rub, change in position.

compartment syndrome — Insufficient arterial perfusion to an extremity caused by trauma or stasis; leads to ischemia and tissue necrosis if not reversed.

compatibility — The quality or state of existing together in harmony. The formation of a stable chemical or biochemical system, specifically in medication, so that two or more drugs can be administered at same time without producing side effects.

compliance — Fulfillment by the client of the caregiver's prescribed course of treatment.

compound — A substance composed of two or more different elements, chemically combined, that cannot be separated by physical means.

compress — Soft pad of gauze or cloth used to apply heat, cold, or medications to the surface of a body part.

concreteness — Communication that includes specific feelings, behaviors, and experiences or situations; communication that is not vague.

conduction — Mechanism of heat transfer involving flow of heat from one object to another with which it is in contact.

conduit — An artificially created channel for drainage of urine, (e.g., ileoloop).

congruent — Harmonious and consistent; the verbal and nonverbal message is congruent when the nonverbal message is the same or consistent with the verbal message.

conjunctiva — Mucous membrane lining the inner surfaces of the eyelids and anterior part of the sclera.

conjunctivitis — A highly contagious eye infection. The crusty drainage that collects on eyelid margins can easily spread from one eye to the other.

conscious sedation — An anesthetic procedure in which analgesia and anesthesia are accomplished without loss of consciousness.

consensual light reflex — Constriction of the pupil of one eye when the other eye is illuminated.

constipation — Condition characterized by difficulty in passing stool, or an infrequent passage of hard stool.

consultation — A process in which the help of a specialist is sought to identify ways to handle problems in client management or in the planning and implementation of health care programs.

contact lens — A small, transparent, curved glass or plastic lens shaped to fit over a person's cornea; the lens floats on a precorneal tear film.

contaminated — Being soiled, stained, touched, or otherwise exposed to harmful agents, such as by entry of potentially infectious microorganisms into or on a previously clean or sterile environment.

contamination — The introduction of infectious material on normally clean or sterile sites.

continent ostomy or diversion — Results from a surgical procedure that leaves the client with an internal pouch where either stool or urine is temporarily stored and the effluent is removed by intubation through the external stoma. It is continent because the effluent does not drain spontaneously from the stoma; instead a catheter must be inserted through the stoma to drain the effluent from the internal pouch.

continuous subcutaneous infusion (CSQI or CSCI) — A method of medication administration in which medication is administered continuously into the subcutaneous tissue using a medication infusion pump.

contracture — Abnormal condition of a joint, characterized by flexion and fixation and caused by atrophy and shortening of muscle fibers or by loss of normal elasticity of the skin.

coping — An individual's ability to manage stressful situations.

core temperature — Temperature of deep body tissues and organs.

costovertebral (CVA) angle tenderness — Palpation over this region can elicit tenderness. Tenderness is common with kidney infection or trauma to the region.

cough — Forced exhalation following this normal series of events: (a) partial or full inhalation; (b) closure of the glottis; (c) active contraction of expiratory muscles; and (d) rapid glottic opening.

countertraction — Use of client's body weight or other weights, ropes, and pulleys to counter the pull of the traction weight.

crackle — Fine bubbling sound heard on auscultation of the lung.

crepitation — The sound and/or feeling produced when bone ends rub against each other. The client describes the sound and feeling.

critical pathway — A schedule of critical care medical and nursing procedures, including diagnostic tests, medications, and consultations designed to effect an efficient coordinated program of treatment.

crutch gait — Gait assumed by a person on crutches by alternately bearing weight on one or both legs and on the crutches.

crutch palsy — Temporary or permanent loss of sensation or movement resulting from pressure on axilla from crutch.

cryotherapy — Therapy in which the skin is exposed to cool or cold temperatures; used to treat localized inflammatory responses.

cuff — A plastic, air or foam and air-filled, balloonlike attachment on the distal end of the endotracheal tube or tracheostomy tube that prevents loss of air from the lung and inhalation of foreign bodies around the tube.

culture — Laboratory test involving the cultivation of microorganisms or cells in a special growth medium.

cutaneous stimulation — Stimulation of the skin.

cuticle — A thin edge of cornified epithelium at the base of a nail.

CVA tenderness — Diagnostic sign of kidney inflammation. Tenderness is elicited during light percussion of the costal vertebral angle (CVA).

cyanosis — Bluish discoloration of the skin and mucous membranes caused by an excess of deoxygenated hemoglobin in the blood or a structural defect in the hemoglobin molecule.

cycloplegic — Pertaining to a drug that paralyzes ciliary muscles of the eye, causing pupillary dilation for ophthalmological examination or surgery.

cystectomy — The surgical removal of the bladder.

cytology — The study of cells, including their formation, origin, structure, function, biochemical activities, and pathology.

Dacron cuff — A sheath of Dacron surrounding an atrial or venous catheter to prevent ascending infections and accidental displacement of the catheter.

dandruff — Scaly material composed of dead, keratinized epithelium shed from the scalp. May also be a mild form of seborrheic dermatitits.

dangling — To sit on the side of a bed with legs dependent or feet on the floor.

dead space — A cavity remaining in a wound.

debride — To remove dead or damaged tissue from a wound; to remove dirt, foreign objects, damaged tissue, and cellular debris from a wound or burn in order to prevent infection and promote healing.

debridement — Removal of dead tissue in a wound.

decompression — Removal of pressure as from gas and fluid in the stomach and intestinal tract.

de-escalation — A communication strategy involving the reduction of anxious and/or agitated behaviors exhibited verbally or nonverbally by the client; using a calm yet firm approach diffuses the client's increasing anxiety and/or agitated state, thereby minimizing potentially violent outbursts.

defecation — Passage of feces from the digestive tract through the rectum.

dehiscence — The separation or opening of wound layers.

dementia — A term used to describe a group of symptoms related to a loss or impairment of mental powers. These symptoms appear in a person who is awake and are demonstrated by symptoms of mental confusion, memory loss, disorientation, intellectual impairment, or similar problems.

dental caries — Chalky white discoloration of teeth or presence of brown or black discoloration.

dentifrice — A pharmaceutical compound used with a toothbrush for cleaning and polishing teeth.

dependent position — The lowest position of an extremity or body.

dermatitis — An inflammatory condition of the skin characterized by erythema and pain or pruritus.

dermatological — Pertaining to the skin.

devitalized — Tissues with reduced oxygen supply and blood flow.

dextrose — The hydrated form of glucose.

diagnosis-related groups (DRGs) — Groups of diseases or conditions classified on the basis of primary and secondary diagnosis, primary and secondary procedure, and client age. The assigned length of stay for each DRG is part of the formula used in determining a medical facility's reimbursement for each DRG.

dialysis — A procedure that removes fluid and solid wastes from the blood or lymph.

diaphoresis — Secretion of sweat typically associated with hyperthermia, physical exertion, and emotional stress.

diastolic pressure — The lower blood pressure measurement, which reflects the pressure consistently exerted within the arterial system during the period of ventricular relaxation.

diluent — Agent that makes a solution or mixture thinner or more liquid by admixture.

discharge planning — The process by which the nurse plans for a client's eventual release from a health care agency; the process begins on a client's admission to the agency.

distraction — A pain-reduction technique that diverts an individual's attention away from the pain sensation.

don — To put on.

dorsal — Pertaining to the back or posterior.

dorsiflexion — Flexion toward the back, as accomplished by a muscle (e.g., in the hand or foot).

dorsum — The back of the hand.

double-void — A procedure of discarding the first urine specimen and testing the second urine specimen that was obtained 30 to 45 minutes later; this procedure gives a more accurate amount of glucose being spilled into the urine at that particular time.

drawsheet — A special sheet placed over the regular sheet on a bed and used to move a person in bed.

drop factor — Refers to the calibration of IV tubing (IV infusion set) in drops per milliliter. For example, the drop factor of microdrip IV tubing is 60 gtt/ml.

drug abuse — Use of a drug to obtain effects for which it is not prescribed. May lead to physical, social, and psychological harm.

drug addiction — Inability to control a drive or craving for a chemical substance.

drug dependence — Psychological or physiological reliance on a chemical substance.

drug interaction — The pharmacological interaction of drugs taken concurrently, which may result in an antagonistic, synergistic, or lethal response.

drug plateau — Blood serum concentration reached and maintained after repeated, fixed doses of a medication.

drug polymorphism — A variation in response to a drug.

drug tolerance — A decreased physiological response after repeated administration of a drug or a chemically related substance.

duration — A characteristic used in assessing a symptom; the length of time a symptom lasts.

duration of action — Length of time during which a drug is present in a concentration great enough to produce a therapeutic effect.

dysphagia — Difficulty swallowing.

dyspnea — Difficulty in breathing.

dysrhythmia — An irregularity or deviation from the normal pattern of a heartbeat.

dysuria — Pain or burning on urination, may also be accompanied with difficulty in urination. Usually indicates an urinary tract infection.

ecchymosis — Discoloration of an area of the skin or mucous membrane resulting from extravasation of blood into the subcutaneous tissues as a result of trauma to the underlying blood vessels or of fragility of the vessel walls.

eczema — Superficial dermatitis of unknown cause.

edema — Abnormal accumulation of fluid in interstitial spaces of tissues.

effective osmolality — Osmolality that causes water to move from one cell compartment to another. Effective osmolality is dependent on the number of solutes and on the permeability of the cell membrane to these solutes. Also referred to as tonicity.

effleurage — A type of massage stroke that glides without manipulating deep muscles, smoothes and extends muscles, increases nutrient absorption, and improves lymphatic and venous circulation.

effluent — The drainage that is normally expected from an ostomy.

egophony — A change in the voice sound as heard on auscultation of a client with pleural effusion. When client is asked to make e-e-e sounds, the sound is heard over the peripheral chest wall as a-a-a.

elastic bandage — Bandage of elasticized fabric that provides support and allows movement.

electrolyte — An element or compound that, when melted or dissolved in water or another solvent, dissociates into ions and is able to carry an electric current.

electronic infusion device (EID) — Used to infuse IV fluid at a prescribed rate. There are two types: an infusion pump, which is designed to deliver a measured amount of fluid over a period of time, and an IV controller, which delivers fluid with the aid of gravity.

embolus (emboli) — A foreign object, a quantity of air or gas, a bit of tissue or tumor, or a piece of thrombus that circulates in the bloodstream until it becomes lodged in a vessel.

empathy — Ability to recognize and to some extent share the emotions and state of mind of another and to understand the meaning and significance of that person's behavior.

end-of-life-care — Care given a terminally ill client.

endotracheal tube — Artificial airway inserted through the mouth into the trachea.

enema — Procedure involving introduction of a solution into the rectum for cleansing or therapeutic purposes.

enteral nutrition — The administration of nutrition via the gastrointestinal tract (i.e., by mouth, tube feeding, or oral supplement).

enteral tube feeding — The introduction of food or nutritive material directly into the digestive tract by nasogastric or gastric tube.

enteric coated — Tablets coated with a substance that does not dissolve until reaching the intestine. Used when drug constituents are irritating to oral and gastric mucosa.

enterostomy — Surgical procedure that produces an artificial anus or fistula in the intestine by incision through the abdominal wall.

enucleation — Removal of the eyeball, performed in cases of malignancy, severe infection, extensive trauma, or to control pain in glaucoma.

epidemiology — Study of the occurrence, distribution, and causes of disease.

epidural analgesia — Administration of local anesthetic by way of a catheter into the epidural space of the spinal column. Designed to produce anesthesia of the pelvic, abdominal, or genital areas.

episiotomy — A surgical procedure in which an incision is made in a woman's perineum to enlarge her vaginal opening for delivery of an infant; procedure prevents tearing of perineum.

epithelialization — The process by which epidermal cells migrate (move) over the wound's surface to close the top or "resurface" the wound.

erythema — Redness or inflammation of the skin or mucous membranes, result of dilatation and congestion of superficial capillaries.

eschar — Scab or dry crust that results from excoriation of the skin.

evaporation — Mechanism of heat loss whereby moisture from the body's surface changes to vapor and transfers heat to the surrounding air.

eversion — Turning outward or inside out, such as turning the foot outward at the ankle.

evidence-based practice — Recommended nursing interventions that have been shown to be effective when tested in clinical research.

evisceration — The separation of wound layers with the protrusion of abdominal organs through the wound layers.

excoriation — An injury to the surface of the skin or other part of the body caused by scratching or abrasion.

excretion — The process of eliminating, shedding, or getting rid of substances by body organs or tissues.

exercise — Performance of any physical activity for the purpose of conditioning the body, improving health, maintaining fitness, or as a therapeutic measure.

exit site — Point at which a catheter leaves a body site.

exophthalmos — Abnormal protrusion of one or both eyeballs caused by trauma, intracranial lesions, intraorbital disorders, or systemic disease, most commonly hyperthyroidism.

expectorant — An agent that facilitates removal of bronchopulmonary secretions.

expectorate — The act of coughing and spitting out mucous from the respiratory tract. Maneuver is useful in assisting to clear a client's airways of pulmonary secretions.

expectoration — Expulsion of mucus or sputum from the mouth or lungs.

exploratory laparotomy — The surgical exploration or examination of an abdominal organ or part.

extended care facility — An institution that provides medical, nursing, and/or custodial care for an individual over a prolonged period, as during the course of a chronic disease or during the rehabilitation phase after an acute illness.

extension — Movement increasing the angle between two adjoining bones.

external air leak — The presence of air originating from outside of the closed chest drainage system.

external fixation — Skeletal traction applied through the use of pins attached to a frame rather than weights.

external jugular vein — One of a pair of large vessels in the neck that receive most of the blood from the exterior of the cranium and the deep tissues of the face.

external rotation — Rotation of a joint outward.

external urethral sphincter — Voluntary muscle that must relax in order for the client to void or completely empty the bladder.

extravasation — The inadvertent infiltration of intravenous fluids or medications into the subcutaneous tissues surrounding the infusion site.

extremity restraints — Restraints used to immobilize one or all extremities.

exudate — Any fluid that has been extruded from a tissue or its capillaries, more specifically because of injury or inflammation. It is characteristically high in protein and white blood cells.

Fahrenheit — Temperature scale in which 32 degrees is the freezing point of water and 212 degrees is the boiling point of water at sea level.

fascia — Fibrous connective tissue.

febrile — Pertaining to or characterized by fever or an elevation in body temperature.

feces — The waste material excreted by the rectum after digestion; stool.

fenestrated drape — A drape with a round or slitlike opening in the center.

fenestrated tracheostomy tube — A tracheostomy tube containing a hole (fenestration) on the posterior aspect of the outer cannula that allows airflow over the vocal cords and speech in spontaneously breathing clients.

fenestration — Surgical procedure in which an opening is created to gain access to the cavity within an organ or a bone.

fever — An abnormal elevation of body temperature.

fiberoptic — Pertaining to fiberoptics; referring to the transmission of an image along flexible bundles of coated glass or plastic fibers having special optical properties.

flatulence — Condition characterized by the accumulation of gas within the lumen of the intestines.

flexion — Movement decreasing the angle between two adjoining bones; bending of a limb.

floor stock — A term applied to medications that are distributed by the pharmacy to the nursing unit in bulk. Generally, floor stock medications are ones that are commonly used and are often obtainable as over-the-counter preparations. Examples include, Tylenol, Milk of Magnesia, antacids, and stool softeners.

flora — Microorganisms that reside on and within the body to compete with disease-producing microorganisms to provide a natural immunity against certain infections.

flossing — Mechanical cleansing of tooth surfaces with the use of stringlike waxed or unwaxed dental floss.

flotation device — A foam mattress with a gel-like pad located in its center, designed to protect bony prominences and distribute pressure more evenly against the skin's surface.

flotation pad — A device constructed of foam or a silicone or polyvinal chloride gel encased in a vinyl-covered square, protects bony prominences and distributes pressure more evenly against the skin's surface.

flow sheet — A recording form used to document the same type of repeated measurements, procedures, or observations over time. Data on flow sheets allow the user to see trends over time.

fluid volume deficit (FVD) — An alteration characterized by the loss of fluids and electrolytes in an isotonic fashion.

fluid volume excess (FVE) — An alteration characterized by the abnormal retention of fluids and electrolytes in an isotonic fashion.

focus charting — A charting methodology for structuring progress notes according to the focus of the note, for example, symptoms and nursing diagnosis. Each note includes data, action, and client response.

fontanel — A space covered by tough membranes between the bones of an infant's cranium.

footboard — Board placed perpendicular to the mattress, parallel to and touching the plantar surface of the client's feet and used to maintain dorsiflexion of the feet.

footdrop — A falling or dragging of the foot from paralysis of the flexors of the ankle.

foramen magnum — The large opening in the anterior and inferior part of the occipital bone, interconnecting the vertebral canal and cranial cavity.

foreign body airway obstruction maneuver (FBAOM) — One of three methods used to remove a foreign object that is obstructing the airway.

four-poster cast — Cast placed over the shoulders; contains four vertical posts or poles on the anterior and posterior lateral sides of the head to immobilize the cervical vertebrae.

Fowler's position — Posture assumed by a client when the head of the bed is raised approximately 45 to 90 degrees, as though the client is sitting upright.

fracture pan — A bedpan designed for clients with body or leg casts or clients restricted from raising their hips. It has a shallow upper end that slips easily under a client.

frail elderly — An older adult over the age of 85 who may have physical or mental disabilities that interfere with independent performance of ADLs.

frequency — Symptom of urinary disorder involving repetitive voidings over a fixed time period.

friction — Effect of rubbing, or the resistance that a moving body meets from the surface on which it moves; a force that occurs in a direction to oppose movement; in massage, technique in which deeper tissues are stroked or rubbed, usually through strong circular movements of the hand.

friction rub — Dry grating sound heard during auscultation, caused by rubbing of tissue surfaces.

full liquid diet — A diet consisting of only liquids and foods that liquefy at body temperature.

gag reflex — A normal neural reflex elicited by touching the soft palate or posterior pharynx, the response being the elevation of the palate, retraction of the tongue, and contraction of the pharyngeal muscles. Tests for function of the vagus and glossopharyngeal nerves.

gait — Manner or style of walking, including rhythm, cadence, and speed.

gait belt — A leather or heavy canvas belt that encircles the client's waist, it may or may not have handles. The purpose of the belt is for the nurse to hold when ambulating the unsteady client, to reduce risk of fall.

gastrostomy feeding tube — Long, hollow, flexible tube inserted into the stomach through a stab wound in the upper left abdominal quadrant.

genuineness — Communication of authenticity or sincerity.

gingivae — The gums of the mouth.

gingivitis — Inflammatory condition in which the gums are red, swollen, and bleeding.

glaucoma — An abnormal condition of elevated pressure within the anterior chamber of an eye that occurs as a result of the obstruction of outflow of aqueous humor.

glucose monitoring — A diagnostic test to determine the blood glucose level.

granulation — The presence of red, granular, moist tissue that appears during the healing of open wounds; type of tissue containing new blood vessels that bleed readily.

granulation tissue — Soft, pink, fleshy projection of tissue that forms during the healing process in a wound not healing by primary intention.

gravity — The heaviness or weight of an object resulting from the effect of the attraction between any body of matter and any planetary body.

grief — Form of sorrow involving the person's thoughts, feelings, and behaviors, occurring as a response to an actual or perceived loss.

guaiac test — Diagnostic test to detect blood in the stool.

guided imagery — Technique in which client focuses on an image, becoming less aware of pain.

gurgle — Abnormal coarse sound heard during auscultation of the lung; produced by air entering large mucus-containing airways.

gypsum — Plaster of Paris; material used for casts as it becomes hard and rigid.

halitosis — Offensive breath resulting from poor oral hygiene, dental or oral infections, ingestion of certain foods, or systemic diseases.

hand roll — Cylindrical roll of cloth or gauze placed against the palmar surface of a client's hand to maintain hand, thumb, and fingers in a functional position.

Harris splint — Expandable splint that supports the thigh in skeletal traction.

hazards of immobility — Health problems resulting from a decrease in physical mobility or activity.

head tilt–chin lift — A method for opening the airway in which the rescuer places one hand on the victim's forehead and applies firm backward pressure with the palm to tilt the head back. At the same time, with the other hand the rescuer places the fingers of the hand under the bony part of the lower jaw near the chin and lifts.

Healing ridge — Induration of collagen deposits beneath the skin extending to about 1 cm on each side of the wound.

heatstroke — Condition characterized by core body temperature of 47° C (113 F).

heave — A lift or thrust felt during palpation of the heart.

Heimlich maneuver — A method by which a foreign body can be dislodged from the larynx or trachea.
hematemesis — Vomiting of blood.
hematology — The study of blood cells.
hematoma — Collection of extravasated blood trapped in the tissues of the skin or in an organ; results from trauma or incomplete coagulation.
hematopoiesis — The formation and development of blood cells in bone marrow.
hematuria — Abnormal presence of blood in the urine.
hemiparesis — Muscular weakness of one half of the body.
hemiplegia — Paralysis of one side of the body.
hemoconcentration — The concentration of red blood cells in one area.
hemodialysis — A procedure in which impurities or wastes are removed from the blood; used in treating renal insufficiency and various toxic conditions.
hemodynamics — The study of movements of the blood and of the forces concerned therein.
hemolysis — The destruction of red blood cells.
hemopneumothorax — An accumulation of both air and blood in the intrapleural space. This condition is characterized by the signs and symptoms listed with pneumothorax and hemothorax.
hemoptysis — Coughing up of blood from the respiratory tract.
hemorrhoids — A varicosity in the lower rectum or anus caused by congestion in the hemorrhoidal veins.
hemostasis — Termination of bleeding by mechanical or chemical means or by the coagulation process of the body.
hemothorax — An accumulation of blood in the intrapleural space caused by a pulmonary infarction, tissue damage that occurs as a result of lung cancer or other chest trauma, or a complication of anticoagulant therapy after chest surgery.
Hemovac drain — A type of closed drain system.
heparin lock — An intravenous needle connected to a small "well" that allows for the intermittent injection of medication without the need for repeated venipuncture.
herniation — The abnormal protrusion of an organ or other body structure through a defect or natural opening in a covering, membrane, muscle, or bone.
high Fowler's position — Placement of a client in a semisitting position by raising the head of the bed up more than 45-60 degrees.
hirsutism — Excessive body hair in a masculine distribution, caused by heredity, hormonal dysfunction, or medication.
Homan's sign — In the presence of phlebitis or when phlebitis is suspected, dorsiflexion of the foot elicits pain in the calf.
homeostasis — The state of equilibrium (balance between opposing pressures) in the internal environment of the body, naturally maintained by adaptive responses that promote healthy survival.
Hoyer lift — Mechanical device that uses a canvas sling to easily lift dependent clients for transferring.
Huber needle — Special needle with a deflected point designed to prevent damage to the silicone septum of implanted infusion ports.
hydrocolloid — An adhesive, moldable wafer made of a carbohydrate-based material, usually with a waterproof backing. This dressing usually is impermeable to oxygen, water, and water vapor and has some absorptive properties.
hydrogel — A water-based, nonadherent, polymer-based dressing that has some absorptive properties.
hygiene — The science of health. Self-care measures people use to maintain their health are called personal hygiene.
hypercalcemia — Greater than normal amounts of calcium in the blood.
hypercapnia — Elevated arterial pCO_2 greater than 45 mm Hg, also called hypercarbia.
hyperemia — Increased blood flow in part of the body, as in the inflammatory response, local relaxation of arterioles, or obstruction of the outflow of blood from an area.
hyperextension — Movement of a body part beyond its normal resting extended position.
hyperkalemia — Refers to solutions with potassium concentrations greater than 5.0 mEq/L.
hypermagnesemia — Refers to solutions with magnesium concentrations greater than 2.5 mEq/L.
hypernatremia — Refers to solutions with sodium concentrations greater than 147 mEq/L.
hyperopia — A refractive error of the eye in which parallel rays of light focus behind the retina; causes difficulty seeing near objects.
hyperphosphatemia — Refers to a higher than normal range of serum phosphorus. Normal range for serum phosphorus is 2.5 to 4.5 mg/100 ml (1.7–2.6 mEq/L).
hyperpigmentation — Unusual darkening of the skin.
hypertension — Condition characterized by an elevated blood pressure persistently exceeding 150/90 mm Hg.
hyperthermia — Condition characterized by body temperature over 38° C (100.4° F).
hypertonic — Having a greater concentration of solute than another solution, hence exerting more osmotic pressure.
hypertonic — A solution with a total electrolyte content of 375 mEq/L or greater.
hypodermoclysis — The injection of an isotonic or hypotonic solution into subcutaneous tissue to supply a continuous and large amount of fluid, electrolytes, and nutrients.
hypokalemia — Refers to solutions with potassium concentrations less than 3.5 mEq/L.
hypomagnesemia — Refers to solutions with magnesium concentrations less than 1.5 mEq/L.
hyponatremia — Refers to solutions with sodium concentrations less than 137 mEq/L.
hypoosmolar — State in which there is an abnormal gain in water or loss of sodium-rich fluids with replacement by water only. As a result, there is a low concentration of solutes in the body fluids.
hypophosphatemia — Refers to a lower than normal range of serum phosphorus. Normal range of serum phosphorus is 2.5 to 4.5 mg/100 ml (1.7 to 2.6 mEq/L).
hypotension — Condition characterized by a low blood pressure that is inadequate to perfuse and oxygenate body tissue.
hypothermia — Condition characterized by body temperature below 36° C (96.8° F).
hypothermia therapy — Techniques used to reduce elevated body temperature.
hypotonic — Having a smaller concentration of solute than another solution, hence exerting less osmotic pressure.
hypovolemic shock — State of physical collapse caused by massive blood loss, circulatory dysfunction, and inadequate tissue perfusion.
hypoxemia — Abnormal deficiency of oxygen in arterial blood.
hypoxia — Insufficient oxygen available to meet the metabolic needs of tissues and cells.
idiosyncratic reaction — A response to a medication or therapy that is unique to an individual.
ileal conduit — A method of urinary diversion through intestinal tissue. Ureters are implanted in a section of dissected ileum that is then sewed to an ostomy in the abdominal wall.
ileostomy — Surgical formation of an opening of the ileum onto the surface of the abdomen, through which fecal matter is emptied.

immobility — Pertaining to the inability of a body part or limb to be moved.
immunocompromised — A state of defective or failed immune response that makes a person more likely to acquire an infection.
impaction — Presence of large or hard fecal mass in the rectum or colon.
implanted infusion port — A self-sealing silicone septum encased in a metal or plastic case with an attached silicone catheter threaded into a large vein. Used to administer chemotherapy and other irritating intravenous medications.
incentive spirometer — Individual client device used to encourage full lung expansion. Reduces the risk of atelectasis in the immobilized or postoperative client.
incentive spirometry — Method of deep breathing providing visual feedback to clients concerning their inspiratory volume.
incident report — Confidential document that describes any client accident while the person is on the premises of a health care agency.
incompatibility — Describes two medications of different chemical makeup that cannot be mixed together.
incontinence — Inability to control urination or defecation.
induration — Hardening of a tissue, particularly the skin.
infection — The invasion and reproduction of microorganisms in a body tissue that can result in a local or systemic clinical response such as cellulitis or fever.
infiltration — Presence of intravenous fluids within the subcutaneous space surrounding a venipuncture site.
informed consent — Permission obtained from a client to perform a specific test or procedure.
infusate — Volume of parenteral fluid infused into a client over an established period of time.
infusion — Introduction of a fluid such as a drug, electrolyte, or nutrient directly into a vein by means of gravity flow.
infusion pump — Device designed to deliver a measured amount of fluid over a period of time.
injection — Act of forcing a liquid into the body by means of a syringe.
injection cap — A rubber diaphragm covering a plastic cap. Permits needle insertion into a catheter or vial.
in-line suction catheter — See closed system suction catheter.
insertion site — Site of large vein into which a catheter is threaded.
inspection — A physical examination skill involving the examiner's looking at external and internal body parts for physical characteristics.
insulation — 1. The act of insulating. 2. A nonconducting substance that offers a barrier to the passage of heat or electricity.
insulator — A substance that conducts temperatures poorly used to protect skin and tissues from hot or cold therapies.
intake — Measurement of the ingestion or infusion of liquids into the body, including all liquids and semiliquids, liquid medications, enteral tube feedings, intravenous therapy, blood components, and parenteral nutrition.
intake/output record — Measuring and recording of all liquid intake and output over a 24-hour period of time.
integument — Skin and its appendages: hair, nails, and sweat and sebaceous glands.
intercostal space — Space found between adjoining ribs.
internal rotation — Rotation of a joint inward.
interviewing — The process of conducting an organized, systematic conversation with a client. Designed to gather information regarding a client's level of health, response to care, or perception of symptoms or events.
intestinal obstruction — Any obstruction that results in failure of the contents of the intestine to pass through the lumen of the bowel.
intraabdominal pressure — Amount of tension within the abdominal cavity.
intracavitary — Within a body cavity.
intracellular fluid — Liquid within the cell membrane.
intraclavicular fossa — Small pocket area or indentation just below the clavicle on both sides of the neck.
intracranial pressure — Pressure exerted by cerebrospinal fluid within the subarachnoid space surrounding the brain and spinal cord.
intradermal (ID) injection — Form of injection in which a solution is introduced into the dermal skin layer.
intramuscular (IM) injection — Form of injection in which a solution is introduced into the body of a muscle.
intrapleural — Pertaining to, or affecting, the potential space between the parietal and visceral pleurae.
intrapulmonic — Pertaining to, or affecting, the spaces within the lungs.
intraspinal — Referring to both the epidural and intrathecal routes of medication administration.
intrathecal — Of or pertaining to a structure, process, or substance within a sheath, as within the spinal canal.
intravenous (IV) injection — Form of injection in which a solution is introduced into a vein.
intravenous conscious sedation (IVCS) — The intravenous administration of pharmacological agents to provide a minimally depressed level of consciousness to provide comfort during diagnostic or treatment procedures.
introitus — An entrance or orifice into a cavity.
intubation — Passage of a tube into a body aperture.
invasive — Referring to procedures that involve puncture, incision, or insertion of a foreign object into the body.
invasive procedure — A procedure in which the normal protective barrier of the skin or mucus membrane is broken or compromised, (e.g., an intravenous puncture or a bladder catheterization).
inversion — Turning something upside down.
irrigate — To flush with a fluid, usually with a slow, steady pressure on a syringe plunger. Done to cleanse a wound or clear tubing.
irrigation — Gentle washing of an area with a stream of solution.
ischemia — A decreased supply of oxygenated blood to a body organ or part.
isolation — Infection control and prevention methods such as barrier technique that are used to decrease the transmission of microorganisms.
isometric contraction — Increased muscle tension without muscle shortening.
isometric exercise — The tightening or tensing of muscles without moving body parts.
iso-osmotic solution — A solution with electrolytes that will exert the same osmotic pressure as the solution it is being compared with (e.g., peripheral vein solution and RBCs).
isotonic — A solution with a total electrolyte content of approximately 310 mEq/L.
isotonic contraction — Increased muscle tension resulting in muscle contraction and muscle shortening.
isotonic exercises — Dynamic, muscle-strengthening exercises that cause muscle contraction and change in muscle length (e.g., walking or aerobics).
isotonic solution — Having the same concentration of solute as another solution, hence exerting the same amount of osmotic pressure as the solution.
IV plug — A small rubber or plastic cap that connects to the open end of a client's IV access catheter. Also referred to as injection cap because a needle can be inserted into the rubber cap for the administration or aspiration of fluids.

jacket restraint — Vestlike restraint that usually crosses in the back of the client but may also cross in the front.

Jackson-Pratt drain — A closed drain system.

jejunostomy — A hollow tube inserted into the jejunum through the abdominal wall for administration of liquefied foods.

joint — Any one of the connections between bones.

Joint Commission on Accreditation of Healthcare Organizations (JCAHO) — A private, nongovernmental agency that establishes guidelines for the operation of health care facilities. The guidelines are the basis of accreditation, generally required for Medicare reimbursement.

Kardex — Trade name for card filing system that allows quick reference to the particular need of the client for certain aspects of nursing care.

keloid — An overgrowth of scar tissue at the site of skin injury, such as a wound or surgical incision.

ketones — An organic chemical compound with two compounds attached to it.

kilogram — The metric conversion for a pound; weight (lb.) × 2.2 = kilograms.

kinesthetic — Related to the ability to perceive the existence or direction of weight or movement.

knee exercise — Mechanical apparatus for passive exercises of the knee joint.

knee sling — Support in sling form used under the knee for Russell traction.

laryngospasm — Spasm of the muscles surrounding the larynx causing airway narrowing and stridorous breathing.

lavage — The irrigation or washing out of an organ or cavity.

lateral flexion — A range of joint motion exercise during which the head is tilted as far as possible toward each shoulder, maintains neck mobility.

latex allergy reaction — Allergic response to products containing latex (e.g., gloves, medical devices). Can present as contact dermatitis, allergic rhinitis, or immediate life-threatening reactions leading to urticaria, bronchospasm, edema, etc.

let-down reflex — A normal reflex in a lactating woman often elicited by tactile stimulation of the nipple, resulting in release of milk from the glands of the breast.

leukopenia — A decrease in circulating white blood cells.

leverage — Occurs when specific bones, such as the humerus, ulna, and radius, and the associated joints, such as the elbow joint, act together as a lever.

line of gravity — An imaginary line that goes from the center of gravity to the base of support.

lipid emulsion — A soybean oil.

lipodystrophy — Any abnormality in metabolism and deposition of fat.

logrolling — Maneuver used to turn a reclining client from one side to the other or completely over without flexing the spinal column.

loss — Absence of a significant other, object, or state of health to which the person must adapt through the grieving process.

lotion — Liquid preparation applied externally to protect the skin or treat a dermatologic disorder.

lower airway respiratory system — All respiratory structures below the epiglottis, including trachea, bronchi, and alveoli.

lumen — The hollow channel within a tube.

lunula — A semilunar structure, such as the crescent-shaped pale area at the base of the nail of a finger or toe.

MAC — Mid–upper arm circumference. Measurement midpoint between tip of acromion process of scapula and olecranon process of ulna. Measurement value denotes muscle wasting.

macerate — To soften, usually by soaking in water.

maceration — Skin that becomes abnormally soft and breaks down because of prolonged exposure to moisture.

maculopapular — Discolored elevated lesions on the skin.

malabsorption — Impaired absorption of nutrients from the GI tract.

malignant hyperthermia — An autosomal dominant trait characterized by often fatal hyperthermia with rigidity of the muscles occuring in affected people exposed to certain anesthetic agents.

malnutrition — Any disorder of nutrition.

MAMC — Mid-arm muscle circumference. Calculation obtained by subtracting the triceps skin fold (TSF) from the mid–upper arm circumference (MAC) measurement. Value assists in denoting muscle wasting.

manometer — An instrument for measuring pressure or tension of liquids or gases.

massage — A form of cutaneous stimulation that involves the application of touch and movement to muscles, tendons, and ligaments.

mastication — Chewing, tearing, or grinding food with the teeth while it mixes with saliva.

meatus — Any opening or tunnel through any part of the body (e.g., the point at which the urethra opens to the skin).

mediastinal shift — A condition in which the mediastinal contents move toward the unaffected side in the presence of a pneumothorax, hemothorax, or hemopneumothorax. The mediastinal shift causes compression of the organs and is a life-threatening situation.

medical asepsis — The techniques used to reduce and prevent the spread of microorganisms (clean technique).

medicated enema — Administration of a medication via an enema. Usually used preoperatively with clients scheduled for bowel surgery.

medullary — Of or pertaining to the medulla of the brain.

megakaryocyte — Precursor of platelets found in blood marrow.

melanin — Black or dark brown pigment that occurs naturally in the skin, hair, and iris.

melanocyte — A body cell capable of producing melanin, the pigment of the skin.

melena — Darkening of the feces by blood pigments.

metastasis — Process by which tumor cells are spread to distant parts of the body.

metered dose inhaler (MDI) — A device designed to deliver a measured dose of an inhalation drug.

microorganism — Any microscopic entity capable of sustaining living processes, such as bacteria, virus, fungi, only some of which typically cause human disease.

microvasculature — The portion of the circulatory system composed of the capillary network.

micturition — Urination; act of passing or expelling urine voluntarily through the urethra.

midarm circumference (MAC) — A measurement of the circumference of the upper arm used to estimate muscle mass.

midstream collection — Procedure in which the client initiates a stream of urine, inserts a sterile collection cup into the stream, and then withdraws the cup before the stream of urine stops.

milliequivalent per liter (mEq/L) — Number of grams of a specific electrolyte dissolved in 1 liter of plasma.

Minerva jacket — Cast encasing the head (with face and ears exposed), continuing over the thorax and back to the iliac crests.

minute ventilation — The volume of air expired per minute.

mitered corner — A triangular folded corner of a bedsheet, used to prevent the sheet from pulling out from the mattress.

mitten restraints — Thumbless mitten devices used to restrain a client's hands.

mobility — The amount and quality of physical activity.
moleskin — Adhesive-backed tape used for some forms of skin traction.
morbid obesity — Pathological state in which an individual weighs greater than 100 pounds (44.5 kg) over ideal weight.
morgue — A unit of a hospital with facilities for the storage and autopsy of the dead.
mucociliary transport — Process in which cilia lining the tracheobronchial tree sweep mucus upward toward the esophagus to keep airways clear of inhaled particulate.
mucopurulent — Characteristic of a combination of mucus and pus.
mummy restraint — Blanket or sheet folded in such a manner as to restrain a small child or infant.
mydriasis — Dilation of the pupil of the eye caused by contraction of dilator muscles of the iris.
mydriatics — Ophthalmic preparations that stimulate the sympathetic nerve fibers or block parasympathetic nerve fibers of the eye, temporarily paralyzing the iris sphincter muscle.
myelosuppression — A decrease in the cellular components of the bone marrow.
myopia — A refractive error of the eye in which parallel rays of light focus in front of the retina; causes difficulty seeing far objects clearly.
nares — The pairs of anterior and posterior openings in the nose that allow for passage of air to the pharynx and lungs.
nasal — Of or pertaining to the nose and nasal cavity.
nasal airway — Flexible, curved piece of rubber or plastic with one wide or trumpetlike end and one narrow end that is inserted through the nose into the pharynx.
nasal cannula — A device for delivering oxygen by way of two small, short tubes that are inserted into the nares.
nasal catheter — A flexible, small-bore tube inserted into the oropharynx by way of the nose.
nasogastric (NG) feeding tube — A small tube that is passed via the nares into the stomach.
nasointestinal (NI) feeding tube — Tungsten-weighted tube inserted through the naris to allow natural peristaltic movement of the tube through the pyloric sphincter into the duodenum or jejunum.
nebulization — Vaporization or dispersion of a liquid in a fine spray.
nebulizer — Device used to distribute medication throughout nasal passages and tracheobronchial airway.
necrosis — Localized tissue death.
necrotic — Related to death of a portion of tissue.
negative pressure — Pressure, measured in mm Hg, that is less than atmospheric pressure.
negative pressure ventilation — Therapy used for clients with primary neuromuscular illnesses that interfere with normal respiratory muscle function. The client is fitted with a poncho or shell that is connected to the ventilator. Air is removed from between the client's chest wall and the interior wall of the poncho or shell, causing the client to inhale.
negligence — Omission of care.
neovascular assessment — Series of eight observations required to measure neurologic and circulatory status of a client's peripheral tissue.
neovascularization — The process by which the vascular network in a wound is generated. This can also be called angiogenesis.
neurological — Pertaining to the study and treatment of the nervous system.
neuropathy — An abnormal condition characterized by inflammation and degeneration of the peripheral nerves.
neurovascular assessment — Series of eight observations (assessments) required to measure neurological and circulatory status of a client's peripheral tissues.
neutropenia — An abnormal decrease in the number of neutrophils in the blood.
neutropenic — Having an abnormal decrease in the number of neutrophils, white blood cells, in the blood.
nitroglycerin — Medication that causes dilation of coronary arteries.
noncontinent (incontinent) ostomy/diversion — Results from a surgical procedure that leaves the client with an external stoma through which either stool or urine drains. It is noncontinent/incontinent because the effluent drains spontaneously from the stoma and the client must continuously wear an external ostomy pouch over the stoma.
noncoring Huber needle — a specially designed needle (straight or a 90 degree needle) intended for use with a vascular access device. This needle permits penetration into the chamber of the vascular access device without causing damage, and thus permits repeated administration of medication directly into the client's blood stream.
noncoring needle — Needle used to access implanted venous access device; it does not result in coring of the rubber diaphragm.
nonopioids — analgesics that do not contain opioids.
nonpharmacological aids — Interventions used to prevent illness and promote health without the use of or in addition to the use of medications.
nosocomial (hospital acquired) infection — An infection that developed during a stay or work in a health care facility and was not present or incubating at the time of admission.
noxious — Harmful, injurious, or detrimental to health.
NPO — Nothing to be taken or given by mouth.
nursing home — Type of extended-care facility that is licensed to provide nursing and custodial care for persons over a prolonged period of time. Some nursing homes have living quarters that allow residents to continue normal living routines under staff supervision.
nutritional risk — The potential to become malnourished because of factors that are primary (e.g., inadequate intake), or secondary (e.g., disease).
nutritional support nursing practice — The care of individuals with potential or known nutrition alterations. The goal is to assist individuals to restore and maintain optimal nutritional health.
objective data — Data obtained by an observer (nurse) through direct physical examination, including observation, palpation, and auscultation, and by laboratory analyses and radiological and other studies.
obstipation — The absolute inability to pass stool.
obturator — Small dull-pointed introducer inserted in outer cannula that facilitates insertion of tracheostomy tube by gradually widening or dilating stoma to width of tracheostomy tube.
occult blood — Blood that appears from a nonspecific source, with obscure signs and symptoms. May be detected by means of a chemical test or microscopic examination.
ocular — Of or pertaining to the eye.
O.D. — Abbreviation for *oculus dexter,* a Latin phrase meaning "right eye."
oil-retention enema — An enema containing a small volume (200 to 250 ml) of an oil-based solution; used to soften fecal mass.
ointment — A semisolid externally applied preparation, usually containing a drug.
olfaction — The sense of smell.
Omnibus Budget Reconciliation Act (OBRA) — Act passed by the U.S. legislature that set reductions in Medicare payments for physician services.
oncology — A branch of medicine regarding the study of tumors.

onset of drug action — Period of time after a drug is administered for it to produce a response.

opening pressure — The amount of tension measured in a manometer following insertion of a spinal needle into the subarachnoid space.

ophthalmic — Of or pertaining to the eye.

ophthalmologist — A medical doctor whose practice is limited to diseases, conditions, and trauma to the eyes. An ophthalmologist also prescribes corrective lenses for clients whose visual acuity is impaired.

opioids — Pertaining to natural and synthetic chemicals that have opiumlike effects although they are not derived from opium.

opposition — The relation between the thumb and the other digits of the hand for the purpose of grasping objects between the thumb and fingers. This maneuver is used during range of joint motion exercises to maintain grasping ability of the client.

optometrist — A person who practices optometry, tests the eyes for visual acuity, prescribes corrective lenses, and recommends eye exercises.

oral airway — Minimally flexible curved piece of plastic extending from the exterior of the lips over the tongue to the pharynx.

organ procurement agency (OPA) — Community-based agency whose focus is to obtain donated organs for transplantation.

organ tissue donation — Families and significant others are offered the option of organ and/or tissue donation. This process includes, but is not limited to, the donation of heart, lung, kidneys, liver, corneal tissue, and bone.

orientation phase — Period in the nurse-client relationship when the nurse and client first meet and set the tone for the rest of their relationship, assessing the client's situation and setting goals.

orifice — Entrance or outlet of any cavity in the body.

orthopedic — Pertaining to the skeletal system.

orthopedics — Branch of medicine devoted to the study and treatment of the skeletal system, its joints, muscles, and associated structures.

orthopnea — An abnormal condition in which a person must sit or stand to breathe deeply or comfortably.

orthostatic hypotension — A drop in blood pressure of 15 mm Hg or more when an individual rises from a sitting to a standing position.

O.S. — Abbreviation for *oculus sinister,* a Latin phrase meaning "left eye."

osmolality — The characteristics of a solution determined by the ionic concentration of the solvent.

osteoblastic — Physiological activity that leads to the formation of specific bone tissue, osteoblasts.

osteoblasts — Osteoblasts synthesize the collagen and glycoproteins to form the matrix for bone formation.

osteoclastic — Physiological activity producing osteoclast bone cells that function in the development and periods of bone growth and repair, such as the breakdown and resorption of osseous tissue.

ostomy — A surgical procedure where the elimination of stool or urine is re-routed from the usual exiting part of the client. Instead the stool or urine exits the body through a surgically created opening called a stoma.

otic — Of or pertaining to the ear.

otitis media — Inflammation or infection of the middle ear, a common childhood affliction.

ototoxic — Having a harmful effect on the eighth cranial nerve or the organs of hearing and balance.

O.U. — Abbreviation for *oculus uterque,* a Latin phrase meaning "each eye."

outer cannula — Main portion of tracheostomy tube through which client breathes that stays in place at all times. The pilot balloon and faceplate are connected to the outer cannula.

output — Includes all liquids excreted, such as urine, vomitus, and diarrhea, and drainage from wounds, fistulas, and suction equipment.

overdose — Oral or parenteral ingestion of an excessive quantity of a medication or drug.

over-the-counter drug (OTC) — Drug available to a consumer without a prescription.

over-the-needle catheter (ONC) — A type of angiocatheter. The needle used for peripheral IV access is encased in a catheter made of Teflon, plastic, or another flexible material. After the needle pierces the skin, the catheter is threaded into a vein and the needle is withdrawn. The catheter remains in the vein for the instillation of fluid.

oximetry — Procedure used to measure amount of oxygenated hemoglobin.

oxygen mask — A flexible mask that fits snugly and securely over the client's nose and mouth for delivery of oxygen.

oxygen saturation — Amount of hemoglobin that is fully saturated with oxygen expressed as percent of total available hemoglobin.

oxygen therapy — Administration of oxygen by any route to a client, to prevent or relieve hypoxia.

oxygen toxicity — Administration of oxygen level greater than 50% for greater than 24 hours resulting in increased permeability of the alveolar wall, alveolar-capillary leakage, noncardiogenic pulmonary edema, decreased lung compliance, and respiratory failure.

pain — Subjective, unpleasant sensation caused by noxious stimulation of sensory nerve endings.

pain intensity — The degree or extent of pain perceived by an individual.

pain threshold — The amount of pain stimulus required to produce a physical or psychological response.

pain tolerance — Point at which a person is not willing to accept pain of greater severity or duration.

pallor — Unnatural paleness or absence of color in the skin.

palpate — To feel with the hand.

palpation — A technique used in physical examination in which the examiner feels the texture, size, consistency, and location of certain parts of the body with the hands.

palpebra — Portion of the conjunctiva that lines the inner surface of the eyelids; it is thick, opaque, and highly vascular.

paralysis — An abnormal condition characterized by loss of muscle function or the loss of sensation.

paralytic ileus — A decrease in or absence of intestinal paralysis that may occur after abdominal surgery, illness, or trauma.

paraphrase — Transform the client's words into the nurse's words, keeping the meaning intact.

parenteral — Not in or through the digestive system.

parenteral nutrition (PN) — The administration of nutrition into the vascular system.

paresis — Slight or partial paralysis related in some cases to local neuritis.

parietal pleura — The pleural membrane that lines the thoracic cavity.

passive range of motion — Exercises of the joints performed for an individual by someone else.

patency — Absence of obstruction such as clots within an intravenous needle or kinks within intravenous tubing.

patent — Open and unblocked.

pathogen — Microorganism capable of producing disease.

pathogenic microorganisms — Those capable of producing an infection or disease.

patient care profile (PCP) — A report that is automatically updated each shift within a computerized medical record.

Patient Self-Determination Act — Legislation that requires all Medicare and Medicaid recipient hospitals to provide clients with information on advance directives and their right to accept or reject medical treatment.

patient-controlled analgesia — Technique that allows clients to self-administer small, continuous doses of IV or subcutaneous opioids as they feel the need.

A Patient's Bill of Rights — A list of patient's rights promulgated by the American Hospital Association; it offers some guidance and protection to clients by stating the responsibilities that a hospital and its staff have toward clients and families during hospitalization; it is not a legally binding document.

peak action — Time it takes for a drug to reach its highest effective concentration.

peak airway pressure — The highest amount of positive pressure needed to inflate the lung.

peak expiratory flow rate (PEFR) — The maximal flow rate, measured in liters, that can be generated during a forced expiratory maneuver.

peak level — Highest effective concentration in the body of a drug.

Pearson's attachment — The support used under the leg in balanced suspension skeletal traction.

pediculosis — Infestation of the integument with blood-sucking lice.

PEH — Acronym for "pseudoepithelioma-tous hyperplasia"; maceration of skin surrounding the stoma.

pelvic belt — Girdle-shaped cotton belt or support that fits around the hips, lumbosacral area, and abdomen for attaching ropes and weights in pelvic belt traction.

pelvic sling — A hammocklike sling that fits under the client's lumbosacral area and hips and is then connected to ropes and weights; it suspends the pelvis off the bed as treatment for fractures of pelvic bones.

Penrose drain — An open drain system.

perception — The conscious recognition and interpretation of sensory stimuli through unconscious associations, especially memory, that serve as a basis for understanding, learning, and knowing, or for the motivation of a particular action or reaction.

percussion — A technique in physical examination used to assess the size, borders, and consistency of some of the internal organs and to discover the presence and to evaluate the amount of fluid in a cavity of the body.

percutaneous — Performed through the skin, such as a biopsy or the aspiration of fluid from a space below the skin using a needle, catheter, and syringe.

perfusion — Effect of pulmonary circulation in moving blood to and from the blood-gas barrier so gas exchange can occur.

periodontal — Referring to tissues surrounding the teeth, such as the gums and buccal mucosa.

periodontitis — Receding gum lines, inflammation, gaps between teeth.

perioperative — Related to the entire surgical experience.

peripherally inserted central catheter (PICC) — A peripherally inserted catheter that extends to the superior vena cava or right atrium.

peristalsis — The coordinated, rhythmical, serial contraction of smooth muscle that forces food through the digestive tract.

peristomal — Referring to the area of skin surrounding a surgically created stoma.

peritoneal fluid — Substance in the abdominal cavity for lubrication of peritoneal membrane and internal organs.

peritonitis — Inflammation of peritoneum produced by bacteria or irritating substances introduced into the abdominal cavity by a penetrating wound or perforation of an organ in the gastrointestinal or reproductive tract.

PERRLA — Acronym for "pupils equal, round, reactive to light, and accommodation"; the acronym is recorded in the physical examination if pupil assessment is normal.

petaling — Finishing the raw or ragged edges of a plaster cast to prevent skin irritation or pressure.

petrissage — A massage technique in which the skin is gently lifted and squeezed.

pH — Reflection of the hydrogen ion concentration of a liquid.

pharmacological agents — Oral, parenteral, or topical substances used to alleviate symptoms and treat or control illness.

pharynx — The throat.

phlebitis — Inflammation of a vein.

phlebitis solution — A hypertonic solution capable of causing inflammation of a vein.

phlebothrombosis — Blood clot formation.

phlebotomy — The incision of a vein for the letting of blood, as in collecting blood from a donor.

physical dependence — A physiological state in which abrupt cessation of a drug results in a withdrawal syndrome.

physical restraint — Any device, garment, material, or object that restricts a person's freedom of movement or access to one's body.

Physicians' Desk Reference (PDR) — A compendium, compiled annually, containing information about drugs supplied by manufacturers.

PIE — An acronym for "problem, intervention, and evaluation," used as an organizing framework for narrative nurses' notes.

piggyback infusion — Method for administering intravenous medications intermittently; a piggyback IV set is a supplementary set that connects with the primary IV tubing.

pillating device — Commercial device that contains a sharp blade used to cut tablets in half.

piloerection — Erection of the hairs of the skin in response to a chilly environment, emotional stimulus, or irritation of the skin.

plantar flexion — Flexion of the foot and toes toward the sole.

plaque (dental) — A thin film on teeth made up of mucin and colloidal material found in saliva and often secondarily invaded by bacteria.

plasmaphoresis — Laboratory procedure in which the plasma proteins are separated by electrophoresis for identification and evaluation of the proportions of the various proteins.

plateau — Blood serum concentration reached and maintained after repeated, fixed doses of a drug.

platelet — Formed particle found in blood that relates directly to the ability of the blood to clot.

pleura — Delicate serous membrane enclosing the lung.

pleural cavity — Space between visceral and parietal pleurae; pressure within the cavity is negative when compared with atmospheric pressure.

pleural fluid — Substance contained between visceral and parietal pleurae for lubrication of the membranes.

pneumonitis — Inflammation of the lung; may be caused by a virus, or may be a hypersensitivity reaction that occurs as a result of allergy to chemical or organic dusts.

pneumothorax — An accumulation of air in the intrapleural space caused by a severe blow to the chest, extremely forceful cough, chest trauma, or open chest surgery.

podiatrist — A health care professional trained to diagnose and treat diseases and disorders of the feet.

point of maximal impulse (PMI) — Point at which the heartbeat can most easily be palpated through the chest wall, usually along the left-midclavicular line at the fourth or fifth intercostal space.

polypharmacy — Concurrent prescription, administration, or use of multiple medications, some of which may not be indicated clinically.

POMR — An acronym for "problem-oriented medical record," used as an organizing framework for a client's complete medical record.

portal hypertension — An increased venous pressure in the portal circulation caused by compression or by occlusion at the portal or hepatic vascular system.

positive pressure — Pressure, measured in mm Hg, that is greater than atmospheric pressure.

positive pressure ventilation — Mechanical ventilation that delivers compressed gas to the airways at greater than ambient pressure.

Postanesthesia care unit (PACU) — Post-surgical recovery area where clients are closely monitored and stabilized before discharge to a specific nursing unit, or in the case of same day surgery to home.

postcast care — Nursing interventions performed for and with clients in casts or after cast removal.

postoperative — Period of time after completion of a surgical procedure wherein the nurse monitors the client's recovery.

postural — Position of body, usually refers to change of position from supine to sitting, sitting to standing.

postural drainage — Gravitational clearance of airway secretions by assumption of one or more of 10 different body positions for 5 to 15 minutes each; each posture corresponds to specific segments of bronchi in the lung.

postural hypotension — Condition in which a normotensive person becomes lightheaded or dizzy and experiences low blood pressure when rising to an upright position.

posture — Position of the body in relation to the surrounding space.

prealbumin — A plasma protein with a half-life of only 2 days used as a marker of nutritional status.

precordial — Of or pertaining to the precordium, which forms the region over the heart and the lower part of the thorax.

premature ventricular contraction (PVC) — A cardiac dysrhythmia characterized by a ventricular contraction preceding the expected contraction; it appears on an electrocardiogram as an early, wide QRS complex without a preceding P wave.

preoperative — The period of time preceding induction of anesthesia and the beginning of a surgical procedure.

preoperative checklist — Agency-specific list of guidelines for ensuring completion of nursing interventions. This list includes items to be assessed or verified, for example, verification that preoperative orders are written and completed, laboratory work is in the client's medical record, the client has voided, current vital signs are documented, etc.

presbycusis — Loss of hearing sensitivity and speech intelligibility, associated with aging.

presbyopia — Farsightedness resulting from a loss of elasticity of the lens of the eye. The condition commonly develops with advancing age.

pressure cycled ventilation — Mechanical ventilation in which gas delivery is limited by a preset pressure to achieve a tidal volume.

pressure ulcer — A lesion that develops in the skin as a result of prolonged, unrelieved pressure.

primary dressing — A dressing that comes in direct contact with the wound bed.

primary intention — Primary union of the edges of a wound, progressing to complete scar formation with granulation.

prn — Abbreviation for *pro re nata,* a Latin phrase meaning "as needed." The times of administration are determined by the needs of the client.

problem-oriented medical record (POMR) — Method of recording data about the health status of a client that fosters a collaborative problem-solving approach by all members of the health care team.

pronation — Movement of a body part so the front or ventral surface faces downward.

proprioception — Sensation that is achieved through stimuli originating from within the body regarding spatial position and muscular activity.

prospective reimbursement — A method of payment to an agency for health care services to be delivered based on predictions of what the agency's costs will be for the coming year.

prosthesis — An artificial replacement for a missing part of the body.

pruritus — The symptom of itching.

Pseudomonas — A genus of gram-negative bacteria that includes several free-living species of soil and water and some opportunistic pathogens, isolated from wounds and sputum; may produce blue and yellow pigments.

pulley — Mechanical round, grooved disks over which ropes can move freely for traction pull.

pulmonary edema — Accumulation of extracellular fluid in a client's lung tissue and alveoli, commonly caused by left-sided heart failure, fluid overload.

pulse deficit — Condition characterized by difference between apical pulse rate and peripheral pulse rate that results in a lack of peripheral perfusion.

quality assurance — In health care, any evaluation of services provided and of the results achieved as compared with accepted standards.

radial flexion — A range of motion exercise during which there is a bending of the wrist medially toward the thumb, maintains wrist mobility.

radiopaque — Not permitting the passage of x-rays or other radiant energy. Bones are relatively radiopaque and therefore show as white areas on an exposed x-ray film.

random voided specimen — A urine specimen obtained at any point of a 24-hour period.

reagent — Chemical used to indicate the presence of a particular substance.

rectal tube — Flexible tube inserted into the rectum to assist in relief of flatus.

rectum — Portion of the large intestine, about 12 cm long, continuous with the descending sigmoid colon, just proximal to the anal canal.

reduction — The alignment of fracture fragments through manipulation. Closed reduction is accomplished through manual manipulation and casting or traction.

reflection — A cognitive strategy that involves reappraisal of one's actions to evaluate outcomes. A communication strategy used to clarify what a client is feeling and to affirm that the client's feelings are acceptable.

refractive error — Condition in which parallel rays of light are not brought to focus on the retina.

refractometer — Device used to measure urinary specific gravity by measuring the amount of light that can pass through a drop of urine.

registered dietician — A health care professional who has successfully completed an examination and maintains continuing education requirements in nutritional care for individuals and groups.

registered nurse first assistant — A nurse with advanced education who assists the surgeon with surgical procedures, performing a combination of nursing and medical functions.

reinfusion device — An apparatus that is placed, usually intraoperatively during orthopedic or vascular procedures, into a space where significant blood loss is anticipated. This device collects the blood, filters it, and is then used to reinfuse that blood intravascularly.

relaxation — A cognitive strategy that provides mental and physical pain relief or reduces pain.

relaxation exercise — Pain relief treatment in which clients perform controlled breathing and relaxation exercises and concentrate on a pleasant situation when a noxious stimulus is applied.

reminiscence — A form of therapy for older adults that provides a life review. Individual talks about remote memories, expression of related feelings, and recognition of positive experiences, as well as conflicts.

remission — The partial or complete disappearance of the clinical and subjective characteristics of a chronic or malignant disease.

renal — Pertaining to the kidney.

renal insufficiency — Partial kidney failure characterized by less than normal urinary excretion and abnormal urinary laboratory results (e.g., creatinine, blood urea nitrogen level).

resident — A client in a long-term or extended care facility.

residual urine — The volume of urine in the bladder after a normal voiding.

resistive isometric exercise — Contracting of muscles while pushing against a stationary object or resisting the movement of an object.

respect — Communication of esteem, honor, or consideration of another.

respiratory arrest — Cessation of respirations.

respiratory distress — Difficulty breathing that may be associated with abnormal blood oxygen or carbon dioxide levels and may require supportive measures to preserve life.

respite care — Provision of short-term relief or time off for people providing home care to an ill, disabled, or frail older adult.

restatement — A communication strategy involving the reiteration of the client's verbal statements and/or questions using similar words; this affirms that the message was acknowledged by the nurse.

restating — The process of verbally clarifying information provided by the client or family.

restraint — Device used to immobilize a client or an extremity.

reverse Trendelenburg's position — Position in which the lower extremities are low and the body and head are elevated on an inclined plane.

rib shaking — Step in chest physiotherapy involving constant downward pressure with an intermittent shaking motion of the hands on the rib cage over the area being drained; it is done with the flat part of the palm of the hand during 4 to 12 prolonged exhalations through pursed lips.

rib vibration — Step in chest physiotherapy involving a downward vibrating pressure done only during exhalation by the flat part of the palm of the hand over the lung segment being drained; usually done during 4 to 12 prolonged exhalations through pursed lips over each segment drained.

right atrial catheter — An indwelling intravenous catheter inserted centrally or peripherally and threaded into the superior vena cava or right atrium.

rigidity — Condition of hardness, stiffness, or inflexibility.

rigor mortis — The rigid stiffening of skeletal and cardiac muscle shortly after death.

rooting reflex — A normal response in newborns when the cheek is touched or stroked along the side of the mouth to turn the head toward the stimulated side and begin to suck.

rotation — A basic range of joint motion allowed by various joints: the rotation of a bone around its central axis, such as shoulder rotation.

Rotokinetic bed — A special bed equipped with an automatic turning device that completely immobilizes clients while rotating them from 90 to 270 degrees along a horizontal axis.

S_1 — Symbol for the first heart sound in the cardiac cycle occurring with ventricular systole; it is associated with the closure of the mitral and tricuspid valves.

S_2 — Symbol for the second heart sound in the cardiac cycle; it is associated with closure of the aortic and pulmonary valves just before ventricular diastole.

saline lock — See heparin lock.

saliva — A digestive secretion emitted from the salivary glands in the mouth.

sclerosis — Condition characterized by hardening of tissue resulting from any of several causes, including inflammation, the deposit of mineral salts, and infiltration of connective tissue cells.

scrubbed team members — Includes the surgeon and scrub nurse or technician and assisting physicians who are scrubbed.

Scrub nurse — Provides the surgeon with instruments and supplies, which requires strict surgical asepsis. In addition, this nurse along with the circulating nurse disposes of soiled sponges and accounts for sponges, needles, and instruments on the surgical field.

sebaceous gland — One of the small glands in the dermis that secretes an oily substance (sebum) on the skin's surface and in the hair.

seborrheic dermatitis — A common and chronic, inflammatory skin disease characterized by dry or moist greasy scales and yellow crusts.

sebum — Oily secretion of the sebaceous glands of the skin. When combined with sweat, sebum forms a moist, oily, acidic film that is antibacterial and antifungal and protects the skin against drying.

secondary dressing — A dressing used to cover or hold primary dressings in place.

secondary intention — Wound closure in which the edges are separated, granulation tissue develops to fill the gap, and, finally, epithelium grows in over the granulation, producing a larger scar than results with primary intention.

secretion — A product produced by a gland of the body.

seizure — A hyperexcitation of neurons in the brain leading to a sudden, violent, involuntary series of muscle contractions that may be paroxysmal and episodic, as in a seizure disorder, or transient and acute, as in after a head injury.

seizure precautions — Measures that protect the client from injury during a seizure.

self-catheterization — The ability of individuals to insert a urinary catheter into their urinary meatus.

semi-Fowler's position — Placement of client in an inclined position, with the upper half of the body raised by elevating the head of the bed approximately 30 to 45 degrees.

sensitivity — Laboratory test used in conjunction with culture; it measures the response of microorganisms to antibiotics that have been placed on a culture plate.

sepsis — Infection, contamination.

serology — Branch of medicine dealing with serum and blood products.

shaking — Physiotherapy technique in which a concurrent, compressive force is supplied to the chest wall.

sharps container — A puncture-proof container that is used for the disposal of any used sharp items such as needles, disposable scissors, and scalpels.

shearing — Pressure exerted against the surface and layers of the skin as tissues slide underneath the body as it moves against a surface.
shearing force — An applied force or pressure exerted against the surface and layers of the skin as tissues slide in opposite but parallel planes.
sheet wadding — Stretchable sheets of cotton padding used to cover skin before a cast is applied.
side effect — An effect caused by a drug that is different from the therapeutic (desired) action; the effect may be harmless or injurious.
sigmoid colon — The part of the large intestine that extends from the descending colon to the rectum.
sign — Objective finding perceived by an examiner, such as a fever, rash, abnormal reflex, or abnormal breath sound.
silicone septum — Silicone partition that covers the port chamber housed in the metal or plastic body of the implanted infusion port.
sitz bath — Special bath in which only the hips and buttocks are immersed in fluid.
skin barrier — An artificial layer of skin, made of plastic or vinyl-like material, applied to skin before application of tape or ostomy drainage bags. Protects skin from chronic irritation.
sling — Used to support or limit movement, enhance circulation, and prevent edema of the arm, hand, or wrist.
slough — Necrotic (dead) tissue in the process of separating from viable portions of the body.
SOAP — Acronym for "subjective, objective, assessment, and plan," the four parts of the written account of a client's health problem in a problem-oriented record.
solute — A substance dissolved in a solution.
solute solution — Solutes are dissolved particles and are either electrolytes or nonelectrolytes. Solute solution refers to these particles when they are found in body fluids or plasma (i.e., solution).
solution — A mixture of one or more substances dissolved in another substance.
spasm — Involuntary muscle contraction.
specific gravity — The ratio between the density of a solution and that of water.
speculum — A retractor used to separate the walls of a cavity (e.g., the vaginal cavity).
sphygmomanometer — Device used for noninvasive measurement of arterial blood pressure consisting of cuff, air bladder, inflation bulb, and gauge to indicate amount of air pressure being exerted.
spica cast — An orthopedic cast applied to immobilize part or all of the trunk of the body and part or all of one or more extremities.
splinting — Supporting the abdominal area to reduce pain caused by coughing or sneezing after surgery.
sponge — Gauze dressing used to absorb blood in a surgical wound.
spore — An inactive but viable state of microorganisms.
spreader bar — A metal bar with curved hoop areas for attaching hooks or pins for traction.
sputum — Lung mucus; normally thin, watery, and white or clear and watery.
standard precautions — Techniques used to reduce the risk of the transmission of blood-borne pathogens or microorganisms present in moist body substances regardless of the client's diagnosis or infection status.
standardized care plan — Documentation that uses the nursing process format in specifying the plan of care for client problems.
staples — Stainless steel wire used to close a surgical wound.
stent — A straw or tubelike device that is placed through the stoma into bowel to keep open the flow of effluent.
sterile — Free from all life forms, including spores.
sterile conscience — One's personal principles and morals that guide them to maintain strict asepsis and sterile techniques at all times.
sterile field — A specified area, such as within a tray or a sterile drape, that is considered free from microorganisms.
sterilization — Process by which microorganisms, including spores, are killed.
stockinette — Stretchable cotton materials of various sizes and widths used immediately over the skin to protect tissues from the irritation of felt or plaster.
stoma — Surgically created opening between a body cavity and the body's surface, such as a colostomy.
stomatitis — Any inflammatory condition of the mouth.
stopcock — A valve that controls the flow of fluid or air through a tube.
strike through — Source of contamination by which moisture permeates a sterile field or barrier.
stroke volume — The volume of blood ejected from the left ventricle with each ventricular contraction.
subarachnoid space — Situated or occurring between the arachnoid and the pia mater membranes, which cover the brain and spinal cord.
subcutaneous emphysema — The presence of free air or gas in the subcutaneous tissues.
subcutaneous (SQ or SC) injection — Form of injection in which a solution is introduced into subcutaneous tissues.
subcutaneous tunnel — A tunnel under the skin between the exit site of a catheter and the entrance into a body cavity (such as the epidural space) or vein.
subjective data — Data collected from a client.
sublingual — Route for administering a drug beneath the tongue.
suction — The act of sucking up a substance by reducing air pressure over its surface.
suction catheter — Thin plastic or rubber tubing used to remove secretions.
summarization — Reworking a lengthy interaction or discussion into a few brief sentences.
summarizing — A process in which an interviewer organizes and condenses information provided, and clarifies with the client that the information is correctly interpreted.
supination — Movement of a body part so the front or ventral surface faces upward.
suppository — A solid form of medication inserted into a body cavity (e.g., the rectum or vagina). The drug is absorbed after it dissolves in the cavity.
surgical asepsis — Practices or techniques designed to render and maintain objects and areas free from pathogenic microorganisms. Also referred to as sterile techniques.
surgical scrub — Process of removing as many microorganisms as possible from the hands and arms by mechanical washing and chemical antisepsis.
suspension — A liquid in which small particles of a solid are dispersed, but not dissolved, and in which the dispersal is maintained by stirring or shaking the mixture.
sympathomimetic — A pharmacological agent that mimics the effects of stimulation of organs and structures by the sympathetic nervous system.
synergistic reaction — An undesired reaction that occurs when one drug potentiates the effect of another.
systemic — Of or pertaining to the whole body rather than to a localized area.
systolic pressure — The higher blood pressure measurement; reflects pressure within the arterial system during the period of ventricular contraction (systole).
T binder — Bandage in the shape of a letter T; used to support perineal dressing.
T tube — A T-shaped device that is attached to an endotracheal or tracheostomy tube for delivery of humidified air.

tachycardia — An abnormality in heart rate in which the myocardium contracts regularly, but at a rate over 100 beats per minute.

tachypnea — Condition characterized by respiratory rate greater than 20 breaths per minute.

tartar — A hard, gritty deposit that collects on the teeth.

telephone order — A physician or nurse practitioner's order for a medication or other therapy that is received by telephone to a nurse to be entered into the client's medical records.

TENS — Transcutaneous electrical nerve stimulation. A mild electrical stimulation that interferes with the transmission of painful stimuli.

tepid — Moderately warm to the touch.

termination phase — The period in the nurse-client relationship when the nurse and client examine and evaluate their relationship and its goals and results; the time when they deal with the emotional content involved in saying good-bye.

tertiary intention — Wound healing that occurs when surgical wounds are not closed immediately, but left open for 3 to 5 days to allow edema or infection to diminish.

therapeutic — Treatments or interventions implemented to prevent illness and/or promote health.

therapeutic silence — The use of silence that encourages verbal description and reflection; avoidance of premature verbal communication that may be due to the nurse's anxiety.

thermoregulation — Ability to control temperature within acceptable range.

third party payor — An insurance plan, HMO, or PPO that reimburses for health care services.

Thomas splint — A long splint with a half or full ring at one end; covered with towels and lined with felt or other soft material, it is used to suspend the thigh in skeletal traction.

thrill — A fine vibration felt by an examiner's hand on the body of a client over the site of an aneurysm or on the precordium.

thrombocytopenia — A decrease in circulating platelets.

thrombophlebitis — Inflammation of a vein, often accompanied by formation of a clot.

thrombosis — An abnormal vascular condition in which thrombus develops within a blood vessel of the body.

thrombus — Accumulation of platelets, fibrin, clotting factors, and the cellular elements of the blood attached to the interior wall of a vein or artery, sometimes occluding the lumen of the vessel.

tidal volume — Amount, in ml, of air inhaled with each breath. Spontaneous tidal volume is 5 to 10 ml/kg body weight.

tidaling — A normal gentle rocking of fluid in a chest tube water-seal system or in the diagnostic indicator of waterless units. Indicates that the system is functioning properly.

timed collection — The collection of a substance such as urine or stool for a specific period of time.

tinnitus — Ringing heard in one or both ears.

tissue ischemia — Decreased blood supply to body tissues.

TLC — 1. Abbreviation for total lung capacity. 2. Informal abbreviation for tender loving care.

tolerance — A phenomenon by which the body becomes increasingly resistant to a drug or other substance through continued exposure to the substance.

tongue-thrust reflex — An immature form of swallowing in which the tongue is projected forward instead of retracted during swallowing.

topical — Of or pertaining to a drug or treatment applied to the surface of a body part.

topical agents — Pertaining to a drug or treatment applied to the surface part of the body.

tourniquet — An item used for the compression of blood vessels.

toxic effects — Severe and progressive negative effects of drugs.

tracheal stenosis — Narrowing of the trachea that occurs as a result of scarring.

tracheo-esophageal fistula — A hole in the posterior wall of the trachea that extends into the anterior wall of the esophagus and permits aspiration of gastric contents into the lung.

tracheobronchial tree — Anatomical divisions of the respiratory tract, including the combination of trachea, bifurcations into the right and left mainstem bronchi, and subsequent bifurcations into smaller bronchi and bronchioles.

tracheomalacia — An abnormal softening or sponginess of the tracheal tissue.

tracheostomy — Opening through the neck into the trachea with an indwelling tube inserted; created surgically to produce an airway.

tracheostomy collar — Curved oxygen delivery device with an adjustable neck strap that fits around the tracheostomy.

traction — Force or pull applied to limbs, bones, or other tissues to pull the tissues apart, often for realignment.

traction boot — A foam rubber boot shaped to fit a forearm or leg, used for a type of skin traction.

transdermal — Refers to a form of medication that is applied to the skin's surface and is absorbed across the dermal or outer skin layer.

transfusion reaction — Systemic response by the body to the administration of blood incompatible with that of the recipient.

transmission-based precautions — Techniques used to prevent the transmission of microorganisms from clients documented or suspected to be infected with highly transmissible pathogens for which additional precautions are needed beyond standard precautions. The three types are Airborne, Droplet, and Contact Precautions.

transtracheal oxygen therapy (**TTOT**) — A method of administering oxygen to a client by establishing a low-flow catheter route directly in the trachea.

Trendelenburg position — Position in which the head is low and the body and legs are elevated.

triceps skinfold (**TSF**) — A measurement, with calipers, of the skinfold over the triceps muscle. The measurement is used to estimate body fat stores.

trocar — A sharp, pointed rod that fits inside a tube; used to pierce the skin and the wall of a cavity or canal in the body to aspirate fluids, to instill a medication or solution, or to guide the placement of a soft catheter.

TSF — Triceps skinfold. Useful in denoting muscle wasting.

tuberculosis — A chronic granulomatous infection caused by an acid-fast bacillus, *Mycobacterium tuberculosis,* generally transmitted by the inhalation or ingestion of infected droplets and usually affecting the lungs.

turning sheet — Bedsheet folded in half, placed under the client between shoulders and below the hips. Used by health care providers to lift, turn, and position the client.

tympanic — Pertaining to a structure that resonates when struck; drumlike.

ulnar flexion — A range of motion exercise during which there is a lateral bending of the wrist toward the fifth finger, maintains wrist mobility.

undermining — Condition of a wound in which the loss of underlying tissues is greater than the loss of the skin.

unit-dose system — System of drug distribution in which a portable cart containing a drawer for each client's medications is prepared by the pharmacy with a 24-hour supply of medications.

unscrubbed team members — Includes the anesthesiologist or anesthetist and the circulating nurse, who wear surgical attire but are not gowned or gloved.
upper airway — The mouth, throat, and larynx.
upper airway respiratory system — All respiratory structures above the epiglottis, including nose, sinuses, mouth, and pharynx.
ureterostomy — An ostomy site in which one or both ureters are surgically brought to the abdominal surface for the excretion of urine.
uretheral sphincter — Voluntary muscle at the neck of the bladder that relaxes to allow micturition.
urethral meatus — The opening to the canal for the discharge of urine.
urgency — The need to void immediately.
urinal — Plastic or metal receptacle for urine.
urinary diversion — A surgical procedure in which the ureters are removed from the urinary bladder and surgically anastomosed directly to the skin or to either a conduit or internal pouch made of bowel with the other end brought out onto the client's skin as a stoma so that the urine can exit the body.
urinary retention — Inability to empty the bladder resulting from a number of possible causes.
urinary tract infection — Greater than normal level of pathogens in the urinary tract.
urine — Fluid secreted by the kidneys, transported by the ureters, stored in the bladder, and voided through the urethra.
urine specific gravity — Measurement of the degree of concentration of the urine.
urinometer — Device used for determining specific gravity of urine.
urostomy — The diversion of urine away from a diseased or defective bladder through a surgically created opening, or stoma, in the skin.
Vacutainer tube — A glass tube with a rubber stopper; air has been removed to create a vacuum.
valgus — An abnormal position in which a part of a limb is bent or twisted outward, away from the midline, such as the heel of the foot.
Valsalva maneuver — Any forced expiratory effort against a closed airway, as when an individual holds the breath and tightens the muscles in a concerted, strenuous effort to move a heavy object or to change position in a bed.
variance — Positive or negative changes in client progress toward expected outcomes on a critical pathway. Deviations from the critical path plan most often used in the case management model of delivering health care.
varices — Tortuous, dilated veins.
varus — An abnormal position in which a part of a limb is turned inward toward the midline, such as the heel and foot.
vascular access device (VAD) — An indwelling catheter, cannula, or other instrumentation used to obtain venous or arterial access.
vasoconstriction — Narrowing of the lumen of any blood vessel, especially the arterioles and the veins in the blood reservoirs of the skin and abdominal viscera.
vasodilation — An increase in the diameter of a blood vessel caused by inhibition of its vasoconstrictor nerves or stimulation of dilator nerves.
vein lumen — Central opening through which blood flows in a vein.
vellus — Soft, fine hair covering all parts of the body except the palms, soles, and areas where other types of hair are normally found.
venipuncture — Technique in which a vein is punctured transcutaneously by a sharp rigid stylet (such as a butterfly needle), a cannula (such as an angiocatheter that contains a flexible plastic catheter), or a needle attached to a syringe.
venous thrombosis — A condition characterized by the presence of a clot in a vein in which the wall of the vessel is not inflamed.
ventilation — Respiratory process by which gases are moved into and out of the lungs.
ventral — Of or pertaining to an anterior position, toward the abdomen.
verbal order — A physician or nurse practitioner's order for a medication or other therapy that is spoken to the RN to be entered into the client's medical records.
vertigo — A sensation of faintness or an inability to maintain normal balance in a standing or seated position, sometimes associated with giddiness, mental confusion, nausea, and weakness.
vesicant — A drug capable of causing tissue necrosis when extravasated.
vial — Glass container with a metal-enclosed rubber seal.
vibration — Physiotherapy technique performed by contracting all the muscles in the caregiver's upper extremities to cause vibration while applying pressure to the chest wall.
viscera — The internal organs enclosed within a body cavity, primarily the abdominal organs.
visceral pleura — A serous membrane lining both lungs.
visceral protein status — The amount of protein that pertains to the internal organs (e.g., abdominal).
vital signs — Physiological parameters that reflect key body processes; refers to temperature, blood pressure, heart rate, respiratory rate, and oxygen saturation.
void — The process of emptying the bladder of urine; urinate; micturate.
volume-cycled ventilation — A specific tidal volume delivered the client on a ventilator within a preset pressure range.
walking belt — Leather device with handles that enables the nurse to help a client walk.
walking heel — Plastic or rubber heel placed in the sole of a leg cast to allow weight bearing.
webril — Stretchable cotton material applied over the skin to protect from plaster irritation.
weight — Force exerted on a body by the gravity of the earth.
weight holder — A metal, T-shaped bar that holds weights for traction.
weights — Filled bags or metal disks of varying poundage used for traction.
whispered pectoriloquy — The transmission of a whisper through the pulmonary structures so that it is heard as normal audible speech on auscultation.
windowing — Cutting a small area of a cast to permit inspection of the tissues below.
working phase — The period in the nurse-client relationship when the focus is on communication strategies, interventions for problem resolution, and enhancement of self-concept.
Yankauer suction — A large filter-tipped rigid plastic suction catheter used mainly in the mouth or other large body cavity.
Z-track method — Method for injecting irritating medications into muscle without tracking residual medication through sensitive tissues.

INDEX

B

D

F

J

K

N

O

S

T

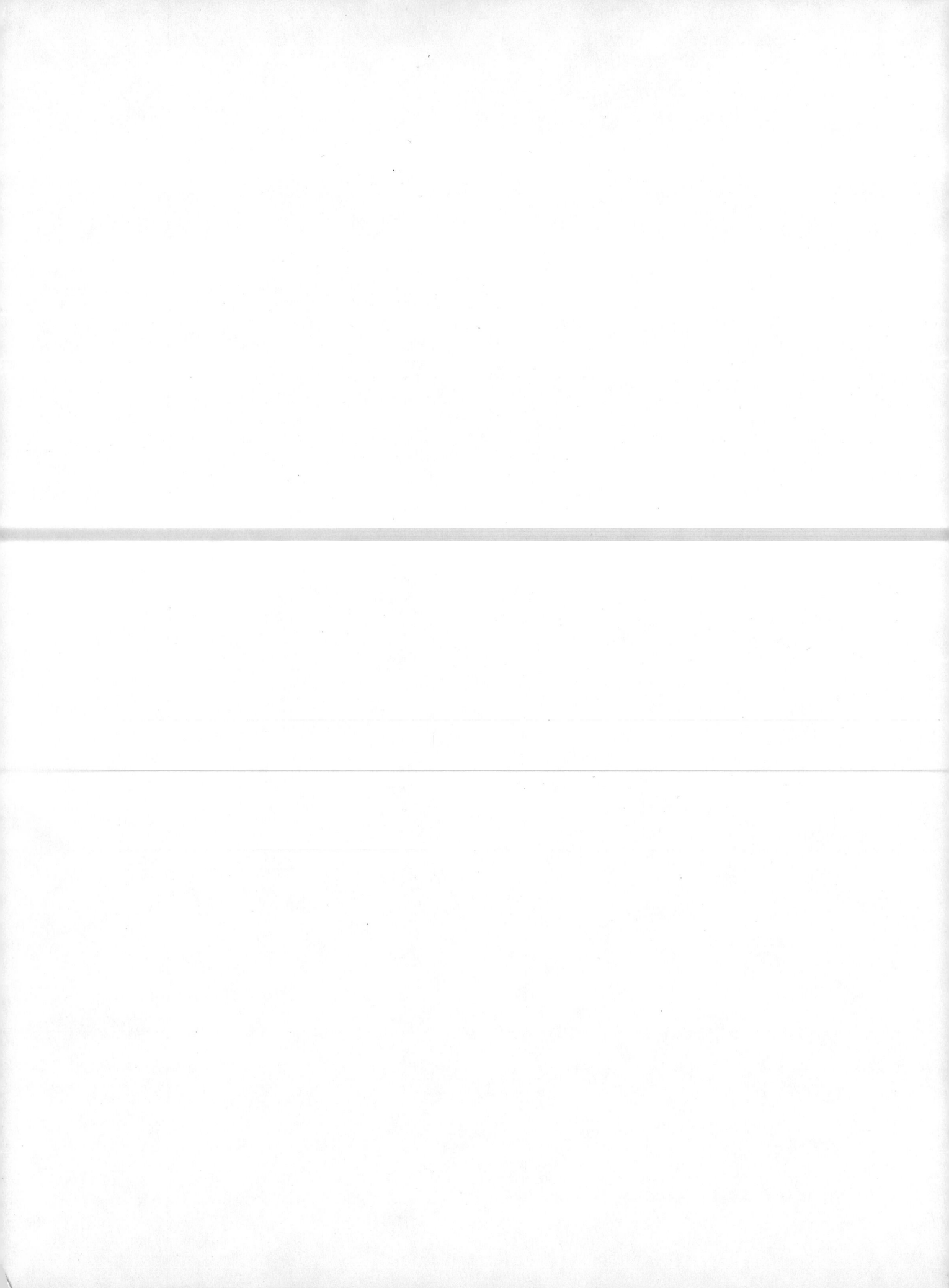

INDEX OF SKILLS